Understanding and Treating Depressive Disorders

Jacob Raber • Franklin Sunzeri
Jennifer M. Loftis • J. Wesson Ashford
Editors

Understanding and Treating Depressive Disorders

An Introduction

Springer

Editors
Jacob Raber
OHSU
Portland, OR, USA

Franklin Sunzeri
Heather Hills Consulting
Coos Bay, OR, USA

Jennifer M. Loftis
VA Portland Health Care System
Portland, OR, USA

J. Wesson Ashford
VA Palo Alto Health Care System
War Related Illness and Injury Study Center
(WRIISC)
Palo Alto, CA, USA

ISBN 978-3-032-14464-5 ISBN 978-3-032-14465-2 (eBook)
https://doi.org/10.1007/978-3-032-14465-2

This Springer imprint is published by the registered company Springer Nature Switzerland AG
The registered company address is: Gewerbestrasse 11, 6330 Cham, Switzerland

We dedicate this volume to all of those whose compassion beckons them to help others overcome clinical depression. May you find the tools you need to support yourself along the way.

Preface

A number of years ago, the NIH funded a Phase 1 Small Business Innovation Research grant that was the inception of our project in behavioral medicine called *Behavioral Medicine: A Research Compendium.* This project is a collaboration between professors at Oregon Health & Science University (OHSU), Stanford University, and the small business, Heather Hills Consulting.

Its objective is to revolutionize interdisciplinary learning among college-level graduate and medical students, faculty, and practitioners in allied behavioral medicine fields. We are doing so by eliminating obstacles to interdisciplinary collaboration that have been recognized within the NIH Roadmap for Medical Research and 2021–2025 Strategic Plan.

Behavioral medicine is the interdisciplinary field concerned with development and integration of behavioral, psychosocial, and biomedical science knowledge and techniques relevant to the understanding of health and illness, and the application of this knowledge and these techniques to prevention, diagnosis, treatment, and rehabilitation.

A wide range of consumers and health professionals are involved in behavioral medicine research and practice, including cardiologists, counselors, epidemiologists, exercise physiologists, family physicians, health educators, internists, nurses, nutritionists, pediatricians, psychiatrists, psychologists, and sociologists.

Behavioral medicine is taught through a variety of university programs. These include programs such as integrative biology that aims to discover complex interrelationships between organisms and the physical and biological environment in which they live and the highly integrative field of translational medicine. Integrative biology combines fields of genetics, genomics, physiology, ecology, systematics, and evolutionary biology to address critical problems related to the environment, ecosystems, human and animal health. There are literally hundreds of behavioral-medicine related programs at universities.

Unfortunately, resources for these courses are often ill defined and ad hoc. Based on the need for a comprehensive and tailored resource, the Compendium was developed.

The Compendium consists of a background science volume, volumes of applied science that cover areas of concentrated knowledge, and an interactive website. The Compendium begins by presenting a foundation in behavioral medicine. The focused volumes highlight a particular clinically relevant disorder. These include topics such as depression, anxiety disorders, post-traumatic stress disorder (PTSD), cardiovascular disease, cancer, autoimmune disorders, obesity, addictions, and violence.

This is the first of the focus volumes. Its goal is to shine light on the relationships discovered by the latest scientific investigations into understanding and treating depressive disorders. The volume *Understanding and Treating Depressive Disorders: An Introduction* includes a chapter on the neuroanatomical view for understanding, preventing, and treating mood disorders by Dr. Ashford, and a chapter on immune mechanisms and anti-inflammatory treatment strategies for mood disorders by Dr. Loftis.

To serve the greatest range of users, the most essential information germane to clinical depression is presented in this applied science focus volume. We begin with etiological considerations underpinning possible relationships between psychosocial variables and health. These include, but are not limited to, communication in the brain, molecular aspects, stress responses, heritability, and disease-associated immune responses. Next, factors relative to the ability to modify behaviors are considered. These include topics such as epigenetics, neuroplasticity, conditioning, therapy genetics, critical periods, and motivation. Then, evidence for efficacy of treatment approaches is presented. These include such interventions as pharmacotherapy, psychotherapy, complementary interventions, and self-medication. We hope that with this approach, clinicians, researchers, and students with diverse experiences will acquire sufficient information to better understand and apply biopsychosocial theory and techniques.

Social interaction is an important part of this endeavor. For this reason, we have created an ancillary website offered to users of the Compendium. There are discussion boards to facilitate learning and dissemination of information, and to foster creativity. A window for feedback and input is part of the online website.

In summary, the Compendium aims to (1) facilitate an understanding of complex, interrelated issues despite users lacking knowledge of, or familiarity with, all the related science; (2) provide rigorously investigated citations and balanced narratives where conflicts in findings exist; and (3) use digital state-of-the-art technology to enhance the learning experience.

We want to acknowledge the very valuable contribution of Abigail O'Niel, a graduate student in the Behavioral Neuroscience graduate program in the laboratory of Dr. Raber at OHSU. She not only created the figures that appear in this focus volume, but she also provided the graduate student perspective and editorial feedback so important for the success of this project. We also want to acknowledge the support of the Springer Nature team, including Kiruthika Andappan, Julia Andrews, Margaret Moore, and Richard Lansing.

We thank Dr. Peter Kaufmann, formerly of the NHLBI division of the NIH, which sponsored the SBIR grant that provided the opportunity to initiate this project, for his belief in the goal of this project and who gave us the confidence to pursue it.

Editor in Chief: Dr. Jacob Raber, Professor of Behavioral Neuroscience, Neurology, and Radiation Medicine, Affiliate Scientist, Division of Neuroscience, ONPRC, OHSU

Editor: Dr. Franklin Sunzeri, Research Immunologist Heather Hills Consulting Services, Coos Bay Oregon

Collaborating Editors: Drs. Jennifer M. Loftis, Professor of Behavioral Neuroscience and Psychiatrist, OHSU, and Research Scientist at the Portland VA Medical Center; and J. Wesson Ashford, Clinical Professor of Psychiatry and Behavioral Sciences, Stanford University, Director the War Related Illness and Injury Study Center at the VA Palo Alto Health Care System and Senior Research Scientist at the Stanford/VA Aging and Alzheimer's Disease Clinical Research Centers

Writers: Dr. Franklin Sunzeri, Elizabeth Sunzeri MS LMFT, Jeffery J. Sunzeri MS, Dr. Jennifer M. Loftis, and Dr. J. Wesson Ashford

Illustrator and provider of graduate student perspective and editorial feedback: Abigail O'Niel

Portland, OR, USA	Jacob Raber
Coos Bay, OR, USA	Franklin Sunzeri
Portland, OR, USA	Jennifer M. Loftis
Palo Alto, CA, USA	J. Wesson Ashford
September 2025	

About the Book

This behavioral medicine textbook is an introduction to understanding and treating clinical depressive disorders.

Behavioral medicine is the interdisciplinary field concerned with development and integration of behavioral, psychosocial, and biomedical science knowledge and techniques relevant to the understanding of health and illness, and the application of this knowledge and these techniques to prevention, diagnosis, treatment, and rehabilitation. Therefore, the objective of this text is to support interdisciplinary learning among college-level graduate and medical students, faculty, and practitioners in allied behavioral medicine fields as they engage in making a difference in depression.

To do this, first etiological considerations underpinning possible relationships between psychosocial variables and health including but not limited to communication in the brain, molecular aspects, stress responses, heritability, and disease associated immune responses are presented. Next, factors relative to ability to change behavior are considered. These include topics such as epigenetics, neuroplasticity, conditioning, therapygenetics, critical periods, and motivation. Then, evidence for efficacy of treatment approaches is presented. These include such interventions as pharmacotherapy, psychotherapy, complementary interventions, and self-medication.

With this comprehensive yet tailored approach, we hope that clinicians, researchers, or students with diverse experiences can acquire sufficient information to understand and apply biopsychosocial theory and techniques to increase understanding and optimize treatments for clinical depression.

Contents

Editors and Contributors

About the Editors

Jacob Raber, PhD is a Professor of Behavioral Neuroscience, Neurology, and Radiation Medicine, and an Affiliate Scientist in the Division of Neuroscience, ONPRC, at the Oregon Health & Science University (OHSU), and a Courtesy Professor in the College of Pharmacy at the Oregon State University (OSU). After completing his Bachelor of Science degree in Chemistry at the Free University of Amsterdam, his master's degree in Pharmacochemistry at the Free University of Amsterdam, he completed his PhD in Molecular Genetics and Virology at the Weizmann Institute of Science. Following a post-doctoral fellowship in the laboratory of Dr. Floyd E. Bloom at the Scripps Research Institute, he joined the Gladstone Institutes and the Department of Neurology at UCSF. In 2001, he joined OHSU. He was an Ellison Medical Foundation New Scholar in Aging from 2002 to 2006. His research is devoted to characterizing effects of environmental and genetic factors on brain function, identifying of affected pathways, and developing treatments to antagonize detrimental effects. As environmental factors, the focus is on irradiation, a high-fat diet, stress, second-hand smoke, and related behavioral and cognitive changes. For the genetic factors, the focus is on isoform-dependent effects of apolipoprotein E. The three major human apoE isoforms (E2, E3, and E4) differ in their risk to develop cognitive impairments with age and following various environmental challenges. He has published 249 peer-reviewed primary publications, 56 book chapters and invited reviews, and 3 editorials on effects of genetic and environmental factors on the brain. He is the contact MPI of the National Institute on Aging funded "Neuroscience of Aging, Neurodegeneration and Alzheimer's Disease" T32 training grant.

Franklin Sunzeri, MD, PhD is a research immunologist. He was an undergraduate major in psychobiology at UC Santa Cruz. He began medical school at CEUX and then participated in the University of California San Francisco's (UCSF) Central San Joaquin Rural Medical Education Program. At UCSF, he received honors in radiology/nuclear medicine and pathology clerkships and was given one-on-one clinicals in pediatrics and psychiatry. He also found pleasure in clinical rotations in the Public Health Service Hospital in the Navajo Area Indian Health Service in Tuba City Arizona. He was a Special Assistant in the UC Berkeley Disabled Students Program where he provided physical and psychological support to students.

After his PhD in immunology from UC Berkeley, he enjoyed a postdoc at Irwin Memorial Blood Centers working on developing methods for rapid detection of viral DNA fragments using PCR and capillary electrophoresis. These developments have been useful for screening the blood supply for viruses and for DNA and mRNA forensic analyses. He then began a career as a principal scientist at Advanced Molecular Systems where he was the PI on a small business innovation research (SBIR) grant in molecular diagnostics. The SBIR grant was focused on developing a multiple capillary instrument for rapid nucleotide analysis. Developments led to affinity capillary electrophoresis to assay protein-ligand interactions for association/binding constants for drugs and ligands; aptamer-based affinity capillary electrophoresis for analysis of specific affinity reagents, binding, separation, and detection of analytes, and other assays.

He left the Silicon Valley, became a consulting immunologist, and moved to Coos Bay Oregon where he wrote an SBIR grant for an Online Encyclopedia of Behavioral Medicine funded by the NHLBI of the NIH. It was the inception of this current venture.

Jennifer M. Loftis, PhD is a Research Scientist at the VA Portland Health Care System, Professor in the Departments of Psychiatry and Behavioral Neuroscience, and Core Faculty in the Clinical Psychology PhD Program at Oregon Health & Science University (OHSU). Her translational research program studies the psychoneuroimmunological mechanisms contributing to mood disorders, cognitive impairments, and addiction and tests immunotherapeutic strategies to treat these conditions. This work includes investigating the impact of hepatitis C and other viral infections on immune response and neural circuits; testing hypotheses regarding the effects of inflammatory factors on central nervous system and psychiatric function; and evaluating interventions to reduce depression and anxiety, enhance cognition, and improve substance use disorder recovery outcomes. To support this research, she has been awarded grants from the Department of Veterans Affairs, National Institutes of Health, and local foundations. She has authored over 95 peer-reviewed publications in the fields of psychiatry, neuroscience, and immunology. She has served as a mentor for the National Science Foundation's STEM program and is currently a mentor in the VA Mentorship program, OHSU's Partnership for Scientific Inquiry, and Saturday Academy's Apprenticeships in Science & Engineering program. In addition to her research expertise, she has clinical experience, which she acquired during the years she worked as a mental health provider in community clinics, hospitals, and addiction treatment programs. Her goal as a scientist is to maintain a productive research program, one that allows for the pursuit of research, teaching, and community service and one that contributes to our understanding of the mechanisms associated with neuropsychiatric impairments and inflammation in order to improve mental health and quality of life.

J. Wesson Ashford, MD, PhD is a Psychiatrist and Neuroscientist. After completing his Bachelor of Science degree at UC Berkeley, he completed his MD, a Psychiatry Residency, and a PhD in Neuroscience at UCLA. During his Chief Residency on the UCLA Geriatric Psychiatry Unit, he developed a focus on Alzheimer's disease, which led to his participating in numerous research projects at Southern Illinois University, UC Davis, University of Kentucky, and Stanford. He has published over 200 peer-reviewed papers listed on PubMed, including articles on brain imaging, measurement of dementia and depression severity, the genetics of Alzheimer's disease, and the neurophysiology, neurochemistry, and treatment of Alzheimer's disease, depression, and post-traumatic stress disorder (PTSD). He is currently a Clinical Professor (affiliated) in the Department of Psychiatry & Behavioral Sciences at Stanford University and the Director of the War Related Illness & Injury Study Center (WRIISC) at the VA Palo Alto Health Care System.

Other Contributors

Elizabeth Sunzeri, MS, LMFT is a Licensed Marriage and Family Therapist in a rural area of the southern Oregon Coast where she specializes in evidence-based psychotherapy for clients with chronic or serious physical health issues, including depression, obesity, PTSD, cancer, heart disease, and autoimmune disorders. She is a former nurse and a past president of the Oregon Association of Marriage and Family Therapists and was on the Steering Committee for the American Association of Marriage and Family Therapists. She was a Collaborating Field Investigator for DSM-5 field trials in routine clinical practice settings where she was assigned to the depression and PTSD section. She was a task force member for Bay Bariatrics, and on the Pain Management Team for Bay Area Hospital. While at UC Berkeley, she was on the team that discovered BRCA1. She has designed and facilitated a variety of training programs for groups.

Jeffery J. Sunzeri, MS is a sociologist and a member of the Alpha Kappa Delta International Honor Society of Sociology. His academic training in social research methodology led to a career beginning as a data analyst in a medical review organization. This position then dovetailed into a decades-long career as a software development consultant where he developed business, scientific, and analytical software for a variety of successful businesses, including Amfac Pharmaceutical Distribution Systems, Hewlett Packard (several business divisions), Royal Saudi Arabian Air Forces, and Smith Dennis & Gaylord Medical Systems. He holds a patent in an innovative digital imaging application that has been used in sociology research.

Abbreviations

5-HT	Serotonin
5-HTTLPR	Serotonin Transporter Linked Polymorphic Region
ABCD	Adolescent Brain Cognitive Development
ACC	Anterior Cingulate Cortex
ACT	Acceptance and Commitment Therapy
ACTH	Adrenocorticotropic Hormone
ADHD	Attention-Deficit/Hyperactivity Disorder
AN	Anorexia Nervosa
AOR	Adjusted Odds Ratio
APA	American Psychiatric Association
ASR	Age-Standardized Incidence Rate
AUD	Alcohol Use Disorder
AVP/ADH	Arginine Vasopressin/Antidiuretic Hormone
BA	Behavioral Activation
BDI	Beck Depression Inventory
BDNF	Brain-Derived Neurotrophic Factor
BMI	Body Mass Index
BN	Bulimia Nervosa
BPD	Borderline Personality Disorder
CBC	Complete Blood Count
CBCL/DP	Child Behavior Checklist-Dysregulation Profile
CBG	Corticosteroid-Binding Globulin
CBT	Cognitive-Behavioral Therapy
CBT-I	Cognitive-Behavioral Therapy for Insomnia
CCMD	Chinese Classification of Mental Disorders
CDC	Centers for Disease Control and Prevention
CES-D	Center for Epidemiologic Studies-Depression Scale
CI	Confidence Interval
CINAHL	Cumulative Index to Nursing and Allied Health Literature
CNS	Central Nervous System
CNV	Copy Number Variation
COMT	Catechol-O-Methyltransferase
CONSORT	Consolidated Standards of Reporting Trials
CRF	Corticotropin Releasing Factor
CRH	Corticotropin Releasing Hormone
CrI	Credible Interval
CRP	C-Reactive Protein
CUD	Cannabis Use Disorder
DALYs	Disability-Adjusted Life Years
DAT	Dopamine Transporter
DBT	Dialectical Behavior Therapy
DDDAMD	Depressive Disorder Due to Another Medical Condition

DLPFC	Dorsolateral Prefrontal Cortex
DMDD	Disruptive Mood Dysregulation Disorder
DRD1/DRD2/DRD4	Dopamine Receptors D1/D2/D4
DSM-5	Diagnostic and Statistical Manual of Mental Disorders, 5th Edition
DSM-5 CC	DSM-5 Cross-Cutting Symptom Measures
DSM-5-TR	Diagnostic and Statistical Manual of Mental Disorders, 5th Edition, Text Revision
DSM-III-R	Diagnostic and Statistical Manual of Mental Disorders, 3rd Edition, Revised
DSM-IV	Diagnostic and Statistical Manual of Mental Disorders, 4th Edition
EAPC	Estimated Annual Percentage Change
ECT	Electroconvulsive Therapy
EMA	Ecological Momentary Assessment
ENCODE	Encyclopedia of DNA Elements
ENIGMA	Enhancing NeuroImaging Genetics Through Meta-Analysis
ENS	Enteric Nervous System
E-Risk	Environmental Risk Longitudinal Twin Study
FDA	Food and Drug Administration
FFM	Five-Factor Model
fMRI	Functional MRI
GABA	Gamma-Aminobutyric Acid
GAD	Generalized Anxiety Disorder
GAD-7	Generalized Anxiety Disorder 7-Item Scale
GBD	Global Burden of Disease
GDS	Geriatric Depression Scale
GIDS	Gender Inclusive Depression Scale
GIGA	Global Imaging Genetics of Adolescents
GMDS	Gotland Male Depression Scale
GRN	Gene Regulatory Network
GTEx	Genotype-Tissue Expression
GWA	Genome-Wide Analysis
GWAS	Genome-Wide Association Study
HADS	Hospital Anxiety and Depression Scale
HAM-D	Hamilton Depression Scale
HAMD/HDRS	Hamilton Depression Rating Scale
HPA	Hypothalamic-Pituitary-Adrenal axis
ICD-10	International Classification of Diseases, 10th Revision
ICD-10/11	International Classification of Diseases, 10th/11th Edition
ICD-10/ICD-11	International Classification of Diseases, 10th/11th Revision
ICD-11	International Classification of Diseases, 11th Revision
IFN-α	Interferon-alpha
IL-6	Interleukin-6
IPT	Interpersonal Psychotherapy
LILACS	Latin American and Caribbean Health Sciences Literature – Database
MADD	Mixed Anxiety and Depression Disorder
MADRS	Montgomery–Åsberg Depression Rating Scale
MADRS-S	Montgomery–Åsberg Depression Rating Scale, Self-Report
MAO	Monoamine Oxidase

MAO/MAOA	Monoamine Oxidase (A)
MAOI	Monoamine Oxidase Inhibitor
MBCT	Mindfulness-Based Cognitive Therapy
MBSR	Mindfulness-Based Stress Reduction
MDAD	Mixed Depressive and Anxiety Disorder
MDD	Major Depressive Disorder
MDS	Masculine Depression Scale
Medline, Embase, PsycINFO, Scopus, ProQuest, CINAHL, LILACS	Biomedical literature databases
MR/GR	Mineralocorticoid/Glucocorticoid Receptor
MRI	Magnetic Resonance Imaging
MRI/fMRI (Functional)	Magnetic Resonance Imaging
MSS	Male Symptoms Scale
NAc	Nucleus Accumbens
NaSSA	Noradrenergic and Specific Serotonergic Antidepressant
NCS-A	National Comorbidity Survey Adolescent Supplement
NCS-R	National Comorbidity Survey Replication
NCS-R/NCS-A	National Comorbidity Survey Replication/Adolescent Supplement
NDA	National Institute of Mental Health Data Archive
NDRI	Norepinephrine-Dopamine Reuptake Inhibitor
NESARC	National Epidemiologic Survey on Alcohol and Related Conditions
NESARC-III	National Epidemiologic Survey on Alcohol and Related Conditions III
NHANES	National Health and Nutrition Examination Survey
NIH	National Institutes of Health
NIMH	National Institute of Mental Health
NK	Natural Killer cells
NNT	Number Needed to Treat
NRC	National Research Council
NSDUH	National Survey on Drug Use and Health
NSSI	Non-Suicidal Self-Injury
OCD	Obsessive-Compulsive Disorder
OR	Odds Ratio
PDD	Persistent Depressive Disorder
PDyD	Premenstrual Dysphoric Disorder
PET	Positron Emission Tomography
PFC	Prefrontal Cortex
PGC	Psychiatric Genomics Consortium
PHQ	Patient Health Questionnaire
PHQ-9	Patient Health Questionnaire-9
PHT-CM	Pharmacotherapy with Clinical Management
PID-5	Personality Inventories for DSM-5
PNI	Psychoneuroimmunology
PNS	Peripheral Nervous System
PRIME-MD	Primary Care Evaluation of Mental Disorders
PRISMA	Preferred Reporting Items for Systematic Reviews and Meta-Analyses
PTSD	Post-Traumatic Stress Disorder
QTL	Quantitative Trait Locus
RCT	Randomized Controlled Trial

RDoC	Research Domain Criteria
RR	Relative Risk
rTMS	Repetitive Transcranial Magnetic Stimulation
SAD	Seasonal Affective Disorder
SARI	Serotonin Antagonist and Reuptake Inhibitor
SD	Standard Deviation
SE	Standard Error
SERT	Serotonin Transporter
SES	Socioeconomic Status
SLC6A4	Serotonin Transporter Gene
SMD	Standardized Mean Difference
SMIDD	Substance/Medication-Induced Depressive Disorder
SNP	Single Nucleotide Polymorphism
SNRI	Serotonin-Norepinephrine Reuptake Inhibitor
SSRI	Selective Serotonin Reuptake Inhibitor
STPP	Short-Term Psychodynamic Psychotherapy
TAU	Treatment As Usual
TCA	Tricyclic Antidepressant
tDCS	Transcranial Direct-Current Stimulation
TEDS	Twins Early Development Study
TNF-α	Tumor Necrosis Factor-alpha
TRD	Treatment-Resistant Depression
TSH	Thyroid Stimulating Hormone
VTA	Ventral Tegmental Area
WGs	Working Groups
WHO	World Health Organization
WHODAS 2.0	World Health Organization Disability Assessment Schedule, Version 2.0
WMD	Weighted Mean Difference
WPA	World Psychiatric Association
YLDs	Years Lived with Disability

List of Figures

Introduction

1

Franklin Sunzeri

Raison d'être

Time is of the essence for busy practitioners. Applying discoveries in epigenetics and psychobiology to clinical practice with precision and avoiding misinformation is a worthy but often daunting goal.

It is our mission to provide a concise and practical guide in as few pages as possible. To do this, we have used sparse language and hyperlinks for more in-depth resources.

One difficult decision has been selecting which references among many excellent papers to include in the reference links. This has been particularly challenging due to the vastness, diversity, and complexity of behavioral medicine as it pertains to depressive disorders.

However, we believe that if you follow the PubMed links back to the articles that we included, you will find more information that links to those other citations.

Environment plays at least an equal part with genetics in determining many of our characteristics including depression [3, 4], substance abuse [5], eating disorders [6], our perception of stress [7], general health [8], parenting and later psychopathology [9, 10], coping [11], and even personality [12, 13]. See Fig. 1.1.

Experiences at critical times early in life may result in stable epigenetic programming including the glucocorticoid receptor gene expression in the hippocampus and may have long-term effects on depression [14–21]. However, even though the environment can induce persistent changes in chromatin, these changes are dynamic and might have the potential to be reversed [22–26]. It is noteworthy that perceived stress, childhood adversities, major depressive disorder, educational attainment, physical activity, and sleep duration may influence telomere length and disease risk [21, 27–29]. And even these telomeric changes may be reversible through behavioral modifications [30, 31].

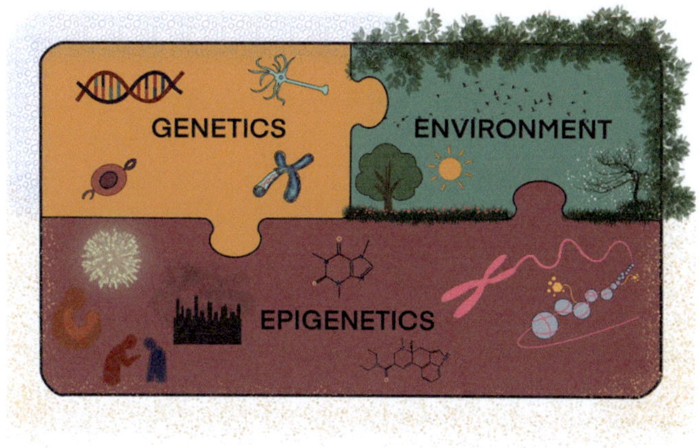

Fig. 1.1 Interplay of genetics, environment, and epigenetics across the lifespan. Genetics and environment form the foundational layers, with epigenetics emerging at their intersection—shaped by inherited traits, parental exposures, and life experiences. Genetic influences include parental genotypes, mutations, and lifestyle-driven changes, while environmental constraints span from preconception to death, encompassing socioeconomic conditions, stressors, and access to resources. Epigenetic mechanisms reflect both ancestral environments and individual trajectories, illustrating how biology and context coalesce to shape vulnerability and resilience

Behavioral medicine research has several goals. One of these is to understand how the behavior and body interaction works and then to apply what has been learned to prevent or lessen the grip of disease [32–34]. However, these interactions are complex: a product of the interdisciplinary nature of behavioral medicine [27, 35, 36].

Cause and effect are sometimes difficult to determine in the behavioral sciences. Many of the psychological concepts such as stress and depression, mood and affect are often nebulous in practice. Although scales have been routinely used to measure such concepts in experimental protocols, it is still unclear what physiological correlates may be involved in a given individual. Ultimately, we need to remember that psychosocial support treats an individual, not a group. One size does not fit all.

F. Sunzeri (✉)
Heather Hills Consulting, Coos Bay, OR, USA

J. Raber et al. (eds.), *Understanding and Treating Depressive Disorders*, https://doi.org/10.1007/978-3-032-14465-2_1

We are stochastic [22, 37–41] and together we make up a set of probabilities. That any one of us will experience and react in a predictable fashion is based upon how closely we fit to that norm. And that is a product of genes, psychosocial environment, and choices we have made and continue to make that reflect our individuality.

We have considerable latitude for psychosocial choices. Nevertheless, it should be pointed out that this environment may have already limited some of our choices [42]. For example, dysfunctional families may have had pathological influences in our formative years on our self-image, perception of stress, and our coping mechanisms [43–46].

The choices we make are further constrained by our mobility, physical limitations, monetary resources, the attitudes, and social mores of the society or even the country in which we were born or live. And sometimes the capriciousness of fate steps in. Given all these considerations, it behooves us to arm ourselves with the best evidence for making our health-related choices. This then is the overall goal of behavioral medicine.

Connections between the classical physiological systemic divisions are mediated by itinerant cells, fixed or semi-fixed hard wiring of nerves and vessels, and messengers that commute in these vessels and cells. Fundamental to understanding this system is to accept the premise that this heterarchy is cognitive and self-organizing [1].

We use cognition as defined by Irun Cohen [2]. That is, a cognitive system combines three principal attributes: (1) It makes decisions, (2) it carries with it a memory of its environment, and (3) it builds upon memories to modify or build its machinery to cope with its environment.

Our experiences, emotions, expectations, physical limitations, language abilities, and intelligence, all combine to make us changeable individuals. We need to adjust temporally and spatially to cope with our environment. From this cognition comes individuality. Individuality that is superimposed upon the uniqueness imparted by our genes and epigenetic effects, and that is expressed in our behavior. Yet, we are always constrained by the conserved part of our genetic code that makes us human.

If we can identify what we can change, whether it is by altering our thought processes or taking therapeutics, we may be able to change ourselves to maximize our potential for health. What appears in the following pages is a nano review of current evidence-based behavioral medicine as it relates to depressive disorders and carries us toward identifying what we can change and how we might be able to do so.

How to Use This Manual

This is an eBook; as such, hyperlinks to digitized information are in the reference lists so that you can reference evidence-based sources for more information.

As an eBook, common digital tools are active. Search functions are especially handy in exploring various concepts for more information that is found in this text. Annotating and making comments are facilitated. You can use the search function to link to any information present in this guide.

What Difference Can We Make?

The answers rest upon the contributing factors to the disorders, genetic, epigenetic, and environmental factors, identifying ways to modulate the effects of epigenetic and environmental factors, the willingness and ability of patients to make those changes, and the ability of the medical practitioners to assist in making those changes.

After this brief introduction, let us look at the evidence for each of these.

We hope that this e-book will help you to provide useful information to your patients and guide them on a safe and stimulating path to maximum wellness.

Enjoy your journey!

References

1. Pert C. Molecules of emotion. New York: Scribner; 1997.
2. Cohen IR. Tending Adam's garden, evolving the cognitive immune self. San Diego: Academic; 2002.
3. Bierut LJ, Heath AC, Bucholz KK, Dinwiddie SH, Madden PA, Statham DJ, Dunne MP, Martin NG. Major depressive disorder in a community-based twin sample: are there different genetic and environmental contributions for men and women? Arch Gen Psychiatry. 1999;56(6):557–63. PMID: 10359473. http://www.ncbi.nlm.nih.gov/pubmed/10359473.
4. Kendler KS, Prescott CA. A population-based twin study of lifetime major depression in men and women. Arch Gen Psychiatry. 1999;56(1):39–44. PMID: 9892254. http://www.ncbi.nlm.nih.gov/pubmed/9892254.
5. Rhee SH, Hewitt JK, Young SE, Corley RP, Crowley TJ, Stallings MC. Genetic and environmental influences on substance initiation, use, and problem use in adolescents. Arch Gen Psychiatry. 2003;60(12):1256–64. PMID: 14662558. http://www.ncbi.nlm.nih.gov/pubmed/9892254.
6. Kortegaard LS, Hoerder K, Joergensen J, Gillberg C, Kyvik KO. A preliminary population-based twin study of self-reported eating disorder. Psychol Med. 2001;31(2):361–5. PMID: 11232922. http://www.ncbi.nlm.nih.gov/pubmed/11232922.
7. Federenko IS, Schlotz W, Kirschbaum C, Bartels M, Hellhammer DH, Wüst S. The heritability of perceived stress. Psychol Med. 2006;36(3):375–85. PMID: 16393364. http://www.ncbi.nlm.nih.gov/pubmed/16393364.

8. Rijsdijk FV, Snieder H, Ormel J, Sham P, Goldberg DP, Spector TD. Genetic and environmental influences on psychological distress in the population: general health questionnaire analyses in UK twins. Psychol Med. 2003;33(5):793–801. PMID: 12877394. http://www.ncbi.nlm.nih.gov/pubmed/12877394.
9. Kendler KS. Parenting: a genetic-epidemiologic perspective. Am J Psychiatry. 1996;153(1):11–20. PMID: 8540566. http://www.ncbi.nlm.nih.gov/pubmed/8540566.
10. Rinehart DJ, Becker MA, Buckley PR, Dailey K, Reichardt CS, Graeber C, Van DeMark NR, Brown E. The relationship between mothers' child abuse potential and current mental health symptoms: implications for screening and referral. J Behav Health Serv Res. 2005;32(2):155–66. PMID: 15834265. http://www.ncbi.nlm.nih.gov/pubmed/15834265.
11. Wang X, Trivedi R, Treiber F, Snieder H. Genetic and environmental influences on anger expression, John Henryism, and stressful life events: the Georgia cardiovascular twin study. Psychosom Med. 2005;67(1):16–23. PMID: 15673619. http://www.ncbi.nlm.nih.gov/pubmed/15673619.
12. Taylor J, Loney BR, Bobadilla L, Iacono WG, McGue M. Genetic and environmental influences on psychopathy trait dimensions in a community sample of male twins. J Abnorm Child Psychol. 2003;31(6):633–45. PMID: 14658743. http://www.ncbi.nlm.nih.gov/pubmed/14658743.
13. Jang KL, Livesley WJ, Vernon PA. Heritability of the big five personality dimensions and their facets: a twin study. J Pers. 1996;64(3):577–91. PMID: 8776880. http://www.ncbi.nlm.nih.gov/pubmed/8776880.
14. Weaver ICG, Meaney MJ, Szyf M. Maternal care effects on the hippocampal transcriptome and anxiety-mediated behaviors in the offspring that are reversible in adulthood. Proc Natl Acad Sci USA. 2006;103(9):3480–5. PMCID: PMC1413873. http://www.ncbi.nlm.nih.gov/pubmed/16484373.
15. Seckl JR, Holmes MC. Mechanisms of disease: glucocorticoids, their placental metabolism and fetal "programming" of adult pathophysiology. Nat Clin Pract Endocrinol Metab. 2007;3(6):479–88. PMID: 17515892. http://www.ncbi.nlm.nih.gov/pubmed/17515892.
16. Seckl JR. Prenatal glucocorticoids and long-term programming. Eur J Endocrinol. 2004;151(Suppl 3):U49–62. PMID: 15554887. http://www.ncbi.nlm.nih.gov/pubmed/15554887.
17. Lupien SJ, King S, Meaney MJ, McEwen BS. Child's stress hormone levels correlate with mother's socioeconomic status and depressive state. Biol Psychiatry. 2000;48(10):976–80. PMID: 11082471. http://www.ncbi.nlm.nih.gov/pubmed/11082471.
18. Slavich GM, Cole SW. The emerging field of human social genomics. Clin Psychol Sci. 2013;1(3):331–48. PMCID: PMC3707393. http://www.ncbi.nlm.nih.gov/pubmed/23853742.
19. Vialou V, Feng J, Robison AJ, Nestler EJ. Epigenetic mechanisms of depression and antidepressant action. Annu Rev Pharmacol Toxicol. 2013;53:59–87. PMCID: PMC3711377. http://www.ncbi.nlm.nih.gov/pubmed/23020296.
20. Reul JMHM. Making memories of stressful events: a journey along epigenetic, gene transcription, and signaling pathways. Front Psychiatry. 2014;5:5. PMCID: PMC3897878. http://www.ncbi.nlm.nih.gov/pubmed/24478733.
21. Hanssen LM, Schutte NS, Malouff JM, Epel ES. The relationship between childhood psychosocial stressor level and telomere length: a meta-analysis. Health Psychol Res. 2017;5(1):6378. PMCID: PMC5452631. http://www.ncbi.nlm.nih.gov/pubmed/28603779.
22. Meaney MJ, Szyf M. Environmental programming of stress responses through DNA methylation: life at the interface between a dynamic environment and a fixed genome. Dialogues Clin Neurosci. 2005;7(2):103–23. PMCID: PMC3181727. http://www.ncbi.nlm.nih.gov/pubmed/16262207.
23. Weder N, Zhang H, Jensen K, Yang BZ, Simen A, Jackowski A, Lipschitz D, Douglas-Palumberi H, Ge M, Perepletchikova F, O'Loughlin K, Hudziak JJ, Gelernter J, Kaufman J. Child abuse, depression, and methylation in genes involved with stress, neural plasticity, and brain circuitry. J Am Acad Child Adolesc Psychiatry. 2014;53(4):417–424.e5. PMCID: PMC4126411. http://www.ncbi.nlm.nih.gov/pubmed/24655651.
24. Nabeshima T, Kim HC. Involvement of genetic and environmental factors in the onset of depression. Exp Neurobiol. 2013;22(4):235–43. PMCID: PMC3897684. http://www.ncbi.nlm.nih.gov/pubmed/24465138.
25. Mayer SE, Prather AA, Puterman E, Lin J, Arenander J, Coccia M, Shields GS, Slavich GM, Epel ES. Cumulative lifetime stress exposure and leukocyte telomere length attrition: the unique role of stressor duration and exposure timing. Psychoneuroendocrinology. 2019;104:210–8. PMCID: PMC6518420. http://www.ncbi.nlm.nih.gov/pubmed/30884304.
26. Meier HCS, Hussein M, Needham B, Barber S, Lin J, Seeman T, Diez Roux A. Cellular response to chronic psychosocial stress: ten-year longitudinal changes in telomere length in the multiethnic study of atherosclerosis. Psychoneuroendocrinology. 2019;107:70–81. PMCID: PMC6635040. http://www.ncbi.nlm.nih.gov/pubmed/31112903.
27. Starkweather AR, Alhaeeri AA, Montpetit A, Brumelle J, Filler K, Montpetit M, Mohanraj L, Lyon DE, Jackson-Cook CK. An integrative review of factors associated with telomere length and implications for biobehavioral research. Nurs Res. 2014;63(1):36–50. PMCID: PMC4112289. http://www.ncbi.nlm.nih.gov/pubmed/24335912.
28. Boccardi M, Boccardi V. Psychological wellbeing and healthy aging: focus on telomeres. Geriatrics (Basel). 2019;4(1):25. PMCID: PMC6473912. http://www.ncbi.nlm.nih.gov/pubmed/31023993
29. Chilton W, O'Brien B, Charchar F. Telomeres, aging and exercise: guilty by association? Int J Mol Sci. 2017;18(12):2573. PMCID: PMC5751176. http://www.ncbi.nlm.nih.gov/pubmed/29186077.
30. Epel E. How "reversible" is telomeric aging? Cancer Prev Res (Phila). 2012;5(10):1163–8. PMID: 23041472. http://www.ncbi.nlm.nih.gov/pubmed/23041472.
31. Conklin QA, Crosswell AD, Saron CD, Epel ES. Meditation, stress processes, and telomere biology. Curr Opin Psychol. 2019;28:92–101. PMCID: PMC6526075. http://www.ncbi.nlm.nih.gov/pubmed/30553080.
32. Meissner HI, Glasgow RE, Vinson CA, Chambers D, Brownson RC, Green LW, Ammerman AS, Weiner BJ, Mittman B. The U.S. training institute for dissemination and implementation research in health. Implement Sci. 2013;8:12. PMCID: PMC3564839. http://www.ncbi.nlm.nih.gov/pubmed/23347882.
33. Glasgow RE, Chambers DA, Cynkin L. News from the NIH: highlights in implementation science from the National Cancer Institute and the National Institute of Mental Health. Transl Behav Med. 2013;3(4):335–7. PMCID: PMC3830018. http://www.ncbi.nlm.nih.gov/pubmed/24294320.
34. Kerner J, Rimer B, Emmons K. Introduction to the special section on dissemination: dissemination research and research dissemination: how can we close the gap? Health Psychol. 2005;24(5):443–6. PMID: 16162037. http://www.ncbi.nlm.nih.gov/pubmed/16162037.
35. Fisher EB, Fitzgibbon ML, Glasgow RE, Haire-Joshu D, Hayman LL, Kaplan RM, Nanney MS, Ockene JK. Behavior matters. Am J Prev Med. 2011;40(5):e15–30. PMCID: PMC3137947. http://www.ncbi.nlm.nih.gov/pubmed/21496745.
36. Glasgow RE. What types of evidence are most needed to advance behavioral medicine? Ann Behav Med. 2008;35(1):19–25. PMID: 18347901. http://www.ncbi.nlm.nih.gov/pubmed/18347901.

37. Robins J, Greenland S. The probability of causation under a stochastic model for individual risk. Biometrics. 1989;45(4):1125–38. PMID: 2611320. http://www.ncbi.nlm.nih.gov/pubmed/2611320.
38. Audley RJ. A stochastic model for individual choice behavior. Psychol Rev. 1960;67:1–15. PMID: 13795057. http://www.ncbi.nlm.nih.gov/pubmed/13795057.
39. Champagnat N, Ferrière R, Méléard S. Unifying evolutionary dynamics: from individual stochastic processes to macroscopic models. Theor Popul Biol. 2006;69(3):297–321. PMID: 16460772. http://www.ncbi.nlm.nih.gov/pubmed/16460772.
40. Lipniacki T, Paszek P, Brasier AR, Luxon BA, Kimmel M. Stochastic regulation in early immune response. Biophys J. 2006;90(3):725–42. PMCID: PMC1367099. http://www.ncbi.nlm.nih.gov/pubmed/16284261.
41. Neufeld RWJ, Vollick D, Carter JR, Boksman K, Jetté J. Application of stochastic modeling to the assessment of group and individual differences in cognitive functioning. Psychol Assess. 2002;14(3):279–98. PMID: 12214434. http://www.ncbi.nlm.nih.gov/pubmed/12214434.
42. Eaton DK, Kann L, Kinchen S, Ross J, Hawkins J, Harris WA, Lowry R, McManus T, Chyen D, Shanklin S, Lim C, Grunbaum JA, Wechsler H. Youth risk behavior surveillance–United States, 2005. MMWR Surveill Summ. 2006;55(5):1–108. PMID: 16760893. http://www.ncbi.nlm.nih.gov/pubmed/16760893.
43. Bush TL. Extraskeletal effects of estrogen and the prevention of atherosclerosis. Osteoporos Int. 1991;2(1):5–11. PMID: 1790422. http://www.ncbi.nlm.nih.gov/pubmed/1790422.
44. Gerra G, Zaimovic A, Garofano L, Ciusa F, Moi G, Avanzini P, Talarico E, Gardini F, Brambilla F, Manfredini M, Donnini C. Perceived parenting behavior in the childhood of cocaine users: relationship with genotype and personality traits. Am J Med Genet B Neuropsychiatr Genet. 2007;144B(1):52–7. PMID: 16972224. http://www.ncbi.nlm.nih.gov/pubmed/16972224.
45. Mullen PE, Martin JL, Anderson JC, Romans SE, Herbison GP. The effect of child sexual abuse on social, interpersonal and sexual function in adult life. Br J Psychiatry. 1994;165(1):35–47. PMID: 7953055. http://www.ncbi.nlm.nih.gov/pubmed/7953055.
46. Szili I, György S. The role of mother-child relationship in development of self-image, dysfunctional attitudes and coping strategies. Psychiatr Hung. 2005;20(2):126–40. PMID: 16389782. http://www.ncbi.nlm.nih.gov/pubmed/16389782.

Diagnosis of Depression

2

Franklin Sunzeri and Elizabeth Sunzeri

Introduction

Diagnosis of the various mood disorders is based upon the symptoms and signs. Screening may be facilitated by any of a variety of brief questionnaires. The clinical criteria for diagnosis of specific mood disorders are met by correspondence with the *Diagnostic and Statistical Manual of Mental Disorders (DSM-5)* [1] and the *International Classification of Diseases (ICD-10)* [2, 3].[1] Depression has a diversity of presentations and is clinically defined on the basis of timing and degrees of affective symptoms such as sadness, apathy, desperation, anhedonia, and discomfort that can influence interest in daily activities [5].

In 2017, Clark et al. published an in-depth comparison of the three approaches to understanding and classifying mental disorders [6]. They reviewed the two major diagnostic manuals: the *WHO's ICD-11* and the *American Psychiatric Association's DSM 5* both of which offer classifications that are useful for clinical diagnoses, research applications, public health, and specific research. Then they contrasted the *National Institute of Mental Health Research Domain Criteria (RDoC)*. The RDOC is a useful research framework for new approaches to investigating mental disorders. The RDoC emphasizes integration of basic behavioral and neuroscience research to advance understanding of mental disorders. Clark et al. suggest that although they share a common goal, the ICD-11, the DSM5 and the RDoC have some differences.

Severity of depression is assessed by the amount of disability (physical, social, or occupational) and the duration of symptoms. Depressive disorders were the fourth leading cause of the burden of disease in 1990 [7], and the third leading cause of disease burden and the principal cause of disability in 2000 [8]. The *Global Burden of Diseases, Injuries, and Risk Factors Study 2017 (GBD 2017)* found that from 1990 to 2017 three chronic noncommunicable diseases (low back pain, headache disorders, and depressive disorders) prevailed as three of the top four leading causes of *years lived with disability (YLDs)* [9] Collectively, worldwide they caused 162 million YLDs and accounted for 20% of global YLDs.

Published in 2019, major depressive disorder (MDD) global prevalence and incidence was meta-analyzed to quantify the burden in the *Global Burden of Disease (GBD) 2017 Study*[2] [10]. Results from 1990 were compared to those in 2017 [13]. During that time, incident cases of depression increased worldwide from 172 million to 258 million: an increase of almost 50%. The largest increase was in Qatar

[1] In March of 2022, a new edition of the DSM-5 was published. It is *The Diagnostic and Statistical Manual of Mental Disorders, Fifth Edition, Text Revision (DSM-5-TR)* [1]. Quoted from the APA Website: "The revised version includes a new diagnosis (prolonged grief disorder), clarifying modifications to the criteria sets for more than 70 disorders, addition of International Classification of Diseases, Tenth Revision, Clinical Modification (ICD-10-CM) symptom codes for suicidal behavior and nonsuicidal self-injury, and updates to descriptive text for most disorders based on extensive review of the literature. In addition, DSM-5-TR includes a comprehensive review of the impact of racism and discrimination on the diagnosis and manifestations of mental disorders". Updates to the DSM-5-TR can be found at [4] .

[2] *The Global Burden of Disease (GBD)* is "an effort to measure epidemiological levels and trends worldwide. It is the product of a global research collaborative and quantifies the impact of hundreds of diseases, injuries, and risk factors in countries around the world." [10]. GBD is led by The *Institute for Health Metrics and Evaluation (IHME)* an independent global health research center at the University of Washington [11]. It is an international consortium of thousands of researchers. Their goal is to quantify health loss from hundreds of diseases, injuries, and risk factors, so that health systems can be improved, and disparities can be eliminated. Their websites contains powerful interactive tools to access and display data [12]. This tool allows users to explore and compare causes and risks for different geographies, patterns and trends by location, age, sex, and year, and changes in disease patterns over time.

F. Sunzeri (✉) · E. Sunzeri
Heather Hills Consulting, Coos Bay, OR, USA

J. Raber et al. (eds.), *Understanding and Treating Depressive Disorders*, https://doi.org/10.1007/978-3-032-14465-2_2

[559.33%). The number of incident cases of depression decreased the most in Latvia (−30.99%), followed by Bosnia and Herzegovina (−25.75%) and Georgia (−23.98%). The number of people with depression increased in all geographical regions and by the most in Central sub-Saharan Africa (124.56%), followed by Western sub-Saharan Africa (124.42%) and Oceania (107.19%).

In 2017, the *age-standardized incidence rate (ASR)*[3] varied widely between the 195 countries and regions that were analyzed. The lowest ASR was in Myanmar (1.28 per 1000) and highest in Lesotho (6.59 per 1000). The ASR increased the most in Belgium (*estimated annual percentage change (EAPC)*[4] = 0.88) and decreased the most in Cuba (EAPC = −1.26). The ASR increased significantly in regions with a high sociodemographic index, such as high-income North America (EAPC = 0.41) and decreased significantly in South Asia (EAPC = −0.63).

In 2017, depression global percentage of *DALYS*[5] had changed 0.28% per year to become 1.72%. In the USA, the percentage of DALYS was 2.5%.

The majority (93.7%) of patients with depression in 2017 had MDD; 6.3% of the patients with depression had dysthymia in 2017.

According to the WHO in 2006, the three leading causes of burden of disease in 2030 are projected to include HIV/AIDS, unipolar depressive disorders, and ischemic heart disease in the baseline and pessimistic scenarios [18].

Diagnostic Classifications

There are two major diagnostic manuals: the WHO's *International Classification of Diseases (ICD-11)* and the American Psychiatric Association's *Diagnostic and Statistical Manual of Mental Disorders (DSM 5)* both of which offer classifications that are useful for clinical diagnoses, research applications, public health, and specific research.

The National Institute of Mental Health (NIMH) has been attempting to achieve its strategic goal of developing new methods to classify mental disorders for research purposes [19]. The *National Institute of Mental Health Research Domain Criteria (RDoC)* is the result of that goal. The RDOC is a useful research framework for new approaches to investigating mental disorders. The RDoC's primary goal is precision medicine for psychiatry [20]. The RDoC emphasizes integration of basic behavioral and neuroscience research to advance understanding of mental disorders.

Clark et al. suggest that although they share a common goal, the ICD-11, the DSM5, and the RDoC have some differences [6]. Based on their purposes, there are four areas that are key challenges in understanding and classifying mental disorders. Those four areas are etiology, relevant factors: are they discrete categories or dimensions, thresholds of disease, and comorbidity. Briefly, they suggest the following

Etiology Psychopathology generally is the result of a complex interplay of multiple biological, behavioral, psychosocial, and cultural factors, influenced by each individual's unique life experience. The result of these interactions and factors is not clearly delimited diseases, rather they are mixtures of psychological difficulties.

Categories and Dimensions Categories are useful for us to handle the complexities of psychopathologies, but the boundaries are not distinct and are perhaps artificial. Dimensions are a recognition that psychopathology is not an all or none; instead, it is graded in its manifestations.

Thresholds For clinical purposes, thresholds are useful but should be considered as arbitrary unless proven by further research to be otherwise.

Comorbidity Comorbidity is perhaps the rule rather than the exception. It may be an artifact of an imperfect classification system.

Diagnostic and Statistical Manual of Mental Disorders (DSM 5)

As research in behavioral medicine has progressed, the definitions of depressive disorders have become more refined. Evidence for these changes can be seen in revised versions of the DSM. Advances in the sciences of psychobiology have resulted in significant changes in the current edition of the DSM, the DSM-5, and DSM-5-TR.

Although all clinicians are by necessity familiar with the DSM-5, a quick look at Depressive Disorders classifications will underscore the temperamental, genetic, and physiological contributions to the differential diagnoses of the depressive disorders. So, let us peek.

[3] *Age-standardized incidence rate (ASR)* is the incidence rate of a particular disease in a population if that population had a standard age structure. This standardization allows populations to be compared when the population profiles are different. [14, 15].

[4] The *annual percent change (APC)* measures trends in disease and mortality rates. A common estimator uses a linear model on the log of the age-standardized rates [16].

[5] Quoted from the WHO Global Health Observatory website: "The overall burden of disease is assessed using the disability-adjusted life year (*DALY*), a time-based measure that combines years of life lost due to premature mortality (*YLLs*) and years of life lost due to time lived in states of less than full health, or years of healthy life lost due to disability (*YLDs*). One DALY represents the loss of the equivalent of one year of full health" [17].

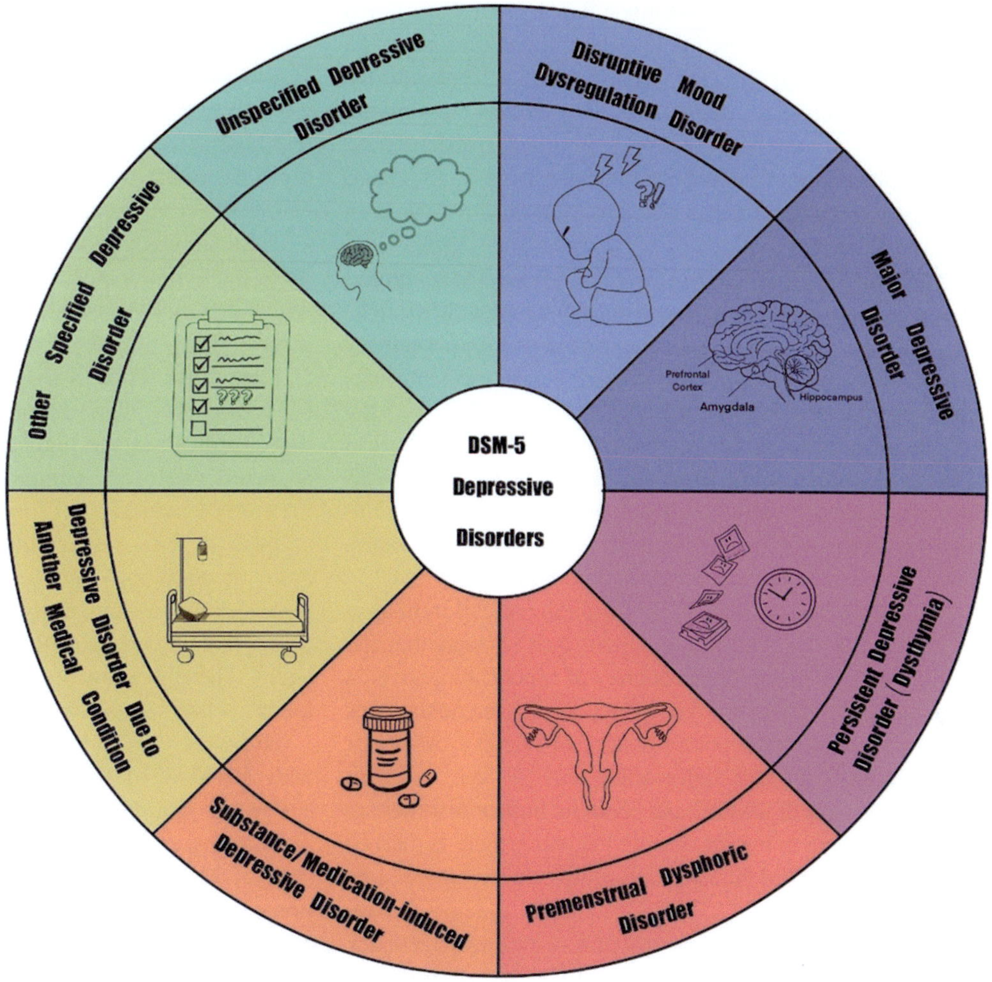

Fig. 2.1 DSM-5 wheel depicting the various mood disorders discussed in this chapter

The DSM-5 categorizes Depressive Disorders as including disruptive mood dysregulation disorder, major depressive disorder, persistent depressive disorder (dysthymia), premenstrual dysphoric disorder, substance/medication-induced depressive disorder, depressive disorder due to another medical condition, other specified depressive disorder, and unspecified depressive disorder. See Fig. 2.1.

It should be worth mentioning that some criticisms have been leveled at the new DSM-5 [21]. It has been said that the new disorders and broader diagnostic criteria may lead to exploitation by pharmaceutical companies. Diagnosis of subthreshold cases and prescription of chemical therapeutics may be promoted by industry-funded key opinion leaders. Online self-diagnoses and expansion of *not otherwise specified* categories may feed into it. A case in point is the epidemic of pediatric bipolar disorder (BD) diagnosis within DSM-IV criteria [22–26]. Indeed, the new diagnostic category disruptive mood dysregulation disorder was proposed to reduce the rate of false bipolar diagnoses in youngsters [27].

Comorbid mental disorders were assessed in a nationally representative sample of adults who participated in the 2008-2012 *Mental Health Surveillance Study* [28]. The results showed that approximately one-third of adults who had a diagnosis of a mood or anxiety disorder suffered from a comorbid mental disorder at the same time. Associated factors were being young, being of non-Hispanic white race/ethnicity, having low family income, and living in a large metropolitan area. They had higher estimates of past-year perceived unmet need for care (21.7% vs. 11.6%, $P < .01$). They were more likely than those with a single mental disorder to be lower functioning and were more likely to have been treated in the last year.

Disruptive Mood Dysregulation Disorder

Disruptive mood dysregulation disorder (DMDD) is chronic, severe, persistent irritability characterized by frequent temper outbursts and chronic persistent irritable or angry mood that is present between outbursts [29–34]. Symptoms will have been present before 10 years of age and the diagnosis is reserved for children between the ages of 7 and 18. The inter-outburst anger is one of the defining characteristics that separate DMDD from bipolar disorder. Bipolar rates are much lower than DMDD before adolescence. Rates of conversion to bipolar are quite low, but there is a significant risk for developing unipolar depressive or anxiety disorders. Comorbidity is very high, with the strongest overlap being oppositional defiant disorder. Irritability, especially as related to mood dysregulation, has been prominently reviewed in [35].

In terms of temperament, DMDD is frequently accompanied by symptoms meeting the criteria for oppositional defiant disorder, anxiety, and attention-deficit/hyperactivity disorder. Familial rates of DMDD, unipolar depression, substance use, anxiety disorders, and bipolar disorders are very similar. Information processing deficits overlap with several of these disorders, while there are also some distinct cognitive differences. There is a greater prevalence of DMDD in males, whereas with bipolar disorders there is approximately equal prevalence between males and females.

Analyses of 82 consecutively hospitalized children, ages 5–12 years, on a children's inpatient unit showed that the DMDD does decrease the frequency of bipolar diagnosis in children [27]. However, the reduction in diagnosis rates depends upon parent-reported history of manic episodes or observations on the inpatient ward.

Consequences of DMDD and pediatric bipolar disorder are very similar. Due to low frustration tolerance, there is marked disruption in peer and family relationships. Severe aggression, dangerous behavior, and suicide ideation and attempts are frequent. Children with DMDD respond to negative feedback with frustration [36]. Frustration seems to reduce attention flexibility especially in severely irritable children. These children demonstrate abnormally reduced activity in areas of the brain involved in emotion, attention, and reward processing. These are the left amygdala, the left and right striatum, the parietal cortex, and the posterior cingulate.

Many of the studies that have produced data suggestive of the diagnostic utility of DMDD have used the *Child Behavior Checklist-Dysregulation Profile (CBCL/DP)*. It is a useful tool to identify youth at increased risk for significant psychopathology [37, 38]. Genetic architecture and biological correlates have suggested distinct patterns of neural dysfunctions underpinning the CBCL/DP [39, 40]. For example, a genome-wide association study of children with attention-deficit/hyperactivity disorder (ADHD) has found developmentally expressed genes operant in hippocampal dependent memory and learning associated with psychopathology results of the CBCL-DP [41]. Electroencephalography and cognitive profiles associated with increased hyperactive/impulsive symptoms, disruptive behavior, mood, and anxiety comorbidities are identifiable.

In one study, children who rated highly on the CBCL-DP for anxiety and disruptive behavior disorders were associated with increased rates of adult anxiety disorders, mood disorders, disruptive behavior disorders, and drug abuse 14 years later [42].

Positive CBCL-DP scores for severe affective and behavioral dysregulation have been associated with subclinical hypothyroidism as represented by elevation of basal serum thyroid-stimulating hormone levels but not serum fT3 and fT4 levels compared to controls [43].

A Dutch study of 489 youth (47% boys) found that activity of the hypothalamic pituitary adrenal (HPA) axis in youth with behavioral dysregulation profile was blunted in response to stress [44].

Data from three 3 community studies involving 7881 observations of 3258 participants, ages from 2 to 17, revealed that DMDD has the highest rates in preschoolers and co-occurred with all common psychiatric disorders [45]. Prevalence rates ranged from 0.8% to 3.3%. Co-occurrence of DMDD with another disorder was 62%–92% and with both an emotional and behavioral disorder 32% to 68%. Oppositional defiant disorder (OR[6] = 52.9 to 103.0) and depressive disorders (OR: 9.9 to 23.5) were the most frequent. There were increased rates of poverty, social impairments, school suspension, and service use.

However, using a sample of 706 children aged 6–12 years who enrolled in the *Longitudinal Assessment of Manic Symptoms (LAMS) study* and DSM-IV criteria, the DMDD diagnosis seemed to be of little diagnostic use [46]. In that study, DMDD could not be discriminated between oppositional defiant disorder and conduct disorder and was not associated with present, future-onset, or parental history of mood or anxiety disorders.

Major Depressive Disorder

Major depressive disorder (MDD) is characterized by persistent symptoms of depressed mood or loss of interest or pleasure that is a change from previous functions [47–52]. Five out of nine symptoms must be present during the same 2-week period. Those symptoms include sleep disturbances, weight changes, psychomotor changes, fatigue, feelings of diminished self-worth, difficulty in thinking, and death-related thoughts [53]. Significant distress in social functioning occurs [54]. It is not attributable to another mental or

[6]Odds ratio (OR) is a way to represent the odds that an outcome will result when a given exposure to a variable of interest occurs compared to when the exposure does not occur. OR quantifies the strength of the association between two events. An OR greater than 1 indicates a positive association or that exposure to that variable increases the odds of that outcome. An OR less than one indicates a negative relationship between two events. An OR of 1 suggests no relationship between two events. An OR is frequently accompanied by a 95% confidence interval (CI). CI is a measure of precision of the OR. The smaller the CI the higher precision as long as it does not overlap OR =1. For more information, see the Chap. 4 on evidence basics in this text.

physical condition, or substance use, and there is no history of mania that would suggest bipolarity.

The temperament of negative affectivity (neuroticism) predisposes to MDD in response to stress [55]. Childhood adversity is powerfully associated [56, 57]. Targeted rejection and other major psychosocial stressors are highly associated with MDD [58–61]. There is a two to four-fold higher risk of MDD when a first-degree relative has MDD [55, 62]. Heritability is approximately 40%. The risk of depression is increased by substance abuse, anxiety, borderline personality disorder and other major non-mood disorders, as well as chronic or disabling physical conditions [63–67]. Although the prevalence is higher in females, there does not seem to be significant differences in the nature or course of MDD. Suicide attempts are greater while completion is lower in females with MDD [68–70]. However, this sex difference is not as great as in the population as a whole.

A systematic review of DSM-IV-based studies for subtypes of MDD referenced in MEDLINE, PsycINFO, and Embase in May 2012 failed to find compelling evidence for the existence of depressive symptoms subtypes [71]. However, other later studies have found evidence for subtypes [72, 73]. A 2018 published cross-sectional study presented a database structure capable of identifying distinct subtypes that denote "specific, coherent, meaningful associations between symptoms, behavior, and brain function, and observable real-world function" [74]. This framework allowed identification of transdiagnostic subtypes of major depressive disorder, panic disorder, and posttraumatic stress disorder. The diagnostic criteria used for the study were that defined by the DSM-IV, but the study's authors suggest that it should be applicable to DSM 5 diagnoses.

For the discovery of data-driven subtypes within a single diagnostic category, stratification has been based on symptom type or severity and behavior within that category [71, 75–77]. Heterogeneity and overlap of symptoms across diagnostic categories have just begun to be analyzed in cohorts of adults who have comorbid mood, anxiety, and trauma disorders with diverse functioning levels [74]. Data was from the *Brain Research and Integrative Neuroscience Network Foundation Database* collected at the University of Sydney and University of Adelaide between 2006 and 2010 and replicated at Stanford University between 2013 and 2017 [74, 78]. The *Brain Resource International Database* is said to be the largest available library of human brain health information acquired using standardized measures, so that multiple sources of data are available on the same individuals [78].

The database for their study included 420 individuals who had a primary diagnosis of major depressive disorder, panic disorder, PTSD, or no disorder. They had a mean age of 39.8 (SD14.1) and 61.0% were female.

They found six *distinct subtypes* characterized by tension (19%), anxious arousal (13%), general anxiety (9%), anhedonia (7%), melancholia (9%), and normative mood (43%). Subtypes were expressed through differences in cognitive control, working memory, electroencephalography-recorded β power[7] in a resting paradigm, electroencephalography-recorded β power in an emotional paradigm, social functional capacity, and emotional resilience.

In participants with a primary diagnosis of MDD, comorbid conditions included post-traumatic stress disorder (PTSD) (12%), panic disorder (14%), generalized anxiety disorder (36%), and attention-deficit/hyperactivity disorder (1%).

In participants with PTSD, comorbid conditions included MDD (36%) and generalized anxiety disorder (9%).

In participants with panic disorder, comorbid conditions included MDD (13%), PTSD (28%), generalized anxiety disorder (9%), dysthymia (6%), obsessive-compulsive disorder (25%), and seasonal affective disorder (59%).

Data from the *National Comorbidity Survey Adolescent Supplement* and the *National Comorbidity Survey Replication* (adult data) samples were used to identify and compare subtypes of MDD in adolescents and adults [75]. Published in 2012, results using DSM-IV criteria identified three subtypes of depression among adolescents and four subtypes among adults.

The *adolescent subtypes* were moderate typical, moderate atypical, severe typical, and atypical. *Moderate typical subtype* (39.9% prevalence) was characterized by decreased appetite and insomnia. It had the lowest proportions of people with thoughts of suicide. The *severe typical subtype* (34.6% prevalence) showed typical symptoms including weight loss. *Atypical subtype* (25.5% prevalence) had increased appetite, weight gain, and fatigue.

For adolescents, a few of the highlights are as follows: severe typical class had double the prevalence rate of agoraphobia compared with the other two classes. Binge eating disorder was highest in the atypical class and lowest in the moderate class. No difference in treatment between the subtypes was seen and no difference in disability was found. The atypical class had the highest BMI. The percentage of adolescents who were overweight or obese was also highest in the atypical group. There were more females in the atypical subtype 80.2% (4.0)[8] severe typical (70.8% (2.7)) and moderate typical (60.4% (3.9)). The number of symptoms was highest in severe typicals. Symptom severity was highest in

[7] A discussion of β power can be found here [80–82]. Beta waves are high-frequency, low-amplitude brain waves common to being awake, and consciously thinking. In high anxiety states beta waves are prominent. In depression, ADHD, dreaming and poor cognitive states, beta waves are suppressed. Lower frequency beta waves are associated with introverted concentration. Middle range beta waves are associated with increased anxiety, energy and performance. High frequency beta waves are associated with higher levels of stress, high arousal, anxiety and high energy.

[8] Female, weighted % (standard error.)

the atypical subtype. A positive family history of depression was seen in severe typical (32.0% (4.7)), atypical (41.8 % (7.1)), and moderate typical (18.8% (4.0))

In adults, the *moderate subtype* (14.6% prevalence) showed moderately severe symptoms. The *moderate typical subtype* (24.8 % prevalence) experienced weight loss, decreased appetite, and insomnia. *Severe typical subtype* (44.9% prevalence) showed a typical symptom pattern but with higher symptom probabilities and proportions of adults with insomnia and suicidal thoughts than the moderate typical class of adolescents. The *atypical subtype* (15.6% prevalence) had a distinct pattern of increased appetite and weight gain.

In adults, females were 51.9% (4.0) of moderates, 57.5% (3.6) of moderate typicals, 66.5% (3.0) of severe typicals, and 79.4% (3.6) of atypicals. The severe typical class had the highest mean number of symptoms and severity scores, followed by the atypical class. The moderate typicals had the fewest number of episodes and the highest percentage of onset before 12 years of age. No differences were seen in the family history of depression. The severe typicals had a more frequent family history of mania. The highest rates of mania were seen in the atypical subtype. The highest rate of hypomania was seen in the severe typical class and the lowest in the atypical class. Social phobia, agoraphobia, and specific phobia had significantly higher prevalence in the severe typical subtype. Typical subtype had the highest BMI and the highest percentage of subjects with BMI greater than 25 kg/m^2 (77.6% vs. 54.2–59.2% in other subtypes). The highest amount of disability was seen in the severe typical subtype.

Severe typical (adults 45%, adolescents 35%) and atypical subtype (adults 16%, adolescents 26%) were subtypes common to both. Sociodemographic data and correlates are presented in [75].

A 2019 systematic review of data-driven biological subtypes of depression concluded that methodological differences across studies and lack of replication do not allow at this time to make definitive conclusions about the existence of clinically useful and generalizable biological subtypes [72].

Functional neural imaging techniques have suggested that the core feature of abnormal emotion processing in MDD involves particular areas of the brain [83–85]. Automatic emotion regulation processes principally involve medial prefrontal cortical areas, the hippocampus and parahippocampus. Voluntary regulation includes lateral prefrontal cortex areas in addition to those areas involved in automatic emotion regulation. People with MDD appear to be deficient in activity in lateral prefrontal areas when explicitly voluntarily attempting to control emotional experience. When these same folks are automatically trying to control the early stages of emotion regulation, they can be successful by recruiting additional lateral prefrontal neural areas, that may be mediated by medial prefrontal, especially rostral/dorsal anterior cingulate gyrus, functioning.

Functional magnetic resonance imaging has shown differences in regions involved in emotion processing during a dynamic emotional faces task between depressed individuals with bipolar disorder (BD) and those with MDD, and in comparison, to normal controls. [86]. Compared to adults with BD, adults with MDD demonstrated significantly greater activity in the left amygdala in response to anger portrayals. Whole-brain analyses showed adults with BD responded to sad faces with greater activity in the temporoparietal regions, especially in the left hemisphere. Adults with MDD vs. BD had greater activity in response to faces demonstrating anger, fear, and happiness. Greater activity for mood-incongruent (fear, anger, happy) faces was seen in MDD, whereas greater activity was seen for mood-congruent (sad) faces in BD.

MDD is associated with widespread impairment in many aspects of executive functions [87, 88]. A meta-analysis conducted in 2012 has revealed effect sizes of impairment ranging from 0.32 to 0.97 [89]. Slower motor processing speed is seen in MDD but that does not seem to be the main association. Age associations were not clear, but deficits appeared to be greater in those who were taking psychotropic medications and who had more severe MDD symptoms.

Major depressive disorder with psychotic (MDDP) features and schizophrenia share a number of attributes. MDDP is a subcategory of MDD that has delusions and/or hallucinations [90, 91]. MDDP has a worse prognosis and greater severity than MDD without psychosis [92]. Neuroimaging studies using positron emission tomography (PET) and functional magnetic resonance imaging (fMRI) have shown that areas involved in emotional processing and psychotic symptoms, such as the hippocampus, insula, and lateral prefrontal cortex, show both similarities and differences in folks with MDDP and MDD [93]. Similar functional and structural abnormalities have been seen in the subgenual cingulate cortex in MDDP and MDD.

Persistent Depressive Disorder (Dysthymia)

Persistent depressive disorder (dysthymia) (PDD) is a conflation of the DSM-IV categories of chronic major depressive disorder and dysthymic disorder [94–99]. The hallmark of PDD is depressed mood ("feeling sad or down in the dumps") that persists for most of the day, for more days than not, for at least 2 years or at least 1 year for non-adults. PDD and MDD may coexist or MDD may precede PDD.

Twelve-month prevalence in the USA is 0.5%. Comorbidity and covariance of PDD over time with borderline personality disorder have suggested a common source. Onset before 21 years of age is associated with higher risks of personality disorders and substance abuse. As with MDD, a neurotic temperament augurs a worse prognosis. Anxiety disorders, conduct disorders, and poorer global functions suggest a worse outcome. Parental loss or separation is prominent among childhood risk factors. Underpinning the lumping in PDD, illness development, course and family history appear to be the same between the DSM-IV categories of chronic major depressive disorder and dysthymic disorder. PDD seems to involve the prefrontal cortex, anterior cingulate, amygdala, and hippocampus. Early onset PDD is highly associated with DSM-IV cluster B and C personality disorders. There is a higher risk of anxiety disorders and substance abuse, and other psychiatric comorbidities.

Premenstrual Dysphoric Disorder

Premenstrual dysphoric disorder (PDyD) is mood lability, irritability, dysphoria, and anxiety starting after the follicular phase and ending around the beginning of menses [100–106]. It must be present for at least 1 year during most of the menstrual cycles, and the follicular phase must be symptom free. Behavioral and physical symptoms vary with social/cultural factors. Prevalence appears to be between 1.3 and 1.8%.

Stress, interpersonal trauma, seasonal changes, and sociocultural aspects of female sexual and gender roles are associated with the expression of PDyD. PDyD heritability is not clear; however, estimates for premenstrual symptoms are between 30% and 80%. Use of oral contraceptives seems to decrease the symptoms. Premenstrual syndrome is considered to be less severe than PDyD. Premenstrual exacerbations of various physical or mental disorders are common.

Substance/Medication-Induced Depressive Disorder

Substance/medication-induced depressive disorder (SMIDD) includes the symptoms of a depressive disorder such as MDD, but the symptoms are associated with the use of a substance and the symptoms persist past the expected duration of the physiological effects, intoxication, and withdrawal [107–111]. The SMIDD should have begun within a month after use of that substance.

Substances that can induce SMIDD include illicit and prescribed drugs: e.g., steroids, stimulants, central nervous system drugs (sedatives, hypnotics, and anxiolytics), dermatological agents, L-dopa, immunological preparations, alcohol, and oral contraceptives [112, 113].

Common risk factors include a history of MDD, psychosocial stressors, previous drug-induced depression, and underlying drug abuse disorders. Specific risk factors relate to the activity of the specific substance itself, for example, interferon-α-induced depression, high doses of corticosteroids, or high estrogen/progesterone concentrations in oral contraceptives.

Psychosocial risk factors in the USA include males, Black, high school diploma or less, no insurance, and low family income. Family history of substance use disorders, antisocial behavior, increased stress in the preceding year, and greater number of MDD criteria are common.

In terms of comorbidity, pathological gambling, paranoid, histrionic, and antisocial personality disorders are more common, while there is less likelihood of PDD.

Depressive Disorder Due to Another Medical Condition

Depressive disorder due to another medical condition (DDDAMD) relates to prominent and persistent depressed mood or manifestly diminished interest in all or almost all activities that is thought to be the direct physiological effects of another medical condition. Temporal association between the onset, exacerbation, or remission of the other medical condition and the symptoms of depression suggests a connection [114–116]. A further consideration is symptoms that are not typical of depressive disorders such as age of onset or lack of family history [117].

Stroke, Huntington's disease, Parkinson's disease, traumatic brain injury, hypothyroidism, Cushing's disease, systemic lupus erythematosus, and multiple sclerosis are some of the diseases that may be associated with DDDAMD [118]. Depressive symptoms may precede the more prominent motor and cognitive impairments of Parkinson's and Huntington's diseases. In the case of a stroke, depression may follow within a day (especially with a stroke of the left frontal lobe) to months and may last an average of 9–11 months [119]. Metabolic disorders (e.g., electrolyte imbalances), cirrhosis of the liver, cardiovascular disease, chronic obstructive pulmonary disease (COPD), cancer, diabetes [120, 121] and rheumatoid arthritis [122] are a few more of the diseases associated with depression [13, 123]. Herpes zoster is a risk factor for MDD and any depressive disorder [124]. Atopic dermatitis is associated with the onset of depression later in life [125].

Psychosocial risk factors and comorbidity seem to relate to those associated with the underlying medical condition. To rule out physical disorders that could cause depression may require screening by a physician using a CBC panel, especially looking at TSH, folate, B12 and B6 levels [126].

Perinatal Depression

Perinatal depression is defined as depression in pregnancy, around childbirth or within the first-year postpartum [127]. A systematic review of perinatal depression was published in

2005 [128]. The combined point prevalence estimates for major and minor depression from meta-analyses ranged from 6.5% to 12.9% at different trimesters of pregnancy and months in the first postpartum year. For MDD alone, it was 1.0-5.6%. The combined period prevalence revealed as many as 19.2% (MDD alone was 7.1%) of women have a depressive episode during the first 3 months postpartum with most of these episodes begin following delivery. The 95% confidence intervals showed significant uncertainty. Suicide rates increase in women with postpartum depression [129]. Around 20% of postnatal deaths in women are a result of suicide.

Another systematic review states that peripartum depression usually has its onset during the third trimester of pregnancy or in the postpartum and is one of the most common medical complications in new mothers [130].

A 2017 systematic review and meta-regression further examined the prevalence and incidence of perinatal depression [131]. They found that prevalence was significantly higher in women from low- and middle-income countries versus women from high-income countries (OR = 1.8; 95% CI: 1.4 to 2.2). Pooled prevalence was 11.9% of women during the perinatal period (95% CI: 11.4 to 12.5).

Obstetrical and neonatal complications are highly associated with depression during pregnancy [132–139]. Depression during pregnancy is a considerable risk for postnatal depression [140]. Postnatal depression can adversely affect infant and childhood temperament [134], developmental delay and IQ [141] and attachment insecurity [142].

Others

Other specified depressive disorder and *other unspecified depressive disorder* encompass symptoms that do not meet the full criteria for any of the disorders in the depressive disorder classification.

Specifiers for depressive episodes include those with anxious distress, mixed features, melancholic features, psychotic features, catatonia, peripartum onset, and seasonal pattern.

Mixed anxiety and depression disorders (MADD) disappeared in the DSM-5 [143] but have been retained in the ICD-11 as *mixed depressive and anxiety disorder (MDAD)* [3]. MADD was a useful category that included a combination of symptoms of anxiety and depression severe enough to warrant a psychiatric diagnosis, but not severe enough to justify the full syndrome of an anxiety or depressive disorder [143–145]. The prevalence of MADD in primary care had been reported to be quite high [146–148]. However, the proposed DSM-5 diagnostic criteria was not sufficiently reliable and produced divergent results and diagnostic instability [149, 150]. On the other hand, using different criteria than the DSM-5 field trials, a *World Psychiatric Association* and WHO survey among about 5000 psychiatrists in 44 countries showed that MADD was the 4th most frequently used diagnostic category; however, the criteria were among the most difficult to use and hence had very low accuracy [151]. The ICD-10 folks decided to add more explicit diagnostic criteria and continue with the MADD category [2, 152]. In the research leading to the ICD-11, results showed that the comorbid MADD ICD-11 is clinical rather than subclinical, is more common than depression or anxiety in the general population, and was associated with high levels of functional impairment and somatization [153].

Chinese Classification of Mental Disorders is a system that is very similar in criteria to the DSM and ICD systems and has been included in some meta-analyses [154].

Diagnostic and Assessment Tools

A 2018 Canadian study found that most patients with depression do not receive even minimally adequate treatment, and this may be a result of physicians not recognizing up to half of all patients who have depression [155–158].

Assessment scales can perform analogous functions to laboratory tests in physical medicine. They are valuable adjuncts to comprehensive clinical evaluation. In addition, they are convenient ways of tracking clinical symptoms and response to treatment. Scales are brief clinician and/or patient-rated measures that can promote mental health. Patient use of scales provides systematic tracking and feedback that can encourage self-management and adherence to treatment.

The book *Assessment Scales in Depression, Mania and Anxiety* is a user-friendly collection of rating scales with commentaries and scoring for busy clinicians [159]. Many of the scales are in the book and others are referenced to the source where they can be acquired. An online list of psychiatric rating scales for depression can be found in this link [160].

In addition, assessment scales are the principal interview tools that are used in research studies on depression. Unstructured interviews with poor reliability were the bane of research in psychiatric disorders until the 1980s [161, 162]. Now, validated semistructured and fully structured diagnostic interviews have found their place in research but are not always used [163–166].

Highly structured interviews and questionnaires are used in qualitative epidemiology and most health services research [167]. In less structured interviews, the person interviewed is more a participant in conveying the meaning of responses rather than just a conduit [168, 169]. Semistructured interviews are ones in which a researcher has some predefined questions or topics but then probes deeper as the participant responds [170]. A systematic methodological review has suggested guidelines for conducting qualitative semistructured interviews [171].

A 2006 journal article detailing *limitations and pitfalls of rating scales* in depression can be found in [172]. A 2016 meta-analysis of the diagnostic accuracy of 21 meta-analyses of depression screening tools concluded that the methodological quality of most meta-analyses of the diagnostic test accuracy of depression screening tools is suboptimal [173]. A review of meta-analyses of accuracy of depression diagnostic tools stated that database searches for studies of diagnostic test accuracy are notoriously difficult to filter, highly resource-intensive, and a potential barrier to quality evidence synthesis [174].

Values expressed in meta-analyses of depression may be reporting higher prevalence rates than the actual prevalence due to the impaired ability of some assessments to detect false positives [175]. Most meta-analyses combine estimates from studies that used screening tools instead of validated diagnostic interviews. Further, most abstracts do not disclose that fact and describe results as the prevalence of depressive disorders and depression. When published in high-impact journals [176], high prevalence rates based upon inadequate collection methods or overinterpretation can be particularly influential [175]. It seems that most clinicians do not venture past the abstracts of research articles [177–180]. Frequently, this appears to reflect limited time, appraisal skills, or access to the complete article [181–183].

The most frequently used observer-rated depression scale is the Hamilton Depression Rating Scale [184–186]. When Hamilton designed the HAM-D, he envisioned it as a scale measuring the severity of depressive states and not as a diagnostic tool [187]. The HAM-D has been the subject of several studies evaluating its validity and suitability for depression measurements. The results of those analyses have generally found the HAM-D to be reliable and valid [188, 189].

The Beck Depression Inventory (BDI) is the most frequently used self-report scale of depression [185, 190]. But the BDI can be used by observers as well [191]. The BDI has been generally shown to be valuable and sensitive worldwide for self-reporting depression in a variety of disorders [192, 193]. The BDI has gone through multiple revisions since its inception in 1961 [194]. The BDI-II, published in 1996, is considerably revised from the original [194].

A comparison study found that the BDI-II used as a self-rating or as an interview-based observer-rating scale can result in different total scores in healthy older adults [191]. In that comparison study, the self-rated BDI-II gave a significantly higher total score than when it was interview rated. There was a moderate correlation between the total scores from each of the methods of administration.

One study found that the BDI, while excellent in detecting moderate to severe depression, does not do so well in identifying mild MDD [195].

A conversion table between the HAM-D and the BDI can be found in [185].

A preliminary review of the BDI-II in veterans questions if new norms and cut scores are needed [196].

The BDI-II and the *Center for Epidemiologic Studies-Depression (CES-D)* Scale seem to do well in Arab adolescents in countries where there is growing social and political unrest [197]. However, they do not always indicate the same cases.

Although the BDI is widely used for assessing adolescent's psychological health, the results sometimes diverge from clinical diagnostic assessments, which may be a reflection of the wide array of adolescents' psychological development challenges [198].

The BDI does not seem to do as well as the *Geriatric Depression Scale and the Geriatric Depression Scale-15* in cognitively intact or mildly impaired patients over 65 years of age [199, 200]. For geriatric patients, the 30-item *Geriatric Depression Scale (GDS-30)* and the shorter *GDS-15, GDS-5, and GDS-4* have been recommended as the best depression screening tools [155, 200, 201].

In primary care, the most frequently used screening tool for depression is the Patient Health Questionnaire (PHQ) [202]. The PHQ is an abbreviated form of the *Primary Care Evaluation of Mental Disorders (PRIME-MD)* [203]. The PRIME-MD took too much time for routine use. The PHQ is more efficient and appears to have comparable validity. The PHQ has been used as a screening and diagnostic tool for mental health disorders of depression, anxiety, alcohol, eating, and somatoform disorders [204]. It can be self-administered, or health care provider administered.

The PHQ is available in the public domain in over 20 languages. All the forms have been validated internationally in a variety of populations [204–208].

There are several versions of the PHQ [209]. These include PHQ-2, PHQ-4, PHQ-8, PHQ-9, PHQ-15, generalized anxiety disorder (GAD)-7, patient health questionnaire somatic, anxiety, and depressive symptom scales (PHQ-SADS), and PHQ-A. The PHQ-2 and PHQ-4 are very brief screening tools that consist of 2 or 4 questions, respectively, from the PHQ [210]. The results of these can help determine if the more complete versions should be used. The GAD-7 is used to assess anxiety symptoms [211]. The PHQ-8 screens for depression but without the PHQ-9 question about suicide [212, 213]. The PHQ-SADS combines the PHQ-9 [214], GAD-7, and the PHQ-15 to screen for somatic, anxiety, and depressive symptoms [205]. The PHQ-A is a version for adolescents [215].

It has been suggested that neither the PHQ-2 nor the PHQ-9 can be used to confirm a clinical diagnosis [202]. However, a 2019 meta-analysis concluded that the PHQ-9 sensitivity compared with semistructured diagnostic interviews was greater than had been calculated in previous conventional meta-analyses that combined reference standards [216].

In 2018, a systematic review identified 23 other tools besides the PHQ that are capable of being used in primary practice [217].

Computerized depression screening instruments that are interfaced or integrated into electronic format may become more common [218]. There appear to be quite a few web-based mental health screening tools that show promise [219]. A 2016 systematic review found 56 studies on 62 online instruments that measured depression, anxiety, stress, self-harm, or suicide ideation [220]. Of the 62, 29 assessed symptoms of depression. The most frequently and well-studied were the *Center for Epidemiological Studies Depression (CES-D)* [221–228] and the *Montgomery–Åsberg Depression Rating Scale Self Report* [229, 230]. The online version of the *Hospital Anxiety and Depression Scale* was the only instrument that had been analyzed in both general and patient populations [231–233]. Analyses have suggested that it demonstrates adequate psychometrics [232, 234, 235].

The CES-D also has a seven-item short form CES-D-SF and a 10-item short form (CES-D-10) that also have been shown to have acceptable psychometric properties [236, 237].

Associations have been seen between displayed depression symptoms on Facebook and self-reported depression symptoms using the PHQ-9 [238].

The American Psychiatric Association (APA) offers several "emerging measures" in *Section III of DSM–5* [1]. They are designed to be used at initial patient intake and to monitor treatment progress. These tools are freely available and can be found on the APA website [239].

The APA DSM-5 Task Force and Work Groups have produced cross-cutting tools (*DSM-5 Cross-Cutting (CC) Symptom Measures (DSM-5 CC)*) based upon the research that went into their DSM-5 [240]. Cross-cutting refers to the presence of co-occurring symptoms across mental disorders [241–245]. Categorical diagnosis often does not reflect the true mental states of patients. For example, patients with MDD may also be experiencing anxiety or even subthreshold psychotic symptoms and may also be abusing drugs [246]

The DSM-5 CC is designed to be self- or observer-administered to anyone coming in for a mental health evaluation and treatment. It assesses the presence and severity of psychiatric symptoms that cut across diagnostic boundaries [241]. These symptoms are depression, anger, mania, anxiety, somatic symptoms, sleep disturbance, psychosis, obsessive thoughts and behaviors, suicidal thoughts and behaviors, substance use (e.g., alcohol, nicotine, prescription medication, and illicit substance use), personality functioning, dissociation, and cognition/memory problems in adults. Assessments for children and adolescents add inattention and irritability, and eliminate personality functioning, dissociation, and cognition/memory problems.

The measures are designed to help in a comprehensive mental status examination and enhance decisions but not to be the only basis for clinical diagnosis. They have been field tested and have shown mostly good-to-excellent reliability [241, 247] and very good clinical usefulness from both patients and clinicians.

Identifying the severity and presence of these cross-cutting symptoms can significantly alter the treatment and prognosis of mental disorders [244, 248, 249]. To accomplish that goal, APA DSM-5 emerging measures include Level 1 and Level 2 Cross-Cutting Symptoms Measures, Disorder-Specific Severity Measures, Disability Measures, Personal Inventories, and Early Development and Home Background Forms.

Level 1 Cross-Cutting Symptoms Measures is the brief 23 question survey. *Level 2 Cross-Cutting Symptoms Measures* follow up with a greater depth into some of the symptoms that have been revealed in Level 1.

Disorder-Specific Severity Measures correspond to criteria that define a particular disorder [250].

The disability measurement is assessed via *The World Health Organization Disability Assessment Schedule, Version 2.0 (WHODAS 2.0)* [251]. It assesses ability to understand and communicate, get around, self-care, get along with people, participate in life activities (e.g., household, work/school), and participate in society. The WHODAS measures the impact of health conditions, monitors effectiveness of interventions, and estimates burden of mental and physical disorders across different populations [252].

The *Personality Inventories for DSM-5 (DSM-5 (PID-5))* measures five maladaptive personality traits: negative affect, detachment, antagonism, disinhibition, and psychoticism [253, 254].

Early Development and Home Background Forms are culturally responsive [255].

A *transdiagnostic approach to psychiatric classifications* has been proposed as an alternative to ICD/DSM categories [256]. Transdiagnostic approaches are designed "to cut across existing categorical diagnoses and go beyond them, to improve the way we classify and treat mental disorders."

Transdiagnostic approaches began from cognitive behavioral treatments for eating disorders [257], anxiety [258], and depression [259].

Instead of the conventional explanation of psychiatric disorders based upon internalizing, externalizing, and thought disorder, proponents of the transdiagnostics believe that a general psychopathology "p" factor is a better explanation [260]. High p is associated with less healthy brain development early in life, greater family association, and worse general life functioning. They argued that many disorders share a common etiology, cognitive-affective, interpersonal, and behavioral features, and risk factors, and comorbidity is high [259, 261]. Focusing on a narrow disorder-specific treatment may be an impediment to robust treatment that is the foundation of cognitive behavioral therapy [259].

A 2019 systematic review and comprehensive guide with suggestions for research into transdiagnostics is presented in [256]. They concluded that the current state of transdiagnostics is heterogeneous and intrinsically incoherent encompassing different and frequently conflicting concepts. They make 6 recommendations for transdiagnostic research in psychiatry.

They suggest that there are 3 conceptual weaknesses in transdiagnostic research. First, the original DSM-IV disclaimer "there is no assumption that each category of mental disorder is a completely discrete entity with absolute boundaries dividing it from other mental disorders" needs to be rediscovered. Second, transdiagnostic research has converted complex symptoms into an illusion of continuity. Third, boundaries between transdiagnostic and diagnosis-specific cognitive behavioral therapy (CBT) are blurry [262]. Their principal conclusion is that there is considerable conceptual bias and that there is no paradigm shift at play. They believe the best hope will be for transdiagnostic research to complement, refine and improve current ways of classifying and treating mental disorders [263, 264].

It seems that transdiagnostic criteria apply to some existing approaches to precision medicine (q.v.). The DSM-5 cross-cutting approach is both categorical (specific diagnosis) and dimensional (continuous or transdiagnostic) [265]. The *Research Domain Criteria (RDoC)* initiative is a transdiagnostic approach [266]. Staging models are transdiagnostic that acknowledge links between biomarkers, clinical phenotypes, and disease extension, and promote a stratified approach to treatment planning [267].

Direct-to-consumer genetic testing includes a variety of tests related to risk for psychiatric illnesses such as MDD, bipolar disorder, schizophrenia, and obsessive-compulsive disorder [268]. In addition, there are tests to predict individual's response to psychotropic medication. However, these tests all have uncertain clinical validity and utility.

Male Compared to Female Depression Tools

In both Western and non-Western studies [269, 270], women are diagnosed with depressive disorders at approximately twice the rate of men. Men die by suicide 3.5 to 4 times more often than women do [271]. However, this diagnostic rate may not reflect the true state of masculine depression [272, 273]. Gender differences in diagnosis largely disappear when male-typical expression of depression are recognized. Males have been conditioned by gendered societal processes to express their emotions differently than females [274].

Addis has suggested *four alternative conceptual frameworks* for understanding the role of gender in the way men experience, express, and react to depression [275, 276]. Addis calls these the *(1) sex differences framework, (2) masked depression framework, (3) masculine depression framework, and (4) gendered response framework.*

The sex difference approach relies on the idea that men and women have the same variables but differ based on sex. The masked depression suggests men are more likely to express their emotional and psychological distress in the form of depressive equivalents as it is socially unacceptable to admit emotional weakness or sadness. The masculine depression framework posits that in a struggle against masculine norms, men are likely to experience an alternative expression that manifests in externalizing symptoms. The gendered response hypothesizes that men are limited in responses to negative affect such as grief, depression, and sadness [277]. And as such, they either adhere to socially dictated roles of masculinity or reject that role.

These possibilities might result in males reacting to emotional pain by less control over impulses and more hyperactivity manifesting in irritability, anger, self-destructive behavior, self-distraction, or numbing of pain with substance use, gambling, womanizing, and workaholism [276, 278–280].

Martin et al. suggest, however, that a more comprehensive approach to understanding depression is a combination of alternative and conventional symptoms [278]. They find masked depression framework difficult to use in practice as it is difficult to identify depressive equivalents [281]. So, they developed two new scales that combined Addis's externalizing symptoms scales with traditional depression symptoms [278]. They used the *Gotland Male Depression Scale (GMDS)* [269, 282, 283] and *Masculine Depression Scale* [284, 285] for externalizing symptoms. The GMDS has also been validated in women [286].

The first scale is called the *Male Symptoms Scale (MSS)* which exclusively includes alternative male-type symptoms of depression. The second scale combines the symptoms from the MSS with traditional depression items to produce the *Gender Inclusive Depression Scale (GIDS)*. With their new scales, they analyzed data from the *National Comorbidity Survey Replication* [287]. Men compared to women showed higher rates of anger attacks/aggression, substance abuse, and risk taking. Using the MSS revealed that a higher proportion of men (26.3%) than women (21.9%) ($P = .007$) met criteria for depression. And the GIDS found that men and women met criteria for depression in equal proportions: 30.6% of men and 33.3% of women ($P = .57$). It is also noteworthy that the male-type symptoms are fairly common in women.

Summary

This chapter introduced the diagnostic classifications of depressive disorders. Then, the diagnostic tools used by clinicians to make differential diagnoses were described.

Diagnosis of mood disorders is based upon symptoms and signs. Screening makes use of a variety of brief questionnaires. Clinical criteria for the diagnosis of specific mood disorders are met by correspondence with the DSM. As research in behavioral medicine has progressed, the definitions of depressive disorders have become more refined as reflected in changes in categories and criteria from the DSM III through the DSM-5-TR. Challenges exist in attempts to meaningfully classify mental disorders. Psychopathology generally is the result of a complex interplay of multiple biological, behavioral, psychosocial, and cultural factors, influenced by each individual's unique life experience. The result of these interactions and factors is not clearly delimited diseases, instead they are mixtures of psychological difficulties. Categories are useful for us to handle the complexities of psychopathologies, but the boundaries are not distinct and are perhaps artificial. Dimensions are a recognition that psychopathology is not an all or none; instead, it is graded in its manifestations. For clinical purposes, thresholds are useful but should be considered as arbitrary unless proven by further research to be otherwise. Comorbidity is perhaps the rule rather than the exception. It may be an artifact of an imperfect classification system.

The Global Burden of Disease (GBD) 2017 Study has homed in on the incidence, prevalence, and comorbidity of depressive disorders. Some of their conclusions are touched upon in this chapter and will be discussed in more detail in other chapters.

Some of the temperamental, genetic, and physiological contributions to the differential diagnoses of the depressive disorders are presented in this chapter. They too will be reviewed in much more detail in later chapters.

References

1. Psychiatry.org – DSM. https://www.psychiatry.org/dsm5.
2. ICD-11. https://icd.who.int/en.
3. International Classification of Diseases (ICD). https://www.who.int/standards/classifications/classification-of-diseases.
4. Psychiatry.org – Updates to DSM Criteria, Text and ICD-10 Codes. https://www.psychiatry.org/psychiatrists/practice/dsm/updates-to-dsm.
5. Ferrari AJ, Charlson FJ, Norman RE, Patten SB, Freedman G, Murray CJL, Vos T, Whiteford HA. Burden of depressive disorders by country, sex, age, and year: findings from the global burden of disease study 2010. PLoS Med. 2013;10(11):e1001547. PMCID: PMC3818162. http://www.ncbi.nlm.nih.gov/pubmed/24223526.
6. Clark LA, Cuthbert B, Lewis-Fernández R, Narrow WE, Reed GM. Three approaches to understanding and classifying mental disorder: ICD-11, DSM-5, and the National Institute of Mental Health's Research Domain Criteria (RDoC). Psychol Sci Publ Int. 2017;18(2):72–145. PMID: 29211974. http://www.ncbi.nlm.nih.gov/pubmed/29211974.
7. Murray CJL, Lopez AD, editors. The global burden of disease: a comprehensive assessment of mortality and disability from diseases, injuries, and risk factors in 1990 and projected to 2020. World Health Organization, Harvard School of Public Health, World Bank; 1996. https://digitallibrary.un.org/record/195443.
8. Ustün TB, Ayuso-Mateos JL, Chatterji S, Mathers C, Murray CJL. Global burden of depressive disorders in the year 2000. Br J Psychiatry. 2004;184:386–92. PMID: 15123501. http://www.ncbi.nlm.nih.gov/pubmed/15123501.
9. GBD 2017 Disease and Injury Incidence and Prevalence Collaborators. Global, regional, and national incidence, prevalence, and years lived with disability for 354 diseases and injuries for 195 countries and territories, 1990-2017: a systematic analysis for the Global Burden of Disease Study 2017. Lancet. 2018;392(10159):1789–858. PMCID: PMC6227754. http://www.ncbi.nlm.nih.gov/pubmed/30496104.
10. Liu Q, He H, Yang J, Feng X, Zhao F, Lyu J. Changes in the global burden of depression from 1990 to 2017: findings from the Global Burden of Disease study. J Psychiatr Res. 2020;126:134–40. PMID: 31439359. http://www.ncbi.nlm.nih.gov/pubmed/31439359.
11. Homepage | Institute for Health Metrics and Evaluation. https://www.healthdata.org/.
12. VizHub – GBD Compare. https://vizhub.healthdata.org/gbd-compare/.
13. Global Health Data Exchange | GHDx. https://ghdx.healthdata.org/.
14. Age standardized rate CI5volX-07 (1).pdf. C:\Users\Franklin Sunzeri\Downloads\CI5volX-07 (1).pdf.
15. Age-standardized mortality rate (per 100 000 population). https://www.who.int/data/gho/indicator-metadata-registry/imr-details/78.
16. 16. Fay MP, Tiwari RC, Feuer EJ, Zou Z. Estimating average annual percent change for disease rates without assuming constant change. Biometrics. 2006;62(3):847–54. PMID: 16984328. http://www.ncbi.nlm.nih.gov/pubmed/16984328.
17. 17. Disability-adjusted life years (DALYs). https://www.who.int/data/gho/indicator-metadata-registry/imr-details/158#:~:text=The%20overall%20burden%20of%20disease,due%20to%20disability%20(YLDs).
18. Mathers CD, Loncar D. Projections of global mortality and burden of disease from 2002 to 2030. PLoS Med. 2006;3(11):e442. PMCID: PMC1664601. http://www.ncbi.nlm.nih.gov/pubmed/17132052.
19. Morris SE, Cuthbert BN. Research Domain Criteria: cognitive systems, neural circuits, and dimensions of behavior. Dialogues Clin Neurosci. 2012;14(1):29–37. PMCID: PMC3341647. http://www.ncbi.nlm.nih.gov/pubmed/22577302.
20. The NIMH Research Domain Criteria (RDoC) Project: Precision Medicine for Psychiatry. Am J Psychiatry. https://psychiatryonline.org/doi/10.1176/appi.ajp.2014.14020138.
21. Raven M, Parry P. Psychotropic marketing practices and problems: implications for DSM-5. J Nerv Ment Dis. 2012;200(6):512–6. PMID: 22833879. http://www.ncbi.nlm.nih.gov/pubmed/22833879.
22. Jenkins MM, Youngstrom EA, Youngstrom JK, Feeny NC, Findling RL. Generalizability of evidence-based assessment recommendations for pediatric bipolar disorder. Psychol Assess. 2012;24(2):269–81. PMCID: PMC3752420. http://www.ncbi.nlm.nih.gov/pubmed/22004538.
23. Jenkins MM, Youngstrom EA, Washburn JJ, Youngstrom JK. Evidence-based strategies improve assessment of pediatric bipolar disorder by community practitioners. Prof Psychol Res Pr.

2011;42(2):121–9. PMCID: PMC3100552. http://www.ncbi.nlm.nih.gov/pubmed/21625392.
24. Correll CU, Kratochvil CJ, March JS. Developments in pediatric psychopharmacology: focus on stimulants, antidepressants, and antipsychotics. J Clin Psychiatry. 2011;72(5):655–70. PMID: 21658348. http://www.ncbi.nlm.nih.gov/pubmed/21658348.
25. Jairam R, Prabhuswamy M, Dullur P. Do we really know how to treat a child with bipolar disorder or one with severe mood dysregulation? Is there a magic bullet? Depress Res Treat. 2012;2012:967302. PMCID: PMC3235717. http://www.ncbi.nlm.nih.gov/pubmed/22203894.
26. Amaladoss A, Roberts N, Amaladoss F. Evidence for use of mood stabilizers and anticonvulsants in the treatment of nonaffective disorders in children and adolescents. Clin Neuropharmacol. 2010;33(6):303–11. PMID: 21079456. http://www.ncbi.nlm.nih.gov/pubmed/21079456
27. Margulies DM, Weintraub S, Basile J, Grover PJ, Carlson GA. Will disruptive mood dysregulation disorder reduce false diagnosis of bipolar disorder in children? Bipolar Disord. 2012;14(5):488–96. PMID: 22713098. http://www.ncbi.nlm.nih.gov/pubmed/22713098.
28. Forman-Hoffman VL, Batts KR, Hedden SL, Spagnola K, Bose J. Comorbid mental disorders among adults in the mental health surveillance survey. Ann Epidemiol. 2018;28(7):468–74. PMID: 29602518. http://www.ncbi.nlm.nih.gov/pubmed/29602518.
29. Sagar-Ouriaghli I, Milavic G, Barton R, Heaney N, Fiori F, Lievesley K, Singh J, Santosh P. Comparing the DSM-5 construct of Disruptive Mood Dysregulation Disorder and ICD-10 Mixed Disorder of Emotion and Conduct in the UK Longitudinal Assessment of Manic Symptoms (UK-LAMS) Study. Eur Child Adolesc Psychiatry. 2018;27(9):1095–104. PMCID: PMC6133106. http://www.ncbi.nlm.nih.gov/pubmed/29730721.
30. Mayes SD, Mathiowetz C, Kokotovich C, Waxmonsky J, Baweja R, Calhoun SL, Bixler EO. Stability of disruptive mood dysregulation disorder symptoms (irritable-angry mood and temper outbursts) throughout childhood and adolescence in a general population sample. J Abnorm Child Psychol. 2015;43(8):1543–9. PMID: 26004122. http://www.ncbi.nlm.nih.gov/pubmed/26004122.
31. Tang MH, Pinsky EG. Mood and affect disorders. Pediatr Rev. 2015;36(2):52–60; quiz 61. PMID: 25646309. http://www.ncbi.nlm.nih.gov/pubmed/25646309.
32. Rao U. DSM-5: disruptive mood dysregulation disorder. Asian J Psychiatr. 2014;11:119–23. PMCID: PMC4254488. http://www.ncbi.nlm.nih.gov/pubmed/25453714.
33. Roy AK, Lopes V, Klein RG. Disruptive mood dysregulation disorder: a new diagnostic approach to chronic irritability in youth. Am J Psychiatry. 2014;171(9):918–24. PMCID: PMC4390118. http://www.ncbi.nlm.nih.gov/pubmed/25178749.
34. Baweja R, Mayes SD, Hameed U, Waxmonsky JG. Disruptive mood dysregulation disorder: current insights. Neuropsychiatr Dis Treat. 2016;12:2115–24. PMCID: PMC5003560. http://www.ncbi.nlm.nih.gov/pubmed/27601906.
35. Stringaris A. Irritability in children and adolescents: a challenge for DSM-5. Eur Child Adolesc Psychiatry. 2011;20(2):61–6. PMID: 21298306. http://www.ncbi.nlm.nih.gov/pubmed/21298306.
36. Deveney CM, Connolly ME, Haring CT, Bones BL, Reynolds RC, Kim P, Pine DS, Leibenluft E. Neural mechanisms of frustration in chronically irritable children. Am J Psychiatry. 2013;170(10):1186–94. PMCID: PMC3938281. http://www.ncbi.nlm.nih.gov/pubmed/23732841.
37. Holtmann M, Buchmann AF, Esser G, Schmidt MH, Banaschewski T, Laucht M. the child behavior checklist-dysregulation profile predicts substance use, suicidality, and functional impairment: a longitudinal analysis. J Child Psychol Psychiatry. 2011;52(2):139–47. PMID: 20854363. http://www.ncbi.nlm.nih.gov/pubmed/20854363.
38. De Caluwé E, Decuyper M, De Clercq B. The child behavior checklist dysregulation profile predicts adolescent DSM-5 pathological personality traits 4 years later. Eur Child Adolesc Psychiatry. 2013;22(7):401–11. PMID: 23381573. http://www.ncbi.nlm.nih.gov/pubmed/26004122.
39. Masi G, Pisano S, Milone A, Muratori P. Child behavior checklist dysregulation profile in children with disruptive behavior disorders: a longitudinal study. J Affect Disord. 2015;186:249–53. PMID: 26254616. http://www.ncbi.nlm.nih.gov/pubmed/26254616.
40. Miller M, Iosif AM, Young GS, Bell LJ, Schwichtenberg AJ, Hutman T, Ozonoff S. The dysregulation profile in preschoolers with and without a family history of autism spectrum disorder. J Child Psychol Psychiatry. 2019;60(5):516–23. PMCID: PMC6458078. http://www.ncbi.nlm.nih.gov/pubmed/30506566.
41. Mick E, McGough J, Loo S, Doyle AE, Wozniak J, Wilens TE, Smalley S, McCracken J, Biederman J, Faraone SV. Genome-wide association study of the child behavior checklist dysregulation profile. J Am Acad Child Adolesc Psychiatry. 2011;50(8):807–817.e8. PMCID: PMC3143361. http://www.ncbi.nlm.nih.gov/pubmed/21784300.
42. Althoff RR, Verhulst FC, Rettew DC, Hudziak JJ, van der Ende J. Adult outcomes of childhood dysregulation: a 14-year follow-up study. J Am Acad Child Adolesc Psychiatry. 2010;49(11):1105–16. PMCID: PMC2965164. http://www.ncbi.nlm.nih.gov/pubmed/20970698.
43. Holtmann M, Duketis E, Goth K, Poustka L, Boelte S. Severe affective and behavioral dysregulation in youth is associated with increased serum TSH. J Affect Disord. 2010;121(1–2):184–8. PMID: 19564046. http://www.ncbi.nlm.nih.gov/pubmed/19564046.
44. Ayer L, Greaves-Lord K, Althoff RR, Hudziak JJ, Dieleman GC, Verhulst FC, van der Ende J. Blunted HPA axis response to stress is related to a persistent Dysregulation Profile in youth. Biol Psychol. 2013;93(3):343–51. PMCID: PMC3714851. http://www.ncbi.nlm.nih.gov/pubmed/23603315.
45. Copeland WE, Angold A, Costello EJ, Egger H. Prevalence, comorbidity, and correlates of DSM-5 proposed disruptive mood dysregulation disorder. Am J Psychiatry. 2013;170(2):173–9. PMCID: PMC3573525. http://www.ncbi.nlm.nih.gov/pubmed/23377638.
46. 46. Axelson D, Findling RL, Fristad MA, Kowatch RA, Youngstrom EA, Horwitz SM, Arnold LE, Frazier TW, Ryan N, Demeter C, Gill MK, Hauser-Harrington JC, Depew J, Kennedy SM, Gron BA, Rowles BM, Birmaher B. Examining the proposed disruptive mood dysregulation disorder diagnosis in children in the Longitudinal Assessment of Manic Symptoms study. J Clin Psychiatry. 2012;73(10):1342–50. PMCID: PMC3581334. http://www.ncbi.nlm.nih.gov/pubmed/23140653.
47. Bains N, Abdijadid S. Major depressive disorder. In: StatPearls [Internet]. Treasure Island: StatPearls Publishing; 2023. p. 2025. PMID: 32644504.
48. Uher R, Payne JL, Pavlova B, Perlis RH. Major depressive disorder in DSM-5: implications for clinical practice and research of changes from DSM-IV. Depress Anxiety. 2014;31(6):459–71. PMID: 24272961. http://www.ncbi.nlm.nih.gov/pubmed/24272961.
49. Katzman MA, Anand L, Furtado M, Chokka P. Food for thought: understanding the value, variety and usage of management algorithms for major depressive disorder. Psychiatry Res. 2014;220(Suppl 1):S3–14. PMID: 25539872. http://www.ncbi.nlm.nih.gov/pubmed/25539872.
50. Evans VC, Iverson GL, Yatham LN, Lam RW. The relationship between neurocognitive and psychosocial functioning in major depressive disorder: a systematic review. J Clin Psychiatry.

2014;75(12):1359–70. PMID: 25551235. http://www.ncbi.nlm.nih.gov/pubmed/25551235.

51. Hirschfeld RM. Differential diagnosis of bipolar disorder and major depressive disorder. J Affect Disord. 2014;169(Suppl 1):S12–6. PMID: 25533909. http://www.ncbi.nlm.nih.gov/pubmed/25533909.
52. Soleimani L, Lapidus KAB, Iosifescu DV. Diagnosis and treatment of major depressive disorder. Neurol Clin. 2011;29(1):177–193, ix. PMID: 21172578. http://www.ncbi.nlm.nih.gov/pubmed/21172578.
53. Hays RD, Wells KB, Sherbourne CD, Rogers W, Spritzer K. Functioning and well-being outcomes of patients with depression compared with chronic general medical illnesses. Arch Gen Psychiatry. 1995;52(1):11–9. PMID: 7811158. http://www.ncbi.nlm.nih.gov/pubmed/7811158.
54. Grant BF. Comorbidity between DSM-IV drug use disorders and major depression: results of a national survey of adults. J Subst Abuse. 1995;7(4):481–97. PMID: 8838629. http://www.ncbi.nlm.nih.gov/pubmed/8838629.
55. Genetics of Personality Consortium, de Moor MHM, van den Berg SM, Verweij KJH, Krueger RF, Luciano M, Arias Vasquez A, Matteson LK, Derringer J, Esko T, Amin N, Gordon SD, Hansell NK, Hart AB, Seppälä I, Huffman JE, Konte B, Lahti J, Lee M, Miller M, Nutile T, Tanaka T, Teumer A, Viktorin A, Wedenoja J, Abecasis GR, Adkins DE, Agrawal A, Allik J, Appel K, Bigdeli TB, Busonero F, Campbell H, Costa PT, Davey Smith G, Davies G, de Wit H, Ding J, Engelhardt BE, Eriksson JG, Fedko IO, Ferrucci L, Franke B, Giegling I, Grucza R, Hartmann AM, Heath AC, Heinonen K, Henders AK, Homuth G, Hottenga JJ, Iacono WG, Janzing J, Jokela M, Karlsson R, Kemp JP, Kirkpatrick MG, Latvala A, Lehtimäki T, Liewald DC, Madden PAF, Magri C, Magnusson PKE, Marten J, Maschio A, Medland SE, Mihailov E, Milaneschi Y, Montgomery GW, Nauck M, Ouwens KG, Palotie A, Pettersson E, Polasek O, Qian Y, Pulkki-Råback L, Raitakari OT, Realo A, Rose RJ, Ruggiero D, Schmidt CO, Slutske WS, Sorice R, Starr JM, St Pourcain B, Sutin AR, Timpson NJ, Trochet H, Vermeulen S, Vuoksimaa E, Widen E, Wouda J, Wright MJ, Zgaga L, Porteous D, Minelli A, Palmer AA, Rujescu D, Ciullo M, Hayward C, Rudan I, Metspalu A, Kaprio J, Deary IJ, Räikkönen K, Wilson JF, Keltikangas-Järvinen L, Bierut LJ, Hettema JM, Grabe HJ, van Duijn CM, Evans DM, Schlessinger D, Pedersen NL, Terracciano A, McGue M, Penninx BWJH, Martin NG, Boomsma DI. Meta-analysis of Genome-wide Association Studies for Neuroticism, and the Polygenic Association with Major Depressive Disorder. JAMA Psychiatry. 2015;72(7):642–50. PMCID: PMC4667957. http://www.ncbi.nlm.nih.gov/pubmed/25993607.
56. Teicher MH, Samson JA. Childhood maltreatment and psychopathology: a case for ecophenotypic variants as clinically and neurobiologically distinct subtypes. Am J Psychiatry. 2013;170(10):1114–33. PMCID: PMC3928064. http://www.ncbi.nlm.nih.gov/pubmed/23982148.
57. Kendler KS, Hettema JM, Butera F, Gardner CO, Prescott CA. Life event dimensions of loss, humiliation, entrapment, and danger in the prediction of onsets of major depression and generalized anxiety. Arch Gen Psychiatry. 2003;60(8):789–96. PMID: 12912762. http://www.ncbi.nlm.nih.gov/pubmed/12912762.
58. Toda H, Inoue T, Tsunoda T, Nakai Y, Tanichi M, Tanaka T, Hashimoto N, Nakato Y, Nakagawa S, Kitaichi Y, Mitsui N, Boku S, Tanabe H, Nibuya M, Yoshino A, Kusumi I. The structural equation analysis of childhood abuse, adult stressful life events, and temperaments in major depressive disorders and their influence on refractoriness. Neuropsychiatr Dis Treat. 2015;11:2079–90. PMCID: PMC4540121. http://www.ncbi.nlm.nih.gov/pubmed/26316754.
59. Slavich GM, Thornton T, Torres LD, Monroe SM, Gotlib IH. Targeted rejection predicts hastened onset of major depression. J Soc Clin Psychol. 2009;28(2):223–43. PMCID: PMC2847269. http://www.ncbi.nlm.nih.gov/pubmed/20357895.
60. Monroe SM, Slavich GM, Torres LD, Gotlib IH. Major life events and major chronic difficulties are differentially associated with history of major depressive episodes. J Abnorm Psychol. 2007;116(1):116–24. PMCID: PMC3631311. http://www.ncbi.nlm.nih.gov/pubmed/17324022.
61. Heim C, Newport DJ, Mletzko T, Miller AH, Nemeroff CB. The link between childhood trauma and depression: insights from HPA axis studies in humans. Psychoneuroendocrinology. 2008;33(6):693–710. PMID: 18602762. http://www.ncbi.nlm.nih.gov/pubmed/18602762.
62. Giniatullina A, Maroteaux G, Geerts CJ, Koopmans B, Loos M, Klaassen R, Chen N, van der Schors RC, van Nierop P, Li KW, de Jong J, Altrock WD, Cornelisse LN, Toonen RF, van der Sluis S, Sullivan PF, Stiedl O, Posthuma D, Smit AB, Groffen AJ, Verhage M. Functional characterization of the PCLO p.Ser4814Ala variant associated with major depressive disorder reveals cellular but not behavioral differences. Neuroscience. 2015;300:518–38. PMID: 26045179. http://www.ncbi.nlm.nih.gov/pubmed/26045179.
63. Boden JM, Fergusson DM. Alcohol and depression. Addiction. 2011;106(5):906–14. PMID: 21382111. http://www.ncbi.nlm.nih.gov/pubmed/21382111.
64. Cottencin O. Severe depression and addictions. Encephale. 2009;35(Suppl 7):S264–8. PMID: 20141784. http://www.ncbi.nlm.nih.gov/pubmed/20141784.
65. Kessler RC, Nelson CB, McGonagle KA, Liu J, Swartz M, Blazer DG. Comorbidity of DSM-III-R major depressive disorder in the general population: results from the US National Comorbidity Survey. Br J Psychiatry Suppl. 1996;30:17–30. PMID: 8864145. http://www.ncbi.nlm.nih.gov/pubmed/8864145.
66. Hirschfeld RMA. The comorbidity of major depression and anxiety disorders: recognition and management in primary care. Prim Care Companion J Clin Psychiatry. 2001;3(6):244–54. PMCID: PMC181193. http://www.ncbi.nlm.nih.gov/pubmed/15014592.
67. Bair MJ, Robinson RL, Katon W, Kroenke K. Depression and pain comorbidity: a literature review. Arch Intern Med. 2003;163(20):2433–45. PMID: 14609780. http://www.ncbi.nlm.nih.gov/pubmed/14609780.
68. Hawton K, Casañas I, Comabella C, Haw C, Saunders K. Risk factors for suicide in individuals with depression: a systematic review. J Affect Disord. 2013;147(1–3):17–28. PMID: 23411024. http://www.ncbi.nlm.nih.gov/pubmed/23411024.
69. Miret M, Ayuso-Mateos JL, Sanchez-Moreno J, Vieta E. Depressive disorders and suicide: epidemiology, risk factors, and burden. Neurosci Biobehav Rev. 2013;37(10 Pt 1):2372–4. PMID: 23313644. http://www.ncbi.nlm.nih.gov/pubmed/23313644.
70. Dalca IM, McGirr A, Renaud J, Turecki G. Gender-specific suicide risk factors: a case-control study of individuals with major depressive disorder. J Clin Psychiatry. 2013;74(12):1209–16. PMID: 24434089. http://www.ncbi.nlm.nih.gov/pubmed/24434089.
71. van Loo HM, de Jonge P, Romeijn JW, Kessler RC, Schoevers RA. Data-driven subtypes of major depressive disorder: a systematic review. BMC Med. 2012;10:156. PMCID: PMC3566979. http://www.ncbi.nlm.nih.gov/pubmed/23210727.
72. Beijers L, Wardenaar KJ, van Loo HM, Schoevers RA. Data-driven biological subtypes of depression: systematic review of biological approaches to depression subtyping. Mol Psychiatry. 2019;24(6):888–900. PMID: 30824865. http://www.ncbi.nlm.nih.gov/pubmed/30824865.
73. Rantala MJ, Luoto S, Krams I, Karlsson H. Depression subtyping based on evolutionary psychiatry: proximate mechanisms and ultimate functions. Brain Behav Immun. 2018;69:603–17. PMID: 29051086. http://www.ncbi.nlm.nih.gov/pubmed/29051086.

74. Grisanzio KA, Goldstein-Piekarski AN, Wang MY, Rashed Ahmed AP, Samara Z, Williams LM. Transdiagnostic symptom clusters and associations with brain, behavior, and daily function in mood, anxiety, and trauma disorders. JAMA Psychiatry. 2018;75(2):201–9. PMCID: PMC5838569. http://www.ncbi.nlm.nih.gov/pubmed/29197929.
75. Lamers F, Burstein M, Jian-Ping H, Avenevoli S, Angst J, Merikangas KR. Structure of major depressive disorder in adolescents and adults in the US general population. Br J Psychiatry. 2012;201(2):143–50. PMCID: PMC3409428. http://www.ncbi.nlm.nih.gov/pubmed/22700082.
76. Rhebergen D, Lamers F, Spijker J, de Graaf R, Beekman ATF, Penninx BWJH. Course trajectories of unipolar depressive disorders identified by latent class growth analysis. Psychol Med. 2012;42(7):1383–96. PMID: 22053816. http://www.ncbi.nlm.nih.gov/pubmed/22053816.
77. Milaneschi Y, Lamers F, Peyrot WJ, Abdellaoui A, Willemsen G, Hottenga JJ, Jansen R, Mbarek H, Dehghan A, Lu C, CHARGE inflammation working group, Boomsma DI, Penninx BWJH. Polygenic dissection of major depression clinical heterogeneity. Mol Psychiatry. 2016;21(4):516–22. PMCID: PMC5546325. http://www.ncbi.nlm.nih.gov/pubmed/26122587.
78. BRAINnet: a standardized global human brain project | Request PDF. https://www.researchgate.net/publication/266139746_BRAINnet_a_standardized_global_human_brain_project.
79. Gordon E, Cooper N, Rennie C, Hermens D, Williams LM. Integrative neuroscience: the role of a standardized database. Clin EEG Neurosci. 2005;36(2):64–75. PMID: 15999901. http://www.ncbi.nlm.nih.gov/pubmed/15999901.
80. Cellular Substrates of Brain Rhythms. Niedermeyer's Electroencephalography: basic principles, clinical applications, and related fields Oxford Academic (oup.com). https://academic.oup.com/book/35515/chapter-abstract/305245903?redirectedFrom=fulltext&login=false.
81. https://www.sciencedirect.com/book/9780128044902/introduction-to-eeg-and-speech-based-emotion-recognition.
82. https://www.sciencedirect.com/topics/medicine-and-dentistry/beta-wave.
83. Rive MM, van Rooijen G, Veltman DJ, Phillips ML, Schene AH, Ruhé HG. Neural correlates of dysfunctional emotion regulation in major depressive disorder. A systematic review of neuroimaging studies. Neurosci Biobehav Rev. 2013;37(10 Pt 2):2529–53. PMID: 23928089. http://www.ncbi.nlm.nih.gov/pubmed/23928089.
84. Phillips LK, Seidman LJ. Emotion processing in persons at risk for schizophrenia. Schizophr Bull. 2008;34(5):888–903. PMCID: PMC2518637. http://www.ncbi.nlm.nih.gov/pubmed/18644853.
85. Ladouceur CD, Almeida JRC, Birmaher B, Axelson DA, Nau S, Kalas C, Monk K, Kupfer DJ, Phillips ML. Subcortical gray matter volume abnormalities in healthy bipolar offspring: potential neuroanatomical risk marker for bipolar disorder? J Am Acad Child Adolesc Psychiatry. 2008;47(5):532–9. PMCID: PMC2711512. http://www.ncbi.nlm.nih.gov/pubmed/18356765.
86. Fournier JC, Keener MT, Almeida J, Kronhaus DM, Phillips ML. Amygdala and whole-brain activity to emotional faces distinguishes major depressive disorder and bipolar disorder. Bipolar Disord. 2013;15(7):741–52. PMCID: PMC3864629. http://www.ncbi.nlm.nih.gov/pubmed/23911154.
87. Dybedal GS, Tanum L, Sundet K, Gaarden TL, Bjølseth TM. Neuropsychological functioning in late-life depression. Front Psychol. 2013;4:381. PMCID: PMC3694218. http://www.ncbi.nlm.nih.gov/pubmed/23818887.
88. Bortolato B, Carvalho AF, McIntyre RS. Cognitive dysfunction in major depressive disorder: a state-of-the-art clinical review. CNS Neurol Disord Drug Targets. 2014;13(10):1804–18. PMID: 25470396. http://www.ncbi.nlm.nih.gov/pubmed/25470396.
89. Snyder HR. Major depressive disorder is associated with broad impairments on neuropsychological measures of executive function: a meta-analysis and review. Psychol Bull. 2013;139(1):81–132. PMCID: PMC3436964. http://www.ncbi.nlm.nih.gov/pubmed/22642228.
90. Keller J, Schatzberg AF, Maj M. Current issues in the classification of psychotic major depression. Schizophr Bull. 2007;33(4):877–85. PMCID: PMC2632329. http://www.ncbi.nlm.nih.gov/pubmed/17548842.
91. Gaudiano BA, Dalrymple KL, Zimmerman M. Prevalence and clinical characteristics of psychotic versus nonpsychotic major depression in a general psychiatric outpatient clinic. Depress Anxiety. 2009;26(1):54–64. PMCID: PMC3111977. http://www.ncbi.nlm.nih.gov/pubmed/18781658.
92. Tohen M, Khalsa HMK, Salvatore P, Vieta E, Ravichandran C, Baldessarini RJ. Two-year outcomes in first-episode psychotic depression the McLean-Harvard First-Episode Project. J Affect Disord. 2012;136(1–2):1–8. PMID: 21943929. http://www.ncbi.nlm.nih.gov/pubmed/21943929.
93. Busatto GF. Structural and functional neuroimaging studies in major depressive disorder with psychotic features: a critical review. Schizophr Bull. 2013;39(4):776–86. PMCID: PMC3686460. http://www.ncbi.nlm.nih.gov/pubmed/23615813.
94. Rhebergen D, Graham R. The re-labelling of dysthymic disorder to persistent depressive disorder in DSM-5: old wine in new bottles? Curr Opin Psychiatry. 2014;27(1):27–31. PMID: 24270481. http://www.ncbi.nlm.nih.gov/pubmed/24270481.
95. Markkula N, Suvisaari J, Saarni SI, Pirkola S, Peña S, Saarni S, Ahola K, Mattila AK, Viertiö S, Strehle J, Koskinen S, Härkänen T. Prevalence and correlates of major depressive disorder and dysthymia in an eleven-year follow-up-results from the Finnish Health 2011 Survey. J Affect Disord. 2015;173:73–80. PMID: 25462399. http://www.ncbi.nlm.nih.gov/pubmed/25462399.
96. Wu W, Wang Z, Wei Y, Zhang G, Shi S, Gao J, Li Y, Tao M, Zhang K, Wang X, Gao C, Yang L, Li K, Shi J, Wang G, Liu L, Zhang J, Du B, Jiang G, Shen J, Liu Y, Liang W, Sun J, Hu J, Liu T, Wang X, Miao G, Meng H, Li Y, Hu C, Li Y, Huang G, Li G, Ha B, Deng H, Mei Q, Zhong H, Gao S, Sang H, Zhang Y, Fang X, Yu F, Yang D, Liu T, Chen Y, Hong X, Wu W, Chen G, Cai M, Song Y, Pan J, Dong J, Pan R, Zhang W, Shen Z, Liu Z, Gu D, Wang X, Liu X, Zhang Q, Li Y, Chen Y, Kendler KS, Flint J, Zhang Z. Clinical features of patients with dysthymia in a large cohort of Han Chinese women with recurrent major depression. PLoS One. 2013;8(12):e83490. PMCID: PMC3873934. http://www.ncbi.nlm.nih.gov/pubmed/24386213.
97. Sansone RA, Sansone LA. Dysthymic disorder: forlorn and overlooked? Psychiatry (Edgmont). 2009;6(5):46–51. PMCID: PMC2719439. http://www.ncbi.nlm.nih.gov/pubmed/19724735.
98. Griffiths J, Ravindran AV, Merali Z, Anisman H. Dysthymia: a review of pharmacological and behavioral factors. Mol Psychiatry. 2000;5(3):242–61. PMID: 10889527. http://www.ncbi.nlm.nih.gov/pubmed/10889527.
99. Devanand DP. Dysthymic disorder in the elderly population. Int Psychogeriatr. 2014;26(1):39–48. PMID: 24152873. http://www.ncbi.nlm.nih.gov/pubmed/24152873.
100. Hantsoo L, Epperson CN. Premenstrual dysphoric disorder: epidemiology and treatment. Curr Psychiatry Rep. 2015;17(11):87. PMCID: PMC4890701. http://www.ncbi.nlm.nih.gov/pubmed/26377947.
101. Czajkowska M, Drosdzol-Cop A, Gałązka I, Naworska B, Skrzypulec-Plinta V. Menstrual cycle and the prevalence of premenstrual syndrome/premenstrual dysphoric disorder in adolescent athletes. J Pediatr Adolesc Gynecol. 2015;28(6):492–8. PMID: 26233292. http://www.ncbi.nlm.nih.gov/pubmed/26233292.
102. Bosman RC, Jung SE, Miloserdov K, Schoevers RA, aan het Rot M. Daily symptom ratings for studying premenstrual dysphoric

disorder: a review. J Affect Disord. 2016;189:43–53. PMID: 26406968. http://www.ncbi.nlm.nih.gov/pubmed/26406968.

103. Reed SC, Levin FR, Evans SM. Changes in mood, cognitive performance and appetite in the late luteal and follicular phases of the menstrual cycle in women with and without PMDD (premenstrual dysphoric disorder). Horm Behav. 2008;54(1):185–93. PMCID: PMC2491904. http://www.ncbi.nlm.nih.gov/pubmed/18413151.
104. Mehta N, Mehta S. Premenstrual dysphoric disorder in the diagnostic and statistical manual of mental disorders, fifth edition: contributions from Asia. East Asian Arch Psychiatry. 2014;24(4):174–7. PMID: 25482838. http://www.ncbi.nlm.nih.gov/pubmed/25482838.
105. Di Giulio G, Reissing ED. Premenstrual dysphoric disorder: prevalence, diagnostic considerations, and controversies. J Psychosom Obstet Gynaecol. 2006;27(4):201–10. PMID: 17225621. http://www.ncbi.nlm.nih.gov/pubmed/17225621.
106. Maharaj S, Trevino K. A comprehensive review of treatment options for premenstrual syndrome and premenstrual dysphoric disorder. J Psychiatr Pract. 2015;21(5):334–50. PMID: 26352222. http://www.ncbi.nlm.nih.gov/pubmed/26352222.
107. Patten SB, Lavorato DH. Medication use and major depressive syndrome in a community population. Compr Psychiatry. 2001;42(2):124–31. PMID: 11244148. http://www.ncbi.nlm.nih.gov/pubmed/11244148.
108. Celano CM, Freudenreich O, Fernandez-Robles C, Stern TA, Caro MA, Huffman JC. Depressogenic effects of medications: a review. Dialogues Clin Neurosci. 2011;13(1):109–25. PMCID: PMC3181967. http://www.ncbi.nlm.nih.gov/pubmed/21485751.
109. Huffman JC, Stern TA. Neuropsychiatric consequences of cardiovascular medications. Dialogues Clin Neurosci. 2007;9(1):29–45. PMCID: PMC3181843. http://www.ncbi.nlm.nih.gov/pubmed/17506224.
110. Terada K, Kojima Y, Watanabe T, Izumo N, Chiba K, Karube Y. Inhibition of nerve growth factor-induced neurite outgrowth from PC12 cells by dexamethasone: signaling pathways through the glucocorticoid receptor and phosphorylated Akt and ERK1/2. PLoS One. 2014;9(3):e93223. PMCID: PMC3965538. http://www.ncbi.nlm.nih.gov/pubmed/24667984.
111. Kelly SG, Taiwo BO, Wu Y, Bhatia R, Kettering CS, Gao Y, Li S, Hutten R, Ragin AB. Early suppressive antiretroviral therapy in HIV infection is associated with measurable changes in the corpus callosum. J Neurovirol. 2014;20(5):514–20. PMCID: PMC4206660. http://www.ncbi.nlm.nih.gov/pubmed/24965253.
112. Patten SB. Non-psychiatric therapeutic medications in the etiology of organic depression. Psychiatr J Univ Ott. 1990;15(3):150–5. PMID: 2147064. http://www.ncbi.nlm.nih.gov/pubmed/2147064.
113. Patten SB, Love EJ. Can drugs cause depression? A review of the evidence. J Psychiatry Neurosci. 1993;18(3):92–102. PMCID: PMC1188504. http://www.ncbi.nlm.nih.gov/pubmed/8499431.
114. Alderson SL, Foy R, Glidewell L, McLintock K, House A. How patients understand depression associated with chronic physical disease–a systematic review. BMC Fam Pract. 2012;13:41. PMCID: PMC3439302. http://www.ncbi.nlm.nih.gov/pubmed/22640234.
115. Alderson SL, Foy R, House A. Understanding depression associated with chronic physical illness: a Q-methodology study in primary care. Br J Gen Pract. 2015;65(635):e401–8. PMCID: PMC4439830. http://www.ncbi.nlm.nih.gov/pubmed/26009535.
116. Health Quality Ontario. Screening and management of depression for adults with chronic diseases: an evidence-based analysis. Ont Health Technol Assess Ser. 2013;13(8):1–45. PMCID: PMC3797467. http://www.ncbi.nlm.nih.gov/pubmed/24133570.
117. Diagnosing, Screening, and Monitoring Depression in the Elderly: A Review of Guidelines [Internet]. Ottawa: Canadian Agency for Drugs and Technologies in Health; 2015. [cited 2024 Dec 22]. Available from: http://www.ncbi.nlm.nih.gov/books/NBK321379/ PMID: 26468558.
118. Katon W, Lin EHB, Kroenke K. The association of depression and anxiety with medical symptom burden in patients with chronic medical illness. Gen Hosp Psychiatry. 2007;29(2):147–55. PMID: 17336664. http://www.ncbi.nlm.nih.gov/pubmed/17336664.
119. Brunner EJ, Shipley MJ, Britton AR, Stansfeld SA, Heuschmann PU, Rudd AG, Wolfe CDA, Singh-Manoux A, Kivimaki M. Depressive disorder, coronary heart disease, and stroke: dose-response and reverse causation effects in the Whitehall II cohort study. Eur J Prev Cardiol. 2014;21(3):340–6. PMID: 24491401. http://www.ncbi.nlm.nih.gov/pubmed/24491401.
120. Fiore V, Marci M, Poggi A, Giagulli VA, Licchelli B, Iacoviello M, Guastamacchia E, De Pergola G, Triggiani V. The association between diabetes and depression: a very disabling condition. Endocrine. 2015;48(1):14–24. PMID: 24927794. http://www.ncbi.nlm.nih.gov/pubmed/24927794.
121. Fava GA, Sonino N, Morphy MA. Major depression associated with endocrine disease. Psychiatr Dev. 1987;5(4):321–48. PMID: 3328199. http://www.ncbi.nlm.nih.gov/pubmed/3328199.
122. Wang SL, Chang CH, Hu LY, Tsai SJ, Yang AC, You ZH. Risk of developing depressive disorders following rheumatoid arthritis: a nationwide population-based study. PLoS One. 2014;9(9):e107791. PMCID: PMC4166666. http://www.ncbi.nlm.nih.gov/pubmed/25226167.
123. Warmenhoven F, Bor H, Lucassen P, Vissers K, van Weel C, Prins J, Schers H. Depressive disorder in the last phase of life in patients with cardiovascular disease, cancer, and COPD: data from a 20-year follow-up period in general practice. Br J Gen Pract. 2013;63(610):e303–8. PMCID: PMC3635575. http://www.ncbi.nlm.nih.gov/pubmed/23643227.
124. Chen MH, Wei HT, Su TP, Li CT, Lin WC, Chang WH, Chen TJ, Bai YM. Risk of depressive disorder among patients with herpes zoster: a nationwide population-based prospective study. Psychosom Med. 2014;76(4):285–91. PMID: 24804885. http://www.ncbi.nlm.nih.gov/pubmed/24804885.
125. Cheng CM, Hsu JW, Huang KL, Bai YM, Su TP, Li CT, Yang AC, Chang WH, Chen TJ, Tsai SJ, Chen MH. Risk of developing major depressive disorder and anxiety disorders among adolescents and adults with atopic dermatitis: a nationwide longitudinal study. J Affect Disord. 2015;178:60–5. PMID: 25795537. http://www.ncbi.nlm.nih.gov/pubmed/25795537.
126. Moorthy D, Peter I, Scott TM, Parnell LD, Lai CQ, Crott JW, Ordovás JM, Selhub J, Griffith J, Rosenberg IH, Tucker KL, Troen AM. Status of vitamins B-12 and B-6 but not of folate, homocysteine, and the methylenetetrahydrofolate reductase C677T polymorphism are associated with impaired cognition and depression in adults. J Nutr. 2012;142(8):1554–60. PMCID: PMC3397340. http://www.ncbi.nlm.nih.gov/pubmed/22739363.
127. Muzik M, Borovska S. Perinatal depression: implications for child mental health. Ment Health Fam Med. 2010;7(4):239–47. PMCID: PMC3083253. http://www.ncbi.nlm.nih.gov/pubmed/22477948.
128. Gavin NI, Gaynes BN, Lohr KN, Meltzer-Brody S, Gartlehner G, Swinson T. Perinatal depression: a systematic review of prevalence and incidence. Obstet Gynecol. 2005;106(5 Pt 1):1071–83. PMID: 16260528. http://www.ncbi.nlm.nih.gov/pubmed/16260528.
129. Lindahl V, Pearson JL, Colpe L. Prevalence of suicidality during pregnancy and the postpartum. Arch Womens Ment Health. 2005;8(2):77–87. PMID: 15883651. http://www.ncbi.nlm.nih.gov/pubmed/15883651.
130. Serati M, Redaelli M, Buoli M, Altamura AC. Perinatal major depression biomarkers: a systematic review. J Affect Disord. 2016;193:391–404. PMID: 26802316. http://www.ncbi.nlm.nih.gov/pubmed/26802316.
131. Woody CA, Ferrari AJ, Siskind DJ, Whiteford HA, Harris MG. A systematic review and meta-regression of the preva-

lence and incidence of perinatal depression. J Affect Disord. 2017;219:86–92. PMID: 28531848. http://www.ncbi.nlm.nih.gov/pubmed/28531848.
132. Santos H, Tan X, Salomon R. Heterogeneity in perinatal depression: how far have we come? A systematic review. Arch Womens Ment Health. 2017;20(1):11–23. PMCID: PMC5507213. http://www.ncbi.nlm.nih.gov/pubmed/27796597.
133. Bodnar LM, Wisner KL, Moses-Kolko E, Sit DKY, Hanusa BH. Prepregnancy body mass index, gestational weight gain, and the likelihood of major depressive disorder during pregnancy. J Clin Psychiatry. 2009;70(9):1290–6. PMCID: PMC2760651. http://www.ncbi.nlm.nih.gov/pubmed/19607761.
134. Britton JR. Infant temperament and maternal anxiety and depressed mood in the early postpartum period. Women Health. 2011;51(1):55–71. PMID: 21391161. http://www.ncbi.nlm.nih.gov/pubmed/21391161.
135. Gentile S, Fusco ML. Untreated perinatal paternal depression: effects on offspring. Psychiatry Res. 2017;252:325–32. PMID: 28314228. http://www.ncbi.nlm.nih.gov/pubmed/28314228.
136. Cripe SM, Frederick IO, Qiu C, Williams MA. Risk of preterm delivery and hypertensive disorders of pregnancy in relation to maternal co-morbid mood and migraine disorders during pregnancy. Paediatr Perinat Epidemiol. 2011;25(2):116–23. PMCID: PMC3756187. http://www.ncbi.nlm.nih.gov/pubmed/21281324.
137. Grote NK, Bridge JA, Gavin AR, Melville JL, Iyengar S, Katon WJ. A meta-analysis of depression during pregnancy and the risk of preterm birth, low birth weight, and intrauterine growth restriction. Arch Gen Psychiatry. 2010;67(10):1012–24. PMCID: PMC3025772. http://www.ncbi.nlm.nih.gov/pubmed/20921117.
138. Jablensky AV, Morgan V, Zubrick SR, Bower C, Yellachich LA. Pregnancy, delivery, and neonatal complications in a population cohort of women with schizophrenia and major affective disorders. Am J Psychiatry. 2005;162(1):79–91. PMID: 15625205. http://www.ncbi.nlm.nih.gov/pubmed/15625205.
139. Pearlstein T. Depression during pregnancy. Best Pract Res Clin Obstet Gynaecol. 2015;29(5):754–64. PMID: 25976080. http://www.ncbi.nlm.nih.gov/pubmed/25976080.
140. Gotlib IH, Whiffen VE, Wallace PM, Mount JH. Prospective investigation of postpartum depression: factors involved in onset and recovery. J Abnorm Psychol. 1991;100(2):122–32. PMID: 2040762. http://www.ncbi.nlm.nih.gov/pubmed/2040762.
141. Deave T, Heron J, Evans J, Emond A. The impact of maternal depression in pregnancy on early child development. BJOG. 2008;115(8):1043–51. PMID: 18651886. http://www.ncbi.nlm.nih.gov/pubmed/18651886.
142. Forman DR, O'Hara MW, Stuart S, Gorman LL, Larsen KE, Coy KC. Effective treatment for postpartum depression is not sufficient to improve the developing mother-child relationship. Dev Psychopathol. 2007;19(2):585–602. PMID: 17459185. http://www.ncbi.nlm.nih.gov/pubmed/17459185.
143. Möller HJ, Bandelow B, Volz HP, Barnikol UB, Seifritz E, Kasper S. The relevance of "mixed anxiety and depression" as a diagnostic category in clinical practice. Eur Arch Psychiatry Clin Neurosci. 2016;266(8):725–36. PMCID: PMC5097109. http://www.ncbi.nlm.nih.gov/pubmed/27002521.
144. World Health Organization, editor. International statistical classification of diseases and related health problems: alphabetical index. ICD-11 World Health Organization; 2024. https://www.who.int/standards/classifications/classification-of-diseases.
145. Wittchen HU, Schuster P, Lieb R. Comorbidity and mixed anxiety-depressive disorder: clinical curiosity or pathophysiological need? Hum Psychopharmacol. 2001;16(S1):S21–30. PMID: 12404532. http://www.ncbi.nlm.nih.gov/pubmed/12404532.
146. Demyttenaere K, Bruffaerts R, Posada-Villa J, Gasquet I, Kovess V, Lepine JP, Angermeyer MC, Bernert S, de Girolamo G, Morosini P, Polidori G, Kikkawa T, Kawakami N, Ono Y, Takeshima T, Uda H, Karam EG, Fayyad JA, Karam AN, Mneimneh ZN, Medina-Mora ME, Borges G, Lara C, de Graaf R, Ormel J, Gureje O, Shen Y, Huang Y, Zhang M, Alonso J, Haro JM, Vilagut G, Bromet EJ, Gluzman S, Webb C, Kessler RC, Merikangas KR, Anthony JC, Von Korff MR, Wang PS, Brugha TS, Aguilar-Gaxiola S, Lee S, Heeringa S, Pennell BE, Zaslavsky AM, Ustun TB, Chatterji S, WHO World Mental Health Survey Consortium. Prevalence, severity, and unmet need for treatment of mental disorders in the World Health Organization World Mental Health Surveys. JAMA. 2004;291(21):2581–90. PMID: 15173149. http://www.ncbi.nlm.nih.gov/pubmed/15173149.
147. Boulenger JP, Fournier M, Rosales D, Lavallée YJ. Mixed anxiety and depression: from theory to practice. J Clin Psychiatry. 1997;58(Suppl 8):27–34. PMID: 9236733. http://www.ncbi.nlm.nih.gov/pubmed/9236733.
148. Wittchen HU, Essau CA. Comorbidity and mixed anxiety-depressive disorders: is there epidemiologic evidence? J Clin Psychiatry. 1993;54(Suppl):9–15. PMID: 8425875. http://www.ncbi.nlm.nih.gov/pubmed/8425875.
149. Regier DA, Narrow WE, Clarke DE, Kraemer HC, Kuramoto SJ, Kuhl EA, Kupfer DJ. DSM-5 field trials in the United States and Canada, Part II: test-retest reliability of selected categorical diagnoses. Am J Psychiatry. 2013;170(1):59–70. PMID: 23111466. http://www.ncbi.nlm.nih.gov/pubmed/23111466.
150. Clarke DE, Narrow WE, Regier DA, Kuramoto SJ, Kupfer DJ, Kuhl EA, Greiner L, Kraemer HC. DSM-5 field trials in the United States and Canada, Part I: study design, sampling strategy, implementation, and analytic approaches. Am J Psychiatry. 2013;170(1):43–58. PMID: 23111546. http://www.ncbi.nlm.nih.gov/pubmed/23111546.
151. Reed GM, Mendonça Correia J, Esparza P, Saxena S, Maj M. The WPA-WHO global survey of psychiatrists' attitudes towards mental disorders classification. World Psychiatry. 2011;10(2):118–31. PMCID: PMC3105474. http://www.ncbi.nlm.nih.gov/pubmed/21633689.
152. icd11factsheet_en.pdf. https://icd.who.int/en/docs/icd11factsheet_en.pdf.
153. Shevlin M, Hyland P, Nolan E, Owczarek M, Ben-Ezra M, Karatzias T. ICD-11 "mixed depressive and anxiety disorder" is clinical rather than sub-clinical and more common than anxiety and depression in the general population. Br J Clin Psychol. 2022;61(1):18–36. PMCID: PMC9291022. http://www.ncbi.nlm.nih.gov/pubmed/34273110.
154. Zheng YP, Lin KM, Zhao JP, Zhang MY, Yong D. Comparative study of diagnostic systems: Chinese classification of mental disorders-second edition versus DSM-III-R. Compr Psychiatry. 1994;35(6):441–9. PMID: 7867317. http://www.ncbi.nlm.nih.gov/pubmed/7867317.
155. Benedetti A, Wu Y, Levis B, Wilchesky M, Boruff J, Ioannidis JPA, Patten SB, Cuijpers P, Shrier I, Gilbody S, Ismail Z, McMillan D, Mitchell N, Ziegelstein RC, Thombs BD. Diagnostic accuracy of the Geriatric Depression Scale-30, Geriatric Depression Scale-15, Geriatric Depression Scale-5 and Geriatric Depression Scale-4 for detecting major depression: protocol for a systematic review and individual participant data meta-analysis. BMJ Open. 2018;8(12):e026598. PMCID: PMC6286470. http://www.ncbi.nlm.nih.gov/pubmed/30518594.
156. Duhoux A, Fournier L, Nguyen CT, Roberge P, Beveridge R. Guideline concordance of treatment for depressive disorders in Canada. Soc Psychiatry Psychiatr Epidemiol. 2009;44(5):385–92. PMID: 18946624. http://www.ncbi.nlm.nih.gov/pubmed/18946624.
157. Starkes JM, Poulin CC, Kisely SR. Unmet need for the treatment of depression in Atlantic Canada. Can J Psychiatry. 2005;50(10):580–90. PMID: 16276848. http://www.ncbi.nlm.nih.gov/pubmed/16276848.

158. Vasiliadis HM, Lesage A, Adair C, Wang PS, Kessler RC. Do Canada and the United States differ in prevalence of depression and utilization of services? Psychiatr Serv. 2007;58(1):63–71. PMID: 17215414. http://www.ncbi.nlm.nih.gov/pubmed/17215414.
159. Lam RW, Michalak EE, Swinson RP. Assessment scales in depression, mania and anxiety. London: Taylor and Francis; 2005.
160. Psychiatric Rating Scales for Depression – Neurotransmitter.net. https://www.neurotransmitter.net/depressionscales.html.
161. Robins LN, Helzer JE, Croughan J, Ratcliff KS. National Institute of Mental Health Diagnostic Interview Schedule. Its history, characteristics, and validity. Arch Gen Psychiatry. 1981;38(4):381–9. PMID: 6260053 http://www.ncbi.nlm.nih.gov/pubmed/6260053
162. Grove WM, Andreasen NC, McDonald-Scott P, Keller MB, Shapiro RW. Reliability studies of psychiatric diagnosis. Theory and practice. Arch Gen Psychiatry. 1981;38(4):408–13. PMID: 7212971. http://www.ncbi.nlm.nih.gov/pubmed/7212971.
163. Miller PR. Inpatient diagnostic assessments: 2. Interrater reliability and outcomes of structured vs. unstructured interviews. Psychiatry Res. 2001;105(3):265–71. PMID: 11814545. http://www.ncbi.nlm.nih.gov/pubmed/11814545.
164. Spitzer RL, Williams JB, Gibbon M, First MB. The Structured Clinical Interview for DSM-III-R (SCID). I: history, rationale, and description. Arch Gen Psychiatry. 1992;49(8):624–9. PMID: 1637252. http://www.ncbi.nlm.nih.gov/pubmed/1637252.
165. Wittchen HU. Reliability and validity studies of the WHO–Composite International Diagnostic Interview (CIDI): a critical review. J Psychiatr Res. 1994;28(1):57–84. PMID: 8064641. http://www.ncbi.nlm.nih.gov/pubmed/8064641.
166. Sowicz TJ, Sefcik JS, Teng HL, Irani E, Kelly TA, Bradway C. The use of closing questions in qualitative research: results of a web-based survey. Nurs Res. 2019;68(6):E8–E12. PMCID: PMC6852793. http://www.ncbi.nlm.nih.gov/pubmed/31693558.
167. Dicicco-Bloom B, Crabtree BF. The qualitative research interview. Med Educ. 2006;40(4):314–21. PMID: 16573666. http://www.ncbi.nlm.nih.gov/pubmed/16573666.
168. Dearnley C. A reflection on the use of semi-structured interviews. Nurse Res. 2005;13(1):19–28. PMID: 16220838. http://www.ncbi.nlm.nih.gov/pubmed/16220838.
169. Doody O, Noonan M. Preparing and conducting interviews to collect data. Nurse Res. 2013;20(5):28–32. PMID: 23687846. http://www.ncbi.nlm.nih.gov/pubmed/23687846.
170. Peters K, Halcomb E. Interviews in qualitative research. Nurse Res. 2015;22(4):6–7. PMID: 25783145. http://www.ncbi.nlm.nih.gov/pubmed/25783145.
171. Kallio H, Pietilä AM, Johnson M, Kangasniemi M. Systematic methodological review: developing a framework for a qualitative semi-structured interview guide. J Adv Nurs. 2016;72(12):2954–65. PMID: 27221824. http://www.ncbi.nlm.nih.gov/pubmed/27221824.
172. Bech P. Rating scales in depression: limitations and pitfalls. Dialogues Clin Neurosci. 2006;8(2):207–15. PMCID: PMC3181766. http://www.ncbi.nlm.nih.gov/pubmed/16889106.
173. Rice DB, Shrier I, Kloda LA, Benedetti A, Thombs BD. Methodological quality of meta-analyses of the diagnostic accuracy of depression screening tools. J Psychosom Res. 2016;84:84–92. PMID: 27095164. http://www.ncbi.nlm.nih.gov/pubmed/27095164.
174. Rice DB, Kloda LA, Levis B, Qi B, Kingsland E, Thombs BD. Are MEDLINE searches sufficient for systematic reviews and meta-analyses of the diagnostic accuracy of depression screening tools? A review of meta-analyses. J Psychosom Res. 2016;87:7–13. PMID: 27411746. http://www.ncbi.nlm.nih.gov/pubmed/27411746.
175. Levis B, Yan XW, He C, Sun Y, Benedetti A, Thombs BD. Comparison of depression prevalence estimates in meta-analyses based on screening tools and rating scales versus diagnostic interviews: a meta-research review. BMC Med. 2019;17(1):65. PMCID: PMC6427845. http://www.ncbi.nlm.nih.gov/pubmed/30894161.
176. Top 100 journals with impact factor in 2022 (Highest To Lowest) – Journal Impact Factor. https://impactfactorforjournal.com/journals-with-impact-factor/.
177. Saint S, Christakis DA, Saha S, Elmore JG, Welsh DE, Baker P, Koepsell TD. Journal reading habits of internists. J Gen Intern Med. 2000;15(12):881–4. PMCID: PMC1495716. http://www.ncbi.nlm.nih.gov/pubmed/11119185.
178. Dal-Ré R, Castell MV, García-Puig J. If the results of an article are noteworthy, read the entire article; do not rely on the abstract alone. Rev Clin Esp (Barc). 2015;215(8):454–7. PMID: 26165166. http://www.ncbi.nlm.nih.gov/pubmed/26165166.
179. Read MEDLINE abstracts with a pinch of salt. Lancet. 2006;368(9545):1394. PMID: 17055921. http://www.ncbi.nlm.nih.gov/pubmed/17055921.
180. Burke DT, Judelson AL, Schneider JC, DeVito MC, Latta D. Reading habits of practicing physiatrists. Am J Phys Med Rehabil. 2002;81(10):779–87. PMID: 12362119. http://www.ncbi.nlm.nih.gov/pubmed/12362119.
181. Kahwati L, Carmody D, Berkman N, Sullivan HW, Aikin KJ, DeFrank J. Prescribers' knowledge and skills for interpreting research results: a systematic review. J Contin Educ Health Prof. 2017;37(2):129–36. PMCID: PMC8218608. http://www.ncbi.nlm.nih.gov/pubmed/28562502.
182. Tsujimoto Y, Aoki T, Shinohara K, So R, Suganuma AM, Kimachi M, Yamamoto Y, Furukawa TA. Physician characteristics associated with proper assessment of overstated conclusions in research abstracts: a secondary analysis of a randomized controlled trial. PLoS One. 2019;14(1):e0211206. PMCID: PMC6347200. http://www.ncbi.nlm.nih.gov/pubmed/30682128.
183. Zwolsman S, te Pas E, Hooft L, Wieringa-de Waard M, van Dijk N. Barriers to GPs' use of evidence-based medicine: a systematic review. Br J Gen Pract. 2012;62(600):e511–21. PMCID: PMC3381277. http://www.ncbi.nlm.nih.gov/pubmed/22781999.
184. HAMILTON DEPRESSION RATING SCALE. http://www.medafile.com/cln/HDRS.html.
185. Furukawa TA, Reijnders M, Kishimoto S, Sakata M, DeRubeis RJ, Dimidjian S, Dozois DJA, Hegerl U, Hollon SD, Jarrett RB, Lespérance F, Segal ZV, Mohr DC, Simons AD, Quilty LC, Reynolds CF, Gentili C, Leucht S, Engel RR, Cuijpers P. Translating the BDI and BDI-II into the HAMD and vice versa with equipercentile linking. Epidemiol Psychiatr Sci. 2019;29:e24. PMCID: PMC8061209. http://www.ncbi.nlm.nih.gov/pubmed/30867082.
186. Hamilton M. Rating depressive patients. J Clin Psychiatry. 1980;41(12 Pt 2):21–4. PMID: 7440521. http://www.ncbi.nlm.nih.gov/pubmed/7440521.
187. Hamilton M. Development of a rating scale for primary depressive illness. Br J Soc Clin Psychol. 1967;6(4):278–96. PMID: 6080235. http://www.ncbi.nlm.nih.gov/pubmed/6080235.
188. Lin CH, Park C, McIntyre RS. Early improvement in HAMD-17 and HAMD-7 scores predict response and remission in depressed patients treated with fluoxetine or electroconvulsive therapy. J Affect Disord. 2019;253:154–61. PMID: 31035216. http://www.ncbi.nlm.nih.gov/pubmed/31035216.
189. Lin HS, Lin CH. Early improvement in HAMD-17 and HAMD-6 scores predicts ultimate response and remission for depressed patients treated with fluoxetine or ECT. J Affect Disord. 2019;245:91–7. PMID: 30368075. http://www.ncbi.nlm.nih.gov/pubmed/30368075.
190. Measures of depression and depressive symptoms: Beck Depression Inventory-II (BDI-II), Center for Epidemiologic Studies Depression Scale (CES-D), Geriatric Depression Scale (GDS), Hospital Anxiety and Depression Scale (HADS), and

Patient Health Questionnaire-9 (PHQ-9). https://acrjournals.onlinelibrary.wiley.com/doi/epdf/10.1002/acr.20556.
191. Stepankova Georgi H, Horakova Vlckova K, Lukavsky J, Kopecek M, Bares M. Beck Depression Inventory-II: self-report or interview-based administrations show different results in older persons. Int Psychogeriatr. 2019;31(5):735–42. PMID: 30298795. http://www.ncbi.nlm.nih.gov/pubmed/30298795.
192. Pop-Jordanova N. BDI in the assessment of depression in different medical conditions. Pril (Makedon Akad Nauk Umet Odd Med Nauki). 2017;38(1):103–11. PMID: 28593888. http://www.ncbi.nlm.nih.gov/pubmed/28593888.
193. Freedland KE, Steinmeyer BC, Carney RM, Rubin EH, Rich MW. Use of the PROMIS® depression scale and the beck depression inventory in patients with heart failure. Health Psychol. 2019;38(5):369–75. PMCID: PMC6499487. http://www.ncbi.nlm.nih.gov/pubmed/31045419.
194. Beck AT, Ward CH, Mendelson M, Mock J, Erbaugh J. An inventory for measuring depression. Arch Gen Psychiatry. 1961;4:561–71. PMID: 13688369. http://www.ncbi.nlm.nih.gov/pubmed/13688369.
195. Simpson N. Treating hyperhidrosis. Br Med J (Clin Res Ed). 1988;296(6633):1345. PMCID: PMC2545820. http://www.ncbi.nlm.nih.gov/pubmed/3134977.
196. Reis DJ, Namekata MS, Oehlert ME, King N. A preliminary review of the Beck Depression Inventory-II (BDI-II) in veterans: are new norms and cut scores needed? Psychol Serv. 2020;17(3):363–71. PMID: 30869975. http://www.ncbi.nlm.nih.gov/pubmed/30869975.
197. Dardas LA, Shoqirat N, Xu H, Al-Khayat A, Bani Ata S, Shawashreh A, Simmons LA. Comparison of the performance of the Beck Depression Inventory-II and the center for epidemiologic studies-depression scale in Arab adolescents. Public Health Nurs. 2019;36(4):564–74. PMID: 31037762. http://www.ncbi.nlm.nih.gov/pubmed/31037762.
198. Savilahti EM, Haravuori H, Rytilä-Manninen M, Lindberg N, Kettunen K, Marttunen M. High Beck Depression Inventory 21 scores in adolescents without depression are associated with negative self-image and immature defense style. Psychiatry Res. 2018;263:61–8. PMID: 29502039. http://www.ncbi.nlm.nih.gov/pubmed/29502039.
199. Balsamo M, Cataldi F, Carlucci L, Padulo C, Fairfield B. Assessment of late-life depression via self-report measures: a review. Clin Interv Aging. 2018;13:2021–44. PMCID: PMC6199213. http://www.ncbi.nlm.nih.gov/pubmed/30410319.
200. Pocklington C, Gilbody S, Manea L, McMillan D. The diagnostic accuracy of brief versions of the Geriatric Depression Scale: a systematic review and meta-analysis. Int J Geriatr Psychiatry. 2016;31(8):837–57. PMID: 26890937. http://www.ncbi.nlm.nih.gov/pubmed/26890937.
201. Mitchell AJ, Bird V, Rizzo M, Meader N. Which version of the geriatric depression scale is most useful in medical settings and nursing homes? Diagnostic validity meta-analysis. Am J Geriatr Psychiatry. 2010;18(12):1066–77. PMID: 21155144. http://www.ncbi.nlm.nih.gov/pubmed/21155144.
202. Mitchell AJ, Yadegarfar M, Gill J, Stubbs B. Case finding and screening clinical utility of the Patient Health Questionnaire (PHQ-9 and PHQ-2) for depression in primary care: a diagnostic meta-analysis of 40 studies. BJPsych Open. 2016;2(2):127–38. PMCID: PMC4995584. http://www.ncbi.nlm.nih.gov/pubmed/27703765.
203. Spitzer RL, Kroenke K, Williams JB. Validation and utility of a self-report version of PRIME-MD: the PHQ primary care study. Primary care evaluation of mental disorders. Patient Health Questionnaire. JAMA. 1999;282(18):1737–44. PMID: 10568646. http://www.ncbi.nlm.nih.gov/pubmed/10568646.
204. Tsai FJ, Huang YH, Liu HC, Huang KY, Huang YH, Liu SI. Patient health questionnaire for school-based depression screening among Chinese adolescents. Pediatrics. 2014;133(2):e402–9. PMID: 24446447. http://www.ncbi.nlm.nih.gov/pubmed/24446447.
205. Kroenke K, Spitzer RL, Williams JBW, Löwe B. The patient health questionnaire somatic, anxiety, and depressive symptom scales: a systematic review. Gen Hosp Psychiatry. 2010;32(4):345–59. PMID: 20633738. http://www.ncbi.nlm.nih.gov/pubmed/20633738.
206. Chen TM, Huang FY, Chang C, Chung H. Using the PHQ-9 for depression screening and treatment monitoring for Chinese Americans in primary care. Psychiatr Serv. 2006;57(7):976–81. PMID: 16816282. http://www.ncbi.nlm.nih.gov/pubmed/16816282.
207. Adewuya AO, Ola BA, Afolabi OO. Validity of the patient health questionnaire (PHQ-9) as a screening tool for depression amongst Nigerian university students. J Affect Disord. 2006;96(1–2):89–93. PMID: 16857265. http://www.ncbi.nlm.nih.gov/pubmed/16857265.
208. Levis B, Benedetti A, Thombs BD, DEPRESsion Screening Data (DEPRESSD) Collaboration. Accuracy of Patient Health Questionnaire-9 (PHQ-9) for screening to detect major depression: individual participant data meta-analysis. BMJ. 2019;365:l1476. PMCID: PMC6454318. http://www.ncbi.nlm.nih.gov/pubmed/30967483.
209. Kroenke K, Spitzer RL, Williams JB. The PHQ-9: validity of a brief depression severity measure. J Gen Intern Med. 2001;16(9):606–13. PMCID: PMC1495268. http://www.ncbi.nlm.nih.gov/pubmed/11556941.
210. Whooley MA, Avins AL, Miranda J, Browner WS. Case-finding instruments for depression. Two questions are as good as many. J Gen Intern Med. 1997;12(7):439–45. PMCID: PMC1497134. http://www.ncbi.nlm.nih.gov/pubmed/9229283.
211. Spitzer RL, Kroenke K, Williams JBW, Löwe B. A brief measure for assessing generalized anxiety disorder: the GAD-7. Arch Intern Med. 2006;166(10):1092–7. PMID: 16717171. http://www.ncbi.nlm.nih.gov/pubmed/16717171.
212. Kroenke K, Strine TW, Spitzer RL, Williams JBW, Berry JT, Mokdad AH. The PHQ-8 as a measure of current depression in the general population. J Affect Disord. 2009;114(1–3):163–73. PMID: 18752852. http://www.ncbi.nlm.nih.gov/pubmed/18752852.
213. Wu Y, Levis B, Riehm KE, Saadat N, Levis AW, Azar M, Rice DB, Boruff J, Cuijpers P, Gilbody S, Ioannidis JPA, Kloda LA, McMillan D, Patten SB, Shrier I, Ziegelstein RC, Akena DH, Arroll B, Ayalon L, Baradaran HR, Baron M, Bombardier CH, Butterworth P, Carter G, Chagas MH, Chan JCN, Cholera R, Conwell Y, de Man-van Ginkel JM, Fann JR, Fischer FH, Fung D, Gelaye B, Goodyear-Smith F, Greeno CG, Hall BJ, Harrison PA, Härter M, Hegerl U, Hides L, Hobfoll SE, Hudson M, Hyphantis T, Inagaki M, Jetté N, Khamseh ME, Kiely KM, Kwan Y, Lamers F, Liu SI, Lotrakul M, Loureiro SR, Löwe B, McGuire A, Mohd-Sidik S, Munhoz TN, Muramatsu K, Osório FL, Patel V, Pence BW, Persoons P, Picardi A, Reuter K, Rooney AG, Santos IS, Shaaban J, Sidebottom A, Simning A, Stafford L, Sung S, Tan PLL, Turner A, van Weert HC, White J, Whooley MA, Winkley K, Yamada M, Benedetti A, Thombs BD. Equivalency of the diagnostic accuracy of the PHQ-8 and PHQ-9: a systematic review and individual participant data meta-analysis. Psychol Med. 2020;50(8):1368–80. PMCID: PMC6954991. http://www.ncbi.nlm.nih.gov/pubmed/31298180.
214. Wittkampf KA, Naeije L, Schene AH, Huyser J, van Weert HC. Diagnostic accuracy of the mood module of the Patient Health Questionnaire: a systematic review. Gen Hosp Psychiatry. 2007;29(5):388–95. PMID: 17888804 http://www.ncbi.nlm.nih.gov/pubmed/17888804

215. Allgaier AK, Pietsch K, Frühe B, Sigl-Glöckner J, Schulte-Körne G. Screening for depression in adolescents: validity of the patient health questionnaire in pediatric care. Depress Anxiety. 2012;29(10):906–13. PMID: 22753313. http://www.ncbi.nlm.nih.gov/pubmed/22753313.
216. He C, Levis B, Riehm KE, Saadat N, Levis AW, Azar M, Rice DB, Krishnan A, Wu Y, Sun Y, Imran M, Boruff J, Cuijpers P, Gilbody S, Ioannidis JPA, Kloda LA, McMillan D, Patten SB, Shrier I, Ziegelstein RC, Akena DH, Arroll B, Ayalon L, Baradaran HR, Baron M, Beraldi A, Bombardier CH, Butterworth P, Carter G, Chagas MHN, Chan JCN, Cholera R, Clover K, Conwell Y, de Man-van Ginkel JM, Fann JR, Fischer FH, Fung D, Gelaye B, Goodyear-Smith F, Greeno CG, Hall BJ, Harrison PA, Härter M, Hegerl U, Hides L, Hobfoll SE, Hudson M, Hyphantis TN, Inagaki M, Ismail K, Jetté N, Khamseh ME, Kiely KM, Kwan Y, Lamers F, Liu SI, Lotrakul M, Loureiro SR, Löwe B, Marsh L, McGuire A, Mohd-Sidik S, Munhoz TN, Muramatsu K, Osório FL, Patel V, Pence BW, Persoons P, Picardi A, Reuter K, Rooney AG, da Silva Dos Santos IS, Shaaban J, Sidebottom A, Simning A, Stafford L, Sung S, PLL T, Turner A, van Weert HCPM, White J, Whooley MA, Winkley K, Yamada M, Thombs BD, Benedetti A. The accuracy of the patient health questionnaire-9 algorithm for screening to detect major depression: an individual participant data meta-analysis. Psychother Psychosom. 2020;89(1):25–37. PMCID: PMC6960351. http://www.ncbi.nlm.nih.gov/pubmed/31593971.
217. Mulvaney-Day N, Marshall T, Downey Piscopo K, Korsen N, Lynch S, Karnell LH, Moran GE, Daniels AS, Ghose SS. Screening for behavioral health conditions in primary care settings: a systematic review of the literature. J Gen Intern Med. 2018;33(3):335–46. PMCID: PMC5834951. http://www.ncbi.nlm.nih.gov/pubmed/28948432.
218. Lakkis NA, Mahmassani DM. Screening instruments for depression in primary care: a concise review for clinicians. Postgrad Med. 2015;127(1):99–106. PMID: 25526224. http://www.ncbi.nlm.nih.gov/pubmed/25526224.
219. Alfonsson S, Maathz P, Hursti T. Interformat reliability of digital psychiatric self-report questionnaires: a systematic review. J Med Internet Res. 2014;16(12):e268. PMCID: PMC4275488. http://www.ncbi.nlm.nih.gov/pubmed/25472463.
220. van Ballegooijen W, Riper H, Cuijpers P, van Oppen P, Smit JH. Validation of online psychometric instruments for common mental health disorders: a systematic review. BMC Psychiatry. 2016;16:45. PMCID: PMC4766750. http://www.ncbi.nlm.nih.gov/pubmed/26915661.
221. Walters SJ, Stern C, Robertson-Malt S. The measurement of collaboration within healthcare settings: a systematic review of measurement properties of instruments. JBI Database System Rev Implement Rep. 2016;14(4):138–97. https://doi.org/10.11124/JBISRIR-2016-2159. https://pubmed.ncbi.nlm.nih.gov/27532315/
222. Schulze M, Donadio JV, Pruchno CJ, Baker PJ, Johnson RJ, Stahl RA, Watkins S, Martin DC, Wurzner R, Gotze O. Elevated urinary excretion of the C5b-9 complex in membranous nephropathy. Kidney Int. 1991;40(3):533–8. PMID: 1787650. http://www.ncbi.nlm.nih.gov/pubmed/1787650.
223. Donker T, van Straten A, Marks I, Cuijpers P. Brief self-rated screening for depression on the Internet. J Affect Disord. 2010;122(3):253–9. PMID: 19679358. http://www.ncbi.nlm.nih.gov/pubmed/19679358.
224. Fortson BL, Scotti JR, Del Ben KS, Chen YC. Reliability and validity of an Internet traumatic stress survey with a college student sample. J Trauma Stress. 2006;19(5):709–20. PMID: 17075908. http://www.ncbi.nlm.nih.gov/pubmed/17075908.
225. Leykin Y, Torres LD, Aguilera A, Muñoz RF. Factor structure of the CES-D in a sample of Spanish- and English-speaking smokers on the Internet. Psychiatry Res. 2011;185(1–2):269–74. PMCID: PMC4165607. http://www.ncbi.nlm.nih.gov/pubmed/20684849.
226. Yu SC, Yu MN. Comparison of Internet-based and paper-based questionnaires in Taiwan using multisample invariance approach. Cyberpsychol Behav. 2007;10(4):501–7. PMID: 17711357. http://www.ncbi.nlm.nih.gov/pubmed/17711357.
227. James C, Powell M, Seixas A, Bateman A, Pengpid S, Peltzer K. Exploring the psychometric properties of the CES-D-10 and its practicality in detecting depressive symptomatology in 27 low- and middle-income countries. Int J Psychol. 2020;55(3):435–45. PMID: 31441518. http://www.ncbi.nlm.nih.gov/pubmed/31441518.
228. Alexandrowicz RW, Jahn R, Wancata J. Assessing the dimensionality of the CES-D using multi-dimensional multi-level Rasch models. PLoS One. 2018;13(5):e0197908. PMCID: PMC5969764. http://www.ncbi.nlm.nih.gov/pubmed/29799866.
229. Wikberg C, Westman J, Petersson EL, Larsson MEH, André M, Eggertsen R, Thorn J, Ågren H, Björkelund C. Use of a self-rating scale to monitor depression severity in recurrent GP consultations in primary care – does it really make a difference? A randomised controlled study. BMC Fam Pract. 2017;18(1):6. PMCID: PMC5244530. http://www.ncbi.nlm.nih.gov/pubmed/28103816.
230. Hedman E, Ljótsson B, Blom K, El Alaoui S, Kraepelien M, Rück C, Andersson G, Svanborg C, Lindefors N, Kaldo V. Telephone versus internet administration of self-report measures of social anxiety, depressive symptoms, and insomnia: psychometric evaluation of a method to reduce the impact of missing data. J Med Internet Res. 2013;15(10):e229. PMCID: PMC3806436. http://www.ncbi.nlm.nih.gov/pubmed/24140566.
231. Andersson G, Kaldo-Sandström V, Ström L, Strömgren T. Internet administration of the Hospital Anxiety and Depression Scale in a sample of tinnitus patients. J Psychosom Res. 2003;55(3):259–62. PMID: 12932800. http://www.ncbi.nlm.nih.gov/pubmed/12932800.
232. McCue P, Buchanan T, Martin CR. Screening for psychological distress using internet administration of the Hospital Anxiety and Depression Scale (HADS) in individuals with chronic fatigue syndrome. Br J Clin Psychol. 2006;45(Pt 4):483–98. PMID: 17076959. http://www.ncbi.nlm.nih.gov/pubmed/17076959.
233. Whitehead L. Methodological issues in Internet-mediated research: a randomized comparison of internet versus mailed questionnaires. J Med Internet Res. 2011;13(4):e109. PMCID: PMC3278095. http://www.ncbi.nlm.nih.gov/pubmed/22155721.
234. McCue P, Martin C, Buchanan T, Rodgers J, Scholey A. An investigation into the psychometric properties of the Hospital Anxiety and Depression Scale in individuals with chronic fatigue syndrome. Psychol Health Med. 2003;8(4):425–39. PMID: 21974733. http://www.ncbi.nlm.nih.gov/pubmed/21974733.
235. Thorén ES, Andersson G, Lunner T. The use of research questionnaires with hearing impaired adults: online vs. paper-and-pencil administration. BMC Ear Nose Throat Disord. 2012;12:12. PMCID: PMC3528487. http://www.ncbi.nlm.nih.gov/pubmed/23107440.
236. Levine SZ. Evaluating the seven-item Center for Epidemiologic Studies depression scale short-form: a longitudinal U.S. community study. Soc Psychiatry Psychiatr Epidemiol. 2013;48(9):1519–26. PMID: 23299927. http://www.ncbi.nlm.nih.gov/pubmed/23299927.
237. Mohebbi M, Nguyen V, JJ MN, Woods RL, Nelson MR, Shah RC, Storey E, Murray AM, Reid CM, Kirpach B, Wolfe R, Lockery JE, Berk M, ASPREE Investigator Group. Psychometric properties of a short form of the Center for Epidemiologic Studies Depression (CES-D-10) scale for screening depressive symptoms in healthy community dwelling older adults. Gen Hosp Psychiatry. 2018;51:118–25. PMCID: PMC6178798. http://www.ncbi.nlm.nih.gov/pubmed/28890280.

238. Moreno MA, Christakis DA, Egan KG, Jelenchick LA, Cox E, Young H, Villiard H, Becker T. A pilot evaluation of associations between displayed depression references on Facebook and self-reported depression using a clinical scale. J Behav Health Serv Res. 2012;39(3):295–304. PMCID: PMC3266445. http://www.ncbi.nlm.nih.gov/pubmed/21863354.
239. Psychiatry.org – DSM-5-TR Online Assessment Measures. https://www.psychiatry.org/psychiatrists/practice/dsm/educational-resources/assessment-measures.
240. Clarke DE, Kuhl EA. DSM-5 cross-cutting symptom measures: a step towards the future of psychiatric care? World Psychiatry. 2014;13(3):314–6. PMCID: PMC4219074. http://www.ncbi.nlm.nih.gov/pubmed/25273306.
241. Narrow WE, Clarke DE, Kuramoto SJ, Kraemer HC, Kupfer DJ, Greiner L, Regier DA. DSM-5 field trials in the United States and Canada, Part III: development and reliability testing of a cross-cutting symptom assessment for DSM-5. Am J Psychiatry. 2013;170(1):71–82. PMID: 23111499. http://www.ncbi.nlm.nih.gov/pubmed/23111499.
242. Merikangas KR, He JP, Burstein M, Swanson SA, Avenevoli S, Cui L, Benjet C, Georgiades K, Swendsen J. Lifetime prevalence of mental disorders in U.S. adolescents: results from the National Comorbidity Survey Replication–Adolescent Supplement (NCS-A). J Am Acad Child Adolesc Psychiatry. 2010;49(10):980–9. PMCID: PMC2946114. http://www.ncbi.nlm.nih.gov/pubmed/20855043.
243. Berry EA, Heaton PT, Kelton CML. National estimates of the inpatient burden of pediatric bipolar disorder in the United States. J Ment Health Policy Econ. 2011;14(3):115–23. PMID: 22116169. http://www.ncbi.nlm.nih.gov/pubmed/22116169.
244. Loga S, Loga-Zec S. Comorbidity in psychiatry: its impact on psychopharmacological treatment. Psychiatr Danub. 2009;21(3):347–9. PMID: 19794354. http://www.ncbi.nlm.nih.gov/pubmed/19794354.
245. Samet S, Nunes EV, Hasin D. Diagnosing comorbidity: concepts, criteria, and methods. Acta Neuropsychiatr. 2004;16(1):9–18. PMID: 26983872. http://www.ncbi.nlm.nih.gov/pubmed/26983872.
246. Helzer JE, Kraemer HC, Krueger RF, et al., editors. Dimensional approaches in diagnostic classification: refining the research agenda for DSM-V. Washington: American Psychiatric Association; 2008. https://psycnet.apa.org/record/2008-05669-000.
247. Clarke DE, Wilcox HC, Miller L, Cullen B, Gerring J, Greiner LH, Newcomer A, McKitty MV, Regier DA, Narrow WE. Feasibility and acceptability of the DSM-5 Field Trial procedures in the Johns Hopkins Community Psychiatry Programs. Int J Methods Psychiatr Res. 2014;23(2):267–78. PMCID: PMC4047142. http://www.ncbi.nlm.nih.gov/pubmed/24615761.
248. Mościcki EK, Clarke DE, Kuramoto SJ, Kraemer HC, Narrow WE, Kupfer DJ, Regier DA. Testing DSM-5 in routine clinical practice settings: feasibility and clinical utility. Psychiatr Serv. 2013;64(10):952–60. PMID: 23852272. http://www.ncbi.nlm.nih.gov/pubmed/23852272.
249. Landheim AS, Bakken K, Vaglum P. Impact of comorbid psychiatric disorders on the outcome of substance abusers: a six year prospective follow-up in two Norwegian counties. BMC Psychiatry. 2006;6:44. PMCID: PMC1626456. http://www.ncbi.nlm.nih.gov/pubmed/17054775.
250. Zimmerman M, Morgan TA, Stanton K. The severity of psychiatric disorders. World Psychiatry. 2018;17(3):258–75. PMCID: PMC6127765. http://www.ncbi.nlm.nih.gov/pubmed/30192110.
251. Ustün TB, Chatterji S, Kostanjsek N, Rehm J, Kennedy C, Epping-Jordan J, Saxena S, von Korff M, Pull C, WHO/NIH Joint Project. Developing the World Health Organization Disability Assessment Schedule 2.0. Bull World Health Organ. 2010;88(11):815–23. PMCID: PMC2971503. http://www.ncbi.nlm.nih.gov/pubmed/21076562.
252. Federici S, Bracalenti M, Meloni F, Luciano JV. World Health Organization disability assessment schedule 2.0: an international systematic review. Disabil Rehabil. 2017;39(23):2347–80. PMID: 27820966. http://www.ncbi.nlm.nih.gov/pubmed/27820966.
253. Al-Dajani N, Gralnick TM, Bagby RM. A psychometric review of the personality inventory for DSM-5 (PID-5): current status and future directions. J Pers Assess. 2016;98(1):62–81. PMID: 26619968. http://www.ncbi.nlm.nih.gov/pubmed/26619968.
254. Oldham JM. DSM models of personality disorders. Curr Opin Psychol. 2018;21:86–8. PMID: 29065382. http://www.ncbi.nlm.nih.gov/pubmed/29065382.
255. APA_DSM5_Early-Development-and-Home-Background-Form-Parent-of-Child-Age-6-to-17.pdf. https://www.psychiatry.org/File%20Library/Psychiatrists/Practice/DSM/APA_DSM5_Early-Development-and-Home-Background-Form-Parent-of-Child-Age-6-to-17.pdf.
256. Fusar-Poli P, Solmi M, Brondino N, Davies C, Chae C, Politi P, Borgwardt S, Lawrie SM, Parnas J, McGuire P. Transdiagnostic psychiatry: a systematic review. World Psychiatry. 2019;18(2):192–207. PMCID: PMC6502428. http://www.ncbi.nlm.nih.gov/pubmed/31059629.
257. Fairburn CG, Cooper Z, Shafran R. Cognitive behaviour therapy for eating disorders: a "transdiagnostic" theory and treatment. Behav Res Ther. 2003;41(5):509–28. PMID: 12711261. http://www.ncbi.nlm.nih.gov/pubmed/12711261.
258. Norton PJ, Philipp LM. Transdiagnostic approaches to the treatment of anxiety disorders: a quantitative review. Psychotherapy (Chic). 2008;45(2):214–26. PMID: 22122418. http://www.ncbi.nlm.nih.gov/pubmed/22122418.
259. Clark DA. Cognitive behavioral therapy for anxiety and depression: possibilities and limitations of a transdiagnostic perspective. Cogn Behav Ther. 2009;38(Suppl 1):29–34. PMID: 22946137. http://www.ncbi.nlm.nih.gov/pubmed/22946137.
260. Caspi A, Houts RM, Belsky DW, Goldman-Mellor SJ, Harrington H, Israel S, Meier MH, Ramrakha S, Shalev I, Poulton R, Moffitt TE. The p factor: one general psychopathology factor in the structure of psychiatric disorders? Clin Psychol Sci. 2014;2(2):119–37. PMCID: PMC4209412. http://www.ncbi.nlm.nih.gov/pubmed/25360393.
261. Newby JM, McKinnon A, Kuyken W, Gilbody S, Dalgleish T. Systematic review and meta-analysis of transdiagnostic psychological treatments for anxiety and depressive disorders in adulthood. Clin Psychol Rev. 2015;40:91–110. PMID: 26094079. http://www.ncbi.nlm.nih.gov/pubmed/26094079.
262. Pearl SB, Norton PJ. Transdiagnostic versus diagnosis specific cognitive behavioural therapies for anxiety: a meta-analysis. J Anxiety Disord. 2017;46:11–24. PMID: 27466074. http://www.ncbi.nlm.nih.gov/pubmed/27466074.
263. Fulford KWM, Handa A. Categorical and/or continuous? Learning from vascular surgery. World Psychiatry. 2018;17(3):304–5. PMCID: PMC6127798. http://www.ncbi.nlm.nih.gov/pubmed/30192107.
264. Maj M. Why the clinical utility of diagnostic categories in psychiatry is intrinsically limited and how we can use new approaches to complement them. World Psychiatry. 2018;17(2):121–2. PMCID: PMC5980436. http://www.ncbi.nlm.nih.gov/pubmed/29856539.
265. Strickland CM, Hopwood CJ, Bornovalova MA, Rojas EC, Krueger RF, Patrick CJ. Categorical and dimensional conceptions of personality pathology in DSM-5: toward a model-based synthesis. J Pers Disord. 2019;33(2):185–213. PMID: 29505383. http://www.ncbi.nlm.nih.gov/pubmed/29505383.
266. Cuthbert BN. The RDoC framework: facilitating transition from ICD/DSM to dimensional approaches that integrate neuroscience and psychopathology. World Psychiatry. 2014;13(1):28–35.

PMCID: PMC3918011. http://www.ncbi.nlm.nih.gov/pubmed/24497240.
267. Scott J, Leboyer M, Hickie I, Berk M, Kapczinski F, Frank E, Kupfer D, McGorry P. Clinical staging in psychiatry: a cross-cutting model of diagnosis with heuristic and practical value. Br J Psychiatry. 2013;202(4):243–5. PMID: 23549937. http://www.ncbi.nlm.nih.gov/pubmed/23549937.
268. Wilde A, Mitchell PB, Meiser B, Schofield PR. Implications of the use of genetic tests in psychiatry, with a focus on major depressive disorder: a review. Depress Anxiety. 2013;30(3):267–75. PMID: 22987566. http://www.ncbi.nlm.nih.gov/pubmed/22987566.
269. Kessler RC, McGonagle KA, Swartz M, Blazer DG, Nelson CB. Sex and depression in the National Comorbidity Survey. I: lifetime prevalence, chronicity and recurrence. J Affect Disord. 1993;29(2–3):85–96. PMID: 8300981. http://www.ncbi.nlm.nih.gov/pubmed/8300981.
270. Depressive disorder (depression). https://www.who.int/news-room/fact-sheets/detail/depression.
271. Suicide statistics | AFSP. https://afsp.org/suicide-statistics/;.
272. Swetlitz N. Depression's problem with men. AMA J Ethics. 2021;23(7):E586–9. PMID: 34351273. http://www.ncbi.nlm.nih.gov/pubmed/34351273.
273. Call JB, Shafer K. Gendered manifestations of depression and help seeking among men. Am J Mens Health. 2018;12(1):41–51. PMCID: PMC5734537. http://www.ncbi.nlm.nih.gov/pubmed/26721265.
274. Men and depression: clinical and empirical perspectives. https://psycnet.apa.org/record/2000-07046-000.
275. Addis ME. Gender and depression in men. Clin Psychol Sci Pract. 2008;15(3):153. https://psycnet.apa.org/record/2008-11982-001.
276. Diamond J. The irritable male syndrome: understanding and managing the 4 key causes of depression and aggression. Emmaus: Rodale Books; 2005. https://psycnet.apa.org/record/2005-09049-000.
277. Levant RF. Research in the psychology of men and masculinity using the gender role strain paradigm as a framework. Am Psychol. 2011;66(8):765–76. PMID: 22082409. http://www.ncbi.nlm.nih.gov/pubmed/22082409.
278. Martin LA, Neighbors HW, Griffith DM. The experience of symptoms of depression in men vs women: analysis of the National Comorbidity Survey Replication. JAMA Psychiatry. 2013;70(10):1100–6. PMID: 23986338. http://www.ncbi.nlm.nih.gov/pubmed/23986338.
279. Newman JL, Fuqua DR, Gray EA, Simpson DB. Gender differences in the relationship of anger and depression in a clinical sample. J Couns Dev. 2006;84(2):157–62. https://eric.ed.gov/?id=EJ742120.
280. Winkler D, Pjrek E, Kasper S. Anger attacks in depression–evidence for a male depressive syndrome. Psychother Psychosom. 2005;74(5):303–7. PMID: 16088268. http://www.ncbi.nlm.nih.gov/pubmed/16088268.
281. Lynch J, Kilmartin C. The pain behind the mask: overcoming masculine depression. New York, NY: Haworth Press; 1999. https://www.taylorfrancis.com/books/mono/10.4324/9781315821665/pain-behind-mask-john-lynch-christopher-kilmartin.
282. McKay JR, Rutherford MJ, Cacciola JS, Kabasakalian-McKay R, Alterman AI. Gender differences in the relapse experiences of cocaine patients. J Nerv Ment Dis. 1996;184(10):616–22. PMID: 8917159. http://www.ncbi.nlm.nih.gov/pubmed/8917159.
283. Greenley JR, Mechanic D. Social selection in seeking help for psychological problems. J Health Soc Behav. 1976;17(3):249–62. PMID: 1002965. http://www.ncbi.nlm.nih.gov/pubmed/1002965.
284. Magovcevic M, Addis ME. The masculine depression scale: development and psychometric evaluation. Psychol Men Masc. 2008;9(3):117. https://psycnet.apa.org/record/2008-09203-001.
285. Möller-Leimkühler AM, Bottlender R, Strauss A, Rutz W. Is there evidence for a male depressive syndrome in inpatients with major depression? J Affect Disord. 2004;80(1):87–93. PMID: 15094262. http://www.ncbi.nlm.nih.gov/pubmed/15094262.
286. Zierau F, Bille A, Rutz W, Bech P. The Gotland Male Depression Scale: a validity study in patients with alcohol use disorder. Nord J Psychiatry. 2002;56(4):265–71. PMID: 12470317. http://www.ncbi.nlm.nih.gov/pubmed/12470317.
287. Pennell BE, Bowers A, Carr D, Chardoul S, Cheung GQ, Dinkelmann K, Gebler N, Hansen SE, Pennell S, Torres M. The development and implementation of the National Comorbidity Survey Replication, the National Survey of American Life, and the National Latino and Asian American Survey. Int J Methods Psychiatr Res. 2004;13(4):241–69. PMCID: PMC6878451. http://www.ncbi.nlm.nih.gov/pubmed/15719531.

Etiology: Contributing Factors

3

Franklin Sunzeri

Introduction

There have been a number of changes to diagnostic classifications and criteria in the Diagnostic and Statistical Manual of Mental Disorders Fifth Edition (DSM-5) published in 2013 and updated in the DSM-5 Text Revision (DSM-5-TR) in 2022. These changes reflect understanding that has emerged from progress in cognitive neuroscience, brain imaging, epidemiology, molecular biology, genetic and epigenetics [172].

One of the important recognitions in the DSM-5 is that boundaries between many disorder categories are more fluid than had previously been realized. Many of the symptoms assigned in previous DSM editions to a particular disorder occur in various degrees of severity in many other disorders. In addition, cognitive functions, behaviors, personality traits, combinations of symptoms, temporality, and physical signs appear to represent shared neural substrates, genetic and environmental risk factors.

Nevertheless, in the DSM-5 and DSM-5TR, classification of bipolar and related disorders is separated from the depressive disorders, and anxiety disorders are in their own category. This categorization is the result of 6 years of intensive reviews and secondary analyses, and comprehensive field trials, followed by public, professional, and expert reviews to ascertain the value of that work. From the standpoint of genetics, family history and symptoms, bipolar and related disorders appear to be a "bridge" between schizophrenic spectrum and other psychotic disorders and depressive disorders. However, the prominent presence of depression in the bipolar spectrum makes it a tempting target to discuss in this Introduction to Evidence-Based Depressive Disorders Treatment. Moreover, comorbidity is so high between depressive disorders and anxiety that it is difficult not to feel the temptation to consider anxiety in this monograph too.

We will only briefly touch upon bipolar and anxiety-related disorders to the degree that we need to in discussing depressive disorders. We will leave those two subjects to further monographs in this series.

Definitions

We will begin by offering some basic definitions. Although we all use these terms, we have frequently found that communication is enhanced by reviewing terms that may have taken on different meanings over time or may have different meanings to different folks. Checking around in respected sources on the Internet, there are varieties of definitions of psychological phenomena that are sometimes at odds with the popular conceptions. Perhaps more importantly, scientific journals, possibly reflecting differing specialties, seem to use psychological terms in ways that can differ from journal to journal.

Emotion is the most fundamental definition that warrants clarification. We prefer the definition offered by the American Psychological Association [173]. To wit: Emotions are conscious mental reactions (such as anger or fear) subjectively experienced as strong feelings usually directed toward a specific object and typically accompanied by physiological and behavioral changes in the body. Emotions are intimately related to personality, temperament, character, disposition, mood, affect, and motivation. Emotions are biologically conserved coordinated responses [1]. They represent identifiable and consistent responses to stimuli that are relevant to an organism. In the neurophysiological realm, emotions heavily involve cognition-based interpretations of stimuli [2]. As mentioned above, *cognition* is information processing that includes attention and memory, which produces learning, reasoning, decision-making, and problem solving. The popular belief in a dichotomy between cognition vs. emotions in determining behavior is probably a misconception based upon temporality [2]. We will have more to say about this relationship in a later section. Varying levels of neuroendo-

F. Sunzeri (✉)
Heather Hills Consulting, Coos Bay, OR, USA

J. Raber et al. (eds.), *Understanding and Treating Depressive Disorders*, https://doi.org/10.1007/978-3-032-14465-2_3

crine transmitters such as dopamine, serotonin, norepinephrine, cortisol, oxytocin, gamma-aminobutyric acid (GABA), and neuromodulators such as estrogen influence emotions. Emotions are often the drive behind motivation [3, 4, 9, 18].

Motivation arouses an individual to work toward a desired goal. In such a quest, motivation is the psychological driving force that provokes, controls, and sustains specific goal-directed behavior. Motivation may be intrinsic (driven from within) or extrinsic (driven from external stimuli). Attributes and qualities of motivation are influenced by genetic, physiological, social, behavioral, and cognitive factors. Commonly ascribed motivators include specific physical needs such as eating, sleeping, and sex. More nebulous motivators include a drive to decrease pain (physical or psychological), to maximize pleasure, and maximize well-being. Expectations, needs, beliefs, and environment modify both the quality and magnitude of our motivation [11–14]. An understanding of an individual's motivation is vital in successfully making long-lasting changes in maladaptive behavior [15–17].

Physiological aspects of emotions are intimately associated with nervous system *arousal*, such as in fear reactions. Arousal is the physiological state and psychological state of being awake or reactive to stimuli. *Feelings* are subjective, conscious, and intuitive. They are subjective representations of emotions that are private to the individual who is experiencing them [2].

From the psychological viewpoint, a particularly suitable definition of *mood* from the American Psychological Association is a "disposition to respond emotionally in a particular way that may last for hours, days, or even weeks, perhaps at a low level and without the person knowing what prompted the state. Moods differ from emotions in lacking an object" [174]. It is also important to compare mood to affect and feelings. It has been said that *affect* is like emotional weather in contrast to emotional climate for mood. Unfortunately, ambiguity exists in the use of the term affect. Affect is frequently interchanged with emotion, and it has also been suggested that affect encompasses emotions, feelings, and moods. Therefore, when reading articles related to emotions and affect, it will be necessary to discern the meaning from the context.

Perhaps the most frequent and useful description that relates affect and mood is where affect is described as the experience of feeling an emotion relative to a specific stimulus; whereas mood is a state of emotion that frequently is a reaction to diffuse triggers and has no specific cause [176]. If we use that distinction as a starting point, it can be said that mood can persist for hours or days, while affect is the result of an instant reaction and lasts a short time. Because mood is diffuse and generalizes, it is harder to change than affect where a stimulus can be resolved. Moods are usually less intense than affect. Affects may communicate mood through body language, especially facial expressions, posture, and subtle or non-subtle oral communication.

Temperament, character, and personality traits also differ from moods and are longer lasting [19]. *Temperament* is a dominant or prevailing quality of mind that characterizes an individual. It appears that most experts believe that temperament is genetically determined but modified by the environment and through maturation [5–7, 20]. Important influences on temperament include unique (nonshared) environment, parenting [21], genetic continuity, and environmental changes during development [23]. Temperament is an early-appearing variation in emotional reactivity [22].

A number of internal and external factors appear to moderate or mediate effects of temperament upon psychopathology [24]. Temperament and character dimensions are related to major depression and panic disorder [25]. For example, meta-analysis of studies up to 2011 has shown strong associations of high harm avoidance and low self-directedness with depression and anxiety symptoms [25]. Classifications of temperament are numerous, but none have reached consensus [5–7].

Character and personality are often confused with each other. *Personality* emerges from the hardware of temperament and the software of character. *Character* is an arrangement and interaction (a configuration) of habits, a disposition to behave in a certain way. Temperament is a configuration of inclinations or a predisposition [7]. Character emerges from the interaction of temperament with the environment. If the environment does not interfere, individuals will develop character commensurate with their temperament.

Personality is immediately noticeable in the way that we present ourselves to others: what others can perceive on the outside. Character is a configuration of morals and beliefs that constrain how we treat other beings, our environment, and ourselves. It is the foundation upon which all our thinking, decisions, and actions are predicated. It is our scale that we use to weigh what is wrong and what is right.

Mood disorders were previously known as *affective disorders* perhaps because anxiety and irritability are commonly involved, or more likely that it reflects the changing understanding of affect and mood. It is interesting to consider these word choices in light of the definitions that we discussed above. Mood disorders are said to be the most prevalent of all psychiatric illnesses [26]. They appear to represent 10% of all nonpsychiatric consultations, 25% of all patients in mental facilities, and 65% of all psychiatric outpatients [8]. The two basic affective components of mood disorders are *clinical depression* and *mania*.

Most mood disorders are *unipolar major depressive disorders* (MDDs) and its variants. Being female is the greatest known risk factor for unipolar depression [234]. Depression that is less severe is known as *dysthymic disorder*. Prevalence of one or more mood disorders (major depression, bipolar 1, or dysthymia) among adults in the USA 2008–2012 was 5.4% for females and 9.3% for males [234]. In 2022, about 22% of adults were suffering from depression [8].

Mania is a condition of psychomotor acceleration manifested as abnormally elevated or irritable mood, arousal, and/or energy levels [27]. Mental status is typically characterized by feelings of euphoria, lack of inhibitions, flight of ideas (aka racing thoughts), talkativeness, poor judgment, risk taking, decreased need for sleep, and irritability.

Mania covers a range of intensities from *hypomania*, which is mild, to *severe mania* that has features of psychoses such as delusions of grandeur, hallucinations, aggression, suspiciousness, catatonia, and preoccupation with activities that may result in self-neglect [10]. Significant activation of the left amygdala and reduced bilateral activation in the lateral orbitofrontal cortex can be seen during manic episodes [28].

Incidence of *bipolar disease* (mania and depression) in the general population may be about 4% to 5%. However, by definition of bipolar disorders, in order to be classified as bipolar, it is not necessary for depressive episodes to have occurred; just that mania has been expressed [29]. Bipolar disease is about equally distributed between the sexes, whereas twice as many women as men seem to have clinical depression. In bipolar disease, more women have predominantly depressive symptoms and men seem to have predominantly manic symptoms. Bipolar tendencies that are less severe are often called *cyclothymic*.

There are additional nuanced classifications and subtypes of depression and bipolar groupings, whose definitions have changed over the decades [10].

The following definitions are ones that can be found in some form in many relevant texts, such as in the following reference [10]. Again, we believe it is handy to briefly mention these here to avoid confusion.

Depression can range from a sinking of spirits to frank clinical mood disorders. There are several levels on which to consider depression: descriptive, symptomatic, epidemiological, and etiological. Depression is multifaceted with complex and probably differing etiologies reflecting the various types. Many factors have been identified including genetics, acute and chronic stress at especially vulnerable times, and somatic disorders [30, 31]. Some types of depression are associated with genetic polymorphisms of various genes related to the neuroendocrine system [32–35]. Epigenetic processes acting through pre-, peri-, and early postnatal strain all the way through adult adversity are involved in depression [36–39].

Dysphoria is a state of feeling acutely hopeless, uncomfortable, and unhappy.

Sadness is normal depression that we all get now and then. It is a reaction to adverse events and may be adaptive in that it allows us to withdraw from an energy-draining circumstance. Sadness related to the first two-postpartum weeks, premenstrual phases, anniversary reactions, or holidays is within normal limits.

Reactive depression is a reaction to meaningful losses or separations (for example, death, divorce, emigration, loss of a relationship, natural disasters). What is commonly called *grief* is the normal manifestation of reactive depression. This includes autonomic nervous system hyperactivity, insomnia, anxiety, and inability to concentrate. A special type of reactive depression is *anaclitic depression* that occurs when an infant is separated from its mother. It is characterized by anorexia, listlessness, and withdrawal, and results in impaired physical, intellectual, and emotional development.

Paradoxical depression may occur after positive incidents. *Elation*, which is generally associated with success, is sometimes viewed as a defense against depression, and in some people, it may lead to mania, which is excessive.

Melancholy has been used in two ways. One way is a name for sluggish and uncomfortable thought processes and low spirits associated with other conditions. The other is a severe form of depression characterized by symptoms of clinical depression. When sadness or grief is excessively intense and lasts significantly longer than is expected by the nature of the stressor, or when it occurs without the association of a stressor, it is diagnosed as *clinical depression*. In contrast to normal emotional reactions, there is significant crippling of physical or social functioning, and work ability.

Irritability may be defined as a "deficit in filtering environmental stimuli combined with a faulty inhibitory capacity, leading to impulsive and exaggerated reactions to common situations" [40]. It relates to interindividual differences in disposition to anger that may reach a pathological level [41]. Longitudinal studies indicate that irritability is remarkably stable and is specifically associated with depression and anxiety [41]. Genetic factors appear to make irritability moderately heritable and underpin its relationship with depression. Compared to controls, persistent irritability is associated with differences in activity in the amygdala, striatum, and frontal areas. It has been suggested that irritability is a mood, and anger is its expression [42]. Two components of irritability are 1) phasic which is manifested as developmentally inappropriate temper outbursts, and 2) tonic, which is the negative affect that continues between these outbursts.

Depressive Disorders are categorized in the DSM-5 as including disruptive mood dysregulation disorder, major depressive disorder, persistent depressive disorder (dysthymia), premenstrual dysphoric disorder, substance/medication-induced depressive disorder, depressive disorder due to another medical condition, other specified depressive disorder, and unspecified depressive disorder [175]. We cover definitions for these categories in a later section.

Considerations and Associations

Race, culture, and socioeconomic class have been variably associated with the diagnosis of depression [44–49] . We will be discussing each of these associations in succeeding chapters.

Diagnosis and treatment of depression seem to vary significantly with the training of the diagnostician [43]. More training may be needed in recognizing depression, especially in recognizing social from clinical attributes and in differentiating dementia symptoms from those of depression. Potential biases may be associated with diagnosing depression in women, in people with cognitive impairment or illness, and in African Americans. An intriguing analysis of a simple random sample of 270 residents from 6 randomly selected nursing homes underscores that perception [50]. Various staff positions tended to have different awareness of depressive symptoms in these residents. Psychiatrists generally saw African Americans as having fewer depressive symptoms than residents of other ethnicities have. Nurse's aides seemed to be the most valid source of information on depression, perhaps uninfluenced by demographics or because they had more or closer contact with the residents. Nurses tended to over-recognize depression in African Americans. Social workers over-recognized depression in African Americans, and they under-recognized depression in women or in residents who were cognitively compromised and/or who had Parkinson's disease.

Comorbidity

The psychosocial burden of depression includes cognitive and psychosomatic difficulties such as fatigue, poor concentration, low mood, loss of pleasure, and loss of sexual desire [51, 52]. Overall, emotional functions, energy, and drive are often compromised [53]. Comorbid conditions such as anxiety [54] and panic attacks are frequent [55–57]. Comorbidity prevalence between anxiety disorder and major depressive disorder has been reported to be as high as 60% in the USA and may be even higher if subsyndromal symptoms are included [58–60]. About half of patients with panic disorders will develop depression, and about half of patients with depression will develop panic disorder. Approximately, one-third of patients with depression present with panic disorder [59]. The risk of suicide in patients with depression and comorbid panic disorder may be increased sevenfold [61, 62].

In attempting to self-medicate these symptoms, abuse of alcohol [63], smoking [64–67], obesity [68–70], and use of recreational drugs [54] are common [71]. Neglect of health may be prominent, leading to progression of diseases that may be linked to poor health practices or to immune system dysfunctions arising from depression itself.

Perhaps due to effects of immune mediators like cytokines [72], and changes in autonomic nervous system functions [73] there is increased risk of several diseases including cardiovascular diseases [74–76], dementia [77], diabetes [78], and cancer [79–81].

Pathological gambling and internet addiction may be more likely [82]. Overall, folks with depression may live 15 to 30 years less than the general population [76].

Depressed patients seem to be less likely to seek medical help and less likely to take prescribed medications [83]. They are more likely than nondepressed people to smoke and are less likely to quit [84].

Major Depressive Disorder Prevalence

Major depressive disorder (MDD) is one of the most common psychiatric disorders. It can cause considerable havoc to social functioning, seriously compromise holding a job, and result in physical disabilities [85]. According to the *US National Comorbidity Survey* (published in 1994 and over 25 years old), 10.3% of the population in the USA had suffered a major depressive episode (as defined by the DSM-III-R) in the last 12 months and 17.1% of the population suffers from a major depressive episode at some point in their lifetime [86]. According to this same study, women were approximately twice as likely to experience a major depressive episode as men were: 21.3% for women and 12.7% for men. Depression seems to cluster in families, but the rates and the relative proportion of genetic influences to environmental influences seem to differ by definitions and in different reports [87–89].

The National Epidemiologic Survey on Alcohol and Related Conditions III analyzed 2016–2017 data that was collected from April 2012 to June 2013, from the [90]. Using DSM-5 criteria, they found 12-month and lifetime prevalence of MDD were 10.4% and 20.6%, respectively. The data showed:

- Odds of 12-month MDD were significantly lower in men (OR =[1] 0.5; 95% CI: 0.46 to 0.55) and in African American (OR = 0.6; 95% CI, 0.54 to 0.68), Asian/Pacific Islander

[1] Odds ratio (OR) is a way to represent the odds that an outcome will result when a given exposure to a variable of interest occurs compared to when the exposure does not occur. OR quantifies the strength of the association between two events. An OR greater than 1 indicates a positive association or that exposure to that variable increases the odds of that outcome. An OR less than one indicates a negative relationship between two events. An OR of 1 suggests no relationship between two events. An OR is frequently accompanied by a 95% confidence interval (CI). CI is a measure of precision of the OR. The smaller the CI the higher precision as long as it does not overlap OR = 1. For more information, see the Chap. 4 on evidence basics in this text.

(OR = 0.6; 95% CI: 0.45 to 0.67), and Hispanic (OR = 0.7; 95% CI: 0.62 to 0.78) adults than in white adults.

- Odds of 12-month MDD were higher in younger adults (age range, 18–29 years; OR = 3.0; 95% CI: 2.48 to 3.55).
- Odds of 12-month MDD were higher in those with low incomes ($19,999 or less; OR = 1.7; 95% CI: 1.49 to 2.04).
- In the DSM diagnostic criteria, 74.6% of the MDD cases were positive for the anxious/distressed specifier, and 15.5% had the mixed-features specifier. When severity was controlled, both were associated with early onset, poor course and functioning, and suicidality.
- The majority of lifetime MDD sufferers had severe (49.5%) or moderate (39.7%) symptoms.
- Those who had severe MDD functioned about 1 standard deviation below the national mean.
- In 12.9% of those with lifetime MDD, all symptoms manifested immediately after the death of someone significant and persisted for less than 2 months.
- Approximately 70% of the lifetime MDD patients had received some form of treatment.
- Psychiatric disease associations of MDD were for specific phobia (OR = 2.1; 95% CI: 1.84 to 2.35), generalized anxiety disorder (OR = 5.7; 95% CI: 4.98 to 6.50).
- MDD associations with substance use disorders for alcohol had an OR of 1.8 (95% CI: 1.63 to 2.01) and for any drug had an OR of 3.0 (95% CI: 2.57 to 3.55).

The prevalence, course, sociodemographic correlates, and societal costs of major depression all over the world in 2013 can be found in reference [91].

In 2012 in China, current, 12-month, and lifetime prevalence of MDD were 1.6%, 2.3%, and 3.3%, respectively. Males showed a lower rate than females (1.3% vs. 2.1%), and rural a greater risk than urban residents (2.0% vs. 1.7%) [238]. Current prevalence of MDD diagnosed with the Structured Clinical Interview for DSM-IV was 1.8% and that diagnosed with the Composite International Diagnostic Interview was 1.1%.

The clinical course of unipolar major depressive disorders as described in 1997 can be found in reference [92]. Attempts at predicting the naturalistic course of depression from a wide range of clinical, psychological, and biological data can be seen in a 2018 reference [93].

Major Depressive Disorder Relationships

Depression is commonly associated with immune system derangements, and other health problems [94]. As both cause and effect, the bidirectional psychoneuroimmunological-depression connection is heavily involved.

One of the assumptions in depression research is that stressful events and chronic difficulties, including illness, can instigate depression in certain genetically predisposed individuals [95–98]. Some researchers have proposed that stress triggers depression through an epigenetic-genomic action of glucocorticoids, glucocorticoid receptors, and hypothalamic pituitary adrenal (HPA) activation [99–101]. In humans who have major depression, it is common to find changes in the hypothalamic pituitary adrenal (HPA) axis [102].

Typically, *acute* depression is associated with elevated secretion of corticotropin-releasing hormone from the hypothalamus, adrenal corticotropic hormone (ACTH) from the pituitary, and cortisol from the adrenal cortex.

In *chronic* depression, the adrenal gland is more sensitive to ACTH and the hypothalamus and pituitary are more sensitive to the negative feedback of cortisol. On balance, this results in elevated cortisol with relatively less ACTH. There is some evidence that abnormal metabolism of adrenal corticosteroids might be involved in perpetuating some types of depression [103].

Chronic stress accompanied by elevations of cortisol might lead to neuroendocrine changes such as increased serotonin uptake both at rest and during stimulation, which might trigger depression symptoms [104, 105].

It has been hypothesized that when confronted by a stressor, activation of negative schema decreases activity in prefrontal areas, via decreased serotonin metabolism controlled by the HPA axis, with resulting impaired attenuation of subcortical areas such as the amygdala [106]. Proponents of the hypothesis believe this process results in increased vulnerability after an episode of depression.

Ruminative brooding (persistent, repetitive, and self-focused criticism) is common in major depression [107]. Brain images have shown that self-referential processing in MDD appears to be associated with abnormally increased activity of anterior cortical midline structures.

The limbic system is implicated in reduced motivation and anhedonia, the fundamental symptoms of depression. In particular, the reward circuit, the ventral tegmental area (VTA) and nucleus accumbens (NAc) are involved [108]. Stress can impair the ability of the hippocampus and amygdala to control the HPA axis [109]. The prefrontal cortex (PFC), hippocampus, and amygdala are implicated in two more of the frequent symptoms of depression, impaired attention, and cognitive dysfunction [109]. The NAc integrates glutamatergic signals from the PFC, hippocampus, and amygdala, and dopaminergic projections from the VTA.

The amygdala, hippocampus, and the mesocorticolimbic system are almost always involved in interpreting the nature of stressors and influencing our responses to them [110]. They are epigenetically programmed beginning even before birth, perhaps as part of transgenerational effects. These epigenetic modifications are superimposed upon polymorphisms of genes that are involved in our stress management systems.

Epigenetic-genomic activity in our stress-reacting neuroendocrine systems seems to underpin the molecular susceptibility and severity of mood disorders [99, 100].

Whereas some *antidepressants* can normalize cytokine levels, other effective antidepressants such as SNRIs do not [111]. However, this does not negate the possibility that inflammatory cytokine effects on the brain are blocked by antidepressants.

Stratified, Precision, and Personalized Medicine

In reading the literature pertaining to depression, the terms stratified medicine, precision medicine, and personalized medicine are frequently encountered.

Stratified, precision, and personalized medicine share overlapping and shifting meanings [112]. A reasonable attempt at discriminating between the three is as follows.

Stratified medicine begins by identifying subgroups of patients who have distinct disease mechanisms or specific responses to treatments. Then it categorizes a population into the most biologically appropriate groupings to determine the optimal therapeutic response.

Precision medicine relies on a more discriminating subclassification of disease, adding repeated monitoring of disease markers to enable designing and modifying treatment to fit individual responses. See Fig. 3.1.

Personalized medicine recognizes the unique characteristics of each individual. The individual phenotype profile (i.e., genetics, epigenetics, clinical symptoms, observable biomarker changes, and environmental factors) [113]. It incorporates precision and stratification along with patient participation and preference to both treat and prevent disease [112].

The National Research Council (NRC)[2] states:

"Precision medicine refers to the tailoring of medical treatment to the individual characteristics of each patient. It does not literally mean the creation of drugs or medical devices that are unique to a patient, but rather the ability to classify individuals into subpopulations that differ in their susceptibility to a particular disease…or in their response to a specific treatment. Although the term "personalized medicine" is also used to convey this meaning, that term is sometimes misinterpreted as implying that unique treatments can be designed for each individual. It should be emphasized that in "precision medicine," the word "precision" is being used in a colloquial sense, to mean both "accurate" and "precise." [10, 114].

Use of the term precision has commonly been replacing personalized in the literature [177]. This is what you appear to have in the text. The process of precision medicine is well

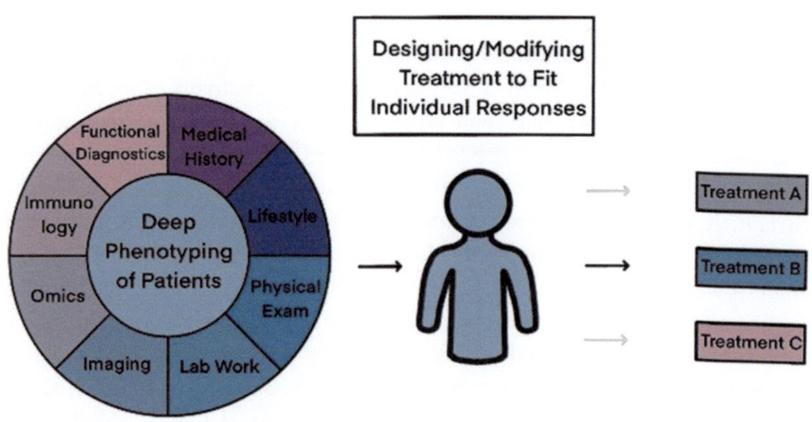

Fig. 3.1 Illustrating the framework of precision medicine, which tailors medical treatment selection based on individual variability in genes, environment, and lifestyle

[2]"**The National Research Council** was organized by the **National Academy of Sciences** in 1916 to associate the broad community of science and technology with the Academy's purposes of furthering knowledge and advising the federal government. Functioning in accordance with general policies determined by the Academy, the Council has become the principal operating agency of both the National Academy of Sciences and the National Academy of Engineering in providing services to the government, the public, and the scientific and engineering communities. The Council is administered jointly by both Academies and the Institute of Medicine" [195, 196].

illustrated in Fig. 3.1 [112, 115]. More on precision medicine can be found in the following references [116–122].

Endophenotypes are quantitative neurobehavioral traits that index genetic susceptibility for a psychiatric disorder [123].

Biomarkers are "a defined characteristic that is measured as an indicator of normal biological processes, pathogenic processes, or responses to an exposure or intervention, including therapeutic interventions" [124]. A *biosignature* relative to psychiatry is a set of biomarkers that when used in systems biology will yield a better diagnosis and prognosis, and a more precisely targeted intervention for better outcomes [125].

Databases

Attempts to bring the power of modern investigative techniques to bear upon precision medicine rely upon various databases. Frequently used sources include Medline [178], Embase [179], PsycINFO [180], Scopus [181], ProQuest [182], Cochrane Central Register of Controlled Trials [183], LILACS: Latin American and Caribbean Health Sciences Literature—database [184], CINAHL: Cumulative Index to Nursing and Allied Health Literature [185], ClinicalTrials.gov [186], WHO International Clinical Trials Registry Platform [187], and other websites of regulatory agencies, and international registers for published and unpublished, double-blind, randomized controlled trials.

To identify prenatal, perinatal, and childhood influences on physical, behavioral, and cognitive development, prospective birth cohort databases have been developed. These include the Avon Longitudinal Study of Parents and Children [188] and the Generation R study [189]. The Adolescent Brain Cognitive Development [190] targets ages 5 to 25.

Longitudinal twin studies are gathering genetic and environment information. These include Twins Early Development Study [191]; and the Environmental Risk Longitudinal Twin Study (E-Risk) [192].

The Global Imaging Genetics of Adolescents initiative is a "collaboration between several major cohorts in UK, Europe, USA, China, and India who investigate health outcomes in children and adolescents via behavioral and imaging genetic studies. Its aim is to enable comparative research on brain development and behavior in different cultures, environments, and ethnic groups, both in industrialized nations and low- and medium-income countries." [194].

The neuroimaging-genetics (IMAGEN) study [193] is a longitudinal neuro*imag*ing-*gen*etics study.

Centers for Disease Control and Prevention provides reports and other products that can be resources for public health officials and other health professionals who need up-to-date statistics and data sources around mental health and mental illness [197].

The BrainSpan Atlas is database that is an atlas of developmental data of the human brain. It is a foundational resource for studying transcriptional mechanisms involved in the developing human brain [219].

The 1000 Genomes Project was finished in 2015. Its mission was to provide a comprehensive description of common human genetic variation by applying whole-genome sequencing to a diverse set of individuals from multiple populations [220]. They reconstructed the genomes of 2504 individuals from 26 populations and characterized a broad spectrum of genetic variation, in total over 88 million variants (84.7 million single-nucleotide polymorphisms (SNPs), 3.6 million short insertions/deletions (indels), and 60,000 structural variants[3]), all phased onto high-quality haplotypes. Their data includes >99% of SNP variants with a frequency of >1% for a variety of ancestries. Their 2015 paper *A global reference for human genetic variation* and *An integrated map of structural variation in 2504 human genomes* describes the distribution of genetic variation across the global sample and discusses the implications for common disease studies [153, 154].

The Disease Ontology is a computable structure linking evidence-based inheritable, environmental, and infectious origins of human disease to facilitate the connection of genetic data, clinical data, and symptoms through the lens of human disease [155, 156, 221].

In 2012, a data fusion project began to fuse all available molecular interactions and ontology data [155]. Results in 2013 had already shown 14 disease-disease associations that were not present at that time in the Disease Ontology databank. Genetic interactions appear to be the most important predictor of a link between diseases [155].

Other molecular data repositories for diseases are hitting their stride. These include *BioDatome* [222]. *The NHGRI-EBI Catalog* of published genome-wide association studies [223]; *Multiplex Diseasome Communities* [224].

A *transcriptome database* for astrocytes, neurons, and oligodendrocytes was published in 2008 [157]: "Their transcriptome database of acutely isolated purified astrocytes, neurons, and oligodendrocytes provides a resource to the neuroscience community by providing improved cell-type-specific markers and for better understanding of neural development, function, and disease."

[3] *Structural variants* are the variations in structure of an organism's chromosome. They are defined as DNA segments larger than 1 kilo base (kb). Structural variants include "microscopic and, more commonly, submicroscopic variants, which include deletions, duplications and large-scale copy-number variants - collectively termed copy-number variants or copy-number polymorphisms - as well as insertions, inversions and translocations" [235, 236].

Below are a few of the larger databases that relate to mental health. Links to other databases will be found in various places in the text.

National Institute of Mental Health (NIMH) Research Domain Criteria

In 2008, the National Institute of Mental Health came up with a strategic plan to prevent and cure mental illness by taking advantage of innovative research [198]. Part of that plan was to develop *The National Institute of Mental Health Research Domain Criteria (RDoC).* The RDoC is said to be a useful research framework for new approaches to investigating mental disorders. It is the centerpiece of NIMH's attempt to reach its strategic goal to develop new methods to classify mental disorders for research purposes [126]. The RDoC's primary goal is precision medicine for psychiatry [199].

Quoted from the NIMH website:

> [The RDoC] integrates many levels of information (from genomics and circuits to behavior and self-reports) in order to explore basic dimensions of functioning that span the full range of human behavior from normal to abnormal. RDoC is not meant to serve as a diagnostic guide, nor is it intended to replace current diagnostic systems. The goal is to understand the nature of mental health and illness in terms of varying degrees of dysfunctions in general psychological/biological systems. [200].

The RDoC is constructed around six major domains of human functioning. These are negative valence systems, positive valence systems, cognitive systems, social processes systems, arousal/regulatory systems, and sensorimotor systems [201].

Constructs are each of the domains constructed of behavioral elements, processes, mechanisms, and responses.. Each of these constructs exists in and is affected by environmental and neurodevelopmental factors. Measurements that are used to understand how these constructs participate in the domains are assessments of molecular, genetic, neurocircuit, and behavioral factors. These are referred to as *units of analysis*. Some of the constructs have designated *subconstructs.*

Negative valence systems are primarily responsible for responses to aversive situations or context, such as fear, anxiety, and loss. They are constructed by acute threat (fear), potential threat (anxiety), sustained threat, loss, and frustrative nonreward.

Positive valence systems are primarily responsible for responses to positive motivational situations or contexts, such as reward seeking, consummatory behavior, and reward/habit learning. They are constructed by reward responsiveness (which has the subconstructs of reward anticipation, initial response to reward, and reward anticipation); reward learning (which has the subconstructs of probabilistic and reinforcement learning, reward prediction error, and habit); and reward valuation (which has the subconstructs of reward (ambiguity/risk), delay, and effort).

Cognitive systems are responsible for various cognitive processes. Cognitive systems are constructed by attention, perception (with subconstructs visual perception, auditory perception, and olfactory/somatosensory/multimodal perception), declarative memory, language, cognitive control (with subconstructs goal selection, updating, representation and maintenance; response selection (inhibition/suppression), and performance monitoring), and working memory (with subconstructs of active maintenance, flexible updating, limited capacity, and inference control).

Systems for social processes mediate responses in interpersonal settings of various types including perception and interpretation of others' actions. They are constructed by affiliation and attachment, social communication (with subconstructs of reception of facial communication, production of facial communication, reception of nonfacial communication, and production of non-facial communication), perception and understanding of self (with subconstructs of agency and self-knowledge), and perception and understanding of others (with subconstructs of animacy perception, action perception, and understanding mental states).

Arousal/regulatory systems are responsible for generating activation of neural systems as appropriate for various contexts and providing appropriate homeostatic regulation of such systems as energy balance and sleep. This domain has the constructs arousal, circadian rhythms, and sleep and wakefulness.

Sensorimotor systems are primarily responsible for the control and execution of motor behaviors, and their refinement during learning and development. They are constructed by motor actions (with subconstructs of action planning and selection, sensorimotor dynamics, initiation, execution, and inhibition and termination), agency and ownership, habit, and innate motor patterns.

The National Institute of Mental Health Data Archive (NDA) is a repository of results generated through the use of the RDoC [202]. "The NDA makes available human subjects data collected from hundreds of research projects across many scientific domains. NDA provides infrastructure for sharing research data, tools, methods, and analyses enabling collaborative science and discovery. De-identified human subjects' data, harmonized to a common standard, are available to qualified researchers. Summary data are available to all."

The NDA is one example of participant-centered initiatives that use social media technologies. A discussion about the benefits and potential pitfalls of these initiatives can be found in the following references [127–132].

A NIMH webinar on the RDoC can be found here on the NIMH website [203]. A 2016 special issue of the *International*

Journal of Psychophysiology [204] has included a number of empirical and review articles relating to the RDoC.

A 2019 paper in the journal *Molecular Neuropsychiatry* offers a critique of the strengths and weaknesses of the RDoC [205]. Ross and Margolis suggest that the RDoC approaches normal human behavior, emotion and cognition as dimensional, with mental illnesses as dimensional extremes. But, they argue that this concept is of little utility for most of the serious mental illnesses. And that results as of 2019 were narrow and of limited impact on the field of mental illness [133].

They find some positives, chief among which is systematizing normal human mental function and attempting to associate underlying psychological constructs of cognition and emotion with specific neural circuitry. In addition, they believe the RDoC calls attention to the phenotypic overlap of many psychiatric disorders, and the RDoC is useful to describe psychiatric disorders that have too much or too little of a normal trait. Examples would include personality disorders, PTSD, and some forms of MDD [134, 135].

They take issue with two claims about the value of the RDoC. First, they believe that the DSM-5 has a stronger focus on neurobiology than the RDoC. Second, they believe that the RDoC has focused on well-established molecular pathways and diverted attention away from molecules newly implicated as risk factors for major mental illness.

They suggest at least 4 major conceptual flaws in the RDoC system. First, they believe the matrix structure and elements are arbitrary and problematic. Second, they assert, "major mental illnesses are best conceptualized as categorically distinct from normal dimensional variation and most effectively using the disease model." Third, RDoC does not "address the natural history of disease, which typically involves initiating, sustaining, and homeostatic processes that change with time, leading to different phenotypic manifestations of the same disease at different stages in its evolution." Fourth, they believe that a top-down approach to mental disorder research is not as helpful as bottom-up approaches.

Top-down approaches start by breaking down complex problems into smaller parts (submodules) and analyzing those until there is no longer a need to reduce further. It goes from the abstract to the concrete. A bottom-up approach is the opposite. It depends upon testing interactions between the submodules at each level until the final result is obtained. Top-down deals with layers of abstractions, bottom-up deals with testing of fundamental properties. They assert that the medical model of disease is bottom-up. They say that medical research begins by looking into etiological factors and then determining how the combination of those factors leads to pathogenic pathways and ultimately to clinical diseases.

In order to move up the chain of causality, they believe that starting at the molecular and genetic level by first examining individual genetic variation, moving through altered gene expression, and splicing in both placental genes and brain genes, then examining effects on cell biology and neuronal signaling (therapeutic targets), and progressing through hypothetical circuit disruptions will arrive at clinical syndromes redefined as biotypes or subbiotypes.

More about top-down and bottom-up in medicine can be found in [136–138]. The benefits of a combination of top-down and bottom-up approaches in pharmacology are discussed in [137].

Other authors have suggested other issues with the RDoC. These include the matrix structure, no consideration of time course, lack of attention to differential response to psychotropic medicines, and no inclusion of references to success or failure [139–142].

Discussions of the background issues and utility of the RDoC can be found in [126, 143–146]. Comparison of the DSM-5 and RDoC can be found in [147, 148].

In 2017, Clark et al *published an in-depth comparison* of the three approaches to understanding and classifying mental disorders [148]. They reviewed the two major diagnostic manuals: the WHO's *International Classification of Diseases (ICD-11)* and the American Psychiatric Association's *Diagnostic and Statistical Manual of Mental Disorders (DSM 5)* both of which offer classifications that are useful for clinical diagnoses, research applications, public health, and specific research. Then they contrasted the *RDoC* that emphasizes integration of basic behavioral and neuroscience research to advance understanding of mental disorders.

Clark et al. suggest that although they share a common goal, the ICD-11, the DSM5 and the RDoC have some differences. Based on their purposes, there are four areas that are key challenges in understanding and classifying mental disorders. Those four areas are etiology, relevant factors: are they discrete categories or dimensions, thresholds of disease, and comorbidity.

The executive summary in their paper contains salient points to consider when attempting to treat or research mental illnesses. Briefly, with respect to each of the four points:

Etiology: Psychopathology generally is the result of a complex interplay of multiple biological, behavioral, psychosocial, and cultural factors, influenced by each individual's unique life experience. The result of these interactions and factors is not clearly delimited diseases, rather they are mixtures of psychological difficulties.

Categories and dimensions: Categories are useful for us to handle the complexities of psychopathologies, but the boundaries are not distinct and are perhaps artificial. Dimensions are a recognition that psychopathology is not an all or none; instead, it is graded in its manifestations.

Thresholds: For clinical purposes, thresholds are useful but should be considered as arbitrary unless proven by further research to be otherwise.

Comorbidity: Comorbidity is perhaps the rule rather than the exception. It may be an artifact of an imperfect classification system.

Psychiatric Genomics Consortium (PGC)

The purpose of the Psychiatric Genomics Consortium (PGC) is to unite investigators around the world to conduct meta- and mega-analyses of genome-wide genomic data for psychiatric disorders. Their website provides information about the organization, implementation, and results of the PGC [206].

The PGC began in 2007 as a collaborative confederation of most of the investigators in the field of psychiatric genome analyses. The PGC includes over 800 investigators from 38 countries. As of 2019, they had more than 900,000 individuals being analyzed. The PGC describes itself as "the largest consortium and the largest biological experiment in the history of psychiatry."

The PGC consists of a coordinating committee, nine disorder working groups, a statistical analysis group (with a pathway analysis subgroup), and a cross-disorder group. The working groups each have a single focus on either autism spectrum disorder, attention-deficit hyperactivity disorder, bipolar disorder, major depressive disorder, or schizophrenia. Several powerful papers have been produced by the PGC. Especially noteworthy was their genome-wide association study on schizophrenia.

Results of their landmark paper on MDD that was published in 2018 [207] are discussed later in this text. PGC has created a video textbook to give a comprehensive review of the current state of the art of research and resources for analyzing psychiatric genetics [208].

PsychENCODE

In 2015, the NIH founded the PsychENCODE Consortium to provide an enhanced framework of regulatory genomic elements in individuals with neuropsychiatric disorders. The collaboration is between researchers at 17 research institutes (as of 2023) [209]. Their collective goal is to accelerate the discovery of noncoding functional genomic elements in the human brain and reveal their involvement in molecular pathophysiology of psychiatric disorders [210].

Although noncoding DNA sequences appear to make up more than 90% of the human genome and their roles in regulating gene expression are well known, they have not been completely characterized [149, 150]. Many human non-protein-coding sequences may be transcribed into noncoding RNAs or may be functional cis-regulatory elements (e.g., promoters, enhancers, and insulators).

They appear to frequently function in a cell- and tissue-specific manner [151]. Common genetic variations associated with human diseases cluster in putative regulatory regions [150, 152]. Noncoding genetic variation is associated with expression differences across various human tissues. Genetic variants associated with psychiatric disorders tend to be located primarily in regulatory regions [152].

"The PsychENCODE project is attempting to produce multidimensional genomic data using tissue- and cell type–specific samples from approximately 1000 phenotypically well-characterized, high-quality healthy and disease-affected human post-mortem brains, as well as functionally characterize disease-associated regulatory elements and variants in model systems." [152].

By 2018, PsychENCODE had generated data sets including bulk transcriptome, chromatin, genotype, and *Hi-C data-sets*[4] and single-cell transcriptomic data from ~32,000 cells for major brain regions. They merged that data with data from *Genotype-Tissue Expression (GTEx),*[5] *ENCODE,*[6] *Roadmap Epigenomics,*[7] and single-cell analyses. They were able to survey functional genomics data on the brain in over 1866 individuals.

They used this data to create lists of brain-expressed genes, coexpression modules, and single-cell expression profiles for many brain cell types; ~79,000 brain-active enhancers[8] with associated Hi-C loops and topologically associating domains; and ~ 2.5 million expression *quantitative-trait loci (QTLs)*[9] comprising ~238,000 linkage-disequilibrium–independent single-nucleotide polymorphisms and of other types of QTLs associated with splice isoforms, cell fractions, and chromatin activity.

[4] *Hi-C* is a proximity ligation method based on Chromosome Conformation Capture to detect chromatin interactions in the mammalian nuclei [211].

[5] The *GTEx (Genotype-Tissue Expression)* Project identified genetic variants that influence how genes are turned on and off in human tissues and organs. Genetic variants that influence how genes behave are called *expression quantitative trait loci (eQTLs)*. These eQTLs regulate the behavior of genes. [212]

[6] The *Encyclopedia of DNA Elements (ENCODE) Consortium* is an ongoing international collaboration of research groups funded by the *National Human Genome Research Institute (NHGRI)*. The goal of ENCODE is to build a comprehensive parts list of functional elements in the human genome, including elements that act at the protein and RNA levels, and regulatory elements that control cells and circumstances in which a gene is active. [213].

[7] *The NIH Roadmap Epigenomics Mapping Consortium* was launched with the goal of producing a public resource of human epigenomic data to catalyze basic biology and disease-oriented research. [214].

[8] *Enhancers* are DNA regions that promote gene expression [149].

[9] A *quantitative trait locus (QTL)* is a region of DNA associated with a particular phenotypic trait, which varies in degree, and which can be attributed to polygenic effects and their environment [215]. A quantitative trait has measurable phenotypic variation owing to genetic and/or environmental influences. Among complex diseases frequently there are thresholds that must be crossed for the phenotype to be expressed.

They discovered that more than 88% of the cross-population variation in brain gene expression can be accounted for by cell fraction changes and that several disorders and aging are associated with changes in cell-type proportions. They found that the brain has distinct expression and epigenetic patterns, including a greater extent of non-coding transcription than other tissues.

Integrative networks based upon this data include a full *gene regulatory network (GRN)* for the brain, linking transcription factors, enhancers, and target genes from merging of the QTLs, generalized element-activity correlations, and Hi-C data. They used these networks to link disease genes *to genome-wide association study (GWAS)* variants for psychiatric disorders. For schizophrenia, they were able to produce an approximately six-fold improvement in predicting psychiatric phenotypes.

Results highlighted key genes and pathways associated with disorder prediction, including immunological, synaptic, and metabolic pathways, recapitulating de novo results from more targeted analyses. They suggest that additional data such as neuroimaging and micro-RNA can become an even greater predictor of disease risk.

By 2024, the Consortium had produced a set of fourteen manuscripts in *Science, Science Translational Medicine,* and *Science Advances* [209]. These articles make major contributions to understanding the biology of the human brain based on analysis of transcriptomic, epigenomic, and genomic data from post-mortem adult and developing human brains, and human cellular model systems. The consortium considers three manuscripts to be the flagship for the project. They are (1) *Integrative functional genomic analysis of human brain development and neuropsychiatric risks* [216]. (2) Transcriptome-wide isoform-level dysregulation in autism spectrum disorder (ASD), schizophrenia, and bipolar disorder [217]. (3) *Comprehensive functional genomic resource and integrative model for the human brain* [218].

New Investigatory Techniques

Preclinical animal models of depression in rodents have explored the importance of sex as a biological variable and the controversial idea of intergenerational and transgenerational transmission of depressive-like traits [158–160]. Rodent models manipulate the environment during development or modify the biological matrix. Chronic unpredictable mild stress as of 2018 is currently the most often used rodent model of depression and is strongly associated with anhedonic behavior in rodents [161]. However, high heterogeneity exists apparently due to differences in protocols.

A *3-level meta-analysis* of rodent studies has revealed phenotypes relative to early life adversity (ELA) [162]. Results indicate that, especially in males, ELA enhances memory formation during stressful learning while harming non-stressful learning. ELA increases anxiety-like behavior and decreases social behavior. A 3-level mixed-effect meta-analysis is a flexible model that accounts for the dependency of observations.[10]

Optogenetic [237][11] *and chemogenetic*[12] *techniques* are being used to explore cell-type-specific control of neurons and behavior by targeting deletion or overexpression of genes in specific neuronal areas [160, 163]. These influences are designed to change biology and behavior associated with pathophysiology and symptoms of MDD. Optogenetics is used for controlling biological functions of target cells using light. It has become one of the most advanced neuroscience experimental techniques providing precise control on target cells and rapidly and specifically altering neuronal activity in vivo and ex vivo. It may have potential clinical applications [164, 165].

Optogenetic and chemogenetic approaches have underscored the previously described roles of *cortico-limbic* structures in depression. These areas include medial prefrontal cortex, anterior cingulate cortex, amygdala, nucleus accumbens, ventral tegmental area, hippocampus and raphe nuclei, and the less frequently associated areas the lateral habenula, or medial dorsal thalamus [160].

Predictive biomarkers may be able to discriminate between the initial episode of bipolar and unipolar depression based on blood proteomic profiling [166]. Profiles of concentrations of different proteins, peptides, and small molecules have been used to construct an algorithm that was able to discriminate depressed bipolar patients from MDD patients with an accuracy of 67%.

ENIGMA (Enhancing NeuroImaging Genetics through Meta Analysis) Consortium is a global alliance of more than 1400 scientists across 43 countries, and 50 working groups (WGs) studying the human brain in health and disease [231].

Beginning in 2010, ENIGMA built upon large-scale genetic studies that discovered the first robustly replicated genetic loci associated with brain metrics. Quoted from their website: "Most ENIGMA WGs focus on specific psychiatric and neurological conditions, other WGs study normal variation due to sex and gender differences, or development and aging; still other WGs develop methodological pipelines and

[10]The authors of that 3-layer meta-analysis state that they applied a novel, machine-learning based analysis *(MetaForest)* to identify the most important moderators of ELA effects on behavior. Based upon that analysis they evaluated the translational potential of ELA rodent models. They used a specially developed web-based tool *MaBapp (Meta-Analysis of Behavior application)* [225]. They also state that interested researchers can perform their own meta-analysis and retrieve valuable ad hoc information for experimental design and power calculations.

[11]Good reviews on optogenetics include [226–228].

[12]Good reviews on chemogenetics include [229, 230].

tools to facilitate harmonized analyses of "big data" (i.e., genetic, and epigenetic data, multimodal MRI, and electroencephalography data).

These international efforts have yielded the largest neuroimaging studies to date in schizophrenia, bipolar disorder, major depressive disorder, post-traumatic stress disorder, substance use disorders, obsessive-compulsive disorder, attention-deficit/hyperactivity disorder, autism spectrum disorders, epilepsy, and 22q11.2 deletion syndrome.

More recent ENIGMA WGs have formed to study anxiety disorders, suicidal thoughts and behavior, sleep and insomnia, eating disorders, irritability, brain injury, antisocial personality and conduct disorder, and dissociative identity disorder."

The following are results of a few ENIGMA studies related to MDD.

Widespread cortical abnormalities were seen in adults and adolescents with major depression based on brain scans from 20 cohorts worldwide in the ENIGMA Major Depressive Disorder Working Group [170]. Results suggest that MDD may impact brain structure in a highly dynamic way, with different patterns of alterations at different stages of life.

Lower hippocampal volume altered cortical structures and decreased integrity of white matter connecting those cortical and subcortical regions (suggesting a disconnection syndrome) are frequent in MDD patients [167–171].

For example, one ENIGMA study revealed subcortical brain alterations including smaller hippocampal volumes in MDD patients (26122586). Mean age, proportion of antidepressant users and proportion of remitted patients, and methodological characteristics did not significantly moderate alterations in brain volumes in MDD. No differences were seen between the first episodes and controls. Smaller hippocampal volume, a trend toward smaller amygdalas, and larger lateral ventricles were seen in patients who had an age of onset less than 21 years of age. Severity of symptoms at onset was not associated with any regional brain volumes. Larger caudate volumes were seen in proportion to the antipsychotic medication use.

Subtle but widespread differences have been seen in white matter microstructure in adult MDD, suggesting structural dysconnectivity[13] in MDD (32198361). The corpus callosum and corona radiata showed the largest differences. Recurrent MDD and adult onset of depression were associated with the largest differences.

An ENIGMA Consortium Analysis showed that there are no alterations of brain structural asymmetry in MDD [232].

[13]Dysconnectivity is used instead of disconnectivity. This is following the meaning of abnormal not decreased [233].

Summary

The DSM-5 and its revision, the DSM-5-TR, released in 2013 and 2022, respectively, reflect an evolving comprehension of mental disorders shaped by cognitive neuroscience, genetics, and epidemiology. These updates acknowledge the fluid boundaries between disorder categories and the shared neural substrates and risk factors among them. While bipolar and related disorders are classified separately from depressive and anxiety disorders, extensive review and analysis position bipolar disorders as a bridge between schizophrenia and depressive disorders due to genetics and symptomatology.

Depressive disorders in the DSM-5 encompass various subtypes, influenced by factors such as race, culture, and socioeconomic status, impacting diagnostic accuracy. Depression often co-occurs with anxiety and panic disorders, alongside substance abuse, exacerbating its impact on physical and mental health, including increased risk of cardiovascular diseases and dementia. Suicidal tendencies are heightened, complicating treatment adherence and health-seeking behaviors.

Depression's association with immune system dysregulation, neuroendocrine system influence, and brain structures like the amygdala and hippocampus underscores the importance of understanding these connections in managing mood disorders. Stratified, precision, and personalized medicine approaches in depression research aim to tailor treatments based on individual characteristics, supported by initiatives like the Research Domain Criteria (RDoC) and collaborative efforts such as the Psychiatric Genomics Consortium (PGC) and PsychENCODE.

Preclinical research employing rodent models, optogenetic, and chemogenetic techniques investigates sex differences, intergenerational transmission, and biomarkers to distinguish bipolar and unipolar depression. The ENIGMA Consortium further enhances understanding through global studies of brain structure abnormalities in depression.

Understanding the complex etiology of depressive disorders will provide a foundation for the possibilities of prevention and successful treatment of depression.

References

1. Fox E. Emotion science: an integration of cognitive and neuroscientific approaches. Palgrave MacMillan; 2008. Emotion Science: Cognitive and Neuroscientific Approaches to Understanding ... - Elaine Fox - Google Books
2. Ekman P. Basic emotions. In: Dalgleish T, Power MJ, editors. Handbook of cognition and emotion. Wiley; 1999. p. 45–60. https://doi.org/10.1002/0470013494.ch3.
3. Gaulin SJC, McBurney DH. Chapter 6. In: Evolutionary psychology. Prentice Hall; 2003. p. 121–42. Evolutionary psychology by Steven J. C. Gaulin | Open Library.

4. Schacter DL. Psychology. 5th ed. New York: Worth Publishers; 2020.
5. Development of Temperament Symposium. 2008. Philoctetes Center, New York; with panelists Sue Carter, Francis Champagne, Susan Coates, Ed Nercessian, Donald Pfaff, Daniel Schechter, Nadia Bruschweiler Stern.
6. Kagan J. Temperament. Encyclopedia on Early Childhood Development 2019. Temperament: Early childhood development | Encyclopedia on Early Childhood Development
7. Keirsey D. Please understand me II: temperament character intelligence. Prometheus Nemesis Book Company; 1998.
8. Depression in the U.S. – Statistics & Facts | Statista
9. Semple D. Oxford handbook of psychiatry. Oxford Press, Oxford Handbook of Psychiatry | Oxford Academic.
10. National Research Council (US) Committee on A Framework for Developing a New Taxonomy of Disease. Toward precision medicine: building a knowledge network for biomedical research and a new taxonomy of disease. Washington, DC: National Academies Press (US); 2011. Available from: https://www.ncbi.nlm.nih.gov/books/NBK91503/ https://pubmed.ncbi.nlm.nih.gov/22536618/
11. Cosmides L, Tooby J. Evolutionary psychology: new perspectives on cognition and motivation. Annu Rev Psychol. 2013;64:201–29. PMID: 23282055. http://www.ncbi.nlm.nih.gov/pubmed/23282055
12. Galtress T, Marshall AT, Kirkpatrick K. Motivation and timing: clues for modeling the reward system. Behav Process. 2012;90(1):142–53. PMCID: PMC3335954. http://www.ncbi.nlm.nih.gov/pubmed/22421220
13. McCall C, Singer T. The animal and human neuroendocrinology of social cognition, motivation and behavior. Nat Neurosci. 2012;15(5):681–8. PMID: 22504348. http://www.ncbi.nlm.nih.gov/pubmed/22504348
14. Shohamy D. Learning and motivation in the human striatum. Curr Opin Neurobiol. 2011;21(3):408–14. PMID: 21658933. http://www.ncbi.nlm.nih.gov/pubmed/21658933
15. Frank MJ, Fossella JA. Neurogenetics and pharmacology of learning, motivation, and cognition. Neuropsychopharmacology. 2011;36(1):133–52. PMCID: PMC3055524. http://www.ncbi.nlm.nih.gov/pubmed/20631684
16. Gaitan-Sierra C, Hyland ME. Nonspecific mechanisms that enhance well-being in health-promoting behaviors. Health Psychol. 2011;30(6):793–6. PMID: 21942748. http://www.ncbi.nlm.nih.gov/pubmed/21942748
17. Hyland ME. Motivation and placebos: do different mechanisms occur in different contexts? Philos Trans R Soc Lond B Biol Sci. 2011;366(1572):1828–37. PMCID: PMC3130400. http://www.ncbi.nlm.nih.gov/pubmed/21576140
18. Lövheim H. A new three-dimensional model for emotions and monoamine neurotransmitters. Med Hypotheses. 2012;78(2):341–8. PMID: 22153577. http://www.ncbi.nlm.nih.gov/pubmed/22153577
19. Sayin A, Aslan S. The relationship between mood disorders and temperament, character and personality. Turk Psikiyatri Derg. 2005;16(4):276–83. PMID: 16362847. http://www.ncbi.nlm.nih.gov/pubmed/16362847
20. Cheung RW, Austerberry C, Fearon P, Hayiou-Thomas ME, Leve LD, Shaw DS, Ganiban JM, Natsuaki MN, Neiderhieser JM, Reiss D. Disentangling genetic and environmental influences on early language development: the interplay of genetic propensity for negative emotionality and surgency, and parenting behavior effects on early language skills in an adoption study. Child Dev. 2024;95(3):699–720. PMCID: PMC11023813 http://www.ncbi.nlm.nih.gov/pubmed/37947162
21. Kiff CJ, Lengua LJ, Zalewski M. Nature and nurturing: parenting in the context of child temperament. Clin Child Fam Psychol Rev. 2011;14(3):251–301. PMCID: PMC3163750. http://www.ncbi.nlm.nih.gov/pubmed/21461681
22. Behrendt HF, Wade M, Bayet L, Nelson CA, Bosquet Enlow M. Pathways to social-emotional functioning in the preschool period: the role of child temperament and maternal anxiety in boys and girls. Dev Psychopathol. 2020;32(3):961–74. PMCID: PMC6982599. http://www.ncbi.nlm.nih.gov/pubmed/31345275
23. Saudino KJ. Behavioral genetics and child temperament. J Dev Behav Pediatr. 2005;26(3):214–23. PMCID: PMC1188235. http://www.ncbi.nlm.nih.gov/pubmed/15956873
24. Rettew DC, McKee L. Temperament and its role in developmental psychopathology. Harv Rev Psychiatry. 2005;13(1):14–27. PMCID: PMC3319036. http://www.ncbi.nlm.nih.gov/pubmed/15804931
25. Mochcovitch MD, Nardi AE, Cardoso A. Temperament and character dimensions and their relationship to major depression and panic disorder. Braz J Psychiatry. 2012;34(3):342–51. PMID: 23429781. http://www.ncbi.nlm.nih.gov/pubmed/23429781
26. Rakofsky J, Rapaport M. Mood disorders. Continuum (Minneap Minn). 2018;24(3, Behavioral Neurology and Psychiatry):804–827. PMID: 29851879. http://www.ncbi.nlm.nih.gov/pubmed/29851879.
27. Berrios GE. Of Mania: introduction (Classic text no 57). Hist Psychiatry. 2004;15(57 Pt 1):105–24. PMID: 15104084. http://www.ncbi.nlm.nih.gov/pubmed/15104084
28. Altshuler L, Bookheimer S, Proenza MA, Townsend J, Sabb F, Firestine A, Bartzokis G, Mintz J, Mazziotta J, Cohen MS. Increased amygdala activation during mania: a functional magnetic resonance imaging study. Am J Psychiatry. 2005;162(6):1211–3. PMID: 15930074. http://www.ncbi.nlm.nih.gov/pubmed/15930074
29. Altman E, Hedeker D, Peterson JL, Davis JM. A comparative evaluation of three self-rating scales for acute mania. Biol Psychiatry. 2001;50(6):468–71. PMID: 11566165. http://www.ncbi.nlm.nih.gov/pubmed/11566165
30. Bach A, Boehrer H, Schmidt H, Geiss HK. Nosocomial sinusitis in ventilated patients. Nasotracheal versus orotracheal intubation. Anaesthesia. 1992;47(4):335–9. PMID: 1519688. http://www.ncbi.nlm.nih.gov/pubmed/1519688
31. Claes SJ. Corticotropin-releasing hormone (CRH) in psychiatry: from stress to psychopathology. Ann Med. 2004;36(1):50–61. PMID: 15000347. http://www.ncbi.nlm.nih.gov/pubmed/15000347
32. Caspi A, Sugden K, Moffitt TE, Taylor A, Craig IW, Harrington H, McClay J, Mill J, Martin J, Braithwaite A, Poulton R. Influence of life stress on depression: moderation by a polymorphism in the 5-HTT gene. Science. 2003;301(5631):386–9. PMID: 12869766. http://www.ncbi.nlm.nih.gov/pubmed/12869766
33. Kendler KS, Kuhn JW, Vittum J, Prescott CA, Riley B. The interaction of stressful life events and a serotonin transporter polymorphism in the prediction of episodes of major depression: a replication. Arch Gen Psychiatry. 2005;62(5):529–35. PMID: 15867106. http://www.ncbi.nlm.nih.gov/pubmed/15867106
34. Schlauder GG, Leverenz GJ, Amann CW, Lesniewski RR, Peterson DA. Detection of the hepatitis C virus genome in acute and chronic experimental infection in chimpanzees. J Clin Microbiol. 1991;29(10):2175–9. PMCID: PMC270293. http://www.ncbi.nlm.nih.gov/pubmed/1658034
35. Lucae S, Salyakina D, Barden N, Harvey M, Gagné B, Labbé M, Binder EB, Uhr M, Paez-Pereda M, Sillaber I, Ising M, Brückl T, Lieb R, Holsboer F, Müller-Myhsok B. P2RX7, a gene coding for a purinergic ligand-gated ion channel, is associated with major depressive disorder. Hum Mol Genet. 2006;15(16):2438–45. PMID: 16822851. http://www.ncbi.nlm.nih.gov/pubmed/16822851

36. Lolak S, Suwannarat P, Lipsky RH. Epigenetics of depression. Prog Mol Biol Transl Sci. 2014;128:103–37. PMID: 25410543. http://www.ncbi.nlm.nih.gov/pubmed/25410543
37. Lockwood LE, Su S, Youssef NA. The role of epigenetics in depression and suicide: a platform for gene-environment interactions. Psychiatry Res. 2015;228(3):235–42. PMID: 26163724. http://www.ncbi.nlm.nih.gov/pubmed/26163724
38. Dalton VS, Kolshus E, McLoughlin DM. Epigenetics and depression: return of the repressed. J Affect Disord. 2014;155:1–12. PMID: 24238955. http://www.ncbi.nlm.nih.gov/pubmed/24238955
39. Heim C, Binder EB. Current research trends in early life stress and depression: review of human studies on sensitive periods, gene-environment interactions, and epigenetics. Exp Neurol. 2012;233(1):102–11. PMID: 22101006. http://www.ncbi.nlm.nih.gov/pubmed/22101006
40. Toohey MJ, DiGiuseppe R. Defining and measuring irritability: construct clarification and differentiation. Clin Psychol Rev. 2017;53:93–108. PMID: 28284170. http://www.ncbi.nlm.nih.gov/pubmed/28284170
41. Vidal-Ribas P, Brotman MA, Valdivieso I, Leibenluft E, Stringaris A. The status of irritability in psychiatry: a conceptual and quantitative review. J Am Acad Child Adolesc Psychiatry. 2016;55(7):556–70. PMCID: PMC4927461. http://www.ncbi.nlm.nih.gov/pubmed/27343883
42. Copeland WE, Brotman MA, Costello EJ. Normative irritability in youth: developmental findings from the Great Smoky Mountains study. J Am Acad Child Adolesc Psychiatry. 2015;54(8):635–42. PMCID: PMC4515775. http://www.ncbi.nlm.nih.gov/pubmed/26210332
43. Kales HC, DiNardo AR, Blow FC, McCarthy JF, Ignacio RV, Riba MB. International medical graduates and the diagnosis and treatment of late-life depression. Acad Med. 2006;81(2):171–5. PMID: 16436580 http://www.ncbi.nlm.nih.gov/pubmed/16436580
44. Kales HC, Mellow AM. Race and depression: does race affect the diagnosis and treatment of late-life depression? Geriatrics. 2006;61(5):18–21. PMID: 16649814. http://www.ncbi.nlm.nih.gov/pubmed/16649814
45. Kales HC, Neighbors HW, Blow FC, Taylor KKK, Gillon L, Welsh DE, Maixner SM, Mellow AM. Race, gender, and psychiatrists' diagnosis and treatment of major depression among elderly patients. Psychiatr Serv. 2005;56(6):721–8. PMID: 15939950. http://www.ncbi.nlm.nih.gov/pubmed/15939950
46. Kales HC, Neighbors HW, Valenstein M, Blow FC, McCarthy JF, Ignacio RV, Taylor KKK, Gillon L, Mellow AM. Effect of race and sex on primary care physicians' diagnosis and treatment of late-life depression. J Am Geriatr Soc. 2005;53(5):777–84. PMID: 15877552. http://www.ncbi.nlm.nih.gov/pubmed/15877552
47. Knox S, Barnes A, Kiefe C, Lewis CE, Iribarren C, Matthews KA, Wong ND, Whooley M. History of depression, race, and cardiovascular risk in CARDIA. Int J Behav Med. 2006;13(1):44–50. PMID: 16503840. http://www.ncbi.nlm.nih.gov/pubmed/16503840
48. Riolo SA, Nguyen TA, Greden JF, King CA. Prevalence of depression by race/ethnicity: findings from the National Health and nutrition examination survey III. Am J Public Health. 2005;95(6):998–1000. PMCID: PMC1449298. http://www.ncbi.nlm.nih.gov/pubmed/15914823
49. Harris PA. The impact of age, gender, race, and ethnicity on the diagnosis and treatment of depression. J Manag Care Pharm. 2004;10(2 Suppl):S2–7. PMID: 15046544. http://www.ncbi.nlm.nih.gov/pubmed/15046544
50. Teresi JA, Abrams R, Holmes D, Ramirez M, Shapiro C, Eimicke JP. Influence of cognitive impairment, illness, gender, and African-American status on psychiatric ratings and staff recognition of depression. Am J Geriatr Psychiatry. 2002;10(5):506–14. PMID: 12213684. http://www.ncbi.nlm.nih.gov/pubmed/12213684
51. Godard J, Baruch P, Grondin S, Lafleur MF. Psychosocial and neurocognitive functioning in unipolar and bipolar depression: a 12-month prospective study. Psychiatry Res. 2012;196(1):145–53. PMID: 22370154. http://www.ncbi.nlm.nih.gov/pubmed/22370154
52. Godard J, Grondin S, Baruch P, Lafleur MF. Psychosocial and neurocognitive profiles in depressed patients with major depressive disorder and bipolar disorder. Psychiatry Res. 2011;190(2–3):244–52. PMID: 21764461. http://www.ncbi.nlm.nih.gov/pubmed/21764461
53. Cabello M, Mellor-Marsá B, Sabariego C, Cieza A, Bickenbach J, Ayuso-Mateos JL. Psychosocial features of depression: a systematic literature review. J Affect Disord. 2012;141(1):22–33. PMID: 22209189. http://www.ncbi.nlm.nih.gov/pubmed/22209189
54. Simon NM. Generalized anxiety disorder and psychiatric comorbidities such as depression, bipolar disorder, and substance abuse. J Clin Psychiatry. 2009;70(Suppl 2):10–4. PMID: 19371501. http://www.ncbi.nlm.nih.gov/pubmed/19371501
55. Batelaan NM, Spijker J, de Graaf R, Cuijpers P. Mixed anxiety depression should not be included in DSM-5. J Nerv Ment Dis. 2012;200(6):495–8. PMID: 22652614. http://www.ncbi.nlm.nih.gov/pubmed/22652614
56. Johnson MR, Lydiard RB. Comorbidity of major depression and panic disorder. J Clin Psychol. 1998;54(2):201–10. PMID: 9467764. http://www.ncbi.nlm.nih.gov/pubmed/9467764
57. Srinivasa K, Neerakal I. A study of panic patients with and without depression. Indian J Psychiatry. 2002;44(3):246–52. PMCID: PMC2954395. http://www.ncbi.nlm.nih.gov/pubmed/21206579
58. Kessler RC, Chiu WT, Demler O, Merikangas KR, Walters EE. Prevalence, severity, and comorbidity of 12-month DSM-IV disorders in the National Comorbidity Survey Replication. Arch Gen Psychiatry. 2005;62(6):617–27. PMCID: PMC2847357. http://www.ncbi.nlm.nih.gov/pubmed/15939839
59. Kaufman J, Charney D. Comorbidity of mood and anxiety disorders. Depress Anxiety. 2000;12(Suppl 1):69–76. PMID: 11098417. http://www.ncbi.nlm.nih.gov/pubmed/11098417
60. Allen LB, White KS, Barlow DH, Shear MK, Gorman JM, Woods SW. Cognitive-behavior therapy (CBT) for panic disorder: relationship of anxiety and depression comorbidity with treatment outcome. J Psychopathol Behav Assess. 2010;32(2):185–92. PMCID: PMC2855025. http://www.ncbi.nlm.nih.gov/pubmed/20421906
61. Sareen J, Houlahan T, Cox BJ, Asmundson GJG. Anxiety disorders associated with suicidal ideation and suicide attempts in the National Comorbidity Survey. J Nerv Ment Dis. 2005;193(7):450–4. PMID: 15985839. http://www.ncbi.nlm.nih.gov/pubmed/15985839
62. Pilowsky DJ, Olfson M, Gameroff MJ, Wickramaratne P, Blanco C, Feder A, Gross R, Neria Y, Weissman MM. Panic disorder and suicidal ideation in primary care. Depress Anxiety. 2006;23(1):11–6. PMCID: PMC3631348. http://www.ncbi.nlm.nih.gov/pubmed/16245304
63. Boden JM, Fergusson DM. Alcohol and depression. Addiction. 2011;106(5):906–14. PMID: 21382111. http://www.ncbi.nlm.nih.gov/pubmed/21382111
64. Park S, Romer D. Associations between smoking and depression in adolescence: an integrative review. Taehan Kanho Hakhoe Chi. 2007;37(2):227–41. PMID: 17435408. http://www.ncbi.nlm.nih.gov/pubmed/17435408
65. Chaiton MO, Cohen JE, O'Loughlin J, Rehm J. A systematic review of longitudinal studies on the association between depression and smoking in adolescents. BMC Public Health. 2009;9:356. PMCID: PMC2758872. http://www.ncbi.nlm.nih.gov/pubmed/19772635
66. Paperwalla KN, Levin TT, Weiner J, Saravay SM. Smoking and depression. Med Clin North Am. 2004;88(6):1483–94. x–xi. PMID: 15464109. http://www.ncbi.nlm.nih.gov/pubmed/15464109

67. Shiesha S. Selections from current literature: smoking and depression. Fam Pract. 1999;16(2):202–5. PMID: 10381030. http://www.ncbi.nlm.nih.gov/pubmed/10381030
68. Arterburn D, Westbrook EO, Ludman EJ, Operskalski B, Linde JA, Rohde P, Jeffery RW, Simon GE. Relationship between obesity, depression, and disability in middle-aged women. Obes Res Clin Pract. 2012;6(3):e197–206. PMCID: PMC3418708. http://www.ncbi.nlm.nih.gov/pubmed/22905068
69. Mazzeschi C, Pazzagli C, Buratta L, Reboldi GP, Battistini D, Piana N, Pippi R, Fatone C, De Feo P. Mutual interactions between depression/quality of life and adherence to a multidisciplinary lifestyle intervention in obesity. J Clin Endocrinol Metab. 2012;97(12):E2261–5. PMID: 23007686. http://www.ncbi.nlm.nih.gov/pubmed/23007686
70. Dave DM, Tennant J, Colman G. Isolating the effect of major depression on obesity: role of selection bias. J Ment Health Policy Econ. 2011;14(4):165–86. PMID: 22345359http://www.ncbi.nlm.nih.gov/pubmed/22345359
71. Gilman SE, Trinh NH, Smoller JW, Fava M, Murphy JM, Breslau J. Psychosocial stressors and the prognosis of major depression: a test of Axis IV. Psychol Med. 2013;43(2):303–16. PMCID: PMC3721739. http://www.ncbi.nlm.nih.gov/pubmed/22640506
72. Kop WJ, Stein PK, Tracy RP, Barzilay JI, Schulz R, Gottdiener JS. Autonomic nervous system dysfunction and inflammation contribute to the increased cardiovascular mortality risk associated with depression. Psychosom Med. 2010;72(7):626–35. PMCID: PMC3059072. http://www.ncbi.nlm.nih.gov/pubmed/20639389
73. Carney RM, Freedland KE, Veith RC. Depression, the autonomic nervous system, and coronary heart disease. Psychosom Med. 2005;67(Suppl 1):S29–33. PMID: 15953797. http://www.ncbi.nlm.nih.gov/pubmed/15953797
74. Kemp AH, Quintana DS, Felmingham KL, Matthews S, Jelinek HF. Depression, comorbid anxiety disorders, and heart rate variability in physically healthy, unmedicated patients: implications for cardiovascular risk. PLoS One. 2012;7(2):e30777. PMCID: PMC3280258. http://www.ncbi.nlm.nih.gov/pubmed/22355326
75. Larsen KK, Vestergaard M, Søndergaard J, Christensen B. Screening for depression in patients with myocardial infarction by general practitioners. Eur J Prev Cardiol. 2013;20(5):800–6. PMID: 22496274. http://www.ncbi.nlm.nih.gov/pubmed/22496274
76. Saravane D, Feve B, Frances Y, Corruble E, Lancon C, Chanson P, Maison P, Terra JL, Azorin JM, avec le soutien institutionnel du laboratoire Lilly. Drawing up guidelines for the attendance of physical health of patients with severe mental illness. Encephale. 2009;35(4):330–9. PMID: 19748369. http://www.ncbi.nlm.nih.gov/pubmed/19748369
77. Wint D. Depression: a shared risk factor for cardiovascular and Alzheimer disease. Cleve Clin J Med. 2011;78(Suppl 1):S44–6. PMID: 21972330. http://www.ncbi.nlm.nih.gov/pubmed/21972330
78. Rustad JK, Musselman DL, Nemeroff CB. The relationship of depression and diabetes: pathophysiological and treatment implications. Psychoneuroendocrinology. 2011;36(9):1276–86. PMID: 21474250. http://www.ncbi.nlm.nih.gov/pubmed/21474250
79. Reiche EMV, Morimoto HK, Nunes SMV. Stress and depression-induced immune dysfunction: implications for the development and progression of cancer. Int Rev Psychiatry. 2005;17(6):515–27. PMID: 16401550. http://www.ncbi.nlm.nih.gov/pubmed/16401550
80. Penninx BW, Guralnik JM, Pahor M, Ferrucci L, Cerhan JR, Wallace RB, Havlik RJ. Chronically depressed mood and cancer risk in older persons. J Natl Cancer Inst. 1998;90(24):1888–93. PMID: 9862626. http://www.ncbi.nlm.nih.gov/pubmed/9862626
81. Li M, Fitzgerald P, Rodin G. Evidence-based treatment of depression in patients with cancer. J Clin Oncol. 2012;30(11):1187–96. PMID: 22412144. http://www.ncbi.nlm.nih.gov/pubmed/22412144
82. Barrault S, Varescon I. Psychopathology in online pathological gamblers: a preliminary study. Encéphale. 2012;38(2):156–63. PMID: 22516274. http://www.ncbi.nlm.nih.gov/pubmed/22516274
83. Whooley MA, Browner WS. Association between depressive symptoms and mortality in older women. Study of Osteoporotic Fractures Research Group. Arch Intern Med. 1998;158(19):2129–35. PMID: 9801180. http://www.ncbi.nlm.nih.gov/pubmed/9801180
84. Wulsin LR, Vaillant GE, Wells VE. A systematic review of the mortality of depression. Psychosom Med. 1999;61(1):6–17. PMID: 10024062. http://www.ncbi.nlm.nih.gov/pubmed/10024062
85. Wells KB, Stewart A, Hays RD, Burnam MA, Rogers W, Daniels M, Berry S, Greenfield S, Ware J. The functioning and well-being of depressed patients. Results from the Medical Outcomes Study. JAMA. 1989;262(7):914–9. PMID: 2754791. http://www.ncbi.nlm.nih.gov/pubmed/2754791
86. Kessler RC, McGonagle KA, Zhao S, Nelson CB, Hughes M, Eshleman S, Wittchen HU, Kendler KS. Lifetime and 12-month prevalence of DSM-III-R psychiatric disorders in the United States. Results from the National Comorbidity Survey. Arch Gen Psychiatry. 1994;51(1):8–19. PMID: 8279933. http://www.ncbi.nlm.nih.gov/pubmed/8279933
87. Tsuang MT, Winokur G, Crowe RR. Morbidity risks of schizophrenia and affective disorders among first degree relatives of patients with schizophrenia, mania, depression and surgical conditions. Br J Psychiatry. 1980;137:497–504. PMID: 7214104. http://www.ncbi.nlm.nih.gov/pubmed/7214104
88. Gershon ES, Bunney WE, Leckman JF, Eerdewegh M, DeBauche BA. The inheritance of affective disorders: a review of data and of hypotheses. Behav Genet. 1976;6(3):227–61. PMID: 1086088. http://www.ncbi.nlm.nih.gov/pubmed/1086088
89. Kendler KS, Neale MC, Kessler RC, Heath AC, Eaves LJ. A population-based twin study of major depression in women. The impact of varying definitions of illness. Arch Gen Psychiatry. 1992;49(4):257–66. PMID: 1558459. http://www.ncbi.nlm.nih.gov/pubmed/1558459
90. Hasin DS, Sarvet AL, Meyers JL, Saha TD, Ruan WJ, Stohl M, Grant BF. Epidemiology of adult DSM-5 major depressive disorder and its specifiers in the United States. JAMA Psychiatr. 2018;75(4):336–46. PMCID: PMC5875313. http://www.ncbi.nlm.nih.gov/pubmed/29450462
91. Kessler RC, Bromet EJ. The epidemiology of depression across cultures. Annu Rev Public Health. 2013;34:119–38. PMCID: PMC4100461. http://www.ncbi.nlm.nih.gov/pubmed/23514317
92. Judd LL. The clinical course of unipolar major depressive disorders. Arch Gen Psychiatry. 1997;54(11):989–91. PMID: 9366654. http://www.ncbi.nlm.nih.gov/pubmed/9366654
93. Dinga R, Marquand AF, Veltman DJ, Beekman ATF, Schoevers RA, van Hemert AM, Penninx BWJH, Schmaal L. Predicting the naturalistic course of depression from a wide range of clinical, psychological, and biological data: a machine learning approach. Transl Psychiatry. 2018;8(1):241. PMCID: PMC6218451. http://www.ncbi.nlm.nih.gov/pubmed/30397196
94. Kiecolt-Glaser JK, Glaser R. Depression and immune function: central pathways to morbidity and mortality. J Psychosom Res. 2002;53(4):873–6. PMID: 12377296. http://www.ncbi.nlm.nih.gov/pubmed/12377296
95. Cohen S, Murphy MLM, Prather AA. Ten surprising facts about stressful life events and disease risk. Annu Rev Psychol. 2019;70:577–97. PMCID: PMC6996482. http://www.ncbi.nlm.nih.gov/pubmed/29949726

96. Checkley S. Neuroendocrine mechanisms and the precipitation of depression by life events. Br J Psychiatry Suppl. 1992;15:7–17. PMID: 1356360. http://www.ncbi.nlm.nih.gov/pubmed/1356360
97. Heinrichs M, Gaab J. Neuroendocrine mechanisms of stress and social interaction: implications for mental disorders. Curr Opin Psychiatry. 2007;20(2):158–62. PMID: 17278915. http://www.ncbi.nlm.nih.gov/pubmed/17278915
98. Meyer SE, Chrousos GP, Gold PW. Major depression and the stress system: a life span perspective. Dev Psychopathol. 2001;13(3):565–80. PMID: 11523848. http://www.ncbi.nlm.nih.gov/pubmed/11523848
99. Pariante CM. Depression, stress and the adrenal axis. J Neuroendocrinol. 2003;15(8):811–2. PMID: 12834443. http://www.ncbi.nlm.nih.gov/pubmed/12834443
100. Barden N. Implication of the hypothalamic-pituitary-adrenal axis in the physiopathology of depression. J Psychiatry Neurosci. 2004;29(3):185–93. PMCID: PMC400688. http://www.ncbi.nlm.nih.gov/pubmed/15173895
101. Smart C, Strathdee G, Watson S, Murgatroyd C, McAllister-Williams RH. Early life trauma, depression and the glucocorticoid receptor gene–an epigenetic perspective. Psychol Med. 2015;45(16):3393–410. PMID: 26387521. http://www.ncbi.nlm.nih.gov/pubmed/26387521
102. Parker KJ, Schatzberg AF, Lyons DM. Neuroendocrine aspects of hypercortisolism in major depression. Horm Behav. 2003;43(1):60–6. PMID: 12614635. http://www.ncbi.nlm.nih.gov/pubmed/12614635
103. Murphy BE, Ghadirian AM, Dhar V. Neuroendocrine responses to inhibitors of steroid biosynthesis in patients with major depression resistant to antidepressant therapy. Can J Psychiatry. 1998;43(3):279–86. PMID: 9561317. http://www.ncbi.nlm.nih.gov/pubmed/9561317.
104. Tafet GE, Smolovich J. Psychoneuroendocrinological studies on chronic stress and depression. Ann N Y Acad Sci. 2004;1032:276–8. PMID: 15677427. http://www.ncbi.nlm.nih.gov/pubmed/15677427
105. Tafet GE, Bernardini R. Psychoneuroendocrinological links between chronic stress and depression. Prog Neuro-Psychopharmacol Biol Psychiatry. 2003;27(6):893–903. PMID: 14499305
106. De Raedt R, Koster EHW. Understanding vulnerability for depression from a cognitive neuroscience perspective: a reappraisal of attentional factors and a new conceptual framework. Cogn Affect Behav Neurosci. 2010;10(1):50–70. PMID: 20233955. http://www.ncbi.nlm.nih.gov/pubmed/20233955
107. Nejad AB, Fossati P, Lemogne C. Self-referential processing, rumination, and cortical midline structures in major depression. Front Hum Neurosci. 2013;7:666. PMCID: PMC3794427. http://www.ncbi.nlm.nih.gov/pubmed/24124416
108. Russo SJ, Nestler EJ. The brain reward circuitry in mood disorders. Nat Rev Neurosci. 2013;14(9):609–25. PMCID: PMC3867253. http://www.ncbi.nlm.nih.gov/pubmed/23942470
109. Seo JS, Wei J, Qin L, Kim Y, Yan Z, Greengard P. Cellular and molecular basis for stress-induced depression. Mol Psychiatry. 2017;22(10):1440–7. PMCID: PMC5269558. http://www.ncbi.nlm.nih.gov/pubmed/27457815
110. Pervanidou P, Chrousos GP. Metabolic consequences of stress during childhood and adolescence. Metabolism. 2012;61(5):611–9. PMID: 22146091. http://www.ncbi.nlm.nih.gov/pubmed/22146091
111. Hannestad J, DellaGioia N, Bloch M. The effect of antidepressant medication treatment on serum levels of inflammatory cytokines: a meta-analysis. Neuropsychopharmacology. 2011;36(12):2452–9. PMCID: PMC3194072. http://www.ncbi.nlm.nih.gov/pubmed/21796103
112. Day S, Coombes RC, McGrath-Lone L, Schoenborn C, Ward H. Stratified, precision or personalised medicine? Cancer services in the "real world" of a London hospital. Sociol Health Illn. 2017;39(1):143–58. PMID: 27460935. http://www.ncbi.nlm.nih.gov/pubmed/27460935
113. Ozomaro U, Wahlestedt C, Nemeroff CB. Personalized medicine in psychiatry: problems and promises. BMC Med. 2013;11:132. PMCID: PMC3668172. http://www.ncbi.nlm.nih.gov/pubmed/23680237
114. Toward precision medicine: building a knowledge network for biomedical research and a new taxonomy of disease [internet]. Washington, D.C.: National Academies Press; 2011 [cited 2024 Dec 16]. p. 13284. Available from: http://www.nap.edu/catalog/13284
115. König IR, Fuchs O, Hansen G, von Mutius E, Kopp MV. What is precision medicine? Eur Respirat Soc [Internet]. 2017;50(4):1700391. Available from: http://erj.ersjournals.com/content/erj/50/4/1700391.abstract
116. Rubin MA. Health: make precision medicine work for cancer care. Nature. 2015;520(7547):290–1. PMID: 25877189. http://www.ncbi.nlm.nih.gov/pubmed/25877189
117. Khoury MJ. Planning for the future of epidemiology in the era of big data and precision medicine. Am J Epidemiol. 2015;182(12):977–9. PMCID: PMC4681267. http://www.ncbi.nlm.nih.gov/pubmed/26628513
118. Robinson PN. Deep phenotyping for precision medicine. Hum Mutat. 2012;33(5):777–80. PMID: 22504886. http://www.ncbi.nlm.nih.gov/pubmed/22504886
119. Hamburg MA, Collins FS. The path to personalized medicine. N Engl J Med. 2010;363(4):301–4. PMID: 20551152. http://www.ncbi.nlm.nih.gov/pubmed/20551152
120. Aalto H, Juhola M, Pyykkö I. Visual stimulator using laser beam for eye-movement studies - PubMed. Med Biol Eng Comput. 1989;27(3):332–5. PMID: 2601459.
121. Aronson SJ, Rehm HL. Building the foundation for genomics in precision medicine. Nature. 2015;526(7573):336–42. PMCID: PMC5669797. http://www.ncbi.nlm.nih.gov/pubmed/26469044
122. Schumann G, Benegal V, Yu C, Tao S, Jernigan T, Heinz A, Araya R, Yu L, Calhoun V, Global imaging genetics in adolescents consortium. Precision medicine and global mental health. Lancet Glob Health. 2019;7(1):e32. PMCID: PMC7313318. http://www.ncbi.nlm.nih.gov/pubmed/30554758
123. Iacono WG. Endophenotypes in psychiatric disease: prospects and challenges. Genome Med. 2018;10(1):11. PMCID: PMC5824588 http://www.ncbi.nlm.nih.gov/pubmed/29471866
124. Biomarkers Definitions Working Group. Biomarkers and surrogate endpoints: preferred definitions and conceptual framework. Clin Pharmacol Ther. 2001;69(3):89–95. PMID: 11240971. http://www.ncbi.nlm.nih.gov/pubmed/11240971
125. Tretter F, Gebicke-Haerter PJ. Systems biology in psychiatric research: from complex data sets over wiring diagrams to computer simulations. Methods Mol Biol. 2012;829:567–92. PMID: 22231839. http://www.ncbi.nlm.nih.gov/pubmed/22231839
126. Morris SE, Cuthbert BN. Research domain criteria: cognitive systems, neural circuits, and dimensions of behavior. Dialogues Clin Neurosci. 2012;14(1):29–37. PMCID: PMC3341647. https://www.tandfonline.com/doi/pdf/10.31887/DCNS.2012.14.1/smorris
127. Kaye J, Curren L, Anderson N, Edwards K, Fullerton SM, Kanellopoulou N, Lund D, MacArthur DG, Mascalzoni D, Shepherd J, Taylor PL, Terry SF, Winter SF. From patients to partners: participant-centric initiatives in biomedical research. Nat Rev Genet. 2012;13(5):371–6. PMCID: PMC3806497 https://pmc.ncbi.nlm.nih.gov/articles/PMC3806497/pdf/nihms509935.pdf

128. Fiske A, Prainsack B, Buyx A. Meeting the needs of underserved populations: setting the agenda for more inclusive citizen science of medicine. J Med Ethics. 2019;45(9):617–22. PMCID: PMC6817991. http://www.ncbi.nlm.nih.gov/pubmed/31300487
129. Fiske A, Prainsack B, Buyx A. Data work: meaning-making in the era of data-rich medicine. J Med Internet Res. 2019;21(7):e11672. PMCID: PMC6647753 http://www.ncbi.nlm.nih.gov/pubmed/31290397
130. Beier K, Schweda M, Schicktanz S. Taking patient involvement seriously: a critical ethical analysis of participatory approaches in data-intensive medical research. BMC Med Inform Decis Mak. 2019;19(1):90. PMCID: PMC6482526 http://www.ncbi.nlm.nih.gov/pubmed/31023321
131. McGuire AL, Majumder MA, Villanueva AG, Bardill J, Bollinger JM, Boerwinkle E, Bubela T, Deverka PA, Evans BJ, Garrison NA, Glazer D, Goldstein MM, Greely HT, Kahn SD, Knoppers BM, Koenig BA, Lambright JM, Mattison JE, O'Donnell C, Rai AK, Rodriguez LL, Simoncelli T, Terry SF, Thorogood AM, Watson MS, Wilbanks JT, Cook-Deegan R. Importance of participant-centricity and Trust for a Sustainable Medical Information Commons. J Law Med Ethics. 2019;47(1):12–20. PMCID: PMC6738947. http://www.ncbi.nlm.nih.gov/pubmed/30994067
132. Boeckhout M, Scheltens P, Manders P, Smit C, Bredenoord AL, Zielhuis GA. Patients to learn from: on the need for systematic integration of research and care in academic health care. J Clin Transl Res. 2018;3(Suppl 3):401–6. PMCID: PMC6412601. http://www.ncbi.nlm.nih.gov/pubmed/30873488
133. Carcone D, Ruocco AC. Six years of research on the National Institute of Mental Health's research domain criteria (RDoC) initiative: a systematic review. Front Cell Neurosci. 2017;11:46. PMCID: PMC5334510. http://www.ncbi.nlm.nih.gov/pubmed/28316565
134. Van Dam NT, O'Connor D, Marcelle ET, Ho EJ, Cameron Craddock R, Tobe RH, Gabbay V, Hudziak JJ, Xavier Castellanos F, Leventhal BL, Milham MP. Data-driven phenotypic categorization for neurobiological analyses: beyond DSM-5 labels. Biol Psychiatry. 2017;81(6):484–94. PMCID: PMC5402759 http://www.ncbi.nlm.nih.gov/pubmed/27667698
135. Kaufman J. Unraveling the genetics of major depression and stress-related psychiatric disorders: is it time for a paradigm shift? Biol Psychiatry. 2018;84(2):82–4. PMID: 31178063 http://www.ncbi.nlm.nih.gov/pubmed/31178063
136. Jamei M, Dickinson GL, Rostami-Hodjegan A. A framework for assessing inter-individual variability in pharmacokinetics using virtual human populations and integrating general knowledge of physical chemistry, biology, anatomy, physiology and genetics: a tale of "bottom-up" vs "top-down" recognition of covariates. Drug Metab Pharmacokinet. 2009;24(1):53–75. PMID: 19252336. http://www.ncbi.nlm.nih.gov/pubmed/19252336
137. Taylor AG, Goehler LE, Galper DI, Innes KE, Bourguignon C. Top-down and bottom-up mechanisms in mind-body medicine: development of an integrative framework for psychophysiological research. Explore (NY). 2010;6(1):29–41. PMCID: PMC2818254. http://www.ncbi.nlm.nih.gov/pubmed/20129310
138. Nicholson AA, Friston KJ, Zeidman P, Harricharan S, McKinnon MC, Densmore M, Neufeld RWJ, Théberge J, Corrigan F, Jetly R, Spiegel D, Lanius RA. Dynamic causal modeling in PTSD and its dissociative subtype: bottom-up versus top-down processing within fear and emotion regulation circuitry. Hum Brain Mapp. 2017;38(11):5551–61. PMCID: PMC6866710. http://www.ncbi.nlm.nih.gov/pubmed/28836726
139. Casey BJ, Craddock N, Cuthbert BN, Hyman SE, Lee FS, Ressler KJ. DSM-5 and RDoC: progress in psychiatry research? Nat Rev Neurosci. 2013;14(11):810–4. PMCID: PMC4372467. http://www.ncbi.nlm.nih.gov/pubmed/24135697
140. Lilienfeld SO. The research domain criteria (RDoC): an analysis of methodological and conceptual challenges. Behav Res Ther. 2014;62:129–39. PMID: 25156396. http://www.ncbi.nlm.nih.gov/pubmed/25156396
141. Lilienfeld SO, Treadway MT. Clashing diagnostic approaches: DSM-ICD versus RDoC. Annu Rev Clin Psychol. 2016;12:435–63. PMCID: PMC5154554. http://www.ncbi.nlm.nih.gov/pubmed/26845519
142. Frances A. RDoC is necessary, but very oversold. World Psychiatry 2014;13(1):47–49. PMCID: PMC3918019 http://www.ncbi.nlm.nih.gov/pubmed/24497248
143. Sanislow CA, Ferrante M, Pacheco J, Rudorfer MV, Morris SE. Advancing translational research using NIMH research domain criteria and computational methods. Neuron. 2019;101(5):779–82. PMID: 30844398. http://www.ncbi.nlm.nih.gov/pubmed/30844398
144. Sanislow CA. Connecting psychopathology meta-structure and mechanisms. J Abnorm Psychol. 2016;125(8):1158–65. PMID: 27819475 http://www.ncbi.nlm.nih.gov/pubmed/27819475
145. Kozak MJ, Cuthbert BN. The NIMH research domain criteria initiative: background, issues, and pragmatics. Psychophysiology. 2016;53(3):286–97. PMID: 26877115 http://www.ncbi.nlm.nih.gov/pubmed/26877115
146. Garvey M, Avenevoli S, Anderson K. The National Institute of Mental Health research domain criteria and clinical research in child and adolescent psychiatry. J Am Acad Child Adolesc Psychiatry. 2016;55(2):93–8. PMCID: PMC4724376 http://www.ncbi.nlm.nih.gov/pubmed/26802775
147. Gore WL, Widiger TA. Negative emotionality across diagnostic models: RDoC, DSM-5 section III, and FFM. Personal Disord. 2018;9(2):155–64. PMID: 29578748. http://www.ncbi.nlm.nih.gov/pubmed/29578748
148. Clark LA, Cuthbert B, Lewis-Fernández R, Narrow WE, Reed GM. Three approaches to understanding and classifying mental disorder: ICD-11, DSM-5, and the National Institute of Mental Health's research domain criteria (RDoC). Psychol Sci Public Interest. 2017;18(2):72–145. PMID: 29211974 http://www.ncbi.nlm.nih.gov/pubmed/29211974
149. Visel A, Rubin EM, Pennacchio LA. Genomic views of distant-acting enhancers. Nature. 2009;461(7261):199–205. PMCID: PMC2923221. http://www.ncbi.nlm.nih.gov/pubmed/19741700
150. Lee TI, Young RA. Transcriptional regulation and its misregulation in disease. Cell. 2013;152(6):1237–51. PMCID: PMC3640494 http://www.ncbi.nlm.nih.gov/pubmed/23498934
151. PsychENCODE Consortium, Akbarian S, Liu C, Knowles JA, Vaccarino FM, Farnham PJ, Crawford GE, Jaffe AE, Pinto D, Dracheva S, Geschwind DH, Mill J, Nairn AC, Abyzov A, Pochareddy S, Prabhakar S, Weissman S, Sullivan PF, State MW, Weng Z, Peters MA, White KP, Gerstein MB, Amiri A, Armoskus C, Ashley-Koch AE, Bae T, Beckel-Mitchener A, Berman BP, Coetzee GA, Coppola G, Francoeur N, Fromer M, Gao R, Grennan K, Herstein J, Kavanagh DH, Ivanov NA, Jiang Y, Kitchen RR, Kozlenkov A, Kundakovic M, Li M, Li Z, Liu S, Mangravite LM, Mattei E, Markenscoff-Papadimitriou E, Navarro FCP, North N, Omberg L, Panchision D, Parikshak N, Poschmann J, Price AJ, Purcaro M, Reddy TE, Roussos P, Schreiner S, Scuderi S, Sebra R, Shibata M, Shieh AW, Skarica M, Sun W, Swarup V, Thomas A, Tsuji J, van Bakel H, Wang D, Wang Y, Wang K, Werling DM, Willsey AJ, Witt H, Won H, Wong CCY, Wray GA, Wu EY, Xu X, Yao L, Senthil G, Lehner T, Sklar P, Sestan N. The PsychENCODE project. Nat Neurosci. 2015;18(12):1707–12. PMCID: PMC4675669 http://www.ncbi.nlm.nih.gov/pubmed/26605881

152. Ward LD, Kellis M. Interpreting noncoding genetic variation in complex traits and human disease. Nat Biotechnol. 2012;30(11):1095–106. PMCID: PMC3703467. http://www.ncbi.nlm.nih.gov/pubmed/23138309
153. 1000 Genomes Project Consortium, Auton A, Brooks LD, Durbin RM, Garrison EP, Kang HM, Korbel JO, Marchini JL, McCarthy S, McVean GA, Abecasis GR. A global reference for human genetic variation. Nature. 2015;526(7571):68–74. PMCID: PMC4750478 http://www.ncbi.nlm.nih.gov/pubmed/26432245
154. Sudmant PH, Rausch T, Gardner EJ, Handsaker RE, Abyzov A, Huddleston J, Zhang Y, Ye K, Jun G, Fritz MHY, Konkel MK, Malhotra A, Stütz AM, Shi X, Casale FP, Chen J, Hormozdiari F, Dayama G, Chen K, Malig M, Chaisson MJP, Walter K, Meiers S, Kashin S, Garrison E, Auton A, Lam HYK, Mu XJ, Alkan C, Antaki D, Bae T, Cerveira E, Chines P, Chong Z, Clarke L, Dal E, Ding L, Emery S, Fan X, Gujral M, Kahveci F, Kidd JM, Kong Y, Lameijer EW, McCarthy S, Flicek P, Gibbs RA, Marth G, Mason CE, Menelaou A, Muzny DM, Nelson BJ, Noor A, Parrish NF, Pendleton M, Quitadamo A, Raeder B, Schadt EE, Romanovitch M, Schlattl A, Sebra R, Shabalin AA, Untergasser A, Walker JA, Wang M, Yu F, Zhang C, Zhang J, Zheng-Bradley X, Zhou W, Zichner T, Sebat J, Batzer MA, McCarroll SA, 1000 Genomes Project Consortium, Mills RE, Gerstein MB, Bashir A, Stegle O, Devine SE, Lee C, Eichler EE, Korbel JO. An integrated map of structural variation in 2,504 human genomes. Nature. 2015;526(7571):75–81. PMCID: PMC4617611 http://www.ncbi.nlm.nih.gov/pubmed/26432246
155. Žitnik M, Janjić V, Larminie C, Zupan B, Pržulj N. Discovering disease-disease associations by fusing systems-level molecular data. Sci Rep. 2013;3:3202. PMCID: PMC3828568 http://www.ncbi.nlm.nih.gov/pubmed/24232732
156. Younesi E, Hofmann-Apitius M. From integrative disease modeling to predictive, preventive, personalized and participatory (P4) medicine. EPMA J. 2013;4(1):23. PMCID: PMC3832251. http://www.ncbi.nlm.nih.gov/pubmed/24195840
157. Cahoy JD, Emery B, Kaushal A, Foo LC, Zamanian JL, Christopherson KS, Xing Y, Lubischer JL, Krieg PA, Krupenko SA, Thompson WJ, Barres BA. A transcriptome database for astrocytes, neurons, and oligodendrocytes: a new resource for understanding brain development and function. J Neurosci. 2008;28(1):264–78. PMCID: PMC6671143. http://www.ncbi.nlm.nih.gov/pubmed/18171944
158. Gururajan A, Reif A, Cryan JF, Slattery DA. The future of rodent models in depression research. Nat Rev Neurosci. 2019;20(11):686–701. PMID: 31578460. http://www.ncbi.nlm.nih.gov/pubmed/31578460
159. Planchez B, Surget A, Belzung C. Animal models of major depression: drawbacks and challenges. J Neural Transm (Vienna). 2019;126(11):1383–408. PMCID: PMC6815270. http://www.ncbi.nlm.nih.gov/pubmed/31584111
160. Biselli T, Lange SS, Sablottny L, Steffen J, Walther A. Optogenetic and chemogenetic insights into the neurocircuitry of depression-like behaviour: a systematic review. Eur J Neurosci. 2021;53(1):9–38. PMID: 31633833. http://www.ncbi.nlm.nih.gov/pubmed/31633833
161. Antoniuk S, Bijata M, Ponimaskin E, Wlodarczyk J. Chronic unpredictable mild stress for modeling depression in rodents: meta-analysis of model reliability. Neurosci Biobehav Rev. 2019;99:101–16. PMID: 30529362. http://www.ncbi.nlm.nih.gov/pubmed/30529362
162. Bonapersona V, Kentrop J, Van Lissa CJ, van der Veen R, Joëls M, Sarabdjitsingh RA. The behavioral phenotype of early life adversity: a 3-level meta-analysis of rodent studies. Neurosci Biobehav Rev. 2019;102:299–307. PMID: 31047892. http://www.ncbi.nlm.nih.gov/pubmed/31047892
163. Muir J, Lopez J, Bagot RC. Wiring the depressed brain: optogenetic and chemogenetic circuit interrogation in animal models of depression. Neuropsychopharmacology. 2019;44(6):1013–26. PMCID: PMC6461994. http://www.ncbi.nlm.nih.gov/pubmed/30555161
164. Cheng Z, Cui R, Ge T, Yang W, Li B. Optogenetics: what it has uncovered in potential pathways of depression. Pharmacol Res. 2020;152:104596. PMID: 31838082. http://www.ncbi.nlm.nih.gov/pubmed/31838082
165. Camporeze B, Manica BA, Bonafé GA, Ferreira JJC, Diniz AL, de Oliveira CTP, Mathias Junior LR, de Aguiar PHP, Ortega MM. Optogenetics: the new molecular approach to control functions of neural cells in epilepsy, depression and tumors of the central nervous system. Am J Cancer Res. 2018;8(10):1900–18. PMCID: PMC6220144. http://www.ncbi.nlm.nih.gov/pubmed/30416844
166. Kittel-Schneider S, Hahn T, Haenisch F, McNeill R, Reif A, Bahn S. Proteomic profiling as a diagnostic biomarker for discriminating between bipolar and unipolar depression. Front Psychiatry. 2020;11:189. PMCID: PMC7184109. http://www.ncbi.nlm.nih.gov/pubmed/32372978
167. Thompson PM, Jahanshad N, Ching CRK, Salminen LE, Thomopoulos SI, Bright J, Baune BT, Bertolín S, Bralten J, Bruin WB, Bülow R, Chen J, Chye Y, Dannlowski U, de Kovel CGF, Donohoe G, Eyler LT, Faraone SV, Favre P, Filippi CA, Frodl T, Garijo D, Gil Y, Grabe HJ, Grasby KL, Hajek T, Han LKM, Hatton SN, Hilbert K, Ho TC, Holleran L, Homuth G, Hosten N, Houenou J, Ivanov I, Jia T, Kelly S, Klein M, Kwon JS, Laansma MA, Leerssen J, Lueken U, Nunes A, Neill JO, Opel N, Piras F, Piras F, Postema MC, Pozzi E, Shatokhina N, Soriano-Mas C, Spalletta G, Sun D, Teumer A, Tilot AK, Tozzi L, van der Merwe C, Van Someren EJW, van Wingen GA, Völzke H, Walton E, Wang L, Winkler AM, Wittfeld K, Wright MJ, Yun JY, Zhang G, Zhang-James Y, Adhikari BM, Agartz I, Aghajani M, Aleman A, Althoff RR, Altmann A, Andreassen OA, Baron DA, Bartnik-Olson BL, Marie Bas-Hoogendam J, Baskin-Sommers AR, Bearden CE, Berner LA, Boedhoe PSW, Brouwer RM, Buitelaar JK, Caeyenberghs K, Cecil CAM, Cohen RA, Cole JH, Conrod PJ, De Brito SA, de Zwarte SMC, Dennis EL, Desrivieres S, Dima D, Ehrlich S, Esopenko C, Fairchild G, Fisher SE, Fouche JP, Francks C, Frangou S, Franke B, Garavan HP, Glahn DC, Groenewold NA, Gurholt TP, Gutman BA, Hahn T, Harding IH, Hernaus D, Hibar DP, Hillary FG, Hoogman M, Hulshoff Pol HE, Jalbrzikowski M, Karkashadze GA, Klapwijk ET, Knickmeyer RC, Kochunov P, Koerte IK, Kong XZ, Liew SL, Lin AP, Logue MW, Luders E, Macciardi F, Mackey S, Mayer AR, McDonald CR, McMahon AB, Medland SE, Modinos G, Morey RA, Mueller SC, Mukherjee P, Namazova-Baranova L, Nir TM, Olsen A, Paschou P, Pine DS, Pizzagalli F, Rentería ME, Rohrer JD, Sämann PG, Schmaal L, Schumann G, Shiroishi MS, Sisodiya SM, Smit DJA, Sønderby IE, Stein DJ, Stein JL, Tahmasian M, Tate DF, Turner JA, van den Heuvel OA, van der Wee NJA, van der Werf YD, van Erp TGM, van Haren NEM, van Rooij D, van Velzen LS, Veer IM, Veltman DJ, Villalon-Reina JE, Walter H, Whelan CD, Wilde EA, Zarei M, Zelman V, ENIGMA Consortium. ENIGMA and global neuroscience: A decade of large-scale studies of the brain in health and disease across more than 40 countries. Transl Psychiatry. 2020;10(1):100. PMCID: PMC7083923. http://www.ncbi.nlm.nih.gov/pubmed/32198361
168. Schmaal L, Veltman DJ, van Erp TGM, Sämann PG, Frodl T, Jahanshad N, Loehrer E, Tiemeier H, Hofman A, Niessen WJ, Vernooij MW, Ikram MA, Wittfeld K, Grabe HJ, Block A, Hegenscheid K, Völzke H, Hoehn D, Czisch M, Lagopoulos J, Hatton SN, Hickie IB, Goya-Maldonado R, Krämer B, Gruber O, Couvy-Duchesne B, Rentería ME, Strike LT, Mills NT, de Zubicaray GI, McMahon KL, Medland SE, Martin NG, Gillespie

NA, Wright MJ, Hall GB, MacQueen GM, Frey EM, Carballedo A, van Velzen LS, van Tol MJ, van der Wee NJ, Veer IM, Walter H, Schnell K, Schramm E, Normann C, Schoepf D, Konrad C, Zurowski B, Nickson T, McIntosh AM, Papmeyer M, Whalley HC, Sussmann JE, Godlewska BR, Cowen PJ, Fischer FH, Rose M, Penninx BWJH, Thompson PM, Hibar DP. Subcortical brain alterations in major depressive disorder: findings from the ENIGMA major depressive disorder working group. Mol Psychiatry. 2016;21(6):806–12. PMCID: PMC4879183. http://www.ncbi.nlm.nih.gov/pubmed/26122586

169. Liao Y, Huang X, Wu Q, Yang C, Kuang W, Du M, Lui S, Yue Q, Chan RCK, Kemp GJ, Gong Q. Is depression a disconnection syndrome? Meta-analysis of diffusion tensor imaging studies in patients with MDD. J Psychiatry Neurosci. 2013;38(1):49–56. PMCID: PMC3529219. http://www.ncbi.nlm.nih.gov/pubmed/22691300

170. Schmaal L, Hibar DP, Sämann PG, Hall GB, Baune BT, Jahanshad N, Cheung JW, van Erp TGM, Bos D, Ikram MA, Vernooij MW, Niessen WJ, Tiemeier H, Hofman A, Wittfeld K, Grabe HJ, Janowitz D, Bülow R, Selonke M, Völzke H, Grotegerd D, Dannlowski U, Arolt V, Opel N, Heindel W, Kugel H, Hoehn D, Czisch M, Couvy-Duchesne B, Rentería ME, Strike LT, Wright MJ, Mills NT, de Zubicaray GI, McMahon KL, Medland SE, Martin NG, Gillespie NA, Goya-Maldonado R, Gruber O, Krämer B, Hatton SN, Lagopoulos J, Hickie IB, Frodl T, Carballedo A, Frey EM, van Velzen LS, Penninx BWJH, van Tol MJ, van der Wee NJ, Davey CG, Harrison BJ, Mwangi B, Cao B, Soares JC, Veer IM, Walter H, Schoepf D, Zurowski B, Konrad C, Schramm E, Normann C, Schnell K, Sacchet MD, Gotlib IH, MacQueen GM, Godlewska BR, Nickson T, McIntosh AM, Papmeyer M, Whalley HC, Hall J, Sussmann JE, Li M, Walter M, Aftanas L, Brack I, Bokhan NA, Thompson PM, Veltman DJ. Cortical abnormalities in adults and adolescents with major depression based on brain scans from 20 cohorts worldwide in the ENIGMA Major Depressive Disorder Working Group. Mol Psychiatry. 2017;22(6):900–909. PMCID: PMC5444023. http://www.ncbi.nlm.nih.gov/pubmed/27137745

171. Thompson PM, Stein JL, Medland SE, Hibar DP, Vasquez AA, Renteria ME, Toro R, Jahanshad N, Schumann G, Franke B, Wright MJ, Martin NG, Agartz I, Alda M, Alhusaini S, Almasy L, Almeida J, Alpert K, Andreasen NC, Andreassen OA, Apostolova LG, Appel K, Armstrong NJ, Aribisala B, Bastin ME, Bauer M, Bearden CE, Bergmann O, Binder EB, Blangero J, Bockholt HJ, Bøen E, Bois C, Boomsma DI, Booth T, Bowman IJ, Bralten J, Brouwer RM, Brunner HG, Brohawn DG, Buckner RL, Buitelaar J, Bulayeva K, Bustillo JR, Calhoun VD, Cannon DM, Cantor RM, Carless MA, Caseras X, Cavalleri GL, Chakravarty MM, Chang KD, Ching CRK, Christoforou A, Cichon S, Clark VP, Conrod P, Coppola G, Crespo-Facorro B, Curran JE, Czisch M, Deary IJ, de Geus EJC, den Braber A, Delvecchio G, Depondt C, de Haan L, de Zubicaray GI, Dima D, Dimitrova R, Djurovic S, Dong H, Donohoe G, Duggirala R, Dyer TD, Ehrlich S, Ekman CJ, Elvsåshagen T, Emsell L, Erk S, Espeseth T, Fagerness J, Fears S, Fedko I, Fernández G, Fisher SE, Foroud T, Fox PT, Francks C, Frangou S, Frey EM, Frodl T, Frouin V, Garavan H, Giddaluru S, Glahn DC, Godlewska B, Goldstein RZ, Gollub RL, Grabe HJ, Grimm O, Gruber O, Guadalupe T, Gur RE, Gur RC, Göring HHH, Hagenaars S, Hajek T, Hall GB, Hall J, Hardy J, Hartman CA, Hass J, Hatton SN, Haukvik UK, Hegenscheid K, Heinz A, Hickie IB, Ho BC, Hoehn D, Hoekstra PJ, Hollinshead M, Holmes AJ, Homuth G, Hoogman M, Hong LE, Hosten N, Hottenga JJ, Hulshoff Pol HE, Hwang KS, Jack CR, Jenkinson M, Johnston C, Jönsson EG, Kahn RS, Kasperaviciute D, Kelly S, Kim S, Kochunov P, Koenders L, Krämer B, Kwok JBJ, Lagopoulos J, Laje G, Landen M, Landman BA, Lauriello J, Lawrie SM, Lee PH, Le Hellard S, Lemaître H, Leonardo CD, Li CS, Liberg B, Liewald DC, Liu X, Lopez LM, Loth E, Lourdusamy A, Luciano M, Macciardi F, Machielsen MWJ, Macqueen GM, Malt UF, Mandl R, Manoach DS, Martinot JL, Matarin M, Mather KA, Mattheisen M, Mattingsdal M, Meyer-Lindenberg A, McDonald C, McIntosh AM, McMahon FJ, McMahon KL, Meisenzahl E, Melle I, Milaneschi Y, Mohnke S, Montgomery GW, Morris DW, Moses EK, Mueller BA, Muñoz Maniega S, Mühleisen TW, Müller-Myhsok B, Mwangi B, Nauck M, Nho K, Nichols TE, Nilsson LG, Nugent AC, Nyberg L, Olvera RL, Oosterlaan J, Ophoff RA, Pandolfo M, Papalampropoulou-Tsiridou M, Papmeyer M, Paus T, Pausova Z, Pearlson GD, Penninx BW, Peterson CP, Pfennig A, Phillips M, Pike GB, Poline JB, Potkin SG, Pütz B, Ramasamy A, Rasmussen J, Rietschel M, Rijpkema M, Risacher SL, Roffman JL, Roiz-Santiañez R, Romanczuk-Seiferth N, Rose EJ, Royle NA, Rujescu D, Ryten M, Sachdev PS, Salami A, Satterthwaite TD, Savitz J, Saykin AJ, Scanlon C, Schmaal L, Schnack HG, Schork AJ, Schulz SC, Schür R, Seidman L, Shen L, Shoemaker JM, Simmons A, Sisodiya SM, Smith C, Smoller JW, Soares JC, Sponheim SR, Sprooten E, Starr JM, Steen VM, Strakowski S, Strike L, Sussmann J, Sämann PG, Teumer A, Toga AW, Tordesillas-Gutierrez D, Trabzuni D, Trost S, Turner J, Van den Heuvel M, van der Wee NJ, van Eijk K, van Erp TGM, van Haren NEM, van 't Ent D, van Tol MJ, Valdés Hernández MC, Veltman DJ, Versace A, Völzke H, Walker R, Walter H, Wang L, Wardlaw JM, Weale ME, Weiner MW, Wen W, Westlye LT, Whalley HC, Whelan CD, White T, Winkler AM, Wittfeld K, Woldehawariat G, Wolf C, Zilles D, Zwiers MP, Thalamuthu A, Schofield PR, Freimer NB, Lawrence NS, Drevets W, Alzheimer's Disease Neuroimaging Initiative, EPIGEN Consortium, IMAGEN Consortium, Saguenay Youth Study (SYS) Group. The ENIGMA Consortium: large-scale collaborative analyses of neuroimaging and genetic data. Brain Imaging Behav. 2014;8(2):153–82. PMCID: PMC4008818. http://www.ncbi.nlm.nih.gov/pubmed/24399358.

172. APA – DSM – Diagnostic and Statistical Manual of Mental Disorders
173. Emotions
174. APA Dictionary of Psychology
175. APA – Depressive Disorders
176. Difference Between Mood and Affect | Difference Between | Mood vs Affect
177. Toward Precision Medicine – Google Books
178. MEDLINE Overview.
179. Embase | The comprehensive medical research database | Elsevier
180. APA PsycInfo
181. Scopus preview – Scopus – Welcome to Scopus
182. ProQuest | Better research, better learning, better insights
183. Cochrane Controlled Register of Trials (CENTRAL) | Cochrane Library
184. | LILACS – Literatura Latino-Americana e do Caribe em Ciências da Saúde – Informação e evidência científica e técnica em saúde da América Latina e Caribe – BIREME/OPAS/OMS – LILACS – Información y evidencia científica y técnica en salud de América Latina y el Caribe | LILACS – Scientific and technic information and evidence of Latin-american and Caribbean Countries
185. EBSCO Information Services.
186. Home | ClinicalTrials.gov
187. International Clinical Trials Registry Platform (ICTRP)
188. Avon Longitudinal Study of Parents and Children | Avon Longitudinal Study of Parents and Children | University of Bristol
189. Researchers – Generation R
190. ABCD Study.
191. The Twins Early Development Study (TEDS)Home
192. The Environmental Risk (E-Risk) Longitudinal Twin Study erisk-study.com

193. The IMAGEN study: a decade of imaging genetics in adolescents | Molecular Psychiatry
194. Precision Medicine and Global Mental Health – PMC
195. THE NATIONAL ACADEMIES – Toward Precision Medicine – NCBI Bookshelf
196. Home | National Academies
197. CDC Data and Statistics
198. The National Institute of Mental Health Strategic Plan – National Institute of Mental Health (NIMH)
199. The NIMH Research Domain Criteria (RDoC) Project: Precision Medicine for Psychiatry | American Journal of Psychiatry
200. Research Domain Criteria (RDoC) – National Institute of Mental Health (NIMH)
201. Definitions of the RDoC Domains and Constructs – National Institute of Mental Health (NIMH)
202. NIMH Data Archive – NDA
203. RDoC Resources: Webinar Series – National Institute of Mental Health (NIMH)
204. Morris SE, Vaidyanathan U, Cuthbert BN. Psychophysiological science and the research domain criteria: a commentary. Int J Psychophysiol. 2015;98(2 Pt 2):378–80. PMCID: PMC4687014. http://www.ncbi.nlm.nih.gov/pubmed/26546860
205. Ross CA, Margolis RL. Research domain criteria: strengths, weaknesses, and potential alternatives for future psychiatric research. Mol Neuropsychiatry. 2019;5(4):218–36. PMCID: PMC6873013. http://www.ncbi.nlm.nih.gov/pubmed/31768375
206. PGC – Psychiatric Genomics Consortium
207. Major Depressive Disorder Working Group of the Psychiatric GWAS Consortium, Ripke S, Wray NR, Lewis CM, Hamilton SP, Weissman MM, Breen G, Byrne EM, Blackwood DHR, Boomsma DI, Cichon S, Heath AC, Holsboer F, Lucae S, Madden PAF, Martin NG, McGuffin P, Muglia P, Noethen MM, Penninx BP, Pergadia ML, Potash JB, Rietschel M, Lin D, Müller-Myhsok B, Shi J, Steinberg S, Grabe HJ, Lichtenstein P, Magnusson P, Perlis RH, Preisig M, Smoller JW, Stefansson K, Uher R, Kutalik Z, Tansey KE, Teumer A, Viktorin A, Barnes MR, Bettecken T, Binder EB, Breuer R, Castro VM, Churchill SE, Coryell WH, Craddock N, Craig IW, Czamara D, De Geus EJ, Degenhardt F, Farmer AE, Fava M, Frank J, Gainer VS, Gallagher PJ, Gordon SD, Goryachev S, Gross M, Guipponi M, Henders AK, Herms S, Hickie IB, Hoefels S, Hoogendijk W, Hottenga JJ, Iosifescu DV, Ising M, Jones I, Jones L, Jung-Ying T, Knowles JA, Kohane IS, Kohli MA, Korszun A, Landen M, Lawson WB, Lewis G, Macintyre D, Maier W, Mattheisen M, McGrath PJ, McIntosh A, McLean A, Middeldorp CM, Middleton L, Montgomery GM, Murphy SN, Nauck M, Nolen WA, Nyholt DR, O'Donovan M, Oskarsson H, Pedersen N, Scheftner WA, Schulz A, Schulze TG, Shyn SI, Sigurdsson E, Slager SL, Smit JH, Stefansson H, Steffens M, Thorgeirsson T, Tozzi F, Treutlein J, Uhr M, van den Oord EJCG, Van Grootheest G, Völzke H, Weilburg JB, Willemsen G, Zitman FG, Neale B, Daly M, Levinson DF, Sullivan PF. A mega-analysis of genome-wide association studies for major depressive disorder. Mol Psychiatry. 2013;18(4):497–511. PMCID: PMC3837431. http://www.ncbi.nlm.nih.gov/pubmed/22472876
208. Psychiatric Genome Consortium PGC Video Textbook
209. PsychENCODE
210. PsychENCODE Consortium | NRGR
211. Belton JM, McCord RP, Gibcus JH, Naumova N, Zhan Y, Dekker J. Hi-C: a comprehensive technique to capture the conformation of genomes. Methods. 2012;58(3):268–76. PMCID: PMC3874846 http://www.ncbi.nlm.nih.gov/pubmed/22652625
212. Genotype-Tissue Expression (GTEx) | NIH Common Fund
213. ENCODE
214. NIH Roadmap Epigenomics – GEO – NCBI
215. Abiola O, Angel JM, Avner P, Bachmanov AA, Belknap JK, Bennett B, Blankenhorn EP, Blizard DA, Bolivar V, Brockmann GA, Buck KJ, Bureau JF, Casley WL, Chesler EJ, Cheverud JM, Churchill GA, Cook M, Crabbe JC, Crusio WE, Darvasi A, de Haan G, Dermant P, Doerge RW, Elliot RW, Farber CR, Flaherty L, Flint J, Gershenfeld H, Gibson JP, Gu J, Gu W, Himmelbauer H, Hitzemann R, Hsu HC, Hunter K, Iraqi FF, Jansen RC, Johnson TE, Jones BC, Kempermann G, Lammert F, Lu L, Manly KF, Matthews DB, Medrano JF, Mehrabian M, Mittlemann G, Mock BA, Mogil JS, Montagutelli X, Morahan G, Mountz JD, Nagase H, Nowakowski RS, O'Hara BF, Osadchuk AV, Paigen B, Palmer AA, Peirce JL, Pomp D, Rosemann M, Rosen GD, Schalkwyk LC, Seltzer Z, Settle S, Shimomura K, Shou S, Sikela JM, Siracusa LD, Spearow JL, Teuscher C, Threadgill DW, Toth LA, Toye AA, Vadasz C, Van Zant G, Wakeland E, Williams RW, Zhang HG, Zou F, Complex trait consortium. The nature and identification of quantitative trait loci: a community's view. Nat Rev Genet. 2003;4(11):911–6. PMCID: PMC2063446. http://www.ncbi.nlm.nih.gov/pubmed/14634638
216. Integrative functional genomic analysis of human brain development and neuropsychiatric risks | Science
217. Transcriptome-wide isoform-level dysregulation in ASD, schizophrenia, and bipolar disorder | Science
218. Comprehensive functional genomic resource and integrative model for the human brain | Science
219. Home:: BrainSpan: Atlas of the Developing Human Brain
220. 1000 Genomes | A Deep Catalog of Human Genetic Variation
221. Disease Ontology DO
222. dataome.mensxmachina.org
223. GWAS Catalog
224. GitHub – r-duh/MultiplexDiseasomeCommunities
225. OSF | The behavioral phenotype of early life adversity: a 3-level meta-analysis of rodent studies
226. Chen W, Li C, Liang W, Li Y, Zou Z, Xie Y, Liao Y, Yu L, Lin Q, Huang M, Li Z, Zhu X. The roles of Optogenetics and Technology in Neurobiology: a review. Front Aging Neurosci. 2022;14:867863. PMCID: PMC9063564 http://www.ncbi.nlm.nih.gov/pubmed/35517048
227. Tan P, He L, Huang Y, Zhou Y. Optophysiology: illuminating cell physiology with optogenetics. Physiol Rev. 2022;102(3):1263–325. PMCID: PMC8993538. http://www.ncbi.nlm.nih.gov/pubmed/35072525
228. Emiliani V, Entcheva E, Hedrich R, Hegemann P, Konrad KR, Lüscher C, Mahn M, Pan ZH, Sims RR, Vierock J, Yizhar O. Optogenetics for light control of biological systems. Nat Rev Methods Primers. 2022;2:55. PMCID: PMC10627578. http://www.ncbi.nlm.nih.gov/pubmed/37933248
229. Poth KM, Texakalidis P, Boulis NM. Chemogenetics: beyond lesions and electrodes. Neurosurgery. 2021;89(2):185–95. PMCID: PMC8279839. http://www.ncbi.nlm.nih.gov/pubmed/33913505
230. Song J, Patel RV, Sharif M, Ashokan A, Michaelides M. Chemogenetics as a neuromodulatory approach to treating neuropsychiatric diseases and disorders. Mol Ther. 2022;30(3):990–1005. PMCID: PMC8899595. http://www.ncbi.nlm.nih.gov/pubmed/34861415
231. ENIGMA
232. de Kovel CGF, Aftanas L, Aleman A, Alexander-Bloch AF, Baune BT, Brack I, Bülow R, Busatto Filho G, Carballedo A, Connolly CG, Cullen KR, Dannlowski U, Davey CG, Dima D, Dohm K, Erwin-Grabner T, Frodl T, Fu CHY, Hall GB, Glahn DC, Godlewska B, Gotlib IH, Goya-Maldonado R, Grabe HJ, Groenewold NA, Grotegerd D, Gruber O, Harris MA, Harrison BJ, Hatton SN, Hickie IB, Ho TC, Jahanshad N, Kircher T, Krämer B, Krug A, Lagopoulos J, Leehr EJ, Li M, MacMaster

FP, MacQueen G, McIntosh AM, McLellan Q, Medland SE, Mueller BA, Nenadic I, Osipov E, Papmeyer M, Portella MJ, Reneman L, Rosa PGP, Sacchet MD, Schnell K, Schrantee A, Sim K, Simulionyte E, Sindermann L, Singh A, Stein DJ, Ubani BN, Van der Wee NJA, Van der Werff SJA, Veer IM, Vives-Gilabert Y, Völzke H, Walter H, Walter M, Schreiner MW, Whalley H, Winter N, Wittfeld K, Yang TT, Yüksel D, Zaremba D, Thompson PM, Veltman DJ, Schmaal L, Francks C. No alterations of brain structural asymmetry in major depressive disorder: an ENIGMA consortium analysis. Am J Psychiatry. 2019;176(12):1039–49. PMID: 31352813. http://www.ncbi.nlm.nih.gov/pubmed/31352813

233. Stephan KE, Baldeweg T, Friston KJ. Synaptic plasticity and dysconnection in schizophrenia. Biol Psychiatry. 2006;59(10):929–39. PMID: 16427028. http://www.ncbi.nlm.nih.gov/pubmed/16427028

234. Mood disorders prevalence U.S. adults by gender 2008–2012 | Statista

235. Feuk L, Carson AR, Scherer SW. Structural variation in the human genome. Nat Rev Genet. 2006;7(2):85–97. PMID: 16418744. http://www.ncbi.nlm.nih.gov/pubmed/16418744

236. Overview of Structural Variation

237. Deisseroth K, Feng G, Majewska AK, Miesenböck G, Ting A, Schnitzer MJ. Next-generation optical technologies for illuminating genetically targeted brain circuits. J Neurosci. 2006;26(41):10380–6. PMCID: PMC2820367. http://www.ncbi.nlm.nih.gov/pubmed/17035522

238. Gu L, Xie J, Long J, Chen Q, Chen Q, Pan R, Yan Y, Wu G, Liang B, Tan J, Xie X, Wei B, Su L. Epidemiology of major depressive disorder in mainland China: a systematic review. PLoS One. 2013;8(6):e65356. PMCID: PMC3681935. http://www.ncbi.nlm.nih.gov/pubmed/23785419

Evidence Basics

4

Franklin Sunzeri

Introduction

To appreciate the evidence behind the evidence-based random clinical trials and meta-analyses that appear in this text, it is helpful to take a very cursory review of some of the principles that guide evidence-based research. There are many excellent references on biostatistics [1–6]. We have used two of them for general references [7, 8]. When we have felt that a more tailored exposition to mental health might be warranted, we have referred to additional resources, many of which are online.

Hypothesis

After making careful observations and positing a question, the next step is to set up a testable hypothesis to answer the question. In doing so, we usually look ahead to being able to test the *null hypothesis*. The null hypothesis states that the results of an experimental comparison or correlation are due to chance. Practically speaking, the null hypothesis is the logical antithesis of the hypothesis that is being examined. Whenever a statistical analysis is performed, the null hypothesis is being tested.

It is important to remember that the null hypothesis is not a measurement of proof. Instead, when applied to a set of data, that data can only be used to reject a null hypothesis or fail to reject it. For example, if analysis of the data between two treatment groups shows no statistically different results between them, this simply means that there is not sufficient evidence to reject the null hypothesis based upon the data of that experiment. It does not mean that there is no real difference between the groups.

On the other side of the coin, if there appears to be insufficient evidence to reject the hypothesis, this does not prove the hypothesis. In some instances, false positives can be difficult to detect.

F. Sunzeri (✉)
Heather Hills Consulting, Coos Bay, OR, USA

Results

If a difference is seen in results, it could be due to *sampling variation or chance*. If the results are very different or very much alike, there is little questioning that it is not due to sampling variation. However, if the observed differences are not as apparent, it is useful to determine what the probability is that the differences are due to chance.

From probability theory, for every defined number of experiments made for statistical significance, there is a chance that the results will appear to be statistically significant when they are not really significant. This type of error is a *false positive* called a *type 1 error* or *alpha error (α-error)*. The *alpha level (α-level)* is commonly set at 0.01, 0.05, or 0.10. For example, if investigators accept that there is a 5% chance of concluding incorrectly that an intervention is effective when it has no true effect, then the alpha level will be set at 0.05. If the results of data analysis show less chance, say 1/40 or 0.025, the probability of falsely not rejecting the null hypothesis is deemed to be significant.

The *alpha score* is the set and acceptable probability that the null hypothesis is true. Psychologists usually set their alpha score to 0.05. So, probabilities are said to not be due to sampling error if the alpha score is less than 0.05.

Also from the probability field, a comparison or relationship is said to be *statistically significant* if the chance of its having occurred purely by a sampling accident is less than an agreed-upon threshold, for example, 1 out of 20 (or less than 5 out of 100; or <5%). This is expressed as $p < 0.05$. This 1 in 20 chance relates to the false positive or type 1 error rates referred to above. If the probability of it occurring by chance is $0.10 > p > 0.05$, it is considered to show a *statistical trend.*

Significant heterogeneity [an important concept in the interpretation of meta-analyses q.i] arises from clinical or methodological diversity [9]. Significant heterogeneity is usually said to be present when $p < 0.05$ of there *not* being heterogeneity. A 1 in 20 chance is the same as odds of 19 to 1 [10]. Significant heterogeneity is present when there are

J. Raber et al. (eds.), *Understanding and Treating Depressive Disorders*, https://doi.org/10.1007/978-3-032-14465-2_4

significant differences in outcomes between studies that attempt to measure the same effect.

As mentioned above, and as bears repeating here, it is important to remember that the null hypothesis is not a measurement of proof. Instead, when applied to a set of data, that data can only be used to reject a null hypothesis or fail to reject it. For example, if analysis of the data between two treatment groups shows no statistically different results between them, this simply means that there is not sufficient evidence to reject the null hypothesis based upon the data of that experiment. It does not mean that there is no real difference between the groups.

On the other side of the coin, if there appears to be insufficient evidence to reject the hypothesis, this does not prove the hypothesis.

Data Interpretation

Frequency distributions of results can be demonstrated by graphs with one of the variables on one axis and the number of subjects on the other axis. A common shape of such a graph is the *bell-shaped curve (normal distribution or Gaussian curve)*. It is frequently seen when the number of subjects or *sample size (N)* is very large and the variable has many determinants. A good example is pulse rates. The curve is symmetrical around the mean, which is equal to the mode and median on such a curve. Most frequency distributions in research do not have a normal distribution: they are *skewed* to the left or right. A *positive skew* is when the mean is on the left of the curve with the *tail* on the right and vice versa for a *negative skew*. *Bimodal distributions* occur when there is no clustering around the mean, and there are two separate tendencies in the sample. *Kurtosis* is the acuteness or flatness of the graph.

Experimental results are real for the subjects in an experiment. But, the goal of most experiments is to predict how the rest of the population might respond to a similar treatment or relate to the test situation. In the real world, there is always a degree of uncertainty in this prediction. Deviation from the mean or the *variability* of test values that diverge from the mean gives an important insight into the occurrence of those results in the population. *Range* is the most common measure of that deviation. Range is the difference between the highest and lowest values. It can be expressed in whatever value the results are expressed. For example, a range of test scores could be 65–98%, or 600 out of 800–800 out of 800.

Another way to help cope with this uncertainty is the use of confidence levels and confidence intervals (CIs). *Confidence levels* are the levels where statistical results or estimates are calculated. The most common level is the 95% confidence level, but 99% and 90% levels are sometimes used. This means that if the experiment were repeated a sufficient number of times in another population, 95% of the results would lie between the upper and lower limits of the *confidence interval (CI)*. A confidence interval is a way of quantifying the range of uncertainty surrounding a result. It is the analysis most often used by the *Cochrane Collaboration*, which is an international endeavor by researchers, health practitioners, and consumers to search through research on health care, and then to prepare, maintain, and publish systematic reviews of their findings [11]. The Collaboration is considered the platinum standard in this effort. See Fig. 4.1.

The CI extends between the lowest possible result that other members of the population could experience and the highest possible result that they could experience. The mean is somewhere in between. The CI is quite useful for numerically and graphically representing statistical significance and precision. Whether or not the limits in the CI are above or below 1 will determine if the results are significant. If the limits are both on the same side of 1, they are significant; if one limit is on one side of 1 and the other is on the opposite side of 1, the result is not significant. To show how this works, let us first look at *point estimates,* more commonly known as *relative risk (RR or risk ratio)* and *odds ratios (OR)*.

Relative risk (RR) is perhaps the most common method of expressing the estimated risk of experiencing a result. RR compares the probability of a specific outcome in the treatment group with that of a control group. When an RR is greater than 1, there seems to be an increased risk of an event. When the RR is less than 1, there appears to be a decreased risk of experiencing an event. If the RR is 1, there is no apparent risk. If the RR = 5, it is 5 times more likely to occur than in the control group. If the RR = 0.5, it is half as likely to happen as in the control group.

Odds ratios (OR) are another way of estimating the effect of a treatment (q.i.). OR compares the probability of a spe-

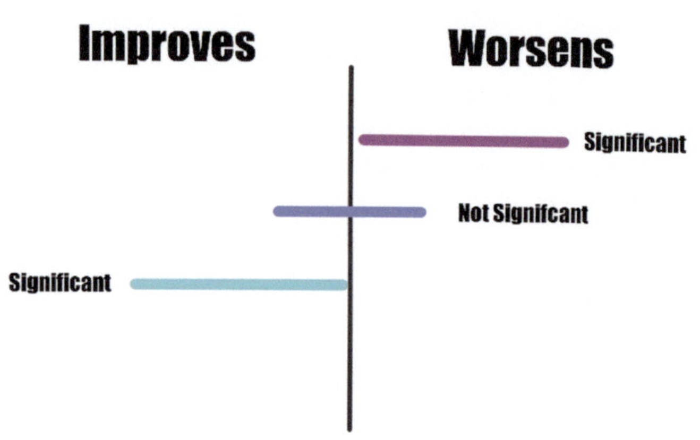

Fig. 4.1 This simplified illustration presents a confidence interval depicting the positional relationship and its upper and lower limits. The horizontal line segment represents the range of plausible values. Labels clarify the positional meaning of the CI, enhancing interpretation of statistical uncertainty and variability in a dataset

cific outcome in the treatment group (*t*) with the outcome of a control group (*c*). It is computed by the formula, [*%t* ÷ (1 − *%t*)] [*%c* ÷ (1 − *%c*)]. For example, if in a given clinical trial, the probability of death in the treatment group was 5% (*%t*) and in the control group it was 20% (*%c*), the OR of surviving is [0.05 ÷ (1 − 0.05)] [0.20 ÷ (1 − 0.20)] = 0.20.

If the OR equals 1, there is no apparent effect. If an OR is greater than 1, the treatment is expected to increase the odds (probability) of something occurring. If it is less than 1, the odds are decreased. The OR is often expressed in terms of 95% confidence intervals as with RR. OR is similar, but not exactly the same as RR.

Now back to CI significance. For example, if the RR for an event is 5.0 and the 95% confidence level goes from 1.5 to 7.0, the results are significant. This is written as RR 5.0 (95% CI: 1.5–7.0). But if the range was 0.5–7.0 (RR 5.0 (95% CI: 0.5–7.0)), it would not be significant. *Precision* in applying the results to others is demonstrated as the narrowness of the range, i.e., the power of the ability (confidence) to predict an individual real-world event is based upon the narrowness of the dispersion. For example, a CI of 2–4 is more precise than 0.2–0.6.

Graphically, a CI can be represented as a horizontal line relative to a vertical line. The line drawn to scale represents the CI range or precision. Its position, also to scale, represents its significance. If all of the horizontal line is on one side of the vertical line, it is significant. If it crosses the vertical line, it is not significant. In general, if the total line is on the left of the vertical line, the intervention improves the situation. If the total line is on the right, the intervention makes the situation worse. This graphic is also handy for representing results of multiple studies on the same intervention: here, horizontal lines are presented relative to one vertical line and each horizontal line represents the results of one study. In fact, such a representation is found in the logo for the Cochrane Collaboration.

Bayesian statistics is a statistical theory based upon a degree of belief in the probability of an event [12]. Belief is grounded on previous experience such as knowledge of situation-specific prior distribution of previous experiments, or on personal beliefs about the event. A *credible interval (CrI)* characterizes a probability distribution wherein a particular unobserved event has the probability of occurring within that interval. The intervals may be predictive probabilities or posterior probabilities. A *credible set* is a generalization.

In contradistinction to frequentist confidence intervals, Bayesian credible intervals base the probability on prior knowledge and treat their boundaries as fixed and the estimated event as random or uncertain [13]. Their target is the analysis of the uncertainty of the target parameter. On the other hand, the frequentist confidence intervals consider their boundaries as random variables and the event as a fixed value. So, confidence intervals refer to the randomness of the confidence intervals based upon a given number of repeated trials. In confidence intervals, a sufficiently large number of repeated samples would ensure a 95% chance that the interval would include the true fixed value of the random sample.

Effect size or *treatment effect* is a scale-free standardized evaluation of the effect of an intervention. It measures the difference in outcome between intervention groups (or experimental intervention and control). Or put another way, the signal-to-noise ratio: the difference in the group means divided by the variability of the groups. It has found its greatest use for quantifying effects measured on arbitrary or unfamiliar scales and for comparing the relative effects from different studies [14]. It is most easily used on normal distributions of controls and experimental groups. One problem with significance tests such as t tests expressed in probabilities is that results depend on both the size of the effect and the size of the sample. This may be important because a very large sample size with only a very small effect could show a similar significance, as could a very large effect with a very small sample. It is of course important to know the statistical significance so that firm conclusions are not drawn on results from a small data set where confidence is not warranted. However, statistical significance does *not* tell us the most important thing, which is the size of the effect.

Effect size is most frequently expressed as correlations (RR or OR) for dichotomous results and as a difference in means for continuous results. The simplest effect size equation is the quantity of the mean of the experimental group minus the mean of the control group, this quantity divided by the standard deviation (see below). Effect sizes coupled with CI carry the same information as tests of statistical significance but with the priority on the significance rather than the sample size.

Effect sizes derived from *meta-analysis* are in its simplest form expressed as *Cohen's d* the *standard difference,* which is the mean difference between groups in standard form, which is the ratio of the difference between the means to the standard deviation [7, 15]. However, in meta-analysis, when comparing effect sizes across groups, conversion of *F* values (q.i.), *p* values, and *t* values to RR or RR is said to be easier than for "*d*." *Hedges' g* scores are another measure of effect size also based upon the difference between the means. Hedges g scores are interpreted very similar to Cohen's d scores [16, 17].

Conventional values for the effect size expressed as *d* or *g* are: small: $d = 0.20$, medium: $d = 0.50$, large: $d = 0.80$ [43, 2, 10). Effects size values are perhaps the easiest to comprehend in terms of the average percentile ranking of the experimental group compared to that of the control group. If the sample has a normal distribution, an effect size of $d = 0.0$ says that the mean of the experimental group is comparable to the 50th percentile of the control group. If $d = 0.5$, the mean of the experimental group is comparable to the 69th percentile of the control. If $d = 0.8$, it is comparable to the 79th percentile. If $d = 1.3$ it is comparable to the 90th percentile. If $d = 2.0$ it is equivalent to the 97.7th percentile. If $d = 3.0$, it is equivalent to the 99.9th percentile.

However, the magnitude of the effect size depends on the subject matter [18]. For example, if a size of effect of 0.04 occurs in drug research, it may be strong enough to save even 4 more lives, then it may warrant further research [19].

One of the powers of meta-analyses is pointing out heterogeneity in effect sizes across studies. When they are not homogeneous, it can point the way to moderators that can be investigated for their influence on the heterogeneity [10].

Standardized mean difference (SMD) and *weighted mean difference (WMD)* are used in meta-analyses to compare the results of randomized controlled trial (RCTs) [20]. When results of the mean differences are pooled after weighting for precision, it is called the WMD. When the results of RCTs are expressed in different units, the mean differences cannot be pooled. In that case, mean differences can be divided by their respective SDs. This gives the SMD. When the SD of the devisor is the pooled SD, the SMD is Cohen's d. Continuous data using the same scale can be evaluated and summarized using WMD and the 95% CI. The weighted mean is similar to the arithmetic mean except that some of the data points contribute more to the mean than others [21].

Risk reduction or risk difference is the difference in risk between two groups. For example, if the incidence for AIDS is 5% in one group and 2% in another group, the risk difference is 3%.

Absolute risk reduction compares the mean or probability of the treatment effect of the outcome on a control vs. a treatment group. It is defined as $\%t - \%c$ or where μ = the mean: $\mu t - \mu c$. For example, in an intervention where the percentage of death in the control group was 20% and the percentage of death in the treatment group was 10%, the risk reduction would be $0.20 - 0.10 = 0.10$. One common use of RR is in assessing *relative risk reduction*; in that case, the formula would be $(\%c - \%t) \div \%c$. For example, if in a given clinical trial, the probability of death in the treatment group was 5% ($\%t$) and in the control group it was 20% ($\%c$), the RR reduction is $(0.20 - 0.05) \div (0.20) = 0.75$.

Another very common measure of deviation from the mean is the *standard deviation from the mean* (σ) which is usually better than the range in taking into account the deviation from the mean of every measurement and is therefore less influenced by rare very high or very low values. The standard deviation is given by the square root of the resultant value obtained by the sum of the squares of the differences between each value and the mean, divided by the number of measurements minus one. In a normal distribution of values, 68% of the measurements lie between −1 and +1 standard deviations from the mean; 95% are between −2 and +2 standard deviations; and 99% lie between −3 and +3 standard deviations from the mean. *Z scores* are based upon how many deviations a value is above or below the mean. *Standard error of the mean (SE)* is the standard deviation divided by the square root of the number of people sampled [22]. It measures the accuracy with which a sample distribution represents a population. SE is the variation between the calculated mean of the population and one which is accepted as accurate. The SE tends to decrease with the more data points of the mean.

An *F-test* compares variances to determine if the ratios of variances among multiple samples are significantly different [23]. It is an important test to determine if the null hypothesis should be rejected or not.

Chi squared is used to ascertain the significance between two or more percentages. Heterogeneity between comparable studies is often assessed using Chi-square tests and visual inspection of graphic presentation of results.

When results of different studies on the same subject are similar or consistent, they are called *homogeneous*. When the results from different studies on the same subject diverge or are conflicting, they are called *heterogeneous*. Remember that *significant heterogeneity* indicates that the results are not "relevantly significant" [24, 25]. In other words, if the p-value for the χ^2 test of heterogeneity is less than 0.05 in a pooled survey (i.e., probability that the results are *not* due to heterogeneity), this means that the results indicate significant heterogeneity, and the results of the various studies are inconsistent. Sometimes the bar is set higher than <0.05. Before combining results of different studies, one should ask if the studies are so clinically heterogeneous that it makes no sense to try to combine them [26]. One problem with meta-analyses is pooling too few studies, which may lead to spurious results [27]. *Forest plots* are a graphical summary of a meta-analysis, including effect size for each study, the 95% CI, the differentiation of effect sizes, outliers, and the pooled effect size [28].

Meta-analysis, a critical element of systematic reviews [29, 30], is a powerful tool to *pool data* or summarize the results of several studies into a single estimate of their combined significance. *Doing meta-analysis in mental health research a practical guide* by Pim Cuijpers is a very lucid exposition on the utility of meta-analysis for health care providers [31]. Meta-analysis is the method used to produce the graphs of confidence intervals of all the studies such as is found in the Cochrane Collaboration's logo. There are two phases to meta-analyses. The first phase computes effect sizes for the different studies. As mentioned above, effect sizes express the magnitude of the relationship between two variables. For example, effect sizes can express the size of the differences in immune responses between the group receiving an intervention and the control group. Importantly, this is independent of the size of the samples. In the second phase, the effect sizes of the individual studies are pooled in a way that reflects an aggregate difference in response between the two groups relative to those variables and that response. So, if there are several immune responses that are analyzed, there could be several affect sizes that are calculated. One of the powers of meta-analyses is pointing out heterogeneity in effect sizes across studies. When they are not homogeneous, it can point the way to moderators that can be investigated for their influence on the heterogeneity [10]. See Fig. 4.2.

I^2-statistic is an indicator of heterogeneity in percentages. As mentioned above, when the results from different studies on the same subject diverge or are conflicting, they are called *heterogeneous* A value of 0% indicates no observed heterogeneity, and larger values indicate increasing heterogeneity, with 25% as low, 50% as moderate, and 75% as high heterogeneity [10]. A 95% confidence interval around I^2 is frequently used [32, 33]. Often, the prediction interval is expressed, which indicates the range in which the true effect size of 95% of all populations will fall.

Secondary studies are studies of studies (*primary studies*). In meta-analyses, to ensure studies with most precise estimates contribute more to the ultimate estimation of effect, the inverse of variance is used to weight each study. Meta-analysis software is available using Review Manger 4.0.4 software from the Cochrane Collaboration. *Fixed effect analysis* and *random effect analysis* are two types of meta-analyses [34].

Network meta-analysis (NMA) compares multiple treatments simultaneously in a single analysis by combining direct and indirect evidence within a network of RCTs. Network meta-analysis may assist in assessing comparative effectiveness of different treatments regularly used in clinical practice [35–37].

Mixed-effects meta-analysis [38] and *three-level meta-analysis* are powerful meta-analyses [39].

In meta-analysis, of binary studies with rare events, the *Peto odds ratio (POR)* method has become the relative effect estimator of choice [40]. However, the POR can cause biased results for the OR when treatment effects are large or there are large group size differences between the control and the

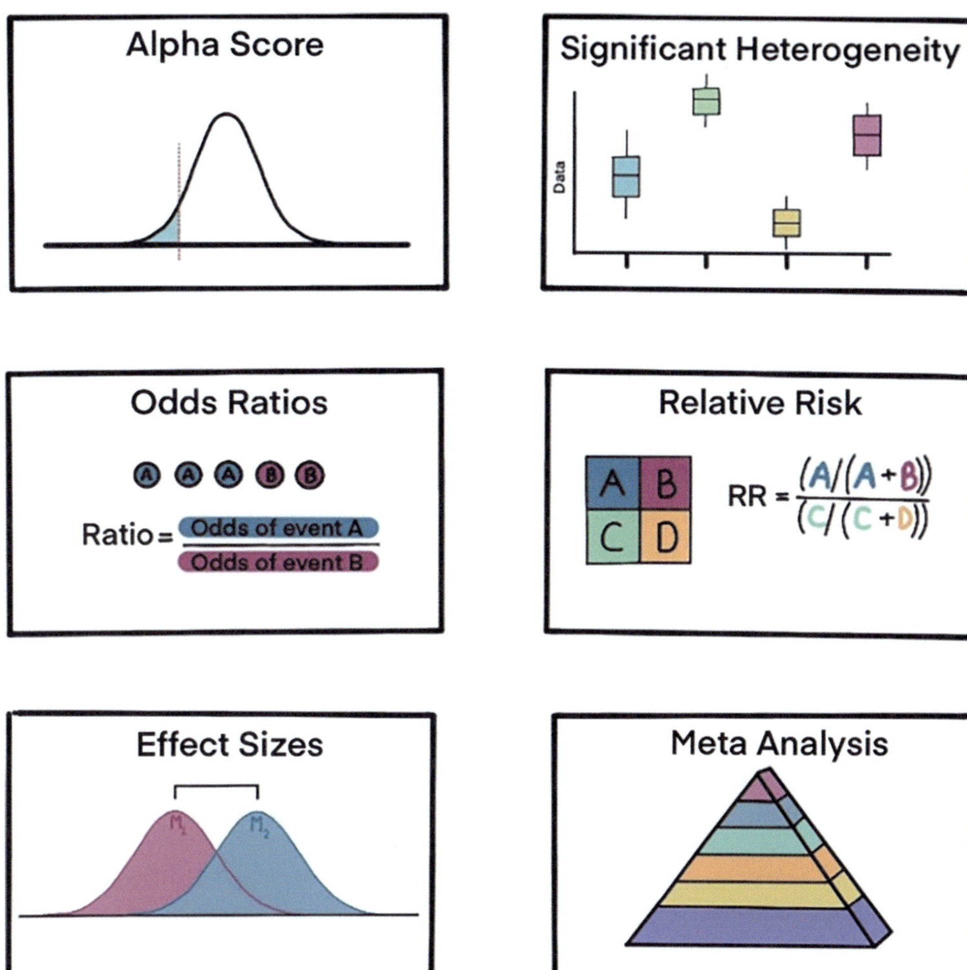

Fig. 4.2 This illustration depicts key concepts in meta-analysis, including alpha level thresholds, indicators of significant heterogeneity, and visual cues for odds ratios, relative risk, and effect sizes across studies. Together, these elements highlight the statistical landscape of evidence synthesis and the variability inherent in pooled data analysis

treatment group. But, the POR can be quite useful in many circumstances [41, 42].

Outcomes may be *mutually exclusive* if one occurs, the other cannot occur. An *exhaustive set* is one in which one of the outcomes must occur and a *mutually exclusive exhaustive set* is one in which one must occur but only one in a single trial. There are *independent events* if the occurrence or non-occurrence of one does not affect the probability of occurrence of the other.

Prevalence rates are the number of cases at a given point in time divided by the number of persons in the population at that time. It is often expressed as a percentage or expressed per 100,000. *Incidence rates* are the number of new cases occurring during a given time divided by the total or average number of people in the population during that time. The time is usually 1 year. *Endemic* refers to a condition that is continuously present in a population. *Epidemics* result when the number of cases exceeds the number of cases expected for that time for a defined population. In contrast to endemics, the disease is introduced from the outside and is not continuously present. *Pandemics* are epidemics afflicting a large geographic area.

Validity is the measure of how well or accurately an experiment (test or procedure) measures what it claims to. *Internal validity* is the degree that a study measures what it was designed to measure. *External validity* is the degree of generalizability of the results to others who were not in the study. *Concurrent validity* is how well a test predicts the performance of or agrees with another measurement by another means performed at the same or about the same time. *Content validity* is the degree to which an experiment is representing that which is to be measured. *Criterion-related validity* or *predictive validity* is the degree to which performance on an experiment accurately predicts real-life results. *Face validity* is the degree to which the experiment appears to sample that which it is supposed to measure.

A *construct* is a hypothetical variable that is being measured [43]. When administering an evaluation survey, it is important to be assured that the tool that is being used to evaluate a construct will elicit reliable and consistent responses, even if the questions in the survey are replaced by similar questions. If a variable is generated by a set of questions that have been shown to elicit such a consistent and stable response, the variable is said to be *reliable*. The central issue then is how well a group of variables (items) measures a latent construct.

Reliability is measured by repeatability and reproducibility. *Repeatability* is the ability to get the same result from the same subject or very similar subjects for the same experiment when repeated by the same researcher. *Reproducibility* is the ability to get the same result from the same or very similar subjects for the same experiment when repeated by a different researcher in a different space/time. *Inter-rater reliability* is the degree to which two researchers agree upon the test outcome. It is frequently measured by a *weighted kappa* score [44].

People are inconsistent and poor subjects for experiments. As test takers, we can make errors on many levels. We can be inattentive, easily distracted, hate repetition, want to please, misinterpret… As test givers or observers, we can be equally unreliable. We have our own prejudices, tend to daydream, lose our focus, misinterpret… All this adds up to questionable reliability and can confound interpretation of experimental results.

Reliability should not be confused with *dependability*, which is more akin to measurement validity although embodying reliability too. Reliability when used in research is a measure that, if assuming that what we are measuring is not changing, will be the same every time we take it. It is most frequently used as synonymous with repeatability or consistency. It is also important to realize that we can never actually compute reliability: we can only estimate it [45]. This is true because we can never calculate the *variance* of the true score. According to *True Score Theory*, when we make an observation of a score for what we are measuring, we never actually see the true score or actual value for the person we are measuring or for that matter the error in measuring it [45]. For example, the person may have had an atypical day: perhaps the person did not understand the question, had an argument before, been distracted, or otherwise produced a value that was not typical. Given human nature, the score is more often likely to have been lower than higher.

The measures of reliability tell us what portion of the *variability* in the measured value is due to the true score. So, reliability is a ratio. It is the ratio of the variance of the true score to the variance of the measure. Variance as stated earlier is the sum of the squared deviations of the scores from their mean, divided by the number of scores. Because we cannot see true scores, we need to use our observed scores and assume that the observed scores are related by the amount that they both share the same true scores. Therefore, to estimate the correlation between two observed scores we look at their *covariance* (shared variance). Then, the covariance is an estimate of the variance in true scores.

Simplifying this, reliability can be calculated as the ratio of the variance of the true scores to the variance of the observed scores (which is the sum of the variance of the true score and the variance of the error). Reliability estimates range between 0 and 1. In estimates of reliability, a value of zero means the measure is entirely in error and there is no true score. A value of one means that there is no error in measurement, and we are seeing only the true score. A value of 0.5 means that an estimated 50% of what we are measuring is due to error. A value of 0.9 means that 90% of the variance of the observed score is due to the truth and 10% due to measurement error.

Trochim has pointed out four general classes of reliability estimates [46]. *Inter-rater or interobserver reliability* is a way of rating the raters. If observations are assigned to categories, one can compare the amount of agreement in assignments to each category. If the measurement is continuous, raters' observations could be compared at regular time intervals. When a measurement is an observation, it is considered one of the best ways to estimate reliability. But it requires multiple observers. *Test-retest reliability* is estimated by giving the same test to the same or quite similar sample on different occasions. The drawback is that the longer the period between retesting, the greater the likelihood that the construct will have changed. This test is often used in experimental studies with a no-treatment control group. *Parallel-forms reliability* is tested by creating two independent forms or sets of questions that are administered one after another to the same sample of people. Usually, the tests are randomly assigned so that one part of the sample gets one of the tests first, and the other part of the sample gets the other test first. It is most often used when researchers intend to use two different tests to measure the same thing. It can be difficult in complex or subjective constructs to produce enough test items to measure the same construct. *Internal-consistency reliability* uses a single test instrument administered once to the same group of people. The basic idea is to determine if different items in the instrument that are set up to determine the same aspect of the construct yield the same results. This type of reliability may be the most commonly assessed and it is most often used when there are many items to be evaluated. Because inter-rater and test-retest tests involve either more than one observer or differing times, their reliability scores are often lower than parallel-forms and internal-consistency.

There are a fair number of vehicles that can be used to measure internal consistency [46]. The *average inter-item correlation* is the mean of all the correlations between each and all of the test items used to measure the same construct. The *average-item total correlation* uses the same data as the average interitem correlation but adds another variable that is the mean of the total correlations for each of those items. In *split-half correlations*, the whole test is given to the same group of people. Then, the items used to measure the same construct are randomly divided in half and the estimated correlation is the correlation between the total scores for each half. *Cronbach's alpha* is a mathematically clever way of averaging all possible randomly created split-half estimates.

Cronbach's alpha [47] is also sometimes known as a *scale reliability coefficient*. From each survey item, a score is computed, and an overall rating known as a scale is derived as the sum of these scores for all the survey items. The reliability (α) is defined as the square of the correlation between the measured scale and the underlying factor that the scale was designed to measure. Cronbach's alpha coefficient ranges between 0 and 1. It is used to estimate the reliability of factors derived from dichotomous (questions with only two possible answers) or multipoint type questionnaires or rating scales. The closer that the alpha coefficient is to 1, the greater the reliability of the generated result is. Although the literature sometimes uses lower acceptable values, it is generally thought that 0.7 or higher is an acceptable reliability coefficient [48].

Number needed to treat (NNT) is a useful measure of the number of people needed to be treated before a beneficial outcome can be anticipated. Number needed to treat is the inverse of absolute risk reduction. For example, if trial results indicated that the probability of an adverse reaction in the treatment group was 10% (*%t*) and in the control group was 30% (*%c*), then the number needed to treat would be $1 \div (\%c - \%t) = 1.0 \div (0.30 - 0.10) = 5$ patients. Another perspective on NNT would be, if, for example, 15 people needed to take a heart attack-preventing drug before one heart attack was prevented, the NNT would be 15 [49].

Association is a known link or a statistical connection between two or more variables. A *positive association* is one wherein the incidence of one variable increases if the other variable increases. A *negative association* is one wherein the incidence of one variable decreases if the other variable decreases. *Inverse associations* are ones where if one variable increases, the other variable decreases; or if one decreases, the other increases.

Regression to the mean is the tendency for random decreases or increases to be followed by values or observations closer to the mean.

Surrogate measures are ones that are substituted for another measure during an experiment, for example, measuring respiratory rates instead of lung capacity.

Stratification is the division of a group of subjects by various criteria. For example, a study population may be subgrouped based on age, socioeconomics, gender, etc. Comparisons and contrasts within the results of an experiment may be made on such strata to find differences in response to treatment.

Heritability is a term that has been inconsistently applied and interpreted [50–54]. Heritability is cogently defined by Rose as "an estimate of the genetic and environmental contributions to the variance of any phenotypic measure around the mean for a given population" [51]. *Variance* is the term that describes how far apart the individual measurements are. Because heritability is defined for a given population in a specific environment, if the environment changes, the heritability changes. This limits extrapolation from one population to another.

If the environment were held constant, heritability would refer to the genetic contribution to the variance. Heritability does not address causes for differences between populations. It measures the amount of *variation* in a trait that can be ascribed to genes *not the amount caused by genes.* If the environment changes in a way that has a differential impact on individuals in that population, then the heritability of that trait might change [55].

Twin studies are frequently used to examine heritability. These studies usually discuss three influences on variations of a trait. These are additive genetic influences, nonshared environmental influences, and shared environmental influences [48]. *Additive genetic influences* are the net result of the sum of the individual alleles that contribute to variation of a trait. *Non-shared environmental influences* are those parts of the environment with which siblings have a different interaction, i.e., they are not correlated (e.g., taking ballet lessons or not). *Shared environmental influences* are aspects of the home environment that are shared, i.e., perfectly correlated (e.g., access to the same food at home).

Heritability ranges from 0 to 1 with 1 taken as indicating that all the *variations* of the particular trait are genetic, and 0 as none of the variations are due to genetics. It is also fairly common to express heritability in percentages.

Caveats

There are many subjects and studies that will be discussed in the following chapters. It will not always be clear whether divergent results are due to methodological errors, fallacies, pseudoscience, or merely the normal vicissitudes to be expected in reproducibility. So, it is wise for us to be on our guard. Producing and interpreting data is subject to uncertainty due to its relationship to our biases and fallacies that may influence our pursuit of the "truth."

Biases

A comprehensive list of dozens of biases can be found in the following website [56]. Their broad categories are decision-making, belief, and behavioral biases; social biases; and memory errors and biases. We will only touch upon a few of these that may be relevant to the current discussion.

There are a number of caveats that need to be considered when evaluating experimental results. One of those is the use of clinically relevant, ecologically valid, and provocative stressors (such as the *Trier Social Stress Test*) instead of sad music or negative slides [57]. The stressors that most frequently cause a depressive episode are ones that are interpersonal and often related to rejection, loss, or other forms of social evaluation [58–61].

Davidson et al. have pointed out the importance of considering time course of emotional reactions [62–64]. They suggest that emotional reactivity and regulation in response to a stressor can be before, during, or after exposure to the stressor. In some mood and anxiety disorders, there may be a failure to quickly terminate a response and/or a dysfunctionally early onset of the response.

Research allegiance (RA) can be prominent especially in comparative outcome research [65–67]. Indeed, a 2013 meta-meta-analysis of all available meta-analytic estimates of the RA-outcome in psychotherapy research found a moderate effect size and a substantial and robust association [68]. Moderating variables included characteristics of treatment, populations, and the type of RA assessment.

Ludwig and Kabat-Zinn have pointed out some potential pitfalls in mindfulness-based stress reduction research that can apply to psychotherapy studies in general [69]. These hazards include few participants, no active control groups, using only subjective endpoints, no details of participant characteristics that could be used to generalize results, inadequately detailed treatment methods, inadequate documentation of participant's protocol adherence, and infrequent use of biologic measures.

There are difficulties with evidence-based double-blinding of psychotherapy clinical trials especially for cognitive-behavioral therapy (CBT) [70]. Subjective endpoint ratings by the subjects involved in psychotherapy major depressive disorder (MDD) clinical trials contradict the possibility of double blindness [71, 72]. Even if the reviewers do not know the allocations, the subjects know what treatment they received [73, 74]. Single blindness in a trial actually refers to the subjects not knowing what they are receiving, so these studies are not even single blinded [74]. It has been suggested that a better term to describe psychotherapeutic trials for MDD would be "*partially-controlled clinical data*" [70]. Spontaneous improvement of depression symptoms due to the placebo effect may be significant [75, 76].

It appears that placebo use by primary care physicians is prevalent [77]. It also appears that placebos do not have to be deceptive for them to work. It is said that "*open label placebos*" can be ethically used. As of 2019, 14 small-scale clinical and experimental trials using open-label placebos have been performed. Mechanisms and effects of placebos in psychological treatment appear to be largely unexplored [78].

One of the confounders in evaluating psychotherapeutic treatments is experimenter's allegiance (EA) [68, 79]. Experimenter's allegiance denotes an experimenter's personal belief in the superiority of a specific psychotherapeutic treatment [79]. EA has sometimes been linked to larger treatment effects. Analysis of 30 meta-analyses including 240 RCTs found significant allegiance effects for all forms of psychotherapy except for CBT [79]. In addition, out of 146 eligible meta-analyses that evaluated data from 1198 unique RCTs, only 17.2% of the meta-analyses reported EA and 4.1% controlled for its influence on results [80]. Out of the 1198 unique RCTs, 66.3% showed EA while 3.2% reported their allegiance and only one (0.2%) controlled its effect.

Attrition bias happens when those who dropped out of the study are not reported. RCTs that include only those who completed the study produce higher effects than those that include all randomized participants in the analyses [81].

Findings on studies use a variety of depression assessment tools. *Beck Depression Inventory (BDI)* that is universally among the most used self-rating scales for measuring depression has advantages and disadvantages [82].

Use of *Hamilton Depression Rating Scale (HAMD)* has multiple problems including different versions with different sensitivities. For example, in evaluating combined treatment of interpersonal psychotherapy and Nefazodone, no differences between treatments were found on the HAMD. However, using the *Montgomery-Åsberg Depression Rating Scale (MADRS)* the combination was more effective in reducing depression symptoms compared to medication alone, but not to psychotherapy alone or interpersonal therapy (IPT) with pill-placebo [83]. It has been suggested that it is a good idea to replace the Hamilton Depression Rating Scale as the primary outcome measure in treatment studies of depression [84, 85].

Combining results of studies that used different assessments such as the MADRS [86] that are more sensitive to treatment effect than the HAMD [86] and the BDI which correlates weakly with the Hamilton Depression Rating Scale (HDRS) [87] may be fraught with pitfalls.

Waiting list controls can be problematic, as these patients do not experience placebo effects. As a result, when waiting list controls are used in active treatment studies, treatment effects can seem to be artificially high. Placebo effects in double-blind antidepressant studies can average 35–40% [88, 89]. That is 35–40% of the control group can respond to a placebo with a 50% reduction in symptoms. As a result, the influence of placebo is very difficult to calculate when the control is merely waiting and not blind.

The *sex of experimenters* can affect apparent baseline responses in behavioral experiments [90]. Experiments found that exposure of mice and rats to male but not female experimenters caused a robust physiological stress response and related analgesia [90]. They also found that T-shirts worn by men, compounds from the human male axilla, and bedding material from intact and unfamiliar male mammals produced similar results. This stress response not only diminishes physical pain but also alters behavior and hormone levels. Lack of replication and reproducibility in some research involving rodent behavior might be related to such responses.

How might this relate to experiments with human behavior?

Other difficulties with interpreting results include the following. Lack of intention to treat analysis may enter a risk of bias. Some treatment effects are evaluated after periods that may be too short to gain the best effect [91]. Other variables include publication bias and clarity, remission and response definitions, manualized vs. nonmanualized, adherence to protocol, Western vs. Eastern, dates of studies, small number of studies, highly heterogeneous population of studies, allocation kept from assessors, and how allocation was randomized [92, 93]. And there is the *file-drawer effect*. The File-drawer effect is the practice of filing away or not publishing negative results or nonconfirmatory results [94, 95].

A *trim and fit* approach to deal with *publication bias* has been suggested and is frequently implemented in dealing with meta-analyses [96]. It is a nonparametric[1] method for estimating the number of missing studies that might exist in a meta-analysis and the effect that these studies might have had on their outcome [94]. Publication bias occurs in clinical studies because studies with favorable results are more likely to be published than are those with unfavorable results, which thereby exaggerate the synthesized evidence in meta-analyses [23, 95, 98].

Systematic Reviews

Systematic reviews attempt to find, select, and collate all available evidence that fits a clear prespecified criteria in an attempt to answer a clearly formulated research question. Through the use of rigorous systematic methods, these reviews attempt to reduce bias and arrive at useful and reliable findings that can be the basis for drawing conclusions and making decisions [99–101].

A *review of systematic reviews* provides easy access to a comprehensive review of interventions, and compiles evidence from all appropriate sources. It has been asserted that more than half of systematic reviews are out of date 5.5 years after publication [102]. *Qualitative indicators* for being out of date include substantial differences in characterizations of effectiveness, new information about harm, and caveats about the previously reported findings that would affect clinical decision making. *Quantitative indications* for the need to update are changes in statistical significance or relative changes in effect magnitude of at least 50% involving one of the primary outcomes of the original systematic review or any mortality outcome. Living systematic reviews have been proposed to ensure timely updates [103].

Although reviews of systematic reviews can be powerful, they have several limitations [104]. They can draw their conclusions only from interventions that have been assessed by systematic reviews, so some RCTs that have not been systematically reviewed will not be included. Those RCTs that

[1] IBM succinctly states, "Parametric statistics are *based on assumptions about the distribution of population from which the sample was taken*. Nonparametric statistics are not based on assumptions, that is, the data can be collected from a sample that does not follow a specific distribution" [93].

do get reviewed may not supply a complete set of variables and stratifications. It is more difficult to provide quality control when the review relies on the investigatory biases and techniques of the original reviewers. Often, characteristics of the populations, interventions, comparators, and outcomes may be less than optimal or incompletely described. Reliability of results is dependent upon the number and quality of available studies.

The *AMSTAR (Assessing Methodological quality of Systematic Reviews)* is a reliable and valid measurement tool to assess the methodological quality (risk of bias, etc.) of systematic reviews [105].

Now, a few more words about bias assessment in clinical trials. Definitions about RCT bias can be found in the *Cochrane Handbook for Systematic Reviews of Interventions* [9]. Typically, the following domains are evaluated: allocation sequence generation, allocation concealment, blinding of participants and personnel, blinding of outcome assessors, incomplete outcome data, selective outcome reporting, for-profit bias and other bias. RCTs that are analyzed to have "uncertain risk of bias" or "high risk of bias" in one or more of these specified domains are considered trials at "high risk of bias." If trials are found to have a "low risk of bias" in all of those domains, then it is considered to be "trials at low risk of bias." In behavioral interventions, it is usually not possible to mask the allocation, so blinding is not possible. In such circumstances, the risks in the other domains are reported.

The risk of bias can be assessed by the *Cochrane risk of bias tool for randomized trials* [106]. The tool particularly emphasizes how to deal with adequate sequence generation, allocation concealment, blinding, incomplete outcome data addressed, selective reporting, and other potential threats to validity. *Funnel plots* can facilitate looking for publication bias or small sample bias but need to be interpreted with caution [107].

Standardized mean difference [SMD] is a measure of effect size in meta-analyses when the studies all assess the same outcome but measure it in a variety of ways [108]. In systematic reviews, the SMD is the mean difference in depression score between the intervention and control groups divided by the pooled SD at follow-up. This gives a unit-free effect size. The conventional SMD effects sizes of 0.2 (small), 0.5 (medium), and 0.8 (large) are used. Dichotomous variables are usually expressed as risk ratio with a 95% CI.

Even though low "p" values suggest that it is possible to reject the null hypothesis, it is a bit more complicated in meta-analysis. If the actual measured differences in effects of the compared interventions are the result of reasoning or knowledge which proceeds from theoretical deduction (a priori) rather than from "true" observation or experience, this needs to be factored in. To do this the *Bayes factor* is implemented [25416419]. The Bayes factor is the ratio of the p-value probabilities of the meta-analysis result divided by the probability of the anticipated effect, or "true" effect. An eight-step approach has been suggested to better validate meta-analytical results in systematic reviews [109]. If a Bayes factor is less than 0.1and there is a low p value, and if bias can be ruled out, then the observed result is compatible with the a priori expected effect. But, if the Bayes factor is greater than 0.1, the result is not compatible with the a priori expected effect and the effect may actually be lower.

The potential of missing data (which is incomplete outcome data bias) can be assessed by procedures described in reference [109] and intention-to-treat analysis in reference [110].

Another problem is that large heterogeneity can be driven by small studies inflating the effects of random-effects analysis [111]. Study design characteristics may lead to exaggeration of intervention effect estimates and increases in between-trial heterogeneity in trials reporting subjectively assessed outcomes [112].

The *CONSORT (Consolidated Standards of Reporting Trials) Statement* was developed to help biomedical researchers report RCTs transparently [113]. An extension to the CONSORT 2010 was published in 2018 to help behavioral and social scientists report RCTs transparently; it is called the statement for social and psychological interventions (*CONSORT-SPI 2018)* [114, 115].

To help improve the content and quality of protocols, an international group of stakeholders developed the *SPIRIT 2013 Statement (Standard Protocol Items: Recommendations for Interventional Trials)*. The SPIRIT statement provides guidance in the form of a checklist of recommended items to include in a clinical trial protocol [116].

Best Treatment Considerations

The following studies have revealed important considerations to keep in mind when assessing the best treatment for a given patient.

In a multivariate metaregression analysis, controlling for major characteristics of the participants, interventions and study designs, psychotherapies appeared to be equally efficacious in younger and older adults (older adults: $d = 0.74$; 95% CI: 0.49–0.99; younger adults: $d = 0.67$; 95% CI: 0.58–0.76) [117].

An early study has suggested that reminiscence and life review may have a significant effect on depression symptoms in the elderly [118]. An overall effect size of 0.84 (95% CI: 0.31–1.37). A larger effect size was seen in those who were more depressed ($d = 1.23$) vs less depressed ($d = 0.37$).

Data from the *1995–2006 Health and Retirement Study*, which sampled 17,196 Americans over 50 years of age with up to six repeated observations, were used to identify distinct courses of depressive symptoms among middle-aged and older Americans and to discover how these changes relate to race or ethnicity [119]. They identified six principal trajectories "(1) minimal depressive symptoms (15.9%), (2) low depressive symptoms (36.3%), (3) moderate and stable depressive symptoms (29.2%), (4) high but decreasing depressive symptoms (6.6%), (5) moderate but increasing depressive symptoms (8.3%), and (6) persistently high depressive symptoms (3.6%)." Hispanics and blacks were significantly more likely than whites to belong to one of the trajectories with greater depression symptoms and were more likely to experience both increasing and decreasing symptoms. Socioeconomic status, marital status, and health status partially mediated these differences.

A 2012 systematic review found four articles that they used to investigate whether depressed patients with *comorbid chronic somatic illnesses* are a high risk for recurrence of depression [120]. They concluded that there is no evidence of an association between an increased risk for recurrence of depression and chronic somatic illness.

There is evidence that most patients with psychotic disorders have sought help for mood or anxiety disorders or substance use before the onset of psychosis [121].

Self-criticism may predict different responses to treating MDD [122]. Participants (n = 102) who received either cognitive-behavioral therapy (CBT), interpersonal therapy (IPT), or pharmacotherapy with clinical management (PHT-CM) were evaluated for self-criticism, dependency, and treatment outcome. Self-criticism predicted poorer treatment response to IPT based upon symptom severity and showed a trend to better treatment response to PHT-CM. There was a trend for dependency to predict worse treatment response to CBT.

A 2013 metaregression analysis attempted to analyze how *amount, frequency, and intensity* of *therapy* are related to psychotherapeutic effects in treating adult depression [123]. They found 70 studies (92 comparisons) with 5403 patients that compared individual psychotherapy with controls. They found no significant association between effect size and number of sessions, total contact time, or duration of therapy. On the other hand, they did find a strong association between effect size and number of sessions per week. Increasing the number of sessions from one to two per week increased the effect size ($g = 0.45$), which suggested concentrating the sessions might be beneficial.

Stepped care may be as beneficial to those patients who are severely depressed as it is to people who are less severely depressed [124]. A meta-analysis of 16 data sets including 2470 depressed patients was performed. Low-intensity interventions (guided self-help by means of written materials and limited professional support, and internet-delivered interventions) appeared to have a larger effect size on those who were severely depressed at baseline (−0.1; 95% CI: −0.19–0.002). It was unclear to the study's authors if this was a clinically significant difference.

Self-report measures and clinician-rated instruments for adult depression are not necessarily equivalent [125]. A 2010 meta-analysis of 48 studies including 2462 participants showed that clinician ratings demonstrated significantly higher effect sizes than self-reports from the same studies.

Five levels of evidence have been summarized by the Oxford Centre for Evidence-Based Medicine OCEBM Levels of Evidence Working Group [126].

Summary

Adhering to sound investigative methodology is the foundation for constructing useful data. Cognitive biases across decision-making, social, and memory realms are important considerations when interpreting results and providing therapy. Placebos, experimenter bias, and methodological flaws affect depression studies. Systematic reviews face updating challenges. RCT bias evaluation is crucial.

We have briefly reviewed these considerations. They are vital in evaluating the best treatment for any individual. With them, we are prepared in succeeding chapters to evaluate evidence for individual psychotherapies, pharmacotherapies, and complementary and alternative therapies.

References

1. Sawilowsky S. New effect size rules of thumb. J Mod Appl Stat Methods. 2009;8(2):467–74.
2. https://academic.oup.com/innovateage/article/3/4/igz036/5560156.
3. https://www.researchgate.net/publication/301815425_Metaanalyses_in_mental_health_research_A_practical_guide.
4. What is effect size? A guide for users Robert Coe: www Version. 2000. http://www.cemcentre.org/renderpage.asp?linkid=30325016.
5. Lakens D. Calculating and reporting effect sizes to facilitate cumulative science: a practical primer for t-tests and ANOVAs. Front Psychol. 2013;4:863. PMCID: PMC3840331. http://www.ncbi.nlm.nih.gov/pubmed/24324449.
6. Shen J, He X. Generalized F test and generalized deviance test in two-way ANOVA models for randomized trials. J Biopharm Stat. 2014;24(3):523–34. https://doi.org/10.1080/10543406.2014.888435. PMID: 24697334. Generalized F test and generalized deviance test in two-way ANOVA models for randomized trials – PubMed.
7. Forthofer RN, Lee ES. Introduction to biostatistics: a guide to design, analysis and discovery. Academic Press; 1998.
8. Norman GR, Streiner DL. Biostatistics: the bare essentials. BC Decker; 2000.
9. Cochrane Handbook for Systematic Reviews of Interventions | Cochrane Training.
10. Higgins JPT, Thompson SG, Deeks JJ, Altman DG. Measuring inconsistency in meta-analyses. BMJ. 2003;327(7414):557–60.

PMCID: PMC192859. http://www.ncbi.nlm.nih.gov/pubmed/12958120.
11. A network for patients and carers within Cochrane | Cochrane Consumer Network.
12. Bolstad WM, Curran JM. Comparing Bayesian and frequentist inferences for mean. In: Introduction to Bayesian statistics. 3rd ed. Wiley; 2016. p. 237–53. Introduction to Bayesian Statistics, Third Edition | Wiley Online Books.
13. Gelman A, Carlin JB, Stern HS, Dunson DB, Vehtari A, Rubin DB. Bayesian data analysis. 3rd ed. Chapman and Hall/CRC; 2013. ISBN 978-1-4398-4095-5. Bayesian Data Analysis | Andrew Gelman, John B. Carlin, Hal S. Stern.
14. https://www.sciencedirect.com/topics/medicine-and-dentistry/funnel-plot.
15. Cohen J. Statistical power analysis for the behavioral sciences. 2nd ed. Hillsdale: Lawrence Erlbaum Associates; 1988.
16. Hedges LV, Olkin I. Overlap between treatment and control distributions as an effect size measure in experiments. Psychol Methods. 2016;21(1):61–8. PMID: 26523436. http://www.ncbi.nlm.nih.gov/pubmed/26523436.
17. Hedges' g: Definition, Formula – Statistics How To.
18. cem.org/hs-search-results?term=effect+size.
19. Effect size and meta-analysis.
20. Andrade C. Mean difference, Standardized Mean Difference (SMD), and their use in meta-analysis: as simple as it gets. J Clin Psychiatry. 2020;81(5):20f13681. https://doi.org/10.4088/JCP.20f13681. PMID: 32965803. Mean Difference, Standardized Mean Difference (SMD), and Their Use in Meta-Analysis: As Simple as It Gets – PubMed.
21. Weighted Mean: Formula: How to Find Weighted Mean – Statistics How To.
22. Standard Error (SE) Definition: Standard Deviation in Statistics Explained.
23. Strech D, Weissgerber T, Dirnagl U, QUEST Group. Improving the trustworthiness, usefulness, and ethics of biomedical research through an innovative and comprehensive institutional initiative. PLoS Biol. 2020;18(2):e3000576. PMCID: PMC7012388. http://www.ncbi.nlm.nih.gov/pubmed/32045410.
24. Fletcher J. What is heterogeneity and is it important? BMJ. 2007;334(7584):94–6. PMCID: PMC1767262. http://www.ncbi.nlm.nih.gov/pubmed/17218716.
25. Ressing M, Blettner M, Klug SJ. Systematic literature reviews and meta-analyses: part 6 of a series on evaluation of scientific publications. Dtsch Arztebl Int. 2009;106(27):456–63. PMCID: PMC2719096. http://www.ncbi.nlm.nih.gov/pubmed/19652768.
26. Tonelli M, Hackam D, Garg AX. Primer on systematic review and meta-analysis. In: Methods Mol Biol, vol. 473; 2009. p. 217–33. PMID: 19160741. http://www.ncbi.nlm.nih.gov/pubmed/19160741.
27. Kontopantelis E, Springate DA, Reeves D. A re-analysis of the Cochrane Library data: the dangers of unobserved heterogeneity in meta-analyses. PLoS One. 2013;8(7):e69930. PMCID: PMC3724681. http://www.ncbi.nlm.nih.gov/pubmed/23922860.
28. Hatcher L. A step-by-step approach to using the SAS(R) system for factor analysis and structural equation modeling. Cary: SAS Institute; 1994.
29. Cochrane and systematic reviews | Cochrane Consumer Network.
30. Welcome! | Doing Meta-Analysis in R.
31. (PDF) Meta-analyses in mental health research: A practical guide.
32. Ioannidis JPA, Patsopoulos NA, Evangelou E. Uncertainty in heterogeneity estimates in meta-analyses. BMJ. 2007;335(7626):914–6. PMCID: PMC2048840. http://www.ncbi.nlm.nih.gov/pubmed/17974687.
33. Ioannidis JPA, Patsopoulos NA, Evangelou E. Heterogeneity in meta-analyses of genome-wide association investigations. PLoS One. 2007;2(9):e841. PMCID: PMC1950790. http://www.ncbi.nlm.nih.gov/pubmed/17786212.
34. Balduzzi S, Rücker G, Schwarzer G. How to perform a meta-analysis with R: a practical tutorial. Evid Based Ment Health. 2019;22(4):153–60. PMCID: PMC10231495. http://www.ncbi.nlm.nih.gov/pubmed/31563865.
35. Rouse B, Chaimani A, Li T. Network meta-analysis: an introduction for clinicians. Intern Emerg Med. 2017;12(1):103–11. PMCID: PMC5247317. http://www.ncbi.nlm.nih.gov/pubmed/27913917.
36. Mavridis D, Giannatsi M, Cipriani A, Salanti G. A primer on network meta-analysis with emphasis on mental health. Evid Based Ment Health. 2015;18(2):40–6. PMCID: PMC11234956. http://www.ncbi.nlm.nih.gov/pubmed/25908686.
37. Lu G, Ades AE. Combination of direct and indirect evidence in mixed treatment comparisons. Stat Med. 2004;23(20):3105–24. PMID: 15449338. http://www.ncbi.nlm.nih.gov/pubmed/15449338.
38. Mixed-Effects Meta Analysis (MEMA) | afni.nimh.nih.gov.
39. Three-level meta-analysis | Request PDF.
40. Brockhaus AC, Bender R, Skipka G. The Peto odds ratio viewed as a new effect measure. Stat Med. 2014;33(28):4861–74. https://doi.org/10.1002/sim.6301. Epub 2014 Sep 22. PMID: 25244540. The Peto odds ratio viewed as a new effect measure – PubMed.
41. Efthimiou O. Statistics in pills: meta-analysis of rare events. Evid Based Ment Health. 2019;22(3):102. https://doi.org/10.1136/ebmental-2019-300103. Epub 2019 Jul 13. PMID: 31302610; PMCID: PMC10270378. Statistics in pills: meta-analysis of rare events – PubMed.
42. Peto Odds Ratio Meta-analysis – StatsDirect.
43. Santos JRA, Lippke L, Pope P. PROC FACTOR: a tool for extracting hidden gems from a mountain of variables. In: Proceedings of the 23rd annual SAS Users Group International conference. Cary: SAS Institute Inc.; 1998.
44. Tang W, Hu J, Zhang H, Wu P, He H. Kappa coefficient: a popular measure of rater agreement. Shanghai Arch Psychiatry. 2015;27(1):62–7. PMCID: PMC4372765. http://www.ncbi.nlm.nih.gov/pubmed/25852260.
45. True Score Theory – Research Methods Knowledge Base.
46. Trochim WM. The research methods knowledge base. 2nd ed. Internet www page, at URL: http://www.socialresearchmethods.net/.
47. Cronbach LJ. Coefficient alpha and the internal structure of tests. Psychometrika. 1951;16:297–334.
48. Nunnaly J. Psychometric theory. New York: McGraw-Hill; 1978.
49. Number Needed to Treat (NNT) Calculator.
50. Vineis P, Pearce NE. Genome-wide association studies may be misinterpreted: genes versus heritability. Carcinogenesis. 2011;32(9):1295–8. PMID: 21565827. http://www.ncbi.nlm.nih.gov/pubmed/21565827.
51. Rose SPR. Commentary: heritability estimatesDOUBLE-HYPHENlong past their sell-by date. Int J Epidemiol. 2006;35(3):525–7. PMID: 16645027. http://www.ncbi.nlm.nih.gov/pubmed/16645027.
52. Vinkhuyzen AAE, van der Sluis S, Maes HHM, Posthuma D. Reconsidering the heritability of intelligence in adulthood: taking assortative mating and cultural transmission into account. Behav Genet. 2012;42(2):187–98. PMCID: PMC3276760. http://www.ncbi.nlm.nih.gov/pubmed/21969232.
53. Tal O. The impact of gene-environment interaction and correlation on the interpretation of heritability. Acta Biotheor. 2012;60(3):225–37. PMID: 21863336. http://www.ncbi.nlm.nih.gov/pubmed/21863336.
54. Kohler HP, Behrman JR, Schnittker J. Social science methods for twins data: integrating causality, endowments, and heritability. Biodemography Soc Biol. 2011;57(1):88–141. PMCID: PMC3158495. http://www.ncbi.nlm.nih.gov/pubmed/21845929.

55. Johnson W, Turkheimer E, Gottesman II, Bouchard TJ. Beyond heritability: twin studies in behavioral research. Curr Dir Psychol Sci. 2010;18(4):217–20. PMCID: PMC2899491. http://www.ncbi.nlm.nih.gov/pubmed/20625474.
56. The Cognitive Biases List: A Visual of 180+ Heuristics.
57. Kirschbaum C, Pirke KM, Hellhammer DH. The 'Trier Social Stress Test'–a tool for investigating psychobiological stress responses in a laboratory setting. Neuropsychobiology. 1993;28(1–2):76–81. PMID: 8255414. http://www.ncbi.nlm.nih.gov/pubmed/8255414.
58. Kendler KS, Hettema JM, Butera F, Gardner CO, Prescott CA. Life event dimensions of loss, humiliation, entrapment, and danger in the prediction of onsets of major depression and generalized anxiety. Arch Gen Psychiatry. 2003;60(8):789–96. PMID: 12912762. http://www.ncbi.nlm.nih.gov/pubmed/12912762.
59. Kendler KS, Karkowski LM, Prescott CA. Causal relationship between stressful life events and the onset of major depression. Am J Psychiatry. 1999;156(6):837–41. PMID: 10360120. http://www.ncbi.nlm.nih.gov/pubmed/10360120.
60. Slavich GM, Irwin MR. From stress to inflammation and major depressive disorder: a social signal transduction theory of depression. Psychol Bull. 2014;140(3):774–815. PMCID: PMC4006295. http://www.ncbi.nlm.nih.gov/pubmed/24417575.
61. Segal ZV, Kennedy S, Gemar M, Hood K, Pedersen R, Buis T. Cognitive reactivity to sad mood provocation and the prediction of depressive relapse. Arch Gen Psychiatry. 2006;63(7):749–55. PMID: 16818864. http://www.ncbi.nlm.nih.gov/pubmed/16818864.
62. Davidson RJ. Affective neuroscience and psychophysiology: toward a synthesis. Psychophysiology. 2003;40(5):655–65. PMID: 14696720. http://www.ncbi.nlm.nih.gov/pubmed/14696720.
63. Davidson RJ, Jackson DC, Kalin NH. Emotion, plasticity, context, and regulation: perspectives from affective neuroscience. Psychol Bull. 2000;126(6):890–909. PMID: 11107881. http://www.ncbi.nlm.nih.gov/pubmed/11107881.
64. Davidson RJ, Pizzagalli D, Nitschke JB, Putnam K. Depression: perspectives from affective neuroscience. Annu Rev Psychol. 2002;53:545–74. PMID: 11752496. http://www.ncbi.nlm.nih.gov/pubmed/11752496.
65. Munder T, Flückiger C, Gerger H, Wampold BE, Barth J. Is the allegiance effect an epiphenomenon of true efficacy differences between treatments? A meta-analysis. J Couns Psychol. 2012;59(4):631–7. PMID: 22946981. http://www.ncbi.nlm.nih.gov/pubmed/22946981.
66. Falkenström F, Markowitz JC, Jonker H, Philips B, Holmqvist R. Can psychotherapists function as their own controls? Meta-analysis of the crossed therapist design in comparative psychotherapy trials. J Clin Psychiatry. 2013;74(5):482–91. PMCID: PMC3683365. http://www.ncbi.nlm.nih.gov/pubmed/23146326.
67. Budd R, Hughes I. The Dodo Bird Verdict–controversial, inevitable and important: a commentary on 30 years of meta-analyses. Clin Psychol Psychother. 2009;16(6):510–22. PMID: 19728292. http://www.ncbi.nlm.nih.gov/pubmed/19728292.
68. Munder T, Brütsch O, Leonhart R, Gerger H, Barth J. Researcher allegiance in psychotherapy outcome research: an overview of reviews. Clin Psychol Rev. 2013;33(4):501–11. PMID: 23500154. http://www.ncbi.nlm.nih.gov/pubmed/23500154.
69. Ludwig DS, Kabat-Zinn J. Mindfulness in medicine. JAMA. 2008;300(11):1350–2. PMID: 18799450. http://www.ncbi.nlm.nih.gov/pubmed/18799450.
70. Berger D. Double-blinding and bias in medication and cognitive-behavioral therapy trials for major depressive disorder. F1000Res. 2015;4:638. PMCID: PMC4732552. http://www.ncbi.nlm.nih.gov/pubmed/26870318.
71. Wood L, Egger M, Gluud LL, Schulz KF, Jüni P, Altman DG, Gluud C, Martin RM, Wood AJG, Sterne JAC. Empirical evidence of bias in treatment effect estimates in controlled trials with different interventions and outcomes: meta-epidemiological study. BMJ. 2008;336(7644):601–5. PMCID: PMC2267990. http://www.ncbi.nlm.nih.gov/pubmed/18316340.
72. Schulz KF, Grimes DA. Blinding in randomised trials: hiding who got what. Lancet. 2002;359(9307):696–700. PMID: 11879884. http://www.ncbi.nlm.nih.gov/pubmed/11879884.
73. https://encyclopedia.pub/entry/36058#:~:text=In%20the%20philosophy%20of%20science,but%20neither%20is%20directly%20observable.
74. Piantadosi S. Clinical trials: a methodologic perspective. 2nd ed. New York: Wiley-Interscience; 2005. https://doi.org/10.1002/0471740136.
75. Rutherford BR, Mori S, Sneed JR, Pimontel MA, Roose SP. Contribution of spontaneous improvement to placebo response in depression: a meta-analytic review. J Psychiatr Res. 2012;46(6):697–702. PMCID: PMC3509755. http://www.ncbi.nlm.nih.gov/pubmed/22410207.
76. Wampold BE, Minami T, Tierney SC, Baskin TW, Bhati KS. The placebo is powerful: estimating placebo effects in medicine and psychotherapy from randomized clinical trials. J Clin Psychol. 2005;61(7):835–54. PMID: 15827993. http://www.ncbi.nlm.nih.gov/pubmed/15827993.
77. Blease CR, Bernstein MH, Locher C. Open-label placebo clinical trials: is it the rationale, the interaction or the pill? BMJ Evid Based Med. 2020;25(5):159–65. PMCID: PMC6930978. http://www.ncbi.nlm.nih.gov/pubmed/31243047.
78. Gaab J, Kossowsky J, Ehlert U, Locher C. Effects and components of placebos with a psychological treatment rationale – three randomized-controlled studies. Sci Rep. 2019;9(1):1421. PMCID: PMC6363794. http://www.ncbi.nlm.nih.gov/pubmed/30723231.
79. Dragioti E, Dimoliatis I, Fountoulakis KN, Evangelou E. A systematic appraisal of allegiance effect in randomized controlled trials of psychotherapy. Ann Gen Psychiatry. 2015;14:25. PMCID: PMC4570291. http://www.ncbi.nlm.nih.gov/pubmed/26379758.
80. Dragioti E, Dimoliatis I, Evangelou E. Disclosure of researcher allegiance in meta-analyses and randomised controlled trials of psychotherapy: a systematic appraisal. BMJ Open. 2015;5(6):e007206. PMCID: PMC4458582. http://www.ncbi.nlm.nih.gov/pubmed/26033943.
81. Cuijpers P, van Straten A, Bohlmeijer E, Hollon SD, Andersson G. The effects of psychotherapy for adult depression are overestimated: a meta-analysis of study quality and effect size. Psychol Med. 2010;40(2):211–23. PMID: 19490745. http://www.ncbi.nlm.nih.gov/pubmed/19490745.
82. Richter P, Werner J, Heerlein A, Kraus A, Sauer H. On the validity of the Beck Depression Inventory. A review. Psychopathology. 1998;31(3):160–8. PMID: 9636945. http://www.ncbi.nlm.nih.gov/pubmed/9636945.
83. Blom MBJ, Jonker K, Dusseldorp E, Spinhoven P, Hoencamp E, Haffmans J, van Dyck R. Combination treatment for acute depression is superior only when psychotherapy is added to medication. Psychother Psychosom. 2007;76(5):289–97. PMID: 17700049. http://www.ncbi.nlm.nih.gov/pubmed/17700049.
84. Zimmerman M, Posternak MA, Chelminski I. Is it time to replace the Hamilton Depression Rating Scale as the primary outcome measure in treatment studies of depression? J Clin Psychopharmacol. 2005;25(2):105–10. PMID: 15738740. http://www.ncbi.nlm.nih.gov/pubmed/15738740.
85. Bagby RM, Ryder AG, Schuller DR, Marshall MB. The Hamilton Depression Rating Scale: has the gold standard become a lead weight? Am J Psychiatry. 2004;161(12):2163–77. PMID: 15569884 http://www.ncbi.nlm.nih.gov/pubmed/15569884.
86. Santen G, Danhof M, Della Pasqua O. Sensitivity of the Montgomery Asberg Depression Rating Scale to response and its consequences for the assessment of efficacy. J Psychiatr Res.

2009;43(12):1049–56. PMID: 19344914. http://www.ncbi.nlm.nih.gov/pubmed/19344914.
87. Schotte CK, Maes M, Cluydts R, De Doncker D, Cosyns P. Construct validity of the Beck Depression Inventory in a depressive population. J Affect Disord. 1997;46(2):115–25. PMID: 9479615. http://www.ncbi.nlm.nih.gov/pubmed/9479615.
88. Furukawa TA, Cipriani A, Atkinson LZ, Leucht S, Ogawa Y, Takeshima N, Hayasaka Y, Chaimani A, Salanti G. Placebo response rates in antidepressant trials: a systematic review of published and unpublished double-blind randomised controlled studies. Lancet Psychiatry. 2016;3(11):1059–66. PMID: 27726982. http://www.ncbi.nlm.nih.gov/pubmed/27726982.
89. Zhu Z, Zhang L, Jiang J, Li W, Cao X, Zhou Z, Zhang T, Li C. Comparison of psychological placebo and waiting list control conditions in the assessment of cognitive behavioral therapy for the treatment of generalized anxiety disorder: a meta-analysis. Shanghai Arch Psychiatry. 2014;26(6):319–31. PMCID: PMC4311105. http://www.ncbi.nlm.nih.gov/pubmed/25642106.
90. Sorge RE, Martin LJ, Isbester KA, Sotocinal SG, Rosen S, Tuttle AH, Wieskopf JS, Acland EL, Dokova A, Kadoura B, Leger P, Mapplebeck JCS, McPhail M, Delaney A, Wigerblad G, Schumann AP, Quinn T, Frasnelli J, Svensson CI, Sternberg WF, Mogil JS. Olfactory exposure to males, including men, causes stress and related analgesia in rodents. Nat Methods. 2014;11(6):629–32. PMID: 24776635. http://www.ncbi.nlm.nih.gov/pubmed/24776635.
91. Martin SD, Martin E, Rai SS, Richardson MA, Royall R. Brain blood flow changes in depressed patients treated with interpersonal psychotherapy or venlafaxine hydrochloride: preliminary findings. Arch Gen Psychiatry. 2001;58(7):641–8. PMID: 11448369. http://www.ncbi.nlm.nih.gov/pubmed/11448369.
92. Mitchell AJ, Ferguson DW, Gill J, Paul J, Symonds P. Depression and anxiety in long-term cancer survivors compared with spouses and healthy controls: a systematic review and meta-analysis. Lancet Oncol. 2013;14(8):721–32. PMID: 23759376. http://www.ncbi.nlm.nih.gov/pubmed/23759376.
93. Hagedoorn M, Sanderman R, Bolks HN, Tuinstra J, Coyne JC. Distress in couples coping with cancer: a meta-analysis and critical review of role and gender effects. Psychol Bull. 2008;134(1):1–30. PMID: 18193993. http://www.ncbi.nlm.nih.gov/pubmed/18193993.
94. Shi L, Lin L. The trim-and-fill method for publication bias: practical guidelines and recommendations based on a large database of meta-analyses. Medicine (Baltimore). 2019;98(23):e15987. PMCID: PMC6571372. http://www.ncbi.nlm.nih.gov/pubmed/31169736.
95. Franco A, Malhotra N, Simonovits G. Social science. Publication bias in the social sciences: unlocking the file drawer. Science. 2014;345(6203):1502–5. PMID: 25170047. http://www.ncbi.nlm.nih.gov/pubmed/25170047.
96. Duval S, Tweedie R. Trim and fill: a simple funnel-plot-based method of testing and adjusting for publication bias in meta-analysis. Biometrics. 2000;56(2):455–63. PMID: 10877304. http://www.ncbi.nlm.nih.gov/pubmed/10877304.
97. Statistics – parametric and nonparametric – IBM Documentation.
98. Bernard R, Weissgerber TL, Bobrov E, Winham SJ, Dirnagl U, Riedel N. fiddle: a tool to combat publication bias by getting research out of the file drawer and into the scientific community. Clin Sci (Lond). 2020;134(20):2729–39. PMCID: PMC7593522. http://www.ncbi.nlm.nih.gov/pubmed/33111948.
99. Chapter 1: Starting a review | Cochrane Training.
100. Home page | Systematic Reviews.
101. The role of systematic reviews in evidence-based research.
102. Shojania KG, Sampson M, Ansari MT, Ji J, Doucette S, Moher D. How quickly do systematic reviews go out of date? A survival analysis. Ann Intern Med. 2007;147(4):224–33. PMID: 17638714. http://www.ncbi.nlm.nih.gov/pubmed/17638714.
103. Millard T, Synnot A, Elliott J, Green S, McDonald S, Turner T. Feasibility and acceptability of living systematic reviews: results from a mixed-methods evaluation. Syst Rev. 2019;8(1):325. PMCID: PMC6911272. http://www.ncbi.nlm.nih.gov/pubmed/31837703.
104. Gartlehner G, Wagner G, Matyas N, Titscher V, Greimel J, Lux L, Gaynes BN, Viswanathan M, Patel S, Lohr KN. Pharmacological and non-pharmacological treatments for major depressive disorder: review of systematic reviews. BMJ Open. 2017;7(6):e014912. PMCID: PMC5623437. http://www.ncbi.nlm.nih.gov/pubmed/28615268.
105. Shea BJ, Hamel C, Wells GA, Bouter LM, Kristjansson E, Grimshaw J, Henry DA, Boers M. AMSTAR is a reliable and valid measurement tool to assess the methodological quality of systematic reviews. J Clin Epidemiol. 2009;62(10):1013–20. PMID: 19230606. http://www.ncbi.nlm.nih.gov/pubmed/19230606.
106. Risk of bias tools – RoB 2 tool.
107. Friedman LM, Furgerg CD, DeMets DL. Fundamentals of clinical trials. 3rd ed. Springer; 1998.
108. Standardized Mean Differences in meta-analysis: a tutorial | Cochrane Methods.
109. Jakobsen JC, Wetterslev J, Winkel P, Lange T, Gluud C. Thresholds for statistical and clinical significance in systematic reviews with meta-analytic methods. BMC Med Res Methodol. 2014;14:120. PMCID: PMC4251848. http://www.ncbi.nlm.nih.gov/pubmed/25416419.
110. Hollis S, Campbell F. What is meant by intention to treat analysis? Survey of published randomised controlled trials. BMJ. 1999;319(7211):670–4. PMCID: PMC28218. http://www.ncbi.nlm.nih.gov/pubmed/10480822.
111. Poole C, Greenland S. Random-effects meta-analyses are not always conservative. Am J Epidemiol. 1999;150(5):469–75. PMID: 10472946. http://www.ncbi.nlm.nih.gov/pubmed/10472946.
112. Savović J, Jones HE, Altman DG, Harris RJ, Jüni P, Pildal J, Als-Nielsen B, Balk EM, Gluud C, Gluud LL, Ioannidis JPA, Schulz KF, Beynon R, Welton NJ, Wood L, Moher D, Deeks JJ, Sterne JAC. Influence of reported study design characteristics on intervention effect estimates from randomized, controlled trials. Ann Intern Med. 2012;157(6):429–38. PMID: 22945832. http://www.ncbi.nlm.nih.gov/pubmed/22945832.
113. Schulz KF, Altman DG, Moher D, CONSORT Group. CONSORT 2010 statement: updated guidelines for reporting parallel group randomized trials. Ann Intern Med. 2010;152(11):726–32. PMID: 20335313. http://www.ncbi.nlm.nih.gov/pubmed/20335313.
114. Grant S, Mayo-Wilson E, Montgomery P, Macdonald G, Michie S, Hopewell S, Moher D, on behalf of the CONSORT-SPI Group. CONSORT-SPI 2018 explanation and elaboration: guidance for reporting social and psychological intervention trials. Trials. 2018;19(1):406. PMCID: PMC6066913. http://www.ncbi.nlm.nih.gov/pubmed/30060763.
115. Montgomery P, Grant S, Mayo-Wilson E, Macdonald G, Michie S, Hopewell S, Moher D, CONSORT-SPI Group. Reporting randomised trials of social and psychological interventions: the CONSORT-SPI 2018 Extension. Trials. 2018;19(1):407. PMCID: PMC6066921. http://www.ncbi.nlm.nih.gov/pubmed/30060754.
116. Chan AW, Tetzlaff JM, Gøtzsche PC, Altman DG, Mann H, Berlin JA, Dickersin K, Hróbjartsson A, Schulz KF, Parulekar WR, Krleza-Jeric K, Laupacis A, Moher D. SPIRIT 2013 explanation and elaboration: guidance for protocols of clinical trials. BMJ. 2013;346:e7586. PMCID: PMC3541470. http://www.ncbi.nlm.nih.gov/pubmed/23303884.
117. Cuijpers P, van Straten A, Smit F, Andersson G. Is psychotherapy for depression equally effective in younger and older adults? A meta-

regression analysis. Int Psychogeriatr. 2009;21(1):16–24. PMID: 19040783. http://www.ncbi.nlm.nih.gov/pubmed/19040783.
118. Bohlmeijer E, Smit F, Cuijpers P. Effects of reminiscence and life review on late-life depression: a meta-analysis. Int J Geriatr Psychiatry. 2003;18(12):1088–94. PMID: 14677140. http://www.ncbi.nlm.nih.gov/pubmed/14677140.
119. Liang J, Xu X, Quiñones AR, Bennett JM, Ye W. Multiple trajectories of depressive symptoms in middle and late life: racial/ethnic variations. Psychol Aging. 2011;26(4):761–77. PMCID: PMC3495237. http://www.ncbi.nlm.nih.gov/pubmed/21875216.
120. Kok GD, Bockting CLH, Burger H, Hannig W, Pijnenborg GHM, Cuijpers P, Hollon SD. Double trouble: does co-morbid chronic somatic illness increase risk for recurrence in depression? A systematic review. PLoS One. 2013;8(3):e57510. PMCID: PMC3589395. http://www.ncbi.nlm.nih.gov/pubmed/23472087.
121. Rietdijk J, Hogerzeil SJ, van Hemert AM, Cuijpers P, Linszen DH, van der Gaag M. Pathways to psychosis: help-seeking behavior in the prodromal phase. Schizophr Res. 2011;132(2–3):213–9. PMID: 21907547. http://www.ncbi.nlm.nih.gov/pubmed/21907547.
122. Marshall MB, Zuroff DC, McBride C, Bagby RM. Self-criticism predicts differential response to treatment for major depression. J Clin Psychol. 2008;64(3):231–44. PMID: 18302208. http://www.ncbi.nlm.nih.gov/pubmed/18302208.
123. Cuijpers P, Huibers M, Ebert DD, Koole SL, Andersson G. How much psychotherapy is needed to treat depression? A metaregression analysis. J Affect Disord. 2013;149(1–3):1–13. PMID: 23528438. http://www.ncbi.nlm.nih.gov/pubmed/23528438.
124. Bower P, Kontopantelis E, Sutton A, Kendrick T, Richards DA, Gilbody S, Knowles S, Cuijpers P, Andersson G, Christensen H, Meyer B, Huibers M, Smit F, van Straten A, Warmerdam L, Barkham M, Bilich L, Lovell K, Liu ETH. Influence of initial severity of depression on effectiveness of low intensity interventions: meta-analysis of individual patient data. BMJ. 2013;346:f540. PMCID: PMC3582703. http://www.ncbi.nlm.nih.gov/pubmed/23444423.
125. Cuijpers P, Li J, Hofmann SG, Andersson G. Self-reported versus clinician-rated symptoms of depression as outcome measures in psychotherapy research on depression: a meta-analysis. Clin Psychol Rev. 2010;30(6):768–78. PMID: 20619943. http://www.ncbi.nlm.nih.gov/pubmed/20619943.
126. The Centre for Evidence-Based Medicine | Evidence Service to support the COVID-19 response.

5 The Sociology of Depression

Jeffery J. Sunzeri

Introduction

Today, major depressive disorder is described as the leading cause of disability in the United States for people between the ages of 15 and 44. A central aspect of major depressive disorder is described in remarkably social terms as feeling lonely, which is caused by things such as becoming cut off from your family and friends. Therapies for dealing with depression focus on the individual and his or her temperament and behaviors and involve psychotherapies, drugs, genes, and biological factors. An indication of how important a sociological perception of the disorder might be is that a diagnosis of depression is based solely on behavioral symptoms, and treatments are most often not specific to an underlying disease pathology.

The sociological perspective on depression is different. The sociological approach differs from the psychological and biological emphasis on personal characteristics, brain functions, and genetics by emphasizing social conditions, roles, social functions, social structures, and culture. Sociology tells us that the determinants of good mental health don't solely depend on the individual and their personalities but vary with the social conditions they live in, and that the variation of these conditions is key to understanding depression.

The sociological approach to depression emphasizes that mental health is not only rooted in the individual characteristics and etiologies but is equally formed from social factors and circumstances. Those social factors include objective cultural affiliations, social roles, economic conditions, life events, social structures, belongingness, and the historical period in which we live.

Sociological conditions affect the likelihood of an individual's feelings of depression, definitions of depression, and resultant desire or need to seek help for the condition.

J. J. Sunzeri (✉)
Sunzeri Consulting, Hollister, CA, USA

Finally, the success of many interventions for depression is tightly tied to social factors of health care, accessibility, quality, and amount of care that is available.

Sociology, Social Psychology, and Psychosocial: What Is the Difference?

In our discussion of the sociology of depression, we will be guided by the tenets of the biopsychosocial model of health and illness, medical sociology, and the sociology of health and well-being.

The *biopsychosocial model of health and illness* operates on the premise that health and wellness is a complex dynamic interaction of biological, psychological, and social factors [48, 49] As such, interventions are comprehensive [47]. The biopsychosocial research separates, defines, and measures detailed interrelationship among these factors [50].

Medical sociology focuses on human social behavior, patterns of social relationships, and social interactions that affect medical practice both at a micro and macro level [43–45].

Sociology of health and well-being acknowledges that our way of approaching well-being is a social construct and our interactions with our medical institutions are social constructs and are socially interpreted [42, 46, 51].

Where *Sociology* and sociologists engage in the scientific study of groups of individuals, *Social Psychology* engages the perspective of studying the individual as found in a social group. Examples of the Social-Psychological perspective would be studies of changing individual behavior to fit in with a group, prejudicial behavior and stereotypes, the bystander effect (not helping in an emergency when others are present), peer influence, and discrimination based on group membership. While deeply meaningful, such perspectives of the individual in groups are outside the *Sociological viewpoint*. We will be discussing the social-psychological perspective in the next chapter in this monograph.

J. Raber et al. (eds.), *Understanding and Treating Depressive Disorders*, https://doi.org/10.1007/978-3-032-14465-2_5

Perspective

Depression is the most common mental illness worldwide [52]. Lifetime risk for major depression is said to be about 17% in the United States, and up to 10% suffer from depression in any given year [53]. Globally, it has been said that major depression comprises 4.4% of the disease burden [41, 54, 55].

In 2017, the WHO reported that depression is the leading cause of ill health and disability worldwide. with more than 300 million people living with depression, an increase of more than 18% between 2005 and 2015 [58].

A systematic analysis of the *Global Burden of Disease Study 2019* revealed that depression was ranked 13th out of the top 25 causes of *disability-adjusted life-years (DALYS)* [56]. Depression was second in the *years lived with disability (YLDs)*. In mental disorders, depression was ranked the highest in all age groups except for the 0–14 age group, where conduct disorders were the leading cause of DALYS.

In 2020, the National Institute of Mental Health (NIMH) reported that in the USA an estimated 8.4%, or 21.0 million adults, aged 18 and older had at least one major depressive episode [59]. Prevalence of major depression was 10.5% for females and 6.2% for males. Highest prevalence was in the age group of 18 to 25 (17.0%). In the age group of 12–17, 17% had at least one major depressive episode. In adolescents, 25.2% of females and 9.2% of adults had a major depressive episode. Of those 18 years of age or older, 66.0% of those who had a major depressive episode were treated in the past year. An estimated 71.0% of those who had a major depressive episode with severe impairment were treated in the past year.[1]

In 2013, depression in older folks was predicted to hit 6.5 million out of the 35 million Americans aged 65 and older [57–61].

Higher socioeconomic status as measured by income, education, and occupation is inversely related to hostility, depressive symptoms, and major depression [62].

The *National Health and Nutrition Examination Survey, 2013–2016* was updated and published in 2018. The Centers for Disease Control and Prevention (CDC) states: "All material appearing in this report is in the public domain and may be reproduced or copied without permission." Key points appear in the footnote below along with a link to the full CDC report.[2]

A non-CDC report using data from the *National Survey on Drug Use and Health (NSDUH)* [63] says that from 2005 to 2015 prevalence of depression increased significantly in the USA [64]. Among youth, the rate of increase was significantly more rapid than for older groups. In addition, significant increases were seen for the lowest and the highest income groups, and those with the most education.

The *Midlife in the United States (MIDUS)* study showed increasing distress (e.g., sadness, hopelessness, and worthlessness) and decreasing well-being (e.g., happiness, fulfillment and life satisfaction) across the age span for those of low relative socioeconomic position, compared to little decline or modest improvement for persons of high relative position [65].

Published in 2017, a random sample of an urban area ($n = 3720$) showed a lifetime prevalence of 15.2% for persistent depressive disorders (PDD) with Persistent Major Depressive Episode, 3.3% for PDD with pure dysthymia, 28.2% for major depressive disorder (MDD), and 9.1% for other specified depressive disorders [66].

In 2014, Medicaid emerged as the largest health insurance program in the USA [67]. Behavioral and mood disorders in 2012 were the most frequently diagnosed reasons for Medicaid-covered and uninsured hospitalization in the USA [68]. In 2011, mood disorders were the most frequent reasons for hospital readmissions in 18 states in the USA [71].

A fundamental question in understanding and preventing mood disorders is what makes the difference between individual susceptibility or resistance to disease. The answers may lie in our ability to adapt to a changing environment. That adaptation is based on a balance of habituation and facilitation. That balance is predicated on both genetic and environmental factors, some constraining and some enabling. Habituation is the progressive diminishing response to repeated stimuli which are often psychosocial. Facilitation is the capacity to enhance or remain responsive to stimuli [72]. A deeper discussion on stress, resilience, and coping can be found in the Background Volume of the Compendium.

The Sociological Process

Sociologists study depression in a social context. That is to say that the sociologist will view and research conditions that exist in the living settings where the individual is found. Social evaluation and research take place in the community made up of the family, city, neighborhood, school, and work-

[1] Statistical methods and caveats can be found in [116].

[2] Key findings Data from the National Health and Nutrition Examination Survey

- During 2013–2016, 8.1% of American adults aged 20 and over had depression in a given 2-week period.
- Women (10.4%) were almost twice as likely as were men (5.5%) to have had depression.
- Depression was lower among non-Hispanic Asian adults, compared with Hispanic, non-Hispanic black, or non-Hispanic white adults.
- The prevalence of depression decreased as family income levels increased.
- About 80% of adults with depression reported at least some difficulty with work, home, and social activities because of their depression.
- From 2007–2008 to 2015–2016, the percentage of American adults with depression did not change significantly over time. [117].

place. This is in contrast to the clinical setting that comprises the basis for research conducted by mental health care professionals.

In a clinical setting where a person would seek care for depression, the professional would evaluate the patient in search of a diagnosis, or lack of same. A person presents behaviors and symptoms that are measured against standards and guidelines and thus is diagnosed with depression or not.

Rather than seeking to diagnose the individual, the sociologist seeks to study and research varying levels of mental health-related circumstances and conditions. The instruments and methods that the sociologist uses are most often social scales that measure and describe aspects of mental health.

Because people present a wide ranges of symptoms, feelings, behaviors, and actions that are not easily observed, assessment scales are often used by mental health professionals in making determinations of depression. These scales are often the result of social research and have a long history of utility in sociological thought.

Rather than utilizing a diagnostic that determines a dichotomy, or an either/or diagnosis, we find sociologists seeking to define an overall measure of personal distress. Rather than a decision that one does or does not have a condition, the sociologist prefers to demonstrate that the individual presents a relative spectrum of a condition. An excellent example of a scalar method is the *Center for Epidemiologic Studies–Depression scale (CES-D)*.[3] This scale was published in 1977, prior to the development of the clinical diagnosis of major depressive disorder in 1987. The CES-D is a 20-question instrument designed to measure symptoms associated with depression. The scale can be self-administered or administered by a clinician resulting in a dimensional assessment of depression (as opposed to a categorical measure).

Sociological studies of dimensions of mental health have been in use since at least the mid-twentieth century when studies were carried out shortly after World War II. These dimensional assessments are often contrasted with the dichotomous or categorical. The two methods of assessment and study have proponents citing their understanding of the underlying assumptions around mental disorders. It is most likely that measures utilizing both methods will derive the best likelihood of meaningful study and understanding.

[3]CES-D has withstood the test of time. Systematic reviews have shown CES-D to be useful for children, adolescents, adults and geriatric populations. For older adults, the CES-D has shown similar useful predictive value as the Geriatric Depression Scale [121]. The CES-D appears to be valuable for screening depression in children and adolescents in Western countries [122]. However, it is uncertain how valuable the CES-D may be for other cultural or ethnic groups [123]. CES-D appears to be useful in first stage screening for major depression in community-indwelling adults, patients with chronic diseases, and psychiatric patients [120].

The Social Components of Mental Health

The determinants of mental health and depression for sociologists are qualities of social conditions. Rather than focusing on the psycho-social (combined influence of psychological factors and the surrounding social environment) and biological aspects which are the mainstay of psychiatry, psychological and medical practitioners, sociologists often measure social conditions (relationships, family and community networks) and circumstances. See Fig. 5.1.

Sociologists have historically developed the paradigm of an individual isolated from society and its functions, creating a dysfunctional and potentially harmful state. The *feeling of belongingness* of the individual to society is a core principle in sociology.

Social Networks Crucially, we find evidence of a link between an individual's feelings and social context. Social feelings connect subjective experiences with social interactions to create the concepts in sociology that help us to understand socially functional mechanisms. Those mechanisms include affiliation, parent-offspring attachment, moral sentiments, norms, and social identity. There is in fact a neurological as well as sociological basis to connect well-being, cognition, emotion, and behavior as the essentials of mental health [77]. We will have more to say about the biological

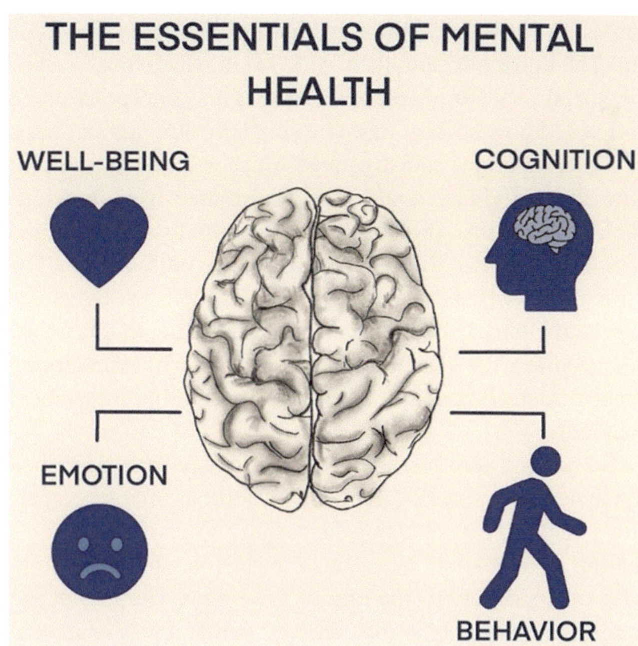

Fig. 5.1 This illustration highlights the interconnected neurological and sociological roots of mental health, showing how well-being, cognition, emotion, and behavior form a unified framework. These elements, both biologically grounded and socially shaped, serve as core pillars in understanding individual mental wellness

understanding of the neuroscience of social feelings in the chapter on Psychobiology.

Often thought to be the first to relate sociology to mental health, Emile Durkheim in 1897 described in "Suicide: A study in sociology" [3] how suicide was the result of the individual being removed from social forces and impacts, in effect being isolated. The forces he described are social integration and moral regulation. He described a state of *anomie* where a person would be in a state of feeling normlessness—a disconnection from society and its norms—and how anomie contributed to isolation and social alienation. Durkheim found data supporting the relationship of social connections to mental health in several instances. Fundamentally, his data showed that strong social ties had the lowest rates of suicide, while the socially isolated showed a high rate of suicides. Data also showed married people had lower suicide rates than the unmarried, and married people with children were especially unlikely to commit suicide. Likewise, members of religions such as Catholicism that shared common practices and beliefs committed a smaller number of suicides than members of Protestant groups that permitted more free inquiry among their congregants. In addition, Durkheim discovered that few people commit suicide during wars and revolutions because of the intensity of shared collective experiences in such periods.

Discussing economic and social conditions, Karl Marx in "Das Kapital" [9] talked about the concept of an individual's alienation and isolation from society due to those social forces. In 1904, Max Weber published "The Protestant Ethic and The Spirit of Capitalism" [13, 14] in which he described the social concept of *rationalization.* This concept explored and stated how society moved to implement a rational basis of social functions and structures which resulted in a shift of how the individual could now be isolated from previous social forces that previously had sought to integrate and socialize. George Simmel writing in a 1908 essay "The Stranger" [11], speaks about social relationship dynamics especially in early twentieth century urban life. In this essay, he introduces the idea of how an individual will experience a sense of detachment and isolation in known but impersonal societies.

So we see that historically, sociologists have described the dynamics of social forces and institutions affecting a person's feelings of inclusion in society. Overall, a person's feeling of affiliation, acceptance, inclusion, and connection with others describes the idea of *belonging*. The loss of the feeling of belonging is then directly tied to a loss of mental health and the occurrence of depression.

It has been suggested that desire for suicide arises when individuals have intractable feelings of burdensomeness, thwarted *belongingness,* and painful and provocative events. This is known as the *Interpersonal-Psychological Theory of Suicide (ITS)* [78–80]. Core constructs and specific hypotheses of the ITS can be found in references [23, 81].

A 2017 systematic review and meta-analysis of a decade of cross-national research [78] in general found support that thwarted belongingness and perceived burdensomeness were significant correlates of suicidal ideation severity, and thwarted belongingness, perceived burdensomeness, and capability for suicide were significantly associated with suicide attempt history. However, the effect sizes were insufficient to show more than a modest clinical significance. Additionally, they found a lack of evidence supporting specific ITS hypotheses, such as predicting death by suicide, as well as the difficulty of managing belonginess and perceived burdensomeness in suicidal desire.

The interpersonal constructs are frequently examined by the Interpersonal Needs Questionnaire [82, 83] and the *Acquired Capability for Suicide Scale (ACSS)* [84–86]. There have been some concerns about the use of the ACSS with combat veterans [84]. These have included a high risk of bias, inconsistent use, and lack of sample heterogeneity yielding mixed results [87].

Many sociological studies demonstrate the importance and dynamic interplay of the social indicators described in the following paragraphs and an individual's mental health. In describing and discussing the following social factors related to depression, it is vitally important to state that it is beyond this essay to ascribe causality of any of these variables. Indeed, it is a ripe area for detailed sociological modeling and study to determine which of these components are causal and the degree to which depression may be either a dependent or independent variable in relation to the social forces.

Social Indicators

Demographic Identity

When we discuss the frequency, importance, and prevalence of depression, it is almost always in terms of individual identification categories. These categories are often age, education level, ethnicity, gender, birth location, income, religious affiliations, nationality, career, and others.[4]

[4]Demography is the study of populations and deep structures and forces that shape both global and personal opportunities and constraints. [147]. Sources for medical demographic data include government agencies such as the National Center for Health Statistics [148]; the US Department of Health and Human Services' website [149] and the NIH Library [150]. An example of a state agency medical demographics database is the Oregon Health Authority [151]. An example of an academic demographic data base for depression is that operated by OHSU that catalogues depression among Oregonians with disabilities [152].

The purpose of collecting and representing the demographic qualities of populations derives from an attempt to ascribe an objective truth or objective quality to the people and conditions being studied so as to develop at least an appearance of causality. So when we say that "major depressive disorder is the leading cause of disability in the United States for people between the ages of 15 and 44" there is meant to be an association of understood causal relationship between the age demographic and major depressive disorder.

Questions arise around the meaningfulness of demographics when examined on a number of levels. In the above example, what is behind the choice of the age range '15 and 44'? How was this range chosen or selected for reporting? Are there behavioral similarities that outweigh differences within this category? Demographic indicators are excellent at descriptors, but are they useful?

Questioning the utility of demographic descriptors becomes increasingly important when we realize the nature of assigning the values of these categories [38–40].

A major quality of demographic categories is whether they are self-reported or objectively derived. Of course, self-reported values may be objectively reported, but as often they may not be representative of an objective truth or reality. For example, ethnicity is an often-used demographic and whether it is reported by the individual being questioned (self-reported), or by a trained investigator, ethnicity may easily be objectively incorrectly reported. Excellent examples of mistaken ethnic identity can be found in reporting of American Indian ethnicity where a number of confounding factors present themselves so as to confuse the objective reality. Essentially, almost any demographic category that is self-reported is subject to objective questioning.[5]

So, when sociologists see a representation of "The prevalence of major depressive episode was highest among those who report having multiple (two or more) races (13.9%)" [59] we must immediately question the validity as well as the reliability of how the demographic was determined and therefore the meaningfulness of any causality inferred.

A Discussion of the Social Construct of Race and Sociology

Although there are phenotypical differences between peoples, science has found that there is more genetic variation within racially defined groups than between them. In sociology, there are many social constructs created and defined by societal agreement, norms, and social systems and race is one of these. Further substantiation that race is a construct and not a fixed attribute is the fact that definition of any one race varies across time and cultures. Indeed, today race is most often simply a matter of self-reporting on a questionnaire.

While racial identity is meaningful in many ways, its lack of fixed biological basis and clearly objective indicators limits its utility in scientific analysis, particularly in inferring the fundamental qualities of independent or dependent variability.

As an invented way of categorizing individuals, the power of racial identity is undeniable. However, as powerful and invasive an identity may be, it is not useful for scientific analysis if the objective underpinnings of the identity are unclear. If an individual chooses on a nonindependently confirmed questionnaire to be identified as Asian, are they categorically the same as a native, Korean-born national? The core question then becomes, how valid is our data? If the validity of our data is in question, then the reliability is in question. When both validity and reliability of data are in question, what is our responsibility in scientific inquiry?

There is no doubt that power structures and social forces surround racial identities in many different ways. However, it does little to advance knowledge and defeat prejudice born of ignorance to apply nonobjective measures to study objective outcomes.

There is room and a need for sociological study of racial identities. Those studies must be well constructed, clearly defined with unimpeachable data validity matched to the social importance of the subject.

Life Events

Long a staple sociological thought, perception, and execution of life events such as marriage, inter-familial death, birth, career change, change in home location, and stressful events in general are often cited in many studies of mental health and risk of mental health.

As with many well-studied sociological concepts, a scale was developed to measure the relationship between life events and their resulting stress levels, and risk of depression. Created in 1967, the *Holmes and Rahe Stress Scale* also called the *Social Readjustment Rating Scale (SRRS)* is the result of studying the links between stress and mental health issues [5]. The SRRS has been revised and validated many times since its inception [15]. In 2023, the SRRS was updated and modernized while still allowing for cross comparisons of prior studies [87]. That revision is an interesting read on changes in societal norms and stressors in the decades since the original SSRS was formulated. For example, on average, adults find SRRS events more taxing than in 1967. However, there are several items that are particularly stressful in the

[5] *Best practices* for demographic data collection and reporting [153].

An Ethics and Social Justice Approach to Collecting and Using Demographic Data for Psychological Researchers [154].

2020s that were not present in the 1960s and still are not on the new list. These include computer-related issues, involvement in court proceedings, being a victim of crime and being a caregiver for a relative.

The SRRS can be self-administered or used by healthcare professionals in a clinical setting. It measures 43 life events deemed meaningful, producing a scalar assessment score of *Life Change Units (LCU)* associated with either positive or negative events, such as marriage or death.

The scores are tallied based on experiences over the past year. Examples of the events would be: death of a spouse, divorce, major personal injury, marriage, job loss, and pregnancy. Score discrimination results in thresholds that indicate moderate stress, high stress and very high stress leading to health issues.

Further accentuating the sociological perspective of life events affecting depression, the following are some of the studies emphasizing life events and their roles in depression.

- The *Heinz Nixdorf Recall* study participants reported experiencing a significant life event in the previous 6 months and showed higher depression scores [88].
- Various meta-analyses showed that both acute and chronic life events are associated with the onset and worsening of depressive disorder symptoms [89–92].
- A population-based twin study evaluated 18 stressful life events, including violent and economic ones, which were then associated with an increased risk of depression [2, 93].
- An *American Journal of Psychiatry* study found that stressful life events have a substantial causal relationship with the onset of major depression [6].
- In 2000, Hammen, Henry, and Daley found that women who experienced more childhood adversities showed more depressive reactions to low levels of stress than women who experienced fewer adversities [4, 94].

Social Structures

The paradigm of sociology is that of the interplay of social structure and social function. Social structures are developed to carry out social functions, and social functions create social structures within which to exist. For example, marriage is developed to carry out the function of family. Understanding the social structures leads us to a framework within which we can measure functionality, functionality being key to health.

Fitting well into the social structure involves measures of an individual's power, status, belongingness, and resources. This is how the social structure determines levels of mental health in the individual.

A large body of research shows that people that fit and belong well into society have better mental health than those who don't. Specifically, studies show that people who are, or feel that they are more powerful, of high status and high wealth demonstrate better mental health compared to those whose experience is on the other end of the spectrum, feeling powerless, of low status and living in poverty [95–98].

Evidence exists that *sociometric status* (the respect and admiration one has in face-to-face groups such as friends and coworkers) matters more to their subjective well-being than does their socioeconomic status [107].

In aging, feeling that what one does in life is worthwhile and meaningful can predict social, economic, health, and behavioral outcomes [108, 109].

An excellent example of the social structure and the individual's integration into the structure is represented in the *Berkman-Syme Social Network Index* [1, 110]. This index, developed in 1979, is a self-reported scale that measures social integration and isolation. Although not specifically an indicator of depression, the index highlights the relationship between specific social factors and health outcomes. A systematic review on the association between social relationships and depression found that the strongest and most consistent findings were significant protective effects of perceived emotional support, perceived instrumental support, and large, diverse social networks [111]. In older individuals with and without health challenges, loneliness. social engagement, religiosity, and living arrangements are significant factors in depression [112–117].

The *Evolutionary Theory of Loneliness* that predicts a lack of social connectedness will have long-term mental and physical health consequences is supported by evidence from a study that showed social support partially mediated the relationship between loneliness and anxiety, depression, and somatic symptoms [118].

Inequality

It is an overriding assumption that society is a creation of unequal parts. Most social institutions exist with inequality yet arrive at equitable arrangements. For example, the institute of marriage seldom exists with perfectly equal partners, yet marriage executes its social functions of child rearing and familial associations equitably among participants. Inequality exists in the workplace, yet work remains a meaningfully important aspect of society. However, as social inequality exists, so does inequity of mental health outcomes based on inequality in social institutions [119–122].

Perhaps the most obvious example of how inequality of social factors affects mental health outcomes and thus the incidence of depression is how income inequality affects depression [123–125]. Recent studies show that a higher risk of the incidence of depression is correlated to a high rate of income inequality [126, 127].

Even though depression is a leading cause of disability in adolescents [128], there is a large disparity between the number of studies in the incidence of adolescent depression and the income of countries [129, 130]. This is especially telling when one considers that about 90% of the world's adolescents live in low- and middle-income countries yet the vast majority of studies are conducted in high-income countries [131].[6]

Another example of inequality as a social factor is how access to health care is tied to outcomes for mental disability. The *National Health and Nutrition Examination Survey* taken in 2009–2012 showed that people below the poverty level were nearly 2½ times more likely to have depression than those at or above the poverty level [16]. In the USA, the *National Survey of Drug Use and Health (NSDUH),* has shown an estimated 9.8 million adults aged 18 or older in the U.S. had a serious mental illness (SMI), including 2.5 million adults living below the poverty line [17]. The percentage of SMI in individuals 18 years of age or older living below the poverty line was 6.8 compared to 4.3 at the poverty line and 3.3 over the poverty line. Mental illness and poverty are a complicated two-way street. Mental illness increases the likelihood of poverty and poverty increases the chances of mental illness [18, 19].

A study of the prevalence of depression in 2019 revealed that the prevalence of a major depressive episode was almost 1.5 times greater among women (9.6%) compared to men (6.0%) [20]. At least in the USA, girls until 13–15 are not more likely to be depressed than boys, then they increase to about twice as likely [12, 132, 133]. The differences that emerge are usually attributed to females experiencing greater life stressors, such as gender inequalities and the role of childbearing [21, 151, 156]. An affective, biological, and cognitive model has been proposed suggesting that beginning in adolescence, negative events combine with affective vulnerability, genetic vulnerability, pubertal hormones, pubertal timing and development, cognitive style, objectified body consciousness and rumination may account for the gender differences [138, 139].

In both Western and non-Western studies [140, 141], even though women are diagnosed with depressions at half the rate of men, men die by suicide 3.5–4 times more often than women do [137]. However, this diagnostic rate may not reflect the true state of masculine depression [142, 143]. Gender differences in diagnosis largely disappear when male-typical expression of depression are recognized [144]. Males have been conditioned by gendered societal processes to express their emotions differently than females [31]. Males tend to react to emotional pain by less control over impulses and more hyperactivity manifesting in irritability, anger, self-destructive behavior, self-distraction, or numbing of pain with substance use, gambling, womanizing, and workaholism [29, 30, 145].

Dissociating and acting out or externalizing suppressed feelings can have a radiating traumatic effect on family members [28]. Angry responses and violence can be especially traumatic on family members. Self-destructive symptoms such as substance abuse can lead to detachment, withdrawal, and abandonment of their children resulting in mismodeling appropriate social functioning such as sensitivity, nurturing, warmth, and engagement [146, 147].

Depression prevalence increases with socioeconomic changes that occur with disasters [148] including pandemics [149] and economic recessions [150]. And health conditions, such as obesity, hypertension, and diabetes, smoking, education, and income status are identified risk factors for increased incidence of depression and its severity [151–153].

Low-income people are subject to higher crime rates [22], less access to medical services [154, 155], less healthy food environments [157], and adverse neighborhood characteristics such as neighborhood socioeconomic status, physical conditions, services/amenities, social capital, and social disorder [158–160]. Additional stressors adding to depression include homelessness and housing insecurities [161], food insecurities [162], retirement loss of income, and social interaction [162]. Chronic health conditions are often associated in a circular fashion with depression [163, 164]. Poverty, depression and anxiety are reviewed in [165]. Along with financial insecurity can come shame, self-blame, and social isolation [159, 160, 162].

Income and income inequality drive depressive symptoms in adults living in the USA [166]. According to the *National Center for Health Statistics, Centers for Disease Control and Prevention; 2019*[7] between 2013 and 2016 about 3.5% of adults 20 years and older living at or above 400% of the federal poverty line were depressed, compared to 16% of those living below the federal poverty line [167].

Data from the 2005-2016 *National Health and Nutrition Examination Survey (NHANES)* [168] was evaluated by *the Patient Health Questionnaire-9 (PHQ-9)* measurement tool [169] to produce scores of 5, 10, 15, or 20 that represent mild, moderate, moderately severe, and severe depression based upon the Diagnostic and Statistical Manual of Mental Disorders (DSM-IV), 4th edition scale [170]. The main independent variable was the *Poverty Income Ratio (PIR)* which was calculated by dividing family income or individual income

[6] [182–184].

[7] [6]

by the poverty guidelines for each survey year. Results were described in three categories: low-PIR (0–1.16), medium-PIR (1.17–2.82), and high-PIR (2.83–5.00). Results indicated that depression is highest among low-PIR men and women with a higher distribution among women. Low-income people compared to high-income people were more likely to score 10 or higher on the PHQ-9. Income distribution was more unequal in women than in men and might relate to inequalities in income and wages [171–173] and occupational risks [174].

Results of the *National Longitudinal Survey of Youth* 1979 cohort on socioeconomic status, incidence and persistence of depression have shown that income is significantly associated with depression [175, 176]. Closer examination shows that ratio of debts to assets and employment status but not income itself are casually related to depression.

Other studies show a more complex picture. For example, one meta-analysis showed that individuals with low income had increased odds (1.81) of depression compared with higher income categories [177]. A large cross-sectional epidemiological study, *US Collaborative Psychiatric Epidemiologic Survey* did not find an association between household income and any anxiety or mood disorder, but they did find that suicide attempts and substance use disorder tracked with decreasing income [178]. However, those associations varied among non-Hispanic white, Hispanic, Asian American, black, and other race categories. Non-Hispanic white people showed a strong negative correlation between income and suicidal ideation (OR=2.15; 95% CI: 1.66 to 2.80) and was much weaker for the other races.

The largest longitudinal, population-based mental health survey to date: *the US National Epidemiologic Survey of Alcohol and Related Conditions* [178–180] has shown that low levels of household income associate with several lifetime mental disorders and suicide attempts [181]. In addition, household income associates with increased risk for incident mental disorders.

Different Depression Experiences by Social Interactions

While we may have arrived at an agreed definition of major depression, it remains that there is no universal cause of the disorder. Just as there are rates of severity in the manifestation of depression, so too are there manifold differences in the social conditions, individual traits, interactions of conditions and traits, which vary with the incidence and severity of mental depression. We see that life events, social structure interactions, social inequalities all interact to form a characterization of the incidence of mental depression.

Of course, it is in human nature to see, seek, and divine patterns and relations in situations. It is this nature that leads us to understand a condition and with diligence and insight prepare and deliver treatments and solutions. It is so with depression as a disorder. As illustrated earlier, Durkheim sought to understand suicide by correlating data with frequencies and this effort persists today in the study of depression.

Sociological Interventions for Depression

It is clear that depression (also known as major depression, major depressive disorder, or clinical depression) is tightly interwoven with sociological conditions. The presence of depression in the population is a meaningfully large social problem on many levels. Given this, what measures can be taken to reduce not only the occurrence of depression, but also lessen the effects of depression both individually as well as on society? What is the interplay between the clinical and social methods and practices that will positively affect the occurrences and outcomes of depression?

How to Define and Thus Respond to Depression

Since this article deals with the sociological perspective and paradigm of social influences on the depression medical disorder, it is natural to introduce the concept of medicalization. *Medicalization* was first described by sociologist Jesse Pitts [10] in 1968 in reference to the idea of social forces seeking and succeeding to control individuals and social actions. Social control in this context would be exercised fundamentally by first defining a social condition as a medical condition.

Having been defined as a medical condition, depression in this case, can then be the subject of study, diagnosis, treatment, and prevention, once medicalized. Used cynically and at times pejoratively by social scientists indicating a social model of behaviors being hijacked by a medical model of conditions, medicalization is also referred to as *'pathologization' and 'disease mongering'* [8]. Medicalization then provides us with a social condition that becomes a medical disease in need of treatment.

While the idea of assuming control over the management of an individual's life condition is anathema to a life of free will, bodily autonomy, feminist ideology, and many other aspects of an individual's personal autonomy and freedom, medicalization brings positive aspects. Once a disease is defined and codified, medicalization benefits society as the symptoms, conditions and behavioral traits can then be treated thus bettering our quality of life.

Medicalization of depression is particularly important as the disorder does not present itself in strictly medical or biological indicators. Many sociologists point out that historically, medical thought and authorities had always sought to define and control social conditions and behaviors in order to achieve social control. Particularly relatable to the course of depression using the concept and term "medicalization" in 1975 the book *Limits to Medicine: Medical Nemesis* the term "*iatrogenesis*" is described as a process where illnesses unintentionally increase as a result of medical intervention [182–185]. The effect of "iatrogenesis" is that medicalized life leaves individuals and society less able to deal with natural social processes such as aging and dying [186].

Medicalization and depression specifically are addressed in a 2007 article that argues that major depression is not served beneficially by medicalization. Further, Roger Mulder in "*An Epidemic of Depression or the Medicalization of Distress?*" [187] proposes that the apparent increase in major depression results from "confusing those who are ill with those who share their symptoms; the surveying of symptoms out of context; the benefits that accrue from such a diagnosis to drug companies, researchers, and clinicians; and changing social constructions around sadness and distress." He argues that the major depression category and treatments thereof should be replaced by an acknowledgement of the continuous distribution of depressive symptoms.

Etiopathogenesis of Depression

Regardless of whether depression is a specific individual medical disorder, or a manifestation of sociological conditions and a continuum of behaviors, we find today that depression is treatable. Not only is the condition treatable but is often reversable in whatever population as long as it is recognized early enough, and appropriate treatments are applied. We also recognize the relationship of depression to other diseases and conditions. Left untreated, depression may result in social dysfunction, social impairment, physical and cognitive issues as well as suicide.

Positive indications of medical treatment outcomes do exist thus indicating that not only is medical treatment beneficial as a preventative, but diagnosis and treatment may also prevent worsening of known cases of major depression.

Social Factors and Brain Structure

Beyond more traditional therapies for depression based in psychotherapy and psychiatry, medicalization and resultant studies by the medical community have resulted in establishing a relationship between *social factors and conditions, and the brain structure*. Neuronal studies of regions in the brain show specific activities that are then related to life events, accumulations of life events and social conditions. These activities are then monitored along with treatments to indicate positively the effects of various medical treatment methodologies.

As a model for maternal social isolation and depression influences on adult offspring, rodent experiments have shown that learning and memory networks in the offspring involving the hippocampus and amygdala are particularly vulnerable to maternal social isolation and can occur in the absence of elevated maternal stress hormone levels, anxiety, or altered mothering [188].

Maladaptive acute psychosocial stress neural recovery has been correlated with altered activity in the anterior cingulate, anterior insula, hippocampus, and striatum [189]. A study of 6- to 8-year-old offspring of depressed parents compared to lower risk peers showed blunted fMRI response to happy faces in the dorsal striatum [190]. In addition, lower activity in the dorsolateral prefrontal cortex was related to lower behavioral reward seeking, but only in high-risk children.

Neuroanatomical studies of major depression have shown diminishing thickness of areas important for social interaction such as salience [191, 192], internal mentation [193], and switching between internal thoughts and executive control [193].

Whole cortex mapping of genetic and environmental associations between brain and behavior that reflects a genetic vulnerability to depression seems to involve executive and social functioning in a distributed process across various regions of the brain [194]. Results seem to underscore the variation in heritability within brain regions [194, 197, 198]. Genome-wide association studies have identified dozens of risk variants and have refined the genetic architecture of major depression including areas associated with lower education attainment [195]. Additionally, genetic susceptibility to major depression appears to differ between early-onset and late-onset depression [196].

Social Processing

Poorer social processing including lack of emotional understanding in social contexts, lack of empathy, callousness and unemotionality may be a mechanism behind sustaining or severity of depression [199–202]. Coinheritance of callousness and depression appears to be likely [203].

Further demonstrating the physical-personal interplay between the individual and social conditions and experiences, in "The reciprocal interaction between serotonin and social behaviour" [7, 204], we find a review of papers demonstrating the relationship of social factors to antidepressive treatments. Using serotonin as a marker for antidepression, the researchers find that serotonin levels are strongly linked to social conditions. While not at the level of dependent and independent variable, this relationship does clearly demonstrate at least one mechanism whereby social conditions and life experiences manifest themselves in the behaviors of the individual.

Urban Versus Rural Environments

There are contradictory reports about the effect of urban vs rural environments on mental health. Most frequently, studies suggest that there is a greater risk of mental health problems in urban environments [205] especially of anxiety and depression [206, 207]. Other reports suggest that might not be so [208]. Questions abound upon what factors contribute to possible associations. Proposals have included lack of green spaces [209], socioeconomic factors, pollution, and individual genetic variations and susceptibilities [36, 37, 210, 211].

A systematic review in 2020 found that urbanization may affect depression differentially across geographic regions and income levels [212]. Out of 11 studies, 4 found adverse effects of urban living on depression. Three studies in China found protective effects of urbanization on depression. Two showed no effects. And two that were stratified by urbanicity found that greenspaces inversely associated with depression in highly populated urban areas.

Research indicates that urbanicity has a synergistic effect with genetic vulnerability to neurobiological stressors that may be conducive to depression [213, 214]. Social-related precursors to depression in urban settings include increased exposure to noise, light and air pollution, poor quality housing, reduced diet quality, physical inactivity, economic strain, and diminished social networks [215].

An intriguing study attempted to capture the complexity of urban living environments and socioeconomic factors on psychiatric symptoms [216]. They suggest that, " different environmental profiles of urban living may influence specific psychiatric symptom groups through distinct neurobiological pathways." In their study, they found correlations with three profiles. The first two profiles were more highly associated than the third.

The first profile encompasses high degrees of social deprivation, air pollution, street network, and urban land-use density and lack of green space. It showed a positive correlation with increased affective symptoms of depression. This profile was mediated by brain volume differences involved in reward processing, and moderated by genes enriched for stress response, including CRHR1. CRHR1is a critical regulator of the hypothalamic and behavioral extrahypothalamic stress response.

The second profile is dominated by green spaces and long distances to waste processing and energy facilities, and proximity to lakes, rivers, and the sea. All of these had a protective effect against symptoms of anxiety. Brain regions involved were those involved in emotion regulation and moderated by reduced volume in the inferior frontal regions, amygdala, and cerebellar regions that are involved in fear and anxiety regulation.

The third urban environmental profile was a correlation of the density of land use and urban infrastructure with a group of emotional instability symptoms. These effects were mediated by the frontal pole, amygdala, precentral gyrus, insular cortex, and cerebellum.

As we have noted elsewhere, the diagnosis for major depression is keyed to the presence of individual behaviors and life experiences. In this way, we see the manifestation of beneficial aspects of a sociological perspective driving the individual-centric viewpoint. It seems quite understandable that a coalition of working perspectives would be the most effective path to treating depression.

Access to Resources

Having defined a paradigm for the nature of depression and ascertained the need for treatments as well as developing paths for effective treatments, it is then necessary to understand the sociological structures and functions that effectively deliver solutions to and for those societies and members of society most affected by depression.

For successful social progress in relation to better social health-care activities, clearly we must not only have the required social structures and functions within our societies, but they must be available. And not only must these components be available, but they must also be available to all who actively participate in the social structures. It is not good enough to have a learned and capable medical community if that community does not serve all of society. Likewise, it does no good to have a mature and well-equipped medical and social service community if their services and expertise are restricted by such social failures as affordability, poor commerce, communication failures, political strife, and ineffective social regulation.

It seems obvious that to access social structures and utilize social functions, we are discussing a lack of barriers, at a minimum. In addition to a lack of barriers, however, we must construct methods and pathways of facilitation. By discussing specific structures and functions of society, we illustrate the interventions that support understanding and treatments for major depression.

Social Structural Support

Beyond the institutions themselves, the major social functions that support good mental health are emotional and physical support. Some of our emotional needs are companionship, a sense of history, shared interests and like-minded support. Some physical functions would be romantic partnerships, community network memberships, and ritual practices.

Historically, social structures encompass such things as family, medical practitioners, educational institutions, and political structures. In the past few decades, a perfect example of a new social structure has emerged in the form of the *internet* [217, 218].

As a social structure, the internet is well suited to support, as well as to deny, access of societies' members to all sorts of elements and services germane to mental health-care [219–222]. Not only do medical professionals deliver care via the internet, but potential patients find care as well as general information, confirm biases, learn of trends, learn of themselves by learning of others and so on. Of course, this structure requires a certain level of understanding and competency of the individual, and a level of learned social acceptance. As an example of a social structure that supports access and utility of mental health-care, the internet is difficult to underplay

Systematic reviews of *social media* and its connection to mental health were published in 2020 through 2023 [223–226]. Their main conclusions were that social media is responsible for aggravating mental health problems especially anxiety and depression, but in a gender nuanced fashion. However, they found mixed evidence for that influence. Nevertheless, evidence compiled from cross-sectional, longitudinal, and empirical studies showed that smartphone and social media use among teenagers associates with increased mental distress, self-harming behaviors, and suicidality [225]. Among their conclusions were that age does not have an effect and females were much more likely to experience mental health issues related to social media [226, 227].

Some social theories attempt to explain social media effect on mental health. Among these are the *Displaced Behavior Theory* that suggests those who spend more time on social media have less time on face-to-face interactions. Although generally believed to be negative, the adverse impact has been debated [32, 228]. For example, expanded opportunities of social support on social media may buffer adverse effects of geographic isolation and loneliness, whereas negative experiences including cyberbullying are associated with depression [224, 229]. Social media may also influence positive mental health by using the internet and social media to find critical information on mental health [230]. Some studies have found no relationships between time spent on social media, or number of online friends and selfies and depression [33]. Another study found no relationship between frequency of social media use and depression.

Males use of social media has been linked to higher self-concept, practicing of social skills and self-esteem, but over-investment in social media was associated with lower self-esteem and increased depression [34]. Females who had a social media profile had significantly higher levels of depression and lower self-esteem. Females more than males tend to be more addicted to social media [35], and reading posts is more strongly associated with depression than making posts [231]. Overall, it appears that frequency of social media use has less influence on depression than family functioning and interpersonal trust [33].

In addition to the *Social networks* like Facebook, Twitter (Now X), Instagram, and Snapchat, there are *Media sharing applications* such as WhatsApp, Instagram, YouTube, Snapchat, and TikTok; *Messengers* including Facebook Messenger, WhatsApp, Telegram, Viber, and iMessage; *Blogging platforms* including WordPress, and Wikipedia; *Discussion forums* like Reddit and Twitter (X); and *Fitness and lifestyle applications* such as Fitbit. As of 2020, there was a gender-based distribution of social media audiences worldwide on different platforms. At that point in time, there was a female preponderance on Twitter (X), LinkedIn, and Facebook; and equal distribution on Instagram, and a male preponderance on Snapchat.

Religious Beliefs

Religious beliefs and the social aspects of joint worship may help some people to cope with uncertainty [232]. Around the world, religion and religious coping are more prevalent in those over 40 compared to younger folks [26, 27, 233]. Women are generally more religious than men, especially among Christians, in spite of the male dominance in positions of authority in many of the world's religions [234]. However, the history of religions and intolerance of those who do not belong to a particular religion is fraught.

The public role of religion has been changing in secularized countries. Religious intolerance practiced by dominant religions and associated governments often has the effect of marginalizing and stressing those who are not part of the majority group. This intolerance and harassment are increasing [235]. These clashes may take various forms including interreligious tension and violence, hostilities to religious norms, harassment by social groups or individuals and organized violence.[8]

On the other hand, when one is a member of a religious group, there may be significant benefits derived from that affiliation [237–239]. Of course, social isolation often means estrangement from religious institutions. When faced with serious stressful challenges, religious coping strategies may have positive or negative effects on depression [239]. There is a complex relationship between positive/negative religious coping styles and depressive symptoms [239]. Positive

[8] The Pew-Templeton Global Religious Futures project, analyzes religious change and its impact on societies around the world [236].

religious coping is based upon a trusting and secure relationship with a loving and supporting God [24, 240, 241]. Negative religious coping is based upon a feeling of desolation and being punished by their God [242, 243]. Most studies find that negative religious coping styles are associated with increased depressive symptoms [244–246]. But, this is predominately in those who chronically use negative religious coping [247]. However, a divine struggle to understand "why" bad things happen and not divine punishment appears to be the factor associated with depression [248]. Positive religious coping seems to be associated with protective effects against depression [249–251]. Although most of these studies were conducted in Christian religion groups, similar findings have been seen in Jews [25] and Muslims [252, 253]. Adding to the complexity is that cultural and religious competence in clinical practice is a challenge [254].

In order to counteract a sense of isolation and lack of integration into society, the individual must be accepted and feel a sense of belongingness. A nonexhaustive list of social structures that are key to delivering a sense of belonging to the individual would consist of: family, cultural organizations, voluntary groups and networks (self-help groups), schools, friends and peers, workmates, pet ownership and neighborhood groups. While all of these groups can function to disillusion the individual, close ties to any or all of these may be key to good mental health.

Social Functional Support

Within the social groups that may provide belongingness, there are functions that these groups should deliver to the people who belong to them. An obvious example would be the core family structure that provides role models, behavioral rules, attachment, behavioral guidelines and most of our early childhood experiences.

The functions we come to expect and those that we need in order to fulfill a mentally healthy life are not always the same, but it may be important to say that if society provides expectations for functions that are not met, that is unhealthy. For example, it is incumbent upon a healthy family function to provide parental and gender role models that coincide with external societal norms. Not meeting this familial function may leave the individual without a sense of normalcy, and with a feeling of alienation, constituents of depression.

Gender Roles, Youth and Adolescence, and Depression

A meta-analysis of the epidemiological literature prior to 2011 revealed that *childhood maltreatment* was associated with increased risk of developing recurrent and persistent depressive episodes (OR = 2.27; 95% CI: 1.80 to 2.87)[9]. In addition, a meta-analysis of clinical trials prior to 2011 indicated that childhood maltreatment was associated with deficiencies of response or remission during treatment for depression (OR=1.43; 95% CI=1.11–1.83).

A 19-year longitudinal study followed the 15% most inhibited and the 15% most aggressive children at 4–6 years of age until they reached 23 years of age [255]. Results indicated that for most of the male and female inhibited children, there were delayed social transitions but few internalizing problems. The most aggressive children had a significant long-term risk of externalizing, were educational and occupational underachievers, and had a higher adult delinquency rate than the controls, independent of sex and socioeconomics. Social anxieties in middle school, self-directed coping strategies, and social withdrawal-disengagement have been independently directly linked with increased peer victimization for boys [256].

Rather than perpetuation across generations, children who were maltreated or witnessed violence are more likely to be victimized as an adult [257]. Although symptoms of depression are associated with *intimate partner violence (IPV)* perpetration and victimization, there are multitudes of socioeconomic and psychosocial risk factors that paint a complex picture [2013 review 258]. These factors include (1) partnership context (demographic, neighborhood, community, and school factors), (2) partner's development and behavior (including family, peer, psychological, behavioral, and cognitive influences), and (3) relationship factors and interactional patterns [258].

Early antisocial behavior increases the risk for IPV, perpetration, and victimization [258, 259], In addition, exposure of children to their parents' IPV predisposes them to increased levels of depression, emotional expressivity, aggression, and hostile reactivity. Child antisocial behavior is associated with parental psychopathology, parenting practices, and child self-regulation in a circular fashion. IPV increases the probability of parental PTSD and alcohol abuse, but not of parental MDD.

Effects on children who were crime victims upon moving to low-poverty neighborhoods show differences between boys and girls [260]. Adolescent girls from families experiencing recent violent crime victimization were significantly

[9]Odds ratio (OR) is a way to represent the odds that an outcome will result when a given exposure to a variable of interest occurs compared to when the exposure does not occur. OR quantifies the strength of the association between two events. An OR greater than 1 indicates a positive association or that exposure to that variable increases the odds of that outcome. An OR less than one indicates a negative relationship between two events. An OR of 1 suggests no relationship between two events. An OR is frequently accompanied by a 95% confidence interval (CI). CI is a measure of precision of the OR. The smaller the CI the higher precision as long as it does not overlap OR =1. For more information, see the Chap. 4 on evidence basics in this text.

less likely to gain mental health benefits in terms of relief from distress, behavioral problems and major depression from the move than were girls from homes where there was no crime. Boys in families where there was crime victimization were actually harmed by moving to the low-poverty neighborhoods. Childhood stress affects development and adult responses to current stresses, influencing mood disorders, aggressive/impulsive traits, and suicidal behavior [261, 262].

The interpersonal role of *food offering* between parents and child in *empathic emotion regulation* has been examined by Hamburg et al. [263]. Empathic emotion regulation is an empathic response to another's emotional state that aims to regulate emotion in the provider and between the interaction partners. Offering food is motivated by the recipient's and the provider's emotional state such that its objective is to increase positive affect for both. Sharing of food resources and food as support increases interpersonal closeness. It is also suggested that if food offering becomes a substitute for other support behaviors, children may learn to use food as the principal way to soothe themselves and others. This may feed into eating disorders and foster an abbreviated set of coping behaviors.

This theme of food sharing and empathic emotion regulation has been discussed and critiqued from an evolutionary perspective by Alley [264].

Social Resources for Treating Depression

Recognizing the progress made over the past decades in understanding the sociological needs and impacts of depression, especially with formalized diagnostics and public acceptance of the social nature of the disorder, a number of specific resources for and about treating depression have arisen. The key to these resources is that they work within a social framework and encompass community resources, social institutions, and social networks.

Some of the available resources for treating mental depression are in the following list.

Peer Support Groups: These groups of individuals that share similar life experiences provide mutual support. Typically, these groups provide a space and setting within which members can share strategies, challenges, and receive emotional support in order to cope with depression.

Examples of peer Support Groups would be

- National Alliance on Mental Illness (NAMI) support groups [265].
- Depression and Bipolar Support Alliance groups [266].

Online Support Communities: Providing anonymity and good accessibility, virtual forums and online support groups allow individuals to connect with others confronted with like-challenges.

Examples of Online Groups:

- 7 Cups of Tea [267].

Community Mental Health Services: Often in both urban and suburban areas, these centers offer a variety of medical and social services including counseling, crisis intervention, therapy both individual and group, and medication management.

Community Mental Health Services are often funded by local governments and listed in local directories as health-care centers and mental health clinics. For example, [268].

Crisis Hotlines and Helplines: Provided by phone line on a 24-h availability, these provide immediate emotional support and guidance to the caller. These lines are available both in voice mode as well as text mode.

Examples of Crisis Hotlines

- National Suicide Prevention Lifeline (988) [269].
- Crisis Text Line (text HOME to 7417410) [270].

Educational and Preventative Programs: Targeting the general public, these programs aim to educate and inform the public about mental health issues with the aim of promoting early intervention and reducing stigma and reluctance to treatment.

Examples of Educational Programs are

- Mental Health First Aid campaigns. [271].
- School-based programs found in public schools typically provide counseling and offer resources to students and their families via school counselors and antibullying programs.

Social and Recreational Activity Groups: Longstanding institutions, social clubs and sport-centered groups offer activities and social interactions to enhance feelings of engagement and belongingness and being connected to the community. Besides participation as a member of social and sporting groups, these clubs and institutions also provide nonpaid volunteering opportunities to serve the memberships as well as special needs groups. Volunteering provides a means of connecting with others as well as a sense of purpose in serving.

Examples are

- YMCA [272].
- YWCA group [273].
- Most public school systems and public-funded recreational groups offer volunteer opportunities as well.

Health and Wellness Programs: Centered often on the relationship between physical activity and mental health, these programs are made up of fitness classes and exercise groups. Promoting connectivity and awareness, these often emphasize social support, nutrition, and overall health through access to physical health.

Examples of Health and Wellness Programs would be

- Classes offered by community school-based programs, health-club fitness classes, and walking groups often targeting mature age groups.

Family and Caregiver Support: Involving family members in therapy groups offers improved communication and enhances support systems while bettering the groups understanding of mental health issues.

Examples of Family and Caregiver Support would be found by searching for

Family Counseling services and Family Support Groups.

Local Caregiver Support Groups for those caring for individuals with mental health issues include

- Family First [274]
- Respite Care [275]
- A Place for Mom [276]

Workplace Mental Health Programs: Business workplaces may offer *Employee Assistance Programs,* often associated with their employee insurance programs they provide resources, support services, and confidential counseling to employees dealing with mental health issues.

Examples would be

- Counseling services and mental health workshops
- A resource for Workplace Mental Health by the American Psychiatric Association [277]

Social Services and Advocacy Organizations: Social Service Agencies, often government-funded in the USA, provide assistance such as housing, health insurance and health care, as well as financial assistance.

Examples of Social Service and Advocacy Organizations are

- California Association of Social Rehabilitation Agencies [278]
- Mental Health America [279]
- Anxiety and Depression Association of America [280]
- The National Alliance on Mental Illness [281]

Collectively standing on the social structures and functions inherent in the sociological model, the foregoing resources describe the support system for those dealing with depressive disorder, aside from the broader medical-institutional model. Integration of and access to these resources enhances and improves mental health outcomes.

A systematic literature review of available devices used to monitor user's social behavior focused on mental health concluded that there are ubiquitous promising assistance tools for patients and mental health professionals. However, they identified limitations that are still to be overcome [282].

Summary

The exploration of depression from a sociological perspective demonstrates a complex interaction between the individual and society that influences mental health. While traditional psychological and medical approaches focus on the individual's biology and behavior, sociology emphasizes the crucial role of social conditions, cultural contexts, and structural inequalities in forming mental health outcomes.

Depression is not solely an individual's burden, but a societal issue influenced by factors such as social roles, economic conditions, cultural affiliations, and life events. Historical sociologists like Durkheim and Marx have shown that isolation from social forces and societal integration are fundamental to understanding mental health. Modern sociological research continues to validate the significance of social determinants in mental health, highlighting the importance of belonging, social support, and accessible healthcare.

Sociological concepts of social indicators, structures, and functions show us a picture of depression and its relationship to life events that exist not only on a spectrum, but also in different manifestation based on a number of social influences. Parental control, lifestyle and stage of life all appear to be related to the incidence of depression. We show some examples highlighting different aspects of the incidence of depression.

Effective interventions for depression must integrate both individual and social perspectives. A comprehensive approach involves medicalization to diagnose and treat the disorder and addressing the social structures and functions that support mental health. This includes enhancing access to mental health resources, fostering social support networks, and addressing societal inequalities. We list a number of social structures and functions that are available and central to the treatment and understanding of depression in society.

In conclusion, understanding and addressing depression requires a multifaceted approach that incorporates the insights of sociology. By recognizing the sociological roots of depression and implementing interventions that consider these factors, we can create a more supportive and inclusive environment that promotes mental well-being for all individuals.

References

1. Berkman LF, Syme SL. Social networks, host resistance, and mortality: a nine-year follow-up study of Almeda County residents. Am J Epidemiol. 1979;109(2):186–204.
2. Bjorndal, et al. Stressful life events increase the risk of major depressive episodes: a population-based twin study. Psychol Med. 2022; https://doi.org/10.1017/S0033291722002227.
3. Durkheim É. Suicide: a study in sociology. Free Press; 1897.
4. Hammen C, Henry R, Daley S. Childhood adversity and adult depression: the role of stress and vulnerability. J Abnorm Psychol. 2000;109(3):455–64.
5. Holmes TH, Rahe RH. The social readjustment rating scale. J Psychosom Res. 1967;11(2):213–8. PMID: 6059863. http://www.ncbi.nlm.nih.gov/pubmed/6059863.
6. Kendler KS, Karkowski LM, Prescott CA. Causal relationship between stressful life events and the onset of major depression. Am J Psychiatry. 1999;156(6):837–41. PMID: 10360120. http://www.ncbi.nlm.nih.gov/pubmed/10360120.
7. Kiser, et al. (2012) Reviews, Volume, February 2012, Pages 786–798. PloS One, (2022). Published online 2022, July 20.
8. Liebert R. Pathologization. In: Teo T, editor. Encyclopedia of critical psychology. New York, NY: Springer; 2014.
9. Marx K. Das Kapital: Kritik der politischen Oekonomie; herausgegeben von Friedrich Engels. Vol. 3: Der Gesamtprozess der kapitalistischen Produktion. 1st ed. Hamburg: Verlag von Otto Meissner; 1894. https://doi.org/10.3931/e-rara-25739.
10. Pitts JR. Medicalization and social control. Am J Sociol. 1968;73(4):363–72.
11. Simmel G. Soziologie: Untersuchungen über die Formen der Vergesellschaftung. Leipzig: Duncker & Humblot. The third and most recent translation of the text was published in a collection edited by Donald Levine ("The Stranger." In Georg Simmel: On Individuality and Social Forms, Chicago: Univ. of Chicago Press, 1971, pp. 143–50). 1908.
12. Data and Statistics on Children's Mental Health | CDC.
13. Sunzeri J. Youth and alienation. Master's Research Thesis. San Jose State University. 1979.
14. Weber M, Baehr PR, Wells GC. The Protestant ethic and the "spirit" of capitalism and other writings. Penguin; 2002. ISBN 978-0-14-043921-2.
15. Hobson CJ, Delunas L. National norms and life-event frequencies for the revised social readjustment rating scale. Int J Stress Manag. 2001;8:299–314.
16. Depression in the U.S. Household Population, 2009–2012 Products – Data Briefs – Number 172 – December 2014 (cdc.gov).
17. Serious Mental Illness Among Adults Below the Poverty Line Serious Mental Illness Among Adults Below the Poverty Line (samhsa.gov).
18. Hudson CG. Socioeconomic status & mental illness: tests of the social causation and selection hypotheses. Am J Orthopsychiatr. 2005;75(1):3–18.
19. Anakwenze U, Zuberi D. Mental health and poverty in the Inner City. Health Soc Work. 2013;38(3):147–57.
20. Abuse S. Key substance use and mental health indicators in the United States: results from the 2019 National Survey on Drug Use and Health. 2020.
21. Belle D, Doucet J. Poverty, inequality, and discrimination as sources of depression among US women. Psychol Women Q. 2003;27(2):101–13.
22. Lee Y, Eck JEOS, Martinez NN. How concentrated is crime at places? A systematic review from 1970 to 2015. Crime Sci. 2017;6:1–16.
23. Joiner TE Jr, Silva C. Why people die by suicide: further development and tests of the interpersonal-psychological theory of suicidal behavior. In: Shaver PR, Mikulincer M, editors. Meaning, mortality, and choice: the social psychology of existential concerns. American Psychological Association; 2012. p. 325–36. Why people die by suicide: Further development and tests of the interpersonal-psychological theory of suicidal behavior. (apa.org).
24. Wilt JA, Stauner N, Harriott VA, Exline JJ, Pargament KI. Partnering with God: Religious coping and perceptions of divine intervention predict spiritual transformation in response to religious– spiritual struggle. Psychol Relig Spiritual. 2019;11(3):278.
25. Rosmarin DH, Pargament KI, Flannelly KJ. Do spiritual struggles predict poorer physical/mental health among Jews? Int J Psychol Relig. 2009;19(4):244–58.
26. Wink P, Dillon M. Spiritual development across the adult life course: findings from a longitudinal study. J Adult Dev. 2002;9:79–94.
27. Idler EL, Musick MA, Ellison CG, George LK, Krause N, Ory MG, et al. Measuring multiple dimensions of religion and spirituality for health research: conceptual background and findings from the 1998 general social survey. Res Aging. 2003;25(4):327–65.
28. Lynch J, Kilmartin C. The pain behind the mask: overcoming masculine depression. Routledge; 2013.
29. Addis ME. Gender and depression in men. Clin Psychol Sci Pract. 2008;15(3):153.
30. Martin LA, Neighbors HW, Griffith DM. The experience of symptoms of depression in men vs women: analysis of the National Comorbidity Survey Replication. JAMA Psychiatry. 2013;70(10):1100–6. https://doi.org/10.1001/jamapsychiatry.2013.1985.
31. Cochran SV, Rabinowitz FE. Men and depression: clinical and empirical perspectives. Elsevier; 1999.
32. Coyne SM, Rogers AA, Zurcher JD, Stockdale L, Booth M. Does time spent using social media impact mental health?: An eight year longitudinal study. Comput Hum Behav. 2020;104:106160.
33. Marwick AE, Boyd D. Networked privacy: how teenagers negotiate context in social media. New Media Soc. 2014;16(7):1051–67.
34. Blomfield Neira CJ, Barber BL. Social networking site use: linked to adolescents' social self-concept, self-esteem, and depressed mood. Aust J Psychol. 2014;66(1):56–64.
35. Wartberg L, Kriston L, Thomasius R. Internet gaming disorder and problematic social media use in a representative sample of German adolescents: prevalence estimates, comorbid depressive symptoms and related psychosocial aspects. Comput Hum Behav. 2020;103:31–6.
36. Pluess M. Individual differences in environmental sensitivity. Child Dev Perspect. 2015;9(3):138–43.
37. Duncan GJ, Magnuson K, Votruba-Drzal E. In: Bornstein MH, et al., editors. Handbook of child psychology and developmental science, Ecological settings and processes, vol. 4. Wiley; 2015. p. 534–73.
38. Rethinking and updating demographic questions: Guidance to improve descriptions of research samples. (apa.org).
39. Demographics: What, Why, and How Evaluators Use the Information—Theories of Evaluation.
40. Introduction to Applied Demography | SpringerLink.
41. Rolak. Neurology secrets. Elsevier Health Science; 2001.
42. Annandale E. The sociology of health and medicine: a critical introduction. 2nd ed. Cambridge; 2014. ISBN 978–0–7456-3461-6. OCLC 885445027.
43. Cockerham WC. Medical sociology. Taylor & Francis; 2017. ISBN 978-1-317-21171-6.
44. Rogers A. In: Rogers A, Pilgrim D, editors. Sociology of mental health and illness. 6th ed. London; 2021. ISBN 978-0-335-24849-0. OCLC 1232510.

45. Cockerham WC. The Wiley Blackwell companion to medical sociology. Wiley; 2021. ISBN 978-1-119-63375-4.
46. Nettleton S. The sociology of health and illness. 3rd ed. Cambridge: Polity; 2013. ISBN 978-0-7456-4600-8. OCLC 819519790.
47. Newman MC, Lawless JJ, Gelo F. Family-oriented patient care. Am Fam Physician. 2007;75(9):1306–10. PMID: 17508523. http://www.ncbi.nlm.nih.gov/pubmed/17508523.
48. Kusnanto H, Agustian D, Hilmanto D. Biopsychosocial model of illnesses in primary care: a hermeneutic literature review. J Family Med Prim Care. 2018;7(3):497–500. PMCID: PMC6069638. http://www.ncbi.nlm.nih.gov/pubmed/30112296.
49. Wade DT, Halligan PW. The biopsychosocial model of illness: a model whose time has come. Clin Rehabil. 2017;31(8):995–1004. PMID: 28730890. http://www.ncbi.nlm.nih.gov/pubmed/28730890.
50. Karunamuni N, Imayama I, Goonetilleke D. Pathways to well-being: untangling the causal relationships among biopsychosocial variables. Soc Sci Med 2021;272:112846. PMID: 32089388. http://www.ncbi.nlm.nih.gov/pubmed/32089388.
51. Conrad P, Barker KK. The social construction of illness: key insights and policy implications. J Health Soc Behav. 2010;51(Suppl):S67–79. PMID: 20943584. http://www.ncbi.nlm.nih.gov/pubmed/20943584.
52. Liu Q, He H, Yang J, Feng X, Zhao F, Lyu J. Changes in the global burden of depression from 1990 to 2017: findings from the global burden of disease study. J Psychiatr Res. 2020;126:134–40. PMID: 31439359. http://www.ncbi.nlm.nih.gov/pubmed/31439359.
53. Bloom BS. Prevalence and economic effects of depression. Manag Care. 2004;13(6 Suppl Depression):9–16. PMID: 15293766. http://www.ncbi.nlm.nih.gov/pubmed/15293766.
54. Ustün TB. The global burden of mental disorders. Am J Public Health. 1999;89(9):1315–8. PMCID: PMC1508755. http://www.ncbi.nlm.nih.gov/pubmed/10474545.
55. Murray CJL, Vos T, Lozano R, Naghavi M, Flaxman AD, Michaud C, Ezzati M, Shibuya K, Salomon JA, Abdalla S, Aboyans V, Abraham J, Ackerman I, Aggarwal R, Ahn, Memish ZA, et al. Disability-adjusted life years (DALYs) for 291 diseases and injuries in 21 regions, 1990-2010: a systematic analysis for the global burden of disease study 2010. Lancet. 2012;380(9859):2197–223. PMID: 23245608. http://www.ncbi.nlm.nih.gov/pubmed/23245608.
56. GBD 2019 Mental Disorders Collaborators. Global, regional, and national burden of 12 mental disorders in 204 countries and territories, 1990–2019: a systematic analysis for the Global Burden of Disease Study 2019. Lancet Psychiatry. 2022;9(2):137–50. PMCID: PMC8776563. http://www.ncbi.nlm.nih.gov/pubmed/35026139.
57. The Depression Boom: As US Population Ages, Mental Illness Rises.
58. "Depression: let's talk" says WHO, as depression tops list of causes of ill health.
59. Major Depression—National Institute of Mental Health (NIMH).
60. Chang-Quan H, Xue-Mei Z, Bi-Rong D, Zhen-Chan L, Ji-Rong Y, Qing-Xiu L. Health status and risk for depression among the elderly: a meta-analysis of published literature. Age Ageing. 2010;39(1):23–30. PMID: 19903775. http://www.ncbi.nlm.nih.gov/pubmed/19903775.
61. Zhao KX, Huang CQ, Xiao Q, Gao Y, Liu QX, Wang ZR, Li YH, Xie YZ. Age and risk for depression among the elderly: a meta-analysis of the published literature. CNS Spectr. 2012;17(3):142–54. PMID: 22892113. http://www.ncbi.nlm.nih.gov/pubmed/22892113.
62. Adler N, Matthews K. Health psychology: why do some people get sick and some stay well? Annu Rev Psychol. 1994;45:229–59. PMID: 8135503. http://www.ncbi.nlm.nih.gov/pubmed/8135503.
63. National Survey on Drug Use and Health.
64. Weinberger AH, Gbedemah M, Martinez AM, Nash D, Galea S, Goodwin RD. Trends in depression prevalence in the USA from 2005 to 2015: widening disparities in vulnerable groups. Psychol Med. 2018;48(8):1308–15. PMID: 29021005. http://www.ncbi.nlm.nih.gov/pubmed/29021005.
65. Goldman N, Glei DA, Weinstein M. Declining mental health among disadvantaged Americans. Proc Natl Acad Sci U S A. 2018;115(28):7290–5. PMCID: PMC6048554. http://www.ncbi.nlm.nih.gov/pubmed/29915079.
66. Vandeleur CL, Fassassi S, Castelao E, Glaus J, Strippoli MPF, Lasserre AM, Rudaz D, Gebreab S, Pistis G, Aubry JM, Angst J, Preisig M. Prevalence and correlates of DSM-5 major depressive and related disorders in the community. Psychiatry Res 2017;250:50–58. PMID: 28142066. http://www.ncbi.nlm.nih.gov/pubmed/28142066.
67. Medicaid.gov: The Official U.S. Government Site for Medicaid and CHIP Services | Medicaid.
68. Most frequent conditions in U.S. Hospitals, 2011 #162.
69. 2020 Methodological Summary and Definitions | CBHSQ Data.
70. Products – Data Briefs – Number 303 – February 2018.
71. Conditions With the Largest Number of Adult Hospital Readmissions by Payer, 2011 – Statistical Brief #172.
72. Research – Bhatnagar Lab.
73. Park SH, Yu HY. How useful is the center for epidemiologic studies depression scale in screening for depression in adults? An updated systematic review and meta-analysis. Psychiatry Res. 2021;302:114037. PMID: 34098160. http://www.ncbi.nlm.nih.gov/pubmed/34098160.
74. Park SH, Lee H. Is the center for epidemiologic studies depression scale as useful as the geriatric depression scale in screening for late-life depression? A systematic review. J Affect Disord. 2021;292:454–63. PMID: 34144371. http://www.ncbi.nlm.nih.gov/pubmed/34144371.
75. Park SH, Kwon YM. Can the Center for Epidemiologic Studies Depression Scale be Used to screen for depression in children and adolescents? An updated systematic review. Child Psychiatry Hum Dev. 2023; PMID: 37354303. http://www.ncbi.nlm.nih.gov/pubmed/37354303.
76. Blodgett JM, Lachance CC, Stubbs B, Co M, Wu YT, Prina M, Tsang VWL, Cosco TD. A systematic review of the latent structure of the Center for Epidemiologic Studies Depression Scale (CES-D) amongst adolescents. BMC Psychiatry. 2021;21(1):197. PMCID: PMC8054366. http://www.ncbi.nlm.nih.gov/pubmed/33874939.
77. Eslinger PJ, Anders S, Ballarini T, Boutros S, Krach S, Mayer AV, Moll J, Newton TL, Schroeter ML, de Oliveira-Souza R, Raber J, Sullivan GB, Swain JE, Lowe L, Zahn R. The neuroscience of social feelings: mechanisms of adaptive social functioning. Neurosci Biobehav Rev. 2021;128:592–620. PMCID: PMC8388127. http://www.ncbi.nlm.nih.gov/pubmed/34089764.
78. Chu C, Buchman-Schmitt JM, Stanley IH, Hom MA, Tucker RP, Hagan CR, Rogers ML, Podlogar MC, Chiurliza B, Ringer FB, Michaels MS, Patros CHG, Joiner TE. The interpersonal theory of suicide: a systematic review and meta-analysis of a decade of cross-national research. Psychol Bull. 2017;143(12):1313–45. PMCID: PMC5730496. http://www.ncbi.nlm.nih.gov/pubmed/29072480.
79. King CA, Brent D, Grupp-Phelan J, Page K, Czyz E, McGuire TC, Mahabee-Gittens EM, Block L, Casper TC. A prospective examination of the interpersonal-psychological theory of suicidal behavior in adolescents. J Clin Child Adolesc Psychol. 2024;53(6):922–34. PMCID: PMC11436474. http://www.ncbi.nlm.nih.gov/pubmed/38547387.
80. Joiner TE, Jeon ME, Lieberman A, Janakiraman R, Duffy ME, Gai AR, Dougherty SP. On prediction, refutation, and explanatory reach: a consideration of the interpersonal theory of suicidal behavior. Prev Med 2021;152(Pt 1):106453. PMID: 34538380. http://www.ncbi.nlm.nih.gov/pubmed/34538380.

81. Van Orden KA, Witte TK, Cukrowicz KC, Braithwaite SR, Selby EA, Joiner TE. The interpersonal theory of suicide. Psychol Rev. 2010;117(2):575–600. PMCID: PMC3130348. http://www.ncbi.nlm.nih.gov/pubmed/20438238.
82. Conrad K, Forkmann T, Schreiber D, Teismann T, Glaesmer H, Spangenberg L, Schönfelder A, Hallensleben N, Paashaus L, Juckel G, Höller I. Understanding suicidal ideation-a network analysis of the interpersonal needs questionnaire. PLoS One. 2023;18(11):e0293026. PMCID: PMC10642825. http://www.ncbi.nlm.nih.gov/pubmed/37956124.
83. Gutierrez PM, Pease J, Matarazzo BB, Monteith LL, Hernandez T, Osman A. Evaluating the psychometric properties of the interpersonal needs questionnaire and the acquired capability for suicide scale in military veterans. Psychol Assess. 2016;28(12):1684–94. PMID: 26998894. http://www.ncbi.nlm.nih.gov/pubmed/26998894.
84. Kramer EB, Gaeddert LA, Jackson CL, Harnke B, Nazem S. Use of the acquired capability for suicide scale (ACSS) among United States military and veteran samples: a systematic review. J Affect Disord. 2020;267:229–42. PMID: 32217223. http://www.ncbi.nlm.nih.gov/pubmed/32217223.
85. Rogers ML, Bauer BW, Gai AR, Duffy ME, Joiner TE. Examination of measurement invariance of the acquired capability for suicide scale. Psychol Assess. 2021;33(5):464–70. PMID: 33705162. http://www.ncbi.nlm.nih.gov/pubmed/33705162.
86. Van Orden KA, Cukrowicz KC, Witte TK, Joiner TE. Thwarted belongingness and perceived burdensomeness: construct validity and psychometric properties of the interpersonal needs questionnaire. Psychol Assess. 2012;24(1):197–215. PMCID: PMC3377972. http://www.ncbi.nlm.nih.gov/pubmed/21928908.
87. Gronewold J, Duman EE, Engel M, Engels M, Siegrist J, Erbel R, Jöckel KH, Hermann DM. Association between life events and later depression in the population-based Heinz Nixdorf recall study-the role of sex and optimism. PLoS One. 2022;17(7):e0271716. PMCID: PMC9299341
88. Monroe SM, Harkness KL. Major depression and its recurrences: life course matters. Annu Rev Clin Psychol. 2022;18:329–57. PMID: 35216520. http://www.ncbi.nlm.nih.gov/pubmed/35216520.
89. Ding X, Liang M, Wang H, Song Q, Guo X, Su W, Li N, Liu H, Ma S, Zhou X, Sun Y. Prenatal stressful life events increase the prevalence of postpartum depression: evidence from prospective cohort studies. J Psychiatr Res. 2023;160:263–71. PMID: 36889197. http://www.ncbi.nlm.nih.gov/pubmed/36889197.
90. Buckman JEJ, Saunders R, Arundell LL, Oshinowo ID, Cohen ZD, O'Driscoll C, Barnett P, Stott J, Ambler G, Gilbody S, Hollon SD, Kendrick T, Watkins E, Eley TC, Skelton M, Wiles N, Kessler D, DeRubeis RJ, Lewis G, Pilling S. Life events and treatment prognosis for depression: a systematic review and individual patient data meta-analysis. J Affect Disord 2022;299:298–308. PMCID: PMC9113943. http://www.ncbi.nlm.nih.gov/pubmed/34920035.
91. Coventry PA, Meader N, Melton H, Temple M, Dale H, Wright K, Cloitre M, Karatzias T, Bisson J, Roberts NP, Brown JVE, Barbui C, Churchill R, Lovell K, McMillan D, Gilbody S. Psychological and pharmacological interventions for posttraumatic stress disorder and comorbid mental health problems following complex traumatic events: systematic review and component network meta-analysis. PLoS Med 2020;17(8):e1003262. PMCID: PMC7446790. http://www.ncbi.nlm.nih.gov/pubmed/32813696.
92. Rnic K, Santee AC, Hoffmeister JA, Liu H, Chang KK, Chen RX, Neufeld RWJ, Machado DA, Starr LR, Dozois DJA, LeMoult J. The vicious cycle of psychopathology and stressful life events: a meta-analytic review testing the stress generation model. Psychol Bull. 2023;149(5–6):330–69. PMID: 37261747. http://www.ncbi.nlm.nih.gov/pubmed/37261747.
93. Bjørndal LD, Kendler KS, Reichborn-Kjennerud T, Ystrom E. Stressful life events increase the risk of major depressive episodes: a population-based twin study. Psychol Med 2023;53(11):5194–5202. PMCID: PMC10476058. http://www.ncbi.nlm.nih.gov/pubmed/35920242.
94. Hammen C, Henry R, Daley SE. Depression and sensitization to stressors among young women as a function of childhood adversity. J Consult Clin Psychol. 2000;68(5):782–7. PMID: 11068964. http://www.ncbi.nlm.nih.gov/pubmed/11068964.
95. Jaeggi AV, Blackwell AD, von Rueden C, Trumble BC, Stieglitz J, Garcia AR, Kraft TS, Beheim BA, Hooper PL, Kaplan H, Gurven M. Do wealth and inequality associate with health in a small-scale subsistence society? elife 2021;10:e59437. PMCID: PMC8225390. http://www.ncbi.nlm.nih.gov/pubmed/33988506.
96. Undurraga EA, Nyberg C, Eisenberg DTA, Magvanjav O, Reyes-García V, Huanca T, Leonard WR, McDade TW, Tanner S, Vadez V, Godoy R, TAPS Bolivia Study Team. Individual wealth rank, community wealth inequality, and self-reported adult poor health: a test of hypotheses with panel data (2002–2006) from native Amazonians, Bolivia. Med Anthropol Q. 2010;24(4):522–48. PMID: 21322409. http://www.ncbi.nlm.nih.gov/pubmed/21322409.
97. Kondo N. Socioeconomic disparities and health: impacts and pathways. J Epidemiol 2012;22(1):2–6. PMCID: PMC3798573. http://www.ncbi.nlm.nih.gov/pubmed/22156290.
98. Xu KQ, Aw JYH, Payne CF. Inequalities in mortality in the Asia-Pacific: a cross-National Comparison of socioeconomic gradients. J Gerontol B Psychol Sci Soc Sci. 2024;79(4):gbad193. PMCID: PMC10948962. http://www.ncbi.nlm.nih.gov/pubmed/38195098.
99. Home—Department of Demography.
100. Search Results | CDC.
101. HealthData.gov
102. NIH LIBRARY | NIH Library.
103. Oregon Health Authority: Data and Statistics: Data and Statistics: State of Oregon.
104. BRFSSdepressionreport_1.2.19.pdf.
105. demographic-data-collection-and-reporting_brief.pdf.
106. Call CC, Eckstrand KL, Kasparek SW, Boness CL, Blatt L, Jamal-Orozco N, Novacek DM, Foti D, Scholars for elevating equity and diversity (SEED). An ethics and social-justice approach to collecting and using demographic data for psychological researchers. Perspect Psychol Sci 2023;18(5):979–995. PMCID: PMC10235209. http://www.ncbi.nlm.nih.gov/pubmed/36459692.
107. Anderson C, Kraus MW, Galinsky AD, Keltner D. The local-ladder effect: social status and subjective Well-being. Psychol Sci. 2012;23(7):764–71. PMID: 22653798. http://www.ncbi.nlm.nih.gov/pubmed/22653798.
108. Steptoe A, Fancourt D. Leading a meaningful life at older ages and its relationship with social engagement, prosperity, health, biology, and time use. Proc Natl Acad Sci USA 2019;116(4):1207–1212. PMCID: PMC6347683. http://www.ncbi.nlm.nih.gov/pubmed/30617082.
109. Hoi LV, Chuc NT, Lindholm L. Health-related quality of life, and its determinants, among older people in rural Vietnam. BMC Public Health. 2010;10:549. PMCID: PMC2944376. http://www.ncbi.nlm.nih.gov/pubmed/20831822.
110. Berkman LF, Syme SL. Social networks, host resistance, and mortality: a nine-year follow-up study of Alameda County residents. Am J Epidemiol. 1979;109(2):186–204. PMID: 425958. http://www.ncbi.nlm.nih.gov/pubmed/425958.
111. Santini ZI, Koyanagi A, Tyrovolas S, Mason C, Haro JM. The association between social relationships and depression: a systematic review. J Affect Disord. 2015;175:53–65. PMID: 25594512. http://www.ncbi.nlm.nih.gov/pubmed/25594512.
112. Barman P, Rahut DB, Mishra R. Mediating role of social disengagement and loneliness in the nexus between functional

health and mental Well-being in older individuals. Sci Rep. 2024;14(1):16232. PMCID: PMC11247097. http://www.ncbi.nlm.nih.gov/pubmed/39004615.
113. Nagargoje VP, James KS, Muhammad T. Moderation of marital status and living arrangements in the relationship between social participation and life satisfaction among older Indian adults. Sci Rep. 2022;12(1):20604. PMCID: PMC9708669. http://www.ncbi.nlm.nih.gov/pubmed/36446850.
114. Muhammad T, Maurya P. Social support moderates the association of functional difficulty with major depression among community-dwelling older adults: evidence from LASI, 2017-18. BMC Psychiatry. 2022;22(1):317. PMCID: PMC9066756. http://www.ncbi.nlm.nih.gov/pubmed/35509005.
115. Vaish K, Patra S, Chhabra P. Functional disability among elderly: a community-based cross-sectional study. J Family Med Prim Care. 2020;9(1):253–8. PMCID: PMC7014891. http://www.ncbi.nlm.nih.gov/pubmed/32110600.
116. Grenade L, Boldy D. Social isolation and loneliness among older people: issues and future challenges in community and residential settings. Aust Health Rev. 2008;32(3):468–78. PMID: 18666874. http://www.ncbi.nlm.nih.gov/pubmed/18666874.
117. Domènech-Abella J, Lara E, Rubio-Valera M, Olaya B, Moneta MV, Rico-Uribe LA, Ayuso-Mateos JL, Mundó J, Haro JM. Loneliness and depression in the elderly: the role of social network. Soc Psychiatry Psychiatr Epidemiol. 2017;52(4):381–90. PMID: 28154893. http://www.ncbi.nlm.nih.gov/pubmed/28154893.
118. Hutten E, Jongen EMM, Vos AECC, van den Hout AJHC, van Lankveld JJDM. Loneliness and mental health: the mediating effect of perceived social support. Int J Environ Res Public Health. 2021;18(22):11963. PMCID: PMC8619017. http://www.ncbi.nlm.nih.gov/pubmed/34831717.
119. Stansfeld SA, Head J, Fuhrer R, Wardle J, Cattell V. Social inequalities in depressive symptoms and physical functioning in the Whitehall II study: exploring a common cause explanation. J Epidemiol Community Health. 2003;57(5):361–7. PMCID: PMC1732450. http://www.ncbi.nlm.nih.gov/pubmed/12700221.
120. Jester DJ, Kohn JN, Tibiriçá L, Thomas ML, Brown LL, Murphy JD, Jeste DV. Differences in social determinants of health underlie racial/ethnic disparities in psychological health and Well-being: study of 11,143 older adults. Am J Psychiatry. 2023;180(7):483–94. PMCID: PMC10329971. http://www.ncbi.nlm.nih.gov/pubmed/23245608.
121. Rhee TG, Lee K, Schensul JJ. Black-white disparities in social and behavioral determinants of health index and their associations with self-rated health and functional limitations in older adults. J Gerontol A Biol Sci Med Sci. 2021;76(4):735–40. PMCID: PMC8011702. http://www.ncbi.nlm.nih.gov/pubmed/33049033.
122. Chiao C, Weng LJ. Mid-life socioeconomic status, depressive symptomatology and general cognitive status among older adults: inter-relationships and temporal effects. BMC Geriatr. 2016;16:88. PMCID: PMC4839082. http://www.ncbi.nlm.nih.gov/pubmed/27099153.
123. Fernández-Niño JA, Manrique-Espinoza BS, Bojorquez-Chapela I, Salinas-Rodríguez A. Income inequality, socioeconomic deprivation and depressive symptoms among older adults in Mexico. PLoS One. 2014;9(9):e108127. PMCID: PMC4176015. http://www.ncbi.nlm.nih.gov/pubmed/25250620.
124. Rai D, Zitko P, Jones K, Lynch J, Araya R. Country- and individual-level socioeconomic determinants of depression: multilevel cross-national comparison. Br J Psychiatry. 2013;202(3):195–203. PMID: 23349294. http://www.ncbi.nlm.nih.gov/pubmed/23349294.
125. Kim KM, Kim D, Chung US. Investigation of the trend in adolescent mental health and its related social factors: a multi-year cross-sectional study for 13 years. Int J Environ Res Public Health. 2020;17(15):5405. PMCID: PMC7432642. http://www.ncbi.nlm.nih.gov/pubmed/32727147.
126. Sturm R, Gresenz CR. Relations of income inequality and family income to chronic medical conditions and mental health disorders: national survey. BMJ. 2002;324(7328):20–3. PMCID: PMC61653. http://www.ncbi.nlm.nih.gov/pubmed/11777799.
127. Menezes PR. Commentary: epidemiological mental health research: contribution from low- and middle-income countries is essential. Int J Epidemiol. 2014;43(2):301–3. PMID: 24681527. http://www.ncbi.nlm.nih.gov/pubmed/24681527.
128. Thapar A, Collishaw S, Pine DS, Thapar AK. Depression in adolescence. Lancet. 2012;379(9820):1056–67. PMCID: PMC3488279. http://www.ncbi.nlm.nih.gov/pubmed/22305766.
129. Battel L, Cunegatto F, Viduani A, Fisher HL, Kohrt BA, Mondelli V, Swartz JR, Kieling C. Mind the brain gap: the worldwide distribution of neuroimaging research on adolescent depression. Neuroimage. 2021;231:117865. PMCID: PMC8328473. http://www.ncbi.nlm.nih.gov/pubmed/33592242.
130. Kieling C, Baker-Henningham H, Belfer M, Conti G, Ertem I, Omigbodun O, Rohde LA, Srinath S, Ulkuer N, Rahman A. Child and adolescent mental health worldwide: evidence for action. Lancet. 2011;378(9801):1515–25. PMID: 22008427. http://www.ncbi.nlm.nih.gov/pubmed/22008427.
131. Kieling C, Rohde LA. Child and adolescent mental health research across the globe. J Am Acad Child Adolesc Psychiatry. 2012;51(9):945–7. PMID: 22917207. http://www.ncbi.nlm.nih.gov/pubmed/22917207.
132. Keenan K, Hipwell AE. Preadolescent clues to understanding depression in girls. Clin Child Fam Psychol Rev. 2005;8(2):89–105. PMCID: PMC2848388. http://www.ncbi.nlm.nih.gov/pubmed/15984082.
133. Khesht-Masjedi MF, Shokrgozar S, Abdollahi E, Golshahi M, Sharif-Ghaziani Z. Comparing depressive symptoms in teenage boys and girls. J Family Med Prim Care. 2017;6(4):775–9. PMCID: PMC5848397. http://www.ncbi.nlm.nih.gov/pubmed/29564262.
134. World Bank Country and Lending Groups—World Bank Data Help Desk.
135. GNI, Atlas method (current US$) | Data.
136. Population, total | Data.
137. Suicide statistics | AFSP.
138. Hyde JS, Mezulis AH, Abramson LY. The ABCs of depression: integrating affective, biological, and cognitive models to explain the emergence of the gender difference in depression. Psychol Rev. 2008;115(2):291–313. PMID: 18426291. http://www.ncbi.nlm.nih.gov/pubmed/18426291.
139. Hyde JS, Mezulis AH. Gender differences in depression: biological, affective, cognitive, and sociocultural factors. Harv Rev Psychiatry. 2020;28(1):4–13. PMID: 31913978. http://www.ncbi.nlm.nih.gov/pubmed/31913978.
140. Bebbington PE. Sex and depression. Psychol Med. 1998;28(1):1–8. PMID: 9483678. http://www.ncbi.nlm.nih.gov/pubmed/9483678.
141. Kessler RC, McGonagle KA, Swartz M, Blazer DG, Nelson CB. Sex and depression in the National Comorbidity Survey. I: lifetime prevalence, chronicity and recurrence. J Affect Disord. 1993;29(2–3):85–96. PMID: 8300981. http://www.ncbi.nlm.nih.gov/pubmed/8300981.
142. Swetlitz N. Depression's problem with men. AMA J Ethics. 2021;23(7):E586–9. PMID: 34351273. http://www.ncbi.nlm.nih.gov/pubmed/34351273.
143. Call JB, Shafer K. Gendered manifestations of depression and help seeking among men. Am J Mens Health. 2018;12(1):41–51. PMCID: PMC5734537. http://www.ncbi.nlm.nih.gov/pubmed/26721265.

144. Martin LA, Neighbors HW, Griffith DM. The experience of symptoms of depression in men vs women: analysis of the National Comorbidity Survey Replication. JAMA Psychiatr. 2013;70(10):1100–6. PMID: 23986338. http://www.ncbi.nlm.nih.gov/pubmed/23986338.
145. Winkler D, Pjrek E, Kasper S. Anger attacks in depression–evidence for a male depressive syndrome. Psychother Psychosom. 2005;74(5):303–7. PMID: 16088268. http://www.ncbi.nlm.nih.gov/pubmed/16088268.
146. Arenas ML, Greif GL. Issues of fatherhood and recovery for VA substance abuse patients. J Psychoactive Drugs. 2000;32(3):339–41. PMID: 11061686. http://www.ncbi.nlm.nih.gov/pubmed/11061686.
147. Wilson S, Durbin CE. Effects of paternal depression on fathers' parenting behaviors: a meta-analytic review. Clin Psychol Rev. 2010;30(2):167–80. PMID: 19926376. http://www.ncbi.nlm.nih.gov/pubmed/19926376.
148. Goldmann E, Galea S. Mental health consequences of disasters. Annu Rev Public Health. 2014;35:169–83. PMID: 24159920. http://www.ncbi.nlm.nih.gov/pubmed/24159920.
149. Ettman CK, Abdalla SM, Cohen GH, Sampson L, Vivier PM, Galea S. Prevalence of depression symptoms in US adults before and during the COVID-19 pandemic. JAMA Netw Open. 2020;3(9):e2019686. PMCID: PMC7489837. http://www.ncbi.nlm.nih.gov/pubmed/32876685.
150. Frasquilho D, Matos MG, Salonna F, Guerreiro D, Storti CC, Gaspar T, Caldas-de-Almeida JM. Mental health outcomes in times of economic recession: a systematic literature review. BMC Public Health. 2016;16:115. PMCID: PMC4741013. http://www.ncbi.nlm.nih.gov/pubmed/26847554.
151. Salk RH, Hyde JS, Abramson LY. Gender differences in depression in representative national samples: meta-analyses of diagnoses and symptoms. Psychol Bull. 2017;143(8):783–822. PMCID: PMC5532074. http://www.ncbi.nlm.nih.gov/pubmed/31913978.
152. Freeman A, Tyrovolas S, Koyanagi A, Chatterji S, Leonardi M, Ayuso-Mateos JL, Tobiasz-Adamczyk B, Koskinen S, Rummel-Kluge C, Haro JM. The role of socio-economic status in depression: results from the COURAGE (aging survey in Europe). BMC Public Health. 2016;16(1):1098. PMCID: PMC5069819. http://www.ncbi.nlm.nih.gov/pubmed/27760538.
153. Fluharty M, Taylor AE, Grabski M, Munafò MR. The Association of Cigarette Smoking with Depression and Anxiety: a systematic review. Nicotine Tob Res. 2017;19(1):3–13. PMCID: PMC5157710. http://www.ncbi.nlm.nih.gov/pubmed/27199385.
154. Cummings JR, Allen L, Clennon J, Ji X, Druss BG. Geographic access to specialty mental health care across high- and low-income US communities. JAMA Psychiatr. 2017;74(5):476–84. PMCID: PMC5693377. http://www.ncbi.nlm.nih.gov/pubmed/28384733.
155. Lazar M, Davenport L. Barriers to health care access for low income families: a review of literature. J Community Health Nurs. 2018;35(1):28–37. PMID: 29323941. http://www.ncbi.nlm.nih.gov/pubmed/29323941.
156. Ge X, Conger RD, Elder GH. Pubertal transition, stressful life events, and the emergence of gender differences in adolescent depressive symptoms. Dev Psychol. 2001;37(3):404–17. PMID: 11370915. http://www.ncbi.nlm.nih.gov/pubmed/11370915.
157. Hilmers A, Hilmers DC, Dave J. Neighborhood disparities in access to healthy foods and their effects on environmental justice. Am J Public Health. 2012;102(9):1644–54. PMCID: PMC3482049. http://www.ncbi.nlm.nih.gov/pubmed/22813465.
158. Kim D. Blues from the neighborhood? Neighborhood characteristics and depression. Epidemiol Rev. 2008;30:101–17. PMID: 18753674. http://www.ncbi.nlm.nih.gov/pubmed/18753674.
159. Patel V, Burns JK, Dhingra M, Tarver L, Kohrt BA, Lund C. Income inequality and depression: a systematic review and meta-analysis of the association and a scoping review of mechanisms. World Psychiatry. 2018;17(1):76–89. PMCID: PMC5775138. http://www.ncbi.nlm.nih.gov/pubmed/29352539.
160. Lynch JW, Smith GD, Kaplan GA, House JS. Income inequality and mortality: importance to health of individual income, psychosocial environment, or material conditions. BMJ. 2000;320(7243):1200–4. PMCID: PMC1127589. http://www.ncbi.nlm.nih.gov/pubmed/10784551.
161. Padgett DK. Homelessness, housing instability and mental health: making the connections. BJPsych Bull. 2020;44(5):197–201. PMCID: PMC7525583. http://www.ncbi.nlm.nih.gov/pubmed/32538335.
162. Leung CW, Epel ES, Willett WC, Rimm EB, Laraia BA. Household food insecurity is positively associated with depression among low-income supplemental nutrition assistance program participants and income-eligible nonparticipants. J Nutr. 2015;145(3):622–7. PMID: 25733480. http://www.ncbi.nlm.nih.gov/pubmed/25733480.
163. Adler NE, Rehkopf DH. U.S. disparities in health: descriptions, causes, and mechanisms. Annu Rev Public Health. 2008;29:235–52. PMID: 18031225. http://www.ncbi.nlm.nih.gov/pubmed/18031225.
164. Katon W, Lin EHB, Kroenke K. The association of depression and anxiety with medical symptom burden in patients with chronic medical illness. Gen Hosp Psychiatry. 2007;29(2):147–55. PMID: 17336664. http://www.ncbi.nlm.nih.gov/pubmed/17336664.
165. Ridley M, Rao G, Schilbach F, Patel V. Poverty, depression, and anxiety: causal evidence and mechanisms. Science. 2020;370(6522):eaay0214. PMID: 33303583. http://www.ncbi.nlm.nih.gov/pubmed/33303583.
166. Zare H, Meyerson NS, Nwankwo CA, Thorpe RJ. How income and income inequality drive depressive symptoms in U.S. adults, does sex matter: 2005-2016. Int J Environ Res Public Health. 2022;19(10):6227. PMCID: PMC9140340. http://www.ncbi.nlm.nih.gov/pubmed/35627767.
167. Brody DJ, Pratt LA, Hughes JP. Prevalence of depression among adults aged 20 and over: United States, 2013–2016. NCHS Data Brief. 2018;303:1–8. PMID: 29638213. http://www.ncbi.nlm.nih.gov/pubmed/29638213.
168. About NHANES | National Health and Nutrition Examination Survey | CDC.
169. NCHS Data Brief, Number 303, February 2018.
170. Hammen C. Risk factors for depression: An autobiographical review. Annu Rev Clin Psychol. 2018;14:1–28. PMID: 29328780 http://www.ncbi.nlm.nih.gov/pubmed/29328780.
171. Health, Income, & Poverty: Where We Are & What Could Help | Health Affairs.
172. Is the Gender Pay Gap Closing or Has Progress Stalled? – WSJ.
173. Busch F. Gender segregation, occupational sorting, and growth of wage disparities between women. Demography. 2020;57(3):1063–88. PMID: 32572788. http://www.ncbi.nlm.nih.gov/pubmed/32572788.
174. Steege AL, Baron SL, Marsh SM, Menéndez CC, Myers JR. Examining occupational health and safety disparities using national data: a cause for continuing concern. Am J Ind Med. 2014;57(5):527–38. PMCID: PMC4556419. http://www.ncbi.nlm.nih.gov/pubmed/24436156.
175. Index to the NLSY79 Cohort | National Longitudinal Surveys.
176. Zimmerman FJ, Katon W. Socioeconomic status, depression disparities, and financial strain: what lies behind the income-depression relationship? Health Econ. 2005;14(12):1197–215. PMID: 15945040 http://www.ncbi.nlm.nih.gov/pubmed/15945040.
177. Lorant V, Deliège D, Eaton W, Robert A, Philippot P, Ansseau M. Socioeconomic inequalities in depression: a meta-analysis. Am J Epidemiol. 2003;157(2):98–112. PMID: 12522017 http://www.ncbi.nlm.nih.gov/pubmed/12522017.

178. McMillan KA, Enns MW, Asmundson GJG, Sareen J. The association between income and distress, mental disorders, and suicidal ideation and attempts: findings from the collaborative psychiatric epidemiology surveys. J Clin Psychiatry. 2010;71(9):1168–75. PMID: 20441719 http://www.ncbi.nlm.nih.gov/pubmed/20441719.
179. Compton WM, Grant BF, Colliver JD, Glantz MD, Stinson FS. Prevalence of marijuana use disorders in the United States: 1991–1992 and 2001–2002. JAMA. 2004;291(17):2114–21. PMID: 15126440 http://www.ncbi.nlm.nih.gov/pubmed/15126440.
180. Ruan WJ, Goldstein RB, Chou SP, Smith SM, Saha TD, Pickering RP, Dawson DA, Huang B, Stinson FS, Grant BF. The alcohol use disorder and associated disabilities interview schedule-IV (AUDADIS-IV): reliability of new psychiatric diagnostic modules and risk factors in a general population sample. Drug Alcohol Depend. 2008;92(1–3):27–36. PMCID: PMC2246381. http://www.ncbi.nlm.nih.gov/pubmed/17706375.
181. Sareen J, Afifi TO, McMillan KA, Asmundson GJG. Relationship between household income and mental disorders: findings from a population-based longitudinal study. Arch Gen Psychiatry. 2011;68(4):419–27. PMID: 21464366. http://www.ncbi.nlm.nih.gov/pubmed/21464366.
182. Killeen RN. A review of Illich's medical nemesis. West J Med. 1976;125(1):67–9. PMCID: PMC1237194. http://www.ncbi.nlm.nih.gov/pubmed/18747743.
183. O'Mahony S. Medical nemesis 40 years on: the enduring legacy of Ivan Illich. J R Coll Physicians Edinb. 2016;46(2):134–9. PMID: 27929580. http://www.ncbi.nlm.nih.gov/pubmed/27929580.
184. Illich I. Medical nemesis. 1974. J Epidemiol Community Health. 2003;57(12):919–22. PMCID: PMC1732343. http://www.ncbi.nlm.nih.gov/pubmed/14652247.
185. Babich B. Ivan Illich's medical nemesis and the "age of the show": on the expropriation of death. Nurs Philos. 2018;19(1) PMID: 29271600. http://www.ncbi.nlm.nih.gov/pubmed/29271600.
186. Peer RF, Shabir N. Iatrogenesis: a review on nature, extent, and distribution of healthcare hazards. J Family Med Prim Care. 2018;7(2):309–14. PMCID: PMC6060929. http://www.ncbi.nlm.nih.gov/pubmed/30090769.
187. Mulder RT. An epidemic of depression or the medicalization of distress? Perspect Biol Med. 2008;51(2):238–50. PMID: 18453728. http://www.ncbi.nlm.nih.gov/pubmed/18453728.
188. McDonald RJ, Hong NS, Trow JS, Kaupp C, Balog RJ, Gokarn L, Falkenberg EA, McCreary KJ, Soltanpour N, Witbeck C, McKenna A, Metz GAS. Effects of maternal social isolation on adult rodent offspring cognition. Sci Rep. 2023;13(1):7748. PMCID: PMC10177704. http://www.ncbi.nlm.nih.gov/pubmed/37173349.
189. Murray RJ, Apazoglou K, Celen Z, Dayer A, Aubry JM, Ville DVD, Vuilleumier P, Piguet C. Maladaptive emotion regulation traits predict altered corticolimbic recovery from psychosocial stress. J Affect Disord. 2021;280(Pt A):54–63. PMID: 33202338. http://www.ncbi.nlm.nih.gov/pubmed/33202338.
190. Morgan JK, Silk JS, Woods BK, Forbes EE. Differential neural responding to affective stimuli in 6- to 8-year old children at high familial risk for depression: associations with behavioral reward seeking. J Affect Disord. 2019;257:445–53. PMCID: PMC6711822. http://www.ncbi.nlm.nih.gov/pubmed/31310906.
191. Uddin LQ. Salience processing and insular cortical function and dysfunction. Nat Rev Neurosci. 2015;16(1):55–61. PMID: 25406711. http://www.ncbi.nlm.nih.gov/pubmed/25406711.
192. Schmaal L, Hibar DP, Sämann PG, Hall GB, Baune BT, Jahanshad N, Cheung JW, van Erp TGM, Bos D, Ikram MA, Vernooij MW, Niessen WJ, Tiemeier H, Hofman A, Wittfeld K, Grabe HJ, Janowitz D, Bülow R, Selonke M, Völzke H, Grotegerd D, Dannlowski U, Arolt V, Opel N, Heindel W, Kugel H, Hoehn D, Czisch M, Couvy-Duchesne B, Rentería ME, Strike LT, Wright MJ, Mills NT, de Zubicaray GI, McMahon KL, Medland SE, Martin NG, Gillespie NA, Goya-Maldonado R, Gruber O, Krämer B, Hatton SN, Lagopoulos J, Hickie IB, Frodl T, Carballedo A, Frey EM, van Velzen LS, Penninx BWJH, van Tol MJ, van der Wee NJ, Davey CG, Harrison BJ, Mwangi B, Cao B, Soares JC, Veer IM, Walter H, Schoepf D, Zurowski B, Konrad C, Schramm E, Normann C, Schnell K, Sacchet MD, Gotlib IH, MacQueen GM, Godlewska BR, Nickson T, McIntosh AM, Papmeyer M, Whalley HC, Hall J, Sussmann JE, Li M, Walter M, Aftanas L, Brack I, Bokhan NA, Thompson PM, Veltman DJ. Cortical abnormalities in adults and adolescents with major depression based on brain scans from 20 cohorts worldwide in the ENIGMA Major Depressive Disorder Working Group. Mol Psychiatry. 2017;22(6):900–9. PMCID: PMC5444023. http://www.ncbi.nlm.nih.gov/pubmed/27137745.
193. Andrews-Hanna JR, Reidler JS, Sepulcre J, Poulin R, Buckner RL. Functional-anatomic fractionation of the brain's default network. Neuron. 2010;65(4):550–62. PMCID: PMC2848443. http://www.ncbi.nlm.nih.gov/pubmed/20188659.
194. Hatoum AS, Reineberg AE, Smolker HR, Hewitt JK, Friedman NP. Whole-cortex mapping of common genetic influences on depression and a social deficits dimension. Transl Psychiatry. 2019;9(1):299. PMCID: PMC6856353. http://www.ncbi.nlm.nih.gov/pubmed/31727881.
195. Wray NR, Ripke S, Mattheisen M, Trzaskowski M, Byrne EM, Abdellaoui A, Adams MJ, Agerbo E, Air TM, Andlauer TMF, Bacanu SA, Bækvad-Hansen M, Beekman AFT, Bigdeli TB, Binder EB, Blackwood DRH, Bryois J, Buttenschøn HN, Bybjerg-Grauholm J, Cai N, Castelao E, Christensen JH, Clarke TK, Coleman JIR, Colodro-Conde L, Couvy-Duchesne B, Craddock N, Crawford GE, Crowley CA, Dashti HS, Davies G, Deary IJ, Degenhardt F, Derks EM, Direk N, Dolan CV, Dunn EC, Eley TC, Eriksson N, Escott-Price V, Kiadeh FHF, Finucane HK, Forstner AJ, Frank J, Gaspar HA, Gill M, Giusti-Rodríguez P, Goes FS, Gordon SD, Grove J, Hall LS, Hannon E, Hansen CS, Hansen TF, Herms S, Hickie IB, Hoffmann P, Homuth G, Horn C, Hottenga JJ, Hougaard DM, Hu M, Hyde CL, Ising M, Jansen R, Jin F, Jorgenson E, Knowles JA, Kohane IS, Kraft J, Kretzschmar WW, Krogh J, Kutalik Z, Lane JM, Li Y, Li Y, Lind PA, Liu X, Lu L, MacIntyre DJ, MacKinnon DF, Maier RM, Maier W, Marchini J, Mbarek H, McGrath P, McGuffin P, Medland SE, Mehta D, Middeldorp CM, Mihailov E, Milaneschi Y, Milani L, Mill J, Mondimore FM, Montgomery GW, Mostafavi S, Mullins N, Nauck M, Ng B, Nivard MG, Nyholt DR, O'Reilly PF, Oskarsson H, Owen MJ, Painter JN, Pedersen CB, Pedersen MG, Peterson RE, Pettersson E, Peyrot WJ, Pistis G, Posthuma D, Purcell SM, Quiroz JA, Qvist P, Rice JP, Riley BP, Rivera M, Saeed Mirza S, Saxena R, Schoevers R, Schulte EC, Shen L, Shi J, Shyn SI, Sigurdsson E, Sinnamon GBC, Smit JH, Smith DJ, Stefansson H, Steinberg S, Stockmeier CA, Streit F, Strohmaier J, Tansey KE, Teismann H, Teumer A, Thompson W, Thomson PA, Thorgeirsson TE, Tian C, Traylor M, Treutlein J, Trubetskoy V, Uitterlinden AG, Umbricht D, Van der Auwera S, van Hemert AM, Viktorin A, Visscher PM, Wang Y, Webb BT, Weinsheimer SM, Wellmann J, Willemsen G, Witt SH, Wu Y, Xi HS, Yang J, Zhang F, eQTLGen, 23andMe, Arolt V, Baune BT, Berger K, Boomsma DI, Cichon S, Dannlowski U, de Geus ECJ, DePaulo JR, Domenici E, Domschke K, Esko T, Grabe HJ, Hamilton SP, Hayward C, Heath AC, Hinds DA, Kendler KS, Kloiber S, Lewis G, Li QS, Lucae S, Madden PFA, Magnusson PK, Martin NG, McIntosh AM, Metspalu A, Mors O, Mortensen PB, Müller-Myhsok B, Nordentoft M, Nöthen MM, O'Donovan MC, Paciga SA, Pedersen NL, Penninx BWJH, Perlis RH, Porteous DJ, Potash JB, Preisig M, Rietschel M, Schaefer C, Schulze TG, Smoller JW, Stefansson K, Tiemeier H, Uher R, Völzke H, Weissman MM, Werge T, Winslow AR, Lewis CM, Levinson DF, Breen G, Børglum AD, Sullivan PF, Major

Depressive Disorder Working Group of the Psychiatric Genomics Consortium. Genome-wide association analyses identify 44 risk variants and refine the genetic architecture of major depression. Nat Genet. 2018;50(5):668–81. PMCID: PMC5934326. http://www.ncbi.nlm.nih.gov/pubmed/29700475.
196. Power RA, Tansey KE, Buttenschøn HN, Cohen-Woods S, Bigdeli T, Hall LS, Kutalik Z, Lee SH, Ripke S, Steinberg S, Teumer A, Viktorin A, Wray NR, Arolt V, Baune BT, Boomsma DI, Børglum AD, Byrne EM, Castelao E, Craddock N, Craig IW, Dannlowski U, Deary IJ, Degenhardt F, Forstner AJ, Gordon SD, Grabe HJ, Grove J, Hamilton SP, Hayward C, Heath AC, Hocking LJ, Homuth G, Hottenga JJ, Kloiber S, Krogh J, Landén M, Lang M, Levinson DF, Lichtenstein P, Lucae S, MacIntyre DJ, Madden P, Magnusson PKE, Martin NG, McIntosh AM, Middeldorp CM, Milaneschi Y, Montgomery GW, Mors O, Müller-Myhsok B, Nyholt DR, Oskarsson H, Owen MJ, Padmanabhan S, Penninx BWJH, Pergadia ML, Porteous DJ, Potash JB, Preisig M, Rivera M, Shi J, Shyn SI, Sigurdsson E, Smit JH, Smith BH, Stefansson H, Stefansson K, Strohmaier J, Sullivan PF, Thomson P, Thorgeirsson TE, Van der Auwera S, Weissman MM, CONVERGE Consortium, CARDIoGRAM Consortium, GERAD1 Consortium, Breen G, Lewis CM. Genome-wide Association for Major Depression Through Age at Onset Stratification: Major Depressive Disorder Working Group of the Psychiatric Genomics Consortium. Biol Psychiatry. 2017;81(4):325–35. PMCID: PMC5262436 http://www.ncbi.nlm.nih.gov/pubmed/27519822.
197. Sunkin SM, Ng L, Lau C, Dolbeare T, Gilbert TL, Thompson CL, Hawrylycz M, Dang C. Allen brain atlas: an integrated spatio-temporal portal for exploring the central nervous system. Nucleic Acids Res. 2013;41(Database issue):D996–D1008. PMCID: PMC3531093. http://www.ncbi.nlm.nih.gov/pubmed/23193282.
198. Yarkoni T, Poldrack RA, Nichols TE, Van Essen DC, Wager TD. Large-scale automated synthesis of human functional neuroimaging data. Nat Methods. 2011;8(8):665–70. PMCID: PMC3146590. http://www.ncbi.nlm.nih.gov/pubmed/21706013.
199. Kimonis ER, Frick PJ, Skeem JL, Marsee MA, Cruise K, Munoz LC, Aucoin KJ, Morris AS. Assessing callous-unemotional traits in adolescent offenders: validation of the inventory of callous-unemotional traits. Int J Law Psychiatry. 2008;31(3):241–52. PMID: 18514315. http://www.ncbi.nlm.nih.gov/pubmed/18514315.
200. Byrd AL, Kahn RE, Pardini DA. A validation of the inventory of callous-unemotional traits in a community sample of Young adult males. J Psychopathol Behav Assess. 2013;35(1):20. PMCID: PMC3864815. http://www.ncbi.nlm.nih.gov/pubmed/24357894.
201. Ladegaard N, Larsen ER, Videbech P, Lysaker PH. Higher-order social cognition in first-episode major depression. Psychiatry Res. 2014;216(1):37–43. PMID: 24524945. http://www.ncbi.nlm.nih.gov/pubmed/24524945.
202. Lamers F, de Jonge P, Nolen WA, Smit JH, Zitman FG, Beekman ATF, Penninx BWJH. Identifying depressive subtypes in a large cohort study: results from The Netherlands Study of Depression and Anxiety (NESDA). J Clin Psychiatry. 2010;71(12):1582–9. PMID: 20673552. http://www.ncbi.nlm.nih.gov/pubmed/20673552.
203. Sullivan PF, Neale MC, Kendler KS. Genetic epidemiology of major depression: review and meta-analysis. Am J Psychiatry. 2000;157(10):1552–62. PMID: 11007705. http://www.ncbi.nlm.nih.gov/pubmed/26721265.
204. Duerler P, Vollenweider FX, Preller KH. A neurobiological perspective on social influence: serotonin and social adaptation. J Neurochem. 2022;162(1):60–79. PMCID: PMC9322456. http://www.ncbi.nlm.nih.gov/pubmed/35274296.
205. Peen J, Schoevers RA, Beekman AT, Dekker J. The current status of urban-rural differences in psychiatric disorders. Acta Psychiatr Scand. 2010;121(2):84–93. PMID: 19624573. http://www.ncbi.nlm.nih.gov/pubmed/19624573.
206. Gruebner O, Rapp MA, Adli M, Kluge U, Galea S, Heinz A. Cities and mental health. Dtsch Arztebl Int. 2017;114(8):121–7. PMCID: PMC5374256. http://www.ncbi.nlm.nih.gov/pubmed/28302261.
207. Lederbogen F, Kirsch P, Haddad L, Streit F, Tost H, Schuch P, Wüst S, Pruessner JC, Rietschel M, Deuschle M, Meyer-Lindenberg A. City living and urban upbringing affect neural social stress processing in humans. Nature. 2011;474(7352):498–501. PMID: 21697947. http://www.ncbi.nlm.nih.gov/pubmed/21697947.
208. Breslau J, Marshall GN, Pincus HA, Brown RA. Are mental disorders more common in urban than rural areas of the United States? J Psychiatr Res. 2014;56:50–5. PMID: 24857610. http://www.ncbi.nlm.nih.gov/pubmed/24857610.
209. Tost H, Reichert M, Braun U, Reinhard I, Peters R, Lautenbach S, Hoell A, Schwarz E, Ebner-Priemer U, Zipf A, Meyer-Lindenberg A. Neural correlates of individual differences in affective benefit of real-life urban green space exposure. Nat Neurosci. 2019;22(9):1389–93. PMID: 31358990. http://www.ncbi.nlm.nih.gov/pubmed/31358990.
210. Uher R, Zwicker A. Etiology in psychiatry: embracing the reality of poly-gene-environmental causation of mental illness. World Psychiatry. 2017;16(2):121–9. PMCID: PMC5428165. http://www.ncbi.nlm.nih.gov/pubmed/28498595.
211. Tost H, Champagne FA, Meyer-Lindenberg A. Environmental influence in the brain, human welfare and mental health. Nat Neurosci. 2015;18(10):1421–31. PMID: 26404717. http://www.ncbi.nlm.nih.gov/pubmed/26404717.
212. Sampson L, Ettman CK, Galea S. Urbanization, urbanicity, and depression: a review of the recent global literature. Curr Opin Psychiatry. 2020;33(3):233–44. PMID: 32040041. http://www.ncbi.nlm.nih.gov/pubmed/32040041.
213. Lecic-Tosevski D. Is urban living good for mental health? Curr Opin Psychiatry. 2019;32(3):204–9. PMID: 30695002. http://www.ncbi.nlm.nih.gov/pubmed/30695002.
214. Lambert KG, Nelson RJ, Jovanovic T, Cerdá M. Brains in the city: neurobiological effects of urbanization. Neurosci Biobehav Rev. 2015;58:107–22. PMCID: PMC4774049. http://www.ncbi.nlm.nih.gov/pubmed/25936504.
215. Hoare E, Jacka F, Berk M. The impact of urbanization on mood disorders: an update of recent evidence. Curr Opin Psychiatry. 2019;32(3):198–203. PMID: 30676331. http://www.ncbi.nlm.nih.gov/pubmed/30676331.
216. Xu J, Liu N, Polemiti E, Garcia-Mondragon L, Tang J, Liu X, Lett T, Yu L, Nöthen MM, Feng J, Yu C, Marquand A, Schumann G, the environMENTAL Consortium. Effects of urban living environments on mental health in adults. Nat Med. 2023;29(6):1456–67. PMCID: PMC10287556. http://www.ncbi.nlm.nih.gov/pubmed/37322117.
217. Sharma MK, John N, Sahu M. Influence of social media on mental health: a systematic review. Curr Opin Psychiatry. 2020;33(5):467–75. PMID: 32639362. http://www.ncbi.nlm.nih.gov/pubmed/32639362.
218. Wang Q, Zhang W, An S. A systematic review and meta-analysis of internet-based self-help interventions for mental health among adolescents and college students. Internet Interv. 2023;34:100690. PMCID: PMC10654252. http://www.ncbi.nlm.nih.gov/pubmed/38023965.
219. Sander LB, Beisemann M, Doebler P, Micklitz HM, Kerkhof A, Cuijpers P, Batterham P, Calear A, Christensen H, De Jaegere E, Domhardt M, Erlangsen A, Eylem-van Bergeijk O, Hill R, Mühlmann C, Österle M, Pettit J, Portzky G, Steubl L, van Spijker B, Tighe J, Werner-Seidler A, Büscher R. The effects of internet-based cognitive behavioral therapy for suicidal ideation or behaviors on depression, anxiety, and hopelessness in individuals with

suicidal ideation: systematic review and meta-analysis of individual participant data. J Med Internet Res. 2023;25:e46771. PMCID: PMC10337381. http://www.ncbi.nlm.nih.gov/pubmed/37358893.
220. Igelström H, Carlsson M, Hauffman A, von Essen L, Grönqvist H, Johansson B, Olsson EMG. Long-term effects on depression and anxiety of an internet-based stepped care intervention for patients with cancer and symptoms of depression and anxiety. The U-CARE AdultCan trial. Internet Interv. 2023;32:100625. PMCID: PMC10235429. http://www.ncbi.nlm.nih.gov/pubmed/37273929.
221. Taple BJ, Chapman R, Schalet BD, Brower R, Griffith JW. The impact of education on depression assessment: differential item functioning analysis. Assessment. 2022;29(2):272–84. PMCID: PMC9060911. http://www.ncbi.nlm.nih.gov/pubmed/33218257.
222. Rahman T, Hossain MM, Bristy NN, Hoque MZ, Hossain MM. Influence of cyber-victimization and other factors on depression and anxiety among university students in Bangladesh. J Health Popul Nutr. 2023;42(1):119. PMCID: PMC10629170. http://www.ncbi.nlm.nih.gov/pubmed/37932869.
223. Karim F, Oyewande AA, Abdalla LF, Chaudhry Ehsanullah R, Khan S. Social media use and its connection to mental health: a systematic review. Cureus. 2020;12(6):e8627. PMCID: PMC7364393. http://www.ncbi.nlm.nih.gov/pubmed/32685296.
224. Health care for the aged: a sense of urgency is growing. Hospitals. 1980;54(10):61–2. PMID: 7364393. http://www.ncbi.nlm.nih.gov/pubmed/7364393.
225. Khalaf AM, Alubied AA, Khalaf AM, Rifaey AA. The impact of social media on the mental health of adolescents and Young adults: a systematic review. Cureus. 2023;15(8):e42990. PMCID: PMC10476631. http://www.ncbi.nlm.nih.gov/pubmed/37671234.
226. Iannotti RJ, Janssen I, Haug E, Kololo H, Annaheim B, Borraccino A, HBSC Physical Activity Focus Group. Interrelationships of adolescent physical activity, screen-based sedentary behaviour, and social and psychological health. Int J Public Health. 2009;54(Suppl 2):191–8. PMCID: PMC2732761. http://www.ncbi.nlm.nih.gov/pubmed/19639256.
227. Muris P, Steerneman P. The revised version of the Screen for Child Anxiety Related Emotional Disorders (SCARED–R): first evidence for its reliability and validity in a clinical sample. Br J Clin Psychol. 2001;40(1):35–44. PMID: 11317947. http://www.ncbi.nlm.nih.gov/pubmed/11317947.
228. O'Reilly M. Social media and adolescent mental health: the good, the bad and the ugly. J Ment Health. 2020;29(2):200–6. PMID: 31989847. http://www.ncbi.nlm.nih.gov/pubmed/31989847.
229. Escobar-Viera CG, Whitfield DL, Wessel CB, Shensa A, Sidani JE, Brown AL, Chandler CJ, Hoffman BL, Marshal MP, Primack BA. For better or for worse? A systematic review of the evidence on social media use and depression among lesbian, gay, and bisexual minorities. JMIR Ment Health. 2018;5(3):e10496. PMCID: PMC6079300. http://www.ncbi.nlm.nih.gov/pubmed/30037786.
230. O'Reilly M, Dogra N, Hughes J, Reilly P, George R, Whiteman N. Potential of social media in promoting mental health in adolescents. Health Promot Int. 2019;34(5):981–91. PMCID: PMC6904320. http://www.ncbi.nlm.nih.gov/pubmed/30060043.
231. Odgers CL, Jensen MR. Annual research review: adolescent mental health in the digital age: facts, fears, and future directions. J Child Psychol Psychiatry. 2020;61(3):336–48. PMCID: PMC8221420. http://www.ncbi.nlm.nih.gov/pubmed/31951670.
232. Howell AN, Carleton RN, Horswill SC, Parkerson HA, Weeks JW, Asmundson GJG. Intolerance of uncertainty moderates the relations among religiosity and motives for religion, depression, and social evaluation fears. J Clin Psychol. 2019;75(1):95–115. PMID: 30238465. http://www.ncbi.nlm.nih.gov/pubmed/30238465.
233. Moberg DO. Research in spirituality, religion and aging. J Gerontol Soc Work. 2005;45(1–2):11–40. PMID: 16172060. http://www.ncbi.nlm.nih.gov/pubmed/16172060.
234. The Gender Gap in Religion Around the World | Pew Research Center
235. How Religious Restrictions Have Risen Around the World | Pew Research Center
236. Key Findings From the Global Religious Futures Project | Pew Research Center
237. Henry NL, Gilley N. Spiritual Assessment. StatPearls [Internet]. Treasure Island (FL): StatPearls Publishing; 2024 [cited 2024 Dec 23]. Available from: http://www.ncbi.nlm.nih.gov/books/NBK599554/ PMID: 38261680 http://www.ncbi.nlm.nih.gov/pubmed/38261680.
238. Brewer G, Robinson S, Sumra A, Tatsi E, Gire N. The influence of religious coping and religious social support on health behaviour, health status and health attitudes in a British Christian sample. J Relig Health. 2015;54(6):2225–34. PMID: 25343948. http://www.ncbi.nlm.nih.gov/pubmed/25343948.
239. Desmet L, Dezutter J, Vandenhoeck A, Dillen A. Religious coping styles and depressive symptoms in geriatric patients: understanding the relationship through experiences of integrity and despair. Int J Environ Res Public Health. 2022;19(7):3835. PMCID: PMC8997691. http://www.ncbi.nlm.nih.gov/pubmed/35409519.
240. Koenig HG, Pargament KI, Nielsen J. Religious coping and health status in medically ill hospitalized older adults. J Nerv Ment Dis. 1998;186(9):513–21. PMID: 9741556. http://www.ncbi.nlm.nih.gov/pubmed/9741556.
241. Pargament KI, Koenig HG, Perez LM. The many methods of religious coping: development and initial validation of the RCOPE. J Clin Psychol. 2000;56(4):519–43. PMID: 10775045. http://www.ncbi.nlm.nih.gov/pubmed/10775045.
242. McConnell KM, Pargament KI, Ellison CG, Flannelly KJ. Examining the links between spiritual struggles and symptoms of psychopathology in a national sample. J Clin Psychol. 2006;62(12):1469–84. PMID: 17019672. http://www.ncbi.nlm.nih.gov/pubmed/17019672.
243. Hayward RD, Krause N. Classes of individual growth trajectories of religious coping in older adulthood: patterns and predictors. Res Aging. 2016;38(5):554–79. PMID: 26187618. http://www.ncbi.nlm.nih.gov/pubmed/26187618.
244. Ano GG, Vasconcelles EB. Religious coping and psychological adjustment to stress: a meta-analysis. J Clin Psychol. 2005;61(4):461–80. PMID: 15503316. http://www.ncbi.nlm.nih.gov/pubmed/15503316.
245. Pargament KI, Koenig HG, Tarakeshwar N, Hahn J. Religious coping methods as predictors of psychological, physical and spiritual outcomes among medically ill elderly patients: a two-year longitudinal study. J Health Psychol. 2004;9(6):713–30. PMID: 15367751. http://www.ncbi.nlm.nih.gov/pubmed/15367751.
246. Smith TB, ME MC, Poll J. Religiousness and depression: evidence for a main effect and the moderating influence of stressful life events. Psychol Bull. 2003;129(4):614–36. PMID: 12848223. http://www.ncbi.nlm.nih.gov/pubmed/12848223.
247. Bosworth HB, Park KS, McQuoid DR, Hays JC, Steffens DC. The impact of religious practice and religious coping on geriatric depression. Int J Geriatr Psychiatry. 2003;18(10):905–14. PMID: 14533123. http://www.ncbi.nlm.nih.gov/pubmed/14533123.
248. Sherman AC, Simonton-Atchley S, O'Brien CE, Campbell D, Reddy RM, Guinee B, Wagner LD, Anderson PJ. Associations between religious/spiritual coping and depression among adults with cystic fibrosis: a 12-month longitudinal study. J Relig Health. 2021;60(4):2646–61. PMID: 33575892. http://www.ncbi.nlm.nih.gov/pubmed/33575892.
249. Santos PR, Capote Júnior JRFG, Cavalcante Filho JRM, Ferreira TP, Dos Santos Filho JNG, da Silva Oliveira S. Religious coping methods predict depression and quality of life among end-stage renal disease patients undergoing hemodialysis: a cross-sectional

study. BMC Nephrol. 2017;18(1):197. PMCID: PMC5474022. http://www.ncbi.nlm.nih.gov/pubmed/28623903.
250. Terreri CJ, Glenwick DS. The relationship of religious and general coping to psychological adjustment and distress in urban adolescents. J Relig Health. 2013;52(4):1188–202. PMID: 22130582. http://www.ncbi.nlm.nih.gov/pubmed/22130582.
251. Bjørkløf GH, Engedal K, Selbæk G, Kouwenhoven SE, Helvik AS. Coping and depression in old age: a literature review. Dement Geriatr Cogn Disord. 2013;35(3–4):121–54. PMID: 23392253. http://www.ncbi.nlm.nih.gov/pubmed/23392253.
252. Francis B, Gill JS, Yit Han N, Petrus CF, Azhar FL, Ahmad Sabki Z, Said MA, Ong Hui K, Chong Guan N, Sulaiman AH. Religious coping, religiosity, depression and anxiety among medical students in a multi-religious setting. Int J Environ Res Public Health. 2019;16(2):259. PMCID: PMC6352239. http://www.ncbi.nlm.nih.gov/pubmed/30658450.
253. Braam AW, Schrier AC, Tuinebreijer WC, Beekman ATF, Dekker JJM, de Wit MAS. Religious coping and depression in multicultural Amsterdam: a comparison between native Dutch citizens and Turkish, Moroccan and Surinamese/Antillean migrants. J Affect Disord. 2010;125(1–3):269–78. PMID: 20334926. http://www.ncbi.nlm.nih.gov/pubmed/20334926.
254. Swihart DL, Yarrarapu SNS, Martin RL. Cultural Religious Competence in Clinical Practice. StatPearls [Internet]. Treasure Island (FL): StatPearls Publishing; 2024 [cited 2024 Dec 23]. Available from: http://www.ncbi.nlm.nih.gov/books/NBK493216/ PMID: 29630268 http://www.ncbi.nlm.nih.gov/pubmed/29630268.
255. Asendorpf JB, Denissen JJA, van Aken MAG. Inhibited and aggressive preschool children at 23 years of age: personality and social transitions into adulthood. Dev Psychol. 2008;44(4):997–1011. PMID: 18605830. http://www.ncbi.nlm.nih.gov/pubmed/18605830.
256. Erath SA, Flanagan KS, Bierman KL. Social anxiety and peer relations in early adolescence: behavioral and cognitive factors. J Abnorm Child Psychol. 2007;35(3):405–16. PMID: 17265192. http://www.ncbi.nlm.nih.gov/pubmed/17265192.
257. Renner LM, Slack KS. Intimate partner violence and child maltreatment: understanding intra- and intergenerational connections. Child Abuse Negl. 2006;30(6):599–617. PMID: 16782195. http://www.ncbi.nlm.nih.gov/pubmed/16782195.
258. Capaldi DM, Knoble NB, Shortt JW, Kim HK. A systematic review of risk factors for intimate partner violence. Partn Abus. 2012;3(2):231–80. PMCID: PMC3384540. http://www.ncbi.nlm.nih.gov/pubmed/22754606.
259. Ehrensaft MK, Cohen P. Contribution of family violence to the intergenerational transmission of externalizing behavior. Prev Sci. 2012;13(4):370–83. PMID: 21720783. http://www.ncbi.nlm.nih.gov/pubmed/21720783.
260. Mair C, Cunradi CB, Todd M. Adverse childhood experiences and intimate partner violence: testing psychosocial mediational pathways among couples. Ann Epidemiol. 2012;22(12):832–9. PMCID: PMC3508260. http://www.ncbi.nlm.nih.gov/pubmed/23084843.
261. Osypuk TL, Schmidt NM, Bates LM, Tchetgen-Tchetgen EJ, Earls FJ, Glymour MM. Gender and crime victimization modify neighborhood effects on adolescent mental health. Pediatrics. 2012;130(3):472–81. PMCID: PMC3428753. http://www.ncbi.nlm.nih.gov/pubmed/22908105.
262. Currier D, Mann JJ. Stress, genes and the biology of suicidal behavior. Psychiatr Clin North Am. 2008;31(2):247–69. PMCID: PMC2710608. http://www.ncbi.nlm.nih.gov/pubmed/18439448.
263. Hamburg ME, Finkenauer C, Schuengel C. Food for love: the role of food offering in empathic emotion regulation. Front Psychol. 2014;5:32. PMCID: PMC3907771. http://www.ncbi.nlm.nih.gov/pubmed/24550860.
264. Alley TR. Food sharing and empathic emotion regulation: an evolutionary perspective. Front Psychol. 2014;5:121. PMCID: PMC3933786. http://www.ncbi.nlm.nih.gov/pubmed/24611057.
265. Support Groups | NAMI
266. DBSA—Depression and Bipolar Support Alliance
267. Free Online Therapist & Counseling | 7 Cups
268. Mental Health Facilities in Oregon | Inpatient & Residential Treatment
269. 988 Lifeline – If you need emotional support, reach out to the national mental health hotline: 988
270. Crisis Text Line | Text HOME to 741741 Free, 24/7 Mental Health Support
271. Mental Health First Aid
272. YMCA of the USA—A Leading Nonprofit Organization
273. YWCA
274. Homepage | Families First
275. Senior Advisor
276. APFM—Respite Care
277. Workplace Mental Health—Home
278. California Association of Social Rehabilitation Agencies | CASRA
279. Mental Health America | Homepage | Mental Health America
280. Anxiety and Depression Association of America, ADAA | Anxiety and Depression Association of America, ADAA
281. NAMI: National Alliance on Mental Illness | SAMHSA
282. Moura I, Teles A, Silva F, Viana D, Coutinho L, Barros F, Endler M. Mental health ubiquitous monitoring supported by social situation awareness: a systematic review. J Biomed Inform. 2020;107:103454. PMID: 32562895. http://www.ncbi.nlm.nih.gov/pubmed/32562895.

Social Psychology Factors of Depression

6

Elizabeth Sunzeri and Jeffery J. Sunzeri

Introduction

A popular definition of social psychology is that by Gordon Alport which is seconded by the American Psychological Association [41, 42]. That is, social psychology is the study of how an individual's thoughts, feelings, and actions are affected by the actual, imagined, or symbolically represented presence of other people. In a complex relationship, an individual's thoughts and behavior are shaped by social interactions.

Social psychology engages the perspective of studying the individual as found in a social group. Sociology studies groups of people.

There are several fundamental assumptions in explaining social psychology phenomena [43, 44].[1] (1) Through processes of attribution, categorization and cognitive biases, individuals construct their social reality. (2) Social environment or context interacts with personalities and dispositions to create significant variability in behavior. (3) Social behavior is shaped by cultural attributes (e.g., beliefs, values, traditions) and physiological processes (e.g., genes, epigenes, hormones). (4) Understanding of the social context of human behavior can be made tractable by scientific pursuit, such that it can be predicted, and potentially influenced. (5) Understanding of reality is subjective, influenced by experience and social norms. As a result, it is subject to biases and distortions. Objectivity is difficult to attain. (6) Humans have an innate social drive: a need to belong to groups and form relationships. (7) Humans are motivated to maintain and enhance a positive self-image. (8) A complex and bidirectional drive exists between our attitudes and our behavior. (9) A drive exists for consistency in beliefs and behaviors.

Topics that are particularly germane to understanding the social psychology factors that relate to depression include the following [43, 44]:

1. Relationship conflict, including compliance, obedience, and conformance. Conflict in relationships is core to the understanding of the interplay between individual attitudes and an individual's behavior, a paradigm in social psychology.
2. Discrimination and perceived social stigma. Feeling and experiencing prejudice and or discrimination as well as feeling judged and stigmatized for mental health issues may strongly affect treatment availability and outcomes.
3. Self-esteem and social comparisons may result in negative self-views resulting in feelings of depression.
4. Social isolation and a lack of social support. Increasing the risk of depression is the individual's separation from others and the support mechanisms provided during times of personal stress and vulnerability.
5. Stressful life events such as bereavement, job loss, a major move, weather phenomena may all trigger feelings of depression.
6. A lack of social skills. Social skills especially in comparison to significant others in personal relationships such as may be found in parent-offspring, unequal marriages, and otherwise marginalized individuals can lead to difficulty in creating or maintaining social interactions, thus leading to depression.

We will look at the theoretical underpinnings for these assumptions and then some of the research that relates these principles to depressive disorders.

[1] A comprehensive list of textbooks that target introductory to advanced general information on social psychology as well as specific research areas that address some of the ramifications of these fundamental assumptions can be found here [141].

E. Sunzeri (✉)
Heather Hills Consulting, Coos Bay, OR, USA

J. J. Sunzeri
Sunzeri Consulting, Hollister, CA, USA

J. Raber et al. (eds.), *Understanding and Treating Depressive Disorders*, https://doi.org/10.1007/978-3-032-14465-2_6

Theoretical Perspectives

Social Support Theory

The heart of social support theory is the idea that sufficient social support and relationships can assist with an individual's coping strategies, quality of life, and overall health [46, 47]. Types of support during challenging times can be companionship, emotional, informational, and instrumental. That support can include sources such as family, friends, acquaintances, pets, and community organizations [54]. However, it should not be lost sight of, in order for the recipient to receive health benefits from social support, that support must be based on the preferences of the individual who needs that support [79, 86–90]. Cultural differences can modify both the giving and receiving of social support [117–130].

Companionship provides the comfort of engaging in shared social activities. It provides a sense of social belonging [48, 49, 88]. *Emotional support* is warmth and nurturance. It is showing concern, caring, encouraging, accepting, letting a person know that he or she is valued [46, 50]. *Informational support* is providing useful information, guidance, advise and suggestions to assist someone to solve their problem [51, 52]. *Instrumental support* is tangible concrete assistance such as financial or providing service [53].

Support has been conceived of as structural or functional; perceived or received. *Structural* refers to the integration of the individual into a social network [55, 59]. *Functional* refers to the specific services provided [47, 48]. *Perceived* support is the belief that a provider has or will supply support [54]. *Received* support is the support that has been given by the provider [56]. Received support has not been consistently linked to health benefits [71, 72].

There are *two main hypotheses* that address the association between social support and health. They are the direct effects and the buffering hypothesis. *Direct effects hypothesis* suggests that regardless of stress, people who have a high level of social support are in better health than people with low social support [61]. Consistent direct effects are seen for mental health benefits [45]. Structural support and perceived support are associated with the main effects [71, 72]. The *buffering hypothesis* posits that social support protects individuals from bad effects of stressors [71]. Buffering seems to be more correlated to perceived support than structural or received support [71].

Theories that guide social support research and research methods are tailored to test these hypotheses. The principal theoretical perspectives on social support research relative to health include the stress and coping perspective, the social constructionist perspective, the relationship perspective, and the life-span theory [45]. *Stress and coping* suggest that support helps protect people from stress [61, 71, 73–76]. It is the theory that supports the buffering hypothesis. It is based upon changing how people adapt their conscious appraisal of the stressful situation to develop a way to cope. Stress and coping theory is the most popular theory.

Social constructionist theory suggests that irrespective of stress, social support directly influences health via promoting self-esteem and self-regulation.

Relationship regulation theory suggests that relationship processes including companionship and intimacy that frequently occur with support is inseparable from health effects of social support. Relationship regulation theory supports the direct effects hypothesis between support and mental health [73, 77, 78]. Regulation suggests that perceived support and mental health are linked by people regulating their emotions by experiencing ordinary activities rather than by conversations directly about coping with stress.

Life span theory suggests that social support develops over the life time [72–77]. Perceived and received support interact to develop adaptable personality traits, social and coping strategies. These traits promote adopting healthy relationships and practices and prevent unhealthy stressful situations.

Social psychological biological pathways linking support to health have been identified [72, 79]. As we have discussed in many places in this text, neuroendocrine, immune, and circulatory systems are constantly interacting with each other. Social support decreases activity in stress related systems in the brain such as the hypothalamic-pituitary-adrenal (HPA) axis, which results in decreased cortisol levels [79–81]. Social integration is correlated with better immune system function [82–84]. Social support can improve cardiovascular reactivity to stress [84, 85]. See Fig. 6.1.

Social support can buffer stress that *effects mental health* through providing tangible and emotional support [54]. People who have high support have fewer symptoms of mental health issues including depression and anxiety than those who have lower social support [60–64, 67]. In addition, they have fewer alcohol and drug problems and less suicidal ideation [65–67]. Social support for eating issues may make a difference in binge eating disorders but people with eating disorders may be reluctant to seek that help due to perceived stigma [68]. For single mothers, supportive relationships with friends and co-workers, rather than task-related support from family, has a greater positive impact on psychological health [70]. Social support between coworkers for work related distress can buffer psychological effects [69]. Higher social support has been associated with less cognitive decline with age [109–115].

Social support is also powerfully linked to *physical health* and its direct and indirect influence on mental health [91–96, 98]. However, direct relationships with social support are hard to ferret out of the complex combination of variables

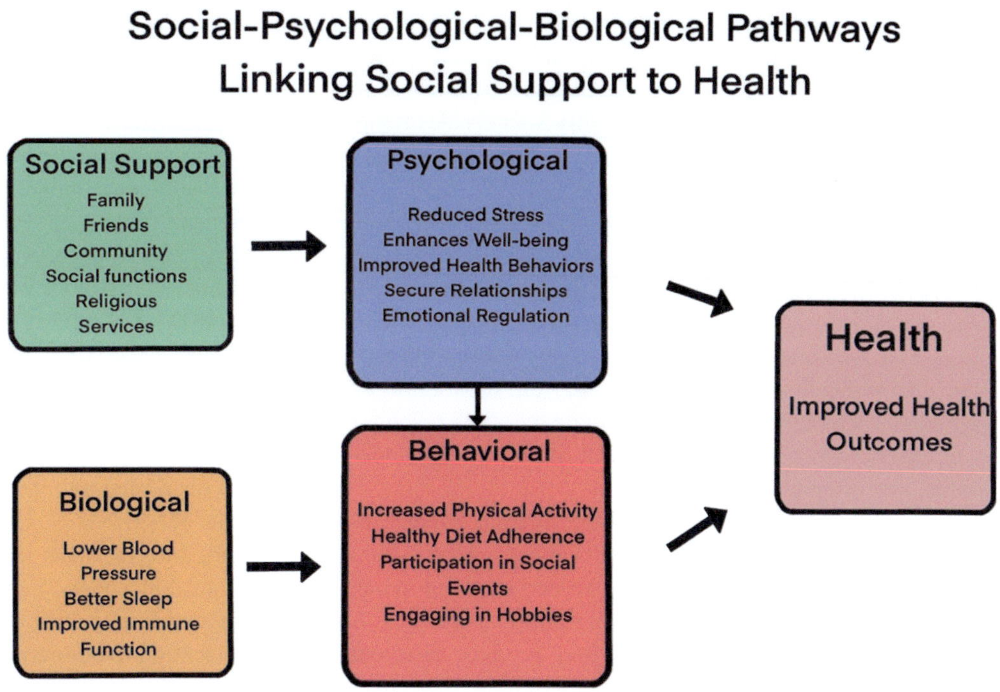

Fig. 6.1 This flow chart illustrates the interconnected social, psychological, biological, and behavioral mechanisms through which social support influences health

involved [87, 97]. Low social support is linked to significantly higher risk of death from some of the most pernicious diseases [47, 72]. For example, low levels of social support have been highly correlated to increase cardiovascular disease [99–103]. Higher social support may be associated with better outcomes of some diseases. Two prominent examples are diabetes [104–108] and cancer [91, 116–121].

Attribution Theory

Attribution theory proposes processes wherein we ascribe motives to our own or other's behavior and whether these motives are internal or external [42]. Internal motivations are also called personal motivations or dispositional attributes. External motivations are also called circumstantial or situational motivations.

Our perceptions are fundamentally influenced by our selection of observables, their classification into schema, and our interpretation based upon our learning and memory of similar experiences [44]. Our interpersonal perception is also skewed by first and last impressions.

Most often we are not aware of our attributions and we are error prone. Many of our attribution errors are caused by negative or positive biases that may result in stereotyping, fundamental vs situational attributional errors, and actor-observer bias. We tend to attribute our own behavior to external forces and attribute other people's behavior to internal dispositions. Self-serving bias is the tendency to attribute our own internal disposition to positive behavioral outcomes and to attribute external forces to unfavorable outcomes.

The progenitor of attribution theory is the balance theory by Heider [131]. It suggests that motivation to change is provided by an interaction between comfortable situations [balanced] and uncomfortable situations (unbalanced]. He conceived of a triad relationship between the observing person, a second person who shares a relationship with the observer, and an event, idea, object, or a third person. Between each member of the triad are a balance or imbalance of either liking, disliking, or neutral. He believed that the relationship is balanced if all of the interactions are liking or there is an even number of disliking. If the overall relationship is imbalanced there is the drive to change.

The most well accepted model of attribution theory is that of Kelley [132]. He postulated three *underlying principles for motivation*. They are covariance, discounting, and augmenting. *Covariance* means that the behavior occurs only when a specific cause is in effect. He divides covariance into personal causes (dispositional), environmental, and unique circumstances. To determine if an attribution is likely to be correct and that it can be predicted, he suggest that we need to examine the consistency, consensus, and distinctiveness of the behavior [133]. *Discounting* means that one needs to examine if the cause of the behavior occurs in any other circumstances, if it does then the attribution to a specific cause is not as likely to be accurate. *Augmenting* says that if a behavior is performed when the known or anticipated costs are great, then their motivation must be stronger than the reasons not to do it [134].

The *theory of correspondent inference* was developed by Jones and Davis as an attempt to understand if a behavior could be explained by correspondence with personality of the actor vs by noncorresponding interference [135]. They believe that the behavior is more likely to be corresponding to a personality or disposition if the behavior is made with free choice, if the behavior is not highly socially desirable, and if the behavior does not appear to have multiple plausible common causes.

Stressful Life Events Models

Stress may be most often defined as a physical or psychological stimulus that produces disequilibrium or strain in an individual such that the body must initiate the stress response to restore homeostasis [142]. Stressful life events are undesirable, and often uncontrollable.

When the brain determines that the internal balance of perceived resources to perceived demands of a given situation has been disrupted, it regulates the nervous, endocrine, and immune systems to restore equilibrium [143–145].

Different psychosocial stressors may produce different levels of stress in different people. For example, there may be differences in individual resources including time, money, friends, information, training, tools, or physical objects. These differences along with sex, age, pregnancy, lactation, and lifestyle variables (such as alcohol, tobacco, and caffeine use], our genes and epigenetic programming, and our life experiences (especially early childhood experiences] help to determine how stressful we perceive a situation to be [146].

Psychosocial stress (particularly stress resulting from interpersonal relationships and navigating one's place in the social hierarchy] can have deleterious effects on immune function, and mental and physical health. For example, chronic job-related stressors such as unemployment [147], job burnout [147–149], and job strain [150] have all been linked to a variety of immune alterations. Psychological factors associated with chronic stress are risk factors for depression [151–153].

Psychosocial stressors in our closest social relationships have the greatest effects. Chronic stress among caregivers of parents or spouses has been shown to have a negative effect on endocrine and immune function leading to poor health, including delayed wound healing and blunted vaccine responses [154–161]. Negative marital functioning not only appears to have an indirect influence on health outcomes through depression and health habits, but also directly affects cardiovascular, endocrine, immune, neurosensory, and other physiological mechanisms [86].

Low socioeconomic status (SES) is associated with a multitude of chronic stressors and is strongly correlated with most causes of morbidity and mortality across various populations [162–166]. Depression, obesity, and diabetes are particularly related to low SES, and those who are the most socioeconomically disadvantaged have the greatest risk for poor mental and physical health. Effects of low SES are cumulative, begin in childhood, and tend to persist and cross cultures [167, 168].

There are two primary pathways through which psychosocial stressors may impact physical health and/or influence physiological processes. First, people are more likely to engage in maladaptive health behaviors or habits such as smoking, excess alcohol consumption, drug abuse, decreased exercise, lack of sleep, and poor eating habits [169–171] when they are under stress. Depressed patients are less likely to seek medical help and less likely to take prescribed medications [172]. These behaviors put individuals at additional risk for the consequences of stress, which may result in compromised endocrine and immune responses and altered cardiovascular functions.

Second, our thoughts and perceptions of a particular stressor are connected to immune and endocrine function through those areas of the central nervous system that deal with higher cognitive functions. The prefrontal cortex, which integrates cognition and affect, interfaces with the limbic system (amygdala, cingulate gyrus) and with the paraventricular nucleus of the hypothalamus, which controls the hypothalamic pituitary adrenal and the sympathetic adrenal medullary axes. See Fig. 6.2.

Social Cognitive Theory

The *social cognitive theory*, an extension of Bandura's social learning theory, integrates the psychosocial milieu with biological constraints to try to explain the multiplex, intricate, and multifaceted way in which behavior arises from the cognitive interaction of self-regulation, motivation, and experiences, to guide our interactions from birth to death [136, 138, 140].

In the field of health, the theory posits that beliefs of self-efficacy interact with goals, impediments, and outcome expectations to regulate motivation, well-being, and behavior. Bandura says that the triad of behavior, environment, and personal factors are the heart of the social cognitive theory [137]. Behavior is related to learning from the consequences of the behavior. Environment is the setting in which the activity occurs. Whether it is conducive to repetition or not. Personal factors are internal factors that influence one's behavior. Importantly, these include attributes such as attitudes and beliefs. Equally importantly, in these interactions, humans can also influence the environment.

Self-efficacy is said to come from physiological states, accomplishments, verbal persuasion, and vicarious experiences [139].

In the chapter on change in this text, we have a deeper discussion of social cognitive theory.

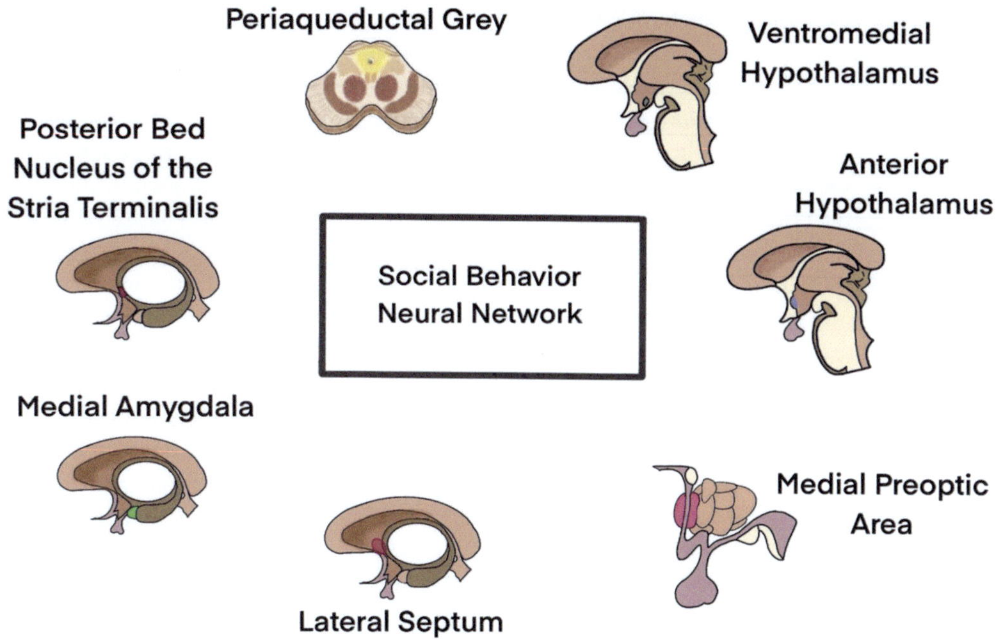

Fig. 6.2 Neural Substrates of the Social Behavior Network. This illustration highlights core brain regions comprising the social behavior neural network, including the periaqueductal grey, posterior bed nucleus of the stria terminalis, medial amygdala, lateral septum, medial preoptic area, anterior hypothalamus, and ventromedial hypothalamus. These interconnected structures modulate a range of social behaviors, integrating sensory, emotional, and hormonal cues to shape context-specific responses

Putting the Pieces Together

Precarious and unsafe family environments can interact with genetic factors in children and result in maladaptive emotional, cognitive, neuroendocrine, and immune system processes [177, 178], psychosocial dysfunction [58, 173], malfunctioning stress regulation [177], and hazardous health behaviors [174–176]. The result may be increased risk for substance abuse, obesity, chronic health disorders, mental health problems, and early mortality.

Effects of environmental factors during early development may modify epigenetics of expression of several psychopathologies including depression and schizophrenia [179]. Prenatal stressors also influence gene expression that may predispose to depression [180].

In this chapter, we will not explore the physiological basis of these associations in depth, as those discussions are reserved for other chapters that provide a more detailed analysis.

Here we will present studies that provide some insights into the relationship between social psychology factors and depression. These studies have frequently been based on investigations designed to test the hypotheses in the context of the theories mentioned above.

Parent–Child Experiences

Adolescent depression has the potential for a lifetime of hurt. For example, it increases the risks for poor academic performance, substance abuse, strained parent–child relationships and suicide [376]. Fortunately, adolescents appear to be resistant to some of the common social factors that might lead to depression. Things such as parental economic status, peer pressure, and feelings of anomie are not always related to rates of depression in adolescents [3, 181].

There are subtleties. For example, there is mixed evidence for *depression socialization*, a process wherein friends influence each other's nonclinical levels of depression [181, 182]. Evidence is suggestive that influence of depressive symptoms may relate only to true same-gender best friends [182]. A *selection de-selection process* in adolescence proposes that adolescents tend to select friends with similar levels of depression, and friends may increase each other's depressive symptoms when relationships last [1, 2, 183, 184].

Parent-child emotional interactions are related to the rates of depression in both children and parents [185–187]. Maternal but not paternal harsh treatment of girls but not boys may result in rumination, which is in turn associated with increased anxiety and depression symptoms [187]. Sampling of elementary and middle school children showed that depression symptoms were mediated by associations between peer victimization and perceived social threat vs social acceptance, as well as associations between harsh parenting and feelings of personal failure vs global self-worth [185]. A lack of positive reinforcement of positive behavior in children can result in future depression risk [188]. Parental behaviors that reinforce depressive behavior or reciprocate aggression and do not reinforce positive behavior have been associated with youth depression.

A study of 4- to 9-year-old children in single-mother households showed that socioeconomic effects of poverty is mediated directly through maternal depression influences on children's socioemotional problems as well as indirectly through physical punishment [189]. Data from the *National Longitudinal Survey of Youth*, sample of 4- to 9-year-old children, in two-parent families shows that the effect of poverty on the socioemotional problems in children may be mediated by maternal depression and marital conflict. [190, 366]. Depressed mothers use *corporal punishment* more frequently and have higher levels of marital conflict, which directly relates to their using corporal punishment [367–370]. Better educated and younger mothers spank their children less frequently. Children who are more frequently spanked show more socioemotional problems including depression [191]. Higher adverse childhood experiences, adverse childhood experience score, and several socio-demographic determinants were associated with a higher likelihood of probable depression and probable anxiety [192]. There appears to be a graded dose response relationship between adverse childhood experiences including spanking and the probability of moderate to heavy drinking, drug use, depressed affect, and suicide attempts in adulthood [193]. Childhood adversities and depression in adulthood are reviewed in reference [194].

Disturbance in positive affect not just negative affect are common in adolescent depression [195–197]. Blunted reward responses are seen in adolescents with major depression and those at high risk for major depression [198]. Reduced activation of positive valence systems is seen in high-risk children of depressed mothers and predict future pathologies [199].

At various times during adolescence, internalizing and externalizing difficulties leads to interpersonal problems with peers [200]. This may result in perceived rejection and rejection sensitivity following depression and/or aggression in a bidirectional relationship.

Lifestyle patterns and behaviors appear to be responsible for an increase in the incidence of depression. "*Lifestyle Medicine*," a change in physical activity, diet, adequate sleep and social interaction, meditation techniques, and the reduction in recreational substances such as nicotine, drugs, and alcohol may enhance mental well-being [201].

Parental socialization of racial messages to Black adolescents can alter the effect of cultural racism on depression symptoms [202, 373–375]. In one study, adolescents who reported higher private regard and more cultural pride messages, showed attenuation of the negative effects of cultural racism on depression [202]. Whereas, those adolescents who reported lower private regard and lower cultural pride messages, showed an increase in the negative effects of cultural racism. Higher public regard and low alertness to discrimination messages also exacerbated the symptoms of depression.

In communities with low neighborhood cohesion, parental racial discrimination experiences have been associated with more cultural socialization messages about racial pride and history for boys and with more promotion of mistrust messages for both boys and girls [373]. Black parents vary in their racial socialization messages based on their family's contexts and experiences [374]. Parents who worked in jobs with fewer Black people were more likely to prepare their children for bias messages vs those Black parents who worked with more Black people.

Despite the high risk of significant exposure to racism-related stress and discrimination, most Black youth do not develop mental health problems [375]. Social-ecological protective factors such as internal assets, mother-adolescent communication, and community cohesion if available to Black adolescents may mitigate depressive symptoms. In particular, effective mother-adolescent communication reduces the risk of adversity driving depressive symptoms.

Geriatric Depression

Further confusing the concept of a straight line between definition and treatment is the occurrence of Geriatric Depression. Geriatric depression prevalence rates in the USA and Europe vary widely from about 10% to 65% [203–206]. Late-life depression triggers include such things that are more common as we age. For example, loneliness, lack of social support, loss of loved ones, illness, frailty, disability and accumulation of negative life events [207–210].

Geriatric Depression differs in that the symptoms are different from those presented in younger people. As major depression is often assessed and diagnosed by using the CES-D scale, the disorder of Geriatric Depression is assessed by a different scale due to the differing nature of the disorder. The *Geriatric Depression Scale (GDS)* [211–213] is applicable to the population aged 65 and older as depressive disorder at that age appears more commonly than in earlier years [214]. Indeed, a diagnostic scale would not be indicated unless the meaning and manifestation of depression were not different for this age group [215].

It could easily be understood then that a disorder that presents so differently as to require a different scalar tool may not represent the same disease, but a different stage of a continuum that represents social processes rather than a specific medical condition [215]. Because of this differential, depression later in life will often go un-diagnosed, or misdiagnosed [213, 216, 217]. To facilitate more rapid screening, much shorter versions of the 30 question GDS, the *GDS-4 and GDS-5 versions*, have been created and systematically analyzed but have fallen short on sensitivity and specificity [216]. However, the *GDS-15 and GDS-10 scales* have been found to be more sensitive and specific than the GDS-30 [218]. Perhaps this speaks to a continuum of life experiences as we age.

Social Psychology of Family Interactions

Family structure can have a profound effect on children's development of self-concept [219, 220], physical and mental health [221], and depression and social adjustment [222–226]. Sources of support at critical times may be important for students to achieve social competence [57]. Especially from teachers and school personnel [58].

Heritability

A complex relationship exists between nature and nurture. It is well established that major depression runs in families as a combination of genetic and environmental influences (i.e., is *heritable*) [227–229]. The question of how much of the variations in the depression syndemic are due to family interactions may not be answerable. However, the following are some of the studies that might shed light on the subject.

A study of 115 second- and third-generation offspring at high or low risk for depression based on the presence or absence of major depressive disorder in the first generation found that high-risk individuals had lower putamen volume and altered neuronal density and mood-modulated function [230]. A scoping review found that children of parents with major depressive disorder (MDD) and bipolar disorders, or elevated anxiety symptoms show alterations in a range of brain regions [231]. The most frequently altered were the amygdala, hippocampal volumes, fusiform thickness, and thickness in temporoparietal regions. Differences in amygdala volumes among children exposed to postnatal as well as persistent maternal depressive symptoms have been seen [232].

A mother's history of major depressive disorder— and, to a lesser extent, a father's— is one of the strongest predictors of depression in adolescent offspring [233–236].

There is some evidence of focal areas of thinner cortical gray matter in high-risk daughters of recurrently depressed mothers [237]. And the location, direction, and extent of the neural anomalies are in concordance with the symptoms.

Sex-specific contributions are suggested by the results of a study that showed psychotic symptoms among offspring of mothers and fathers with depression: bipolar disorder and schizophrenia were significantly more prevalent among daughters of affected fathers and sons of affected mothers than among offspring of the same sex as their affected parent [238]. These results may suggest X-chromosome-linked genetic transmission or inherited chromosomal modifications.

A testament to the complexity of associations is the indirect influences from parents that can make its way to depression in offspring via substance use related problems [239, 240]. For example, paternal smoking before pregnancy and paternal psychiatric disorders, but not maternal smoking, may act as modifiers in elevating the risk of substance-use-related problems among offspring. [241]. Substance use problems later in life are associated with increases in risk of anxiety, depression, and substance abuse disorders in young adulthood [242–244]. Although not examined for depression, of note is that father's smoking can cause DNA sequence mutations and epigenetic modifications in the sperm, which can then be transmitted to the embryo and may potentially associate with diseases in offspring [245].

Twin studies of heritability of depressive symptoms generally indicate a significant heritability but not always [246]. Samples from the *Colorado Adoption Project* found that for both the sibling adoption and the parent-offspring designs, heritability irrespective of child gender was negligible, shared environment was modest, and non-shared environment was substantial [247]. Significant family effects of anxiety and depression have been seen on environmental transmission from mothers, but not from fathers to their children [248]. Sisters shared the greatest effects. It was lower in brothers and nonexistent in siblings of the opposite sex. Correlations decreased with increasing age differences between relatives. Estimated heritability was between 0 and 0.20.[2]

A French study examined roles of various socioeconomic factors in adolescent multi-morbidity (cumulated number of mental health, behavioral, and school difficulties) [249]. Multimorbidity was common. Insufficient income and non-intact families were the most heavily implicated, although being immigrant, low parents' education, and low fathers' occupations in early adolescence were also strong players. A Canadian study indicated that in offspring exposed to maternal depressive symptoms, the adjusted rates of incident *suicide-related thoughts (SRT)* and *suicide attempts (SA)* and of recurrent SRT and SA were significantly elevated compared to non-exposed offspring, but only in females not in males [250].

Mothers with persistent psychological distress had daughters with 2.5 times risk of depressive disorders and had sons with no extra risk related to maternal depression, but the sons did have depressive symptoms related to a lower educational attainment [251].

It is difficult to fit in and adapt to a predominant ethnic society that is different from one's own parents. Complicating that desire to belong is the impact that parental cultural

[2] *Heritability* can range between 0 (genetics explains nothing about the trait) and 1 (genetics explains everything) [263]. It is important, however, to keep in mind that heritability estimates can be misleading [264].

socialization, preparation for bias, and promotion of mistrust has upon children. Ethnic socialization practices can have different mental health effects on adolescents based upon whether the mother or the father is promoting distrust [252]. In a Mexican-American study, father's but not mother's promotion of mistrust but not cultural socialization or preparation of bias by either the father or mother exacerbated adolescent discrimination-depression [252].

Exposure in the offspring to maternal anxiety or depression *in utero* is associated with a greater risk for emotional and behavioral problems in childhood and clinical levels of anxiety and depression in adulthood [253–256]. Maternal depression and recent stress may independently associate with brain age and the pace of aging, respectively, in young adulthood of their offspring [257]. *Brain age* refers to the estimated difference between neuroanatomical age and chronological age as assessed through an MRI scan [258]. And direct transmission of genetic/epigenetic risks for depression is possible. Many of the wide range of neurobiological disturbances in the structure and function of cortical and subcortical gray matter and dysregulation of the HPA axis in major depression are found in never-depressed offspring of adults with recurrent depression [259].

High-frequency heart rate variability (HF-HRV) is frequently used as an experimental indicator of parasympathetic (vagal) function [26, 260]. HF-HRV is related to depression, stress, emotion regulation, and social engagement [261].[3] If heart rate is highly variable (that is greater variance between beats), this is usually evidence that the cardiovascular system is functioning well, and the body can adapt to many kinds of changes. So, highly variable heart rate is often an indication of low stress and happiness. In healthy mother-daughter dyads, vagal responses are often synchronous indicating a reciprocal social engagement that speaks of secure emotional bonding and healthy emotional regulation. When mothers have major depression, there is a discordant and diminished vagal response in the dyad.

Bridge symptoms between cooccurring depression within families after having a baby and emotional symptoms in children in early adolescence have been identified [262]. Feeling guilty and self-harm ideation reinforced depression symptoms in mother and father. Mother's symptoms of feeling guilty, and symptoms of anhedonia, panic, and sadness were highly connected with child emotional difficulties. Father's symptoms of feeling overwhelmed were associated with child's emotional difficulties. Indirect associations were seen between guilt and anhedonia in fathers and children's emotional difficulties.

The *Year-15 survey of the Fragile Families and Child Wellbeing Study*,[4] which follows a cohort of children born in large U.S. cities, primarily to unmarried parents, revealed that the relationship between maternal depression and adolescent internalizing symptoms [e.g., mood and anxiety disturbances] is substantially larger for daughters compared to sons [267].

Psychological wellbeing can mean the hedonic subjective well-being in the pursuit of pleasure and the presence of a sense of life satisfaction [32] or *eudaimonic well-being*,[5] which refers to optimal human functioning and the endeavor to achieve meaningful goals in life [36–40, 268, 269]. Various dimensions of eudaimonic well-being that protects mental and physical health have been proposed. These include the Carol Ryff eudaimonic model that has been found to be negatively associated with depressive symptoms in adolescents [270, 271], adults [37, 272–274], and older folks [275, 276].

Ryff's model proposes six dimensions: autonomy, a feeling of purpose or meaning in life, positive relationships with others, self-acceptance, personal growth and development, and environmental mastery [269]. A balance between challenges and acceptances in those dimensions may be conducive to psychological well-being.

A study of a large cohort of older adults found that lack of positive well-being is a substantial risk factor for depression [271]. In that cohort, people with low levels of well-being after controlling for personality, negative functioning, prior depression, demographic, economic, and physical heath variables were more than twice as likely to be depressed 10 years later.

A systematic review of *scales used for measuring eudaimonic well-being* found that Mental Health Continuum, Flourishing Scale, General Causality Orientations Scale, and Orientations to Happiness Subscales were the most used for clinical populations [277]. Results of studies using those scales indicated that autonomy was important in pursuing treatment for depression.

[3]The vagus nerves influence beat-to-beat variations in heart rate, and it modulates expression of emotions and receptivity of social engagement by regulating muscles of facial expressions, eye gaze, vocalizations, and head orientation [265]. More on the vagal nerve and autonomic reactivity can be seen in [266].

[4]*The Fragile Families and Child Wellbeing Study (FFCWS)*, (a.k.a. *The Future of Families and Child Wellbeing Study*) is a nationally sampled longitudinal cohort of U.S. urban births with a large share of disadvantaged families. It is a good database for looking at effects of internalizing symptoms, as internalizing symptoms are much more common among disadvantaged adolescents [295, 370].

[5]*Eudaimonia* is a Greek word meaning good spirit and most commonly understood as happiness [296].

Maternal Depression and Effects on Their Children

A 2012 study using data from the *Fragile Families and Child Well-being Study* [370] suggests that about 38% of mothers have symptoms of depression during the first 8 years of their child's life [278]. Prevalence estimates of depression in disadvantaged mothers may be higher [279–281] and may be lower in the general population [282].

Stability and change in maternal depression are most heavily associated with the sociodemographic variables of employment status, relationship status, and fathers' depression [283–288]. Unmarried mothers are especially vulnerable [34, 284, 289]. Unwanted or mistimed pregnancy, not having breast fed, and poor child health are related to increased depression symptoms but not to persistence [290].

It is common for mothers with subclinical or major depression to have a pervasive psychosocial dysfunction [291]. These burdens include increased strain in the home, social irritably, poor health, less activity, more days in bed, and decreased physical and job functioning with resultant financial strain [291, 292]. These mothers are at risk for lower confidence in their child-rearing ability [293] and decreased bonding with their infants [294].

Maternal depression not only takes a substantial toll on the mothers but may also have radiating effects on the whole family [292] and especially the children [278]. These children are at great risk for compromised cognitive, behavioral, and health effects from infancy through adulthood [299–303]. Effective parenting may be limited such that interactions of depressed mothers with their children may be withdrawn, negative, or hostile, and the home environment may be stressful [297, 298]. Young children are particularly vulnerable as they are dependent upon their mothers [35].

The interactive experience between infant and a depressed mother is constantly awash in negative affect and has a long-term compromising effect on both infant-mother relationship and childhood development [304]. This effect occurs in acutely and severely depressed mothers and in mothers who have high levels of depression symptoms. Consequences of this interaction include development of infant negative affect states that skews their interactions and worsens their affective difficulties. Male infants may be more susceptible than females to maternal depression [304].

Children frequently have social, psychological, and physiological difficulties [305]. Social problems include attachment insecurity [306] and aggression [307]. Psychological difficulties include depression [308–310], and anxiety and disruptive disorders that begin early and persist into adulthood [311, 312]. Physiological differences between infants of depressed vs non-depressed mothers include significantly higher cortisol and norepinephrine and significantly lower dopamine levels [313]. For example, maternal depression symptoms positively correlate with her infant's cortisol stress response [305].

Maternal depression effects extend beyond the postpartum period into early and middle childhood [290, 314] and into adulthood [312]. A 20-year study suggests that children of depressed parents compared to children of non-depressed parents have a more than three-fold increased risk of anxiety disorders, major depression, and substance dependence [315]. Interestingly, this study found that for children of *non-depressed* parents, parental affectionless control and family discord were associated with nearly a five-fold increased risk of major depressive disorder and greater than a 14-fold increased risk of substance use disorders [312].

In addition, cortisol in mother's milk may significantly contribute to infant temperament [305, 316, 317]. Breastfed infants fear behavior is significantly associated with maternal breast milk cortisol levels [316]. The negative affectivity association with maternal breast milk cortisol may be stronger in females [317]. Cortisol synchrony may be influenced by factors such as time of day, household income, physical interaction, and shared environment [318].

Adults who have experienced childhood stressors have specific epigenetic changes found in adult diseases such as major depression and cardiovascular disease [319]. Stress in preschool children increases cortisol and causes loss of DNA methylation in *short interspersed nuclear elements (SINEs*; a type of retrotransposon) and genes (such as a *zinc-finger transcription factor, ZNF263*) important for calcium transport commonly affected in stress-related diseases and in biological aging [319].

In childhood, the incidence of depression is about equal between boys and girls; however, during adolescence the rates of depression become about 2 to 1 in females vs males [320]. Before puberty, boys are more likely to be depressed than girls, but between 11 and 13 years of age, the reverse becomes true [321]. By the age of 15, girls are about twice as likely to be depressed, and this trend continues until 50–55 years of age. However as mentioned above, this statistic may be the result of different expressions of depression in males [322, 323]. Gender differences in diagnosis largely disappear when male-typical expression of depression are recognized [324].

Prevention or early treatment of psychiatric disorders is appropriate to start at an early age. Between February 2001 and April 2003, the *National Comorbidity Survey Replication* study was conducted in the USA. Data were used to assess lifetime prevalence and age-of-onset distributions of DSM-IV lifetime anxiety, mood, impulse-control, and substance use disorders [325]. Lifetime prevalence for anxiety disorders was 28.8%; for mood disorders 20.8%; for impulse-control disorders 24.8%; for substance use disorders 14.6%; and for any disorder 46.4%. Half of all these cases started by 14 years of age and 75% were identified by 24 years of age.

The median age of onset was 11 for anxiety and impulse-control disorders, 20 for substance use, and 30 for mood disorders. Advanced age of onset appeared more related to comorbidity. Lifetime prevalence overall was 46.4% and lifetime risk of any psychiatric disorder by 75 years of age was 50.8%.

Data from the *Sequenced Treatment Alternatives to Relieve Depression (STAR*D)* trial found that *age at onset (AAO)* makes a difference in symptoms in adolescent, young adult, and middle age [326]. Earlier AAO associated with more severe symptoms, except for sleep, which increased with AAO. Loss of libido, psychomotor disturbance, and appetite-weight disturbance did not vary with AAO. Child AAO symptom network differed significantly in strength from middle age AAO. Adolescent AAO symptom network significantly differed from young adult and middle age AAO networks in structure and strength.

A meta-analysis of the epidemiological literature prior to 2011 revealed that *childhood maltreatment* was associated with increased risk of developing recurrent and persistent depressive episodes (OR[6] =2.27; 95% CI: 1.80 to 2.87) [327]. In addition, a meta-analysis of clinical trials prior to 2011 indicated that childhood maltreatment was associated with deficiencies of response or remission during treatment for depression (OR=1.43; 95% CI=1.11–1.83).

A 19-year longitudinal study followed the 15% most inhibited and the 15% most aggressive children at 4–6 years of age until they reached 23 years of age [328]. Results indicated that for most of the male and female inhibited children, there were delayed social transitions but few internalizing problems. The most aggressive children had significant long-term risk of externalizing, were educational and occupational underachievers, and had a higher adult delinquency rate than the controls, independent of sex and socioeconomics. Social anxieties in middle school, self-directed coping strategies, and social withdrawal-disengagement have been independently directly linked with increased peer victimization for boys [329].

Rather than perpetuation across generations, children who were maltreated or witnessed violence are more likely to be victimized as an adult [330]. Although symptoms of depression are associated with *intimate partner violence (IPV)* perpetration and victimization, there are multitudes of socioeconomic and psychosocial risk factors that paint a complex picture [331]. These factors include (1) partnership context (demographic, neighborhood, community, and school factors), (2) partner's development and behavior (including family, peer, psychological, behavioral, and cognitive influences), and (3) relationship factors and interactional patterns [331].

Early antisocial behavior increases the risk for IPV, perpetration, and victimization [331–333]. In addition, exposure of children to their parents' IPV predisposes them to increased levels of depression, emotional expressivity, aggression, and hostile reactivity. Child anti-social behavior is associated with parental psychopathology, parenting practices, and child self-regulation in a circular fashion. IPV increases the probability of parental posttraumatic stress disorder (PTSD) and alcohol abuse, but not of parental MDD.

Effects on children who were crime victims upon moving to low-poverty neighborhoods show differences between boys and girls [334]. Adolescent girls from families experiencing recent violent crime victimization were significantly less likely to gain mental health benefits in terms of relief from distress, behavioral problems, and major depression from the move than were girls from homes where there was no crime. Boys in families where there was crime victimization were actually harmed by moving to the low-poverty neighborhoods. Childhood stress affects development and adult responses to current stresses influencing mood disorders, aggressive/impulsive traits, and suicidal behavior [335].

The interpersonal role of *food offering* between parents and child in *empathic emotion regulation* has been examined by Hamburg et al [336]. Empathic emotion regulation is an empathic response to another's emotional state that aims to regulate emotion in the provider and between the interaction partners. Offering food is motivated by the recipient's and the provider's emotional state such that its objective is to increase positive affect for both. Sharing of food resources and food as support increases interpersonal closeness. It is also suggested that if food offering becomes a substitute for other support behaviors, children may learn to use food as the principal way to soothe themselves and others. This may feed into eating disorders and foster an abbreviated set of coping behaviors.

This theme of food sharing and empathic emotion regulation has been discussed and critiqued from an evolutionary perspective by Alley [337].

In 2007, it was reported that estimates of combined childhood and adolescent depression in the USA varied between approximately 3 and 5% [338]. *The National Comorbidity Survey-Adolescent Supplement NCS-A* of 13- and 18-year-olds in the continental USA found that anxiety disorders

[6]Odds ratio (OR) is a way to represent the odds that an outcome will result when a given exposure to a variable of interest occurs compared to when the exposure does not occur. OR quantifies the strength of the association between two events. An OR greater than 1 indicates a positive association or that exposure to that variable increases the odds of that outcome. An OR less than one indicates a negative relationship between two events. An OR of 1 suggests no relationship between two events. An OR is frequently accompanied by a 95% confidence interval (CI). CI is a measure of precision of the OR. The smaller the CI, the higher the precision as long as it does not overlap OR =1. For more information, see chapter 4 on evidence basics in this text.

were the most common condition (31.9%), followed by behavior disorders (19.1%), mood disorders (14.3%), and substance use disorders (11.4%) [339]. Approximately 40% lifetime comorbidity was identified. Prevalence of severe distress was 11.2% with mood disorders, 8.3% with anxiety disorders, and 9.6% with behavior disorders. Median onset for anxiety was 6 years, for behavioral disorders 11 years, for mood disorders 13 years, and for substance use disorders 15 years.

There is some evidence that depressive symptoms in 13–18 years of age group may lead to early adulthood depressive disorders (major depression and dysthymia), comorbidity, psychosocial impairment, and alcohol abuse [340]. Risk factors include a family history of depression, childhood abuse or neglect, female sex, stressful life events, and chronic illness [338].

Association between depressive symptoms and alcohol use during adolescence may relate to shared genetic and environmental influences and causal influences [339, 341]. In a study of identical twins, early environment influenced relationships throughout adolescence between internalizing symptoms and alcohol intoxication frequency, whereas genetics demonstrated no correlation [342].

Risks for mood disorders depend upon predisposition provided by genetics and epigenetic set points programmed during critical periods as well as stochastic events [343, 344]. The timing of environmental influences on depression during adolescence depends upon pubertal development [345].

Disrupted sleep actually does not seem to have a direct causal impact on anxiety or depression [346].

The fall 2008 *National College Health Assessment (NCHA)* assessed *non-medically prescribed drug use (NMPDU)* (antidepressants, painkillers, sedatives, and stimulants) [348]. Both symptoms of depression and suicidality were significantly associated with increased likelihood of any NMPDU. The strongest correlation, especially for females, was painkiller use. Overall, about 13% reported NMPDU, with reports of hopelessness, sadness, depression, and suicidality being 1.22–1.31 times more likely to report NMPDU ($p < 0.05$). Hopelessness and depression were associated with 1.44– 1.91 times more likelihood to have used antidepressants.

A 2013 article reviewed the literature on predictors of outcome in psychotherapy of children and adolescents treated for anxiety and depression [347]. Most of the studies showed no relationship between gender and age and treatment outcome. For anxiety, most studies showed no relationships between demographic (age, gender, ethnicity, IQ) and clinical factors (duration, type of diagnosis, pre-treatment severity, comorbidity) and treatment outcome. However, depression baseline severity of symptoms and comorbid anxiety did influence treatment response.

Additional Sex and Gender Differences

As mentioned above, almost twice as many adult women as men suffer from the typical symptoms of depression [33, 349]. However, males have been conditioned by gendered societal processes to express their emotions differently than females [31]. Males tend to react to emotional pain by less control over impulses and more hyperactivity manifesting in irritability, anger, self-destructive behavior, self-distraction, or numbing of pain with substance use, gambling, womanizing, and workaholism [28–30, 350].[7] Influences of sociocultural relationships, current and early experiences as well as family relationships may make a significant contribution to depression [349]. Gender roles and beliefs have been said to foster and perpetuate depression in men and women [351–353].

Negative feelings and mood along with baseline hypersecretion of dehydroepiandrosterone but not cortisol have been associated with predicting within 12 months the first onset of major depression in a group of adolescents [354].

Twin studies and/or adoption studies are usually informative in teasing out genetic and environmental components to disorders. Prevalence of major depressive disorder (MDD) in men vs women was investigated in a community-based twin sample [355]. Genetic model fitting was used to evaluate genetic and environmental contributions in 2662 volunteer pairs of Australian twins. The mean age for women was 44 years (range = 28–89 years; SD =12.35), and for men, the mean age was 42 years (range = 28–84 years; SD = 11.23). Three different criteria sets were used to define depression: *DSM-III-R* major depressive disorder (the broadest definition), *DSM-IV* major depressive disorder, and *severe DSM-IV* major depressive disorder (the narrowest definition). Lifetime prevalence using the DSM-III-R, DSM-IV, and severe DSM-IV for women and men were respectively 31% and 24%; 22% and 16%; 9% and 3%.

For both sexes, the relative contribution of environment and genetics were stable for each definition. For women, it seems that genetic factors and unique environmental factors contribute to development of MDD: genetic heritability estimates range from 36% to 44%. For men, environmental factors appear to play a much larger role: heritability estimates range was 1% for the narrowest definition to 24% for the broadest, but because of such a small prevalence of depression by the narrow definition, this range may be illusory. Familial aggregation of MDD was moderately seen in women and was mostly explained by genetics. In men, familial aggregation of MDD was only modest. As defined by the broader definition of the DSM-III, MDD was more heritable

[7] A question is how to reconcile the definitions of depression to accommodate these male manifestations.

for women. For both sexes, the environment made a large contribution to MDD.

The female preponderance in depression begins to emerge around the age of 13. To explain this sex difference, a developmentally sensitive, elaborated, *cognitive vulnerability-transactional stress model of depression* has been proposed [356]. It goes something like this. Negative events contribute to a general elevation of negative affect. Genetic cognitive vulnerability factors modulate the probability that the negative effect will turn into depression. Then, increases in depression can transactionally lead to more self-generated negative life events and more input to perpetuate the cycle.

In addition, there may be sex differences in the pathways to depression. A study investigated the relationship of *cognitive diathesis-stress factors* to depression [357] *Diathesis–stress* is a term that suggests that a disorder may occur when an underlying vulnerability is coupled with a triggering event. Men were less likely to have experienced a match between a cognitive diathesis-stress and a pre-onset negative stressor than women. Stress variables were different for men and women. Depressed women had a greater probability of having experienced a severely negative event before the depression began. They also had more occurrences of negative interpersonal events. Cognitive variables were the same for men and women.

Sex differences in symptoms of depression have been seen in depressed and nondepressed elderly men and women [358]. From a family study, 326 people, 50 years old or more, with a lifetime diagnosis of major depression, and 357 general population controls age and sex matched were evaluated with the *Composite International Diagnostic Interview*. Women controls had more symptoms of depression than men did, less joy, and more appetite disturbances. Sex differences in depressive symptoms in the general population could be entirely attributed to employment status and sex differences in the family. In the subjects with major depression, men were more agitated, and women had more disturbances with appetite. These differences were not attributable to psychosocial factors.

Gender role expectations and identities, and the economic and social environment dynamically interact. Parental child-rearing gender-role attitudes can significantly impact social adjustment. For example, children from single parent families are at higher risk for depression [222, 359, 360].

A socioeconomic study of white working middle class families identified three *gender role attitude patterns*: egalitarian parents and children, traditional parents and children, and a divergent pattern, with parents more traditional and children more egalitarian [361]. Results indicated that these patterns related to socioeconomic status, parents' time spent in gendered household tasks and with children, and the sex constellation of sibling dyads. The most family conflict occurred in the traditional family patterns.

In advocating for gender equality—which remains sorely lacking in many parts of the world—it is essential to understand the origins of societal attitudes and how they can be changed to create more chances for equal opportunities in mental health [16].

People, who have higher educational attainment and greater income, express more egalitarian gender role orientations [362]. *Gender role attitudes* are socially accepted gender-typical expectations and characteristics [22]. These attitudes are frequently passed on to children [4, 5]. However, development of gender attitudes varies with contextual and personal characteristics [363]. Development of gender role attitudes have shown associations with a variety of familial socioeconomic characteristics including parents' attitudes, family roles, and mother's employment [17–20, 23–25].

Individual identity, world view, and gender role attitudes shift during adolescence from parents to friends, peers, and classmates [13–15]. Data from a *German National Educational Panel Study* have shown that more egalitarian adolescent attitudes relate to attending a school with a higher socioeconomic status, a lower proportion of female classmates, and more egalitarian classmates' gender role attitudes [13]. Males more than females were affected by classmates gender role attitudes. Male adolescents seem to be more susceptible to peer pressure than female adolescents [21].

Not surprisingly, given gender biases, parents frequently have significantly different expectations for boys and girls regarding the expressing, thinking, knowledge acquisition, concentration, and hands-on competencies [6–9, 27]. They often expect males to be more competent in STEM competency and females to be more competent in languages and reading [10–12]. Emphasis on STEM varies with parent's education and culture [364, 365].

A systematic review of *interventions designed to shift attitudes* and behavior of gendered stereotypes and norms suggests six strategies across several outcomes of gender inequality including violence against women and sexual and reproductive health [377]. These are increasing knowledge and awareness of gendered stereotypes or norms; peer engagement; addressing multiple levels of the ecological framework, developing agents of change, modelling/role models; and co-design of interventions with participants or target populations.[8]

[8]Acknowledging the importance of women in the process of economic development, individual health, and societal advancement, a series of papers on women's entrepreneurship and culture, *Gender role expectations and identities, societal culture, and the entrepreneurial environment*, explores the dynamic and complex interactions in different economic and societal systems throughout the world [371]. Many barriers and constraints on women are gender specific and are results of cultural norms, values, and customs [51–53, 55, 372].

Summary

Through processes of attribution, categorization, and cognitive biases, we all construct our social reality. Social environment interacts with personalities and dispositions to create significant variability in behavior. Social behavior is shaped by beliefs, values, and traditions as well as physiological processes.

We have an innate social drive to belong to groups and form relationships. We are motivated to achieve a positive self-image. Our attitudes and our behavior are influenced by experience and social norms. Even though we all strive for consistency in our beliefs and behaviors, our sense of reality is beset by biases and distortions. Objectivity is difficult to attain.

Nevertheless, we do believe that if we can understand our social behavior, we may be able to make predictions and change that behavior.

Sufficient social support and relationships can assist with an individual's coping strategies, quality of life, and overall health. But that social support can take many forms and must be tailored to the recipient's needs and abilities to receive it.

Attribution theory tells us the factors that we use to ascribe motives to our own or other's behavior. Most often we are not aware of our attributions and we are error prone due to our experiences and biases.

Stressful life events may be the tipping point for manifestations of mental or physical diseases such as depressive disorders.

Social cognitive theories attempt to describe the way in which behavior arises from the cognitive interactions of self-regulation, motivation, and experiences in order to guide us throughout our lives.

Critical stages for psychosocial influences on our mental and physical health begin at birth and are influenced by family dynamics and socioeconomic conditions. Childhood bullying and maladaptive behavior can be difficult to overcome. Stressors as adults can have profound interactive effects on mental and physical health leading to depression and reduced quality of life. Late-life depression can be triggered by loneliness, lack of social support, loss of loved ones, illness, frailty, disability and accumulation of negative life events.

In the next chapter, we will discuss communication in the brain. It is a peak under the covers of what is going on anatomically and physiologically during our social psychological interactions. In other chapters, we will consider what and how we can change ourselves based upon our psychosocial milieu.

References

1. Neal JW, Veenstra R. Network selection and influence effects on children's and adolescents' internalizing behaviors and peer victimization: a systematic review. Dev Rev. 2021;59:100944.
2. Stone LL, Giletta M, Brendgen M, Otten R, Engels RC, Janssens JM. Friendship similarities in internalizing problems in early childhood. Early Child Res Q. 2013;28(2):210–7.
3. Sunzeri J. Youth and alienation. Master's Research Thesis. San Jose State University; 1979.
4. Ruble DN, Martin CL, Damon W, Eisenberg N. Handbook of child psychology: Vol. 3. Social, emotional, and personality development. Wiley; 1998.
5. Eccles JS. Understanding women's educational and occupational choices: Applying the Eccles et al. Model of achievement-related choices. Psychol Women Q. 1994;18(4):585–609.
6. Zhan Z, Li Y, Mei H, et al. Key competencies acquired from STEM education: gender-differentiated parental expectations | Humanities and Social Sciences Communications. Humanit Soc Sci Commun. 2023;10:464.
7. Eccles JS, Jacobs JE, Harold RD. Gender role stereotypes, expectancy effects, and parents' socialization of gender differences. J Soc Issues. 1990;46(2):183–201.
8. Eccles JS. Gendered socialization of STEM interests in the family. Int J Gend Sci Technol. 2015;7(2):116–32.
9. Jhang FH, Lee YT. The role of parental involvement in academic achievement trajectories of elementary school children with southeast Asian and Taiwanese mothers. Int J Educ Res. 2018;89:68–79.
10. To grab and to hold: Cultivating communal goals to overcome cultural and structural barriers in first-generation college students' science interest. (apa.org).
11. The Roles of Teachers, Classroom Experiences, and Finding Balance: A Qualitative Perspective on the Experiences and Expectations of Females Within STEM and Non-STEM Careers | International Journal of Gender, Science and Technology (open.ac.uk).
12. Why they leave: the impact of stereotype threat on the attrition of women and minorities from science, math and engineering majors | Social Psychology of Education (springer.com).
13. Taraszow T, Gresch C, Kempert S. The role of school context factors for gender role attitudes: general and differential associations between female and male adolescents. Youth Soc. 2024;56(5):967–91.
14. Hurrelmann K, Quenzel G. Developmental tasks in adolescence. Routledge; 2018.
15. Erikson EH. Identity youth and crisis (No. 7). WW Norton & company; 1968.
16. Dotti Sani GM, Quaranta M. The best is yet to come? Attitudes toward gender roles among adolescents in 36 countries. Sex Roles. 2017;77(1):30–45.
17. Farré L, Vella F. The intergenerational transmission of gender role attitudes and its implications for female labour force participation. Economica. 2013;80(318):219–47.
18. Tenenbaum HR, Leaper C. Are parents' gender schemas related to their children's gender-related cognitions? A meta-analysis. Dev Psychol. 2002;38(4):615.
19. Van De Vijver FJ. Cultural and gender differences in gender-role beliefs, sharing household task and child-care responsibilities, and Well-being among immigrants and majority members in The Netherlands. Sex Roles. 2007;57:813–24.
20. Wolter I, Braun E, Hannover B. Reading is for girls!? The negative impact of preschool teachers' traditional gender role attitudes on boys' reading related motivation and skills. Front Psychol. 2015;6:1267.
21. Halimi M, Davis SN, Consuegra E. The power of peers? Early adolescent gender typicality, peer relations, and gender role attitudes in Belgium. Gend Issues. 2021;38(2):210–37.
22. Knight CR, Brinton MC. One egalitarianism or several? Two decades of gender-role attitude change in Europe. Am J Sociol. 2017;122(5):1485–532.
23. Khandelwal P, Sehgal A. Exploring work-family interface for Indian women entrepreneurs. Gender Manag Int J. 2018;33(3):203–16.

24. Baughn CC, Chua BL, Neupert KE. The normative context for women's participation in entrepreneurship: a multicountry study. Entrep Theory Pract. 2006;30(5):687–708.
25. Bullough A, Renko M, Abdelzaher D. Women's business ownership: operating within the context of institutional and in-group collectivism. J Manag. 2017;43(7):2037–64.
26. Appelhans BM, Luecken LJ. Heart rate variability as an index of regulated emotional responding. Rev Gen Psychol. 2006;10(3):229–40.
27. Fussy DS, Iddy H, Amani J, Mkimbili ST. Girls' participation in science education: structural limitations and sustainable alternatives. Int J Sci Educ. 2023;45(14):1141–61.
28. Lynch J, Kilmartin C. The pain behind the mask: overcoming masculine depression. Routledge; 2013.
29. Addis ME. Gender and depression in men. Clin Psychol Sci Pract. 2008;15(3):153.
30. Martin LA, Neighbors HW, Griffith DM. The experience of symptoms of depression in men vs women: analysis of the National Comorbidity Survey Replication. JAMA Psychiatry. 2013;70(10):1100–6. https://doi.org/10.1001/jamapsychiatry.2013.1985.
31. Cochran SV, Rabinowitz FE. Men and depression: clinical and empirical perspectives. Elsevier; 1999.
32. Diener E, Heintzelman SJ, Kushlev K, Tay L, Wirtz D, Lutes LD, Oishi S. Findings all psychologists should know from the new science on subjective Well-being. Can Psychol. 2017;58(2):87.
33. Rolak. Neurology secrets. Elsevier Health Science; 2001.
34. Sigle-Rushton W, McLanahan S. Father absence and child well-being: a critical review. In: Moynihan DP, Smeeding TE, Rainwater L, editors. The future of the family. New York: Russell Sage Foundation; 2004. p. 116–55.
35. Radke-Yarrow M, Klimes-Dougan B. Parental depression and offspring disorders: a developmental perspective. In: Goodman SH, Gotlib IH, editors. Children of depressed parents: mechanisms of risk and implications for treatment. Washington, DC: American Psychological Association; 2002. p. 155–74.
36. Huta V, Waterman AS. Eudaimonia and its distinction from hedonia: developing a classification and terminology for understanding conceptual and operational definitions. J Happiness Stud. 2014;15:1425–56.
37. Ruini C, Albieri E, Vescovelli F. Well-being therapy: state of the art and clinical exemplifications. J Contemp Psychother. 2015;45:129–36.
38. Russell D. Eudaimonia. In: Michalos AC, editor. Encyclopedia of quality of life and Well-being research. Dordrecht: Springer; 2014. https://doi.org/10.1007/978-94-007-0753-5_928.
39. Ryff CD. Happiness is everything, or is it? Explorations on the meaning of psychological Well-being. J Pers Soc Psychol. 1989;57(6):1069–81.
40. LeBar M. The value of living well. Oxford University Press; 2013.
41. Allport GW. The historical background of social psychology. In: Lindzey G, Aronson E, editors. The handbook of social psychology. New York: McGraw Hill; 1985. p. 5.
42. APA Dictionary of Psychology.
43. Fiske ST, Gilbert DT, Lindzey G. Handbook of social psychology. 5th ed. Wiley; 2010.
44. Deb S, Gireesan A, Prabhavalkar P, Deb S. Social psychology: theories and applications. 1st ed. Routledge India; 2023.
45. Lakey B, Cohen S. Social support theory and measurement. In: Cohen S, Underwood LG, Gottlieb BH, editors. Social support measurement and intervention: a guide for health and social scientists. Oxford University; 2000. p. 29–52.
46. Wills TA. Social support and interpersonal relationships. In: Margaret C, editor. Prosocial behavior, review of personality and social psychology, vol. 12. Sage Publications; 1991. p. 265–89.
47. Uchino B. Social Support and physical health: understanding the health consequences of relationships. New Haven: Yale University Press; 2004. p. 16–7.
48. Uchino BN. Social support and health: a review of physiological processes potentially underlying links to disease outcomes. J Behav Med. 2006;29(4):377–87. https://doi.org/10.1007/s10865-006-9056-5. Epub 2006 Jun 7
49. Wills TA. Supportive functions of interpersonal relationships. In: Cohen S, Syme L, editors. Social support and health. Orlando: Academic Press; 1985. p. 61–82.
50. Slevin ML, Nichols SE, Downer SM, Wilson P, Lister TA, Arnott S, Maher J, Souhami RL, Tobias JS, Goldstone AH, Cody M. Emotional support for cancer patients: what do patients really want? Br J Cancer. 1996;74(8):1275–9. PMCID: PMC2075927. http://www.ncbi.nlm.nih.gov/pubmed/8883417.
51. Langford CP, Bowsher J, Maloney JP, Lillis PP. Social support: a conceptual analysis. J Adv Nurs. 1997;25(1):95–100. PMID: 900401. http://www.ncbi.nlm.nih.gov/pubmed/9004016.
52. Hupcey JE. Clarifying the social support theory-research linkage. J Adv Nurs. 1998;27(6):1231–41. PMID: 9663875. http://www.ncbi.nlm.nih.gov/pubmed/9663875.
53. Tilden VP, Weinert C. Social support and the chronically ill individual. Nurs Clin North Am. 1987;22(3):613–20. PMID: 3649795. http://www.ncbi.nlm.nih.gov/pubmed/3649795.
54. Heaney CA, Israel BA. Social networks and social support. In: Glanz K, Rimer BK, Viswanath K, editors. Health behavior and health education: theory, research, and practice. 4th ed. San Francisco: Jossey-Bass; 2008.
55. Taylor SE. Social support: a review. In: Friedman MS, editor. The handbook of health psychology. New York: Oxford University Press; 2011. p. 189–214.
56. Wills TA. Social support. In: Blechman EA, Brownell KD, editors. Behavioral medicine and women: a comprehensive handbook. New York: Guilford Press; 1998. p. 118–28.
57. Gurung RAR. Coping and social support. In: Health psychology: a cultural approach. Belmont: Thomson Wadsworth; 2006. p. 131–71.
58. Repetti RL, Taylor SE, Seeman TE. Risky families: family social environments and the mental and physical health of offspring. Psychol Bull. 2002;128(2):330–66. PMID: 11931522. http://www.ncbi.nlm.nih.gov/pubmed/11931522.
59. Chu PS, Saucier DA, Hafner E. Meta-analysis of the relationships between social support and Well-being in children and adolescents. J Soc Clin Psychol. 2010;29(6):624–45.
60. Lakey B, Cronin A. Low social support and major depression: research, theory, and methodological issues. In: Dobson KS, Dozois D, editors. Risk factors for depression. Academic; 2008. p. 385–408.
61. Cohen S, Wills TA. Stress, social support, and the buffering hypothesis. Psychol Bull. 1985;98(2):310–57.
62. Brewin CR, Andrews B, Valentine JD. Meta-analysis of risk factors for posttraumatic stress disorder in trauma-exposed adults. J Consult Clin Psychol. 2000;68(5):748–66. PMID: 11068961. http://www.ncbi.nlm.nih.gov/pubmed/11068961.
63. Klein DN, Taylor EB, Dickstein S, Harding K. Primary early-onset dysthymia: comparison with primary nonbipolar nonchronic major depression on demographic, clinical, familial, personality, and socioenvironmental characteristics and short-term outcome. J Abnorm Psychol. 1988;97(4):387–98. PMID: 3204224. http://www.ncbi.nlm.nih.gov/pubmed/3204224.
64. Casey PR, Dunn G, Kelly BD, Birkbeck G, Dalgard OS, Lehtinen V, Britta S, Ayuso-Mateos JL, Dowrick C, ODIN Group. Factors associated with suicidal ideation in the general population: five-Centre analysis from the ODIN study. Br J Psychiatry. 2006;189:410–5. PMID: 17077430. http://www.ncbi.nlm.nih.gov/pubmed/17077430.

65. Stice E, Barrera M, Chassin L. Prospective differential prediction of adolescent alcohol use and problem use: examining the mechanisms of effect. J Abnorm Psychol. 1998;107(4):616–28. PMID: 9830249. http://www.ncbi.nlm.nih.gov/pubmed/9830249.
66. Wiegel C, Sattler S, Göritz AS, Diewald M. Work-related stress and cognitive enhancement among university teachers. Anxiety Stress Coping. 2016;29(1):100–17. PMID: 25747817. http://www.ncbi.nlm.nih.gov/pubmed/25747817.
67. Stice E, Presnell K, Spangler D. Risk factors for binge eating onset in adolescent girls: a 2-year prospective investigation. Health Psychol. 2002;21(2):131–8. PMID: 11950103. http://www.ncbi.nlm.nih.gov/pubmed/11950103.
68. Akey JE, Rintamaki LS, Kane TL. Health belief model deterrents of social support seeking among people coping with eating disorders. J Affect Disord. 2013;145(2):246–52. PMID: 22840616. http://www.ncbi.nlm.nih.gov/pubmed/22840616.
69. Patterson GT. Examining the effects of coping and social support on work and life stress among police officers. J Crim Just. 2003;31(3):215–26.
70. D'Ercole A. Single mothers: stress, coping, and social Support. J Community Psychol. 1988;16:41–54.
71. Barrera M. Distinctions between social support concepts, measures, and models. Am J Community Psychol. 1986;14(4):413–45.
72. Uchino BN. Understanding the links between social Support and physical health: a life-span perspective with emphasis on the separability of perceived and received support. Perspect Psychol Sci. 2009;4(3):236–55. PMID: 26158961. http://www.ncbi.nlm.nih.gov/pubmed/26158961.
73. Lakey B, Orehek E. Relational regulation theory: a new approach to explain the link between perceived social support and mental health. Psychol Rev. 2011;118(3):482–95. PMID: 21534704. http://www.ncbi.nlm.nih.gov/pubmed/21534704.
74. Thoits PA. Social support as coping assistance. J Consult Clin Psychol. 1986;54(4):416–23. PMID: 3745593. http://www.ncbi.nlm.nih.gov/pubmed/3745593.
75. Lazarus RS, Folkman S. Stress, appraisal, and coping. New York: Springer; 1984.
76. Corsi F, Sartani A, Galli D, Alineri S, Uccelli M, Fontana A, Foschi D. Usefulness of preoperative diagnosis with magnetic resonance imaging for conservative surgery in Paget's disease of the breast. Breast Care (Basel). 2010;5(1):26–8. PMCID: PMC3357163. http://www.ncbi.nlm.nih.gov/pubmed/22619638.
77. Lakey B. Social support: basic research and new strategies for intervention. In: Maddux JE, Tangney JP, editors. Social psychological foundations of clinical psychology. New York: Guildford; 2010. p. 177–94.
78. Wethington E, Kessler RC. Perceived support, received support, and adjustment to stressful life events. J Health Soc Behav. 1986;27(1):78–89. PMID: 3711634. http://www.ncbi.nlm.nih.gov/pubmed/3711634.
79. Eslinger PJ, Anders S, Ballarini T, Boutros S, Krach S, Mayer AV, Moll J, Newton TL, Schroeter ML, de Oliveira-Souza R, Raber J, Sullivan GB, Swain JE, Lowe L, Zahn R. The neuroscience of social feelings: mechanisms of adaptive social functioning. Neurosci Biobehav Rev. 2021;128:592–620. PMCID: PMC8388127. http://www.ncbi.nlm.nih.gov/pubmed/34089764.
80. Turner-Cobb JM, Sephton SE, Koopman C, Blake-Mortimer J, Spiegel D. Social support and salivary cortisol in women with metastatic breast cancer. Psychosom Med. 2000;62(3):337–45. PMID: 10845347. http://www.ncbi.nlm.nih.gov/pubmed/10845347.
81. Eisenberger NI, Taylor SE, Gable SL, Hilmert CJ, Lieberman MD. Neural pathways link social support to attenuated neuroendocrine stress responses. Neuroimage. 2007;35(4):1601–12. PMCID: PMC2710966. http://www.ncbi.nlm.nih.gov/pubmed/17395493.
82. Herbert TB, Cohen S. Stress and immunity in humans: a meta-analytic review. Psychosom Med. 1993;55(4):364–79. PMID: 8416086. http://www.ncbi.nlm.nih.gov/pubmed/8416086.
83. Loucks EB, Berkman LF, Gruenewald TL, Seeman TE. Relation of social integration to inflammatory marker concentrations in men and women 70 to 79 years. Am J Cardiol. 2006;97(7):1010–6. PMID: 16563907. http://www.ncbi.nlm.nih.gov/pubmed/16563907.
84. Uchino BN. Social support and health: a review of physiological processes potentially underlying links to disease outcomes. J Behav Med. 2006;29(4):377–87. PMID: 16758315. http://www.ncbi.nlm.nih.gov/pubmed/16758315.
85. Undén AL, Orth-Gomér K, Elofsson S. Cardiovascular effects of social support in the work place: twenty-four-hour ECG monitoring of men and women. Psychosom Med. 1991;53(1):50–60. PMID: 2011650. http://www.ncbi.nlm.nih.gov/pubmed/2011650.
86. Kiecolt-Glaser JK, Newton TL. Marriage and health: his and hers. Psychol Bull. 2001;127(4):472–503. PMID: 11439708. http://www.ncbi.nlm.nih.gov/pubmed/11439708.
87. Callaghan P, Morrissey J. Social support and health: a review. J Adv Nurs. 1993;18(2):203–10. PMID: 8436711. http://www.ncbi.nlm.nih.gov/pubmed/8436711.
88. Wills TA, Shinar O. Measuring perceived and received social support. In: Social support measurement and intervention: a guide for health and social scientists. New York: Oxford University Press; 2000. p. 86–135.
89. Thurn T, Brandstätter M, Fensterer V, Küchenhoff H, Fegg MJ. Existential behavioral therapy for informal caregivers of palliative patients: barriers and promoters of support utilization. Palliat Support Care. 2015;13(3):757–66. https://doi.org/10.1017/S1478951514000546. Epub 2014 Jun 6. PMID: 24905397. http://www.ncbi.nlm.nih.gov/pubmed/24195840.
90. Loureiro F, Peças D, Neves AC, Antunes AV. Coping strategies and social support in nursing students during clinical practice: a scoping review. Nurs Open. 2024;11(2):e2112. https://doi.org/10.1002/nop2.2112. PMID:; PMCID: PMC10879724. http://www.ncbi.nlm.nih.gov/pubmed/38379350.
91. Nausheen B, Gidron Y, Peveler R, Moss-Morris R. Social support and cancer progression: a systematic review. J Psychosom Res. 2009;67(5):403–15. PMID: 19837203. http://www.ncbi.nlm.nih.gov/pubmed/19837203.
92. Dzhambov AM, Lercher P, Vincens N, Persson Waye K, Klatte M, Leist L, Lachmann T, Schreckenberg D, Belke C, Ristovska G, Kanninen KM, Botteldooren D, Van Renterghem T, Jeram S, Selander J, Arat A, White K, Julvez J, Clark C, Foraster M, van Kamp I. Protective effect of restorative possibilities on cognitive function and mental health in children and adolescents: a scoping review including the role of physical activity. Environ Res. 2023;233:116452. PMID: 37339694. http://www.ncbi.nlm.nih.gov/pubmed/37339694.
93. Thoits PA. Mechanisms linking social ties and support to physical and mental health. J Health Soc Behav. 2011;52(2):145–61. PMID: 21673143. http://www.ncbi.nlm.nih.gov/pubmed/21673143.
94. Ring D. Mental and social health are inseparable from physical health. J Bone Joint Surg Am. 2021;103(11):951–2. PMID: 33877056. http://www.ncbi.nlm.nih.gov/pubmed/11068961.
95. Kim S, Thomas PA. Direct and indirect pathways from social support to health? J Gerontol B Psychol Sci Soc Sci. 2019;74(6):1072–80. PMID: 29106661. http://www.ncbi.nlm.nih.gov/pubmed/29106661.
96. Suanet B, Aartsen MJ, Hoogendijk EO, Huisman M. The social Support-health Link unraveled: pathways linking social Support to functional capacity in later life. J Aging Health. 2020;32(7–8):616–26. PMID: 30983471. http://www.ncbi.nlm.nih.gov/pubmed/30983471.

97. Uchino BN, Bowen K, Carlisle M, Birmingham W. Psychological pathways linking social support to health outcomes: a visit with the "ghosts" of research past, present, and future. Soc Sci Med. 2012;74(7):949–57. PMCID: PMC3298603. http://www.ncbi.nlm.nih.gov/pubmed/22326104.
98. Uchino BN, Carlisle M, Birmingham W, Vaughn AA. Social support and the reactivity hypothesis: conceptual issues in examining the efficacy of received support during acute psychological stress. Biol Psychol. 2011;86(2):137–42. PMCID: PMC2928410. http://www.ncbi.nlm.nih.gov/pubmed/20398724.
99. Mannoh I, Hussien M, Commodore-Mensah Y, Michos ED. Impact of social determinants of health on cardiovascular disease prevention. Curr Opin Cardiol. 2021;36(5):572–9. PMID: 34397464. http://www.ncbi.nlm.nih.gov/pubmed/34397464.
100. Golaszewski NM, LaCroix AZ, Godino JG, Allison MA, Manson JE, King JJ, Weitlauf JC, Bea JW, Garcia L, Kroenke CH, Saquib N, Cannell B, Nguyen S, Bellettiere J. Evaluation of social isolation, loneliness, and cardiovascular disease among older women in the US. JAMA Netw Open. 2022;5(2):e2146461. PMCID: PMC8811637. http://www.ncbi.nlm.nih.gov/pubmed/35107574.
101. Freak-Poli R, Hu J, Phyo AZZ, Barker SF. Social isolation and social Support influence health service utilisation and survival after a cardiovascular disease event: a systematic review. Int J Environ Res Public Health. 2023;20(6):4853. PMCID: PMC10049557. http://www.ncbi.nlm.nih.gov/pubmed/36981761.
102. Clayton C, Motley C, Sakakibara B. Enhancing social Support among people with cardiovascular disease: a systematic scoping review. Curr Cardiol Rep. 2019;21(10):123. PMID: 31485908. http://www.ncbi.nlm.nih.gov/pubmed/31485908.
103. Datta BK, Coughlin SS, Gummadi A, Mehrabian D, Ansa BE. Perceived social Support and cardiovascular risk among nonelderly adults in the United States. Am J Cardiol. 2023;209:146–53. PMID: 37865124. http://www.ncbi.nlm.nih.gov/pubmed/37865124.
104. Fernandez-Luque L, Mejova Y, Mayer MA, Hasvold PE, Joshi S. Panel: big data & social media for empowering patients with diabetes. Stud Health Technol Inform. 2016;225:607–9. PMID: 27332274. http://www.ncbi.nlm.nih.gov/pubmed/27332274.
105. Wang X, Zhang F, Ge Y, Ding Y, Liu T. The associations between social support, self-regulatory fatigue, and health-promoting behaviors among people with type 2 diabetes mellitus: a cross-sectional survey. Front Public Health. 2023;11:1281065. PMCID: PMC10752976. http://www.ncbi.nlm.nih.gov/pubmed/38155890.
106. Stenberg J, Hjelm K. Social support as perceived, provided and needed by family-members of migrants with type 2 diabetes—a qualitative study. BMC Public Health. 2024;24(1):1612. PMCID: PMC11181519. http://www.ncbi.nlm.nih.gov/pubmed/38886671.
107. Kim M, Kim B, Park S. Social Support, eHealth literacy, and mHealth use in older adults with diabetes: moderated mediating effect of the perceived importance of app design. Comput Inform Nurs. 2024;42(2):136–43. PMCID: PMC11444354. http://www.ncbi.nlm.nih.gov/pubmed/38129323.
108. Chen W, Maimaitituerxun R, Xiang J, Xie Y, Xiao F, Wu IX, Chen L, Yang J, Liu A, Dai W. Social Support, coping strategies, depression, anxiety, and cognitive function among people with type 2 diabetes mellitus: a path analysis. Psychiatry Investig. 2024;21(9):1033–44. PMCID: PMC11421914. http://www.ncbi.nlm.nih.gov/pubmed/39219380.
109. Seeman TE, Lusignolo TM, Albert M, Berkman L. Social relationships, social support, and patterns of cognitive aging in healthy, high-functioning older adults: MacArthur studies of successful aging. Health Psychol. 2001;20(4):243–55. PMID: 11515736. http://www.ncbi.nlm.nih.gov/pubmed/11515736.
110. Yang M, Li J, Fu Y, Wang G, Liu M, Chen J, Liu J. Association of childhood trauma, social support, cognition, and suicidality in females with bipolar disorder. BMC Psychiatry. 2024;24(1):243. PMCID: PMC10986031. http://www.ncbi.nlm.nih.gov/pubmed/38566037.
111. Zhang H, Hu Z, Jiang S, Hao M, Li Y, Liu Y, Jiang XY, Jin L, Wang X. Social frailty and the incidence of motoric cognitive risk syndrome in older adults. Alzheimers Dement. 2024;20(4):2329–39. PMCID: PMC11032557. http://www.ncbi.nlm.nih.gov/pubmed/38284799.
112. Arenaza-Urquijo EM, Boyle R, Casaletto K, Anstey KJ, Vila-Castelar C, Colverson A, Palpatzis E, Eissman JM, Kheng Siang Ng T, Raghavan S, Akinci M, Vonk JMJ, Machado LS, Zanwar PP, Shrestha HL, Wagner M, Tamburin S, Sohrabi HR, Loi S, Bartrés-Faz D, Dubal DB, Vemuri P, Okonkwo O, Hohman TJ, Ewers M, Buckley RF, Reserve, Resilience and Protective Factors Professional Interest Area, Sex and Gender Professional Interest area and the ADDRESS! Special Interest Group. Sex and gender differences in cognitive resilience to aging and Alzheimer's disease. Alzheimers Dement. 2024;20(8):5695–719. PMCID: PMC11350140. http://www.ncbi.nlm.nih.gov/pubmed/38967222.
113. Moorman SM, Pai M. Social Support from family and friends, educational attainment, and cognitive function. J Appl Gerontol. 2024;43(4):396–401. PMID: 37859405. http://www.ncbi.nlm.nih.gov/pubmed/37859405.
114. Ebner NC, Horta M, El-Shafie D. New directions for studying the aging social-cognitive brain. Curr Opin Psychol. 2024;56:101768. PMCID: PMC10939782. http://www.ncbi.nlm.nih.gov/pubmed/38104362.
115. Zide BS, Donovan NJ, Lee S, Nag S, Bennett DA, Jacobs HIL. Social activity mediates locus coeruleus tangle-related cognition in older adults. Mol Psychiatry. 2024;29(7):2001–8. PMCID: PMC11408254. http://www.ncbi.nlm.nih.gov/pubmed/38355788.
116. Falagas ME, Zarkadoulia EA, Ioannidou EN, Peppas G, Christodoulou C, Rafailidis PI. The effect of psychosocial factors on breast cancer outcome: a systematic review. Breast Cancer Res. 2007;9(4):R44. PMCID: PMC2206717. http://www.ncbi.nlm.nih.gov/pubmed/17640330.
117. Bybee SG, Waters AR, Smith K, Warner EL. Misalignment of social support in the social media posts of young adult cancer caregivers. Cancer Rep (Hoboken). 2024;7(2):e1998. PMCID: PMC10884617. http://www.ncbi.nlm.nih.gov/pubmed/38389399.
118. Wang F, Simon MS, Kroenke CH, Krok-Schoen J, Jung SY, Chlebowski R, Ballinger TJ, Pichardo MS, Coday M, Garcia L, Luo J. Social support, social strain, stressful life events and mortality among postmenopausal women with breast cancer. Psychooncology. 2024;33(11):e70013. PMID: 39520665. http://www.ncbi.nlm.nih.gov/pubmed/39520665.
119. Zhao M, Na N, Xing N, Zhu H, Wu G, Xu G, Jiang Y. The impact of social support on benefit finding among patients with advanced lung cancer and their caregivers: based on actor-partner interdependence mediation model. Support Care Cancer. 2024;32(5):287. PMID: 38619660. http://www.ncbi.nlm.nih.gov/pubmed/38619660.
120. Marín-Chollom AM, Rillamas-Sun E, Koch PA, Contento IR, Gaffney AO, Ulanday KT, Hershman DL, Greenlee H. Social Support, diet, and physical activity among Latina/Hispanic women breast cancer survivors. J Immigr Minor Health. 2024;26(6):1053–61. PMID: 38954235. http://www.ncbi.nlm.nih.gov/pubmed/38954235.
121. Li H, Lyu M, Wang A, Yin Y, Zhang J, Li P. Social Support and life satisfaction in women with cervical cancer: a serial multiple mediation model. Cancer Nurs. 2024;47(1):64–71. PMID: 36322694. http://www.ncbi.nlm.nih.gov/pubmed/36322694.
122. Hansford M, Jobson L. Sociocultural context and the post-traumatic psychological response: considering culture, social support, and posttraumatic stress disorder. Psychol Trauma.

2022;14(4):669–79. PMID: 33507796. http://www.ncbi.nlm.nih.gov/pubmed/33507796.
123. Chen JM, Kim HS, Mojaverian T, Morling B. Culture and social support provision: who gives what and why. Pers Soc Psychol Bull. 2012;38(1):3–13. PMID: 22214884. http://www.ncbi.nlm.nih.gov/pubmed/22214884.
124. Kim HS, Sherman DK, Taylor SE. Culture and social support. Am Psychol. 2008;63(6):518–26. PMID: 18793039. http://www.ncbi.nlm.nih.gov/pubmed/18793039.
125. Sherman DK, Kim HS, Taylor SE. Culture and social support: neural bases and biological impact. Prog Brain Res. 2009;178:227–37. PMID: 19874973. http://www.ncbi.nlm.nih.gov/pubmed/19874973.
126. Kim HS, Sherman DK, Ko D, Taylor SE. Pursuit of comfort and pursuit of harmony: culture, relationships, and social support seeking. Pers Soc Psychol Bull. 2006;32(12):1595–607. PMID: 17122173. http://www.ncbi.nlm.nih.gov/pubmed/17122173.
127. Taylor SE, Sherman DK, Kim HS, Jarcho J, Takagi K, Dunagan MS. Culture and social support: who seeks it and why? J Pers Soc Psychol. 2004;87(3):354–62. PMID: 15382985. http://www.ncbi.nlm.nih.gov/pubmed/15382985.
128. Stevens JH. Social support, locus of control, and parenting in three low-income groups of mothers: black teenagers, black adults, and white adults. Child Dev. 1988;59(3):635–42. PMID: 3383672. http://www.ncbi.nlm.nih.gov/pubmed/39520665.
129. Lindblad-Goldberg M, Dukes JL. Social support in black, low-income, single-parent families: normative and dysfunctional patterns. Am J Orthopsychiatry. 1985;55(1):42–58. PMID: 3970150. http://www.ncbi.nlm.nih.gov/pubmed/3970150.
130. Park J, Kitayama S, Karasawa M, Curhan K, Markus HR, Kawakami N, Miyamoto Y, Love GD, Coe CL, Ryff CD. Clarifying the links between social support and health: culture, stress, and neuroticism matter. J Health Psychol. 2013;18(2):226–35. PMCID: PMC3556221. http://www.ncbi.nlm.nih.gov/pubmed/22419414.
131. Heider F. The psychology of interpersonal relations. New York: Wiley; 1958.
132. Kelley HH. Attribution theory in social psychology. In: Levine D, editor. Nebraska symposium on motivation, vol. 15. Lincoln: University of Nebraska Press; 1967. p. 192–238.
133. Kelley HH, Michela JL. Attribution theory and research. Annu Rev Psychol. 1980;31:457–501. PMID: 20809783. http://www.ncbi.nlm.nih.gov/pubmed/20809783.
134. Fauth EB, Novak JR, Gossner J, Aller TB, Kelley HH, Levin ME. Family caregivers' Progress toward values moderates the associations between behavioral symptoms of dementia, caregiver burden, and depressive symptoms. Int J Aging Hum Dev. 2024:914150241240115. PMID: 38839099. http://www.ncbi.nlm.nih.gov/pubmed/38839099.
135. Jones EE, Davis KE. From acts to dispositions: the attribution process in social psychology. In: Berkowitz L, editor. Advances in experimental social psychology, vol. 2. New York: Academic Press; 1965. p. 219–66.
136. Bandura A. Health promotion by social cognitive means. Health Educ Behav. 2004;31(2):143–64. PMID: 15090118. http://www.ncbi.nlm.nih.gov/pubmed/15090118.
137. Bandura A. Media effects: advances in theory and research. 3rd ed. Florence: Routledge; 2009. p. 94–124.
138. Bandura A, National Inst of Mental Health. Social foundations of thought and action: A social cognitive theory. Prentice-Hall, Inc; 1986.
139. Bandura A. Perceived self-efficacy in cognitive development and functioning. Educ Psychol. 1993;28(2):117–48.
140. McAlister AL, Perry CL, Parcel GS. How individuals, environments, and health behaviors interact: social cognitive theory. In: Health behavior and health education: theory, research, and practice 4th Edition. San Francisco: Wiley; 2008. p. 169–88.
141. Social Psychology Textbooks.
142. Steinman L. Elaborate interactions between the immune and nervous systems. Nat Immunol. 2004;5(6):575–81. PMID: 15164017. http://www.ncbi.nlm.nih.gov/pubmed/15164017.
143. Lashani E, Larsen IG, Kanske P, Rosendahl J, Blasberg JU, Engert V. Witnessing their mother's acute and prolonged stress affects executive functioning in children. Commun Psychol. 2024;2(1):98. PMCID: PMC11500099. http://www.ncbi.nlm.nih.gov/pubmed/39443663.
144. Hendry E, McCallister B, Elman DJ, Freeman R, Borsook D, Elman I. Validity of mental and physical stress models. Neurosci Biobehav Rev. 2024;158:105566. PMCID: PMC11082879. http://www.ncbi.nlm.nih.gov/pubmed/38307304.
145. Bower JE, Kuhlman KR. Psychoneuroimmunology: an introduction to immune-to-brain communication and its implications for clinical psychology. Annu Rev Clin Psychol. 2023;19:331–59. PMID: 36791765. http://www.ncbi.nlm.nih.gov/pubmed/36791765.
146. Kudielka BM, Hellhammer DH, Wüst S. Why do we respond so differently? Reviewing determinants of human salivary cortisol responses to challenge. Psychoneuroendocrinology. 2009;34(1):2–18. PMID: 19041187. http://www.ncbi.nlm.nih.gov/pubmed/19041187.
147. Arnetz BB, Brenner SO, Levi L, Hjelm R, Petterson IL, Wasserman J, Petrini B, Eneroth P, Kallner A, Kvetnansky R. Neuroendocrine and immunologic effects of unemployment and job insecurity. Psychother Psychosom. 1991;55(2–4):76–80. PMID: 1891571. http://www.ncbi.nlm.nih.gov/pubmed/1891571.
148. Lerman Y, Melamed S, Shragin Y, Kushnir T, Rotgoltz Y, Shirom A, Aronson M. Association between burnout at work and leukocyte adhesiveness/aggregation. Psychosom Med. 1999;61(6):828–33. PMID: 10593635. http://www.ncbi.nlm.nih.gov/pubmed/10593635.
149. Melamed S, Ugarten U, Shirom A, Kahana L, Lerman Y, Froom P. Chronic burnout, somatic arousal and elevated salivary cortisol levels. J Psychosom Res. 1999;46(6):591–8. PMID: 10454175. http://www.ncbi.nlm.nih.gov/pubmed/10454175.
150. Kawakami N, Tanigawa T, Araki S, Nakata A, Sakurai S, Yokoyama K, Morita Y. Effects of job strain on helper-inducer (CD4+CD29+) and suppressor-inducer (CD4+CD45RA+) T cells in Japanese blue-collar workers. Psychother Psychosom. 1997;66(4):192–8. PMID: 9259042. http://www.ncbi.nlm.nih.gov/pubmed/9259042.
151. Southwick SM, Vythilingam M, Charney DS. The psychobiology of depression and resilience to stress: implications for prevention and treatment. Annu Rev Clin Psychol. 2005;1:255–91. PMID: 17716089
152. Ming Q, Zhong X, Zhang X, Pu W, Dong D, Jiang Y, Gao Y, Wang X, Detre JA, Yao S, Rao H. State-independent and dependent neural responses to psychosocial stress in current and remitted depression. Am J Psychiatry. 2017;174(10):971–9. PMID: 28618857. http://www.ncbi.nlm.nih.gov/pubmed/28618857.
153. Morris MC, Rao U, Garber J. Cortisol responses to psychosocial stress predict depression trajectories: social-evaluative threat and prior depressive episodes as moderators. J Affect Disord. 2012;143(1–3):223–30. PMCID: PMC3489962. http://www.ncbi.nlm.nih.gov/pubmed/22858210.
154. Schulz R, Beach SR. Caregiving as a risk factor for mortality: the caregiver health effects study. JAMA. 1999;282(23):2215–9. PMID: 10605972. http://www.ncbi.nlm.nih.gov/pubmed/10605972.

155. Vitaliano PP, Scanlan JM, Zhang J, Savage MV, Hirsch IB, Siegler IC. A path model of chronic stress, the metabolic syndrome, and coronary heart disease. Psychosom Med. 2002;64(3):418–35. PMID: 12021416. http://www.ncbi.nlm.nih.gov/pubmed/12021416.
156. Vedhara K, Cox NK, Wilcock GK, Perks P, Hunt M, Anderson S, Lightman SL, Shanks NM. Chronic stress in elderly carers of dementia patients and antibody response to influenza vaccination. Lancet. 1999;353(9153):627–31. PMID: 10030328. http://www.ncbi.nlm.nih.gov/pubmed/10030328.
157. Wu H, Wang J, Cacioppo JT, Glaser R, Kiecolt-Glaser JK, Malarkey WB. Chronic stress associated with spousal caregiving of patients with Alzheimer's dementia is associated with downregulation of B-lymphocyte GH mRNA. J Gerontol A Biol Sci Med Sci. 1999;54(4):M212–5. PMID: 10219013. http://www.ncbi.nlm.nih.gov/pubmed/10219013.
158. Kiecolt-Glaser JK, Glaser R, Shuttleworth EC, Dyer CS, Ogrocki P, Speicher CE. Chronic stress and immunity in family caregivers of Alzheimer's disease victims. Psychosom Med. 1987;49(5):523–35. PMID: 3671639. http://www.ncbi.nlm.nih.gov/pubmed/3671639.
159. Kiecolt-Glaser JK, Preacher KJ, RC MC, Atkinson C, Malarkey WB, Glaser R. Chronic stress and age-related increases in the proinflammatory cytokine IL-6. Proc Natl Acad Sci USA. 2003;100(15):9090–5. PMCID: PMC166443. http://www.ncbi.nlm.nih.gov/pubmed/12840146.
160. Kiecolt-Glaser JK, McGuire L, Robles TF, Glaser R. Psychoneuroimmunology: psychological influences on immune function and health. J Consult Clin Psychol. 2002;70(3):537–47. PMID: 12090368. http://www.ncbi.nlm.nih.gov/pubmed/12090368.
161. Esterling BA, Kiecolt-Glaser JK, Glaser R. Psychosocial modulation of cytokine-induced natural killer cell activity in older adults. Psychosom Med. 1996;58(3):264–72. PMID: 8771626. http://www.ncbi.nlm.nih.gov/pubmed/8771626.
162. Buka SL. Disparities in health status and substance use: ethnicity and socioeconomic factors. Public Health Rep. 2002;117(Suppl 1):S118–25. PMCID: PMC1913692. http://www.ncbi.nlm.nih.gov/pubmed/12435835.
163. Adler NE, Newman K. Socioeconomic disparities in health: pathways and policies. Health Aff Millwood. 2002;21(2):60–76. PMID: 11900187. http://www.ncbi.nlm.nih.gov/pubmed/11900187.
164. Adler NE, Ostrove JM. Socioeconomic status and health: what we know and what we don't. Ann NY Acad Sci. 1999;896:3–15. PMID: 10681884. http://www.ncbi.nlm.nih.gov/pubmed/10681884.
165. Marmot M, Feeney A. General explanations for social inequalities in health. IARC Sci Publ. 1997;138:207–28. PMID: 9353666. http://www.ncbi.nlm.nih.gov/pubmed/9353666.
166. Taylor SE, Repetti RL, Seeman T. Health psychology: what is an unhealthy environment and how does it get under the skin? Annu Rev Psychol. 1997;48:411–47. PMID: 9046565. http://www.ncbi.nlm.nih.gov/pubmed/9046565.
167. Everson SA, Maty SC, Lynch JW, Kaplan GA. Epidemiologic evidence for the relation between socioeconomic status and depression, obesity, and diabetes. J Psychosom Res. 2002;53(4):891–5. PMID: 12377299. http://www.ncbi.nlm.nih.gov/pubmed/12377299.
168. Zimmerman FJ, Katon W. Socioeconomic status, depression disparities, and financial strain: what lies behind the income-depression relationship? Health Econ. 2005;14(12):1197–215. PMID: 15945040. http://www.ncbi.nlm.nih.gov/pubmed/15945040.
169. Kiecolt-Glaser JK, McGuire L, Robles TF, Glaser R. Emotions, morbidity, and mortality: new perspectives from psychoneuroimmunology. Annu Rev Psychol. 2002;53:83–107. PMID: 11752480. http://www.ncbi.nlm.nih.gov/pubmed/11752480.
170. Lindquist TL, Beilin LJ, Knuiman MW. Influence of lifestyle, coping, and job stress on blood pressure in men and women. Hypertension. 1997;29(1 Pt 1):1–7. PMID: 9039072. http://www.ncbi.nlm.nih.gov/pubmed/9039072.
171. Kiecolt-Glaser JK, Glaser R. Methodological issues in behavioral immunology research with humans. Brain Behav Immun. 1988;2(1):67–78. PMID: 3052653. http://www.ncbi.nlm.nih.gov/pubmed/3052653.
172. Whooley MA, Browner WS. Association between depressive symptoms and mortality in older women. Study of Osteoporotic Fractures Research Group. Arch Intern Med. 1998;158(19):2129–35. PMID: 9801180. http://www.ncbi.nlm.nih.gov/pubmed/9801180.
173. Dozier M, Peloso E. The role of early stressors in child health and mental health outcomes. Arch Pediatr Adolesc Med. 2006;160(12):1300–1. PMID: 17146029. http://www.ncbi.nlm.nih.gov/pubmed/17146029.
174. Anda RF, Felitti VJ, Bremner JD, Walker JD, Whitfield C, Perry BD, Dube SR, Giles WH. The enduring effects of abuse and related adverse experiences in childhood. A convergence of evidence from neurobiology and epidemiology. Eur Arch Psychiatry Clin Neurosci. 2006;256(3):174–86. PMCID: PMC3232061. https://pmc.ncbi.nlm.nih.gov/articles/PMC3232061/pdf/nihms340170.pdf.
175. Dube SR, Felitti VJ, Dong M, Giles WH, Anda RF. The impact of adverse childhood experiences on health problems: evidence from four birth cohorts dating back to 1900. Prev Med. 2003;37(3):268–77. PMID: 12914833. http://www.ncbi.nlm.nih.gov/pubmed/12914833.
176. Lissau I, Sørensen TI. Parental neglect during childhood and increased risk of obesity in young adulthood. Lancet. 1994;343(8893):324–7. PMID: 7905145. http://www.ncbi.nlm.nih.gov/pubmed/7905145.
177. Charmandari E, Kino T, Souvatzoglou E, Chrousos GP. Pediatric stress: hormonal mediators and human development. Horm Res. 2003;59(4):161–79. PMID: 12649570. http://www.ncbi.nlm.nih.gov/pubmed/12649570.
178. Wyman PA, Moynihan J, Eberly S, Cox C, Cross W, Jin X, Caserta MT. Association of family stress with natural killer cell activity and the frequency of illnesses in children. Arch Pediatr Adolesc Med. 2007;161(3):228–34. PMID: 17339503. http://www.ncbi.nlm.nih.gov/pubmed/17339503.
179. Grossman AW, Churchill JD, McKinney BC, Kodish IM, Otte SL, Greenough WT. Experience effects on brain development: possible contributions to psychopathology. J Child Psychol Psychiatry. 2003;44(1):33–63. PMID: 12553412. http://www.ncbi.nlm.nih.gov/pubmed/12553412.
180. Lo CL, Zhou FC. Environmental alterations of epigenetics prior to the birth. Int Rev Neurobiol. 2014;115:1–49. PMCID: PMC4158947. http://www.ncbi.nlm.nih.gov/pubmed/25131541.
181. Bernasco EL, van der Graaff J, Nelemans SA, Kaufman TML, Branje S. Depression socialization in early adolescent friendships: the role of baseline depressive symptoms and autonomous functioning. J Youth Adolesc. 2023;52(7):1417–32. PMCID: PMC10155137. http://www.ncbi.nlm.nih.gov/pubmed/37133557.
182. Giletta M, Scholte RHJ, Burk WJ, Engels RCME, Larsen JK, Prinstein MJ, Ciairano S. Similarity in depressive symptoms in adolescents' friendship dyads: selection or socialization? Dev Psychol. 2011;47(6):1804–14. PMCID: PMC3349236. http://www.ncbi.nlm.nih.gov/pubmed/21639621.
183. Van Zalk MHW, Kerr M, Branje SJT, Stattin H, Meeus WHJ. It takes three: selection, influence, and de-selection processes of depression in adolescent friendship networks. Dev Psychol. 2010;46(4):927–38. PMID: 20604612. http://www.ncbi.nlm.nih.gov/pubmed/20604612.

184. Schwartz-Mette RA, Rose AJ. Co-rumination mediates contagion of internalizing symptoms within youths' friendships. Dev Psychol. 2012;48(5):1355–65. PMCID: PMC3371303. http://www.ncbi.nlm.nih.gov/pubmed/22369336.
185. Cole DA, Sinclair-McBride KR, Zelkowitz R, Bilsk SA, Roeder K, Spinelli T. Peer victimization and harsh parenting predict cognitive diatheses for depression in children and adolescents. J Clin Child Adolesc Psychol. 2016;45(5):668–80. PMCID: PMC4564367. http://www.ncbi.nlm.nih.gov/pubmed/25751612.
186. Cole DA, Martin NC, Sterba SK, Sinclair-McBride K, Roeder KM, Zelkowitz R, Bilsky SA. Peer victimization (and harsh parenting) as developmental correlates of cognitive reactivity, a diathesis for depression. J Abnorm Psychol. 2014;123(2):336–49. PMID: 24886008. http://www.ncbi.nlm.nih.gov/pubmed/24886008.
187. Iselin AMR, DiGiunta L, Lunetti C, Lansford JE, Eisenberg N, Dodge KA, Pastorelli C, Tirado LMU, Bacchini D, Thartori E, Fiasconaro I, Gliozzo G, Favini A, Basili E, Cirimele F, Remondi C, Skinner AT. Pathways from maternal harsh discipline through rumination to anxiety and depression symptoms: gender and Normativeness of harsh discipline as moderators. Res Child Adolesc Psychopathol 2022;50(10):1313–1326. PMCID: PMC9979779. http://www.ncbi.nlm.nih.gov/pubmed/35870036.
188. Watling R, Schwartz IS. Understanding and implementing positive reinforcement as an intervention strategy for children with disabilities. Am J Occup Ther. 2004;58(1):113–6. PMID: 14763644. http://www.ncbi.nlm.nih.gov/pubmed/14763644.
189. Eamon MK, Zuehl RM. Maternal depression and physical punishment as mediators of the effect of poverty on socioemotional problems of children in single-mother families. Am J Orthopsychiatry. 2001;71(2):218–26. PMID: 11347362. http://www.ncbi.nlm.nih.gov/pubmed/11347362.
190. Eamon MK. Antecedents and socioemotional consequences of physical punishment on children in two-parent families. Child Abuse Negl. 2001;25(6):787–802. PMID: 11525526. http://www.ncbi.nlm.nih.gov/pubmed/11525526.
191. Collin-Vézina D, Cyr M, Pauzé R, McDuff P. The role of depression and dissociation in the link between childhood sexual abuse and later parental practices. J Trauma Dissociation. 2005;6(1):71–97. PMID: 16150686. http://www.ncbi.nlm.nih.gov/pubmed/16150686.
192. Craig A, Rochat T, Naicker SN, Mapanga W, Mtintsilana A, Dlamini SN, Ware LJ, Du Toit J, Draper CE, Richter L, Norris SA. The prevalence of probable depression and probable anxiety, and associations with adverse childhood experiences and socio-demographics: a national survey in South Africa. Front Public Health. 2022;10:986531. PMCID: PMC9650309. http://www.ncbi.nlm.nih.gov/pubmed/36388391.
193. Merrick MT, Ports KA, Ford DC, Afifi TO, Gershoff ET, Grogan-Kaylor A. Unpacking the impact of adverse childhood experiences on adult mental health. Child Abuse Negl. 2017;69:10–9. PMCID: PMC600780. http://www.ncbi.nlm.nih.gov/pubmed/28419887.
194. Liu RT. Childhood adversities and depression in adulthood: current findings and future directions. Clin Psychol (New York). 2017;24(2):140–53. PMCID: PMC5600284. http://www.ncbi.nlm.nih.gov/pubmed/28924333.
195. Forbes EE. Editorial: missing the pull of life's rewards? Attention shifting and the development of depression. J Am Acad Child Adolesc Psychiatry. 2019;58(3):313–4. PMID: 30832902. http://www.ncbi.nlm.nih.gov/pubmed/30832902.
196. Gilbert KE, Luking KR, Pagliaccio D, Luby L, J, Barch DM. Dampening positive affect and neural reward responding in healthy children: implications for affective inflexibility. J Clin Child Adolesc Psychol. 2019;48(1):120–30. PMCID: PMC5420488. http://www.ncbi.nlm.nih.gov/pubmed/27819484.
197. Gibb BE. Editorial: evidence for transactional relations between reward processing and depressive symptoms in adolescence. J Am Acad Child Adolesc Psychiatry. 2023;62(7):726–7. PMID: 36898604. http://www.ncbi.nlm.nih.gov/pubmed/36898604.
198. Luking KR, Pagliaccio D, Luby JL, Barch DM. Reward processing and risk for depression across development. Trends Cogn Sci. 2016;20(6):456–68. PMCID: PMC4875800. http://www.ncbi.nlm.nih.gov/pubmed/27131776.
199. Burkhouse KL, Dao A, Argiros A, Granros M, Cárdenas E, Dickey L, Feurer C, Hill K, Pegg S, Venanzi L, Kujawa A. Corrigendum to "Targeting positive valence systems function in children of mothers with depressive symptoms: A pilot randomized trial of an RDoC-informed preventive intervention" [Behav. Res. Ther. 168 (September 2023) 104–384]. Behav Res Ther. 2024;173:104465. PMID: 38129267. http://www.ncbi.nlm.nih.gov/pubmed/38129267.
200. Beeson CML, Brittain H, Vaillancourt T. The temporal precedence of peer rejection, rejection sensitivity, depression, and aggression across adolescence. Child Psychiatry Hum Dev. 2020;51(5):781–91. PMID: 32462359. http://www.ncbi.nlm.nih.gov/pubmed/32462359.
201. Sarris J, O'Neil A, Coulson CE, Schweitzer I, Berk M. Lifestyle medicine for depression. BMC Psychiatry. 2014;14:107. PMCID: PMC3998225. http://www.ncbi.nlm.nih.gov/pubmed/24721040.
202. Gibson SM, Bouldin BM, Stokes MN, Lozada FT, Hope EC. Cultural racism and depression in black adolescents: examining racial socialization and racial identity as moderators. J Res Adolesc. 2022;32(1):41–8. PMID: 34874089. http://www.ncbi.nlm.nih.gov/pubmed/34874089.
203. Dennis M, Kadri A, Coffey J. Depression in older people in the general hospital: a systematic review of screening instruments. Age Ageing. 2012;41(2):148–54. PMID: 22236655. http://www.ncbi.nlm.nih.gov/pubmed/22236655.
204. Kurlowicz LH, Streim JE. Measuring depression in hospitalized, medically ill, older adults. Arch Psychiatr Nurs. 1998;12(4):209–18. PMID: 9714940. http://www.ncbi.nlm.nih.gov/pubmed/9714940.
205. Weinberger MI, Raue PJ, Meyers BS, Bruce ML. Predictors of new onset depression in medically ill, disabled older adults at 1 year follow-up. Am J Geriatr Psychiatry. 2009;17(9):802–9. PMCID: PMC2836732. http://www.ncbi.nlm.nih.gov/pubmed/19700952.
206. Reichardt LA, van Seben R, Aarden JJ, van der Esch M, van der Schaaf M, Engelbert RHH, Twisk JWR, Bosch JA, Buurman BM, Hospital-ADL study group. Trajectories of cognitive-affective depressive symptoms in acutely hospitalized older adults: the hospital-ADL study. J Psychosom Res. 2019;120:66–73. PMID: 30929710. http://www.ncbi.nlm.nih.gov/pubmed/30929710.
207. Jongenelis K, Pot AM, Eisses AMH, Beekman ATF, Kluiter H, Ribbe MW. Prevalence and risk indicators of depression in elderly nursing home patients: the AGED study. J Affect Disord. 2004;83(2–3):135–42. PMID: 15555706. http://www.ncbi.nlm.nih.gov/pubmed/15555706.
208. Prince MJ, Harwood RH, Thomas A, Mann AH. A prospective population-based cohort study of the effects of disablement and social milieu on the onset and maintenance of late-life depression. The Gospel Oak Project VII. Psychol Med. 1998;28(2):337–50. PMID: 9572091. http://www.ncbi.nlm.nih.gov/pubmed/9572091.
209. Wilson K, Mottram P, Sixsmith A. Depressive symptoms in the very old living alone: prevalence, incidence and risk factors. Int J Geriatr Psychiatry. 2007;22(4):361–6. PMID: 17044137. http://www.ncbi.nlm.nih.gov/pubmed/17044137.
210. Borges MK, Aprahamian I, Romanini CV, Oliveira FM, Mingardi SVB, Lima NA, Cecato JF, Petrella M, Oude Voshaar RC. Depression as a determinant of frailty in late life. Aging Ment Health. 2021;25(12):2279–85. PMID: 33307781. http://www.ncbi.nlm.nih.gov/pubmed/33307781.

211. Yesavage JA, Brink TL, Rose TL, Lum O, Huang V, Adey M, Leirer VO. Development and validation of a geriatric depression screening scale: a preliminary report. J Psychiatr Res 1982. 1983;17(1):37–49. PMID: 7183759. http://www.ncbi.nlm.nih.gov/pubmed/7183759.
212. Park SH, Kwak MJ. Performance of the geriatric depression Scale-15 with older adults Aged over 65 years: an updated review 2000-2019. Clin Gerontol. 2021;44(2):83–96. PMID: 33164674. http://www.ncbi.nlm.nih.gov/pubmed/33164674.
213. Pocklington C, Gilbody S, Manea L, McMillan D. The diagnostic accuracy of brief versions of the geriatric depression scale: a systematic review and meta-analysis. Int J Geriatr Psychiatry. 2016;31(8):837–57. PMID: 26890937. http://www.ncbi.nlm.nih.gov/pubmed/26890937.
214. Cai H, Jin Y, Liu R, Zhang Q, Su Z, Ungvari GS, Tang YL, Ng CH, Li XH, Xiang YT. Global prevalence of depression in older adults: a systematic review and meta-analysis of epidemiological surveys. Asian J Psychiatr. 2023;80:103417. PMID: 36587492. http://www.ncbi.nlm.nih.gov/pubmed/36587492.
215. Park SH, Lee H. Is the center for epidemiologic studies depression scale as useful as the geriatric depression scale in screening for late-life depression? A systematic review. J Affect Disord. 2021;292:454–63. PMID: 34144371. http://www.ncbi.nlm.nih.gov/pubmed/34144371.
216. Brañez-Condorena A, Soriano-Moreno DR, Navarro-Flores A, Solis-Chimoy B, Diaz-Barrera ME, Taype-Rondan A. Accuracy of the geriatric depression scale (GDS)-4 and GDS-5 for the screening of depression among older adults: a systematic review and meta-analysis. PLoS One. 2021;16(7):e0253899. PMCID: PMC8248624. http://www.ncbi.nlm.nih.gov/pubmed/34197527.
217. Zenebe Y, Akele B, W/Selassie M, Necho M. Prevalence and determinants of depression among old age: a systematic review and meta-analysis. Ann Gen Psychiatry. 2021;20(1):55. PMCID: PMC8684627. http://www.ncbi.nlm.nih.gov/pubmed/34922595.
218. Krishnamoorthy Y, Rajaa S, Rehman T. Diagnostic accuracy of various forms of geriatric depression scale for screening of depression among older adults: systematic review and meta-analysis. Arch Gerontol Geriatr. 2020;87:104002. PMID: 31881393. http://www.ncbi.nlm.nih.gov/pubmed/31881393.
219. van Dijk R, van der Valk IE, Deković M, Branje S. A meta-analysis on interparental conflict, parenting, and child adjustment in divorced families: examining mediation using meta-analytic structural equation models. Clin Psychol Rev. 2020;79:101861. PMID: 32512420. http://www.ncbi.nlm.nih.gov/pubmed/32512420.
220. van Dijk R, van der Valk IE, Deković M, Branje S. Corrigendum to "A meta-analysis on interparental conflict, parenting, and child adjustment in divorced families: Examining mediation using meta-analytic structural equation models" [Clinical Psychology Review 79 (2020) 101861]. Clin Psychol Rev. 2021;88:102060. PMID: 34183202. http://www.ncbi.nlm.nih.gov/pubmed/34183202.
221. Hannighofer J, Foran H, Hahlweg K, Zimmermann T. Impact of relationship status and quality (family type) on the mental health of mothers and their children: a 10-year longitudinal study. Front Psychiatry. 2017;8:266. PMCID: PMC5712550. http://www.ncbi.nlm.nih.gov/pubmed/29238312.
222. Zeiders KH, Roosa MW, Tein JY. Family structure and family processes in Mexican-American families. Fam Process. 2011;50(1):77–91. PMCID: PMC3077030. http://www.ncbi.nlm.nih.gov/pubmed/21361925.
223. Barrett AE, Turner RJ. Family structure and mental health: the mediating effects of socioeconomic status, family process, and social stress. J Health Soc Behav. 2005;46(2):156–69. PMID: 16028455. http://www.ncbi.nlm.nih.gov/pubmed/16028455.
224. Williams DH. The epidemiology of mental illness in Afro-Americans. Hosp Community Psychiatry. 1986;37(1):42–9. PMID: 3510954. http://www.ncbi.nlm.nih.gov/pubmed/3510954.
225. Malatras JW, Israel AC. The influence of family stability on self-control and adjustment. J Clin Psychol. 2013;69(7):661–70. PMID: 23124588. http://www.ncbi.nlm.nih.gov/pubmed/23124588.
226. Deater-Deckard K, Pickering K, Dunn JF, Golding J. Family structure and depressive symptoms in men preceding and following the birth of a child. The Avon longitudinal study of pregnancy and childhood study team. Am J Psychiatry. 1998;155(6):818–23. PMID: 9619156. http://www.ncbi.nlm.nih.gov/pubmed/9619156.
227. Weavers B, Riglin L, Martin J, Anney R, Collishaw S, Heron J, Thapar A, Thapar A, Rice F. Characterising depression trajectories in young people at high familial risk of depression. J Affect Disord. 2023;337:66–74. PMCID: PMC10824668. http://www.ncbi.nlm.nih.gov/pubmed/37224886.
228. Rice F, Harold G, Thapar A. The genetic aetiology of childhood depression: a review. J Child Psychol Psychiatry. 2002;43(1):65–79. PMID: 11848337. http://www.ncbi.nlm.nih.gov/pubmed/11848337.
229. Rice F, Harold GT, Shelton KH, Thapar A. Family conflict interacts with genetic liability in predicting childhood and adolescent depression. J Am Acad Child Adolesc Psychiatry. 2006;45(7):841–8. PMID: http://www.ncbi.nlm.nih.gov/pubmed/16832321.
230. Talati A, van Dijk MT, Pan L, Hao X, Wang Z, Gameroff M, Dong Z, Kayser J, Shankman S, Wickramaratne PJ, Posner J, Weissman MM. Putamen structure and function in familial risk for depression: a multimodal imaging study. Biol Psychiatry. 2022;92(12):932–41. PMCID: PMC9872322. http://www.ncbi.nlm.nih.gov/pubmed/36038379.
231. Kemp JVA, Bernier E, Lebel C, Kopala-Sibley DC. Associations between parental mood and anxiety psychopathology and offspring brain structure: a scoping review. Clin Child Fam Psychol Rev. 2022;25(1):222–47.
232. Pellowski JA, Wedderburn CJ, Groenewold NA, Roos A, Subramoney S, Hoffman N, Fouche JP, Joshi SH, Woods RP, Narr KL, Zar HJ, Donald KA, Stein DJ. Maternal perinatal depression and child brain structure at 2-3 years in a South African birth cohort study. Transl Psychiatry. 2023;13(1):96. PMCID: PMC10027817. http://www.ncbi.nlm.nih.gov/pubmed/36941258.
233. Connell AM, Goodman SH. The association between psychopathology in fathers versus mothers and children's internalizing and externalizing behavior problems: a meta-analysis. Psychol Bull. 2002;128(5):746–73. PMID: 12206193. http://www.ncbi.nlm.nih.gov/pubmed/12206193.
234. Lieb R, Isensee B, Höfler M, Pfister H, Wittchen HU. Parental major depression and the risk of depression and other mental disorders in offspring: a prospective-longitudinal community study. Arch Gen Psychiatry. 2002;59(4):365–74. PMID: 11926937. http://www.ncbi.nlm.nih.gov/pubmed/11926937.
235. Beardslee WR, Versage EM, Gladstone TR. Children of affectively ill parents: a review of the past 10 years. J Am Acad Child Adolesc Psychiatry. 1998;37(11):1134–41. PMID: 9808924. http://www.ncbi.nlm.nih.gov/pubmed/9808924.
236. Williamson DE, Birmaher B, Axelson DA, Ryan ND, Dahl RE. First episode of depression in children at low and high familial risk for depression. J Am Acad Child Adolesc Psychiatry. 2004;43(3):291–7. PMID: 15076262. http://www.ncbi.nlm.nih.gov/pubmed/15076262.
237. Foland-Ross LC, Behzadian N, LeMoult J, Gotlib IH. Concordant patterns of brain structure in mothers with recurrent depression and their never-depressed daughters. Dev Neurosci. 2016;38(2):115–23. PMCID: PMC4927380. http://www.ncbi.nlm.nih.gov/pubmed/27198667.
238. Aylott A, Zwicker A, MacKenzie LE, Cumby J, Propper L, Abidi S, Bagnell A, Fisher HL, Pavlova B, Alda M, Uher R. Like father like daughter: sex-specific parent-of-origin effects in the transmis-

sion of liability for psychotic symptoms to offspring. J Dev Orig Health Dis. 2019;10(1):100–7. PMID: 30156170. http://www.ncbi.nlm.nih.gov/pubmed/30156170.
239. Goldschmidt L, Cornelius MD, Day NL. Prenatal cigarette smoke exposure and early initiation of multiple substance use. Nicotine Tob Res. 2012;14(6):694–702. PMCID: PMC3430468. http://www.ncbi.nlm.nih.gov/pubmed/22180590.
240. Niemelä S, Räisänen A, Koskela J, Taanila A, Miettunen J, Ramsay H, Veijola J. The effect of prenatal smoking exposure on daily smoking among teenage offspring. Addiction. 2017;112(1):134–43. PMID: 27444807. http://www.ncbi.nlm.nih.gov/pubmed/27444807.
241. Sarala M, Mustonen A, Alakokkare AE, Salom C, Miettunen J, Niemelä S. Parental smoking and young adult offspring psychosis, depression and anxiety disorders and substance use disorder. Eur J Public Health. 2022;32(2):254–60. PMCID: PMC9090280. http://www.ncbi.nlm.nih.gov/pubmed/35092289.
242. Boden JM, Fergusson DM, Horwood LJ. Cigarette smoking and depression: tests of causal linkages using a longitudinal birth cohort. Br J Psychiatry. 2010;196(6):440–6. PMID: 20513853. http://www.ncbi.nlm.nih.gov/pubmed/20513853.
243. Moylan S, Gustavson K, Karevold E, Øverland S, Jacka FN, Pasco JA, Berk M. The impact of smoking in adolescence on early adult anxiety symptoms and the relationship between infant vulnerability factors for anxiety and early adult anxiety symptoms: the TOPP Study. PLoS One. 2013;8(5):e63252. PMCID: PMC3655993. http://www.ncbi.nlm.nih.gov/pubmed/23696803.
244. Salom CL, Betts KS, Williams GM, Najman JM, Alati R. Predictors of comorbid polysubstance use and mental health disorders in young adults-a latent class analysis. Addiction. 2016;111(1):156–64. PMID: 26190689. http://www.ncbi.nlm.nih.gov/pubmed/26190689.
245. Fullston T, McPherson NO, Zander-Fox D, Lane M. The most common vices of men can damage fertility and the health of the next generation. J Endocrinol. 2017;234(2):F1–6. PMID: 28500085. http://www.ncbi.nlm.nih.gov/pubmed/28500085.
246. Shadrina M, Bondarenko EA, Slominsky PA. Genetics factors in major depression disease. Front Psychiatry. 2018;9:334. PMCID: PMC6065213. http://www.ncbi.nlm.nih.gov/pubmed/30083112.
247. Eley TC, Deater-Deckard K, Fombonne E, Fulker DW, Plomin R. An adoption study of depressive symptoms in middle childhood. J Child Psychol Psychiatry. 1998;39(3):337–45. PMID: 9670089. http://www.ncbi.nlm.nih.gov/pubmed/9670089.
248. Tambs K, Moum T. Low genetic effect and age-specific family effect for symptoms of anxiety and depression in nuclear families, halfsibs and twins. J Affect Disord. 1993;27(3):183–95. PMID: 8478506. http://www.ncbi.nlm.nih.gov/pubmed/8478506.
249. Chau K, Baumann M, Chau N. Socioeconomic inequities patterns of multi-morbidity in early adolescence. Int J Equity Health. 2013;12:65. PMCID: PMC3765191. http://www.ncbi.nlm.nih.gov/pubmed/23962097.
250. Goodday SM, Bondy S, Sutradhar R, Brown HK, Rhodes A. Exposure to maternal depressive symptoms in childhood and suicide-related thoughts and attempts in Canadian youth: test of effect-modifying factors. Soc Psychiatry Psychiatr Epidemiol. 2019;54(2):191–200. PMID: 30357436. http://www.ncbi.nlm.nih.gov/pubmed/30357436.
251. Ensminger ME, Hanson SG, Riley AW, Juon HS. Maternal psychological distress: adult sons' and daughters' mental health and educational attainment. J Am Acad Child Adolesc Psychiatry. 2003;42(9):1108–15. PMID: 12960711. http://www.ncbi.nlm.nih.gov/pubmed/12960711.
252. Park IJK, Du H, Wang L, Williams DR, Alegría M. The role of parents' ethnic-racial socialization practices in the discrimination-depression Link among Mexican-origin adolescents. J Clin Child Adolesc Psychol. 2020;49(3):391–404. PMCID: PMC6661225. http://www.ncbi.nlm.nih.gov/pubmed/30689432.
253. O'Donnell KJ, Glover V, Barker ED, O'Connor TG. The persisting effect of maternal mood in pregnancy on childhood psychopathology. Dev Psychopathol. 2014;26(2):393–403. PMID: 24621564. http://www.ncbi.nlm.nih.gov/pubmed/24621564.
254. O'Donnell KJ, Meaney MJ. Fetal origins of mental health: the developmental origins of health and disease hypothesis. Am J Psychiatry. 2017;174(4):319–28. PMID: 27838934. http://www.ncbi.nlm.nih.gov/pubmed/27838934.
255. Meaney MJ. Perinatal maternal depressive symptoms as an issue for population health. Am J Psychiatry. 2018;175(11):1084–93. PMID: 30068258. http://www.ncbi.nlm.nih.gov/pubmed/30068258.
256. Monk C, Lugo-Candelas C, Trumpff C. Prenatal developmental origins of future psychopathology: mechanisms and pathways. Annu Rev Clin Psychol. 2019;15:317–44. PMCID: PMC7027196. http://www.ncbi.nlm.nih.gov/pubmed/30795695.
257. Mareckova K, Marecek R, Jani M, Zackova L, Andryskova L, Brazdil M, Nikolova YS. Association of Maternal Depression during Pregnancy and Recent Stress with Brain age among Adult Offspring. JAMA Netw Open. 2023;6(1):e2254581. PMCID: PMC9887495. http://www.ncbi.nlm.nih.gov/pubmed/36716025.
258. Franke K, Ziegler G, Klöppel S, Gaser C, Alzheimer's Disease Neuroimaging Initiative. Estimating the age of healthy subjects from T1-weighted MRI scans using kernel methods: exploring the influence of various parameters. Neuroimage. 2010;50(3):883–92. PMID: 20070949. http://www.ncbi.nlm.nih.gov/pubmed/20070949.
259. Foland-Ross LC, Hardin MG, Gotlib IH. Neurobiological markers of familial risk for depression. Curr Top Behav Neurosci. 2013;14:181–206. PMID: 22573472. http://www.ncbi.nlm.nih.gov/pubmed/22573472.
260. Cyranowski JM, Hofkens TL, Swartz HA, Salomon K, Gianaros PJ. Cardiac vagal control in nonmedicated depressed women and nondepressed controls: impact of depression status, lifetime trauma history, and respiratory factors - PubMed. Psychosom Med. 2011;73(4):336–43. PMCID: PMC3090496
261. Libet JM, Lewinsohn PM. Concept of social skill with special reference to the behavior of depressed persons. J Consult Clin Psychol. 1973;40(2):304–12. PMID: 4694208. http://www.ncbi.nlm.nih.gov/pubmed/4694208.
262. Martin AF, Maughan B, Konac D, Barker ED. Mother and father depression symptoms and child emotional difficulties: a network model. Br J Psychiatry. 2023;222(5):204–11. PMCID: PMC10895513. http://www.ncbi.nlm.nih.gov/pubmed/36942415.
263. Tenesa A, Haley CS. The heritability of human disease: estimation, uses and abuses. Nat Rev Genet. 2013;14(2):139–49. PMID: 23329114. http://www.ncbi.nlm.nih.gov/pubmed/23329114.
264. Benchek PH, Morris NJ. How meaningful are heritability estimates of liability? Hum Genet. 2013;132(12):1351–60. PMCID: PMC3843952. http://www.ncbi.nlm.nih.gov/pubmed/23867980.
265. Porges SW. Social engagement and attachment: a phylogenetic perspective. Ann N Y Acad Sci. 2003;1008:31–47. PMID: 14998870. http://www.ncbi.nlm.nih.gov/pubmed/14998870.
266. Porges SW. The polyvagal perspective. Biol Psychol. 2007;74(2):116–43. PMCID: PMC1868418. http://www.ncbi.nlm.nih.gov/pubmed/17049418.
267. Livings MS. The gendered relationship between maternal depression and adolescent internalizing symptoms. Soc Sci Med. 2021;291:114464. PMID: 34666277. http://www.ncbi.nlm.nih.gov/pubmed/34666277.
268. Ruini C, Cesetti G. Spotlight on eudaimonia and depression. A systematic review of the literature over the past 5 years. Psychol Res Behav Manag. 2019;12:767–92. PMCID: PMC6720155. http://www.ncbi.nlm.nih.gov/pubmed/31507332.

269. Ryff CD. Psychological Well-being revisited: advances in the science and practice of eudaimonia. Psychother Psychosom. 2014;83(1):10–28. PMCID: PMC4241300. http://www.ncbi.nlm.nih.gov/pubmed/24281296.
270. Ruini C, Ottolini F, Tomba E, Belaise C, Albieri E, Visani D, Offidani E, Caffo E, Fava GA. School intervention for promoting psychological well-being in adolescence. J Behav Ther Exp Psychiatry. 2009;40(4):522–32. PMID: 19683703. http://www.ncbi.nlm.nih.gov/pubmed/19683703.
271. Wood AM, Joseph S. The absence of positive psychological (eudemonic) well-being as a risk factor for depression: a ten year cohort study. J Affect Disord. 2010;122(3):213–7. PMID: 19706357. http://www.ncbi.nlm.nih.gov/pubmed/19706357.
272. Ryff CD, Singer B. Psychological well-being: meaning, measurement, and implications for psychotherapy research. Psychother Psychosom. 1996;65(1):14–23. PMID: 8838692
273. Fava GA, Ruini C, Rafanelli C, Finos L, Conti S, Grandi S. Six-year outcome of cognitive behavior therapy for prevention of recurrent depression. Am J Psychiatry. 2004;161(10):1872–6. PMID: 15465985. http://www.ncbi.nlm.nih.gov/pubmed/15465985.
274. Fava GA, Ruini C, Rafanelli C. Sequential treatment of mood and anxiety disorders. J Clin Psychiatry. 2005;66(11):1392–400. PMID: 16420076. http://www.ncbi.nlm.nih.gov/pubmed/16420076.
275. Friedman EM, Ruini C, Foy R, Jaros L, Sampson H, Ryff CD. Lighten UP! A community-based group intervention to promote psychological well-being in older adults. Aging Ment Health. 2017;21(2):199–205. PMCID: PMC5636191. http://www.ncbi.nlm.nih.gov/pubmed/26460594.
276. Cesetti G, Vescovelli F, Ruini C. The promotion of well-being in aging individuals living in nursing homes: a controlled pilot intervention with Narrative strategies. Clin Gerontol. 2017;40(5):380–91. PMID: 28452650. http://www.ncbi.nlm.nih.gov/pubmed/28452650.
277. Brandel M, Vescovelli F, Ruini C. Beyond Ryff's scale: comprehensive measures of eudaimonic Well-being in clinical populations. A systematic review. Clin Psychol Psychother. 2017;24(6):O1524–46. PMID: 28770559. http://www.ncbi.nlm.nih.gov/pubmed/28770559.
278. Turney K. Prevalence and correlates of stability and change in maternal depression: evidence from the fragile families and child wellbeing study. PLoS One. 2012;7(9):e45709. PMCID: PMC3447862. http://www.ncbi.nlm.nih.gov/pubmed/23029194.
279. Hall LA. Prevalence and correlates of depressive symptoms in mothers of young children. Public Health Nurs. 1990;7(2):71–9. PMID: 2100981. http://www.ncbi.nlm.nih.gov/pubmed/2100981.
280. Mulvaney C, Kendrick D. Depressive symptoms in mothers of pre-school children–effects of deprivation, social support, stress and neighbourhood social capital. Soc Psychiatry Psychiatr Epidemiol. 2005;40(3):202–8. PMID: 15742225. http://www.ncbi.nlm.nih.gov/pubmed/15742225.
281. McLanahan S. Fragile families and the reproduction of poverty. Ann Am Acad Pol Soc Sci. 2009;621(1):111–31. PMCID: PMC2831755. http://www.ncbi.nlm.nih.gov/pubmed/20204078.
282. Lanzi RG, Pascoe JM, Keltner B, Ramey SL. Correlates of maternal depressive symptoms in a national head start program sample. Arch Pediatr Adolesc Med. 1999;153(8):801–7. PMID: 10437751. http://www.ncbi.nlm.nih.gov/pubmed/10437751.
283. Kessler RC, Berglund P, Demler O, Jin R, Koretz D, Merikangas KR, Rush AJ, Walters EE, Wang PS, National Comorbidity Survey Replication. The epidemiology of major depressive disorder: results from the National Comorbidity Survey Replication (NCS-R). JAMA. 2003;289(23):3095–105. PMID: 12813115. http://www.ncbi.nlm.nih.gov/pubmed/12813115.
284. DeKlyen M, Brooks-Gunn J, McLanahan S, Knab J. The mental health of married, cohabiting, and non-coresident parents with infants. Am J Public Health. 2006;96(10):1836–41. PMCID: PMC1586128. http://www.ncbi.nlm.nih.gov/pubmed/16571717.
285. Weissman MM. Advances in psychiatric epidemiology: rates and risks for major depression. Am J Public Health. 1987;77(4):445–51. PMCID: PMC1646931. http://www.ncbi.nlm.nih.gov/pubmed/3826462.
286. Kessler RC, Akiskal HS, Ames M, Birnbaum H, Greenberg P, Hirschfeld RMA, Jin R, Merikangas KR, Simon GE, Wang PS. Prevalence and effects of mood disorders on work performance in a nationally representative sample of U.S. workers. Am J Psychiatry. 2006;163(9):1561–8. PMCID: PMC1924724. http://www.ncbi.nlm.nih.gov/pubmed/16946181.
287. Phelan JC, Link BG. Who are "the homeless"? Reconsidering the stability and composition of the homeless population. Am J Public Health. 1999;89(9):1334–8. PMCID: PMC1508759. http://www.ncbi.nlm.nih.gov/pubmed/10474549.
288. Pascoe JM, Stolfi A, Ormond MB. Correlates of mothers' persistent depressive symptoms: a national study. J Pediatr Health Care. 2006;20(4):261–9. PMID: 16831634. http://www.ncbi.nlm.nih.gov/pubmed/16831634.
289. Martin JA, Hamilton BE, Sutton PD, Ventura SJ, Mathews TJ, Osterman MJK. Births: final data for 2008. Natl Vital Stat Rep. 2010;59(1):3–71. PMID: 22145497. http://www.ncbi.nlm.nih.gov/pubmed/22145497.
290. JD ML, Kotelchuck M, Cho H. Prevalence, persistence, and correlates of depressive symptoms in a national sample of mothers of toddlers. J Am Acad Child Adolesc Psychiatry. 2001;40(11):1316–23. PMID: 11699806. http://www.ncbi.nlm.nih.gov/pubmed/11699806.
291. Judd LL, Paulus MP, Wells KB, Rapaport MH. Socioeconomic burden of subsyndromal depressive symptoms and major depression in a sample of the general population. Am J Psychiatry. 1996;153(11):1411–7. PMID: 8890673. http://www.ncbi.nlm.nih.gov/pubmed/8890673.
292. Letourneau NL, Dennis CL, Benzies K, Duffett-Leger L, Stewart M, Tryphonopoulos PD, Este D, Watson W. Postpartum depression is a family affair: addressing the impact on mothers, fathers, and children. Issues Ment Health Nurs. 2012;33(7):445–57. PMID: 22757597. http://www.ncbi.nlm.nih.gov/pubmed/22757597.
293. Weinberg MK, Tronick EZ, Beeghly M, Olson KL, Kernan H, Riley JM. Subsyndromal depressive symptoms and major depression in postpartum women. Am J Orthopsychiatry. 2001;71(1):87–97. PMID: 11271721. http://www.ncbi.nlm.nih.gov/pubmed/11271721.
294. Letourneau N, Tryphonopoulos P, Giesbrecht G, Dennis CL, Bhogal S, Watson B. Narrative and meta-analytic review of interventions aiming to improve maternal-child attachment security. Infant Ment Health J. 2015;36(4):366–87. PMID: 26112776. http://www.ncbi.nlm.nih.gov/pubmed/26112776.
295. Future of Families and Child Wellbeing Study | Center for Research on Child and Family Wellbeing.
296. Search (Stanford Encyclopedia of Philosophy).
297. Downey G, Coyne JC. Children of depressed parents: an integrative review. Psychol Bull. 1990;108(1):50–76. PMID: 2200073. http://www.ncbi.nlm.nih.gov/pubmed/2200073.
298. Lovejoy MC, Graczyk PA, O'Hare E, Neuman G. Maternal depression and parenting behavior: a meta-analytic review. Clin Psychol Rev. 2000;20(5):561–92. PMID: 10860167. http://www.ncbi.nlm.nih.gov/pubmed/10860167.
299. Augustine JM, Crosnoe R. Mothers' depression and educational attainment and their children's academic trajectories. J Health Soc Behav. 2010;51(3):274–90. PMCID: PMC5555847. http://www.ncbi.nlm.nih.gov/pubmed/20943590.

300. Brennan PA, Hammen C, Andersen MJ, Bor W, Najman JM, Williams GM. Chronicity, severity, and timing of maternal depressive symptoms: relationships with child outcomes at age 5. Dev Psychol. 2000;36(6):759–66. PMID: 11081699. http://www.ncbi.nlm.nih.gov/pubmed/11081699.
301. Civic D, Holt VL. Maternal depressive symptoms and child behavior problems in a nationally representative normal birthweight sample. Matern Child Health J. 2000;4(4):215–21. PMID: 11272341. http://www.ncbi.nlm.nih.gov/pubmed/11272341.
302. Kiernan KE, Huerta MC. Economic deprivation, maternal depression, parenting and children's cognitive and emotional development in early childhood. Br J Sociol. 2008;59(4):783–806. PMID: 19035922. http://www.ncbi.nlm.nih.gov/pubmed/19035922.
303. Petterson SM, Albers AB. Effects of poverty and maternal depression on early child development. Child Dev. 2001;72(6):1794–813. PMID: 11768146. http://www.ncbi.nlm.nih.gov/pubmed/11768146.
304. Tronick E, Reck C. Infants of depressed mothers. Harv Rev Psychiatry. 2009;17(2):147–56. PMID: 19373622. http://www.ncbi.nlm.nih.gov/pubmed/19373622.
305. Khoury JE, Gonzalez A, Levitan R, Masellis M, Basile V, Atkinson L. Maternal self-reported depressive symptoms and maternal cortisol levels interact to predict infant cortisol levels. Infant Ment Health J. 2016;37(2):125–39. PMID: 26939829. http://www.ncbi.nlm.nih.gov/pubmed/26939829.
306. Campbell SB, Brownell CA, Hungerford A, Spieker SI, Mohan R, Blessing JS. The course of maternal depressive symptoms and maternal sensitivity as predictors of attachment security at 36 months. Dev Psychopathol. 2004;16(2):231–52. PMID: 15487594. http://www.ncbi.nlm.nih.gov/pubmed/15487594.
307. Campbell SB, Spieker S, Vandergrift N, Belsky J, Burchinal M, NICHD Early Child Care Research Network. Predictors and sequelae of trajectories of physical aggression in school-age boys and girls. Dev Psychopathol. 2010;22(1):133–50. PMCID: PMC4520547. http://www.ncbi.nlm.nih.gov/pubmed/20102652.
308. Weissman MM, Wickramaratne P, Pilowsky DJ, Poh E, Batten LA, Hernandez M, Flament MF, Stewart JA, McGrath P, Blier P, Stewart JW. Treatment of maternal depression in a medication clinical trial and its effect on children. Am J Psychiatry. 2015;172(5):450–9. PMCID: PMC4417045. http://www.ncbi.nlm.nih.gov/pubmed/25615566,
309. Weissman MM, Wickramaratne P, Pilowsky DJ, Poh E, Hernandez M, Batten LA, Flament MF, Stewart JW, Blier P. The effects on children of depressed mothers' remission and relapse over 9 months. Psychol Med. 2014;44(13):2811–24. PMCID: PMC4174338. http://www.ncbi.nlm.nih.gov/pubmed/25065614.
310. Pilowsky DJ, Wickramaratne P, Poh E, Hernandez M, Batten LA, Flament MF, Stewart JW, Blier P, Weissman MM. Psychopathology and functioning among children of treated depressed fathers and mothers. J Affect Disord. 2014;164:107–11. PMCID: PMC4152938. http://www.ncbi.nlm.nih.gov/pubmed/24856562.
311. Weissman MM, Pilowsky DJ, Wickramaratne PJ, Talati A, Wisniewski SR, Fava M, Hughes CW, Garber J, Malloy E, King CA, Cerda G, Sood AB, Alpert JE, Trivedi MH, Rush AJ, STAR*D-Child Team. Remissions in maternal depression and child psychopathology: a STAR*D-child report. JAMA. 2006;295(12):1389–98. PMID: 16551710. http://www.ncbi.nlm.nih.gov/pubmed/16551710.
312. Pilowsky DJ, Wickramaratne P, Nomura Y, Weissman MM. Family discord, parental depression, and psychopathology in offspring: 20-year follow-up. J Am Acad Child Adolesc Psychiatry. 2006;45(4):452–60. PMID: 16601650. http://www.ncbi.nlm.nih.gov/pubmed/16601650.
313. Field T, Diego M, Hernandez-Reif M, Vera Y, Gil K, Schanberg S, Kuhn C, Gonzalez-Garcia A. Prenatal maternal biochemistry predicts neonatal biochemistry. Int J Neurosci. 2004;114(8):933–45. PMID: 15527200. http://www.ncbi.nlm.nih.gov/pubmed/15527200.
314. Letourneau N, Salmani M, Duffett-Leger L. Maternal depressive symptoms and parenting of children from birth to 12 years. West J Nurs Res. 2010;32(5):662–85. PMID: 20693340. http://www.ncbi.nlm.nih.gov/pubmed/20693340.
315. Weissman MM, Wickramaratne P, Nomura Y, Warner V, Pilowsky D, Verdeli H. Offspring of depressed parents: 20 years later. Am J Psychiatry. 2006;163(6):1001–8. PMID: 16741200. http://www.ncbi.nlm.nih.gov/pubmed/16741200.
316. Glynn LM, Davis EP, Schetter CD, Chicz-Demet A, Hobel CJ, Sandman CA. Postnatal maternal cortisol levels predict temperament in healthy breastfed infants. Early Hum Dev. 2007;83(10):675–81. PMID: 173360021. http://www.ncbi.nlm.nih.gov/pubmed/17336002.
317. Grey KR, Davis EP, Sandman CA, Glynn LM. Human milk cortisol is associated with infant temperament. Psychoneuroendocrinology. 2013;38(7):1178–85. PMCID: PMC4777694. http://www.ncbi.nlm.nih.gov/pubmed/23265309.
318. Benjamin Neelon SE, Stroo M, Mayhew M, Maselko J, Hoyo C. Correlation between maternal and infant cortisol varies by breastfeeding status. Infant Behav Dev. 2015;40:252–8. PMCID: PMC4544873. http://www.ncbi.nlm.nih.gov/pubmed/26196472.
319. Nätt D, Johansson I, Faresjö T, Ludvigsson J, Thorsell A. High cortisol in 5-year-old children causes loss of DNA methylation in SINE retrotransposons: a possible role for ZNF263 in stress-related diseases. Clin Epigenetics. 2015;7(1):91. PMCID: PMC4559301. http://www.ncbi.nlm.nih.gov/pubmed/26339299.
320. Angold A, Worthman CW. Puberty onset of gender differences in rates of depression: a developmental, epidemiologic and neuroendocrine perspective. J Affect Disord. 1993;29(2–3):145–58. PMID: 8300975. http://www.ncbi.nlm.nih.gov/pubmed/8300975.
321. Cyranowski JM, Frank E, Young E, Shear MK. Adolescent onset of the gender difference in lifetime rates of major depression: a theoretical model. Arch Gen Psychiatry. 2000;57(1):21–7. PMID: 10632229. http://www.ncbi.nlm.nih.gov/pubmed/10632229.
322. Slee AM, Wuonola MA, McRipley RJ, Zajac I, Zawada MJ, Bartholomew PT, Gregory Worbes M. Oxazolidinones, a new class of synthetic antibacterial agents: in vitro and in vivo activities of DuP 105 and DuP 721. Antimicrob Agents Chemother. 1987;31(11):1791–7. PMCID: PMC175041. http://www.ncbi.nlm.nih.gov/pubmed/3435127.
323. Call JB, Shafer K. Gendered manifestations of depression and help seeking among men. Am J Mens Health. 2018;12(1):41–51. PMCID: PMC5734537. http://www.ncbi.nlm.nih.gov/pubmed/26721265.
324. Martin LA, Neighbors HW, Griffith DM. The experience of symptoms of depression in men vs women: analysis of the National Comorbidity Survey Replication. JAMA Psychiatr. 2013;70(10):1100–6. PMID: 23986338. http://www.ncbi.nlm.nih.gov/pubmed/23986338.
325. Kessler RC, Berglund P, Demler O, Jin R, Merikangas KR, Walters EE. Lifetime prevalence and age-of-onset distributions of DSM-IV disorders in the National Comorbidity Survey Replication. Arch Gen Psychiatry. 2005;62(6):593–602. PMID: 15939837. http://www.ncbi.nlm.nih.gov/pubmed/15939837.
326. Baez LM, Heller AS. Impact of age at onset on the phenomenology of depression in treatment-seeking adults in the STAR*D trial. J Affect Disord. 2020;262:381–8. PMCID: PMC6917830. http://www.ncbi.nlm.nih.gov/pubmed/31740109.
327. Nanni V, Uher R, Danese A. Childhood maltreatment predicts unfavorable course of illness and treatment outcome in depression: a meta-analysis. Am J Psychiatry. 2012;169(2):141–51. PMID: 22420036. http://www.ncbi.nlm.nih.gov/pubmed/28924333.

328. Asendorpf JB, Denissen JJA, van Aken MAG. Inhibited and aggressive preschool children at 23 years of age: personality and social transitions into adulthood. Dev Psychol. 2008;44(4):997–1011. PMID: 18605830. http://www.ncbi.nlm.nih.gov/pubmed/18605830.
329. Erath SA, Flanagan KS, Bierman KL. Social anxiety and peer relations in early adolescence: behavioral and cognitive factors. J Abnorm Child Psychol. 2007;35(3):405–16. PMID: 17265192. http://www.ncbi.nlm.nih.gov/pubmed/17265192.
330. Renner LM, Slack KS. Intimate partner violence and child maltreatment: understanding intra- and intergenerational connections. Child Abuse Negl. 2006;30(6):599–617. PMID: 16782195. http://www.ncbi.nlm.nih.gov/pubmed/16782195.
331. Capaldi DM, Knoble NB, Shortt JW, Kim HK. A systematic review of risk factors for intimate partner violence. Partn Abus. 2012;3(2):231–80. PMCID: PMC3384540. http://www.ncbi.nlm.nih.gov/pubmed/22754606.
332. Ehrensaft MK, Cohen P. Contribution of family violence to the intergenerational transmission of externalizing behavior. Prev Sci. 2012;13(4):370–83. PMID: 21720783. http://www.ncbi.nlm.nih.gov/pubmed/21720783.
333. Mair C, Cunradi CB, Todd M. Adverse childhood experiences and intimate partner violence: testing psychosocial mediational pathways among couples. Ann Epidemiol. 2012;22(12):832–9. PMCID: PMC3508260. http://www.ncbi.nlm.nih.gov/pubmed/23084843.
334. Osypuk TL, Schmidt NM, Bates LM, Tchetgen-Tchetgen EJ, Earls FJ, Glymour MM. Gender and crime victimization modify neighborhood effects on adolescent mental health. Pediatrics. 2012;130(3):472–81. PMCID: PMC3428753. http://www.ncbi.nlm.nih.gov/pubmed/22908105.
335. Currier D, Mann JJ. Stress, genes and the biology of suicidal behavior. Psychiatr Clin North Am. 2008;31(2):247–69. PMCID: PMC2710608. http://www.ncbi.nlm.nih.gov/pubmed/18439448.
336. Hamburg ME, Finkenauer C, Schuengel C. Food for love: the role of food offering in empathic emotion regulation. Front Psychol. 2014;5:32. PMCID: PMC3907771. http://www.ncbi.nlm.nih.gov/pubmed/24550860.
337. Alley TR. Food sharing and empathic emotion regulation: an evolutionary perspective. Front Psychol. 2014;5:121. PMCID: PMC3933786. http://www.ncbi.nlm.nih.gov/pubmed/24611057.
338. Bhatia SK, Bhatia SC. Childhood and adolescent depression. Am Fam Physician. 2007;75(1):73–80. PMID: 17225707. http://www.ncbi.nlm.nih.gov/pubmed/17225707.
339. Aho HJ, Hopsu-Havu VK. Expression of the 43 kDa papain inhibitor during human fetal skin development. J Dermatol Sci. 1990;1(3):157–65. PMID: 2085504. http://www.ncbi.nlm.nih.gov/pubmed/2085504.
340. Aalto-Setälä T, Marttunen M, Tuulio-Henriksson A, Poikolainen K, Lönnqvist J. Depressive symptoms in adolescence as predictors of early adulthood depressive disorders and maladjustment. Am J Psychiatry. 2002;159(7):1235–7. PMID: 12091207. http://www.ncbi.nlm.nih.gov/pubmed/12091207.
341. Edwards AC, Sihvola E, Korhonen T, Pulkkinen L, Moilanen I, Kaprio J, Rose RJ, Dick DM. Depressive symptoms and alcohol use are genetically and environmentally correlated across adolescence. Behav Genet. 2011;41(4):476–87. PMCID: PMC3085050. http://www.ncbi.nlm.nih.gov/pubmed/20890653.
342. Edwards AC, Larsson H, Lichtenstein P, Kendler KS. Early environmental influences contribute to covariation between internalizing symptoms and alcohol intoxication frequency across adolescence. Addict Behav. 2011;36(3):175–82. PMCID: PMC3052998. http://www.ncbi.nlm.nih.gov/pubmed/21051153.
343. Natsuaki MN, Klimes-Dougan B, Ge X, Shirtcliff EA, Hastings PD, Zahn-Waxler C. Early pubertal maturation and internalizing problems in adolescence: sex differences in the role of cortisol reactivity to interpersonal stress. J Clin Child Adolesc Psychol. 2009;38(4):513–24. PMCID: PMC3061854. http://www.ncbi.nlm.nih.gov/pubmed/20183638.
344. Silberg J, Pickles A, Rutter M, Hewitt J, Simonoff E, Maes H, Carbonneau R, Murrelle L, Foley D, Eaves L. The influence of genetic factors and life stress on depression among adolescent girls. Arch Gen Psychiatry. 1999;56(3):225–32. PMID: 10078499. http://www.ncbi.nlm.nih.gov/pubmed/10078499.
345. Edwards AC, Rose RJ, Kaprio J, Dick DM. Pubertal development moderates the importance of environmental influences on depressive symptoms in adolescent girls and boys. J Youth Adolesc. 2011;40(10):1383–93. PMCID: PMC3091957. http://www.ncbi.nlm.nih.gov/pubmed/21136145.
346. Gillespie NA, Gehrman P, Byrne EM, Kendler KS, Heath AC, Martin NG. Modeling the direction of causation between cross-sectional measures of disrupted sleep, anxiety and depression in a sample of male and female Australian twins. J Sleep Res. 2012;21(6):675–83. PMCID: PMC3461239. http://www.ncbi.nlm.nih.gov/pubmed/22738694.
347. Nilsen TS, Eisemann M, Kvernmo S. Predictors and moderators of outcome in child and adolescent anxiety and depression: a systematic review of psychological treatment studies. Eur Child Adolesc Psychiatry. 2013;22(2):69–87. PMID: 22923065. http://www.ncbi.nlm.nih.gov/pubmed/22923065.
348. Zullig KJ, Divin AL. The association between non-medical prescription drug use, depressive symptoms, and suicidality among college students. Addict Behav. 2012;37(8):890–9. PMID: 22541802. http://www.ncbi.nlm.nih.gov/pubmed/22541802.
349. Bloom BS. Prevalence and economic effects of depression. Manag Care. 2004;13(6 Suppl Depression):9–16. PMID: 15293766. http://www.ncbi.nlm.nih.gov/pubmed/15293766.
350. Winkler D, Pjrek E, Kasper S. Anger attacks in depression–evidence for a male depressive syndrome. Psychother Psychosom. 2005;74(5):303–7. PMID: 16088268. http://www.ncbi.nlm.nih.gov/pubmed/16088268.
351. Schmitt DP, Long AE, McPhearson A, O'Brien K, Remmert B, Shah SH. Personality and gender differences in global perspective. Int J Psychol. 2017;52(Suppl 1):45–56. PMID: 27000535. http://www.ncbi.nlm.nih.gov/pubmed/27000535.
352. Neitzke AB. An illness of power: gender and the social causes of depression. Cult Med Psychiatry. 2016;40(1):59–73. PMID: 26215590. http://www.ncbi.nlm.nih.gov/pubmed/26215590.
353. Juster RP, Pruessner JC, Desrochers AB, Bourdon O, Durand N, Wan N, Tourjman V, Kouassi E, Lesage A, Lupien SJ. Sex and gender roles in relation to mental health and Allostatic load. Psychosom Med. 2016;78(7):788–804. PMID: 27359170. http://www.ncbi.nlm.nih.gov/pubmed/27359170.
354. Goodyer IM, Herbert J, Tamplin A, Altham PM. First-episode major depression in adolescents. Affective, cognitive and endocrine characteristics of risk status and predictors of onset. Br J Psychiatry. 2000;176:142–9. PMID: 10755051. http://www.ncbi.nlm.nih.gov/pubmed/10755051.
355. Bierut LJ, Heath AC, Bucholz KK, Dinwiddie SH, Madden PA, Statham DJ, Dunne MP, Martin NG. Major depressive disorder in a community-based twin sample: are there different genetic and environmental contributions for men and women? Arch Gen Psychiatry. 1999;56(6):557–63. PMID: 10359473. http://www.ncbi.nlm.nih.gov/pubmed/10359473.
356. Hankin BL, Abramson LY. Development of gender differences in depression: an elaborated cognitive vulnerability-transactional stress theory. Psychol Bull. 2001;127(6):773–96. PMID: 11726071. http://www.ncbi.nlm.nih.gov/pubmed/11726071.
357. Spangler DL, Simons AD, Monroe SM, Thase ME. Gender differences in cognitive diathesis-stress domain match: implica-

tions for differential pathways to depression. J Abnorm Psychol. 1996;105(4):653–7. PMID: 8952199. http://www.ncbi.nlm.nih.gov/pubmed/8952199.

358. Kockler M, Heun R. Gender differences of depressive symptoms in depressed and nondepressed elderly persons. Int J Geriatr Psychiatry. 2002;17(1):65–72. PMID: 11802233. http://www.ncbi.nlm.nih.gov/pubmed/11802233.
359. Compas BE, Williams RA. Stress, coping, and adjustment in mothers and young adolescents in single- and two-parent families. Am J Community Psychol. 1990;18(4):525–45. PMID: 2075890. http://www.ncbi.nlm.nih.gov/pubmed/2075890.
360. Markowitz AJ, Ryan RM. Father absence and adolescent depression and delinquency: a comparison of siblings approach. J Marriage Fam. 2016;78(5):1300–14. PMCID: PMC5082431. http://www.ncbi.nlm.nih.gov/pubmed/27795578.
361. Marks J, Bun LC, McHale SM. Family patterns of gender role attitudes. Sex Roles. 2009;61(3–4):221–34. PMCID: PMC3270818. http://www.ncbi.nlm.nih.gov/pubmed/22308059.
362. Crompton R, Lyonette C. The new gender essentialism--domestic and family "choices" and their relation to attitudes. Br J Sociol. 2005;56(4):601–20. PMID: 16309438. http://www.ncbi.nlm.nih.gov/pubmed/16309438.
363. Crouter AC, Whiteman SD, McHale SM, Osgood DW. Development of gender attitude traditionality across middle childhood and adolescence. Child Dev. 2007;78(3):911–26. PMID: 17517012. http://www.ncbi.nlm.nih.gov/pubmed/17517012.
364. Hsieh TY, Simpkins SD. Longitudinal associations between parent degree/occupation, parent support, and adolescent motivational beliefs in STEM. J Adolesc. 2022;94(5):728–47. PMID: 35695089. http://www.ncbi.nlm.nih.gov/pubmed/35695089.
365. Puente K, Simpkins SD, Eccles JS. Longitudinal associations between Latine parents' support and their adolescents' science motivation and STEM career expectations. J Adolesc. 2024;96(6):1182–97. PMID: 38616412. http://www.ncbi.nlm.nih.gov/pubmed/38616412.
366. National Longitudinal Surveys Home Page: U.S. Bureau of Labor Statistics (bls.gov).
367. Physical Punishment (aacap.org).
368. Wiggers M, Paas F. Harsh physical discipline and externalizing behaviors in children: a systematic review. Int J Environ Res Public Health. 2022;19(21):14385. PMCID: PMC9656315. http://www.ncbi.nlm.nih.gov/pubmed/36361265.
369. Avezum MDM de M, Altafim ERP, Linhares MBM. Spanking and corporal punishment parenting practices and child development: a systematic review. Trauma Violence Abuse. 2023;24(5):3094–111. PMID: 36177799. http://www.ncbi.nlm.nih.gov/pubmed/36177799.
370. FFCWS changes name to The Future of Families and Child Wellbeing Study | Center for Research on Child and Family Wellbeing.
371. Bullough A, Guelich U, Manolova TS, Schjoedt L. Women's entrepreneurship and culture: gender role expectations and identities, societal culture, and the entrepreneurial environment. Small Bus Econ (Dordr). 2022;58(2):985–96. PMCID: PMC7794635. http://www.ncbi.nlm.nih.gov/pubmed/38624690.
372. Eagly AH, Karau SJ. Role congruity theory of prejudice toward female leaders. Psychol Rev. 2002;109(3):573–98. PMID: 12088246. http://www.ncbi.nlm.nih.gov/pubmed/12088246.
373. Saleem FT, English D, Busby DR, Lambert SF, Harrison A, Stock ML, Gibbons FX. The Impact of African American Parents' Racial Discrimination Experiences and Perceived Neighborhood Cohesion on their Racial Socialization Practices. J Youth Adolesc. 2016;45(7):1338–49. https://doi.org/10.1007/s10964-016-0499-x. Epub 2016 May 17. PMID: 27189721; PMCID: PMC5192560.
374. Scott LE, Varner F. Who, what, and where? How racial composition and gender influence the association between racial discrimination and racial socialization messages. Cultur Divers Ethnic Minor Psychol. 2023;29(4):447–58. https://doi.org/10.1037/cdp0000611. Epub 2023 Jun 29. PMID: 37384443; PMCID: PMC10543602
375. Thomsen KN, Howell KH, Gilliam HC, Ahmed AM, Thurston IB. Social-ecological protective and risk factors associated with depressive symptoms among black adolescents. Res Child Adolesc Psychopathol. 2025;53(3):317–29. https://doi.org/10.1007/s10802-024-01266-x. Epub 2024 Nov 26. PMID: 39589651.
376. Bernaras E, Jaureguizar J, Garaigordobil M. Child and adolescent depression: a review of theories, evaluation instruments, prevention programs, and treatments. Front Psychol. 2019;10:543. https://doi.org/10.3389/fpsyg.2019.00543. PMID: 30949092; PMCID: PMC6435492.
377. Stewart R, Wright B, Smith L, Roberts S, Russell N. Gendered stereotypes and norms: a systematic review of interventions designed to shift attitudes and behaviour. Heliyon. 2021;7(4):e06660. https://doi.org/10.1016/j.heliyon.2021.e06660. PMID: 33912699; PMCID: PMC8066375.

Communication in the Depressed Brain

7

Franklin Sunzeri

Psychoneuroimmunology and Depression

Communication in the brain exists between neurons, glial cells, immune cells, and endocrine cells. This is a classical *psychoneuroimmunological* interaction. Anatomic and physiologic evidence for the interconnection of the neuroendocrine and immune systems shows that immune system cells have receptors for hormones and neurotransmitters [1]. Moreover, certain areas of the brain express receptors for immune system cytokines and complement [2, 3].

Hormones of the neuroendocrine system and direct innervation of the sensory [4] and autonomic nervous system modulate the functioning of bone marrow [5] and other immune organs, as well as important immune system cells, such as the macrophages and lymphocytes [6–9].

Immunohistochemical staining of tissues in the skin has revealed neuropeptides in cutaneous nerve fibers and in all the cutaneous cells that were examined [10, 11]. These cells include Langerhans cells, fibroblasts, lymphocytes, endothelial cells, and keratinocytes. These neuropeptides include neurotransmitters, hormones, neuromodulators, and growth factors.

In addition to having receptors for input from other systems, cells of the nervous, endocrine, and immune systems can produce each other's products [1]. Immune system cells can produce neuropeptides, and nerve cells can produce immune system cytokines [12]. Endorphins and adrenocorticotropic hormone (ACTH) are produced in several non-hormonal tissues [13, 14]. One important immune system cell, the mast cell, is found in almost all tissues including the brain, and produces at least 50 mediators including biogenic amines that may function as neuromodulators (e.g., epinephrine, serotonin, and dopamine) or peptides that may function as hormones (e.g., corticotropin-releasing hormone (CRH), somatostatin, substance P, and vasoactive intestinal peptide) [15].

The intimate link between the neuroendocrine and immune systems is further illustrated in the presence of systemic infections. The immune system releases proinflammatory soluble molecules, which interact with cells of the blood–brain barrier and circumventricular organs [16]. These cells then release prostaglandins that influence autonomic functions, such as glucocorticoid release, essential for homeostasis and negative feedback to the immune system [9].

There are about an equal number of glial cells as neurons in the brain (~90 billion each) [17]. Gliotransmitters, several of which are classic neurotransmitters, are affected by and affect both pre- and postsynaptic neurons [18–20]. Glial cells are involved in central nervous system processing, transfer, and storage of information [21].

It is now generally acknowledged that the nervous, endocrine, and immune systems are an integrated system of adaptive processes responsible in part for regulating homeostasis in the organism [22]. The integrative neuro-, endocrine-, immune system has generally been described as two principal pathways, the hypothalamic pituitary adrenal (HPA) axis, which results in cortisol production, and the sympathetic adrenal medullary (SAM) system, which results in catecholamine production. However, this integration is more than that. A deeper discussion is beyond the purpose of this e-text.

Nervous System Basic Interactions in the Brain

A quick refresher brought to you by the synapse: The communication junction between neurons is called synapse, whereas connections between neurons and other cells are usually called neuroeffector junctions but are also frequently referred to as synapses [23].

Neuromuscular junctions involve motor neurons, skeletal muscle fibers, and Schwann cells [24–27]. The autonomic nervous system interfaces with a myriad of tissue receptors and provides the neural control of all of the body with the

F. Sunzeri (✉)
Heather Hills Consulting, Coos Bay, OR, USA

J. Raber et al. (eds.), *Understanding and Treating Depressive Disorders*, https://doi.org/10.1007/978-3-032-14465-2_7

exception of skeletal muscles [28, 29]. In turn, the neurons receive signals both directly and indirectly by chemical and physical factors produced by the target tissues. Neuroimmune regulation uses a variety of receptors to fine-tune immune responses and reciprocal synaptic plasticity from development through adulthood, with both long-range and short-range interactions [30]. In many cases, neurons and immune system cells share similar receptors and produce similar effector molecules.

There are an estimated 100–500 trillion synapses in the human brain. A typical neuron has several thousands of synapses with other neurons or with other cells [31, 32]. Most connections are axon to dendrites, axon to cell body, axon to axon, or dendrite to dendrites. However, there are other important not as widely known synapses that are important for altering epigenetic states [33]. For example, axonic cilia connections are found in neurons and glial cells in human brains [34, 35].[1]

These synapses actually are *quadripartite* which is elaborated upon in Chap. 10. There are two major types of synapses: the chemical and the electrical synapse [38]. However, there are other types of neuronal communication. There are combination chemical and electrical synapses [39]. And even more exotic, there are non-synaptic *ephaptic* (from the Greek for tangential) coupling using indirect electric biomagnetic fields to communicate between glial cells and neurons that can influence synchronization of action potentials [40–42]. Ephaptic transmission is very fast and may provide communication across distant cortical neurons [43]. Then there are the *autapse* (self-synapse), which is the synapse that forms between the axon and dendrites of the same neuron and may play a significant role in time-delayed self-feedback or resonance of neural circuits [44, 45]. Graphic representations of each of these types and their functions can be found in the referenced articles.

Synaptic adhesion molecules (SAMs) stabilize synapses [46]. Excitatory synapses are driven by an influx of sodium ions in the cation channels of the postsynaptic neuron, depolarizing and pushing the neuron closer to reaching the action potential threshold. Inhibitory synapses open either K+ or Cl- channels, causing the postsynaptic membranes to become less depolarized.

Most mammalian synapses are chemical. Chemical synapses use neurotransmitters and modulators to propagate signals that must cross a gap of 20–40 nm, which means there is a time delay of 0.5–1 milliseconds [47]. Although they may seem insignificant, electrical synapses operate with remarkable speed. They do not use neurotransmitters or modulators and have a gap junction of about 3.8 nm and virtually no time delay in propagating signals. Electrical synapses are found throughout the brain and are important in neural connections that need to be as fast as possible, like in defense and escape reactions. Both chemical and electrical synapses are capable of plasticity and modifications [48].

Electrical synapses are bidirectional and continuously on [38, 40]. They are responsible for complicated synchronization or chaotic dynamics [40, 49]. These electrical gap junctions are mostly composed of *connexins*. They can be modulated to provide plasticity [49].The gap junctions have pores that are 1.2–2 nm wide. This is wide enough that ions and medium-sized molecules can pass from the cytoplasm of adjacent cells [47, 50]. See Fig. 7.1.

Chemical transmission consists of synthesis, release, receptor activation, and signal termination. The neurotransmitters are most usually either neuropeptides or small molecules [51]. See Fig. 7.2.

The *small molecules are synthesized* in the neuron cell body and transported to the presynaptic terminal, where they are modified and then released into the synaptic cleft.

Synthesis of neuropeptides uses the protein synthesis and translation pathways of the neuron cell body. They are packaged into a dense vesicle along with a protease. These vesicles are transported in microtubules to the presynaptic terminal. At the terminal are a collection of terminal *SNARE* (t-SNARE) proteins [52] that combine with vesicle SNAREs (v-SNAREs). When an action potential reaches the presynaptic terminal, it causes a rapid influx of calcium, which causes the SNAREs to change conformation and fuse the vesicle with the terminal membrane, resulting in the release of the vesicle contents into the synaptic cleft. Upon release, the vesicle membrane is endocytosed.

Upon reaching the postsynaptic neuron, the neurotransmitter may interact with either a ligand-gated ion channel or a G-protein-coupled receptor. The *ligand-gated receptors* are fast, direct acting and terminate quickly. These may be excitatory or inhibitory receptors. *G-protein coupled receptors* will bind to a G-protein heterotrimer (a family of guanine nucleotide-binding proteins), which in turn hydrolyzes GTP to GDP to activate a cascade of secondary messengers to either open or close ion channels (exciting or inhibiting) [53]. This process is relatively slow but effects last from seconds to minutes.

Neurotransmitters may also be classified as having metabotropic (Greek: metabo = metabolism + tropic = turning) and/or ionotropic properties depending upon the characteristics of the neurotransmitter receptors. *Metabotropic receptors* rely upon signal transduction and are often G-protein coupled and do not form ion channels directly

[1] *Primary cilia* are nonmotile key integrators of extracellular ligand-based signaling, regulating neuronal cell differentiation and effects on a myriad of behaviors including appetite and obesity [36, 37]. Primary cilia are microtubule-based, membrane-bound proteins extending a few microns from the basal body of most vertebrate cell types into the extracellular space [34]. Cilia are present in most of the mature neurons and glia in the human brain [35].

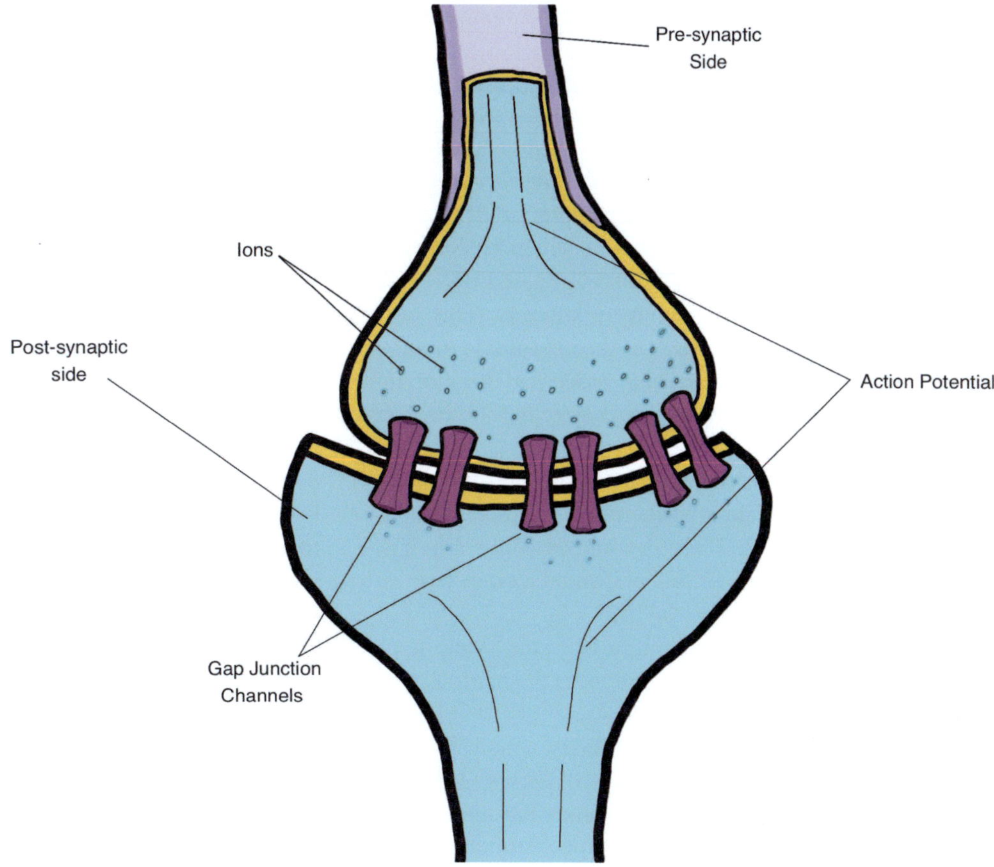

Fig. 7.1 This simplified depiction showcases the core features of an electrical synapse, where ions flow directly between adjacent neurons via gap junctions. The cartoon highlights bidirectional signal transmission and rapid communication enabled by these specialized intercellular channels

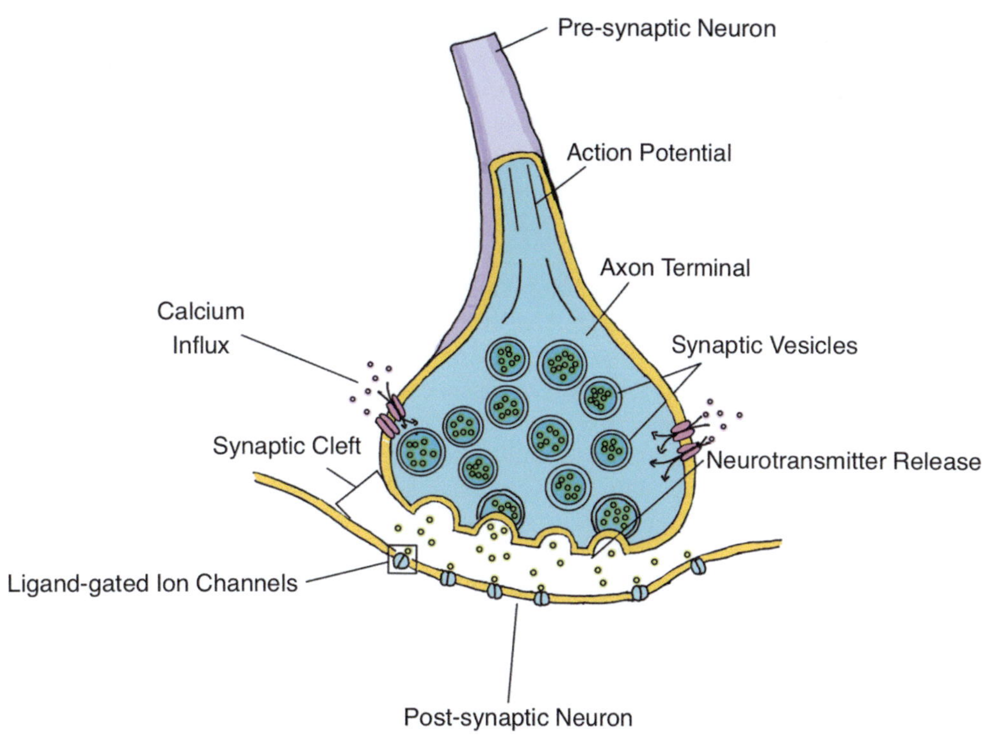

Fig. 7.2 Cartoon depiction of a chemical synapse. This illustration shows the essential components of a chemical synapse, highlighting neurotransmitter release from the presynaptic neuron, receptor binding on the postsynaptic membrane, and the synaptic cleft as the communication bridge

[54–56]. *Ionotropic receptors* more directly open ion channels in response to the signal [57, 58].

The ionotropic glutamate receptors are the most abundant excitatory receptors in the central nervous system of mammals [59]. However, there are also inhibitory glutamate receptors that are closely related to the ionotropic gamma-aminobutyric (GABA) and glycine receptors [60].

Termination of the signal occurs by several mechanisms. Small-molecule transmitters can be eliminated by *reuptake* into the presynaptic neuron or by glial cells. This allows recycling. Small molecules such as the neurotoxic glutamate are reuptaken by glial cells and processed to glutamine before being transferred to the presynaptic neuron for future use.

The primary way that dopamine is removed from the cleft in the CNS is via the integral membrane protein *dopamine transporter (DAT)* [61]. There is some evidence that a *norepinephrine transporter* in the prefrontal cortex may also play a role in dopamine removal [62].

Diffusion of the neurotransmitter from the synaptic cleft and into the circulation gradually reduces the neurotransmitter effects

Enzymatic *degradation* is the primary source for terminating peptide molecules. *Monoamine oxidases (MAOs)* use oxygen to remove the amine group from the monoamines. MAOs are found in the outer membrane of mitochondria in both neurons and astroglia. MAO-A[2] operates on serotonin, melatonin, norepinephrine, epinephrine, dopamine, tyramine, and tryptamine. MAO-B will degrade dopamine, tyramine, tryptamine, phenethylamine, and benzylamine.

Catechol-O-Methyltransferase (COMT) breaks down catecholamines, including dopamine, epinephrine, and norepinephrine [65]. COMT is active intracellularly postsynaptically in neurons and glia and extracellularly in the cleft [66]. COMT polymorphisms are associated with depression [67, 68].

Each of these steps is capable of being modified by the members of the quadripartite synapse. That is the pre- and postsynaptic neurons, microglia, and astrocytes. Information processing and plasticity in the synapses are dependent upon dynamic states of the presynaptic and postsynaptic neurons, astrocytes, and microglia. The astrocytes enfold the synapses in a heteromorphic embrace, while the microglia in a functionally dependent fashion animatedly interact with the synapse.

Combinations of chemical and electrical synapses combine fast and slow signal transmission [69, 70].

It is important to note that propagation and relaying of impulses in a single nerve cell are not all or none [71]. There is a definite sophisticated time-space continuum of integration and differentiation of shading described by complex wave equations based upon multiple facilitating and inhibitory impulses from different sources impinging upon that single cell [72, 73]. Therefore, various patterns of firing can be produced.

Since the mid-1980s, dozens of neurotransmitters (as of 2019, *more than 100 neurotransmitters and neuromodulators were identified in the brain) have been discovered* (only four were well known in the 1970s) [74, 75]. There are at least 18 major neurotransmitters. The neurotransmitters are stored in synaptic vesicles that are membrane-bound vacuoles, generally only on the presynaptic side. However, some synapses contain neurotransmitter vesicles on the postsynaptic side as well, implying that transmission may also occur post- to presynaptically. Vesicles protect neurotransmitters from degradation by intracellular enzymes and permit fusion to the axonal membrane to release the neurotransmitters. Each vesicle stores a quantum of neurotransmitters (usually several thousand molecules) [22, 76, 77].

One of the most *convenient ways to classify and study neurotransmitters* is by dividing them into amino acids, monoamines, trace amines, peptides, purines, gasotransmitters, and others. *Amino acids* examples include glutamate, aspartate, glycine, gamma-aminobutyric acid (GABA), and serine. *Monoamine* examples include the catecholamines (dopamine, norepinephrine, epinephrine), indolamine (serotonin, melatonin), and histamine. *Trace amines* are represented by tyramine and phenethylamine (found in chocolate and other places) [78]. *Neuropeptides* are numerous and diverse small proteins. These include peptides such as oxytocin, endorphins, opioids, somatostatin, adrenocorticotropic hormone (ACTH), glucagon-like peptide-1, cocaine- and amphetamine-regulated transcript (CART), insulin, and glucagon. *Purines* include adenosine and adenosine triphosphate. *Gasotransmitters* include nitric oxide, carbon monoxide, and hydrogen sulfide. *Others* include *acetylcholine* and some *single elements*, such as zinc, that function as neurotransmitters in fear conditioning pathways [79]. *Lipids* such as anandamide (a derivative of arachidonic acid and found in the reward system) can activate cannabinoid receptors [80].

Most of the well-characterized neurotransmitters are monoamines or amino acids. The most studied neurotransmitters are acetylcholine, epinephrine, norepinephrine, serotonin, glycine, histamine, dopamine, glutamic acid, taurine, and gamma-aminobutyric acid (GABA). The number of transmitters released may be a few hundred to a few thousand. Neuromuscular junctions of skeletal muscles involve the release of multimolecular packets (quanta) of acetylcholine.

Testosterone, progesterone, pregnenolone, and dehydroepiandrosterone have also been identified as *neuromodulators* [81, 82]. Their fluctuations throughout life may have

[2]Elevated MAO-A density is associated with excessive monoamine lowering activity in major depression [63, 64].

significant influences on mood disorders in genetically predisposed individuals [74, 83–85].

Originally, it had been thought that each neuron had only one type of chemical transmitter. It is now known that in many neurons, such as those that release serotonin or norepinephrine, there is an assortment of other neurotransmitters as well [86, 87]. In addition, there is evidence that two different neurotransmitters released from the same presynaptic cell may act upon the same postsynaptic receptor (e.g., GABA and glycine) [87].

Most rapid signaling appears to rely on amino acids such as glycine, glutamic acid, and GABA. The most common *inhibitory neurotransmitter* in the brain is GABA. About 1/3 of all the synapses in the brain are thought to involve GABA. A deficiency in GABA appears to be the cause of Huntington's chorea. Glutamate and aspartate are the principal *excitatory neurotransmitters* in the CNS, and are found in the cerebral cortex, cerebellum, and spinal cord. Glycine, which is similar in activity to GABA, is found principally in the interneurons of the spinal cord. In reality, the type of neurotransmitter is not the determinant of resultant excitation or inhibition. This is the province of the postsynaptic cell. The same neurotransmitter may produce excitation or inhibition depending upon the properties of the receptor cell. Indeed, a single postsynaptic neuron can modify and balance excitatory and inhibitory signals from more than one presynaptic neuron [88].

Many neurons secrete neuropeptides in addition to the classical neurotransmitters [89]. These include endorphins, vasopressin, oxytocin, and gastrin. These neuropeptides are active outside of the synapse, and their effects may last hours to days. Although they are stored in a different type of vesicle, they are released in a calcium-dependent fashion like the classic transmitters.

Of the more than 100 identified *neurotransmitters and neuromodulators*, the most heavily studied classic neurotransmitters are probably the *catecholamines* (meaning that they are *pyrocatechol* derivatives with an alkylamine side chain). The catecholamines dopamine, norepinephrine, and epinephrine are produced sequentially in the same pathway starting with the amino acid L-tyrosine. The rate-limiting synthesis step is tyrosine hydroxylase, which catalyzes the first step in the pathway converting L-tyrosine to L-DOPA. Excess catecholamines in the axon terminal inhibit tyrosine hydroxylase. A deficiency stimulates tyrosine hydroxylase. Epinephrine is principally a neurohormone and as such will not be discussed here. Noradrenaline is the old name for norepinephrine; adrenalin is the old name for epinephrine. We will briefly present an overview of some of the most discussed neurotransmitters.

Dopamine is found in some peripheral nervous system neurons and is the transmitter of choice in the neurons of the substancia nigra (part of the basal ganglia) that project to two parts of the corpus striatum: the putamen (Latin = that which falls off in pruning) and caudate nuclei (two of the basal ganglia), and to the frontal cortex. The primary function of these parts of the basal ganglia is smooth integration of skeletal muscle movement. So, when there is a degeneration or malfunction of the nigrostriatal dopaminergic pathway, the classic symptoms of Parkinson's disease occur. Parkinson's is the second most common neurodegenerative disease of the elderly [90, 91]. These symptoms include slow movement, shuffling gate, festination (breaking into a run to keep from falling), drooling, resting rhythmic or pill-rolling tremors, mask-like expressionless faces, and rigidity. Because of the frontal lobe involvement, depression can occur [92–94]. Prevalence of depression in Parkinson's has been reported to be between 2.7% and 90% with about 35% having clinically significant depressive symptoms [95]. Some antipsychotic drugs, neuroleptics, may block the dopamine receptors and create a pseudo and reversible Parkinson's disease. Levodopa, the metabolic precursor to dopamine, can help reduce the symptoms. Tyrosine hydroxylase and monoamine oxidase regulate nerve terminal dopamine levels.

Dopaminergic neurons are also found in the arcuate nucleus of the hypothalamus, which sends axons to the venous sinuses of the pituitary. Here the dopamine inhibits the secretion of the pituitary hormone prolactin, the hormone that prompts breast milk release. Once again, the neuroleptic dopamine blockers can create a side effect. Occasionally, they can prompt the release of breast milk in a nonpregnant woman.

Dopamine is a vital neurotransmitter in the *mesocorticolimbic dopaminergic system*, which is part of the anticipatory and reward pathways. Dopamine is the principle neurotransmitter that signals *motivational salience* toward or away from an outcome [96–98].

Norepinephrine-containing neurons are called noradrenergic from the word noradrenaline, a synonym for norepinephrine, which belies its original characterization in the adrenal medulla. The location in the brain with the highest number of noradrenergic neuronal cell bodies is the locus coeruleus (Latin = blue place), located bilaterally in the floor of the pons varolii. It contains over half of all norepinephrine-containing neurons in the CNS. Axons from these neurons connect with thousands of neurons in the cerebellum, cerebral cortex, thalamus, and hypothalamus. It is the mediator of most postganglionic sympathetic fibers. Tyrosine hydroxylase and monoamine oxidase regulate nerve-terminal norepinephrine levels.

Serotonin (5-hydroxytryptamine (5-HT)) is produced from the decarboxylation of 5-hydroxytryptophan, which is produced from the hydrolysis of tryptophan. Concentrations are controlled by tryptophan uptake and intraneuronal monoamine oxidase. High concentrations are found in the basal ganglia and the hypothalamus. The group of median raphe nuclei surrounding the midbrain aqueduct and midline neurons of the pons varolii and upper brain stem produce the most 5-HT. Those 5-HT neurons connected to the cerebral cortex and hypothalamus are associated with REM sleep; those connected to the limbic system relate to aggression and depression; and those connected to the spinal column are associated with sensitivity to pain.

Serotonin occurs in quite a few peripheral tissues and in some carcinoid tumors. It is also a vasoconstrictor stored in platelets, which actively concentrates it from plasma; it inhibits gastric secretions and stimulates the contraction of smooth muscle. Serotonin may also act as a neuromodulator or fine-tuner in the CNS by release from swellings (varicosities) along the axon. Fascinating reviews of serotonin can be found in [99, 100]. Serotonin does not cross the blood–brain barrier, but its production and therefore some behaviors can be moderated by dietary intake of tryptophan (q.i). Suppression of 5-HT reuptake and disruption of the serotonin system may result from the recreational use of methamphetamines, MDMA (ecstasy), and cocaine.

Acetylcholine is synthesized from choline and acetyl coenzyme A, derived from mitochondria. Acetylcholine levels are regulated by choline esterase and reuptake of choline. Acetylcholine is the principal neurotransmitter of the bulbospinal (from the medulla oblongata to the spine) nerves, preganglionic to ganglionic synapse for both the sympathetic and parasympathetic systems, and from the parasympathetic postganglionic fibers to target organs, basal ganglia to the cerebral cortex, hippocampus, and other parts of the limbic system. Also, the nucleus basalis of Meynert and the globus pallidus use acetylcholine neurons to contact the cerebral cortex. Acetylcholine is critical in memory processes. Indeed, delirium is a possible side effect of anticholinergic drugs (e.g., atropine and scopolamine), along with neuroleptics and tricyclic antidepressants.

Gamma amino-butyric acid (GABA) as mentioned above is the major inhibitory neurotransmitter in the brain. GABA comes from the decarboxylation of glutamic acid. After its interaction with the postsynaptic cell receptor, GABA is actively pumped back up by the presynaptic cell and metabolized. Inhibition is thought to be due to increased permeability of chloride ions. GABA neurons are short-range and locally acting as opposed to long-distance catecholamines. *Glycine* has analogous activity to GABA and is the principal interneuron inhibitor of the spinal nerves. It appears to be derived from serine.

L-Glutamic acid is the primary excitatory neurotransmitter in the brain.

Endorphins are polypeptides that bind to the same receptors that opioid narcotic analgesics bind. They activate many CNS neurons, especially in the hypothalamus, thalamus, amygdala, and locus coeruleus. The dorsal horn of the spinal tract is a location where they inhibit the pain-relaying sensory neurons. These endorphin neurons produce a large polypeptide precursor *(pro-opiomelanocortin (POMC))* that is transported down the axon, where it is cleaved into several endorphins including α-, β-, and γ- endorphins. The most common endorphin appears to be β-endorphin. Under stress, β-endorphin is released from the anterior pituitary. Peptidases hydrolyze β-endorphins into inactive amino acids and oligopeptides after interaction with the opioid receptors.

Enkephalins are oligopeptides that can be found in many CNS neurons, especially in the globus pallidus, thalamus, and caudate nuclei. These enkephalin neurons produce a polypeptide precursor (proenkephalin) that is transported down the axon, where it is cleaved into met- and leu-enkephalins, each of these is 5-amino acids with a terminal methionine or a terminal leucine, respectively. *Dynorphins are* a family of seven peptides with related amino acid sequences. They appear to share locations and activities with enkephalins. Peptidases hydrolyze enkephalins and dynorphins into inactive amino acids and oligopeptides after interaction with the opioid receptors.

Substance P is an eleven-amino acid peptide that is released by intense afferent pain stimulation. It is found in high concentrations in the dorsal root ganglia of the spinal column, substancia nigra, hypothalamus, basal ganglia, medulla oblongata, and the habenula (Latin = frenulum; a cell mass in the dorsomedial thalamus). It is also found in the smooth muscle of the intestine and is one of the most potent stimulators of smooth muscles in dilating blood vessels and contracting intestines.

Neurotransmitter Systems

Although most neurotransmitters, such as GABA, glutamate, and glycine, are not concentrated in one part of the brain, there are some families of neurotransmitters that act together in particular areas. These are known as *neurotransmitter systems* [101].

The most frequently investigated neurotransmitter systems are the dopamine system, norepinephrine system, serotonin system, histamine system, acetylcholine system, and adrenaline system. We will just briefly highlight some of the targets and effects of these pathways. Excellent figures illustrating the pathways, etc., can be found in the references that we cite.

Dopamine System

The dopamine system consists of six principle pathways [102, 103]. They are the mesolimbic pathway and the mesocortical pathway (aka the mesocorticolimbic dopamine system), the nigrostriatal pathway, the tuberoinfundibular pathway, the hypothalamospinal tract, and the incertohypothalamic pathway. Dopamine is a principal actor in behavioral and physiological processes such as moving, executive functioning, cognitive processing, eating, motivating, and controlling neuroendocrine activities. The *mesocorticolimbic pathway* is involved in learning, motivation, reward, pleasure, memory, and movement [104–107]. The *mesocortical pathway* from the ventral tegmental area (VTA) to the prefrontal cortex is involved in executive functions such as working memory, attention, and planning [108]. The *mesolimbic pathway* from the VTA to the ventral striatum (nucleus accumbens and olfactory tubercle) is often called the reward pathway [109, 110]. The *nigrostriatal pathway* is involved in movement and motivation [111, 112]. The dorsal striatum is involved in reward and decision making [113]. The substancia nigra is associated with motor functioning [114]. The *tuberoinfundibular pathway* from the arcuate nucleus of the hypothalamus to the pituitary is active in regulating hormonal balance [115]. The *cortico-basal ganglia-thalamo-cortical loop* [116, 117] is composed of the *hypothalamospinal tract*, which has motor functions, and the *incertohypothalamic pathway*, which has visceral and sensorimotor functions [118].

Norepinephrine System

The overarching function of the *norepinephrine system* is to mobilize us for action, especially in the face of danger [119, 120]. In the CNS, norepinephrine heightens awareness and focuses attention, and along with dopamine, enhances memory formation and retrieval. As side effects of this arousal, it can increase restlessness and anxiety. Not surprisingly, stimuli are mostly the same to alert the brain and the sympathetic nervous system. Norepinephrine increases energy availability by hepatic glycogenolysis or gluconeogenesis to release glucose and by lipolysis in adipose tissue [121]. It prepares the body for action by increasing heart rate and blood pressure, thereby increasing blood flow and delivering energy to skeletal muscles while decreasing gastrointestinal activity and urination [122, 123]. Norepinephrine is the main neurotransmitter of the sympathetic ganglia and it is also the adrenal medullary hormone. In a complex interaction, the sympathetic component interacts with immune system tissues such as the thymus, bone marrow, and spleen [124, 125]. But back to the brain. There are comparatively few neurons whose primary neurotransmitter is norepinephrine, but they send projections to every major part of the brain and spinal cord and have profound influences [126]. There are several notable norepinephrine cell groups. These include the *solitary nucleus* in the brain stem that plays roles in cognitive and behavioral functions such as stress responses and eating [119]. The *locus coeruleus (LC)* is the most extensively studied group, with its norepinephrine-producing cells estimated to number approximately 15,000 [120, 127]. Its activity follows the need to be alert. The LC idles during most of the day, decreases to a very low level during sleep stages and springs into action when stimulated by unpleasant stimuli. Intense fear or pain accelerates LC activity to a very high level. In the brain, the LC interacts with multiple cell types, such as astrocytes and glial cells, to regulate neuroinflammation and optimize and modulate both rapid and slow performance [128]. The LC appears to be heavily involved in age-associated pathophysiology and Alzheimer's disease [129].

Serotonin System

The *serotonin system* is thought to be involved in many physiological and behavioral processes [130, 131]. These include depression[3], anxiety, social behavior, sexual activity, eating, sleep, biological rhythms, learning, and memory [140–142]. The serotonin system is a widely expansive neurochemical network in the CNS of vertebrates [100]. The *raphe nuclei* neurons along the midline of the brainstem and centered on the reticular formation are the main source for releasing serotonin in the brain [143]. *Caudal nuclei of the raphe* project to the cerebral cortex, thalamus, caudate nucleus, nucleus accumbens, cerebellum, and spinal cord. *Rostral nuclei of the raphe* project to the hypothalamus, thalamus, amygdala, cingulate cortex, neocortex, ventral tegmental area, and septum. Serotonin may interact directly or indirectly with other parts of the brain to influence aggression and other social behaviors [144–146]. Serotonin is involved via the *midbrain inferior colliculus* in auditory processing in social interactions [147–149].

Histaminergic System

The histaminergic system in the brain consists of histamine-producing neurons exclusively located in the tuberomammillary nucleus and four types of G-protein-coupled histamine receptors that are tissue-specific but spread through most of the brain [101, 150, 151]. It has been suggested that histamine may increase excitability throughout the brain [152].

Histamine is a pleiotropic monoamine that has key functions in immune response, cell growth and differentiation, and nutrition, as well as being a neurotransmitter and neuro-

[3]A 2023 umbrella meta-analysis, however, found no consistent evidence of an association between serotonin and depression and no evidence that depression is caused by lowered serotonin activity or concentration [132, 133]. However, those findings are debated [134–139]. We will have more to say about that debate. It is important not to confuse association with causality.

modulator [153, 154]. The principal histaminergic CNS pathways are from the *tuberomammillary nucleus* to the cerebral cortex, hippocampus, amygdala, hypothalamus, neostriatum, and nucleus accumbens [155]. *Histamine N-methyltransferase* inactivates brain histamine [156]. The histamine system is involved in the etiopathogenesis of neuropsychiatric disorders [157]. Histamine metabolism connects many complex metabolic and homeostatic processes [158–160]. Diffuse connections promote wakefulness and vigilance in various environmental and behavioral conditions [161, 162]. Histamine stimulates serotonin, norepinephrine, and especially dopamine transmission in the brain [163]. Histamine may be a unifying factor that links monoamines to cytokines [164]. In the brain, histamine regulates glial and neuron interactions [165]. Outside of the brain, histamine is involved in autoimmune disorders, gastric acid secretion, and hematopoiesis. Histamine is found in all tissues but is highly concentrated in basophils, mast cells, and lungs. Histamine release from basophils and mast cells are said to be involved in almost two dozen different physiological actions [101, 166].

Acetylcholine System

A coordinated *acetylcholine system* in the CNS is vital for flexible cognitive functions. In addition, acetylcholine is the primary neurotransmitter in neuromuscular junctions and is the main neurotransmitter in the end organs of the parasympathetic system, where it modulates endocrine activity.

Acetylcholine in the brain may act through the long-timescale extrasynaptic volume transmission and through conventional rapid point-to-point neurotransmission [167, 168]. The acetylcholine system modulates the time course of potential behaviors to adapt to environmental changes by enhancing some responses and minimizing others [167, 169]. Acetylcholine contributes to endogenous brain rhythms and synchronicity of the limbic system [170, 171]. Basal forebrain acetylcholine neurons can corelease GABA [172], and those in the striatum can corelease glutamate [173]. Through nicotinic receptors and muscarinic receptors, acetylcholine can modulate the mesolimbic dopamine reward functions [174, 175].

The acetylcholine system in the brain consists of three cholinergic pathways [167, 176]. They are the path from the *basal forebrain cholinergic nuclei* to the hippocampus, cerebral cortex, limbic cortex, and sensory cortex. The *striatal* tonically active cholinergic neurons connect to the medium spiny neurons. The *brainstem cholinergic nuclei* connect to the ventral tegmental area and the thalamus. The principal functions of these are modulation of cognition, especially attention, arousal, short-term memory, motivational salience, learning, emotions, mood, and motor functions [177–180]. The modulation of the nicotinic and muscarinic receptors is controlled by these circuits to affect sensory plasticity [181]. The cholinergic attention system is influenced by sex differences and is hormonally regulated [179]. Active forgetting of unwanted memories involves the acetylcholine system [182].

Homeostatic regulation of the acetylcholine system is critical for mood regulation and reaction to stress [183, 184]. Optimal levels of acetylcholine in the brain are necessary for sustained attention and facilitated learning and memory, but increased levels of acetylcholine are seen in the brain during depressive episodes [185]. When the breakdown of acetylcholine is impaired, symptoms of anxiety, depression, and stress reactions can increase [186, 187]. Interaction between noradrenergic and cholinergic signals in the amygdala can regulate depression and anxiety symptoms [188].

Adrenaline System

The *adrenaline system* connects the *rostral ventrolateral medulla (RVLM)* to the spinal cord, the rest of the brain stem, and the hypothalamus [189–191]. Via catecholamine projections to the sympathetic preganglionic neurons, the RVLM is responsible for basal and reflex control of the sympathetic nervous system [192, 193]. *C1 neurons* of the RVLM innervate sympathetic and parasympathetic preganglionic neurons, the hypothalamic paraventricular nucleus, and numerous brain structures involved in autonomic regulation, stress, and arousal [190]. C1 neurons use glutamate as a fast transmitter and synthesize catecholamines and neuropeptides [189]. Depending on the nature of stressors, C1 cell mediation may be allostatic or homeostatic. There are both direct and indirect complex routes whereby the C1 cells influence the hypothalamic-pituitary axis. Adrenaline facilitates encoding of emotionally loaded events that lead to higher fear-related arousal and lead to pathologies such as PTSD [194, 195].

The actions of adrenaline as a hormone are well known [196]. It should be noted that all behaviors involve both the endocrine and nervous systems [197, 198]. Adrenaline does not readily cross the blood–brain barrier [199, 200]. However, it would appear that circulating epinephrine from the adrenal medulla may connect with the CNS stress circuits via the vagal nerve β-adrenergic receptors to release norepinephrine, which could stimulate the release of catecholamines from the nucleus tractus solitarius and locus coeruleus [199]. The basal lateral amygdala may stimulate a sequence of afferents through the hypothalamus, neocortex, hippocampus, caudate nucleus, etc. In this fashion, adrenaline may have both a short-term and long-term effect in regulating stress and stress-related reactions.

These systems may act in consort to produce *volume transmission effects* [201]. Neurotransmitters may diffuse through the extracellular fluid to local or remote parts of the brain where they may interact with extra-synaptic receptors [202]. This interaction, called *tonic transmission*, may last longer than the *phasic transmission* from single synapses [203, 204].Volume transmission effects in neurotransmitter systems appear to underlie the pharmaceutical effects (both adverse and beneficial) of many drugs.

Endocannabinoid System

The endocannabinoid system (eCBS)[4] is conserved in all vertebrates where it is involved in physiological processes such as appetite, cancer, cardiovascular diseases, fertility, immune functions, memory, neuroprotection, and pain modulation [208, 209]. Physiological systems associated with emotional reward, cognition, and response to stress that are dysregulated in depression are heavily invested in endocannabinoid receptors.

The endocannabinoids (eCBs) mediate both long-term and short-term plasticity. They are synthesized and released on demand postsynaptically into the extracellular space. The retrograde effects appear to act locally or at a distance. Inactivation of the eCBs is primarily through triggering microglia to produce a variety of lipid-based molecules. The most bioactive eCBs are anandamide (arachidonylethanolamide; AEA) and 2-arachidonoylglycerol (2-AG) [207][5].

There are two main cannabinoid receptors (CBRs): CB1R mainly present in the central nervous system [210] but also in several non-neuronal cells and tissues [211]; and CB2R, mainly distributed in peripheral and immune cells [212] but also in the brain stem [213] and in neuronal cells upon exogenous insults [214]. GPR55 (CB3R) is often considered to be a third cannabinoid receptor [215]; it is highly expressed in large dorsal root ganglion neurons [216].

Physiological systems associated with emotional reward, cognition, and response to stress that are dysregulated in depression are heavily invested with endocannabinoid receptors [217, 218].

Decreased activity in the eCBS is frequently found in animal depression models [219], and depression like behavior has been seen when blocking CB1Rs in rats [220].

Decreased eCB signaling is seen in "depressed" mice when confronted with chronic unpredictable stress (CUS) [221]. However, cortical and subcortical structures are differently altered [222]. Even though the CUS model produces a decrease in AEA, there is a compensatory increase in CB1R binding site density in the prefrontal cortex and a decrease in CB1R binding site density in the hippocampus, hypothalamus, and ventral striatum [223] and decreased CB1R functions in the nucleus accumbens [224].

Increased CB1R in the prefrontal cortex has been reported in post-mortem studies of depressed individuals and depressed suicide victims compared to controls [225, 226].

Decreased depression-like behavior has been seen in conditions where fatty acid amide hydrolase (FAAH), which catalyzes the intracellular hydrolysis of AEA, has been blocked, resulting in AEA being elevated in mice [227–230].

In mice with increased expression of CB2Rs, resistance to depression has been seen when confronted with stress [231].

The eCBS is active via CB1Rs in basal tonic regulation of the HPA axis [232]. The eCBS suppresses HPA activity through actions within the prefrontal cortex, amygdala, and hypothalamus, and has distinct roles to play in response to acute stress and glucocorticoid negative feedback. Disruption of CB1Rs increases corticosterone levels [233, 234] and CB1R knockout mice have depression-like symptoms and elevated basal ACTH levels [235].

The idea that depression and anxiety result from impaired adult neurogenesis and restoration of adult neurogenesis leads to recovery has been tested frequently, but results are heterogeneous [236]. Such is the case with the eCBS. Nevertheless, CB2Rs are involved in all important stages of neural progenitor cell cycle proliferation, differentiation, and migration [237, 238]. Decreased BDNF in the hippocampus is frequently seen in MDD and in animal models of depression [239–241]. Experiments where CB1R is blocked decreased BDNF in the hippocampus and suppressed dentate gyrus progenitor proliferation [220, 239]. Increased eCB signaling increases BDNF levels and stimulates neurogenesis [242–244].

As to the use of exogenous cannabinoids, consistent use of marijuana is associated with decreased CB1R expression [245] and a reduction in hippocampal neuronal density [246].

Cannabis can be both pro- and antidepressant depending upon a variety of factors [247]. Some studies have found that recreational cannabis use can diminish the perception of negative depressive behaviors [248, 249]. Results of an internet-based epidemiological study suggested that frequent cannabis users showed a more positive affect and less depressed mood when compared to non-users [250]. Those who used it once per week or less reported less depressed mood, more positive affect, and fewer somatic complaints than non-users. Daily users had less depressed mood and more positive affect than non-users. In the same study, medi-

[4]A 2019 review is Cannabinoid Receptors and the Endocannabinoid System: Signaling and Function in the Central Nervous System [204]. Additional reviews are the 2016 Neurobiological Interactions Between Stress and the Endocannabinoid System [205] and the 2012 The Endocannabinoid System: an Overview [206].

[5]Additional eCBs include virodhamine, noladin ether, and *N*-arachidonoyldopamine (NADA), homo-linolenylethanolamide (HEA), docosatetraenylethanolamide (DEA), and other cognate compounds such as palmitoylethanolamide (PEA) and oleoylethanolamide (OEA) [206].

cal marijuana users reported a more depressed mood and more somatic complaints than recreational users.

A few studies have suggested that cannabis use is associated with antidepressant effects in some people with MDD [251]. A comprehensive review of the potential use of cannabis for treatment of anxiety, mood, and related disorders was published in 2017 [252].

Use of endocannabinoids has been suggested as a potential treatment for MDD [253, 254]. Self-medication with cannabinoids is discussed in the Treatment chapter.

Neurotransmitter Receptors

Neurotransmitter receptors are transmembrane protein complexes.[6] A precise level of neurotransmission control is maintained by a combination of the most common postsynaptic receptors and far less common presynaptic receptors. This is in contrast to *intracellular receptors* for many hormones, such as thyroid hormones and steroid hormones, including glucocorticoids, mineralocorticoids, and the sex steroid hormones [256, 257].

To maintain a harmonious regulation of tissue function, downregulation, decreased or hyposensitivity to stimulation, occurs in receptors that are continuously stimulated by neurotransmitters or drugs (agonists). Upregulation, increased or hypersensitivity, occurs in receptors that are chronically under-stimulated (such as those blocked by drugs or other antagonists). Tolerance and physical dependence, along with withdrawal rebound phenomena, can readily occur as a result of changes to receptor density or affinity.

Many of the receptors that have been characterized are classified into divisions based upon the neurotransmitters that bind to them, and into subtypes based upon the response or location.[7] Neurotransmission can be increased or decreased to adapt to changes in physiology. Once propagation has been instigated, the amount of neurotransmitters released can be modified by various factors, including drugs, toxins (e.g., botulinum), and antibodies (e.g., myasthenia gravis).

A few neurotransmitter molecules are always leaking from the synapse, but it is an insufficient amount to transmit an impulse to the next cell. When the action potential reaches the axon terminal, a channel is opened for the influx of *calcium* ions, which leads to the fusion of many synaptic vesicles containing the neurotransmitters with the axonal synaptic membrane. This fusion results in the release of the neurotransmitters into the synapse in a process called *exocytosis*.

[6] Some receptors (*ionotropes*) are multimeric, ion-channel permeability-enhancing proteins acting by second messengers or by directly changing ion conductance [254]. Others (*metabotropes*) are monomers coupled to second messengers and consist of three parts. The exterior part is glycosylated, the transmembrane part is where the neurotransmitter presumably acts, and the inner cytoplasmic part is where phosphorylation of the messenger or G-protein binding occurs. *G proteins* are GTPases, so called due to their ability to bind to and enzymatically hydrolyze guanosine triphosphate (GTP) to guanosine diphosphate (GDP). When bound to GTP, they are "on"', and when they are bound to GDP, they are "off".

[7] *Dopaminergic receptors* are identified as D_1, D_2, D_3, D_4, and D_5. D_2 receptors control the extrapyramidal system. D_3 and D_4 receptors limit the negative symptoms of schizophrenia and seem to be involved in the control of thoughts.

Adrenergic receptors react to the catecholamines epinephrine and norepinephrine. Adrenergic receptors include the reactive components of the effector tissues, most of which are activated by postganglionic adrenergic sympathetic neurons. Based on their response to various activators and blockers, receptors are categorized into α_1, which occurs postsynaptically in the sympathetic system, and α_2, which occurs presynaptically in the sympathetic system and postsynaptically in the brain. Some physiological responses include contraction of pilomotor muscles (erect hairs), mydriasis (pupil dilation), and increased vascular constriction. β_1 occurs in the heart, and responses include an increase in cardiac rate and force of contraction. β_2 is in other non-cardiac sympathetically innervated tissues, and responses include vascular and bronchial smooth muscle relaxation.

Serotoninergic (5-HT) receptors include at least 15 types. The 6 major types are the 4 subtypes of $5\text{-}HT_1$, $5\text{-}HT_2$, *and* $5\text{-}HT_3$. Modulation of *adenyl cyclase* is induced by $5\text{-}HT_{1A}$ receptors postsynaptically in the hippocampus and by inhibition of uptake of adenyl cyclase presynaptically in the raphe nucleus. $5\text{-}HT_2$ receptors in the 4th cortical layer are associated with *phosphoinositol* hydrolysis. *5-HT3* receptors can be found presynaptically in the *nucleus tractus solitarius*. Many psychoactive drugs use the 5-HT receptors. These include LSD and the *entheogens* psilocybin (from psychedelic mushrooms) and dimethyltryptamine (DMT).

Cholinergic receptors are categorized as *nicotinic 1* (N_1) in the autonomic ganglia and in the adrenal medulla; and *nicotinic 2* (N_2) in skeletal muscle, and *muscarinic 1* (M_1) in the cerebral cortex, corpus striatum, hippocampus, and autonomic nervous system, and *muscarinic 2* (M_2) in the heart, intestinal smooth muscle, rhombencephalon, cerebellum, and autonomic nervous system [258]. *Muscarinic 3* (M_3) receptors are widely distributed including many glands [259, 260]. *Muscarinic 4* (M_4) receptors seem to be inhibitory [261]. *Muscarinic 5* (M_5) receptors seem to be involved in circuits involving dopamine; otherwise, very little is presently known about its physiological role [262, 263]. Briefly, the *nicotinic receptors* are composed of five units wrapped around a central cavity [264]. These receptors are classified as either muscular or neuronal types based on the tissues in which they are expressed. A 2018 comprehensive review of the structure and function of nicotinic acetylcholine receptors can be found in [265].

GABA receptors are classified as $GABA_A$, which activate chloride channels, and $GABA_B$, which induce cyclic AMP formation. Benzodiazepines act on $GABA_A$. More about $GABA_A$ can be found in the discussion about benzodiazepines below.

Glutamate excitatory receptors are usually classified into three types. (1) NMDA receptors that bind NMDA, glycine, magnesium ions, and zinc. (2) Non-NMDA receptors that are permeable to sodium and potassium but not calcium ions. (3) Receptors that bind phencyclidine (PCP or angel dust) and influence the influx of sodium, potassium, and calcium ions. Another classification scheme suggests 4 types: NMDA receptors, quisqualate/AMPA receptors, kainate receptors, and the AMPA metabotropic receptors. Each of these has distinctive properties and differences in speed and strength of signal transmission.

Three Possibilities Can Now Occur

1. The neurotransmitter may be degraded by an enzyme, or it diffuses into the surrounding tissues.
2. It may be reuptaken by the presynaptic cell.
3. If it is bound to a receptor on the body, dendrite, or axon of the postsynaptic cell, neurotransmission may result, but only if sufficient neurotransmitters are bound in an appropriate time and space continuum to reach a threshold effect on the postsynaptic cell.

These first two will not result in neurotransmission. Whichever interaction occurs, the neurotransmitter-receptor interaction ends quickly to allow for a subsequent transmission.

In the *presynaptic* cell, two transportation systems work in tandem. One system is a *plasma membrane pump*. It is dependent on ATP to provide energy for the active reuptake of neurotransmitters from the synaptic cleft once the neurotransmitter has been secreted. This recycling helps to terminate the activation of the postsynaptic cell, restocks the neurotransmitter supply, and, when the transmitter is glutamate, it prevents toxicity that could be caused by a surfeit of glutamate. The second system is a *vesicle-bound pump* deriving energy from cytoplasmic pH and a voltage gradient across the vesicular membrane. It concentrates the neurotransmitter into the vesicle for future exocytosis. Problems with the vesicular pump can occur when a lack of oxygen or blood supply occurs to the neuron. The result can be a leaky vesicle such that glutamate can reach a toxic intracellular level.

Neurotransmitter transportation for regulation, endocytosis, and recycling is closely controlled by sodium and chloride-dependent transporters in the SLC6 gene family [266]. Apparently, constitutively and in response to psychological stimulation, neuronal activity, and receptor activation, the levels of expression of the membrane transporters are dynamically changed.

A detailed discussion about the tripartite synapse can be found at [267].

The Limbic System

The *limbic system* is a heterogeneous collection of *pairs* of structures near the border (Latin limbus = border) of the medial wall of the temporal lobe, at the junction of the hemispheres with the diencephalon and the brain stem. See Fig. 7.3.

In clinical studies and experimental reports, there is a prodigious amount of reference to limbic functions, structures, and systems. The concept of limbic system functions is one of the bedrocks of behavioral medicine. Functionally, it is a system considered to be integral to control and modulation of affect, memory, motivation, and reward. However, over

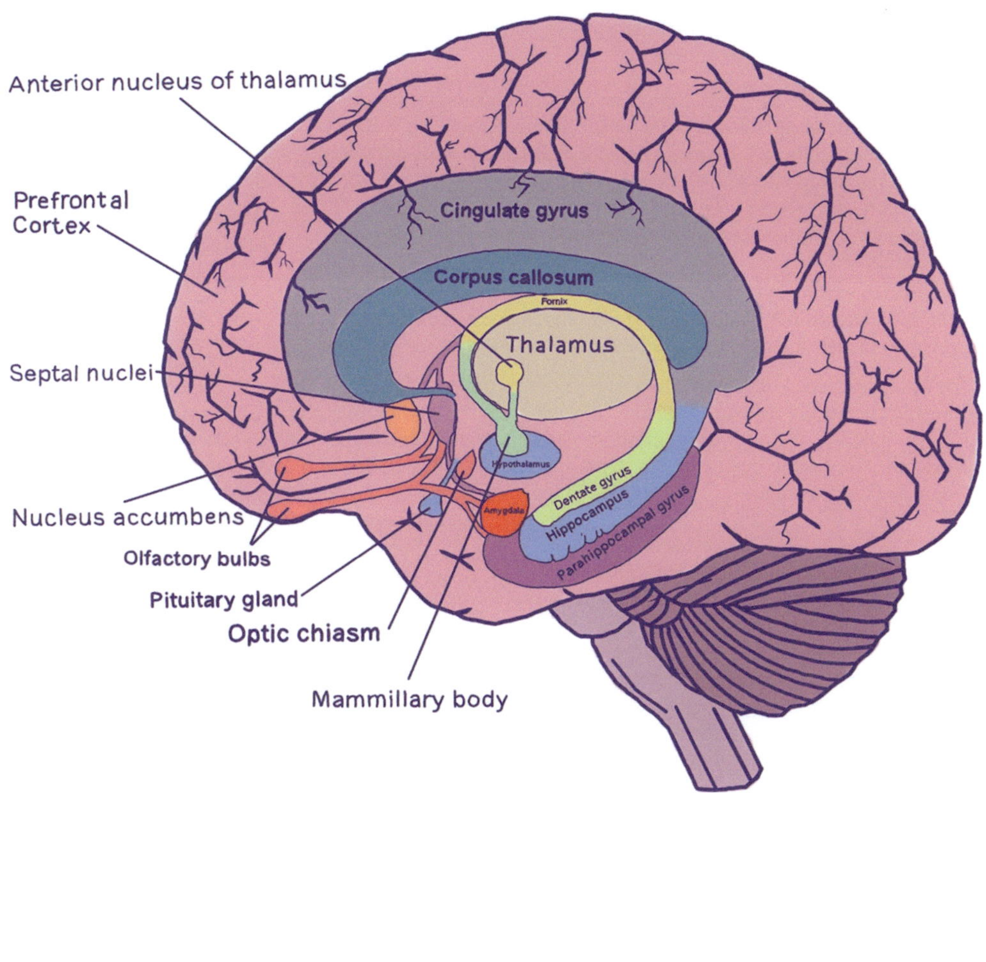

Fig. 7.3 Key structures of the limbic system. This illustration highlights major components of the limbic system, including the anterior nucleus of the thalamus, prefrontal cortex, septal nuclei, nucleus accumbens, olfactory bulbs, pituitary gland, optic chiasm, and mammillary body. These interconnected structures support emotional regulation, reward processing, memory formation, and neuroendocrine signaling, reflecting the integrative role of the limbic system in linking cognitive and affective states

the last several decades, advances in methodological research and attributions of structure to function have resulted in rather imprecise, divergent, partially unrelated, and partially contradictory definitions [268, 269]. [8]

The limbic system has also been said to integrate emotions by mediating between the hypothalamic monitoring and responding to internal cues, and the cerebral cortex cognitive component.

For our purposes, we will take a bit deeper look at the amygdala and the hippocampus.

The *hippocampus* (Greek = seahorse) and *amygdala* (Greek = almond, Latin = tonsil) have similar, but not identical, functions. The hippocampus and the amygdala can pinch hit for each other in learning object recognition; however, the hippocampus seems to be more important for learning spatial arrangements. The word most often associated with the *hippocampus* is probably *memory*. Memory loss can occur with damage to the hippocampus. The hippocampus is vital for *declarative memory (*long-term conscious memory of facts and knowledge), but it is not needed for *memory storage*, *procedural memory* (long-term unconscious memory of things such as skills), or *working memory*.[9]

It has been frequently said that the one word to associate with the *amygdala* is *fear*. It is responsible for associating a learned sensory stimulus with an adaptive response, for example, driving a car in an area of intermittent black ice. The amygdala receives somewhat highly processed sensory input from all the cortical sensory systems so that it can recognize the dangerous elements. Most of this information comes via the visual, auditory, and somatosensory cortices. For our example: Its cold, it's winter, it's still dark, here comes a bridge over a creek, we hear tires crunching on the pavement, and we can feel the car start to slide. The outputs relative to the amygdala are to the autonomic nervous system to ramp up sympathetic response via the hypothalamus and brainstem nuclei. Our physical response is our heart rate speeds up, we sweat, our pupils dilate, and more blood rushes to our muscles. And the amygdala, via its direct and extensive connections with the frontal cortex, medial striatum, and the mediodorsal thalamus, is involved in conscious emotional responses and mood. Indeed, the same areas of the amygdala that receive sensory input relay messages to the hypothalamus where it seems to influence mood and motivation. In our example, depending upon the efficiency of our reactions, we might feel panic, and later, relief mixed with heightened alert or anxiety and dread.

The amygdala connects to the thalamus via a memory-related system and may mediate the association of memories that have been received through the potpourri of sensory input. In 2003, a review was published on the types of stimuli that bring the amygdala online and the functional consequences of its involvement [277]. Their conclusions are as follows:

1. Exposure to aversive stimuli from multiple sensory modes engages the amygdala.
2. Adverse stimuli consistently engage the amygdala. Positive stimuli engage the amygdala much less consistently.

[8]According to the *Encyclopedia of the Neurological Sciences 2014* [270], the following structures are most frequently said to be *components of the limbic system*:

- Cingulate gyrus with cingulum bundle
- Hippocampus, including indusium griseum, dentate gyrus, and fornix (Latin for arch)
- Parahippocampal gyrus, including the entorhinal cortex
- Amygdala
- Septal nuclei
- Parts of the thalamus and hypothalamus (specifically those connected with the above structures).

Components such as gyrus fornicatus and olfactory systems are commonly considered together with other limbic categories. Some experts believe that both the structural and functional concepts are too vague and too comprehensive to serve any useful purpose [271–274]. But the controversy seems to be more about the formulation of heuristic ideas and precise terminology rather than the existence of a limbic system [275, 276].

So, Kotter, writing in the *Encyclopedia of the Neurological Sciences 2003* [269], makes the following well-considered recommendations, based upon the latest research, for using limbic system terminology:

1. Identify the exact structures, functions, or mechanisms that are meant when using the word "limbic."
2. When possible, use a different, more precise term than limbic. For example, for limbic inputs, use the term afferents from the amygdala and hippocampus.
3. Be on the lookout for limbic being used as a popular catch phrase or as shorthand in titles and abstracts. Look to see if it is being used as a global term for a unimodal description.
4. Do not invoke a limbic system concept to explain or build new hypotheses. Often, the underlying areas and their relationships to functions are not sufficiently understood to be used in precise hypotheses.
5. It would be a mistake to equate the limbic system concepts with detailed scientific explanations. Their best use may be to guide us to unanswered questions in brain research, for example, mechanisms of emotions, consciousness, or the self.

[9]The hippocampus is usually considered to be divided into 5 or more sections. There are the *cornu ammones* (L. horn of a ram) designated *CA1*, *CA2*, and *CA3*; the *dentate gyrus*, and the *subiculum*. The subiculum is at the base of the hippocampus and is continuous with the *entorhinal cortex*, which is part of the *parahippocampal gyrus*. Memory is born somewhere in a loop from the sensory cortex through the hippocampus and back to the sensory cortex. The *perforant path* is the point of input to the hippocampus. It is so named as it perforates the area between the dentate gyrus and the subiculum. These fibers then synapse on the neurons of the dentate nucleus which sends axons (*mossy fibers*: neurons with bulbous terminals) to synapse on the CA3 which sends axons (called *Schaeffer collaterals*) to CA1 which sends axons to the subiculum. The exit point of information from the hippocampus is the subiculum. The subiculum sends axons via the fornix to the mammillary bodies and directly to the hypothalamus. And the subiculum sends axons to the entorhinal cortex, which connects back to the sensory cortex.

3. Arousal level, hedonic strength, and current motivational value of the stimulus modulate amygdala responses.
4. Amygdala responses rapidly habituate (i.e., diminish response to repeated stimuli).
5. Subject populations and stimulus categories determine the temporal characteristics of the amygdala response.
6. We do not need to be conscious of emotionally charged stimuli for the amygdala to become engaged.
7. Conscious hedonic appraisals do not need amygdala engagement.
8. When the amygdala is engaged, it is associated with the modulation of autonomic functions, motor preparedness, and cognitive processes such as attention and memory.
9. Traditional models of lateralization of emotions do not apply to amygdala activation.
10. Factors such as psychiatric status, gender, and personality influence the extent and laterality of amygdala activations.

Executive Functions: Prefrontal Cortex and Anterior Cingulate Gyrus

The *prefrontal cortex* is involved in expressing personality, implementing socially correct behavior, and planning complex cognitive actions [278]. Its divisions are the lateral, orbitofrontal, and medial prefrontal areas, each of which appears to have distinctive functions [279]. Histologically, it is composed principally of internal granular layer IV. The prefrontal cortex is extensively interconnected with the reticular activating system and the limbic system. This suggests reliance on alertness and important interactions with emotional centers of the brain.

The central *executive function* describes the functions of the prefrontal cortex. These functions include thinking flexibly, problem solving, planning, concept formation, abstract thinking, creativity, inhibition, and impulse control [280]. Working memory and attention are usually considered to be essential for proper executive functioning [281, 282]. The prefrontal cortex is involved in working memory in humans [283] and is often considered to be a cognitive executive that, in general, controls and manages the selection of actions and other cognitive processes [284]. Lesions of the prefrontal cortex often interfere with the ability to delay gratification.

The *anterior cingulate gyrus* is associated with the executive functions and has extensive connections to the frontal, temporal, and parietal cortices, as well as the entorhinal association cortexes and the amygdala. The anterior cingulate cortex is often considered to be an interface between emotion and cognition [285]. The anterior cingulate cortex is the area where emotions are integrated with emotional self-control, focused problem solving, recognition of errors, and adapting responses to fit changing conditions.

Depression and the Stress Response

Hans Selye first used the word stress to describe a syndrome produced by "Diverse Nocuous Agents" or insults that might perturb the balance of the body's internal milieu or homeostasis [101]. Although ambiguity exists in the definition of *stress* in biological systems, stress may be most often defined as a physical or psychological stimulus that produces disequilibrium or strain in an individual such that the body must initiate the stress response in an attempt to restore homeostasis.

The Brain's Role

Real-world stress can be as mild as standing up from a seated position or as intense as a life-threatening assault. For both physical stress and psychological stress, the brain is the master and commander [286]. The brain determines when the internal balance has been disrupted, and the brain regulates the nervous, endocrine, and immune systems to restore equilibrium. [10]

In the case of psychological stress as well as physical stress, the brain is monitoring a state of internal balance. However, what the brain is monitoring relative to psychological stress is the balance of perceived resources to perceived demands of a given situation [288–294].

For example, if a student has a major exam that will require 20 h of studying to do well (demand), and she only has 6 h to study (resources), she will feel stressed. Make the demands greater (her chances of getting a good grade in the class and going to graduate school depend on it) or the resources less (she also must work 2 h at her work-study job during the 6 h she has to study), and the stress becomes greater.

[10]For example, to sense a remote immune response to a novel antigen (e.g., a virus or vaccine), the brain has receptors for cytokines, such as interleukin 1 (IL-1), released by monocytes when they first encounter and phagocytose the antigen for presentation to T cells. These cytokines travel to the brain, where, based upon information such as the dose of cytokines, the brain may then determine if a systemic response is warranted. If a response is needed, the brain communicates via the autonomic nervous system to immune system organs, and by way of neurotransmitters (such as acetylcholine, norepinephrine, and histamine) modifies the activity of immune system cells. In addition, neuroendocrine molecules such as substance P, leptin, and corticotropin-releasing hormone regulate cytokine production. Results of this type of communication may include inducing fever, promoting production of heat shock proteins or acute phase reactants, or recruitment of additional immune system cells [287].

For several reasons, different stressors may produce different levels of stress in different people. For example, there may be differences in individual resources, including time, money, friends, information, training, tools, or physical objects. These differences, coupled with sex, age, pregnancy, lactation, and lifestyle variables (such as alcohol, tobacco, and caffeine use), our genes and epigenetic programming, and our life experiences (especially early childhood experiences), help to determine how stressful we perceive a situation to be [295].

Acute and Chronic Stress

Another important factor influencing one's experience or perception of a stressor is the duration and course of the stressor (e.g., discrete or acute vs. continuous or chronic). Both acute stress and chronic stress seem to depress some measures of immune response [296]. However, the type and duration of stressor (acute vs. chronic) can have different effects on the immune system [297, 298]. Many acute stressors that last for only a few minutes may produce adaptive increases in some parts of innate immunity, but a decrease in some measures of adaptive immunity. Chronic stressors in general seem to suppress both cellular and humoral immunity.

Chronic stressors, combined with genetic variances among individuals (e.g., single nucleotide polymorphisms of glucocorticoid receptors [299]], may result in initiation of disease or exacerbation of an already existing illness. Chronic stressors appear to interact with genetic and epigenetic factors to increase the risk of depression [218, 300–308].

The effects of stress on immunity and neuroendocrine modulation of the immune system have been studied in relationship to disease onset and progression [22, 309–311]. For example, several studies have shown that chronic stress can contribute to the etiology of or exacerbate cardiovascular disease, type 2 diabetes, arthritis, periodontal disease, Alzheimer's disease, osteoporosis, and frailty with aging. Chronic stress has also been shown to increase the risk of particular infections (e.g., reactivation of latent herpes virus) and even some cancers (e.g., ovarian [312] and squamous cell carcinoma [313]) [22, 314].

How does stress influence the above effects on the human body and on disease onset and progression? Some of the effects of stress on the human body and on disease onset and progression are discussed below in terms of interactions between the peripheral stress system, the central stress system, critical development periods, psychosocial aspects, immune responses, and genetics [315, 316].

Stress Systems

The *stress system* includes a complex interplay of interconnected areas of the brain [317]. The primary areas involved in the stress response are the hypothalamus, amygdala, and hippocampus. This system receives input from the higher cortical centers, somatic and visceral afferents. Its output to the neuroendocrine and immune systems is principally through the hypothalamus (especially the hypothalamic pituitary adrenal axis) and the autonomic nervous system.

A web of integrative structures in the brain generates the stress response [315–320]. *The principal generators* are subregions of the hypothalamus (e.g., the paraventricular nucleus), the amygdala, and the periaqueductal gray matter. *Input* to these structures comes from various sources: cortical areas, somatic and visceral afferents, and from fluid sources of blood and lymph. The main cortical areas include the medial prefrontal cortex and subregions of the insular cortex and the anterior cingulate. *Output* from the generators flows to the pituitary and the nuclei of the pontomedullary area. The pituitary mediates neuroendocrine communication with the rest of the body. And, the pontomedullary nuclei mediate autonomic output.

Feedback to the generators is accomplished via neural signals and products carried in the circulatory system. Monoadrenergic fibers ascend from various pontomedullary nuclei, especially from the noradrenergic nuclei (e.g., the locus coeruleus) and serotonergic nuclei (e.g., the raphe nuclei). Circulating molecules such as glucocorticoids and corticotropin-releasing hormone (CRH), and cytokines from various sources interact with receptors in various parts of the CNS. This includes glucocorticoid receptors in the hippocampus and prefrontal cortex.

To look a bit deeper, we will discuss the stress response, input, and output in terms of the artificial constructs of a peripheral stress system and a central stress system.

Peripheral Stress System

The *peripheral stress system* in response to environmental perturbation (e.g., a virus enters the body, a threat is perceived) is engaged in part via neurosensory and limbic signals carried by molecules in the circulatory system. The peripheral stress system is composed of the *hypothalamic-pituitary-adrenal (HPA) axis, systemic adrenomedullary system (SAS)*, and the *sympathetic nervous system (SNS)*. The SAS and SNS are often lumped together as the *sympathetic adrenal medullary (SAM) system.*

Back in the 1970s, the pituitary was considered the master gland. Today, many endocrinologists recognize a new master. It is the *hypothalamus*. The hypothalamus is usually spoken of as part of the triumvirate consisting of the hypothalamus-pituitary-adrenal axis, but it is more powerful than that association. Through its relationship with the entire central nervous system (CNS) and the pituitary, it has much more influence than just control of the adrenal functions. In addition to its role with the endocrine system, it activates and controls that part of the nervous system that is in charge of vegetative body functions.

The *hypothalamus* (Greek: hypo = below, thalamus = bed (room)) is the smaller part of the diencephalon and right above the mesencephalon (you may wish to refer to the *Compendium Background Volume* [*Link*] section on the nervous system for explanations of the diencephalon and mesencephalon). It receives information from all the CNS, massages it, and sends pertinent information to the pituitary gland and other tissues. Its ventral surface has, from top to bottom, the *optic chiasma*, the *infundibulum* (Latin = funnel) that connects to the *posterior lobe of the pituitary*, and the *mammillary bodies*. The hypothalamus influences moods, sexual development, sleep, and motivational states. Stimulation of the *lateral hypothalamus* may result in anger, dilation of skin blood vessels, and decreased shivering, resulting in lowered body temperature. The lateral hypothalamus also contains the feeding center. The *medial hypothalamus* contains the satiety center. Stimulation of the *posterior hypothalamus* generates and conserves heat. The *suprachiasmatic nucleus* influences circadian rhythms.

The *pituitary* (Latin for phlegm) is also called the *hypophysis* (Greek for undergrowth) as it is suspended by the infundibulum from the base of the hypothalamus. The pituitary is a tiny gland about the size of a pea. It is divided into the anterior and the posterior lobes or hypophyses.

Through its *neurological link* with the *posterior hypophysis (neurohypophysis)*, the hypothalamus is vitally involved with autonomic nervous system functions, such as, regulation of heart rate, body temperature, and metabolism. Indeed, the neurohypophysis is a collection of axons that arise from cell bodies located in the hypothalamus. Some of these axons also store two neuropeptide hormones *vasopressin (antidiuretic hormone (ADH) or arginine vasopressin (AVP))*, and *oxytocin* that are produced in the *supraoptic* and *paraventricular* nuclei of the hypothalamus.

ADH enhances water conservation and, at high concentrations, causes vasoconstriction. Its main stimulus is the increased osmotic pressure of body water sensed by *osmoreceptors* in the hypothalamus. Secondarily, volume depletion is sensed by *baroreceptors* in the aortic arch, left atrium, carotid sinus, and pulmonary veins, and transmitted to the brainstem and the hypothalamus via vagal and glossopharyngeal nerves. ADH release is stimulated by dopamine and angiotensin II. ADH release is inhibited by opioid peptides. Norepinephrine, depending upon the context, can either stimulate or inhibit ADH release.

ADH-containing neurons also project to the brainstem, forebrain, and to the median eminence of the adenohypophysis, where they facilitate the release of *adrenocorticotropic hormone (ACTH)*. ADH is also found in several non-nervous system tissues, including the thymus.

In addition to the hypothalamus and pituitary, *oxytocin* is found in other regions of the CNS, for example, in the pineal gland. And it is also produced in non-CNS tissue, such as the thymus and the gonads. Oxytocin is not found in the same neurons as ADH. Both catecholamine and cholinergic neurons can affect oxytocin release, but their effects are dependent upon the receptors being activated. For example, norepinephrine stimulation of α receptors increases oxytocin release, whereas stimulation of β receptors decreases release. The most familiar and predominant stimulus for oxytocin release is suckling.

The hypothalamus is involved with the pituitary via *special vascular connections* with the *anterior lobe of the pituitary hypophysis (adenohypophysis)*. It regulates both the production and secretion of the major peptide hormones of the adenohypophysis. The adenohypophysis then regulates many of the other endocrine glands. Several of these regulators are also produced in the peripheral tissues, especially in the gastrointestinal tract, where they have paracrine effects (e.g., vasoactive intestinal peptide, which stimulates water and electrolyte secretion, and inhibits gastrin secretion). Several of the hypothalamic regulators control more than one pituitary hormone.

The *major* six adenohypophyseal hormones are *adrenocorticotropic hormone (ACTH), thyroid-stimulating hormone (TSH), luteinizing hormone (LH), follicle-stimulating hormone (FSH), growth hormone (GH), and prolactin*. A feedback loop exists between the hypothalamus-adenohypophysis system and the products of the target tissues (e.g., thyroid, gonads, and adrenal cortex). Several of these peptide hormones are formed from a precursor called *pro-opiomelanocortin (POMC)*. These hormones include *ACTH, melanocyte-stimulating hormone (MSH), endorphins,* and *enkephalins*. The endorphins and enkephalins can bind to and activate various opioid receptors throughout the CNS and can ease perception of pain. LH, FSH, TSH, and *human chorionic gonadotropin* are all glycoproteins composed of two subunits: an identical α unit and differing β unit.

Adrenal glands are two triangular structures, one on top of each kidney. Functionally, they are two glands in one. The outer portion, the *adrenal cortex,* produces three steroid hormones. The inner portion, the *adrenal medulla*, is sometimes considered a part of the sympathetic nervous system. The adrenal medulla produces *catecholamines* such as epinephrine, which increases heart rate and blood pressure when we feel stress. The steroids produced by the cortex are the mineralocorticoids, the glucocorticoids, and the gonadotropins. The most potent *mineralocorticoid* is *aldosterone*. Mineralocorticoids control the balance of water and minerals, principally by increasing potassium and hydrogen loss in exchange for sodium reabsorption in the kidney. The principal and most potent *glucocorticoid* is *cortisol (hydrocortisone)*. Cortisol controls many aspects of metabolism and buffers stress, such as those arising from infections, hemorrhaging, and trauma. Most glucocorticoids have some mineralocorticoid activity as well, and vice versa. *Gonadotropins,* principally adrenal androgens, are hormones involved in sexual functions and may contribute to the beginning of puberty.

The HPA and SAM systems increase arousal and attention, alert the amygdala, which is involved in fear, and stimulate the mesocorticolimbic dopaminergic system, which is part of the anticipatory and reward pathways but helps the individual to cognitively cope with stress [321]. The HPA axis and SAM system produce stress-related hormones, including the catecholamines (epinephrine and norepinephrine), cortisol, ACTH and the proopiomelanocortin-derived peptides (alpha-melanocyte-stimulating hormone and the endorphins), growth hormone, arginine vasopressin, and prolactin [319]. Many of these stress-related hormones have a direct influence on the immune system. The overall and localized effects of these hormones may be negative or positive depending on a space-time context [298].

Cortisol and CRH

Elevated cortisol levels in response to stress have been found to adversely affect several immune system functions [322, 323]. Cortisol directly inhibits pituitary gonadotropin, growth hormone, and thyrotropin secretion and induces a resistant state in the target tissues of these hormones [324]. Cortisol, in its role as a glucocorticoid, also inhibits insulin actions on skeletal muscle and increases insulin activity on adipose tissue, along with increasing hepatic gluconeogenesis. In addition, cortisol directly inhibits osteoblastic functions and promotes osteoporosis. Some researchers believe that once cortisol levels rise, they can initiate, maintain, or magnify depression and depression associated symptoms, such as poor memory, poor quality sleep, and anxiety [325].

However, cortisol functions are complex, such that depending upon the target, permissive, stimulative, and inhibitive properties of cortisol are dependent upon both context and timing [218, 298–327].

Pregnancy and postpartum are times of high susceptibility to MDD and other mood disorders [328]. A 2016 systematic review of perinatal maternal depression and cortisol function in pregnancy and the postpartum period found that the *cortisol awakening response*[11] is positively associated with momentary mood states but is blunted in MDD [335]. Data suggested that hypercortisolemia is linked to transient depressive states and hypocortisolemia is related to chronic postpartum depression.

Infants exposed to both low and high levels of antenatal maternal depression showed, in a "U" shaped curve, greater cortisol reactivity to immunizations [336].[12] A 2014 prospective longitudinal study of a possible association between salivary cortisol and subsequent depression has concluded that their findings do not support the hypothesis that elevated salivary cortisol increases the short-term risk of subsequent depressive illness [337].

Corticotropin-releasing hormone (CRH: also called corticotropin-releasing factor (CRF) is a critical regulatory element integrating and controlling much of neuroendocrine, autonomic, and behavioral responses to both normal living and physical and psychological stress [338–341]. People who have genetic or epigenetic imbalances in this network may be predisposed to various diseases when they encounter adversity [342–344]. These include depression, anxiety, addictions, neurodegenerative diseases, neuroendocrine and immunological disorders [345].

CRH, as a neuromodulator, does not modify synaptic strength or efficacy. Instead, it facilitates or depresses the effects of neurotransmitters within specific neuronal circuits [346, 347]. In addition to its role in the HPA axis, CRH neurons connect to the hippocampus and amygdala, directly affecting anxiety and depression [348]. Overexpression of CRH can induce stress and an anxiety phenotype [349] while

[11] The *cortisol awakening response* (CAR) is the pronounced increase in cortisol secretion over the first 30–45 min after morning awakening [329]. It has been associated with a wide range of psychosocial, physical, and mental health parameters. It appears to be influenced by factors that include gender, health status, and health behavior or stress perception [330]. Greater depressive symptoms have been associated with a greater CAR. However, depressive symptoms were linked to a shorter sleep time [331]. While greater depressive symptoms were associated with an elevated CAR among females, they were associated with a blunted CAR among males [332]. Sleep quality has a complex relationship with CAR [333]. In some sleep studies, due to at-home sampling, sample timing inaccuracies may plague results [334].

[12] The production of corticotropin-releasing hormone (CRH) during stress inhibits immune, reproduction, growth, and thyroid functions by inhibiting gonadotropin-releasing hormone secretion, growth hormone (via increasing somatostatin), and thyrotropin (via decreasing thyroid-releasing hormone) [322, 323]. However, in some localized responses, CRH can provoke pro-inflammatory cytokine production and stimulation of mast cells to release histamines [298]. CRH can also have a direct effect on the limbic system and may influence its effects on the HPA axis [346].

suppressing CRH can be anxiolytic [350, 351]. Environmental factors such as stress and diet can, through a complex network, result in the DNA sequences that control the expression of CRH being exposed for a shorter or longer time for transcription [352][13].

Transcription is a temporal-spatial-based phenomenon. In acute stress responses, transcription factors and nuclear regulatory proteins may turn on or off CRH and CRH receptors in different targets and last only a matter of hours or days before being reset. In prolonged stress, epigenetic mechanisms may change the set point of the switches to leave them on or off for a longer duration.

SNS Innervation

It has long been known that every immune organ in the body, including the bone marrow, is highly innervated by the SNS [353–357], and that this innervation has functional significance, tightly regulating (enhancing or suppressing) immune function. [14]

Increased stress is associated with increased salivary monoamine oxidase (MAO) A and B inhibitory activity [359]. MAO inhibitors inhibit the activity of monoamine oxidase that would normally break down the monoamine neurotransmitters, such as epinephrine, norepinephrine, serotonin, and the trace amines. Thus, with the inhibition of MAO, these neurotransmitters are functionally more available in the synapse.

It has been speculated that the stress-related increased incidence of chronic inflammatory diseases and susceptibility to infections may be due to dysregulations of the neuroendocrine system with increased activity of the HPA axis and the SAM axis, and decreased sex hormones [360]. Of course, there is a dose-response relationship between stress and these effects; however, the nature of this relationship is not yet transparent [360–363]. It is possible that epigenetic and genetic vulnerability will account for much of the variance in individual susceptibility [299]. Another source of variance in individual susceptibility is exposure to stressors during critical developmental periods [364].

[13]A 2017 detailed review of CRH can be found in Endocrinology and the brain: corticotropin-releasing hormone signaling [329].

[14]For example, SNS innervation of bone marrow happens immediately before the onset of hematopoiesis in utero [353], and growth of early hematopoietic progenitor cells is impaired in patients with spinal cord injury who have interrupted transmission of SNS activity below the site of the injury [358]. Animal studies have shown that sympathetic innervation of the bone marrow modulates proliferation and mobilization of hematopoietic stem cells in the bone marrow microenvironment [5]. Taken together, these data provide strong evidence that alterations in SNS tone (e.g., in response to a stressor) may influence proliferation and mobilization of hematopoietic stem cells.

Central Stress System

The *central stress system* is those areas of the CNS dealing with cognitive higher functions that influence the peripheral system [320, 365]. These areas include the prefrontal cortex that integrates and mediates cognition and affects [365–367]. The prefrontal cortex interfaces with the paraventricular nucleus of the hypothalamus, which controls the HPA axis and the SAM axis.

When the central stress system is shifted to a higher level by stress, it results in behavioral and peripheral responses that favor survival and that are critical for adaptive psychosocial functioning and health. However, when the central stress system operates at an excessively high level, malfunctions may occur. For example, malfunctioning stress responses have been linked to inadequate growth and development, and mental health disorders [368]. Manifestations of disease are generally the result of environment, genetic vulnerability, and timing.

Inescapable stress resulting in conditions, such as excessive worry, anxiety, and depression, is often associated with problems in neuroendocrine and immune responses. For example, worry may affect the immune response to phobic fear. In one study, subjects with high scores of worry did not show a normal circadian rise in NK cells [369]. In affective disorders such as depression and anxiety in humans, there is persistent HPA activation, often measured by elevated urinary corticosteroid over a 24-h period [370].

Further evidence from studies in rats suggests that neuroendocrine changes persist for days rather than hours following intense stressors [371]. In rats, 24-h elevation of urinary corticosterone persists for 3 days after intense stress [372]. After single or repeated exposures to mild restraint and inescapable tail shock, circadian trough corticosterone levels were elevated for 3–5 days, adrenal and prolactin levels were persistently elevated for 24 h, and thyroid and reproductive hormones were inhibited for 24 h. The effects were not assessed for a longer.

The concept of *limbic system functions* is one of the foundations of behavioral medicine. Functionally, it is a system considered to be integral to control and modulation of affect, memory, motivation, and reward. It is a heterogeneous collection of structures that have been variously defined. It is usually said to include the cingulate gyrus, hippocampus, parahippocampal nuclei, amygdala, septal nuclei, and parts of the thalamus and hypothalamus. The limbic system appears to integrate emotions by mediating between the hypothalamic functions of monitoring and responding to internal cues and the cognitive component of the cerebral cortex.

The *septal region of the basal forebrain* appears to have at least two principal roles [373]. The septal nuclei facilitate a variety of cognitive functions that involve the hippocampus.

It does this by changing the excitability of the hippocampus, and thereby aiding the plasticity of hippocampal circuits. In so doing, it lessens the possibility of the hippocampus becoming abnormally excited.

When the central stress system is shifted to a higher level by stress, it results in behavioral and peripheral responses that favor survival. HPA and SAM systems increase arousal and attention, alert the amygdala, which is involved in fear, and stimulate the mesocorticolimbic dopaminergic system, which is part of the anticipatory and reward pathways but helps the individual to cognitively cope with the stress [321].

Corticotropin-releasing hormone (CRH) organizes and orchestrates endocrine, autonomic, behavioral, and immune responses to stress [317]. In addition, CRH integrates central nervous system responses to stress by acting as a neurotransmitter or neuromodulator in the amygdala, dorsal raphe nucleus, hippocampus, and locus coeruleus.

During stress, CRH inhibits reproduction, growth, and thyroid functions by inhibiting gonadotropin-releasing hormone secretion, growth hormone (via somatostatin), and thyrotropin (via thyroid-releasing hormone). Cortisol directly inhibits pituitary gonadotropin, growth hormone, and thyrotropin secretion and induces a resistant state in the target tissues of these hormones [324]. Cortisol, in its role as a glucocorticoid, also inhibits insulin actions on skeletal muscle and increases insulin activity on adipose tissue, along with increasing hepatic gluconeogenesis. Cortisol directly inhibits osteoblastic functions and promotes osteoporosis. Glucocorticoids may suppress CRH in the hypothalamus, while they may stimulate CRH in the amygdala. And CRH and cortisol may act synergistically (e.g., in acoustic startle responses). CRH has been said to have strong *kindling* properties, while cortisol has potent *consolidating* abilities in producing stress-related disorders [368, 374]. Kindling is the phenomenon of producing a relatively profound change in brain function from repetitive electrical or chemical stimulation. It was first applied to the experimental production of epilepsy. Here, it refers to sensitizing the related targets to the effects of stress or starting the fire, while cortisol is the fuel that maintains the fire. As a consolidator, once cortisol levels rise, they may, as mentioned above, initiate, maintain, or magnify depression and depression associated symptoms such as poor memory, poor quality sleep, and anxiety [325].

Of course, there is a dose-response relationship between stress and these effects. Genetic vulnerability may account for much of the variance in susceptibility [299].

It has been speculated that the increased incidence of chronic inflammatory diseases and susceptibility to infections may be due to dysregulations of the endocrine system with increased activity of the HPA axis and decreased sex hormones [360]. One experiment has shown that in elderly men, stress-induced increases in cortisol did not differ significantly between groups, but *sensitivity* to glucocorticoids increased significantly in young controls and testosterone-treated elderly men, while it decreased in non-treated elderly men (F[15] = 5.28, $p<0.01$). The researchers suggest that increased sensitivity to glucocorticoids after stress may protect us from stress-induced pro-inflammatory cytokines, and that this mechanism is disturbed in elderly men and is partially restored by testosterone.

Salivary *monoamine oxidase (MAO) A and B inhibitory activities* correlate with stress. MAO inhibitors inhibit the activity of monoamine oxidase that would normally break down the monoamine neurotransmitters such as epinephrine, norepinephrine, serotonin, and the trace amines. Thus, with the inhibition of MAO, the neurotransmitters are functionally more available in the synapse. Increased stress is associated with increased MAO A and B inhibitory activity [359]. In a stress experiment, MAO A inhibitory activity peaked at the end of the stress, and cortisol levels peaked 12 minutes after the end of the stress [375]. The amount of MAO inhibitory activity positively predicted the subsequent amount of cortisol rise. It is possible that increased monoamines due to the inhibition of their main metabolic enzyme for central monoamines can activate the HPA axis in the stress response [376]. Salivary IgA shows a similar circadian variation to that of cortisol [377]. Upon waking, salivary IgA and MAO inhibitor peaks, followed within the first ½ hour by cortisol [376]. Salivary IgA begins to fall as cortisol rises and becomes stable 6 h after awakening. Urinary output of endogenous MAO inhibitory activity is related to daily stress: increased MAO inhibitory activity in the urine in normal healthy people seems to be indicative of a relatively enduring state of everyday stress [378].

Psychological modulation of the HPA axis is chiefly by way of neocortical and limbic influences on the CRH and arginine vasopressin (AVP) neurons in the paraventricular nucleus (PVN) of the hypothalamus [379].

AVP seems to have a dynamic role in cortisol release, whereas CRH is permissive; that is, AVP increases CRH stimulation of ACTH [380]. ACTH stimulates cortisol synthesis and release by interacting with *melanocortin 2 receptors (MC2R)* in the adrenal cortex. Moreover, independent of the adrenal cortex, ACTH regulates the expression of genes involved in the synthesis of norepinephrine in the sympathetic preganglionic neurons in the spinal cord [381, 382].

In depression or stress-related disorders, norepinephrine or neuropeptide Y may supersede the negative feedback of cortisol on the PVN and may stimulate an increased AVP/CRH ratio, which stimulates preganglionic sympathetic spi-

[15]An *F-test* compares variances to determine if the ratios of variances among multiple samples are significantly different. It is an important test to determine if the null hypothesis should be rejected or not. For more information, see Chap. 4 Evidence Basics.

nal neurons that increase cortisol output by the adrenal cortex [381, 383, 384].

A general assumption is that there would be a covariance with stress between activation of the CRH/AVP neurons in the PVN and linear release of ACTH and subsequent cortisol release by the adrenal cortex, but that is not what happens [385, 386]. Instead, covariance between psychological measurements of stress and levels of salivary cortisol appears to be attributable to interactions between the AVP/CRH neurons, ACTH, sympathetic nervous system activation, and norepinephrine containing neurons of the nucleus coeruleus and the superior cervical ganglia [379].

When the central stress system is shifted to a higher level by stress, it results in behavioral and peripheral responses that favor survival and that are critical for adaptive psychosocial functioning and health. However, when the central stress system is running at a level that is too high, malfunctions may result. For example, malfunctioning stress responses have been linked to inadequate growth and development, and mental health disorders [368]. Manifestations of disease are generally the result of environment, genetic vulnerability, and timing.

Inescapable stress resulting in conditions, such as excessive worry, anxiety, and depression, is often associated with problems in neuroendocrine and immune responses [369]. In affective disorders such as depression and anxiety in humans, there is persistent HPA activation, often measured by elevated urinary corticosteroid over a 24-h period [372]. [16]

Norepinephrine, locus coeruleus, and stress: Norepinephrine is a hormone, neurotransmitter, and neuromodulator. Overall, its role is to marshal the forces of the body and brain for action. During stressful situations, norepinephrine reaches high levels, often preparing for the classical fight-or-flight response. During sleep, it is at its nadir [127]. The rest of the time, norepinephrine responds with relative output to match the conditions. Norepinephrine increases heart rate and blood pressure, releases glucose from storage, and increases circulation to skeletal muscles. At the same time, norepinephrine decreases circulation to the gastrointestinal tract, decreases gastrointestinal mobility, and decreases bladder voiding of urine. In the brain, norepinephrine is arousing, increasing alertness, vigilance, and focusing attention to prepare for action. In so doing, it increases memory formation and retrieval [387]. When norepinephrine reaches higher levels, it can increase restlessness and anxiety. And if it becomes uncoupled from an appropriate response, it may lead to anxiety disorders [388] and/ or depression [389].

During intensely unpleasant conditions such as extreme fear or pain, the locus coeruleus is highly aroused [120]. This increased activity and concomitant autonomic response can arise as a spontaneous reaction or, importantly, from a behavioral adaptation standpoint, may be a conditioned response to behaviorally salient stimuli. Of note, increased activity in the locus coeruleus occurs when encountering situations that are perceived to be threatening, whether real or not.

During the experience of any situation that threatens us, the two most frequently activated systems are the hypothalamic-pituitary-adrenal system, the sympathetic nervous system, and the locus-coeruleus system [315]. Norepinephrine is central to these responses both in positive and negative feedback loops. These include the HPA sympathetic stimulation of the adrenal medulla to produce norepinephrine, and cortisol produced in the adrenal cortex that stimulates enzymatic activity to produce norepinephrine (and epinephrine).

Sustained levels of norepinephrine, such as in chronic stress, may be central to creating damage to various organs and their functions. When norepinephrine directs resources toward action, it may compromise recuperation. Results may be decreased immune responses, depression, vulnerability to addiction, decreased sleep, stunted growth, especially in children, and gastrointestinal problems [390–392]. Particularly important is the relationship between the locus coeruleus and the shift from acute to chronic pain in stress-related disorders, such as major depression and anxiety [393]. Activation and deactivation of specific projection neurons play an important role. In acute pain, the locus coeruleus-mediated ascending efferent response produces analgesia, aversion, and vigilance, whereas in chronic pain, the locus coeruleus facilitates pain via anxiety, aversive memory, and despair through its influences on the amygdala, prefrontal cortex, and medulla.

Psychosocial Aspects

A large body of evidence indicates that psychosocial stress (particularly stress resulting from interpersonal relationships and navigating one's place in the social hierarchy) can have deleterious effects on immune function and physical health. For example, chronic job-related stressors such as unemployment [394], job burnout [395, 396], and job strain [397] have all been linked to a variety of immune alterations. Job stress, social isolation, and interpersonal conflict may also influence coronary artery disease and its progression to coronary heart disease (CHD) [398], in part because sympathetic systolic reactivity to stress is associated with atherosclerosis

[16]Further evidence has been seen in rats that neuroendocrine changes persist for days, not hours, after intense stressors [370]. In rats, 24-h elevation of urinary corticosterone persists for 3 days after intense stress [371]. After single or repeated exposures to mild restraint and inescapable tail shock, circadian trough corticosterone levels were elevated for 3–5 days, adrenal and prolactin levels were persistently elevated for 24 h, and thyroid and reproductive hormones were inhibited for 24 h. The effects were not assessed for a longer time.

and hypertension. These factors may also contribute to the etiology of stroke, especially ischemic stroke [399].

Stressors in our closest social relationships have the greatest effects [400]. Chronic stress among caregivers of parents or spouses has been shown to have a negative effect on endocrine and immune function (e.g., NK cell cytotoxicity), leading to poor health, including delayed wound healing and blunted vaccine responses [401–408]. Negative marital functioning appears to have an indirect influence on health outcomes through depression and health habits, but also directly affects cardiovascular, endocrine, immune, neurosensory, and other physiological mechanisms [409].

Low *socioeconomic status (SES)* is associated with a multitude of chronic stressors and is strongly correlated with most causes of morbidity and mortality across various populations [410–414]. Obesity, depression, and diabetes are particularly related to low SES, and those who are the most socioeconomically disadvantaged have the greatest risk for poor mental and physical health. Pooled data from four large epidemiological studies found that the effects of low SES are cumulative, begin in childhood, and tend to persist and cross cultures [415]. An additional study showed that childhood socioeconomic position was associated with adult psychosocial problems of cynical hostility and hopelessness, but not depression [416]. However, in terms of cognitive function, it appears that a disadvantaged childhood can be overcome somewhat by upward mobility later in life [417, 418]. Cognitive functions in middle age and late in life may be products of unique contributions of socioeconomic conditions at various life stages.

The likelihood of repeated episodes of MDD increases with every subsequent episode [419, 420]. For example, in one series, the risk of recurrence increased by 16% with each successive recurrence [421]. Earlier episodes are more likely than later episodes to be triggered by major stressors [422, 423]. In other words, it takes less stress to trigger a subsequent episode of MDD after each episode.

Various hypotheses have attempted to explain why this increase occurs and why some people are more likely to get depressed [424–430]. Progressive vulnerability (*diathesis*) to negative life events (aka *diathesis stress*) is commonly posited [80, 81, 431, 432]. This *kindling* [422, 433] *or stress sensitization* [422, 434, 435] refers to intra-individual and inter-individual differences in thresholds of stress needed to elicit the same response and changes in magnitude of response to the same trigger. This phenomenon, called *cognitive reactivity,* is thought to be the result of activating latent negative information processing biases as a reaction to negative affect that can escalate the negative affect into the symptoms of MDD [82].

Diathesis stress is thought to arise from inadequate control of the limbic system by the prefrontal cortex, with the consequential protracted activation of the sympathetic nervous system and the amygdala as a response to stressors [436–442].

The result of this preloading is progressive, prolonged, or intensified negative affect in response to stressors (*emotional reactivity*) that may increase the risk for recurrence of MDD [429, 443]. Increased emotional reactivity to daily stress has been associated with a tendency towards depression [443–445] and poor response to treatment [446]. Inability to rebound quickly from transient negative affect following daily life stressors is associated with the development of depression symptoms [443, 447].

Postpartum depression can afflict between 10% and 18% of mothers in the Western world [448, 449]. Devastating effects can occur on the infant–mother relationship if not treated [449, 450]. Adverse developmental and behavioral effects can result [451]. SSRIs or SNRIs are often the treatment of choice [452].

When nursing mothers take antidepressants, it is unclear if they pose a risk to nursing infants [453]. Infant doses from breast milk of less than 10% of the maternal weight-adjusted dose are generally considered safe [141, 454]. Paroxetine (Paxil) and sertraline (Zoloft) reach 0.5–3% in infants' sera; however, fluoxetine (Prozac), citalopram (Celexa), and desvenlafaxine [455] appear in levels close to or above 10% [456–459]. A 2013 review states, "Newer antidepressants transfer into breast milk in low amounts and have not been associated with serious adverse events" [460, 461]. A 2017 review updates this information [462]. We will have more to say in a later section on antidepressants.

DNA methylation patterns related to hippocampal synaptic plasticity may be involved in postpartum depression as a consequence of altered sensitivity to estrogen-mediated epigenetic changes [449, 463]. It seems that postpartum depression can be predicted before birth using blood DNA methylation biomarkers related to estradiol responses in maternal blood [449].

Pathways

There are two primary pathways through which psychosocial stressors may impact physical health and/or influence physiological processes. First, people are more likely to engage in maladaptive health behaviors or habits such as smoking, excess alcohol consumption, drug abuse, decreased exercise, lack of sleep, and poor eating habits [314, 464, 465] when they are under stress. These behaviors further serve to put individuals at additional risk for the consequences of stress, which may result in compromised endocrine and immune responses and altered cardiovascular functions.

Second, our thoughts and perceptions of a particular stressor are connected to immune and endocrine function through those areas of the central nervous system that deal with higher cognitive functions. The prefrontal cortex, which integrates cognition and affect, interfaces with the limbic system (especially the amygdala and hippocampus), the cingulate gyrus, and the paraventricular nucleus of the hypothalamus, which controls the HPA and SAM axes.

Effects of Psychological Stress: Wound Healing and Cardiovascular Disease

Several studies have assessed the effects of psychological stress on wound healing [466, 467]. Negative emotions, such as feeling depressed and anxious as a reaction to stress, can increase production of proinflammatory cytokines [468–474]. Higher levels of anxiety (fear and distress) prior to surgery have been linked to more complicated and slower recovery. Part of the explanation for that connection is delayed wound healing associated with stress. Additionally, the adverse effects of pain on the endocrine and immune systems may play a role in recovery [475]. Even relatively benign stress, such as mid-term examinations in students, can have significant effects on wound healing [476].

Acute and chronic stress have also long been known to influence the course of cardiovascular disease [477, 478]. Generally, such cardiac symptoms as arrhythmias (an irregularity of the heartbeat) and tachycardia (fast heartbeats) are thought to be associated with increased sympathetic stimulation or a reflexive response to histamine-induced hypotension (low blood pressure). Recently an additional possibility has emerged: acute stress has also been shown to stimulate cardiac-associated mast cells to release hista mine and IL-6 [479–481]. Mast cells are abundant in the hypothalamus and thalamus and may be implicated in exacerbations of mast cell-related disorders during stressful times [482, 483]. This mast cell activation may be involved in acute stress-triggered myocardial infarction and unstable angina [484–486].

Extensive literature also suggests that psychological factors associated with chronic stress are risk factors for coronary artery disease, including depression, hostility, low social support, and low socioeconomic status [487]. Hostility has been shown to be an independent and significant risk factor for all-cause mortality and coronary heart disease (CHD) [488]. And a significant relationship has been shown between expressed anger and incident stroke [489]. Here too, the immune system plays a key mediating role in the relationship between stress and coronary artery disease (CAD). The proinflammatory cytokine IL-6 has been shown to be an important player in CAD and the acute coronary syndrome [490, 491]. Psychological distress can also directly provoke pro-inflammatory cytokine production in the absence of injury or invasion by a pathogen [492–494].

Immune Responses

Many distressed or anxious people have derangements in immune responses. In 2004, Segerstrom and Miller published a now-classical meta-analysis of 30 years of empirical articles on the relationships of stress and the immune system in humans [297]. In general, they concluded that acute stressors that lasted just a few minutes resulted in potentially adaptive increases in some aspects of innate immunity and a decrease in some parameters of adaptive immunity. Examinations and other brief natural stressors tended to decrease cellular immunity and leave humoral immunity alone. Chronic stressors tended to suppress both cellular and humoral immunity. The type of stressor such as bereavement or trauma affected the type of immune response.

Genetics

Despite statistically significant associations between stress and heredity, relatively few studies have actually examined the genes that might be involved. In 2006, a particularly comprehensive review was published on the genetics of stress response and stress-related disorders [299]. They conclude that there are significant associations between human stress responses and specific alleles, including single-nucleotide polymorphisms (SNPs), of glucocorticoid receptors and stress inhibitory genes.

As in any new branch of science, there are many questions that need to be answered. One of the more salient yet one of the more difficult questions to answer is, "What is the influence of individual genetics on susceptibility to stress?" Providing a few clues, some research has shown that *gender, age, and reproductive status mediated in part by hormonal effects on disease susceptibility genes may modify inhibitory stress responses of the immune* system [495]. For example, in systemic lupus erythematosus (SLE), recent evidence shows that estrogen enhances and testosterone suppresses autoantibody production, which may help to explain the female sex prevalence in SLE [496]. Animal models also indicate that many autoimmune disease regulatory genes are sex influenced [22, 495, 497–499]. Depression and Alzheimer's have shared immune pathways with overlapping neuroanatomical features [500].

A variety of socio-behavioral factors associated with depression risk can modify vulnerability to inflammation-induced depressed mood [501]. These might include baseline levels of perceived stress, anxiety, and sensitivity to social disconnection, but not early life stress, social status, social support, neuroticism, or sleep disturbance.

In 2010, an exciting paper opened the door to identifying genetic factors that interact with social environments to influence human health [502]. They used a clever bioinformatic strategy to couple expression array-based detection of environmentally responsive transcription factors to a computer-based detection of regulatory polymorphisms in order to predict genes that modulate transcription as a response to environmental stressors. Their model predicted that social adversity-induced alteration of β-adrenergic activation of a GATA1 polymorphism in association with individual IL-6 genotypes can change human health risk. The *GATA family of transcription factors* shares the ability to bind to GATA DNA sequences [503]. GATA1 is involved in several processes, including cell growth, overall body homeostasis [504], and cancer [505].

Validation of their prediction was provided by (1) in vitro biochemical analyses that showed β-adrenergic stimulation increased activation of GATA1, (2) in vivo animal models that showed increased transcription of GATA1 target genes, and (3) human epidemiological data that showed an association between adverse social conditions and increased transcription of GATA1 targets in primary neural, immune, and cancer cells. Epidemiologically, they documented an increased 10-year mortality risk associated with later-life depression symptoms that were present only in homozygous carriers of the GATA1-sensitive G allele of rs1800795. And this IL-6-associated risk was solely related to increased chronic inflammation and inflammation-related deaths.

In 2015, a genome-wide study in China identified two genetic loci on chromosome 10 contributing to the risk of major depressive disorder (MDD): one near the SIRT1 gene and the other in an intron of the LHPP gene [506, 507]. A severe subtype of MDD, melancholia, was highly associated with the SIRT1 locus. However, the interpretation of these associations is subject to debate [508].

A 2019 study of university students checked for a relationship between early-life adversity and depressive symptoms and cytokine single-nucleotide polymorphisms (SNPs) of the inflammatory cytokines IL-1β rs16944, IL-6 rs1800795 SNP, and TNF-α rs1800629 [509]. There are indications that in the setting of early life adversity, genetic variations of IL-1β functioning may associate with a male and female variance in susceptibility to depression symptoms. For females, greater maltreatment in childhood is associated with increased symptoms of depression without regard to the genetic variations of IL-1β. For males, this association was quite strong for the GG genotype of the IL-1β SNP.

Commensurate with increases in depression symptoms during late adolescence, an increased expression of inflammation-related genes and decreased expression of antiviral-related genes has been documented in adolescents with higher levels of depression compared to their peers with lower levels of depression [510]. The researchers suggest that these differences may be mediated by greater activity of the pro-inflammatory transcription factor, nuclear factor-kappa B (NF-κB), and reduced activity of glucocorticoid receptors (GRs) and interferon response factors (IRFs). They also suggest that monocytes, B cells, and dendritic cells may be the primary source of these cytokines.

It has also been seen that inflammatory physiology moderates relationships between recent stressful life events and subsequent depressive symptoms in adolescence [511]. Adolescents with recent stressful life events who had moderate and high levels of IL-6 and C-reactive protein (CRP) following these stressors had an increased risk for more severe depressive symptoms after about one year since the event.

Macrophage heterogeneity and cytokine-induced neuroinflammation in major depressive disorder have been reviewed in 2019 [512].

Mental stress-induced myocardial ischemia (MSIMI) is associated with increased risk of dangerous cardiovascular outcomes [513] and is associated with acute increases in several inflammatory markers [514]. Researchers measured inflammatory responses to acute laboratory mental stress of public speaking in patients with CAD and the inflammatory association with MSIMI [515]. Mental stress resulted in significant increases of interleukin-6 (IL-6), monocyte chemoattractant protein-1 (MCP-1), matrix metallopeptidase 9 (MMP-9), and high-sensitivity C-reactive protein (hsCRP) 90 min after mental stress. Nevertheless, neither the baseline inflammatory status nor the magnitude of the inflammatory response to mental stress is significantly associated with MSIMI.

In 2009, Oitzl and colleagues reviewed *possible roles of glucocorticoids and their receptors in determining why some individuals perish while others flourish when faced with similar stress* [516]. They believe that the determining factors are interactions between genetics and cognitive/emotional inputs in which glucocorticoids and their receptors perform critical functions. Concentration-dependent activity of glucocorticoids may be due in large part to differential intracellular binding to ligand-inducible *high-affinity type I mineralocorticoid receptors (MRs)* or *low-affinity type II glucocorticoid receptors (GRs)* [517]. They have reviewed four hypotheses that might help to explain how individual coping mechanisms may change from protective to harmful.

1. The *Glucocorticoid Cascade Hypothesis* proposes that inability to cope with chronic stress begins a feed-forward cycle of excessive glucocorticoids accompanied by downregulation of hippocampal GRs and a cascade of degeneration and disease [518, 519]. This hypothesis is weak and has not been substantiated.
2. The *Balance Hypothesis of MR/GR* proposes that limbic MR/GR imbalance may cause alteration in information processing in circuits that deal with fear, reward, social behavior, and resilience, such that dysregulation of the HPA axis and dysfunctional behavioral adaptation may

result [520, 521]. Imbalances may be caused by gene variants of the MR and GR receptors coupled with life experiences that may provoke epigenetic changes that affect their expression.
3. The *Maternal Mediation Hypothesis* focuses upon the maternal role in influencing the epigenetic changes that are part of the Balance Hypothesis.
4. The *Predictive Adaptation Hypothesis* builds upon the Balance and Maternal hypotheses to question how adaptable to future demands is the result of perinatal gene–environment interactions that permute the MR/GR balance.

During baseline and low stress levels (i.e., during the permissive phase), glucocorticoid effects are predominantly mediated by the MRs. During high stress, the effects are largely mediated through the GRs, and suppression (except in the CNS) predominates. Moderate stress levels and ratios of MR/GR binding appear to be associated with varied effects of stimulation. This modulation occurs as the MR is the first to be occupied, such that at baseline levels, only a relatively few GRs are bound. As stress increases, the MRs become saturated and the number of GRs that are bound increases. At high levels of stress, the GRs finally become saturated.

GRs are found everywhere in the brain and are most common in the hypothalamic CRH neurons and pituitary corticotropes (cells in the anterior pituitary that produce ACTH and MSH) [522]. Although MRs are expressed in the hypothalamus by a wide margin, the highest concentration of MRs is found in the hippocampus. The hippocampus, as part of the limbic system, is intimately involved in learning, memory, and the stress response.

The balance of occupancy of MRs and GRs in the hippocampus (and probably other areas) may have substantial influences on neuronal soundness [523, 524] and function [525] associated with differences in neuroendocrine regulation [526] and behavior [527].

Context is critical in determining the output of a cell during stress [517, 528, 529]. To begin with, the glucocorticoids must reach the cell. This is influenced by molecules that carry the glucocorticoids in the circulation. *Corticosteroid-binding globulin (CBG)* is the principal transport molecule. It is regulated by various signals, including estrogens [530, 531] and is downregulated by glucocorticoids and stress [532]. This is important because the part of circulating glucocorticoids that is not bound (<5%) is the fraction that is biologically available.

Once the glucocorticoids are in the cell, the interconversion of cortisol and corticosterone changes the availability of active glucocorticoids. In the section on targets, we discuss this regulation by 11β-hydroxysteroid dehydrogenases (11βHSD). In the hippocampus, only the 11βHSD type 1 (which converts inactive hydrocortisone to active cortisol) is found, but its role is unclear [517].

Next, the cellular profile of expression of MR and GR receptors, and their variants [533] will determine the cell's ability to bind the glucocorticoid. Then, the cellular context and physiological conditions will determine if the effects on the cell will enhance or repress gene transcription. Part of this response is determined by the activity of other neuroendocrine and cytokine factors that may have influenced the expression of NFκB, AP-1, or cAMP-response element binding protein [517]. Ultimately, temporal-spatial organization relative to cellular differentiation and cell cycle stages may control access of the glucocorticoid to the nucleus [534].

Manipulation of MR and GR expression in inbred mice has demonstrated individual differences in stress, emotions, and cognition, and the ability to successfully adapt to challenges [535–538].

During aging, MR is downregulated, and age-related functions of the HPA axis may be partly attributable to these changes in MR expression in the hippocampus [539]. In addition, MR is involved in regulating the circadian nadir and peak activity of the HPA axis, and these rhythms tend to change with age [540]. Experiments in rhesus monkeys have shown significant intergroup and age differences in feedback regulation of the HPA axis [541]. The researchers believe that this is due to unequal individual and age-related changes in the activity of MC and GC receptors in the brain structures involved. Decreased negative feedback regulation of the HPA was seen in the older individuals with depression-associated behavior.

MR and GR variants are not the only variant genes that affect HPA-related stress responses. Common influential gene variants have been found in the GABA(A) receptor, the μ-opioid receptor, the serotonin transporter, catechol O-methyltransferase (COMT), monoamine oxidase (MAOA), the α(2)-adrenergic receptor, brain-derived neurotrophic factor, and the angiotensin-converting enzyme [542].

Early-life adversity can induce some epigenetically regulated changes in hippocampal dopaminergic molecular pathways, which either alleviate or aggravate depression-like symptoms later in life [543]. In a mouse model, behavioral and neurobiological consequences of long-term separation stress (LTSS) and short-term separation stress (STSS) were tested. LTSS induced depression-like behavior. STSS reduced depressive-like behavioral symptoms. STSS exposure elevated dopamine receptor D1 (DRD1) gene expression and decreased gene expression of its downstream modulator DARPP-32 (32-kDa dopamine- and cAMP-regulated phosphoprotein), which was paralleled by decreased H3 acetylation at its gene promoter region. On the other hand, LTSS elevated DARPP-32 gene expression, which was not paralleled by changes in histone acetylation and DRD1 gene expression.

People under stress tend to adopt maladaptive health habits such as excess alcohol consumption, drug abuse, decreased exercise, lack of sleep, and poorer eating habits. These bad habits put them at additional risk for the consequences of stress. This may result in compromised endocrine and immune responses, and improper cardiovascular functions. Many distressed or anxious people have delayed or weaker immune responses.

In general, acute stressors that last just a few minutes result in potentially adaptive increases in some aspects of innate immunity and a decrease in some parameters of adaptive immunity. Examinations and other brief natural stressors tend to decrease cellular immunity and leave humoral immunity alone. Chronic stressors tend to suppress both cellular and humoral immunity responses. But chronic stress and depression are often associated with increased systemic inflammation with leukocytosis and increased circulating neutrophils. Symptoms of depression are frequently associated with these conditions.

Summary

A fundamental question is why some people are resilient and others are susceptible to the adverse effects of chronic stress. This chapter has outlined the interaction of genetics, epigenetics, and the environment in determining our responses to stress and the possible outcome of depressive disorders. Focus has been on both the genes and control of their products, especially as they modify the stress-related psychoneuroimmunological pathways. Stress exposure during critical periods such as the prenatal and early postnatal periods can make a lifetime difference. Often, this difference is reflected in the balance of habituation and resilience.

Although this chapter deals with communication in the depressed brain, it is important to realize that adaptation and reinforcement of pathways that are associated with depression involve the whole body. In later chapters, we will discuss some of these changes as they relate to the immune system and the gut-liver-brain axis.

References

1. Blalock JE, Smith EM. Conceptual development of the immune system as a sixth sense. Brain Behav Immun. 2007;21(1):23–33. PMID: 17088044. http://www.ncbi.nlm.nih.gov/pubmed/17088044.
2. Farooqui AA, Horrocks LA, Farooqui T. Modulation of inflammation in brain: a matter of fat. J Neurochem. 2007;101(3):577–99. PMID: 17257165. http://www.ncbi.nlm.nih.gov/pubmed/17257165.
3. Barnum SR. Complement biosynthesis in the central nervous system. Crit Rev Oral Biol Med. 1995;6(2):132–46. PMID: 7548620. http://www.ncbi.nlm.nih.gov/pubmed/7548620.
4. Roosterman D, Goerge T, Schneider SW, Bunnett NW, Steinhoff M. Neuronal control of skin function: the skin as a neuroimmunoendocrine organ. Physiol Rev. 2006;86(4):1309–79. PMID: 17015491. http://www.ncbi.nlm.nih.gov/pubmed/17015491.
5. Katayama Y, Battista M, Kao WM, Hidalgo A, Peired AJ, Thomas SA, Frenette PS. Signals from the sympathetic nervous system regulate hematopoietic stem cell egress from bone marrow. Cell. 2006;124(2):407–21. PMID: 16439213. http://www.ncbi.nlm.nih.gov/pubmed/16439213.
6. Falaschi P, Martocchia A, Proietti A, Pastore R, D'Urso R, Barnaba V. Neuroendocrinoimmunology. Ann Ital Med Int. 1994;9(2):96–9. PMID: 7917767. http://www.ncbi.nlm.nih.gov/pubmed/7917767.
7. Mix E, Goertsches R, Zettl UK. Immunology and neurology. J Neurol. 2007;254 Suppl 2:II2–7. PMID: 17503123. http://www.ncbi.nlm.nih.gov/pubmed/17503123.
8. Petrovsky N. Towards a unified model of neuroendocrine-immune interaction. Immunol Cell Biol. 2001;79(4):350–7. PMID: 11488982. http://www.ncbi.nlm.nih.gov/pubmed/11488982.
9. Turrin NP, Rivest S. Unraveling the molecular details involved in the intimate link between the immune and neuroendocrine systems. Exp Biol Med (Maywood). 2004;229(10):996–1006. PMID: 15522835. http://www.ncbi.nlm.nih.gov/pubmed/15522835.
10. Jahr J, Grände PO. Pulmonary and haemodynamic effects of extracorporeal circulation in the cat and the beneficial effects of prostacyclin. Intensive Care Med. 1992;18(2):118–22. PMID: 1613191. http://www.ncbi.nlm.nih.gov/pubmed/1613191.
11. Luger TA. Neuromediators–a crucial component of the skin immune system. J Dermatol Sci. 2002;30(2):87–93. PMID: 12413763. http://www.ncbi.nlm.nih.gov/pubmed/12413763.
12. Pert CB, Dreher HE, Ruff MR. The psychosomatic network: foundations of mind-body medicine. Altern Ther Health Med. 1998;4(4):30–41. PMID: 9656499. http://www.ncbi.nlm.nih.gov/pubmed/9656499.
13. Hadley ME, Haskell-Luevano C. The proopiomelanocortin system. Ann N Y Acad Sci. 1999;885:1–21. PMID: 10816638. http://www.ncbi.nlm.nih.gov/pubmed/10816638.
14. Bhardwaj RS, Luger TA. Proopiomelanocortin production by epidermal cells: evidence for an immune neuroendocrine network in the epidermis. Arch Dermatol Res. 1994;287(1):85–90. PMID: 7726641. http://www.ncbi.nlm.nih.gov/pubmed/7726641.
15. Theoharides TC. Mast cells and stress–a psychoneuroimmunological perspective. J Clin Psychopharmacol. 2002;22(2):103–8. PMID: 11910253. http://www.ncbi.nlm.nih.gov/pubmed/11910253.
16. Cutler R, Westcott D, Ringrose D. Antibiotic prophylaxis and hysterectomy. Dimens Health Serv. 1976;53(12):34–5. PMID: 992236. http://www.ncbi.nlm.nih.gov/pubmed/992236.
17. Azevedo FAC, Carvalho LRB, Grinberg LT, Farfel JM, Ferretti REL, Leite REP, Jacob Filho W, Lent R, Herculano-Houzel S. Equal numbers of neuronal and nonneuronal cells make the human brain an isometrically scaled-up primate brain. J Comp Neurol. 2009;513(5):532–41. PMID: 19226510. http://www.ncbi.nlm.nih.gov/pubmed/19226510.
18. Navarrete M, Perea G, Maglio L, Pastor J, García de Sola R, Araque A. Astrocyte calcium signal and gliotransmission in human brain tissue. Cereb Cortex. 2013;23(5):1240–6. PMID: 22581850. http://www.ncbi.nlm.nih.gov/pubmed/22581850.
19. Perea G, Araque A. GLIA modulates synaptic transmission. Brain Res Rev. 2010;63(1–2):93–102. PMID: 19896978. http://www.ncbi.nlm.nih.gov/pubmed/19896978.
20. Perea G, Navarrete M, Araque A. Tripartite synapses: astrocytes process and control synaptic information. Trends Neurosci. 2009;32(8):421–31. PMID: 19615761. http://www.ncbi.nlm.nih.gov/pubmed/19615761.

21. Alvarellos-González A, Pazos A, Porto-Pazos AB. Computational models of neuron-astrocyte interactions lead to improved efficacy in the performance of neural networks. Comput Math Methods Med. 2012;2012:476324. PMCID: PMC3357509. http://www.ncbi.nlm.nih.gov/pubmed/22649480.
22. Wiederholt. Neurology for non-neurologists. 4th ed. Elsevier Health Science; 2000.
23. Südhof TC. The cell biology of synapse formation. J Cell Biol. 2021;220(7):e202103052. PMCID: PMC8186004. http://www.ncbi.nlm.nih.gov/pubmed/34086051.
24. Kouyoumdjian JA, de Estephan EP. Electrophysiological evaluation of the neuromuscular junction: a brief review. Arq Neuropsiquiatr. 2023;81(12):1040–52. PMCID: PMC10756823. http://www.ncbi.nlm.nih.gov/pubmed/38157872.
25. Wang Q, Cui C, Zhang N, Lin W, Chai S, Chow SKH, Wong RMY, Hu Y, Law SW, Cheung WH. Effects of physical exercise on neuromuscular junction degeneration during ageing: a systematic review. J Orthop Translat. 2024;46:91–102. PMCID: PMC11137388. http://www.ncbi.nlm.nih.gov/pubmed/38817243.
26. Li L, Xiong WC, Mei L. Neuromuscular junction formation, aging, and disorders. Annu Rev Physiol. 2018;80:159–88. PMID: 29195055. http://www.ncbi.nlm.nih.gov/pubmed/29195055.
27. Barik A, Li L, Sathyamurthy A, Xiong WC, Mei L. Schwann cells in neuromuscular junction formation and maintenance. J Neurosci. 2016;36(38):9770–81. PMCID: PMC5030347. http://www.ncbi.nlm.nih.gov/pubmed/27656017.
28. Wehrwein EA, Orer HS, Barman SM. Overview of the anatomy, physiology, and pharmacology of the autonomic nervous system. Compr Physiol. 2016;6(3):1239–78. PMID: 27347892. http://www.ncbi.nlm.nih.gov/pubmed/27347892.
29. Gutmann JL, Fava LR. Perspectives on periradicular healing using Sealapex: a case report. Int Endod J. 1991;24(3):135–8. PMID: 1778626. http://www.ncbi.nlm.nih.gov/pubmed/1778626.
30. Dantzer R. Neuroimmune interactions: from the brain to the immune system and vice versa. Physiol Rev. 2018;98(1):477–504. PMCID: PMC5866360. http://www.ncbi.nlm.nih.gov/pubmed/29351513.
31. Herculano-Houzel S. The human brain in numbers: a linearly scaled-up primate brain. Front Hum Neurosci. 2009;3:31. PMCID: PMC2776484. http://www.ncbi.nlm.nih.gov/pubmed/19915731.
32. Drachman DA. Do we have brain to spare? Neurology. 2005;64(12):2004–5. PMID: 15985565. http://www.ncbi.nlm.nih.gov/pubmed/15985565.
33. Sheu SH, Upadhyayula S, Dupuy V, Pang S, Deng F, Wan J, Walpita D, Pasolli HA, Houser J, Sanchez-Martinez S, Brauchi SE, Banala S, Freeman M, Xu CS, Kirchhausen T, Hess HF, Lavis L, Li Y, Chaumont-Dubel S, Clapham DE. A serotonergic axon-cilium synapse drives nuclear signaling to alter chromatin accessibility. Cell. 2022;185(18):3390–3407.e18. PMCID: PMC9789380. http://www.ncbi.nlm.nih.gov/pubmed/36055200.
34. Anvarian Z, Mykytyn K, Mukhopadhyay S, Pedersen LB, Christensen ST. Cellular signalling by primary cilia in development, organ function and disease. Nat Rev Nephrol. 2019;15(4):199–219. PMCID: PMC6426138. http://www.ncbi.nlm.nih.gov/pubmed/30733609.
35. Guemez-Gamboa A, Coufal NG, Gleeson JG. Primary cilia in the developing and mature brain. Neuron. 2014;82(3):511–21. PMCID: PMC4104280. http://www.ncbi.nlm.nih.gov/pubmed/24811376.
36. Shalata A, Ramirez MC, Desnick RJ, Priedigkeit N, Buettner C, Lindtner C, Mahroum M, Abdul-Ghani M, Dong F, Arar N, Camacho-Vanegas O, Zhang R, Camacho SC, Chen Y, Ibdah M, DeFronzo R, Gillespie V, Kelley K, Dynlacht BD, Kim S, Glucksman MJ, Borochowitz ZU, Martignetti JA. Morbid obesity resulting from inactivation of the ciliary protein CEP19 in humans and mice. Am J Hum Genet. 2013;93(6):1061–71. PMCID: PMC3852924. http://www.ncbi.nlm.nih.gov/pubmed/24268657.
37. Berbari NF, Pasek RC, Malarkey EB, Yazdi SMZ, McNair AD, Lewis WR, Nagy TR, Kesterson RA, Yoder BK. Leptin resistance is a secondary consequence of the obesity in ciliopathy mutant mice. Proc Natl Acad Sci USA. 2013;110(19):7796–801. PMCID: PMC3651481. http://www.ncbi.nlm.nih.gov/pubmed/23599282.
38. Borroto-Escuela DO, Gonzalez-Cristo E, Ochoa-Torres V, Serra-Rojas EM, Ambrogini P, Arroyo-García LE, Fuxe K. Understanding electrical and chemical transmission in the brain. Front Cell Neurosci. 2024;18:1398862. PMCID: PMC11233782. http://www.ncbi.nlm.nih.gov/pubmed/38988663.
39. Thomas D, Recabal-Beyer A, Senecal JM, Serletis D, Lynn BD, Jackson MF, Nagy JI. Association of connexin36 with adherens junctions at mixed synapses and distinguishing electrophysiological features of those at mossy fiber terminals in rat ventral hippocampus. Int J Physiol Pathophysiol Pharmacol. 2024;16(3):28–54. PMCID: PMC11249852. http://www.ncbi.nlm.nih.gov/pubmed/39021415.
40. Vaughn MJ, Haas JS. On the diverse functions of electrical synapses. Front Cell Neurosci. 2022;16:910015. PMCID: PMC9219736. http://www.ncbi.nlm.nih.gov/pubmed/35755782.
41. Martinez-Banaclocha M. Ephaptic coupling of cortical neurons: possible contribution of Astroglial magnetic fields? Neuroscience. 2018;370:37–45. PMID: 2879323. http://www.ncbi.nlm.nih.gov/pubmed/28793233.
42. Pinotsis DA, Miller EK. In vivo ephaptic coupling allows memory network formation. Cereb Cortex. 2023;33(17):9877–95. PMCID: PMC10472500. http://www.ncbi.nlm.nih.gov/pubmed/37420330.
43. Ruffini G, Salvador R, Tadayon E, Sanchez-Todo R, Pascual-Leone A, Santarnecchi E. Realistic modeling of mesoscopic ephaptic coupling in the human brain. PLoS Comput Biol. 2020;16(6):e1007923. PMCID: PMC7289436. http://www.ncbi.nlm.nih.gov/pubmed/32479496.
44. Qi C, Li Y, Gu H, Yang Y. Nonlinear mechanism for the enhanced bursting activities induced by fast inhibitory autapse and reduced activities by fast excitatory autapse. Cogn Neurodyn. 2023;17(4):1093–113. PMCID: PMC10374520. http://www.ncbi.nlm.nih.gov/pubmed/37522049.
45. Yilmaz E, Ozer M, Baysal V, Perc M. Autapse-induced multiple coherence resonance in single neurons and neuronal networks. Sci Rep. 2016;6:30914. PMCID: PMC4969620. http://www.ncbi.nlm.nih.gov/pubmed/27480120.
46. Missler M, Südhof TC, Biederer T. Synaptic cell adhesion. Cold Spring Harb Perspect Biol. 2012;4(4):a005694. PMCID: PMC3312681. http://www.ncbi.nlm.nih.gov/pubmed/22278667.
47. Bennett MVL, Zukin RS. Electrical coupling and neuronal synchronization in the Mammalian brain. Neuron. 2004;41(4):495–511. PMID: 14980200. http://www.ncbi.nlm.nih.gov/pubmed/14980200.
48. Pereda AE, Curti S, Hoge G, Cachope R, Flores CE, Rash JE. Gap junction-mediated electrical transmission: regulatory mechanisms and plasticity. Biochim Biophys Acta. 2013;1828(1):134–46. PMCID: PMC3437247. http://www.ncbi.nlm.nih.gov/pubmed/22659675.
49. Curti S, Davoine F, Dapino A. Function and plasticity of electrical synapses in the mammalian brain: role of non-Junctional mechanisms. Biology (Basel). 2022;11(1):81. PMCID: PMC8773336. http://www.ncbi.nlm.nih.gov/pubmed/35053079.
50. Hormuzdi SG, Filippov MA, Mitropoulou G, Monyer H, Bruzzone R. Electrical synapses: a dynamic signaling system that shapes the activity of neuronal networks. Biochim Biophys Acta. 2004;1662(1–2):113–37. PMID: 15033583. http://www.ncbi.nlm.nih.gov/pubmed/15033583.
51. Südhof TC. The presynaptic active zone. Neuron. 2012;75(1):11–25. PMCID: PMC3743085 PubMed entry

[Internet]. [cited 2024 Dec 24]. Available from: http://www.ncbi.nlm.nih.gov/pubmed/22794257.
52. Malsam J, Söllner TH. Organization of SNAREs within the Golgi stack. Cold Spring Harb Perspect Biol. 2011;3(10):a005249. PMCID: PMC3179334. http://www.ncbi.nlm.nih.gov/pubmed/21768609.
53. Hurowitz EH, Melnyk JM, Chen YJ, Kouros-Mehr H, Simon MI, Shizuya H. Genomic characterization of the human heterotrimeric G protein alpha, beta, and gamma subunit genes. DNA Res. 2000;7(2):111–20. PMID: 10819326. http://www.ncbi.nlm.nih.gov/pubmed/10819326.
54. Ferraguti F, Crepaldi L, Nicoletti F. Metabotropic glutamate 1 receptor: current concepts and perspectives. Pharmacol Rev. 2008;60(4):536–81. PMID: 19112153. http://www.ncbi.nlm.nih.gov/pubmed/19112153.
55. Durand D, Pampillo M, Caruso C, Lasaga M. Role of metabotropic glutamate receptors in the control of neuroendocrine function. Neuropharmacology. 2008;55(4):577–83. PMID: 18616955. http://www.ncbi.nlm.nih.gov/pubmed/18616955.
56. D'Antoni S, Berretta A, Bonaccorso CM, Bruno V, Aronica E, Nicoletti F, Catania MV. Metabotropic glutamate receptors in glial cells. Neurochem Res. 2008;33(12):2436–43. PMID: 18438710. http://www.ncbi.nlm.nih.gov/pubmed/18438710.
57. Brockie PJ, Maricq AV. Ionotropic glutamate receptors: genetics, behavior and electrophysiology. WormBook. 2006:1–16. PMCID: PMC4781458. http://www.ncbi.nlm.nih.gov/pubmed/18050468.
58. Oswald RE. Ionotropic glutamate receptor recognition and activation. Adv Protein Chem. 2004;68:313–49. PMID: 15500865. http://www.ncbi.nlm.nih.gov/pubmed/15500865.
59. Oswald RE, Ahmed A, Fenwick MK, Loh AP. Structure of glutamate receptors. Curr Drug Targets. 2007;8(5):573–82. PMID: 17504102. http://www.ncbi.nlm.nih.gov/pubmed/17504102.
60. Cleland TA. Inhibitory glutamate receptor channels. Mol Neurobiol. 1996;13(2):97–136. PMID: 8938647. http://www.ncbi.nlm.nih.gov/pubmed/8938647.
61. Schultz W. Predictive reward signal of dopamine neurons. J Neurophysiol. 1998;80(1):1–27. PMID: 9658025. http://www.ncbi.nlm.nih.gov/pubmed/9658025.
62. Carboni E, Tanda GL, Frau R, Di Chiara G. Blockade of the noradrenaline carrier increases extracellular dopamine concentrations in the prefrontal cortex: evidence that dopamine is taken up in vivo by noradrenergic terminals. J Neurochem. 1990;55(3):1067–70. PMID: 2117046. http://www.ncbi.nlm.nih.gov/pubmed/2117046.
63. Meyer JH, Ginovart N, Boovariwala A, Sagrati S, Hussey D, Garcia A, Young T, Praschak-Rieder N, Wilson AA, Houle S. Elevated monoamine oxidase a levels in the brain: an explanation for the monoamine imbalance of major depression. Arch Gen Psychiatry. 2006;63(11):1209–16. PMID: 17088501. http://www.ncbi.nlm.nih.gov/pubmed/17088501.
64. Zhang K, He L, Li Z, Ding R, Han X, Chen B, Cao G, Ye JH, Li T, Fu R. Bridging neurobiological insights and clinical biomarkers in postpartum depression: a narrative review. Int J Mol Sci. 2024;25(16):8835. PMCID: PMC11354679. http://www.ncbi.nlm.nih.gov/pubmed/39201521.
65. Schacht JP. COMT val158met moderation of dopaminergic drug effects on cognitive function: a critical review. Pharmacogenomics J. 2016;16(5):430–8. PMCID: PMC5028240. http://www.ncbi.nlm.nih.gov/pubmed/27241058.
66. Chen J, Song J, Yuan P, Tian Q, Ji Y, Ren-Patterson R, Liu G, Sei Y, Weinberger DR. Orientation and cellular distribution of membrane-bound catechol-O-methyltransferase in cortical neurons: implications for drug development. J Biol Chem. 2011;286(40):34752–60. PMCID: PMC318643. http://www.ncbi.nlm.nih.gov/pubmed/21846718.
67. Wang Y, Li S, Niu L, Ma Y, Qiu Y, Li S, Guobule N, Cao H, Li J. Polymorphisms of COMT and CREB1 are associated with treatment-resistant depression in a Chinese Han population. J Neural Transm (Vienna). 2022;129(1):85–93. PMID: 34767111. http://www.ncbi.nlm.nih.gov/pubmed/34767111.
68. Tosato S, Bonetto C, De Santi K, Lasalvia A, Gennarelli M, Cristofalo D, Bertani M, Ruggeri M, On Behalf Of The Picos-Veneto Group null. COMT but Not 5HTTLPR gene is associated with depression in first-episode psychosis: the role of stressful life events. Genes (Basel). 2023;14(2):350. PMCID: PMC9956580 http://www.ncbi.nlm.nih.gov/pubmed/36833277.
69. Nagy JI, Pereda AE, Rash JE. On the occurrence and enigmatic functions of mixed (chemical plus electrical) synapses in the mammalian CNS. Neurosci Lett. 2019;695:53–64. PMCID: PMC5845811. http://www.ncbi.nlm.nih.gov/pubmed/28911821.
70. Gutiérrez R. Gap junctions in the brain: hardwired but functionally versatile. Neuroscientist. 2023;29(5):554–68. PMID: 36125001. http://www.ncbi.nlm.nih.gov/pubmed/36125001.
71. Zhang D, Li Y, Rasch MJ, Wu S. Nonlinear multiplicative dendritic integration in neuron and network models. Front Comput Neurosci. 2013;7:56. PMCID: PMC3647120. http://www.ncbi.nlm.nih.gov/pubmed/23658543.
72. Feng J. Is the integrate-and-fire model good enough?–a review. Neural Netw. 2001;14(6–7):955–75. PMID: 11665785. http://www.ncbi.nlm.nih.gov/pubmed/11665785.
73. Zhou D, Li S, Zhang X, hui, Cai D. Phenomenological incorporation of nonlinear dendritic integration using integrate-and-fire neuronal frameworks. PLoS One. 2013;8(1):e53508. PMCID: PMC3538611. http://www.ncbi.nlm.nih.gov/pubmed/23308241.
74. Westberg L, Eriksson E. Sex steroid-related candidate genes in psychiatric disorders. J Psychiatry Neurosci. 2008;33(4):319–30. PMCID: PMC2440794. http://www.ncbi.nlm.nih.gov/pubmed/18592033.
75. Fricker LD, Devi LA. Orphan neuropeptides and receptors: novel therapeutic targets. Pharmacol Ther. 2018;185:26–33. PMCID: PMC5899030. http://www.ncbi.nlm.nih.gov/pubmed/29174650.
76. Guyton. Textbook of medical physiology. 11th ed. Elsevier Health Science; 2006.
77. Rolak. Neurology secrets. Elsevier Health Science; 2001.
78. Pei Y, Asif-Malik A, Canales JJ. Trace amines and the trace amine-associated receptor 1: pharmacology, neurochemistry, and clinical implications. Front Neurosci. 2016;10:148. PMCID: PMC4820462. http://www.ncbi.nlm.nih.gov/pubmed/27092049.
79. Kodirov SA, Takizawa S, Joseph J, Kandel ER, Shumyatsky GP, Bolshakov VY. Synaptically released zinc gates long-term potentiation in fear conditioning pathways. Proc Natl Acad Sci USA. 2006;103(41):15218–23. PMCID: PMC1622803. http://www.ncbi.nlm.nih.gov/pubmed/17005717.
80. Martin BR, Mechoulam R, Razdan RK. Discovery and characterization of endogenous cannabinoids. Life Sci. 1999;65(6–7):573–95. PMID: 10462059. http://www.ncbi.nlm.nih.gov/pubmed/10462059.
81. Soares CN, Phillips SD. Hormones in the treatment of depression. Womens Health (Lond). 2006;2(3):435–45. PMID: 19803915. http://www.ncbi.nlm.nih.gov/pubmed/19803915.
82. Steiner M, Dunn E, Born L. Hormones and mood: from menarche to menopause and beyond. J Affect Disord. 2003;74(1):67–83. PMID: 12646300. http://www.ncbi.nlm.nih.gov/pubmed/12646300.
83. ter Horst JP, de Kloet ER, Schächinger H, Oitzl MS. Relevance of stress and female sex hormones for emotion and cognition. Cell Mol Neurobiol. 2012;32(5):725–35. PMCID: PMC3377901. http://www.ncbi.nlm.nih.gov/pubmed/22113371.
84. Watson CS, Alyea RA, Cunningham KA, Jeng YJ. Estrogens of multiple classes and their role in mental health disease mechanisms. Int J Women's Health. 2010;2:153–66. PMCID: PMC2971739. http://www.ncbi.nlm.nih.gov/pubmed/21072308.

85. Barron ML, Flick LH, Cook CA, Homan SM, Campbell C. Associations between psychiatric disorders and menstrual cycle characteristics. Arch Psychiatr Nurs. 2008;22(5):254–65. PMCID: PMC2588420. http://www.ncbi.nlm.nih.gov/pubmed/18809118.
86. Trudeau LE. Glutamate co-transmission as an emerging concept in monoamine neuron function. J Psychiatry Neurosci. 2004;29(4):296–310. PMCID: PMC446224. http://www.ncbi.nlm.nih.gov/pubmed/15309046.
87. Singer JH. GABA is an endogenous ligand for synaptic glycine receptors. Neuron. 2008;57(4):475–7. PMID: 18304476. http://www.ncbi.nlm.nih.gov/pubmed/18304476.
88. Neuropeptide Functions and Regulation – Basic Neurochemistry – NCBI Bookshelf.
89. Neuropeptides I: classification, synthesis and co-localization with classical neurotransmitters (Chapter 11) – An Introduction to Neuroendocrinology.
90. Lauretani F. Parkinson's disease in the elderly and the comprehensive geriatric assessment. Niger Med J. 2013;54(2):146–7. PMCID: PMC3687868. http://www.ncbi.nlm.nih.gov/pubmed/23798803.
91. Mhyre TR, Boyd JT, Hamill RW, Maguire-Zeiss KA. Parkinson's disease. Subcell Biochem 2012;65:389–455. PMCID: PMC4372387. http://www.ncbi.nlm.nih.gov/pubmed/23225012.
92. Marsh L. Depression and Parkinson's disease: current knowledge. Curr Neurol Neurosci Rep. 2013;13(12):409. PMCID: PMC4878671. http://www.ncbi.nlm.nih.gov/pubmed/24190780.
93. Schrag A, Taddei RN. Depression and anxiety in Parkinson's disease. Int Rev Neurobiol. 2017;133:623–55. PMID: 28802935. http://www.ncbi.nlm.nih.gov/pubmed/28802935.
94. Rihmer Z, Gonda X, Döme P. Depression in Parkinson's disease. Ideggyogy Sz. 2014;67(7–8):229–36. PMID: 25509363. http://www.ncbi.nlm.nih.gov/pubmed/25509363.
95. Timmer MHM, van Beek MHCT, Bloem BR, Esselink RAJ. What a neurologist should know about depression in Parkinson's disease. Pract Neurol. 2017;17(5):359–68. PMID: 28739866. http://www.ncbi.nlm.nih.gov/pubmed/28739866.
96. Wenzel JM, Rauscher NA, Cheer JF, Oleson EB. A role for phasic dopamine release within the nucleus accumbens in encoding aversion: a review of the neurochemical literature. ACS Chem Neurosci. 2015;6(1):16–26. PMCID: PMC5820768. http://www.ncbi.nlm.nih.gov/pubmed/25491156.
97. Puglisi-Allegra S, Ventura R. Prefrontal/accumbal catecholamine system processes high motivational salience. Front. Behav Neurosci. 2012;6:31. PMCID: PMC3384081. http://www.ncbi.nlm.nih.gov/pubmed/22754514.
98. Baliki MN, Mansour A, Baria AT, Huang L, Berger SE, Fields HL, Apkarian AV. Parceling human accumbens into putative core and shell dissociates encoding of values for reward and pain. J Neurosci. 2013;33(41):16383–93. PMCID: PMC3792469. http://www.ncbi.nlm.nih.gov/pubmed/24107968.
99. Törk I. Anatomy of the serotonergic system. Ann N Y Acad Sci. 1990;600:9–34; discussion 34–35. PMID: 2252340. http://www.ncbi.nlm.nih.gov/pubmed/2252340.
100. Jacobs BL, Azmitia EC. Structure and function of the brain serotonin system. Physiol Rev. 1992;72(1):165–229. PMID: 1731370. http://www.ncbi.nlm.nih.gov/pubmed/1731370.
101. Malenka RC, Nestler EJ, Hyman SE. Chapter 6: Widely projecting systems: monoamines, acetylcholine, and Orexin. In: Sydor A, Brown RY, editors. Molecular neuropharmacology: a foundation for clinical neuroscience. 2nd ed. New York: McGraw-Hill Medical; 2009.
102. Alcaro A, Huber R, Panksepp J. Behavioral functions of the mesolimbic dopaminergic system: an affective neuroethological perspective. Brain Res Rev. 2007;56(2):283–321. PMCID: PMC2238694. http://www.ncbi.nlm.nih.gov/pubmed/17905440.
103. Ikemoto S. Brain reward circuitry beyond the mesolimbic dopamine system: a neurobiological theory. Neurosci Biobehav Rev. 2010;35(2):129–50. PMCID: PMC2894302. http://www.ncbi.nlm.nih.gov/pubmed/20149820.
104. Reynolds LM, Flores C. Mesocorticolimbic dopamine pathways across adolescence: diversity in development. Front Neural Circuits. 2021;15:735625. PMCID: PMC8456011. http://www.ncbi.nlm.nih.gov/pubmed/34566584.
105. Yamaguchi T, Wang HL, Li X, Ng TH, Morales M. Mesocorticolimbic glutamatergic pathway. J Neurosci. 2011;31(23):8476–90. PMCID: PMC6623324. http://www.ncbi.nlm.nih.gov/pubmed/21653852.
106. Seib DR, Tobiansky DJ, Meitzen J, Floresco SB, Soma KK. Neurosteroids and the mesocorticolimbic system. Neurosci Biobehav Rev. 2023;153:105356. PMID: 37567491. http://www.ncbi.nlm.nih.gov/pubmed/37567491.
107. Blum K, Gondré-Lewis M, Steinberg B, Elman I, Baron D, Modestino EJ, Badgaiyan RD, Gold MS. Our evolved unique pleasure circuit makes humans different from apes: reconsideration of data derived from animal studies. J Syst Integr Neurosci. 2018;4:(1). PMCID: PMC6446569. http://www.ncbi.nlm.nih.gov/pubmed/30956812.
108. Floresco SB, Magyar O. Mesocortical dopamine modulation of executive functions: beyond working memory. Psychopharmacology. 2006;188(4):567–85. PMID: 16670842. http://www.ncbi.nlm.nih.gov/pubmed/16670842.
109. Salamone JD, Correa M. The mysterious motivational functions of mesolimbic dopamine. Neuron. 2012;76(3):470–85. PMCID: PMC4450094. http://www.ncbi.nlm.nih.gov/pubmed/23141060.
110. Berridge KC, Kringelbach ML. Pleasure systems in the brain. Neuron. 2015;86(3):646–64. PMCID: PMC4425246. http://www.ncbi.nlm.nih.gov/pubmed/25950633.
111. Balleine BW, Delgado MR, Hikosaka O. The role of the dorsal striatum in reward and decision-making. J Neurosci. 2007;27(31):8161–5. PMCID: PMC6673072. http://www.ncbi.nlm.nih.gov/pubmed/17670959.
112. Haber SN, Kim KS, Mailly P, Calzavara R. Reward-related cortical inputs define a large striatal region in primates that interface with associative cortical connections, providing a substrate for incentive-based learning. J Neurosci. 2006;26(32):8368–76. PMCID: PMC6673798. http://www.ncbi.nlm.nih.gov/pubmed/16899732.
113. Haber SN. Corticostriatal circuitry. Dialogues Clin Neurosci. 2016;18(1):7–21. PMCID: PMC4826773. http://www.ncbi.nlm.nih.gov/pubmed/27069376.
114. Mariani E, Frabetti F, Tarozzi A, Pelleri MC, Pizzetti F, Casadei R. Meta-analysis of Parkinson's disease Transcriptome data using TRAM software: whole Substantia Nigra tissue and single dopamine neuron differential gene expression. PLoS One. 2016;11(9):e0161567. PMCID: PMC5017670. http://www.ncbi.nlm.nih.gov/pubmed/27611585.
115. Jiang-Xie LF, Yin L, Zhao S, Prevosto V, Han BX, Dzirasa K, Wang F. A common neuroendocrine substrate for diverse general Anesthetics and sleep. Neuron. 2019;102(5):1053–1065.e4. PMCID: PMC6554048. http://www.ncbi.nlm.nih.gov/pubmed/31006556.
116. Baladron J, Hamker FH. Habit learning in hierarchical cortex-basal ganglia loops. Eur J Neurosci. 2020;52(12):4613–38. PMID: 32237250. http://www.ncbi.nlm.nih.gov/pubmed/32237250.
117. Foster NN, Barry J, Korobkova L, Garcia L, Gao L, Becerra M, Sherafat Y, Peng B, Li X, Choi JH, Gou L, Zingg B, Azam S, Lo D, Khanjani N, Zhang B, Stanis J, Bowman I, Cotter K, Cao C, Yamashita S, Tugangui A, Li A, Jiang T, Jia X, Feng Z, Aquino S, Mun HS, Zhu M, Santarelli A, Benavidez NL, Song M, Dan G, Fayzullina M, Ustrell S, Boesen T, Johnson DL, Xu H, Bienkowski MS, Yang XW, Gong H, Levine MS, Wickersham I, Luo Q, Hahn JD, Lim BK, Zhang LI, Cepeda C, Hintiryan H, Dong HW. The mouse cortico-basal ganglia-thalamic network.

Nature. 2021;598(7879):188–94. PMCID: PMC8494639. http://www.ncbi.nlm.nih.gov/pubmed/34616074.
118. Lam S, Langevin JP, Malkasian D, Gorgulho A, DeSalles A. Deep brain stimulator-induced diaphoresis in Parkinson's disease patients. J Clin Neurosci. 2014;21(4):676–8. PMID: 24210802. http://www.ncbi.nlm.nih.gov/pubmed/24210802.
119. Rinaman L. Hindbrain noradrenergic A2 neurons: diverse roles in autonomic, endocrine, cognitive, and behavioral functions. Am J Physiol Regul Integr Comp Physiol. 2011;300(2):R222–35. PMCID: PMC3043801. http://www.ncbi.nlm.nih.gov/pubmed/20962208.
120. Sara SJ, Bouret S. Orienting and reorienting: the locus coeruleus mediates cognition through arousal. Neuron. 2012;76(1):130–41. PMID: 23040811. http://www.ncbi.nlm.nih.gov/pubmed/23040811.
121. Thorp AA, Schlaich MP. Relevance of sympathetic nervous system activation in obesity and metabolic syndrome. J Diabetes Res. 2015;2015:341583. PMCID: PMC4430650. http://www.ncbi.nlm.nih.gov/pubmed/26064978.
122. Tank AW, Lee WD. Peripheral and central effects of circulating catecholamines. Compr Physiol. 2015;5(1):1–15. PMID: 25589262. http://www.ncbi.nlm.nih.gov/pubmed/25589262.
123. Konturek SJ, Konturek JW, Pawlik T, Brzozowski T. Brain-gut axis and its role in the control of food intake. J Physiol Pharmacol. 2004;55(1 Pt 2):137–54. PMID: 15082874. http://www.ncbi.nlm.nih.gov/pubmed/15082874.
124. Kenney MJ, Ganta CK. Autonomic nervous system and immune system interactions. Compr Physiol. 2014;4(3):1177–200. PMCID: PMC4374437. http://www.ncbi.nlm.nih.gov/pubmed/24944034.
125. Shouman K, Benarroch EE. Peripheral neuroimmune interactions: selected review and some clinical implications. Clin Auton Res. 2021;31(4):477–89. PMCID: PMC7914391. http://www.ncbi.nlm.nih.gov/pubmed/33641054.
126. Dahlstroem A, Fuxe K. Evidence for the existence of monoamine-containing neurons in the central nervous system. I. Demonstration of monoamines in the cell bodies of brain stem neurons. Acta Physiol Scand Suppl. 1964;SUPPL 232:1–55. PMID: 14229500. http://www.ncbi.nlm.nih.gov/pubmed/14229500.
127. Berridge CW, Schmeichel BE, España RA. Noradrenergic modulation of wakefulness/arousal. Sleep Med Rev. 2012;16(2):187–97. PMCID: PMC3278579. http://www.ncbi.nlm.nih.gov/pubmed/22296742.
128. O'Donnell J, Zeppenfeld D, McConnell E, Pena S, Nedergaard M. Norepinephrine: a neuromodulator that boosts the function of multiple cell types to optimize CNS performance. Neurochem Res. 2012;37(11):2496–512. PMCID: PMC3548657. http://www.ncbi.nlm.nih.gov/pubmed/22717696.
129. Satoh A, Iijima KM. Roles of tau pathology in the locus coeruleus (LC) in age-associated pathophysiology and Alzheimer's disease pathogenesis: potential strategies to protect the LC against aging. Brain Res. 2019;1702:17–28. PMID: 29274876. http://www.ncbi.nlm.nih.gov/pubmed/29274876.
130. Dayer A. Serotonin-related pathways and developmental plasticity: relevance for psychiatric disorders. Dialogues Clin Neurosci. 2014;16(1):29–41. PMCID: PMC3984889. http://www.ncbi.nlm.nih.gov/pubmed/24733969.
131. Helton SG, Lohoff FW. Serotonin pathway polymorphisms and the treatment of major depressive disorder and anxiety disorders. Pharmacogenomics. 2015;16(5):541–53. PMID: 25916524. http://www.ncbi.nlm.nih.gov/pubmed/25916524.
132. Moncrieff J, Cooper RE, Stockmann T, Amendola S, Hengartner MP, Horowitz MA. The serotonin theory of depression: a systematic umbrella review of the evidence. Mol Psychiatry. 2023;28(8):3243–56. PMCID: PMC10618090. http://www.ncbi.nlm.nih.gov/pubmed/35854107.
133. Möller HJ, Falkai P. Is the serotonin hypothesis/theory of depression still relevant? Methodological reflections motivated by a recently published umbrella review. Eur Arch Psychiatry Clin Neurosci. 2023;273(1):1–3. PMCID: PMC9957868. http://www.ncbi.nlm.nih.gov/pubmed/36790577.
134. Jauhar S, Arnone D, Baldwin DS, Bloomfield M, Browning M, Cleare AJ, Corlett P, Deakin JFW, Erritzoe D, Fu C, Fusar-Poli P, Goodwin GM, Hayes J, Howard R, Howes OD, Juruena MF, Lam RW, Lawrie SM, McAllister-Williams H, Marwaha S, Matuskey D, McCutcheon RA, Nutt DJ, Pariante C, Pillinger T, Radhakrishnan R, Rucker J, Selvaraj S, Stokes P, Upthegrove R, Yalin N, Yatham L, Young AH, Zahn R, Cowen PJ. A leaky umbrella has little value: evidence clearly indicates the serotonin system is implicated in depression. Mol Psychiatry. 2023;28(8):3149–52. PMCID: PMC10618084. http://www.ncbi.nlm.nih.gov/pubmed/37322065.
135. Moncrieff J, Cooper RE, Stockmann T, Amendola S, Hengartner MP, Plöderl M, Horowitz MA. The serotonin hypothesis of depression: both long discarded and still supported? Mol Psychiatry. 2023;28(8):3160–3. PMID: 37322064. http://www.ncbi.nlm.nih.gov/pubmed/37322064.
136. El-Mallakh RS, Doroodgar M, Elsayed OH, Kidambi N. The serotonin theory of depression. Mol Psychiatry. 2023;28(8):3157. PMID: 37322061. http://www.ncbi.nlm.nih.gov/pubmed/37322061.
137. Almulla AF, Maes M. Although serotonin is not a major player in depression, its precursor is. Mol Psychiatry. 2023;28(8):3155–6. PMID: 37322063. http://www.ncbi.nlm.nih.gov/pubmed/37322063.
138. Arnone D, Wise T, Fitzgerald PB, Harmer CJ. The involvement of serotonin in major depression: nescience in disguise? Mol Psychiatry. 2024;29(1):200–2. PMID: 38374356. http://www.ncbi.nlm.nih.gov/pubmed/38374356.
139. Ahmed DR. Letter to the editor concerning: "The serotonin theory of depression: a systematic umbrella review of the evidence". Mol Psychiatry. 2024;29(1):205. PMID: 38374358. http://www.ncbi.nlm.nih.gov/pubmed/38374358.
140. Mohammad-Zadeh LF, Moses L, Gwaltney-Brant SM. Serotonin: a review. J Vet Pharmacol Ther. 2008;31(3):187–99. PMID: 18471139. http://www.ncbi.nlm.nih.gov/pubmed/18471139.
141. Cespuglio R. Serotonin: its place today in sleep preparation, triggering or maintenance. Sleep Med. 2018;49:31–9. PMID: 30029993. http://www.ncbi.nlm.nih.gov/pubmed/30029993.
142. Vaseghi S, Arjmandi-Rad S, Eskandari M, Ebrahimnejad M, Kholghi G, Zarrindast MR. Modulating role of serotonergic signaling in sleep and memory. Pharmacol Rep. 2022;74(1):1–26. PMID: 34743316. http://www.ncbi.nlm.nih.gov/pubmed/34743316.
143. Frazer A, Hensler JG. Understanding the neuroanatomical organization of serotonergic cells in the brain provides insight into the functions of this neurotransmitter. In: Siegel GJ, Agranoff BW, Fisher SK, Albers RW, Uhler MD, editors. Basic neurochemistry. 6th ed. Lippincott Williams & Wilkins; 1999.
144. Bacqué-Cazenave J, Bharatiya R, Barrière G, Delbecque JP, Bouguiyoud N, Di Giovanni G, Cattaert D, De Deurwaerdère P. Serotonin in animal cognition and behavior. Int J Mol Sci. 2020;21(5):1649. PMCID: PMC7084567. http://www.ncbi.nlm.nih.gov/pubmed/32121267.
145. Sanchez CL, Biskup CS, Herpertz S, Gaber TJ, Kuhn CM, Hood SH, Zepf FD. The role of serotonin (5-HT) in Behavioral control: findings from animal research and clinical implications. Int J Neuropsychopharmacol. 2015;18(10):pyv050. PMCID: PMC4648158. http://www.ncbi.nlm.nih.gov/pubmed/25991656.
146. Huber R, Smith K, Delago A, Isaksson K, Kravitz EA. Serotonin and aggressive motivation in crustaceans: altering the decision to retreat. Proc Natl Acad Sci USA. 1997;94(11):5939–42. PMCID: PMC20885. http://www.ncbi.nlm.nih.gov/pubmed/9159179.

147. Hood KE, Hurley LM. Listening to your partner: serotonin increases male responsiveness to female vocal signals in mice. Front Hum Neurosci. 2023;17:1304653. PMCID: PMC10847236. http://www.ncbi.nlm.nih.gov/pubmed/38328678.
148. Petersen CL, Hurley LM. Putting it in context: linking auditory processing with social behavior circuits in the vertebrate brain. Integr Comp Biol. 2017;57(4):865–77. PMCID: PMC6251620. http://www.ncbi.nlm.nih.gov/pubmed/28985384.
149. Keesom SM, Sloss BG, Erbowor-Becksen Z, Hurley LM. Social experience alters socially induced serotonergic fluctuations in the inferior colliculus. J Neurophysiol. 2017;118(6):3230–41. PMID: 28855293. http://www.ncbi.nlm.nih.gov/pubmed/28855293.
150. Panula P, Nuutinen S. The histaminergic network in the brain: basic organization and role in disease. Nat Rev Neurosci. 2013;14(7):472–87. PMID: 23783198. http://www.ncbi.nlm.nih.gov/pubmed/23783198.
151. Histamine Actions in the Central Nervous System – Basic Neurochemistry – NCBI Bookshelf.
152. Wada H, Inagaki N, Yamatodani A, Watanabe T. Is the histaminergic neuron system a regulatory center for whole-brain activity? Trends Neurosci. 1991;14(9):415–8. PMID: 1720584. http://www.ncbi.nlm.nih.gov/pubmed/1720584.
153. Iwańczuk W, Guźniczak P. Neurophysiological foundations of sleep, arousal, awareness and consciousness phenomena. Part 1. Anaesthesiol Intensive Ther. 2015;47(2):162–7. PMID: 25940332. http://www.ncbi.nlm.nih.gov/pubmed/25940332.
154. Branco ACCC, Yoshikawa FSY, Pietrobon AJ, Sato MN. Role of histamine in modulating the immune response and inflammation. Mediat Inflamm. 2018;2018:9524075. PMCID: PMC6129797. http://www.ncbi.nlm.nih.gov/pubmed/30224900.
155. Riccio D, Andersen HH, Arendt-Nielsen L. Antipruritic effects of transient heat stimulation on histaminergic and nonhistaminergic itch. Br J Dermatol. 2019;181(4):786–95. PMID: 30802929. http://www.ncbi.nlm.nih.gov/pubmed/30802929.
156. Naganuma F, Yoshikawa T. Organic Cation transporters in brain histamine clearance: physiological and psychiatric implications. Handb Exp Pharmacol. 2021;266:169–85. PMID: 33641029. http://www.ncbi.nlm.nih.gov/pubmed/33641029.
157. Szukiewicz D. Histaminergic system activity in the central nervous system: the role in neurodevelopmental and neurodegenerative disorders. Int J Mol Sci. 2024;25(18):9859. PMCID: PMC11432521. http://www.ncbi.nlm.nih.gov/pubmed/39337347.
158. Moya-García AA, Pino-Ángeles A, Sánchez-Jiménez F, Urdiales JL, Medina MÁ. Histamine, metabolic remodelling and angiogenesis: a systems level approach. Biomolecules. 2021;11(3):415. PMCID: PMC8000605. http://www.ncbi.nlm.nih.gov/pubmed/33799732.
159. Chazot P. Molecular biology of histamine system, volume 1. Int J Mol Sci. 2022;23(9):5026. PMCID: PMC9104633 http://www.ncbi.nlm.nih.gov/pubmed/35563417.
160. Patel RH, Mohiuddin SS. Biochemistry, Histamine. In: StatPearls [Internet]. Treasure Island (FL): StatPearls Publishing; 2024. [cited 2024 Dec 25]. Available from: http://www.ncbi.nlm.nih.gov/books/NBK557790/ PMID: 32491722 http://www.ncbi.nlm.nih.gov/pubmed/32491722.
161. Arrigoni E, Fuller PM. The role of the central Histaminergic system in Behavioral state control. Curr Top Behav Neurosci. 2022;59:447–68. PMID: 34595740. http://www.ncbi.nlm.nih.gov/pubmed/34595740.
162. Scammell TE, Jackson AC, Franks NP, Wisden W, Dauvilliers Y. Histamine: neural circuits and new medications. Sleep. 2019;42(1):zsy183. PMCID: PMC6335869. http://www.ncbi.nlm.nih.gov/pubmed/30239935.
163. Flik G, Folgering JHA, Cremers TIHF, Westerink BHC, Dremencov E. Interaction between brain histamine and serotonin, norepinephrine, and dopamine systems: in vivo microdialysis and Electrophysiology Study. J Mol Neurosci. 2015;56(2):320–8. PMID: 25820671. http://www.ncbi.nlm.nih.gov/pubmed/25820671.
164. Hersey M, Hashemi P, Reagan LP. Integrating the monoamine and cytokine hypotheses of depression: is histamine the missing link? Eur J Neurosci. 2022;55(9–10):2895–911. PMID: 34265868. http://www.ncbi.nlm.nih.gov/pubmed/34265868.
165. Iida T, Yanai K, Yoshikawa T. Histamine and Microglia. Curr Top Behav Neurosci. 2022;59:241–59. PMID: 35538301. http://www.ncbi.nlm.nih.gov/pubmed/35538301.
166. Noszal B, Kraszni M, Racz A. Histamine: fundamentals of biological chemistry. In: Falus A, Grosman N, Darvas Z, editors. Histamine: biology and medical aspects. SpringMed: Budapest; 2004. p. 15–28.
167. Picciotto MR, Higley MJ, Mineur YS. Acetylcholine as a neuromodulator: cholinergic signaling shapes nervous system function and behavior. Neuron. 2012;76(1):116–29. PMCID: PMC3466476. http://www.ncbi.nlm.nih.gov/pubmed/23040810.
168. Sarter M, Parikh V, Howe WM. Phasic acetylcholine release and the volume transmission hypothesis: time to move on. Nat Rev Neurosci. 2009;10(5):383–90. PMCID: PMC2699581. http://www.ncbi.nlm.nih.gov/pubmed/19377503.
169. Picciotto MR. Nicotine as a modulator of behavior: beyond the inverted U. Trends Pharmacol Sci. 2003;24(9):493–9. PMID: 12967775. http://www.ncbi.nlm.nih.gov/pubmed/12967775.
170. Hasselmo ME, Giocomo LM. Cholinergic modulation of cortical function. J Mol Neurosci. 2006;30(1–2):133–5. PMID: 17192659. http://www.ncbi.nlm.nih.gov/pubmed/17192659.
171. Hasselmo ME, McGaughy J. High acetylcholine levels set circuit dynamics for attention and encoding and low acetylcholine levels set dynamics for consolidation. Prog Brain Res. 2004;145:207–31. PMID: 14650918. http://www.ncbi.nlm.nih.gov/pubmed/14650918.
172. Saunders A, Granger AJ, Sabatini BL. Corelease of acetylcholine and GABA from cholinergic forebrain neurons. elife. 2015;4:e06412. PMCID: PMC4371381. http://www.ncbi.nlm.nih.gov/pubmed/25723967.
173. Gras C, Amilhon B, Lepicard EM, Poirel O, Vinatier J, Herbin M, Dumas S, Tzavara ET, Wade MR, Nomikos GG, Hanoun N, Saurini F, Kemel ML, Gasnier B, Giros B, El Mestikawy S. The vesicular glutamate transporter VGLUT3 synergizes striatal acetylcholine tone. Nat Neurosci. 2008;11(3):292–300. PMID: 18278042. http://www.ncbi.nlm.nih.gov/pubmed/18278042.
174. Mark GP, Shabani S, Dobbs LK, Hansen ST. Cholinergic modulation of mesolimbic dopamine function and reward. Physiol Behav. 2011;104(1):76–81. PMCID: PMC4495915. http://www.ncbi.nlm.nih.gov/pubmed/21549724.
175. Teles-Grilo Ruivo LM, Baker KL, Conway MW, Kinsley PJ, Gilmour G, Phillips KG, Isaac JTR, Lowry JP, Mellor JR. Coordinated acetylcholine release in prefrontal cortex and hippocampus is associated with arousal and reward on distinct timescales. Cell Rep. 2017;18(4):905–17. PMCID: PMC5289927. http://www.ncbi.nlm.nih.gov/pubmed/28122241.
176. Hasselmo ME, Sarter M. Modes and models of forebrain cholinergic neuromodulation of cognition. Neuropsychopharmacology. 2011;36(1):52–73. PMCID: PMC2992803. http://www.ncbi.nlm.nih.gov/pubmed/20668433.
177. Runyon K, Bui T, Mazanek S, Hartle A, Marschalko K, Howe WM. Distinct cholinergic circuits underlie discrete effects of reward on attention. Front Mol Neurosci. 2024;17:1429316. PMCID: PMC11390659. http://www.ncbi.nlm.nih.gov/pubmed/39268248.
178. Rolls ET. Emotion, motivation, decision-making, the orbitofrontal cortex, anterior cingulate cortex, and the amygdala. Brain Struct Funct. 2023;228(5):1201–57. PMCID: PMC10250292. http://www.ncbi.nlm.nih.gov/pubmed/37178232.

179. Parikh V, Bangasser DA. Cholinergic Signaling dynamics and cognitive control of attention. Curr Top Behav Neurosci. 2020;45:71–87. PMCID: PMC10771779. http://www.ncbi.nlm.nih.gov/pubmed/32447715.
180. de Castro BM, Pereira GS, Magalhães V, Rossato JI, De Jaeger X, Martins-Silva C, Leles B, Lima P, Gomez MV, Gainetdinov RR, Caron MG, Izquierdo I, Cammarota M, Prado VF, Prado MAM. Reduced expression of the vesicular acetylcholine transporter causes learning deficits in mice. Genes Brain Behav. 2009;8(1):23–35. PMID: 18778400. http://www.ncbi.nlm.nih.gov/pubmed/18778400.
181. Kunnath AJ, Gifford RH, Wallace MT. Cholinergic modulation of sensory perception and plasticity. Neurosci Biobehav Rev. 2023;152:105323. PMCID: PMC10424559. http://www.ncbi.nlm.nih.gov/pubmed/37467908.
182. Costanzi M, Cianfanelli B, Santirocchi A, Lasaponara S, Spataro P, Rossi-Arnaud C, Cestari V. Forgetting unwanted memories: active forgetting and implications for the development of psychological disorders. J Pers Med. 2021;11(4):241. PMCID: PMC8066077. http://www.ncbi.nlm.nih.gov/pubmed/33810436.
183. Picciotto MR, Addy NA, Mineur YS, Brunzell DH. It is not "either/or": activation and desensitization of nicotinic acetylcholine receptors both contribute to behaviors related to nicotine addiction and mood. Prog Neurobiol. 2008;84(4):329–42. PMCID: PMC2390914. http://www.ncbi.nlm.nih.gov/pubmed/18242816.
184. Mineur YS, Picciotto MR. Nicotine receptors and depression: revisiting and revising the cholinergic hypothesis. Trends Pharmacol Sci. 2010;31(12):580–6. PMCID: PMC2991594. http://www.ncbi.nlm.nih.gov/pubmed/20965579.
185. Mineur YS, Picciotto MR. The role of acetylcholine in negative encoding bias: too much of a good thing? Eur J Neurosci. 2021;53(1):114–25. PMCID: PMC7282966. http://www.ncbi.nlm.nih.gov/pubmed/31821620.
186. Kaufer D, Friedman A, Seidman S, Soreq H. Acute stress facilitates long-lasting changes in cholinergic gene expression. Nature. 1998;393(6683):373–7. PMID: 9620801. http://www.ncbi.nlm.nih.gov/pubmed/9620801.
187. Kaufer D, Friedman A, Seidman S, Soreq H. Anticholinesterases induce multigenic transcriptional feedback response suppressing cholinergic neurotransmission. Chem Biol Interact. 1999;119–120:349–60. PMID: 10421471. http://www.ncbi.nlm.nih.gov/pubmed/10421471.
188. Mineur YS, Cahuzac EL, Mose TN, Bentham MP, Plantenga ME, Thompson DC, Picciotto MR. Interaction between noradrenergic and cholinergic signaling in amygdala regulates anxiety- and depression-related behaviors in mice. Neuropsychopharmacology. 2018;43(10):2118–25. PMCID: PMC6098039. http://www.ncbi.nlm.nih.gov/pubmed/29472646.
189. Guyenet PG, Stornetta RL, Bochorishvili G, Depuy SD, Burke PGR, Abbott SBG. C1 neurons: the body's EMTs. Am J Physiol Regul Integr Comp Physiol. 2013;305(3):R187–204. PMCID: PMC3743001. http://www.ncbi.nlm.nih.gov/pubmed/23697799.
190. Stornetta RL, Guyenet PG. C1 neurons: a nodal point for stress? Exp Physiol. 2018;103(3):332–6. PMCID: PMC5832554. http://www.ncbi.nlm.nih.gov/pubmed/29080216.
191. Kumagai H, Oshima N, Matsuura T, Iigaya K, Imai M, Onimaru H, Sakata K, Osaka M, Onami T, Takimoto C, Kamayachi T, Itoh H, Saruta T. Importance of rostral ventrolateral medulla neurons in determining efferent sympathetic nerve activity and blood pressure. Hypertens Res. 2012;35(2):132–41. PMCID: PMC3273996. http://www.ncbi.nlm.nih.gov/pubmed/22170390.
192. Pace SA, Myers B. Hindbrain adrenergic/noradrenergic control of integrated endocrine and autonomic stress responses. Endocrinology. 2023;165(1):bqad178. PMID: 38015813. http://www.ncbi.nlm.nih.gov/pubmed/38015813.
193. Mischel NA, Subramanian M, Dombrowski MD, Llewellyn-Smith IJ, Mueller PJ. (In)activity-related neuroplasticity in brainstem control of sympathetic outflow: unraveling underlying molecular, cellular, and anatomical mechanisms. Am J Physiol Heart Circ Physiol. 2015;309(2):H235–43. PMCID: PMC4504968. http://www.ncbi.nlm.nih.gov/pubmed/25957223.
194. Toth M, Ziegler M, Sun P, Gresack J, Risbrough V. Impaired conditioned fear response and startle reactivity in epinephrine-deficient mice. Behav Pharmacol. 2013;24(1):1–9. PMCID: PMC3558035. http://www.ncbi.nlm.nih.gov/pubmed/23268986.
195. Cahill L, Alkire MT. Epinephrine enhancement of human memory consolidation: interaction with arousal at encoding. Neurobiol Learn Mem. 2003;79(2):194–8. PMID: 12591227. http://www.ncbi.nlm.nih.gov/pubmed/12591227.
196. Motiejunaite J, Amar L, Vidal-Petiot E. Adrenergic receptors and cardiovascular effects of catecholamines. Ann Endocrinol (Paris). 2021;82(3–4):193–7. PMID: 32473788. http://www.ncbi.nlm.nih.gov/pubmed/32473788.
197. James KA, Stromin JI, Steenkamp N, Combrinck MI. Understanding the relationships between physiological and psychosocial stress, cortisol and cognition. Front Endocrinol (Lausanne). 2023;14:1085950. PMCID: PMC10025564. http://www.ncbi.nlm.nih.gov/pubmed/36950689.
198. Tseng YT, Schaefke B, Wei P, Wang L. Defensive responses: behaviour, the brain and the body. Nat Rev Neurosci. 2023;24(11):655–71. PMID: 37730910. http://www.ncbi.nlm.nih.gov/pubmed/37730910.
199. Wong DL, Tai TC, Wong-Faull DC, Claycomb R, Meloni EG, Myers KM, Carlezon WA Jr, Kvetnansky R. Epinephrine: a short- and long-term regulator of stress and development of illness : a potential new role for epinephrine in stress. Cell Mol Neurobiol. 2012;32(5):737–48. https://doi.org/10.1007/s10571-011-9768-0. PMID: 22090159. PMCID: PMC11498570. http://www.ncbi.nlm.nih.gov/pubmed/22090159.
200. Zhao Y, Gan L, Ren L, Lin Y, Ma C, Lin X. Factors influencing the blood-brain barrier permeability. Brain Res. 2022;1788:147937. https://doi.org/10.1016/j.brainres.2022.147937. Epub 2022 May 11. PMID: 35568085. http://www.ncbi.nlm.nih.gov/pubmed/35568085.
201. Taber KH, Hurley RA. Volume transmission in the brain: beyond the synapse. J Neuropsychiatry Clin Neurosci. 2014;26(1):iv, 1–4. PMID: 24515717. http://www.ncbi.nlm.nih.gov/pubmed/24515717.
202. Castañeda-Hernández GC, Bach-y-Rita P. Volume transmission and pain perception. ScientificWorldJournal. 2003;3:677–83. PMCID: PMC5974734. http://www.ncbi.nlm.nih.gov/pubmed/12920309.
203. Dreyer JK, Herrik KF, Berg RW, Hounsgaard JD. Influence of phasic and tonic dopamine release on receptor activation. J Neurosci. 2010;30(42):14273–83. PMCID: PMC6634758. http://www.ncbi.nlm.nih.gov/pubmed/20962248.
204. Goto Y, Otani S, Grace AA. The Yin and Yang of dopamine release: a new perspective. Neuropharmacology. 2007;53(5):583–7. PMCID: PMC2078202. http://www.ncbi.nlm.nih.gov/pubmed/17709119.
205. Zou S, Kumar U. Cannabinoid receptors and the Endocannabinoid system: Signaling and function in the central nervous system. Int J Mol Sci. 2018;19(3):833. PMCID: PMC5877694. http://www.ncbi.nlm.nih.gov/pubmed/29533978.
206. Morena M, Patel S, Bains JS, Hill MN. Neurobiological interactions between stress and the Endocannabinoid system. Neuropsychopharmacology. 2016;41(1):80–102. PMCID: PMC4677118. http://www.ncbi.nlm.nih.gov/pubmed/26068727.
207. Battista N, Di Tommaso M, Bari M, Maccarrone M. The endocannabinoid system: an overview. Front. Behav Neurosci.

2012;6:9. PMCID: PMC3303140. http://www.ncbi.nlm.nih.gov/pubmed/22457644.
208. Ligresti A, Petrosino S, Di Marzo V. From endocannabinoid profiling to "endocannabinoid therapeutics". Curr Opin Chem Biol. 2009;13(3):321–31. PMID: 19497779. http://www.ncbi.nlm.nih.gov/pubmed/19497779.
209. Maccarrone M, Dainese E, Oddi S. Intracellular trafficking of anandamide: new concepts for signaling. Trends Biochem Sci. 2010;35(11):601–8. PMID: 20570522. http://www.ncbi.nlm.nih.gov/pubmed/20570522.
210. Herkenham M, Lynn AB, Johnson MR, Melvin LS, de Costa BR, Rice KC. Characterization and localization of cannabinoid receptors in rat brain: a quantitative in vitro autoradiographic study. J Neurosci. 1991;11(2):563–83. PMCID: PMC6575215. http://www.ncbi.nlm.nih.gov/pubmed/1992016.
211. Gong JP, Onaivi ES, Ishiguro H, Liu QR, Tagliaferro PA, Brusco A, Uhl GR. Cannabinoid CB2 receptors: immunohistochemical localization in rat brain. Brain Res. 2006;1071(1):10–23. PMID: 16472786. http://www.ncbi.nlm.nih.gov/pubmed/16472786.
212. Munro S, Thomas KL, Abu-Shaar M. Molecular characterization of a peripheral receptor for cannabinoids. Nature. 1993;365(6441):61–5. PMID: 7689702. http://www.ncbi.nlm.nih.gov/pubmed/7689702.
213. Van Sickle MD, Duncan M, Kingsley PJ, Mouihate A, Urbani P, Mackie K, Stella N, Makriyannis A, Piomelli D, Davison JS, Marnett LJ, Di Marzo V, Pittman QJ, Patel KD, Sharkey KA. Identification and functional characterization of brainstem cannabinoid CB2 receptors. Science. 2005;310(5746):329–32. PMID: 16224028. http://www.ncbi.nlm.nih.gov/pubmed/16224028.
214. Viscomi MT, Oddi S, Latini L, Pasquariello N, Florenzano F, Bernardi G, Molinari M, Maccarrone M. Selective CB2 receptor agonism protects central neurons from remote axotomy-induced apoptosis through the PI3K/Akt pathway. J Neurosci. 2009;29(14):4564–70. PMCID: PMC6665736. http://www.ncbi.nlm.nih.gov/pubmed/19357281.
215. Chiocchetti R, Galiazzo G, Tagliavia C, Stanzani A, Giancola F, Menchetti M, Militerno G, Bernardini C, Forni M, Mandrioli L. Cellular distribution of canonical and putative cannabinoid receptors in canine cervical dorsal root ganglia. Front Vet Sci. 2019;6:313. PMCID: PMC6761858. http://www.ncbi.nlm.nih.gov/pubmed/31608295.
216. Lauckner JE, Jensen JB, Chen HY, Lu HC, Hille B, Mackie K. GPR55 is a cannabinoid receptor that increases intracellular calcium and inhibits M current. Proc Natl Acad Sci USA. 2008;105(7):2699–704. PMCID: PMC2268199. http://www.ncbi.nlm.nih.gov/pubmed/18263732.
217. Gorzalka BB, Hill MN. Putative role of endocannabinoid signaling in the etiology of depression and actions of antidepressants. Prog Neuro-Psychopharmacol Biol Psychiatry. 2011;35(7):1575–85. PMID: 21111017. http://www.ncbi.nlm.nih.gov/pubmed/21111017.
218. Hill MN, Hellemans KGC, Verma P, Gorzalka BB, Weinberg J. Neurobiology of chronic mild stress: parallels to major depression. Neurosci Biobehav Rev. 2012;36(9):2085–117. PMCID: PMC4821201. http://www.ncbi.nlm.nih.gov/pubmed/22776763.
219. Valverde O, Torrens M. CB1 receptor-deficient mice as a model for depression. Neuroscience. 2012;204:193–206. PMID: 21964469. http://www.ncbi.nlm.nih.gov/pubmed/21964469.
220. Beyer CE, Dwyer JM, Piesla MJ, Platt BJ, Shen R, Rahman Z, Chan K, Manners MT, Samad TA, Kennedy JD, Bingham B, Whiteside GT. Depression-like phenotype following chronic CB1 receptor antagonism. Neurobiol Dis. 2010;39(2):148–55. PMID: 20381618. http://www.ncbi.nlm.nih.gov/pubmed/20381618.
221. Willner P. Chronic mild stress (CMS) revisited: consistency and behavioural-neurobiological concordance in the effects of CMS. Neuropsychobiology. 2005;52(2):90–110. PMID: 16037678. http://www.ncbi.nlm.nih.gov/pubmed/16037678.
222. Hill MN, Carrier EJ, McLaughlin RJ, Morrish AC, Meier SE, Hillard CJ, Gorzalka BB. Regional alterations in the endocannabinoid system in an animal model of depression: effects of concurrent antidepressant treatment. J Neurochem. 2008;106(6):2322–36. PMCID: PMC2606621. http://www.ncbi.nlm.nih.gov/pubmed/18643796.
223. McLaughlin RJ, Hill MN, Dang SS, Wainwright SR, Galea LAM, Hillard CJ, Gorzalka BB. Upregulation of CB_1 receptor binding in the ventromedial prefrontal cortex promotes proactive stress-coping strategies following chronic stress exposure. Behav Brain Res. 2013;237:333–7. PMCID: PMC3501995. http://www.ncbi.nlm.nih.gov/pubmed/23047058.
224. Wang W, Sun D, Pan B, Roberts CJ, Sun X, Hillard CJ, Liu Q, song. Deficiency in endocannabinoid signaling in the nucleus accumbens induced by chronic unpredictable stress. Neuropsychopharmacology. 2010;35(11):2249–61. PMCID: PMC3055309. http://www.ncbi.nlm.nih.gov/pubmed/20664582.
225. Choi K, Le T, McGuire J, Xing G, Zhang L, Li H, Parker CC, Johnson LR, Ursano RJ. Expression pattern of the cannabinoid receptor genes in the frontal cortex of mood disorder patients and mice selectively bred for high and low fear. J Psychiatr Res. 2012;46(7):882–9. PMID: 22534181. http://www.ncbi.nlm.nih.gov/pubmed/22534181.
226. Hungund BL, Vinod KY, Kassir SA, Basavarajappa BS, Yalamanchili R, Cooper TB, Mann JJ, Arango V. Upregulation of CB1 receptors and agonist-stimulated [35S]GTPgammaS binding in the prefrontal cortex of depressed suicide victims. Mol Psychiatry. 2004;9(2):184–90. PMID: 14966476. http://www.ncbi.nlm.nih.gov/pubmed/14966476.
227. Bortolato M, Mangieri RA, Fu J, Kim JH, Arguello O, Duranti A, Tontini A, Mor M, Tarzia G, Piomelli D. Antidepressant-like activity of the fatty acid amide hydrolase inhibitor URB597 in a rat model of chronic mild stress. Biol Psychiatry. 2007;62(10):1103–10. PMID: 17511970. http://www.ncbi.nlm.nih.gov/pubmed/17511970.
228. Gobbi G, Bambico FR, Mangieri R, Bortolato M, Campolongo P, Solinas M, Cassano T, Morgese MG, Debonnel G, Duranti A, Tontini A, Tarzia G, Mor M, Trezza V, Goldberg SR, Cuomo V, Piomelli D. Antidepressant-like activity and modulation of brain monoaminergic transmission by blockade of anandamide hydrolysis. Proc Natl Acad Sci USA. 2005;102(51):18620–5. PMCID: PMC1317988. http://www.ncbi.nlm.nih.gov/pubmed/16352709.
229. Vinod KY, Xie S, Psychoyos D, Hungund BL, Cooper TB, Tejani-Butt SM. Dysfunction in fatty acid amide hydrolase is associated with depressive-like behavior in Wistar Kyoto rats. PLoS One. 2012;7(5):e36743. PMCID: PMC3351478. http://www.ncbi.nlm.nih.gov/pubmed/22606285.
230. García-Gutiérrez MS, Pérez-Ortiz JM, Gutiérrez-Adán A, Manzanares J. Depression-resistant endophenotype in mice overexpressing cannabinoid CB(2) receptors. Br J Pharmacol. 2010;160(7):1773–84. PMCID: PMC2936848. http://www.ncbi.nlm.nih.gov/pubmed/20649579.
231. Bahi A, Al Mansouri S, Al Memari E, Al Ameri M, Nurulain SM, Ojha S. β-Caryophyllene, a CB2 receptor agonist produces multiple behavioral changes relevant to anxiety and depression in mice. Physiol Behav. 2014;135:119–24. PMID: 24930711. http://www.ncbi.nlm.nih.gov/pubmed/24930711.
232. Hill MN, Tasker JG. Endocannabinoid signaling, glucocorticoid-mediated negative feedback, and regulation of the hypothalamic-pituitary-adrenal axis. Neuroscience. 2012;204:5–16. PMCID: PMC3288468. http://www.ncbi.nlm.nih.gov/pubmed/22214537.

233. Wade MR, Degroot A, Nomikos GG. Cannabinoid CB1 receptor antagonism modulates plasma corticosterone in rodents. Eur J Pharmacol. 2006;551(1–3):162–7. PMID: 17030030. http://www.ncbi.nlm.nih.gov/pubmed/17030030.
234. Patel S, Roelke CT, Rademacher DJ, Cullinan WE, Hillard CJ. Endocannabinoid signaling negatively modulates stress-induced activation of the hypothalamic-pituitary-adrenal axis. Endocrinology. 2004;145(12):5431–8. PMID: 15331569. http://www.ncbi.nlm.nih.gov/pubmed/15331569.
235. Barna I, Zelena D, Arszovszki AC, Ledent C. The role of endogenous cannabinoids in the hypothalamo-pituitary-adrenal axis regulation: in vivo and in vitro studies in CB1 receptor knockout mice. Life Sci. 2004;75(24):2959–70. PMID: 15454346. http://www.ncbi.nlm.nih.gov/pubmed/15454346.
236. Miller BR, Hen R. The current state of the neurogenic theory of depression and anxiety. Curr Opin Neurobiol. 2015;30:51–8. PMCID: PMC4293252. http://www.ncbi.nlm.nih.gov/pubmed/25240202.
237. Palazuelos J, Ortega Z, Díaz-Alonso J, Guzmán M, Galve-Roperh I. CB2 cannabinoid receptors promote neural progenitor cell proliferation via mTORC1 signaling. J Biol Chem. 2012;287(2):1198–209. PMCID: PMC3256884. http://www.ncbi.nlm.nih.gov/pubmed/22102284.
238. Galve-Roperh I, Chiurchiù V, Díaz-Alonso J, Bari M, Guzmán M, Maccarrone M. Cannabinoid receptor signaling in progenitor/stem cell proliferation and differentiation. Prog Lipid Res. 2013;52(4):633–50. PMID: 24076098. http://www.ncbi.nlm.nih.gov/pubmed/16472786.
239. Lee S, Kim DH, Yoon SH, Ryu JH. Sub-chronic administration of rimonabant causes loss of antidepressive activity and decreases doublecortin immunoreactivity in the mouse hippocampus. Neurosci Lett. 2009;467(2):111–6. PMID: 19819298. http://www.ncbi.nlm.nih.gov/pubmed/19819298.
240. Santarelli L, Saxe M, Gross C, Surget A, Battaglia F, Dulawa S, Weisstaub N, Lee J, Duman R, Arancio O, Belzung C, Hen R. Requirement of hippocampal neurogenesis for the behavioral effects of antidepressants. Science. 2003;301(5634):805–9. PMID: 12907793. http://www.ncbi.nlm.nih.gov/pubmed/12907793.
241. Sheline YI, Wang PW, Gado MH, Csernansky JG, Vannier MW. Hippocampal atrophy in recurrent major depression. Proc Natl Acad Sci USA. 1996;93(9):3908–13. PMCID: PMC39458. http://www.ncbi.nlm.nih.gov/pubmed/8632988.
242. Jiang W, Zhang Y, Xiao L, Van Cleemput J, Ji SP, Bai G, Zhang X. Cannabinoids promote embryonic and adult hippocampus neurogenesis and produce anxiolytic- and antidepressant-like effects. J Clin Invest. 2005;115(11):3104–16. PMCID: PMC1253627. http://www.ncbi.nlm.nih.gov/pubmed/16224541.
243. Duman RS, Monteggia LM. A neurotrophic model for stress-related mood disorders. Biol Psychiatry. 2006;59(12):1116–27. PMID: 16631126. http://www.ncbi.nlm.nih.gov/pubmed/16631126.
244. Wyrofsky R, McGonigle P, Van Bockstaele EJ. Drug discovery strategies that focus on the endocannabinoid signaling system in psychiatric disease. Expert Opin Drug Discov. 2015;10(1):17–36. PMCID: PMC4696509. http://www.ncbi.nlm.nih.gov/pubmed/25488672.
245. Hirvonen J, Goodwin RS, Li CT, Terry GE, Zoghbi SS, Morse C, Pike VW, Volkow ND, Huestis MA, Innis RB. Reversible and regionally selective downregulation of brain cannabinoid CB1 receptors in chronic daily cannabis smokers. Mol Psychiatry. 2012;17(6):642–9. PMCID: PMC3223558. http://www.ncbi.nlm.nih.gov/pubmed/21747398.
246. Landfield PW, Cadwallader LB, Vinsant S. Quantitative changes in hippocampal structure following long-term exposure to delta 9-tetrahydrocannabinol: possible mediation by glucocorticoid systems. Brain Res. 1988;443(1–2):47–62. PMID: 2834017. http://www.ncbi.nlm.nih.gov/pubmed/2834017.
247. Poleszak E, Wośko S, Sławińska K, Szopa A, Wróbel A, Serefko A. Cannabinoids in depressive disorders. Life Sci. 2018;213:18–24. PMID: 30290188. http://www.ncbi.nlm.nih.gov/pubmed/30290188.
248. Schnelle M, Grotenhermen F, Reif M, Gorter RW. Results of a standardized survey on the medical use of cannabis products in the German-speaking area. Forsch Komplementmed. 1999;6(Suppl 3):28–36. PMID: 10575286. http://www.ncbi.nlm.nih.gov/pubmed/10575286.
249. Prentiss D, Power R, Balmas G, Tzuang G, Israelski DM. Patterns of marijuana use among patients with HIV/AIDS followed in a public health care setting. J Acquir Immune Defic Syndr. 2004;35(1):38–45. PMID: 14707790. http://www.ncbi.nlm.nih.gov/pubmed/14707790.
250. Denson TF, Earleywine M. Decreased depression in marijuana users. Addict Behav. 2006;31(4):738–42. PMID: 15964704. http://www.ncbi.nlm.nih.gov/pubmed/15964704.
251. Gruber AJ, Pope HG, Brown ME. Do patients use marijuana as an antidepressant? Depression. 1996;4(2):77–80. PMID: 9160645. http://www.ncbi.nlm.nih.gov/pubmed/9160645.
252. Turna J, Patterson B, Van Ameringen M. Is cannabis treatment for anxiety, mood, and related disorders ready for prime time? Depress Anxiety. 2017;34(11):1006–17. PMID: 28636769. http://www.ncbi.nlm.nih.gov/pubmed/28636769.
253. Hill MN, Hillard CJ, Bambico FR, Patel S, Gorzalka BB, Gobbi G. The therapeutic potential of the endocannabinoid system for the development of a novel class of antidepressants. Trends Pharmacol Sci. 2009;30(9):484–93. PMID: 19732971. http://www.ncbi.nlm.nih.gov/pubmed/19732971.
254. Hill MN, Gorzalka BB. Is there a role for the endocannabinoid system in the etiology and treatment of melancholic depression? Behav Pharmacol. 2005;16(5–6):333–52. PMID: 16148438. http://www.ncbi.nlm.nih.gov/pubmed/16148438.
255. Ligand-Gated Ion Channel database – Ligand-Gated Ion Channel Database.
256. Evans RM. The steroid and thyroid hormone receptor superfamily. Science. 1988;240(4854):889–95. PMCID: PMC6159881. http://www.ncbi.nlm.nih.gov/pubmed/3283939.
257. Olefsky JM. Nuclear receptor minireview series. J Biol Chem. 2001;276(40):36863–4. PMID: 11459855. http://www.ncbi.nlm.nih.gov/pubmed/11459855.
258. Bradley SJ, Tobin AB, Prihandoko R. Muscarinic acetylcholine receptors in the central nervous system. Neuropharmacology. 2018;136(Pt C):361. PMID: 29894772. http://www.ncbi.nlm.nih.gov/pubmed/29894772.
259. Nahorski SR, Tobin AB, Willars GB. Muscarinic M3 receptor coupling and regulation. Life Sci. 1997;60(13–14):1039–45. PMID: 9121345. http://www.ncbi.nlm.nih.gov/pubmed/9121345.
260. Gautam D, Jeon J, Li JH, Han SJ, Hamdan FF, Cui Y, Lu H, Deng C, Gavrilova O, Wess J. Metabolic roles of the M3 muscarinic acetylcholine receptor studied with M3 receptor mutant mice: a review. J Recept Signal Transduct Res. 2008;28(1–2):93–108. PMID: 18437633. http://www.ncbi.nlm.nih.gov/pubmed/18437633.
261. Nawaratne V, Leach K, Suratman N, Loiacono RE, Felder CC, Armbruster BN, Roth BL, Sexton PM, Christopoulos A. New insights into the function of M4 muscarinic acetylcholine receptors gained using a novel allosteric modulator and a DREADD (designer receptor exclusively activated by a designer drug). Mol Pharmacol. 2008;74(4):1119–31. PMID: 18628403. http://www.ncbi.nlm.nih.gov/pubmed/18628403.
262. Yamada M, Basile AS, Fedorova I, Zhang W, Duttaroy A, Cui Y, Lamping KG, Faraci FM, Deng CX, Wess J. Novel insights into M5 muscarinic acetylcholine receptor function by the use of gene targeting technology. Life Sci. 2003;74(2–3):345–53. PMID: 14607263. http://www.ncbi.nlm.nih.gov/pubmed/14607263.

263. Caulfield MP, Birdsall NJ. International Union of Pharmacology. XVII. Classification of muscarinic acetylcholine receptors. Pharmacol Rev. 1998;50(2):279–90. PMID: 9647869. http://www.ncbi.nlm.nih.gov/pubmed/9647869.
264. Albuquerque EX, Pereira EFR, Alkondon M, Rogers SW. Mammalian nicotinic acetylcholine receptors: from structure to function. Physiol Rev. 2009;89(1):73–120. PMCID: PMC2713585. http://www.ncbi.nlm.nih.gov/pubmed/19126755.
265. Wonnacott S, Bermudez I, Millar NS, Tzartos SJ. Nicotinic acetylcholine receptors. Br J Pharmacol. 2018;175(11):1785–8. PMCID: PMC5979630. http://www.ncbi.nlm.nih.gov/pubmed/29878346.
266. Melikian HE. Neurotransmitter transporter trafficking: endocytosis, recycling, and regulation. Pharmacol Ther. 2004;104(1):17–27. PMID: 15500906. http://www.ncbi.nlm.nih.gov/pubmed/15500906.
267. Arizono M, Nägerl UV. Deciphering the functional nano-anatomy of the tripartite synapse using stimulated emission depletion microscopy. Glia. 2022;70(4):607–18. PMID: 34664734. http://www.ncbi.nlm.nih.gov/pubmed/34664734.
268. Rolls ET. Limbic systems for emotion and for memory, but no single limbic system. Cortex. 2015;62:119–57. PMID: 24439664. http://www.ncbi.nlm.nih.gov/pubmed/24439664.
269. Torrico TJ, Abdijadid S. Neuroanatomy, limbic system. In: StatPearls [Internet]. Treasure Island (FL): StatPearls Publishing; 2024. [cited 2024 Dec 25]. Available from: http://www.ncbi.nlm.nih.gov/books/NBK538491/ PMID: 30860726 http://www.ncbi.nlm.nih.gov/pubmed/30860726.
270. Kotter R. Limbic system. In: In the Encyclopedia of the neurological sciences. Elsevier Science; 2014.
271. Kamali A, Milosavljevic S, Gandhi A, Lano KR, Shobeiri P, Sherbaf FG, Sair HI, Riascos RF, Hasan KM. The Cortico-limbo-Thalamo-cortical circuits: an update to the original Papez circuit of the human limbic system. Brain Topogr. 2023;36(3):371–89. PMCID: PMC10164017. http://www.ncbi.nlm.nih.gov/pubmed/37148369.
272. Heather Ashton. Protracted withdrawal symptoms from benzodiazepines. In: Comprehensive handbook of drug & alcohol addiction; 2004. http://www.benzo.org.uk/pws04.htm.
273. Rajmohan V, Mohandas E. The limbic system. Indian J Psychiatry. 2007;49(2):132–9. PMCID: PMC2917081. http://www.ncbi.nlm.nih.gov/pubmed/20711399.
274. Catani M, Dell'acqua F, Thiebaut de Schotten M. A revised limbic system model for memory, emotion and behaviour. Neurosci Biobehav Rev. 2013;37(8):1724–37. PMID: 23850593. http://www.ncbi.nlm.nih.gov/pubmed/23850593.
275. Semple D, Smyth R, Burns J, Darjee R, McIntosh A. [2005]. "13". Oxford Handbook of psychiatry. Oxford University Press; 2007. p. 540.
276. Cooper ML. Motivations for alcohol use among adolescents: development and validation of a four-factor model. Psychol Assess. 1994;6:117–28.
277. Zald DH. The human amygdala and the emotional evaluation of sensory stimuli. Brain Res Brain Res Rev. 2003;41(1):88–123. PMID: 12505650. http://www.ncbi.nlm.nih.gov/pubmed/12505650.
278. Degar S, Prince AM, Pascual D, Lavie G, Levin B, Mazur Y, Lavie D, Ehrlich LS, Carter C, Meruelo D. Inactivation of the human immunodeficiency virus by hypericin: evidence for photochemical alterations of p24 and a block in uncoating. AIDS Res Hum Retrovir. 1992;8(11):1929–36. PMID: 1283309. http://www.ncbi.nlm.nih.gov/pubmed/1283309.
279. Nachev P. Cognition and medial frontal cortex in health and disease. Curr Opin Neurol. 2006;19(6):586–92. PMCID: PMC2658463. http://www.ncbi.nlm.nih.gov/pubmed/17102698.
280. Homack S, Lee D, Riccio CA. Test review: delis-Kaplan executive function system. J Clin Exp Neuropsychol. 2005;27(5):599–609. PMID: 16019636. http://www.ncbi.nlm.nih.gov/pubmed/16019636.
281. Sánchez-Carpintero R, Narbona J. Executive system: a conceptual review and its study in children with attention deficit hyperactivity disorder. Rev Neurol. 2001;33(1):47–53. PMID: 11562861. http://www.ncbi.nlm.nih.gov/pubmed/11562861.
282. Kilmer W. A thalamo-cortical model of the executive attention system. Biol Cybern. 2001;84(4):279–89. PMID: 11324339. http://www.ncbi.nlm.nih.gov/pubmed/11324339.
283. D'Esposito M, Detre JA, Alsop DC, Shin RK, Atlas S, Grossman M. The neural basis of the central executive system of working memory. Nature. 1995;378(6554):279–81. PMID: 7477346. http://www.ncbi.nlm.nih.gov/pubmed/7477346.
284. Hazy TE, Frank MJ, O'reilly RC. Towards an executive without a homunculus: computational models of the prefrontal cortex/basal ganglia system. Philos Trans R Soc Lond Ser B Biol Sci. 2007;362(1485):1601–13. PMCID: PMC2440774. http://www.ncbi.nlm.nih.gov/pubmed/17428778.
285. Allman JM, Hakeem A, Erwin JM, Nimchinsky E, Hof P. The anterior cingulate cortex. The evolution of an interface between emotion and cognition. Ann N Y Acad Sci. 2001;935:107–17. PMID: 11411161. http://www.ncbi.nlm.nih.gov/pubmed/11411161.
286. Steinman L. Elaborate interactions between the immune and nervous systems. Nat Immunol. 2004;5(6):575–81. PMID: 15164017. http://www.ncbi.nlm.nih.gov/pubmed/15164017.
287. Fleshner M, Laudenslager ML. Psychoneuroimmunology: then and now. Behav Cogn Neurosci Rev. 2004;3(2):114–30. PMID: 15537988. http://www.ncbi.nlm.nih.gov/pubmed/15537988.
288. Day TA, Walker FR, More appraisal please: a commentary on Pfaff et al. Relations between mechanisms of CNS arousal and mechanisms of stress. Stress. 2007;10(4):311–3; discussion 314–315. PMID: 17999347. http://www.ncbi.nlm.nih.gov/pubmed/17999347.
289. Pfaff DW, Martin EM, Ribeiro AC. Relations between mechanisms of CNS arousal and mechanisms of stress. Stress. 2007;10(4):316–25. PMID: 17999349. http://www.ncbi.nlm.nih.gov/pubmed/17999349.
290. Gaab J, Rohleder N, Nater UM, Ehlert U. Psychological determinants of the cortisol stress response: the role of anticipatory cognitive appraisal. Psychoneuroendocrinology. 2005;30(6):599–610. PMID: 15808930. http://www.ncbi.nlm.nih.gov/pubmed/15808930.
291. Schlotz W, Kumsta R, Layes I, Entringer S, Jones A, Wüst S. Covariance between psychological and endocrine responses to pharmacological challenge and psychosocial stress: a question of timing. Psychosom Med. 2008;70(7):787–96. PMID: 18725434. http://www.ncbi.nlm.nih.gov/pubmed/18725434.
292. Aldwin CM, Sutton KJ, Chiara G, Spiro A. Age differences in stress, coping, and appraisal: findings from the Normative Aging Study. J Gerontol B Psychol Sci Soc Sci. 1996;51(4):P179–88. PMID: 8673639. http://www.ncbi.nlm.nih.gov/pubmed/8673639.
293. Bohus B, Koolhaas JM, Heijnen CJ, de Boer O. Immunological responses to social stress: dependence on social environment and coping abilities. Neuropsychobiology. 1993;28(1–2):95–9. PMID: 8255418. http://www.ncbi.nlm.nih.gov/pubmed/8255418.
294. Borysenko M, Borysenko J. Stress, behavior, and immunity: animal models and mediating mechanisms. Gen Hosp Psychiatry. 1982;4(1):59–67. PMID: 6281128. http://www.ncbi.nlm.nih.gov/pubmed/6281128.
295. Kudielka BM, Hellhammer DH, Wüst S. Why do we respond so differently? Reviewing determinants of human salivary cortisol responses to challenge. Psychoneuroendocrinology. 2009;34(1):2–18. PMID: 19041187. http://www.ncbi.nlm.nih.gov/pubmed/19041187.

296. Hiramoto RN, Solvason HB, Hsueh CM, Rogers CF, Demissie S, Hiramoto NS, Gauthier DK, Lorden JF, Ghanta VK. Psychoneuroendocrine immunology: perception of stress can alter body temperature and natural killer cell activity. Int J Neurosci. 1999;98(1–2):95–129. PMID: 10395364. http://www.ncbi.nlm.nih.gov/pubmed/10395364.
297. Segerstrom SC, Miller GE. Psychological stress and the human immune system: a meta-analytic study of 30 years of inquiry. Psychol Bull. 2004;130(4):601–30. PMCID: PMC1361287. http://www.ncbi.nlm.nih.gov/pubmed/15250815.
298. Elenkov IJ, Chrousos GP. Stress system–organization, physiology and immunoregulation. Neuroimmunomodulation. 2006;13(5–6):257–67. PMID: 17709947. http://www.ncbi.nlm.nih.gov/pubmed/17709947.
299. Ising M, Holsboer F. Genetics of stress response and stress-related disorders. Dialogues Clin Neurosci. 2006;8(4):433–44. PMCID: PMC3181835. http://www.ncbi.nlm.nih.gov/pubmed/17290801.
300. Moriam S, Sobhani ME. Epigenetic effect of chronic stress on dopamine signaling and depression. Genet Epigenet. 2013;5:11–6. PMCID: PMC4222332. http://www.ncbi.nlm.nih.gov/pubmed/25512703.
301. Tafet GE, Bernardini R. Psychoneuroendocrinological links between chronic stress and depression. Prog Neuro-Psychopharmacol Biol Psychiatry. 2003;27(6):893–903. PMID: 14499305. http://www.ncbi.nlm.nih.gov/pubmed/14499305.
302. Checkley S. The neuroendocrinology of depression and chronic stress. Br Med Bull. 1996;52(3):597–617. PMID: 8949260. http://www.ncbi.nlm.nih.gov/pubmed/8949260.
303. Tabak BA, Vrshek-Schallhorn S, Zinbarg RE, Prenoveau JM, Mineka S, Redei EE, Adam EK, Craske MG. Interaction of CD38 variant and chronic interpersonal stress prospectively predicts social anxiety and depression symptoms over six years. Clin. Psychol Sci. 2016;4(1):17–27. PMCID: PMC4779340. http://www.ncbi.nlm.nih.gov/pubmed/26958455.
304. Conway CC, Rutter LA, Brown TA. Chronic environmental stress and the temporal course of depression and panic disorder: a trait-state-occasion modeling approach. J Abnorm Psychol. 2016;125(1):53–63. PMCID: PMC4701646. http://www.ncbi.nlm.nih.gov/pubmed/26595465.
305. Vrshek-Schallhorn S, Stroud CB, Mineka S, Hammen C, Zinbarg RE, Wolitzky-Taylor K, Craske MG. Chronic and episodic interpersonal stress as statistically unique predictors of depression in two samples of emerging adults. J Abnorm Psychol. 2015;124(4):918–32. PMCID: PMC4948584. http://www.ncbi.nlm.nih.gov/pubmed/26301973.
306. Papadopoulou A, Siamatras T, Delgado-Morales R, Amin ND, Shukla V, Zheng YL, Pant HC, Almeida OFX, Kino T. Acute and chronic stress differentially regulate cyclin-dependent kinase 5 in mouse brain: implications to glucocorticoid actions and major depression. Transl. Psychiatry. 2015;5(6):e578. PMCID: PMC4490283. http://www.ncbi.nlm.nih.gov/pubmed/26057048.
307. Starr LR, Hammen C. Genetic moderation of the association between adolescent romantic involvement and depression: contributions of serotonin transporter gene polymorphism, chronic stress, and family discord. Dev Psychopathol. 2016;28(2):447–57. PMCID: PMC5546886. http://www.ncbi.nlm.nih.gov/pubmed/26037034.
308. Franceschelli A, Herchick S, Thelen C, Papadopoulou-Daifoti Z, Pitychoutis PM. Sex differences in the chronic mild stress model of depression. Behav Pharmacol. 2014;25(5–6):372–83. PMID: 25025701. http://www.ncbi.nlm.nih.gov/pubmed/25025701.
309. Glaser R. Stress-associated immune dysregulation and its importance for human health: a personal history of psychoneuroimmunology. Brain Behav Immun. 2005;19(1):3–11. PMID: 15581732. http://www.ncbi.nlm.nih.gov/pubmed/15581732.
310. Ramachandruni S, Handberg E, Sheps DS. Acute and chronic psychological stress in coronary disease. Curr Opin Cardiol. 2004;19(5):494–9. PMID: 15316459. http://www.ncbi.nlm.nih.gov/pubmed/15316459.
311. Li J, Nørgard B, Precht DH, Olsen J. Psychological stress and inflammatory bowel disease: a follow-up study in parents who lost a child in Denmark. Am J Gastroenterol. 2004;99(6):1129–33. PMID: 15180736. http://www.ncbi.nlm.nih.gov/pubmed/15180736.
312. Thaker PH, Lutgendorf SK, Sood AK. The neuroendocrine impact of chronic stress on cancer. Cell Cycle. 2007;6(4):430–3. PMID: 17312398. http://www.ncbi.nlm.nih.gov/pubmed/17312398.
313. Saul AN, Oberyszyn TM, Daugherty C, Kusewitt D, Jones S, Jewell S, Malarkey WB, Lehman A, Lemeshow S, Dhabhar FS. Chronic stress and susceptibility to skin cancer. J Natl Cancer Inst. 2005;97(23):1760–7. PMCID: PMC3422720. http://www.ncbi.nlm.nih.gov/pubmed/16333031.
314. Kiecolt-Glaser JK, McGuire L, Robles TF, Glaser R. Emotions, morbidity, and mortality: new perspectives from psychoneuroimmunology. Annu Rev Psychol. 2002;53:83–107. PMID: 11752480. http://www.ncbi.nlm.nih.gov/pubmed/11752480.
315. Chrousos GP. Stress and disorders of the stress system. Nat Rev Endocrinol. 2009;5(7):374–81. PMID: 19488073. http://www.ncbi.nlm.nih.gov/pubmed/19488073.
316. Chrousos GP. Stress, chronic inflammation, and emotional and physical well-being: concurrent effects and chronic sequelae. J Allergy Clin Immunol. 2000;106(5 Suppl):S275–91. PMID: 11080744. http://www.ncbi.nlm.nih.gov/pubmed/11080744.
317. Carrasco GA, Van de Kar LD. Neuroendocrine pharmacology of stress. Eur J Pharmacol. 2003;463(1–3):235–72. PMID: 12600714. http://www.ncbi.nlm.nih.gov/pubmed/12600714.
318. McEwen BS. Physiology and neurobiology of stress and adaptation: central role of the brain. Physiol Rev. 2007;87(3):873–904. PMID: 17615391. http://www.ncbi.nlm.nih.gov/pubmed/17615391.
319. Charmandari E, Tsigos C, Chrousos G. Endocrinology of the stress response. Annu Rev Physiol. 2005;67:259–84. PMID: 15709959. http://www.ncbi.nlm.nih.gov/pubmed/15709959.
320. Stratakis CA, Chrousos GP. Neuroendocrinology and pathophysiology of the stress system. Ann N Y Acad Sci. 1995;771:1–18. PMID: 8597390. http://www.ncbi.nlm.nih.gov/pubmed/8597390.
321. Pani L, Porcella A, Gessa GL. The role of stress in the pathophysiology of the dopaminergic system. Mol Psychiatry. 2000;5(1):14–21. PMID: 10673764. http://www.ncbi.nlm.nih.gov/pubmed/10673764.
322. Vedhara K, Tuinstra J, Miles JNV, Sanderman R, Ranchor AV. Psychosocial factors associated with indices of cortisol production in women with breast cancer and controls. Psychoneuroendocrinology. 2006;31(3):299–311. PMID: 16183206. http://www.ncbi.nlm.nih.gov/pubmed/16183206.
323. Greaves-Lord K, Ferdinand RF, Oldehinkel AJ, Sondeijker FEPL, Ormel J, Verhulst FC. Higher cortisol awakening response in young adolescents with persistent anxiety problems. Acta Psychiatr Scand. 2007;116(2):137–44. PMID: 17650276. http://www.ncbi.nlm.nih.gov/pubmed/17650276.
324. Chrousos GP. The role of stress and the hypothalamic-pituitary-adrenal axis in the pathogenesis of the metabolic syndrome: neuro-endocrine and target tissue-related causes. Int J Obes Relat Metab Disord. 2000;24(Suppl 2):S50–5. PMID: 10997609. http://www.ncbi.nlm.nih.gov/pubmed/10997609.
325. Wolkowitz OM, Reus VI. Treatment of depression with antiglucocorticoid drugs. Psychosom Med. 1999;61(5):698–711. PMID: 10511017. http://www.ncbi.nlm.nih.gov/pubmed/10511017.
326. Elenkov IJ, Iezzoni DG, Daly A, Harris AG, Chrousos GP. Cytokine dysregulation, inflammation and well-being.

Neuroimmunomodulation. 2005;12(5):255–69. PMID: 16166805. http://www.ncbi.nlm.nih.gov/pubmed/16166805.
327. Elenkov IJ. Glucocorticoids and the Th1/Th2 balance. Ann N Y Acad Sci. 2004;1024:138–46. PMID: 15265778. http://www.ncbi.nlm.nih.gov/pubmed/15265778.
328. Szpunar MJ, Parry BL. A systematic review of cortisol, thyroid-stimulating hormone, and prolactin in peripartum women with major depression. Arch Womens Ment Health. 2018;21(2):149–61. PMCID: PMC5857206. http://www.ncbi.nlm.nih.gov/pubmed/29022126.
329. Inda C, Armando NG, Dos Santos Claro PA, Silberstein S. Endocrinology and the brain: corticotropin-releasing hormone signaling. Endocr Connect. 2017;6(6):R99–R120. PMCID: PMC5551434. http://www.ncbi.nlm.nih.gov/pubmed/28710078.
330. Stalder T, Kirschbaum C, Kudielka BM, Adam EK, Pruessner JC, Wüst S, Dockray S, Smyth N, Evans P, Hellhammer DH, Miller R, Wetherell MA, Lupien SJ, Clow A. Assessment of the cortisol awakening response: expert consensus guidelines. Psychoneuroendocrinology. 2016;63:414–32. PMID: 26563991. http://www.ncbi.nlm.nih.gov/pubmed/26563991.
331. Fries E, Dettenborn L, Kirschbaum C. The cortisol awakening response (CAR): facts and future directions. Int J Psychophysiol. 2009;72(1):67–73. PMID: 18854200. http://www.ncbi.nlm.nih.gov/pubmed/18854200.
332. Vargas I, Mayer S, Lopez-Duran N. The cortisol awakening response and depressive symptomatology: the moderating role of sleep and gender. Stress Health. 2017;33(3):199–210. PMID: 27465684. http://www.ncbi.nlm.nih.gov/pubmed/27465684.
333. Fekedulegn D, Innes K, Andrew ME, Tinney-Zara C, Charles LE, Allison P, Violanti JM, Knox SS. Sleep quality and the cortisol awakening response (CAR) among law enforcement officers: the moderating role of leisure time physical activity. Psychoneuroendocrinology. 2018;95:158–69. PMCID: PMC6401560. http://www.ncbi.nlm.nih.gov/pubmed/29864672.
334. Smyth N, Thorn L, Hucklebridge F, Clow A, Evans P. Assessment of the cortisol awakening response: real-time analysis and curvilinear effects of sample timing inaccuracy. Psychoneuroendocrinology. 2016;74:380–6. PMID: 27750142. http://www.ncbi.nlm.nih.gov/pubmed/27750142.
335. Seth S, Lewis AJ, Galbally M. Perinatal maternal depression and cortisol function in pregnancy and the postpartum period: a systematic literature review. BMC Pregnancy Childbirth. 2016;16(1):124. PMCID: PMC4886446. http://www.ncbi.nlm.nih.gov/pubmed/27245670.
336. Fernandes M, Stein A, Srinivasan K, Menezes G, Ramchandani PG. Foetal exposure to maternal depression predicts cortisol responses in infants: findings from rural South India. Child Care Health Dev. 2015;41(5):677–86. PMID: 25131942. http://www.ncbi.nlm.nih.gov/pubmed/25131942.
337. Carnegie R, Araya R, Ben-Shlomo Y, Glover V, O'Connor TG, O'Donnell KJ, Pearson R, Lewis G. Cortisol awakening response and subsequent depression: prospective longitudinal study. Br J Psychiatry. 2014;204(2):137–43. PMCID: PMC3909839. http://www.ncbi.nlm.nih.gov/pubmed/24311550.
338. de Kloet ER, Joëls M, Holsboer F. Stress and the brain: from adaptation to disease. Nat Rev Neurosci. 2005;6(6):463–75. PMID: 15891777. http://www.ncbi.nlm.nih.gov/pubmed/15891777.
339. Bale TL, Vale WW. CRF and CRF receptors: role in stress responsivity and other behaviors. Annu Rev Pharmacol Toxicol. 2004;44:525–57. PMID: 14744257. http://www.ncbi.nlm.nih.gov/pubmed/14744257.
340. Smith GW, Aubry JM, Dellu F, Contarino A, Bilezikjian LM, Gold LH, Chen R, Marchuk Y, Hauser C, Bentley CA, Sawchenko PE, Koob GF, Vale W, Lee KF. Corticotropin releasing factor receptor 1-deficient mice display decreased anxiety, impaired stress response, and aberrant neuroendocrine development. Neuron. 1998;20(6):1093–102. PMID: 9655498. http://www.ncbi.nlm.nih.gov/pubmed/9655498.
341. Korosi A, Baram TZ. The central corticotropin releasing factor system during development and adulthood. Eur J Pharmacol. 2008;583(2–3):204–14. PMCID: PMC2329668. http://www.ncbi.nlm.nih.gov/pubmed/18275957.
342. Maras PM, Baram TZ. Sculpting the hippocampus from within: stress, spines, and CRH. Trends Neurosci. 2012;35(5):315–24. PMCID: PMC3423222. http://www.ncbi.nlm.nih.gov/pubmed/22386641.
343. Paez-Pereda M, Hausch F, Holsboer F. Corticotropin releasing factor receptor antagonists for major depressive disorder. Expert Opin Investig Drugs. 2011;20(4):519–35. PMID: 21395482. http://www.ncbi.nlm.nih.gov/pubmed/21395482.
344. Sanders J, Nemeroff C. The CRF system as a therapeutic target for neuropsychiatric disorders. Trends Pharmacol Sci. 2016;37(12):1045–54. PMCID: PMC5121012. http://www.ncbi.nlm.nih.gov/pubmed/27717506.
345. Lozovaya N, Miller AD. Chemical neuroimmunology: health in a nutshell bidirectional communication between immune and stress (limbic-hypothalamic-pituitary-adrenal) systems. Chembiochem. 2003;4(6):466–84. PMID: 12794857. http://www.ncbi.nlm.nih.gov/pubmed/12794857.
346. Gallagher JP, Orozco-Cabal LF, Liu J, Shinnick-Gallagher P. Synaptic physiology of central CRH system. Eur J Pharmacol. 2008;583(2-3):215–25. https://doi.org/10.1016/j.ejphar.2007.11.075. Epub 2008 Feb 1. PMID: 18342852; PMCID: PMC2424315. Synaptic physiology of central CRH system- PubMed.
347. Owens MJ, Nemeroff CB. Physiology and pharmacology of corticotropin-releasing factor. Pharmacol Rev. 1991;43(4):425–73. PMID: 1775506. http://www.ncbi.nlm.nih.gov/pubmed/1775506.
348. Swaab DF, Bao AM, Lucassen PJ. The stress system in the human brain in depression and neurodegeneration. Ageing Res Rev. 2005;4(2):141–94. PMID: 15996533. http://www.ncbi.nlm.nih.gov/pubmed/15996533.
349. van Gaalen MM, Stenzel-Poore MP, Holsboer F, Steckler T. Effects of transgenic overproduction of CRH on anxiety-like behaviour. Eur J Neurosci. 2002;15(12):2007–15. PMID: 1209990. http://www.ncbi.nlm.nih.gov/pubmed/12099906.
350. Griebel G, Holsboer F. Neuropeptide receptor ligands as drugs for psychiatric diseases: the end of the beginning? Nat Rev Drug Discov. 2012;11(6):462–78. PMID: 22596253. http://www.ncbi.nlm.nih.gov/pubmed/22596253.
351. Keck ME, Holsboer F. Hyperactivity of CRH neuronal circuits as a target for therapeutic interventions in affective disorders. Peptides. 2001;22(5):835–44. PMID: 11337098. http://www.ncbi.nlm.nih.gov/pubmed/11337098.
352. Jawahar MC, Murgatroyd C, Harrison EL, Baune BT. Epigenetic alterations following early postnatal stress: a review on novel aetiological mechanisms of common psychiatric disorders. Clin. Epigenetics. 2015;7:122. PMCID: PMC4650349. http://www.ncbi.nlm.nih.gov/pubmed/26583053.
353. Afan AM, Broome CS, Nicholls SE, Whetton AD, Miyan JA. Bone marrow innervation regulates cellular retention in the murine haemopoietic system. Br J Haematol. 1997;98(3):569–77. PMID: 9332309. http://www.ncbi.nlm.nih.gov/pubmed/9332309.
354. Felten DL, Felten SY, Carlson SL, Olschowka JA, Livnat S. Noradrenergic and peptidergic innervation of lymphoid tissue. J Immunol. 1985;135(2 Suppl):755s–65s. PMID: 2861231. http://www.ncbi.nlm.nih.gov/pubmed/2861231.
355. Felten SY, Felten DL, Bellinger DL, Carlson SL, Ackerman KD, Madden KS, Olschowka JA, Livnat S. Noradrenergic sympathetic

innervation of lymphoid organs. Prog Allergy. 1988;43:14–36. PMID: 3059356.
356. Bellinger DL, Lorton D, Felten SY, Felten DL. Innervation of lymphoid organs and implications in development, aging, and autoimmunity. Int J Immunopharmacol. 1992;14(3):329–44. PMID: 1319962. http://www.ncbi.nlm.nih.gov/pubmed/1319962.
357. Felten SY, Felten DL. Neural-immune interactions. Prog Brain Res. 1994;100:157–62. PMID: 7938514. http://www.ncbi.nlm.nih.gov/pubmed/7938514.
358. Iversen PO, Hjeltnes N, Holm B, Flatebo T, Strom-Gundersen I, Ronning W, Stanghelle J, Benestad HB. Depressed immunity and impaired proliferation of hematopoietic progenitor cells in patients with complete spinal cord injury. Blood. 2000;96(6):2081–3. PMID: 10979951. http://www.ncbi.nlm.nih.gov/pubmed/10979951.
359. Doyle A, Hucklebridge F, Evans P, Clow A. Salivary monoamine oxidase A and B inhibitory activities correlate with stress. Life Sci. 1996;59(16):1357–62. PMID: 8876665. http://www.ncbi.nlm.nih.gov/pubmed/8876665.
360. Rohleder N, Kudielka BM, Hellhammer DH, Wolf JM, Kirschbaum C. Age and sex steroid-related changes in glucocorticoid sensitivity of pro-inflammatory cytokine production after psychosocial stress. J Neuroimmunol. 2002;126(1–2):69–77. PMID: 12020958. http://www.ncbi.nlm.nih.gov/pubmed/12020958.
361. Rozman KK, Doull J. Scientific foundations of hormesis. Part 2. Maturation, strengths, limitations, and possible applications in toxicology, pharmacology, and epidemiology. Crit Rev Toxicol. 2003;33(3–4):451–62. PMID: 12809434. http://www.ncbi.nlm.nih.gov/pubmed/12809434.
362. Calabrese EJ. Stress biology and hormesis: the Yerkes-Dodson law in psychology–a special case of the hormesis dose response. Crit Rev Toxicol. 2008;38(5):453–62. PMID: 18568865. http://www.ncbi.nlm.nih.gov/pubmed/18568865.
363. Hoffmann GR. A perspective on the scientific, philosophical, and policy dimensions of hormesis. Dose Response. 2009;7(1):1–51. PMCID: PMC2664639. http://www.ncbi.nlm.nih.gov/pubmed/19343115.
364. Nestler EJ, Peña CJ, Kundakovic M, Mitchell A, Akbarian S. Epigenetic basis of mental illness. Neuroscientist. 2016;22(5):447–63. PMCID: PMC4826318. http://www.ncbi.nlm.nih.gov/pubmed/26450593.
365. Hänsel A, von Känel R. The ventro-medial prefrontal cortex: a major link between the autonomic nervous system, regulation of emotion, and stress reactivity? Biopsychosoc Med. 2008;2:21. PMCID: PMC2590602. http://www.ncbi.nlm.nih.gov/pubmed/18986513.
366. Cerqueira JJ, Almeida OFX, Sousa N. The stressed prefrontal cortex. Left? Right! Brain Behav Immun. 2008;22(5):630–8. PMID: 18281193. http://www.ncbi.nlm.nih.gov/pubmed/18281193.
367. Radley JJ, Williams B, Sawchenko PE. Noradrenergic innervation of the dorsal medial prefrontal cortex modulates hypothalamo-pituitary-adrenal responses to acute emotional stress. J Neurosci. 2008;28(22):5806–16. PMCID: PMC2796223. http://www.ncbi.nlm.nih.gov/pubmed/18509042.
368. Charmandari E, Kino T, Souvatzoglou E, Chrousos GP. Pediatric stress: hormonal mediators and human development. Horm Res. 2003;59(4):161–79. PMID: 12649570. http://www.ncbi.nlm.nih.gov/pubmed/12649570.
369. Segerstrom SC, Glover DA, Craske MG, Fahey JL. Worry affects the immune response to phobic fear. Brain Behav Immun. 1999;13(2):80–92. PMID: 10373274. http://www.ncbi.nlm.nih.gov/pubmed/10373274.
370. Mizoguchi K, Shoji H, Ikeda R, Tanaka Y, Tabira T. Persistent depressive state after chronic stress in rats is accompanied by HPA axis dysregulation and reduced prefrontal dopaminergic neurotransmission. Pharmacol Biochem Behav. 2008;91(1):170–5. PMID: 18675292. http://www.ncbi.nlm.nih.gov/pubmed/18675292.
371. Servatius RJ, Natelson BH, Moldow R, Pogach L, Brennan FX, Ottenweller JE. Persistent neuroendocrine changes in multiple hormonal axes after a single or repeated stressor exposures. Stress. 2000;3(4):263–74. PMID: 11342392. http://www.ncbi.nlm.nih.gov/pubmed/11342392.
372. Brennan FX, Ottenweller JE, Seifu Y, Zhu G, Servatius RJ. Persistent stress-induced elevations of urinary corticosterone in rats. Physiol Behav. 2000;71(5):441–6. PMID: 11239661. http://www.ncbi.nlm.nih.gov/pubmed/11239661.
373. Colom LV, Garrido-Sanabria E. Modulation of normal and altered hippocampal excitability states by septal networks. J Neurosci Res. 2007;85(13):2839–43. PMID: 17393499. http://www.ncbi.nlm.nih.gov/pubmed/17393499.
374. Florio P, Zatelli MC, Reis FM, degli Uberti EC, Petraglia F. Corticotropin releasing hormone: a diagnostic marker for behavioral and reproductive disorders? Front Biosci. 2007;12:551–60. PMID: 17127316. http://www.ncbi.nlm.nih.gov/pubmed/17127316.
375. Clow A, Patel S, Najafi M, Evans PD, Hucklebridge F. The cortisol response to psychological challenge is preceded by a transient rise in endogenous inhibitor of monoamine oxidase. Life Sci. 1997;61(5):567–75. PMID: 9247326. http://www.ncbi.nlm.nih.gov/pubmed/9247326.
376. Hucklebridge F, Sen S, Evans PD, Clow A. The relationship between circadian patterns of salivary cortisol and endogenous inhibitor of monoamine oxidase A. Life Sci. 1998;62(25):2321–8. PMID: 9651121. http://www.ncbi.nlm.nih.gov/pubmed/9651121.
377. Hucklebridge F, Clow A, Evans P. The relationship between salivary secretory immunoglobulin A and cortisol: neuroendocrine response to awakening and the diurnal cycle. Int J Psychophysiol. 1998;31(1):69–76. PMID: 9934622. http://www.ncbi.nlm.nih.gov/pubmed/9934622.
378. Doyle A, Hucklebridge F, Evans P, Clow A. Urinary output of endogenous monoamine oxidase inhibitory activity is related to everyday stress. Life Sci. 1996;58(20):1723–30. PMID: 8637396. http://www.ncbi.nlm.nih.gov/pubmed/8637396.
379. Chrousos GP, Kino T. Glucocorticoid action networks and complex psychiatric and/or somatic disorders. Stress. 2007;10(2):213–9. PMID: 17514590. http://www.ncbi.nlm.nih.gov/pubmed/17514590.
380. Plotsky PM. Pathways to the secretion of adrenocorticotropin: a view from the portal*. J Neuroendocrinol. 1991;3(1):1–9. PMID: 19215439. http://www.ncbi.nlm.nih.gov/pubmed/19215439.
381. Engeland WC, Arnhold MM. Neural circuitry in the regulation of adrenal corticosterone rhythmicity. Endocrine. 2005;28(3):325–32. PMID: 16388123. http://www.ncbi.nlm.nih.gov/pubmed/16388123.
382. Serova LI, Gueorguiev V, Cheng SY, Sabban EL. Adrenocorticotropic hormone elevates gene expression for catecholamine biosynthesis in rat superior cervical ganglia and locus coeruleus by an adrenal independent mechanism. Neuroscience. 2008;153(4):1380–9. PMCID: PMC2586879. http://www.ncbi.nlm.nih.gov/pubmed/18440707.
383. Liu JP, Clarke IJ, Funder JW, Engler D. Studies of the secretion of corticotropin-releasing factor and arginine vasopressin into the hypophysial-portal circulation of the conscious sheep. II. The central noradrenergic and neuropeptide Y pathways cause immediate and prolonged hypothalamic-pituitary-adrenal activation. Potential involvement in the pseudo-Cushing's syndrome of endogenous depression and anorexia nervosa. J Clin Invest.

1994;93(4):1439–50. PMCID: PMC294157. http://www.ncbi.nlm.nih.gov/pubmed/8163648.

384. Bornstein SR, Engeland WC, Ehrhart-Bornstein M, Herman JP. Dissociation of ACTH and glucocorticoids. Trends Endocrinol Metab. 2008;19(5):175–80. PMID: 18394919. http://www.ncbi.nlm.nih.gov/pubmed/18394919.
385. Carlson DE, Chiu WC, Fiedler SM, Hoffman GE. Central neural distribution of immunoreactive Fos and CRH in relation to plasma ACTH and corticosterone during sepsis in the rat. Exp Neurol. 2007;205(2):485–500. PMCID: PMC1950276. http://www.ncbi.nlm.nih.gov/pubmed/17462630.
386. Watts AG. Glucocorticoid regulation of peptide genes in neuroendocrine CRH neurons: a complexity beyond negative feedback. Front Neuroendocrinol. 2005;26(3–4):109–30. PMID: 16289311. http://www.ncbi.nlm.nih.gov/pubmed/16289311.
387. Sara SJ. Locus Coeruleus in time with the making of memories. Curr Opin Neurobiol. 2015;35:87–94. PMID: 26241632. http://www.ncbi.nlm.nih.gov/pubmed/26241632.
388. Daviu N, Bruchas MR, Moghaddam B, Sandi C, Beyeler A. Neurobiological links between stress and anxiety. Neurobiol Stress. 2019;11:100191. PMCID: PMC6712367. http://www.ncbi.nlm.nih.gov/pubmed/31467945.
389. Perrelli M, Goparaju P, Postolache TT, Del Bosque-Plata L, Gragnoli C. Stress and the CRH system, norepinephrine, depression, and type 2 diabetes. Biomedicine. 2024;12(6):1187. PMCID: PMC11200886. http://www.ncbi.nlm.nih.gov/pubmed/38927393.
390. Gold PW. The organization of the stress system and its dysregulation in depressive illness. Mol Psychiatry. 2015;20(1):32–47. PMID: 25486982. http://www.ncbi.nlm.nih.gov/pubmed/25486982.
391. Malta MB, Martins J, Novaes LS, Dos Santos NB, Sita L, Camarini R, Scavone C, Bittencourt J, Munhoz CD. Norepinephrine and glucocorticoids modulate chronic unpredictable stress-induced increase in the type 2 CRF and glucocorticoid receptors in brain structures related to the HPA Axis activation. Mol Neurobiol. 2021;58(10):4871–85. PMID: 34213722. http://www.ncbi.nlm.nih.gov/pubmed/34213722.
392. Wood SK, Valentino RJ. The brain norepinephrine system, stress and cardiovascular vulnerability. Neurosci Biobehav Rev. 2017;74(Pt B):393–400. PMCID: PMC5083238. http://www.ncbi.nlm.nih.gov/pubmed/27131968.
393. Suárez-Pereira I, Llorca-Torralba M, Bravo L, Camarena-Delgado C, Soriano-Mas C, Berrocoso E. The role of the locus Coeruleus in pain and associated stress-related disorders. Biol Psychiatry. 2022;91(9):786–97. PMID: 35164940. http://www.ncbi.nlm.nih.gov/pubmed/35164940.
394. Arnetz BB, Brenner SO, Levi L, Hjelm R, Petterson IL, Wasserman J, Petrini B, Eneroth P, Kallner A, Kvetnansky R. Neuroendocrine and immunologic effects of unemployment and job insecurity. Psychother Psychosom. 1991;55(2–4):76–80. PMID: 1891571. http://www.ncbi.nlm.nih.gov/pubmed/1891571.
395. Lerman Y, Melamed S, Shragin Y, Kushnir T, Rotgoltz Y, Shirom A, Aronson M. Association between burnout at work and leukocyte adhesiveness/aggregation. Psychosom Med. 1999;61(6):828–33. PMID: 10593635. http://www.ncbi.nlm.nih.gov/pubmed/10593635.
396. Melamed S, Ugarten U, Shirom A, Kahana L, Lerman Y, Froom P. Chronic burnout, somatic arousal and elevated salivary cortisol levels. J Psychosom Res. 1999;46(6):591–8. PMID: 10454175. http://www.ncbi.nlm.nih.gov/pubmed/10454175.
397. Kawakami N, Tanigawa T, Araki S, Nakata A, Sakurai S, Yokoyama K, Morita Y. Effects of job strain on helper-inducer (CD4+CD29+) and suppressor-inducer (CD4+CD45RA+) T cells in Japanese blue-collar workers. Psychother Psychosom. 1997;66(4):192–8. PMID: 9259042. http://www.ncbi.nlm.nih.gov/pubmed/9259042.
398. Smith TW, Ruiz JM. Psychosocial influences on the development and course of coronary heart disease: current status and implications for research and practice. J Consult Clin Psychol. 2002;70(3):548–68. PMID: 12090369. http://www.ncbi.nlm.nih.gov/pubmed/12090369.
399. Everson SA, Lynch JW, Kaplan GA, Lakka TA, Sivenius J, Salonen JT. Stress-induced blood pressure reactivity and incident stroke in middle-aged men. Stroke. 2001;32(6):1263–70. PMID: 11387485. http://www.ncbi.nlm.nih.gov/pubmed/11387485.
400. Wood SK, Bhatnagar S. Resilience to the effects of social stress: evidence from clinical and preclinical studies on the role of coping strategies. Neurobiol Stress. 2015;1:164–73. PMCID: PMC4286805. http://www.ncbi.nlm.nih.gov/pubmed/25580450.
401. Schulz R, Beach SR. Caregiving as a risk factor for mortality: the caregiver health effects study. JAMA. 1999;282(23):2215–9. PMID: 10605972. http://www.ncbi.nlm.nih.gov/pubmed/10605972.
402. Vitaliano PP, Scanlan JM, Zhang J, Savage MV, Hirsch IB, Siegler IC. A path model of chronic stress, the metabolic syndrome, and coronary heart disease. Psychosom Med. 2002;64(3):418–35. PMID: 12021416. http://www.ncbi.nlm.nih.gov/pubmed/12021416.
403. Vedhara K, Cox NK, Wilcock GK, Perks P, Hunt M, Anderson S, Lightman SL, Shanks NM. Chronic stress in elderly carers of dementia patients and antibody response to influenza vaccination. Lancet. 1999;353(9153):627–31. PMID: 10030328. http://www.ncbi.nlm.nih.gov/pubmed/10030328.
404. Wu H, Wang J, Cacioppo JT, Glaser R, Kiecolt-Glaser JK, Malarkey WB. Chronic stress associated with spousal caregiving of patients with Alzheimer's dementia is associated with downregulation of B-lymphocyte GH mRNA. J Gerontol A Biol Sci Med Sci. 1999;54(4):M212–5. PMID: 10219013. http://www.ncbi.nlm.nih.gov/pubmed/10219013.
405. Kiecolt-Glaser JK, Glaser R, Shuttleworth EC, Dyer CS, Ogrocki P, Speicher CE. Chronic stress and immunity in family caregivers of Alzheimer's disease victims. Psychosom Med. 1987;49(5):523–35. PMID: 3671639. http://www.ncbi.nlm.nih.gov/pubmed/3671639.
406. Kiecolt-Glaser JK, Preacher KJ, MacCallum RC, Atkinson C, Malarkey WB, Glaser R. Chronic stress and age-related increases in the proinflammatory cytokine IL-6. Proc Natl Acad Sci USA. 2003;100(15):9090–5. PMCID: PMC166443. http://www.ncbi.nlm.nih.gov/pubmed/12840146.
407. Kiecolt-Glaser JK, McGuire L, Robles TF, Glaser R. Psychoneuroimmunology: psychological influences on immune function and health. J Consult Clin Psychol. 2002;70(3):537–47. PMID: 12090368. http://www.ncbi.nlm.nih.gov/pubmed/12090368.
408. Esterling BA, Kiecolt-Glaser JK, Glaser R. Psychosocial modulation of cytokine-induced natural killer cell activity in older adults. Psychosom Med. 1996;58(3):264–72. PMID: 8771626. http://www.ncbi.nlm.nih.gov/pubmed/8771626.
409. Kiecolt-Glaser JK, Newton TL. Marriage and health: his and hers. Psychol Bull. 2001;127(4):472–503. PMID: 11439708. http://www.ncbi.nlm.nih.gov/pubmed/11439708.
410. Buka SL. Disparities in health status and substance use: ethnicity and socioeconomic factors. Public Health Rep. 2002;117(Suppl 1):S118–25. PMCID: PMC1913692. http://www.ncbi.nlm.nih.gov/pubmed/12435835.
411. Adler NE, Newman K. Socioeconomic disparities in health: pathways and policies. Health Aff (Millwood). 2002;21(2):60–76. PMID: 11900187. http://www.ncbi.nlm.nih.gov/pubmed/11900187.
412. Adler NE, Ostrove JM. Socioeconomic status and health: what we know and what we don't. Ann NY Acad Sci. 1999;896:3–15. PMID: 10681884. http://www.ncbi.nlm.nih.gov/pubmed/10681884.

413. Marmot M, Feeney A. General explanations for social inequalities in health. IARC Sci Publ. 1997;138:207–28. PMID: 9353666. http://www.ncbi.nlm.nih.gov/pubmed/9353666.
414. Taylor SE, Repetti RL, Seeman T. Health psychology: what is an unhealthy environment and how does it get under the skin? Annu Rev Psychol. 1997;48:411–47. PMID: 9046565. http://www.ncbi.nlm.nih.gov/pubmed/9046565.
415. Everson SA, Maty SC, Lynch JW, Kaplan GA. Epidemiologic evidence for the relation between socioeconomic status and depression, obesity, and diabetes. J Psychosom Res. 2002;53(4):891–5. PMID: 12377299. http://www.ncbi.nlm.nih.gov/pubmed/12377299.
416. Christensen U, Lund R, Damsgaard MT, Holstein BE, Ditlevsen S, Diderichsen F, Due P, Iversen L, Lynch J. Cynical hostility, socioeconomic position, health behaviors, and symptom load: a cross-sectional analysis in a Danish population-based study. Psychosom Med. 2004;66(4):572–7. PMID: 15272105. http://www.ncbi.nlm.nih.gov/pubmed/15272105.
417. Turrell G, Lynch JW, Kaplan GA, Everson SA, Helkala EL, Kauhanen J, Salonen JT. Socioeconomic position across the lifecourse and cognitive function in late middle age. J Gerontol B Psychol Sci Soc Sci. 2002;57(1):S43–51. PMID: 11773232. http://www.ncbi.nlm.nih.gov/pubmed/11773232.
418. Kaplan GA, Turrell G, Lynch JW, Everson SA, Helkala EL, Salonen JT. Childhood socioeconomic position and cognitive function in adulthood. Int J Epidemiol. 2001;30(2):256–63. PMID: 11369724. http://www.ncbi.nlm.nih.gov/pubmed/11369724.
419. Judd LL. The clinical course of unipolar major depressive disorders. Arch Gen Psychiatry. 1997;54(11):989–91. PMID: 9366654. http://www.ncbi.nlm.nih.gov/pubmed/9366654.
420. Mueller TI, Leon AC, Keller MB, Solomon DA, Endicott J, Coryell W, Warshaw M, Maser JD. Recurrence after recovery from major depressive disorder during 15 years of observational follow-up. Am J Psychiatry. 1999;156(7):1000–6. PMID: 10401442. http://www.ncbi.nlm.nih.gov/pubmed/10401442.
421. Solomon DA, Keller MB, Leon AC, Mueller TI, Lavori PW, Shea MT, Coryell W, Warshaw M, Turvey C, Maser JD, Endicott J. Multiple recurrences of major depressive disorder. Am J Psychiatry. 2000;157(2):229–33. PMID: 10671391. http://www.ncbi.nlm.nih.gov/pubmed/10671391.
422. Post RM. Transduction of psychosocial stress into the neurobiology of recurrent affective disorder. Am J Psychiatry. 1992;149(8):999–1010. PMID: 1353322. http://www.ncbi.nlm.nih.gov/pubmed/1353322.
423. Stroud CB, Davila J, Moyer A. The relationship between stress and depression in first onsets versus recurrences: a meta-analytic review. J Abnorm Psychol. 2008;117(1):206–13. PMID: 18266498. http://www.ncbi.nlm.nih.gov/pubmed/18266498.
424. Hammen C. Stress and depression. Annu Rev Clin Psychol. 2005;1:293–319. PMID: 17716090. http://www.ncbi.nlm.nih.gov/pubmed/17716090.
425. Kendler KS, Thornton LM, Gardner CO. Stressful life events and previous episodes in the etiology of major depression in women: an evaluation of the "kindling" hypothesis. Am J Psychiatry. 2000;157(8):1243–51. PMID: 10910786. http://www.ncbi.nlm.nih.gov/pubmed/10910786.
426. Post RM. Mechanisms of illness progression in the recurrent affective disorders. Neurotox Res. 2010;18(3–4):256–71. PMID: 20390474. http://www.ncbi.nlm.nih.gov/pubmed/20390474.
427. Segal ZV, Gemar M, Williams S. Differential cognitive response to a mood challenge following successful cognitive therapy or pharmacotherapy for unipolar depression. J Abnorm Psychol. 1999;108(1):3–10. PMID: 10066988. http://www.ncbi.nlm.nih.gov/pubmed/10066988.
428. Segal ZV, Kennedy S, Gemar M, Hood K, Pedersen R, Buis T. Cognitive reactivity to sad mood provocation and the prediction of depressive relapse. Arch Gen Psychiatry. 2006;63(7):749–55. PMID: 16818864. http://www.ncbi.nlm.nih.gov/pubmed/16818864.
429. Segal ZV, Williams JM, Teasdale JD, Gemar M. A cognitive science perspective on kindling and episode sensitization in recurrent affective disorder. Psychol Med. 1996;26(2):371–80. PMID: 8685293. http://www.ncbi.nlm.nih.gov/pubmed/8685293.
430. Mitchell PB, Parker GB, Gladstone GL, Wilhelm K, Austin MPV. Severity of stressful life events in first and subsequent episodes of depression: the relevance of depressive subtype. J Affect Disord. 2003;73(3):245–52. PMID: 12547293. http://www.ncbi.nlm.nih.gov/pubmed/12547293.
431. Hankin BL. Cognitive vulnerability-stress model of depression during adolescence: investigating depressive symptom specificity in a multi-wave prospective study. J Abnorm Child Psychol. 2008;36(7):999–1014. PMCID: PMC2763423. http://www.ncbi.nlm.nih.gov/pubmed/18437551.
432. Hankin BL, Abramson LY. Development of gender differences in depression: an elaborated cognitive vulnerability-transactional stress theory. Psychol Bull. 2001;127(6):773–96. PMID: 11726071. http://www.ncbi.nlm.nih.gov/pubmed/11726071.
433. Monroe SM, Harkness KL. Life stress, the "kindling" hypothesis, and the recurrence of depression: considerations from a life stress perspective. Psychol Rev. 2005;112(2):417–45. PMID: 15783292. http://www.ncbi.nlm.nih.gov/pubmed/15783292.
434. Stroud CB, Davila J, Hammen C, Vrshek-Schallhorn S. Severe and nonsevere events in first onsets versus recurrences of depression: evidence for stress sensitization. J Abnorm Psychol. 2011;120(1):142–54. PMID: 21171724. http://www.ncbi.nlm.nih.gov/pubmed/21171724.
435. Morris MC, Ciesla JA, Garber J. A prospective study of stress autonomy versus stress sensitization in adolescents at varied risk for depression. J Abnorm Psychol. 2010;119(2):341–54. PMCID: PMC2869472. http://www.ncbi.nlm.nih.gov/pubmed/20455607.
436. Siegle GJ, Thompson W, Carter CS, Steinhauer SR, Thase ME. Increased amygdala and decreased dorsolateral prefrontal BOLD responses in unipolar depression: related and independent features. Biol Psychiatry. 2007;61(2):198–209. PMID: 17027931. http://www.ncbi.nlm.nih.gov/pubmed/17027931.
437. Siegle GJ, Steinhauer SR, Thase ME, Stenger VA, Carter CS. Can't shake that feeling: event-related fMRI assessment of sustained amygdala activity in response to emotional information in depressed individuals. Biol Psychiatry. 2002;51(9):693–707. PMID: 11983183. http://www.ncbi.nlm.nih.gov/pubmed/11983183.
438. Ochsner KN, Gross JJ. The cognitive control of emotion. Trends Cogn Sci. 2005;9(5):242–9. PMID: 15866151. http://www.ncbi.nlm.nih.gov/pubmed/15866151.
439. Davidson RJ, Pizzagalli D, Nitschke JB, Putnam K. Depression: perspectives from affective neuroscience. Annu Rev Psychol. 2002;53:545–74. PMID: 11752496. http://www.ncbi.nlm.nih.gov/pubmed/11752496.
440. Ochsner KN, Bunge SA, Gross JJ, Gabrieli JDE. Rethinking feelings: an FMRI study of the cognitive regulation of emotion. J Cogn Neurosci. 2002;14(8):1215–29. PMID: 12495527. http://www.ncbi.nlm.nih.gov/pubmed/12495527.
441. Drevets WC. Neuroimaging and neuropathological studies of depression: implications for the cognitive-emotional features of mood disorders. Curr Opin Neurobiol. 2001;11(2):240–9. PMID: 11301246. http://www.ncbi.nlm.nih.gov/pubmed/11301246.
442. Johnstone T, van Reekum CM, Urry HL, Kalin NH, Davidson RJ. Failure to regulate: counterproductive recruitment of top-down

prefrontal-subcortical circuitry in major depression. J Neurosci. 2007;27(33):8877–84. PMCID: PMC6672169. http://www.ncbi.nlm.nih.gov/pubmed/17699669.
443. Cohen LH, Gunthert KC, Butler AC, O'Neill SC, Tolpin LH. Daily affective reactivity as a prospective predictor of depressive symptoms. J Pers. 2005;73(6):1687–713. PMID: 16274450. http://www.ncbi.nlm.nih.gov/pubmed/16274450.
444. Myin-Germeys I, Peeters F, Havermans R, Nicolson NA, DeVries MW, Delespaul P, Van Os J. Emotional reactivity to daily life stress in psychosis and affective disorder: an experience sampling study. Acta Psychiatr Scand. 2003;107(2):124–31. PMID: 12534438. http://www.ncbi.nlm.nih.gov/pubmed/12534438.
445. Pine DS, Cohen P, Brook JS. Emotional reactivity and risk for psychopathology among adolescents. CNS Spectr. 2001;6(1):27–35. PMID: 17008830. http://www.ncbi.nlm.nih.gov/pubmed/17008830.
446. Cohen LH, Gunthert KC, Butler AC, Parrish BP, Wenze SJ, Beck JS. Negative affective spillover from daily events predicts early response to cognitive therapy for depression. J Consult Clin Psychol. 2008;76(6):955–65. PMID: 19045964. http://www.ncbi.nlm.nih.gov/pubmed/19045964.
447. Jarrett RB, Minhajuddin A, Borman PD, Dunlap L, Segal ZV, Kidner CL, Friedman ES, Thase ME. Cognitive reactivity, dysfunctional attitudes, and depressive relapse and recurrence in cognitive therapy responders. Behav Res Ther. 2012;50(5):280–6. PMCID: PMC3336865. http://www.ncbi.nlm.nih.gov/pubmed/22445946.
448. Gaynes BN, Gavin N, Meltzer-Brody S, Lohr KN, Swinson T, Gartlehner G, Brody S, Miller WC. Perinatal depression: prevalence, screening accuracy, and screening outcomes. Evid Rep Technol Assess (Summ). 2005;119:1–8. PMCID: PMC4780910. http://www.ncbi.nlm.nih.gov/pubmed/15760246.
449. Guintivano J, Arad M, Gould TD, Payne JL, Kaminsky ZA. Antenatal prediction of postpartum depression with blood DNA methylation biomarkers. Mol Psychiatry. 2014;19(5):560–7. PMCID: PMC7039252. http://www.ncbi.nlm.nih.gov/pubmed/23689534.
450. Moehler E, Brunner R, Wiebel A, Reck C, Resch F. Maternal depressive symptoms in the postnatal period are associated with long-term impairment of mother-child bonding. Arch Womens Ment Health. 2006;9(5):273–8. PMID: 16937313. http://www.ncbi.nlm.nih.gov/pubmed/16937313.
451. Grace SL, Evindar A, Stewart DE. The effect of postpartum depression on child cognitive development and behavior: a review and critical analysis of the literature. Arch Womens Ment Health. 2003;6(4):263–74. PMID: 14628179. http://www.ncbi.nlm.nih.gov/pubmed/14628179.
452. Lam RW, Kennedy SH, Grigoriadis S, McIntyre RS, Milev R, Ramasubbu R, Parikh SV, Patten SB, Ravindran AV. Canadian Network for Mood and Anxiety Treatments (CANMAT). Canadian Network for Mood and Anxiety Treatments (CANMAT) clinical guidelines for the management of major depressive disorder in adults. III. Pharmacotherapy. J Affect Disord. 2009;117(Suppl 1):S26–43. PMID: 19674794. http://www.ncbi.nlm.nih.gov/pubmed/19674794.
453. Weissman AM, Levy BT, Hartz AJ, Bentler S, Donohue M, Ellingrod VL, Wisner KL. Pooled analysis of antidepressant levels in lactating mothers, breast milk, and nursing infants. Am J Psychiatry. 2004;161(6):1066–78. PMID: 15169695. http://www.ncbi.nlm.nih.gov/pubmed/15169695.
454. Ito S. Drug therapy for breast-feeding women. N Engl J Med. 2000;343(2):118–26. PMID: 10891521. http://www.ncbi.nlm.nih.gov/pubmed/10891521.
455. Rampono J, Teoh S, Hackett LP, Kohan R, Ilett KF. Estimation of desvenlafaxine transfer into milk and infant exposure during its use in lactating women with postnatal depression. Arch Womens Ment Health. 2011;14(1):49–53. PMID: 20960017. http://www.ncbi.nlm.nih.gov/pubmed/20960017.
456. Berle JØ, Spigset O. Antidepressant use during breastfeeding. Curr Womens Health Rev. 2011;7(1):28–34. PMCID: PMC3267169. http://www.ncbi.nlm.nih.gov/pubmed/22299006.
457. Ilett KF, Watt F, Hackett LP, Kohan R, Teoh S. Assessment of infant dose through milk in a lactating woman taking amisulpride and desvenlafaxine for treatment-resistant depression. Ther Drug Monit. 2010;32(6):704–7. PMID: 20926994. http://www.ncbi.nlm.nih.gov/pubmed/20926994.
458. Moretti M. Breastfeeding and the use of antidepressants. J Popul Ther Clin Pharmacol. 2012;19(3):e387–90. PMID: 23075497. http://www.ncbi.nlm.nih.gov/pubmed/23075497.
459. Fitelson E, Kim S, Baker AS, Leight K. Treatment of postpartum depression: clinical, psychological and pharmacological options. Int J Women's Health. 2010;3:1–14. PMCID: PMC3039003. http://www.ncbi.nlm.nih.gov/pubmed/21339932.
460. O'Hara MW, McCabe JE. Postpartum depression: current status and future directions. Annu Rev Clin Psychol. 2013;9:379–407. PMID: 23394227. http://www.ncbi.nlm.nih.gov/pubmed/23394227.
461. Chad L, Pupco A, Bozzo P, Koren G. Update on antidepressant use during breastfeeding. Can Fam Physician. 2013;59(6):633–4. PMCID: PMC3681447. http://www.ncbi.nlm.nih.gov/pubmed/23766044.
462. Carvalho AF, Sharma MS, Brunoni AR, Vieta E, Fava GA. The safety, tolerability and risks associated with the use of newer generation antidepressant drugs: a critical review of the literature. Psychother Psychosom. 2016;85(5):270–88. PMID: 27508501. http://www.ncbi.nlm.nih.gov/pubmed/27508501.
463. Mehta D, Newport DJ, Frishman G, Kraus L, Rex-Haffner M, Ritchie JC, Lori A, Knight BT, Stagnaro E, Ruepp A, Stowe ZN, Binder EB. Early predictive biomarkers for postpartum depression point to a role for estrogen receptor signaling. Psychol Med. 2014;44(11):2309–22. PMID: 24495551. http://www.ncbi.nlm.nih.gov/pubmed/24495551.
464. Lindquist TL, Beilin LJ, Knuiman MW. Influence of lifestyle, coping, and job stress on blood pressure in men and women. Hypertension. 1997;29(1 Pt 1):1–7. PMID: 9039072. http://www.ncbi.nlm.nih.gov/pubmed/9039072.
465. Kiecolt-Glaser JK, Glaser R. Methodological issues in behavioral immunology research with humans. Brain Behav Immun. 1988;2(1):67–78. PMID: 3052653. http://www.ncbi.nlm.nih.gov/pubmed/3052653.
466. Rozlog LA, Kiecolt-Glaser JK, Marucha PT, Sheridan JF, Glaser R. Stress and immunity: implications for viral disease and wound healing. J Periodontol. 1999;70(7):786–92. PMID: 10440641. http://www.ncbi.nlm.nih.gov/pubmed/10440641.
467. Glaser R, Kiecolt-Glaser JK, Marucha PT, MacCallum RC, Laskowski BF, Malarkey WB. Stress-related changes in proinflammatory cytokine production in wounds. Arch Gen Psychiatry. 1999;56(5):450–6. PMID: 10232300. http://www.ncbi.nlm.nih.gov/pubmed/10232300.
468. Song C, Kenis G, van Gastel A, Bosmans E, Lin A, de Jong R, Neels H, Scharpé S, Janca A, Yasukawa K, Maes M. Influence of psychological stress on immune-inflammatory variables in normal humans. Part II. Altered serum concentrations of natural anti-inflammatory agents and soluble membrane antigens of monocytes and T lymphocytes. Psychiatry Res. 1999;85(3):293–303. PMID: 10333381. http://www.ncbi.nlm.nih.gov/pubmed/10333381.
469. Maes M, Lin AH, Delmeire L, Van Gastel A, Kenis G, De Jongh R, Bosmans E. Elevated serum interleukin-6 (IL-6) and IL-6 receptor concentrations in posttraumatic stress disorder following accidental man-made traumatic events. Biol Psychiatry.

1999;45(7):833–9. PMID: 10202570. http://www.ncbi.nlm.nih.gov/pubmed/10202570.
470. Maes M, Song C, Lin A, De Jongh R, Van Gastel A, Kenis G, Bosmans E, De Meester I, Benoy I, Neels H, Demedts P, Janca A, Scharpé S, Smith RS. The effects of psychological stress on humans: increased production of pro-inflammatory cytokines and a Th1-like response in stress-induced anxiety. Cytokine. 1998;10(4):313–8. PMID: 9617578. http://www.ncbi.nlm.nih.gov/pubmed/9617578.
471. Maes M, Bosmans E, Ombelet W. In the puerperium, primiparae exhibit higher levels of anxiety and serum peptidase activity and greater immune responses than multiparae. J Clin Psychiatry. 2004;65(1):71–6. PMID: 14744172. http://www.ncbi.nlm.nih.gov/pubmed/14744172.
472. Dentino AN, Pieper CF, Rao MK, Currie MS, Harris T, Blazer DG, Cohen HJ. Association of interleukin-6 and other biologic variables with depression in older people living in the community. J Am Geriatr Soc. 1999;47(1):6–11. PMID: 9920223. http://www.ncbi.nlm.nih.gov/pubmed/9920223.
473. Lutgendorf SK, Logan H, Costanzo E, Lubaroff D. Effects of acute stress, relaxation, and a neurogenic inflammatory stimulus on interleukin-6 in humans. Brain Behav Immun. 2004;18(1):55–64. PMID: 14651947. http://www.ncbi.nlm.nih.gov/pubmed/14651947.
474. Nicholson RA, Houle TT, Rhudy JL, Norton PJ. Psychological risk factors in headache. Headache. 2007;47(3):413–26. PMCID: PMC2408884. http://www.ncbi.nlm.nih.gov/pubmed/17371358.
475. Kiecolt-Glaser JK, Page GG, Marucha PT, MacCallum RC, Glaser R. Psychological influences on surgical recovery. Perspectives from psychoneuroimmunology. Am Psychol. 1998;53(11):1209–18. PMID: 9830373. http://www.ncbi.nlm.nih.gov/pubmed/9830373.
476. Marucha PT, Kiecolt-Glaser JK, Favagehi M. Mucosal wound healing is impaired by examination stress. Psychosom Med. 1998;60(3):362–5. PMID: 9625226. http://www.ncbi.nlm.nih.gov/pubmed/9625226.
477. Hassan M, Mela A, Li Q, Brumback B, Fillingim RB, Conti JB, Sheps DS. The effect of acute psychological stress on QT dispersion in patients with coronary artery disease. Pacing Clin Electrophysiol. 2009;32(9):1178–83. PMCID: PMC2739112. http://www.ncbi.nlm.nih.gov/pubmed/19719496.
478. James PR, Taggart P, McNally ST, Newman SP, Sproton SC, Hardman SM. Acute psychological stress and the propensity to ventricular arrhythmias; evidence for a linking mechanism. Eur Heart J. 2000;21(12):1023–8. PMID: 10901515. http://www.ncbi.nlm.nih.gov/pubmed/10901515.
479. Huang M, Pang X, Karalis K, Theoharides TC. Stress-induced interleukin-6 release in mice is mast cell-dependent and more pronounced in Apolipoprotein E knockout mice. Cardiovasc Res. 2003;59(1):241–9. PMID: 12829195. http://www.ncbi.nlm.nih.gov/pubmed/12829195.
480. Huang M, Pang X, Letourneau R, Boucher W, Theoharides TC. Acute stress induces cardiac mast cell activation and histamine release, effects that are increased in Apolipoprotein E knockout mice. Cardiovasc Res. 2002;55(1):150–60. PMID: 12062718. http://www.ncbi.nlm.nih.gov/pubmed/12062718.
481. Pang X, Alexacos N, Letourneau R, Seretakis D, Gao W, Boucher W, Cochrane DE, Theoharides TC. A neurotensin receptor antagonist inhibits acute immobilization stress-induced cardiac mast cell degranulation, a corticotropin-releasing hormone-dependent process. J Pharmacol Exp Ther. 1998;287(1):307–14. PMID: 9765351. http://www.ncbi.nlm.nih.gov/pubmed/9765351.
482. Pang X, Letourneau R, Rozniecki JJ, Wang L, Theoharides TC. Definitive characterization of rat hypothalamic mast cells. Neuroscience. 1996;73(3):889–902. PMID: 8809807. http://www.ncbi.nlm.nih.gov/pubmed/8809807.
483. Kovács P, Hernádi I, Wilhelm M. Mast cells modulate maintained neuronal activity in the thalamus in vivo. J Neuroimmunol. 2006;171(1–2):1–7. PMID: 16300831. http://www.ncbi.nlm.nih.gov/pubmed/16300831.
484. Jiang W, Babyak M, Krantz DS, Waugh RA, Coleman RE, Hanson MM, Frid DJ, McNulty S, Morris JJ, O'Connor CM, Blumenthal JA. Mental stress–induced myocardial ischemia and cardiac events. JAMA. 1996;275(21):1651–6. PMID: 8637138. http://www.ncbi.nlm.nih.gov/pubmed/8637138.
485. Deanfield JE, Shea M, Kensett M, Horlock P, Wilson RA, de Landsheere CM, Selwyn AP. Silent myocardial ischaemia due to mental stress. Lancet. 1984;2(8410):1001–5. PMID: 6149394. http://www.ncbi.nlm.nih.gov/pubmed/6149394.
486. Bairey CN, Krantz DS, Rozanski A. Mental stress as an acute trigger of ischemic left ventricular dysfunction and blood pressure elevation in coronary artery disease. Am J Cardiol. 1990;66(16):28G–31G. PMID: 2239710. http://www.ncbi.nlm.nih.gov/pubmed/2239710.
487. Krantz DS, McCeney MK. Effects of psychological and social factors on organic disease: a critical assessment of research on coronary heart disease. Annu Rev Psychol. 2002;53:341–69. PMID: 11752489. http://www.ncbi.nlm.nih.gov/pubmed/11752489.
488. Miller TQ, Smith TW, Turner CW, Guijarro ML, Hallet AJ. A meta-analytic review of research on hostility and physical health. Psychol Bull. 1996;119(2):322–48. PMID: 8851276. http://www.ncbi.nlm.nih.gov/pubmed/8851276.
489. Everson SA, Kaplan GA, Goldberg DE, Lakka TA, Sivenius J, Salonen JT. Anger expression and incident stroke: prospective evidence from the Kuopio ischemic heart disease study. Stroke. 1999;30(3):523–8. PMID: 10066846. http://www.ncbi.nlm.nih.gov/pubmed/10066846.
490. Papanicolaou DA, Wilder RL, Manolagas SC, Chrousos GP. The pathophysiologic roles of interleukin-6 in human disease. Ann Intern Med. 1998;128(2):127–37. PMID: 9441573. http://www.ncbi.nlm.nih.gov/pubmed/9441573.
491. Mälarstig A, Wallentin L, Siegbahn A. Genetic variation in the interleukin-6 gene in relation to risk and outcomes in acute coronary syndrome. Thromb Res. 2007;119(4):467–73. PMID: 16782174. http://www.ncbi.nlm.nih.gov/pubmed/16782174.
492. Bierhaus A, Wolf J, Andrassy M, Rohleder N, Humpert PM, Petrov D, Ferstl R, von Eynatten M, Wendt T, Rudofsky G, Joswig M, Morcos M, Schwaninger M, McEwen B, Kirschbaum C, Nawroth PP. A mechanism converting psychosocial stress into mononuclear cell activation. Proc Natl Acad Sci USA. 2003;100(4):1920–5. PMCID: PMC149934. http://www.ncbi.nlm.nih.gov/pubmed/12578963.
493. Hänsel A, Hong S, Cámara RJA, von Känel R. Inflammation as a psychophysiological biomarker in chronic psychosocial stress. Neurosci Biobehav Rev. 2010;35(1):115–21. PMID: 20026349. http://www.ncbi.nlm.nih.gov/pubmed/20026349.
494. Miller GE, Rohleder N, Cole SW. Chronic interpersonal stress predicts activation of pro- and anti-inflammatory signaling pathways 6 months later. Psychosom Med. 2009;71(1):57–62. PMCID: PMC2720615. http://www.ncbi.nlm.nih.gov/pubmed/19073750.
495. Wilder RL. Neuroimmunoendocrinology of the rheumatic diseases: past, present, and future. Ann N Y Acad Sci. 2002;966:13–9. PMID: 12114254. http://www.ncbi.nlm.nih.gov/pubmed/12114254.
496. Rider V, Abdou NI. Gender differences in autoimmunity: molecular basis for estrogen effects in systemic lupus erythematosus. Int Immunopharmacol. 2001;1(6):1009–24. PMID: 11407298. http://www.ncbi.nlm.nih.gov/pubmed/11407298.
497. Becker KG, Simon RM, Bailey-Wilson JE, Freidlin B, Biddison WE, McFarland HF, Trent JM. Clustering of non-major histocompatibility complex susceptibility candidate loci in human autoim-

mune diseases. Proc Natl Acad Sci USA. 1998;95(17):9979–84. PMCID: PMC21447. http://www.ncbi.nlm.nih.gov/pubmed/9707586.

498. Furuya T, Salstrom JL, McCall-Vining S, Cannon GW, Joe B, Remmers EF, Griffiths MM, Wilder RL. Genetic dissection of a rat model for rheumatoid arthritis: significant gender influences on autosomal modifier loci. Hum Mol Genet. 2000;9(15):2241–50. PMID: 11001927. http://www.ncbi.nlm.nih.gov/pubmed/11001927.

499. Gubbels MR, Jørgensen TN, Metzger TE, Menze K, Steele H, Flannery SA, Rozzo SJ, Kotzin BL. Effects of MHC and gender on lupus-like autoimmunity in Nba2 congenic mice. J Immunol. 2005;175(9):6190–6. PMID: 16237116. http://www.ncbi.nlm.nih.gov/pubmed/16237116.

500. Herman FJ, Simkovic S, Pasinetti GM. Neuroimmune nexus of depression and dementia: shared mechanisms and therapeutic targets. Br J Pharmacol. 2019;176(18):3558–84. PMCID: PMC6715609. http://www.ncbi.nlm.nih.gov/pubmed/30632147.

501. Irwin MR, Cole S, Olmstead R, Breen EC, Cho JJ, Moieni M, Eisenberger NI. Moderators for depressed mood and systemic and transcriptional inflammatory responses: a randomized controlled trial of endotoxin. Neuropsychopharmacology. 2019;44(3):635–41. PMCID: PMC6333799. http://www.ncbi.nlm.nih.gov/pubmed/30391995.

502. Cole SW, Arevalo JMG, Takahashi R, Sloan EK, Lutgendorf SK, Sood AK, Sheridan JF, Seeman TE. Computational identification of gene-social environment interaction at the human IL6 locus. Proc Natl Acad Sci USA. 2010;107(12):5681–6. PMCID: PMC2851818. http://www.ncbi.nlm.nih.gov/pubmed/20176930.

503. Ko LJ, Engel JD. DNA-binding specificities of the GATA transcription factor family. Mol Cell Biol. 1993;13(7):4011–22. PMCID: PMC359950. http://www.ncbi.nlm.nih.gov/pubmed/8321208.

504. Ciovacco WA, Raskind WH, Kacena MA. Human phenotypes associated with GATA-1 mutations. Gene. 2008;427(1–2):1–6. PMCID: PMC2601579. http://www.ncbi.nlm.nih.gov/pubmed/18930124.

505. GATA1 GATA binding protein 1 [Homo sapiens (human)] – Gene – NCBI.

506. CONVERGE consortium. Sparse whole-genome sequencing identifies two loci for major depressive disorder. Nature. 2015;523(7562):588–91. PMCID: PMC4522619. http://www.ncbi.nlm.nih.gov/pubmed/26176920.

507. Rivera M, McGuffin P. The successful search for genetic loci associated with depression. Genome Med. 2015;7(1):92. PMCID: PMC4548917. http://www.ncbi.nlm.nih.gov/pubmed/26302953.

508. Sancho-Balsells A, Borràs-Pernas S, Flotta F, Chen W, Del Toro D, Rodríguez MJ, Alberch J, Relano-Gines A, Blivet G, Touchon J, Xifró X, Giralt A. Corrigendum to "Brain-gut photobiomodulation restores cognitive alterations in chronically stressed mice through the regulation of Sirt1 and neuroinflammation" J Affect Disord. 354 (2024) 574–588 10.1016/j.jad.2024.03.075 (Jun 1, Epub 2024 Mar 14, PMID: 38490587). J Affect Disord. 2024;361:799. PMID: 38969582. http://www.ncbi.nlm.nih.gov/pubmed/38969582.

509. McQuaid RJ, Gabrys RL, McInnis OA, Anisman H, Matheson K. Understanding the relation between early-life adversity and depression symptoms: the moderating role of sex and an interleukin-1β gene variant. Front Psychiatry. 2019;10:151. PMCID: PMC6438954. http://www.ncbi.nlm.nih.gov/pubmed/30967802.

510. Chiang JJ, Cole SW, Bower JE, Irwin MR, Taylor SE, Arevalo J, Fuligni AJ. Depressive symptoms and immune transcriptional profiles in late adolescents. Brain Behav Immun. 2019;80:163–9. PMCID: PMC6710012. http://www.ncbi.nlm.nih.gov/pubmed/30851376.

511. Kautz MM, Coe CL, McArthur BA, Mac Giollabhui N, Ellman LM, Abramson LY, Alloy LB. Longitudinal changes of inflammatory biomarkers moderate the relationship between recent stressful life events and prospective symptoms of depression in a diverse sample of urban adolescents. Brain Behav Immun. 2020;86:43–52. PMCID: PMC6710165. http://www.ncbi.nlm.nih.gov/pubmed/30822466.

512. Dey A, Hankey Giblin PA. Insights into macrophage heterogeneity and cytokine-induced neuroinflammation in major depressive disorder. Pharmaceuticals (Basel). 2018;11(3):64. PMCID: PMC6160985. http://www.ncbi.nlm.nih.gov/pubmed/29941796.

513. Liu MY, Yang Y, Zhang LJ, Pu LH, He DF, Liu JY, Hafeez A, Ding YC, Ma H, Geng QS. Potential predictors for mental stress-induced myocardial ischemia in patients with coronary artery disease. Chin Med J. 2019;132(12):1390–9. PMCID: PMC6629334. http://www.ncbi.nlm.nih.gov/pubmed/31205095.

514. Lima BB, Hammadah M, Wilmot K, Pearce BD, Shah A, Levantsevych O, Kaseer B, Obideen M, Gafeer MM, Kim JH, Sullivan S, Lewis TT, Weng L, Elon L, Li L, Bremner JD, Raggi P, Quyyumi A, Vaccarino V. Posttraumatic stress disorder is associated with enhanced interleukin-6 response to mental stress in subjects with a recent myocardial infarction. Brain Behav Immun. 2019;75:26–33. PMCID: PMC6279471. http://www.ncbi.nlm.nih.gov/pubmed/30172946.

515. Hammadah M, Sullivan S, Pearce B, Al Mheid I, Wilmot K, Ramadan R, Tahhan AS, O'Neal WT, Obideen M, Alkhoder A, Abdelhadi N, Mohamed Kelli H, Ghafeer MM, Pimple P, Sandesara P, Shah AJ, Hosny KM, Ward L, Ko YA, Sun YV, Weng L, Kutner M, Bremner JD, Sheps DS, Esteves F, Raggi P, Vaccarino V, Quyyumi AA. Inflammatory response to mental stress and mental stress induced myocardial ischemia. Brain Behav Immun. 2018;68:90–7. PMCID: PMC5808921. http://www.ncbi.nlm.nih.gov/pubmed/28986223.

516. Oitzl MS, Champagne DL, van der Veen R, de Kloet ER. Brain development under stress: hypotheses of glucocorticoid actions revisited. Neurosci Biobehav Rev. 2010;34(6):853–66. PMID: 19631685. http://www.ncbi.nlm.nih.gov/pubmed/19631685.

517. De Kloet ER, Vreugdenhil E, Oitzl MS, Joëls M. Brain corticosteroid receptor balance in health and disease. Endocr Rev. 1998;19(3):269–301. PMID: 9626555. http://www.ncbi.nlm.nih.gov/pubmed/9626555.

518. Stein-Behrens BA, Sapolsky RM. Stress, glucocorticoids, and aging. Aging (Milano). 1992;4(3):197–210. PMID: 1420403. http://www.ncbi.nlm.nih.gov/pubmed/1420403.

519. Sapolsky RM, Krey LC, McEwen BS. The neuroendocrinology of stress and aging: the glucocorticoid cascade hypothesis. Endocr Rev. 1986;7(3):284–301. PMID: 3527687. http://www.ncbi.nlm.nih.gov/pubmed/3527687.

520. Ferguson D, Sapolsky R. Overexpression of mineralocorticoid and transdominant glucocorticoid receptor blocks the impairing effects of glucocorticoids on memory. Hippocampus. 2008;18(11):1103–11. PMID: 18651616. http://www.ncbi.nlm.nih.gov/pubmed/18651616.

521. Mitra R, Ferguson D, Sapolsky RM. Mineralocorticoid receptor overexpression in basolateral amygdala reduces corticosterone secretion and anxiety. Biol Psychiatry. 2009;66(7):686–90. PMID: 19500777. http://www.ncbi.nlm.nih.gov/pubmed/19500777.

522. McEwen BS, De Kloet ER, Rostene W. Adrenal steroid receptors and actions in the nervous system. Physiol Rev. 1986;66(4):1121–88. PMID: 3532143. http://www.ncbi.nlm.nih.gov/pubmed/3532143.

523. McEwen BS. Corticosteroids and hippocampal plasticity. Ann N Y Acad Sci. 1994;746:134–42; discussion 142–144, 178–179. PMID: 7825871. http://www.ncbi.nlm.nih.gov/pubmed/7825871.

524. Gould E, McEwen BS, Tanapat P, Galea LA, Fuchs E. Neurogenesis in the dentate gyrus of the adult tree shrew is regulated by psychosocial stress and NMDA receptor activation. J Neurosci. 1997;17(7):2492–8. PMCID: PMC6573503. http://www.ncbi.nlm.nih.gov/pubmed/9065509.
525. Joëls M, de Kloet ER. Control of neuronal excitability by corticosteroid hormones. Trends Neurosci. 1992;15(1):25–30. PMID: 1374954. http://www.ncbi.nlm.nih.gov/pubmed/1374954.
526. Jacobson L, Sapolsky R. The role of the hippocampus in feedback regulation of the hypothalamic-pituitary-adrenocortical axis. Endocr Rev. 1991;12(2):118–34. PMID: 2070776. http://www.ncbi.nlm.nih.gov/pubmed/2070776.
527. Oitzl MS, de Kloet ER. Selective corticosteroid antagonists modulate specific aspects of spatial orientation learning. Behav Neurosci. 1992;106(1):62–71. PMID: 1313244. http://www.ncbi.nlm.nih.gov/pubmed/1313244.
528. Beato M, Sánchez-Pacheco A. Interaction of steroid hormone receptors with the transcription initiation complex. Endocr Rev. 1996;17(6):587–609. PMID: 8969970. http://www.ncbi.nlm.nih.gov/pubmed/8969970.
529. van Steensel B, Jenster G, Damm K, Brinkmann AO, van Driel R. Domains of the human androgen receptor and glucocorticoid receptor involved in binding to the nuclear matrix. J Cell Biochem. 1995;57(3):465–78. PMID: 7768981. http://www.ncbi.nlm.nih.gov/pubmed/7768981.
530. White T, Ozel B, Jain JK, Stanczyk FZ. Effects of transdermal and oral contraceptives on estrogen-sensitive hepatic proteins. Contraception. 2006;74(4):293–6. PMID: 16982228. http://www.ncbi.nlm.nih.gov/pubmed/16982228.
531. Dodig-Curkovic K, Kurbel S, Matic VC. Can incidence of depression in women be linked to estrogen dependent secretion of various hormone binding proteins? Med Hypotheses. 2009;72(2):211–2. PMID: 18996648. http://www.ncbi.nlm.nih.gov/pubmed/18996648.
532. Smith CL, Hammond GL. Hormonal regulation of corticosteroid-binding globulin biosynthesis in the male rat. Endocrinology. 1992;130(4):2245–51. PMID: 1547738. http://www.ncbi.nlm.nih.gov/pubmed/1547738.
533. Manenschijn L, van den Akker ELT, Lamberts SWJ, van Rossum EFC. Clinical features associated with glucocorticoid receptor polymorphisms. An overview. Ann N Y Acad Sci. 2009;1179:179–98. PMID: 19906240. http://www.ncbi.nlm.nih.gov/pubmed/19906240.
534. de Kloet ER, Fitzsimons CP, Datson NA, Meijer OC, Vreugdenhil E. Glucocorticoid signaling and stress-related limbic susceptibility pathway: about receptors, transcription machinery and microRNA. Brain Res. 2009;1293:129–41. PMID: 19332027. http://www.ncbi.nlm.nih.gov/pubmed/19332027.
535. Brinks V, Berger S, Gass P, de Kloet ER, Oitzl MS. Mineralocorticoid receptors in control of emotional arousal and fear memory. Horm Behav. 2009;56(2):232–8. PMID: 19447109. http://www.ncbi.nlm.nih.gov/pubmed/19447109.
536. Brinks V, de Kloet ER, Oitzl MS. Corticosterone facilitates extinction of fear memory in BALB/c mice but strengthens cue related fear in C57BL/6 mice. Exp Neurol. 2009;216(2):375–82. PMID: 19162011. http://www.ncbi.nlm.nih.gov/pubmed/19162011.
537. Brinks V, van der Mark M, de Kloet R, Oitzl M. Emotion and cognition in high and low stress sensitive mouse strains: a combined neuroendocrine and behavioral study in BALB/c and C57BL/6J mice. Front. Behav Neurosci. 2007;1:8. PMCID: PMC2525853. http://www.ncbi.nlm.nih.gov/pubmed/18958190.
538. Brinks V, de Kloet ER, Oitzl MS. Strain specific fear behaviour and glucocorticoid response to aversive events: modelling PTSD in mice. Prog Brain Res. 2008;167:257–61. PMID: 18037021. http://www.ncbi.nlm.nih.gov/pubmed/18037021.
539. Giordano R, Bo M, Pellegrino M, Vezzari M, Baldi M, Picu A, Balbo M, Bonelli L, Migliaretti G, Ghigo E, Arvat E. Hypothalamus-pituitary-adrenal hyperactivity in human aging is partially refractory to stimulation by mineralocorticoid receptor blockade. J Clin Endocrinol Metab. 2005;90(10):5656–62. PMID: 16014406. http://www.ncbi.nlm.nih.gov/pubmed/16014406.
540. Heuser I, Deuschle M, Weber A, Kniest A, Ziegler C, Weber B, Colla M. The role of mineralocorticoid receptors in the circadian activity of the human hypothalamus-pituitary-adrenal system: effect of age. Neurobiol Aging. 2000;21(4):585–9. PMID: 10924776. http://www.ncbi.nlm.nih.gov/pubmed/10924776.
541. Goncharova N, Chigarova O, Rudenko N, Oganyan T. Glucocorticoid negative feedback in regulation of the hypothalamic-pituitary-adrenal Axis in rhesus monkeys with various types of adaptive behavior: individual and age-related differences. Front Endocrinol (Lausanne). 2019;10:24. PMCID: PMC6381009. http://www.ncbi.nlm.nih.gov/pubmed/30814974.
542. Derijk RH. Single nucleotide polymorphisms related to HPA axis reactivity. Neuroimmunomodulation. 2009;16(5):340–52. PMID: 19571595. http://www.ncbi.nlm.nih.gov/pubmed/19571595.
543. Köhler JC, Gröger N, Lesse A, Guara Ciurana S, Rether K, Fegert J, Bock J, Braun K. Early-life adversity induces epigenetically regulated changes in hippocampal dopaminergic molecular pathways. Mol Neurobiol. 2019;56(5):3616–25. PMCID: PMC6476847. http://www.ncbi.nlm.nih.gov/pubmed/30173406.

Molecular Aspects of Depressive Disorders

8

Franklin Sunzeri

Introduction

Complex traits, infinitesimal models, missing heritability, epistasis, gene–gene interactions, polygeneity, omnigeneity, gene–environment interactions, and the dark matter inside us all: epigenetics and noncoding variants…

Our understanding of the molecular contributions to complex diseases is constantly evolving [7]. Overly simplified: Mendel's work came first focusing on monogenic phenotypes. Then came *Fisher's infinitesimal model* [1] that showed that as the number of genes that control a trait grows, the contribution of each gene gets smaller, and as the number grows, the random sampling of alleles produces a continuous normally distributed phenotype in a population [2]. *Genome-wide association studies* and exome-sequencing showed that even the most salient loci have small effect sizes and that the cumulative effects of multiple loci do not explain very much of the genetic variance: the *missing heritability* [8]. Next, the missing heritability was found [9, 10]. It was asserted that variance can be explained by considering all SNPs simultaneously because the individual effects are too small to pass stringent significance tests. Additionally heritability is thought to be due to incomplete *linkage disequilibrium*[1] between causal variants and genotyped SNPs, exacerbated by causal variants of unexplored SNPs having lower and rarer minor allele frequency but possibly having larger effect sizes [11–13].

Following these insights was the realization that, instead of Mendelian diseases that are mainly caused by alterations in protein coding, complex diseases are frequently caused by *regulatory noncoding variants* [14–18]. The model for complex disease manifestation then became that complex disease is a result of the summation of weak effects on key genes and regulatory pathways [19, 20]. As a corollary, Boyle et al. suggest an *omnigenic hypothesis* that due to the interconnectedness of regulatory networks, disease-causing variants do not have to cluster in key pathways, "…all genes expressed in disease-relevant cells are liable to affect the functions of core disease-related genes and that most heritability can be explained by effects on genes outside core pathways" [7].

In the typical *genome-wide association study*, each naturally occurring genetic variant is checked against a complex disease trait, and then all the effects of all the variants are added to determine the effects of those DNA polymorphisms on that trait [21]. An underlying assumption is that these effects are independent of the genetic background. However, if the effect of one variant is dependent upon the effect of another variant, then this assumption does not hold [24]. This dependence is called *epistasis*[2] [25–29]. Epistasis makes it difficult to actually gauge the influence of a genetic variant on a complex disease trait.

Phenotypes are almost always controlled by multiple genes with two or more alleles [31]. Genes may be turned on sequentially, such as in ontogeny, or they may function synergistically to produce complex phenotypes. Genes can also interfere or modify the expression of other genes.

A useful definition is that epistasis refers to interactions between genes in which the contribution of one gene to a phenotype depends on the genotype at another locus, or more broadly, the genetic background of the organism [32], i.e., *gene–gene interactions* [31]. A comprehensive review of how epistasis can affect human health and disease and how it can be detected in population-based studies, along with implications of epistasis for personal genetics, is presented in [31].

[1] Linkage disequilibrium is where alleles (DNA markers) occur together more often than can be accounted for by chance because of their physical proximity on a chromosome [22, 23].

[2] Modifications include such things as masking, inhibiting, or suppressing by the expression of one or more other genes [30].

F. Sunzeri (✉)
Heather Hills Consulting, Coos Bay, OR, USA

J. Raber et al. (eds.), *Understanding and Treating Depressive Disorders*, https://doi.org/10.1007/978-3-032-14465-2_8

In some of the earlier literature, epistasis referred only to masking. The allele or gene doing the masking is the epistatic gene or allele. The alleles or genes that are being masked are called *hypostatic*. Sometimes, the nature of epistasis is the dysfunction of a gene in a pathway in a way that downstream or upstream genes in the pathway cannot be properly expressed. It is also epistasis when a dominant allele masks the expression of a different gene, or in a reciprocal relationship where if either of two genes is dominant, the phenotype is the same. When any single characteristic shows a phenotype ratio of 16 to 1, it is likely the product of two nonlinked genes interacting.

It has been argued that epistasis and *pleiotropy* (one mutation causes multiple phenotypes) are ubiquitous and inherent properties of biomolecular networks and should be treated as fundamental components of genetic analyses [32].

When reading genotype-to-phenotype relationships studies, it is important to remember that statistical epistasis at a population level is different from epistasis at the cellular level [24, 33]. *Statistical epistasis* is defined as deviation from additivity in a mathematical model, summarizing the relationship between multilocus genotypes and phenotypic variation in a population [24]. When biological epistasis and statistical epistasis cross paths is discussed in Moore and Williams reference [24]: "Traversing the conceptual divide between biological and statistical epistasis: systems biology and a more modern synthesis."

A detailed analysis of *genetic association studies* suggests that interpretations of disease markers (highly associated SNPs), even with replicated highly significant odds ratios, may not be good at sorting out the constituent relationships [34]. Nevertheless, they can be very valuable in pointing the way to new etiological hypotheses previously not considered.

In addition, it has been suggested that it is perilous to analyze disease risk based upon odds ratios or p values for associations that are the discovery phase statistical measures [35]. Measures like sensitivity, specificity, and positive and negative predictive values may be more useful when proposing a genetic profile for risk prediction.

Molecular Hypotheses

Several hypotheses have attempted to explain the molecular basis of depression [36, 37]. These include the *monoamine dysregulation hypothesis* [38] the *dysregulation of the hypothalamic-pituitary-adrenal axis* [39], and the *macrophage excessive secretion of monokines hypothesis* [40]. It is quite likely that there is an intimate relationship between these hypotheses, with different balances determining different degrees and types of depression [41].

Within these hypotheses is the *bidirectional psychoneuroimmunology-depression connection* [42, 43]. A *cytokine hypothesis of depression* suggests that proinflammatory cytokines functioning as modulators of neural interactions are the key elements in the central mediation of neuroendocrine,+ neurochemical, and behavioral aspects of major depression [43–45].

Major depression may be a significant life-threatening complication of various endocrine diseases [46]. These include Cushing's syndrome, Addison's disease, hyperthyroidism, hypothyroidism, and hyperprolactinemic amenorrhea. It is unclear whether cytokines are causes of depression or associated phenomena. Nevertheless, evidence has accumulated along epidemiological and experimental lines. Cytokines may activate the tryptophan and serotonin metabolizing enzyme indoleamine-2,3-dioxygenase (IDO), resulting in reduced levels of tryptophan, the precursor to serotonin, and thereby producing the reduced levels of serotonin often found in major depression [47]. Cytokines may interfere with negative feedback inhibition of the HPA axis and account for the hyperactive hypothalamic-pituitary-adrenal (HPA) axis often found in depression.

Depression is associated with several chronic inflammatory diseases (e.g., rheumatoid arthritis), and treatment with cytokines often provokes depressive symptoms. One of the most suggestive associations between cytokines and depression is the almost immediate appearance of depression symptoms (especially the symptoms described below for *sickness behavior*) when IFN-α, TNF-α, or IL-2 is administered to patients with hepatitis C [48, 49] or cancer [50]. Accumulating evidence suggests that the immune system may be intimately involved in this depression [51–53]. The prevalence of depression associated with physical illness is so high that in the Diagnostic and Statistical Manual of Mental Disorders, it is a specific diagnosis.

When we get sick, a set of adaptive behaviors occurs to marshal our defenses and reorganize our priorities to cope with disease [54]. Most frequently, they include lethargy, depression, anorexia [55, 56], sleepiness [3, 57], hyperalgesia, difficulty in concentrating [58], and reduction in grooming [59–61]. Sickness behavior is almost identical symptoms of major depression. As such, it has been proposed that major depression is a maladaptive manifestation of sickness behavior as a reaction to circulating cytokines [62–65].

Increased activity in the subgenual anterior cingulate cortex and decreased mesolimbic connectivity are involved both in IL-6-associated responses in immune responses and in depression [66, 67]. During inflammation-associated changes in mood, functional connectivity is decreased between the subgenual anterior cingulate cortex and the superior temporal sulcus, nucleus accumbens, medial prefrontal cortex, and the amygdala [67].

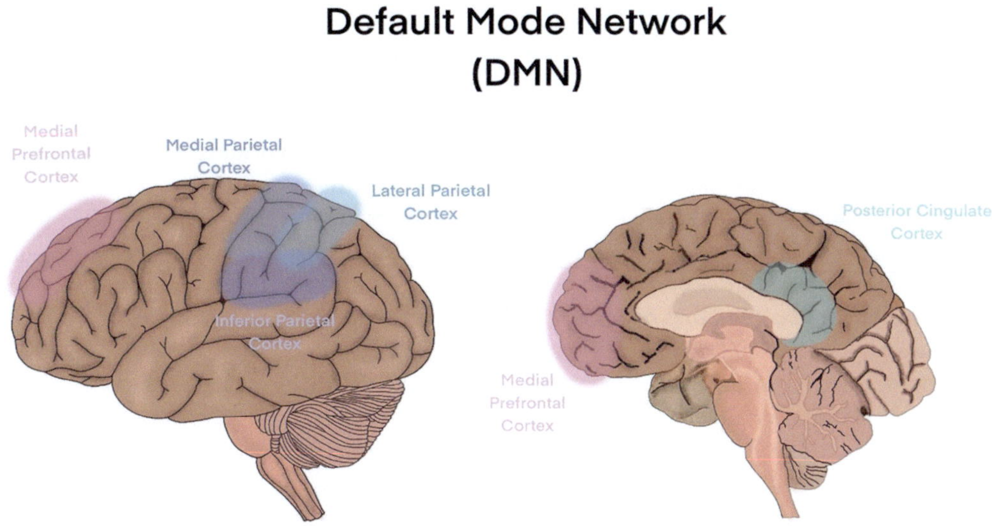

Fig. 8.1 This illustration highlights core regions of the brain's Default Mode Network (DMN) including the medial prefrontal cortex, and medial, lateral, and inferior parietal cortex. The DMN, the most well-characterized intrinsic connectivity network, is predominantly active during rest and self-referential thought and shows reduced activity during externally focused, goal-directed tasks. Disruptions in DMN function are associated with symptoms of mood disorders, reflecting its role in internal cognition and emotional regulation

Many neurological disorders, such as epilepsy, migraine, Alzheimer's disease, Parkinson's disease, essential tremor, and stroke, are associated with psychiatric disorders such as depression [68, 69].

Abnormal functions in *intrinsic connectivity networks (ICNs)* [70, 71], particularly the *Default Mode Network (DMN)* [72, 73], which is the most well-characterized ICN, are associated with symptoms of mood disorders [73–76]. During task-related activities or when executive functions are needed, activity in a variety of brain areas, including the DMN, is reduced. That is, the DMN is predominantly engaged and activated during rest, times when there are self-referential (autobiographical) and spontaneous thoughts, and is quiet when we are undertaking goal-directed, attention-requiring thought [74]. See Fig. 8.1.

These regions include the precuneus/posterior cingulate cortex (PCC), medial prefrontal cortex (MPFC), and medial, lateral, and inferior parietal cortex. Multivariate pattern analysis (MVPA), which has been used to distinguish psychiatric patients from healthy controls using brain imaging, has shown normalization of DMN functions in 30% of MDD patients after antidepressant treatment [77, 78]. Irregularities in DMN functional connectivity and activity are found in several neuropsychiatric disorders and metabolic disorders. Irregularities in particular parts of the DMN are demonstrable in MDD [76]. MDD symptoms of rumination and overgeneral autobiographical memory (OGM) have been associated with alterations in different regions of the DMN. Anterior medial regions of resting-state DMN showed increased functional connectivity in ruminators. Posterior medial regions were associated with decreased functional connectivity in OGM.

Neuroendocrine Hypotheses

Some researchers have proposed that stress triggers depression through an epigenetic-genomic action of glucocorticoids, glucocorticoid receptors, and HPA activation [79, 80]. An outstanding series of 15 reports by *Robert Rubin* and colleagues on the *neuroendocrine aspects of primary endogenous depression* began in 1987 [81] and continued through 1997 [82]. They covered the state of the art at the time of their publication on various aspects, such as cortisol, melatonin, gonadal hormones, prolactin, growth hormone, race, and sex associations with depression. Well worth the read through, more than 25 years of research have since expanded upon the knowledge that they present.

For insight into the biochemistry of depression, the Nobel Prize work of *Paul Greengard* is worth reading by the molecularly inclined. Three papers of special interest relative to dopamine and serotonin are [83–85].

In the 1960s, the original *biological hypothesis of major depression* suggested abnormalities in the serotonin and/or norepinephrine neurotransmitter systems [86, 87]. However, supporting evidence for this hypothesis has been mixed.

For example, levels of norepinephrine metabolites in the cortical spinal fluid of folks with depression vs. normal healthy controls have yielded conflicting results [88–91]. Yet, it does seem that there is evidence for decreased levels of norepinephrine in major depression. It has been hypothesized that polymorphisms of the *norepinephrine transporter* (which terminates norepinephrine action by recycling norepinephrine in the synapse) may be related to such deficiencies [92]. Although it seems that serotonin and norepinephrine are involved in depression, it is likely that their dysfunctions are due to modulation by and of other neurobiological systems [93]. For example, abnormal modulation of cortical-hippocampal-amygdala pathways may dispose to oversensitivity to stress and fear, with possible results of malfunctioning control over affect.

Early investigations of some of the polymorphisms in diverse populations have so far been inconclusive [94–96].

The principal current neuroendocrine-related hypotheses are the *monoamine dysregulation hypothesis* [38] and the *dysregulation of the hypothalamic–pituitary–adrenal axis* [40]. These hypotheses may be mixed with the effects of neurotoxic and neuroprotective processes involving genes such as the brain-derived neurotrophic factor (BDNF) and cytokines produced from the immune system [97, 98].

With respect to the monoamine dysregulation hypothesis, serotonin has perhaps been the most heavily studied monoamine involved in depression [100]. Monoamine depletion studies suggest a link between monoamines (dopamine, serotonin, and norepinephrine) and mood, at least in people afflicted with major depression [100]. Serotonin responses to stress, both chronic and acute, are controlled by a panoply of molecules. These include those that control serotonin neuron development (Pet-1), synthesis (tryptophan hydroxylase 1 and 2 isozymes), packaging (vesicular monoamine transporter 2), activities at presynaptic and postsynaptic receptors (5-HT1A, 5-HT1B, 5-HT2A, 5-HT2C, 5-HT3A, 5-HT4, 5-HT5A, 5-HT6, 5-HT7), reuptake (serotonin transporter), and degradation (monoamine oxidase A) [419]. Differences in serotonin metabolism seem to be associated with a variety of conditions, such as obsessive-compulsive disorder, clinical depression, hypertension, generalized social phobia [418], alcoholism, and romantic love [101].

Genetic polymorphisms in these molecules have been hypothesized to influence functions of neural circuits involved in individual differences in stress responses and hence stress-associated diseases. One of those circuits is the one connecting the amygdala, medial prefrontal cortex, and dorsal raphe nucleus that is involved in fear [102].

Generally, serotonin involvement in depression seems to be impaired neurotransmission rather than changes in sensitivity of post-synaptic serotonin receptors [103]. Extensive literature implicates serotonin in the pathophysiology of affective disorders, but its precise role is unclear [104]. The *serotonin transporter (5-HTT, SERT, SLC6A4)*[3] is frequently implicated in these disorders and is a target of many antidepressants [105, 106]. The serotonin transporter carries the serotonin from the synaptic cleft back into the presynaptic cell, thus terminating the signal.

Genetic variation at the serotonin transporter influences sensitivity to depression causing effects of stressful life events [112]. Additionally, polymorphisms of the serotonin transporter gene appear to be associated with PTSD, sudden infant death syndrome, and aggressive behavior in Alzheimer's disease [113].

The serotonin transporter is a membrane protein of the presynaptic neuron that transports serotonin from the synaptic space back into the presynaptic neuron, thereby terminating the action of serotonin and recycling the used transmitter [113].

Two polymorphisms of the serotonin transporter 5-HTT that modulate transcription have been widely studied. These are a *44-base pair (bp) insertion/deletion in the promoter region (5-HTTLPR)* and a *17 bp variable number of tandem repeats in the second intron (VNTR-2 or STin2)* [114]. See Fig. 8.2.

The expression rate of 5-HTT is controlled by the *serotonin transporter promoter region length polymorphism (5-HTTLPR/SLC6A4)* [115]. The 5-HTTLPR polymorphism is a 44 bp insertion/deletion involving 2 units in a sequence of 16 repeated elements [116]. The 44 bp *deletion* is known as the *short allele,* and the 44 bp *insertion* is known as the *long allele*. It would seem that folks with two short alleles have an increased sensitivity to the impact of mild stressors. Moreover, there may be an interaction between neurotic tendencies and 5-HTT polymorphisms [117]. There may be an epigenetic influence on this interaction, as early life events such as childhood abuse may sensitize individuals to future life stressors [118].

This promoter region is controlled by the binding of various molecules, including cortisol [119]. At least in vitro, the binding of cortisol increases the expression of 5-HTT.

In 2003, a prospective longitudinal study showed that people with one or two copies of the short allele of 5-HTTLPR vs. those who were homozygous for the long allele demonstrated more depressive symptoms, diagnosable depression, and suicidality in relation to stressful life events [120]. In addition, people who are homozygous for short alleles were seen to be much more likely to become depressed in reaction to mild life stressors [112]. Moreover, women were much more likely than men were to become depressed in reaction to severe life stressors.

The functional polymorphism resulting in a short allele causes an approximately 30–40% reduction in the rate of in vitro expression of 5-HTT mRNA [121]. This reduction in transcription efficiency causes a decrease in 5-HT uptake. This reduction has been seen in association studies to explain 3–4% of total variation and 7–9% of inherited variance in anxiety-related personality traits in individuals.

[3]The serotonin transporter gene is designated SLC6A4, which stands for solute carrier family 6 [neurotransmitter transporter, serotonin], member 4. The serotonin transporter molecule is abbreviated 5-HTT for the 5-hydroxytryptamine (serotonin) transporter.

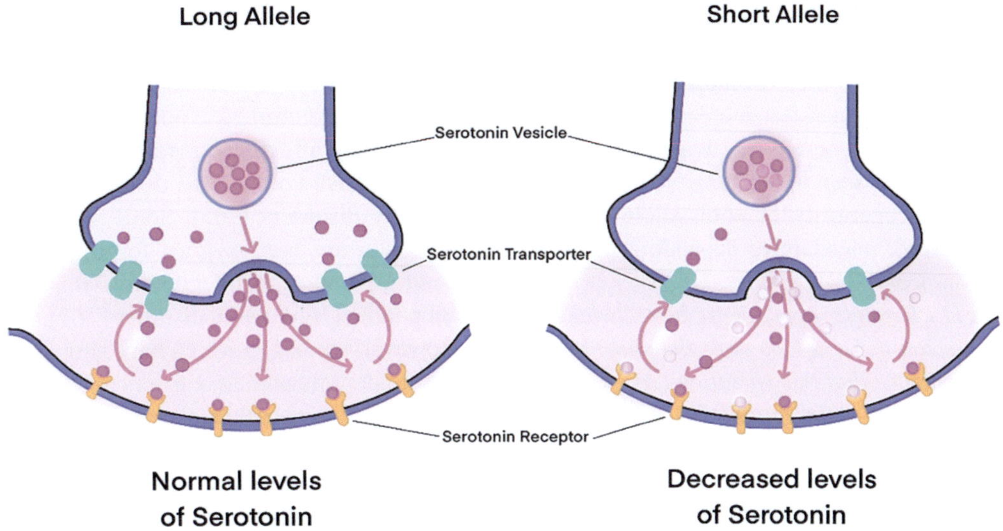

Fig. 8.2 Effects of long and short alleles on synaptic serotonin levels. This diagram illustrates how genetic variation in the serotonin transporter-linked polymorphic region (5-HTTLPR) alleles influences synaptic serotonin levels. The long (L) allele is associated with more efficient serotonin reuptake, maintaining typical levels at the synapse. In contrast, the short (S) allele leads to reduced transporter expression, resulting in decreased serotonin availability in the synaptic cleft—an alteration implicated in mood disorder susceptibility and stress reactivity

However, in vivo, the effect of these polymorphisms on 5-HTT binding is not apparent in healthy subjects [122] or between healthy and depressed individuals [123, 124].

Carriers of the short allele of the 5-HTTLPR/SLC6A4[4] have been shown to be prone to increased anxiety, increased amygdala reactions, and increased likelihood of depression [122]. However, increased amygdala activity in carriers of the short alleles has not been shown to be achieved by current 5-HTT availability, but by a smaller amygdala volume that appears to be dependent upon [epi]genetic influences during neurodevelopment [125]. These carriers had decreased gray matter in the limbic areas (especially the amygdala and the perigenual cingulate) involved in processing negative emotions [122]. These areas appear to be important in feedback control on negative affect [122]. Short allele carriers showed an uncoupling of the negative feedback [122]. The magnitude of the uncoupling associated with this polymorphism predicted almost 30% of the increase in anxiety. The implication is that there is a developmentally determined systemic mechanism relating to emotional reaction and depression susceptibility.

Stressful life events, sex, and race have been shown to moderate associations of the 5-HTTLPR and depression [126, 127]. The short alleles of 5-HTTLPR may be involved in the association between stressful social environments and the risk of harmful cardiovascular reactivity to stress, and there is a sex influence on this reactivity [128]. In addition, the length polymorphism of the 5-HTTLPR may influence tolerance of SSRIs and behavioral symptoms in dementia [129]. Women with unipolar disorder and the homozygosity for the short allele appear to have higher severity of depression [126]. However, some studies have not shown associations between stressful life events and the short alleles [130–132].

There is some evidence that under acute stress, the homozygous short 5-HTTLPR alleles increase cognitive-attentional bias for negative emotional content, which may increase vulnerability for depression [133]. The homozygotes for the long alleles appear to be more resilient and may exhibit increasing emotional control after acute stress.

On the other hand, a good case can be made that the short alleles of 5-HTTLPR probably have evolutionary advan-

[4]*The serotonin transporter (SERT) promoter region* functional length polymorphism (5-HTTLPR; SLC6A4 (the gene that codes for the 5-HTTLPR)) has been associated with several anxiety traits [108]. Hariri et al. have shown that people with one or two copies of the short allele compared to homozygotes for the long allele have reduced expression and function of 5-HTT, increased fear and anxiety-related characteristics, and greater amygdala activity in response to fearful stimuli. Further work has suggested that gene-by-environment interactions in the serotonin system in the amygdala and the ventromedial prefrontal cortex activation may reflect a neural endophenotype that translates genetic and adverse environmental influences into vulnerability for or resilience against developing fear-based affective psychopathology [107].

Homberg has suggested that for carriers, hyperactivity in the corticolimbic areas creates hypervigilance that is found in both anxiety-related traits and cognitive superiority [109]. In addition, the environment will determine if response will be negative (emotional) or positive (cognitive).

Interestingly, an intron (VNTR-2 or STin2) in the SLC6A4 gene, polymorphisms in 5-HTTLPR, and variable number tandem repeats RS1, RS3 and AVR in the AVPR1A (arginine vasopressin receptor 1a) gene have been associated with both behavior and creativity [110, 111].

tages, or they would not be maintained in the population [107, 109]. Humans and nonhuman primates with the short allele outperform individuals who have the long allele in an array of cognitive tasks and manifest increased social conformity [109]. It has been suggested that hypervigilance of the corticolimbic system, as seen in the anxiety-related traits and socially cognitive superiority of short-allele carriers, may either be adaptive or maladaptive depending upon the psychosocial environment.

The long 5-HTTLPR allele appears to have twice the basal level of expression of 5-HTT as does the short allele. There is abundant evidence that this variation has effects on the antidepressant effects of different antidepressants [134, 135]. For example, homozygotes of the short allele appear to have a slower and a selective improvement of core depression and somatic anxiety symptoms [135, 136].

Caucasians with the 5-HTTLPR s/s or s/l genotype are generally found to be at an increased risk of developing adverse events such as dermatologic reactions, weight change, and fatigue while using SSRIs [137–140]. However, opposite or inconsistent results have also been seen [141–146]. In addition, in Asian populations, it sometimes seems that either the short alleles have a more favorable response [147–150], or the long alleles show a better response [151–155], or no discernible differences are seen [156–158].

Table 6 from [134] lists association reports relating 5-HTTLPR variants with antidepressant responses.

Apparently, at least some side effects of SSRIs relate to the short allele of the 5-HTTLPR [134, 144]. These include increased risk of insomnia or agitation with fluoxetine [159].

According to a 2006 meta-analysis, 5-HTTLPR genotypes appear to be linked to a variety of diseases with affective symptoms such as depression, bipolar disorder, anxiety disorders, eating disorders, and substance abuse [160]. These relationships may be moderated at least in part by hippocampal volume and amygdala responses. Allelic differences seem to influence mood disorder characteristics such as age of onset, periodicity, and recurrence, cycling speed, antidepressant response, and reactions to stress [160]. In addition, personality traits and pathological behaviors relevant to stress, anxiety, and impulsiveness appear to be associated. These include addictions such as alcoholism and smoking, eating disorders, suicide, ADHD, and autism [160].

When coupled with low social support, the short allele of 5-HTTLPR has been associated with 4.5 times greater risk of PTSD and major depression following high levels of exposure to a hurricane [161]. These results were independent of age, sex, and ancestry. Similar results have been seen in carriers who have experienced both childhood adversity and adult traumatic events.

In addition, when error processing, the short allele appears to increase the response [164]. Seasonal affective disorder also seems to have an associated increase in frequency in carriers of the short allele [162, 163].

A 2011 study has reviewed evidence of associations between the serotonin gene polymorphism and mental disorders, including affective disorders, post-traumatic stress disorder, obsessive-compulsive disorder, suicide, autism, and personality disorders [165]. Some studies have shown that people who are homozygous for the short alleles do not respond as well to antidepressants that are prescribed for social phobia [166], panic disorder [167], and bulimia [168].

However, studies in Korea have shown better response to some antidepressants in carriers of the short allele. For example, the therapeutic response to the antidepressant escitalopram was better in short allele carriers [169]. Moreover, a meta-analysis and other studies of 5-HTTLPR polymorphisms and panic disorder found no evidence to support an association [170]. Other polymorphisms that were investigated after meta-analysis have shown possible connections. For example, a putative association with panic disorders has been seen with rs3813034, a functional polymorphism in the serotonin transporter, which alters the balance of the two polyadenylation forms of the serotonin transporter [171–173].

Differences have been seen between men and women in reactions to *acute tryptophan* (the precursor to serotonin) *depletion* [174]. Men demonstrated increased impulsiveness and did not show mood reduction. Women demonstrated more caution and mood reduction. Women who are heterozygotes for 5-HTTLPR appeared to be less sensitive to mood imbalances resulting from tryptophan depletion than homozygotes for either the short or the long alleles.

Supporting the roles of serotonin in affective disorders is the response to tryptophan depletion in depressed and normal subjects [104]. Experimentally, tryptophan is depleted in a diet replete with all the other amino acids. This depletion results in a dramatic drop in circulating tryptophan, and in one experiment, it induced a transient return of depressive symptoms in those who had remitted major depression but not in controls ($p < 0.001$) [175]. Those patients who had remitted major depression but not controls showed an increase in regional cerebral glucose utilization in the orbitofrontal cortex, medial thalamus, anterior and posterior cingulate cortices, and ventral striatum.

Interestingly, tryptophan depletion results in decreased morning cortisol levels in both normals and subjects who have OCD or primary insomnia [176].

In a sample of elderly folks, the short allele at the 5-HTTLPR was associated significantly with poor scores on delayed recall and higher waking cortisol levels that negatively affected memory, apparently involving the hippocampal volume [177]. No interactions were seen among the short allele, accumulated life stress, or cortisol. It is suggestive that the influence of the short allele on memory is mediated via the HPA axis. One experiment showed that in caregivers, but not in normal controls, the short allele was associated with poorer sleep quality [178].

Comorbidity with anxiety is so high that it is not surprising that short-allele carriers of 5-HTTLPR polymorphisms are also involved in anxiety and fear-based disorders [179]. As investigation proceeds on the associations with the 5-HTTLPR alleles, the results have become more nuanced. Here are a few examples.

People with two short alleles who have experienced childhood mistreatment appear to be at increased risk of persistent, but not single-episode depression [180]. Additionally, these short alleles seem to confer a higher risk of bullying among individuals with emotional problems [181].

Epigenetic effects on 5-HTT expression were assessed in shift working nurses who are prone to burnout and depression [182]. Results showed that increased environmental stress was concurrent with decreased methylation of 5-HTTLPR/SLC6A4 (i.e., increased expression). Burnout and work stress significantly contributed ($p = 0.038$ and $p < 0.0001$, respectively) to methylation levels. The implication is that it may lead to increased transcription of the transporter gene, increased reuptake of serotonin, and decreased serotonin activity.

Another possibility is that it appears that the short allele may increase risk for depression by its effects on decreasing motivational incentive processing [183].

Animal studies have suggested that the *rh5-HTTLPR* genotype variation and early experience may also increase vulnerability to alcoholism [184]. Animals carrying the short allele appear to be more susceptible. It is thought this might operate via a link between serotonin neurotransmission and limbic-hypothalamic-pituitary-adrenal (LHPA) axis hormones that reinforce alcohol intake. Acute stress or subacute stress may actually be linked to decreased alcohol consumption, whereas chronic stress, especially early in life, may lead to increased propensity for alcoholism [185]. These sensitivities in complex diseases may be a result of genetic and environmental interactions [105].

Epigenetic regulation of serotonin has received a fair amount of attention, often as related to therapeutic drug responses [186]. In macaques, early life stressors experienced by high-risk serotonin transport gene polymorphism promoter (5-HTTLPR) carriers induced 5-HTT CpG methylation that contributed to mood disorders [187]. However, the critical element was the level of methylation, not the actual genotype.

There is some evidence that the short allele of a polymorphism in the promoter region of the serotonin transporter gene (5-HTTLPR) (5-HTTLPR (rs25531) and the monoamine oxidase A-upstream variable number tandem repeat (MAOA-uVNTR) interacts with stress to influence the start of depression [188]. When assessed at 13 and then at 15 years of age, girls frequently showed elevated depressive symptoms when they encountered negative life experiences if they had low-expression MAOA-uVNTR alleles and short 5-HTTLPR alleles. Boys were more likely to express symptoms when they had low-expression MAOA-uVNTR alleles but long 5-HTTLPR alleles.

Nevertheless, a study that genotyped nine polymorphisms in the genes encoding the serotonin transporter, brain-derived neurotrophic factor, catechol-O-methyltransferase, angiotensin converting enzyme, tryptophan hydroxylase, and the serotonin receptors 1A, 2A, and 2C found no relationships between these polymorphisms and stressful life events that influenced antidepressant treatment outcomes in patients experiencing a single episode of depression [189].

Recent reviews suggest that in addition to genetic variants in 5-HTTLPR, variants in VNTR2/STin2, HTR1A, HTR2A, TPH1, and BDNF may also modulate antidepressant response and susceptibility to various psychopathologies [190–192].[5]

For example, in a study of folks with unipolar depression or bipolar disorder, three novel alleles of the *VNTR2/STin2 region of the serotonin transporter* were identified [202]. These were STin2.9, STin2.10, and Stin2.12, containing 9, 10, and 12 copies of the VNTR element,[6] respectively. Results indicated a significantly associated risk of unipolar depression with the STin2.9 allele (odds ratio = 6.95 [95% CI: 1.8–27.2]).

STin2 polymorphisms have also been shown to be synergistic with 5-HTTLPR [15158428]. STin2 is a risk factor in major depression [203] and suicide behavior [204] and

[5] *HTR1A and HTR2A* are two subtypes in the known seven families of serotonin receptors [6, 193, 194]. There are at least 15 different serotonin receptors [195, 196].

HTR1A is the gene that codes for 5-hydroxytryptamine (serotonin) receptor 1A, G protein-coupled [197].

HTR2A is the gene that codes for 5-hydroxytryptamine (serotonin) receptor 2A, G protein-coupled, one of the serotonin receptors. Multiple transcript variants and mutations have been associated with susceptibility to schizophrenia and obsessive-compulsive disorder and are associated with response to the antidepressant citalopram in patients with major depressive disorder [200]

TPH1 is the gene that codes for tryptophan hydroxylase 1. The protein coded by TPH1 catalyzes the first and rate limiting step in the biosynthesis of serotonin. Mutations of TPH1 are associated with increased risk of disorders, including addictions, suicidal behavior, somatic anxiety, anger-related traits, bipolar, and schizophrenia [198].

BDNF is brain-derived neurotrophic factor. It is one of the nerve growth factors. It is produced by cortical neurons and is essential for striatal neurons survival. Reduction in expression is seen in Huntington's disease and Alzheimer's disease. BDNF participates in regulating stress response and moods. Several transcript variants occur, which result in distinct isoforms [199].

[6] *VNTR* stands for variable number tandem repeats. Analysis of VNTRs has become a powerful tool in genetic research. For a discussion of VNTRs in depression, see [201].

is associated with variations in antidepressant responses [205, 206].

Variation in the 5-HTTLPR and another polymorphism in the gene STin4 significantly modified a differential response associated with stressful life events to two types of antidepressants [207]. There was no effect on response to the tricyclic nortriptyline, but there was a significantly better response to SSRI escitalopram.

Also, a polymorphism (rs25531) immediately upstream from the 5-HTTLPR has been associated with modulating the effects of other 5-HTTLPR alleles [208, 209].

Gene–gene interactions have been seen between the *serotonin transporter gene (SLC6A4) 5-HTTLPR/rs25531* haplotype and the *serotonin 2A receptor gene (HTR2A) single-nucleotide polymorphism (SNP) rs7997012* in antidepressant venlafaxine XR treatment outcome in generalized anxiety disorder [210].

Some types of depression are associated with *genetic polymorphisms of several genes related to the neuroendocrine system.* These include tryptophan hydroxylase 2 [211, 212], 5HT-transport [112, 120], glucocorticoid receptor [213], and P2X ligand-gated ion channel 7 [214]. However, recurrent unipolar depression with early age of onset in families does not seem to be linked to some 38 different candidate simple sequence tandem repeat polymorphisms (SSTRPs) from 12 genes associated with neuroendocrine or serotonergic functions [215].

However, it would seem that straightforward associations between genes and mood disorders are probably not there [216, 217]. For example, inconsistent findings investigating associations between major depression disorders (MDD), bipolar disorders (BD), and variations of genes that code for serotonin receptors and transporters prompted a 2003 meta-analysis [218]. There were numerous studies that investigated associations between MDD or BD and 5-HT2A 102 T/C, the 5-HTT promoter 44 bp insertion/deletion and the intron 2 VNTR polymorphisms. They concluded that overall, the associations were not significant (OR[7]=1.08; 95% CI: 0.96–1.22).

A meta-analysis was conducted on associations between personality traits and candidate genes 5HTT LPR, DRD4 c > t, DRD4 length, DRD2 A1/A2, and DRD3 A1/A2 polymorphisms and found no significant associations [219].

Associations, if they exist, may be a result of genes that influence the liability to mood disorders not via a main effect on risk but by effects on sensitivity to environmental influences [216, 217, 220]. For example, variations in specific genes may be associated with personality traits that are associated with a risk for a disease such as depression [221, 222]. These traits may be more highly heritable than the actual disease [223]. A case in point may be an association between a brain-derived neurotrophic factor (BDNF) polymorphism and a small but significant proportion of population variation in neuroticism [224, 225]. Neuroticism as measured by the revised *NEO Personality Inventory (NEO-PI-R)* is characterized by a high frequency of negative emotions, including anxiety, hostility, and low mood [225]. Neuroticism is strongly associated with depression [225–227].

Neuroticism is reported to be 40–50% heritable [228, 229] vs. about 36% for depression [230]. In a longitudinal twin study, shared genetic risk factors accounted for 70% of the correlation between neuroticism and depression risk, whereas 20% was due to shared environmental risk factors, and direct causal effects of major depression on neuroticism were approximately 10% [226]. Additionally, genetic liability for major depression was uniquely 45%, while shared liability with neuroticism was about 55%.

The results regarding BDNF remain ambiguous. For instance, lower serum BDNF is associated with both a dispositional vulnerability to depression and acute depressive states in the general population [231]. Additionally, while BDNF plasma concentration is linked to the Val66Met functional polymorphism of the BDNF gene, a recent study found that in men—but not in women—this polymorphism was associated with personality traits related to depression [232]. However, the association was in the opposite direction. Lower plasma BDNF levels were seen in men with lower depression scores and less vulnerability to stress, and higher amounts of conscientiousness and extraversion.

However, nonserotonin related polymorphisms have shown some tantalizing associations. For example, associations have been seen between single-nucleotide polymorphisms (SNPs) in the *limbic system-associated membrane protein (LSAMP)* gene and mood and anxiety disorders [233]. A strong association was shown between LSAMP SNPs and major depression disorder, and a suggestive association between LSAMP SNPs and panic disorders.

From an integration of results across 11 human studies, it appears that accelerated aging, as well as functional and biological decline associated with MDD, is reflected in reduced leukocyte telomere length and diminished telomerase activity—likely due to cumulative exposure to the chronic stress of MDD [234].

Although earlier genome-wide studies have not found significant associations between *individual* single nucleotide polymorphisms (SNPs) and MDD [19065144, 21042317], a

[7]Odds ratio (OR) is a way to represent the odds that an outcome will result when a given exposure to a variable of interest occurs compared to when the exposure does not occur. OR quantifies the strength of the association between two events. An OR greater than 1 indicates a positive association or that exposure to that variable increases the odds of that outcome. An OR less than one indicates a negative relationship between two events. An OR of 1 suggests no relationship between two events. An OR is frequently accompanied by a 95% confidence interval (CI). CI is a measure of precision of the OR. The smaller the CI, the higher precision as long as it does not overlap OR = 1. For more information, see the Chap. 4 on evidence basics in this text.

2012 genome-wide study has found that the additive genetic variance of MDD due to *all* SNPs was estimated at 32% (95% CI: [15.0%, 48.8%]) and 28% (95% CI: [16.5%, 39.3%]) using two different methods [235].

In 2015, a genome-wide study in China identified two genetic loci on chromosome 10 contributing to the risk of major depressive disorder (MDD): one near the SIRT1 gene and the other in an intron of the LHPP gene [236, 237]. A severe subtype of MDD, melancholia, was highly associated with the SIRT1 locus. However, the interpretation of these associations is subject to debate [238–240].

The SIRT1 gene family regulates epigenetic gene silencing and suppresses recombination of rDNA [241]. The LHPP gene functions are not clear [242].

Anatomical Associations

Increasing evidence from functional neuroimaging studies suggests that major depression and bipolar disorders may be neurological disorders with psychiatric symptoms [99, 243, 417]. These imaging studies have revealed abnormal blood flow and metabolic activity, and decreased volumes of several frontal lobe areas, the hippocampi, amygdala, entorhinal cortex, and basal ganglia.

A seminal paper from the National Institute of Mental Health was published in 2005 that demonstrated the 5-HTTLPR polymorphism has an influence on human cingulate-amygdala interactions and is a genetic susceptibility mechanism for depression [122]. As mentioned above, the short allele carriers seem to have increased anxiety-related temperamental traits, increased amygdala reactivity and a greater risk of depression. Morphometrical (size and shape) analyses revealed a reduction in gray matter volume in short-allele carriers in limbic regions essential for processing negative emotion, particularly in the *perigenual cingulate*[8] and amygdala. Functional analyses showed that those regions, while processing fearful stimuli, demonstrated a robust feedback circuit that was involved in extinguishing negative affect. Carriers of the short allele demonstrated deficiencies in coupling within that circuit. Significantly, the amount of coupling between the cingulate and the amygdala predicted an inverse relationship to almost 30% of variations in temperamental anxiety. They concluded that these anatomical and functional alterations are dependent upon developmental systems level mechanisms that underpin normal emotional reactions and genetic susceptibility for depression.

[8] *The perigenual cingulate* is involved in the modulation of emotional behavior in an extended "visceromotor network" of autonomic/neuroendocrine responses and transmission in the neural processing of reward, fear, and stress [66, 252].

Involvement of hippocampi in human depression and post-traumatic stress disorder (PTSD) has been well demonstrated [244, 245]. Derangements of the hypothalamic-pituitary-adrenal axis (HPA) with elevated glucocorticoids are very prominent in depression. Repeated stress with concomitant exposure to glucocorticoids is highly associated with atrophy of the hippocampus in rodents. In humans, some neuroimaging studies have shown a reduction in total and posterior hippocampus volume in folks with major depression [246], and post-mortem decreased serotonin 5-HT(1A) mRNA [247]. It is unclear if the atrophy precedes the manifestation of depression or predisposes to depression. This hippocampal atrophy has been associated with cognitive deficits characteristic of PTSD and major depression. See Fig. 8.3.

Meta-analysis has shown that the total number of depressive episodes in folks with unipolar depression was significantly correlated to reduced volume of the right but not left hippocampus [248].

Depressed elderly folks with hippocampal atrophy are more likely to experience cognitive decline [20808107]. Smaller hippocampal volume occurs with increased length of depression, and antidepressants may afford some protection against volume loss [249]. In that study, which was conducted on females, the critical time point appeared to be after about 1000 days of depression. A cohort of males with bipolar I had showed a significant correlation between duration of illness and neuronal loss/dysfunction in the right but not the left hippocampus [250]. Major depression in adolescents may be associated with earlier changes in hippocampi, and these changes at least in one study seem to be much more strongly associated with the left rather than the right hippocampus [251]. MRIs of 21 women with borderline personality disorder and early traumas showed 16% smaller volumes of the hippocampus ($P < 0.001$) and 8% smaller volumes of the amygdala ($P < 0.05$) than controls [253]. However, the associations of decreased volumes with trauma were unclear.

Human studies implicate additional nonhippocampal areas [254]. Various studies have shown atrophy in various areas, including the lateral and third ventricles, basal ganglia, frontal lobes, temporal lobes, as well as amygdala/hippocampi [248, 255, 256]. Other neuroimaging studies of major depression have shown abnormal prefrontal serotonin-rich areas, especially Brodmann area 25 of the midline subgenual anterior cingulate cortex [257], and atrophy of the subgenual anterior cingulate cortex, particularly in the subcallosal area, as an effective auxiliary means of diagnosis for major depressive disorder. This area is involved in mediating emotional and autonomic responses to socially provocative stimuli, and in modulating neurotransmitter systems that are influenced by pharmacological antidepressants. Hypermetabolic states in rostral anterior cingulate

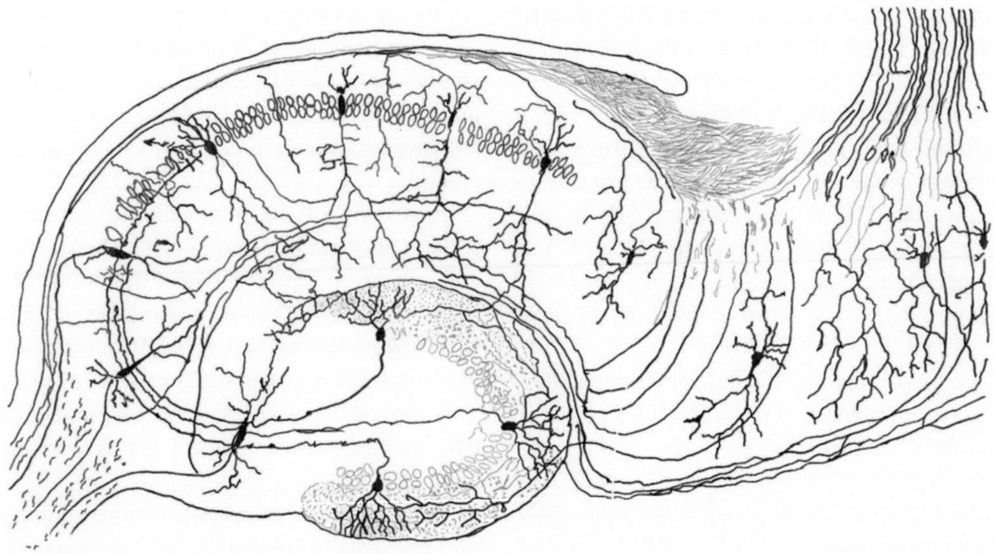

Fig. 8.3 Artistic rendering of the hippocampus inspired by Ramón y Cajal's neuroanatomical sketches. This illustration draws inspiration from Ramón y Cajal's pioneering work, depicting the layered architecture and neuronal diversity of the hippocampus. Highlighted are principal cells such as pyramidal neurons of the CA regions and granule cells of the dentate gyrus, with intricate dendritic arborizations echoing Cajal's inked motifs. The figure emphasizes the hippocampus's cytoarchitecture and connectivity—key to its role in learning, memory, and emotional regulation

areas have been seen in depressed folks who responded to antidepressants, and hypometabolic states were seen in non-responders [258].

PET scans in humans were used to evaluate reciprocal limbic-neocortical functions and sadness [259]. Transient and chronic increases in negative mood were accompanied by increased metabolism (blood flow) in limbic-paralimbic areas (Brodmann area 25: subgenual cingulate and anterior insula) and decreased metabolism (blood flow) in neocortical areas (right dorsolateral prefrontal and inferior parietal). The opposite pattern was seen upon recovery from depression.

Dysregulation of the fronto-limbic network, specifically hyperactivation of limbic areas, leads to increased attention toward and processing of emotional information, especially biases toward negative input [260]. Internal self-focus resulting in pathological rumination over emotionally salient events is facilitated by baseline neuroactivation in that network. The insular cortex, in light of its widespread connections to the fronto-limbic network, may be at the heart of integrating emotional, visceromotor, autonomic, and interoceptive data [260].

Meta-analyses have shown that the total number of depressive episodes in folks with unipolar depression was significantly correlated to reduced volume of the right, but not left, hippocampus [248, 256, 261]. Both cell size and number decrease. Stress can lead to both rapid and prolonged reductions in cell proliferation, resulting in slowed neurogenesis and decreased synaptic connectivity [262]. It is of interest that hippocampal atrophy is also found in PTSD, schizophrenia, and Alzheimer's disease [263]. Indeed, there is evidence that the behavioral effects of antidepressants are mediated via stimulation of neurogenesis in the hippocampus [264–266]. Meta-analyses have also shown significant decreases in anterior cingulate/paracingulate gyrus, inferior frontal gyrus, and insula activation after psychotherapy for depression and anxiety [267].

And speaking of atrophy relative to stressors: Chronic back pain has also been associated with decreased density of gray matter bilaterally in the prefrontal lobes and the right thalamus [268]. The pattern of atrophy showed distinct patterns relative to neuropathic or non-neuropathic origins. A 24-year study of women indicated that overweight and obesity throughout adult life might contribute to the development of atrophy of the temporal lobe [269].

In clinical depression, the orbital and medial prefrontal cortexes appear to have specific functional and cellular changes (including activity, volume, and number of glial cells) that relate to establishing mood [270].

It has been hypothesized that when confronted by a stressor, activation of negative schema decreases activity in prefrontal areas, via decreased serotonin metabolism controlled by the HPA axis, with resulting impaired attenuation of subcortical areas such as the amygdala [271]. It is suggested that this process results in increased vulnerability after an episode of depression.

Ruminative brooding (persistent, repetitive, and self-focused criticism) is common in major depression [272]. Brain images have shown that self-referential processing in MDD appears to be associated with abnormally increased activity of anterior cortical midline structures.

Neuroendocrine aberrations as responses to neurotransmitters in depression have been reported to involve the HPA axis [273], *thyroid hormones [17353866], growth hormone* [274], *and prolactin* [276]. It is also possible that there is a linked interaction of the various axes [275–278].

A common thread that runs through many mood and anxiety disorders is changes in the hypothalamic-pituitary-adrenal (HPA) axis [279–281]. These disorders include major depressive disorder, general anxiety disorder, panic disorders, PTSD, ADHD, borderline personality disorder, and bipolar disorder. Functional disorders where the HPA axis is also implicated include chronic fatigue syndrome, alcoholism, irritable bowel syndrome, and fibromyalgia [282].

One of the assumptions in depression research is that stressful events and chronic difficulties can instigate depression in certain genetically predisposed individuals [283]. In humans who have major depression, it is common to find changes in the HPA axis [273]. Typically, acute depression is associated with elevated secretion of corticotropin-releasing hormone (CRH) from the hypothalamus, adrenal corticotropic hormone (ACTH) from the pituitary, and cortisol from the adrenal cortex. In chronic depression, the adrenal gland is more sensitive to ACTH, and the hypothalamus and pituitary are more sensitive to the negative feedback of cortisol. In sum, this balance results in elevated cortisol with relatively less ACTH. There is some evidence that abnormal metabolism of adrenal corticosteroids might be involved in perpetuating some types of depression [284].

Hypersecretion of CRH in the central nervous system may be an important risk factor for major depression [285, 286]. The bioavailability of CRH is regulated by corticotropin-releasing-hormone binding protein (CRHBP) [285]. CRH is a neuroregulator that functions in a complex neuroendocrine and endocrine system to integrate and adapt behavior relative to stress [287]. Overactive and maladaptive CRH networks are frequently associated with neuroendocrine and stress-associated disorders such as depression and anxiety.

In humans, CRH and vasopressin (aka arginine vasopressin or AVP) are the main neuropeptide regulators of the HPA. Vasopressin increases CRH-induced ACTH release. Desmopressin is a synthetic analogue of vasopressin [288]. Vasopressin receptor V3 specifically mediates the stimulatory effect of vasopressin on ACTH release. People suffering from major depression have been shown to have increased ACTH and cortisol responses to desmopressin, which suggests increased anterior pituitary vasopressin V3 receptors [289]. CRH also has direct effects on the limbic system [286]. For a comprehensive review of the central CRH system in relation to stress, you might want to refer to reference [286].

Chronic stress accompanied by elevations of cortisol might lead to neuroendocrine changes such as increased serotonin uptake both at rest and during stimulation, which might trigger depression symptoms [290, 291]. Neuroendocrine changes induced by stress have an impact on the immune system and production of cytokines, which may be strategically involved in depression.

Cortisol modulation of the expression of corticosteroid-responsive genes can last for hours to days [292].

Some types of depression are associated with genetic polymorphisms of several genes related to the neuroendocrine system. These include tryptophan hydroxylase 2 [211, 212], 5HT-transport [112], glucocorticoid receptor [213], and P2X ligand-gated ion channel 7 [214]. Nevertheless, recurrent unipolar depression with early age of onset in families does not show linkage to any of 38 different candidate simple sequence tandem repeat polymorphisms (SSTRPs) from 12 genes associated with neuroendocrine or serotonergic functions [215].

Genes and proteins that relate to the HPA axis have been associated with PTSD, anxiety, bipolar disorder, and major depression [293]. For example, FKBP5 (FK506-binding protein 5) SNPs interact with childhood trauma in a way that moderates the severity of adult-onset PTSD [294–297]. FKBP5 is a co-chaperone of hsp90, which regulates glucocorticoid receptor sensitivity [293]. When FKBP5 binds to the receptor complex, cortisol has less binding affinity to the receptor and propagation of the response is less efficient. Increased expression of FKBP5 after trauma interferes with feedback control and prolongs stress hormone system activation after exposure to stress.

Another example is the variation in the corticotropin-releasing hormone receptor (CRHR1) gene that can interact with childhood trauma to predict adult depression [298]. The CRHR1 rs110402 and rs242924 polymorphisms appear to increase cortisol reaction to stress. It has been suggested that this increased activation may dispose to increased anxiety and depression symptoms. Cortisol and catecholamines are frequently elevated in depressed or anxious persons, and growth hormone is often depressed [299]. Elevated catecholamines in acute stress can be beneficial, but in chronic stress, they can result in immune downregulation. As important as long-term changes in hormone levels are, the possible effects upon circadian and ultradian rhythms may be equally important [300–302]. Clinical depression is well documented to be associated with elevated levels of cortisol in the blood [303].

Glucocorticoid receptor (Nuclear Receptor Subfamily 3, Group C, Member 1; NR3C1) polymorphisms can influence corticosteroid sensitivity to stress and changes in metabolism and cardiovascular control [213, 292]. For example, BclI and ER22/23EK polymorphisms have been associated with susceptibility to major depression, and ER22/23EK polymorphism has been linked to a faster clinical response to at least some antidepressants [304]. Other polymorphisms that occur in the 5′ region of the NR3C1 gene may also play a role in the genetic vulnerability for MDD [305].

A variety of genetic variations (e.g. (BclI, ER22/23EK, N363S) of the *glucocorticoid receptor gene NR3C1* affect cortisol sensitivity and increased [306–308] or decreased risk [309] for depression. Gene–environment interaction between common variants of *NR3C1* and childhood adversity creates vulnerability for developing clinically relevant depressive symptoms in old age [310].

Hypermethylation of the *low-affinity type II glucocorticoid receptor* (GR) promoter is more common in suicide victims who have experienced neglect or abuse [311–313]. In one study, no epigenetic marking of the hippocampus was seen in suicide victims who did not have childhood adversity or MDD [314]. Epigenetic changes to the HPA axis introduced by early adversity can adversely affect the sensitivity and set points in the HPA axis and may lead to mood disorders [315–318].

An association has been seen between premenopausal women with both major depression and the GG genotype of the Bcl1 polymorphism and greater abdominal obesity compared with non-GG carriers [319].

Stress Hormones

Major depression may be thought of as a manifestation of a *dysfunctional stress response syndrome* [303, 320]. There may be important genetic factors at work. In adolescents, baseline sleep-related growth hormone levels were predictive of subsequent depression [321]. First-degree relatives of people suffering from depression appear to have significantly depressed HPA responses compared to folks who are not related by first degree to someone so afflicted. HPA functions and central serotonin functions show an interesting contrast between depression and chronic fatigue syndrome (CFS) [322]. CFS seems to be accompanied by elevated central serotonin transmission and low cortisol, while depression is associated with decreased central serotonin transmission and increased cortisol. Baseline plasma levels of cortisol were the lowest in the CFS group, highest in the depressed group, and intermediate in the controls ($p = 0.01$). The selective serotonin-releasing agent d-fenfluramine produced the highest prolactin response in the CFS group, the lowest in the depressed group, and intermediate in the control group ($p = 0.01$). Marked inverse relations were seen between prolactin and cortisol responses and baseline cortisol levels.

Abuse and neglect, especially in early childhood, increase the risk for cognitive impairment, emotional and social problems, physical, and neuropsychiatric disorders [323, 324]. A 2010 review [323] found that a common thread appears to be early adversity and atypical structural and functional development of the HPA stress response. The most prominent structural changes that have been identified are in the corpus callosum in children and the hippocampus in adults. Atypical functional activity is seen in several brain regions, including decreased activity of the prefrontal cortex.

PTSD sufferers demonstrate smaller cerebral and cerebellar volumes in proportion to the duration and earlier onset of abuse [325, 326], and abnormal functions in the prefrontal cortex [327, 328]. Decreased cortisol reactivity may result from childhood emotional abuse that accumulates [316].

Hippocampal dysfunction related to early stressors and persistence of adult stressors may continue and may affect the development of reward systems [330, 331]. Mood disorders, daily activity, stressors, trauma, sleep patterns, seasonal variation, and health influence the morning awakening increase in cortisol [329]. Within half hour of rising, cortisol increases 50% to 75%. Higher basal morning cortisol levels are seen in folks with mood disorders.

Job stress and general stress increase morning cortisol rise, whereas fatigue and burnout decrease morning cortisol rise [332]. Salivary cortisol levels are influenced by sex, age, awakening time, working day, sampling month, sleep duration, smoking, physical activity, and cardiovascular disease [333]. In adolescents, waking cortisol levels, bedtime cortisol levels, the size of the cortisol awakening response, average cortisol, and the slope of the diurnal cortisol rhythm across the waking day are significant prospective risk factors for the development of MDD in young adults [334].

People who have a parental history of depression or anxiety may have a higher cortisol-awakening curve, similar to that of people with depression or anxiety disorders [335].

Meta-analysis of reactions to stressors by sufferers of MDD and nondepressed (ND) individuals has shown that MDD and ND individuals had similar baseline and stress cortisol levels; however, MDD patients showed much higher cortisol levels during recovery than their ND people [336]. When stressors were encountered in the afternoon, those with MDD more frequently experienced higher baseline cortisol levels, blunted stress reactivity, and impaired recovery. This was especially true for older and more depressed people.

Improved responses to dexamethasone/corticotropin-releasing hormone tests during inpatient antidepressant treatment of MDD may predict beneficial treatment response after 5 weeks and a higher remission rate at the end of hospitalization [337]. Relapse of MDD may be predicted by higher post-treatment maximal cortisol levels on the dexamethasone/corticotropin-releasing hormone test [338, 339].

Elevated cortisol levels are associated with mood disorders, abdominal obesity, type 2 diabetes, osteoporosis, and cardiovascular disease [340]. Serum, saliva, and urine cortisol levels measure cortisol at a defined point in time. Measurement of cortisol in scalp hair can be used to evaluate long-term levels [340]. Cortisol levels in scalp hair are elevated in people with chronic stress [341].

A 2012 systematic review focusing on nonmedicated *maternal prenatal depression* and effects on the offspring has concluded that prepartum depression is highly prevalent and is associated with negative outcomes in offspring [342]. They also concluded that effects are understudied. Maternal cortisol promotes the secretion of placental CRH, and high levels of CRH are one of the important triggers for parturition [343]. Second-trimester CRH concentrations and mean evening salivary cortisol concentrations may be significantly elevated in depressed pregnant women.

The cerebellum has reciprocal monosynaptic connections to the hypothalamus and has a high density of glucocorticoid-binding sites [344].

Circadian rhythms of ACTH and cortisol are frequently changed in depressed women [345], as are the sizes of the pituitary and adrenals [346].

Hypothyroid conditions appear to reduce central serotonin activity and reduce the threshold for developing depression [347]. In one study, attenuation of the thyrotropin (TSH) response to thyrotropin-releasing hormone (TRH) injection was seen in 33% of 54 depressed patients but in none of the normal patients [348]. *Dexamethasone suppression escape*[9] was seen in 43% of the 54 depressed patients but only 11% of the normal patients. There were only 6 out of the 54 patients that showed abnormal responses to both tests. This would seem to indicate that abnormalities in the HPA and *hypothalamic-pituitary-thyroid (HPT) axis* are independent. Combined sensitivity of the two tests for detecting major depressive disorder was 67% with 92% specificity.

In another HPT challenge, 47 patients with DSM-III criteria for MDD with melancholia, 16 of the depressed patients, and none of the normal controls showed blunted responses to TRH, and 8 of the depressed patients (all women) and none of the controls showed increased responses to TRH [349]. The patients who showed blunted TRH responses (but none of the other participants) also showed blunted prolactin responses to TRH.

In another study, persistent neuroendocrine dysregulation of the HPA and HPT axes in MDD at the time of symptomatic improvement predicted early relapse [350].

Growth hormone (GH) regulation may be improper in folks with depression. Norepinephrine, dopamine, acetylcholine, and somatomedin, and negative feedback from insulin-like growth factor-1 control *growth hormone-releasing hormone (GHRH)* to regulate growth hormone release [351]. The most widely supported abnormalities in this control system during major depression relate to noradrenergic-mediated GH release, acetylcholine-induced GH release through the somatostatin system, GABA, and GHRH-stimulated release. Eleven out of 18 adults who had growth hormone deficiency were found to have atypical depression (but none of the adults with childhood onset growth hormone deficiency: 0 of 7), and this depression was improved significantly by growth hormone treatment [352].

Depressed Japanese patients who relapsed within 6 months after completing treatment demonstrated significantly lower growth hormone responses to growth hormone-releasing hormone at the time of discharge [274].

Sex-related differences have been seen in the effects of GH-releasing hormone on sleep-endocrine activity in depressed patients [353].

Sex Differences in Stress Reactions

As might be expected from the above synopses, which indicate that depressed men and women differ in several important ways, it is likely that gender or sex differences may exist in responses to pharmacotherapeutic or psychotherapeutic treatments. Indeed, this has been shown to be the case in one study of differences in response of depressed men and women to cognitive behavior therapy [354]. Reported in 1994, 44 women and 40 men were interviewed with the Schedule for Affective Disorders and Schizophrenia and diagnosed according to the Research Diagnostic Criteria and DSM III R criteria. Then they received cognitive behavioral therapy according to a standardized protocol. Every other week, they were assessed with the Hamilton Depression Rating Scale, Beck Depression Inventory, and Global Assessment Scale. Several significant pretreatment differences between men and women were seen, and the men attended significantly fewer therapy sessions. For those who had worse pretreatment symptoms, the results were not as good, especially for women. But, for those men and women who had similar symptoms, the results were comparable.

[9]The dexamethasone suppression test assesses aberrations in the production of cortisol [356]. Dexamethasone is a synthetic steroid that negatively feeds back to the glucocorticoid receptors in the pituitary to suppress secretion of ACTH and CRH [355]. For example, in conjunction with circadian rhythms, many depressed patients escape in the afternoon from dexamethasone suppression. As will be discussed later on, the two principal physiological systems that regulate the stress response is the hypothalamus-pituitary-adrenal (HPA) axis and the sympathetic nervous system (SNS). The suppression tests can tease out their individual contributions (22701740).

The *neurobiological effects of estrogen* have received increasing attention beginning in the late 1980s. Estrogen, similar to other neural growth factors, influences neurogenesis, neuronal differentiation, and neuronal survival throughout all the stages of life [357, 358]. When the brain is damaged or is estrogen deprived, such as in aging, it appears that re-expression of developmental estrogen effects can occur [358]. Estrogen has multiple neuro-protective effects on neurons and neurotransmitters in the brain. Estrogens maintain the function of essential structures, such as the hippocampus and the basal forebrain, and their wide-ranging dopaminergic, serotonergic, and noradrenergic neurotransmission systems [357]. Estrogens also have an anti-toxic effect, perhaps as a free radical scavenging system [357].

During adolescence, in girls, pubertal development interacts with environmental influences on symptoms of depression [359–361]. Increasing estrogen levels may be involved [362].

When estrogens are significantly decreased due to ovarian suppression by *gonadotropin-releasing hormone (GnRH)* agonists or due to natural or surgical menopause, there is a generally reversible diminishing of declarative memory and motor functions that can respond to estrogen therapy [3, 363–365]. Estrogen's effects on the nigrostriatal dopaminergic system are likely involved in motor changes, while its impact on the hippocampus may explain memory changes. Mood changes and perimenopausal depression may be tied to estrogen effects [366, 367].

Estrogens influence the development and aging of several regions of the brain that are involved in higher cognitive functions. Many of the estrogen effects are different both in quality and in quantity between males and females [357]. These differences may reflect variance in sexual differentiation in the development of the brain or may reflect a reaction to a different circulating hormonal milieu. Estrogen receptors are found, of course, in the hypothalamus, but they are also present, although at lower levels, in the amygdala, hippocampus, cingulate cortex, locus coeruleus, midbrain raphe nuclei, and central gray matter [368]. Receptor expression may be stable or transient, and apparently developmentally regulated [368].

Perhaps the most telling effect of estrogens on cognitive functions is their influence on memory [369]. One of the more studied structures involved in memory is the *hippocampus.* The hippocampus is a part of the limbic system, important in affective and vegetative states, and is heavily involved in declarative, spatial, and contextual memory, and the perception of pain [3, 370, 371]. It also provides a cognitive function or context to a range of desirable (e.g., reward or motivation) or aversive stimuli [4, 5].

The hippocampus is a major target for and is quite sensitive to circulating adrenal glucocorticoids secreted during their circadian rhythm and during chronic stress [55, 370]. The hippocampus can adapt to the adrenal steroids if they are not elevated for too long, and adrenal corticoids may actually modulate excitability in the hippocampus in a protective fashion. But when stress is repeated or the hypothalamic-pituitary-adrenal axis is dysregulated, the hippocampus can be damaged. This process is known as *allostatic load.*

In severe stress, high levels of adrenal corticoids can reversibly damage declarative memory. It is hypothesized that the hippocampus exhibits structural plasticity and can adapt to and protect itself from repeated stress, but if the imbalance in critical mediators is not resolved, it is possible that changes in the hippocampus brought on by allostatic loads may alter memory functions and perception of chronic pain [370].

Depression in premenopausal women appears to be highly correlated with hormonal changes found in menopause, and these changes involve *gonadal hormones* (significantly lower estradiol and significantly higher follicle-stimulating hormone) and serotonin deficiency [372]. Baseline cortisol, but not prolactin, was seen in one study to be significantly elevated in these depressed women.

The *Harvard Study of Moods and Cycles* has suggested earlier menopause is associated with a history of depression [373].

Because women are living longer than they used to, more of a woman's life is spent in a state of relatively low estrogen. With this in mind, a comprehensive review of *neuroendocrinology in the aging female brain* was conducted using MEDLINE for English-language references between 1970 and June 2004 [374]. They used the search terms cognition, immune function, aging, mood, neuroendocrinology, gonadotropins, cardiovascular disease, depression, estrogens, neurotransmitters, osteoporosis, and ovarian steroids. Here are their main conclusions:

1. It is likely that during middle age, temporal patterns of neural signals are altered, which leads to the end of reproductive cycles, and the complex interactions of ovarian, hypothalamic, and pituitary pacemakers become more erratic with age, finally resulting in menopause.
2. Lack of estrogen is associated with low mood.
3. Estrogen therapy seems to be associated with decreased depression and improvements in various measures of well-being.
4. The effects of estrogen on mood, depression and feelings of well-being are likely to be mediated by changes in the metabolism of serotonin and norepinephrine.
5. Estrogen seems to have specific effects on cognitive functions in women, especially enhancing characteristics of verbal memory, abstract reasoning, and information processing.

6. Both humoral and cellular immunity show significant gender dimorphism.
7. Estrogen deficiency increases the risk of osteoporosis in both men and women.
8. Estrogen effects on the cardiovascular system are complex, with current evidence showing a negative effect of oral estrogen in primary and secondary prevention of cardiovascular events, including increased risk of stroke.

Lest males feel left out of the estrogen depletion picture, it is important to note that testosterone is converted to estrogens for use in male brains and testosterone has many important functions in the brain [375]. Moreover, male climacteric or andropause is a real phenomenon where testosterone levels decrease with age [376]. What effects this decline in testosterone has on estrogen levels in the male brain are not well researched [377–379]. The etiology of depressive symptoms associated with partial androgen deficiency appears to be multifactorial [380, 381]. Other hormones (such as melatonin, dehydroepiandrosterone, growth hormone, insulin-like growth factor, and thyroxine) also decrease with age [382, 383]. What effects these all have on male mentation with age is unclear [384]. For reviews of andropause and depression in aging males, see the following [385–389].

Substance Use Effects

A variety of substances can also induce mood disorders [17960298]. These include alcohol [390–393] and benzodiazepines [394]. Stimulants such as methamphetamines and cocaine can induce hypomanic, manic, depressive, and mixed episodes [395–398]. Alcohol can induce independent bipolar, panic, and social phobic disorders [393]. Benzodiazepines may have similar effects as alcohol on the brain and can induce major depression both during use and during withdrawal [394–400]. SSRIs [401–403] and malignancies [404–407] may contribute to mania or depression. Cannabis associated mortality in folks with mental illnesses such as depression is much higher [408]. Cannabis use and depression-related quality of life show a sex-related association [409–411] with a more severe impact on women. Decreased white matter integration, depression, and apathy are also associated with cannabis use [412].

Withdrawal or intoxication of several pharmacologicals used in internal medicine can induce depression, anxiety, or psychotic symptoms [413]. These medicines include corticosteroids, anabolic steroids, isotretinoin, levo-dopa, interferon-α, and some over-the-counter medications.

Other Molecules and Other Effects

A multifunctional protein p11 (also known as annexin II light chain, S100A10), which binds to 5-HT receptors, in layer II/III neurons of the prelimbic cortex, has been shown to be a strategic molecule in a specific cell type that regulates stress-induced depression [414]. Chronic restraint stress can induce selective loss of p11 and depression-like behaviors in mice. Both of these are capable of being reversed by selective serotonin reuptake inhibitors and tricyclic antidepressants. This seems to work via increasing activity in dopamine D2 receptor-expressing (D2+) glutamatergic neurons.

Transcription factor early growth response 3 (EGR3) is increased in D1 receptor containing nucleus accumbens medium spiny neurons of mice susceptible to social defeat stress [415]. Decreasing Egr 3 levels has prevented depression-like symptoms in susceptible mice.

Short-term calorie restriction has been shown in some basic and clinical studies to induce an antidepressant effect [416]. One hypothesis is that it involves orexin signaling activation, increased CREB phosphorylation and neurotrophic effects, release of endorphin, and ketone production.

Summary

Depression is heavily influenced by genetics and adverse psychosocial circumstances, especially at critical times. Depression varies in severity and probably has differing etiologies. Hyperactivity of the central and peripheral stress systems is common. Cortisol and neuroendocrine changes, such as decreased available serotonin, may be implicated in depression symptoms. Immune system derangements are common and may be effects and causes of depression. Depression may alter the immune response in some illnesses and increase risks for conditions such as cardiovascular disease, some cancers, arthritis, type 2 diabetes, hypertension, inflammatory bowel disease, frailty, periodontal disease, wound healing, and suicide.

Consensus from molecular, behavioral, electrophysiological, and pharmacological studies concludes that depression is the result of maladaptive neuroplastic processes in emotional processing circuits, including those of the prefrontal cortex, hippocampus, amygdala, and ventral striatum.

Glucocorticoids, BDNF, and other biogenic amines alter astrocyte and microglia functions; some antidepressant treatments (as we will discuss further on) improve glial function while also ameliorating depressive-like symptoms.

It seems reasonable to think of depression as the result of alterations of the quadripartite synapse in the frontolimbic area. Information processing and plasticity in the synapses are dependent upon dynamic states of the presynaptic and postsynaptic neurons, astrocytes, and microglia. The astrocytes enfold the synapses in a heteromorphic embrace, while the microglia in a functionally dependent fashion animatedly interact with the synapse.

Astrocytes regulate the base levels of glutamate, ATP, and potassium ion concentration. These establish the basal excitability of the neurons and, via the extracellular levels of glutamate, help to establish the density of post-synaptic NMDA receptors and AMPA receptors. NMDA triggers alterations of synaptic plasticity. AMPA membrane receptors sustain synaptic plasticity alterations.

Learning and memory are based upon suitable programming of long-term potentiation (LTP) and long-term depression (LTD) of neuronal transmission (neuronal plasticity), which are dependent upon the appropriate functioning of the glial cells. In a complex dynamic ever-changing context, microglia are regulators of this plasticity.

During clinical depression, astroglial cells become hypertrophic and hypofunctional with decreased complexity. Microglia shift toward a proinflammatory profile with decreased microglia-derived BDNF release. In such a state, the astrocytes cannot buffer K+ and clear extracellular glutamate. The result is increased noisy excitability with an imbalance of NMDA and AMPA receptors and less BDNF than is needed for neuronal health.

These finely tuned neuroplastic processes can become sloppy when inflammation is increased, such as during intense short-term stress, infections, stroke, trauma, autoimmune, or neurodegenerative diseases. Or when the astroglia and microglia become damaged during conditions such as chronic unpredictable stress exposure, aging, and inadequate nutrition. In such a state, decreased neuroplasticity and less neurogenesis can occur and lead to symptoms of depression.

Genome-wide association meta-analyses found that all of us carry different degrees of genetic risk factors for MDD. These genes relate to all the other risk factors mentioned in this section. That we vary on the amount of strain that we can tolerate before developing symptoms of depression relies upon the resiliency or susceptibility of our coping systems, which are a product of genetics, epigenetic programming, and our immediate psychosocial environment.

Depression is a dynamic process, and for the first time, a recent advance in real-time imaging techniques has revealed correlations between changing affective states and cellular activity in specific areas of the brain. High-speed imaging with millisecond slices of brain activity in a rodent model of stress-induced changes in affective states demonstrated a neurophysiological circuit for those changes. They followed stressful stimulus-provoked activity as it worked its way through the dentate gyrus into the hippocampus and watched the induced changes in affect. Will this new technique help to answer the roles of various pathways as they react to environmental cues in the manifestation of depressive disorders?

The next question will be how do environmentally induced changes in our neurophysiology interact with our genetic material to shape our behavior? This is the focus of our next chapter: Heritability.

References

1. Fisher RA. The correlation between relatives on the supposition of Mendelian inheritance. Trans R Soc Edinburgh. 1918;52(02):399–433.
2. Barton NH, Etheridge AM, Veber A. The infinitesimal model. BioRxiv 039768 2016.
3. Gray J. Précis of the neuropsychology of anxiety: an enquiry into the functions of the septo-hippocampal system. Behav Brain Sci. 1982;5:469–534.
4. LeDoux JE. The emotional brain. New York: Simon and Schuster; 1996.
5. McEwen BS, Sakai RR, Spencer RL. Adrenal steroid effects on the brain: versatile hormones with good and bad effects. In: Schulkin J, editor. Hormonally-induced changes in mind and brain. San Diego: Academic; 1993. p. 157–89.
6. Nestler E, Hyman SE, Malenka R. Molecular neuropharmacology: a Foundation for Clinical Neuroscience. 2nd ed. United Kingdom: McGraw-Hill Education; 2009.
7. Boyle EA, Li YI, Pritchard JK. An expanded view of complex traits: from polygenic to Omnigenic. Cell. 2017;169(7):1177–86. PMCID: PMC5536862. http://www.ncbi.nlm.nih.gov/pubmed/28622505.
8. Manolio TA, Collins FS, Cox NJ, Goldstein DB, Hindorff LA, Hunter DJ, McCarthy MI, Ramos EM, Cardon LR, Chakravarti A, Cho JH, Guttmacher AE, Kong A, Kruglyak L, Mardis E, Rotimi CN, Slatkin M, Valle D, Whittemore AS, Boehnke M, Clark AG, Eichler EE, Gibson G, Haines JL, Mackay TFC, McCarroll SA, Visscher PM. Finding the missing heritability of complex diseases. Nature. 2009;461(7265):747–53. PMCID: PMC2831613. http://www.ncbi.nlm.nih.gov/pubmed/19812666.
9. Yang J, Benyamin B, McEvoy BP, Gordon S, Henders AK, Nyholt DR, Madden PA, Heath AC, Martin NG, Montgomery GW, Goddard ME, Visscher PM. Common SNPs explain a large proportion of the heritability for human height. Nat Genet. 2010;42(7):565–9. PMCID: PMC3232052. http://www.ncbi.nlm.nih.gov/pubmed/20562875.
10. Shi H, Kichaev G, Pasaniuc B. Contrasting the genetic architecture of 30 complex traits from summary association data. Am J Hum Genet. 2016;99(1):139–53. PMCID: PMC5005444. http://www.ncbi.nlm.nih.gov/pubmed/27346688.
11. Marouli E, Graff M, Medina-Gomez C, Lo KS, Wood AR, Kjaer TR, Fine RS, Lu Y, Schurmann C, Highland HM, Rüeger S, Thorleifsson G, Justice AE, Lamparter D, Stirrups KE, Turcot V, Young KL, Winkler TW, Esko T, Karaderi T, Locke AE, Masca NGD, Ng MCY, Mudgal P, Rivas MA, Vedantam S, Mahajan A, Guo X, Abecasis G, Aben KK, Adair LS, Alam DS, Albrecht E, Allin KH, Allison M, Amouyel P, Appel EV, Arveiler D, Asselbergs FW, Auer PL, Balkau B, Banas B, Bang LE, Benn M, Bergmann S, Bielak LF, Blüher M, Boeing H, Boerwinkle E, Böger CA, Bonnycastle LL, Bork-Jensen J, Bots ML, Bottinger EP, Bowden DW, Brandslund I, Breen G, Brilliant MH, Broer L, Burt AA, Butterworth AS, Carey DJ, Caulfield MJ, Chambers JC, Chasman DI, Chen YDI, Chowdhury R, Christensen C, Chu

AY, Cocca M, Collins FS, Cook JP, Corley J, Galbany JC, Cox AJ, Cuellar-Partida G, Danesh J, Davies G, de Bakker PIW, de Borst GJ, de Denus S, de Groot MCH, de Mutsert R, Deary IJ, Dedoussis G, Demerath EW, den Hollander AI, Dennis JG, Di Angelantonio E, Drenos F, Du M, Dunning AM, Easton DF, Ebeling T, Edwards TL, Ellinor PT, Elliott P, Evangelou E, Farmaki AE, Faul JD, Feitosa MF, Feng S, Ferrannini E, Ferrario MM, Ferrieres J, Florez JC, Ford I, Fornage M, Franks PW, Frikke-Schmidt R, Galesloot TE, Gan W, Gandin I, Gasparini P, Giedraitis V, Giri A, Girotto G, Gordon SD, Gordon-Larsen P, Gorski M, Grarup N, Grove ML, Gudnason V, Gustafsson S, Hansen T, Harris KM, Harris TB, Hattersley AT, Hayward C, He L, Heid IM, Heikkilä K, Helgeland Ø, Hernesniemi J, Hewitt AW, Hocking LJ, Hollensted M, Holmen OL, Hovingh GK, Howson JMM, Hoyng CB, Huang PL, Hveem K, Ikram MA, Ingelsson E, Jackson AU, Jansson JH, Jarvik GP, Jensen GB, Jhun MA, Jia Y, Jiang X, Johansson S, Jørgensen ME, Jørgensen T, Jousilahti P, Jukema JW, Kahali B, Kahn RS, Kähönen M, Kamstrup PR, Kanoni S, Kaprio J, Karaleftheri M, Kardia SLR, Karpe F, Kee F, Keeman R, Kiemeney LA, Kitajima H, Kluivers KB, Kocher T, Komulainen P, Kontto J, Kooner JS, Kooperberg C, Kovacs P, Kriebel J, Kuivaniemi H, Küry S, Kuusisto J, La Bianca M, Laakso M, Lakka TA, Lange EM, Lange LA, Langefeld CD, Langenberg C, Larson EB, Lee IT, Lehtimäki T, Lewis CE, Li H, Li J, Li-Gao R, Lin H, Lin LA, Lin X, Lind L, Lindström J, Linneberg A, Liu Y, Liu Y, Lophatananon A, Luan J, Lubitz SA, Lyytikäinen LP, Mackey DA, Madden PAF, Manning AK, Männistö S, Marenne G, Marten J, Martin NG, Mazul AL, Meidtner K, Metspalu A, Mitchell P, Mohlke KL, Mook-Kanamori DO, Morgan A, Morris AD, Morris AP, Müller-Nurasyid M, Munroe PB, Nalls MA, Nauck M, Nelson CP, Neville M, Nielsen SF, Nikus K, Njølstad PR, Nordestgaard BG, Ntalla I, O'Connel JR, Oksa H, Loohuis LMO, Ophoff RA, Owen KR, Packard CJ, Padmanabhan S, Palmer CNA, Pasterkamp G, Patel AP, Pattie A, Pedersen O, Peissig PL, Peloso GM, Pennell CE, Perola M, Perry JA, Perry JRB, Person TN, Pirie A, Polasek O, Posthuma D, Raitakari OT, Rasheed A, Rauramaa R, Reilly DF, Reiner AP, Renström F, Ridker PM, Rioux JD, Robertson N, Robino A, Rolandsson O, Rudan I, Ruth KS, Saleheen D, Salomaa V, Samani NJ, Sandow K, Sapkota Y, Sattar N, Schmidt MK, Schreiner PJ, Schulze MB, Scott RA, Segura-Lepe MP, Shah S, Sim X, Sivapalaratnam S, Small KS, Smith AV, Smith JA, Southam L, Spector TD, Speliotes EK, Starr JM, Steinthorsdottir V, Stringham HM, Stumvoll M, Surendran P, 't Hart LM, Tansey KE, Tardif JC, Taylor KD, Teumer A, Thompson DJ, Thorsteinsdottir U, Thuesen BH, Tönjes A, Tromp G, Trompet S, Tsafantakis E, Tuomilehto J, Tybjaerg-Hansen A, Tyrer JP, Uher R, Uitterlinden AG, Ulivi S, van der Laan SW, Van Der Leij AR, van Duijn CM, van Schoor NM, van Setten J, Varbo A, Varga TV, Varma R, Edwards DRV, Vermeulen SH, Vestergaard H, Vitart V, Vogt TF, Vozzi D, Walker M, Wang F, Wang CA, Wang S, Wang Y, Wareham NJ, Warren HR, Wessel J, Willems SM, Wilson JG, Witte DR, Woods MO, Wu Y, Yaghootkar H, Yao J, Yao P, Yerges-Armstrong LM, Young R, Zeggini E, Zhan X, Zhang W, Zhao JH, Zhao W, Zhao W, Zheng H, Zhou W, EPIC-InterAct Consortium, CHD Exome+ Consortium, ExomeBP Consortium, T2D-Genes Consortium, GoT2D Genes Consortium, Global Lipids Genetics Consortium, ReproGen Consortium, MAGIC Investigators, Rotter JI, Boehnke M, Kathiresan S, McCarthy MI, Willer CJ, Stefansson K, Borecki IB, Liu DJ, North KE, Heard-Costa NL, Pers TH, Lindgren CM, Oxvig C, Kutalik Z, Rivadeneira F, Loos RJF, Frayling TM, Hirschhorn JN, Deloukas P, Lettre G. Rare and low-frequency coding variants alter human adult height. Nature. 2017;542(7640):186–90. PMCID: PMC5302847 http://www.ncbi.nlm.nih.gov/pubmed/28146470.

12. De Rubeis S, He X, Goldberg AP, Poultney CS, Samocha K, Cicek AE, Kou Y, Liu L, Fromer M, Walker S, Singh T, Klei L, Kosmicki J, Shih-Chen F, Aleksic B, Biscaldi M, Bolton PF, Brownfeld JM, Cai J, Campbell NG, Carracedo A, Chahrour MH, Chiocchetti AG, Coon H, Crawford EL, Curran SR, Dawson G, Duketis E, Fernandez BA, Gallagher L, Geller E, Guter SJ, Hill RS, Ionita-Laza J, Jimenz Gonzalez P, Kilpinen H, Klauck SM, Kolevzon A, Lee I, Lei I, Lei J, Lehtimäki T, Lin CF, Ma'ayan A, Marshall CR, McInnes AL, Neale B, Owen MJ, Ozaki N, Parellada M, Parr JR, Purcell S, Puura K, Rajagopalan D, Rehnström K, Reichenberg A, Sabo A, Sachse M, Sanders SJ, Schafer C, Schulte-Rüther M, Skuse D, Stevens C, Szatmari P, Tammimies K, Valladares O, Voran A, Li-San W, Weiss LA, Willsey AJ, Yu TW, Yuen RKC, DDD Study, Homozygosity Mapping Collaborative for Autism, UK10K Consortium, Cook EH, Freitag CM, Gill M, Hultman CM, Lehner T, Palotie A, Schellenberg GD, Sklar P, State MW, Sutcliffe JS, Walsh CA, Scherer SW, Zwick ME, Barett JC, Cutler DJ, Roeder K, Devlin B, Daly MJ, Buxbaum JD. Synaptic, transcriptional and chromatin genes disrupted in autism. Nature. 2014;515(7526):209–15. PMCID: PMC4402723 http://www.ncbi.nlm.nih.gov/pubmed/25363760.
13. Purcell SM, Moran JL, Fromer M, Ruderfer D, Solovieff N, Roussos P, O'Dushlaine C, Chambert K, Bergen SE, Kähler A, Duncan L, Stahl E, Genovese G, Fernández E, Collins MO, Komiyama NH, Choudhary JS, Magnusson PKE, Banks E, Shakir K, Garimella K, Fennell T, DePristo M, Grant SGN, Haggarty SJ, Gabriel S, Scolnick EM, Lander ES, Hultman CM, Sullivan PF, McCarroll SA, Sklar P. A polygenic burden of rare disruptive mutations in schizophrenia. Nature. 2014;506(7487):185–90. PMCID: PMC4136494. http://www.ncbi.nlm.nih.gov/pubmed/24463508.
14. Botstein D, Risch N. Discovering genotypes underlying human phenotypes: past successes for mendelian disease, future approaches for complex disease. Nat Genet. 2003;33(Suppl):228–37. PMID: 12610532. http://www.ncbi.nlm.nih.gov/pubmed/12610532.
15. Pickrell JK. Joint analysis of functional genomic data and genome-wide association studies of 18 human traits. Am J Hum Genet. 2014;94(4):559–73. PMCID: PMC3980523. http://www.ncbi.nlm.nih.gov/pubmed/24702953.
16. Li YI, van de Geijn B, Raj A, Knowles DA, Petti AA, Golan D, Gilad Y, Pritchard JK. RNA splicing is a primary link between genetic variation and disease. Science. 2016;352(6285):600–4. PMCID: PMC5182069. http://www.ncbi.nlm.nih.gov/pubmed/27126046.
17. Maurano MT, Humbert R, Rynes E, Thurman RE, Haugen E, Wang H, Reynolds AP, Sandstrom R, Qu H, Brody J, Shafer A, Neri F, Lee K, Kutyavin T, Stehling-Sun S, Johnson AK, Canfield TK, Giste E, Diegel M, Bates D, Hansen RS, Neph S, Sabo PJ, Heimfeld S, Raubitschek A, Ziegler S, Cotsapas C, Sotoodehnia N, Glass I, Sunyaev SR, Kaul R, Stamatoyannopoulos JA. Systematic localization of common disease-associated variation in regulatory DNA. Science. 2012;337(6099):1190–5. PMCID: PMC3771521. http://www.ncbi.nlm.nih.gov/pubmed/22955828.
18. Farh KKH, Marson A, Zhu J, Kleinewietfeld M, Housley WJ, Beik S, Shoresh N, Whitton H, Ryan RJH, Shishkin AA, Hatan M, Carrasco-Alfonso MJ, Mayer D, Luckey CJ, Patsopoulos NA, De Jager PL, Kuchroo VK, Epstein CB, Daly MJ, Hafler DA, Bernstein BE. Genetic and epigenetic fine mapping of causal autoimmune disease variants. Nature. 2015;518(7539):337–43. PMCID: PMC4336207. http://www.ncbi.nlm.nih.gov/pubmed/25363779.
19. Chakravarti A, Turner TN. Revealing rate-limiting steps in complex disease biology: the crucial importance of studying rare, extreme-phenotype families. BioEssays. 2016;38(6):578–86. PMID: 27062178. http://www.ncbi.nlm.nih.gov/pubmed/27062178.
20. Furlong LI. Human diseases through the lens of network biology. Trends Genet. 2013;29(3):150–9. PMID: 23219555. http://www.ncbi.nlm.nih.gov/pubmed/23219555.

21. Cordell HJ. Detecting gene-gene interactions that underlie human diseases. Nat Rev Genet. 2009;10(6):392–404. PMCID: PMC2872761. http://www.ncbi.nlm.nih.gov/pubmed/19434077.
22. Definition of linkage disequilibrium - NCI Dictionary of Genetics Terms - NCI.
23. Linkage Disequilibrium - Genome-Wide Association Studies (GWAS) Explained Simply Part 2.
24. Moore JH, Williams SM. Traversing the conceptual divide between biological and statistical epistasis: systems biology and a more modern synthesis. BioEssays. 2005;27(6):637–46. PMID: 15892116. http://www.ncbi.nlm.nih.gov/pubmed/15892116.
25. Cheverud JM, Routman EJ. Epistasis and its contribution to genetic variance components. Genetics. 1995;139(3):1455–61. PMCID: PMC1206471. http://www.ncbi.nlm.nih.gov/pubmed/7768453.
26. Phillips PC. The language of gene interaction. Genetics. 1998;149(3):1167–71. PMCID: PMC1460246. http://www.ncbi.nlm.nih.gov/pubmed/9649511.
27. Phillips PC. Epistasis—the essential role of gene interactions in the structure and evolution of genetic systems. Nat Rev Genet. 2008;9(11):855–67. PMCID: PMC2689140. http://www.ncbi.nlm.nih.gov/pubmed/18852697.
28. Wade MJ. Epistasis, complex traits, and mapping genes. Genetica. 2001;112–113:59–69. PMID: 11838787. http://www.ncbi.nlm.nih.gov/pubmed/11838787.
29. Cordell HJ. Epistasis: what it means, what it doesn't mean, and statistical methods to detect it in humans. Hum Mol Genet. 2002;11(20):2463–8. PMID: 12351582. http://www.ncbi.nlm.nih.gov/pubmed/12351582.
30. Epistasis.
31. Moore JH, Williams SM. Epistasis and its implications for personal genetics. Am J Hum Genet. 2009;85(3):309–20. PMCID: PMC2771593. http://www.ncbi.nlm.nih.gov/pubmed/19733727.
32. Tyler AL, Asselbergs FW, Williams SM, Moore JH. Shadows of complexity: what biological networks reveal about epistasis and pleiotropy. BioEssays. 2009;31(2):220–7. PMCID: PMC3159922. http://www.ncbi.nlm.nih.gov/pubmed/19204994.
33. Li W, Reich J. A complete enumeration and classification of two-locus disease models. Hum Hered. 2000;50(6):334–49. PMID: 10899752. http://www.ncbi.nlm.nih.gov/pubmed/10899752.
34. Jakobsdottir J, Gorin MB, Conley YP, Ferrell RE, Weeks DE. Interpretation of genetic association studies: markers with replicated highly significant odds ratios may be poor classifiers. PLoS Genet. 2009;5(2):e1000337. PMCID: PMC2629574. http://www.ncbi.nlm.nih.gov/pubmed/19197355.
35. Kraft P, Wacholder S, Cornelis MC, Hu FB, Hayes RB, Thomas G, Hoover R, Hunter DJ, Chanock S. Beyond odds ratios--communicating disease risk based on genetic profiles. Nat Rev Genet. 2009;10(4):264–9. PMID: 19238176. http://www.ncbi.nlm.nih.gov/pubmed/19238176.
36. Roy M, Tapadia MG, Joshi S, Koch B. Molecular and genetic basis of depression. J Genet. 2014;93(3):879–92. PMID: 25572252. http://www.ncbi.nlm.nih.gov/pubmed/25572252.
37. Wray NR, Ripke S, Mattheisen M, Trzaskowski M, Byrne EM, Abdellaoui A, Adams MJ, Agerbo E, Air TM, Andlauer TMF, Bacanu SA, Bækvad-Hansen M, Beekman AFT, Bigdeli TB, Binder EB, Blackwood DRH, Bryois J, Buttenschøn HN, Bybjerg-Grauholm J, Cai N, Castelao E, Christensen JH, Clarke TK, Coleman JIR, Colodro-Conde L, Couvy-Duchesne B, Craddock N, Crawford GE, Crowley CA, Dashti HS, Davies G, Deary IJ, Degenhardt F, Derks EM, Direk N, Dolan CV, Dunn EC, Eley TC, Eriksson N, Escott-Price V, Kiadeh FHF, Finucane HK, Forstner AJ, Frank J, Gaspar HA, Gill M, Giusti-Rodríguez P, Goes FS, Gordon SD, Grove J, Hall LS, Hannon E, Hansen CS, Hansen TF, Herms S, Hickie IB, Hoffmann P, Homuth G, Horn C, Hottenga JJ, Hougaard DM, Hu M, Hyde CL, Ising M, Jansen R, Jin F, Jorgenson E, Knowles JA, Kohane IS, Kraft J, Kretzschmar WW, Krogh J, Kutalik Z, Lane JM, Li Y, Li Y, Lind PA, Liu X, Lu L, MacIntyre DJ, MacKinnon DF, Maier RM, Maier W, Marchini J, Mbarek H, McGrath P, McGuffin P, Medland SE, Mehta D, Middeldorp CM, Mihailov E, Milaneschi Y, Milani L, Mill J, Mondimore FM, Montgomery GW, Mostafavi S, Mullins N, Nauck M, Ng B, Nivard MG, Nyholt DR, O'Reilly PF, Oskarsson H, Owen MJ, Painter JN, Pedersen CB, Pedersen MG, Peterson RE, Pettersson E, Peyrot WJ, Pistis G, Posthuma D, Purcell SM, Quiroz JA, Qvist P, Rice JP, Riley BP, Rivera M, Saeed Mirza S, Saxena R, Schoevers R, Schulte EC, Shen L, Shi J, Shyn SI, Sigurdsson E, Sinnamon GBC, Smit JH, Smith DJ, Stefansson H, Steinberg S, Stockmeier CA, Streit F, Strohmaier J, Tansey KE, Teismann H, Teumer A, Thompson W, Thomson PA, Thorgeirsson TE, Tian C, Traylor M, Treutlein J, Trubetskoy V, Uitterlinden AG, Umbricht D, Van der Auwera S, van Hemert AM, Viktorin A, Visscher PM, Wang Y, Webb BT, Weinsheimer SM, Wellmann J, Willemsen G, Witt SH, Wu Y, Xi HS, Yang J, Zhang F, eQTLGen, 23andMe, Arolt V, Baune BT, Berger K, Boomsma DI, Cichon S, Dannlowski U, de Geus ECJ, DePaulo JR, Domenici E, Domschke K, Esko T, Grabe HJ, Hamilton SP, Hayward C, Heath AC, Hinds DA, Kendler KS, Kloiber S, Lewis G, Li QS, Lucae S, Madden PFA, Magnusson PK, Martin NG, McIntosh AM, Metspalu A, Mors O, Mortensen PB, Müller-Myhsok B, Nordentoft M, Nöthen MM, O'Donovan MC, Paciga SA, Pedersen NL, Penninx BWJH, Perlis RH, Porteous DJ, Potash JB, Preisig M, Rietschel M, Schaefer C, Schulze TG, Smoller JW, Stefansson K, Tiemeier H, Uher R, Völzke H, Weissman MM, Werge T, Winslow AR, Lewis CM, Levinson DF, Breen G, Børglum AD, Sullivan PF, Major Depressive Disorder Working Group of the Psychiatric Genomics Consortium. Genome-wide association analyses identify 44 risk variants and refine the genetic architecture of major depression. Nat Genet. 2018;50(5):668–81. PMCID: PMC5934326 http://www.ncbi.nlm.nih.gov/pubmed/29700475.
38. Levinson DF. The genetics of depression: a review. Biol Psychiatry. 2006;60(2):84–92. PMID: 16300747. http://www.ncbi.nlm.nih.gov/pubmed/16300747.
39. de Mello A, de Mello MF, Carpenter LL, Price LH. Update on stress and depression: the role of the hypothalamic-pituitary-adrenal (HPA) axis. Braz J Psychiatry. 2003;25(4):231–8. PMCID: PMC4479183. http://www.ncbi.nlm.nih.gov/pubmed/15328550.
40. Smith RS. The macrophage theory of depression. Med Hypotheses. 1991;35(4):298–306. PMID: 1943879. http://www.ncbi.nlm.nih.gov/pubmed/1943879.
41. Leonard BE, Song C. Stress and the immune system in the etiology of anxiety and depression. Pharmacol Biochem Behav. 1996;54(1):299–303. PMID: 8728571. http://www.ncbi.nlm.nih.gov/pubmed/8728571.
42. Irwin MR, Miller AH. Depressive disorders and immunity: 20 years of progress and discovery. Brain Behav Immun. 2007;21(4):374–83. PMID: 17360153. http://www.ncbi.nlm.nih.gov/pubmed/17360153.
43. Pucak ML, Kaplin AI. Unkind cytokines: current evidence for the potential role of cytokines in immune-mediated depression. Int Rev Psychiatry. 2005;17(6):477–83. PMID: 16401546. http://www.ncbi.nlm.nih.gov/pubmed/16401546.
44. Schiepers OJG, Wichers MC, Maes M. Cytokines and major depression. Prog Neuro-Psychopharmacol Biol Psychiatry. 2005;29(2):201–17. PMID: 15694227. http://www.ncbi.nlm.nih.gov/pubmed/15694227.
45. Dunn AJ, Swiergiel AH, de Beaurepaire R. Cytokines as mediators of depression: what can we learn from animal studies? - PubMed Neurosci Biobehav Rev. 2005;29(4–5):891–909. PMID: 15885777
46. Fava GA, Sonino N, Morphy MA. Major depression associated with endocrine disease. Psychiatr Dev. 1987;5(4):321–48. PMID: 3328199. http://www.ncbi.nlm.nih.gov/pubmed/3328199.

47. Müller N, Schwarz MJ. The immune-mediated alteration of serotonin and glutamate: towards an integrated view of depression. Mol Psychiatry. 2007;12(11):988–1000. PMID: 17457312. http://www.ncbi.nlm.nih.gov/pubmed/17457312.
48. Meyers CA. Mood and cognitive disorders in cancer patients receiving cytokine therapy. Adv Exp Med Biol. 1999;461:75–81. PMID: 10442168. http://www.ncbi.nlm.nih.gov/pubmed/10442168.
49. Vignau J, Karila L, Costisella O, Canva V. Hepatitis C, interferon a and depression: main physiopathologic hypothesis. Encéphale. 2005;31(3):349–57. PMID: 16142050. http://www.ncbi.nlm.nih.gov/pubmed/16142050.
50. O'Connor MF, Irwin MR, Seldon J, Kwan L, Ganz PA. Pro-inflammatory cytokines and depression in a familial cancer registry. Psychooncology. 2007;16(5):499–501. PMID: 17094069. http://www.ncbi.nlm.nih.gov/pubmed/17094069.
51. Dantzer R, Wollman E, Vitkovic L, Yirmiya R. Cytokines and depression: fortuitous or causative association? Mol Psychiatry. 1999;4(4):328–32. PMID: 10483048. http://www.ncbi.nlm.nih.gov/pubmed/10483048.
52. Yirmiya R, Pollak Y, Morag M, Reichenberg A, Barak O, Avitsur R, Shavit Y, Ovadia H, Weidenfeld J, Morag A, Newman ME, Pollmächer T. Illness, cytokines, and depression. Ann N Y Acad Sci. 2000;917:478–87. PMID: 11268375. http://www.ncbi.nlm.nih.gov/pubmed/11268375.
53. Corcos M, Guilbaud O, Hjalmarsson L, Chambry J, Jeammet P. Cytokines and depression: an analogic approach. Biomed Pharmacother. 2002;56(2):105–10. PMID: 12000135. http://www.ncbi.nlm.nih.gov/pubmed/12000135.
54. Hart BL. Biological basis of the behavior of sick animals. Neurosci Biobehav Rev. 1988;12(2):123–37. PMID: 3050629. http://www.ncbi.nlm.nih.gov/pubmed/3050629.
55. Exton MS. Infection-induced anorexia: active host defence strategy. Appetite. 1997;29(3):369–83. PMID: 9468766. http://www.ncbi.nlm.nih.gov/pubmed/9468766.
56. Murray MJ, Murray AB. Anorexia of infection as a mechanism of host defense. Am J Clin Nutr. 1979;32(3):593–6. PMID: 283688. http://www.ncbi.nlm.nih.gov/pubmed/283688.
57. Konsman JP. So many faces, phases, and facets, sickness behavior beyond disciplines. Front Psych. 2021;12:630331. PMCID: PMC7947683. http://www.ncbi.nlm.nih.gov/pubmed/33716828.
58. Kelley KW, Bluthé RM, Dantzer R, Zhou JH, Shen WH, Johnson RW, Broussard SR. Cytokine-induced sickness behavior. Brain Behav Immun. 2003;17(Suppl 1):S112–8. PMID: 12615196. http://www.ncbi.nlm.nih.gov/pubmed/12615196.
59. Kent S, Bluthe RM, Dantzer R, Hardwick AJ, Kelley KW, Rothwell NJ, Vannice JL. Different receptor mechanisms mediate the pyrogenic and behavioral effects of interleukin 1. Proc Natl Acad Sci USA. 1992;89(19):9117–20. PMCID: PMC50076. http://www.ncbi.nlm.nih.gov/pubmed/1409612.
60. Maier SF, Wiertelak EP, Martin D, Watkins LR. Interleukin-1 mediates the behavioral hyperalgesia produced by lithium chloride and endotoxin. Brain Res. 1993;623(2):321–4. PMID: 8221116. http://www.ncbi.nlm.nih.gov/pubmed/8221116.
61. Yirmiya R, Weidenfeld J, Pollak Y, Morag M, Morag A, Avitsur R, Barak O, Reichenberg A, Cohen E, Shavit Y, Ovadia H. Cytokines, "depression due to a general medical condition," and antidepressant drugs. Adv Exp Med Biol. 1999;461:283–316. PMID: 10442179. http://www.ncbi.nlm.nih.gov/pubmed/10442179.
62. Charlton BG. The malaise theory of depression: major depressive disorder is sickness behavior and antidepressants are analgesic. Med Hypotheses. 2000;54(1):126–30. PMID: 10790737. http://www.ncbi.nlm.nih.gov/pubmed/10790737.
63. Maes M. The cytokine hypothesis of depression: inflammation, oxidative & nitrosative stress (IO&NS) and leaky gut as new targets for adjunctive treatments in depression. Neuro Endocrinol Lett. 2008;29(3):287–91. PMID: 18580840. http://www.ncbi.nlm.nih.gov/pubmed/18580840.
64. Yirmiya R. Endotoxin produces a depressive-like episode in rats. Brain Res. 1996;711(1–2):163–74. PMID: 8680860. http://www.ncbi.nlm.nih.gov/pubmed/8680860.
65. Harrison NA, Brydon L, Walker C, Gray MA, Steptoe A, Dolan RJ, Critchley HD. Neural origins of human sickness in interoceptive responses to inflammation. Biol Psychiatry. 2009;66(5):415–22. PMCID: PMC2885492. http://www.ncbi.nlm.nih.gov/pubmed/19409533.
66. Drevets WC, Savitz J, Trimble M. The subgenual anterior cingulate cortex in mood disorders. CNS Spectr. 2008;13(8):663–81. PMCID: PMC2729429. http://www.ncbi.nlm.nih.gov/pubmed/18704022.
67. Harrison NA, Brydon L, Walker C, Gray MA, Steptoe A, Critchley HD. Inflammation causes mood changes through alterations in subgenual cingulate activity and mesolimbic connectivity. Biol Psychiatry. 2009;66(5):407–14. PMCID: PMC2885494. http://www.ncbi.nlm.nih.gov/pubmed/19423079.
68. Hesdorffer DC. Comorbidity between neurological illness and psychiatric disorders. CNS Spectr. 2016;21(3):230–8. PMID: 26898322. http://www.ncbi.nlm.nih.gov/pubmed/26898322.
69. Coppola G, Operto FF, Matricardi S, Verrotti A. Monitoring and managing depression in adolescents with epilepsy: current perspectives. Neuropsychiatr Dis Treat. 2019;15:2773–80. PMCID: PMC6765392. http://www.ncbi.nlm.nih.gov/pubmed/31576132.
70. Buckner RL, Andrews-Hanna JR, Schacter DL. The brain's default network: anatomy, function, and relevance to disease. Ann N Y Acad Sci. 2008;1124:1–38. PMID: 18400922. http://www.ncbi.nlm.nih.gov/pubmed/18400922.
71. Raichle ME, MacLeod AM, Snyder AZ, Powers WJ, Gusnard DA, Shulman GL. A default mode of brain function. Proc Natl Acad Sci U S A. 2001;98(2):676–82. PMCID: PMC14647. http://www.ncbi.nlm.nih.gov/pubmed/11209064.
72. Raichle ME. The brain's default mode network. Annu Rev Neurosci. 2015;38:433–47. PMID: 25938726. http://www.ncbi.nlm.nih.gov/pubmed/25938726.
73. Mohan A, Roberto AJ, Mohan A, Lorenzo A, Jones K, Carney MJ, Liogier-Weyback L, Hwang S, Lapidus KAB. The significance of the Default Mode Network (DMN) in neurological and neuropsychiatric disorders: a review. Yale J Biol Med. 2016;89(1):49–57. PMCID: PMC4797836
74. Cha DS, De Michele F, Soczynska JK, Woldeyohannes HO, Kaidanovich-Beilin O, Carvalho AF, Malhi GS, Patel H, Sim K, Brietzke E, Mansur R, Dunlop KAM, Alsuwaidan M, Baskaran A, Fagiolini A, Reznikov R, Kudlow PA, McIntyre RS. The putative impact of metabolic health on default mode network activity and functional connectivity in neuropsychiatric disorders. CNS Neurol Disord Drug Targets. 2014;13(10):1750–8. PMID: 25470392. http://www.ncbi.nlm.nih.gov/pubmed/25470392.
75. Gao Y, Wang M, Yu R, Li Y, Yang Y, Cui X, Zheng J. Abnormal default mode network homogeneity in treatment-naive patients with first-episode depression. Front Psych. 2018;9:697. PMCID: PMC6305293. http://www.ncbi.nlm.nih.gov/pubmed/30618871.
76. Zhu X, Wang X, Xiao J, Liao J, Zhong M, Wang W, Yao S. Evidence of a dissociation pattern in resting-state default mode network connectivity in first-episode, treatment-naive major depression patients. Biol Psychiatry. 2012;71(7):611–7. PMID: 22177602. http://www.ncbi.nlm.nih.gov/pubmed/22177602.
77. Qin J, Shen H, Zeng LL, Jiang W, Liu L, Hu D. Predicting clinical responses in major depression using intrinsic functional connectivity. Neuroreport. 2015;26(12):675–80. PMID: 26164454. http://www.ncbi.nlm.nih.gov/pubmed/26164454.
78. He Y, Lim S, Fortunato S, Sporns O, Zhang L, Qiu J, Xie P, Zuo XN. Reconfiguration of cortical networks in MDD uncovered by multiscale community detection with fMRI. Cereb Cortex.

2018;28(4):1383–95. PMCID: PMC6093364. http://www.ncbi.nlm.nih.gov/pubmed/29300840.
79. Pariante CM. Depression, stress and the adrenal axis. J Neuroendocrinol. 2003;15(8):811–2. PMID: 12834443. http://www.ncbi.nlm.nih.gov/pubmed/12834443.
80. Barden N. Implication of the hypothalamic-pituitary-adrenal axis in the physiopathology of depression. J Psychiatry Neurosci. 2004;29(3):185–93. PMCID: PMC400688. http://www.ncbi.nlm.nih.gov/pubmed/15173895.
81. Rubin RT, Poland RE, Lesser IM, Winston RA, Blodgett AL. Neuroendocrine aspects of primary endogenous depression. I. Cortisol secretory dynamics in patients and matched controls. Arch Gen Psychiatry. 1987;44(4):328–36. PMID: 3566455. http://www.ncbi.nlm.nih.gov/pubmed/3566455.
82. Sekula LK, Lucke JF, Heist EK, Czambel RK, Rubin RT. Neuroendocrine aspects of primary endogenous depression. XV: mathematical modeling of nocturnal melatonin secretion in major depressives and normal controls. Psychiatry Res. 1997;69(2–3):143–53. PMID: 9109182. http://www.ncbi.nlm.nih.gov/pubmed/9109182.
83. Svenningsson P, Tzavara ET, Liu F, Fienberg AA, Nomikos GG, Greengard P. DARPP-32 mediates serotonergic neurotransmission in the forebrain. Proc Natl Acad Sci U S A. 2002;99(5):3188–93. PMCID: PMC122494. http://www.ncbi.nlm.nih.gov/pubmed/11880652.
84. Svenningsson P, Tzavara ET, Witkin JM, Fienberg AA, Nomikos GG, Greengard P. Involvement of striatal and extrastriatal DARPP-32 in biochemical and behavioral effects of fluoxetine (Prozac). Proc Natl Acad Sci USA. 2002;99(5):3182–7. PMCID: PMC122493. http://www.ncbi.nlm.nih.gov/pubmed/11880651.
85. Svenningsson P, Greengard P. p11 (S100A10)—an inducible adaptor protein that modulates neuronal functions. Curr Opin Pharmacol. 2007;7(1):27–32. PMID: 17085073. http://www.ncbi.nlm.nih.gov/pubmed/17085073.
86. Bunney WE, Davis JM. Norepinephrine in depressive reactions. A review. Arch Gen Psychiatry. 1965;13(6):483–94. PMID: 5320621. http://www.ncbi.nlm.nih.gov/pubmed/5320621.
87. Schildkraut JJ. The catecholamine hypothesis of affective disorders: a review of supporting evidence. Am J Psychiatry. 1965;122(5):509–22. PMID: 5319766. http://www.ncbi.nlm.nih.gov/pubmed/5319766.
88. Mårtensson B, Wägner A, Beck O, Brodin K, Montero D, Asberg M. Effects of clomipramine treatment on cerebrospinal fluid monoamine metabolites and platelet 3H-imipramine binding and serotonin uptake and concentration in major depressive disorder. Acta Psychiatr Scand. 1991;83(2):125–33. PMID: 1708190. http://www.ncbi.nlm.nih.gov/pubmed/1708190.
89. Sheline Y, Bardgett ME, Csernansky JG. Correlated reductions in cerebrospinal fluid 5-HIAA and MHPG concentrations after treatment with selective serotonin reuptake inhibitors. J Clin Psychopharmacol. 1997;17(1):11–4. PMID: 9004051. http://www.ncbi.nlm.nih.gov/pubmed/9004051.
90. De Bellis MD, Geracioti TD, Altemus M, Kling MA. Cerebrospinal fluid monoamine metabolites in fluoxetine-treated patients with major depression and in healthy volunteers. Biol Psychiatry. 1993;33(8–9):636–41. PMID: 7687151. http://www.ncbi.nlm.nih.gov/pubmed/7687151.
91. Katz MM, Maas JW, Frazer A, Koslow SH, Bowden CL, Berman N, Swann AC, Stokes PE. Drug-induced actions on brain neurotransmitter systems and changes in the behaviors and emotions of depressed patients. Neuropsychopharmacology. 1994;11(2):89–100. PMID: 7530963. http://www.ncbi.nlm.nih.gov/pubmed/7530963.
92. Stöber G, Nöthen MM, Pörzgen P, Brüss M, Bönisch H, Knapp M, Beckmann H, Propping P. Systematic search for variation in the human norepinephrine transporter gene: identification of five naturally occurring missense mutations and study of association with major psychiatric disorders. Am J Med Genet. 1996;67(6):523–32. PMID: 8950409. http://www.ncbi.nlm.nih.gov/pubmed/8950409.
93. Ressler KJ, Nemeroff CB. Role of serotonergic and noradrenergic systems in the pathophysiology of depression and anxiety disorders. Depress Anxiety. 2000;12(Suppl 1):2–19. PMID: 11098410. http://www.ncbi.nlm.nih.gov/pubmed/11098410.
94. Schüle C, Minov C, Behrens S, Rupprecht R, Hegerl U, Möller HJ, Bondy B. Identification of a naturally occurring polymorphism in the promoter region of the norepinephrine transporter and analysis in major depression. Neuropsychopharmacology. 2002;26(4):489–93. PMID: 11927173. http://www.ncbi.nlm.nih.gov/pubmed/11927173.
95. Ryu SH, Lee SH, Lee HJ, Cha JH, Ham BJ, Han CS, Choi MJ, Lee MS. Association between norepinephrine transporter gene polymorphism and major depression. Neuropsychobiology. 2004;49(4):174–7. PMID: 1511835. http://www.ncbi.nlm.nih.gov/pubmed/15118352.
96. Dick W, Traub E, Kraus H, Töllner U, Burghard R, Muck J. General anaesthesia versus epidural anaesthesia for primary caesarean section--a comparative study. Eur J Anaesthesiol. 1992;9(1):15–21. PMID: 1735394. http://www.ncbi.nlm.nih.gov/pubmed/1735394.
97. Roy A, Campbell MK. A unifying framework for depression: bridging the major biological and psychosocial theories through stress. Clin Invest Med. 2013;36(4):E170–90. PMID: 23906489. http://www.ncbi.nlm.nih.gov/pubmed/23906489.
98. Dey A, Hankey Giblin PA. Insights into macrophage heterogeneity and cytokine-induced neuroinflammation in major depressive disorder. Pharmaceuticals (Basel). 2018;11(3):64. PMCID: PMC6160985. http://www.ncbi.nlm.nih.gov/pubmed/29941796.
99. Northoff G. Gene, brains, and environment-genetic neuroimaging of depression. Curr Opin Neurobiol. 2013;23(1):133–42. PMID: 22995550. http://www.ncbi.nlm.nih.gov/pubmed/22995550.
100. Ruhé HG, Mason NS, Schene AH. Mood is indirectly related to serotonin, norepinephrine and dopamine levels in humans: a meta-analysis of monoamine depletion studies. Mol Psychiatry. 2007;12(4):331–59. PMID: 17389902. http://www.ncbi.nlm.nih.gov/pubmed/17389902.
101. Marazziti D, Akiskal HS, Rossi A, Cassano GB. Alteration of the platelet serotonin transporter in romantic love. Psychol Med. 1999;29(3):741–5. PMID: 10405096. http://www.ncbi.nlm.nih.gov/pubmed/10405096.
102. Almada RC, Borelli KG, Albrechet-Souza L, Brandão ML. Serotonergic mechanisms of the median raphe nucleus-dorsal hippocampus in conditioned fear: output circuit involves the prefrontal cortex and amygdala. Behav Brain Res. 2009;203(2):279–87. PMID: 19464321. http://www.ncbi.nlm.nih.gov/pubmed/19464321.
103. Cowen PJ. Serotonin receptor subtypes in depression: evidence from studies in neuroendocrine regulation. Clin Neuropharmacol. 1993;16(Suppl 3):S6–18. PMID: 8131155. http://www.ncbi.nlm.nih.gov/pubmed/8131155.
104. Nugent AC, Neumeister A, Goldman D, Herscovitch P, Charney DS, Drevets WC. Serotonin transporter genotype and depressive phenotype determination by discriminant analysis of glucose metabolism under acute tryptophan depletion. NeuroImage. 2008;43(4):764–74. PMCID: PMC2650221. http://www.ncbi.nlm.nih.gov/pubmed/18718871.
105. Caspi A, Hariri AR, Holmes A, Uher R, Moffitt TE. Genetic sensitivity to the environment: the case of the serotonin transporter gene and its implications for studying complex diseases and traits. Am J Psychiatry. 2010;167(5):509–27. PMCID: PMC2943341. http://www.ncbi.nlm.nih.gov/pubmed/20231323.
106. Serotonin transport in the 21st century | Journal of General Physiology | Rockefeller University Press.

107. Hermann A, Küpper Y, Schmitz A, Walter B, Vaitl D, Hennig J, Stark R, Tabbert K. Functional gene polymorphisms in the serotonin system and traumatic life events modulate the neural basis of fear acquisition and extinction. PLoS One. 2012;7(9):e44352. PMCID: PMC3434167. http://www.ncbi.nlm.nih.gov/pubmed/22957066.
108. Hariri AR, Mattay VS, Tessitore A, Kolachana B, Fera F, Goldman D, Egan MF, Weinberger DR. Serotonin transporter genetic variation and the response of the human amygdala. Science. 2002;297(5580):400–3. PMID: 12130784. http://www.ncbi.nlm.nih.gov/pubmed/12130784.
109. Homberg JR, Lesch KP. Looking on the bright side of serotonin transporter gene variation. Biol Psychiatry. 2011;69(6):513–9. PMID: 21047622. http://www.ncbi.nlm.nih.gov/pubmed/21047622.
110. Morley AP, Narayanan M, Mines R, Molokhia A, Baxter S, Craig G, Lewis CM, Craig I. AVPR1A and SLC6A4 polymorphisms in choral singers and non-musicians: a gene association study. PLoS One. 2012;7(2):e31763. PMCID: PMC3285181. http://www.ncbi.nlm.nih.gov/pubmed/22384070.
111. Ukkola-Vuoti L, Kanduri C, Oikkonen J, Buck G, Blancher C, Raijas P, Karma K, Lähdesmäki H, Järvelä I. Genome-wide copy number variation analysis in extended families and unrelated individuals characterized for musical aptitude and creativity in music. PLoS One. 2013;8(2):e56356. PMCID: PMC3584088. http://www.ncbi.nlm.nih.gov/pubmed/23460800.
112. Kendler KS, Kuhn JW, Vittum J, Prescott CA, Riley B. The interaction of stressful life events and a serotonin transporter polymorphism in the prediction of episodes of major depression: a replication. Arch Gen Psychiatry. 2005;62(5):529–35. PMID: 15867106. http://www.ncbi.nlm.nih.gov/pubmed/15867106.
113. SLC6A4 solute carrier family 6 member 4 [Homo sapiens (human)] - Gene - NCBI.
114. Hranilovic D, Stefulj J, Schwab S, Borrmann-Hassenbach M, Albus M, Jernej B, Wildenauer D. Serotonin transporter promoter and intron 2 polymorphisms: relationship between allelic variants and gene expression. Biol Psychiatry. 2004;55(11):1090–4. PMID: 15158428. http://www.ncbi.nlm.nih.gov/pubmed/15158428.
115. Iurescia S, Seripa D, Rinaldi M. Role of the 5-HTTLPR and SNP promoter polymorphisms on serotonin transporter gene expression: a closer look at genetic architecture and in vitro functional studies of common and uncommon allelic variants. Mol Neurobiol. 2016;53(8):5510–26. PMID: 26464328. http://www.ncbi.nlm.nih.gov/pubmed/26464328.
116. Heils A, Teufel A, Petri S, Stöber G, Riederer P, Bengel D, Lesch KP. Allelic variation of human serotonin transporter gene expression. J Neurochem. 1996;66(6):2621–4. PMID: 8632190. http://www.ncbi.nlm.nih.gov/pubmed/8632190.
117. Jacobs N, Kenis G, Peeters F, Derom C, Vlietinck R, van Os J. Stress-related negative affectivity and genetically altered serotonin transporter function: evidence of synergism in shaping risk of depression. Arch Gen Psychiatry. 2006;63(9):989–96. PMID: 16953001. http://www.ncbi.nlm.nih.gov/pubmed/16953001.
118. Kendler KS, Kuhn JW, Prescott CA. Childhood sexual abuse, stressful life events and risk for major depression in women. Psychol Med. 2004;34(8):1475–82. PMID: 15724878. http://www.ncbi.nlm.nih.gov/pubmed/15724878.
119. Glatz K, Mössner R, Heils A, Lesch KP. Glucocorticoid-regulated human serotonin transporter (5-HTT) expression is modulated by the 5-HTT gene-promotor-linked polymorphic region. J Neurochem. 2003;86(5):1072–8. PMID: 12911615. http://www.ncbi.nlm.nih.gov/pubmed/12911615.
120. Caspi A, Sugden K, Moffitt TE, Taylor A, Craig IW, Harrington H, McClay J, Mill J, Martin J, Braithwaite A, Poulton R. Influence of life stress on depression: moderation by a polymorphism in the 5-HTT gene. Science. 2003;301(5631):386–9. PMID: 12869766. http://www.ncbi.nlm.nih.gov/pubmed/12869766.
121. Lesch KP, Bengel D, Heils A, Sabol SZ, Greenberg BD, Petri S, Benjamin J, Müller CR, Hamer DH, Murphy DL. Association of anxiety-related traits with a polymorphism in the serotonin transporter gene regulatory region. Science. 1996;274(5292):1527–31. PMID: 8929413. http://www.ncbi.nlm.nih.gov/pubmed/8929413.
122. Pezawas L, Meyer-Lindenberg A, Drabant EM, Verchinski BA, Munoz KE, Kolachana BS, Egan MF, Mattay VS, Hariri AR, Weinberger DR. 5-HTTLPR polymorphism impacts human cingulate-amygdala interactions: a genetic susceptibility mechanism for depression. Nat Neurosci. 2005;8(6):828–34. PMID: 15880108. http://www.ncbi.nlm.nih.gov/pubmed/15880108.
123. Shioe K, Ichimiya T, Suhara T, Takano A, Sudo Y, Yasuno F, Hirano M, Shinohara M, Kagami M, Okubo Y, Nankai M, Kanba S. No association between genotype of the promoter region of serotonin transporter gene and serotonin transporter binding in human brain measured by PET. Synapse. 2003;48(4):184–8. PMID: 12687637. http://www.ncbi.nlm.nih.gov/pubmed/12687637.
124. Mann JJ, Huang YY, Underwood MD, Kassir SA, Oppenheim S, Kelly TM, Dwork AJ, Arango V. A serotonin transporter gene promoter polymorphism (5-HTTLPR) and prefrontal cortical binding in major depression and suicide. Arch Gen Psychiatry. 2000;57(8):729–38. PMID: 10920459. http://www.ncbi.nlm.nih.gov/pubmed/10920459.
125. Kobiella A, Reimold M, Ulshöfer DE, Ikonomidou VN, Vollmert C, Vollstädt-Klein S, Rietschel M, Reischl G, Heinz A, Smolka MN. How the serotonin transporter 5-HTTLPR polymorphism influences amygdala function: the roles of in vivo serotonin transporter expression and amygdala structure. Transl Psychiatry. 2011;1(8):e37. PMCID: PMC3309509. http://www.ncbi.nlm.nih.gov/pubmed/22832611.
126. Rucci P, Nimgaonkar VL, Mansour H, Miniati M, Masala I, Fagiolini A, Cassano GB, Frank E. Gender moderates the relationship between mania spectrum and serotonin transporter polymorphisms in depression. Am J Med Genet B Neuropsychiatr Genet. 2009;150B(7):907–13. PMCID: PMC3387576. http://www.ncbi.nlm.nih.gov/pubmed/19125390.
127. Hoefgen B, Schulze TG, Ohlraun S, von Widdern O, Höfels S, Gross M, Heidmann V, Kovalenko S, Eckermann A, Kölsch H, Metten M, Zobel A, Becker T, Nöthen MM, Propping P, Heun R, Maier W, Rietschel M. The power of sample size and homogenous sampling: association between the 5-HTTLPR serotonin transporter polymorphism and major depressive disorder. Biol Psychiatry. 2005;57(3):247–51. PMID: 15691525. http://www.ncbi.nlm.nih.gov/pubmed/15691525.
128. Way BM, Taylor SE. A polymorphism in the serotonin transporter gene moderates cardiovascular reactivity to psychosocial stress. Psychosom Med. 2011;73(4):310–7. PMCID: PMC3090451. http://www.ncbi.nlm.nih.gov/pubmed/21364196.
129. Dombrovski AY, Mulsant BH, Ferrell RE, Lotrich FE, Rosen JI, Wallace M, Houck PR, Mazumdar S, Pollock BG. Serotonin transporter triallelic genotype and response to citalopram and risperidone in dementia with behavioral symptoms. Int Clin Psychopharmacol. 2010;25(1):37–45. PMCID: PMC2887732. http://www.ncbi.nlm.nih.gov/pubmed/19996755.
130. Serretti A, Lilli R, Lorenzi C, Lattuada E, Cusin C, Smeraldi E. Serotonin transporter gene (5-HTTLPR) and major psychoses. Mol Psychiatry. 2002;7(1):95–9. PMID: 11803453. http://www.ncbi.nlm.nih.gov/pubmed/11803453.
131. Mendlewicz J, Massat I, Souery D, Del-Favero J, Oruc L, Nöthen MM, Blackwood D, Muir W, Battersby S, Lerer B, Segman RH, Kaneva R, Serretti A, Lilli R, Lorenzi C, Jakovljevic M, Ivezic S, Rietschel M, Milanova V, Van Broeckhoven C. Serotonin transporter 5HTTLPR polymorphism and affective disorders: no evidence of association in a large European multicenter study. Eur J

Hum Genet. 2004;12(5):377–82. PMID: 14735161. http://www.ncbi.nlm.nih.gov/pubmed/14735161.

132. Surtees PG, Wainwright NWJ, Willis-Owen SAG, Luben R, Day NE, Flint J. Social adversity, the serotonin transporter (5-HTTLPR) polymorphism and major depressive disorder. Biol Psychiatry. 2006;59(3):224–9. PMID: 16154545. http://www.ncbi.nlm.nih.gov/pubmed/16154545.
133. Markus CR, De Raedt R. Differential effects of 5-HTTLPR genotypes on inhibition of negative emotional information following acute stress exposure and tryptophan challenge. Neuropsychopharmacology. 2011;36(4):819–26. PMCID: PMC3055739. http://www.ncbi.nlm.nih.gov/pubmed/21150915.
134. Porcelli S, Drago A, Fabbri C, Gibiino S, Calati R, Serretti A. Pharmacogenetics of antidepressant response. J Psychiatry Neurosci. 2011;36(2):87–113. PMCID: PMC3044192. http://www.ncbi.nlm.nih.gov/pubmed/21172166.
135. Serretti A, Kato M, De Ronchi D, Kinoshita T. Meta-analysis of serotonin transporter gene promoter polymorphism (5-HTTLPR) association with selective serotonin reuptake inhibitor efficacy in depressed patients. Mol Psychiatry. 2007;12(3):247–57. PMID: 17146470. http://www.ncbi.nlm.nih.gov/pubmed/17146470.
136. Serretti A, Mandelli L, Lorenzi C, Pirovano A, Olgiati P, Colombo C, Smeraldi E. Serotonin transporter gene influences the time course of improvement of "core" depressive and somatic anxiety symptoms during treatment with SSRIs for recurrent mood disorders. Psychiatry Res. 2007;149(1–3):185–93. PMID: 17157919. http://www.ncbi.nlm.nih.gov/pubmed/17157919.
137. Smits K, Smits L, Peeters F, Schouten J, Janssen R, Smeets H, van Os J, Prins M. Serotonin transporter polymorphisms and the occurrence of adverse events during treatment with selective serotonin reuptake inhibitors. Int Clin Psychopharmacol. 2007;22(3):137–43. PMID: 17414739. http://www.ncbi.nlm.nih.gov/pubmed/17414739.
138. Smeraldi E, Zanardi R, Benedetti F, Di Bella D, Perez J, Catalano M. Polymorphism within the promoter of the serotonin transporter gene and antidepressant efficacy of fluvoxamine. Mol Psychiatry. 1998;3(6):508–11. PMID: 9857976. http://www.ncbi.nlm.nih.gov/pubmed/9857976.
139. Serretti A, Cusin C, Rossini D, Artioli P, Dotoli D, Zanardi R. Further evidence of a combined effect of SERTPR and TPH on SSRIs response in mood disorders. Am J Med Genet B Neuropsychiatr Genet. 2004;129B(1):36–40. PMID: 15274037. http://www.ncbi.nlm.nih.gov/pubmed/15274037.
140. Crisafulli C, Fabbri C, Porcelli S, Drago A, Spina E, De Ronchi D, Serretti A. Pharmacogenetics of antidepressants. Front Pharmacol. 2011;2:6. PMCID: PMC3108562. http://www.ncbi.nlm.nih.gov/pubmed/21687501.
141. Minov C, Baghai TC, Schüle C, Zwanzger P, Schwarz MJ, Zill P, Rupprecht R, Bondy B. Serotonin-2A-receptor and -transporter polymorphisms: lack of association in patients with major depression. Neurosci Lett. 2001;303(2):119–22. PMID: 11311507. http://www.ncbi.nlm.nih.gov/pubmed/11311507.
142. Maron E, Tammiste A, Kallassalu K, Eller T, Vasar V, Nutt DJ, Metspalu A. Serotonin transporter promoter region polymorphisms do not influence treatment response to escitalopram in patients with major depression. Eur Neuropsychopharmacol. 2009;19(6):451–6. PMID: 19272758. http://www.ncbi.nlm.nih.gov/pubmed/19272758.
143. Oswald P, Souery D, Massat I, Del-Favero J, Linotte S, Papadimitriou G, Dikeos D, Kaneva R, Milanova V, Oruc L, Ivezic S, Serretti A, Lilli R, Van Broeckhoven C, Mendlewicz J. Lack of association between the 5HT2A receptor polymorphism (T102C) and unipolar affective disorder in a multicentric European study. Eur Neuropsychopharmacol. 2003;13(5):365–8. PMID: 12957335. http://www.ncbi.nlm.nih.gov/pubmed/12957335.
144. Hu XZ, Rush AJ, Charney D, Wilson AF, Sorant AJM, Papanicolaou GJ, Fava M, Trivedi MH, Wisniewski SR, Laje G, Paddock S, McMahon FJ, Manji H, Lipsky RH. Association between a functional serotonin transporter promoter polymorphism and citalopram treatment in adult outpatients with major depression. Arch Gen Psychiatry. 2007;64(7):783–92. PMID: 17606812. http://www.ncbi.nlm.nih.gov/pubmed/17606812.
145. Dogan O, Yuksel N, Ergun MA, Yilmaz A, Ilhan MN, Karslioglu HE, Koc A, Menevse A. Serotonin transporter gene polymorphisms and sertraline response in major depression patients. Genet Test. 2008;12(2):225–31. PMID: 18452396. http://www.ncbi.nlm.nih.gov/pubmed/18452396.
146. Wilkie MJV, Smith G, Day RK, Matthews K, Smith D, Blackwood D, Reid IC, Wolf CR. Polymorphisms in the SLC6A4 and HTR2A genes influence treatment outcome following antidepressant therapy. Pharmacogenomics J. 2009;9(1):61–70. PMID: 18253134. http://www.ncbi.nlm.nih.gov/pubmed/18253134.
147. Kang RH, Wong ML, Choi MJ, Paik JW, Lee MS. Association study of the serotonin transporter promoter polymorphism and mirtazapine antidepressant response in major depressive disorder. Prog Neuro-Psychopharmacol Biol Psychiatry. 2007;31(6):1317–21. PMID: 17618721. http://www.ncbi.nlm.nih.gov/pubmed/17618721.
148. Kim DK, Lim SW, Lee S, Sohn SE, Kim S, Hahn CG, Carroll BJ. Serotonin transporter gene polymorphism and antidepressant response. Neuroreport. 2000;11(1):215–9. PMID: 10683861. http://www.ncbi.nlm.nih.gov/pubmed/10683861.
149. Yoshida K, Ito K, Sato K, Takahashi H, Kamata M, Higuchi H, Shimizu T, Itoh K, Inoue K, Tezuka T, Suzuki T, Ohkubo T, Sugawara K, Otani K. Influence of the serotonin transporter gene-linked polymorphic region on the antidepressant response to fluvoxamine in Japanese depressed patients. Prog Neuro-Psychopharmacol Biol Psychiatry. 2002;26(2):383–6. PMID: 11817517. http://www.ncbi.nlm.nih.gov/pubmed/11817517.
150. Kim H, Lim SW, Kim S, Kim JW, Chang YH, Carroll BJ, Kim DK. Monoamine transporter gene polymorphisms and antidepressant response in koreans with late-life depression. JAMA. 2006;296(13):1609–18. PMID: 17018806. http://www.ncbi.nlm.nih.gov/pubmed/17018806.
151. Yu YWY, Tsai SJ, Chen TJ, Lin CH, Hong CJ. Association study of the serotonin transporter promoter polymorphism and symptomatology and antidepressant response in major depressive disorders. Mol Psychiatry. 2002;7(10):1115–9. PMID: 12476327. http://www.ncbi.nlm.nih.gov/pubmed/12476327.
152. Lee MS, Lee HY, Lee HJ, Ryu SH. Serotonin transporter promoter gene polymorphism and long-term outcome of antidepressant treatment. Psychiatr Genet. 2004;14(2):111–5. PMID: 15167699. http://www.ncbi.nlm.nih.gov/pubmed/15167699.
153. Kato M, Ikenaga Y, Wakeno M, Okugawa G, Nobuhara K, Fukuda T, Fukuda K, Azuma J, Kinoshita T. Controlled clinical comparison of paroxetine and fluvoxamine considering the serotonin transporter promoter polymorphism. Int Clin Psychopharmacol. 2005;20(3):151–6. PMID: 15812265. http://www.ncbi.nlm.nih.gov/pubmed/15812265.
154. Kato M, Fukuda T, Wakeno M, Fukuda K, Okugawa G, Ikenaga Y, Yamashita M, Takekita Y, Nobuhara K, Azuma J, Kinoshita T. Effects of the serotonin type 2A, 3A and 3B receptor and the serotonin transporter genes on paroxetine and fluvoxamine efficacy and adverse drug reactions in depressed Japanese patients. Neuropsychobiology. 2006;53(4):186–95. PMID: 16874005. http://www.ncbi.nlm.nih.gov/pubmed/16874005.
155. Hong CJ, Chen TJ, Yu YWY, Tsai SJ. Response to fluoxetine and serotonin 1A receptor (C-1019G) polymorphism in Taiwan Chinese major depressive disorder. Pharmacogenomics J. 2006;6(1):27–33. PMID: 16302021. http://www.ncbi.nlm.nih.gov/pubmed/16302021.

156. Takahashi H, Yoshida K, Ito K, Sato K, Kamata M, Higuchi H, Shimizu T, Ito K, Inoue K, Tezuka T, Suzuki T, Ohkubo T, Sugawara K. No association between the serotonergic polymorphisms and incidence of nausea induced by fluvoxamine treatment. Eur Neuropsychopharmacol. 2002;12(5):477–81. PMID: 12208565. http://www.ncbi.nlm.nih.gov/pubmed/12208565.
157. Yoshida K, Takahashi H, Higuchi H, Kamata M, Ito K, Ichi SK, Naito S, Shimizu T, Itoh K, Inoue K, Suzuki T, Nemeroff CB. Prediction of antidepressant response to milnacipran by norepinephrine transporter gene polymorphisms. Am J Psychiatry. 2004;161(9):1575–80. PMID: 15337646. http://www.ncbi.nlm.nih.gov/pubmed/15337646.
158. Yoshimura R, Umene-Nakano W, Suzuki A, Ueda N, Miyamoto K, Ikenouchi-Sugita A, Hori H, Otani K, Nakamura J. Rapid response to paroxetine is associated with plasma paroxetine levels at 4 but not 8 weeks of treatment and is independent of serotonin transporter promoter polymorphism in Japanese depressed patients. Hum Psychopharmacol. 2009;24(6):489–94. PMID: 19606452. http://www.ncbi.nlm.nih.gov/pubmed/19606452.
159. Perlis RH, Mischoulon D, Smoller JW, Wan YJY, Lamon-Fava S, Lin KM, Rosenbaum JF, Fava M. Serotonin transporter polymorphisms and adverse effects with fluoxetine treatment. Biol Psychiatry. 2003;54(9):879–83. PMID: 14573314. http://www.ncbi.nlm.nih.gov/pubmed/14573314.
160. Serretti A, Calati R, Mandelli L, De Ronchi D. Serotonin transporter gene variants and behavior: a comprehensive review. Curr Drug Targets. 2006;7(12):1659–69. PMID: 17168841. http://www.ncbi.nlm.nih.gov/pubmed/17168841.
161. Kilpatrick DG, Koenen KC, Ruggiero KJ, Acierno R, Galea S, Resnick HS, Roitzsch J, Boyle J, Gelernter J. The serotonin transporter genotype and social support and moderation of posttraumatic stress disorder and depression in hurricane-exposed adults. Am J Psychiatry. 2007;164(11):1693–9. PMID: 17974934. http://www.ncbi.nlm.nih.gov/pubmed/17974934.
162. Sher L, Hardin TA, Greenberg BD, Murphy DL, Li Q, Rosenthal NE. Seasonality associated with the serotonin transporter promoter repeat length polymorphism. Am J Psychiatry. 1999;156(11):1837. PMID: 10553760. http://www.ncbi.nlm.nih.gov/pubmed/10553760.
163. Levitan RD. The chronobiology and neurobiology of winter seasonal affective disorder. Dialogues Clin Neurosci. 2007;9(3):315–24. PMCID: PMC3202491. http://www.ncbi.nlm.nih.gov/pubmed/17969868.
164. Fallgatter AJ, Herrmann MJ, Roemmler J, Ehlis AC, Wagener A, Heidrich A, Ortega G, Zeng Y, Lesch KP. Allelic variation of serotonin transporter function modulates the brain electrical response for error processing. Neuropsychopharmacology. 2004;29(8):1506–11. PMID: 15187981. http://www.ncbi.nlm.nih.gov/pubmed/15187981.
165. Margoob MA, Mushtaq D. Serotonin transporter gene polymorphism and psychiatric disorders: is there a link? Indian J Psychiatry. 2011;53(4):289–99. PMCID: PMC3267339. http://www.ncbi.nlm.nih.gov/pubmed/22303036.
166. Stein MB, Seedat S, Gelernter J. Serotonin transporter gene promoter polymorphism predicts SSRI response in generalized social anxiety disorder. Psychopharmacology. 2006;187(1):68–72. PMID: 16525856. http://www.ncbi.nlm.nih.gov/pubmed/16525856.
167. Perna G, Favaron E, Di Bella D, Bussi R, Bellodi L. Antipanic efficacy of paroxetine and polymorphism within the promoter of the serotonin transporter gene. Neuropsychopharmacology. 2005;30(12):2230–5. PMID: 16034444. http://www.ncbi.nlm.nih.gov/pubmed/16034444.
168. Monteleone P, Santonastaso P, Tortorella A, Favaro A, Fabrazzo M, Castaldo E, Caregaro L, Fuschino A, Maj M. Serotonin transporter polymorphism and potential response to SSRIs in bulimia nervosa. Mol Psychiatry. 2005;10(8):716–8. PMID: 15940301. http://www.ncbi.nlm.nih.gov/pubmed/15940301.
169. Won ES, Chang HS, Lee HY, Ham BJ, Lee MS. Association between serotonin transporter-linked polymorphic region and escitalopram antidepressant treatment response in Korean patients with major depressive disorder. Neuropsychobiology. 2012;66(4):221–9. PMID: 23095326. http://www.ncbi.nlm.nih.gov/pubmed/23095326.
170. Blaya C, Salum GA, Lima MS, Leistner-Segal S, Manfro GG. Lack of association between the Serotonin Transporter Promoter Polymorphism (5-HTTLPR) and Panic Disorder: a systematic review and meta-analysis. Behav Brain Funct. 2007;3:41. PMCID: PMC1994953. http://www.ncbi.nlm.nih.gov/pubmed/17705872.
171. Gyawali S, Subaran R, Weissman MM, Hershkowitz D, McKenna MC, Talati A, Fyer AJ, Wickramaratne P, Adams PB, Hodge SE, Schmidt CJ, Bannon MJ, Glatt CE. Association of a polyadenylation polymorphism in the serotonin transporter and panic disorder. Biol Psychiatry. 2010;67(4):331–8. PMCID: PMC2980348. http://www.ncbi.nlm.nih.gov/pubmed/19969287.
172. Hartley CA, McKenna MC, Salman R, Holmes A, Casey BJ, Phelps EA, Glatt CE. Serotonin transporter polyadenylation polymorphism modulates the retention of fear extinction memory. Proc Natl Acad Sci USA. 2012;109(14):5493–8. PMCID: PMC3325655. http://www.ncbi.nlm.nih.gov/pubmed/22431634.
173. Schumacher J, Deckert J. Serotonin transporter polymorphisms and panic disorder. Genome Med. 2010;2(6):40. PMCID: PMC2905100. http://www.ncbi.nlm.nih.gov/pubmed/20587004.
174. Walderhaug E, Magnusson A, Neumeister A, Lappalainen J, Lunde H, Refsum H, Landrø NI. Interactive effects of sex and 5-HTTLPR on mood and impulsivity during tryptophan depletion in healthy people. Biol Psychiatry. 2007;62(6):593–9. PMID: 17544379. http://www.ncbi.nlm.nih.gov/pubmed/17544379.
175. Neumeister A, Nugent AC, Waldeck T, Geraci M, Schwarz M, Bonne O, Bain EE, Luckenbaugh DA, Herscovitch P, Charney DS, Drevets WC. Neural and behavioral responses to tryptophan depletion in unmedicated patients with remitted major depressive disorder and controls. Arch Gen Psychiatry. 2004;61(8):765–73. PMID: 15289275. http://www.ncbi.nlm.nih.gov/pubmed/15289275.
176. Vielhaber K, Riemann D, Feige B, Kuelz A, Kirschbaum C, Voderholzer U. Impact of experimentally induced serotonin deficiency by tryptophan depletion on saliva cortisol concentrations. Pharmacopsychiatry. 2005;38(2):87–94. PMID: 15744632. http://www.ncbi.nlm.nih.gov/pubmed/15744632.
177. O'Hara R, Schröder CM, Mahadevan R, Schatzberg AF, Lindley S, Fox S, Weiner M, Kraemer HC, Noda A, Lin X, Gray HL, Hallmayer JF. Serotonin transporter polymorphism, memory and hippocampal volume in the elderly: association and interaction with cortisol. Mol Psychiatry. 2007;12(6):544–55. PMCID: PMC2084475. http://www.ncbi.nlm.nih.gov/pubmed/17353910.
178. Brummett BH, Krystal AD, Ashley-Koch A, Kuhn CM, Züchner S, Siegler IC, Barefoot JC, Ballard EL, Gwyther LP, Williams RB. Sleep quality varies as a function of 5-HTTLPR genotype and stress. Psychosom Med. 2007;69(7):621–4. PMCID: PMC2758820. http://www.ncbi.nlm.nih.gov/pubmed/17766685.
179. Agren T, Furmark T, Eriksson E, Fredrikson M. Human fear reconsolidation and allelic differences in serotonergic and dopaminergic genes. Transl. Psychiatry. 2012;2(2):e76. PMCID: PMC3309551. http://www.ncbi.nlm.nih.gov/pubmed/22832813.
180. Uher R, Caspi A, Houts R, Sugden K, Williams B, Poulton R, Moffitt TE. Serotonin transporter gene moderates childhood maltreatment's effects on persistent but not single-episode depression: replications and implications for resolving inconsistent results. J Affect Disord. 2011;135(1–3):56–65. PMCID: PMC3752793. http://www.ncbi.nlm.nih.gov/pubmed/21439648.

181. Sugden K, Arseneault L, Harrington H, Moffitt TE, Williams B, Caspi A. Serotonin transporter gene moderates the development of emotional problems among children following bullying victimization. J Am Acad Child Adolesc Psychiatry. 2010;49(8):830–40. PMCID: PMC2908591. http://www.ncbi.nlm.nih.gov/pubmed/20643316.
182. Alasaari JS, Lagus M, Ollila HM, Toivola A, Kivimäki M, Vahtera J, Kronholm E, Härmä M, Puttonen S, Paunio T. Environmental stress affects DNA methylation of a CpG rich promoter region of serotonin transporter gene in a nurse cohort. PLoS One. 2012;7(9):e45813. PMCID: PMC3461019. http://www.ncbi.nlm.nih.gov/pubmed/23029256.
183. Roiser JP, Blackwell AD, Cools R, Clark L, Rubinsztein DC, Robbins TW, Sahakian BJ. Serotonin transporter polymorphism mediates vulnerability to loss of incentive motivation following acute tryptophan depletion. Neuropsychopharmacology. 2006;31(10):2264–72. PMCID: PMC1852058. http://www.ncbi.nlm.nih.gov/pubmed/16541086.
184. Barr CS, Newman TK, Lindell S, Shannon C, Champoux M, Lesch KP, Suomi SJ, Goldman D, Higley JD. Interaction between serotonin transporter gene variation and rearing condition in alcohol preference and consumption in female primates. Arch Gen Psychiatry. 2004;61(11):1146–52. PMID: 15520362. http://www.ncbi.nlm.nih.gov/pubmed/15520362.
185. Becker HC, Lopez MF, Doremus-Fitzwater TL. Effects of stress on alcohol drinking: a review of animal studies. Psychopharmacology. 2011;218(1):131–56. PMCID: PMC3247761. http://www.ncbi.nlm.nih.gov/pubmed/21850445.
186. Traber DL. Endotoxin: the causative factor of mediator release during sepsis. Prog Clin Biol Res. 1987:236A:377–92. PMID: 3615441. http://www.ncbi.nlm.nih.gov/pubmed/3615441.
187. Kinnally EL, Capitanio JP, Leibel R, Deng L, LeDuc C, Haghighi F, Mann JJ. Epigenetic regulation of serotonin transporter expression and behavior in infant rhesus macaques. Genes Brain Behav. 2010;9(6):575–82. PMCID: PMC2921011. http://www.ncbi.nlm.nih.gov/pubmed/20398062.
188. Priess-Groben HA, Hyde JS. 5-HTTLPR X stress in adolescent depression: moderation by MAOA and gender. J Abnorm Child Psychol. 2013;41(2):281–94. PMID: 22836288. http://www.ncbi.nlm.nih.gov/pubmed/22836288.
189. Bukh JD, Bock C, Vinberg M, Werge T, Gether U, Kessing LV. No interactions between genetic polymorphisms and stressful life events on outcome of antidepressant treatment. Eur Neuropsychopharmacol. 2010;20(5):327–35. PMID: 20022223. http://www.ncbi.nlm.nih.gov/pubmed/20022223.
190. Niitsu T, Fabbri C, Bentini F, Serretti A. Pharmacogenetics in major depression: a comprehensive meta-analysis. Prog Neuro-Psychopharmacol Biol Psychiatry. 2013;45:183–94. PMID: 23733030. http://www.ncbi.nlm.nih.gov/pubmed/23733030.
191. Fabbri C, Marsano A, Serretti A. Genetics of serotonin receptors and depression: state of the art. Curr Drug Targets. 2013;14(5):531–48. PMID: 23547754. http://www.ncbi.nlm.nih.gov/pubmed/23547754.
192. Kato M, Serretti A. Review and meta-analysis of antidepressant pharmacogenetic findings in major depressive disorder. Mol Psychiatry. 2010;15(5):473–500. PMID: 18982004. http://www.ncbi.nlm.nih.gov/pubmed/18982004.
193. Serotonin Receptors - Basic Neurochemistry - NCBI Bookshelf.
194. Hoyer D, Clarke DE, Fozard JR, Hartig PR, Martin GR, Mylecharane EJ, Saxena PR, Humphrey PP. International Union of Pharmacology classification of receptors for 5-hydroxytryptamine (Serotonin). Pharmacol Rev. 1994;46(2):157–203. PMID: 7938165. http://www.ncbi.nlm.nih.gov/pubmed/7938165.
195. Yohn CN, Gergues MM, Samuels BA. The role of 5-HT receptors in depression. Mol Brain. 2017;10(1):28. PMCID: PMC5483313. http://www.ncbi.nlm.nih.gov/pubmed/28646910.
196. Mechanisms of signal transduction by hormones and growth factors. Proceedings of the Second International Symposium on Cellular Endocrinology. Lake Placid, New York, September 8–11, 1986. Prog Clin Biol Res. 1987;249:1–321. PMID: 2823287. http://www.ncbi.nlm.nih.gov/pubmed/2823287.
197. HTR1A 5-hydroxytryptamine receptor 1A [Homo sapiens (human)] - Gene - NCBI.
198. TPH1 tryptophan hydroxylase 1 [Homo sapiens (human)] - Gene - NCBI.
199. BDNF brain derived neurotrophic factor [Homo sapiens (human)] - Gene - NCBI.
200. HTR2A - Gene - NCBI.
201. Gontijo BR, Possatti I, Fratelli CF, Pereira ASR, Bonasser LSS, de Souza Silva CM, Rodrigues da Silva IC. The 3'UTR VNTR SLC6A3 genetic variant and major depressive disorder: a systematic review. Biomedicine. 2023;11(8):2270. PMCID: PMC10452352. http://www.ncbi.nlm.nih.gov/pubmed/37626766.
202. Ogilvie AD, Battersby S, Bubb VJ, Fink G, Harmar AJ, Goodwim GM, Smith CA. Polymorphism in serotonin transporter gene associated with susceptibility to major depression. Lancet. 1996;347(9003):731–3. PMID: 8602004. http://www.ncbi.nlm.nih.gov/pubmed/8602004.
203. Gutiérrez B, Pintor L, Gastó C, Rosa A, Bertranpetit J, Vieta E, Fañanás L. Variability in the serotonin transporter gene and increased risk for major depression with melancholia. Hum Genet. 1998;103(3):319–22. PMID: 9799087. http://www.ncbi.nlm.nih.gov/pubmed/9799087.
204. Lopez de Lara C, Dumais A, Rouleau G, Lesage A, Dumont M, Chawky N, Alda M, Benkelfat C, Turecki G. STin2 variant and family history of suicide as significant predictors of suicide completion in major depression. Biol Psychiatry. 2006;59(2):114–20. PMID: 16125146. http://www.ncbi.nlm.nih.gov/pubmed/16125146.
205. Min W, Li T, Ma X, Li Z, Yu T, Gao D, Zhang B, Yun Y, Sun X. Monoamine transporter gene polymorphisms affect susceptibility to depression and predict antidepressant response. Psychopharmacology. 2009;205(3):409–17. PMID: 19468717. http://www.ncbi.nlm.nih.gov/pubmed/19468717.
206. Peters EJ, Slager SL, McGrath PJ, Knowles JA, Hamilton SP. Investigation of serotonin-related genes in antidepressant response. Mol Psychiatry. 2004;9(9):879–89. PMID: 15052272. http://www.ncbi.nlm.nih.gov/pubmed/15052272.
207. Keers R, Uher R, Huezo-Diaz P, Smith R, Jaffee S, Rietschel M, Henigsberg N, Kozel D, Mors O, Maier W, Zobel A, Hauser J, Souery D, Placentino A, Larsen ER, Dmitrzak-Weglarz M, Gupta B, Hoda F, Craig I, McGuffin P, Farmer AE, Aitchison KJ. Interaction between serotonin transporter gene variants and life events predicts response to antidepressants in the GENDEP project. Pharmacogenomics J. 2011;11(2):138–45. PMID: 20212518. http://www.ncbi.nlm.nih.gov/pubmed/20212518.
208. Smeraldi E, Serretti A, Artioli P, Lorenzi C, Catalano M. Serotonin transporter gene-linked polymorphic region: possible pharmacogenetic implications of rare variants. Psychiatr Genet. 2006;16(4):153–8. PMID: 16829782. http://www.ncbi.nlm.nih.gov/pubmed/16829782.
209. Kraft JB, Slager SL, McGrath PJ, Hamilton SP. Sequence analysis of the serotonin transporter and associations with antidepressant response. Biol Psychiatry. 2005;58(5):374–81. PMID: 15993855. http://www.ncbi.nlm.nih.gov/pubmed/15993855.
210. Lohoff FW, Narasimhan S, Rickels K. Interaction between polymorphisms in serotonin transporter (SLC6A4) and serotonin receptor 2A (HTR2A) genes predict treatment response to venlafaxine XR in generalized anxiety disorder. Pharmacogenomics J. 2013;13(5):464–9. PMID: 22907732. http://www.ncbi.nlm.nih.gov/pubmed/22907732.

211. Zhang X, Gainetdinov RR, Beaulieu JM, Sotnikova TD, Burch LH, Williams RB, Schwartz DA, Krishnan KRR, Caron MG. Loss-of-function mutation in tryptophan hydroxylase-2 identified in unipolar major depression. Neuron. 2005;45(1):11–6. PMID: 15629698. http://www.ncbi.nlm.nih.gov/pubmed/15629698.
212. Gao J, Pan Z, Jiao Z, Li F, Zhao G, Wei Q, Pan F, Evangelou E. TPH2 gene polymorphisms and major depression—a meta-analysis. PLoS One. 2012;7(5):e36721. PMCID: PMC3365065. http://www.ncbi.nlm.nih.gov/pubmed/22693556.
213. van Rossum EFC, Binder EB, Majer M, Koper JW, Ising M, Modell S, Salyakina D, Lamberts SWJ, Holsboer F. Polymorphisms of the glucocorticoid receptor gene and major depression. Biol Psychiatry. 2006;59(8):681–8. PMID: 16580345. http://www.ncbi.nlm.nih.gov/pubmed/16580345.
214. Lucae S, Salyakina D, Barden N, Harvey M, Gagné B, Labbé M, Binder EB, Uhr M, Paez-Pereda M, Sillaber I, Ising M, Brückl T, Lieb R, Holsboer F, Müller-Myhsok B. P2RX7, a gene coding for a purinergic ligand-gated ion channel, is associated with major depressive disorder. Hum Mol Genet. 2006;15(16):2438–45. PMID: 16822851. http://www.ncbi.nlm.nih.gov/pubmed/16822851.
215. Neiswanger K, Zubenko GS, Giles DE, Frank E, Kupfer DJ, Kaplan BB. Linkage and association analysis of chromosomal regions containing genes related to neuroendocrine or serotonin function in families with early-onset, recurrent major depression. Am J Med Genet. 1998;81(5):443–9. PMID: 9754632. http://www.ncbi.nlm.nih.gov/pubmed/9754632.
216. Ørstavik RE, Kendler KS, Røysamb E, Czajkowski N, Tambs K, Reichborn-Kjennerud T. Genetic and environmental contributions to the co-occurrence of depressive personality disorder and DSM-IV personality disorders. J Personal Disord. 2012;26(3):435–51. PMCID: PMC3443639. http://www.ncbi.nlm.nih.gov/pubmed/22686231.
217. Kendler KS, Halberstadt LJ. The road not taken: life experiences in monozygotic twin pairs discordant for major depression. Mol Psychiatry. 2013;18(9):975–84. PMCID: PMC3523211. http://www.ncbi.nlm.nih.gov/pubmed/22641178.
218. Anguelova M, Benkelfat C, Turecki G. A systematic review of association studies investigating genes coding for serotonin receptors and the serotonin transporter: I. Affective disorders. Mol Psychiatry. 2003;8(6):574–91. PMID: 12851635. http://www.ncbi.nlm.nih.gov/pubmed/12851635.
219. Munafò MR, Clark TG, Moore LR, Payne E, Walton R, Flint J. Genetic polymorphisms and personality in healthy adults: a systematic review and meta-analysis. Mol Psychiatry. 2003;8(5):471–84. PMID: 12808427. http://www.ncbi.nlm.nih.gov/pubmed/12808427.
220. Kendler KS, Eaves LJ. Models for the joint effect of genotype and environment on liability to psychiatric illness. Am J Psychiatry. 1986;143(3):279–89. PMID: 3953861. http://www.ncbi.nlm.nih.gov/pubmed/3953861.
221. Lander ES, Schork NJ. Genetic dissection of complex traits. Science. 1994;265(5181):2037–48. PMID: 8091226. http://www.ncbi.nlm.nih.gov/pubmed/8091226.
222. Stoltenberg SF, Burmeister M. Recent progress in psychiatric genetics-some hope but no hype. Hum Mol Genet. 2000;9(6):927–35. PMID: 10767316. http://www.ncbi.nlm.nih.gov/pubmed/10767316.
223. Almasy L, Blangero J. Endophenotypes as quantitative risk factors for psychiatric disease: rationale and study design. Am J Med Genet. 2001;105(1):42–4. PMID: 11424994. http://www.ncbi.nlm.nih.gov/pubmed/11424994.
224. Sen S, Nesse RM, Stoltenberg SF, Li S, Gleiberman L, Chakravarti A, Weder AB, Burmeister M. A BDNF coding variant is associated with the NEO personality inventory domain neuroticism, a risk factor for depression. Neuropsychopharmacology. 2003;28(2):397–401. PMID: 12589394. http://www.ncbi.nlm.nih.gov/pubmed/12589394.
225. Costa PT, McCrae RR. Stability and change in personality assessment: the revised NEO Personality Inventory in the year 2000. J Pers Assess. 1997;68(1):86–94. PMID: 9018844. http://www.ncbi.nlm.nih.gov/pubmed/9018844.
226. Kendler KS, Neale MC, Kessler RC, Heath AC, Eaves LJ. A longitudinal twin study of personality and major depression in women. Arch Gen Psychiatry. 1993;50(11):853–62. PMID: 8215811. http://www.ncbi.nlm.nih.gov/pubmed/8215811.
227. Bagby RM, Young LT, Schuller DR, Bindseil KD, Cooke RG, Dickens SE, Levitt AJ, Joffe RT. Bipolar disorder, unipolar depression and the Five-Factor Model of personality. J Affect Disord. 1996;41(1):25–32. PMID: 8938202. http://www.ncbi.nlm.nih.gov/pubmed/8938202.
228. Lake RI, Eaves LJ, Maes HH, Heath AC, Martin NG. Further evidence against the environmental transmission of individual differences in neuroticism from a collaborative study of 45,850 twins and relatives on two continents. Behav Genet. 2000;30(3):223–33. PMID: 11105396. http://www.ncbi.nlm.nih.gov/pubmed/11105396.
229. Jang KL, Livesley WJ, Vernon PA. Heritability of the big five personality dimensions and their facets: a twin study. J Pers. 1996;64(3):577–91. PMID: 8776880. http://www.ncbi.nlm.nih.gov/pubmed/8776880.
230. Kendler KS, Karkowski LM, Prescott CA. Causal relationship between stressful life events and the onset of major depression. Am J Psychiatry. 1999;156(6):837–41. PMID: 10360120. http://www.ncbi.nlm.nih.gov/pubmed/10360120. http://www.ncbi.nlm.nih.gov/pubmed/10360120.
231. Terracciano A, Lobina M, Piras MG, Mulas A, Cannas A, Meirelles O, Sutin AR, Zonderman AB, Uda M, Crisponi L, Schlessinger D. Neuroticism, depressive symptoms, and serum BDNF. Psychosom Med. 2011;73(8):638–42. PMCID: PMC3188695. http://www.ncbi.nlm.nih.gov/pubmed/21949427.
232. Terracciano A, Martin B, Ansari D, Tanaka T, Ferrucci L, Maudsley S, Mattson MP, Costa PT. Plasma BDNF concentration, Val66Met genetic variant and depression-related personality traits. Genes Brain Behav. 2010;9(5):512–8. PMCID: PMC2907437. http://www.ncbi.nlm.nih.gov/pubmed/20345896.
233. Koido K, Traks T, Balõtšev R, Eller T, Must A, Koks S, Maron E, Tõru I, Shlik J, Vasar V, Vasar E. Associations between LSAMP gene polymorphisms and major depressive disorder and panic disorder. Transl Psychiatry. 2012;2(8):e152. PMCID: PMC3432189. http://www.ncbi.nlm.nih.gov/pubmed/22892717.
234. Kinser PA, Lyon DE. Major depressive disorder and measures of cellular aging: an integrative review. Nurs Res Pract. 2013;2013:469070. PMCID: PMC3649747. http://www.ncbi.nlm.nih.gov/pubmed/23691300.
235. Lubke GH, Hottenga JJ, Walters R, Laurin C, de Geus EJC, Willemsen G, Smit JH, Middeldorp CM, Penninx BWJH, Vink JM, Boomsma DI. Estimating the genetic variance of major depressive disorder due to all single nucleotide polymorphisms. Biol Psychiatry. 2012;72(8):707–9. PMCID: PMC3404250. http://www.ncbi.nlm.nih.gov/pubmed/22520966.
236. CONVERGE consortium. Sparse whole-genome sequencing identifies two loci for major depressive disorder. Nature. 2015;523(7562):588–91. PMCID: PMC4522619. http://www.ncbi.nlm.nih.gov/pubmed/26176920.
237. Rivera M, McGuffin P. The successful search for genetic loci associated with depression. Genome Med. 2015;7(1):92. PMCID: PMC4548917. http://www.ncbi.nlm.nih.gov/pubmed/26302953.
238. Zhang Y, Anoopkumar-Dukie S, Davey AK. SIRT1 and SIRT2 modulators: potential anti-inflammatory treatment for depression? Biomolecules. 2021;11(3):353. PMCID: PMC7996578. http://www.ncbi.nlm.nih.gov/pubmed/33669121.

239. Lei Y, Wang J, Wang D, Li C, Liu B, Fang X, You J, Guo M, Lu XY. SIRT1 in forebrain excitatory neurons produces sexually dimorphic effects on depression-related behaviors and modulates neuronal excitability and synaptic transmission in the medial prefrontal cortex. Mol Psychiatry. 2020;25(5):1094–111. PMCID: PMC7192847. http://www.ncbi.nlm.nih.gov/pubmed/30705425.
240. Wang D, Tang W, Zhao J, Fan W, Zhang Y, Zhang C. A comprehensive analysis of the effect of SIRT1 variation on the risk of Schizophrenia and depressive symptoms. Front Genet. 2020;11:832. PMCID: PMC7413929. http://www.ncbi.nlm.nih.gov/pubmed/32849821.
241. SIRT1 Gene - GeneCards | SIR1 Protein | SIR1 Antibody.
242. WikiGenes - LHPP - phospholysine phosphohistidine inorganic...
243. Kanner AM. Is major depression a neurologic disorder with psychiatric symptoms? Epilepsy Behav. 2004;5(5):636–44. PMID: 15380113. http://www.ncbi.nlm.nih.gov/pubmed/15380113.
244. Sapolsky RM. Glucocorticoids and hippocampal atrophy in neuropsychiatric disorders. Arch Gen Psychiatry. 2000;57(10):925–35. PMID: 11015810. http://www.ncbi.nlm.nih.gov/pubmed/11015810.
245. Krugers HJ, Lucassen PJ, Karst H, Joëls M. Chronic stress effects on hippocampal structure and synaptic function: relevance for depression and normalization by anti-glucocorticoid treatment. Front Synaptic Neurosci. 2010;2:24. PMCID: PMC3059694. http://www.ncbi.nlm.nih.gov/pubmed/21423510.
246. Neumeister A, Wood S, Bonne O, Nugent AC, Luckenbaugh DA, Young T, Bain EE, Charney DS, Drevets WC. Reduced hippocampal volume in unmedicated, remitted patients with major depression versus control subjects. Biol Psychiatry. 2005;57(8):935–7. PMID: 15820716. http://www.ncbi.nlm.nih.gov/pubmed/15820716.
247. López-Figueroa AL, Norton CS, López-Figueroa MO, Armellini-Dodel D, Burke S, Akil H, López JF, Watson SJ. Serotonin 5-HT1A, 5-HT1B, and 5-HT2A receptor mRNA expression in subjects with major depression, bipolar disorder, and schizophrenia. Biol Psychiatry. 2004;55(3):225–33. PMID: 14744462. http://www.ncbi.nlm.nih.gov/pubmed/14744462.
248. Videbech P, Ravnkilde B. Hippocampal volume and depression: a meta-analysis of MRI studies. Am J Psychiatry. 2004;161(11):1957–66. PMID: 15514393. http://www.ncbi.nlm.nih.gov/pubmed/15514393.
249. Sheline YI, Gado MH, Kraemer HC. Untreated depression and hippocampal volume loss. Am J Psychiatry. 2003;160(8):1516–8. PMID: 12900317. http://www.ncbi.nlm.nih.gov/pubmed/12900317.
250. Deicken RF, Pegues MP, Anzalone S, Feiwell R, Soher B. Lower concentration of hippocampal N-acetylaspartate in familial bipolar I disorder. Am J Psychiatry. 2003;160(5):873–82. PMID: 12727690. http://www.ncbi.nlm.nih.gov/pubmed/12727690.
251. MacMaster FP, Kusumakar V. Hippocampal volume in early onset depression. BMC Med. 2004;2:2. PMCID: PMC333436. http://www.ncbi.nlm.nih.gov/pubmed/14969587.
252. Strege MV, Siegle GJ, Richey JA, Krawczak RA, Young K. Cingulate prediction of response to antidepressant and cognitive behavioral therapies for depression: meta-analysis and empirical application. Brain Imaging Behav. 2023;17(4):450–60. PMCID: PMC10329727. http://www.ncbi.nlm.nih.gov/pubmed/36622532.
253. Driessen M, Herrmann J, Stahl K, Zwaan M, Meier S, Hill A, Osterheider M, Petersen D. Magnetic resonance imaging volumes of the hippocampus and the amygdala in women with borderline personality disorder and early traumatization. Arch Gen Psychiatry. 2000;57(12):1115–22. PMID: 11115325. http://www.ncbi.nlm.nih.gov/pubmed/11115325.
254. Niida A, Niida R, Matsuda H, Inada T, Motomura M, Uechi A. Identification of atrophy of the subgenual anterior cingulate cortex, in particular the subcallosal area, as an effective auxiliary means of diagnosis for major depressive disorder. Int J Gen Med. 2012;5:667–74. PMCID: PMC3422897. http://www.ncbi.nlm.nih.gov/pubmed/22924012.
255. Geerlings MI, Sigurdsson S, Eiriksdottir G, Garcia ME, Harris TB, Sigurdsson T, Gudnason V, Launer LJ. Associations of current and remitted major depressive disorder with brain atrophy: the AGES-Reykjavik study. Psychol Med. 2013;43(2):317–28. PMCID: PMC4244840. http://www.ncbi.nlm.nih.gov/pubmed/22647536.
256. Campbell S, Marriott M, Nahmias C, MacQueen GM. Lower hippocampal volume in patients suffering from depression: a meta-analysis. Am J Psychiatry. 2004;161(4):598–607. PMID: 15056502. http://www.ncbi.nlm.nih.gov/pubmed/15056502.
257. Drevets WC, Price JL, Simpson JR, Todd RD, Reich T, Vannier M, Raichle ME. Subgenual prefrontal cortex abnormalities in mood disorders. Nature. 1997;386(6627):824–7. PMID: 9126739. http://www.ncbi.nlm.nih.gov/pubmed/9126739.
258. Mayberg HS, Brannan SK, Mahurin RK, Jerabek PA, Brickman JS, Tekell JL, Silva JA, McGinnis S, Glass TG, Martin CC, Fox PT. Cingulate function in depression: a potential predictor of treatment response. Neuroreport. 1997;8(4):1057–61. PMID: 9141092 PMID: 9141092. http://www.ncbi.nlm.nih.gov/pubmed/9141092.
259. Mayberg HS, Liotti M, Brannan SK, McGinnis S, Mahurin RK, Jerabek PA, Silva JA, Tekell JL, Martin CC, Lancaster JL, Fox PT. Reciprocal limbic-cortical function and negative mood: converging PET findings in depression and normal sadness. Am J Psychiatry. 1999;156(5):675–82. PMID: 10327898. http://www.ncbi.nlm.nih.gov/pubmed/10327898.
260. Sliz D, Hayley S. Major depressive disorder and alterations in insular cortical activity: a review of current functional magnetic imaging research. Front Hum Neurosci. 2012;6:323. PMCID: PMC3512092. http://www.ncbi.nlm.nih.gov/pubmed/23227005.
261. Molendijk ML, Bus BAA, Spinhoven P, Kaimatzoglou A, Oude Voshaar RC, Penninx BWJH, van IJzendoorn MH, Elzinga BM. A systematic review and meta-analysis on the association between BDNF val(66)met and hippocampal volume—a genuine effect or a winners curse? Am J Med Genet B Neuropsychiatr Genet. 2012;159B(6):731–40. PMID: 22815222. http://www.ncbi.nlm.nih.gov/pubmed/22815222.
262. Warner-Schmidt JL, Duman RS. Hippocampal neurogenesis: opposing effects of stress and antidepressant treatment. Hippocampus. 2006;16(3):239–49. PMID: 16425236. http://www.ncbi.nlm.nih.gov/pubmed/16425236.
263. DeCarolis NA, Eisch AJ. Hippocampal neurogenesis as a target for the treatment of mental illness: a critical evaluation. Neuropharmacology. 2010;58(6):884–93. PMCID: PMC2839019. http://www.ncbi.nlm.nih.gov/pubmed/20060007.
264. Santarelli L, Saxe M, Gross C, Surget A, Battaglia F, Dulawa S, Weisstaub N, Lee J, Duman R, Arancio O, Belzung C, Hen R. Requirement of hippocampal neurogenesis for the behavioral effects of antidepressants. Science. 2003;301(5634):805–9. PMID: 12907793. http://www.ncbi.nlm.nih.gov/pubmed/12907793.
265. Schmidt HD, Duman RS. The role of neurotrophic factors in adult hippocampal neurogenesis, antidepressant treatments and animal models of depressive-like behavior. Behav Pharmacol. 2007;18(5–6):391–418. PMID: 17762509. http://www.ncbi.nlm.nih.gov/pubmed/17762509.
266. Hunsberger J, Austin DR, Henter ID, Chen G. The neurotrophic and neuroprotective effects of psychotropic agents. Dialogues Clin Neurosci. 2009;11(3):333–48. PMCID: PMC2804881. http://www.ncbi.nlm.nih.gov/pubmed/19877500.
267. Marwood L, Wise T, Perkins AM, Cleare AJ. Meta-analyses of the neural mechanisms and predictors of response to psychotherapy in depression and anxiety. Neurosci Biobehav Rev. 2018;95:61–72. PMCID: PMC6267850. http://www.ncbi.nlm.nih.gov/pubmed/30278195.

268. Apkarian AV, Sosa Y, Sonty S, Levy RM, Harden RN, Parrish TB, Gitelman DR. Chronic back pain is associated with decreased prefrontal and thalamic gray matter density. J Neurosci. 2004;24(46):10410–5. PMCID: PMC6730296. http://www.ncbi.nlm.nih.gov/pubmed/15548656.
269. Gustafson D, Lissner L, Bengtsson C, Björkelund C, Skoog I. A 24-year follow-up of body mass index and cerebral atrophy. Neurology. 2004;63(10):1876–81. PMID: 15557505. http://www.ncbi.nlm.nih.gov/pubmed/15557505.
270. Ongür D, Price JL. The organization of networks within the orbital and medial prefrontal cortex of rats, monkeys and humans. Cereb Cortex. 2000;10(3):206–19. PMID: 10731217. http://www.ncbi.nlm.nih.gov/pubmed/10731217.
271. De Raedt R, Koster EHW. Understanding vulnerability for depression from a cognitive neuroscience perspective: a reappraisal of attentional factors and a new conceptual framework. Cogn Affect Behav Neurosci. 2010;10(1):50–70. PMID: 20233955. http://www.ncbi.nlm.nih.gov/pubmed/20233955.
272. Nejad AB, Fossati P, Lemogne C. Self-referential processing, rumination, and cortical midline structures in major depression. Front Hum Neurosci. 2013;7:666. PMCID: PMC3794427. http://www.ncbi.nlm.nih.gov/pubmed/24124416.
273. Parker KJ, Schatzberg AF, Lyons DM. Neuroendocrine aspects of hypercortisolism in major depression. Horm Behav. 2003;43(1):60–6. PMID: 12614635. http://www.ncbi.nlm.nih.gov/pubmed/12614635.
274. Owashi T, Otsubo T, Oshima A, Nakagome K, Higuchi T, Kamijima K. Relationships of DEX/CRH and GHRH test results to the outcome of depression--preliminary results suggest the GHRH test may predict relapse after discharge. J Psychiatr Res. 2008;42(5):356–64. PMID: 17412362. http://www.ncbi.nlm.nih.gov/pubmed/17412362.
275. Tichomirowa MA, Keck ME, Schneider HJ, Paez-Pereda M, Renner U, Holsboer F, Stalla GK. Endocrine disturbances in depression. J Endocrinol Investig. 2005;28(1):89–99. PMID: 15816377. http://www.ncbi.nlm.nih.gov/pubmed/15816377.
276. Joyce PR. Neuroendocrine changes in depression. Aust N Z J Psychiatry. 1985;19(2):120–7. PMID: 2413836. http://www.ncbi.nlm.nih.gov/pubmed/2413836.
277. Rupprecht R, Lesch KP. Psychoneuroendocrine research in depression. I. Hormone levels of different neuroendocrine axes and the dexamethasone suppression test. J Neural Transm. 1989;75(3):167–78. PMID: 2538556. http://www.ncbi.nlm.nih.gov/pubmed/2538556.
278. Lesch KP, Müller U, Rupprecht R, Kruse K, Schulte HM. Endocrine responses to growth hormone-releasing hormone, thyrotropin-releasing hormone and corticotropin-releasing hormone in depression. Acta Psychiatr Scand. 1989;79(6):597–602. PMID: 2548370. http://www.ncbi.nlm.nih.gov/pubmed/2548370.
279. Frodl T, O'Keane V. How does the brain deal with cumulative stress? A review with focus on developmental stress, HPA axis function and hippocampal structure in humans. Neurobiol Dis. 2013;52:24–37. PMID: 22426398. http://www.ncbi.nlm.nih.gov/pubmed/22426398.
280. Swaab DF, Bao AM, Lucassen PJ. The stress system in the human brain in depression and neurodegeneration. Ageing Res Rev. 2005;4(2):141–94. PMID: 15996533. http://www.ncbi.nlm.nih.gov/pubmed/15996533.
281. Marković VM, Čupić Ž, Vukojević V, Kolar-Anić L. Predictive modeling of the hypothalamic-pituitary-adrenal (HPA) axis response to acute and chronic stress. Endocr J. 2011;58(10):889–904. PMID: 21852742. http://www.ncbi.nlm.nih.gov/pubmed/21852742.
282. Engelmann M, Landgraf R, Wotjak CT. The hypothalamic-neurohypophysial system regulates the hypothalamic-pituitary-adrenal axis under stress: an old concept revisited. Front Neuroendocrinol. 2004;25(3–4):132–49. PMID: 15589266. http://www.ncbi.nlm.nih.gov/pubmed/15589266.
283. Checkley S. Neuroendocrine mechanisms and the precipitation of depression by life events. Br J Psychiatry Suppl. 1992;(15):7–17. PMID: 1356360. http://www.ncbi.nlm.nih.gov/pubmed/1356360.
284. Murphy BE, Ghadirian AM, Dhar V. Neuroendocrine responses to inhibitors of steroid biosynthesis in patients with major depression resistant to antidepressant therapy. Can J Psychiatr. 1998;43(3):279–86. PMID: 9561317. http://www.ncbi.nlm.nih.gov/pubmed/9561317.
285. Claes SJ. Corticotropin-releasing hormone (CRH) in psychiatry: from stress to psychopathology. Ann Med. 2004;36(1):50–61. PMID: 15000347. http://www.ncbi.nlm.nih.gov/pubmed/15000347.
286. Gallagher JP, Orozco-Cabal LF, Liu J, Shinnick-Gallagher P. Synaptic physiology of central CRH system. Eur J Pharmacol. 2008;583(2–3):215–25. PMCID: PMC2424315. http://www.ncbi.nlm.nih.gov/pubmed/18342852.
287. Bonfiglio JJ, Inda C, Refojo D, Holsboer F, Arzt E, Silberstein S. The corticotropin-releasing hormone network and the hypothalamic-pituitary-adrenal axis: molecular and cellular mechanisms involved. Neuroendocrinology. 2011;94(1):12–20. PMID: 21576930. http://www.ncbi.nlm.nih.gov/pubmed/21576930.
288. Scott LV, Medbak S, Dinan TG. Desmopressin augments pituitary-adrenal responsivity to corticotropin-releasing hormone in subjects with chronic fatigue syndrome and in healthy volunteers. Biol Psychiatry. 1999;45(11):1447–54. PMID: 10356627. http://www.ncbi.nlm.nih.gov/pubmed/10356627.
289. Dinan TG, O'Brien S, Lavelle E, Scott LV. Further neuroendocrine evidence of enhanced vasopressin V3 receptor responses in melancholic depression. Psychol Med. 2004;34(1):169–72. PMID: 14971638. http://www.ncbi.nlm.nih.gov/pubmed/14971638.
290. Tafet GE, Smolovich J. Psychoneuroendocrinological studies on chronic stress and depression. Ann N Y Acad Sci. 2004;1032:276–8. PMID: 15677427. http://www.ncbi.nlm.nih.gov/pubmed/15677427.
291. Tafet GE, Bernardini R. Psychoneuroendocrinological links between chronic stress and depression. Prog Neuro-Psychopharmacol Biol Psychiatry. 2003;27(6):893–903. PMID: 14499305. http://www.ncbi.nlm.nih.gov/pubmed/14499305.
292. DeRijk RH, Schaaf M, de Kloet ER. Glucocorticoid receptor variants: clinical implications. J Steroid Biochem Mol Biol. 2002;81(2):103–22. PMID: 12137800. http://www.ncbi.nlm.nih.gov/pubmed/12137800.
293. Binder EB. The role of FKBP5, a co-chaperone of the glucocorticoid receptor in the pathogenesis and therapy of affective and anxiety disorders. Psychoneuroendocrinology. 2009;34(Suppl 1):S186–95. PMID: 19560279. http://www.ncbi.nlm.nih.gov/pubmed/19560279.
294. Mehta D, Gonik M, Klengel T, Rex-Haffner M, Menke A, Rubel J, Mercer KB, Pütz B, Bradley B, Holsboer F, Ressler KJ, Müller-Myhsok B, Binder EB. Using polymorphisms in FKBP5 to define biologically distinct subtypes of posttraumatic stress disorder: evidence from endocrine and gene expression studies. Arch Gen Psychiatry. 2011;68(9):901–10. PMCID: PMC3686481. http://www.ncbi.nlm.nih.gov/pubmed/21536970.
295. Zou YF, Wang F, Feng XL, Li WF, Tao JH, Pan FM, Huang F, Su H. Meta-analysis of FKBP5 gene polymorphisms association with treatment response in patients with mood disorders. Neurosci Lett. 2010;484(1):56–61. PMID: 20709156. http://www.ncbi.nlm.nih.gov/pubmed/20709156.
296. Binder EB, Bradley RG, Liu W, Epstein MP, Deveau TC, Mercer KB, Tang Y, Gillespie CF, Heim CM, Nemeroff CB, Schwartz AC, Cubells JF, Ressler KJ. Association of FKBP5 polymorphisms and childhood abuse with risk of posttraumatic stress disorder

symptoms in adults. JAMA. 2008;299(11):1291–305. PMCID: PMC2441757. http://www.ncbi.nlm.nih.gov/pubmed/18349090.
297. Pratt WB, Toft DO. Steroid receptor interactions with heat shock protein and immunophilin chaperones. Endocr Rev. 1997;18(3):306–60. PMID: 9183567. http://www.ncbi.nlm.nih.gov/pubmed/9183567.
298. Tyrka AR, Price LH, Gelernter J, Schepker C, Anderson GM, Carpenter LL. Interaction of childhood maltreatment with the corticotropin-releasing hormone receptor gene: effects on hypothalamic-pituitary-adrenal axis reactivity. Biol Psychiatry. 2009;66(7):681–5. PMCID: PMC2881567. http://www.ncbi.nlm.nih.gov/pubmed/17544379.
299. Malarkey WB, Mills PJ. Endocrinology: the active partner in PNI research. Brain Behav Immun. 2007;21(2):161–8. PMCID: PMC2569824. http://www.ncbi.nlm.nih.gov/pubmed/17174524.
300. Dhabhar FS, McEwen BS. Acute stress enhances while chronic stress suppresses cell-mediated immunity in vivo: a potential role for leukocyte trafficking. Brain Behav Immun. 1997;11(4):286–306. PMID: 9512816. http://www.ncbi.nlm.nih.gov/pubmed/9512816.
301. Dhabhar FS, Miller AH, Stein M, McEwen BS, Spencer RL. Diurnal and acute stress-induced changes in distribution of peripheral blood leukocyte subpopulations. Brain Behav Immun. 1994;8(1):66–79. PMID: 8003772. http://www.ncbi.nlm.nih.gov/pubmed/8003772.
302. Dhabhar FS, Miller AH, McEwen BS, Spencer RL. Effects of stress on immune cell distribution. Dynamics and hormonal mechanisms. J Immunol. 1995;154(10):5511–27. PMID: 7730652. http://www.ncbi.nlm.nih.gov/pubmed/7730652.
303. de Kloet ER, Derijk RH, Meijer OC. Therapy Insight: is there an imbalanced response of mineralocorticoid and glucocorticoid receptors in depression? Nat Clin Pract Endocrinol Metab. 2007;3(2):168–79. PMID: 17237843. http://www.ncbi.nlm.nih.gov/pubmed/17237843.
304. van Rossum EFC, Koper JW, Huizenga NATM, Uitterlinden AG, Janssen JAMJL, Brinkmann AO, Grobbee DE, de Jong FH, van Duyn CM, Pols HAP, Lamberts SWJ. A polymorphism in the glucocorticoid receptor gene, which decreases sensitivity to glucocorticoids in vivo, is associated with low insulin and cholesterol levels. Diabetes. 2002;51(10):3128–34. PMID: 12351458. http://www.ncbi.nlm.nih.gov/pubmed/12351458.
305. van West D, Van Den Eede F, Del-Favero J, Souery D, Norrback KF, Van Duijn C, Sluijs S, Adolfsson R, Mendlewicz J, Deboutte D, Van Broeckhoven C, Claes S. Glucocorticoid receptor gene-based SNP analysis in patients with recurrent major depression. Neuropsychopharmacology. 2006;31(3):620–7. PMID: 16192984. http://www.ncbi.nlm.nih.gov/pubmed/16192984.
306. Russcher H, Smit P, van den Akker ELT, van Rossum EFC, Brinkmann AO, de Jong FH, Lamberts SWJ, Koper JW. Two polymorphisms in the glucocorticoid receptor gene directly affect glucocorticoid-regulated gene expression. J Clin Endocrinol Metab. 2005;90(10):5804–10. PMID: 16030164. http://www.ncbi.nlm.nih.gov/pubmed/16030164.
307. Manenschijn L, van den Akker ELT, Lamberts SWJ, van Rossum EFC. Clinical features associated with glucocorticoid receptor polymorphisms. an overview. Ann N Y Acad Sci. 2009;1179:179–98. PMID: 19906240. http://www.ncbi.nlm.nih.gov/pubmed/19906240.
308. van Rossum EFC, Koper JW, van den Beld AW, Uitterlinden AG, Arp P, Ester W, Janssen JAMJL, Brinkmann AO, de Jong FH, Grobbee DE, Pols HAP, Lamberts SWJ. Identification of the BclI polymorphism in the glucocorticoid receptor gene: association with sensitivity to glucocorticoids in vivo and body mass index. Clin Endocrinol. 2003;59(5):585–92. PMID: 14616881. http://www.ncbi.nlm.nih.gov/pubmed/14616881.
309. van Rossum EFC, Feelders RA, van den Beld AW, Uitterlinden AG, Janssen JAMJL, Ester W, Brinkmann AO, Grobbee DE, de Jong FH, Pols HAP, Koper JW, Lamberts SWJ. Association of the ER22/23EK polymorphism in the glucocorticoid receptor gene with survival and C-reactive protein levels in elderly men. Am J Med. 2004;117(3):158–62. PMID: 15276593. http://www.ncbi.nlm.nih.gov/pubmed/15276593.
310. Bet PM, Penninx BWJH, Bochdanovits Z, Uitterlinden AG, Beekman ATF, van Schoor NM, Deeg DJH, Hoogendijk WJG. Glucocorticoid receptor gene polymorphisms and childhood adversity are associated with depression: new evidence for a gene-environment interaction. Am J Med Genet B Neuropsychiatr Genet. 2009;150B(5):660–9. PMID: 19051288. http://www.ncbi.nlm.nih.gov/pubmed/19051288.
311. Menke A, Klengel T, Binder EB. Epigenetics, depression and antidepressant treatment. Curr Pharm Des. 2012;18(36):5879–89. PMID: 22681167. http://www.ncbi.nlm.nih.gov/pubmed/22681167.
312. McGowan PO, Sasaki A, Huang TCT, Unterberger A, Suderman M, Ernst C, Meaney MJ, Turecki G, Szyf M. Promoter-wide hypermethylation of the ribosomal RNA gene promoter in the suicide brain. PLoS One. 2008;3(5):e2085. PMCID: PMC2330072. http://www.ncbi.nlm.nih.gov/pubmed/18461137.
313. McGowan PO, Sasaki A, D'Alessio AC, Dymov S, Labonté B, Szyf M, Turecki G, Meaney MJ. Epigenetic regulation of the glucocorticoid receptor in human brain associates with childhood abuse. Nat Neurosci. 2009;12(3):342–8. PMCID: PMC2944040. http://www.ncbi.nlm.nih.gov/pubmed/19234457.
314. Alt SR, Turner JD, Klok MD, Meijer OC, Lakke EAJF, Derijk RH, Muller CP. Differential expression of glucocorticoid receptor transcripts in major depressive disorder is not epigenetically programmed. Psychoneuroendocrinology. 2010;35(4):544–56. PMID: 19782477. http://www.ncbi.nlm.nih.gov/pubmed/19782477.
315. Spijker AT, van Rossum EFC. Glucocorticoid sensitivity in mood disorders. Neuroendocrinology. 2012;95(3):179–86. PMID: 22076031. http://www.ncbi.nlm.nih.gov/pubmed/22076031.
316. Carpenter LL, Tyrka AR, Ross NS, Khoury L, Anderson GM, Price LH. Effect of childhood emotional abuse and age on cortisol responsivity in adulthood. Biol Psychiatry. 2009;66(1):69–75. PMCID: PMC2696583. http://www.ncbi.nlm.nih.gov/pubmed/19375070.
317. Polanczyk G, Caspi A, Williams B, Price TS, Danese A, Sugden K, Uher R, Poulton R, Moffitt TE. Protective effect of CRHR1 gene variants on the development of adult depression following childhood maltreatment: replication and extension. Arch Gen Psychiatry. 2009;66(9):978–85. PMCID: PMC3750953. http://www.ncbi.nlm.nih.gov/pubmed/19736354.
318. Nugent NR, Tyrka AR, Carpenter LL, Price LH. Gene-environment interactions: early life stress and risk for depressive and anxiety disorders. Psychopharmacology. 2011;214(1):175–96. PMCID: PMC3615637. http://www.ncbi.nlm.nih.gov/pubmed/21225419.
319. Krishnamurthy P, Romagni P, Torvik S, Gold PW, Charney DS, Detera-Wadleigh S, Cizza G, P.O.W.E.R. (Premenopausal, Osteoporosis Women, Alendronate, Depression) Study Group. Glucocorticoid receptor gene polymorphisms in premenopausal women with major depression. Horm Metab Res. 2008;40(3):194–8. PMID: 18246526. http://www.ncbi.nlm.nih.gov/pubmed/18246526.
320. Sternberg EM, Chrousos GP, Wilder RL, Gold PW. The stress response and the regulation of inflammatory disease. Ann Intern Med. 1992;117(10):854–66. PMID: 1416562. http://www.ncbi.nlm.nih.gov/pubmed/1416562.
321. Coplan JD, Wolk SI, Goetz RR, Ryan ND, Dahl RE, Mann JJ, Weissman MM. Nocturnal growth hormone secretion studies in adolescents with or without major depression re-examined:

integration of adult clinical follow-up data. Biol Psychiatry. 2000;47(7):594–604. PMID: 10745051. http://www.ncbi.nlm.nih.gov/pubmed/10745051.
322. Cleare AJ, Bearn J, Allain T, McGregor A, Wessely S, Murray RM, O'Keane V. Contrasting neuroendocrine responses in depression and chronic fatigue syndrome. J Affect Disord. 1995;34(4):283–9. PMID: 8550954. http://www.ncbi.nlm.nih.gov/pubmed/8550954.
323. McCrory E, De Brito SA, Viding E. Research review: the neurobiology and genetics of maltreatment and adversity. J Child Psychol Psychiatry. 2010;51(10):1079–95. PMID: 20546078. http://www.ncbi.nlm.nih.gov/pubmed/20546078.
324. Murgatroyd C, Spengler D. Epigenetics of early child development. Front Psych. 2011;2:16. PMCID: PMC3102328. http://www.ncbi.nlm.nih.gov/pubmed/21647402.
325. De Bellis MD, Kuchibhatla M. Cerebellar volumes in pediatric maltreatment-related posttraumatic stress disorder. Biol Psychiatry. 2006;60(7):697–703. PMID: 16934769. http://www.ncbi.nlm.nih.gov/pubmed/16934769.
326. Lindemer ER, Salat DH, Leritz EC, McGlinchey RE, Milberg WP. Reduced cortical thickness with increased lifetime burden of PTSD in OEF/OIF Veterans and the impact of comorbid TBI. Neuroimage Clin. 2013;2:601–11. PMCID: PMC3777819. http://www.ncbi.nlm.nih.gov/pubmed/24179811.
327. Koenen KC, Driver KL, Oscar-Berman M, Wolfe J, Folsom S, Huang MT, Schlesinger L. Measures of prefrontal system dysfunction in posttraumatic stress disorder. Brain Cogn. 2001;45(1):64–78. PMID: 11161363. http://www.ncbi.nlm.nih.gov/pubmed/11161363.
328. Leaf CD, Wishnok JS, Tannenbaum SR. Mechanisms of endogenous nitrosation. Cancer Surv. 1989;8(2):323–34. PMID: 2696583. http://www.ncbi.nlm.nih.gov/pubmed/2696583.
329. Chida Y, Steptoe A. Cortisol awakening response and psychosocial factors: a systematic review and meta-analysis. Biol Psychol. 2009;80(3):265–78. PMID: 19022335. http://www.ncbi.nlm.nih.gov/pubmed/19022335.
330. Eiland L, McEwen BS. Early life stress followed by subsequent adult chronic stress potentiates anxiety and blunts hippocampal structural remodeling. Hippocampus. 2012;22(1):82–91. PMID: 20848608. http://www.ncbi.nlm.nih.gov/pubmed/20848608.
331. Lopez MF, Doremus-Fitzwater TL, Becker HC. Chronic social isolation and chronic variable stress during early development induce later elevated ethanol intake in adult C57BL/6J mice. Alcohol. 2011;45(4):355–64. PMCID: PMC3013234. http://www.ncbi.nlm.nih.gov/pubmed/20880662.
332. Vreeburg SA, Hoogendijk WJG, van Pelt J, Derijk RH, Verhagen JCM, van Dyck R, Smit JH, Zitman FG, Penninx BWJH. Major depressive disorder and hypothalamic-pituitary-adrenal axis activity: results from a large cohort study. Arch Gen Psychiatry. 2009;66(6):617–26. PMID: 19487626. http://www.ncbi.nlm.nih.gov/pubmed/19487626.
333. Vreeburg SA, Kruijtzer BP, van Pelt J, van Dyck R, DeRijk RH, Hoogendijk WJG, Smit JH, Zitman FG, Penninx BWJH. Associations between sociodemographic, sampling and health factors and various salivary cortisol indicators in a large sample without psychopathology. Psychoneuroendocrinology. 2009;34(8):1109–20. PMID: 19515498. http://www.ncbi.nlm.nih.gov/pubmed/19515498.
334. Adam EK, Doane LD, Zinbarg RE, Mineka S, Craske MG, Griffith JW. Prospective prediction of major depressive disorder from cortisol awakening responses in adolescence. Psychoneuroendocrinology. 2010;35(6):921–31. PMCID: PMC2875344. http://www.ncbi.nlm.nih.gov/pubmed/20079576.
335. Vreeburg SA, Hartman CA, Hoogendijk WJG, van Dyck R, Zitman FG, Ormel J, Penninx BWJH. Parental history of depression or anxiety and the cortisol awakening response. Br J Psychiatry. 2010;197(3):180–5. PMID: 20807961. http://www.ncbi.nlm.nih.gov/pubmed/20807961.
336. Burke HM, Davis MC, Otte C, Mohr DC. Depression and cortisol responses to psychological stress: a meta-analysis. Psychoneuroendocrinology. 2005;30(9):846–56. PMID: 15961250. http://www.ncbi.nlm.nih.gov/pubmed/15961250.
337. Ising M, Horstmann S, Kloiber S, Lucae S, Binder EB, Kern N, Künzel HE, Pfennig A, Uhr M, Holsboer F. Combined dexamethasone/corticotropin releasing hormone test predicts treatment response in major depression - a potential biomarker? Biol Psychiatry. 2007;62(1):47–54. PMID: 17123470. http://www.ncbi.nlm.nih.gov/pubmed/17123470.
338. Appelhof BC, Huyser J, Verweij M, Brouwer JP, van Dyck R, Fliers E, Hoogendijk WJG, Tijssen JGP, Wiersinga WM, Schene AH. Glucocorticoids and relapse of major depression (dexamethasone/corticotropin-releasing hormone test in relation to relapse of major depression). Biol Psychiatry. 2006;59(8):696–701. PMID: 16368077. http://www.ncbi.nlm.nih.gov/pubmed/16368077.
339. Zobel AW, Nickel T, Sonntag A, Uhr M, Holsboer F, Ising M. Cortisol response in the combined dexamethasone/CRH test as predictor of relapse in patients with remitted depression. A prospective study. J Psychiatr Res. 2001;35(2):83–94. PMID: 11377437. http://www.ncbi.nlm.nih.gov/pubmed/11377437.
340. Manenschijn L, Koper JW, Lamberts SWJ, van Rossum EFC. Evaluation of a method to measure long term cortisol levels. Steroids. 2011;76(10–11):1032–6. PMID: 21515299. http://www.ncbi.nlm.nih.gov/pubmed/21515299.
341. Van Uum SHM, Sauvé B, Fraser LA, Morley-Forster P, Paul TL, Koren G. Elevated content of cortisol in hair of patients with severe chronic pain: a novel biomarker for stress. Stress. 2008;11(6):483–8. PMID: 18609301. http://www.ncbi.nlm.nih.gov/pubmed/18609301.
342. Davalos DB, Yadon CA, Tregellas HC. Untreated prenatal maternal depression and the potential risks to offspring: a review. Arch Womens Ment Health. 2012;15(1):1–14. PMID: 22215285. http://www.ncbi.nlm.nih.gov/pubmed/22215285.
343. O'Keane V, Lightman S, Marsh M, Pawlby S, Papadopoulos AS, Taylor A, Moore R, Patrick K. Increased pituitary-adrenal activation and shortened gestation in a sample of depressed pregnant women: a pilot study. J Affect Disord. 2011;130(1–2):300–5. PMID: 21093926. http://www.ncbi.nlm.nih.gov/pubmed/21093926.
344. Schutter DJLG. The cerebello-hypothalamic-pituitary-adrenal axis dysregulation hypothesis in depressive disorder. Med Hypotheses. 2012;79(6):779–83. PMID: 22999737. http://www.ncbi.nlm.nih.gov/pubmed/22999737.
345. Mortola JF, Liu JH, Gillin JC, Rasmussen DD, Yen SS. Pulsatile rhythms of adrenocorticotropin (ACTH) and cortisol in women with endogenous depression: evidence for increased ACTH pulse frequency. J Clin Endocrinol Metab. 1987;65(5):962–8. PMID: 2822756. http://www.ncbi.nlm.nih.gov/pubmed/2822756.
346. Axelson DA, Doraiswamy PM, Boyko OB, Rodrigo Escalona P, McDonald WM, Ritchie JC, Patterson LJ, Ellinwood EH, Nemeroff CB, Krishnan KR. In vivo assessment of pituitary volume with magnetic resonance imaging and systematic stereology: relationship to dexamethasone suppression test results in patients. Psychiatry Res. 1992;44(1):63–70. PMID: 1461948. http://www.ncbi.nlm.nih.gov/pubmed/1461948.
347. Cleare AJ, McGregor A, O'Keane V. Neuroendocrine evidence for an association between hypothyroidism, reduced central 5-HT activity and depression. Clin Endocrinol. 1995;43(6):713–9. PMID: 8736274. http://www.ncbi.nlm.nih.gov/pubmed/8736274.
348. Targum SD, Sullivan AC, Byrnes SM. Neuroendocrine interrelationships in major depressive disorder. Am J Psychiatry.

1982;139(3):282–6. PMID: 6800269. http://www.ncbi.nlm.nih.gov/pubmed/6800269.
349. Targum SD, Sullivan AC, Byrnes SM. Compensatory pituitary-thyroid mechanisms in major depressive disorder. Psychiatry Res. 1982;6(1):85–96. PMID: 6799973. http://www.ncbi.nlm.nih.gov/pubmed/6799973.
350. Targum SD. Persistent neuroendocrine dysregulation in major depressive disorder: a marker for early relapse. Biol Psychiatry. 1984;19(3):305–18. PMID: 6426529. http://www.ncbi.nlm.nih.gov/pubmed/6426529.
351. Dinan TG. Psychoneuroendocrinology of depression. Growth hormone. Psychiatr Clin North Am. 1998;21(2):325–39. PMID: 9670229. http://www.ncbi.nlm.nih.gov/pubmed/9670229.
352. Mahajan T, Crown A, Checkley S, Farmer A, Lightman S. Atypical depression in growth hormone deficient adults, and the beneficial effects of growth hormone treatment on depression and quality of life. Eur J Endocrinol. 2004;151(3):325–32. PMID: 15362961. http://www.ncbi.nlm.nih.gov/pubmed/15362961.
353. Antonijevic IA, Murck H, Frieboes RM, Steiger A. Sexually dimorphic effects of GHRH on sleep-endocrine activity in patients with depression and normal controls - part II: hormone secretion. Sleep Res Online. 2000;3(1):15–21. PMID: 11382895. http://www.ncbi.nlm.nih.gov/pubmed/11382895.
354. Thase ME, Reynolds CF, Frank E, Simons AD, McGeary J, Fasiczka AL, Garamoni GG, Jennings JR, Kupfer DJ. Do depressed men and women respond similarly to cognitive behavior therapy? Am J Psychiatry. 1994;151(4):500–5. PMID: 8147447. http://www.ncbi.nlm.nih.gov/pubmed/8147447.
355. Cole MA, Kim PJ, Kalman BA, Spencer RL. Dexamethasone suppression of corticosteroid secretion: evaluation of the site of action by receptor measures and functional studies. Psychoneuroendocrinology. 2000;25(2):151–67. PMID: 10674279. http://www.ncbi.nlm.nih.gov/pubmed/10674279.
356. Fountoulakis KN, Gonda X, Rihmer Z, Fokas C, Iacovides A. Revisiting the Dexamethasone suppression test in unipolar major depression: an exploratory study. Ann General Psychiatry. 2008;7:22. PMCID: PMC2590593. http://www.ncbi.nlm.nih.gov/pubmed/19014558.
357. McEwen BS. Invited review: Estrogens effects on the brain: multiple sites and molecular mechanisms. J Appl Physiol (1985). 2001;91(6):2785–801. PMID: 11717247. http://www.ncbi.nlm.nih.gov/pubmed/11717247.
358. Toran-Allerand CD. Estrogen and the brain: beyond ER-alpha and ER-beta. Exp Gerontol. 2004;39(11–12):1579–86. PMID: 15582272. http://www.ncbi.nlm.nih.gov/pubmed/15582272.
359. Kolltveit S, Lange-Nielsen II, Thabet AAM, Dyregrov A, Pallesen S, Johnsen TB, Laberg JC. Risk factors for PTSD, anxiety, and depression among adolescents in Gaza. J Trauma Stress. 2012;25(2):164–70. PMID: 22522730. http://www.ncbi.nlm.nih.gov/pubmed/22522730.
360. Edwards AC, Rose RJ, Kaprio J, Dick DM. Pubertal development moderates the importance of environmental influences on depressive symptoms in adolescent girls and boys. J Youth Adolesc. 2011;40(10):1383–93. PMCID: PMC3091957. http://www.ncbi.nlm.nih.gov/pubmed/21136145.
361. Fernandez Castelao C, Kröner-Herwig B. Different trajectories of depressive symptoms in children and adolescents: predictors and differences in girls and boys. J Youth Adolesc. 2013;42(8):1169–82. PMCID: PMC3714554. http://www.ncbi.nlm.nih.gov/pubmed/23160660.
362. Joinson C, Heron J, Araya R, Paus T, Croudace T, Rubin C, Marcus M, Lewis G. Association between pubertal development and depressive symptoms in girls from a UK cohort. Psychol Med. 2012;42(12):2579–89. PMID: 22717026. http://www.ncbi.nlm.nih.gov/pubmed/22717026.
363. Sherwin BB. Estrogen and cognitive functioning in women: lessons we have learned. Behav Neurosci. 2012;126(1):123–7. PMCID: PMC4838456. http://www.ncbi.nlm.nih.gov/pubmed/22004260.
364. Phillips SM, Sherwin BB. Effects of estrogen on memory function in surgically menopausal women. Psychoneuroendocrinology. 1992;17(5):485–95. PMID: 1484915. http://www.ncbi.nlm.nih.gov/pubmed/1484915.
365. Sherwin BB. Estrogen and/or androgen replacement therapy and cognitive functioning in surgically menopausal women. Psychoneuroendocrinology. 1988;13(4):345–57. PMID: 3067252. http://www.ncbi.nlm.nih.gov/pubmed/3067252.
366. Rubinow DR, Schmidt PJ, Roca CA. Estrogen-serotonin interactions: implications for affective regulation. Biol Psychiatry. 1998;44(9):839–50. PMID: 9807639. http://www.ncbi.nlm.nih.gov/pubmed/9807639.
367. Schmidt PJ, Nieman LK, Danaceau MA, Adams LF, Rubinow DR. Differential behavioral effects of gonadal steroids in women with and in those without premenstrual syndrome. N Engl J Med. 1998;338(4):209–16. PMID: 9435325. http://www.ncbi.nlm.nih.gov/pubmed/9435325.
368. McEwen BS, Alves SE. Estrogen actions in the central nervous system. Endocr Rev. 1999;20(3):279–307. PMID: 10368772. http://www.ncbi.nlm.nih.gov/pubmed/10368772.
369. Cutter WJ, Norbury R, Murphy DGM. Oestrogen, brain function, and neuropsychiatric disorders. J Neurol Neurosurg Psychiatry. 2003;74(7):837–40. PMCID: PMC1738534. http://www.ncbi.nlm.nih.gov/pubmed/12810759.
370. McEwen BS. Plasticity of the hippocampus: adaptation to chronic stress and allostatic load. Ann N Y Acad Sci. 2001;933:265–77. PMID: 12000027. http://www.ncbi.nlm.nih.gov/pubmed/12000027.
371. Eichenbaum H, Otto T, Cohen NJ. The hippocampus—what does it do? Behav Neural Biol. 1992;57(1):2–36. PMID: 1567331. http://www.ncbi.nlm.nih.gov/pubmed/1567331.
372. Rajewska J, Rybakowski JK. Depression in premenopausal women: gonadal hormones and serotonergic system assessed by D-fenfluramine challenge test. Prog Neuro-Psychopharmacol Biol Psychiatry. 2003;27(4):705–9. PMID: 12787860. http://www.ncbi.nlm.nih.gov/pubmed/12787860.
373. Harlow BL, Wise LA, Otto MW, Soares CN, Cohen LS. Depression and its influence on reproductive endocrine and menstrual cycle markers associated with perimenopause: the Harvard Study of Moods and Cycles. Arch Gen Psychiatry. 2003;60(1):29–36. PMID: 12511170. http://www.ncbi.nlm.nih.gov/pubmed/12511170.
374. Rehman HU, Masson EA. Neuroendocrinology of female aging. Gend Med. 2005;2(1):41–56. PMID: 16115597. http://www.ncbi.nlm.nih.gov/pubmed/16115597.
375. Höfer P, Lanzenberger R, Kasper S. Testosterone in the brain: neuroimaging findings and the potential role for neuropsychopharmacology. Eur Neuropsychopharmacol. 2013;23(2):79–88. PMID: 22578782. http://www.ncbi.nlm.nih.gov/pubmed/22578782.
376. Lang PO, Samaras D, Samaras N. Testosterone replacement therapy in reversing "andropause": what is the proof-of-principle? Rejuvenation Res. 2012;15(5):453–65. PMID: 22656862. http://www.ncbi.nlm.nih.gov/pubmed/22656862.
377. Moses-Kolko EL, Price JC, Shah N, Berga S, Sereika SM, Fisher PM, Coleman R, Becker C, Mason NS, Loucks T, Meltzer CC. Age, sex, and reproductive hormone effects on brain serotonin-1A and serotonin-2A receptor binding in a healthy population. Neuropsychopharmacology. 2011;36(13):2729–40. PMCID: PMC3230496. http://www.ncbi.nlm.nih.gov/pubmed/21849982.
378. Simpson ER, Mahendroo MS, Means GD, Kilgore MW, Hinshelwood MM, Graham-Lorence S, Amarneh B, Ito Y, Fisher CR, Michael MD. Aromatase cytochrome P450, the

enzyme responsible for estrogen biosynthesis. Endocr Rev. 1994;15(3):342–55. PMID: 8076586. http://www.ncbi.nlm.nih.gov/pubmed/8076586.

379. McCarthy MM. How it's made: organisational effects of hormones on the developing brain. J Neuroendocrinol. 2010;22(7):736–42. PMCID: PMC3170038. http://www.ncbi.nlm.nih.gov/pubmed/20646174.

380. Amore M, Innamorati M, Costi S, Sher L, Girardi P, Pompili M. Partial androgen deficiency, depression, and testosterone supplementation in aging men. Int J Endocrinol. 2012;2012:280724. PMCID: PMC3376477. http://www.ncbi.nlm.nih.gov/pubmed/22719760.

381. Nemeth CL, Harrell CS, Beck KD, Neigh GN. Not all depression is created equal: sex interacts with disease to precipitate depression. Biol Sex Differ. 2013;4(1):8. PMCID: PMC3639119. http://www.ncbi.nlm.nih.gov/pubmed/23594674.

382. Morales A. Andropause (or symptomatic late-onset hypogonadism): facts, fiction and controversies. Aging Male. 2004;7(4):297–303. PMID: 15799125. http://www.ncbi.nlm.nih.gov/pubmed/15799125.

383. Kolovou G, Bilianou H, Marvaki A, Mikhailidis DP. Aging men and lipids. Am J Mens Health. 2011;5(2):152–65. PMID: 20483870. http://www.ncbi.nlm.nih.gov/pubmed/20483870.

384. Mitsiades N, Correa D, Gross CP, Hurria A, Slovin SF. Cognitive effects of hormonal therapy in older adults. Semin Oncol. 2008;35(6):569–81. PMID: 19027461. http://www.ncbi.nlm.nih.gov/pubmed/19027461.

385. Seidman SN. Normative hypogonadism and depression: does "andropause" exist? Int J Impot Res. 2006;18(5):415–22. PMID: 16395322. http://www.ncbi.nlm.nih.gov/pubmed/16395322.

386. Seidman SN. Testosterone deficiency and mood in aging men: pathogenic and therapeutic interactions. World J Biol Psychiatry. 2003;4(1):14–20. PMID: 12582972. http://www.ncbi.nlm.nih.gov/pubmed/12582972.

387. Khosravi S, Ardebili HE, Larijani B, Nedjat S, Nikbakht Nasrabadi A, Ardebili ME, Dabiran S, Samizadeh E. Are andropause symptoms related to depression? Aging Clin Exp Res. 2015;27(6):813–20. PMID: 25762159. http://www.ncbi.nlm.nih.gov/pubmed/25762159.

388. Rodgers S, Grosse Holtforth M, Hengartner MP, Müller M, Aleksandrowicz AA, Rössler W, Ajdacic-Gross V. Serum testosterone levels and symptom-based depression subtypes in men. Front Psych. 2015;6:61. PMCID: PMC4418274. http://www.ncbi.nlm.nih.gov/pubmed/25999864.

389. Moraga-Amaro R, van Waarde A, Doorduin J, de Vries EFJ. Sex steroid hormones and brain function: PET imaging as a tool for research. J Neuroendocrinol. 2018;30(2):e12565. PMCID: PMC5838537. http://www.ncbi.nlm.nih.gov/pubmed/29237239.

390. Fergusson DM, Boden JM, Horwood LJ. Tests of causal links between alcohol abuse or dependence and major depression. Arch Gen Psychiatry. 2009;66(3):260–6. PMID: 19255375. http://www.ncbi.nlm.nih.gov/pubmed/19255375.

391. Falk DE, Yi HY, Hilton ME. Age of onset and temporal sequencing of lifetime DSM-IV alcohol use disorders relative to comorbid mood and anxiety disorders. Drug Alcohol Depend. 2008;94(1–3):234–45. PMCID: PMC2386955. http://www.ncbi.nlm.nih.gov/pubmed/18215474.

392. Schuckit MA, Tipp JE, Bergman M, Reich W, Hesselbrock VM, Smith TL. Comparison of induced and independent major depressive disorders in 2,945 alcoholics. Am J Psychiatry. 1997;154(7):948–57. PMID: 9210745. http://www.ncbi.nlm.nih.gov/pubmed/9210745.

393. Schuckit MA, Tipp JE, Bucholz KK, Nurnberger JI, Hesselbrock VM, Crowe RR, Kramer J. The life-time rates of three major mood disorders and four major anxiety disorders in alcoholics and controls. Addiction. 1997;92(10):1289–304. PMID: 9489046. http://www.ncbi.nlm.nih.gov/pubmed/9489046.

394. Nathan RG, Robinson D, Cherek DR, Davison S, Sebastian S, Hack M. Long-term benzodiazepine use and depression. Am J Psychiatry. 1985;142(1):144–5. PMID: 2857068. http://www.ncbi.nlm.nih.gov/pubmed/2857068.

395. Darke S, Kaye S, McKetin R, Duflou J. Major physical and psychological harms of methamphetamine use. Drug Alcohol Rev. 2008;27(3):253–62. PMID: 18368606. http://www.ncbi.nlm.nih.gov/pubmed/18368606.

396. Wieland DM, Halter MJ, Levine C. Bath salts: they are not what you think. J Psychosoc Nurs Ment Health Serv. 2012;50(2):17–21. PMID: 22439144. http://www.ncbi.nlm.nih.gov/pubmed/22439144.

397. Beaulieu S, Saury S, Sareen J, Tremblay J, Schütz CG, McIntyre RS, Schaffer A. Canadian Network for Mood and Anxiety Treatments (CANMAT) Task Force. The Canadian Network for Mood and Anxiety Treatments (CANMAT) task force recommendations for the management of patients with mood disorders and comorbid substance use disorders. Ann Clin Psychiatry. 2012;24(1):38–55. PMID: 22303521. http://www.ncbi.nlm.nih.gov/pubmed/22303521.

398. Marshall BDL, Werb D. Health outcomes associated with methamphetamine use among young people: a systematic review. Addiction. 2010;105(6):991–1002. PMID: 20659059. http://www.ncbi.nlm.nih.gov/pubmed/20659059.

399. Modell JG. Protracted benzodiazepine withdrawal syndrome mimicking psychotic depression. Psychosomatics. 1997;38(2):160–1. PMID: 9063050. http://www.ncbi.nlm.nih.gov/pubmed/9063050.

400. Lader M. Anxiety or depression during withdrawal of hypnotic treatments. J Psychosom Res. 1994;38(Suppl 1):113–23; discussion 118-123. PMID: 7799243. http://www.ncbi.nlm.nih.gov/pubmed/7799243.

401. Biernacka JM, McElroy SL, Crow S, Sharp A, Benitez J, Veldic M, Kung S, Cunningham JM, Post RM, Mrazek D, Frye MA. Pharmacogenomics of antidepressant induced mania: a review and meta-analysis of the serotonin transporter gene (5HTTLPR) association. J Affect Disord. 2012;136(1–2):e21–9. PMID: 21680025. http://www.ncbi.nlm.nih.gov/pubmed/21680025.

402. Parker S, Nagarsekar BB. Escitalopram induced mania. Indian J Psychiatry. 2007;49(2):121–2. PMCID: PMC2917077. http://www.ncbi.nlm.nih.gov/pubmed/20711395.

403. Baumer FM, Howe M, Gallelli K, Simeonova DI, Hallmayer J, Chang KD. A pilot study of antidepressant-induced mania in pediatric bipolar disorder: characteristics, risk factors, and the serotonin transporter gene. Biol Psychiatry. 2006;60(9):1005–12. PMID: 16945343. http://www.ncbi.nlm.nih.gov/pubmed/16945343.

404. Casey C, Chen L, may, Rabow MW. Symptom management in gynecologic malignancies. Expert Rev Anticancer Ther. 2011;11(7):1077–89. PMID: 21806331. http://www.ncbi.nlm.nih.gov/pubmed/21806331.

405. Pamuk GE, Harmandar F, Ermantaş N, Harmandar O, Turgut B, Demir M, Vural O. EORTC QLQ-C30 assessment in Turkish patients with hematological malignancies: association with anxiety and depression. Ann Hematol. 2008;87(4):305–10. PMID: 18219486. http://www.ncbi.nlm.nih.gov/pubmed/18219486.

406. Dimeo F, Schmittel A, Fietz T, Schwartz S, Köhler P, Böning D, Thiel E. Physical performance, depression, immune status and fatigue in patients with hematological malignancies after treatment. Ann Oncol. 2004;15(8):1237–42. PMID: 15277264. http://www.ncbi.nlm.nih.gov/pubmed/15277264.

407. Wittmann M, Vollmer T, Schweiger C, Hiddemann W. The relation between the experience of time and psychological distress in patients with hematological malignancies. Palliat Support Care.

2006;4(4):357–63. PMID: 17133895. http://www.ncbi.nlm.nih.gov/pubmed/17133895.

408. Hjorthøj C, Østergaard MLD, Benros ME, Toftdahl NG, Erlangsen A, Andersen JT, Nordentoft M. Association between alcohol and substance use disorders and all-cause and cause-specific mortality in schizophrenia, bipolar disorder, and unipolar depression: a nationwide, prospective, register-based study. Lancet Psychiatry. 2015;2(9):801–8. PMID: 26277044. http://www.ncbi.nlm.nih.gov/pubmed/26277044.

409. Aspis I, Feingold D, Weiser M, Rehm J, Shoval G, Lev-Ran S. Cannabis use and mental health-related quality of life among individuals with depressive disorders. Psychiatry Res. 2015;230(2):341–9. PMID: 26388103. http://www.ncbi.nlm.nih.gov/pubmed/26388103.

410. Lev-Ran S, Imtiaz S, Taylor BJ, Shield KD, Rehm J, Le Foll B. Gender differences in health-related quality of life among cannabis users: results from the National Epidemiologic Survey on alcohol and related conditions. Drug Alcohol Depend. 2012;123(1–3):190–200. PMID: 22143039. http://www.ncbi.nlm.nih.gov/pubmed/22143039.

411. Cooper ZD, Haney M. Investigation of sex-dependent effects of cannabis in daily cannabis smokers. Drug Alcohol Depend. 2014;136:85–91. PMCID: PMC4518446. http://www.ncbi.nlm.nih.gov/pubmed/24440051.

412. Shollenbarger SG, Price J, Wieser J, Lisdahl K. Poorer fronto-limbic white matter integrity is associated with chronic cannabis use, FAAH genotype, and increased depressive and apathy symptoms in adolescents and young adults. Neuroimage Clin. 2015;8:117–25. PMCID: PMC4473294. http://www.ncbi.nlm.nih.gov/pubmed/26106535.

413. Casagrande TR. Psychiatric side effects of medications prescribed in internal medicine. Dialogues Clin Neurosci. 2003;5(2):155–65. PMCID: PMC3181628. http://www.ncbi.nlm.nih.gov/pubmed/22034468.

414. Seo JS, Wei J, Qin L, Kim Y, Yan Z, Greengard P. Cellular and molecular basis for stress-induced depression. Mol Psychiatry. 2017;22(10):1440–7. PMCID: PMC5269558. http://www.ncbi.nlm.nih.gov/pubmed/27457815.

415. Francis TC, Chandra R, Gaynor A, Konkalmatt P, Metzbower SR, Evans B, Engeln M, Blanpied TA, Lobo MK. Molecular basis of dendritic atrophy and activity in stress susceptibility. Mol Psychiatry. 2017;22(11):1512–9. PMCID: PMC5747312. http://www.ncbi.nlm.nih.gov/pubmed/28894298.

416. Zhang Y, Liu C, Zhao Y, Zhang X, Li B, Cui R. The effects of calorie restriction in depression and potential mechanisms. Curr Neuropharmacol. 2015;13(4):536–42. PMCID: PMC4790398. http://www.ncbi.nlm.nih.gov/pubmed/26412073.

417. Airan RD, Meltzer LA, Roy M, Gong Y, Chen H, Deisseroth K. High-speed imaging reveals neurophysiological links to behavior in an animal model of depression. Science. 2007;317(5839):819–23. PMID: 17615305. http://www.ncbi.nlm.nih.gov/pubmed/17615305.

418. van der Wee NJ, van Veen JF, Stevens H, van Vliet IM, van Rijk PP, Westenberg HG. Increased serotonin and dopamine transporter binding in psychotropic medication-naive patients with generalized social anxiety disorder shown by 123I-beta-(4-iodophenyl)-tropane SPECT. J Nucl Med. 2008;49(5):757–63. https://doi.org/10.2967/jnumed.107.045518. Epub 2008 Apr 15. PMID: 18413401.

419. Holmes A. Genetic variation in cortico-amygdala serotonin function and risk for stress-related disease. Neurosci Biobehav Rev. 2008;32(7):1293–314. https://doi.org/10.1016/j.neubiorev.2008.03.006. Epub 2008 Mar 26. PMID: 18439676; PMCID: PMC2561331.

Heritability: Genes × Environment

9

Franklin Sunzeri

Introduction

How Different Are We?

In humans, the *cerebrum* is the largest and best developed of the three principal divisions of the brain.[1] The cerebrum consists of two cerebral hemispheres composed of the gray matter [4, 5, 7] of the cerebral cortex [6, 7, 9] and the white matter of the subcortical area [10].

The gray matter is predominantly neuron cell bodies [11] and glial cells [12]. The cerebral cortex is generally classified into four divisions: frontal, temporal, parietal, and occipital lobes [13].

The subcortical deep parts of the brain and superficial areas of the spinal cord are predominantly white matter composed of fibers connecting various areas of gray matter. Within the white matter of the cerebrum are aggregates of gray matter including the basal ganglia and brain stem nuclei such as the cranial nerves [3].

Neurons have a remarkable diversity of morphology and a tremendous number of connections. The human brain has about 85–100 billion neurons; each neuron has been estimated to have 5000–200,000 synapses, for a total of about 1.5×10^{14} synapses in just the human neocortex [14–17]. The *neocortex* is the outer layer of the cerebral hemispheres, composed of six layers that perform higher functions such as sensory perception, motor commands, language, spatial reasoning, and conscious thought. The *allocortex* is the area where the limbic system is. Together, they make up the *cerebral cortex*. In humans, the neocortex may be about 90% of the cerebral cortex.

Glial cells are the primary active partners to neurons in the CNS and PNS [18, 19]. There is an approximate 1:1 ratio of glia to neurons in the entire human brain, and a range of 40–130 billion glial cells [20]. Glial cells have a diversity of functions including important roles in neurotransmission and synaptic connections [21].

Human diploid cells (all cells except haploid egg and sperm cells) contain approximately 6 billion DNA base pairs. Among these, nucleotide differences account for about 0.1% to 0.4% between individuals, compared to a roughly 1% difference between humans and our closest primates [22, 23]. In these base pairs, there are about 24,000 protein-coding genes comprising only about 1.5% of the total genome. The rest of the DNA is *noncoding for protein* (about 98.5%) and performs various biochemical functions such as transcription, noncoding RNA, organization of chromosome architecture, gene expression regulation, and epigenetic inheritance [24, 25]. Although noncoding for protein, more than 90% of the human genome is actively transcribed into RNA [26], see Fig. 9.1.

Noncoding DNA regions (i.e., DNA regions that do not code for protein) include introns, *Long Interspersed Elements (LINEs), Short Interspersed Elements (SINEs),* and other sequences of yet unknown functions [27]. Some of these non-coding DNA regions will code for RNA that perform functional duties such as transfer RNA (tRNA), ribosomal RNA (rRNA), and regulatory RNAs. Other noncoding DNA regions code for RNAs of unknown function. These latter DNA regions include origins of replication, centromeres, and telomeres.

LINEs are *retrotransposons* (a DNA element that is first transcribed into RNA and then reverse-transcribed into DNA and then inserted elsewhere in the genome) that copy and paste themselves into the genome. *LINE-1s* are found in such an amount that they constitute about 17% of the human

[1] Based upon embryogenesis, connectivity, and function, the cerebrum is one of the three divisions of the central nervous system (the cerebellum and the cerebrospinal trunk are the others) [8].

F. Sunzeri (✉)
Heather Hills Consulting, Coos Bay, OR, USA

J. Raber et al. (eds.), *Understanding and Treating Depressive Disorders*, https://doi.org/10.1007/978-3-032-14465-2_9

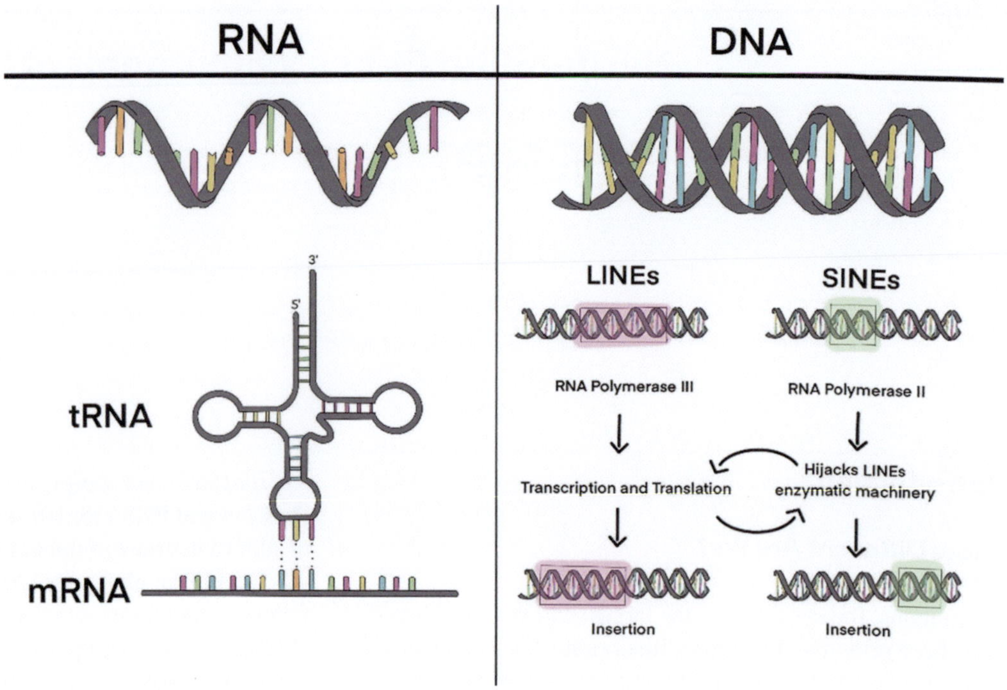

Fig. 9.1 Comparative illustration of RNA and DNA components. This figure contrasts structural and functional elements of RNA and DNA, emphasizing key subtypes: messenger RNA (mRNA), ribosomal RNA (rRNA), and genomic repetitive elements—long interspersed nuclear elements (LINEs) and short interspersed nuclear elements (SINEs). mRNA and rRNA, both transcribed from DNA, play distinct roles in protein synthesis and ribosome structure, respectively. LINEs and SINEs are transposable DNA sequences that contribute to genomic variability and regulatory complexity

genome [28, 29].[2] When they reinsert themselves back into the genome, they influence gene expression and are likely to generate genomic neuronal plasticity in individual cells [34]. It is posited that LINE-1 induced neuronal plasticity is a mechanism for generating diversity in the brain thereby enlarging the spectrum of behavior that is possible from a single genome [35–39].

SINEs are retrotransposons less than 500 bases that compose about 11% of the human genome and have been associated with neuronal processes [40, 41].

The evolution of new human-specific genes and tissue-specific gene expression appears to be tied to transposable elements such as LINEs and SINEs [27, 42–46].

Gene retrocopy insertion polymorphisms (GRIPs) are widespread [47, 48]. For example, researchers found 48 GRIPs in the genomes of one or more humans who were sequenced in the *1000 Genomes Project* [49] and *The Cancer Genome Atlas* [50] that were not in the human reference database [47, 48]. The researchers estimated that novel retrocopy insertions occur at a rate of approximately one per 6000 individuals. Their significance to behavioral disorders is being explored. Most of these are LINEs. Retroposed genes may be functional genes called retrocopies or nonfunctional *pseudogenes (q.i.)* [51].

Another subset of noncoding DNA regions is the *noncoding RNAs (ncRNAs)* (i.e., *RNA that is not transcribed into protein*), which are critical regulators of transcription, epigenetic processes, and gene silencing [26, 52, 53]. It is likely that they evolved to control genomic functions that coordinate tissue- and developmental stage-specific regulation of gene expression [54]. As such, they have a role in neural plasticity and cognition. They are highly expressed in the brain. They contribute to neuropsychiatric disorders, for example, fear [55], addiction, anxiety, and schizophrenia.

There are several classifications of ncRNAs most of which seem to be capable of directing epigenetic processes [56]. The simplest current classification is that of *small ncRNAs*, between 20 and 200 nucleotides, and *long ncRNAs*, defined as any ncRNA over 200 nucleotides. For example, a class of endogenous small ncRNAs, *microRNAs*, is thought to affect up to 60% of protein-coding transcripts [57]. Familiar ncRNAs include tRNA and rRNA.

Many ncRNAs remain silent until the appropriate developmental age or environmental trigger occurs [58]. In addition, different classes of ncRNAs are expressed either in the oocytes (*siRNA*) [59] or in the sperm (*piRNA*) [22541438], which makes them interesting candidates for transgenerational epigenetic controls [52].

---

[2] *Retrotransposons* are a type of *transposable elements* (TEs) [30]. TEs are mobile DNA sequences that can replicate themselves within genomes independently of the host cell DNA [31]. Capacity for inheritance through the germ line is a feature of all TEs.

TEs are usually 100 to 10,000 base pairs that often encode proteins (LINEs and SINEs are exceptions) with several biochemical activities and complex noncoding regulatory sequences that promote their propagation [32]. They are abundant in pro-and eukaryotes interacting with host genomes resulting in evolutionary changes shaping functions and structures.

Retrotransposons are usually classified as long terminal repeat (LTR) containing or non-long terminal repeat (non-LTRs) [33]. Human endogenous retroviruses (HERVs) are LTR retrotransposons. LINEs and SINEs are non-LTR. Most of the human retrotransposons are non-LTRs.

There may be an intimate relationship between retrotransposons like LINEs and SINEs and microRNAs and other ncRNAs [60].

On another level, *sequence variations in the human genome* also include *single-nucleotide polymorphisms (SNPs),* which may be in the coding or non-coding regions but are usually in the noncoding regions [61]. SNPs usually have only two *alleles* (allelomorphs or different forms of a gene that appear at a rate of more than 1%). Even when the SNPs are not in coding regions, they can still have an impact on the regulation or transcription of DNA. SNPs comprise about 90% of all sequence variations and are estimated to occur once in every 100–300 bases [62].

Genomic *copy number variations (CNVs)* are structural genomic variants[3] that arise from duplications, inversions, translocations, or deletions of a genomic region [68]. CNVs can range from 1000 nucleotide bases up to several million bases [63, 64]. Unrelated people differ by about 0.4% in copy numbers and CNVs can be inherited or spontaneously arise [65]. More than SNPs, CNVs contribute to human evolution and intraindividual genetic diversity, and traits [66, 67]. Over 100,000 CNVs at more than 15,000 loci have been identified in the *Database of Genomic Variants* [71]. Some estimates suggest that 12% to 18.8% of the euchromatic human genome is copy number variable [69, 70, 72].

Effects of CNVs can be prominent when they intersect a gene or alter the genomic control environment [73]. It is thought that phenotypic variability, complex behavioral traits, and disease susceptibility are related to having too few or too many copies of dosage-sensitive genes that result from CNV processes [68, 74, 75]. In addition, CNVs may relate to phenotypes of intelligence and height [76–78].

CNVs are thought to have a role in complex diseases [79–81], for example, susceptibility to cancer [82], HIV-1 infection/AIDS [83], Crohn's disease [84], and autoimmune disorders [85, 86].

CNVs have been shown to have an important role in neuropsychiatric disorders [87–91]. An emerging model of diseases suggests a *polygenic heterogeneity* involving CNVs that induce broad susceptibility to a range of neurodevelopmental disorders [92]. Some specific disorders that have been associated with CNVs include schizophrenia [93, 94], epilepsy [95], mental retardation [96], Alzheimer's disease [97], Parkinson's disease [98], autism [99], suicide ideation [100], and major depressive disorder [100–103].

Here are some examples found in the literature. Whole-genome scans of CNVs, including 1693 major depressive disorder (MDD) cases and 4506 controls, revealed that duplication of the SLIT3 locus on 5q35.1 predisposes to MDD [101]. In a large sample, resistance to recurrent depression has been significantly associated with duplication CNVs, whereas susceptibility to recurrent depression was associated with deletion CNVs [102]. In particular, CNVs that delete protein-coding regions were mainly responsible for that association. Prevalence of de novo or rare copy number CNVs in six genomic regions (1q21.1, 2p16.3, 3q29, 15q11.2, 15q13.3, and 16p11.2) has been associated with neuropsychiatric diseases, especially with schizophrenia and intellectual impairment [104]. CNV-associated microdeletions and duplications and SNPs in 16p11.2 in particular have been associated with major depressive disorder [105].

A case-control study using data from the *UK Biobank* study sample of 502,534 individuals living in the United Kingdom showed that some neurodevelopmental CNVs seem to be associated with depression [106]. Effects of inbreeding that are associated with runs of homozygosity, homozygous deletions, and other CNVs on risk for depression and suicide attempt were quantified in an Arab Bedouin Kindred [107]. Runs of homozygosity were not found to be significantly associated with risk. However, one of the CNVs (on 9p24.1) that covers GLDC, which encodes glycine dehydrogenase that binds to glycine and results in its degradation, was found to be significantly associated with depression. Glycine is a co-agonist at N-methyl-D-aspartate (NMDA) glutamate receptors, thereby increasing glutamatergic neurotransmission. Some studies have shown significantly increased glycine levels in depression [108], but others have not [109].

CNVs may not have a substantial role in recurrent depressive disorder. In an association analysis of a Danish cohort, large deletions CNVs were no more frequent in cases than control samples [110]. Data from two genome-wide association studies comprising 1263 Caucasians showed that large rare CNVs do not appear to make a substantial contribution to treatment-resistant depression [111].

Intraindividual neuronal genomes are genetically diverse, and brains are *somatic mosaics (the presence of genetically distinct cells within the same organism or tissue)* [35, 36], resulting from loss or gain of active LINEs [39], whole chromosomes (*aneuploidy*) [37], and genomic copy number variations [38]. Somatic mosaicism contributes to normal and abnormal human brain development [112]. Somatic mutations in the brain have been linked to age-related decline [113].

While mosaicism has been well known to occur in cancer cells [114, 115] and in the normal healthy cells of the immune system, it has only recently come to be appreciated in other normal healthy cells [116]. Indeed, genome rearrangements are common in healthy human cells [117]. These include retrotransposition in neurons [118, 119] and age-related copy number variations (CNVs) in human blood cells [120] and somatic tissues [121]. Independent of replication, human

[3] Structural genomic variants are generally defined as a region of DNA approximately 1 kb and larger in size [74].

somatic cells acquire an average of one nine-base substitution per year and 2–3 mutations per DNA replication [122].

Somatic mutations are mutations that can be passed on to the progeny of a particular cell. In contrast, *germ-line mutations* are inherited genetic changes that occur in sperm or eggs. Somatic mutations that occur in embryonic stages have the potential for the mutations to be shared in tissues that are developing at that time, such that many tissues or organs or the whole body can be affected. For a review of the implications of mosaicism on disease, see [123, 124].

This mosaicism is likely to be missed when using surrogate cells such as using DNA from saliva or blood [125]. DNA is sequenced from populations of cells, so the genetic composition of individual cells is lost. So, mutations and heterogeneity are not easily revealed. Single-cell genome analysis and single-cell RNA analysis can be performed, and more sensitive and automated processes are being developed [126–128]. Simultaneous isolation and parallel sequencing of genomic DNA and total RNA from single cells has also been accomplished [129].

Chimerism is the presence in the body of DNA from two different zygotes. In contradistinction, mosaicism is the presence of differences in DNA that came from only one zygote. During pregnancy, fetal cells enter the mother's circulation and establish *microchimerism* (the presence of genetically distinct cells in a single organism) [130]. For example, in one study, 56% of women carried male cells in their breast tissue for decades and only 21% of women with cancer did so [130]. The correlation with disease is obscure because excess male microchimerism in *hyperchimerism* is also implicated in cancer.

It has been estimated that offspring have about 60 mutations (from the various sources as discussed above) that differ from those of their parents; however, that rate appears to vary greatly from family to family [138]. Among other causes of mutagenesis are DNA repair mistakes, DNA polymerase errors, mobile element insertions, and microsatellites[4] [139]. With innovative technology approaches, it seems that de novo mutation rates may be considerably lower than previous estimates [140]. There is a considerable variation in mutation rates within and between families and with sex, age, and genomic context [141].

In one study, 92% of the observed *germline de novo mutations (DNMs)* in one family came from the paternal germline, while 36% came from the paternal germline in another family [138]. Other studies indicate that the majority of DNMs do come from the paternal lineage and increase with age [139]. In particular, it appears that offspring of older fathers are at greater risk of neurodevelopmental disorders including autism and schizophrenia, but linkage with adult occurrence of depression is unclear [142, 143]. *Four main hypotheses to explain this association* are reviewed in reference [143]. They call these the de novo mutation hypothesis, the hypothesis concerning epigenetic alterations, the selection into late fatherhood hypothesis, and the environmental resource hypothesis.

Throughout our life, our brains are susceptible to somatic mutations. During gestational weeks 4 through 24 neuronal precursor cells divide at more than 10^5 times per minute [144]. When we are newborn, new neurons are being produced at a high rate and find their way in the rostral migratory stream from the subventricular area to the prefrontal cortex [145]. It has been suggested that these neurons are particularly vulnerable at this stage.

As adults, we generate new neurons in the dentate gyrus of the hippocampus, the striatum, and the subventricular zone adjacent to the lateral ventricle [146–148]. It has been estimated that a third of the hippocampal neurons are replaced in our life and about 700 new neurons are added to the hippocampus each day [146]. Declining slightly with age, there may be an annual turnover of about 1.75% of the neurons [146, 149].

During our maturing and aging, somatic mutations appear in neurons [150–153], in mitochondria [152], and in glial cells [154–156].

As an investigation into sources of somatic mutations, a 2012 genome-wide *LINE-1 (L1) retrotransposition insertion profile* of 300 single neurons from the cerebral cortex and caudate nucleus of three normal individuals, came up with an estimate <0.6 unique somatic insertions per neuron, and that most neurons lack detectable somatic insertions [119]. So, their results suggest that L1 is not a major generator of neuronal diversity in the cortex and caudate nucleus.

Somatic deletions and insertions may affect metabolic processes and neuronal development in different ways in different brain regions [157].

Somatic retrotransposition may become activated as cells age [158]. However, calorie restriction, which slows aging, appears to counteract this process.

[4]Repeated elements are usually classified as either *tandem repeats* or *dispersed repeats*. Tandem repeats include gene tandems, ribosomal DNA repeat arrays, and satellite DNA. Satellites are further divided into satellites, minisatellites, and microsatellites. Satellite DNA is areas of tandemly repeating, non-coding DNA. Satellites are the main constituent of functional centromeres [133] and the principal structural component of heterochromatin. They are called satellites due to their appearance as a differently segregating band on density gradient DNA analysis.

Microsatellites have a greater allelic diversity than biallelic SNPs and have important roles in measuring genomic variation in linkage and association studies [131]. Satellites along with SNPs and mitochondria sequencing have gained important roles in forensics [132].

Dispersed repeats include transposons, tRNA genes, and gene paralogues. In the human genome, repeated elements can comprise half of the whole genome. The mechanisms that create and sustain these different repeats appear to be distinct. [131, 134]. *Paralogues* are a pair of genes that derives from the same ancestral gene and now reside at different locations within the same genome [135, 136].

Genome-wide association studies do not look at genes [137].[5] They generally look at SNPs. So, due to SNPs' potential remoteness from genes, it is always a question as to how they relate to what gene [1]. For example, *IRX3* plays a significant role in obesity, but its connection to obesity-associated variants (SNPs) within the fat mass and obesity-related (*FTO*) locus is a long distance [2]. Indeed, the regulatory switches that control the expression of IRX3 are located several hundred thousand base pairs away in the *FTO* locus [159].

Roman-Franco has succinctly put it that over the 3.8 billion years of organic evolution, the human microecosystem of 100 trillion cells and viral elements is not exclusively and irreducibly human [160, 161]. *Homo sapiens* are composed of constituents derived from the archaeal [165, 166], bacterial, and eukaryan domains via endosymbiotic, commensalistic, and mutualistic interactions [161]. Almost 8% of the human genome is constructed of *human endogenous retroviruses (HERVs)* [162–164, 167].[6]

In animals, HERVs cause specific diseases, including cancer; however, in humans, their association with disease has been controversial [175, 176]. However, environmental factors have reproducibly been shown to trigger their expression [168, 177]. There is some evidence that the resulting production of envelope proteins from HERV-W and HERV-K, appears to participate in pathways leading to the pathognomonic features of multiple sclerosis and amyotrophic lateral sclerosis, respectively [168, 178]. Transcription of human endogenous retroviruses in the human brain has shown increased expression of overall HERV, and HERV-W family in samples from both schizophrenia and bipolar disorder patients [179]. A researcher in 2019 at SUNY has suggested two hypotheses linking HERVs and MDD [180]. They are (1) exposure to either exogenous viruses or traumatic experiences can activate HERVs in the brain to cause psychiatric symptoms and (2) that individual differences in vulnerability or resilience to MDD result from the balance of activated HERVs with pathogenic versus protective functions in the brain.

Telomere shortening is a normal process of aging. Telomeres are disposable elements at the end of chromosomes. They become shorter during each cell division. However, the degree of shortening seems to be responsive to environmental factors [181]. There is a relationship between psychosocial, environmental, and behavioral factors and changes in telomere length [182, 183]. Shortening of telomeres is associated with increased morbidity and mortality. Factors that are beginning to be investigated include perceived stress, childhood adversities, major depressive disorder [184], educational attainment, physical activity, and sleep [182, 185–187].[7]

There are promising findings that telomere shortening can be reversed [188]. For example, a multidisciplinary weight loss intervention for 2 months was accompanied by a significant increase in telomere length in overweight/obese adolescents [189].

Environmental and genetic factors modify the rate at which we age [190–192]. There is some evidence that via epigenetic rejuvenation, the aging clock can be slowed and reversed: aged cells may regain some of their youthful characteristics [193]. There is some evidence that adverse social conditions may accelerate biological aging via telomere shortening rates [191, 194].

The *brain age gap estimation (BrainAGE)* method utilizes structural MRI data to directly quantify acceleration or deceleration of individual brain aging [195, 196]. BrainAGE appears to provide individualized biomarkers for the biological age of brain structure especially as it might pertain to the occurrence of age-related cognitive decline and age-related neurodegenerative diseases [197].

The human genome contains over 14,000 *pseudogenes* [198, 199]. "Pseudo" means that the sequence of DNA has lost its original function due to a variation in sequence relative to the parent coding gene [200]. These pseudogenes vary from characteristics of functional genes that may have recently died to dead genes that may have been resurrected as functional non-protein-coding RNA [198, 201]. Pseudogenes may play significant parts in normal and abnormal functioning of cells [200]. They may be classified as processed or nonprocessed [48, 202]. Processed pseudogenes have arisen from retrotransposition of processed mRNAs (LINEs). More than 8000 processed pseudogenes have been catalogued [203]. Processed pseudogenes are approximately one-third more abundant in our X chromosome than in our autosomes [204]. One Swedish study found novel pseudogenes in almost two-thirds of individuals, and some novel pseudogenes were population specific [48].

Nonprocessed pseudogenes arise from gene duplication or unequal crossing followed by mutations that make the copied gene nonfunctional [205].

[5]The key concepts that underlie the genome-wide association studies are discussed in reference [174].

[6]Figure 1 in Küry P, Nath A, Créange et al. [168] shows relative proportions of different types of DNA sequences in the human genome. Remnants of mobile genetic machinery represent almost half of the human genome. Most of these are retrotransposons. A significant portion of these retrotransposons is HERVs. HERV DNA sequences are frequently truncated, containing mutations, insertions, or deletions, and are sometimes complete copies.

[7]Telomeres are protein-DNA complexes that protect chromosome ends from improper ligation and resection [169, 170]. Both short and overly long telomeres have been associated with age related disorders [171, 172]. Some T cells acquire telomeres from antigen presenting cells protecting them from senescence and conferring long-term immune protection [173].

The diversity of neurons can be generated by *stochastic independent expression of autosomal alleles* that leads to functional differences among neurons [206]. An example is the monoallelic expression of the approximately 50 members of the homophilic cell-adhesion proteins clustered protocadherins (Pcdhs). Clustered Pcdhs are critical to the accuracy of axonal projections, synaptic formation, dendritic arborization, and neuronal survival. In addition, the clustered Pcdh members provide a diversity of selective binding sites for neuron-to-neuron interactions.

Heritability is a term that has been inconsistently applied and interpreted [207–213]. Heritability is cogently defined by Rose as "an estimate of the genetic and environmental contributions to the variance of any phenotypic measure around the mean for a given population" [208]. Van Asselt says, "Heritability is defined as the proportion of the total phenotypic variation within a population that can be attributed to the genetic variance. *Variance* is the term that describes how far apart the individual measurements are. In analysis of variance (ANOVA), a commonly used method to compute heritability, the shared variance is attributed to genetic variance, and the nonshared variance is attributed to error, environment, or both" [214].

Because heritability is defined for a given population in a specific environment, if the environment changes, the heritability changes. This limits extrapolation from one population to another. Heritability is specific to a given population at a given point of time.

If the environment were held constant, heritability would refer to the genetic contribution to the variance. *Heritability does not address causes for differences between populations.* It measures the amount of *variation* in a trait that can be ascribed to genes, *not* the amount *caused* by genes. If the environment changes in a way that has a differential impact on individuals in that population, then the heritability of that trait might change [213, 215].

Bailey summarizes fallacies in attempting to use heritability in humans to explain differences in human behavior and cognition [216]. His major points are (1) heritability of a trait does not address the influence of genetic or environmental *changes* upon that trait, so it cannot be used to formulate remediation. (2) Non-additive effects on behavior and cognitive processes such as covariance of genes and environment interaction make heritability estimates inaccurate.

When reading studies that describe heritability for various traits, it is important to keep these admonitions in mind. A good guide to understanding the analytical approaches to evaluating environment-genetic interactions can be found in the publication *Introductory Guide to the Statistics of Molecular Genetics* [217]. *An Introductory Guide to the Language of Molecular Genetics* could be quite helpful as well [218].

Early studies suggested that depression symptoms seem to be largely heritable, and the relative influences vary by genetics and age [219]. Heritability estimates for MDD have been said to vary from about 37% and up to 70% if severity, relapse rate, and age of onset are factored in [221]. Twin study-based models have shown a gradual increase in the liability to depression and rates of change with increasing age [220]. This liability seems to be both genetically determined and environmentally influenced by experiences at different ages. The following studies illustrate some of the variables in estimating heritability of MDD.

Four hundred eleven twin pairs between the ages of 8 and 16 years were evaluated. Over the whole age range, the best data fit was for an additive genetic model. However, for ages 8–11 the symptoms were attributable to shared environmental factors, whereas ages 12–16 showed a strong association with genetic factors.

Effects of heredity and environment on depression were analyzed in 182 prepubertal female, 237 prepubertal male, 314 pubertal female, and 171 pubertal male twin pairs from the *Virginia Twin Study of Adolescent Behavioral Development* [222]. Child self-reported depression was assessed by the Child and Adolescent Psychiatric Interview. Variance due to hereditability was seen only in pubescent girls (28%). Adolescent females seemed to be particularly susceptible to depression via the influence of life events in the year preceding depression. Latent genetic factors seemed to mediate depression and an increase in the influence of life events in this group.

Genetic and environmental contributions to major depression (MD) in males and females were studied in a volunteer sample of 2662 Australian Twins [379]. The mean age for women was 44 years (range = 28–89 years; SD =12.35), and for men the mean age was 42 years (range = 28–84 years; SD = 11.23). Three different criteria sets were used to define depression: DSM-III-R major depressive disorder (the broadest definition), DSM-IV major depressive disorder, and the severity subtype of the DSM-IV qualifier [20056021] for major depressive disorder (the narrowest definition). Lifetime prevalence using the DSM-III-R, DSM-IV, and severe DSM-IV for women and men were, respectively: 31% and 24%; 22% and 16%; 9% and 3%. For both sexes, the relative contribution of environment and genetics was stable for each definition. For women, it seems that genetic factors and unique environmental factors contribute to the development of MD: genetic heritability estimates range from 36% to 44%. For men, environmental factors appear to play a much larger role: heritability estimates range was 1% for the narrowest definition to 24% for the broadest, but because of such a small prevalence of depression by the narrow definition, this range may be illusory. Familial aggregation of MD was moderately seen in women and was mostly explained by genetics. In men, familial aggregation of MD was only modest. As defined by the broader definition of the DSM-III, MD was more heritable for women. For both sexes, the environment made a large contribution to MD.

Lifetime histories of MD were assessed by the DSM-III-R in 3790 male–male, female–female, and male–female twin pairs, and comparisons between the sexes were made [223]. The prevalence of female–female lifetime MD was 35.5% in dizygotes and 31.2% in monozygotes. The prevalence of lifetime MD was 17.0% in male–male dizygotes and 14.9% in monozygotes. And the prevalence of lifetime MD for female–male pairs was 17.8%. Odds ratios for female–female dizygotes and monozygotes were 1.59 and 3.02, respectively. Odds ratios for male–male dizygotes and monozygotes were 1.86 and 3.29, respectively. The odds ratio for male–female dizygotes was 1.39.

Many studies have attempted to determine what contributions specific genetic and environmental factors make to anxiety and depressive disorders [224–228]. Conclusions seem to rest upon studies that parsed childhood symptoms with more specificity [229]. Here are some examples.

Investigations of the environmental and genetic components of biases in recognizing threats and avoidance in anxious children show moderate heritability with heavy influence of nonshared environments [230–232]. It appears that stressful life events, independent of the individual and not appearing to be moderated by 5HTTLPR genotype, are associated with anxiety and depression [233].

A *longitudinal cross-lagged study* of associations between anxiety sensitivity, anxiety, and depression has shown stability over time [234, 235]. However, there were reciprocal relationships that developed in time. Cross-lagged analyses collect longitudinal data so that each observation is recorded at multiple time points. The goal is to estimate the directional influence that variables have on each other as time progresses. The analysis is called crossed as it estimates reciprocal influences. It is called lagged because these relationships are examined at different times. In this study, data were recorded at two points between 15 and 17 years of age. New genetic influences were seen at the second data points, whereas environmental effects seemed to be more time specific. Other time-based analyses have shown genetic factors contributing to continuity of symptoms with new genetic factors emerging over time [238]. Additional nonshared environmental influences emerged over time, while others remained stable.

Stable genetic influences on specific anxiety-related behavior between 7 and 11 years of age may account for 68% of continuity of symptoms [239]. In that same study, shared and nonshared environmental factors contributed about 18% and 28% to changes from one type of anxiety-associated behavior to another type.

In a cross-sectional longitudinal study, a genetic correlation between adolescent irritability and depression showed a significant correlation (r(A) = 0.70, 95% CI: 0.59–0.82) [240].

Negative attributions and depressive symptoms in children seem to be both a latent factor and shared and nonshared aspects of the environment [241]. Meta-analysis suggests that separation anxiety disorder and separation anxiety symptoms appear to be about 43% genetic and 17% environmental, with females having a meta-heritability of 0.52 and males 0.26 [242]. Nonshared environmental effects in females were 0.41 and in males 0.74.

Associations between sleep quality and anxiety and depression seem to be mainly due to genes [243, 244]. In one study, genes explained 74% of anxiety and 58% of depression covariances [245]. Nonshared-environmental factors contributed the rest. Yet, sleep quality seems to be in part dependent upon genetics and/or shared environment [246]. The differences in sleep quality between monozygotic twins for males were significantly tied to general health ($\beta = 1.56$, $p < 0.001$) and for females to relationship satisfaction ($\beta = 1.01$, $p < 0.05$). In young children, dysfunctional beliefs and attitudes about sleep contribute to sleep difficulties [247].

Sleep quality and diurnal preference in young adults have been investigated for associations with 5-HTTLPR, variable-number tandem repeat in the human clock gene PERIOD3 (PER3), and another polymorphism in the clock gene CLOCK 3111 [248–250]. Results have been heterogeneous, with some studies showing poorer sleep quality in homozygotes for the long 5-HTTLPR alleles and others not [248]. Generally, CLOCK and PERs seem to have only population-specific effects.

A 2019 study examined the role of *gene–gene interactions*[8] between several circadian clock genes[9] and mood disorders [251]. They found that single gene associations, TIMELESS rs4630333 and CSNK1E rs135745 were significantly associated with both major depressive disorder and bipolar disorder. And, the CLOCK haplotype was also strongly associated. The two-gene combination of TIMELESS rs4630333 and CSNK1E rs135745 had the most significant association with mood disorders in the two-locus model. BHLHB2 rs2137947 for major depressive disorder and CLOCK rs12649507 for bipolar disorder were the most significant third loci in the three-locus combination model.

Correlation of normative childhood repetitive routines and obsessive-compulsive symptoms has been estimated in one study of 6-year-old twins to be 0.40 (95% CI: 0.27–0.50) and attributable wholly to additive genetic effects [252].

---

[8]Gene–gene interactions (also known as epistasis) are discussed in [235].

[9]They examined the clock genes BHLHB2, CLOCK, CSNK1E, NR1D1, PER2, PER3, and TIMELESS. And allele, genotype, and haplotype associations were tested.

Parenting discipline, friendship quality, and peer group characteristics appear to be moderately to substantially heritable; hence, adolescent genetic propensities may account for the relationship between parental discipline and quality of peer friendship [253].

One study suggests that parental punitive discipline, negative life events and gene–environment interactions are context dependent in influencing externalizing behavior [228]. For example, maternal punitive behavior decreased genetic variance and increased environmental influences. Paternal punitive discipline increased the influence of genetic variance, while negative life events influenced only nonshared environmental influences on externalizing behavior.

Interestingly, it seems that the death of a parent during childhood does not, for the majority of children, result in increased mental health problems, reduced functional limitations, or a greater need for mental health services during adulthood [254].

Of interest, as discussed later in this text, Crisafulli et al. (2011) reviewed data on the pharmacogenetics of antidepressants and found that nearly 60% of depressed patients do not exhibit a complete response to antidepressants, while up to 30% show no response at all [255]. Approximately half of the response appears to be contributed by genetic factors.

The depression associated genetic candidates that have been investigated seem to influence behavior, susceptibility to psychological disorders, and treatment response. Many of these effects seem to be modulated by gene x environment interactions. Those genes include the cytochrome P450 superfamily, the P-glycoprotein (ABCB1), the tryptophan hydroxylase, the catechol-O-methyltransferase, the monoamine oxidase A, the serotonin transporter (5-HTTLPR), the norepinephrine transporter, the dopamine transporter, variants in the 5-hydroxytryptamine receptors (5-HT1A, 5-HT2A, 5-HT3A, 5-HT3B, and 5-HT6), adrenoreceptor beta-1 and alpha-2, the dopamine receptors (D2), the G protein beta 3 subunit, the corticotropin releasing hormone receptors (CRHR1 and CRHR2), the glucocorticoid receptors, the c-AMP response-element binding, and the brain-derived neurotrophic factor (BDNF). In addition, some associations have been seen for angiotensin I converting enzyme, circadian locomotor output cycles kaput protein, glutamatergic system, nitric oxide synthase, and interleukin 1-beta gene [256–258].

We will have more to say about specific genes that may be involved in depression and personalized psychotherapy treatment. A deeper discussion can be found in the section on "Therapygenetics."

In childhood abuse, depending upon the Val/Val versus Met allele of BDNF, the s/s 5-HTTLPR genotype appears to convey either risk or protection relative to depression symptoms [259].

A small sample has shown that genetic susceptibility to family environment has been associated with BDNF Val66met and 5-HTTLPR as an influence on depression [260]. In the presence of those alleles, influences of family dynamics until the age of 15 influenced depression symptoms. However, after 15 years of age the interactions were predictive of depression only in females.

The *differential susceptibility model* of gene–environment interaction suggests that particular genetic polymorphisms predispose to increased sensitivity to environmental factors that can be positive or negative depending on the nature of the environment [261, 262]. In contradistinction, the *diathesis-stress model* suggests that biologically predisposed individuals, when exposed to negative stress, are at risk for negative consequences, but are unaffected by positive environments [260, 263].

Susceptibility to depression after childhood abuse is moderated by epistasis of BDNF Val66Met polymorphism and serotonin transporter (5-HTTLPR) [259].

In families with recurrent, early-onset, major depression, five sex-specific susceptibility loci interacted with the CREB1 locus to influence the development of depression [264].

A 2017 review presents evidence for epistatic interactions in neuropsychiatric disorders [265].

A further level of insight into the constellation of factors that can produce disease may come from the melding of fusion project data with an understanding of *molecular crowding* interactions between intracellular constituents, DNA, and products [266–268]. That is where chemistry and physics interface with biology. Apparently, about 40% of the intracellular volume is composed of a myriad of molecules crowded into a highly structured and complex environment (e.g., in the endoplasmic reticulum, Golgi apparatus, and cytoskeletal structures) [266]. These crowded associations seem to be linked to a variety of constraints on interactions as well as propagation of aberrant reactions [269, 270].

There is some evidence that *mitochondrial function* [271] and depression may be linked [272–274]. Hypotheses revolve around oxidative stress and malfunctioning mitochondria. To power the brain cells, glucose, the obligatory brain energy substrate, goes through an oxidative metabolic process in mitochondria to produce prodigious amounts of adenosine triphosphate (ATP) [236, 275].

In producing energy to power the brain, mitochondria produce reactive oxygen species (ROS) and reactive nitrogen species (RNS) along with abundant ATP [276, 277]. If the mitochondria malfunction and if the antioxidant processes fail to balance ROS/RNS production, oxidative stress grows [278]. Free radical targets include carbohydrates, lipids, proteins, and DNA. Aberrant cell functions and even cell death can occur [279]. This may further impact the mitochondria themselves, the host cell, and the rest of the brain.

Appropriate mitochondrial function is vital for the brain, as neurons cannot store glucose and use a vast quantity of ATP [273]. Although it comprises only 2% of the total body mass, the brain accounts for 25% of the body's total glucose utilization. Functional or quantitative alterations in mitochondria have been shown to negatively impact cell functions [280]. These include brain plasticity, mood, and resiliency [273, 281]. Glutamate, acetylcholine, and gamma-aminobutyric acid production are dependent upon the glucose substrate. Mitochondria also play a role in buffering calcium and amino acid metabolism [289]. In the cortex, most of the synapses are excitatory, and the demand for energy is high for processes such as producing axonal action potentials, cell signaling, presynaptic Ca2+ entry, recycling of neurotransmitters, and releasing synaptic vesicles [282–284].

MDD patients both in resting state and under stress show reduced blood flow and glucose metabolism in the caudate nucleus, anterior cingulate cortex, and prefrontal cortex [285]. In contrast, the orbital cortex, medial thalamus, and amygdala show increased blood flow and glucose metabolism [286].

Compared to controls, MDD patients show an increased proportion of deletions in mitochondrial DNA, decreased mitochondrial ATP production and lower activity levels of mitochondrial enzymes [287, 288]. The glutamatergic system and mitochondrial energy metabolism have also been seen to be compromised [287].

Further associations have been observed between energy imbalance and depression [290]. Proteomic analyses of postmortem brains from patients with schizophrenia (SCZ), bipolar disorder (BPD), and major depressive disorder (MDD) revealed differentially expressed energy-related proteins—41 in MDD, 92 in SCZ, and 95 in BPD [290]. These proteins are ones that are primarily associated with oxidative phosphorylation, and most of them are subunits of cytochrome c, ATP synthase, or NADH dehydrogenase. Some of these proteins of the electron transport chain have also been seen to be reduced in the cerebellum of patients with MDD [291].

It has been suggested that mitochondria may be used in the differential diagnosis of MDD, as biomarkers[10] for exploring the cause of MDD, and as a potential target for therapeutic interventions. When mitochondria are severely stressed, they can traffic between cells, replacing mitochondria in cells with damaged and malfunctioning DNA [292, 293, 296]. When demand is increased, mitochondria change their morphology [280, 294, 295]. Individual mitochondria may fuse into dynamic networks to increase energy output [297]. When there is less demand, excess mitochondria are removed via a process called *mitophagy*. If the mitochondria are damaged, mitophagy removes the damaged parts, and the viable parts are subject to fusion [298].

Interestingly, some antidepressants (e.g., amitriptyline, imipramine, citalopram, and venlafaxine) induce changes in NADH dehydrogenase and cytochrome c oxidase, both components of the electron transport chain in mitochondrial energy production [299].

Because of its intricate and highly connected network, the brain has been studied as a *connectome* [304]. A connectome is a map of connections. The *Human Connectome Project* aims to map all the neural pathways in the human brain [305]. Neurons are conceived of as nodes in this network. Axons and synapses are the connecting pathways. Several groups have been investigating the nodes as either functioning to facilitate information transfer or disrupting transfer [306–309]. MRI, functional MRI, diffusion tensor imaging, and electroencephalography have demonstrated that various brain disorders such as autism and schizophrenia are associated with disrupted neural conductivity [310, 311] as well as dementia in aging [312].

Of particular importance to our subject at hand, relationships between the connectome and depression have begun to be investigated [313–315]. In two groups of depressed patients who had attempted or committed suicide, there was a significant reduction in assortativity and decreased functional connectivity in mainly central and posterior brain networks [313]. Of note is that vulnerability to suicide was seen in relatives of patients who committed suicide. These were weak resilience, poor segregation, and reduced connectivities affecting the ventral and dorsal prefrontal cortex, the anterior cingulate, thalamus, striatum, and possibly the insula, fusiform gyrus, and the cerebellum. Another study used resting-state functional magnetic resonance imaging (rs-fMRI) to identify bilateral differences in the hippocampi and amygdalas in people who had MDD and those who did not [315].

As we have discussed, epigenetic management of neuronal gene expression is the underlying regulatory system for neuronal functions and adaptation to stimuli. Evolving technologies have been revealing the epigenetic molecular basis of behavior and disease [316]. A discussion of epigenetics can be found in the "Epigenetic" chapter in this text.

In 2018, publication of a *powerful genome-wide association (GWA) meta-analysis identified 44 independent risk variants for MDD and refined the genetic architecture of*

[10] A 2016 review addressed several issues related to molecular biomarkers for depression [300]. These included transcriptomic, proteomic, genomic and telomeric biomarkers. In addition, they discussed the main pitfalls, ethical, moral, and legal issues relating to clinical use.

In 2018, a review of biomarkers for MDD was published [301]. Its aim was to evaluate growth factors, cytokines and other inflammatory markers, oxidative stress markers, endocrine markers, energy balance hormones, genetic and epigenetic features, and neuroimaging as possible candidates for biomarkers for MDD. A biomarker has been defined as "a property that can be objectively measured and considered as an indicator of a normal biological process, a pathological process, or a response of an individual to a therapeutic intervention" [302]. An expansion to that frequently used definition was provided in 2017 [237]. The abstract to that review gives a succinct characterization of biomarker properties [237].

The utility of biomarkers in depression is to identify and stratify subtypes of MDD in order to predict the probability of onset or presence of depression and evaluate relationships to severity and treatment response.

MDD (PGC MDD) [317].[11] The meta-analyses involved 135,458 cases and 344,901 controls and associated clinical features and anatomical differences. They found that all of us carry different degrees of genetic risk factors for MDD. Results added to elucidating MDD neurobiology, its relationship to other psychiatric disorders and treatments, and it may possibly point the way to more precise treatment of MDD. An earlier study had found that only a large case study would be sufficient to tease out these relationships, and this mega-analysis seems to fit that criterion [318].

The study presented six major conclusions. First, the best genetic match for MDD vs. controls is gene expression patterns in the prefrontal and anterior cingulate cortex. The genetic differences are in neurons, not microglia or astrocytes. *Second,* genetic associations are in genomic regions highly conserved in placental animals [319]. They were not in exons or coding regions. *Third,* developmental gene regulatory processes seem to be at fault. Splicing regions that generate alternative isoforms may be implicated in changing the proportions of isoforms from a gene. Isoforms frequently have strikingly different biological functions [320, 321]. *Fourth*, independent of IQ, lower educational attainment and higher body mass created increased risk and were apparently causal or correlated to causal risk factors for MDD. There does not seem to be a direct causal correlation from MDD driving decreased educational attainment or higher BMI. *Fifth,* correlations with MDD were seen from all the psychiatric disorders that they studied including those appearing in childhood. Particularly, schizophrenia and MDD have a partially shared biological etiology. The study's authors reason that current classifications of major mental disorders do not align well with the genetic underpinnings of these disorders [341, 342]. Although there is an overlap, there are substantial differences. *Sixth*: MDD had modest genome-wide SNP-heritability (h2SNP (8.7%)), which was expected because MDD is a complex disorder with both genetic and environmental determinants [322, 323].

There was no evidence for any enriched Neanderthal introgressed[12] regions in MDD [324, 325]. Positive correlations were seen with daytime sleepiness, insomnia, and tiredness. Strong correlations were seen with neuroticism, decreased age at menarche, age at first birth, and increased number of children, and with coronary artery disease and lung cancer, and negative correlations with well-being.

Four key genes that were revealed in the PGC MDD mega-analysis to be associated with MDD are as follows:

1. The first two genes *OLFM4* and *NEGR1* are associated with obesity and body mass index [326–329]. These genes play a role in synaptic function, glutamate signaling, insulin secretion/action, energy metabolism, lipid biology, and adipogenesis.
2. *RBFOX1* is a key factor coordinating regulation of both neurodevelopmentally important alternative splicing events and clinically relevant neuronal transcriptional programs in developing human neurons [330, 331]. RNA splicing is critical in programming neuronal differentiation and normal human neurodevelopment. It has been suggested that its disruption may underlie neurodevelopmental and neuropsychiatric disorders. *RBFOX1* may play a part in chronic HPA activation, one of the consistent findings in MDD [332–334].
3. *LRFN5* is involved in presynaptic differentiation [335, 336]. SALM5/Lrfn5 is a synaptic adhesion-like molecule (SALM), one of a family of SALMs that induce presynaptic differentiation in contacting axons. *LRFN5* is also involved in neuroinflammation as a crucial contributor to immune responses in the CNS [337]. It has been shown that SALM5 suppressed lipopolysaccharide-induced inflammatory responses in the CNS and that a SALM-specific monoclonal antibody promoted inflammation in the CNS. This will be an important connection to remember in the discussion about immune responses and MDD which will be discussed in the next section.

Forty-five of 153 significant genes that were identified were found in the extended major histocompatibility complex (MHC) region[13] [338]. Neuronal expression of MHC-I is involved in developmental synaptic plasticity and axonal regeneration in the CNS [339]. The MHC may play a neuroinflammatory role in neurodegenerative diseases [340].

Three of the 153 genes that are outside of the MHC area may be potential targets for antidepressant drug therapy. These genes function in neuronal calcium signaling (*CACNA1E and CACNA2D1*); dopaminergic neurotransmission (*DRD2*), a principal target of antipsychotics; glutamate neurotransmission (*GRIK5 and GRM5*); and presynaptic vesicle trafficking (*PCLO*).

Six of the same loci in the extended MHC region are also associated with schizophrenia. These include transcription factor 4 (TCF4) which is essential for normal brain development.

It has been suggested that complex psychiatric disorders including major depressive disorder involving *complex risk factors aggregate in particular biological pathways* or are

[11] "The purpose of the *Psychiatric Genomics Consortium (PGC)* is to unite investigators around the world to conduct meta-analyses and mega-analyses of genome-wide genomic data for psychiatric disorders." [303].

[12] Introgression is the movement of a gene from one species into the gene pool of another by repeated backcrossing of an interspecific hybrid with one of its parent species [344].

[13] An illustrated review of MHC class I and MHC class II antigen presentation can be found in this 2016 reference [346]. MHC I and MHC II molecules are extremely polymorphic: more than 10,000 different alleles of MHC I molecules had been identified by 2015.

part of a higher order grouping of genes (*gene sets*) that are functionally connected [343, 345]. Their results implicated neuronal, immune, and histone pathways that are common across schizophrenia, bipolar disorder, and major depression.

The genome-wide association studies (GWAS) identified 19 significant pathways, with the following groupings judged as the most significant.

1. *RBFOX1, RBFOX2, RBFOX3, or CELF4 regulatory networks:* The RNA-binding protein, fox homolog (*Rbfox*) family of proteins form homo-and hetero oligomeric complexes to regulate alternative pre-mRNA splicing in various tissues via direct binding to their RNA-binding element [376]. *CELF4* is critical for maintaining mRNA stability and availability for translation [377]. It is expressed primarily in excitatory neurons, and it regulates excitatory but not inhibitory neurotransmission [347]. *CELF4* is developmentally regulated in the brain [348].
2. *Genes whose mRNAs are bound by FMRP:* Fragile X mental retardation protein (*FMRP*) is a polyribosome-associated neuronal RNA binding protein that plays a key role in regulating neuronal translation [349]. Its absence or reduction can cause cognitive impairment [350].
3. *Synaptic genes:* The assembly, function, plasticity, and maintenance of synapses need the coordinated expression of synaptic genes [350]. Hundreds of synaptic genes have been identified, but there are probably many more [351, 352].
4. *Genes involved in neuronal morphogenesis:* Neuronal migration and polarization are essential activities in brain morphogenesis, and both rely on microtubule function [353–355]. Toll-like receptors may also be involved in neuronal morphogenesis [356].
5. *Genes involved in neuron projection:* Interneurons and projection neurons are the two major classes of neocortex neurons [357–359]. The interneurons are generated by progenitor cells in the ventral proliferative zone of the telencephalon.[14] Then they migrate to the neocortex [360, 361]. They make connections locally within the neocortex and are mainly inhibitory. Projection neurons are generated by progenitors in the dorsal proliferative zone of the telencephalon [362, 363]. They send axonal projections to distant targets in the brain and are excitatory.
6. *Genes associated with schizophrenia (at $P < 10^{-4}$):* An earlier PGC GWAS study identified 128 independent associations spanning 108 conservatively defined loci [364]. The study's authors contend that their results point to a fundamental biological process common to MDD, schizophrenia, and other psychiatric disorders.
7. *Genes involved in CNS neuron differentiation:* Some of the processes that control neuron differentiation and survival are described in [365–368].
8. *Genes encoding voltage-gated calcium channels:* L-type voltage-gated calcium channels (L-VGCCs) activity is critical to healthy neurodevelopment and multiple neuronal processes [369, 370]. GWASs have shown that risk loci are found in the L-VGCCs for bipolar disorder, schizophrenia, MDD, anxiety disorders, autism spectrum disorder, and attention-deficit and hyperactivity disorder [369]. Suboptimal concentrations of Vitamin D could alter brain maturation through modulation of L-VGCC signaling [371].
9. *Genes involved in cytokine and immune response:* The psychoneuroimmunological association of MDD is the subject of much discussion in this chapter. It is not surprising to see that the GWAS data underscores this relationship. A 2019 review of chemokines and MDD can be found in [372].
10. *Genes known to bind to the retinoid X receptor:* There is, at this writing in 2024, very little known about genes that bind to the nuclear retinoid X receptors [373–375].

[14] Telencephalon lineage branching [378].

Summary

As we will attempt to substantiate in this monograph, both genes and nonshared environment contribute heavily to the etiology of major depressive disorders. As to the genomic contribution, candidate gene and genome-wide association studies have produced variable results. It has been speculated that uncontrolled environmental factors, in addition to small samples in early studies, gene–gene interactions, population stratification, LINES, SINES, noncoding RNAs, SNPs, CNVs, epigenetic phenomena, rare variation, and phenotypic and allelic heterogeneity may have contributed to this variability.

However, more technically sophisticated molecular techniques and powerful computational algorithms have moved us closer to the goal of understanding depression. The PGC MDD has elucidated structure variants related to MDD. PsychENCODE has pointed out the way to functional mapping of MDD epigenome relations. The 1000 Genomes Project has produced a comprehensive description of common human genetic variation in a diverse set of individuals from multiple populations. The Human Connectome Project has begun to map all the neural pathways in the brain and relate them to brain disorders of faulty connectivity.

Now we are ready for the next chapter: a look at the complex interactions of the immune system with depression.

References

1. Van den Boogaard M, Smemo S, Burnicka-Turek O, Arnolds DE, et al. A common genetic variant within SCN10A modulates cardiacSCN5A expression. J Clin Invest. 2014; https://doi.org/10.1172/JCI73140.
2. Smemo S, Tena JT, Kim K, Gamazon ER, et al. Obesity-associated variants within FTO form long-range functional connections with IRX3. Nature. 2014; https://doi.org/10.1038/nature13138.
3. Vilensky J, Robertson W, Suarez-Quian C. The clinical anatomy of the cranial nerves: the nerves of "On Olympus Towering Top". Ames: Wiley-Blackwell; 2015. ISBN 978-1-118-49201-7.
4. Purves D, Augustine GJ, Fitzpatrick D, Hall WC, LaMantia AS, McNamara JO, White LE. Neuroscience. 4th ed. Sinauer Associates; 2008. p. 15–6.
5. Kolb B, Whishaw IQ. Fundamentals of human neuropsychology. 5th ed. New York: Worth Publishing; 2003. p. 49. ISBN 978-0-7167-5300-1.
6. Saladin K. Human anatomy. 3rd ed. McGraw-Hill; 2011. p. 416–22. ISBN 9780071222075.
7. Liang J, Yu Q, Liu Y, Qiu Y, Tang R, Yan L, Zhou P. Gray matter abnormalities in patients with major depressive disorder and social anxiety disorder: a voxel-based meta-analysis. Brain Imaging Behav. 2023;17(6):749–63. PMCID: PMC10733224. http://www.ncbi.nlm.nih.gov/pubmed/37725323.
8. Brain Map - brain-map.org.
9. Physiology, Cerebral Cortex Functions - StatPearls - NCBI Bookshelf.
10. Filley CM, Fields RD. White matter and cognition: making the connection. J Neurophysiol. 2016;116(5):2093–104. PMCID: PMC5102321. http://www.ncbi.nlm.nih.gov/pubmed/27512019.
11. Brain Basics: The Life and Death of a Neuron | National Institute of Neurological Disorders and Stroke
12. What are glia? - Queensland Brain Institute - University of Queensland.
13. Appan D, Hsu SM, Hsu WH, Chou SJ. Patterning the cerebral cortex into distinct functional domains during development. Curr Opin Neurobiol. 2023;80:102698. PMID: 36893490. http://www.ncbi.nlm.nih.gov/pubmed/36893490.
14. Pakkenberg B, Pelvig D, Marner L, Bundgaard MJ, Gundersen HJG, Nyengaard JR, Regeur L. Aging and the human neocortex. Exp Gerontol. 2003;38(1–2):95–9. PMID: 12543266. http://www.ncbi.nlm.nih.gov/pubmed/12543266.
15. Pakkenberg B, Gundersen HJ. Neocortical neuron number in humans: effect of sex and age. J Comp Neurol. 1997;384(2):312–20. PMID: 9215725. http://www.ncbi.nlm.nih.gov/pubmed/9215725.
16. Williams RW. Mapping genes that modulate mouse brain development: a quantitative genetic approach. Results Probl Cell Differ. 2000;30:21–49. PMID: 10857184. http://www.ncbi.nlm.nih.gov/pubmed/10857184.
17. Silvestri L, Sacconi L, Pavone FS. The connectomics challenge. Funct Neurol. 2013;28(3):167–73. PMCID: PMC3812743. http://www.ncbi.nlm.nih.gov/pubmed/24139653.
18. von Bernhardi R, Eugenín-von Bernhardi J, Flores B, Eugenín LJ. Glial cells and integrity of the nervous system. Adv Exp Med Biol. 2016;949:1–24. PMID: 27714682. http://www.ncbi.nlm.nih.gov/pubmed/27714682.
19. Verkhratsky A, Ho MS, Parpura V. Evolution of neuroglia. Adv Exp Med Biol. 2019;1175:15–44. PMCID: PMC7188604. http://www.ncbi.nlm.nih.gov/pubmed/31583583.
20. von Bartheld CS, Bahney J, Herculano-Houzel S. The search for true numbers of neurons and glial cells in the human brain: a review of 150 years of cell counting. J Comp Neurol. 2016;524(18):3865–95. PMCID: PMC5063692. http://www.ncbi.nlm.nih.gov/pubmed/27187682.
21. Henn RE, Noureldein MH, Elzinga SE, Kim B, Savelieff MG, Feldman EL. Glial-neuron crosstalk in health and disease: a focus on metabolism, obesity, and cognitive impairment. Neurobiol Dis. 2022;170:105766. PMCID: PMC10071699. http://www.ncbi.nlm.nih.gov/pubmed/35584728.
22. Tishkoff SA, Kidd KK. Implications of biogeography of human populations for "race" and medicine. Nat Genet. 2004;36(11 Suppl):S21–7. PMID: 15507999. http://www.ncbi.nlm.nih.gov/pubmed/15507999.
23. Jorde LB, Wooding SP. Genetic variation, classification and "race". Nat Genet. 2004;36(11 Suppl):S28–33. PMID: 15508000. http://www.ncbi.nlm.nih.gov/pubmed/15508000.
24. Pennisi E. Genomics. ENCODE project writes eulogy for junk DNA. Science. 2012;337(6099):1159, 1161. PMID: 22955811. http://www.ncbi.nlm.nih.gov/pubmed/22955811.
25. International Human Genome Sequencing Consortium. Finishing the euchromatic sequence of the human genome. Nature. 2004;431(7011):931–45. PMID: 15496913. http://www.ncbi.nlm.nih.gov/pubmed/15496913.
26. Derrien T, Guigó R, Johnson R. The long non-coding RNAs: a new (P)layer in the "Dark Matter.". Front Genet. 2011;2:107. PMCID: PMC3266617. http://www.ncbi.nlm.nih.gov/pubmed/22303401.
27. Cordaux R, Batzer MA. The impact of retrotransposons on human genome evolution. Nat Rev Genet. 2009;10(10):691–703. PMCID: PMC2884099. http://www.ncbi.nlm.nih.gov/pubmed/19763152.
28. Singer T, McConnell MJ, Marchetto MCN, Coufal NG, Gage FH. LINE-1 retrotransposons: mediators of somatic variation in neuronal genomes? Trends Neurosci. 2010;33(8):345–54. PMCID: PMC2916067. http://www.ncbi.nlm.nih.gov/pubmed/20471112.
29. Lander ES, Linton LM, Birren B, Nusbaum C, Zody MC, Baldwin J, Devon K, Dewar K, Doyle M, FitzHugh W, Funke R, Gage D, Harris K, Heaford A, Howland J, Kann L, Lehoczky J, LeVine R, McEwan P, McKernan K, Meldrim J, Mesirov JP, Miranda C, Morris W, Naylor J, Raymond C, Rosetti M, Santos R, Sheridan A, Sougnez C, Stange-Thomann Y, Stojanovic N, Subramanian A, Wyman D, Rogers J, Sulston J, Ainscough R, Beck S, Bentley D, Burton J, Clee C, Carter N, Coulson A, Deadman R, Deloukas P, Dunham A, Dunham I, Durbin R, French L, Grafham D, Gregory S, Hubbard T, Humphray S, Hunt A, Jones M, Lloyd C, McMurray A, Matthews L, Mercer S, Milne S, Mullikin JC, Mungall A, Plumb R, Ross M, Shownkeen R, Sims S, Waterston RH, Wilson RK, Hillier LW, McPherson JD, Marra MA, Mardis ER, Fulton LA, Chinwalla AT, Pepin KH, Gish WR, Chissoe SL, Wendl MC, Delehaunty KD, Miner TL, Delehaunty A, Kramer JB, Cook LL, Fulton RS, Johnson DL, Minx PJ, Clifton SW, Hawkins T, Branscomb E, Predki P, Richardson P, Wenning S, Slezak T, Doggett N, Cheng JF, Olsen A, Lucas S, Elkin C, Uberbacher E, Frazier M, Gibbs RA, Muzny DM, Scherer SE, Bouck JB, Sodergren EJ, Worley KC, Rives CM, Gorrell JH, Metzker ML, Naylor SL, Kucherlapati RS, Nelson DL, Weinstock GM, Sakaki Y, Fujiyama A, Hattori M, Yada T, Toyoda A, Itoh T, Kawagoe C, Watanabe H, Totoki Y, Taylor T, Weissenbach J, Heilig R, Saurin W, Artiguenave F, Brottier P, Bruls T, Pelletier E, Robert C, Wincker P, Smith DR, Doucette-Stamm L, Rubenfield M, Weinstock K, Lee HM, Dubois J, Rosenthal A, Platzer M, Nyakatura G, Taudien S, Rump A, Yang H, Yu J, Wang J, Huang G, Gu J, Hood L, Rowen L, Madan A, Qin S, Davis RW, Federspiel NA, Abola AP, Proctor MJ, Myers RM, Schmutz J, Dickson M, Grimwood J, Cox DR, Olson MV, Kaul R, Raymond C, Shimizu N, Kawasaki K, Minoshima S, Evans GA, Athanasiou M, Schultz R, Roe BA, Chen F, Pan H, Ramser J, Lehrach H, Reinhardt R, McCombie WR, de la Bastide M, Dedhia N, Blöcker H, Hornischer K, Nordsiek G, Agarwala R, Aravind L, Bailey JA, Bateman A, Batzoglou S, Birney E, Bork P, Brown DG, Burge CB, Cerutti L, Chen HC, Church D,

Clamp M, Copley RR, Doerks T, Eddy SR, Eichler EE, Furey TS, Galagan J, Gilbert JG, Harmon C, Hayashizaki Y, Haussler D, Hermjakob H, Hokamp K, Jang W, Johnson LS, Jones TA, Kasif S, Kaspryzk A, Kennedy S, Kent WJ, Kitts P, Koonin EV, Korf I, Kulp D, Lancet D, Lowe TM, McLysaght A, Mikkelsen T, Moran JV, Mulder N, Pollara VJ, Ponting CP, Schuler G, Schultz J, Slater G, Smit AF, Stupka E, Szustakowki J, Thierry-Mieg D, Thierry-Mieg J, Wagner L, Wallis J, Wheeler R, Williams A, Wolf YI, Wolfe KH, Yang SP, Yeh RF, Collins F, Guyer MS, Peterson J, Felsenfeld A, Wetterstrand KA, Patrinos A, Morgan MJ, de Jong P, Catanese JJ, Osoegawa K, Shizuya H, Choi S, Chen YJ, Szustakowki J, International Human Genome Sequencing Consortium. Initial sequencing and analysis of the human genome. Nature. 2001;409(6822):860–921. PMID: 11237011. http://www.ncbi.nlm.nih.gov/pubmed/11237011.

30. Chesnokova E, Beletskiy A, Kolosov P. The role of transposable elements of the human genome in neuronal function and pathology. Int J Mol Sci. 2022;23(10):5847. PMCID: PMC9148063. http://www.ncbi.nlm.nih.gov/pubmed/35628657.
31. Wells JN, Feschotte C. A field guide to eukaryotic transposable elements. Annu Rev Genet. 2020;54:539–61. PMCID: PMC8293684. http://www.ncbi.nlm.nih.gov/pubmed/32955944.
32. Arkhipova IR, Yushenova IA. Giant transposons in eukaryotes: is bigger better? Genome Biol Evol. 2019;11(3):906–18. PMCID: PMC6431247. http://www.ncbi.nlm.nih.gov/pubmed/30796812.
33. Xiong Y, Eickbush TH. Origin and evolution of retroelements based upon their reverse transcriptase sequences. EMBO J. 1990;9(10):3353–62. PMCID: PMC552073. http://www.ncbi.nlm.nih.gov/pubmed/1698615.
34. Muotri AR, Zhao C, Marchetto MCN, Gage FH. Environmental influence on L1 retrotransposons in the adult hippocampus. Hippocampus. 2009;19(10):1002–7. PMCID: PMC2758700. http://www.ncbi.nlm.nih.gov/pubmed/19771587.
35. Coufal NG, Garcia-Perez JL, Peng GE, Yeo GW, Mu Y, Lovci MT, Morell M, O'Shea KS, Moran JV, Gage FH. L1 retrotransposition in human neural progenitor cells. Nature. 2009;460(7259):1127–31. PMCID: PMC2909034. http://www.ncbi.nlm.nih.gov/pubmed/19657334.
36. Rehen SK, Yung YC, McCreight MP, Kaushal D, Yang AH, Almeida BSV, Kingsbury MA, Cabral KMS, McConnell MJ, Anliker B, Fontanoz M, Chun J. Constitutional aneuploidy in the normal human brain. J Neurosci. 2005;25(9):2176–80. PMCID: PMC6726097. http://www.ncbi.nlm.nih.gov/pubmed/15745943.
37. Rehen SK, McConnell MJ, Kaushal D, Kingsbury MA, Yang AH, Chun J. Chromosomal variation in neurons of the developing and adult mammalian nervous system. Proc Natl Acad Sci U S A. 2001;98(23):13361–6. PMCID: PMC60876. http://www.ncbi.nlm.nih.gov/pubmed/11698687.
38. Bruder CEG, Piotrowski A, Gijsbers AACJ, Andersson R, Erickson S, Diaz de Ståhl T, Menzel U, Sandgren J, von Tell D, Poplawski A, Crowley M, Crasto C, Partridge EC, Tiwari H, Allison DB, Komorowski J, van Ommen GJB, Boomsma DI, Pedersen NL, den Dunnen JT, Wirdefeldt K, Dumanski JP. Phenotypically concordant and discordant monozygotic twins display different DNA copy-number-variation profiles. Am J Hum Genet. 2008;82(3):763–71. PMCID: PMC2427204. http://www.ncbi.nlm.nih.gov/pubmed/18304490.
39. Muotri AR, Chu VT, Marchetto MCN, Deng W, Moran JV, Gage FH. Somatic mosaicism in neuronal precursor cells mediated by L1 retrotransposition. Nature. 2005;435(7044):903–10. PMID: 15959507. http://www.ncbi.nlm.nih.gov/pubmed/15959507.
40. Crepaldi L, Policarpi C, Coatti A, Sherlock WT, Jongbloets BC, Down TA, Riccio A. Binding of TFIIIC to sine elements controls the relocation of activity-dependent neuronal genes to transcription factories. PLoS Genet. 2013;9(8):e1003699. PMCID: PMC3744447. http://www.ncbi.nlm.nih.gov/pubmed/23966877.
41. Volff JN, Brosius J. Modern genomes with retro-look: retrotransposed elements, retroposition and the origin of new genes. Genome Dyn. 2007;3:175–90. PMID: 18753792. http://www.ncbi.nlm.nih.gov/pubmed/18753792.
42. Gotea V, Makałowski W. Do transposable elements really contribute to proteomes? Trends Genet. 2006;22(5):260–7. PMID: 16569458. http://www.ncbi.nlm.nih.gov/pubmed/16569458.
43. Xing J, Wang H, Belancio VP, Cordaux R, Deininger PL, Batzer MA. Emergence of primate genes by retrotransposon-mediated sequence transduction. Proc Natl Acad Sci U S A. 2006;103(47):17608–17613. PMCID: PMC1693794. http://www.ncbi.nlm.nih.gov/pubmed/17101974.
44. Chueh AC, Northrop EL, Brettingham-Moore KH, Choo KHA, Wong LH. LINE retrotransposon RNA is an essential structural and functional epigenetic component of a core neocentromeric chromatin. PLoS Genet. 2009;5(1):e1000354. PMCID: PMC2625447. http://www.ncbi.nlm.nih.gov/pubmed/19180186.
45. Faulkner GJ, Kimura Y, Daub CO, Wani S, Plessy C, Irvine KM, Schroder K, Cloonan N, Steptoe AL, Lassmann T, Waki K, Hornig N, Arakawa T, Takahashi H, Kawai J, Forrest ARR, Suzuki H, Hayashizaki Y, Hume DA, Orlando V, Grimmond SM, Carninci P. The regulated retrotransposon transcriptome of mammalian cells. Nat Genet. 2009;41(5):563–71. PMID: 19377475. http://www.ncbi.nlm.nih.gov/pubmed/19377475.
46. Mätlik K, Redik K, Speek M. L1 antisense promoter drives tissue-specific transcription of human genes. J Biomed Biotechnol. 2006;2006(1):71753. PMCID: PMC1559930. http://www.ncbi.nlm.nih.gov/pubmed/16877819.
47. Ewing AD, Ballinger TJ, Earl D, Broad Institute Genome Sequencing, Program A, Platform HCC, Ding L, Wilson RK, Haussler D. Retrotransposition of gene transcripts leads to structural variation in mammalian genomes. Genome Biol. 2013;14(3):R22. PMCID: PMC3663115. http://www.ncbi.nlm.nih.gov/pubmed/23497673.
48. Berk T, de Boer E, Bilgrav Saether K, Eisfeldt J. Discovery of non-reference processed pseudogenes in the Swedish population. Front Genet. 2023;14:1176626. PMCID: PMC10267823. http://www.ncbi.nlm.nih.gov/pubmed/37323659.
49. 1000 Genomes | A Deep Catalog of Human Genetic Variation.
50. The Cancer Genome Atlas Program (TCGA) - NCI.
51. Kaessmann H, Vinckenbosch N, Long M. RNA-based gene duplication: mechanistic and evolutionary insights. Nat Rev Genet. 2009;10(1):19–31. PMCID: PMC3690669. http://www.ncbi.nlm.nih.gov/pubmed/19030023.
52. Spadaro PA, Bredy TW. Emerging role of non-coding RNA in neural plasticity, cognitive function, and neuropsychiatric disorders. Front Genet. 2012;3:132. PMCID: PMC3395882. http://www.ncbi.nlm.nih.gov/pubmed/22811697.
53. Washietl S, Pedersen JS, Korbel JO, Stocsits C, Gruber AR, Hackermüller J, Hertel J, Lindemeyer M, Reiche K, Tanzer A, Ucla C, Wyss C, Antonarakis SE, Denoeud F, Lagarde J, Drenkow J, Kapranov P, Gingeras TR, Guigó R, Snyder M, Gerstein MB, Reymond A, Hofacker IL, Stadler PF. Structured RNAs in the ENCODE selected regions of the human genome. Genome Res. 2007;17(6):852–64. PMCID: PMC1891344. http://www.ncbi.nlm.nih.gov/pubmed/17568003.
54. Mattick JS. The double life of RNA. Biochimie. 2011;93(11):viii–ix. PMID: 21963144. http://www.ncbi.nlm.nih.gov/pubmed/21963144.
55. Lin Q, Wei W, Coelho CM, Li X, Baker-Andresen D, Dudley K, Ratnu VS, Boskovic Z, Kobor MS, Sun YE, Bredy TW. The brain-specific microRNA miR-128b regulates the formation of fear-extinction memory. Nat Neurosci. 2011;14(9):1115–7. PMID: 21841775. http://www.ncbi.nlm.nih.gov/pubmed/17568003.

56. Mattick JS, Makunin IV. Non-coding RNA. Hum Mol Genet. 2006;15 Spec No 1:R17-29. PMID: 16651366. http://www.ncbi.nlm.nih.gov/pubmed/16651366.
57. Friedman RC, Farh KKH, Burge CB, Bartel DP. Most mammalian mRNAs are conserved targets of microRNAs. Genome Res. 2009;19(1):92–105. PMCID: PMC2612969. http://www.ncbi.nlm.nih.gov/pubmed/18955434.
58. Kretz M, Webster DE, Flockhart RJ, Lee CS, Zehnder A, Lopez-Pajares V, Qu K, Zheng GXY, Chow J, Kim GE, Rinn JL, Chang HY, Siprashvili Z, Khavari PA. Suppression of progenitor differentiation requires the long noncoding RNA ANCR. Genes Dev. 2012;26(4):338–43. PMCID: PMC3289881. http://www.ncbi.nlm.nih.gov/pubmed/22302877.
59. Nejepinska J, Malik R, Filkowski J, Flemr M, Filipowicz W, Svoboda P. dsRNA expression in the mouse elicits RNAi in oocytes and low adenosine deamination in somatic cells. Nucleic Acids Res. 2012;40(1):399–413. PMCID: PMC3245926. http://www.ncbi.nlm.nih.gov/pubmed/21908396.
60. Borchert GM, Holton NW, Williams JD, Hernan WL, Bishop IP, Dembosky JA, Elste JE, Gregoire NS, Kim JA, Koehler WW, Lengerich JC, Medema AA, Nguyen MA, Ower GD, Rarick MA, Strong BN, Tardi NJ, Tasker NM, Wozniak DJ, Gatto C, Larson ED. Comprehensive analysis of microRNA genomic loci identifies pervasive repetitive-element origins. Mob Genet Elem. 2011;1(1):8–17. PMCID: PMC3190270. http://www.ncbi.nlm.nih.gov/pubmed/22016841.
61. Varela MA, Amos W. Heterogeneous distribution of SNPs in the human genome: microsatellites as predictors of nucleotide diversity and divergence. Genomics. 2010;95(3):151–9. PMID: 20026267. http://www.ncbi.nlm.nih.gov/pubmed/20026267.
62. Collins FS, Brooks LD, Chakravarti A. A DNA polymorphism discovery resource for research on human genetic variation. Genome Res. 1998;8(12):1229–31. PMID: 9872978. http://www.ncbi.nlm.nih.gov/pubmed/9872978.
63. Stankiewicz P, Lupski JR. Structural variation in the human genome and its role in disease. Annu Rev Med. 2010;61:437–55. PMID: 20059347. http://www.ncbi.nlm.nih.gov/pubmed/20059347.
64. Stranger BE, Forrest MS, Dunning M, Ingle CE, Beazley C, Thorne N, Redon R, Bird CP, de Grassi A, Lee C, Tyler-Smith C, Carter N, Scherer SW, Tavaré S, Deloukas P, Hurles ME, Dermitzakis ET. Relative impact of nucleotide and copy number variation on gene expression phenotypes. Science. 2007;315(5813):848–53. PMCID: PMC2665772. http://www.ncbi.nlm.nih.gov/pubmed/17289997.
65. Kidd JM, Cooper GM, Donahue WF, Hayden HS, Sampas N, Graves T, Hansen N, Teague B, Alkan C, Antonacci F, Haugen E, Zerr T, Yamada NA, Tsang P, Newman TL, Tüzün E, Cheng Z, Ebling HM, Tusneem N, David R, Gillett W, Phelps KA, Weaver M, Saranga D, Brand A, Tao W, Gustafson E, McKernan K, Chen L, Malig M, Smith JD, Korn JM, McCarroll SA, Altshuler DA, Peiffer DA, Dorschner M, Stamatoyannopoulos J, Schwartz D, Nickerson DA, Mullikin JC, Wilson RK, Bruhn L, Olson MV, Kaul R, Smith DR, Eichler EE. Mapping and sequencing of structural variation from eight human genomes. Nature. 2008;453(7191):56–64. PMCID: PMC2424287. http://www.ncbi.nlm.nih.gov/pubmed/18451855.
66. Zhang F, Gu W, Hurles ME, Lupski JR. Copy number variation in human health, disease, and evolution. Annu Rev Genomics Hum Genet. 2009;10:451–81. PMCID: PMC4472309. http://www.ncbi.nlm.nih.gov/pubmed/19715442.
67. Gross L. A new human genome sequence paves the way for individualized genomics. PLoS Biol. 2007;5(10):e266. PMCID: PMC1964778. http://www.ncbi.nlm.nih.gov/pubmed/20076646.
68. Redon R, Ishikawa S, Fitch KR, Feuk L, Perry GH, Andrews TD, Fiegler H, Shapero MH, Carson AR, Chen W, Cho EK, Dallaire S, Freeman JL, González JR, Gratacòs M, Huang J, Kalaitzopoulos D, Komura D, MacDonald JR, Marshall CR, Mei R, Montgomery L, Nishimura K, Okamura K, Shen F, Somerville MJ, Tchinda J, Valsesia A, Woodwark C, Yang F, Zhang J, Zerjal T, Zhang J, Armengol L, Conrad DF, Estivill X, Tyler-Smith C, Carter NP, Aburatani H, Lee C, Jones KW, Scherer SW, Hurles ME. Global variation in copy number in the human genome. Nature. 2006;444(7118):444–54. PMCID: PMC2669898. http://www.ncbi.nlm.nih.gov/pubmed/17122850.
69. Soto DC, Uribe-Salazar JM, Shew CJ, Sekar A, McGinty SP, Dennis MY. Genomic structural variation: a complex but important driver of human evolution. Am J Biol Anthropol. 2023;181 Suppl 76(Suppl 76):118–44. PMCID: PMC10329998. http://www.ncbi.nlm.nih.gov/pubmed/36794631.
70. Perry GH, Tchinda J, McGrath SD, Zhang J, Picker SR, Cáceres AM, Iafrate AJ, Tyler-Smith C, Scherer SW, Eichler EE, Stone AC, Lee C. Hotspots for copy number variation in chimpanzees and humans. Proc Natl Acad Sci U S A. 2006;103(21):8006–11. PMCID: PMC1472420. http://www.ncbi.nlm.nih.gov/pubmed/16702545.
71. Home - dbVar - NCBI.
72. Database of Genomic Variants [*** v107 ***].
73. Hochstenbach R, Buizer-Voskamp JE, Vorstman J, Ophoff RA. Genome arrays for the detection of copy number variations in idiopathic mental retardation, idiopathic generalized epilepsy and neuropsychiatric disorders: lessons for diagnostic workflow and research. Cytogenet Genome Res. 2011;135(3–4):174–202. PMID: 22056632. http://www.ncbi.nlm.nih.gov/pubmed/22056632.
74. Freeman JL, Perry GH, Feuk L, Redon R, McCarroll SA, Altshuler DM, Aburatani H, Jones KW, Tyler-Smith C, Hurles ME, Carter NP, Scherer SW, Lee C. Copy number variation: new insights in genome diversity. Genome Res. 2006;16(8):949–61. PMID: 16809666. http://www.ncbi.nlm.nih.gov/pubmed/16809666.
75. Lee JA, Lupski JR. Genomic rearrangements and gene copy-number alterations as a cause of nervous system disorders. Neuron. 2006;52(1):103–21. PMID: 17015230. http://www.ncbi.nlm.nih.gov/pubmed/17015230.
76. Li X, Tan L, Liu X, Lei S, Yang T, Chen X, Zhang F, Fang Y, Guo Y, Zhang L, Yan H, Pan F, Zhang Z, Peng Y, Zhou Q, He L, Zhu X, Cheng J, Zhang L, Liu Y, Tian Q, Deng H. A genome wide association study between copy number variation (CNV) and human height in Chinese population. J Genet Genomics. 2010;37(12):779–85. PMID: 21193156. http://www.ncbi.nlm.nih.gov/pubmed/21193156.
77. Dauber A, Yu Y, Turchin MC, Chiang CW, Meng YA, Demerath EW, Patel SR, Rich SS, Rotter JI, Schreiner PJ, Wilson JG, Shen Y, Wu BL, Hirschhorn JN. Genome-wide association of copy-number variation reveals an association between short stature and the presence of low-frequency genomic deletions. Am J Hum Genet. 2011;89(6):751–9. PMCID: PMC3234379. http://www.ncbi.nlm.nih.gov/pubmed/22118881.
78. Yeo RA, Gangestad SW, Liu J, Calhoun VD, Hutchison KE. Rare copy number deletions predict individual variation in intelligence. PloS One. 2011;6(1):e16339. PMCID: PMC3027642. http://www.ncbi.nlm.nih.gov/pubmed/21298096.
79. Wellcome Trust Case Control Consortium, Craddock N, Hurles ME, Cardin N, Pearson RD, Plagnol V, Robson S, Vukcevic D, Barnes C, Conrad DF, Giannoulatou E, Holmes C, Marchini JL, Stirrups K, Tobin MD, Wain LV, Yau C, Aerts J, Ahmad T, Andrews TD, Arbury H, Attwood A, Auton A, Ball SG, Balmforth AJ, Barrett JC, Barroso I, Barton A, Bennett AJ, Bhaskar S, Blaszczyk K, Bowes J, Brand OJ, Braund PS, Bredin F, Breen G, Brown MJ, Bruce IN, Bull J, Burren OS, Burton J, Byrnes J, Caesar S, Clee CM, Coffey AJ, Connell JMC, Cooper JD, Dominiczak AF, Downes K, Drummond HE, Dudakia D, Dunham A, Ebbs B, Eccles D, Edkins S, Edwards C, Elliot A, Emery P, Evans DM, Evans G, Eyre S, Farmer A, Ferrier IN,

Feuk L, Fitzgerald T, Flynn E, Forbes A, Forty L, Franklyn JA, Freathy RM, Gibbs P, Gilbert P, Gokumen O, Gordon-Smith K, Gray E, Green E, Groves CJ, Grozeva D, Gwilliam R, Hall A, Hammond N, Hardy M, Harrison P, Hassanali N, Hebaishi H, Hines S, Hinks A, Hitman GA, Hocking L, Howard E, Howard P, Howson JMM, Hughes D, Hunt S, Isaacs JD, Jain M, Jewell DP, Johnson T, Jolley JD, Jones IR, Jones LA, Kirov G, Langford CF, Lango-Allen H, Lathrop GM, Lee J, Lee KL, Lees C, Lewis K, Lindgren CM, Maisuria-Armer M, Maller J, Mansfield J, Martin P, Massey DCO, McArdle WL, McGuffin P, McLay KE, Mentzer A, Mimmack ML, Morgan AE, Morris AP, Mowat C, Myers S, Newman W, Nimmo ER, O'Donovan MC, Onipinla A, Onyiah I, Ovington NR, Owen MJ, Palin K, Parnell K, Pernet D, Perry JRB, Phillips A, Pinto D, Prescott NJ, Prokopenko I, Quail MA, Rafelt S, Rayner NW, Redon R, Reid DM, Renwick null, Ring SM, Robertson N, Russell E, St Clair D, Sambrook JG, Sanderson JD, Schuilenburg H, Scott CE, Scott R, Seal S, Shaw-Hawkins S, Shields BM, Simmonds MJ, Smyth DJ, Somaskantharajah E, Spanova K, Steer S, Stephens J, Stevens HE, Stone MA, Su Z, Symmons DPM, Thompson JR, Thomson W, Travers ME, Turnbull C, Valsesia A, Walker M, Walker NM, Wallace C, Warren-Perry M, Watkins NA, Webster J, Weedon MN, Wilson AG, Woodburn M, Wordsworth BP, Young AH, Zeggini E, Carter NP, Frayling TM, Lee C, McVean G, Munroe PB, Palotie A, Sawcer SJ, Scherer SW, Strachan DP, Tyler-Smith C, Brown MA, Burton PR, Caulfield MJ, Compston A, Farrall M, Gough SCL, Hall AS, Hattersley AT, Hill AVS, Mathew CG, Pembrey M, Satsangi J, Stratton MR, Worthington J, Deloukas P, Duncanson A, Kwiatkowski DP, McCarthy MI, Ouwehand W, Parkes M, Rahman N, Todd JA, Samani NJ, Donnelly P. Genome-wide association study of CNVs in 16,000 cases of eight common diseases and 3,000 shared controls. Nature. 2010;464(7289):713–20. PMCID: PMC2892339. http://www.ncbi.nlm.nih.gov/pubmed/20360734.

80. Leveziel N, Puche N, Zerbib J, Benlian P, Coscas G, Soubrane G, Souied E. Genetic factors associated with age-related macular degeneration. Med Sci (Paris). 2010;26(5):509–15. PMID: 20510150. http://www.ncbi.nlm.nih.gov/pubmed/20510150.
81. Girirajan S, Campbell CD, Eichler EE. Human copy number variation and complex genetic disease. Annu Rev Genet. 2011;45:203–26. PMCID: PMC6662611. http://www.ncbi.nlm.nih.gov/pubmed/21854229.
82. Frank B, Hemminki K, Meindl A, Wappenschmidt B, Sutter C, Kiechle M, Bugert P, Schmutzler RK, Bartram CR, Burwinkel B. BRIP1 (BACH1) variants and familial breast cancer risk: a case-control study. BMC Cancer. 2007;7:83. PMCID: PMC1887536. http://www.ncbi.nlm.nih.gov/pubmed/17504528.
83. Gonzalez E, Kulkarni H, Bolivar H, Mangano A, Sanchez R, Catano G, Nibbs RJ, Freedman BI, Quinones MP, Bamshad MJ, Murthy KK, Rovin BH, Bradley W, Clark RA, Anderson SA, O'connell RJ, Agan BK, Ahuja SS, Bologna R, Sen L, Dolan MJ, Ahuja SK. The influence of CCL3L1 gene-containing segmental duplications on HIV-1/AIDS susceptibility. Science. 2005;307(5714):1434–40. PMID: 15637236 http://www.ncbi.nlm.nih.gov/pubmed/15637236.
84. Fellermann K, Stange DE, Schaeffeler E, Schmalzl H, Wehkamp J, Bevins CL, Reinisch W, Teml A, Schwab M, Lichter P, Radlwimmer B, Stange EF. A chromosome 8 gene-cluster polymorphism with low human beta-defensin 2 gene copy number predisposes to Crohn disease of the colon. Am J Hum Genet. 2006;79(3):439–48. PMCID: PMC1559531. http://www.ncbi.nlm.nih.gov/pubmed/16909382.
85. McKinney C, Merriman ME, Chapman PT, Gow PJ, Harrison AA, Highton J, Jones PBB, McLean L, O'Donnell JL, Pokorny V, Spellerberg M, Stamp LK, Willis J, Steer S, Merriman TR. Evidence for an influence of chemokine ligand 3-like 1 (CCL3L1) gene copy number on susceptibility to rheumatoid arthritis. Ann Rheum Dis. 2008;67(3):409–13. PMID: 17604289. http://www.ncbi.nlm.nih.gov/pubmed/17604289.
86. Hollox EJ, Huffmeier U, Zeeuwen PLJM, Palla R, Lascorz J, Rodijk-Olthuis D, van de Kerkhof PCM, Traupe H, de Jongh G, den Heijer M, Reis A, Armour JAL, Schalkwijk J. Psoriasis is associated with increased beta-defensin genomic copy number. Nat Genet. 2008;40(1):23–5. PMCID: PMC2447885. http://www.ncbi.nlm.nih.gov/pubmed/18059266.
87. Merikangas AK, Corvin AP, Gallagher L. Copy-number variants in neurodevelopmental disorders: promises and challenges. Trends Genet. 2009;25(12):536–44. PMID: 19910074. http://www.ncbi.nlm.nih.gov/pubmed/19910074.
88. Itsara A, Cooper GM, Baker C, Girirajan S, Li J, Absher D, Krauss RM, Myers RM, Ridker PM, Chasman DI, Mefford H, Ying P, Nickerson DA, Eichler EE. Population analysis of large copy number variants and hotspots of human genetic disease. Am J Hum Genet. 2009;84(2):148–61. PMCID: PMC2668011. http://www.ncbi.nlm.nih.gov/pubmed/18304490.
89. Magri C, Sacchetti E, Traversa M, Valsecchi P, Gardella R, Bonvicini C, Minelli A, Gennarelli M, Barlati S. New copy number variations in schizophrenia. PloS One. 2010;5(10):e13422. PMCID: PMC2954184. http://www.ncbi.nlm.nih.gov/pubmed/20967226.
90. Salyakina D, Cukier HN, Lee JM, Sacharow S, Nations LD, Ma D, Jaworski JM, Konidari I, Whitehead PL, Wright HH, Abramson RK, Williams SM, Menon R, Haines JL, Gilbert JR, Cuccaro ML, Pericak-Vance MA. Copy number variants in extended autism spectrum disorder families reveal candidates potentially involved in autism risk. PloS One. 2011;6(10):e26049. PMCID: PMC3189231. http://www.ncbi.nlm.nih.gov/pubmed/22016809.
91. Karlsson R, Graae L, Lekman M, Wang D, Favis R, Axelsson T, Galter D, Belin AC, Paddock S. MAGI1 copy number variation in bipolar affective disorder and schizophrenia. Biol Psychiatry. 2012;71(10):922–30. PMID: 22381734. http://www.ncbi.nlm.nih.gov/pubmed/22381734.
92. Rucker JJH, McGuffin P. Genomic structural variation in psychiatric disorders. Dev Psychopathol. 2012;24(4):1335–44. PMID: 23062301. http://www.ncbi.nlm.nih.gov/pubmed/23062301.
93. Xu B, Roos JL, Levy S, van Rensburg EJ, Gogos JA, Karayiorgou M. Strong association of de novo copy number mutations with sporadic schizophrenia. Nat Genet. 2008;40(7):880–5. PMID: 18511947. http://www.ncbi.nlm.nih.gov/pubmed/18511947.
94. Helbig I, Mefford HC, Sharp AJ, Guipponi M, Fichera M, Franke A, Muhle H, de Kovel C, Baker C, von Spiczak S, Kron KL, Steinich I, Kleefuss-Lie AA, Leu C, Gaus V, Schmitz B, Klein KM, Reif PS, Rosenow F, Weber Y, Lerche H, Zimprich F, Urak L, Fuchs K, Feucht M, Genton P, Thomas P, Visscher F, de Haan GJ, Møller RS, Hjalgrim H, Luciano D, Wittig M, Nothnagel M, Elger CE, Nürnberg P, Romano C, Malafosse A, BPC K, Lindhout D, Stephani U, Schreiber S, Eichler EE, Sander T. 15q13.3 microdeletions increase risk of idiopathic generalized epilepsy. Nat Genet. 2009;41(2):160–2. PMCID: PMC3026630. http://www.ncbi.nlm.nih.gov/pubmed/19136953.
95. Ibáñez P, Bonnet AM, Débarges B, Lohmann E, Tison F, Pollak P, Agid Y, Dürr A, Brice A. Causal relation between alpha-synuclein gene duplication and familial Parkinson's disease. Lancet. 2004;364(9440):1169–71. PMID: 15451225. http://www.ncbi.nlm.nih.gov/pubmed/15451225.
96. McMullan DJ, Bonin M, Hehir-Kwa JY, de Vries BBA, Dufke A, Rattenberry E, Steehouwer M, Moruz L, Pfundt R, de Leeuw N, Riess A, Altug-Teber O, Enders H, Singer S, Grasshoff U, Walter M, Walker JM, Lamb CV, Davison EV, Brueton L, Riess O, Veltman JA. Molecular karyotyping of patients with unexplained mental retardation by SNP arrays: a multicenter study. Hum

Mutat. 2009;30(7):1082–92. PMID: 19388127. http://www.ncbi.nlm.nih.gov/pubmed/19388127.
97. Rovelet-Lecrux A, Hannequin D, Raux G, Le Meur N, Laquerrière A, Vital A, Dumanchin C, Feuillette S, Brice A, Vercelletto M, Dubas F, Frebourg T, Campion D. APP locus duplication causes autosomal dominant early-onset Alzheimer disease with cerebral amyloid angiopathy. Nat Genet. 2006;38(1):24–6. PMID: 16369530. http://www.ncbi.nlm.nih.gov/pubmed/16369530.
98. Singleton AB, Farrer M, Johnson J, Singleton A, Hague S, Kachergus J, Hulihan M, Peuralinna T, Dutra A, Nussbaum R, Lincoln S, Crawley A, Hanson M, Maraganore D, Adler C, Cookson MR, Muenter M, Baptista M, Miller D, Blancato J, Hardy J, Gwinn-Hardy K. alpha-Synuclein locus triplication causes Parkinson's disease. Science. 2003;302(5646):841. PMID: 14593171. http://www.ncbi.nlm.nih.gov/pubmed/14593171.
99. Weiss LA, Shen Y, Korn JM, Arking DE, Miller DT, Fossdal R, Saemundsen E, Stefansson H, Ferreira MAR, Green T, Platt OS, Ruderfer DM, Walsh CA, Altshuler D, Chakravarti A, Tanzi RE, Stefansson K, Santangelo SL, Gusella JF, Sklar P, Wu BL, Daly MJ, Autism Consortium. Association between microdeletion and microduplication at 16p11.2 and autism. N Engl J Med. 2008;358(7):667–75. PMID: 18184952. http://www.ncbi.nlm.nih.gov/pubmed/18184952.
100. Perlis RH, Ruderfer D, Hamilton SP, Ernst C. Copy number variation in subjects with major depressive disorder who attempted suicide. PloS One. 2012;7(9):e46315. PMCID: PMC3459919. http://www.ncbi.nlm.nih.gov/pubmed/23029476.
101. Glessner JT, Wang K, Sleiman PMA, Zhang H, Kim CE, Flory JH, Bradfield JP, Imielinski M, Frackelton EC, Qiu H, Mentch F, Grant SFA, Hakonarson H. Duplication of the SLIT3 locus on 5q35.1 predisposes to major depressive disorder. PloS One. 2010;5(12):e15463. PMCID: PMC2995745. http://www.ncbi.nlm.nih.gov/pubmed/21152026.
102. Rucker JJH, Breen G, Pinto D, Pedroso I, Lewis CM, Cohen-Woods S, Uher R, Schosser A, Rivera M, Aitchison KJ, Craddock N, Owen MJ, Jones L, Jones I, Korszun A, Muglia P, Barnes MR, Preisig M, Mors O, Gill M, Maier W, Rice J, Rietschel M, Holsboer F, Farmer AE, Craig IW, Scherer SW, McGuffin P. Genome-wide association analysis of copy number variation in recurrent depressive disorder. Mol Psychiatry. 2013;18(2):183–9. PMCID: PMC3939438. http://www.ncbi.nlm.nih.gov/pubmed/22042228.
103. Mollon J, Almasy L, Jacquemont S, Glahn DC. The contribution of copy number variants to psychiatric symptoms and cognitive ability. Mol Psychiatry. 2023;28(4):1480–93. PMCID: PMC10213133. http://www.ncbi.nlm.nih.gov/pubmed/36737482.
104. Van Den Bossche MJ, Johnstone M, Strazisar M, Pickard BS, Goossens D, Lenaerts AS, De Zutter S, Nordin A, Norrback KF, Mendlewicz J, Souery D, De Rijk P, Sabbe BG, Adolfsson R, Blackwood D, Del-Favero J. Rare copy number variants in neuropsychiatric disorders: Specific phenotype or not? Am J Med Genet B Neuropsychiatr Genet. 2012;159B(7):812–22. PMID: 22911887. http://www.ncbi.nlm.nih.gov/pubmed/22911887.
105. Degenhardt F, Priebe L, Herms S, Mattheisen M, Mühleisen TW, Meier S, Moebus S, Strohmaier J, Groß M, Breuer R, Lange C, Hoffmann P, Meyer-Lindenberg A, Heinz A, Walter H, Lucae S, Wolf C, Müller-Myhsok B, Holsboer F, Maier W, Rietschel M, Nöthen MM, Cichon S. Association between copy number variants in 16p11.2 and major depressive disorder in a German case-control sample. Am J Med Genet B Neuropsychiatr Genet. 2012;159B(3):263–73. PMID: 22344817. http://www.ncbi.nlm.nih.gov/pubmed/22344817.
106. Kendall KM, Rees E, Bracher-Smith M, Legge S, Riglin L, Zammit S, O'Donovan MC, Owen MJ, Jones I, Kirov G, Walters JTR. Association of rare copy number variants with risk of depression. JAMA Psychiatry. 2019;76(8):818–25. PMCID: PMC6583866. http://www.ncbi.nlm.nih.gov/pubmed/30994872.
107. Melhem NM, Hamdan S, Klei L, Wood S, Zelazny J, Frisch A, Weizman A, Carmel M, Michaelovsky E, Farbstein I, Wasserman D, El-Heib M, Ferrell R, Apter A, Devlin B, Brent D. Runs of homozygosity, copy number variation, and risk for depression and suicidal behavior in an Arab Bedouin kindred. Psychiatr Genet. 2017;27(5):169–77. PMCID: PMC5572483. http://www.ncbi.nlm.nih.gov/pubmed/28570395.
108. Mitani H, Shirayama Y, Yamada T, Maeda K, Ashby CR, Kawahara R. Correlation between plasma levels of glutamate, alanine and serine with severity of depression. Prog Neuropsychopharmacol Biol Psychiatry. 2006;30(6):1155–8. PMID: 16707201. http://www.ncbi.nlm.nih.gov/pubmed/16707201.
109. Maes M, Verkerk R, Vandoolaeghe E, Lin A, Scharpé S. Serum levels of excitatory amino acids, serine, glycine, histidine, threonine, taurine, alanine and arginine in treatment-resistant depression: modulation by treatment with antidepressants and prediction of clinical responsivity. Acta Psychiatr Scand. 1998;97(4):302–8. PMID: 9570492. http://www.ncbi.nlm.nih.gov/pubmed/9570492.
110. Rucker JJH, Tansey KE, Rivera M, Pinto D, Cohen-Woods S, Uher R, Aitchison KJ, Craddock N, Owen MJ, Jones L, Jones I, Korszun A, Barnes MR, Preisig M, Mors O, Maier W, Rice J, Rietschel M, Holsboer F, Farmer AE, Craig IW, Scherer SW, McGuffin P, Breen G. Phenotypic Association analyses with copy number variation in recurrent depressive disorder. Biol Psychiatry. 2016;79(4):329–36. PMCID: PMC4725574. http://www.ncbi.nlm.nih.gov/pubmed/25861698.
111. O'Dushlaine C, Ripke S, Ruderfer DM, Hamilton SP, Fava M, Iosifescu DV, Kohane IS, Churchill SE, Castro VM, Clements CC, Blumenthal SR, Murphy SN, Smoller JW, Perlis RH. Rare copy number variation in treatment-resistant major depressive disorder. Biol Psychiatry. 2014;76(7):536–41. PMCID: PMC4104153. http://www.ncbi.nlm.nih.gov/pubmed/24529801.
112. D'Gama AM, Walsh CA. Somatic mosaicism and neurodevelopmental disease. Nat Neurosci. 2018;21(11):1504–14. PMID: 30349109. http://www.ncbi.nlm.nih.gov/pubmed/30349109.
113. Lodato MA, Walsh CA. Genome aging: somatic mutation in the brain links age-related decline with disease and nominates pathogenic mechanisms. Hum Mol Genet. 2019;28(R2):R197–206. PMCID: PMC6872434. http://www.ncbi.nlm.nih.gov/pubmed/31578549.
114. Nowell PC. The clonal evolution of tumor cell populations. Science. 1976;194(4260):23–8. PMID: 959840. http://www.ncbi.nlm.nih.gov/pubmed/959840.
115. Croce CM. Oncogenes and cancer. N Engl J Med. 2008;358(5):502–11. PMID: 18234754. http://www.ncbi.nlm.nih.gov/pubmed/18234754.
116. O'Huallachain M, Karczewski KJ, Weissman SM, Urban AE, Snyder MP. Extensive genetic variation in somatic human tissues. Proc Natl Acad Sci U S A. 2012;109(44):18018–23. PMCID: PMC3497787. http://www.ncbi.nlm.nih.gov/pubmed/23043118.
117. Lupski JR. Genetics. Genome mosaicism--one human, multiple genomes. Science. 2013;341(6144):358–9. PMID: 23888031. http://www.ncbi.nlm.nih.gov/pubmed/23888031.
118. Baillie JK, Barnett MW, Upton KR, Gerhardt DJ, Richmond TA, De Sapio F, Brennan PM, Rizzu P, Smith S, Fell M, Talbot RT, Gustincich S, Freeman TC, Mattick JS, Hume DA, Heutink P, Carninci P, Jeddeloh JA, Faulkner GJ. Somatic retrotransposition alters the genetic landscape of the human brain. Nature. 2011;479(7374):534–7. PMCID: PMC3224101. http://www.ncbi.nlm.nih.gov/pubmed/22037309.
119. Evrony GD, Cai X, Lee E, Hills LB, Elhosary PC, Lehmann HS, Parker JJ, Atabay KD, Gilmore EC, Poduri A, Park PJ, Walsh CA. Single-neuron sequencing analysis of L1 retrotransposition and somatic mutation in the human brain. Cell. 2012;151(3):483–96. PMCID: PMC3567441. http://www.ncbi.nlm.nih.gov/pubmed/23101622.

120. Forsberg LA, Rasi C, Razzaghian HR, Pakalapati G, Waite L, Thilbeault KS, Ronowicz A, Wineinger NE, Tiwari HK, Boomsma D, Westerman MP, Harris JR, Lyle R, Essand M, Eriksson F, Assimes TL, Iribarren C, Strachan E, O'Hanlon TP, Rider LG, Miller FW, Giedraitis V, Lannfelt L, Ingelsson M, Piotrowski A, Pedersen NL, Absher D, Dumanski JP. Age-related somatic structural changes in the nuclear genome of human blood cells. Am J Hum Genet. 2012;90(2):217–28. PMCID: PMC3276669. http://www.ncbi.nlm.nih.gov/pubmed/22305530.
121. Piotrowski A, Bruder CEG, Andersson R, Diaz de Ståhl T, Menzel U, Sandgren J, Poplawski A, von Tell D, Crasto C, Bogdan A, Bartoszewski R, Bebok Z, Krzyzanowski M, Jankowski Z, Partridge EC, Komorowski J, Dumanski JP. Somatic mosaicism for copy number variation in differentiated human tissues. Hum Mutat. 2008;29(9):1118–24. PMID: 18570184. http://www.ncbi.nlm.nih.gov/pubmed/18570184.
122. Lynch M. Rate, molecular spectrum, and consequences of human mutation. Proc Natl Acad Sci U S A. 2010;107(3):961–8. PMCID: PMC2824313. http://www.ncbi.nlm.nih.gov/pubmed/20080596.
123. Biesecker LG, Spinner NB. A genomic view of mosaicism and human disease. Nat Rev Genet. 2013;14(5):307–20. PMID: 23594909. http://www.ncbi.nlm.nih.gov/pubmed/23594909.
124. Campbell IM, Shaw CA, Stankiewicz P, Lupski JR. Somatic mosaicism: implications for disease and transmission genetics. Trends Genet. 2015;31(7):382–92. PMCID: PMC4490042. http://www.ncbi.nlm.nih.gov/pubmed/25910407.
125. O'Huallachain M, Weissman SM, Snyder MP. The variable somatic genome. Cell Cycle. 2013;12(1):5–6. PMCID: PMC3570516. http://www.ncbi.nlm.nih.gov/pubmed/23255102.
126. Olsen TK, Baryawno N. Introduction to single-cell RNA sequencing. Curr Protoc Mol Biol. 2018;122(1):e57. PMID: 29851283. http://www.ncbi.nlm.nih.gov/pubmed/29851283.
127. Picelli S. Single-cell RNA-sequencing: the future of genome biology is now. RNA Biol. 2017;14(5):637–50. PMCID: PMC5449089. http://www.ncbi.nlm.nih.gov/pubmed/27442339.
128. Stuart T, Satija R. Integrative single-cell analysis. Nat Rev Genet. 2019;20(5):257–72. PMID: 30696980. http://www.ncbi.nlm.nih.gov/pubmed/30696980.
129. Han KY, Kim KT, Joung JG, Son DS, Kim YJ, Jo A, Jeon HJ, Moon HS, Yoo CE, Chung W, Eum HH, Kim S, Kim HK, Lee JE, Ahn MJ, Lee HO, Park D, Park WY. SIDR: simultaneous isolation and parallel sequencing of genomic DNA and total RNA from single cells. Genome Res. 2018;28(1):75–87. PMCID: PMC5749184. http://www.ncbi.nlm.nih.gov/pubmed/29208629.
130. Dhimolea E, Denes V, Lakk M, Al-Bazzaz S, Aziz-Zaman S, Pilichowska M, Geck P. High male chimerism in the female breast shows quantitative links with cancer. Int J Cancer. 2013;133(4):835–42. PMID: 23390035. http://www.ncbi.nlm.nih.gov/pubmed/23390035.
131. Gulcher J. Microsatellite markers for linkage and association studies. Cold Spring Harb Protoc. 2012;2012(4):425–32. PMID: 22474656. http://www.ncbi.nlm.nih.gov/pubmed/22474656.
132. Bruijns B, Tiggelaar R, Gardeniers H. Massively parallel sequencing techniques for forensics: a review. Electrophoresis. 2018;39(21):2642–54. PMCID: PMC6282972. http://www.ncbi.nlm.nih.gov/pubmed/30101986.
133. Bloom K, Costanzo V. Centromere structure and function. Prog Mol Subcell Biol. 2017;56:515–39. PMCID: PMC6535225. http://www.ncbi.nlm.nih.gov/pubmed/28840251.
134. Richard GF, Kerrest A, Dujon B. Comparative genomics and molecular dynamics of DNA repeats in eukaryotes. Microbiol Mol Biol Rev. 2008;72(4):686–727. PMCID: PMC2593564. http://www.ncbi.nlm.nih.gov/pubmed/19052325.
135. Ibn-Salem J, Muro EM, Andrade-Navarro MA. Co-regulation of paralog genes in the three-dimensional chromatin architecture. Nucleic Acids Res. 2017;45(1):81–91. PMCID: PMC5224500. http://www.ncbi.nlm.nih.gov/pubmed/27634932.
136. Koonin EV. Orthologs, paralogs, and evolutionary genomics. Annu Rev Genet. 2005;39:309–38. PMID: 16285863. http://www.ncbi.nlm.nih.gov/pubmed/16285863.
137. He J, Gai J. Genome-Wide Association Studies (GWAS). Methods Mol Biol. 2023;2638:123–46. PMID: 36781639. http://www.ncbi.nlm.nih.gov/pubmed/36781639.
138. Conrad DF, Keebler JEM, DePristo MA, Lindsay SJ, Zhang Y, Casals F, Idaghdour Y, Hartl CL, Torroja C, Garimella KV, Zilversmit M, Cartwright R, Rouleau GA, Daly M, Stone EA, Hurles ME, Awadalla P, 1000 Genomes Project. Variation in genome-wide mutation rates within and between human families. Nat Genet. 2011;43(7):712–714. PMCID: PMC3322360. http://www.ncbi.nlm.nih.gov/pubmed/21666693.
139. Campbell CD, Eichler EE. Properties and rates of germline mutations in humans. Trends Genet. 2013;29(10):575–84. PMCID: PMC3785239. http://www.ncbi.nlm.nih.gov/pubmed/23684843.
140. Ségurel L, Wyman MJ, Przeworski M. Determinants of mutation rate variation in the human germline. Annu Rev Genomics Hum Genet. 2014;15:47–70. PMID: 25000986. http://www.ncbi.nlm.nih.gov/pubmed/25000986.
141. Ohno M. Spontaneous de novo germline mutations in humans and mice: rates, spectra, causes and consequences. Genes Genet Syst. 2019;94(1):13–22. PMID: 30381610. http://www.ncbi.nlm.nih.gov/pubmed/30381610.
142. Goriely A, McGrath JJ, Hultman CM, Wilkie AOM, Malaspina D. "Selfish spermatogonial selection": a novel mechanism for the association between advanced paternal age and neurodevelopmental disorders. Am J Psychiatry. 2013;170(6):599–608. PMCID: PMC4001324. http://www.ncbi.nlm.nih.gov/pubmed/23639989.
143. de Kluiver H, Buizer-Voskamp JE, Dolan CV, Boomsma DI. Paternal age and psychiatric disorders: a review. Am J Med Genet B Neuropsychiatr Genet. 2017;174(3):202–13. PMCID: PMC5412832. http://www.ncbi.nlm.nih.gov/pubmed/27770494.
144. Insel TR. Brain somatic mutations: the dark matter of psychiatric genetics? Mol Psychiatry. 2014;19(2):156–8. PMID: 24342990. http://www.ncbi.nlm.nih.gov/pubmed/24342990.
145. Sanai N, Nguyen T, Ihrie RA, Mirzadeh Z, Tsai HH, Wong M, Gupta N, Berger MS, Huang E, Garcia-Verdugo JM, Rowitch DH, Alvarez-Buylla A. Corridors of migrating neurons in the human brain and their decline during infancy. Nature. 2011;478(7369):382–6. PMCID: PMC3197903. http://www.ncbi.nlm.nih.gov/pubmed/21964341.
146. Spalding KL, Bergmann O, Alkass K, Bernard S, Salehpour M, Huttner HB, Boström E, Westerlund I, Vial C, Buchholz BA, Possnert G, Mash DC, Druid H, Frisén J. Dynamics of hippocampal neurogenesis in adult humans. Cell. 2013;153(6):1219–27. PMCID: PMC4394608. http://www.ncbi.nlm.nih.gov/pubmed/23746839.
147. Eriksson PS, Perfilieva E, Björk-Eriksson T, Alborn AM, Nordborg C, Peterson DA, Gage FH. Neurogenesis in the adult human hippocampus. Nat Med. 1998;4(11):1313–7. PMID: 9809557. http://www.ncbi.nlm.nih.gov/pubmed/9809557.
148. Ernst A, Alkass K, Bernard S, Salehpour M, Perl S, Tisdale J, Possnert G, Druid H, Frisén J. Neurogenesis in the striatum of the adult human brain. Cell. 2014;156(5):1072–83. PMID: 24561062. http://www.ncbi.nlm.nih.gov/pubmed/24561062.
149. Horgusluoglu-Moloch E, Risacher SL, Crane PK, Hibar D, Thompson PM, Saykin AJ, Nho K. Alzheimer's Disease Neuroimaging Initiative (ADNI). Genome-wide association analysis of hippocampal volume identifies enrichment of neurogenesis-related pathways. Sci Rep. 2019;9(1):14498. PMCID: PMC6787090. http://www.ncbi.nlm.nih.gov/pubmed/31601890.
150. Cai X, Evrony GD, Lehmann HS, Elhosary PC, Mehta BK, Poduri A, Walsh CA. Single-cell, genome-wide sequencing identifies

clonal somatic copy-number variation in the human brain. Cell Rep. 2014;8(5):1280–9. PMCID: PMC4272008. http://www.ncbi.nlm.nih.gov/pubmed/25159146.
151. McConnell MJ, Lindberg MR, Brennand KJ, Piper JC, Voet T, Cowing-Zitron C, Shumilina S, Lasken RS, Vermeesch JR, Hall IM, Gage FH. Mosaic copy number variation in human neurons. Science. 2013;342(6158):632–7. PMCID: PMC3975283. http://www.ncbi.nlm.nih.gov/pubmed/24179226.
152. Williams SL, Mash DC, Züchner S, Moraes CT. Somatic mtDNA mutation spectra in the aging human putamen. PLoS Genet. 2013;9(12):e1003990. PMCID: PMC3854840. http://www.ncbi.nlm.nih.gov/pubmed/24339796.
153. Evrony GD, Lee E, Mehta BK, Benjamini Y, Johnson RM, Cai X, Yang L, Haseley P, Lehmann HS, Park PJ, Walsh CA. Cell lineage analysis in human brain using endogenous retroelements. Neuron. 2015;85(1):49–59. PMCID: PMC4299461. http://www.ncbi.nlm.nih.gov/pubmed/25569347.
154. Gómez-Pinedo U, Sirerol-Piquer MS, Durán-Moreno M, García-Verdugo JM, Matias-Guiu J. Alexander disease mutations produce cells with coexpression of Glial Fibrillary acidic protein and NG2 in neurosphere cultures and inhibit differentiation into mature Oligodendrocytes. Front Neurol. 2017;8:255. PMCID: PMC5459916. http://www.ncbi.nlm.nih.gov/pubmed/28634469.
155. Kaminsky N, Bihari O, Kanner S, Barzilai A. Connecting malfunctioning glial cells and brain degenerative disorders. Genomics Proteomics Bioinformatics. 2016;14(3):155–65. PMCID: PMC4936608. http://www.ncbi.nlm.nih.gov/pubmed/27245308.
156. Biernat W, Aguzzi A, Sure U, Grant JW, Kleihues P, Hegi ME. Identical mutations of the p53 tumor suppressor gene in the gliomatous and the sarcomatous components of gliosarcomas suggest a common origin from glial cells. J Neuropathol Exp Neurol. 1995;54(5):651–6. PMID: 7666053. http://www.ncbi.nlm.nih.gov/pubmed/7666053.
157. Kim J, Shin JY, Kim JI, Seo JS, Webster MJ, Lee D, Kim S. Somatic deletions implicated in functional diversity of brain cells of individuals with schizophrenia and unaffected controls. Sci Rep. 2014;4:3807. PMCID: PMC3897957. http://www.ncbi.nlm.nih.gov/pubmed/24448323.
158. De Cecco M, Criscione SW, Peterson AL, Neretti N, Sedivy JM, Kreiling JA. Transposable elements become active and mobile in the genomes of aging mammalian somatic tissues. Aging (Albany NY). 2013;5(12):867–83. PMCID: PMC3883704. http://www.ncbi.nlm.nih.gov/pubmed/24323947.
159. Smemo S, Tena JJ, Kim KH, Gamazon ER, Sakabe NJ, Gómez-Marín C, Aneas I, Credidio FL, Sobreira DR, Wasserman NF, Lee JH, Puviindran V, Tam D, Shen M, Son JE, Vakili NA, Sung HK, Naranjo S, Acemel RD, Manzanares M, Nagy A, Cox NJ, Hui CC, Gomez-Skarmeta JL, Nóbrega MA. Obesity-associated variants within FTO form long-range functional connections with IRX3. Nature. 2014;507(7492):371–5. PMCID: PMC4113484. http://www.ncbi.nlm.nih.gov/pubmed/24646999.
160. Román-Franco AA. Homo sapiens as physician and patient: a view from Darwinian medicine. P R Health Sci J. 2013;32(3):113–23. PMID: 24133892. http://www.ncbi.nlm.nih.gov/pubmed/24133892.
161. Román-Franco AA. Medicine in the 21st century: towards a Darwinian medical epistemology. P R Health Sci J. 2009;28(4):345–51. PMID: 19999243. http://www.ncbi.nlm.nih.gov/pubmed/19999243.
162. Johnson WE. Origins and evolutionary consequences of ancient endogenous retroviruses. Nat Rev Microbiol. 2019;17(6):355–70. PMID: 30962577. http://www.ncbi.nlm.nih.gov/pubmed/30962577.
163. Griffiths DJ. Endogenous retroviruses in the human genome sequence. Genome Biol. 2001;2(6):REVIEWS1017. PMCID: PMC138943. http://www.ncbi.nlm.nih.gov/pubmed/11423012.
164. Greenwood AD, Ishida Y, O'Brien SP, Roca AL, Eiden MV. Transmission, evolution, and endogenization: lessons learned from recent retroviral invasions. Microbiol Mol Biol Rev. 2018;82(1):e00044–17. PMCID: PMC5813887. http://www.ncbi.nlm.nih.gov/pubmed/29237726.
165. Introduction to the Archaea.
166. Archaea in the Human Microbiome and Potential Effects on Human Infectious Disease - Volume 30, Number 8—August 2024 - Emerging Infectious Diseases journal - CDC.
167. Li Y, Zhang G, Cui J. Origin and deep evolution of human endogenous Retroviruses in Pan-Primates. Viruses. 2022;14(7):1370. PMCID: PMC9323773. http://www.ncbi.nlm.nih.gov/pubmed/35891351.
168. Küry P, Nath A, Créange A, Dolei A, Marche P, Gold J, Giovannoni G, Hartung HP, Perron H. Human endogenous Retroviruses in neurological diseases. Trends Mol Med. 2018;24(4):379–94. PMCID: PMC7185488. http://www.ncbi.nlm.nih.gov/pubmed/29551251.
169. Smith EM, Pendlebury DF, Nandakumar J. Structural biology of telomeres and telomerase. Cell Mol Life Sci. 2020;77(1):61–79. PMCID: PMC6986361. http://www.ncbi.nlm.nih.gov/pubmed/31728577.
170. Jenner LP, Peska V, Fulnečková J, Sýkorová E. Telomeres and their neighbors. Genes (Basel). 2022;13(9):1663. PMCID: PMC9498494. http://www.ncbi.nlm.nih.gov/pubmed/36140830.
171. Armanios M. The role of telomeres in human disease. Annu Rev Genomics Hum Genet. 2022;23:363–81. PMCID: PMC10111244. http://www.ncbi.nlm.nih.gov/pubmed/35609925.
172. Lansdorp PM. Telomeres, aging, and cancer: the big picture. Blood. 2022;139(6):813–21. PMCID: PMC8832478. http://www.ncbi.nlm.nih.gov/pubmed/35142846.
173. Foley JF. Telomeres to go. Sci Signal. 2022;15(752):eade9136.
174. Dehghan A. Genome-Wide Association studies. Methods Mol Biol. 2018;1793:37–49. PMID: 29876890. http://www.ncbi.nlm.nih.gov/pubmed/29876890.
175. Misiak B, Ricceri L, Sąsiadek MM. Transposable elements and their epigenetic regulation in mental disorders: current evidence in the field. Front Genet. 2019;10:580. PMCID: PMC6603224. http://www.ncbi.nlm.nih.gov/pubmed/31293617.
176. Rigogliuso G, Biniossek ML, Goodier JL, Mayer B, Pereira GC, Schilling O, Meese E, Mayer J. A human endogenous retrovirus encoded protease potentially cleaves numerous cellular proteins. Mob DNA. 2019;10:36. PMCID: PMC6707001. http://www.ncbi.nlm.nih.gov/pubmed/31462935.
177. Christensen T. Human endogenous retroviruses in neurologic disease. APMIS. 2016;124(1–2):116–26. PMID: 26818266. http://www.ncbi.nlm.nih.gov/pubmed/26818266.
178. Garcia-Montojo M, Doucet-O'Hare T, Henderson L, Nath A. Human endogenous retrovirus-K (HML-2): a comprehensive review. Crit Rev Microbiol. 2018;44(6):715–38. PMCID: PMC6342650. http://www.ncbi.nlm.nih.gov/pubmed/30318978.
179. Li F, Sabunciyan S, Yolken RH, Lee D, Kim S, Karlsson H. Transcription of human endogenous retroviruses in human brain by RNA-seq analysis. PloS One. 2019;14(1):e0207353. PMCID: PMC6317784. http://www.ncbi.nlm.nih.gov/pubmed/30605476.
180. Canli T. A model of human endogenous retrovirus (HERV) activation in mental health and illness. Med Hypotheses. 2019;133:109404. PMID: 31557593. http://www.ncbi.nlm.nih.gov/pubmed/31557593.
181. Hathorn MK. Respiratory modulation of heart rate in newborn infants. Early Hum Dev. 1989;20(2):81–99. PMID: 2591340. http://www.ncbi.nlm.nih.gov/pubmed/2591340.
182. Starkweather AR, Alhaeeri AA, Montpetit A, Brumelle J, Filler K, Montpetit M, Mohanraj L, Lyon DE, Jackson-Cook CK. An integrative review of factors associated with telomere length and implications for biobehavioral research. Nurs Res.

2014;63(1):36–50. PMCID: PMC4112289. http://www.ncbi.nlm.nih.gov/pubmed/24335912.
183. Shalev I, Entringer S, Wadhwa PD, Wolkowitz OM, Puterman E, Lin J, Epel ES. Stress and telomere biology: a lifespan perspective. Psychoneuroendocrinology. 2013;38(9):1835–42. PMCID: PMC3735679. http://www.ncbi.nlm.nih.gov/pubmed/23639252.
184. Kinser PA, Lyon DE. Major depressive disorder and measures of cellular aging: an integrative review. Nurs Res Pract. 2013;2013:469070. PMCID: PMC3649747. http://www.ncbi.nlm.nih.gov/pubmed/23691300.
185. Price LH, Kao HT, Burgers DE, Carpenter LL, Tyrka AR. Telomeres and early-life stress: an overview. Biol Psychiatry. 2013;73(1):15–23. PMCID: PMC3495091. http://www.ncbi.nlm.nih.gov/pubmed/22831981.
186. Steptoe A, Hamer M, Butcher L, Lin J, Brydon L, Kivimäki M, Marmot M, Blackburn E, Erusalimsky JD. Educational attainment but not measures of current socioeconomic circumstances are associated with leukocyte telomere length in healthy older men and women. Brain Behav Immun. 2011;25(7):1292–8. PMID: 21536122. http://www.ncbi.nlm.nih.gov/pubmed/21536122.
187. Tyrka AR, Price LH, Kao HT, Porton B, Marsella SA, Carpenter LL. Childhood maltreatment and telomere shortening: preliminary support for an effect of early stress on cellular aging. Biol Psychiatry. 2010;67(6):531–4. PMCID: PMC2853238. http://www.ncbi.nlm.nih.gov/pubmed/19828140.
188. Epel E. How "reversible" is telomeric aging? Cancer Prev Res (Phila). 2012;5(10):1163–8. PMID: 23041472. http://www.ncbi.nlm.nih.gov/pubmed/23041472.
189. García-Calzón S, Moleres A, Marcos A, Campoy C, Moreno LA, Azcona-Sanjulián MC, Martínez-González MA, Martínez JA, Zalba G, Marti A, EVASYON Study Group. Telomere length as a biomarker for adiposity changes after a multidisciplinary intervention in overweight/obese adolescents: the EVASYON study. PloS One. 2014;9(2):e89828. PMCID: PMC3933678. http://www.ncbi.nlm.nih.gov/pubmed/24587065.
190. Rossiello F, Jurk D, Passos JF, d'Adda di Fagagna F. Telomere dysfunction in ageing and age-related diseases. Nat Cell Biol. 2022;24(2):135–47. PMCID: PMC8985209. http://www.ncbi.nlm.nih.gov/pubmed/35165420.
191. Mathur MB, Epel E, Kind S, Desai M, Parks CG, Sandler DP, Khazeni N. Perceived stress and telomere length: a systematic review, meta-analysis, and methodologic considerations for advancing the field. Brain Behav Immun. 2016;54:158–69. PMCID: PMC5590630. http://www.ncbi.nlm.nih.gov/pubmed/26853993.
192. Pepper GV, Bateson M, Nettle D. Telomeres as integrative markers of exposure to stress and adversity: a systematic review and meta-analysis. R Soc Open Sci. 2018;5(8):180744. PMCID: PMC6124068. http://www.ncbi.nlm.nih.gov/pubmed/30225068.
193. Rando TA, Chang HY. Aging, rejuvenation, and epigenetic reprogramming: resetting the aging clock. Cell. 2012;148(1–2):46–57. PMCID: PMC3336960. http://www.ncbi.nlm.nih.gov/pubmed/22265401.
194. Rentscher KE, Carroll JE, Mitchell C. Psychosocial stressors and Telomere length: a current review of the science. Annu Rev Public Health. 2020;41:223–45. PMID: 31900099. http://www.ncbi.nlm.nih.gov/pubmed/31900099.
195. Le TT, Kuplicki R, Yeh HW, Aupperle RL, Khalsa SS, Simmons WK, Paulus MP. Effect of Ibuprofen on BrainAGE: a randomized, placebo-controlled, dose-response exploratory study. Biol Psychiatry: Cognit Neurosci Neuroimaging. 2018;3(10):836–43. PMCID: PMC6510235. http://www.ncbi.nlm.nih.gov/pubmed/29941380.
196. Cole JH, Franke K. Predicting age using neuroimaging: innovative brain ageing biomarkers. Trends Neurosci. 2017;40(12):681–90. PMID: 29074032. http://www.ncbi.nlm.nih.gov/pubmed/29074032.
197. Franke K, Gaser C. Ten years of BrainAGE as a neuroimaging biomarker of brain aging: what insights have we gained? Front Neurol. 2019;10:789. PMCID: PMC6702897. http://www.ncbi.nlm.nih.gov/pubmed/31474922.
198. Pei B, Sisu C, Frankish A, Howald C, Habegger L, Mu XJ, Harte R, Balasubramanian S, Tanzer A, Diekhans M, Reymond A, Hubbard TJ, Harrow J, Gerstein MB. The GENCODE pseudogene resource. Genome Biol. 2012;13(9):R51. PMCID: PMC3491395. http://www.ncbi.nlm.nih.gov/pubmed/22951037.
199. Tutar Y. Pseudogenes. Comp Funct Genomics. 2012;2012:424526. PMCID: PMC3352212. http://www.ncbi.nlm.nih.gov/pubmed/22611337.
200. Kovalenko TF, Patrushev LI. Pseudogenes as functionally significant elements of the genome. Biochemistry (Mosc). 2018;83(11):1332–49. PMID: 30482145. http://www.ncbi.nlm.nih.gov/pubmed/30482145.
201. Alexander RP, Fang G, Rozowsky J, Snyder M, Gerstein MB. Annotating non-coding regions of the genome. Nat Rev Genet. 2010;11(8):559–71. PMID: 20628352. http://www.ncbi.nlm.nih.gov/pubmed/20628352.
202. Harrison PM, Zheng D, Zhang Z, Carriero N, Gerstein M. Transcribed processed pseudogenes in the human genome: an intermediate form of expressed retrosequence lacking protein-coding ability. Nucleic Acids Res. 2005;33(8):2374–83. PMCID: PMC1087782. http://www.ncbi.nlm.nih.gov/pubmed/15860774.
203. Millions of Years of Evolution Preserved: A Comprehensive Catalog of the Processed Pseudogenes in the Human Genome.
204. Maranda V, Sunstrum FG, Drouin G. Both male and female gamete generating cells produce processed pseudogenes in the human genome. Gene. 2019;684:70–5. PMID: 30359744. http://www.ncbi.nlm.nih.gov/pubmed/30359744.
205. Vanin EF. Processed pseudogenes: characteristics and evolution. Annu Rev Genet. 1985;19:253–72. PMID: 3909943. http://www.ncbi.nlm.nih.gov/pubmed/23684843.
206. Yagi T. Genetic basis of neuronal individuality in the mammalian brain. J Neurogenet. 2013;27(3):97–105. PMCID: PMC3852966. http://www.ncbi.nlm.nih.gov/pubmed/23808929.
207. Vineis P, Pearce NE. Genome-wide association studies may be misinterpreted: genes versus heritability. Carcinogenesis. 2011;32(9):1295–8. PMID: 21565827. http://www.ncbi.nlm.nih.gov/pubmed/21565827.
208. Rose SPR. Commentary: heritability estimates--long past their sell-by date. Int J Epidemiol. 2006;35(3):525–7. PMID: 16645027. http://www.ncbi.nlm.nih.gov/pubmed/16645027.
209. Lewontin RC. The analysis of variance and the analysis of causes. 1974. Int J Epidemiol. 2006;35(3):520–5. PMID: 16645033. http://www.ncbi.nlm.nih.gov/pubmed/16645033.
210. Vinkhuyzen AAE, van der Sluis S, Maes HHM, Posthuma D. Reconsidering the heritability of intelligence in adulthood: taking assortative mating and cultural transmission into account. Behav Genet. 2012;42(2):187–98. PMCID: PMC3276760. http://www.ncbi.nlm.nih.gov/pubmed/21969232.
211. Tal O. The impact of gene-environment interaction and correlation on the interpretation of heritability. Acta Biotheor. 2012;60(3):225–37. PMID: 21863336. http://www.ncbi.nlm.nih.gov/pubmed/21863336.
212. Kohler HP, Behrman JR, Schnittker J. Social science methods for twins data: integrating causality, endowments, and heritability. Biodemograph Soc Biol. 2011;57(1):88–141. PMCID: PMC3158495. http://www.ncbi.nlm.nih.gov/pubmed/21845929.
213. Pearce N. Epidemiology in a changing world: variation, causation and ubiquitous risk factors. Int J Epidemiol. 2011;40(2):503–12. PMID: 21247886. http://www.ncbi.nlm.nih.gov/pubmed/21247886.

214. van Asselt KM, Kok HS, van der Schouw YT, Peeters PHM, Pearson PL, Grobbee DE. Role of genetic analyses in cardiology: part II: heritability estimation for gene searching in multifactorial diseases. Circulation. 2006;113(8):1136–9. PMID: 16505191. http://www.ncbi.nlm.nih.gov/pubmed/16505191.
215. Johnson W, Turkheimer E, Gottesman II, Bouchard TJ. Beyond heritability: twin studies in behavioral research. Curr Dir Psychol Sci. 2010;18(4):217–20. PMCID: PMC2899491. http://www.ncbi.nlm.nih.gov/pubmed/20625474.
216. Bailey RC. Hereditarian scientific fallacies. Genetica. 1997;99(2–3):125–33. PMID: 9463068. http://www.ncbi.nlm.nih.gov/pubmed/9463068.
217. Eley TC, Rijsdijk F. Introductory guide to the statistics of molecular genetics. J Child Psychol Psychiatry. 2005;46(10):1042–4. PMID: 16178927. http://www.ncbi.nlm.nih.gov/pubmed/16178927.
218. Eley TC, Craig IW. Introductory guide to the language of molecular genetics. J Child Psychol Psychiatry. 2005;46(10):1039–41. PMID: 16178926. http://www.ncbi.nlm.nih.gov/pubmed/16178926.
219. Thapar A, McGuffin P. A twin study of depressive symptoms in childhood. Br J Psychiatry. 1994;165(2):259–65. PMID: 7953041. http://www.ncbi.nlm.nih.gov/pubmed/7953041.
220. Gillespie NA, Eaves LJ, Maes H, Silberg JL. Testing models for the contributions of genes and environment to developmental change in adolescent depression. Behav Genet. 2015;45(4):382–93. PMCID: PMC4459950. https://pmc.ncbi.nlm.nih.gov/articles/PMC4459950/pdf/nihms682982.pdf.
221. Menke A, Klengel T, Binder EB. Epigenetics, depression and antidepressant treatment. Curr Pharm Des. 2012;18(36):5879–89. PMID: 22681167. http://www.ncbi.nlm.nih.gov/pubmed/22681167.
222. Silberg J, Pickles A, Rutter M, Hewitt J, Simonoff E, Maes H, Carbonneau R, Murrelle L, Foley D, Eaves L. The influence of genetic factors and life stress on depression among adolescent girls. Arch Gen Psychiatry. 1999;56(3):225–32. PMID: 10078499. http://www.ncbi.nlm.nih.gov/pubmed/22303401.
223. Kendler KS, Prescott CA. A population-based twin study of lifetime major depression in men and women. Arch Gen Psychiatry. 1999;56(1):39–44. PMID: 9892254. http://www.ncbi.nlm.nih.gov/pubmed/9892254.
224. Lau JYF, Eley TC. The genetics of mood disorders. Annu Rev Clin Psychol. 2010;6:313–37. PMID: 20001729. http://www.ncbi.nlm.nih.gov/pubmed/20001729.
225. Gregory AM, Lau JYF, Eley TC. Finding gene-environment interactions for generalised anxiety disorder. Eur Arch Psychiatry Clin Neurosci. 2008;258(2):69–75. PMID: 18297422. http://www.ncbi.nlm.nih.gov/pubmed/18297422.
226. Lau JYF, Gregory AM, Goldwin MA, Pine DS, Eley TC. Assessing gene-environment interactions on anxiety symptom subtypes across childhood and adolescence. Dev Psychopathol. 2007;19(4):1129–46. PMID: 17931439. http://www.ncbi.nlm.nih.gov/pubmed/17931439.
227. Mortada M, Pancino G, Charpin C, Schlageter MH, Calvo F, Roseto A. Detection of a soluble serum antigen by a new monoclonal antibody ED8 in patients with breast cancer. C R Acad Sci III. 1990;311(2):63–8. PMID: 2119859. http://www.ncbi.nlm.nih.gov/pubmed/2119859.
228. Button TMM, Lau JYF, Maughan B, Eley TC. Parental punitive discipline, negative life events and gene-environment interplay in the development of externalizing behavior. Psychol Med. 2008;38(1):29–39. PMCID: PMC2906398. http://www.ncbi.nlm.nih.gov/pubmed/17803832.
229. Wamboldt MZ. Parsing childhood symptoms with more specificity can clarify differential outcomes. Am J Psychiatry. 2012;169(1):4–6. PMID: 22223006. http://www.ncbi.nlm.nih.gov/pubmed/22223006.
230. Lau JYF, Hilbert K, Goodman R, Gregory AM, Pine DS, Viding EM, Eley TC. Investigating the genetic and environmental bases of biases in threat recognition and avoidance in children with anxiety problems. Biol Mood Anxiety Disord. 2012;2:12. PMCID: PMC3487968. http://www.ncbi.nlm.nih.gov/pubmed/22788754.
231. Brown HM, McAdams TA, Lester KJ, Goodman R, Clark DM, Eley TC. Attentional threat avoidance and familial risk are independently associated with childhood anxiety disorders. J Child Psychol Psychiatry. 2013;54(6):678–85. PMID: 23176633. http://www.ncbi.nlm.nih.gov/pubmed/23176633.
232. Brown HM, Trzaskowski M, Zavos HMS, Rijsdijk FV, Gregory AM, Eley TC. Phenotypic and genetic structure of anxiety sensitivity in adolescence and early adulthood. J Anxiety Disord. 2012;26(6):680–8. PMID: 22721752. http://www.ncbi.nlm.nih.gov/pubmed/22721752.
233. Zavos HMS, Wong CCY, Barclay NL, Keers R, Mill J, Rijsdijk FV, Gregory AM, Eley TC. Anxiety sensitivity in adolescence and young adulthood: the role of stressful life events, 5HTTLPR and their interaction. Depress Anxiety. 2012;29(5):400–8. PMID: 22447535. http://www.ncbi.nlm.nih.gov/pubmed/22447535.
234. de Maio NM, Lampraki C, Marques A, Gouveia ÉR, Adsuar JC, Ihle A. Longitudinal cross-lagged analysis of depression, loneliness, and quality of life in 12 European countries. BMC Public Health. 2024;24(1):1986. PMCID: PMC11270973. http://www.ncbi.nlm.nih.gov/pubmed/39054451.
235. Zavos HMS, Rijsdijk FV, Eley TC. A longitudinal, genetically informative, study of associations between anxiety sensitivity, anxiety and depression. Behav Genet. 2012;42(4):592–602. PMID: 22437876. http://www.ncbi.nlm.nih.gov/pubmed/22437876.
236. Chan DC. Mitochondrial dynamics and its involvement in disease. Annu Rev Pathol. 2020;15:235–59. PMID: 31585519. http://www.ncbi.nlm.nih.gov/pubmed/31585519.
237. Aronson JK, Ferner RE. Biomarkers-a general review. Curr Protoc Pharmacol. 2017;76:9.23.1–9.23.17. PMID: 28306150. http://www.ncbi.nlm.nih.gov/pubmed/28306150.
238. Zavos HMS, Gregory AM, Eley TC. Longitudinal genetic analysis of anxiety sensitivity. Dev Psychol. 2012;48(1):204–12. PMID: 21842987. http://www.ncbi.nlm.nih.gov/pubmed/21842987.
239. Trzaskowski M, Zavos HMS, Haworth CMA, Plomin R, Eley TC. Stable genetic influence on anxiety-related behaviours across middle childhood. J Abnorm Child Psychol. 2012;40(1):85–94. PMCID: PMC3268971. http://www.ncbi.nlm.nih.gov/pubmed/21766214.
240. Stringaris A, Zavos H, Leibenluft E, Maughan B, Eley TC. Adolescent irritability: phenotypic associations and genetic links with depressed mood. Am J Psychiatry. 2012;169(1):47–54. PMCID: PMC3660701. http://www.ncbi.nlm.nih.gov/pubmed/22193524.
241. Lau JYF, Belli SD, Gregory AM, Napolitano M, Eley TC. The role of children's negative attributions on depressive symptoms: an inherited characteristic or a product of the early environment? Dev Sci. 2012;15(4):569–78. PMID: 22709405. http://www.ncbi.nlm.nih.gov/pubmed/22709405.
242. Scaini S, Ogliari A, Eley TC, Zavos HMS, Battaglia M. Genetic and environmental contributions to separation anxiety: a meta-analytic approach to twin data. Depress Anxiety. 2012;29(9):754–61. PMID: 22496044. http://www.ncbi.nlm.nih.gov/pubmed/22496044.
243. Barclay NL, Eley TC, Maughan B, Rowe R, Gregory AM. Associations between diurnal preference, sleep quality and externalizing behaviours: a behavioural genetic analysis. Psychol Med. 2011;41(5):1029–40. PMID: 20836908. http://www.ncbi.nlm.nih.gov/pubmed/20836908.
244. Gregory AM, Rijsdijk FV, Lau JYF, Dahl RE, Eley TC. The direction of longitudinal associations between sleep problems and depression symptoms: a study of twins aged 8 and 10 years.

Sleep. 2009;32(2):189–99. PMCID: PMC2635583. http://www.ncbi.nlm.nih.gov/pubmed/19238806.
245. Gregory AM, Buysse DJ, Willis TA, Rijsdijk FV, Maughan B, Rowe R, Cartwright S, Barclay NL, Eley TC. Associations between sleep quality and anxiety and depression symptoms in a sample of young adult twins and siblings. J Psychosom Res. 2011;71(4):250–5. PMID: 21911103. http://www.ncbi.nlm.nih.gov/pubmed/21911103.
246. Barclay NL, Eley TC, Buysse DJ, Maughan B, Gregory AM. Nonshared environmental influences on sleep quality: a study of monozygotic twin differences. Behav Genet. 2012;42(2):234–44. PMID: 22002163. http://www.ncbi.nlm.nih.gov/pubmed/22002163.
247. Gregory AM, Cox J, Crawford MR, Holland J, Harvey AG, Steps Team. Dysfunctional beliefs and attitudes about sleep in children. J Sleep Res. 2009;18(4):422–6. PMID: 19686237. http://www.ncbi.nlm.nih.gov/pubmed/19686237.
248. Barclay NL, Eley TC, Mill J, Wong CCY, Zavos HMS, Archer SN, Gregory AM. Sleep quality and diurnal preference in a sample of young adults: associations with 5HTTLPR, PER3, and CLOCK 3111. Am J Med Genet B Neuropsychiatr Genet. 2011;156B(6):681–90. PMID: 21714069. http://www.ncbi.nlm.nih.gov/pubmed/21714069.
249. Osland TM, Bjorvatn BR, Steen VM, Pallesen S le. Association study of a variable-number tandem repeat polymorphism in the clock gene PERIOD3 and chronotype in Norwegian university students. Chronobiol Int. 2011;28(9):764–70. PMID: 21919721. http://www.ncbi.nlm.nih.gov/pubmed/21919721.
250. Kishi T, Yoshimura R, Fukuo Y, Kitajima T, Okochi T, Matsunaga S, Inada T, Kunugi H, Kato T, Yoshikawa T, Ujike H, Umene-Nakano W, Nakamura J, Ozaki N, Serretti A, Correll CU, Iwata N. The CLOCK gene and mood disorders: a case-control study and meta-analysis. Chronobiol Int. 2011;28(9):825–33. PMID: 22080789. http://www.ncbi.nlm.nih.gov/pubmed/22080789.
251. Park M, Kim SA, Yee J, Shin J, Lee KY, Joo EJ. Significant role of gene-gene interactions of clock genes in mood disorder. J Affect Disord. 2019;257:510–7. PMID: 31323592. http://www.ncbi.nlm.nih.gov/pubmed/31323592.
252. Bolton D, Rijsdijk F, Eley TC, O'Connor TG, Briskman J, Perrin S. Normative childhood repetitive routines and obsessive compulsive symptomatology in 6-year-old twins. J Child Psychol Psychiatry. 2009;50(9):1139–46. PMID: 19457049. http://www.ncbi.nlm.nih.gov/pubmed/19457049.
253. Pike A, Eley TC. Links between parenting and extra-familial relationships: nature or nurture? J Adolesc. 2009;32(3):519–33. PMID: 18783821. http://www.ncbi.nlm.nih.gov/pubmed/18783821.
254. Stikkelbroek Y, Prinzie P, de Graaf R, Ten Have M, Cuijpers P. Parental death during childhood and psychopathology in adulthood. Psychiatry Res. 2012;198(3):516–20. PMID: 22425472. http://www.ncbi.nlm.nih.gov/pubmed/22425472.
255. Crisafulli C, Fabbri C, Porcelli S, Drago A, Spina E, De Ronchi D, Serretti A. Pharmacogenetics of antidepressants. Front Pharmacol. 2011;2:6. PMCID: PMC3108562. http://www.ncbi.nlm.nih.gov/pubmed/21687501.
256. Shadrina M, Bondarenko EA, Slominsky PA. Genetics factors in major depression disease. Front Psych. 2018;9:334. PMCID: PMC6065213. http://www.ncbi.nlm.nih.gov/pubmed/30083112.
257. Tsang RSM, Mather KA, Sachdev PS, Reppermund S. Systematic review and meta-analysis of genetic studies of late-life depression. Neurosci Biobehav Rev. 2017;75:129–39. PMID: 28137459. http://www.ncbi.nlm.nih.gov/pubmed/28137459.
258. Van der Auwera S, Peyrot WJ, Milaneschi Y, Hertel J, Baune B, Breen G, Byrne E, Dunn EC, Fisher H, Homuth G, Levinson D, Lewis C, Mills N, Mullins N, Nauck M, Pistis G, Preisig M, Rietschel M, Ripke S, Sullivan P, Teumer A, Völzke H, Major Depressive Disorder Working Group of the Psychiatric Genomics Consortium, Boomsma DI, Wray NR, Penninx B, Grabe H. Genome-wide gene-environment interaction in depression: a systematic evaluation of candidate genes: the childhood trauma working-group of PGC-MDD. Am J Med Genet B Neuropsychiatr Genet. 2018;177(1):40–9. PMCID: PMC5726923. http://www.ncbi.nlm.nih.gov/pubmed/29159863.
259. Grabe HJ, Schwahn C, Mahler J, Appel K, Schulz A, Spitzer C, Fenske K, Barnow S, Freyberger HJ, Teumer A, Petersmann A, Biffar R, Rosskopf D, John U, Völzke H. Genetic epistasis between the brain-derived neurotrophic factor Val66Met polymorphism and the 5-HTT promoter polymorphism moderates the susceptibility to depressive disorders after childhood abuse. Prog Neuropsychopharmacol Biol Psychiatry. 2012;36(2):264–70. PMID: 21996278. http://www.ncbi.nlm.nih.gov/pubmed/21996278.
260. Dalton ED, Hammen CL, Najman JM, Brennan PA. Genetic susceptibility to family environment: BDNF Val66met and 5-HTTLPR influence depressive symptoms. J Fam Psychol. 2014;28(6):947–56. PMCID: PMC5510745. http://www.ncbi.nlm.nih.gov/pubmed/25347540.
261. Belsky J, Pluess M. Beyond diathesis stress: differential susceptibility to environmental influences. Psychol Bull. 2009;135(6):885–908. PMID: 19883141. http://www.ncbi.nlm.nih.gov/pubmed/19883141.
262. Belsky J, Pluess M. Beyond risk, resilience, and dysregulation: phenotypic plasticity and human development. Dev Psychopathol. 2013;25(4 Pt 2):1243–61. PMID: 24342838. http://www.ncbi.nlm.nih.gov/pubmed/24342838.
263. Monroe SM, Simons AD. Diathesis-stress theories in the context of life stress research: implications for the depressive disorders. Psychol Bull. 1991;110(3):406–25. PMID: 1758917. http://www.ncbi.nlm.nih.gov/pubmed/1758917.
264. Zubenko GS, Maher B, Hughes HB, Zubenko WN, Stiffler JS, Kaplan BB, Marazita ML. Genome-wide linkage survey for genetic loci that influence the development of depressive disorders in families with recurrent, early-onset, major depression. Am J Med Genet B Neuropsychiatr Genet. 2003;123B(1):1–18. PMID: 14582139. http://www.ncbi.nlm.nih.gov/pubmed/14582139.
265. Webber C. Epistasis in neuropsychiatric disorders. Trends Genet. 2017;33(4):256–65. PMID: 28268034. http://www.ncbi.nlm.nih.gov/pubmed/28268034.
266. Foffi G, Pastore A, Piazza F, Temussi PA. Macromolecular crowding: chemistry and physics meet biology (Ascona, Switzerland, 10-14 June 2012). Phys Biol. 2013;10(4):040301. PMID: 23912807. http://www.ncbi.nlm.nih.gov/pubmed/23912807.
267. Ichi NS, Miyoshi D, Sugimoto N. Effects of molecular crowding on the structures, interactions, and functions of nucleic acids. Chem Rev. 2014;114(5):2733–58. PMID: 24364729. http://www.ncbi.nlm.nih.gov/pubmed/24364729.
268. Breydo L, Reddy KD, Piai A, Felli IC, Pierattelli R, Uversky VN. The crowd you're in with: effects of different types of crowding agents on protein aggregation. Biochim Biophys Acta. 2014;1844(2):346–57. PMID: 24252314. http://www.ncbi.nlm.nih.gov/pubmed/24252314.
269. Yi CW, Xu WC, Chen J, Liang Y. Recent progress in prion and prion-like protein aggregation. Acta Biochim Biophys Sin (Shanghai). 2013;45(6):520–6. PMID: 23709368. http://www.ncbi.nlm.nih.gov/pubmed/23709368.
270. Ma Q, Hu JY, Chen J, Liang Y. The role of crowded physiological environments in prion and prion-like protein aggregation. Int J Mol Sci. 2013;14(11):21339–52. PMCID: PMC3856008. http://www.ncbi.nlm.nih.gov/pubmed/24284393.
271. McBride HM, Neuspiel M, Wasiak S. Mitochondria: more than just a powerhouse. Curr Biol. 2006;16(14):R551–60. PMID: 16860735. http://www.ncbi.nlm.nih.gov/pubmed/16860735.

272. Caruso G, Benatti C, Blom JMC, Caraci F, Tascedda F. The many faces of mitochondrial dysfunction in depression: from pathology to treatment. Front Pharmacol. 2019;10:995. PMCID: PMC6746908. http://www.ncbi.nlm.nih.gov/pubmed/31551791.
273. Allen J, Romay-Tallon R, Brymer KJ, Caruncho HJ, Kalynchuk LE. Mitochondria and Mood: Mitochondrial dysfunction as a key player in the manifestation of depression. Front Neurosci. 2018;12:386. PMCID: PMC5997778. http://www.ncbi.nlm.nih.gov/pubmed/29928190.
274. Koene S, Kozicz TL, Rodenburg RJT, Verhaak CM, de Vries MC, Wortmann S, van de Heuvel L, Smeitink J, Morava E. Major depression in adolescent children consecutively diagnosed with mitochondrial disorder. J Affect Disord. 2009;114(1–3):327–32. PMID: 18692904. http://www.ncbi.nlm.nih.gov/pubmed/18692904.
275. Martin JL, Magistretti PJ, Allaman I. Regulation of neurotrophic factors and energy metabolism by antidepressants in astrocytes. Curr Drug Targets. 2013;14(11):1308–21. PMID: 23469874. http://www.ncbi.nlm.nih.gov/pubmed/23469874.
276. Pizzorno J. Mitochondria-fundamental to life and health. Integr Med (Encinitas). 2014;13(2):8–15. PMCID: PMC4684129. http://www.ncbi.nlm.nih.gov/pubmed/26770084.
277. Johannsen DL, Ravussin E. The role of mitochondria in health and disease. Curr Opin Pharmacol. 2009;9(6):780–6. PMCID: PMC3951182. http://www.ncbi.nlm.nih.gov/pubmed/19796990.
278. Petschner P, Gonda X, Baksa D, Eszlari N, Trivaks M, Juhasz G, Bagdy G. Genes linking Mitochondrial function, cognitive impairment and depression are associated with endophenotypes serving precision medicine. Neuroscience. 2018;370:207–17. PMID: 28987512. http://www.ncbi.nlm.nih.gov/pubmed/28987512.
279. Manji H, Kato T, Di Prospero NA, Ness S, Beal MF, Krams M, Chen G. Impaired mitochondrial function in psychiatric disorders. Nat Rev Neurosci. 2012;13(5):293–307. PMID: 22510887. http://www.ncbi.nlm.nih.gov/pubmed/22510887.
280. Herst PM, Rowe MR, Carson GM, Berridge MV. Functional Mitochondria in health and disease. Front Endocrinol (Lausanne). 2017;8:296. PMCID: PMC5675848. http://www.ncbi.nlm.nih.gov/pubmed/29163365.
281. Quiroz JA, Gray NA, Kato T, Manji HK. Mitochondrially mediated plasticity in the pathophysiology and treatment of bipolar disorder. Neuropsychopharmacology. 2008;33(11):2551–65. PMID: 18235426. http://www.ncbi.nlm.nih.gov/pubmed/18235426.
282. Alle H, Roth A, Geiger JRP. Energy-efficient action potentials in hippocampal mossy fibers. Science. 2009;325(5946):1405–8. PMID: 19745156. http://www.ncbi.nlm.nih.gov/pubmed/19745156.
283. Attwell D, Laughlin SB. An energy budget for signaling in the grey matter of the brain. J Cereb Blood Flow Metab. 2001;21(10):1133–45. PMID: 11598490. http://www.ncbi.nlm.nih.gov/pubmed/11598490.
284. Bélanger M, Allaman I, Magistretti PJ. Brain energy metabolism: focus on astrocyte-neuron metabolic cooperation. Cell Metab. 2011;14(6):724–38. PMID: 22152301. http://www.ncbi.nlm.nih.gov/pubmed/22152301.
285. Videbech P. PET measurements of brain glucose metabolism and blood flow in major depressive disorder: a critical review. Acta Psychiatr Scand. 2000;101(1):11–20. PMID: 10674946. http://www.ncbi.nlm.nih.gov/pubmed/10674946.
286. Drevets WC. Neuroimaging and neuropathological studies of depression: implications for the cognitive-emotional features of mood disorders. Curr Opin Neurobiol. 2001;11(2):240–9. PMID: 11301246. http://www.ncbi.nlm.nih.gov/pubmed/11301246.
287. Abdallah CG, Jiang L, De Feyter HM, Fasula M, Krystal JH, Rothman DL, Mason GF, Sanacora G. Glutamate metabolism in major depressive disorder. Am J Psychiatry. 2014;171(12):1320–7. PMCID: PMC4472484. http://www.ncbi.nlm.nih.gov/pubmed/25073688.
288. Gardner A, Johansson A, Wibom R, Nennesmo I, von Döbeln U, Hagenfeldt L, Hällström T. Alterations of mitochondrial function and correlations with personality traits in selected major depressive disorder patients. J Affect Disord. 2003;76(1–3):55–68. PMID: 12943934. http://www.ncbi.nlm.nih.gov/pubmed/12943934.
289. Clay HB, Sillivan S, Konradi C. Mitochondrial dysfunction and pathology in bipolar disorder and schizophrenia. Int J Dev Neurosci. 2011;29(3):311–24. PMCID: PMC3010320. http://www.ncbi.nlm.nih.gov/pubmed/20833242.
290. Zuccoli GS, Saia-Cereda VM, Nascimento JM, Martins-de-Souza D. The energy metabolism dysfunction in psychiatric disorders postmortem brains: focus on proteomic evidence. Front Neurosci. 2017;11:493. PMCID: PMC5594406. http://www.ncbi.nlm.nih.gov/pubmed/28936160.
291. Ben-Shachar D, Karry R. Neuroanatomical pattern of mitochondrial complex I pathology varies between schizophrenia, bipolar disorder and major depression. PloS One. 2008;3(11):e3676. PMCID: PMC2579333. http://www.ncbi.nlm.nih.gov/pubmed/18989376.
292. Spees JL, Olson SD, Whitney MJ, Prockop DJ. Mitochondrial transfer between cells can rescue aerobic respiration. Proc Natl Acad Sci U S A. 2006;103(5):1283–8. PMCID: PMC1345715. http://www.ncbi.nlm.nih.gov/pubmed/16432190.
293. Berridge MV, Neuzil J. The mobility of mitochondria: Intercellular trafficking in health and disease. Clin Exp Pharmacol Physiol. 2017;44(Suppl 1):15–20. PMID: 28409855. http://www.ncbi.nlm.nih.gov/pubmed/28409855.
294. Chan DC. Fusion and fission: interlinked processes critical for mitochondrial health. Annu Rev Genet. 2012;46:265–87. PMID: 22934639. http://www.ncbi.nlm.nih.gov/pubmed/22934639.
295. Hoitzing H, Johnston IG, Jones NS. What is the function of mitochondrial networks? A theoretical assessment of hypotheses and proposal for future research. Bioessays. 2015;37(6):687–700. PMCID: PMC4672710. http://www.ncbi.nlm.nih.gov/pubmed/25847815.
296. Misgeld T, Schwarz TL. Mitostasis in neurons: maintaining Mitochondria in an extended cellular architecture. Neuron. 2017;96(3):651–66. PMCID: PMC5687842. http://www.ncbi.nlm.nih.gov/pubmed/29096078.
297. Vásquez-Trincado C, García-Carvajal I, Pennanen C, Parra V, Hill JA, Rothermel BA, Lavandero S. Mitochondrial dynamics, mitophagy and cardiovascular disease. J Physiol. 2016;594(3):509–25. PMCID: PMC5341713. http://www.ncbi.nlm.nih.gov/pubmed/26537557.
298. Ikeda Y, Shirakabe A, Brady C, Zablocki D, Ohishi M, Sadoshima J. Molecular mechanisms mediating mitochondrial dynamics and mitophagy and their functional roles in the cardiovascular system. J Mol Cell Cardiol. 2015;78:116–22. PMCID: PMC4268018. http://www.ncbi.nlm.nih.gov/pubmed/25305175.
299. Hroudova J, Fisar Z. Activities of respiratory chain complexes and citrate synthase influenced by pharmacologically different antidepressants and mood stabilizers. Neuro Endocrinol Lett. 2010;31(3):336–42. PMID: 20588251. http://www.ncbi.nlm.nih.gov/pubmed/20588251.
300. Gururajan A, Clarke G, Dinan TG, Cryan JF. Molecular biomarkers of depression. Neurosci Biobehav Rev. 2016;64:101–33. PMID: 26906761. http://www.ncbi.nlm.nih.gov/pubmed/26906761.
301. Hacimusalar Y, Eşel E. Suggested biomarkers for major depressive disorder. Noro Psikiyatr Ars. 2018;55(3):280–90. PMCID: PMC6138223. http://www.ncbi.nlm.nih.gov/pubmed/30224877.
302. Biomarkers Definitions Working Group. Biomarkers and surrogate endpoints: preferred definitions and conceptual framework.

Clin Pharmacol Ther. 2001;69(3):89–95. PMID: 11240971. http://www.ncbi.nlm.nih.gov/pubmed/11240971.
303. PGC – Psychiatric Genomics Consortium.
304. Sporns O, Tononi G, Kötter R. The human connectome: a structural description of the human brain. PLoS Comput Biol 2005;1(4):e42. PMCID: PMC1239902. http://www.ncbi.nlm.nih.gov/pubmed/16201007.
305. Human Connectome Project | Mapping the human brain connectivity.
306. Fornito A, Zalesky A, Breakspear M. The connectomics of brain disorders. Nat Rev Neurosci. 2015;16(3):159–72. PMID: 25697159. http://www.ncbi.nlm.nih.gov/pubmed/25697159.
307. Coalson TS, Harms MP, Jenkinson M, Moeller S, Robinson EC, Sotiropoulos SN, Xu J, Yacoub E, Ugurbil K, Van Essen DC. The Human Connectome Project's neuroimaging approach. Nat Neurosci. 2016;19(9):1175–87. PMCID: PMC6172654. http://www.ncbi.nlm.nih.gov/pubmed/27571196.
308. Brandl F, Meng C, Zimmer C, Sorg C. The role of brain connectome imaging in the estimation of depressive relapse risk. Rofo. 2018;190(11):1036–43. PMID: 30103235. http://www.ncbi.nlm.nih.gov/pubmed/30103235.
309. Preti MG, Bolton TA, Van De Ville D. The dynamic functional connectome: state-of-the-art and perspectives. Neuroimage. 2017;160:41–54. PMID: 28034766. http://www.ncbi.nlm.nih.gov/pubmed/28034766.
310. Fornito A, Bullmore ET. Connectomic intermediate phenotypes for psychiatric disorders. Front Psychiatry. 2012;3:32. PMCID: PMC3329878. http://www.ncbi.nlm.nih.gov/pubmed/22529823.
311. Hahamy A, Behrmann M, Malach R. The idiosyncratic brain: distortion of spontaneous connectivity patterns in autism spectrum disorder. Nat Neurosci. 2015;18(2):302–9. PMID: 25599222. http://www.ncbi.nlm.nih.gov/pubmed/25599222.
312. Toga AW, Thompson PM. Connectopathy in ageing and dementia. Brain. 2014;137(Pt 12):3104–6. PMCID: PMC4240289. http://www.ncbi.nlm.nih.gov/pubmed/25413934.
313. Wagner G, de la Cruz F, Köhler S, Pereira F, Richard-Devantoy S, Turecki G, Bär KJ, Jollant F. Connectomics-based functional network alterations in both depressed patients with suicidal behavior and healthy relatives of suicide victims. Sci Rep. 2019;9(1):14330. PMCID: PMC6778100. http://www.ncbi.nlm.nih.gov/pubmed/31586117.
314. Xia MR, Si TM, He Y. Imaging connectomics in depression. CNS Neurosci Ther. 2018;24(11):991–993. PMCID: PMC6490023. http://www.ncbi.nlm.nih.gov/pubmed/30315642.
315. Chen VCH, Shen CY, Liang SHY, Li ZH, Hsieh MH, Tyan YS, Lu ML, Lee Y, McIntyre RS, Weng JC. Assessment of brain functional connectome alternations and correlation with depression and anxiety in major depressive disorders. PeerJ. 2017;5:e3147. PMCID: PMC5702252. http://www.ncbi.nlm.nih.gov/pubmed/29181274.
316. Telese F, Gamliel A, Skowronska-Krawczyk D, Garcia-Bassets I, Rosenfeld MG. "Seq-ing" insights into the epigenetics of neuronal gene regulation. Neuron. 2013;77(4):606–23. PMCID: PMC3736682. http://www.ncbi.nlm.nih.gov/pubmed/23439116.
317. Wray NR, Ripke S, Mattheisen M, Trzaskowski M, Byrne EM, Abdellaoui A, Adams MJ, Agerbo E, Air TM, Andlauer TMF, Bacanu SA, Bækvad-Hansen M, Beekman AFT, Bigdeli TB, Binder EB, Blackwood DRH, Bryois J, Buttenschøn HN, Bybjerg-Grauholm J, Cai N, Castelao E, Christensen JH, Clarke TK, Coleman JIR, Colodro-Conde L, Couvy- Sullivan PF, et al. Major Depressive Disorder Working Group of the Psychiatric Genomics Consortium. Genome-wide association analyses identify 44 risk variants and refine the genetic architecture of major depression. Nat Genet. 2018;50(5):668–81. PMCID: PMC5934326. http://www.ncbi.nlm.nih.gov/pubmed/29700475.
318. Hek K, Demirkan A, Lahti J, Terracciano A, Teumer A, Cornelis MC, Amin N, Bakshis E, Baumert J, Ding J, Liu Y, Marciante K, Meirelles O, Nalls MA, Sun YV, Vogelzangs N, Yu L, Bandinelli S, Benjamin EJ, Bennett DA, Boomsma D, Cannas A, Coker LH, de Geus et al. Newman AB, Tiemeier H, Murabito J. A genome-wide association study of depressive symptoms. Biol Psychiatry. 2013;73(7):667–78. PMCID: PMC3845085. http://www.ncbi.nlm.nih.gov/pubmed/23290196.
319. Finucane HK, Bulik-Sullivan B, Gusev A, Trynka G, Reshef Y, Loh PR, Anttila V, Xu H, Zang C, Farh K, Ripke S, Day FR, ReproGen Consortium, Schizophrenia Working Group of the Psychiatric Genomics Consortium, RACI Consortium, Purcell S, Stahl E, Lindstrom S, Perry JRB, Okada Y, Raychaudhuri S, Daly MJ, Patterson N, Neale BM, Price AL. Partitioning heritability by functional annotation using genome-wide association summary statistics. Nat Genet. 2015;47(11):1228–35. PMCID: PMC4626285. http://www.ncbi.nlm.nih.gov/pubmed/26414678.
320. Yang X, Coulombe-Huntington J, Kang S, Sheynkman GM, Hao T, Richardson A, Sun S, Yang F, Shen YA, Murray RR, Spirohn K, Begg BE, Duran-Frigola M, MacWilliams A, Pevzner SJ, Zhong Q, Wanamaker SA, Tam S, Ghamsari L, Sahni N, Yi S, Rodriguez MD, Balcha D, Tan G, Costanzo M, Andrews B, Boone C, Zhou XJ, Salehi-Ashtiani K, Charloteaux B, Chen AA, Calderwood MA, Aloy P, Roth FP, Hill DE, Iakoucheva LM, Xia Y, Vidal M. Widespread expansion of protein interaction capabilities by alternative splicing. Cell. 2016;164(4):805–17. PMCID: PMC4882190. http://www.ncbi.nlm.nih.gov/pubmed/26871637.
321. Zhang X, Chen MH, Wu X, Kodani A, Fan J, Doan R, Ozawa M, Ma J, Yoshida N, Reiter JF, Black DL, Kharchenko PV, Sharp PA, Walsh CA. Cell-type-specific alternative splicing governs cell fate in the developing cerebral cortex. Cell. 2016;166(5):1147–1162.e15. PMCID: PMC5248659. http://www.ncbi.nlm.nih.gov/pubmed/27565344.
322. Cross-Disorder Group of the Psychiatric Genomics Consortium, Lee SH, Ripke S, Neale BM, Faraone SV, Purcell SM, Perlis RH, Mowry BJ, Thapar A, Goddard ME, Witte JS, Absher D, Agartz I, Akil H, Amin F, Andreassen OA, Anjorin A, Anney R, Anttila V, Arking DE, Asherson P, Azevedo MH, Backlund L, Badner JA, Bailey AJ, Banaschewski et al. International Inflammatory Bowel Disease Genetics Consortium (IIBDGC). Genetic relationship between five psychiatric disorders estimated from genome-wide SNPs. Nat Genet. 2013;45(9):984–94. PMCID: PMC3800159. http://www.ncbi.nlm.nih.gov/pubmed/23933821.
323. Bulik-Sullivan B, Finucane HK, Anttila V, Gusev A, Day FR, Loh PR, ReproGen Consortium, Psychiatric Genomics Consortium, Genetic Consortium for Anorexia Nervosa of the Wellcome Trust Case Control Consortium 3, Duncan L, Perry JRB, Patterson N, Robinson EB, Daly MJ, Price AL, Neale BM. An atlas of genetic correlations across human diseases and traits. Nat Genet. 2015;47(11):1236–41. PMCID: PMC4797329. http://www.ncbi.nlm.nih.gov/pubmed/26414676.
324. Simonti CN, Vernot B, Bastarache L, Bottinger E, Carrell DS, Chisholm RL, Crosslin DR, Hebbring SJ, Jarvik GP, Kullo IJ, Li R, Pathak J, Ritchie MD, Roden DM, Verma SS, Tromp G, Prato JD, Bush WS, Akey JM, Denny JC, Capra JA. The phenotypic legacy of admixture between modern humans and Neandertals. Science. 2016;351(6274):737–41. PMCID: PMC4849557. http://www.ncbi.nlm.nih.gov/pubmed/26912863.
325. Raveane A, Aneli S, Montinaro F, Athanasiadis G, Barlera S, Birolo G, Boncoraglio G, Di Blasio AM, Di Gaetano C, Pagani L, Parolo S, Paschou P, Piazza A, Stamatoyannopoulos G, Angius A, Brucato N, Cucca F, Hellenthal G, Mulas A, Peyret-Guzzon M, Zoledziewska M, Baali A, Bycroft C, Cherkaoui M, Chiaroni J, Di Cristofaro J, et al. Population structure of modern-day Italians reveals patterns of ancient and archaic ancestries in Southern

Europe. Sci Adv. 2019;5(9):eaaw3492. PMCID: PMC6726452. http://www.ncbi.nlm.nih.gov/pubmed/31517044.

326. Locke AE, Kahali B, Berndt SI, Justice AE, Pers TH, Day FR, Powell C, Vedantam S, Buchkovich ML, Yang J, Croteau-Chonka DC, Esko T, Fall T, Ferreira T, Gustafsson S, Kutalik Z, Luan J, Mägi R, Randall JC, Winkler TW, Wood AR, Workalemahu T, Faul JD, et al. Genetic studies of body mass index yield new insights for obesity biology. Nature. 2015;518(7538):197–206. PMCID: PMC4382211. http://www.ncbi.nlm.nih.gov/pubmed/25673413.

327. Berndt SI, Gustafsson S, Mägi R, Ganna A, Wheeler E, Feitosa MF, Justice AE, Monda KL, Croteau-Chonka DC, Day FR, Esko T, Fall T, Ferreira T, Gentilini D, Jackson AU, et al. Genome-wide meta-analysis identifies 11 new loci for anthropometric traits and provides insights into genetic architecture. Nat Genet. 2013;45(5):501–12. PMCID: PMC3973018. http://www.ncbi.nlm.nih.gov/pubmed/23563607.

328. Speliotes EK, Willer CJ, Berndt SI, Monda KL, Thorleifsson G, Jackson AU, Lango Allen H, Lindgren CM, Luan J, Mägi R, Randall JC, Vedantam S, Winkler TW, Qi L, Workalemahu T, Heid IM, Steinthorsdottir V, Stringham HM, Weedon MN, Wheeler E, Wood AR, Ferreira T, Weyant RJ, Segrè AV, Estrada K, Liang L, Nemesh J, Park JH, Ingelsson E, Loos RJF, et al. Association analyses of 249,796 individuals reveal 18 new loci associated with body mass index. Nat Genet. 2010;42(11):937–48. PMCID: PMC3014648. http://www.ncbi.nlm.nih.gov/pubmed/20935630.

329. Willer CJ, Speliotes EK, Loos RJF, Li S, Lindgren CM, Heid IM, Berndt SI, Elliott AL, Jackson AU, Lamina C, Lettre G, Lim N, Lyon HN, McCarroll SA, Papadakis K, Qi L, Randall JC, Roccasecca RM, Sanna S, Scheet P, Weedon MN, Wheeler E, Zhao JH, Jacobs LC, Prokopenko I, Soranzo N, Tanaka T, Timpson NJ, Almgren P, Bennett A, Bergman RN, Bingham SA, Bonnycastle LL, Brown M, Burtt NP, Chines P, Coin L, Collins FS, Barroso I, Abecasis GR, Hirschhorn JN, et al. Genetic Investigation of ANthropometric Traits Consortium. Six new loci associated with body mass index highlight a neuronal influence on body weight regulation. Nat Genet. 2009;41(1):25–34. PMCID: PMC2695662

330. Fogel BL, Wexler E, Wahnich A, Friedrich T, Vijayendran C, Gao F, Parikshak N, Konopka G, Geschwind DH. RBFOX1 regulates both splicing and transcriptional networks in human neuronal development. Hum Mol Genet. 2012;21(19):4171–86. PMCID: PMC3441119. http://www.ncbi.nlm.nih.gov/pubmed/22730494.

331. Gehman LT, Stoilov P, Maguire J, Damianov A, Lin CH, Shiue L, Ares M, Mody I, Black DL. The splicing regulator Rbfox1 (A2BP1) controls neuronal excitation in the mammalian brain. Nat Genet. 2011;43(7):706–11. PMCID: PMC3125461. http://www.ncbi.nlm.nih.gov/pubmed/21623373.

332. Pariante CM, Lightman SL. The HPA axis in major depression: classical theories and new developments. Trends Neurosci. 2008;31(9):464–8. PMID: 18675469. http://www.ncbi.nlm.nih.gov/pubmed/18675469.

333. Amir-Zilberstein L, Blechman J, Sztainberg Y, Norton WHJ, Reuveny A, Borodovsky N, Tahor M, Bonkowsky JL, Bally-Cuif L, Chen A, Levkowitz G. Homeodomain protein otp and activity-dependent splicing modulate neuronal adaptation to stress. Neuron. 2012;73(2):279–91. PMCID: PMC4387198. http://www.ncbi.nlm.nih.gov/pubmed/22284183.

334. Norris AD, Calarco JA. Emerging roles of alternative pre-mRNA splicing regulation in neuronal development and function. Front Neurosci. 2012;6:122. PMCID: PMC3424503. http://www.ncbi.nlm.nih.gov/pubmed/22936897.

335. Choi Y, Nam J, Whitcomb DJ, Song YS, Kim D, Jeon S, Um JW, Lee SG, Woo J, Kwon SK, Li Y, Mah W, Kim HM, Ko J, Cho K, Kim E. SALM5 trans-synaptically interacts with LAR-RPTPs in a splicing-dependent manner to regulate synapse development. Sci Rep. 2016;6:26676. PMCID: PMC4881023. http://www.ncbi.nlm.nih.gov/pubmed/27225731.

336. Mah W, Ko J, Nam J, Han K, Chung WS, Kim E. Selected SALM (synaptic adhesion-like molecule) family proteins regulate synapse formation. J Neurosci. 2010;30(16):5559–68. PMCID: PMC6632343. http://www.ncbi.nlm.nih.gov/pubmed/20410109.

337. Zhu Y, Yao S, Augustine MM, Xu H, Wang J, Sun J, Broadwater M, Ruff W, Luo L, Zhu G, Tamada K, Chen L. Neuron-specific SALM5 limits inflammation in the CNS via its interaction with HVEM. Sci Adv. 2016;2(4):e1500637. PMCID: PMC4846428. http://www.ncbi.nlm.nih.gov/pubmed/27152329.

338. Cebrián C, Loike JD, Sulzer D. Neuronal MHC-I expression and its implications in synaptic function, axonal regeneration and Parkinson's and other brain diseases. Front Neuroanat. 2014;8:114. PMCID: PMC4195363. http://www.ncbi.nlm.nih.gov/pubmed/25352786.

339. Elmer BM, McAllister AK. Major histocompatibility complex class I proteins in brain development and plasticity. Trends Neurosci. 2012;35(11):660–70. PMCID: PMC3493469. http://www.ncbi.nlm.nih.gov/pubmed/22939644.

340. McAllister AK. Major histocompatibility complex I in brain development and schizophrenia. Biol Psychiatry. 2014;75(4):262–8. PMCID: PMC4354937. http://www.ncbi.nlm.nih.gov/pubmed/24199663.

341. Kendler KS, Prescott CA, Myers J, Neale MC. The structure of genetic and environmental risk factors for common psychiatric and substance use disorders in men and women. Arch Gen Psychiatry. 2003;60(9):929–37. PMID: 12963675. http://www.ncbi.nlm.nih.gov/pubmed/12963675.

342. Kendell RE. The classification of depressions: a review of contemporary confusion. Br J Psychiatry. 1976;129:15–28. PMID: 938800. http://www.ncbi.nlm.nih.gov/pubmed/938800.

343. Network and Pathway Analysis Subgroup of Psychiatric Genomics Consortium. Psychiatric genome-wide association study analyses implicate neuronal, immune and histone pathways. Nat Neurosci. 2015;18(2):199–209. PMCID: PMC4378867. http://www.ncbi.nlm.nih.gov/pubmed/25599223.

344. Avian introgression in the genomic era | Avian Research | Full Text.

345. Rock KL, Reits E, Neefjes J. Present yourself! By MHC class I and MHC class II molecules. Trends Immunol. 2016;37(11):724–37. PMCID: PMC5159193. http://www.ncbi.nlm.nih.gov/pubmed/27614798.

346. Wagnon JL, Briese M, Sun W, Mahaffey CL, Curk T, Rot G, Ule J, Frankel WN. CELF4 regulates translation and local abundance of a vast set of mRNAs, including genes associated with regulation of synaptic function. PLoS Genet. 2012;8(11):e1003067. PMCID: PMC3510034. http://www.ncbi.nlm.nih.gov/pubmed/23209433.

347. Ladd AN, Charlet N, Cooper TA. The CELF family of RNA binding proteins is implicated in cell-specific and developmentally regulated alternative splicing. Mol Cell Biol. 2001;21(4):1285–1296. PMCID: PMC99581 http://www.ncbi.nlm.nih.gov/pubmed/11158314.

348. Darnell JC, Van Driesche SJ, Zhang C, Hung KYS, Mele A, Fraser CE, Stone EF, Chen C, Fak JJ, Chi SW, Licatalosi DD, Richter JD, Darnell RB. FMRP stalls ribosomal translocation on mRNAs linked to synaptic function and autism. Cell. 2011;146(2):247–61. PMCID: PMC3232425. http://www.ncbi.nlm.nih.gov/pubmed/21784246.

349. Arsenault J, Gholizadeh S, Niibori Y, Pacey LK, Halder SK, Koxhioni E, Konno A, Hirai H, Hampson DR. FMRP expression levels in Mouse Central nervous system neurons determine behavioral phenotype. Hum Gene Ther. 2016;27(12):982–96. PMCID: PMC5178026. http://www.ncbi.nlm.nih.gov/pubmed/27604541.

350. Pazos Obregón F, Papalardo C, Castro S, Guerberoff G, Cantera R. Putative synaptic genes defined from a Drosophila whole body

developmental transcriptome by a machine learning approach. BMC Genom. 2015;16(1):694. PMCID: PMC4570697 http://www.ncbi.nlm.nih.gov/pubmed/26370122.
351. Emes RD, Grant SGN. Evolution of synapse complexity and diversity. Annu Rev Neurosci. 2012;35:111–31. PMID: 22715880. http://www.ncbi.nlm.nih.gov/pubmed/22715880.
352. Laßek M, Weingarten J, Volknandt W. The synaptic proteome. Cell Tissue Res. 2015;359(1):255–65. PMID: 25038742. http://www.ncbi.nlm.nih.gov/pubmed/25038742.
353. Sakakibara A, Ando R, Sapir T, Tanaka T. Microtubule dynamics in neuronal morphogenesis. Open Biol. 2013;3(7):130061. PMCID: PMC3728923. http://www.ncbi.nlm.nih.gov/pubmed/23864552.
354. Menon S, Gupton S. Recent advances in branching mechanisms underlying neuronal morphogenesis. F1000Res. 2018;7:F1000 Faculty Rev-1779. PMCID: PMC6234733. http://www.ncbi.nlm.nih.gov/pubmed/30473771.
355. Südhof TC. Towards an understanding of synapse formation. Neuron. 2018;100(2):276–93. PMCID: PMC6226307. http://www.ncbi.nlm.nih.gov/pubmed/30359597.
356. Chen CY, Shih YC, Hung YF, Hsueh YP. Beyond defense: regulation of neuronal morphogenesis and brain functions via Toll-like receptors. J Biomed Sci. 2019;26(1):90. PMCID: PMC6827257. http://www.ncbi.nlm.nih.gov/pubmed/31684953.
357. Parnavelas JG. The origin and migration of cortical neurones: new vistas. Trends Neurosci. 2000;23(3):126–31. PMID: 10675917. http://www.ncbi.nlm.nih.gov/pubmed/10675917.
358. Greig LC, Woodworth MB, Galazo MJ, Padmanabhan H, Macklis JD. Molecular logic of neocortical projection neuron specification, development and diversity. Nat Rev Neurosci. 2013;14(11):755–69. PMCID: PMC3876965. http://www.ncbi.nlm.nih.gov/pubmed/24105342.
359. Leone DP, Srinivasan K, Chen B, Alcamo E, McConnell SK. The determination of projection neuron identity in the developing cerebral cortex. Curr Opin Neurobiol. 2008;18(1):28–35. PMCID: PMC2483251. http://www.ncbi.nlm.nih.gov/pubmed/18508260.
360. Wichterle H, Turnbull DH, Nery S, Fishell G, Alvarez-Buylla A. In utero fate mapping reveals distinct migratory pathways and fates of neurons born in the mammalian basal forebrain. Development. 2001;128(19):3759–71. PMID: 11585802. http://www.ncbi.nlm.nih.gov/pubmed/11585802.
361. Wonders CP, Anderson SA. The origin and specification of cortical interneurons. Nat Rev Neurosci. 2006;7(9):687–96. PMID: 16883309. http://www.ncbi.nlm.nih.gov/pubmed/16883309.
362. Gorski JA, Talley T, Qiu M, Puelles L, Rubenstein JLR, Jones KR. Cortical excitatory neurons and glia, but not GABAergic neurons, are produced in the Emx1-expressing lineage. J Neurosci. 2002;22(15):6309–14. PMCID: PMC6758181. http://www.ncbi.nlm.nih.gov/pubmed/12151506.
363. Molyneaux BJ, Arlotta P, Menezes JRL, Macklis JD. Neuronal subtype specification in the cerebral cortex. Nat Rev Neurosci. 2007;8(6):427–37. PMID: 17514196. http://www.ncbi.nlm.nih.gov/pubmed/17514196.
364. Schizophrenia Working Group of the Psychiatric Genomics Consortium. Biological insights from 108 schizophrenia-associated genetic loci. Nature. 2014;511(7510):421–7. PMCID: PMC4112379. http://www.ncbi.nlm.nih.gov/pubmed/25056061.
365. Adnani L, Han S, Li S, Mattar P, Schuurmans C. Mechanisms of cortical differentiation. Int Rev Cell Mol Biol. 2018;336:223–320. PMID: 29413892. http://www.ncbi.nlm.nih.gov/pubmed/29413892.
366. Pfisterer U, Khodosevich K. Neuronal survival in the brain: neuron type-specific mechanisms. Cell Death Dis. 2017;8(3):e2643. PMCID: PMC5386560. http://www.ncbi.nlm.nih.gov/pubmed/28252642.
367. Xie K, Sheppard A. Dietary micronutrients promote neuronal differentiation by modulating the Mitochondrial-nuclear dialogue. Bioessays. 2018;40(7):e1800051. PMID: 29878388. http://www.ncbi.nlm.nih.gov/pubmed/29878388.
368. Wegner SH, Park JJ, Workman T, Hermsen SAB, Wallace J, Stanaway IB, Kim HY, Griffith WC, Hong S, Faustman EM. Anchoring a dynamic in vitro model of human neuronal differentiation to key processes of early brain development in vivo. Reprod Toxicol. 2020;91:116–30. PMCID: PMC6980388. http://www.ncbi.nlm.nih.gov/pubmed/31740287.
369. Andrade A, Brennecke A, Mallat S, Brown J, Gomez-Rivadeneira J, Czepiel N, Londrigan L. Genetic Associations between voltage-gated calcium channels and psychiatric disorders. Int J Mol Sci. 2019;20(14):3537. PMCID: PMC6679227. http://www.ncbi.nlm.nih.gov/pubmed/31331039.
370. Heyes S, Pratt WS, Rees E, Dahimene S, Ferron L, Owen MJ, Dolphin AC. Genetic disruption of voltage-gated calcium channels in psychiatric and neurological disorders. Prog Neurobiol. 2015;134:36–54. PMCID: PMC4658333. http://www.ncbi.nlm.nih.gov/pubmed/26386135.
371. Gooch H, Cui X, Anggono V, Trzaskowski M, Tan MC, Eyles DW, Burne THJ, Jang SE, Mattheisen M, Hougaard DM, Pedersen BN, Cohen A, Mortensen PB, Sah P, McGrath JJ. 1,25-Dihydroxyvitamin D modulates L-type voltage-gated calcium channels in a subset of neurons in the developing mouse prefrontal cortex. Transl. Psychiatry. 2019;9(1):281. PMCID: PMC6848150. http://www.ncbi.nlm.nih.gov/pubmed/31712549.
372. Milenkovic VM, Stanton EH, Nothdurfter C, Rupprecht R, Wetzel CH. The role of Chemokines in the pathophysiology of major depressive disorder. Int J Mol Sci. 2019;20(9):2283. PMCID: PMC6539240. http://www.ncbi.nlm.nih.gov/pubmed/31075818.
373. Petkovich M, Chambon P. Retinoic acid receptors at 35 years. J Mol Endocrinol. 2022;69(4):T13–24. PMID: 36149754. http://www.ncbi.nlm.nih.gov/pubmed/36149754.
374. Martínez C, Souto JA, de Lera AR. Ligand design for modulation of RXR functions. Methods Mol Biol. 2019;2019:51–72. PMID: 31359388. http://www.ncbi.nlm.nih.gov/pubmed/31359388.
375. de Vera IMS, Zheng J, Novick S, Shang J, Hughes TS, Brust R, Munoz-Tello P, Gardner WJ, Marciano DP, Kong X, Griffin PR, Kojetin DJ. Synergistic regulation of coregulator/nuclear receptor interaction by ligand and DNA. Structure. 2017;25(10):1506–1518.e4. PMCID: PMC5653230. http://www.ncbi.nlm.nih.gov/pubmed/28890360.
376. Choi S, Kim YE, Kim JW, Cho N, Cheon S, Kim KK. Rbfox family proteins make the homo- and hetero-oligomeric complexes. Biochem Biophys Res Commun. 2018;495(1):1022–7. PMID: 29170129. http://www.ncbi.nlm.nih.gov/pubmed/29170129.
377. CELF4 - CUGBP Elav-like family member 4 - Homo sapiens (Human) | UniProtKB | UniProt.
378. Ma L, Du Y, Hui Y, Li N, Fan B, Zhang X, Li X, Hong W, Wu Z, Zhang S, Zhou S, Xu X, Zhou Z, Jiang C, Liu L, Zhang X. Developmental programming and lineage branching of early human telencephalon. EMBO J. 2021;40(21):e107277. PMCID: PMC8561642. http://www.ncbi.nlm.nih.gov/pubmed/34558085.
379. Bierut LJ, Heath AC, Bucholz KK, Dinwiddie SH, Madden PA, Statham DJ, Dunne MP, Martin NG. Major depressive disorder in a community-based twin sample: are there different genetic and environmental contributions for men and women? Arch Gen Psychiatry. 1999;56(6):557–63. https://doi.org/10.1001/archpsyc.56.6.557. PMID: 10359473.

10 Depression and the Immune Responses

Franklin Sunzeri

Introduction

Chronic stress and depression are most often associated with increased systemic inflammation, including overall leukocytosis and increased circulating neutrophils, but with a depressed immune system response [1–8]. Catecholamines, glucocorticoids, cytokines, opioids, and histamines let loose during chronic stress or depression can dampen cellular-mediated immune responses by macrophages, antigen-presenting cells, NK cells, Th1 cells, and cytotoxic T cells, among others. Th2-type responses and humoral immunity are usually little affected [9], see Fig. 10.1.

People under chronic stress or who are depressed tend to have higher basal plasma cortisol, decreased dehydroepiandrosterone, and elevated circulating levels of the complement components C3 and C4 [10], positive acute phase proteins, and antibodies to HSV-1 and EBV [11].

Cytokine responses are generally proinflammatory with increased IL-6 and IL-8, but with decreased Th1-type cytokines (e.g., IL-2, IL-12, IFN-γ, and IL-18/IL-1γ) and

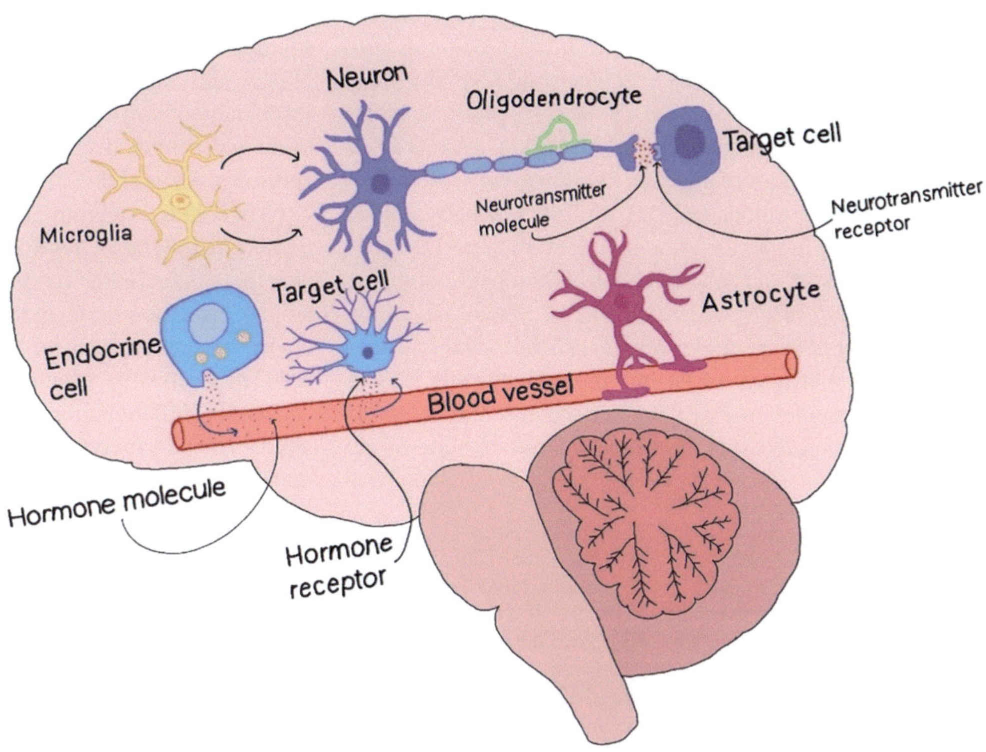

Fig. 10.1 Cartoon representation of brain-immune cell interactions. This illustration depicts key cellular components involved in neuroimmune and neuroendocrine communication. Featured are neurons, microglia, and oligodendrocytes interacting with target cells, highlighting roles in signaling and myelination. An endocrine cell is shown releasing hormones into a blood vessel, which influences distant target cells. An astrocyte wraps around the vessel, emphasizing its role in blood-brain barrier support and homeostasis

F. Sunzeri (✉)
Heather Hills Consulting, Coos Bay, OR, USA

J. Raber et al. (eds.), *Understanding and Treating Depressive Disorders*, https://doi.org/10.1007/978-3-032-14465-2_10

increased Th2-type cytokines and soluble cytokine receptors (e.g., IL-10, TGF-γ, sTNF-αR, sIL-2R, and IL-1 receptor antagonist (IL-1ra)) [7]. These altered balances can dampen the cellular-mediated immune Th1 responses to some infections and cancer [9].

This dampened immune response is also associated with decreased growth hormone secretion secondary to increased IL-6 and increased corticotropin-releasing hormone stimulation of somatostatin and decreased prolactin mRNA expression [4–6, 8].

IL-6 production is enhanced by anxiety, chronic stress, and depression [12, 13]. Elevated circulating IL-6 is a potent stimulator of CRH, which in turn leads to increased HPA activity [14]. Increased circulating IL-6 is associated in an age-related fashion with various cancers, osteoporosis, cardiovascular disease, type-2 diabetes, and arthritis [14, 15].

The Glasers in 2002 reviewed the evidence that depression can directly stimulate production of proinflammatory cytokines in a number of illnesses associated with aging and increased risks for morbidity and mortality [12]. These conditions include cardiovascular disease, osteoporosis, some cancers, arthritis, type 2 diabetes, frailty, periodontal disease, and functional decline. They also pointed out that depression associated with decreased cellular immune response may prolong infections and delay wound healing.

A variety of illnesses are associated with psychological and neuroendocrine attributes of depression. It is generally believed that cytokines are involved in the process as proposed in the *cytokine model of depression*. Cytokines can have significant effects on the CNS. Besides physical symptoms of malaise, lethargy, fatigue, shivering, and *sickness behavior*[1] such as loss of appetite, cytokines may provoke or enhance negative moods [17–21]. In fact, a negative mood may be the first indication of an incipient disease [22].

The process of sickness behavior begins with *pathogen-associated molecular patterns (PAMPs)*, which are recognized by *pattern recognition receptors (PRRs)* on the surface or in the cytoplasm of innate immune system cells [23]. A couple of examples of PRRs are surface *Toll-like receptors (TLRs)*[2] [30] and the cytoplasmic *nucleotide-binding oligomerization domain (Nod)-like receptors* [31] that are found primarily in macrophages and dendritic cells.

After a series of steps, these cells begin an inflammatory response by producing and releasing an assortment of cytokines [31]. If the infection is not in the brain, these cytokines act via both a fast transmission pathway via primary afferent nerves that invest the inflammatory site and a slow pathway via humoral (blood and lymph) transmission [32]. In addition to the cytokines, products of the infectious agent will also be carried to the blood-brain barrier (BBB).

Neuronal impulses may, for example, activate the afferent branch of the vagus nerve, which communicates through the lower brain stem (nucleus tractus solitarius) with higher brain centers including the hypothalamus and amygdala [33].

Humoral carried cytokines and infectious-agent products begin a cytokine response from the vascular endothelium of the BBB of the choroid plexus and circumventricular organs [34]. These cytokines are both newly synthesized at the BBB and carried from the periphery then diffuse into the parenchyma of the brain via *volume transmission*.[3]

All the cells within the brain can initiate cytokine secretion, but microglias are particularly responsive to afferent stimuli [32].

In both healthy and pathological physiological conditions, the neuroimmune system and neuroplasticity mechanisms engage in a strong dialogue [37, 38]. In depression, anti-neuroplastic changes are associated with decreased proliferation of neural stem cells, decreased survival of neuroblasts and immature neurons, impaired neurocircuitry (especially of cortical-striatal-limbic circuits), reduced levels of neurotrophins, decreased long-term potentiation, reduced spine density, and dendritic retraction [39].

When there is a brain-associated immune response (a.k.a. *neuroinflammation*), not only is neuroplasticity reduced, but also there is increased oxidative stress, glucocorticoid insensitivity, and neurotransmitter malfunction including toxic levels of glutamate and catabolites of tryptophan, and reduced levels of serotonin [17, 18, 37, 40–42].

In neuroinflammation, it appears that there is a disturbed ability of the glucocorticoid receptor to translocate to the nucleus, where it normally regulates expression of inflam-

[1]Sickness behavior is the coordinated adapted response to infections that develop during infections. It is the expression of a central motivational state that changes the individual's priorities in order to combat the infection [16]. Sickness behavior is due to effects of proinflammatory cytokines, such as interleukin-1 (IL-1) and tumor necrosis factor-alpha (TNF α), in the brain.

[2]*Toll-like receptors* (TLRs) are a family of highly conserved pattern-recognizing receptors involved in innate immune activity in mammals and in regulating adult hippocampal neurogenesis [24]. Two members of TLRs, TLR2 and TLR4, are expressed on sentinel cells such as macrophages, mast cells, and dendritic cells [25, 26]. In the nervous system, they recognize endogenous ligands of necrotic/injured cells [27] and adult neural stem/progenitor cells (NPCs) and have distinct and opposing functions in NPC proliferation and differentiation [24]. Activation of brain and peripheral TLR4 can trigger sickness behavior and depression [28]. Dysregulation of TLR signaling has been seen in monocytes in MDD and some antidepressants appear to balance this dysregulation [29].

[3]There are two main modes of transmission in the brain. Synaptic transmission and volume transmission. Synaptic transmission is rapid and precise (*phasic transmission*). Volume transmission is the diffusion of neurotransmitters and neuromodulators through extracellular fluid filled channels of the extracellular space, the cerebrospinal fluid filled ventricular space, and sub-arachnoid space. Volume transmission is well suited to modulation and tuning. It lasts longer and is referred to as *tonic transmission* [35, 36].

matory transcription factors including nuclear factor-kappa B (NF-κB) [18].

Neuroinflammatory activation of indoleamine 2,3-dioxygenase (the tryptophan-degrading enzyme) changes tryptophan metabolism into a pathway that produces 3-hydroxykyurenin and quinolinic acid, which are neurotoxins, while at the same time decreasing serotonin synthesis [42–44].

Neuroinflammatory-induced increased activation of serotonin, norepinephrine, and dopamine transporters can also stimulate reuptake of these neurotransmitters from the synapse [45–47].

Acute and chronic stress of neuroinflammation and changes in glucocorticoids may negatively affect glutamate release, glutamate receptors, and glutamate clearance, resulting in glutamate levels becoming neurotoxic, especially in the frontal cortex and the hippocampus [48–50].

Alterations in cells such as *CD4⁺CD25⁺T regulatory cells*, CNS-specific autoreactive CD4⁺T cells, macrophages, microglia, and astrocytes, and humoral factors such as IL-1, IL-6, and TNF-α are implicated in depression.[4] In particular, the neuroprotective M2-type blood-derived macrophages that produce neuroregulatory factors and inflammation-moderating cytokines may be malfunctional in depression [51–54]. Depression is frequently accompanied by reduced levels of important immunoregulatory proteins such as insulin-like growth factor-1 [55, 56], Crohn's disease (CD) 200 modulated by IL-4 [57, 58], and CX3CL1 via increased levels of IL-1β [59–61].

However, the influence of cytokines on depression is not at all settled. Whereas many studies have reported increased cytokines in depression [17, 62–64], others have found that at least some brain cytokines demonstrate antidepressant activity and mediate the influences of the principal serotonin-specific reuptake inhibitor (SSRI) antidepressant drugs [65, 66]. Nonsteroidal anti-inflammatory drugs (NSAIDs) such as ibuprofen appear to block the therapeutic activity of SSRIs by inhibiting the formation of brain cytokines [65, 67]. The putative mechanism relates to intracellular *S100A10 (p11)*, which regulates serotonin receptor activity in psychiatric mood disorders [68].

On the other hand, other authors have not found that to be the case [69]. For example, augmentation of antidepressant effects of aspirin with fluoxetine [70], celecoxib with SSRIs [71], and TNF-α antagonist etanercept decreasing depression in psoriasis sufferers [72]. Indeed, it has been suggested that aspirin may be beneficial for a variety of mental disorders including depression, schizophrenia, bipolar disorder, and Alzheimer's disease [73]. Such results may reflect the complexity of the large variety of cytokines and their interactions with different chemotherapeutics.

A 2011 meta-analysis of the effects of antidepressants on cytokines argues against the idea that resolution of a depressive episode is associated with normalization of levels of circulating inflammatory cytokines [74]. Nevertheless, the data does suggest that inflammatory cytokines might add to depressive symptoms, and antidepressants block inflammatory cytokines effects on the brain. Some antidepressants can normalize cytokine levels, whereas other effective antidepressants—such as SNRIs—do not [74]. However, this does not negate the possibility that inflammatory cytokine effects on the brain are blocked by antidepressants.

The *sequenced treatment alternatives to relieve depression (STAR*D)* prospective cohort study of treatment-resistant depression reported antagonistic effects of anti-inflammatories on antidepressant-induced behaviors [65]. For example, widely used anti-inflammatory drugs antagonized biochemical and behavioral responses to SSRIs. In addition, frontal cortical levels (in contradistinction to serum levels) of TNFα and IFNγ were increased by SSRIs. These observations have fueled the speculation that patient use of nonsteroidal anti-inflammatory drugs may interfere with the potential effects of SSRIs and may explain high treatment-resistant rates [66].

These observations have also led to the suggestion that anti-inflammatory drugs may impede the production of brain-derived cytokines and chemokines that would induce migration of neuroprotective immune cells involved in protective immunosurveillance [52].

It has become clearer *that many neuroimmune factors also offer protection* to the nervous system. Even those cytokines that are commonly considered proinflammatory can be neuroprotective in the appropriate context [52, 53, 75].

For example, TNF-α and IL-6 seem to play a neuroprotective role in memory, learning, and neuroplasticity [37, 76]. Cytokine genotypes of IL-1β and TNF-α may have different effects on cognition [77]. IL-1β-1418C→T polymorphism can be detrimental to memory performance, while TNF-α-308G→A polymorphism may enhance processing speed in elderly individuals.

Some studies have shown that the *IL-6* G-allele of the SNP rs1800795 may have a protective effect on hippocampal volumes [78].[5]

[4]Reduced hippocampal neurogenesis in depressed rodents seems to be tied to stress-activated protein kinase (SAPK)/Janus Kinase (JNK) pathway, hypoxia-inducible factors (HIF)-1α, JAK-Signal Transducer and Activator of Transcription (STAT) pathway, mitogen-activated protein kinase (MAPK)/cAMP responsive element binding protein (CREB) pathway, Ras-MAPK, PI-3 kinase, IKK/nuclear factor (NF)-κB and TGFβ activated kinase-1 (TAK-1) [37, 42].

[5]IL-6 appears to be potentially neuroprotective via various pathways: Janus Kinase (JAK)/Signal Transducer and Activator of Transcription (STAT), Mitogen-activated Protein Kinase (MAPK)/cAMP Response Element-binding (CREB), and Ras-MAPK, Phosphatidylinositol 3-kinases (PI3K) [78, 79].

Other studies on IL-6 have not found positive effects on neurogenesis nor have they found detrimental effects [37]. However, evidence for differences between anti-neurogenic and pro-neurogenic effects of IL-6 seems to be dependent upon at least experimental conditions and concentrations [37].

TNF-α may exert a protective effect via the primarily neuroprotective pathway TNFR2 (vs. TNFR1, which is neurodegenerative), and related signaling pathways [80, 81].[6] TNF-α may enhance cognitive functions and hippocampal neurogenesis in depression [80, 83]. It seems that the balance of whether TNF-α damages or protects is dependent upon the duration of NF-κB activity [83].

In rodents, TNF-α deficiency may impede hippocampal memory and learning [84]. TNF-α-308G→A polymorphism may enhance processing speed in healthy elderly individuals [77] and enhance cognition in healthy youngsters [80].

In response to neurotoxicity, IL-4 from CNS-specific autoreactive CD4+ T cells may be neuroprotective and antidepressive [54]. Binding of IL-4 to receptors on cytotoxic microglial cells [85] can downregulate proinflammatory cytokines, induce BDNF and IGF-1, and enhance neurogenesis [53, 86, 87].

In vitro microglial exposure to IL-4 or low levels of IFN-γ can stimulate neurogenesis and neuronal stem cell differentiation [88]. IL-4 can also stimulate neuroprotective M2-type microglial phenotype [86, 89].

IL-10 may have neuroprotective effects [90]. In a lipopolysaccharide model of sickness behavior in rats, IL-10 was able to prevent emergence of behavioral signs of depression [91]. Deficiency of IL-10 in rodents was associated with greater anxiety and depression [92], and in humans, IL-10 appears to be reduced in depression [93].

Macrophages are the first cellular responders of the innate immune system, responsible for sensing, alerting, removing, and destroying intrinsic and extrinsic pathogens [94–96]. Three principal phenotypes have been characterized. There are those that support bacterial clearance (classical activation M1), parasite defense/tissue repair (alternative activation M2), and anti-inflammation (deactivation). The balance of the three types of macrophages appears to influence the symptoms of sickness behavior [96]. The M1s produce proinflammatory cytokines and sickness behavior [18, 96]. The M2s decrease proinflammatory cytokines and sickness behavior [97, 98]. The role of deactivation macrophages appears to decrease inflammation via uncertain means [99, 100].

It has been suggested that CNS-specific autoreactive CD4+ T cells and blood-derived M2 macrophages are importantly involved in *protective immunosurveillance in the brain* and associated with anxiety and depression [38, 53]. According to this protective immunosurveillance hypothesis, susceptibility to mental disorders may result from a lack of appropriate circulating T cells and their IL-4 which is necessary to combat neuroinflammation and restore healthy brain states [54].

It is thought that CNS-specific autoreactive CD4+ T cells support and recruit, via IL-4 and IFN-γ, the infiltration of neuroprotective M2 macrophages to the sub-arachnoid meningeal spaces and choroid plexus [54, 97, 101]. The M2 macrophages and the microglial cells with whose activity they modulate, downregulate inflammatory associated factors including IL-1β, TNF-α, iNOS, and COX-2, increase BDNF and IGF-1 growth factors, and mop up cellular debris and toxic substances including free radicals [102–110].

There is some criticism of the immunosurveillance idea, principally based on the phenotype of the CNS-specific autoreactive CD4+ T cells [111]. T cell differentiation into the T reg cell type is context-dependent and can either be opposed or enhanced by IL-4 [112]. They suggest that due to the presence of IL-4 and IL-10, the regulatory cell is not always CD25+ and other candidates include Th3, Tr1, Th2, IL-10^{+}TH1, CD8+ reg cells, regulatory Foxp3+ NKT, IL-10^{+}CD56^{bright}NK, or various other IL-10-secreting cell types [113].

Glial cells are the primary active partners to neurons in the CNS and PNS [114, 115]. There is an approximate 1:1 ratio of glia to neurons in the entire human brain, and a range of 40–130 billion glial cells [116]. They occupy about ½ of the volume of the CNS. The ratio of glial cells to neurons varies greatly depending upon the location and the type of glial cells [117]. There are three main types of glial cells. They are oligodendrocytes (45–75% of the total), astrocytes (19–40%), and microglia (around 10% or less). For our purposes, we are considering astrocytes and microglial relationships to depression.

Astrocytes are part of the *tripartite synapse* [118]. This concept refers to the intimate relationship at the synapse between the astrocytes, the presynaptic neuron, and the postsynaptic element. As such, the astrocytes are closely involved in actively controlling synaptic transmission and neuronal activity. There are some reasons to refer to a *quadripartite synapse* instead, the fourth partner being the microglia, which we will discuss in a few paragraphs later [119].

Astrocytes are highly involved in homeostasis and defense of the CNS at multiple levels [120]. Astrocytes are heterogeneous and highly adaptable. They are crucial regulators of immune responses in the brain and contain multiple neurotransmitter receptors [121–123].

They provide metabolic support, regulate extracellular ion concentration [124], modulate synaptic transmission [125], and perform gluconeogenesis and so provide neurons

[6] Related pathways include IκB kinase (IKK)/Nuclear Factor κB (NF-κB), Transforming Growth factor β-activated Kinase 1 (TAK-1), PI3K-PKB-Akt, c-Jun N-terminal kinases (JNK), and IL-6) [80–82].

with glucose [126]. Astrocytes provide neurons with glutamate and the GABA precursor glutamine [127] and ATP [128]. They modulate blood flow [129], drive the circadian clock to trigger brain-state transitions [130–132], promote oligodendrocytic myelination activity [133], affect nervous system repair [134, 135], and enhance memory [136, 137]. Astrocytes have neuroplastic functions which include glutamate recycling and synaptic plasticity [138]. As an important source of trophic molecules during neuronal development, they promote excitatory synapse formation [139–141].

Connections to anxiety and depression-like symptoms in mice appear to involve decreased expression of plasticity genes in astrocytes when confronted with excess stress [142].

Through neurogenesis-dependent and independent mechanisms, hippocampal astrocytes interact with neurons under pharmacological conditions to release BDNF to regulate various aspects of antidepressant-like activities [143].

Astrocytes are vital regulators of CNS adaptive and innate immune responses [121]. In this role, they can either enhance or suppress inflammation and repair depending upon the context [121]. Astrocytes can express MHC class II antigens and B7, and CD40 which are essential for antigen presentation and stimulation of T cells [144]. Indeed, they can produce a wide range of chemokines and cytokines. Astrocytes respond to inflammatory cytokines such as IL-1β, TNF-α, and IL-6, and phagocytose debris [137].

It appears that astrocyte-microglia cross-talk is at the command center for determining immune system reactivity in the CNS [145]. Microglia via an NFκβ-dependent secretome have a critical influence upon astrocyte activation [146]. It also appears that astrocytes have the potential to modify the immune reactivity of microglia [145, 147].

In consort with microglia, astrocytes may actually be neurotoxic under conditions of excess stress [148].

As part of the quadripartite synapse, they are intimately involved in actively controlling neuronal activity and synaptic neurotransmission [118]. Astrocytes have been shown to have a role in learning, memory, and long-term potentiation [149–152].

There is some evidence to support the hypothesis that MDD is a disease of astrocyte pathology [153]. In certain brain regions affected by MDD, astrocytes decrease in number and often undergo degeneration [153, 154]. Major antidepressants have direct effects on astroglia biochemistry and physiology that can be associated with the amelioration of symptoms [154]. On the other hand, the massive GWAS PGC MDD found that genetic differences between MDD sufferers and controls are in neurons, not microglia or astrocytes [155].

Although microglia and astrocytes are the primary immune system cells in the central nervous system, their roles in depression are not very well understood. However, there appear to be context-dependent neuroprotective properties [156–159]. It has been reasoned that all the molecular pathways leading to depression pass through microglia [160, 161].

Microglia cells are the macrophages of the CNS [162, 163]. They are found throughout the CNS. They have a multitude of functions and change their morphology to adapt to their functions [164]. Microglia are the principal immune effector and regulator cells in the CNS responding to immunological, physiological, and psychological strain [160, 165].

- They are very sensitive sentries looking for subtle signs of damaged neurons.
- As antigen-presenting cells, they are the generals orchestrating innate and adaptive immune responses [166].
- As phagocytes, they consume invading pathogens [167], cellular debris, and apoptotic cells.
- They are active in controlling neuron proliferation and differentiation, synaptic connections, and brain homeostasis in development and in the adult brain [160].

Microglia development and colonization of embryonic and postnatal brain are regulated by intrinsic factors such as chemokines and hormones and can be disrupted by external factors including stress and infections [158, 168]. These influences on glial cells may impact neural development and can make a considerable difference in mental health and cognition throughout life [158]. Structure and function of microglia themselves can be damaged by intense inflammation or by senescence, resulting in impaired neuroplasticity and neurogenesis, and depression [169].

During times of excess stress, microglias are implicated in disrupting neuroplasticity and neuroprotection, degenerating hippocampi, organizing neuroinflammation, and exacerbating depression [170]. Microglial morphology and phenotype are affected by excessive glucocorticoids, neuroactive molecules from the gastrointestinal system, and alterations in the genetic expression of various neurotrophic factors, leading to chronic inflammation and symptoms of depression [165]. Malfunctions of microglia can result in microglial phagocytosis of live neurons and have the potential to increase the risk of autoimmune CNS disorders [160, 170]. The effects of chronic stress that upregulate hippocampal microglia create a persistent expression of *receptor for advanced glycation end products (RAGE)* that increases vulnerability to depressive-like behaviors long after the stress has gone [171].

Two-way communication of microglia with neurons and other cells in the brain is accomplished via *fractalkine sig-*

naling[7] [173, 174], characterized by secreted soluble factors and extracellular vesicles [160]. The network of communication with other microglia, astrocytes, neurons, T cells, and endothelial cells is extremely complicated [160, 175]. Microglia are constantly on alert and during chronic stress or under the influence of specific cytokine profiles, they can produce neurotoxic mediators including nitric oxide, PGE2, superoxide anions, and proinflammatory cytokines [158, 176]. For example, microglia may mediate the effects of stress on prefrontal cortex (PFC) neuronal function and PFC-regulated behavior [177–179]. In rodents, restraint stress showed an association between increased microglial activity in the medial PFC and a decline in working memory [180]. A microglial activation inhibitor (minocycline) has been shown to relieve depressive-like behaviors in rats with bone cancer pain by inhibiting microglia activation in the hippocampus [181].

However, in a complex dynamic, ever-changing context, microglia are neuroprotective and support neurogenesis when under the influence of CNS-specific autoreactive CD4+ T cells [158, 182, 183]. It also appears that microglial patterns of activation may be regionally and developmentally specific [158]. Early-life stress appears to prime microglia to respond, especially in the hippocampus, leading to an increased response to later stress [184].

Several types of chronic stresses (chronic unpredictable stress, chronic restraint stress, and chronic social defeat stress) in mice can activate loss of endogenous hippocampal microglia while leaving cortical microglia intact [185]. In that experiment, treatment by stimulators of microglia, lipopolysaccharide, or macrophage colony-stimulating factor reversed the microglia loss and depressive behavior. When minocycline prevented the initial activation of these hippocampal microglia, it prevented both the reduction of these microglia and the depressive behavior that had been induced by those stressors [185].

Dysfunctional microglia may be central to producing depressive symptoms either by directly altering synaptic plasticity [186, 187] or indirectly by their effects on astrocytes [188].

In depression, when astrocyte function decreases, it releases less ATP and adenosine [189, 190]. This decrease causes inadequate astrocyte-to-neuron activation of P2X2 (ATP) receptors and inadequate activation of inhibitory adenosine A1 receptors in neurons [191]. Adenosine A1 receptor numbers decrease under chronic stress [192, 193]. Adenosine A1 receptors are inhibitory and adenosine A2a receptors are facilitatory [193]. Under these conditions, A2a receptors are increased [192, 194]. This increased excitability results in microglia hyper-responsiveness via an increase in expression of microglia P2X7 receptors and deranged plasticity [195–197]. Increasing ATP and adenosine from astrocytes, blocking A2a receptors, enhancing adenosine A1 receptors, and inhibiting microglia activity each can decrease symptoms of depression [192].

Microglia alterations in frontolimbic areas are highly associated with inflammation and depression [169, 198–200]. They are activated by depression-associated glucocorticoids [201], serotonin [202], BDNF [203], dopamine, and norepinephrine [204].

Microglia function may be recovered, and depression symptoms may be lessened by minocycline [205], and antidepressants such as ketamine [206], citalopram [207], and fluoxetine [207].

There are two types of T cells that have the ability to suppress immune responses [208, 209]. These are the naturally occurring and inducible or adaptive *T regulatory cells (Tregs)* [209, 210]. Thymus-derived *CD4+CD25+ Tregs* are about 5–10% of peripheral CD4+ T cells [211]. All Tregs express *Foxp3* (forkhead box 3), which is a master transcription factor in the development and function of Tregs [212].

As with other immune system factors, the context will determine whether the overall effects of Tregs are positive or negative in depression or cognition [111, 213–215].

Treg depletion modulates anxiety and depression-like behaviors in mice [215]. There is some evidence that Treg cells may influence the immune imbalance in patients with major depression and may relate to the 5-HT system [216].

Tregs that are reactive to CNS-associated self-antigens appear to be capable of suppressing endogenous anti-stress attributes in mice [217]. Increased Tregs during antidepressant treatment is associated with decreased cytokine production and decreased depression symptoms [93]. Inhibition of excessive or maladaptive immune responses is also ascribed to Tregs [43, 93]. Decreased IL-10 and TGF-β in depressed humans may be related to reduced Treg function or expression [218–221]. Tregs are essential for maintaining self-tolerance [213].

On the other hand, Tregs have also been shown to inhibit the beneficial effects of CNS-specific autoreactive CD4+ T cells on reducing stress-associated anxiety in rodents [217]. In addition, the microbiota of the gut may also modify the attributes of Tregs and their influence on higher neurocognitive behaviors [111].

Th1, Th2 cells are other subtypes of T cells that appear to be involved in depression. However, the relative contributions of cytokines produced by these subtypes of T cells are open for discussion [111, 222]. Th1 cells are classically associated with producing IFN-γ, IL-2, and TNF-α. Th2 cells commonly produce IL-4, IL-6, and IL-10. Some of the evidence points to a net excess of Th1 cytokines associated

[7] Fractalkine (FKN) is a chemokine constitutively expressed by healthy neurons. It signals to microglia by interacting with the FKN receptor, CX3CR1 [172].

with immune dysfunction in depression, whereas other evidence points to Th2 cytokines being at fault [41, 111, 218].

T-bet, a Th1-specific transcription factor, regulates Th1 cell development through the induction of endogenous Th1 cytokines and IFN-γ [223, 224]. T-bet-deficient mice are resistant to stress-induced neuroinflammation and depression-like behavior [224]. In a Mexican American sample, an SNP of the *T-bet* (*Tbx21*) gene, which is critical for Th1cell function, is associated with susceptibility to major depression [223].

Depression and the Gut–Liver–Brain Axis

The gastrointestinal tract (GI tract or gut), the liver, and the brain are a finely tuned partnership that includes the endocrine, immune, autonomic, and enteric nervous systems [225], see Fig. 10.2.

A truly comprehensive 2023 review of the gut-liver-brain axis details the complex interactions and consequence of derangements and implications for therapeutic intervention in disease [226].

Links in the gut–brain–liver axis involve the circulatory system, enteric nervous system [227], neuroendocrine system [228], immune system [229], and the vagus nerve [230].

Transfer of nutrients from the intestines is controlled in a healthy gut. However, in dysbiosis, the gut barrier is disrupted by uncontrolled bacteria, and their metabolites enter the circulation and find their way to the liver [231–233]. In addition, compounds produced by the intestines and the resident microbiota enter the circulation and interact with the vagal nerves, spinal afferent nerves, and the brain, which then sends messages back to the gut, pancreas, and liver via vagal parasympathetic pathways [234]. Activation of inflammatory pathways can lead to liver damage [235–240].

Regulation of this interaction appears to be provided principally by the *microbiome*[8] and molecules produced by the microbiome organisms [248]. For example, the microbiome controls the intestinal permeability. The microbiome composition is influenced by host factors such as high-fat diet, age, physiological condition, and genetic and epigenetic background [249]. In gut dysbiosis, inflammatory cytokines released from a leaky gut or from the liver can induce structural changes of the blood-brain barrier [250–253] and may play a role in neuropsychiatric disorders [254–256].

The GI tract is the largest endocrine organ in mammals and secretes dozens of communication molecules [257]. These molecules can interact with receptors on immune system cells and vagus nerve terminals thereby establishing the gut to brain axis [257]. This gut-brain pathway often begins by integrating sensory information from the gut that is transformed into neural, hormonal, and immunological signals [265].[9] Microbiome metabolites influence depressive behavior by direct stimulation of CNS receptors, peripheral stimulation of neural, endocrine, and immune intermediaries, and

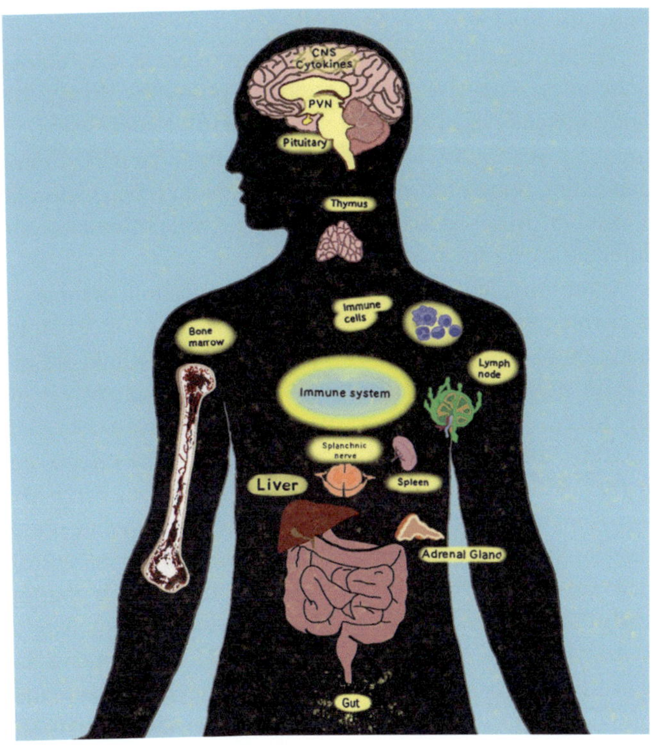

Fig. 10.2 Interconnected dynamics between the brain, gut, and immune-neuroendocrine systems. The figure illustrates the bidirectional relationships among central nervous system components—including the hypothalamic paraventricular nucleus (PVN), pituitary gland, and CNS-derived cytokines—and peripheral structures such as the gut, thymus, lymph nodes, spleen, adrenal glands, and bone marrow. Immune cell trafficking and neuroendocrine signaling mediate systemic feedback loops, highlighting an integrated network critical for maintaining homeostasis under environmental and genetic influences

[8] *The microbiome is the collective genomes* of trillions of bacteria, archaea, viruses, fungi, and other microeukaryotic organisms [241, 242]. For an introduction to the human microbiome, we recommend, The Host Microbiome Regulates and Maintains Human Health: A Primer and Perspective for Non-Microbiologists [241]. And, Demystifying the Manipulation of host Immunity, Metabolism, and Extraintestinal Tumors by the gut Microbiome [243].

In 2007, *The Human Microbiome Project Phase I* began to identify and characterize human microbial flora. It was superseded by the *Integrative Human Microbiome Project* in 2014 [210] with the goal of characterizing the roles of microbes in health and disease. [244–246]. In addition, *The International Human Microbiome Consortium* was formed in 2008 to, "understand the role of the human microbiome in the maintenance of health and causation of disease and to use that knowledge to improve the ability to prevent and treat disease" [216–225, 227–240, 244–264].

[9] A discussion of the immune system pathways relating to the GI tract can be seen in [266, 267]. Neural pathways related to the gut-brain system can be found in [268, 269].

by epigenetic regulation of histone acetylation and DNA methylation [258].

Specialized endoderm-derived epithelial cells (*enteroendocrine cells*) are widely distributed in the GI tract and provide the signaling molecules [259, 260]. Activity of these enteroendocrine cells is modulated by the GI microbiota [261, 262]. Diversity and composition of the microbiota influences this release of signaling molecules. Some of these molecules include glucagon-like peptide [263],[10] neuropeptide Y family [272],[11] cholecystokinin [275],[12] corticotropin-releasing factor [277],[13] oxytocin [279],[14] ghrelin [225],[15] and serotonin (5-HT) [284].

These molecules play an important role in stress-related disorders such as anxiety and depression [225]. Quite a few of these molecules are neuropeptides that have essential functions in the CNS, where they are well known to be involved in anxiety and depression [285]. Alterations in microbiota that induce changes in the expression of these GI tract-derived peptides have been implicated in changes in the gut-brain communication stream [286]. In one experiment, antibiotic-induced gut dysbiosis disrupted microbiota-brain communication and resulted in demonstrable cognitive impairment in mice [286].

Many of these peptides associated with depression play a hypothalamic role in regulating appetite and eating [287]. This relationship may tie into the comorbidity of obesity and psychiatric disorders [288]. Alterations in the GI microbiota can have an impact on disorders ranging from obesity [289] to allergies [290], autoimmune disorders [291], inflammatory bowel disease [292, 293], and irritable bowel syndrome [261], and to psychiatric disorders such as depression [294–297]. In addition to communicating with the CNS to influence host behavior as mentioned above, our microbiome functions include producing vitamins, metabolizing fatty acids, and educating the immune system [298–300].

Our microbiome appears to start before birth [246, 301–306]. The human placenta has been said to have a microbiome very similar to that of the human oral microbiome [301, 307]. However, a study in 2019 disputes those findings [308]. It has been reported that *Enterococcus*, *Streptococcus*, *Staphylococcus*, and *Propionibacterium* can be isolated from umbilical cord blood [309]. Meconium of healthy neonates can contain *Enterococcus* and *Streptococcus* [310]. Amniotic fluid can contain mycoplasma bacteria in midtrimester amniocentesis without always being associated with adverse outcomes [311].

However, a 2017 careful review of the evidence for in utero colonization of the fetal environment concludes, "current scientific evidence does not support the existence of microbiomes within the healthy fetal milieu" [312]. Nevertheless, a 2019 study using high-sensitivity detection methods states that, "bacterial DNA and SCFAs [short-chain fatty acids] are present in utero and have the potential to influence the developing fetal immune system." They found bacterial evidence in meconium and amniotic fluid [313].

Delivery method shapes the acquisition and structure of the initial microbiota across multiple body habitats in newborns [314]. For example, vaginally delivered infants acquired bacterial communities resembling their own mother's vaginal microbiota, whereas C-section infants sheltered bacterial communities similar to those found on the skin surface [314]. Irrespective of delivery method, unlike their mother's highly differentiated bacterial communities, neonates harbor undifferentiated communities across multiple body areas [315].

Within the first 6 weeks after birth, infant microbiota undergoes extensive reorganization, primarily driven by body site and not by delivery method [316]. Nevertheless, in the first year after birth, the gut microbiota still differs depending upon birth mode, and microbiota composition at 1 week of life is associated with the number of respiratory infections over the first year [314].

Over time, the infant microbiome composition assumes a dynamic profile depending upon many factors [302, 317]. In addition to birth delivery mode, these factors include maternal lifestyle including diet, breastfeeding, and age of weaning [318].

Early-life microbial exposure has persistent effects on natural killer T cell function [319]. In addition, early-life exposure to normal gut microbiota appears to modulate brain development and behavior at least in regard to motor control and anxiety [320]. The microbiome-gut-brain axis during early life appears to regulate the hippocampal serotonergic system in a sex-dependent fashion [321]. Experiments in germ-free (GF) animals showed a significant elevation in the hippocampal concentration of 5-HT and 5-hydroxyindoleacetic acid, its main metabolite, compared to control animals. Concentration of plasma tryptophan, the serotonin precursor, was increased in male GF animals but not in female GFs. This abnormal neurotransmission persisted even after the normal gut flora was restored.

The adult microbiome composition is shaped by diet, exercise, disease, antibiotics, host genetics, and epigenetics [322–325]. In addition, social behavior including kissing,

[10]For reviews of Glucagon-like peptide 1 (GLP-1) in stress regulation we recommend [270, 271].

[11]For reviews of the role of neuropeptide Y (NPY) in mood and immune system interactions we recommend the following references [273, 274].

[12]For reviews of the role of cholecystokinin (CCK) in gut brain and anxiety we recommend [276].

[13]Helpful reviews can be seen in [278].

[14]Here are some reviews for oxytocin relative to depression [280–282].

[15]Ghrelin along with growth hormone may be important in formatting the amygdala to exert a fear-exacerbating effect of repeated stress [283]. This action is independent of the classical HPA activation pathways.

grooming, and sexual intercourse may transfer microbes [326]. In addition, there seems to be ethnic affiliation and oral microbiome composition [327].

The first 1000 cultured species of the human gastrointestinal microbiota were presented in a powerful review in 2014 [328]. It is a systematic overview and detailed reference of 1057 intestinal species of eukarya [329], archaea [330–332], and bacteria [333–335]. It is a compendium of prevalence, abundance, stability, physiology, genetics, and their association with human health.[16]

The most prevalent of these eukarya are yeasts [336–338]. There are a few species of parasites that may be a normal part of GI tracts of some humans [339]. In 2022, a catalogue was published of the human associated archaea in the microbiome of the gut [340, 341]. In 1167 genomes, they identified protein clusters with significant associations with sociodemographic characteristics including age groups and lifestyle. Viruses and the microbiome are discussed in reference [342]. Most of the work on health and disease associations is with bacteria [225].

In healthy adults, about 90% of the bacterial microbiome is represented by bacterial phyla *Firmicutes* (60–80%: including *Lactobacillus*, Clostridium, and Enterococcus genera) and *Bacteroidetes* (15–25%: e.g., *Bacteroides* genus) [243, 343, 344]. Another 8% are *Proteobacteria* and *Actinobacteria.* Density and diversity increase from the stomach to the colon [345]. There are about 3.3 million genes in the human microbiome; over 99% are bacterial and each individual harbors at least 150 species out of an estimated 4000–4500 prevalent bacterial species [346]. It is interesting to compare this to our human 20,000–25,000 genes.

A healthy GI tract hosts a diverse and stable microbiome [347]. Its influence on overall human health comes by way of modulating the innate and adaptive immune response [266, 348], directly defending against pathogenic bacteria [349], decreasing metabolic syndrome tendencies [350], modulating bile acid processing [351], producing vitamins [352], polyamines, polyphenols, indoles and choline metabolites [353], and converting nondigestable complex carbohydrates into short-chain fatty acids [285, 354].

For example, *short-chain fatty acids (SCFAs)*[17] bind receptors along the GI tract to regulate energy homeostasis by stimulating leptin production in adipocytes, and secretion of gut peptides from colonic enteroendocrine cells [347, 359]. However, SCFAs can have both obesogenic and anti-obesogenic properties depending upon the specific SCFAs which in turn depend on the microbes available in the gut and the type of fiber ingested [347]. Indeed, the nutrients we ingest, and microbial by-products can change the phenotype and function of the *enteric nervous system (ENS)* both directly and through its stimulation of *enteroendocrine cells (EECs)* [360].

By its effects on short-chain fatty acids, the gut microbiome can influence the amount of serotonin that is synthesized and released by the *enterochromaffin cells (ECs)* which are a specialized type of enteroendocrine cell [361]. ECs have chemosensory receptors and modulate primary afferent nerve fiber signals from the gut to the brain [265]. They can transduce environmental, metabolic, and homeostatic data from the GI tract directly to the nervous system [361, 362].

More than 90% of the human body's production of serotonin is produced in gastrointestinal ECs [361, 363, 364]. Serotonin in the brain represents a separate independently regulated pool using a different gene for tryptophan hydroxylase which catalyzes the rate limiting step in serotonin synthesis [365]; and the blood-brain barrier is relatively impermeable to serotonin [366]. CNS serotonin is synthesized in the raphe nuclei of the brain stem and the pineal gland and involved in the central control of food intake, sleep, and mood [367].[18]

Serotonin signals in the gut, via extrinsic vagal and spinal afferent fibers and paracrine functions, results in slowed gas-

[16] Reference [328] presents the following tables.

Table S1. List of bacterial species that can be members of the human gastrointestinal microbiota, with a reference that provides the link between the species and gastrointestinal tract as ecological niche.

Table S2. List of archaeal species that can be members of the human gastrointestinal microbiota, with a reference that provides the link between the species and gastrointestinal tract as ecological niche.

Table S3. List of eukaryal species that can be members of the human gastrointestinal microbiota, with a reference that provides the link between the species and gastrointestinal tract as ecological niche.

[17] *Short-chain fatty acids* are 1–6 carbon volatile fatty acids straight or branched-chained that is influenced by the type of food intake and diet-mediated changes in the GI tract microbiota. A 2016 review of short-chain fatty acids in the gut can be found in [355]. Bacterial cross-feeding or nutrient sharing is common in the microbiome [356]. Short-term diets composed of entirely plant or animal products can rapidly and reproducibly alter the human gut microbiome [357]. In that study, the animal-based diet increased the quantity of bile-tolerant microorganisms (*Alistipes*, *Bilophila*, and *Bacteroides*) and decreased the number of Firmicutes that metabolize dietary plant polysaccharides (*Roseburia*, *Eubacterium rectale*, and *Ruminococcus bromii*). Increased number and activity of *Bilophila wadsworthia* suggests a link between dietary animal fat, bile acids, and the increase of microorganisms capable of triggering inflammatory bowel disease. The researchers also noted that foodborne microbes (including bacteria, fungi, and viruses) from animal and plant diets transiently colonized the guts.

Diets with reduced carbohydrate and increased protein contents may decrease fecal cancer protective metabolites and increase concentrations of hazardous metabolites that may increase the risk of colorectal disease [358]. These changes associate with decreased proportion of butyrate in fecal SCFA concentrations, and a reduction in the *Roseburia/Eubacterium rectale* bacteria, and significant reduction in fiber-derived, antioxidant phenolic acids.

[18] Other sources of serotonin include the thymus and spleen. Pancreatic β cells produce and use serotonin [368–370]. Adipocytes have a functional system for serotonin synthesis, reuptake, and receptor activation [371]. Osteoclastogenesis is also influenced by locally produced serotonin [372], CNS produced serotonin via increasing SNS tone [373], and gut derived serotonin [372, 374].

tric emptying, pancreatic secretion, vasodilation, satiation, discomfort, nausea, and vomiting [225, 368]. Serotonin modulates immunity/inflammation via 5-HT7 or 5-HT4 receptors, development and maintenance of neurons and Cajal cells; and via platelet serotonin that came from the GI tract it influences hematopoiesis [368] and hemostasis [284].

The signaling molecules of the ENS consist of molecules such as serotonin and a variety of peptides that are found in both the gut and CNS [259, 375–377]. Stimulation of these peptides is elicited by contact of bacterial products with different types of EECs [378]. Upon secretion, the peptides diffuse through the lamina propria where immune cells reside, and reach the bloodstream, where they can stimulate the vagal nerve to signal the brain [379]. The blood-brain barrier then selectively facilitates entry of some of the peptides directly into the brain [225, 380–383].

Peptides that are released from EECs and those that are produced in the CNS can travel to their targets where they are metabolized and do not accumulate in tissues [225, 384, 385]. In humans, there are more than 100 of these peptides identified, many of which play a role in the GI tract where they may have paracrine or endocrine functions [259, 376, 377, 386]. Various subtypes of EECs produce different peptides in the GI tract and several of them can be stimulated by bacterial products that come into contact with these EECs [258, 387].

It might be reasonable to contemplate that some of these gut-derived peptides have an indirect role in remote processes related to neurophysiology and neurobehavioral disorders [257, 388]. Indeed, there is abundant literature that documents bidirectional influences of the GI tract and mental health [225, 388–390]. For example, mental states such as fear, anger, pain, and adverse life experiences can affect physiologic and gastric functions, resulting in GI symptoms such as functional dyspepsia, gastroesophageal reflux disease, inflammatory bowel disease, and peptic ulcer disease [391, 392].

Stressed mental states such as anxiety and depression are frequently associated with changes in gut microbiota, colonic morphology, and physiology [393–395].

As part of the loop, stress-associated disorders can trigger enhanced permeability of the intestinal barrier and release of inimical microbiota products or *bacterial translocation* [396–398] from the GI tract that might prompt a proinflammatory response [399, 400]. This series of events may be responsible for the chronic low-grade inflammation of psychiatric disorders such as depression [399]. Chronic depression is accompanied by increased IgM and IgA responses directed against gram-negative gut commensals [401]. It has been suggested that these bacteria translocate secondary to systemic inflammation in depression and can intensify and perpetuate the primary inflammatory response, or it may be a primary trigger associated with the onset of depression in some susceptible individuals [402].

Alterations in fecal microbiota composition have been seen in patients with MDD [403]. In patients with active MDD but not in MDD patients who were not actively exhibiting MDD symptoms, compared to healthy controls there was increased fecal bacterial *α-diversity*.[19] In active and non-active MDD patients versus healthy controls, there was significantly elevated numbers of *Bacteroidetes* and *Proteobacteria*, and a significant reduction of *Actinobacteria* and *Firmicutes*. Although there were considerable interindividual differences, the MDD patients showed increased levels of *Enterobacteriaceae* and *Alistipes* but reduced levels of *Faecalibacterium*. *Faecalibacterium* levels were negatively correlated with the severity of MDD symptoms.

Fecal transplant of gut microbiota from MDD patients transferred to microbiota-deficient rats induced physiological and behavioral changes in the rats [406]. These changes included altered tryptophan metabolism, anhedonia, and anxiety-like symptoms.

Chronic variable stress-induced depression in rats has been associated with significant changes in relative abundance of bacterial genera [407]. In that experiment, there was a significant relative decrease in abundance of the bacterial genera *Marvinbryantia*, *Corynebacterium*, *Psychrobacter*, *Christensenella*, *Lactobacillus*, *Peptostreptococcaceae incertae sedis*, *Anaerovorax*, *Clostridiales incertae sedis*, and *Coprococcus*. There was a significant increase in *Candidatus*, *Arthromitus*, and *Oscillibacter*. Significant metabolic changes included lesser amounts of amino acids, and fatty acids, and higher amounts of bile acids, hypoxanthine, and stercobilins. The most pronounced associations with altered microbiota were with tryptophan and bile acid metabolites.

Exposures to social disruption stress in mice can change the community structure of gut microbiota and increase circulating inflammatory cytokines [400]. This stressor exposure increased the relative amounts of *Clostridia* while decreasing the relative amounts of *Bacteroides*. The three genera that were most significantly associated with the cytokine increases were *Coprococcus*, *Pseudobutyrivibrio*, and *Dorea*. When the mice were pretreated with antibiotics, the social disruption stress did not elicit cytokine production. This would imply that these members of the microbiome were necessary for their production.

Increases in *Clostridium* (*difficile*) are particularly interesting as they are believed to be implicated in the severity of infections and are frequently altered by microbiome metabolites including tryptophan, phenylalanine, and tyrosine [408,

[19] *α-Diversity* is an ecological descriptor. It is the mean species diversity in sites or habitats at a local scale [404, 405].

409]. The gut microbiota can control 5-HT levels and neuroactive metabolites [410].

Serotonin (5-HT) levels are tightly controlled in the gut, and dysregulation of their control is implicated in a variety of GI clinical disorders [411]. The intestinal 5-HT transporter (5-HTT) is central to controlling the levels of 5-HT [412, 413]. When less 5-HTT is expressed, 5-HT levels increase and are associated with inflammatory disorders such as ulcerative colitis [15188158, 20303355].

Humans who have the short allele of the 5-HTTLPR are more susceptible to early-life stress, as discussed earlier [414, 415], which alters the composition of the gut microbiota [416]. Lower 5-HTT expression has also been shown to be associated with an altered microbiome composition. In one experiment, there was an increase in *Desulfovibrio*, *Mucispirillum*, and *Fusobacterium*, which have been associated with MDD [409]. Some short-chain fatty acids that are metabolized by microbiota are increased by spore-forming microbiota, and they promote increased 5-HT levels in ECs regardless of the 5-HTT form [417].

Some antidepressants and antibiotics can influence GI microbiota, anxiety, and depression [418, 419]. Lithium and some antidepressants appear to interact with eicosanoids, including prostaglandins, to be at once immunostimulating and antimicrobial [420, 421]. Ketamine has both antidepressant and anti-inflammatory properties that seem to be mediated by its modification of specific bacteria in the microbiome [422]. The SSRIs sertraline, fluoxetine, and paroxetine have selective antibiotic effects both alone and combined with some antibiotics [423].

All classes of antimicrobials (e.g., antibiotics, antimycobacterials, antivirals, antifungals, and antiretrovirals), have potential neurotoxic side effects that include headaches, anxiety and depression, confusion, delirium, psychosis, mania, and seizures [424]. For example, fluoroquinolones (e.g., ciprofloxacin) are associated with developing sometimes serious symptoms of anxiety and depression [425–427]. On the other hand, the antibiotic doxycycline is comparable to imipramine in effectively ameliorating lipopolysaccharide-induced depressive-like behavior in rats [428]. Minocycline combined with antidepressants (fluvoxamine, paroxetine, and sertraline) is effective in the treatment of unipolar psychotic depression.

It has been suggested that gut microbiota is functioning as an epigenetic analog [429]. Our microbiome is transgenerationally inherited. It is subject to environmental changes. It can influence developmental regulation and maturation of the immune system. And molecular and behavioral phenotypes can be reversed by external influences.

Gut-microbial products can affect chromatin plasticity within their host's brain which leads to changes in neuronal transcription and eventually alters host behavior [388]. Gut microbiota is an important mediator of gene-environment interactions. Effects of our microbiome on brain epigenetic processes are produced via diverse means, including immunomodulation and neuroactive metabolite secretion [430]. Some bacteria have been identified as being able to modify transcription of their host's genome. They appear to perform such an epigenetic function by secreting protein effectors that mimic host-endogenous transcriptional regulators [431–433]. The factors involved in such modifications have been referred to as *nucleomodulins* [432]. An introductory discussion of the epigenetic properties of these nucleomodulins can be found in reference [429].

Inflammatory Bowel Disease (IBD)

Inflammatory bowel disease (IBD) is a chronic relapsing disease for which there is no current cure [434]. IBD has heterogeneous manifestations, of which Crohn's disease (CD) and ulcerative colitis (UC) are the two principal subtypes of IBD [435, 436].

The global prevalence of IBD is increasing as newly industrialized countries become more westernized [437]. The highest reported prevalence values were in Europe. CD was 322 per 100 000 in Germany. UC was 505 per 100 000 in Norway. In North America, the highest was UC 286 per 100 000 in the USA. CD was 319 per 100 000 in Canada. In western countries, CD incidence may be decreasing or stabilizing.

IBD is characterized by a web of complex, dynamic interplay between susceptibility genes, the environment, the endocrine system, the CNS, the enteric nervous system, epigenetic factors, and the immune system [438, 439]. The microbiome plays an important role, directly and indirectly [440, 441]. And so does stress, anxiety, and depression [395].

The hallmark of IBD is disruption of the integrity of the gut mucosa [442]. There are many stress conditions that can impair the gut epithelium. These include major stressors such as critical illness, trauma, burns, pancreatitis, septic shock, heat stroke, and hemorrhagic shock. In addition, milder stressors of prolonged endurance exercise [443, 444] and chronic psychological stress can damage the gut epithelium [395, 445, 446].

Stress-induced damage can result in acute gastric mucosal hemorrhagic lesions [447, 448]. Psychological factors include long-term depression and perceived stress [449, 450]. Psychosocial distress and other psychosocial factors are also highly prevalent in functional GI disorders such as irritable bowel syndrome [451, 452] and functional dyspepsia [453].

As mentioned in the previous section, Microbiome and Depression, stressed mental states such as anxiety and depression are frequently associated with changes in gut microbiota, colonic morphology, and physiology [394, 395].

As part of the loop, stress-associated disorders can trigger enhanced permeability of the intestinal barrier, weakening of the tight junctions, and release of dangerous microbiota products or bacterial translocation [396, 397] from the GI tract that might prompt a proinflammatory response [399]. Chronic depression is accompanied by increased IgM and IgA responses directed against gram-negative gut commensals [402]. It has been suggested that these bacteria translocate secondary to systemic inflammation in depression and can intensify and perpetuate the primary inflammatory response, or it may be a primary trigger associated with the onset of depression in some susceptible individuals [401, 402].

A more detailed discussion of stress-induced changes in the gut can be found in these references [442, 454, 455].

Anxiety and depression are the most prevalent psychiatric disorders among IBD patients [456]. Depression in IBD is associated with reduced quality of life and more aggressive disease [457]. However, the rates are not consistently determined. Data is generally more supportive of associations between depressive state and subsequent deterioration in disease course in CD rather than UC. It has been suggested that data on baseline IBD activity may be a variable as well as self-reporting [458]. One study suggested that IBD patients with depression were most likely to be female, lack social support, have active disease, be treated with corticosteroids but not TNF-alpha inhibitors, and exhibit reduced positive emotional recognition bias [459]. *Emotional recognition processing bias* is the greater propensity to identify sad than happy facial expressions [460].

There seems to be a significantly higher prevalence of depressive, cyclothymic, and anxiety temperaments in CD patients and significant differences between moods in CD and UC [461]. UC patients seem to be less critical and complaining and less aggressive and dysphoric than controls and CD patients.

There appears to be a definite link between susceptibility of affective temperament to depressive and anxiety disorders [462].

Inherited personality traits that may predispose to becoming extreme manifestations of affective disorders such as MDD is termed *affective temperament* [461–464]. The *Temperament Evaluation of Memphis, Pisa, Paris, and San Diego Autoquestionnaire (TEMPS-A)* was used to assess five affective temperaments in IBD patients compared to controls [465]. The five temperaments are hyperthymic, depressive, irritable, cyclothymic, and anxious.

Depressive temperament is characterized by low energy, non-assertiveness, negative cognition or being shy, highly pessimistic, and gloomy [464, 466].

Cyclothymic temperament manifests tendencies to rapidly shift between high-energy (hyperthymic) and low-energy (depressive) moods [462, 467].

Anxious temperament traits tend to respond to environmental threats by excessive worrying and inability to relax [465, 468].

Hyperthymic temperament seems to be independent of other temperaments [469]. It is characterized by high self-esteem, exuberance, higher sociability, and narcissism [470]. Hyperthymic temperament modified by age and education may have a protective effect on most mental disorders, with the exceptions of separation anxiety, bipolar, substance abuse, and impulse control disorders [471].

Irritable temperament is an unstable mix of dysthymic and hyperthymic characteristics [472–474].

One study found that IBD patients with active but not remitted disease had higher levels of anxiety and depression than the general population [457]. They also found that mental disorders were present in 27.7% when IBD symptoms were slight, 49.3% in those with moderate/severe disease activity, and 11.3% when in remission. The general population control had 10.4% ($P < 0.001$). Another study found that duration of disease and corticosteroid treatment or surgery for IBD were not associated with depression or anxiety [475]. Those who had more severe CD had more severe depression. The severity of UC did not correlate with severity of anxiety or depression in UC.

A large-scale Canadian national health survey, the *Canadian Community Health Survey (CCHS)* analyzed adjusted odds ratios for major depression for various health conditions [476]. The strongest associations were chronic fatigue syndrome (adjusted odds ratio [AOR] 7.2) and fibromyalgia (AOR 3.4). Least strongly associated were hypertension (AOR 1.2), diabetes, heart disease, and thyroid disease (AOR 1.4 in each case). The AOR for bowel disorders, Crohn's and colitis was 2.8. For cancer, the AOR was 2.3, and for COPD, it was 2.7.

Six months of antidepressant drug therapy in patients with Crohn's showed improvement in depression, anxiety, quality of life, and sexual functioning scores, as well as an improvement in Crohn's disease activity index [477]. The control group showed poorer scores on several parameters. The researchers suggested that reasons for the differences may relate to psychological changes that influenced biological processes, but they do not know.

Analysis of clinical and treatment data on 2007 adult participants of the *Swiss Inflammatory Bowel Disease Study* (56% with Crohn's disease [CD], 48% male) performed in Switzerland from 2006 through 2015 found a significant association between symptoms of depression or anxiety and clinical recurrence [478]. For all patients with

IBD, $P = 0.000001$; for subjects with CD, $P = 0.0007$; for subjects with ulcerative colitis, $P = 0.005$. Symptoms of anxiety and clinical recurrence over time in all subjects with IBD were significantly associated ($P = 0.0014$) and in subjects with CD ($P = 0.031$) but not with ulcerative colitis ($P = 0.066$). Additional data presented in 2023 underscored the relevance of lifestyle factors, including a protective effect of physical activity on the onset of IBD [479]. Further data from the Swiss Inflammatory Bowel Disease Study showed that depressive symptoms were a strong predictor of clinical deterioration and that genetic markers may play a part [480].

A 2015 study found that male and female IBD patients with an active disease demonstrated impaired sexual function relative to patients in remission and controls [481]. The study's authors believed that depression was the most important determinant for compromised sexual function in IBD.

A retrospective cohort study including patients with CD and UC without a prior psychiatric diagnosis found female gender, aggressive disease, and disease activity (verified by endoscopic/radiological activity) to be independently associated with the development of depression in IBD [456]. IBD phenotype, exposure to IBD medications, history of a surgical stoma or Seton stitch [482] placement, extra-intestinal manifestations, and laboratory indices were not associated with developing depression.

A prospective, longitudinal, observational study of 60 patients with clinically inactive IBD (Crohn disease, $n = 47$, 78%; ulcerative colitis, $n = 13$, 22%) were followed after a flare of disease [483]. A significant correlation was seen between baseline depression index scores at baseline and the total number of relapses after 12 months ($P < 0.01$) and 18 months ($P < 0.01$) of follow-up. Baseline depression scores correlated with time until the first recurrence of the disease ($P < 0.05$). In addition, a correlation was seen between more frequent relapses and anxiety ($P < 0.05$) and low health-related quality of life $P < 0.01$.

Even during remission, a significant number of IBD patients still present with anxiety and depression [484]. A 2018 Polish study observed significantly higher prevalence of depressive, cyclothymic, and anxiety temperaments in CD patients compared to the control group and to UC patients [461].

Suicide rates are higher in IBD patients [31294727]. In a large US database, suicidal ideation, and suicide/self-inflicted injury among hospitalized adults with IBD occurred in over 1% of the IBD population, and they were increased in CD versus UC [29272476]. A systematic review and meta-analysis published in 2018 assessed the expected number of deaths or standardized mortality ratio (SMR) for suicide in IBD [485]. They found the SMR for suicide in patients with IBD for all studies included was 1.20 (95% confidence interval (CI), 0.94–1.54). The overall pooled SMR for CD and UC were 1.36 (95% CI, 0.98–1.88) and 1.16 (95% CI, 0.8–1.69), respectively.

Baseline depression is associated with a higher risk for aggressive IBD at follow-up [486]. Data from the *Sinai-Helmsley Alliance for Research Excellence* cohort were examined. Adjusted for sex, remission, and disease activity, CD patients with baseline depression had increased risk for relapse (RR[20]: 2.3; 95% confidence interval (CI): 1.9–2.8), surgery, or hospitalization (RR: 1.3; 95% CI: 1.1–1.6) at follow-up. UC patients with baseline depression had increased risk for relapse (RR: 1.3; 95% CI: 0.9–1.7), surgery, or hospitalization (RR: 1.3; 95% CI: 1.1–1.5) at follow-up. The study's authors suggest that the *Patient Health Questionnaire (PHQ-8)* should be used to identify those at greater risk for aggressive disease.

Comprehensive geriatric assessments comprising a somatic, functional, mental, and social assessment of frailty have shown that frailty is associated with adverse health outcomes in IBD patients [487].

Depression may stimulate IBD patients to seek more medical testing, which has been shown to be a risk for CD patients to have greater cumulative radiation exposure [488].

The *Manitoba Inflammatory Bowel Disease Cohort* study of the prevalence of lifetime and 12-month anxiety and mood disorders in direct comparisons with matched controls found the following lifetime prevalence (IBD vs. controls): social anxiety disorder was lower in IBD (6% vs. 11%, OR[21] = 0.52; 95% CI: 0.32–0.85), panic disorder was not significantly different (8.0% vs. 4.7%, OR = 1.59; 95% CI: 0.96–2.63), agoraphobia without panic was not significantly different (1.1% vs. 0.6%, OR = 1.44; 95% CI: 0.37–5.55), but major depression was higher (27.2% vs. 12.3%, OR = 2.20; 95% CI: 1.64–2.95). There was a lower quality of life and earlier onset

[20] *Relative risk (RR)* is perhaps the most common method of expressing the estimated risk of experiencing a result. RR compares the probability of a specific outcome in the treatment group with that of a control group. When an RR is greater than 1, there seems to be an increased risk of an event. When the RR is less than 1, there appears to be a decreased risk of experiencing an event. If the RR is 1, there is no apparent risk. If the RR = 5, it is 5 times more likely to occur than in the control group. If the RR = 0.5, it is half as likely to happen as in the control group. For more information, see Chap. 4.

[21] *Odds ratio (OR)* is a way to represent the odds that an outcome will result when a given exposure to a variable of interest occurs compared to when the exposure does not occur. OR quantifies the strength of the association between two events. An OR greater than 1 indicates a positive association or that exposure to that variable increases the odds of that outcome. An OR less than one indicates a negative relationship between two events. An OR of 1 suggests no relationship between two events. An OR is frequently accompanied by a 95% confidence interval (CI). CI is a measure of precision of the OR. The smaller the CI the higher precision as long as it does not overlap OR = 1. For more information, see the Chap. 4 on evidence basics in this text.

of IBD symptoms, and there was a trend toward earlier IBD diagnosis in those who had anxiety or a mood disorder [489].

In a Korean study, for those who had CD, socioeconomic deprivation was associated with anxiety ($P = 0.03$) [484]. Disease duration ($P = 0.04$) and socioeconomic deprivation ($P = 0.013$) were associated with depression. For those with UC, there was no significant independent predictor of anxiety and/or depression, but low income tended to be associated with depression ($P = 0.096$).

Summary

Depression arises through a complex and dynamic interplay of immune, endocrine, and neural cells and communication molecules. Not all of these are mammalian.

Chronic stress and depression are most often associated with increased systemic inflammation, including overall leukocytosis and increased circulating neutrophils, but with a depressed immune system response.

A variety of illnesses are associated with psychological and neuroendocrine attributes of depression. In both healthy and pathological physiological conditions, the neuroimmune system and neuroplasticity mechanisms engage in a strong dialogue.

The influence of cytokines on depression is not at all settled. Many studies have reported increased cytokines in depression; others have found that at least some brain cytokines demonstrate antidepressant activity and mediate influences of the principal SSRI antidepressant drugs. Many neuroimmune factors also offer protection to the nervous system. Even those cytokines that are commonly considered proinflammatory can be neuroprotective in the appropriate context.

Although microglia and astrocytes are the primary immune system cells in the central nervous system, their roles in depression are not very well understood; however, there appear to be context-dependent neuroprotective properties. Th1, Th2, and other subtypes of T cells appear to be involved in depression. However, the relative contributions of cytokines produced by these subtypes of T cells are open for discussion.

The gastrointestinal tract and the brain are a finely tuned partnership that includes the endocrine, immune, autonomic, and enteric nervous systems. Regulation of this interaction appears to be provided principally by the microbiome and molecules produced by the microbiome organisms. The gut microbiota is functioning as an epigenetic analog. Our microbiome is transgenerationally inherited and is subject to environmental changes. It can influence developmental regulation and maturation of the immune system. Molecular and behavioral phenotypes can be reversed by external influences.

Gut-microbial products can affect chromatin plasticity within their host's brain, which leads to changes in neuronal transcription and eventually alters host behavior. Stressed mental states such as anxiety and depression are frequently associated with changes in gut microbiota, colonic morphology, and physiology.

In the next section, we will discuss some of the psychosocial triggers of depression.

References

1. Dantzer R. Neuroimmune interactions: from the brain to the immune system and vice versa. Physiol Rev. 2018;98(1):477–504. PMCID: PMC5866360. http://www.ncbi.nlm.nih.gov/pubmed/29351513.
2. Najjar S, Pearlman DM, Alper K, Najjar A, Devinsky O. Neuroinflammation and psychiatric illness. J Neuroinflammation. 2013;10:43. PMCID: PMC3626880. http://www.ncbi.nlm.nih.gov/pubmed/23547920.
3. Littrell JL. Taking the perspective that a depressive state reflects inflammation: implications for the use of antidepressants. Front Psychol. 2012;3:297. PMCID: PMC3421432. http://www.ncbi.nlm.nih.gov/pubmed/22912626.
4. Olff M. Stress, depression and immunity: the role of defense and coping styles. Psychiatry Res. 1999;85(1):7–15. PMID: 10195312. http://www.ncbi.nlm.nih.gov/pubmed/10195312.
5. Plotsky PM, Owens MJ, Nemeroff CB. Psychoneuroendocrinology of depression. hypothalamic-pituitary-adrenal axis. Psychiatr Clin North Am. 1998;21(2):293–307. PMID: 9670227. http://www.ncbi.nlm.nih.gov/pubmed/9670227.
6. Black PH. Central nervous system-immune system interactions: psychoneuroendocrinology of stress and its immune consequences. Antimicrob Agents Chemother. 1994;38(1):1–6. PMCID: PMC284388. http://www.ncbi.nlm.nih.gov/pubmed/8141561.
7. Reiche EMV, Morimoto HK, Nunes SMV. Stress and depression-induced immune dysfunction: implications for the development and progression of cancer. Int Rev Psychiatry. 2005;17(6):515–27. PMID: 16401550. http://www.ncbi.nlm.nih.gov/pubmed/16401550.
8. Moynihan JA. Mechanisms of stress-induced modulation of immunity. Brain Behav Immun. 2003;17(Suppl 1):S11–6. PMID: 12615181. http://www.ncbi.nlm.nih.gov/pubmed/12615181.
9. Reiche EMV, Nunes SOV, Morimoto HK. Stress, depression, the immune system, and cancer. Lancet Oncol. 2004;5(10):617–25. PMID: 15465465. http://www.ncbi.nlm.nih.gov/pubmed/15465465.
10. Kronfol Z, House JD. Lymphocyte mitogenesis, immunoglobulin and complement levels in depressed patients and normal controls. Acta Psychiatr Scand. 1989;80(2):142–7. https://doi.org/10.1111/j.1600-0447.1989.tb01316.x. PMID: 2801162.
11. Zorrilla EP, Luborsky L, McKay JR, Rosenthal R, Houldin A, Tax A, McCorkle R, Seligman DA, Schmidt K. The relationship of depression and stressors to immunological assays: a meta-analytic review. Brain Behav Immun. 2001;15(3):199–226. PMID: 11566046. http://www.ncbi.nlm.nih.gov/pubmed/11566046.
12. Kiecolt-Glaser JK, Glaser R. Depression and immune function: central pathways to morbidity and mortality. J Psychosom Res. 2002;53(4):873–6. PMID: 12377296. http://www.ncbi.nlm.nih.gov/pubmed/12377296.
13. Kiecolt-Glaser JK, McGuire L, Robles TF, Glaser R. Emotions, morbidity, and mortality: new perspectives from psychoneuroimmunology. Annu Rev Psychol. 2002;53:83–107. PMID: 11752480. http://www.ncbi.nlm.nih.gov/pubmed/11752480.

14. Kiecolt-Glaser JK, McGuire L, Robles TF, Glaser R. Psychoneuroimmunology: psychological influences on immune function and health. J Consult Clin Psychol. 2002;70(3):537–47. PMID: 12090368. http://www.ncbi.nlm.nih.gov/pubmed/12090368.
15. Kiecolt-Glaser JK, Robles TF, Heffner KL, Loving TJ, Glaser R. Psycho-oncology and cancer: psychoneuroimmunology and cancer. Ann Oncol. 2002;13(Suppl 4):165–9. PMID: 12401684. http://www.ncbi.nlm.nih.gov/pubmed/12401684.
16. Dantzer R. Cytokine-induced sickness behavior: where do we stand? Brain Behav Immun. 2001;15(1):7–24. PMID: 11259077. http://www.ncbi.nlm.nih.gov/pubmed/11259077.
17. Miller AH, Maletic V, Raison CL. Inflammation and its discontents: the role of cytokines in the pathophysiology of major depression. Biol Psychiatry. 2009;65(9):732–41. PMCID: PMC2680424. http://www.ncbi.nlm.nih.gov/pubmed/19150053.
18. Dantzer R, O'Connor JC, Freund GG, Johnson RW, Kelley KW. From inflammation to sickness and depression: when the immune system subjugates the brain. Nat Rev Neurosci. 2008;9(1):46–56. PMCID: PMC2919277. http://www.ncbi.nlm.nih.gov/pubmed/18073775.
19. McAfoose J, Baune BT. Evidence for a cytokine model of cognitive function. Neurosci Biobehav Rev. 2009;33(3):355–66. PMID: 18996146. http://www.ncbi.nlm.nih.gov/pubmed/18996146.
20. Strouse TB. The relationship between cytokines and pain/depression: a review and current status. Curr Pain Headache Rep. 2007;11(2):98–103. PMID: 17367587. http://www.ncbi.nlm.nih.gov/pubmed/17367587.
21. Craddock D, Thomas A. Cytokines and late-life depression. Essent Psychopharmacol. 2006;7(1):42–52. PMID: 16989292. http://www.ncbi.nlm.nih.gov/pubmed/16989292.
22. Leventhal EA, Hansell S, Diefenbach M, Leventhal H, Glass DC. Negative affect and self-report of physical symptoms: two longitudinal studies of older adults. Health Psychol. 1996;15(3):193–9. PMID: 8698033. http://www.ncbi.nlm.nih.gov/pubmed/8698033.
23. Broz P, Monack DM. Newly described pattern recognition receptors team up against intracellular pathogens. Nat Rev Immunol. 2013;13(8):551–65. PMID: 23846113. http://www.ncbi.nlm.nih.gov/pubmed/23846113.
24. Rolls A, Shechter R, London A, Ziv Y, Ronen A, Levy R, Schwartz M. Toll-like receptors modulate adult hippocampal neurogenesis. Nat Cell Biol. 2007;9(9):1081–8. PMID: 17704767. http://www.ncbi.nlm.nih.gov/pubmed/17704767.
25. Takeda K, Akira S. Toll-like receptors. Curr Protoc Immunol. 2015;109:14.12.1–14.12.10. PMID: 25845562. http://www.ncbi.nlm.nih.gov/pubmed/25845562.
26. De Nardo D. Toll-like receptors: activation, signalling and transcriptional modulation. Cytokine. 2015;74(2):181–9. PMID: 25846205. http://www.ncbi.nlm.nih.gov/pubmed/25846205.
27. Paschon V, Takada SH, Ikebara JM, Sousa E, Raeisossadati R, Ulrich H, Kihara AH. Interplay between exosomes, microRNAs and Toll-like receptors in brain disorders. Mol Neurobiol. 2016;53(3):2016–28. PMID: 25862375. http://www.ncbi.nlm.nih.gov/pubmed/25862375.
28. García Bueno B, Caso JR, Madrigal JLM, Leza JC. Innate immune receptor Toll-like receptor 4 signalling in neuropsychiatric diseases. Neurosci Biobehav Rev. 2016;64:134–47. PMID: 26905767. http://www.ncbi.nlm.nih.gov/pubmed/26905767.
29. Hung YY. Antidepressants improve negative regulation of Toll-like receptor signaling in monocytes from patients with major depression. Neuroimmunomodulation. 2018;25(1):42–8. PMID: 29898456. http://www.ncbi.nlm.nih.gov/pubmed/29898456.
30. Beck M, Heard W, Mbengue M, Robatzek S. The INs and OUTs of pattern recognition receptors at the cell surface. Curr Opin Plant Biol. 2012;15(4):367–74. PMID: 22664220. http://www.ncbi.nlm.nih.gov/pubmed/22664220.
31. Krishnaswamy JK, Chu T, Eisenbarth SC. Beyond pattern recognition: NOD-like receptors in dendritic cells. Trends Immunol. 2013;34(5):224–33. PMCID: PMC3646908. http://www.ncbi.nlm.nih.gov/pubmed/23352728.
32. McCusker RH, Kelley KW. Immune-neural connections: how the immune system's response to infectious agents influences behavior. J Exp Biol. 2013;216(Pt 1):84–98. PMCID: PMC3515033. http://www.ncbi.nlm.nih.gov/pubmed/23225871.
33. Konsman JP, Veeneman J, Combe C, Poole S, Luheshi GN, Dantzer R. Central nervous action of interleukin-1 mediates activation of limbic structures and behavioural depression in response to peripheral administration of bacterial lipopolysaccharide. Eur J Neurosci. 2008;28(12):2499–510. PMID: 19087175. http://www.ncbi.nlm.nih.gov/pubmed/19087175.
34. Quan N, Banks WA. Brain-immune communication pathways. Brain Behav Immun. 2007;21(6):727–35. PMID: 17604598. http://www.ncbi.nlm.nih.gov/pubmed/17604598.
35. Dreyer JK, Herrik KF, Berg RW, Hounsgaard JD. Influence of phasic and tonic dopamine release on receptor activation. J Neurosci. 2010;30(42):14273–83. PMCID: PMC6634758. http://www.ncbi.nlm.nih.gov/pubmed/20962248.
36. Castañeda-Hernández GC, Bach-y-Rita P. Volume transmission and pain perception. ScientificWorldJournal. 2003;3:677–83. PMCID: PMC5974734. http://www.ncbi.nlm.nih.gov/pubmed/12920309.
37. Eyre H, Baune BT. Neuroplastic changes in depression: a role for the immune system. Psychoneuroendocrinology. 2012;37(9):1397–416. PMID: 22525700. http://www.ncbi.nlm.nih.gov/pubmed/22525700.
38. Yirmiya R, Goshen I. Immune modulation of learning, memory, neural plasticity and neurogenesis. Brain Behav Immun. 2011;25(2):181–213. PMID: 20970492. http://www.ncbi.nlm.nih.gov/pubmed/20970492.
39. Daugirdas JT. Rapid methods of estimating Kt/V: three formulas compared. ASAIO Trans. 1990;36(3):M362–4. PMID: 2252700. http://www.ncbi.nlm.nih.gov/pubmed/2252700.
40. Robson MJ, Quinlan MA, Blakely RD. Immune system activation and depression: roles of serotonin in the central nervous system and periphery. ACS Chem Neurosci. 2017;8(5):932–42. PMID: 28345868. http://www.ncbi.nlm.nih.gov/pubmed/28345868.
41. Leonard B, Maes M. Mechanistic explanations how cell-mediated immune activation, inflammation and oxidative and nitrosative stress pathways and their sequels and concomitants play a role in the pathophysiology of unipolar depression. Neurosci Biobehav Rev. 2012;36(2):764–85. PMID: 22197082. http://www.ncbi.nlm.nih.gov/pubmed/22197082.
42. Moylan S, Maes M, Wray NR, Berk M. The neuroprogressive nature of major depressive disorder: pathways to disease evolution and resistance, and therapeutic implications. Mol Psychiatry. 2013;18(5):595–606. PMID: 22525486. http://www.ncbi.nlm.nih.gov/pubmed/22525486.
43. Miller AH. Depression and immunity: a role for T cells? Brain Behav Immun. 2010;24(1):1–8. PMCID: PMC2787959. http://www.ncbi.nlm.nih.gov/pubmed/19818725.
44. Dantzer R, O'Connor JC, Lawson MA, Kelley KW. Inflammation-associated depression: from serotonin to kynurenine. Psychoneuroendocrinology. 2011;36(3):426–36. PMCID: PMC3053088. http://www.ncbi.nlm.nih.gov/pubmed/21041030.
45. Morón JA, Zakharova I, Ferrer JV, Merrill GA, Hope B, Lafer EM, Lin ZC, Wang JB, Javitch JA, Galli A, Shippenberg TS. Mitogen-activated protein kinase regulates dopamine transporter surface expression and dopamine transport capacity. J Neurosci. 2003;23(24):8480–8. PMCID: PMC6740378. http://www.ncbi.nlm.nih.gov/pubmed/13679416.
46. Zhu CB, Blakely RD, Hewlett WA. The proinflammatory cytokines interleukin-1beta and tumor necrosis factor-alpha activate serotonin transporters. Neuropsychopharmacology.

2006;31(10):2121–31. PMID: 16452991. http://www.ncbi.nlm.nih.gov/pubmed/16452991.
47. Nakajima A, Yamada K, Nagai T, Uchiyama T, Miyamoto Y, Mamiya T, He J, Nitta A, Mizuno M, Tran MH, Seto A, Yoshimura M, Kitaichi K, Hasegawa T, Saito K, Yamada Y, Seishima M, Sekikawa K, Kim HC, Nabeshima T. Role of tumor necrosis factor-alpha in methamphetamine-induced drug dependence and neurotoxicity. J Neurosci. 2004;24(9):2212–25. PMCID: PMC6730419. http://www.ncbi.nlm.nih.gov/pubmed/14999072.
48. Popoli M, Yan Z, McEwen BS, Sanacora G. The stressed synapse: the impact of stress and glucocorticoids on glutamate transmission. Nat Rev Neurosci. 2011;13(1):22–37. PMCID: PMC3645314. http://www.ncbi.nlm.nih.gov/pubmed/22127301.
49. Hashimoto K. Emerging role of glutamate in the pathophysiology of major depressive disorder. Brain Res Rev. 2009;61(2):105–23. PMID: 19481572. http://www.ncbi.nlm.nih.gov/pubmed/19481572.
50. McNally L, Bhagwagar Z, Hannestad J. Inflammation, glutamate, and glia in depression: a literature review. CNS Spectr. 2008;13(6):501–10. PMID: 18567974. http://www.ncbi.nlm.nih.gov/pubmed/18567974.
51. Schwartz M, Shechter R. Protective autoimmunity functions by intracranial immunosurveillance to support the mind: the missing link between health and disease. Mol Psychiatry. 2010;15(4):342–54. PMID: 20332793. http://www.ncbi.nlm.nih.gov/pubmed/20332793.
52. Schwartz M, Shechter R. Systemic inflammatory cells fight off neurodegenerative disease. Nat Rev Neurol. 2010;6(7):405–10. PMID: 20531383. http://www.ncbi.nlm.nih.gov/pubmed/20531383.
53. Martino G, Pluchino S, Bonfanti L, Schwartz M. Brain regeneration in physiology and pathology: the immune signature driving therapeutic plasticity of neural stem cells. Physiol Rev. 2011;91(4):1281–304. PMCID: PMC3552310. http://www.ncbi.nlm.nih.gov/pubmed/22013212.
54. Ron-Harel N, Cardon M, Schwartz M. Brain homeostasis is maintained by "danger" signals stimulating a supportive immune response within the brain's borders. Brain Behav Immun. 2011;25(5):1036–43. PMID: 21182929. http://www.ncbi.nlm.nih.gov/pubmed/21182929.
55. Park SE, Lawson M, Dantzer R, Kelley KW, McCusker RH. Insulin-like growth factor-I peptides act centrally to decrease depression-like behavior of mice treated intraperitoneally with lipopolysaccharide. J Neuroinflammation. 2011;8:179. PMCID: PMC3264674. http://www.ncbi.nlm.nih.gov/pubmed/22189158.
56. Park SE, Dantzer R, Kelley KW, McCusker RH. Central administration of insulin-like growth factor-I decreases depressive-like behavior and brain cytokine expression in mice. J Neuroinflammation. 2011;8:12. PMCID: PMC3045937. http://www.ncbi.nlm.nih.gov/pubmed/21306618.
57. Lyons A, Downer EJ, Crotty S, Nolan YM, Mills KHG, Lynch MA. CD200 ligand receptor interaction modulates microglial activation in vivo and in vitro: a role for IL-4. J Neurosci. 2007;27(31):8309–13. PMCID: PMC6673084. http://www.ncbi.nlm.nih.gov/pubmed/17670977.
58. Ojo B, Rezaie P, Gabbott PL, Davies H, Colyer F, Cowley TR, Lynch M, Stewart MG. Age-related changes in the hippocampus (loss of synaptophysin and glial-synaptic interaction) are modified by systemic treatment with an NCAM-derived peptide, FGL. Brain Behav Immun. 2012;26(5):778–88. PMID: 21986303. http://www.ncbi.nlm.nih.gov/pubmed/21986303.
59. Rogers JT, Morganti JM, Bachstetter AD, Hudson CE, Peters MM, Grimmig BA, Weeber EJ, Bickford PC, Gemma C. CX3CR1 deficiency leads to impairment of hippocampal cognitive function and synaptic plasticity. J Neurosci. 2011;31(45):16241–50. PMCID: PMC3236509. http://www.ncbi.nlm.nih.gov/pubmed/22072675.
60. Giunti D, Parodi B, Usai C, Vergani L, Casazza S, Bruzzone S, Mancardi G, Uccelli A. Mesenchymal stem cells shape microglia effector functions through the release of CX3CL1. Stem Cells. 2012;30(9):2044–53. PMID: 22821677. http://www.ncbi.nlm.nih.gov/pubmed/22821677.
61. Corona AW, Norden DM, Skendelas JP, Huang Y, O'Connor JC, Lawson M, Dantzer R, Kelley KW, Godbout JP. Indoleamine 2,3-dioxygenase inhibition attenuates lipopolysaccharide induced persistent microglial activation and depressive-like complications in fractalkine receptor (CX(3)CR1)-deficient mice. Brain Behav Immun. 2013;31:134–42. PMCID: PMC3554840. http://www.ncbi.nlm.nih.gov/pubmed/22926082.
62. Dowlati Y, Herrmann N, Swardfager W, Liu H, Sham L, Reim EK, Lanctôt KL. A meta-analysis of cytokines in major depression. Biol Psychiatry. 2010;67(5):446–57. PMID: 20015486. http://www.ncbi.nlm.nih.gov/pubmed/20015486.
63. Pucak ML, Carroll KAL, Kerr DA, Kaplin AI. Neuropsychiatric manifestations of depression in multiple sclerosis: neuroinflammatory, neuroendocrine, and neurotrophic mechanisms in the pathogenesis of immune-mediated depression. Dialogues Clin Neurosci. 2007;9(2):125–39. PMCID: PMC3181849. http://www.ncbi.nlm.nih.gov/pubmed/17726912.
64. Musselman DL, Lawson DH, Gumnick JF, Manatunga AK, Penna S, Goodkin RS, Greiner K, Nemeroff CB, Miller AH. Paroxetine for the prevention of depression induced by high-dose interferon alfa. N Engl J Med. 2001;344(13):961–6. PMID: 11274622. http://www.ncbi.nlm.nih.gov/pubmed/11274622.
65. Warner-Schmidt JL, Vanover KE, Chen EY, Marshall JJ, Greengard P. Antidepressant effects of selective serotonin reuptake inhibitors (SSRIs) are attenuated by antiinflammatory drugs in mice and humans. Proc Natl Acad Sci USA. 2011;108(22):9262–7. PMCID: PMC3107316. http://www.ncbi.nlm.nih.gov/pubmed/21518864.
66. Gallagher PJ, Castro V, Fava M, Weilburg JB, Murphy SN, Gainer VS, Churchill SE, Kohane IS, Iosifescu DV, Smoller JW, Perlis RH. Antidepressant response in patients with major depression exposed to NSAIDs: a pharmacovigilance study. Am J Psychiatry. 2012;169(10):1065–72. PMCID: PMC3787520. http://www.ncbi.nlm.nih.gov/pubmed/23032386.
67. Kouba BR, de Araujo Borba L, Borges de Souza P, Gil-Mohapel J, Rodrigues ALS. Role of inflammatory mechanisms in major depressive disorder: from etiology to potential pharmacological targets. Cells. 2024;13(5):423. PMCID: PMC10931285. http://www.ncbi.nlm.nih.gov/pubmed/38474387.
68. Hedhli N, Falcone DJ, Huang B, Cesarman-Maus G, Kraemer R, Zhai H, Tsirka SE, Santambrogio L, Hajjar KA. The annexin A2/S100A10 system in health and disease: emerging paradigms. J Biomed Biotechnol. 2012;2012:406273. PMCID: PMC3496855. http://www.ncbi.nlm.nih.gov/pubmed/23193360.
69. Uher R, Carver S, Power RA, Mors O, Maier W, Rietschel M, Hauser J, Dernovsek MZ, Henigsberg N, Souery D, Placentino A, Farmer A, McGuffin P. Non-steroidal anti-inflammatory drugs and efficacy of antidepressants in major depressive disorder. Psychol Med. 2012;42(10):2027–35. PMID: 22391106. http://www.ncbi.nlm.nih.gov/pubmed/22391106.
70. Mendlewicz J, Kriwin P, Oswald P, Souery D, Alboni S, Brunello N. Shortened onset of action of antidepressants in major depression using acetylsalicylic acid augmentation: a pilot open-label study. Int Clin Psychopharmacol. 2006;21(4):227–31. PMID: 16687994. http://www.ncbi.nlm.nih.gov/pubmed/16687994.
71. Tinaz AC, Karadag LS, Alaçam T, Mihçioglu T. Evaluation of the smear layer removal effectiveness of EDTA using two techniques: an SEM study. J Contemp Dent Pract. 2006;7(1):9–16. PMID: 16491143. http://www.ncbi.nlm.nih.gov/pubmed/16491143.
72. Tyring S, Gottlieb A, Papp K, Gordon K, Leonardi C, Wang A, Lalla D, Woolley M, Jahreis A, Zitnik R, Cella D, Krishnan R. Etanercept and clinical outcomes, fatigue, and depression in psoriasis: double-blind placebo-controlled randomised phase III trial. Lancet.

2006;367(9504):29–35. PMID: 16399150. http://www.ncbi.nlm.nih.gov/pubmed/16399150.
73. Berk M, Dean O, Drexhage H, McNeil JJ, Moylan S, O'Neil A, Davey CG, Sanna L, Maes M. Aspirin: a review of its neurobiological properties and therapeutic potential for mental illness. BMC Med. 2013;11:74. PMCID: PMC3751197. http://www.ncbi.nlm.nih.gov/pubmed/23506529.
74. Hannestad J, DellaGioia N, Bloch M. The effect of antidepressant medication treatment on serum levels of inflammatory cytokines: a meta-analysis. Neuropsychopharmacology. 2011;36(12):2452–9. PMCID: PMC3194072. http://www.ncbi.nlm.nih.gov/pubmed/21796103.
75. Kokaia Z, Martino G, Schwartz M, Lindvall O. Cross-talk between neural stem cells and immune cells: the key to better brain repair? Nat Neurosci. 2012;15(8):1078–87. PMID: 22837038. http://www.ncbi.nlm.nih.gov/pubmed/22837038.
76. Carlson NG, Wieggel WA, Chen J, Bacchi A, Rogers SW, Gahring LC. Inflammatory cytokines IL-1 alpha, IL-1 beta, IL-6, and TNF-alpha impart neuroprotection to an excitotoxin through distinct pathways. J Immunol. 1999;163(7):3963–8. PMID: 10490998. http://www.ncbi.nlm.nih.gov/pubmed/10490998.
77. Baune BT, Ponath G, Rothermundt M, Riess O, Funke H, Berger K. Association between genetic variants of IL-1beta, IL-6 and TNF-alpha cytokines and cognitive performance in the elderly general population of the MEMO-study. Psychoneuroendocrinology. 2008;33(1):68–76. PMID: 17988804. http://www.ncbi.nlm.nih.gov/pubmed/17988804.
78. Baune BT, Konrad C, Grotegerd D, Suslow T, Birosova E, Ohrmann P, Bauer J, Arolt V, Heindel W, Domschke K, Schöning S, Rauch AV, Uhlmann C, Kugel H, Dannlowski U. Interleukin-6 gene (IL-6): a possible role in brain morphology in the healthy adult brain. J Neuroinflammation. 2012;9:125. PMCID: PMC3464888. http://www.ncbi.nlm.nih.gov/pubmed/22695063.
79. Baune BT, Dannlowski U, Domschke K, Janssen DGA, Jordan MA, Ohrmann P, Bauer J, Biros E, Arolt V, Kugel H, Baxter AG, Suslow T. The interleukin 1 beta (IL1B) gene is associated with failure to achieve remission and impaired emotion processing in major depression. Biol Psychiatry. 2010;67(6):543–9. PMID: 20044070. http://www.ncbi.nlm.nih.gov/pubmed/20044070.
80. Eyre H, Baune BT. Neuroimmunological effects of physical exercise in depression. Brain Behav Immun. 2012;26(2):251–66. PMID: 21986304. http://www.ncbi.nlm.nih.gov/pubmed/21986304.
81. Poon VY, Choi S, Park M. Growth factors in synaptic function. Front Synaptic Neurosci. 2013;5:6. PMCID: PMC3776238. http://www.ncbi.nlm.nih.gov/pubmed/24065916.
82. Pion PD, Kittleson MD, Rogers QR. Taurine deficiency as a cause of dilated cardiomyopathy in cats. Tijdschr Diergeneeskd. 1989;114(Suppl 1):62S–4S. PMID: 2749718. http://www.ncbi.nlm.nih.gov/pubmed/2749718.
83. Santello M, Volterra A. TNFα in synaptic function: switching gears. Trends Neurosci. 2012;35(10):638–47. PMID: 22749718. http://www.ncbi.nlm.nih.gov/pubmed/22749718.
84. Baune BT, Wiede F, Braun A, Golledge J, Arolt V, Koerner H. Cognitive dysfunction in mice deficient for TNF- and its receptors. Am J Med Genet B Neuropsychiatr Genet. 2008;147B(7):1056–64. PMID: 18286589. http://www.ncbi.nlm.nih.gov/pubmed/18286589.
85. Kipnis J, Derecki NC, Yang C, Scrable H. Immunity and cognition: what do age-related dementia, HIV-dementia and "chemo-brain" have in common? Trends Immunol. 2008;29(10):455–63. PMID: 18789764. http://www.ncbi.nlm.nih.gov/pubmed/18789764.
86. Butovsky O, Talpalar AE, Ben-Yaakov K, Schwartz M. Activation of microglia by aggregated beta-amyloid or lipopolysaccharide impairs MHC-II expression and renders them cytotoxic whereas IFN-gamma and IL-4 render them protective. Mol Cell Neurosci. 2005;29(3):381–93. PMID: 15890528. http://www.ncbi.nlm.nih.gov/pubmed/15890528.
87. Lyons A, McQuillan K, Deighan BF, O'Reilly JA, Downer EJ, Murphy AC, Watson M, Piazza A, O'Connell F, Griffin R, Mills KHG, Lynch MA. Decreased neuronal CD200 expression in IL-4-deficient mice results in increased neuroinflammation in response to lipopolysaccharide. Brain Behav Immun. 2009;23(7):1020–7. PMID: 19501645. http://www.ncbi.nlm.nih.gov/pubmed/19501645.
88. Walton NM, Sutter BM, Laywell ED, Levkoff LH, Kearns SM, Marshall GP, Scheffler B, Steindler DA. Microglia instruct subventricular zone neurogenesis. Glia. 2006;54(8):815–25. PMID: 16977605. http://www.ncbi.nlm.nih.gov/pubmed/16977605.
89. Schwartz M, Butovsky O, Brück W, Hanisch UK. Microglial phenotype: is the commitment reversible? Trends Neurosci. 2006;29(2):68–74. PMID: 16406093. http://www.ncbi.nlm.nih.gov/pubmed/16406093.
90. Raison CL, Miller AH. Is depression an inflammatory disorder? Curr Psychiatry Rep. 2011;13(6):467–75. PMCID: PMC3285451. http://www.ncbi.nlm.nih.gov/pubmed/21927805.
91. Bluthé RM, Castanon N, Pousset F, Bristow A, Ball C, Lestage J, Michaud B, Kelley KW, Dantzer R. Central injection of IL-10 antagonizes the behavioural effects of lipopolysaccharide in rats. Psychoneuroendocrinology. 1999;24(3):301–11. PMID: 10101735. http://www.ncbi.nlm.nih.gov/pubmed/10101735.
92. Mesquita AR, Correia-Neves M, Roque S, Castro AG, Vieira P, Pedrosa J, Palha JA, Sousa N. IL-10 modulates depressive-like behavior. J Psychiatr Res. 2008;43(2):89–97. PMID: 18394646. http://www.ncbi.nlm.nih.gov/pubmed/18394646.
93. Himmerich H, Milenović S, Fulda S, Plümäkers B, Sheldrick AJ, Michel TM, Kircher T, Rink L. Regulatory T cells increased while IL-1β decreased during antidepressant therapy. J Psychiatr Res. 2010;44(15):1052–7. PMID: 20413130. http://www.ncbi.nlm.nih.gov/pubmed/20413130.
94. Murray PJ. Macrophage polarization. Annu Rev Physiol. 2017;79:541–66. PMID: 27813830. http://www.ncbi.nlm.nih.gov/pubmed/27813830.
95. Moon ML, McNeil LK, Freund GG. Macrophages make me sick: how macrophage activation states influence sickness behavior. Psychoneuroendocrinology. 2011;36(10):1431–40. PMCID: PMC3199305. http://www.ncbi.nlm.nih.gov/pubmed/21855222.
96. Ginhoux F, Guilliams M. Tissue-resident macrophage ontogeny and homeostasis. Immunity. 2016;44(3):439–49. PMID: 26982352. http://www.ncbi.nlm.nih.gov/pubmed/26982352.
97. Derecki NC, Quinnies KM, Kipnis J. Alternatively activated myeloid (M2) cells enhance cognitive function in immune compromised mice. Brain Behav Immun. 2011;25(3):379–85. PMCID: PMC3039052. http://www.ncbi.nlm.nih.gov/pubmed/21093578.
98. Sherry CL, Kim SS, Dilger RN, Bauer LL, Moon ML, Tapping RI, Fahey GC, Tappenden KA, Freund GG. Sickness behavior induced by endotoxin can be mitigated by the dietary soluble fiber, pectin, through up-regulation of IL-4 and Th2 polarization. Brain Behav Immun. 2010;24(4):631–40. PMCID: PMC2856791. http://www.ncbi.nlm.nih.gov/pubmed/20138982.
99. Wada Y, Nakamachi T, Endo K, Seki T, Ohtaki H, Tsuchikawa D, Hori M, Tsuchida M, Yoshikawa A, Matkovits A, Kagami N, Imai N, Fujisaka S, Usui I, Tobe K, Koide R, Takahashi H, Shioda S. PACAP attenuates NMDA-induced retinal damage in association with modulation of the microglia/macrophage status into an acquired deactivation subtype. J Mol Neurosci. 2013;51(2):493–502. PMID: 23720065. http://www.ncbi.nlm.nih.gov/pubmed/23720065.
100. Valledor AF, Comalada M, Santamaría-Babi LF, Lloberas J, Celada A. Macrophage proinflammatory activation and deactivation: a question of balance. Adv Immunol. 2010;108:1–20. PMID: 21056727. http://www.ncbi.nlm.nih.gov/pubmed/21056727.

101. Derecki NC, Cardani AN, Yang CH, Quinnies KM, Crihfield A, Lynch KR, Kipnis J. Regulation of learning and memory by meningeal immunity: a key role for IL-4. J Exp Med. 2010;207(5):1067–80. PMCID: PMC2867291. http://www.ncbi.nlm.nih.gov/pubmed/20439540.
102. Prinz M, Priller J, Sisodia SS, Ransohoff RM. Heterogeneity of CNS myeloid cells and their roles in neurodegeneration. Nat Neurosci. 2011;14(10):1227–35. PMID: 21952260. http://www.ncbi.nlm.nih.gov/pubmed/21952260.
103. Shechter R, London A, Varol C, Raposo C, Cusimano M, Yovel G, Rolls A, Mack M, Pluchino S, Martino G, Jung S, Schwartz M. Infiltrating blood-derived macrophages are vital cells playing an anti-inflammatory role in recovery from spinal cord injury in mice. PLoS Med. 2009;6(7):e1000113. PMCID: PMC2707628. http://www.ncbi.nlm.nih.gov/pubmed/19636355.
104. Shimizu E, Kawahara K, Kajizono M, Sawada M, Nakayama H. IL-4-induced selective clearance of oligomeric beta-amyloid peptide(1-42) by rat primary type 2 microglia. J Immunol. 2008;181(9):6503–13. PMID: 18941241. http://www.ncbi.nlm.nih.gov/pubmed/18941241.
105. Koronyo-Hamaoui M, Ko MK, Koronyo Y, Azoulay D, Seksenyan A, Kunis G, Pham M, Bakhsheshian J, Rogeri P, Black KL, Farkas DL, Schwartz M. Attenuation of AD-like neuropathology by harnessing peripheral immune cells: local elevation of IL-10 and MMP-9. J Neurochem. 2009;111(6):1409–24. PMID: 19780903. http://www.ncbi.nlm.nih.gov/pubmed/19780903.
106. Rolls A, Schori H, London A, Schwartz M. Decrease in hippocampal neurogenesis during pregnancy: a link to immunity. Mol Psychiatry. 2008;13(5):468–9. PMID: 18421294. http://www.ncbi.nlm.nih.gov/pubmed/18421294.
107. Chiu IM, Chen A, Zheng Y, Kosaras B, Tsiftsoglou SA, Vartanian TK, Brown RH, Carroll MC. T lymphocytes potentiate endogenous neuroprotective inflammation in a mouse model of ALS. Proc Natl Acad Sci USA. 2008;105(46):17913–8. PMCID: PMC2581614. http://www.ncbi.nlm.nih.gov/pubmed/18997009.
108. Shaked I, Tchoresh D, Gersner R, Meiri G, Mordechai S, Xiao X, Hart RP, Schwartz M. Protective autoimmunity: interferon-gamma enables microglia to remove glutamate without evoking inflammatory mediators. J Neurochem. 2005;92(5):997–1009. PMID: 15715651. http://www.ncbi.nlm.nih.gov/pubmed/15715651.
109. Beers DR, Henkel JS, Zhao W, Wang J, Appel SH. CD4+ T cells support glial neuroprotection, slow disease progression, and modify glial morphology in an animal model of inherited ALS. Proc Natl Acad Sci USA. 2008;105(40):15558–63. PMCID: PMC2547419. http://www.ncbi.nlm.nih.gov/pubmed/18809917.
110. Butovsky O, Ziv Y, Schwartz A, Landa G, Talpalar AE, Pluchino S, Martino G, Schwartz M. Microglia activated by IL-4 or IFN-gamma differentially induce neurogenesis and oligodendrogenesis from adult stem/progenitor cells. Mol Cell Neurosci. 2006;31(1):149–60. PMID: 16297637. http://www.ncbi.nlm.nih.gov/pubmed/16297637.
111. Rook GAW, Lowry CA, Raison CL. Lymphocytes in neuroprotection, cognition and emotion: is intolerance really the answer? Brain Behav Immun. 2011;25(4):591–601. PMID: 21167931. http://www.ncbi.nlm.nih.gov/pubmed/21167931.
112. Chapoval S, Dasgupta P, Dorsey NJ, Keegan AD. Regulation of the T helper cell type 2 (Th2)/T regulatory cell (Treg) balance by IL-4 and STAT6. J Leukoc Biol. 2010;87(6):1011–8. PMCID: PMC2872539. http://www.ncbi.nlm.nih.gov/pubmed/20335310.
113. Fujio K, Okamura T, Yamamoto K. The family of IL-10-secreting CD4+ T cells. Adv Immunol. 2010;105:99–130. PMID: 20510731. http://www.ncbi.nlm.nih.gov/pubmed/20510731.
114. von Bernhardi R, Eugenín-von Bernhardi J, Flores B, Eugenín LJ. Glial cells and integrity of the nervous system. Adv Exp Med Biol. 2016;949:1–24. PMID: 27714682. http://www.ncbi.nlm.nih.gov/pubmed/27714682.
115. Verkhratsky A, Ho MS, Parpura V. Evolution of neuroglia. Adv Exp Med Biol. 2019;1175:15–44. PMCID: PMC7188604. https://pmc.ncbi.nlm.nih.gov/articles/PMC7188604/pdf/nihms-1581152.pdf.
116. von Bartheld CS, Bahney J, Herculano-Houzel S. The search for true numbers of neurons and glial cells in the human brain: a review of 150 years of cell counting. J Comp Neurol. 2016;524(18):3865–95. PMCID: PMC5063692. http://www.ncbi.nlm.nih.gov/pubmed/27187682.
117. Azevedo FAC, Carvalho LRB, Grinberg LT, Farfel JM, Ferretti REL, Leite REP, Jacob Filho W, Lent R, Herculano-Houzel S. Equal numbers of neuronal and nonneuronal cells make the human brain an isometrically scaled-up primate brain. J Comp Neurol. 2009;513(5):532–41. PMID: 19226510. http://www.ncbi.nlm.nih.gov/pubmed/19226510.
118. Araque A, Parpura V, Sanzgiri RP, Haydon PG. Tripartite synapses: glia, the unacknowledged partner. Trends Neurosci. 1999;22(5):208–15. PMID: 10322493. http://www.ncbi.nlm.nih.gov/pubmed/10322493.
119. Schafer DP, Lehrman EK, Stevens B. The "quad-partite" synapse: microglia-synapse interactions in the developing and mature CNS. Glia. 2013;61(1):24–36. PMCID: PMC4082974. http://www.ncbi.nlm.nih.gov/pubmed/22829357.
120. Verkhratsky A, Nedergaard M. Physiology of astroglia. Physiol Rev. 2018;98(1):239–389. PMCID: PMC6050349. http://www.ncbi.nlm.nih.gov/pubmed/29351512.
121. Colombo E, Farina C. Astrocytes: key regulators of neuroinflammation. Trends Immunol. 2016;37(9):608–20. PMID: 27443914. http://www.ncbi.nlm.nih.gov/pubmed/27443914.
122. Volterra A, Meldolesi J. Astrocytes, from brain glue to communication elements: the revolution continues. Nat Rev Neurosci. 2005;6(8):626–40. PMID: 16025096. http://www.ncbi.nlm.nih.gov/pubmed/16025096.
123. Haydon PG, Carmignoto G. Astrocyte control of synaptic transmission and neurovascular coupling. Physiol Rev. 2006;86(3):1009–31. PMID: 16816144. http://www.ncbi.nlm.nih.gov/pubmed/16816144.
124. Walz W. Role of astrocytes in the clearance of excess extracellular potassium. Neurochem Int. 2000;36(4–5):291–300. PMID: 10732996. http://www.ncbi.nlm.nih.gov/pubmed/10732996.
125. Piet R, Vargová L, Syková E, Poulain DA, Oliet SHR. Physiological contribution of the astrocytic environment of neurons to intersynaptic crosstalk. Proc Natl Acad Sci USA. 2004;101(7):2151–5. PMCID: PMC357067. http://www.ncbi.nlm.nih.gov/pubmed/14766975.
126. Figley CR, Stroman PW. The role(s) of astrocytes and astrocyte activity in neurometabolism, neurovascular coupling, and the production of functional neuroimaging signals. Eur J Neurosci. 2011;33(4):577–88. PMID: 21314846. http://www.ncbi.nlm.nih.gov/pubmed/21314846.
127. Jourdain P, Bergersen LH, Bhaukaurally K, Bezzi P, Santello M, Domercq M, Matute C, Tonello F, Gundersen V, Volterra A. Glutamate exocytosis from astrocytes controls synaptic strength. Nat Neurosci. 2007;10(3):331–9. PMID: 17310248. http://www.ncbi.nlm.nih.gov/pubmed/17310248.
128. Koizumi S, Fujishita K, Inoue K. Regulation of cell-to-cell communication mediated by astrocytic ATP in the CNS. Purinergic Signal. 2005;1(3):211–7. PMCID: PMC2096541. http://www.ncbi.nlm.nih.gov/pubmed/18404506.
129. Parri R, Crunelli V. An astrocyte bridge from synapse to blood flow. Nat Neurosci. 2003;6(1):5–6. PMID: 12494240. http://www.ncbi.nlm.nih.gov/pubmed/12494240.
130. Brancaccio M, Edwards MD, Patton AP, Smyllie NJ, Chesham JE, Maywood ES, Hastings MH. Cell-autonomous clock of astrocytes drives circadian behavior in mammals. Science. 2019;363(6423):187–92. PMCID: PMC6440650. http://www.ncbi.nlm.nih.gov/pubmed/30630934.

131. Poskanzer KE, Yuste R. Astrocytes regulate cortical state switching in vivo. Proc Natl Acad Sci USA. 2016;113(19):E2675–84. PMCID: PMC4868485. http://www.ncbi.nlm.nih.gov/pubmed/27122314.
132. Paukert M, Agarwal A, Cha J, Doze VA, Kang JU, Bergles DE. Norepinephrine controls astroglial responsiveness to local circuit activity. Neuron. 2014;82(6):1263–70. PMCID: PMC4080721. http://www.ncbi.nlm.nih.gov/pubmed/24945771.
133. Ishibashi T, Dakin KA, Stevens B, Lee PR, Kozlov SV, Stewart CL, Fields RD. Astrocytes promote myelination in response to electrical impulses. Neuron. 2006;49(6):823–32. PMCID: PMC147483. http://www.ncbi.nlm.nih.gov/pubmed/16543131.
134. Zhao YF, Verkhratsky A, Tang Y, Illes P. Astrocytes and major depression: the purinergic avenue. Neuropharmacology. 2022;220:109252. PMID: 36122663. http://www.ncbi.nlm.nih.gov/pubmed/36122663.
135. Anderson MA, Burda JE, Ren Y, Ao Y, O'Shea TM, Kawaguchi R, Coppola G, Khakh BS, Deming TJ, Sofroniew MV. Astrocyte scar formation aids central nervous system axon regeneration. Nature. 2016;532(7598):195–200. PMCID: PMC5243141. http://www.ncbi.nlm.nih.gov/pubmed/27027288.
136. Han X, Chen M, Wang F, Windrem M, Wang S, Shanz S, Xu Q, Oberheim NA, Bekar L, Betstadt S, Silva AJ, Takano T, Goldman SA, Nedergaard M. Forebrain engraftment by human glial progenitor cells enhances synaptic plasticity and learning in adult mice. Cell Stem Cell. 2013;12(3):342–53. PMCID: PMC3700554. http://www.ncbi.nlm.nih.gov/pubmed/23472873.
137. Verkhratsky A, Nedergaard M. The homeostatic astroglia emerges from evolutionary specialization of neural cells. Philos Trans R Soc Lond Ser B Biol Sci. 2016;371(1700):20150428. PMCID: PMC4938028. http://www.ncbi.nlm.nih.gov/pubmed/27377722.
138. Rial D, Lemos C, Pinheiro H, Duarte JM, Gonçalves FQ, Real JI, Prediger RD, Gonçalves N, Gomes CA, Canas PM, Agostinho P, Cunha RA. Depression as a glial-based synaptic dysfunction. Front Cell Neurosci. 2015;9:521. PMCID: PMC4722129. http://www.ncbi.nlm.nih.gov/pubmed/26834566.
139. Allen NJ, Bennett ML, Foo LC, Wang GX, Chakraborty C, Smith SJ, Barres BA. Astrocyte glypicans 4 and 6 promote formation of excitatory synapses via GluA1 AMPA receptors. Nature. 2012;486(7403):410–4. PMCID: PMC3383085. http://www.ncbi.nlm.nih.gov/pubmed/22722203.
140. Christopherson KS, Ullian EM, Stokes CCA, Mullowney CE, Hell JW, Agah A, Lawler J, Mosher DF, Bornstein P, Barres BA. Thrombospondins are astrocyte-secreted proteins that promote CNS synaptogenesis. Cell. 2005;120(3):421–33. PMID: 15707899. http://www.ncbi.nlm.nih.gov/pubmed/15707899.
141. Singh SK, Stogsdill JA, Pulimood NS, Dingsdale H, Kim YH, Pilaz LJ, Kim IH, Manhaes AC, Rodrigues WS, Pamukcu A, Enustun E, Ertuz Z, Scheiffele P, Soderling SH, Silver DL, Ji RR, Medina AE, Eroglu C. Astrocytes assemble thalamocortical synapses by bridging NRX1α and NL1 via hevin. Cell. 2016;164(1–2):183–96. PMCID: PMC4715262. http://www.ncbi.nlm.nih.gov/pubmed/26771491.
142. Simard S, Coppola G, Rudyk CA, Hayley S, McQuaid RJ, Salmaso N. Profiling changes in cortical astroglial cells following chronic stress. Neuropsychopharmacology. 2018;43(9):1961–71. PMCID: PMC6046043. http://www.ncbi.nlm.nih.gov/pubmed/29907879.
143. Quesseveur G, Gardier AM, Guiard BP. The monoaminergic tripartite synapse: a putative target for currently available antidepressant drugs. Curr Drug Targets. 2013;14(11):1277–94. PMID: 24020973. http://www.ncbi.nlm.nih.gov/pubmed/24020973.
144. Dong Y, Benveniste EN. Immune function of astrocytes. Glia. 2001;36(2):180–90. PMID: 11596126. http://www.ncbi.nlm.nih.gov/pubmed/11596126.
145. Jha MK, Jo M, Kim JH, Suk K. Microglia-astrocyte crosstalk: an intimate molecular conversation. Neuroscientist. 2019;25(3):227–40. PMID: 29931997. http://www.ncbi.nlm.nih.gov/pubmed/29931997.
146. Kano SI, Choi EY, Dohi E, Agarwal S, Chang DJ, Wilson AM, Lo BD, Rose IVL, Gonzalez S, Imai T, Sawa A. Glutathione S-transferases promote proinflammatory astrocyte-microglia communication during brain inflammation. Sci Signal. 2019;12(569):eaar2124. PMCID: PMC6637164. http://www.ncbi.nlm.nih.gov/pubmed/30783009.
147. Priego N, Valiente M. The potential of astrocytes as immune modulators in brain tumors. Front Immunol. 2019;10:1314. PMCID: PMC6579886. http://www.ncbi.nlm.nih.gov/pubmed/31244853.
148. Liddelow SA, Guttenplan KA, Clarke LE, Bennett FC, Bohlen CJ, Schirmer L, Bennett ML, Münch AE, Chung WS, Peterson TC, Wilton DK, Frouin A, Napier BA, Panicker N, Kumar M, Buckwalter MS, Rowitch DH, Dawson VL, Dawson TM, Stevens B, Barres BA. Neurotoxic reactive astrocytes are induced by activated microglia. Nature. 2017;541(7638):481–7. PMCID: PMC5404890. http://www.ncbi.nlm.nih.gov/pubmed/28099414.
149. Bracchi-Ricard V, Brambilla R, Levenson J, Hu WH, Bramwell A, Sweatt JD, Green EJ, Bethea JR. Astroglial nuclear factor-kappaB regulates learning and memory and synaptic plasticity in female mice. J Neurochem. 2008;104(3):611–23. PMID: 17953667. http://www.ncbi.nlm.nih.gov/pubmed/17953667.
150. Stellwagen D, Malenka RC. Synaptic scaling mediated by glial TNF-alpha. Nature. 2006;440(7087):1054–9. PMID: 16547515. http://www.ncbi.nlm.nih.gov/pubmed/16547515.
151. Ben Menachem-Zidon O, Avital A, Ben-Menahem Y, Goshen I, Kreisel T, Shmueli EM, Segal M, Ben Hur T, Yirmiya R. Astrocytes support hippocampal-dependent memory and long-term potentiation via interleukin-1 signaling. Brain Behav Immun. 2011;25(5):1008–16. PMID: 21093580. http://www.ncbi.nlm.nih.gov/pubmed/21093580.
152. Garg SK, Banerjee R, Kipnis J. Neuroprotective immunity: T cell-derived glutamate endows astrocytes with a neuroprotective phenotype. J Immunol. 2008;180(6):3866–73. PMID: 18322194. http://www.ncbi.nlm.nih.gov/pubmed/18322194.
153. Wang Q, Jie W, Liu JH, Yang JM, Gao TM. An astroglial basis of major depressive disorder? An overview. Glia. 2017;65(8):1227–50. PMID: 28317185. http://www.ncbi.nlm.nih.gov/pubmed/28317185.
154. Peng L, Verkhratsky A, Gu L, Li B. Targeting astrocytes in major depression. Expert Rev Neurother. 2015;15(11):1299–306. PMID: 26471936. http://www.ncbi.nlm.nih.gov/pubmed/26471936.
155. Wray NR, Ripke S, Mattheisen M, Trzaskowski M, Byrne EM, Abdellaoui A, Adams MJ, Agerbo E, Air TM, Andlauer TMF, Bacanu SA, Bækvad-Hansen M, Beekman AFT, Bigdeli TB, Binder EB, Clarke TK, Coleman JIR, Colodro-Conde L, Sullivan PF, et al. Major Depressive Disorder Working Group of the Psychiatric Genomics Consortium. Genome-wide association analyses identify 44 risk variants and refine the genetic architecture of major depression. Nat Genet. 2018;50(5):668–81. PMCID: PMC5934326. http://www.ncbi.nlm.nih.gov/pubmed/29700475.
156. Wolf SA, Boddeke HWGM, Kettenmann H. Microglia in physiology and disease. Annu Rev Physiol. 2017;79:619–43. PMID: 27959620. http://www.ncbi.nlm.nih.gov/pubmed/27959620.
157. Schwarz JM, Bilbo SD. Sex, glia, and development: interactions in health and disease. Horm Behav. 2012;62(3):243–53. PMCID: PMC3374064. http://www.ncbi.nlm.nih.gov/pubmed/22387107.
158. Ekdahl CT. Microglial activation – tuning and pruning adult neurogenesis. Front Pharmacol. 2012;3:41. PMCID: PMC3297835. http://www.ncbi.nlm.nih.gov/pubmed/22408626.
159. Beumer W, Gibney SM, Drexhage RC, Pont-Lezica L, Doorduin J, Klein HC, Steiner J, Connor TJ, Harkin A, Versnel MA, Drexhage HA. The immune theory of psychiatric diseases: a key role for activated microglia and circulating monocytes. J Leukoc Biol. 2012;92(5):959–75. PMID: 22875882. http://www.ncbi.nlm.nih.gov/pubmed/22875882.

160. Szepesi Z, Manouchehrian O, Bachiller S, Deierborg T. Bidirectional microglia-neuron communication in health and disease. Front Cell Neurosci. 2018;12:323. PMCID: PMC6170615. http://www.ncbi.nlm.nih.gov/pubmed/30319362.
161. Chung WS, Welsh CA, Barres BA, Stevens B. Do glia drive synaptic and cognitive impairment in disease? Nat Neurosci. 2015;18(11):1539–45. PMCID: PMC4739631. http://www.ncbi.nlm.nih.gov/pubmed/26505565.
162. Ginhoux F, Lim S, Hoeffel G, Low D, Huber T. Origin and differentiation of microglia. Front Cell Neurosci. 2013;7:45. PMCID: PMC3627983. http://www.ncbi.nlm.nih.gov/pubmed/23616747.
163. Lawson LJ, Perry VH, Gordon S. Turnover of resident microglia in the normal adult mouse brain. Neuroscience. 1992;48(2):405–15. PMID: 1603325. http://www.ncbi.nlm.nih.gov/pubmed/1603325.
164. Ginhoux F, Prinz M. Origin of microglia: current concepts and past controversies. Cold Spring Harb Perspect Biol. 2015;7(8):a020537. PMCID: PMC4526747. http://www.ncbi.nlm.nih.gov/pubmed/26134003.
165. Singhal G, Baune BT. Microglia: an interface between the loss of neuroplasticity and depression. Front Cell Neurosci. 2017;11:270. PMCID: PMC5596091. http://www.ncbi.nlm.nih.gov/pubmed/28943841.
166. Filiano AJ, Gadani SP, Kipnis J. Interactions of innate and adaptive immunity in brain development and function. Brain Res. 2015;1617:18–27. PMCID: PMC4320678. http://www.ncbi.nlm.nih.gov/pubmed/25110235.
167. Gehrmann J, Matsumoto Y, Kreutzberg GW. Microglia: intrinsic immuneffector cell of the brain. Brain Res Brain Res Rev. 1995;20(3):269–87. PMID: 7550361. http://www.ncbi.nlm.nih.gov/pubmed/7550361.
168. Bilbo SD, Smith SH, Schwarz JM. A lifespan approach to neuroinflammatory and cognitive disorders: a critical role for glia. J Neuroimmune Pharmacol. 2012;7(1):24–41. PMCID: PMC3267003. http://www.ncbi.nlm.nih.gov/pubmed/21822589.
169. Yirmiya R, Rimmerman N, Reshef R. Depression as a microglial disease. Trends Neurosci. 2015;38(10):637–58. PMID: 26442697. http://www.ncbi.nlm.nih.gov/pubmed/26442697.
170. Yanuck SF. Microglial phagocytosis of neurons: diminishing neuronal loss in traumatic, infectious, inflammatory, and autoimmune CNS disorders. Front Psych. 2019;10:712. PMCID: PMC6786049. http://www.ncbi.nlm.nih.gov/pubmed/31632307.
171. Franklin TC, Wohleb ES, Zhang Y, Fogaça M, Hare B, Duman RS. Persistent increase in microglial RAGE contributes to chronic stress-induced priming of depressive-like behavior. Biol Psychiatry. 2018;83(1):50–60. PMCID: PMC6369917. http://www.ncbi.nlm.nih.gov/pubmed/28882317.
172. Mendiola AS, Garza R, Cardona SM, Mythen SA, Lira SA, Akassoglou K, Cardona AE. Fractalkine signaling attenuates perivascular clustering of microglia and fibrinogen leakage during systemic inflammation in mouse models of diabetic retinopathy. Front Cell Neurosci. 2017;10:303. https://www.frontiersin.org/journals/cellular-neuroscience/articles/10.3389/fncel.2016.00303/full.
173. Maciejewski-Lenoir D, Chen S, Feng L, Maki R, Bacon KB. Characterization of fractalkine in rat brain cells: migratory and activation signals for CX3CR-1-expressing microglia. J Immunol. 1999;163(3):1628–35. PMID: 10415068. http://www.ncbi.nlm.nih.gov/pubmed/10415068.
174. Wolf Y, Yona S, Kim KW, Jung S. Microglia, seen from the CX3CR1 angle. Front Cell Neurosci. 2013;7:26. PMCID: PMC3600435. http://www.ncbi.nlm.nih.gov/pubmed/23507975.
175. Rodríguez-Iglesias N, Sierra A, Valero J. Rewiring of memory circuits: connecting adult newborn neurons with the help of microglia. Front Cell Dev Biol. 2019;7:24. PMCID: PMC6411767. http://www.ncbi.nlm.nih.gov/pubmed/30891446.
176. Liu D, Wang Z, Liu S, Wang F, Zhao S, Hao A. Anti-inflammatory effects of fluoxetine in lipopolysaccharide(LPS)-stimulated microglial cells. Neuropharmacology. 2011;61(4):592–9. PMID: 21575647. http://www.ncbi.nlm.nih.gov/pubmed/21575647.
177. Calcia MA, Bonsall DR, Bloomfield PS, Selvaraj S, Barichello T, Howes OD. Stress and neuroinflammation: a systematic review of the effects of stress on microglia and the implications for mental illness. Psychopharmacology. 2016;233(9):1637–50. PMCID: PMC4828495. http://www.ncbi.nlm.nih.gov/pubmed/26847047.
178. Hinwood M, Morandini J, Day TA, Walker FR. Evidence that microglia mediate the neurobiological effects of chronic psychological stress on the medial prefrontal cortex. Cereb Cortex. 2012;22(6):1442–54. PMID: 21878486. http://www.ncbi.nlm.nih.gov/pubmed/21878486.
179. Walker PA, Letourneau PA, Bedi S, Shah SK, Jimenez F, Cox CS. Progenitor cells as remote "bioreactors": neuroprotection via modulation of the systemic inflammatory response. World J Stem Cells. 2011;3(2):9–18. PMCID: PMC3097935. http://www.ncbi.nlm.nih.gov/pubmed/21607132.
180. Möller T, Bard F, Bhattacharya A, Biber K, Campbell B, Dale E, Eder C, Gan L, Garden GA, Hughes ZA, Pearse DD, Staal RGW, Sayed FA, Wes PD, Boddeke HWGM. Critical data-based re-evaluation of minocycline as a putative specific microglia inhibitor. Glia. 2016;64(10):1788–94. PMID: 27246804. http://www.ncbi.nlm.nih.gov/pubmed/27246804.
181. Bassett B, Subramaniyam S, Fan Y, Varney S, Pan H, Carneiro AMD, Chung CY. Minocycline alleviates depression-like symptoms by rescuing decrease in neurogenesis in dorsal hippocampus via blocking microglia activation/phagocytosis. Brain Behav Immun. 2021;91:519–30. PMID: 33176182. http://www.ncbi.nlm.nih.gov/pubmed/33176182.
182. Peruzzotti-Jametti L, Willis CM, Krzak G, Hamel R, Pirvan L, Ionescu RB, Reisz JA, Prag HA, Garcia-Segura ME, Wu V, Xiang Y, Barlas B, Casey AM, van den Bosch AMR, Nicaise AM, Roth L, Bates GR, Huang H, Prasad P, Vincent AE, Frezza C, Viscomi C, Balmus G, Takats Z, Marioni JC, D'Alessandro A, Murphy MP, Mohorianu I, Pluchino S. Mitochondrial complex I activity in microglia sustains neuroinflammation. Nature. 2024;628(8006):195–203. PMCID: PMC10990929. http://www.ncbi.nlm.nih.gov/pubmed/38480879.
183. Ziv Y, Ron N, Butovsky O, Landa G, Sudai E, Greenberg N, Cohen H, Kipnis J, Schwartz M. Immune cells contribute to the maintenance of neurogenesis and spatial learning abilities in adulthood. Nat Neurosci. 2006;9(2):268–75. PMID: 16415867. http://www.ncbi.nlm.nih.gov/pubmed/16415867.
184. Gildawie KR, Orso R, Peterzell S, Thompson V, Brenhouse HC. Sex differences in prefrontal cortex microglia morphology: impact of a two-hit model of adversity throughout development. Neurosci Lett. 2020;738:135381. PMCID: PMC7584734. http://www.ncbi.nlm.nih.gov/pubmed/32927000.
185. Tong L, Gong Y, Wang P, Hu W, Wang J, Chen Z, Zhang W, Huang C. Microglia loss contributes to the development of major depression induced by different types of chronic stresses. Neurochem Res. 2017;42(10):2698–711. PMID: 28434164. http://www.ncbi.nlm.nih.gov/pubmed/28434164.
186. Paolicelli RC, Bolasco G, Pagani F, Maggi L, Scianni M, Panzanelli P, Giustetto M, Ferreira TA, Guiducci E, Dumas L, Ragozzino D, Gross CT. Synaptic pruning by microglia is necessary for normal brain development. Science. 2011;333(6048):1456–8. PMID: 21778362. http://www.ncbi.nlm.nih.gov/pubmed/21778362.
187. Zhan Y, Paolicelli RC, Sforazzini F, Weinhard L, Bolasco G, Pagani F, Vyssotski AL, Bifone A, Gozzi A, Ragozzino D, Gross CT. Deficient neuron-microglia signaling results in impaired functional brain connectivity and social behavior. Nat Neurosci. 2014;17(3):400–6. PMID: 24487234. http://www.ncbi.nlm.nih.gov/pubmed/24487234.
188. Pascual O, Ben Achour S, Rostaing P, Triller A, Bessis A. Microglia activation triggers astrocyte-mediated modula-

tion of excitatory neurotransmission. Proc Natl Acad Sci USA. 2012;109(4):E197–205. PMCID: PMC3268269. http://www.ncbi.nlm.nih.gov/pubmed/22167804.
189. Cao X, Li LP, Wang Q, Wu Q, Hu HH, Zhang M, Fang YY, Zhang J, Li SJ, Xiong WC, Yan HC, Gao YB, Liu JH, Li XW, Sun LR, Zeng YN, Zhu XH, Gao TM. Astrocyte-derived ATP modulates depressive-like behaviors. Nat Med. 2013;19(6):773–7. PMID: 23644515. http://www.ncbi.nlm.nih.gov/pubmed/23644515.
190. Hines DJ, Schmitt LI, Hines RM, Moss SJ, Haydon PG. Antidepressant effects of sleep deprivation require astrocyte-dependent adenosine mediated signaling. Transl Psychiatry. 2013;3(1):e212. PMCID: PMC3566717. http://www.ncbi.nlm.nih.gov/pubmed/23321809.
191. Serchov T, Clement HW, Schwarz MK, Iasevoli F, Tosh DK, Idzko M, Jacobson KA, de Bartolomeis A, Normann C, Biber K, van Calker D. Increased signaling via adenosine A1 receptors, sleep deprivation, imipramine, and ketamine inhibit depressive-like behavior via induction of homer1a. Neuron. 2015;87(3):549–62. PMCID: PMC4803038. http://www.ncbi.nlm.nih.gov/pubmed/26247862.
192. Kaster MP, Machado NJ, Silva HB, Nunes A, Ardais AP, Santana M, Baqi Y, Müller CE, Rodrigues ALS, Porciúncula LO, Chen JF, Tomé ÂR, Agostinho P, Canas PM, Cunha RA. Caffeine acts through neuronal adenosine A2A receptors to prevent mood and memory dysfunction triggered by chronic stress. Proc Natl Acad Sci USA. 2015;112(25):7833–8. PMCID: PMC4485143. http://www.ncbi.nlm.nih.gov/pubmed/26056314.
193. Cunha GMA, Canas PM, Oliveira CR, Cunha RA. Increased density and synapto-protective effect of adenosine A2A receptors upon sub-chronic restraint stress. Neuroscience. 2006;141(4):1775–81. PMID: 16797134. http://www.ncbi.nlm.nih.gov/pubmed/16797134.
194. Silva AC, Lemos C, Gonçalves FQ, Pliássova AV, Machado NJ, Silva HB, Canas PM, Cunha RA, Lopes JP, Agostinho P. Blockade of adenosine A2A receptors recovers early deficits of memory and plasticity in the triple transgenic mouse model of Alzheimer's disease. Neurobiol Dis. 2018;117:72–81. PMID: 29859867. http://www.ncbi.nlm.nih.gov/pubmed/29859867.
195. Batalha VL, Pego JM, Fontinha BM, Costenla AR, Valadas JS, Baqi Y, Radjainia H, Müller CE, Sebastião AM, Lopes LV. Adenosine A(2A) receptor blockade reverts hippocampal stress-induced deficits and restores corticosterone circadian oscillation. Mol Psychiatry. 2013;18(3):320–31. PMID: 22371048. http://www.ncbi.nlm.nih.gov/pubmed/22371048.
196. Liu WX, Wang J, Xie ZM, Xu N, Zhang GF, Jia M, Zhou ZQ, Hashimoto K, Yang JJ. Regulation of glutamate transporter 1 via BDNF-TrkB signaling plays a role in the anti-apoptotic and antidepressant effects of ketamine in chronic unpredictable stress model of depression. Psychopharmacology. 2016;233(3):405–15. PMID: 26514555. http://www.ncbi.nlm.nih.gov/pubmed/26514555.
197. Stokes L, Spencer SJ, Jenkins TA. Understanding the role of P2X7 in affective disorders-are glial cells the major players? Front Cell Neurosci. 2015;9:258. PMCID: PMC4495333. http://www.ncbi.nlm.nih.gov/pubmed/26217184.
198. Setiawan E, Wilson AA, Mizrahi R, Rusjan PM, Miler L, Rajkowska G, Suridjan I, Kennedy JL, Rekkas PV, Houle S, Meyer JH. Role of translocator protein density, a marker of neuroinflammation, in the brain during major depressive episodes. JAMA Psychiatry. 2015;72(3):268–75. PMCID: PMC4836849. http://www.ncbi.nlm.nih.gov/pubmed/25629589.
199. Milior G, Lecours C, Samson L, Bisht K, Poggini S, Pagani F, Deflorio C, Lauro C, Alboni S, Limatola C, Branchi I, Tremblay ME, Maggi L. Fractalkine receptor deficiency impairs microglial and neuronal responsiveness to chronic stress. Brain Behav Immun. 2016;55:114–25. PMID: 26231972. http://www.ncbi.nlm.nih.gov/pubmed/26231972.
200. Schnieder TP, Trencevska I, Rosoklija G, Stankov A, Mann JJ, Smiley J, Dwork AJ. Microglia of prefrontal white matter in suicide. J Neuropathol Exp Neurol. 2014;73(9):880–90. PMCID: PMC4141011. http://www.ncbi.nlm.nih.gov/pubmed/25101704.
201. Ros-Bernal F, Hunot S, Herrero MT, Parnadeau S, Corvol JC, Lu L, Alvarez-Fischer D, Carrillo-de Sauvage MA, Saurini F, Coussieu C, Kinugawa K, Prigent A, Höglinger G, Hamon M, Tronche F, Hirsch EC, Vyas S. Microglial glucocorticoid receptors play a pivotal role in regulating dopaminergic neurodegeneration in parkinsonism. Proc Natl Acad Sci USA. 2011;108(16):6632–7. PMCID: PMC3080980. http://www.ncbi.nlm.nih.gov/pubmed/21467220.
202. Krabbe G, Matyash V, Pannasch U, Mamer L, Boddeke HWGM, Kettenmann H. Activation of serotonin receptors promotes microglial injury-induced motility but attenuates phagocytic activity. Brain Behav Immun. 2012;26(3):419–28. PMID: 22198120. http://www.ncbi.nlm.nih.gov/pubmed/22198120.
203. Gomes C, Ferreira R, George J, Sanches R, Rodrigues DI, Gonçalves N, Cunha RA. Activation of microglial cells triggers a release of brain-derived neurotrophic factor (BDNF) inducing their proliferation in an adenosine A2A receptor-dependent manner: A2A receptor blockade prevents BDNF release and proliferation of microglia. J Neuroinflammation. 2013;10:16. PMCID: PMC3567964. http://www.ncbi.nlm.nih.gov/pubmed/23363775.
204. Färber K, Pannasch U, Kettenmann H. Dopamine and noradrenaline control distinct functions in rodent microglial cells. Mol Cell Neurosci. 2005;29(1):128–38. PMID: 15866053. http://www.ncbi.nlm.nih.gov/pubmed/15866053.
205. Hinwood M, Tynan RJ, Charnley JL, Beynon SB, Day TA, Walker FR. Chronic stress induced remodeling of the prefrontal cortex: structural re-organization of microglia and the inhibitory effect of minocycline. Cereb Cortex. 2013;23(8):1784–97. PMID: 22710611. http://www.ncbi.nlm.nih.gov/pubmed/22710611.
206. Verdonk F, Petit AC, Abdel-Ahad P, Vinckier F, Jouvion G, de Maricourt P, De Medeiros GF, Danckaert A, Van Steenwinckel J, Blatzer M, Maignan A, Langeron O, Sharshar T, Callebert J, Launay JM, Chrétien F, Gaillard R. Microglial production of quinolinic acid as a target and a biomarker of the antidepressant effect of ketamine. Brain Behav Immun. 2019;81:361–73. PMID: 31255681. http://www.ncbi.nlm.nih.gov/pubmed/31255681.
207. Su F, Yi H, Xu L, Zhang Z. Fluoxetine and S-citalopram inhibit M1 activation and promote M2 activation of microglia in vitro. Neuroscience. 2015;294:60–8. PMID: 25711936. http://www.ncbi.nlm.nih.gov/pubmed/25711936.
208. Jonuleit H, Tuettenberg A, Steinbrink K, Working Group Dermatologic Research (Abeitsgemeinschaft Dermatologische Forschung, ADF). Research in practice: regulatory T cells – targets for therapeutic approaches? J Dtsch Dermatol Ges. 2011;9(1):8–11. PMID: 21166772. http://www.ncbi.nlm.nih.gov/pubmed/21166772.
209. Workman CJ, Szymczak-Workman AL, Collison LW, Pillai MR, Vignali DAA. The development and function of regulatory T cells. Cell Mol Life Sci. 2009;66(16):2603–22. PMCID: PMC2715449. http://www.ncbi.nlm.nih.gov/pubmed/19390784.
210. Dasgupta A, Saxena R. Regulatory T cells: a review. Natl Med J India. 2012;25(6):341–51. PMID: 23998865. http://www.ncbi.nlm.nih.gov/pubmed/23998865.
211. Cools N, Ponsaerts P, Van Tendeloo VFI, Berneman ZN. Regulatory T cells and human disease. Clin Dev Immunol. 2007;2007:89195. PMCID: PMC2253668. http://www.ncbi.nlm.nih.gov/pubmed/18317534.
212. Zhang L, Zhao Y. The regulation of Foxp3 expression in regulatory CD4(+)CD25(+)T cells: multiple pathways on the road. J Cell Physiol. 2007;211(3):590–7. PMID: 17311282. http://www.ncbi.nlm.nih.gov/pubmed/17311282.

213. Zhou X, Bailey-Bucktrout S, Jeker LT, Bluestone JA. Plasticity of CD4(+) FoxP3(+) T cells. Curr Opin Immunol. 2009;21(3):281–5. PMCID: PMC2733784. http://www.ncbi.nlm.nih.gov/pubmed/19500966.
214. Kipnis J, Avidan H, Caspi RR, Schwartz M. Dual effect of CD4+CD25+ regulatory T cells in neurodegeneration: a dialogue with microglia. Proc Natl Acad Sci USA. 2004;101 Suppl 2(Suppl 2):14663–9. PMCID: PMC521988. http://www.ncbi.nlm.nih.gov/pubmed/15331781.
215. Kim SJ, Lee H, Lee G, Oh SJ, Shin MK, Shim I, Bae H. CD4+CD25+ regulatory T cell depletion modulates anxiety and depression-like behaviors in mice. PLoS One. 2012;7(7):e42054. PMCID: PMC34091454. http://www.ncbi.nlm.nih.gov/pubmed/22860054.
216. Li Y, Xiao B, Qiu W, Yang L, Hu B, Tian X, Yang H. Altered expression of CD4(+)CD25(+) regulatory T cells and its 5-HT(1a) receptor in patients with major depression disorder. J Affect Disord. 2010;124(1–2):68–75. PMID: 19900711. http://www.ncbi.nlm.nih.gov/pubmed/19900711.
217. Cohen H, Ziv Y, Cardon M, Kaplan Z, Matar MA, Gidron Y, Schwartz M, Kipnis J. Maladaptation to mental stress mitigated by the adaptive immune system via depletion of naturally occurring regulatory CD4+CD25+ cells. J Neurobiol. 2006;66(6):552–63. PMID: 16555237. http://www.ncbi.nlm.nih.gov/pubmed/16555237.
218. Myint AM, Leonard BE, Steinbusch HWM, Kim YK. Th1, Th2, and Th3 cytokine alterations in major depression. J Affect Disord. 2005;88(2):167–73. PMID: 16126278. http://www.ncbi.nlm.nih.gov/pubmed/16126278.
219. Sutcigil L, Oktenli C, Musabak U, Bozkurt A, Cansever A, Uzun O, Sanisoglu SY, Yesilova Z, Ozmenler N, Ozsahin A, Sengul A. Pro- and anti-inflammatory cytokine balance in major depression: effect of sertraline therapy. Clin Dev Immunol. 2007;2007:76396. PMCID: PMC2248234. http://www.ncbi.nlm.nih.gov/pubmed/18317531.
220. Dhabhar FS, Burke HM, Epel ES, Mellon SH, Rosser R, Reus VI, Wolkowitz OM. Low serum IL-10 concentrations and loss of regulatory association between IL-6 and IL-10 in adults with major depression. J Psychiatr Res. 2009;43(11):962–9. PMID: 19552919. http://www.ncbi.nlm.nih.gov/pubmed/19552919.
221. Musil R, Schwarz MJ, Riedel M, Dehning S, Cerovecki A, Spellmann I, Arolt V, Müller N. Elevated macrophage migration inhibitory factor and decreased transforming growth factor-beta levels in major depressionDOUBLEHYPHENno influence of celecoxib treatment. J Affect Disord. 2011;134(1–3):217–25. PMID: 21684012. http://www.ncbi.nlm.nih.gov/pubmed/21684012.
222. Capuron L, Miller AH. Immune system to brain signaling: neuropsychopharmacological implications. Pharmacol Ther. 2011;130(2):226–38. PMCID: PMC3072299. http://www.ncbi.nlm.nih.gov/pubmed/21334376.
223. Wong ML, Dong C, Maestre-Mesa J, Licinio J. Polymorphisms in inflammation-related genes are associated with susceptibility to major depression and antidepressant response. Mol Psychiatry. 2008;13(8):800–12. PMCID: PMC2650233. http://www.ncbi.nlm.nih.gov/pubmed/18504423.
224. Kim SJ, Lee H, Joung HY, Lee G, Lee H-J, Shin MK, Kim SH, Shim I, Bae H. T-bet deficient mice exhibit resistance to stress-induced development of depression-like behaviors. J Neuroimmunol. 2011;240–241:45–51. PMID: 22018704. http://www.ncbi.nlm.nih.gov/pubmed/22018704.
225. Lach G, Schellekens H, Dinan TG, Cryan JF. Anxiety, depression, and the microbiome: a role for gut peptides. Neurotherapeutics. 2018;15(1):36–59. PMCID: PMC5794698. http://www.ncbi.nlm.nih.gov/pubmed/29134359.
226. Yan M, Man S, Sun B, Ma L, Guo L, Huang L, Gao W. Gut liver brain axis in diseases: the implications for therapeutic interventions. Signal Transduct Target Ther. 2023;8(1):443. PMCID: PMC10700720. http://www.ncbi.nlm.nih.gov/pubmed/38057297.
227. Agirman G, Hsiao EY. SnapShot: the microbiota-gut-brain axis. Cell. 2021;184(9):2524–2524.e1. PMID: 33930299. http://www.ncbi.nlm.nih.gov/pubmed/33930299.
228. Farzi A, Fröhlich EE, Holzer P. Gut microbiota and the neuroendocrine system. Neurotherapeutics. 2018;15(1):5–22. PMCID: PMC5794709. http://www.ncbi.nlm.nih.gov/pubmed/29380303.
229. Long-Smith C, O'Riordan KJ, Clarke G, Stanton C, Dinan TG, Cryan JF. Microbiota-gut-brain axis: new therapeutic opportunities. Annu Rev Pharmacol Toxicol. 2020;60:477–502. PMID: 31506009. http://www.ncbi.nlm.nih.gov/pubmed/31506009.
230. Berding K, Vlckova K, Marx W, Schellekens H, Stanton C, Clarke G, Jacka F, Dinan TG, Cryan JF. Diet and the microbiota-gut-brain axis: sowing the seeds of good mental health. Adv Nutr. 2021;12(4):1239–85. PMCID: PMC8321864. http://www.ncbi.nlm.nih.gov/pubmed/33693453.
231. Bauer KC, Littlejohn PT, Ayala V, Creus-Cuadros A, Finlay BB. Nonalcoholic fatty liver disease and the gut-liver axis: exploring an undernutrition perspective. Gastroenterology. 2022;162(7):1858–1875.e2. PMID: 35248539. http://www.ncbi.nlm.nih.gov/pubmed/35248539.
232. Bajaj JS, Ng SC, Schnabl B. Promises of microbiome-based therapies. J Hepatol. 2022;76(6):1379–91. PMCID: PMC9588437. http://www.ncbi.nlm.nih.gov/pubmed/35589257.
233. Brescia P, Rescigno M. The gut vascular barrier: a new player in the gut-liver-brain axis. Trends Mol Med. 2021;27(9):844–55. PMID: 34229973. http://www.ncbi.nlm.nih.gov/pubmed/34229973.
234. Socała K, Doboszewska U, Szopa A, Serefko A, Włodarczyk M, Zielińska A, Poleszak E, Fichna J, Wlaź P. The role of microbiota-gut-brain axis in neuropsychiatric and neurological disorders. Pharmacol Res. 2021;172:105840. PMID: 34450312. http://www.ncbi.nlm.nih.gov/pubmed/34450312.
235. Lang S, Schnabl B. Microbiota and fatty liver disease-the known, the unknown, and the future. Cell Host Microbe. 2020;28(2):233–44. PMCID: PMC7467841. http://www.ncbi.nlm.nih.gov/pubmed/32791115.
236. Allam-Ndoul B, Castonguay-Paradis S, Veilleux A. Gut microbiota and intestinal trans-epithelial permeability. Int J Mol Sci. 2020;21(17):6402. PMCID: PMC7503654. http://www.ncbi.nlm.nih.gov/pubmed/32899147.
237. Chopyk DM, Grakoui A. Contribution of the intestinal microbiome and gut barrier to hepatic disorders. Gastroenterology. 2020;159(3):849–63. PMCID: PMC7502510. http://www.ncbi.nlm.nih.gov/pubmed/32569766.
238. Delgado TC, de Las Heras J, Martínez-Chantar ML. Understanding gut-liver axis nitrogen metabolism in fatty liver disease. Front Endocrinol (Lausanne). 2022;13:1058101. PMCID: PMC9797658. http://www.ncbi.nlm.nih.gov/pubmed/36589817.
239. Meijnikman AS, Davids M, Herrema H, Aydin O, Tremaroli V, Rios-Morales M, Levels H, Bruin S, de Brauw M, Verheij J, Kemper M, Holleboom AG, Tushuizen ME, Schwartz TW, Nielsen J, Brandjes D, Dirinck E, Weyler J, Verrijken A, De Block CEM, Vonghia L, Francque S, Beuers U, Gerdes VEA, Bäckhed F, Groen AK, Nieuwdorp M. Microbiome-derived ethanol in nonalcoholic fatty liver disease. Nat Med. 2022;28(10):2100–6. PMID: 36216942. http://www.ncbi.nlm.nih.gov/pubmed/36216942.
240. Fang J, Yu CH, Li XJ, Yao JM, Fang ZY, Yoon SH, Yu WY. Gut dysbiosis in nonalcoholic fatty liver disease: pathogenesis, diagnosis, and therapeutic implications. Front Cell Infect Microbiol. 2022;12:997018. PMCID: PMC9679376. http://www.ncbi.nlm.nih.gov/pubmed/36425787.
241. Thomas S, Izard J, Walsh E, Batich K, Chongsathidkiet P, Clarke G, Sela DA, Muller AJ, Mullin JM, Albert K, Gilligan JP, DiGuilio K, Dilbarova R, Alexander W, Prendergast GC. The host microbiome regulates and maintains human health: a primer and perspective for non-microbiologists. Cancer Res.

2017;77(8):1783–812. PMCID: PMC5392374. http://www.ncbi.nlm.nih.gov/pubmed/28292977.
242. Human Microbiome Project – NIH Human Microbiome Project Consortium Publication and Presentation Policies. https://commonfund.nih.gov/hmp/presentationpolicies.
243. Zhang Z, Tang H, Chen P, Xie H, Tao Y. Demystifying the manipulation of host immunity, metabolism, and extraintestinal tumors by the gut microbiome. Signal Transduct Target Ther. 2019;4:41. PMCID: PMC6799818. http://www.ncbi.nlm.nih.gov/pubmed/31637019.
244. NIH Human Microbiome Portfolio Analysis Team. A review of 10 years of human microbiome research activities at the US National Institutes of Health, fiscal years 2007-2016. Microbiome. 2019;7(1):31. PMCID: PMC6391833. http://www.ncbi.nlm.nih.gov/pubmed/30808411.
245. Mills S, Stanton C, Lane JA, Smith GJ, Ross RP. Precision nutrition and the microbiome, Part I: Current state of the science. Nutrients. 2019;11(4):923. PMCID: PMC6520976. http://www.ncbi.nlm.nih.gov/pubmed/31022973.
246. Sinha R, Ahsan H, Blaser M, Caporaso JG, Carmical JR, Chan AT, Fodor A, Gail MH, Harris CC, Helzlsouer K, Huttenhower C, Knight R, Kong HH, Lai GY, Hutchinson DLS, Le Marchand L, Li H, Orlich MJ, Shi J, Truelove A, Verma M, Vogtmann E, White O, Willett W, Zheng W, Mahabir S, Abnet C. Next steps in studying the human microbiome and health in prospective studies, Bethesda, MD, May 16-17, 2017. Microbiome. 2018;6(1):210. PMCID: PMC6257978. http://www.ncbi.nlm.nih.gov/pubmed/30477563.
247. IHMS. https://human-microbiome.org/index.php?id=25.
248. Dockray GJ. Gastrointestinal hormones and the dialogue between gut and brain. J Physiol. 2014;592(14):2927–41. PMCID: PMC4214649. http://www.ncbi.nlm.nih.gov/pubmed/24566540.
249. Gérard P. Gut microbiota and obesity. Cell Mol Life Sci. 2016;73(1):147–62. PMCID: PMC11108539. http://www.ncbi.nlm.nih.gov/pubmed/26459447.
250. Andersson EA, Mallard C, Ek CJ. Circulating tight-junction proteins are potential biomarkers for blood-brain barrier function in a model of neonatal hypoxic/ischemic brain injury. Fluids Barriers CNS. 2021;18(1):7. PMCID: PMC7877092. http://www.ncbi.nlm.nih.gov/pubmed/33568200.
251. Braniste V, Al-Asmakh M, Kowal C, Anuar F, Abbaspour A, Tóth M, Korecka A, Bakocevic N, Ng LG, Kundu P, Gulyás B, Halldin C, Hultenby K, Nilsson H, Hebert H, Volpe BT, Diamond B, Pettersson S. The gut microbiota influences blood-brain barrier permeability in mice. Sci Transl Med. 2014;6(263):263ra158. PMCID: PMC4396848. http://www.ncbi.nlm.nih.gov/pubmed/25411471.
252. Takata F, Nakagawa S, Matsumoto J, Dohgu S. Blood-brain barrier dysfunction amplifies the development of neuroinflammation: understanding of cellular events in brain microvascular endothelial cells for prevention and treatment of BBB dysfunction. Front Cell Neurosci. 2021;15:661838. PMCID: PMC8475767. http://www.ncbi.nlm.nih.gov/pubmed/34588955.
253. Sweeney MD, Zhao Z, Montagne A, Nelson AR, Zlokovic BV. Blood-brain barrier: from physiology to disease and back. Physiol Rev. 2019;99(1):21–78. PMCID: PMC6335099. http://www.ncbi.nlm.nih.gov/pubmed/30280653.
254. Anand N, Gorantla VR, Chidambaram SB. The role of gut dysbiosis in the pathophysiology of neuropsychiatric disorders. Cells. 2022;12(1):54. PMCID: PMC9818777. http://www.ncbi.nlm.nih.gov/pubmed/36611848.
255. Nakhal MM, Yassin LK, Alyaqoubi R, Saeed S, Alderei A, Alhammadi A, Alshehhi M, Almehairbi A, Al Houqani S, BaniYas S, Qanadilo H, Ali BR, Shehab S, Statsenko Y, Meribout S, Sadek B, Akour A, Hamad MIK. The microbiota-gut-brain axis and neurological disorders: a comprehensive review. Life. 2024;14(10):1234. PMCID: PMC11508655. http://www.ncbi.nlm.nih.gov/pubmed/39459534.
256. Ribichini E, Scalese G, Mocci C, Severi C. Gut-brain axis and psychopathology: exploring the impact of diet with a focus on the low-FODMAP approach. Nutrients. 2024;16(20):3515. PMCID: PMC11510627. http://www.ncbi.nlm.nih.gov/pubmed/39458509.
257. Latorre R, Sternini C, De Giorgio R, Greenwood-Van Meerveld B. Enteroendocrine cells: a review of their role in brain-gut communication. Neurogastroenterol Motil. 2016;28(5):620–30. PMCID: PMC4842178. http://www.ncbi.nlm.nih.gov/pubmed/26691223.
258. Caspani G, Kennedy S, Foster JA, Swann J. Gut microbial metabolites in depression: understanding the biochemical mechanisms. Microb Cell. 2019;6(10):454–81. PMCID: PMC6780009. http://www.ncbi.nlm.nih.gov/pubmed/31646148.
259. Gribble FM, Reimann F. Enteroendocrine cells: chemosensors in the intestinal epithelium. Annu Rev Physiol. 2016;78:277–99. PMID: 26442437. http://www.ncbi.nlm.nih.gov/pubmed/26442437.
260. Psichas A, Reimann F, Gribble FM. Gut chemosensing mechanisms. J Clin Invest. 2015;125(3):908–17. PMCID: PMC4362249. http://www.ncbi.nlm.nih.gov/pubmed/25664852.
261. De Palma G, Collins SM, Bercik P. The microbiota-gut-brain axis in functional gastrointestinal disorders. Gut Microbes. 2014;5(3):419–29. PMCID: PMC4153782. http://www.ncbi.nlm.nih.gov/pubmed/24921926.
262. Bravo JA, Julio-Pieper M, Forsythe P, Kunze W, Dinan TG, Bienenstock J, Cryan JF. Communication between gastrointestinal bacteria and the nervous system. Curr Opin Pharmacol. 2012;12(6):667–72. PMID: 23041079. http://www.ncbi.nlm.nih.gov/pubmed/23041079.
263. Sasaki-Hamada S, Nakamura R, Nakao Y, Akimoto T, Sanai E, Nagai M, Horiguchi M, Yamashita C, Oka JI. Antidepressant-like effects exerted by the intranasal administration of a glucagon-like peptide-2 derivative containing cell-penetrating peptides and a penetration-accelerating sequence in mice. Peptides. 2017;87:64–70. PMID: 27894924. http://www.ncbi.nlm.nih.gov/pubmed/27894924.
264. Scott AJ, Alexander JL, Merrifield CA, Cunningham D, Jobin C, Brown R, Alverdy J, O'Keefe SJ, Gaskins HR, Teare J, Yu J, Hughes DJ, Verstraelen H, Burton J, O'Toole PW, Rosenberg DW, Marchesi JR, Kinross JM. International Cancer Microbiome Consortium consensus statement on the role of the human microbiome in carcinogenesis. Gut. 2019;68(9):1624–32. PMCID: PMC6709773. http://www.ncbi.nlm.nih.gov/pubmed/31092590.
265. Bellono NW, Bayrer JR, Leitch DB, Castro J, Zhang C, O'Donnell TA, Brierley SM, Ingraham HA, Julius D. Enterochromaffin cells are gut chemosensors that couple to sensory neural pathways. Cell. 2017;170(1):185–198.e16. PMCID: PMC5839326. http://www.ncbi.nlm.nih.gov/pubmed/28648659.
266. Honda K, Littman DR. The microbiota in adaptive immune homeostasis and disease. Nature. 2016;535(7610):75–84. PMID: 27383982. http://www.ncbi.nlm.nih.gov/pubmed/27383982.
267. Ferreira CM, Vieira AT, Vinolo MAR, Oliveira FA, Curi R, Martins FDS. The central role of the gut microbiota in chronic inflammatory diseases. J Immunol Res. 2014;2014:689492. PMCID: PMC4189530. http://www.ncbi.nlm.nih.gov/pubmed/25309932.
268. Carabotti M, Scirocco A, Maselli MA, Severi C. The gut-brain axis: interactions between enteric microbiota, central and enteric nervous systems. Ann Gastroenterol. 2015;28(2):203–9. PMCID: PMC4367209. http://www.ncbi.nlm.nih.gov/pubmed/25830558.
269. Kentish SJ, Page AJ. Plasticity of gastro-intestinal vagal afferent endings. Physiol Behav. 2014;136:170–8. PMID: 24657740. http://www.ncbi.nlm.nih.gov/pubmed/24657740.
270. O'Malley D. Endocrine regulation of gut function – a role for glucagon-like peptide-1 in the pathophysiology of irritable bowel syndrome. Exp Physiol. 2019;104(1):3–10. PMID: 30444291. http://www.ncbi.nlm.nih.gov/pubmed/30444291.

271. Ghosal S, Myers B, Herman JP. Role of central glucagon-like peptide-1 in stress regulation. Physiol Behav. 2013;122:201–7. PMCID: PMC3778098. http://www.ncbi.nlm.nih.gov/pubmed/23623992.
272. Holzer P, Reichmann F, Farzi A. Neuropeptide Y, Peptide YY and pancreatic polypeptide in the gut-brain axis. Neuropeptides. 2012;46(6):261–74. PMCID: PMC3516703. http://www.ncbi.nlm.nih.gov/pubmed/22979996.
273. Wang W, Xu T, Chen X, Dong K, Du C, Sun J, Shi C, Li X, Yang Y, Li H, Xu ZQD. NPY receptor 2 mediates NPY antidepressant effect in the mPFC of LPS rat by suppressing NLRP3 signaling pathway. Mediat Inflamm. 2019;2019:7898095. PMCID: PMC6815592. http://www.ncbi.nlm.nih.gov/pubmed/31736656.
274. Reichmann F, Holzer P. Neuropeptide Y: a stressful review. Neuropeptides. 2016;55:99–109. PMCID: PMC4830398. http://www.ncbi.nlm.nih.gov/pubmed/26441327.
275. Vialou V, Bagot RC, Cahill ME, Ferguson D, Robison AJ, Dietz DM, Fallon B, Mazei-Robison M, Ku SM, Harrigan E, Winstanley CA, Joshi T, Feng J, Berton O, Nestler EJ. Prefrontal cortical circuit for depression- and anxiety-related behaviors mediated by cholecystokinin: role of ΔFosB. J Neurosci. 2014;34(11):3878–87. PMCID: PMC3951691. http://www.ncbi.nlm.nih.gov/pubmed/24623766.
276. Bauer PV, Hamr SC, Duca FA. Regulation of energy balance by a gut-brain axis and involvement of the gut microbiota. Cell Mol Life Sci. 2016;73(4):737–55. PMCID: PMC11108299. http://www.ncbi.nlm.nih.gov/pubmed/26542800.
277. Waters RP, Rivalan M, Bangasser DA, Deussing JM, Ising M, Wood SK, Holsboer F, Summers CH. Evidence for the role of corticotropin-releasing factor in major depressive disorder. Neurosci Biobehav Rev. 2015;58:63–78. PMCID: PMC4828243. http://www.ncbi.nlm.nih.gov/pubmed/26271720.
278. Aubry JM. CRF system and mood disorders. J Chem Neuroanat. 2013;54:20–4. PMID: 24060608. http://www.ncbi.nlm.nih.gov/pubmed/24060608.
279. Moura D, Canavarro MC, Figueiredo-Braga M. Oxytocin and depression in the perinatal period-a systematic review. Arch Womens Ment Health. 2016;19(4):561–70. PMID: 27295067. http://www.ncbi.nlm.nih.gov/pubmed/27295067.
280. Leng G, Ludwig M. Intranasal oxytocin: myths and delusions. Biol Psychiatry. 2016;79(3):243–50. PMID: 26049207. http://www.ncbi.nlm.nih.gov/pubmed/26049207.
281. Olff M, Frijling JL, Kubzansky LD, Bradley B, Ellenbogen MA, Cardoso C, Bartz JA, Yee JR, van Zuiden M. The role of oxytocin in social bonding, stress regulation and mental health: an update on the moderating effects of context and interindividual differences. Psychoneuroendocrinology. 2013;38(9):1883–94. PMID: 23856187. http://www.ncbi.nlm.nih.gov/pubmed/23856187.
282. Norman GJ, Karelina K, Morris JS, Zhang N, Cochran M, Courtney DeVries A. Social interaction prevents the development of depressive-like behavior post nerve injury in mice: a potential role for oxytocin. Psychosom Med. 2010;72(6):519–26. PMID: 20466999. http://www.ncbi.nlm.nih.gov/pubmed/20466999.
283. Meyer RM, Burgos-Robles A, Liu E, Correia SS, Goosens KA. A ghrelin-growth hormone axis drives stress-induced vulnerability to enhanced fear. Mol Psychiatry. 2014;19(12):1284–94. PMCID: PMC3988273. http://www.ncbi.nlm.nih.gov/pubmed/24126924.
284. Mawe GM, Hoffman JM. Serotonin signalling in the gutDOUBLEHYPHENfunctions, dysfunctions and therapeutic targets. Nat Rev Gastroenterol Hepatol. 2013;10(8):473–86. PMCID: PMC4048923. http://www.ncbi.nlm.nih.gov/pubmed/23797870.
285. Burokas A, Arboleya S, Moloney RD, Peterson VL, Murphy K, Clarke G, Stanton C, Dinan TG, Cryan JF. Targeting the microbiota-gut-brain axis: prebiotics have anxiolytic and antidepressant-like effects and reverse the impact of chronic stress in mice. Biol Psychiatry. 2017;82(7):472–87. PMID: 28242013. http://www.ncbi.nlm.nih.gov/pubmed/28242013.
286. Fröhlich EE, Farzi A, Mayerhofer R, Reichmann F, Jačan A, Wagner B, Zinser E, Bordag N, Magnes C, Fröhlich E, Kashofer K, Gorkiewicz G, Holzer P. Cognitive impairment by antibiotic-induced gut dysbiosis: analysis of gut microbiota-brain communication. Brain Behav Immun. 2016;56:140–55. PMCID: PMC5014122. http://www.ncbi.nlm.nih.gov/pubmed/26923630.
287. Cummings DE, Overduin J. Gastrointestinal regulation of food intake. J Clin Invest. 2007;117(1):13–23. PMCID: PMC1716217. http://www.ncbi.nlm.nih.gov/pubmed/17200702.
288. Gariepy G, Wang J, Lesage A, Schmitz N. The interaction of obesity and psychological distress on disability. Soc Psychiatry Psychiatr Epidemiol. 2010;45(5):531–40. PMID: 19575138. http://www.ncbi.nlm.nih.gov/pubmed/19575138.
289. Patterson E, Ryan PM, Cryan JF, Dinan TG, Ross RP, Fitzgerald GF, Stanton C. Gut microbiota, obesity and diabetes. Postgrad Med J. 2016;92(1087):286–300. PMID: 26912499. http://www.ncbi.nlm.nih.gov/pubmed/26912499.
290. Inoue Y, Shimojo N. Microbiome/microbiota and allergies. Semin Immunopathol. 2015;37(1):57–64. PMID: 25326106. http://www.ncbi.nlm.nih.gov/pubmed/25326106.
291. Shamriz O, Mizrahi H, Werbner M, Shoenfeld Y, Avni O, Koren O. Microbiota at the crossroads of autoimmunity. Autoimmun Rev. 2016;15(9):859–69. PMID: 27392501. http://www.ncbi.nlm.nih.gov/pubmed/27392501.
292. Rapozo DCM, Bernardazzi C, de Souza HSP. Diet and microbiota in inflammatory bowel disease: the gut in disharmony. World J Gastroenterol. 2017;23(12):2124–40. PMCID: PMC5374124. http://www.ncbi.nlm.nih.gov/pubmed/28405140.
293. O'Mahony SM, Clarke G, Dinan TG, Cryan JF. Irritable bowel syndrome and stress-related psychiatric co-morbidities: focus on early life stress. Handb Exp Pharmacol. 2017;239:219–46. PMID: 28233180. http://www.ncbi.nlm.nih.gov/pubmed/28233180.
294. Inserra A, Rogers GB, Licinio J, Wong ML. The microbiota-inflammasome hypothesis of major depression. BioEssays. 2018;40(9):e1800027. PMID: 30004130. http://www.ncbi.nlm.nih.gov/pubmed/30004130.
295. Dinan TG, Cryan JF. Melancholic microbes: a link between gut microbiota and depression? Neurogastroenterol Motil. 2013;25(9):713–9. PMID: 23910373. http://www.ncbi.nlm.nih.gov/pubmed/23910373.
296. Koopman M, El Aidy S, MIDtrauma consortium. Depressed gut? The microbiota-diet-inflammation trialogue in depression. Curr Opin Psychiatry. 2017;30(5):369–77. PMID: 28654462. http://www.ncbi.nlm.nih.gov/pubmed/28654462.
297. Neufeld KAM, Kang N, Bienenstock J, Foster JA. Effects of intestinal microbiota on anxiety-like behavior. Commun Integr Biol. 2011;4(4):492–4. PMCID: PMC3181531. http://www.ncbi.nlm.nih.gov/pubmed/21966581.
298. Bäckhed F, Ley RE, Sonnenburg JL, Peterson DA, Gordon JI. Host-bacterial mutualism in the human intestine. Science. 2005;307(5717):1915–20. PMID: 15790844. http://www.ncbi.nlm.nih.gov/pubmed/15790844.
299. Cryan JF, Dinan TG. Mind-altering microorganisms: the impact of the gut microbiota on brain and behaviour. Nat Rev Neurosci. 2012;13(10):701–12. PMID: 22968153. http://www.ncbi.nlm.nih.gov/pubmed/22968153.
300. Rajilić-Stojanović M. Function of the microbiota. Best Pract Res Clin Gastroenterol. 2013;27(1):5–16. PMID: 23768548. http://www.ncbi.nlm.nih.gov/pubmed/23768548.
301. Gomez-Arango LF, Barrett HL, McIntyre HD, Callaway LK, Morrison M, Nitert MD. Contributions of the maternal oral and gut microbiome to placental microbial colonization in overweight

and obese pregnant women. Sci Rep. 2017;7(1):2860. PMCID: PMC5460277. http://www.ncbi.nlm.nih.gov/pubmed/28588199.
302. Moore RE, Townsend SD. Temporal development of the infant gut microbiome. Open Biol. 2019;9(9):190128. PMCID: PMC6769289. http://www.ncbi.nlm.nih.gov/pubmed/31506017.
303. Human Microbiome Project Consortium. Structure, function and diversity of the healthy human microbiome. Nature. 2012;486(7402):207–14. PMCID: PMC3564958. http://www.ncbi.nlm.nih.gov/pubmed/22699609.
304. Aagaard K, Riehle K, Ma J, Segata N, Mistretta TA, Coarfa C, Raza S, Rosenbaum S, Van den Veyver I, Milosavljevic A, Gevers D, Huttenhower C, Petrosino J, Versalovic J. A metagenomic approach to characterization of the vaginal microbiome signature in pregnancy. PLoS One. 2012;7(6):e36466. PMCID: PMC3374618. http://www.ncbi.nlm.nih.gov/pubmed/22719832.
305. Human Microbiome Project Consortium. A framework for human microbiome research. Nature. 2012;486(7402):215–21. PMCID: PMC3377744. http://www.ncbi.nlm.nih.gov/pubmed/22699610.
306. Aagaard K, Petrosino J, Keitel W, Watson M, Katancik J, Garcia N, Patel S, Cutting M, Madden T, Hamilton H, Harris E, Gevers D, Simone G, McInnes P, Versalovic J. The Human Microbiome Project strategy for comprehensive sampling of the human microbiome and why it matters. FASEB J. 2013;27(3):1012–22. PMCID: PMC3574278. http://www.ncbi.nlm.nih.gov/pubmed/23165986.
307. Aagaard K, Ma J, Antony KM, Ganu R, Petrosino J, Versalovic J. The placenta harbors a unique microbiome. Sci Transl Med. 2014;6(237):237ra65. PMCID: PMC4929217. http://www.ncbi.nlm.nih.gov/pubmed/24848255.
308. de Goffau MC, Lager S, Sovio U, Gaccioli F, Cook E, Peacock SJ, Parkhill J, Charnock-Jones DS, Smith GCS. Human placenta has no microbiome but can contain potential pathogens. Nature. 2019;572(7769):329–34. PMCID: PMC6697540. http://www.ncbi.nlm.nih.gov/pubmed/31367035.
309. Jiménez E, Fernández L, Marín ML, Martín R, Odriozola JM, Nueno-Palop C, Narbad A, Olivares M, Xaus J, Rodríguez JM. Isolation of commensal bacteria from umbilical cord blood of healthy neonates born by cesarean section. Curr Microbiol. 2005;51(4):270–4. PMID: 16187156. http://www.ncbi.nlm.nih.gov/pubmed/16187156.
310. Jiménez E, Marín ML, Martín R, Odriozola JM, Olivares M, Xaus J, Fernández L, Rodríguez JM. Is meconium from healthy newborns actually sterile? Res Microbiol. 2008;159(3):187–93. PMID: 18281199. http://www.ncbi.nlm.nih.gov/pubmed/18281199.
311. Nguyen DP, Gerber S, Hohlfeld P, Sandrine G, Witkin SS. Mycoplasma hominis in mid-trimester amniotic fluid: relation to pregnancy outcome. J Perinat Med. 2004;32(4):323–6. PMID: 15346817. http://www.ncbi.nlm.nih.gov/pubmed/15346817.
312. Perez-Muñoz ME, Arrieta MC, Ramer-Tait AE, Walter J. A critical assessment of the "sterile womb" and "in utero colonization" hypotheses: implications for research on the pioneer infant microbiome. Microbiome. 2017;5(1):48. PMCID: PMC5410102. http://www.ncbi.nlm.nih.gov/pubmed/28454555.
313. Stinson LF, Boyce MC, Payne MS, Keelan JA. The not-so-sterile womb: evidence that the human fetus is exposed to bacteria prior to birth. Front Microbiol. 2019;10:1124. PMCID: PMC6558212. http://www.ncbi.nlm.nih.gov/pubmed/31231319.
314. Reyman M, van Houten MA, van Baarle D, Bosch AATM, Man WH, Chu MLJN, Arp K, Watson RL, Sanders EAM, Fuentes S, Bogaert D. Impact of delivery mode-associated gut microbiota dynamics on health in the first year of life. Nat Commun. 2019;10(1):4997. PMCID: PMC6825150. http://www.ncbi.nlm.nih.gov/pubmed/31676793.
315. Dominguez-Bello MG, Costello EK, Contreras M, Magris M, Hidalgo G, Fierer N, Knight R. Delivery mode shapes the acquisition and structure of the initial microbiota across multiple body habitats in newborns. Proc Natl Acad Sci USA. 2010;107(26):11971–5. PMCID: PMC2900693. http://www.ncbi.nlm.nih.gov/pubmed/20566857.
316. Chu DM, Ma J, Prince AL, Antony KM, Seferovic MD, Aagaard KM. Maturation of the infant microbiome community structure and function across multiple body sites and in relation to mode of delivery. Nat Med. 2017;23(3):314–26. PMCID: PMC5345907. http://www.ncbi.nlm.nih.gov/pubmed/28112736.
317. Milani C, Duranti S, Bottacini F, Casey E, Turroni F, Mahony J, Belzer C, Delgado Palacio S, Arboleya Montes S, Mancabelli L, Lugli GA, Rodriguez JM, Bode L, de Vos W, Gueimonde M, Margolles A, van Sinderen D, Ventura M. The first microbial colonizers of the human gut: composition, activities, and health implications of the infant gut microbiota. Microbiol Mol Biol Rev. 2017;81(4):e00036-17. PMCID: PMC5706746. http://www.ncbi.nlm.nih.gov/pubmed/29118049.
318. Olszak T, An D, Zeissig S, Vera MP, Richter J, Franke A, Glickman JN, Siebert R, Baron RM, Kasper DL, Blumberg RS. Microbial exposure during early life has persistent effects on natural killer T cell function. Science. 2012;336(6080):489–93. PMCID: PMC3437652. http://www.ncbi.nlm.nih.gov/pubmed/22442383.
319. Diaz Heijtz R, Wang S, Anuar F, Qian Y, Björkholm B, Samuelsson A, Hibberd ML, Forssberg H, Pettersson S. Normal gut microbiota modulates brain development and behavior. Proc Natl Acad Sci USA. 2011;108(7):3047–52. PMCID: PMC3041077. http://www.ncbi.nlm.nih.gov/pubmed/21282636.
320. Clarke G, Grenham S, Scully P, Fitzgerald P, Moloney RD, Shanahan F, Dinan TG, Cryan JF. The microbiome-gut-brain axis during early life regulates the hippocampal serotonergic system in a sex-dependent manner. Mol Psychiatry. 2013;18(6):666–73. PMID: 22688187. http://www.ncbi.nlm.nih.gov/pubmed/22688187.
321. Sohail MU, Yassine HM, Sohail A, Thani AAA. Impact of physical exercise on gut microbiome, inflammation, and the pathobiology of metabolic disorders. Rev Diabet Stud. 2019;15:35–48. PMCID: PMC6760895. http://www.ncbi.nlm.nih.gov/pubmed/31380886.
322. Das B, Nair GB. Homeostasis and dysbiosis of the gut microbiome in health and disease. J Biosci. 2019;44(5):117. PMID: 31719226. http://www.ncbi.nlm.nih.gov/pubmed/31719226.
323. Welly RJ, Liu TW, Zidon TM, Rowles JL, Park YM, Smith TN, Swanson KS, Padilla J, Vieira-Potter VJ. Comparison of diet versus exercise on metabolic function and gut microbiota in obese rats. Med Sci Sports Exerc. 2016;48(9):1688–98. PMCID: PMC4987217. http://www.ncbi.nlm.nih.gov/pubmed/27128671.
324. Aleksandrova K, Romero-Mosquera B, Hernandez V. Diet, gut microbiome and epigenetics: emerging links with inflammatory bowel diseases and prospects for management and prevention. Nutrients. 2017;9(9):962. PMCID: PMC5622722. http://www.ncbi.nlm.nih.gov/pubmed/28867793.
325. Miro-Blanch J, Yanes O. Epigenetic regulation at the interplay between gut microbiota and host metabolism. Front Genet. 2019;10:638. PMCID: PMC6628876. http://www.ncbi.nlm.nih.gov/pubmed/31338107.
326. Montiel-Castro AJ, González-Cervantes RM, Bravo-Ruiseco G, Pacheco-López G. The microbiota-gut-brain axis: neurobehavioral correlates, health and sociality. Front Integr Neurosci. 2013;7:70. PMCID: PMC3791857. http://www.ncbi.nlm.nih.gov/pubmed/24109440.
327. Mason MR, Nagaraja HN, Camerlengo T, Joshi V, Kumar PS. Deep sequencing identifies ethnicity-specific bacterial signatures in the oral microbiome. PLoS One. 2013;8(10):e77287. PMCID: PMC3806732. http://www.ncbi.nlm.nih.gov/pubmed/24194878.
328. Rajilić-Stojanović M, de Vos WM. The first 1000 cultured species of the human gastrointestinal microbiota. FEMS Microbiol Rev. 2014;38(5):996–1047. PMCID: PMC4262072. http://www.ncbi.nlm.nih.gov/pubmed/24861948.

329. Burki F, Roger AJ, Brown MW, Simpson AGB. The new tree of eukaryotes. Trends Ecol Evol. 2020;35(1):43–55. https://www.cell.com/trends/ecology-evolution/fulltext/S0169-5347(19)30257-5?_returnURL=https%3A%2F%2Flinkinghub.elsevier.com%2Fretrieve%2Fpii%2FS0169534719302575%3Fshowall%3Dtrue.
330. Aparici-Carratalá D, Esclapez J, Bautista V, Bonete M-J, Camacho M. Archaea: current and potential biotechnological applications. Res Microbiol. 2023;174(7):104080. https://www.sciencedirect.com/science/article/pii/S0923250823000554?via%3Dihub.
331. Duller S, Moissl-Eichinger C. Archaea in the human microbiome and potential effects on human infectious disease. Emerg Infect Dis. 2024;30(8):1505–13. https://wwwnc.cdc.gov/eid/article/30/8/24-0181_article.
332. Gaci N, Borrel G, Tottey W, O'Toole PW, Brugère JF. Archaea and the human gut: new beginning of an old story. World J Gastroenterol. 2014;20(43):16062–78. PMCID: PMC4239492. http://www.ncbi.nlm.nih.gov/pubmed/25473158.
333. Verbunt J, Jocken J, Blaak E, Savelkoul P, Stassen F. Gut-bacteria derived membrane vesicles and host metabolic health: a narrative review. Gut Microbes. 2024;16(1):2359515. PMCID: PMC11141482. http://www.ncbi.nlm.nih.gov/pubmed/38808455.
334. Chen Z, Jin W, Hoover A, Chao Y, Ma Y. Decoding the microbiome: advances in genetic manipulation for gut bacteria. Trends Microbiol. 2023;31(11):1143–61. PMID: 37394299. http://www.ncbi.nlm.nih.gov/pubmed/37394299.
335. Nohesara S, Abdolmaleky HM, Zhou JR, Thiagalingam S. Microbiota-induced epigenetic alterations in depressive disorders are targets for nutritional and probiotic therapies. Genes (Basel). 2023;14(12):2217. PMCID: PMC10742434. http://www.ncbi.nlm.nih.gov/pubmed/38137038.
336. Paterson MJ, Oh S, Underhill DM. Host-microbe interactions: commensal fungi in the gut. Curr Opin Microbiol. 2017;40:131–7. PMCID: PMC5733715. http://www.ncbi.nlm.nih.gov/pubmed/29175338.
337. Li J, Chen D, Yu B, He J, Zheng P, Mao X, Yu J, Luo J, Tian G, Huang Z, Luo Y. Fungi in gastrointestinal tracts of human and mice: from community to functions - PubMed. Microb Ecol. 2018;75(4):821–9. PMID: 29110065.
338. Sam QH, Chang MW, Chai LYA. The fungal mycobiome and its interaction with gut bacteria in the host. Int J Mol Sci. 2017;18(2):330. PMCID: PMC5343866. http://www.ncbi.nlm.nih.gov/pubmed/28165395.
339. Scanlan PD, Marchesi JR. Micro-eukaryotic diversity of the human distal gut microbiota: qualitative assessment using culture-dependent and -independent analysis of faeces. ISME J. 2008;2(12):1183–93. PMID: 18670396. http://www.ncbi.nlm.nih.gov/pubmed/18670396.
340. Chibani CM, Mahnert A, Borrel G, Almeida A, Werner A, Brugère JF, Gribaldo S, Finn RD, Schmitz RA, Moissl-Eichinger C. A catalogue of 1,167 genomes from the human gut archaeome. Nat Microbiol. 2022;7(1):48–61. https://doi.org/10.1038/s41564-021-01020-9. Epub 2021 Dec 30. Erratum in: 2022;7(2):339. doi: 10.1038/s41564-022-01061-8. PMID: 34969981; PMCID: PMC8727293. https://pubmed.ncbi.nlm.nih.gov/34969981/.
341. Chibani CM, Mahnert A, Borrel G, Almeida A, Werner A, Brugère JF, Gribaldo S, Finn RD, Schmitz RA, Moissl-Eichinger C. Publisher correction: a catalogue of 1,167 genomes from the human gut archaeome. Nat Microbiol. 2022;7(2):339. https://doi.org/10.1038/s41564-022-01061-8. Erratum for: Nat Microbiol. 2022;7(1):48–61. doi: 10.1038/s41564-021-01020-9. PMID: 35013594; PMCID: PMC8813613. https://pubmed.ncbi.nlm.nih.gov/35013594/.
342. Ungaro F, Massimino L, D'Alessio S, Danese S. The gut virome in inflammatory bowel disease pathogenesis: from metagenomics to novel therapeutic approaches. United European Gastroenterol J. 2019;7(8):999–1007. PMCID: PMC6794698. http://www.ncbi.nlm.nih.gov/pubmed/31662858.
343. Hidalgo-Cantabrana C, Delgado S, Ruiz L, Ruas-Madiedo P, Sánchez B, Margolles A. Bifidobacteria and their health-promoting effects. Microbiol Spectr. 2017;5(3). PMID: 28643627. http://www.ncbi.nlm.nih.gov/pubmed/28643627.
344. Sánchez B, Delgado S, Blanco-Míguez A, Lourenço A, Gueimonde M, Margolles A. Probiotics, gut microbiota, and their influence on host health and disease. Mol Nutr Food Res. 2017;61(1). PMID: 27500859. http://www.ncbi.nlm.nih.gov/pubmed/27500859.
345. Biragyn A, Ferrucci L. Gut dysbiosis: a potential link between increased cancer risk in ageing and inflammaging. Lancet Oncol. 2018;19(6):e295–304. PMCID: PMC6047065. http://www.ncbi.nlm.nih.gov/pubmed/29893261.
346. Nayfach S, Shi ZJ, Seshadri R, Pollard KS, Kyrpides NC. New insights from uncultivated genomes of the global human gut microbiome. Nature. 2019;568(7753):505–10. PMCID: PMC6784871. http://www.ncbi.nlm.nih.gov/pubmed/30867587.
347. Davis HC. Can the gastrointestinal microbiota be modulated by dietary fibre to treat obesity? Ir J Med Sci. 2018;187(2):393–402. PMID: 29038988. http://www.ncbi.nlm.nih.gov/pubmed/29038988.
348. O'Mahony SM, Clarke G, McKernan DP, Bravo JA, Dinan TG, Cryan JF. Differential visceral nociceptive, behavioural and neurochemical responses to an immune challenge in the stress-sensitive Wistar Kyoto rat strain. Behav Brain Res. 2013;253:310–7. PMID: 23872358. http://www.ncbi.nlm.nih.gov/pubmed/23872358.
349. Ostaff MJ, Stange EF, Wehkamp J. Antimicrobial peptides and gut microbiota in homeostasis and pathology. EMBO Mol Med. 2013;5(10):1465–83. PMCID: PMC3799574. http://www.ncbi.nlm.nih.gov/pubmed/24039130.
350. Lippert K, Kedenko L, Antonielli L, Kedenko I, Gemeier C, Leitner M, Kautzky-Willer A, Paulweber B, Hackl E. Gut microbiota dysbiosis associated with glucose metabolism disorders and the metabolic syndrome in older adults. Benef Microbes. 2017;8(4):545–56. PMID: 28701081. http://www.ncbi.nlm.nih.gov/pubmed/28701081.
351. Golubeva AV, Joyce SA, Moloney G, Burokas A, Sherwin E, Arboleya S, Flynn I, Khochanskiy D, Moya-Pérez A, Peterson V, Rea K, Murphy K, Makarova O, Buravkov S, Hyland NP, Stanton C, Clarke G, Gahan CGM, Dinan TG, Cryan JF. Microbiota-related changes in bile acid & tryptophan metabolism are associated with gastrointestinal dysfunction in a mouse model of autism. EBioMedicine. 2017;24:166–78. PMCID: PMC5652137. http://www.ncbi.nlm.nih.gov/pubmed/28965876.
352. Bhat MI, Kapila R. Dietary metabolites derived from gut microbiota: critical modulators of epigenetic changes in mammals. Nutr Rev. 2017;75(5):374–89. PMID: 28444216. http://www.ncbi.nlm.nih.gov/pubmed/28444216.
353. Caspani G, Swann J. Small talk: microbial metabolites involved in the signaling from microbiota to brain. Curr Opin Pharmacol. 2019;48:99–106. PMID: 31525562. http://www.ncbi.nlm.nih.gov/pubmed/31525562.
354. Grosse J, Reimann F, Gribble FM. Short-chain fatty acids stimulate glucagon-like peptide-1 secretion via the G-protein-coupled receptor FFAR2. Diabetes. 2012;61(2):364–71. PMCID: PMC3266401. http://www.ncbi.nlm.nih.gov/pubmed/22190648.
355. Ríos-Covián D, Ruas-Madiedo P, Margolles A, Gueimonde M, de Los Reyes-Gavilán CG, Salazar N. Intestinal short chain fatty acids and their link with diet and human health. Front Microbiol. 2016;7:185. PMCID: PMC4756104. http://www.ncbi.nlm.nih.gov/pubmed/26925050.
356. Milani C, Lugli GA, Duranti S, Turroni F, Mancabelli L, Ferrario C, Mangifesta M, Hevia A, Viappiani A, Scholz M, Arioli S, Sanchez B, Lane J, Ward DV, Hickey R, Mora D, Segata N,

Margolles A, van Sinderen D, Ventura M. Bifidobacteria exhibit social behavior through carbohydrate resource sharing in the gut. Sci Rep. 2015;5:15782. PMCID: PMC4623478. http://www.ncbi.nlm.nih.gov/pubmed/26506949.

357. David LA, Maurice CF, Carmody RN, Gootenberg DB, Button JE, Wolfe BE, Ling AV, Devlin AS, Varma Y, Fischbach MA, Biddinger SB, Dutton RJ, Turnbaugh PJ. Diet rapidly and reproducibly alters the human gut microbiome. Nature. 2014;505(7484):559–63. PMCID: PMC3957428. http://www.ncbi.nlm.nih.gov/pubmed/24336217.
358. Russell WR, Gratz SW, Duncan SH, Holtrop G, Ince J, Scobbie L, Duncan G, Johnstone AM, Lobley GE, Wallace RJ, Duthie GG, Flint HJ. High-protein, reduced-carbohydrate weight-loss diets promote metabolite profiles likely to be detrimental to colonic health. Am J Clin Nutr. 2011;93(5):1062–72. PMID: 21389180. http://www.ncbi.nlm.nih.gov/pubmed/21389180.
359. Simpson HL, Campbell BJ. Review article: dietary fibre-microbiota interactions. Aliment Pharmacol Ther. 2015;42(2):158–79. PMCID: PMC4949558. http://www.ncbi.nlm.nih.gov/pubmed/26011307.
360. Neunlist M, Schemann M. Nutrient-induced changes in the phenotype and function of the enteric nervous system. J Physiol. 2014;592(14):2959–65. PMCID: PMC4214652. http://www.ncbi.nlm.nih.gov/pubmed/24907307.
361. Reigstad CS, Salmonson CE, Rainey JF, Szurszewski JH, Linden DR, Sonnenburg JL, Farrugia G, Kashyap PC. Gut microbes promote colonic serotonin production through an effect of short-chain fatty acids on enterochromaffin cells. FASEB J. 2015;29(4):1395–403. PMCID: PMC4396604. http://www.ncbi.nlm.nih.gov/pubmed/25550456.
362. Martin AM, Sun EW, Rogers GB, Keating DJ. The influence of the gut microbiome on host metabolism through the regulation of gut hormone release. Front Physiol. 2019;10:428. PMCID: PMC6477058. http://www.ncbi.nlm.nih.gov/pubmed/31057420.
363. Bertaccini G. Tissue 5-hydroxytryptamine and urinary 5-hydroxyindoleacetic acid after partial or total removal of the gastro-intestinal tract in the rat. J Physiol. 1960;153(2):239–49. PMCID: PMC1359746. http://www.ncbi.nlm.nih.gov/pubmed/16992061.
364. Grondin JA, Khan WI. Emerging roles of gut serotonin in regulation of immune response, microbiota composition and intestinal inflammation. J Can Assoc Gastroenterol. 2024;7(1):88–96. PMCID: PMC10836984. http://www.ncbi.nlm.nih.gov/pubmed/38314177.
365. Walther DJ, Bader M. A unique central tryptophan hydroxylase isoform. Biochem Pharmacol. 2003;66(9):1673–80. PMID: 14563478. http://www.ncbi.nlm.nih.gov/pubmed/14563478.
366. Côté F, Thévenot E, Fligny C, Fromes Y, Darmon M, Ripoche MA, Bayard E, Hanoun N, Saurini F, Lechat P, Dandolo L, Hamon M, Mallet J, Vodjdani G. Disruption of the nonneuronal tph1 gene demonstrates the importance of peripheral serotonin in cardiac function. Proc Natl Acad Sci USA. 2003;100(23):13525–30. PMCID: PMC263847. http://www.ncbi.nlm.nih.gov/pubmed/14597720.
367. Cirillo C, Vanden Berghe P, Tack J. Role of serotonin in gastrointestinal physiology and pathology. Minerva Endocrinol. 2011;36(4):311–24. PMID: 22322654. http://www.ncbi.nlm.nih.gov/pubmed/22322654.
368. Spohn SN, Mawe GM. Non-conventional features of peripheral serotonin signalling – the gut and beyond. Nat Rev Gastroenterol Hepatol. 2017;14(7):412–20. PMCID: PMC5672796. http://www.ncbi.nlm.nih.gov/pubmed/28487547.
369. Paulmann N, Grohmann M, Voigt JP, Bert B, Vowinckel J, Bader M, Skelin M, Jevsek M, Fink H, Rupnik M, Walther DJ. Intracellular serotonin modulates insulin secretion from pancreatic beta-cells by protein serotonylation. PLoS Biol. 2009;7(10):e1000229. PMCID: PMC2760755. http://www.ncbi.nlm.nih.gov/pubmed/19859528.
370. Kim H, Toyofuku Y, Lynn FC, Chak E, Uchida T, Mizukami H, Fujitani Y, Kawamori R, Miyatsuka T, Kosaka Y, Yang K, Honig G, van der Hart M, Kishimoto N, Wang J, Yagihashi S, Tecott LH, Watada H, German MS. Serotonin regulates pancreatic beta cell mass during pregnancy. Nat Med. 2010;16(7):804–8. PMCID: PMC2921604. http://www.ncbi.nlm.nih.gov/pubmed/20581837.
371. Stunes AK, Reseland JE, Hauso O, Kidd M, Tømmerås K, Waldum HL, Syversen U, Gustafsson BI. Adipocytes express a functional system for serotonin synthesis, reuptake and receptor activation. Diabetes Obes Metab. 2011;13(6):551–8. PMID: 21320265. http://www.ncbi.nlm.nih.gov/pubmed/21320265.
372. Chabbi-Achengli Y, Coudert AE, Callebert J, Geoffroy V, Côté F, Collet C, de Vernejoul MC. Decreased osteoclastogenesis in serotonin-deficient mice. Proc Natl Acad Sci USA. 2012;109(7):2567–72. PMCID: PMC3289318. http://www.ncbi.nlm.nih.gov/pubmed/22308416.
373. Yadav VK, Oury F, Suda N, Liu ZW, Gao XB, Confavreux C, Klemenhagen KC, Tanaka KF, Gingrich JA, Guo XE, Tecott LH, Mann JJ, Hen R, Horvath TL, Karsenty G. A serotonin-dependent mechanism explains the leptin regulation of bone mass, appetite, and energy expenditure. Cell. 2009;138(5):976–89. PMCID: PMC2768582. http://www.ncbi.nlm.nih.gov/pubmed/19737523.
374. Yadav VK, Balaji S, Suresh PS, Liu XS, Lu X, Li Z, Guo XE, Mann JJ, Balapure AK, Gershon MD, Medhamurthy R, Vidal M, Karsenty G, Ducy P. Pharmacological inhibition of gut-derived serotonin synthesis is a potential bone anabolic treatment for osteoporosis. Nat Med. 2010;16(3):308–12. PMCID: PMC2836724. http://www.ncbi.nlm.nih.gov/pubmed/20139991.
375. Furness JB. The enteric nervous system and neurogastroenterology. Nat Rev Gastroenterol Hepatol. 2012;9(5):286–94. PMID: 22392290. http://www.ncbi.nlm.nih.gov/pubmed/22392290.
376. Yoo BB, Mazmanian SK. The enteric network: interactions between the immune and nervous systems of the gut. Immunity. 2017;46(6):910–26. PMCID: PMC5551410. http://www.ncbi.nlm.nih.gov/pubmed/28636959.
377. Mansouri A, Langhans W. Enterocyte-afferent nerve interactions in dietary fat sensing. Diabetes Obes Metab. 2014;16(Suppl 1):61–7. PMID: 25200298. http://www.ncbi.nlm.nih.gov/pubmed/25200298.
378. Lin HV, Frassetto A, Kowalik EJ, Nawrocki AR, Lu MM, Kosinski JR, Hubert JA, Szeto D, Yao X, Forrest G, Marsh DJ. Butyrate and propionate protect against diet-induced obesity and regulate gut hormones via free fatty acid receptor 3-independent mechanisms. PLoS One. 2012;7(4):e35240. PMCID: PMC3323649. http://www.ncbi.nlm.nih.gov/pubmed/22506074.
379. Okano-Matsumoto S, McRoberts JA, Taché Y, Adelson DW. Electrophysiological evidence for distinct vagal pathways mediating CCK-evoked motor effects in the proximal versus distal stomach. J Physiol. 2011;589(Pt 2):371–93. PMCID: PMC3043539. http://www.ncbi.nlm.nih.gov/pubmed/21078593.
380. Banks WA, Tschöp M, Robinson SM, Heiman ML. Extent and direction of ghrelin transport across the blood-brain barrier is determined by its unique primary structure. J Pharmacol Exp Ther. 2002;302(2):822–7. PMID: 12130749. http://www.ncbi.nlm.nih.gov/pubmed/12130749.
381. Nonaka N, Shioda S, Niehoff ML, Banks WA. Characterization of blood-brain barrier permeability to PYY3-36 in the mouse. J Pharmacol Exp Ther. 2003;306(3):948–53. PMID: 12750431. http://www.ncbi.nlm.nih.gov/pubmed/12750431.
382. Whitcomb DC, Taylor IL, Vigna SR. Characterization of saturable binding sites for circulating pancreatic polypeptide in rat brain.

Am J Phys. 1990;259(4 Pt 1):G687–91. PMID: 2221079. http://www.ncbi.nlm.nih.gov/pubmed/2221079.
383. Banks WA. Peptides and the blood-brain barrier. Peptides. 2015;72:16–9. PMCID: PMC5354301. http://www.ncbi.nlm.nih.gov/pubmed/25805003.
384. Fernández-Tomé S, Marin AC, Ortega Moreno L, Baldan-Martin M, Mora-Gutiérrez I, Lanas-Gimeno A, Moreno-Monteagudo JA, Santander C, Sánchez B, Chaparro M, Gisbert JP, Bernardo D. Immunomodulatory effect of gut microbiota-derived bioactive peptides on human immune system from healthy controls and patients with inflammatory bowel disease. Nutrients. 2019;11(11):2605. PMCID: PMC6893616. http://www.ncbi.nlm.nih.gov/pubmed/31683517.
385. Banks WA. The blood-brain barrier in neuroimmunology: tales of separation and assimilation. Brain Behav Immun. 2015;44:1–8. PMCID: PMC4275374. http://www.ncbi.nlm.nih.gov/pubmed/25172555.
386. Berg CJ, Kaunitz JD. Gut chemosensing: implications for disease pathogenesis. F1000Res. 2016;5:2424. PMCID: PMC5054811. http://www.ncbi.nlm.nih.gov/pubmed/27781093.
387. Gao Z, Yin J, Zhang J, Ward RE, Martin RJ, Lefevre M, Cefalu WT, Ye J. Butyrate improves insulin sensitivity and increases energy expenditure in mice. Diabetes. 2009;58(7):1509–17. PMCID: PMC2699871. http://www.ncbi.nlm.nih.gov/pubmed/19366864.
388. Vuong HE, Yano JM, Fung TC, Hsiao EY. The microbiome and host behavior. Annu Rev Neurosci. 2017;40:21–49. PMCID: PMC6661159. http://www.ncbi.nlm.nih.gov/pubmed/28301775.
389. Pinto-Sanchez MI, Hall GB, Ghajar K, Nardelli A, Bolino C, Lau JT, Martin FP, Cominetti O, Welsh C, Rieder A, Traynor J, Gregory C, De Palma G, Pigrau M, Ford AC, Macri J, Berger B, Bergonzelli G, Surette MG, Collins SM, Moayyedi P, Bercik P. Probiotic Bifidobacterium longum NCC3001 reduces depression scores and alters brain activity: a pilot study in patients with irritable bowel syndrome. Gastroenterology. 2017;153(2):448–459.e8. PMID: 28483500. http://www.ncbi.nlm.nih.gov/pubmed/28483500.
390. Gulas E, Wysiadecki G, Strzelecki D, Gawlik-Kotelnicka O, Polguj M. Can microbiology affect psychiatry? A link between gut microbiota and psychiatric disorders. Psychiatr Pol. 2018;52(6):1023–39. PMID: 30659564. http://www.ncbi.nlm.nih.gov/pubmed/30659564.
391. Nardone G, Compare D. The psyche and gastric functions. Dig Dis. 2014;32(3):206–12. PMID: 24732184. http://www.ncbi.nlm.nih.gov/pubmed/24732184.
392. Melinder C, Hiyoshi A, Fall K, Halfvarson J, Montgomery S. Stress resilience and the risk of inflammatory bowel disease: a cohort study of men living in Sweden. BMJ Open. 2017;7(1):e014315. PMCID: PMC5278277. http://www.ncbi.nlm.nih.gov/pubmed/28130207.
393. Bailey MT, Coe CL. Maternal separation disrupts the integrity of the intestinal microflora in infant rhesus monkeys. Dev Psychobiol. 1999;35(2):146–55. PMID: 10461128. http://www.ncbi.nlm.nih.gov/pubmed/10461128.
394. Herd P, Palloni A, Rey F, Dowd JB. Social and population health science approaches to understand the human microbiome. Nat Hum Behav. 2018;2(11):808–15. PMCID: PMC6711373. http://www.ncbi.nlm.nih.gov/pubmed/31457107.
395. Oligschlaeger Y, Yadati T, Houben T, Condello Oliván CM, Shiri-Sverdlov R. Inflammatory bowel disease: a stressed "gut/feeling". Cells. 2019;8(7):659. PMCID: PMC6678997. http://www.ncbi.nlm.nih.gov/pubmed/31262067.
396. Nagpal R, Yadav H. Bacterial translocation from the gut to the distant organs: an overview. Ann Nutr Metab. 2017;71(Suppl 1):11–6. PMID: 28950279. http://www.ncbi.nlm.nih.gov/pubmed/28950279.
397. Browne HP, Neville BA, Forster SC, Lawley TD. Transmission of the gut microbiota: spreading of health. Nat Rev Microbiol. 2017;15(9):531–43. PMCID: PMC5837012. http://www.ncbi.nlm.nih.gov/pubmed/28603278.
398. Zareie M, Johnson-Henry K, Jury J, Yang PC, Ngan BY, McKay DM, Soderholm JD, Perdue MH, Sherman PM. Probiotics prevent bacterial translocation and improve intestinal barrier function in rats following chronic psychological stress. Gut. 2006;55(11):1553–60. PMCID: PMC1860130. http://www.ncbi.nlm.nih.gov/pubmed/16638791.
399. Kelly JR, Kennedy PJ, Cryan JF, Dinan TG, Clarke G, Hyland NP. Breaking down the barriers: the gut microbiome, intestinal permeability and stress-related psychiatric disorders. Front Cell Neurosci. 2015;9:392. PMCID: PMC4604320. http://www.ncbi.nlm.nih.gov/pubmed/26528128.
400. Bailey MT, Dowd SE, Galley JD, Hufnagle AR, Allen RG, Lyte M. Exposure to a social stressor alters the structure of the intestinal microbiota: implications for stressor-induced immunomodulation. Brain Behav Immun. 2011;25(3):397–407. PMCID: PMC3039072. http://www.ncbi.nlm.nih.gov/pubmed/21040780.
401. Maes M, Kubera M, Leunis JC. The gut-brain barrier in major depression: intestinal mucosal dysfunction with an increased translocation of LPS from gram negative enterobacteria (leaky gut) plays a role in the inflammatory pathophysiology of depression. Neuro Endocrinol Lett. 2008;29(1):117–24. PMID: 18283240. http://www.ncbi.nlm.nih.gov/pubmed/18283240.
402. Maes M, Kubera M, Leunis JC, Berk M. Increased IgA and IgM responses against gut commensals in chronic depression: further evidence for increased bacterial translocation or leaky gut. J Affect Disord. 2012;141(1):55–62. PMID: 22410503. http://www.ncbi.nlm.nih.gov/pubmed/22410503.
403. Jiang H, Ling Z, Zhang Y, Mao H, Ma Z, Yin Y, Wang W, Tang W, Tan Z, Shi J, Li L, Ruan B. Altered fecal microbiota composition in patients with major depressive disorder. Brain Behav Immun. 2015;48:186–94. PMID: 25882912. http://www.ncbi.nlm.nih.gov/pubmed/25882912.
404. Whittaker RJ, Willis KJ, Field R. Scale and species richness: towards a general, hierarchical theory of species diversity. J Biogeogr. 2001;28(4):453–70. https://onlinelibrary.wiley.com/doi/abs/10.1046/j.1365-2699.2001.00563.x.
405. Whittaker RH. Evolution and measurement of species diversity. Taxon. 1972;21(2–3):213–51. https://onlinelibrary.wiley.com/doi/abs/10.2307/1218190.
406. Kelly JR, Borre Y, O'Brien C, Patterson E, El Aidy S, Deane J, Kennedy PJ, Beers S, Scott K, Moloney G, Hoban AE, Scott L, Fitzgerald P, Ross P, Stanton C, Clarke G, Cryan JF, Dinan TG. Transferring the blues: depression-associated gut microbiota induces neurobehavioural changes in the rat. J Psychiatr Res. 2016;82:109–18. PMID: 27491067. http://www.ncbi.nlm.nih.gov/pubmed/27491067.
407. Yu M, Jia H, Zhou C, Yang Y, Zhao Y, Yang M, Zou Z. Variations in gut microbiota and fecal metabolic phenotype associated with depression by 16S rRNA gene sequencing and LC/MS-based metabolomics. J Pharm Biomed Anal. 2017;138:231–9. PMID: 28219800. http://www.ncbi.nlm.nih.gov/pubmed/28219800.
408. El-Zaatari M, Chang YM, Zhang M, Franz M, Shreiner A, McDermott AJ, van der Sluijs KF, Lutter R, Grasberger H, Kamada N, Young VB, Huffnagle GB, Kao JY. Tryptophan catabolism restricts IFN-γ-expressing neutrophils and Clostridium difficile immunopathology. J Immunol. 2014;193(2):807–16. PMCID: PMC4091639. http://www.ncbi.nlm.nih.gov/pubmed/24935925.
409. El Aidy S, Ramsteijn AS, Dini-Andreote F, van Eijk R, Houwing DJ, Salles JF, Olivier JDA. Serotonin transporter genotype modulates the gut microbiota composition in young rats, an effect augmented by early life stress. Front Cell Neurosci.

2017;11:222. PMCID: PMC5540888. http://www.ncbi.nlm.nih.gov/pubmed/28824378.
410. O'Mahony SM, Clarke G, Borre YE, Dinan TG, Cryan JF. Serotonin, tryptophan metabolism and the brain-gut-microbiome axis. Behav Brain Res. 2015;277:32–48. PMID: 25078296. http://www.ncbi.nlm.nih.gov/pubmed/25078296.
411. Spiller R. Serotonin and GI clinical disorders. Neuropharmacology. 2008;55(6):1072–80. PMID: 18687345. http://www.ncbi.nlm.nih.gov/pubmed/18687345.
412. Martel F. Recent advances on the importance of the serotonin transporter SERT in the rat intestine. Pharmacol Res. 2006;54(2):73–6. PMID: 16750380. http://www.ncbi.nlm.nih.gov/pubmed/16750380.
413. Gill RK, Pant N, Saksena S, Singla A, Nazir TM, Vohwinkel L, Turner JR, Goldstein J, Alrefai WA, Dudeja PK. Function, expression, and characterization of the serotonin transporter in the native human intestine. Am J Physiol Gastrointest Liver Physiol. 2008;294(1):G254–62. PMCID: PMC4880408. http://www.ncbi.nlm.nih.gov/pubmed/17991706.
414. Olivier JDA, Åkerud H, Skalkidou A, Kaihola H, Sundström-Poromaa I. The effects of antenatal depression and antidepressant treatment on placental gene expression. Front Cell Neurosci. 2014;8:465. PMCID: PMC4292720. http://www.ncbi.nlm.nih.gov/pubmed/25628539.
415. Carola V, Frazzetto G, Pascucci T, Audero E, Puglisi-Allegra S, Cabib S, Lesch KP, Gross C. Identifying molecular substrates in a mouse model of the serotonin transporter x environment risk factor for anxiety and depression. Biol Psychiatry. 2008;63(9):840–6. PMID: 17949690. http://www.ncbi.nlm.nih.gov/pubmed/17949690.
416. Dinan TG, Cryan JF. Regulation of the stress response by the gut microbiota: implications for psychoneuroendocrinology. Psychoneuroendocrinology. 2012;37(9):1369–78. PMID: 22483040. http://www.ncbi.nlm.nih.gov/pubmed/22483040.
417. Yano JM, Yu K, Donaldson GP, Shastri GG, Ann P, Ma L, Nagler CR, Ismagilov RF, Mazmanian SK, Hsiao EY. Indigenous bacteria from the gut microbiota regulate host serotonin biosynthesis. Cell. 2015;161(2):264–76. PMCID: PMC4393509. http://www.ncbi.nlm.nih.gov/pubmed/25860609.
418. Lukić I, Getselter D, Ziv O, Oron O, Reuveni E, Koren O, Elliott E. Antidepressants affect gut microbiota and Ruminococcus flavefaciens is able to abolish their effects on depressive-like behavior. Transl Psychiatry. 2019;9(1):133. PMCID: PMC6456569. http://www.ncbi.nlm.nih.gov/pubmed/30967529.
419. Walsh J, Griffin BT, Clarke G, Hyland NP. Drug-gut microbiota interactions: implications for neuropharmacology. Br J Pharmacol. 2018;175(24):4415–29. PMCID: PMC6255959. http://www.ncbi.nlm.nih.gov/pubmed/29782640.
420. Lieb J. The immunostimulating and antimicrobial properties of lithium and antidepressants. J Infect. 2004;49(2):88–93. PMID: 15236914. http://www.ncbi.nlm.nih.gov/pubmed/15236914.
421. Lieb J. Lithium and antidepressants: stimulating immune function and preventing and reversing infection. Med Hypotheses. 2007;69(1):8–11. PMID: 17287092. http://www.ncbi.nlm.nih.gov/pubmed/17287092.
422. Getachew B, Aubee JI, Schottenfeld RS, Csoka AB, Thompson KM, Tizabi Y. Ketamine interactions with gut-microbiota in rats: relevance to its antidepressant and anti-inflammatory properties. BMC Microbiol. 2018;18(1):222. PMCID: PMC6303954. http://www.ncbi.nlm.nih.gov/pubmed/30579332.
423. Munoz-Bellido JL, Munoz-Criado S, Garcìa-Rodrìguez JA. Antimicrobial activity of psychotropic drugs: selective serotonin reuptake inhibitors. Int J Antimicrob Agents. 2000;14(3):177–80. PMID: 10773485. http://www.ncbi.nlm.nih.gov/pubmed/10773485.
424. Bangert MK, Hasbun R. Neurological and psychiatric adverse effects of antimicrobials. CNS Drugs. 2019;33(8):727–53. PMID: 31321707. http://www.ncbi.nlm.nih.gov/pubmed/31321707.
425. Ahmed AIA, van der Heijden FMMA, van den Berkmortel H, Kramers K. A man who wanted to commit suicide by hanging himself: an adverse effect of ciprofloxacin. Gen Hosp Psychiatry. 2011;33(1):82.e5–7. PMID: 21353135. http://www.ncbi.nlm.nih.gov/pubmed/21353135.
426. Kaur K, Fayad R, Saxena A, Frizzell N, Chanda A, Das S, Chatterjee S, Hegde S, Baliga MS, Ponemone V, Rorro M, Greene J, Elraheb Y, Redd AJ, Bian J, Restaino J, Norris LB, Qureshi ZP, Love BL, Brookstaver B, Georgantopoulos P, Sartor O, Raisch DW, Rao G, Lu K, Ray P, Hrusheshky W, Schulz R, Ablin R, Noxon V, Bennett CL, Southern Network on Adverse Reactions (SONAR) project. Fluoroquinolone-related neuropsychiatric and mitochondrial toxicity: a collaborative investigation by scientists and members of a social network. J Community Support Oncol. 2016;14(2):54–65. PMID: 26955658. http://www.ncbi.nlm.nih.gov/pubmed/26955658.
427. Bennett AC, Bennett CL, Witherspoon BJ, Knopf KB. An evaluation of reports of ciprofloxacin, levofloxacin, and moxifloxacin-association neuropsychiatric toxicities, long-term disability, and aortic aneurysms/dissections disseminated by the Food and Drug Administration and the European Medicines Agency. Expert Opin Drug Saf. 2019;18(11):1055–63. PMCID: PMC9830651. http://www.ncbi.nlm.nih.gov/pubmed/31500468.
428. Mello BSF, Monte AS, McIntyre RS, Soczynska JK, Custódio CS, Cordeiro RC, Chaves JH, Vasconcelos SMM, Nobre HV, Florenço de Sousa FC, Hyphantis TN, Carvalho AF, Macêdo DS. Effects of doxycycline on depressive-like behavior in mice after lipopolysaccharide (LPS) administration. J Psychiatr Res. 2013;47(10):1521–9. PMID: 23835040. http://www.ncbi.nlm.nih.gov/pubmed/23835040.
429. Stilling RM, Dinan TG, Cryan JF. Microbial genes, brain & behaviour – epigenetic regulation of the gut-brain axis. Genes Brain Behav. 2014;13(1):69–86. PMID: 24286462. http://www.ncbi.nlm.nih.gov/pubmed/24286462.
430. Sommer F, Bäckhed F. The gut microbiotaDOUBLEHYPHENmasters of host development and physiology. Nat Rev Microbiol. 2013;11(4):227–38. PMID: 23435359. http://www.ncbi.nlm.nih.gov/pubmed/23435359.
431. Niller HH, Minarovits J. Patho-epigenetics of infectious diseases caused by intracellular bacteria. Adv Exp Med Biol. 2016;879:107–30. PMID: 26659266. http://www.ncbi.nlm.nih.gov/pubmed/26659266.
432. Grabiec AM, Potempa J. Epigenetic regulation in bacterial infections: targeting histone deacetylases. Crit Rev Microbiol. 2018;44(3):336–50. PMCID: PMC6109591. http://www.ncbi.nlm.nih.gov/pubmed/28971711.
433. Schuhmacher MK, Rolando M, Bröhm A, Weirich S, Kudithipudi S, Buchrieser C, Jeltsch A. The Legionella pneumophila methyltransferase RomA methylates also non-histone proteins during infection. J Mol Biol. 2018;430(13):1912–25. PMID: 29733858. http://www.ncbi.nlm.nih.gov/pubmed/29733858.
434. de Souza HSP, Fiocchi C, Iliopoulos D. The IBD interactome: an integrated view of aetiology, pathogenesis and therapy. Nat Rev Gastroenterol Hepatol. 2017;14(12):739–49. PMID: 28831186. http://www.ncbi.nlm.nih.gov/pubmed/28831186.
435. Wehkamp J, Götz M, Herrlinger K, Steurer W, Stange EF. Inflammatory bowel disease. Dtsch Arztebl Int. 2016;113(5):72–82. PMCID: PMC4782273. http://www.ncbi.nlm.nih.gov/pubmed/26900160.
436. Sairenji T, Collins KL, Evans DV. An update on inflammatory bowel disease. Prim Care. 2017;44(4):673–92. PMID: 29132528. http://www.ncbi.nlm.nih.gov/pubmed/29132528.

437. Ng SC, Shi HY, Hamidi N, Underwood FE, Tang W, Benchimol EI, Panaccione R, Ghosh S, Wu JCY, Chan FKL, Sung JJY, Kaplan GG. Worldwide incidence and prevalence of inflammatory bowel disease in the 21st century: a systematic review of population-based studies. Lancet. 2017;390(10114):2769–78. PMID: 29050646. http://www.ncbi.nlm.nih.gov/pubmed/29050646.
438. de Souza HSP. Etiopathogenesis of inflammatory bowel disease: today and tomorrow. Curr Opin Gastroenterol. 2017;33(4):222–9. PMID: 28402995. http://www.ncbi.nlm.nih.gov/pubmed/28402995.
439. Rogler G, Biedermann L, Scharl M. New insights into the pathophysiology of inflammatory bowel disease: microbiota, epigenetics and common signalling pathways. Swiss Med Wkly. 2018;148:w14599. PMID: 29566254. http://www.ncbi.nlm.nih.gov/pubmed/29566254.
440. Nishida A, Inoue R, Inatomi O, Bamba S, Naito Y, Andoh A. Gut microbiota in the pathogenesis of inflammatory bowel disease. Clin J Gastroenterol. 2018;11(1):1–10. PMID: 29285689. http://www.ncbi.nlm.nih.gov/pubmed/29285689.
441. Yue B, Luo X, Yu Z, Mani S, Wang Z, Dou W. Inflammatory bowel disease: a potential result from the collusion between gut microbiota and mucosal immune system. Microorganisms. 2019;7(10):440. PMCID: PMC6843348. http://www.ncbi.nlm.nih.gov/pubmed/31614539.
442. Brzozowski B, Mazur-Bialy A, Pajdo R, Kwiecien S, Bilski J, Zwolinska-Wcislo M, Mach T, Brzozowski T. Mechanisms by which stress affects the experimental and clinical inflammatory bowel disease (IBD): role of brain-gut axis. Curr Neuropharmacol. 2016;14(8):892–900. PMCID: PMC5333596. http://www.ncbi.nlm.nih.gov/pubmed/27040468.
443. Pals KL, Chang RT, Ryan AJ, Gisolfi CV. Effect of running intensity on intestinal permeability. J Appl Physiol. 1997;82(2):571–6. PMID: 9049739. http://www.ncbi.nlm.nih.gov/pubmed/9049739.
444. Tiller NB, Chiesa ST, Roberts JD, Turner LA, Jones S, Romer LM. Physiological and pathophysiological consequences of a 25-day ultra-endurance exercise challenge. Front Physiol. 2019;10:589. PMCID: PMC6530658. http://www.ncbi.nlm.nih.gov/pubmed/31156464.
445. Söderholm JD, Yang PC, Ceponis P, Vohra A, Riddell R, Sherman PM, Perdue MH. Chronic stress induces mast cell-dependent bacterial adherence and initiates mucosal inflammation in rat intestine. Gastroenterology. 2002;123(4):1099–108. PMID: 12360472. http://www.ncbi.nlm.nih.gov/pubmed/12360472.
446. Wei L, Li Y, Tang W, Sun Q, Chen L, Wang X, Liu Q, Yu S, Yu S, Liu C, Ma X. Chronic unpredictable mild stress in rats induces colonic inflammation. Front Physiol. 2019;10:1228. PMCID: PMC6764080. http://www.ncbi.nlm.nih.gov/pubmed/31616319.
447. Whitehead WE, Palsson O, Jones KR. Systematic review of the comorbidity of irritable bowel syndrome with other disorders: what are the causes and implications? Gastroenterology. 2002;122(4):1140–56. PMID: 11910364. http://www.ncbi.nlm.nih.gov/pubmed/11910364.
448. Koloski NA, Jones M, Kalantar J, Weltman M, Zaguirre J, Talley NJ. The brainDOUBLEHYPHENgut pathway in functional gastrointestinal disorders is bidirectional: a 12-year prospective population-based study. Gut. 2012;61(9):1284–90. PMID: 22234979. http://www.ncbi.nlm.nih.gov/pubmed/22234979.
449. Henningsen P, Zimmermann T, Sattel H. Medically unexplained physical symptoms, anxiety, and depression: a meta-analytic review. Psychosom Med. 2003;65(4):528–33. PMID: 12883101. http://www.ncbi.nlm.nih.gov/pubmed/12883101.
450. Graff LA, Walker JR, Bernstein CN. Depression and anxiety in inflammatory bowel disease: a review of comorbidity and management. Inflamm Bowel Dis. 2009;15(7):1105–18. PMID: 19161177. http://www.ncbi.nlm.nih.gov/pubmed/19161177.
451. Pigrau M, Rodiño-Janeiro BK, Casado-Bedmar M, Lobo B, Vicario M, Santos J, Alonso-Cotoner C. The joint power of sex and stress to modulate brain-gut-microbiota axis and intestinal barrier homeostasis: implications for irritable bowel syndrome. Neurogastroenterol Motil. 2016;28(4):463–86. PMID: 26556786. http://www.ncbi.nlm.nih.gov/pubmed/26556786.
452. Qin HY, Cheng CW, Tang XD, Bian ZX. Impact of psychological stress on irritable bowel syndrome. World J Gastroenterol. 2014;20(39):14126–31. PMID: 25339801; PMCID: PMC4202343. https://doi.org/10.3748/wjg.v20.i39.14126.
453. Lackner JM, Ma CX, Keefer L, Brenner DM, Gudleski GD, Satchidanand N, Firth R, Sitrin MD, Katz L, Krasner SS, Ballou SK, Naliboff BD, Mayer EA. Type, rather than number, of mental and physical comorbidities increases the severity of symptoms in patients with irritable bowel syndrome. Clin Gastroenterol Hepatol. 2013;11(9):1147–57. PMCID: PMC3779619. http://www.ncbi.nlm.nih.gov/pubmed/23524278.
454. Dave M, Papadakis KA, Faubion WA. Immunology of inflammatory bowel disease and molecular targets for biologics. Gastroenterol Clin N Am. 2014;43(3):405–24. PMCID: PMC4480636. http://www.ncbi.nlm.nih.gov/pubmed/25110250.
455. Wallace KL, Zheng LB, Kanazawa Y, Shih DQ. Immunopathology of inflammatory bowel disease. World J Gastroenterol. 2014;20(1):6–21. PMCID: PMC3886033. http://www.ncbi.nlm.nih.gov/pubmed/24415853.
456. Panara AJ, Yarur AJ, Rieders B, Proksell S, Deshpande AR, Abreu MT, Sussman DA. The incidence and risk factors for developing depression after being diagnosed with inflammatory bowel disease: a cohort study. Aliment Pharmacol Ther. 2014;39(8):802–10. PMID: 24588323. http://www.ncbi.nlm.nih.gov/pubmed/24588323.
457. Häuser W, Janke KH, Klump B, Hinz A. Anxiety and depression in patients with inflammatory bowel disease: comparisons with chronic liver disease patients and the general population. Inflamm Bowel Dis. 2011;17(2):621–32. PMID: 20848528. http://www.ncbi.nlm.nih.gov/pubmed/20848528.
458. Alexakis C, Kumar S, Saxena S, Pollok R. Systematic review with meta-analysis: the impact of a depressive state on disease course in adult inflammatory bowel disease. Aliment Pharmacol Ther. 2017;46(3):225–35. PMID: 28573652. http://www.ncbi.nlm.nih.gov/pubmed/28573652.
459. Wilkinson B, Trick L, Knight A, Valton V, Goodhand J, Kennedy NA, Heerasing N, Ahmad T, Bland A, Elliott R, Roiser JP, Dickens C. Factors associated with depression in people with inflammatory bowel disease: the relationship between active disease and biases in neurocognitive processing. Neurogastroenterol Motil. 2019;31(8):e13647. PMID: 31267614. http://www.ncbi.nlm.nih.gov/pubmed/31267614.
460. Bourke C, Douglas K, Porter R. Processing of facial emotion expression in major depression: a review. Aust N Z J Psychiatry. 2010;44(8):681–96. PMID: 20636189. http://www.ncbi.nlm.nih.gov/pubmed/20636189.
461. Bieliński M, Lesiewska N, Bielińska J, Liebert A, Mieczkowski A, Sopońska-Brzoszczyk P, Brzoszczyk B, Kłopocka M, Borkowska A. Affective temperament in inflammatory bowel diseases: another brick in the wall of differentiation. PLoS One. 2018;13(11):e0205606. PMCID: PMC6211668. http://www.ncbi.nlm.nih.gov/pubmed/30383791.
462. Mendlowicz MV, Jean-Louis G, Kelsoe JR, Akiskal HS. A comparison of recovered bipolar patients, healthy relatives of bipolar probands, and normal controls using the short TEMPS-A. J Affect Disord. 2005;85(1–2):147–51. PMID: 15780685. http://www.ncbi.nlm.nih.gov/pubmed/15780685.
463. Akiskal HS, Akiskal KK. TEMPS: temperament evaluation of Memphis, Pisa, Paris and San Diego. J Affect Disord.

2005;85(1–2):1–2. PMID: 15780670. http://www.ncbi.nlm.nih.gov/pubmed/15780670.
464. von Zerssen D, Akiskal HS. Personality factors in affective disorders: historical developments and current issues with special reference to the concepts of temperament and character. J Affect Disord. 1998;51(1):1–5. PMID: 9879798. http://www.ncbi.nlm.nih.gov/pubmed/9879798.
465. Akiskal HS, Akiskal KK, Haykal RF, Manning JS, Connor PD. TEMPS-A: progress towards validation of a self-rated clinical version of the temperament evaluation of the Memphis, Pisa, Paris, and San Diego autoquestionnaire. J Affect Disord. 2005;85(1–2):3–16. PMID: 15780671. http://www.ncbi.nlm.nih.gov/pubmed/15780671.
466. Mella LFB, Bértolo MB, Dalgalarrondo P. Depressive symptoms in rheumatoid arthritis. Braz J Psychiatry. 2010;32(3):257–63. PMID: 20694442. http://www.ncbi.nlm.nih.gov/pubmed/20694442.
467. Akiskal HS, Maser JD, Zeller PJ, Endicott J, Coryell W, Keller M, Warshaw M, Clayton P, Goodwin F. Switching from "unipolar" to bipolar II. An 11-year prospective study of clinical and temperamental predictors in 559 patients. Arch Gen Psychiatry. 1995;52(2):114–23. PMID: 7848047. http://www.ncbi.nlm.nih.gov/pubmed/7848047.
468. Shirahama M, Terao T, Ishii N, Hatano K, Hirakawa H, Kohno K. Relationship between anxious temperament and harm avoidance in medical students and staff. Psychiatry Clin Neurosci. 2018;72(5):322–8. PMID: 29286553. http://www.ncbi.nlm.nih.gov/pubmed/29286553.
469. Greenwood TA, Akiskal HS, Akiskal KK, Bipolar Genome Study, Kelsoe JR. Genome-wide association study of temperament in bipolar disorder reveals significant associations with three novel Loci. Biol Psychiatry. 2012;72(4):303–10. PMCID: PMC3925336. http://www.ncbi.nlm.nih.gov/pubmed/22365631.
470. Gois C, Barbosa A, Ferro A, Santos AL, Sousa F, Akiskal H, Akiskal K, Figueira ML. The role of affective temperaments in metabolic control in patients with type 2 diabetes. J Affect Disord. 2011;134(1–3):52–8. PMID: 21641045. http://www.ncbi.nlm.nih.gov/pubmed/21641045.
471. Karam EG, Salamoun MM, Yeretzian JS, Mneimneh ZN, Karam AN, Fayyad J, Hantouche E, Akiskal K, Akiskal HS. The role of anxious and hyperthymic temperaments in mental disorders: a national epidemiologic study. World Psychiatry. 2010;9(2):103–10. PMCID: PMC2911090. http://www.ncbi.nlm.nih.gov/pubmed/20671899.
472. Serafini G, Geoffroy PA, Aguglia A, Adavastro G, Canepa G, Pompili M, Amore M. Irritable temperament and lifetime psychotic symptoms as predictors of anxiety symptoms in bipolar disorder. Nord J Psychiatry. 2018;72(1):63–71. PMID: 29022840. http://www.ncbi.nlm.nih.gov/pubmed/29022840.
473. Taşkesen A, Demirkale I, Taşkesen N, Okumuş M, Can DÖ. Irritable temperament profile prevails among patients with boxer fractures. Eur J Trauma Emerg Surg. 2017;43(6):869–73. PMID: 28224184. http://www.ncbi.nlm.nih.gov/pubmed/28224184.
474. Asik M, Altinbas K, Eroglu M, Karaahmet E, Erbag G, Ertekin H, Sen H. Evaluation of affective temperament and anxiety-depression levels of patients with polycystic ovary syndrome. J Affect Disord. 2015;185:214–8. PMID: 26241866. http://www.ncbi.nlm.nih.gov/pubmed/26241866.
475. Bhamre R, Sawrav S, Adarkar S, Sakaria R, Bhatia SJ. Psychiatric comorbidities in patients with inflammatory bowel disease. Indian J Gastroenterol. 2018;37(4):307–12. PMID: 30196516. http://www.ncbi.nlm.nih.gov/pubmed/30196516.
476. Patten SB, Beck CA, Kassam A, Williams JVA, Barbui C, Metz LM. Long-term medical conditions and major depression: strength of association for specific conditions in the general population. Can J Psychiatr. 2005;50(4):195–202. PMID: 15898458. http://www.ncbi.nlm.nih.gov/pubmed/15898458.
477. Yanartas O, Kani HT, Bicakci E, Kilic I, Banzragch M, Acikel C, Atug O, Kuscu K, Imeryuz N, Akin H. The effects of psychiatric treatment on depression, anxiety, quality of life, and sexual dysfunction in patients with inflammatory bowel disease. Neuropsychiatr Dis Treat. 2016;12:673–83. PMCID: PMC4818049. http://www.ncbi.nlm.nih.gov/pubmed/27069364.
478. Mikocka-Walus A, Pittet V, Rossel JB, von Känel R, Swiss IBD Cohort Study Group. Symptoms of depression and anxiety are independently associated with clinical recurrence of inflammatory bowel disease. Clin Gastroenterol Hepatol. 2016;14(6):829–835.e1. PMID: 26820402. http://www.ncbi.nlm.nih.gov/pubmed/26820402.
479. Lautenschlager SA, Barry MP, Rogler G, Biedermann L, Schreiner P, Siebenhüner AR, Swiss IBD Cohort Study Group. Lifestyle factors associated with inflammatory bowel disease: data from the Swiss IBD cohort study. BMC Gastroenterol. 2023;23(1):71. https://doi.org/10.1186/s12876-023-02692-9. PMID: 36907848; PMCID: PMC10008613. https://pubmed.ncbi.nlm.nih.gov/36907848/.
480. Jordi SBU, Lang BM, Auschra B, von Känel R, Biedermann L, Greuter T, Schreiner P, Rogler G, Krupka N, Sulz MC, Misselwitz B, Begré S, Swiss IBD Cohort Study Group. Depressive symptoms predict clinical recurrence of inflammatory bowel disease. Inflamm Bowel Dis. 2022;28(4):560–71. https://doi.org/10.1093/ibd/izab136. PMID: 34096587. https://pubmed.ncbi.nlm.nih.gov/34096587/.
481. Bel LGJ, Vollebregt AM, Van der Meulen-de Jong AE, Fidder HH, Ten Hove WR, Vliet-Vlieland CW, Ter Kuile MM, de Groot HE, Both S. Sexual dysfunctions in men and women with inflammatory bowel disease: the influence of IBD-related clinical factors and depression on sexual function. J Sex Med. 2015;12(7):1557–67. PMID: 26054013. http://www.ncbi.nlm.nih.gov/pubmed/26054013.
482. Stellingwerf ME, Bak MTJ, de Groof EJ, Buskens CJ, Molenaar CBH, Gecse KB, Nerkens W, Horeman T, Bemelman WA. Knotless seton for perianal fistulas: feasibility and effect on perianal disease activity. Sci Rep. 2020;10:16693. https://www.nature.com/articles/s41598-020-73737-2.pdf.
483. Mittermaier C, Dejaco C, Waldhoer T, Oefferlbauer-Ernst A, Miehsler W, Beier M, Tillinger W, Gangl A, Moser G. Impact of depressive mood on relapse in patients with inflammatory bowel disease: a prospective 18-month follow-up study. Psychosom Med. 2004;66(1):79–84. PMID: 14747641. http://www.ncbi.nlm.nih.gov/pubmed/14747641.
484. Kim MC, Jung YS, Song YS, Lee JI, Park JH, Sohn CI, Choi KY, Park DI. Factors associated with anxiety and depression in Korean patients with inactive inflammatory bowel disease. Gut Liver. 2016;10(3):399–405. PMCID: PMC4849693. http://www.ncbi.nlm.nih.gov/pubmed/26470768.
485. Zhang C, Byrne G, Lee T, Singer J, Giustini D, Bressler B. Incidence of suicide in inflammatory bowel disease: a systematic review and meta-analysis. J Can Assoc Gastroenterol. 2018;1(3):107–14. PMCID: PMC6507288. http://www.ncbi.nlm.nih.gov/pubmed/31294727.
486. Kochar B, Barnes EL, Long MD, Cushing KC, Galanko J, Martin CF, Raffals LE, Sandler RS. Depression is associated with more aggressive inflammatory bowel disease. Am J Gastroenterol. 2018;113(1):80–5. PMCID: PMC5962285. http://www.ncbi.nlm.nih.gov/pubmed/29134965.
487. Asscher VER, Lee-Kong FVY, Kort ED, van Deudekom FJ, Mooijaart SP, Maljaars PWJ. Systematic review: components of a comprehensive geriatric assessment in inflammatory bowel disease – a potentially promising but often neglected risk stratification. J Crohns Colitis. 2019;13(11):1418–32.

PMCID: PMC6821240. http://www.ncbi.nlm.nih.gov/pubmed/31002331.
488. Englund H, Lidén KK, Lind T, Sundström T, Karling P. Radiation exposure in patients with inflammatory bowel disease and irritable bowel syndrome in the years 2001-2011. Scand J Gastroenterol. 2017;52(3):300–5. PMID: 27832710. http://www.ncbi.nlm.nih.gov/pubmed/27832710.
489. Walker JR, Ediger JP, Graff LA, Greenfeld JM, Clara I, Lix L, Rawsthorne P, Miller N, Rogala L, McPhail CM, Bernstein CN. The Manitoba IBD cohort study: a population-based study of the prevalence of lifetime and 12-month anxiety and mood disorders. Am J Gastroenterol. 2008;103(8):1989–97. PMID: 18796096. http://www.ncbi.nlm.nih.gov/pubmed/18796096.

Social Isolation and Depression

11

Jeffery J. Sunzeri

Introduction: Sociology and Isolation

The concept of an individual being removed and isolated from social structures and forces is well described and discussed by the earliest sociologists. It is a fundamental paradigm of sociology that an individual isolated from society is either in or creating a dysfunctional and potentially harmful state.

In 1897, Emile Durkheim described in *Suicide: A Study in Sociology* how suicide was the result of the individual being removed from social forces and impacts, in effect being isolated [1]. The forces he described are social integration and moral regulation. He described a state of *anomie*, where a person would be in a state of feeling normlessness, a disconnection from society and its norms. He described how anomie contributed to isolation and social alienation.

In 1894, Karl Marx in *Das Kapital* talked about the idea of alienation and isolation in relation to capitalism and other social forces [25]. These social forces then resulted in isolation and disconnection from society.

In 1904, Max Weber published *The Protestant Ethic and The Spirit of Capitalism*, in which he described the social concept of *rationalization* [26]. This concept explored and stated how society moved to implement a rational basis of social functions and structures, which resulted in a shift of how the individual could now be isolated from previous social forces that sought to integrate and socialize.

In a 1908 essay "The Stranger," George Simmel speaks about social relationship dynamics, especially in twentieth-century urban life. In this essay, he introduces the idea of how an individual will experience a sense of detachment and isolation in known but impersonal societies [27].

Thus, the foundations of sociology show us that societies are structured in ways that can either foster or hinder social connections. It is suggested and shown that urbanization and modernization have led to increased social fragmentation, with individuals becoming more disconnected from their communities and support networks. The primary benefit of urbanization is an increased level of medical services [42] and sanitation [43]. Education and income levels are frequently higher among urban students than their rural counterparts [38].

The new dominant form of urbanization are *city-regions* which are polycentric networks of multiple cities of assorted sizes [30–32]. These city-regions are highly differentiated and are rife with urban-rural and urban-urban social inequities and social deficiencies that may amplify social isolation. Recent work has shown that this disconnection can contribute to feelings of isolation and loneliness, which are significant risk factors for depression [2, 42–46].

Defining Social Isolation

Social isolation refers to the state of being disconnected from others, both physically and emotionally, leading to a lack of meaningful social relationships and interactions. This phenomenon has significant implications for individual well-being, community cohesion, and broader societal dynamics. See Fig. 11.1.

Sociologists typically define *social isolation* as the absence or insufficiency of social relationships and social integration. It involves a subjective feeling of loneliness and a lack of belongingness within one's social environment [47].

Loneliness and social isolation are frequently used interchangeably, but they are distinct [48]. *Loneliness* is a subjective experience of feeling alone and reflects an individual's dissatisfaction with closeness and frequency of social contacts [2]. *Perceived social isolation* is colloquially referred to as loneliness [49]. *Social isolation* is an objective quantification of social contacts [28]. *Social loneliness* is the absence of a broad network of quality friendships. *Emotional loneliness* is dissatisfaction with one's current social relationships

J. J. Sunzeri (✉)
Sunzeri Consulting, Hollister, CA, USA

J. Raber et al. (eds.), *Understanding and Treating Depressive Disorders*, https://doi.org/10.1007/978-3-032-14465-2_11

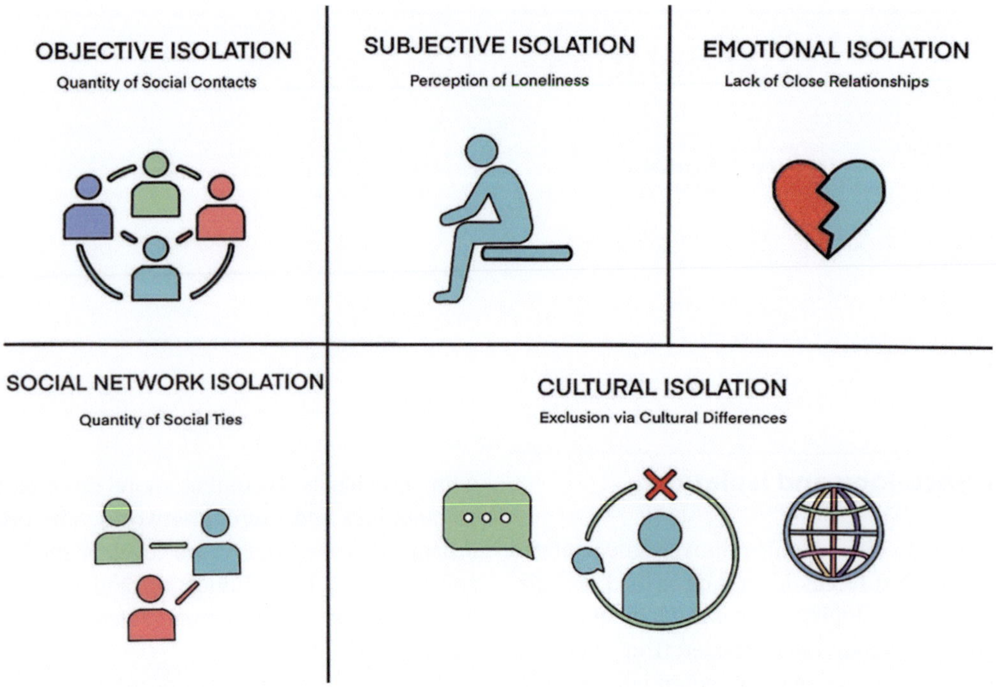

Fig. 11.1 Conceptual illustration of social isolation dimensions. This figure depicts the multifaceted nature of social isolation, distinguishing between objective isolation—defined by the measurable quantity of social contacts—and subjective isolation, which reflects individuals' perceived sense of loneliness. Emotional isolation is represented as the absence of close, emotionally supportive relationships. Social network isolation emphasizes the scarcity or fragmentation of interpersonal ties within broader social systems. Cultural isolation highlights exclusion or detachment resulting from cultural differences or a lack of shared norms. Together, these dimensions illustrate the complex interplay of quantitative and qualitative factors contributing to the experience of isolation

[33]. In the literature, loneliness and social isolation are most frequently examined together [50].

People who are lonely are more likely to be socially isolated, and people who are socially isolated are more likely to be lonely [29, 51, 52].

A systematic review of loneliness, social isolation, cardiovascular disease, and mortality has synthesized the literature up to 2018 and produced a conceptual framework that emphasizes the complexity of associations between loneliness, social isolation, and mortality [53, 54].

Social isolation can occur at different levels—individual, community, or societal—and can be influenced by a range of factors, such as age, gender, socioeconomic status, and cultural norms.

There are several factors that contribute to social isolation [75]. These include demographic factors (e.g., living alone, being unmarried), life transitions (e.g., retirement, migration), economic factors (e.g., poverty, unemployment), health issues (e.g., disability, mental illness), and structural factors (e.g., urbanization, breakdown of community networks) [53].

We can and should differentiate between different types and dimensions of social isolation [34]. For instance, there is a distinction between *objective isolation* (measured by the quantity of social contacts) and *subjective isolation* (based on individuals' perceptions of loneliness). Dimensions may also include *emotional isolation* (lack of close relationships), *social network isolation* (few social ties), and *cultural isolation* (exclusion due to cultural differences).

A systematic review of longitudinal risk factors for loneliness in older adults showed associations with not being married/partnered and partner loss, a limited social network, a low level of social activity, poor self-perceived health, and depression/depressed mood and an increase in depression.

Around one-third of individuals in industrialized countries have been found to be affected by loneliness [55]. Loneliness is contagious, and factors such as income, education, sex, and ethnicity are not protective. Loneliness is associated with a 26% increase in the risk of premature mortality.

Selectively altered attentional, cognitive, and affective processes are the hallmarks of loneliness [2]. Perceived social isolation (loneliness) compared to objective social isolation is associated with a greater than two-fold increase in risk of developing Alzheimer's disease [56].

There are suggestions that loneliness is associated with altered functional connectivity in neural networks associated with tonic alertness and executive control [49]. These changes in functional connectivity may be associated with hypervigilance to social threats and reduced impulse control. A *differential reactivity hypothesis* posits that lonely people respond to social environments differently than nonlonely people do [57].

A number of meta-analyses have indicated that loneliness has a potent effect on all-cause mortality [51, 58–60]. Meta-analyses point to particular interactions with mental health [61–64], including paranoia [68], and physical health, especially cardiovascular disorders [65–67].

It is debatable if there is an inherent predisposition to loneliness, although someone can feel socially isolated even among other people [69–71]. A 2020 review highlights the interplay between loneliness and known and emerging correlations and risk factors from demography; physical health; mental health; cognitive health; brain, biology, and genetics; and socio-environmental factors [72].

A 2019 *genome-wide association study (GWAS)* meta-analysis of loneliness showed significant genetic variants from 16 loci, including four novel loci, and 58 significantly associated genes [73]. This study shows the presence of a genetic predisposition toward loneliness, associated with cardiovascular, psychiatric, and metabolic disorders. There was also an increasing effect of both BMI and body fat on loneliness.

Loneliness is especially formidable in folks with brain disorders, such as alcohol dependency, depression, epilepsy, multiple sclerosis, Parkinson's disease, schizophrenia, and stroke [74].

Cultural and Historical Contexts

We can analyze social isolation within specific cultural and historical contexts. Cultural norms and values shape how individuals perceive and experience social isolation. For instance, individualistic societies may prioritize individuality or *personal autonomy* [76], which can inadvertently contribute to feelings of loneliness and isolation [35–37]. Historical trends, such as urbanization [77–79] and changes in family structures [80–84], also influence the prevalence and nature of social isolation.

History of Social Isolation

Both the flu epidemic of the early twentieth century, often referred to as the Spanish flu, and the COVID-19 pandemic of the twenty-first century have created significant instances of social isolation. The nature and impact of social isolation resulting from these pandemics can be understood through various sociological perspectives, considering factors, such as public health measures, changes in social behaviors, and the broader societal responses to these crises. Let us explore these aspects with references to scholarly work.

Social Isolation During the Spanish Flu Epidemic (1918–1919)

The Spanish flu pandemic, which occurred between 1918 and 1919, was one of the deadliest pandemics in history. The widespread transmission of the virus led to extensive social disruption and isolation for several reasons.

During the Spanish flu, governments implemented measures, such as quarantine, isolation, and the closure of public spaces, to control the spread of the virus [10]. These interventions restricted social interactions and disrupted community life, leading to feelings of isolation among individuals and families.

The fear of contracting the flu and the associated stigma toward infected individuals contributed to social distancing and avoidance behaviors [16]. This fear-induced isolation further impacted social cohesion and community dynamics.

The pandemic disrupted social structures, such as workplaces, schools, and religious institutions. Many people were unable to participate in daily communal activities, leading to a sense of disconnection and isolation [15].

Social Isolation During the COVID-19 Pandemic (2019–Present)

The COVID-19 pandemic has similarly resulted in widespread social isolation, albeit with distinct characteristics and impacts.

Governments worldwide imposed lockdowns and physical distancing measures to curb the spread of the virus [12]. These measures restricted social gatherings, travel, and in-person interactions, leading to increased social isolation.

The pandemic prompted a rapid shift to remote work and online education, altering traditional social interactions in workplaces and schools [14]. This shift, while necessary for public health, contributed to feelings of isolation and loneliness.

Despite physical distancing, technology played a crucial role in maintaining social connections through virtual communication platforms [13]. However, reliance on digital communication also highlighted disparities in access to technology and exacerbated feelings of isolation among certain groups [39, 85].

Worldwide, depression affected 5.7% of people aged 60 years and over before the pandemic and increased by approximately 27.6% (33.6 million to 68.7 million) [86–88]. A systematic review found that loneliness was one of the predominant factors in that age group [89]. Older adults with Alzheimer's disease, related dementias, and subjective cognitive changes were especially hard hit [90–92].

Traditional Perspectives on Pandemic-Induced Social Isolation

We can analyze and understand pandemic-induced social isolation through various theoretical lenses which seek to explain the mechanisms behind the process.

One theoretical framework seeks to explain actions and processes in terms of how the social structure provides functionality. *Structural Functionalism* considers how disruptions in social structures and institutions impact the functions of social integration and cohesion [17]. Pandemics can strain social systems and structures, leading to dysfunction and increased isolation and alienation.

A more individual-oriented approach labeled *Symbolic Interactionism* looks at how individual people interpret and respond to pandemic-related changes in social interactions [11]. Rather than strictly inferring causality in the process of social isolation resulting in incidents of depression in an individual, the stigma associated with infectious and mental diseases can influence social behaviors and contribute to isolation.

A third theoretical perspective, termed *Social Capital Theory*, emphasizes the importance of social networks and community ties in buffering against social isolation at the individual level [18]. Pandemics can erode social capital by disrupting trust and reciprocity among individuals and groups.

Thus, a brief review of social history shows us that both the Spanish flu epidemic of the early twentieth century and the COVID-19 pandemic of the twenty-first century have created significant social isolation due to public health measures, fear and stigma, disruptions in social structures, and shifts in social behaviors. These pandemics have highlighted the impact of infectious diseases on social relationships and community dynamics, at least one result of which would be an increase in the incidence of mental disorders, such as depression [86].

Depression as a Consequence of Social Fractures and Isolation

Beyond speculation and assumptions derived from various social theoretical frameworks, we see that research consistently demonstrates a strong association between social isolation and depression. When individuals experience social fractures and lack adequate social support, they are more vulnerable to developing depressive symptoms. Social isolation can lead to feelings of loneliness, hopelessness, and worthlessness—key components of depression. Studies have shown that loneliness and perceived social isolation are significant predictors of depressive disorders [19].

Loneliness is associated with subtle impairment across several cognitive domains in older adults [93]. Social isolation, limited social networks, lack of social support, and feelings of loneliness are risk factors that contribute to the onset and subsequent mortality after a stroke [67]. There is some evidence that loneliness is associated with the risk of mild cognitive impairment [94, 95].

A significant adverse effect of social isolation on antiviral immune regulation has been seen [96]. Neuroimmune mechanisms of elevated sympathetic nervous system activity and diminished type 1 interferon responses have been seen in monkey models of loneliness [97].

The *evolutionary theory of loneliness* posits an inherited adaptation signaling that health-giving social interactions are endangered, and it is important to reconnect with significant others [98, 99]. Expression of these putative genes is then dependent on epigenetic interaction between social connections [100]. Paradoxically, the desire for self-preservation results in hypervigilance to social threats and decreased trust, and these behaviors may compete with the drive for connection, which may result in motivation for a larger interpersonal distance within intimate space [101]. Additionally the result of a small study suggests that loneliness increases the need for self-preservation and self-centeredness, leading to depression and negative mood followed by loneliness in a repetitive cycle [102]. Just beneath the surface in individuals experiencing loneliness lie the *"4 T" vulnerabilities of territory, threat, trauma, and trust* [103].

Social Determinants of Depression

Social theories emphasize the role of social factors and structures as determinants in shaping mental health outcomes such as depression. Factors such as poverty, unemployment, discrimination, and social exclusion contribute to both social fractures and increased risk of depression. For example, individuals living in economically deprived neighborhoods may experience higher levels of social isolation due to limited access to resources and support networks, which in turn can exacerbate depressive symptoms [21].

Intersection of Social Identity and Depression

Intersectionality is a framework developed by Kimberlé Crenshaw that emphasizes how various social identities (such as race, gender, class, sexual orientation, and disability) intersect and overlap to create unique forms of discrimination and privilege [104]. The framework challenges traditional approaches that often focus on single-axis categories (e.g., only gender or only race) and instead considers how multiple dimensions of identity simultaneously shape individuals' experiences within social structures [105, 106].

The intersectionality framework highlights how social identities intersect with social fractures and isolation to influence depression risk [107]. Marginalized individuals and minority groups often face systemic barriers that contribute to social exclusion and isolation, leading to higher rates of depression [20, 122]. For instance, studies have shown that LGBTQ+ individuals experience elevated levels of social isolation and depression due to stigma and discrimination [22, 108].

Impact of Technology on Social Fractures and Depression

Technological advancements have transformed social interactions which can in some circumstances and populations be beneficial in addressing social isolation and loneliness [109, 110]. However, digital technology may also contribute to new forms of social fractures and isolation [111–113]. There is some evidence that a threshold effect exists between the use of technology in susceptible teenagers and young adults and depression [114].

While digital technologies enable connectivity, they can also lead to feelings of disconnection and superficial relationships [115]. Excessive use of social media, for instance, has been linked to increased loneliness and depressive symptoms among certain populations [23, 116, 117]. These contradictions highlight the complex relationship between technology, social fractures, and mental health outcomes [118]. This complex relationship makes it hard to distinguish between cause and effect on mental health and digital technology [119, 120].

Fractured Conclusion

In summary, the interplay between depression, social fractures, and isolation appears multifaceted and influenced by various social, economic, and cultural factors. Social research has contributed to this understanding by examining how social structures and relationships impact mental health outcomes.

Solutions and Interventions

A meta-analysis of interventions to reduce loneliness has identified four primary intervention strategies: (a) improving social skills, (b) enhancing social support, (c) increasing opportunities for social contact, and (d) addressing maladaptive social cognition [121]. The most successful interventions addressed maladaptive social cognition. Although some "common sense" treatments such as social skills training, and provisions for social support and social contact seem to be ineffective, some community programs, behavioral interventions, and online resources seem promising [55, 121]. By addressing social structures and functions, and promoting social connectedness, researchers and policymakers can work toward reducing the prevalence and impact of depression associated with social fractures and isolation.

The potential efficacy of integrated interventions that combine (social) cognitive behavioral therapy with short-term adjunctive pharmacological treatments is discussed in references [123, 124].

A meta-analysis heavily weighted with Chinese samples indicated that the effect of social support on loneliness is greater from a friend than from family or a significant other [61].

Validated diagnostic scales for loneliness are available, including a brief three-item instrument suitable for telephone administration [125]. Findings from this scale indicate that while quantitative and qualitative aspects of social relationships are related, they represent distinct dimensions of loneliness.

Policy Implications and Interventions

Understanding the interplay between depression, social fractures, and isolation has important implications for public health policies and interventions. Sociologists advocate for policies that address social determinants of mental health, promote social inclusion, and strengthen community resilience. Interventions focusing on building social networks, reducing social inequalities, and enhancing access to mental health services can help mitigate the adverse effects of social fractures on depression [24].

Social Support and Coping Mechanisms

Social support plays a crucial role in buffering individuals from the negative effects of stress and adversity. When individuals lack adequate social support networks, they may struggle to cope with life's challenges, leading to increased vulnerability to depression [3]. This is particularly relevant in contexts where traditional sources of social support, such as extended family or close-knit communities, have eroded due to social isolation.

Stigmatization and Discrimination

Stigma surrounding mental illness can contribute to social isolation by discouraging individuals from seeking help or disclosing their struggles to others [4]. Fear of being judged or marginalized may lead individuals to withdraw from social interactions, further exacerbating feelings of isolation and depression. Recognition of this stigma by non-healthcare professionals, such as clergy, extended family, community leaders, and educators, would then be critical in breaking this chain of events resulting in mental illness.

Digital Connectivity and Social Media

While digital technologies offer new avenues for social connection, they can also contribute to feelings of isolation and depression. Paradoxically, excessive use of social media may lead to superficial relationships and a sense of inadequacy through social comparison [5]. Moreover, cyberbullying and online harassment can exacerbate feelings of loneliness and depression, particularly among vulnerable populations [6].

As mentioned earlier in this chapter, the absence of physical touch, which is not mediated by digital communication, can further exacerbate the feeling of social disconnection and loneliness [126]. The desire for intimate physical interactions has been associated with increased anxiety and loneliness [127, 128]. The use of social media is not sufficient to overcome the desire for interpersonal touch, and to prevent the feeling of social isolation and loneliness [40, 41, 126].

Although increased social media use is often driven by a desire to alleviate loneliness, it does not necessarily lead to greater happiness [129].

Cultural Norms and Expectations

Cultural norms regarding individualism and self-reliance can exacerbate feelings of isolation by promoting the idea that seeking help is a sign of weakness [7]. In societies where self-disclosure is discouraged or mental health issues are stigmatized, individuals may be less likely to reach out for support, leading to prolonged periods of social isolation and depression.

Intersectionality and Marginalization

Intersectional factors such as race, gender, sexuality, and socioeconomic status intersect to shape individuals' experiences of social isolation and depression [8]. Marginalized groups, such as LGBTQ+ individuals or racial minorities, may face additional barriers to social inclusion, further exacerbating their risk of depression.

Community Interventions and Social Policies

We understand that addressing social isolation and depression requires not only individual-level interventions but also systemic changes at the community and policy levels. Initiatives aimed at strengthening social ties, promoting inclusivity, and reducing stigma can help mitigate the adverse effects of social isolation on mental health [9]. Again, awareness by the general population would be key in intervening in processes that may result in poor mental health.

The sociology of social isolation and depression underscores the complex interplay between social structures, interpersonal relationships, cultural norms, and systemic inequalities. Understanding these dynamics is essential for developing holistic approaches to addressing mental health disparities and promoting well-being across the population.

If you or someone you know is struggling with loneliness or is feeling helpless and suicidal, there are many resources out there. If you are in the USA, support can be found at Find a support group | AFSP. *If suicide is in the picture and you need assistance immediately, call 988 or National Suicide Prevention Helpline at 1-800-273-TALK (8255). The Helpline is a free, confidential crisis hotline that is available to everyone 24 hours a day, seven days a week.* National Hotline for Mental Health Crises and Suicide Prevention | NAMI

If you are in another country, you can go to www.befrienders.org *to find a helpline near you.*

Summary

This chapter explores the sociology of isolation, tracing historical perspectives from classical sociologists, such as Emile Durkheim, Karl Marx, Max Weber, and George Simmel. It highlights how urbanization and modernization have contributed to increased social fragmentation, leading to feelings of isolation and loneliness.

The impact of social isolation is analyzed within cultural and historical contexts, considering various factors, such as age, gender, socioeconomic status, and cultural norms. Effects have been examined of pandemics (e.g., Spanish flu, COVID-19) on social isolation and community dynamics, illustrating how public health measures and societal responses shape social interactions.

Connections between social isolation and depression are explored, emphasizing the role of social determinants, intersectionality, and technological advancements in influencing mental health outcomes.

The chapter concludes with discussions on interventions and policy implications aimed at reducing social fractures, promoting social connectedness, and addressing mental health disparities within diverse communities.

References

1. Durkheim, Suicide 1897.
2. Hawkley LC, Cacioppo JT. Loneliness matters: a theoretical and empirical review of consequences and mechanisms. Ann Behav Med. 2010;40(2):218–27.
3. Thoits PA. Mechanisms linking social ties and support to physical and mental health. J Health Soc Behav. 2011;52(2):145–61.
4. Corrigan PW. How stigma interferes with mental health care. Am Psychol. 2004;59(7):614–25.
5. Kross E, Verduyn P, Demiralp E, Park J, Lee DS, Lin N, et al. Facebook use predicts declines in subjective Well-being in young adults. PLoS One. 2013;8(8):e69841.
6. Kowalski RM, Giumetti GW, Schroeder AN, Lattanner MR. Bullying in the digital age: a critical review and meta-analysis of cyberbullying research among youth. Psychol Bull. 2014;140(4):1073–137.
7. Twenge JM, Campbell WK, Freeman EC. Generational differences in young adults' life goals, concern for others, and civic orientation, 1966–2009. J Pers Soc Psychol. 2010;98(5):750–9.
8. Hankivsky O. Intersectionality 101. The Institute for Intersectionality Research and Policy, Simon Fraser University; 2014.
9. Leigh-Hunt N, Bagguley D, Bash K, Turner V, Turnbull S, Valtorta N, Caan W. An overview of systematic reviews on the public health consequences of social isolation and loneliness. Public Health. 2017;152:157–71.
10. Barry JM. The great influenza: the epic story of the deadliest plague in history. Viking Penguin; 2004.
11. Blumer H. Symbolic interactionism: perspective and method. University of California Press; 1969.
12. Brooks SK, Webster RK, Smith LE, Woodland L, Wessely S, Greenberg N, Rubin GJ. The psychological impact of quarantine and how to reduce it: rapid review of the evidence. Lancet. 2020;395(10227):912–20.
13. Fancourt D, Steptoe A, Bu F. Trajectories of anxiety and depressive symptoms during enforced isolation due to COVID-19: longitudinal analyses of 36,520 adults in England. medRxiv. 2020;
14. Fouad NA, Grus CL, Hatcher R, Kaslow NJ, Hutchings PS, Madson MB, et al. COVID-19 impact on research, teaching, and service: a community psychology perspective. Am J Community Psychol. 2021;67(3–4):357–69.
15. Klingaman WK. The year without summer: 1816 and the volcano that darkened the world and changed history. St. Martin's Press; 1989.
16. Kudish N. A crucial misconception: "the eternal return" of the Spanish flu in historical memory. Historia Crítica. 2016;62:153–77.
17. Parsons T. The social system. Free Press; 1951.
18. Putnam RD. Bowling alone: the collapse and revival of American community. Simon and Schuster; 2000.
19. Cacioppo JT, Hawkley LC. Loneliness. In: Fiske ST, Gilbert DT, Lindzey G, editors. Handbook of social psychology, vol. 2. John Wiley & Sons Inc.; 2010. p. 815–38.
20. Hankerson SH, Fenton MC. Racial and ethnic differences in the association between social support and mental health in a national sample of young adults in the United States. J Natl Med Assoc. 2015;107(1):36–48.
21. Lorant V, Deliège D, Eaton W, Robert A, Philippot P, Ansseau M. Socioeconomic inequalities in depression: a meta-analysis. Am J Epidemiol. 2003;157(2):98–112.
22. Meyer IH. Prejudice, social stress, and mental health in lesbian, gay, and bisexual populations: conceptual issues and research evidence. Psychol Bull. 2003;129(5):674–97.
23. Primack BA, Shensa A, Sidani JE, Whaite EO, Lin LY, Rosen D, et al. Social media use and perceived social isolation among young adults in the U.S. Am J Prev Med. 2017;53(1):1–8.
24. Fazel M, Wheeler J. Social determinants of mental health. Int Rev Psychiatry. 2010;22(6):571–83.
25. Marx K. Das Kapital: Kritik der politischen Oekonomie; herausgegeben von Friedrich Engels. Vol. 3: Der Gesamtprozess der kapitalistischen Produktion. 1st ed. Hamburg: Verlag von Otto Meissner; 1894. https://doi.org/10.3931/e-rara-25739.
26. Weber M, Baehr PR, Wells GC. The Protestant ethic and the "spirit" of capitalism and other writings. Penguin; 2002. ISBN 978-0-14-043921-2
27. Simmel G. Soziologie: Untersuchungen über die Formen der Vergesellschaftung. Leipzig: Duncker & Humblot; 1908. The third and most recent translation of the text was published in a collection edited by Donald Levine ("The Stranger." In Georg Simmel: On Individuality and Social Forms, Chicago: Univ. of Chicago Press, 1971, pp. 143–50)
28. McPherson M, Smith-Lovin L, Brashears ME. Social isolation in America: changes in core discussion networks over two decades. Am Sociol Rev. 2006;71(3):353–75.
29. Cacioppo JT, Hawkley LC, Berntson GG. The anatomy of loneliness. Curr Dir Psychol Sci. 2003;12(3):71–4.
30. Rodríguez-PoseA.Theriseofthe"City-region"conceptanditsdevelopment policy implications. Eur Plan Stud. 2008;16(8):1025–46. https://doi.org/10.1080/09654310802315567.
31. Cattaneo A, Girgin S, de By R, et al. Worldwide delineation of multi-tier city–regions. Nat Cities. 2024;1:469–79. https://doi.org/10.1038/s44284-024-00083-z.
32. Roy A. The 21st-century Metropolis: new geographies of theory. Reg Stud. 2009;43(6):819–30. https://doi.org/10.1080/00343400701809665.
33. Weiss R. Loneliness: the experience of emotional and social isolation. MIT Press; 1975.
34. https://nap.nationalacademies.org/read/25663/chapter/1
35. Heu LC, van Zomeren M, Hansen N. Does loneliness thrive in relational freedom or restriction? The culture-loneliness framework. Rev Gen Psychol. 2021;25(1):60–72.
36. Lykes VA, Kemmelmeier M. What predicts loneliness? Cultural difference between individualistic and collectivistic societies in Europe. J Cross-Cult Psychol. 2014;45(3):468–90.
37. Oyserman D, Coon HM, Kemmelmeier M. Rethinking individualism and collectivism: evaluation of theoretical assumptions and meta-analyses. Psychol Bull. 2002;128(1):3–72.
38. Chauvin JP, Glaeser E, Ma Y, Tobio K. What is different about urbanization in rich and poor countries? Cities in Brazil, China, India and the United States. J Urban Econ. 2017;98:17–49.
39. Suh J, Horvitz E, White RW, et al. Disparate impacts on online information access during the Covid-19 pandemic. Nat Commun. 2022;13:7094. https://doi.org/10.1038/s41467-022-34592-z.
40. Twenge JM, Spitzberg BH, Campbell WK. Less in-person social interaction with peers among U.S. adolescents in the 21st century and links to loneliness. J Soc Pers Relat. 2019;36:1892–913. https://doi.org/10.1177/0265407519836170.
41. Triberti S, Brivio E, Galimberti C. On social presence: theories, methodologies, and guidelines for the innovative contexts of computer-mediated learning. In: Marmon M, editor. Enhancing social presence in online learning environments. Hershey: IGI Global; 2018.
42. Wang X, Chen J, Burström B, Burström K. Exploring pathways to outpatients' satisfaction with health care in Chinese public hospitals in urban and rural areas using patient-reported experiences. Int J Equity Health. 2019;18(1):29. PMCID: PMC6366112. http://www.ncbi.nlm.nih.gov/pubmed/30728005
43. Miao J, Wu X. Urbanization, socioeconomic status and health disparity in China. Health Place. 2016;42:87–95. PMID: 27750075. http://www.ncbi.nlm.nih.gov/pubmed/27750075
44. Kelsall-Foreman I, Bucks RS, Weinborn M, Badcock JC. Loneliness and objective social isolation are differentially associated with anomalous perceptions in community-dwelling

older adults. Cogn Neuropsychiatry. 2023;28(2):130–46. PMID: 36744805. http://www.ncbi.nlm.nih.gov/pubmed/36744805

45. Visvalingam S, Magson NR, Newins AR, Norberg MM. Going it alone: examining interpersonal sensitivity and hostility as mediators of the link between perfectionism and social disconnection. J Pers. 2024;92(4):1024–36. PMID: 37519015. http://www.ncbi.nlm.nih.gov/pubmed/37519015
46. Simionato J, Vally H, Archibald D. Circumstances that promote social connectedness in older adults participating in intergenerational programmes with adolescents: a realist review. BMJ Open. 2023;13(10):e069765. PMCID: PMC10583064. http://www.ncbi.nlm.nih.gov/pubmed/37848294
47. Cacioppo JT, Hawkley LC, Norman GJ, Berntson GG. Social isolation. Ann N Y Acad Sci. 2011;1231(1):17–22. PMCID: PMC3166409. http://www.ncbi.nlm.nih.gov/pubmed/21651565
48. Holt-Lunstad J, Smith TB, Baker M, Harris T, Stephenson D. Loneliness and social isolation as risk factors for mortality: a meta-analytic review. Perspect Psychol Sci. 2015;10(2):227–37. PMID: 25910392. http://www.ncbi.nlm.nih.gov/pubmed/25910392
49. Layden EA, Cacioppo JT, Cacioppo S, Cappa SF, Dodich A, Falini A, Canessa N. Perceived social isolation is associated with altered functional connectivity in neural networks associated with tonic alertness and executive control. Neuroimage. 2017;145(Pt A):58–73. PMID: 27664824. http://www.ncbi.nlm.nih.gov/pubmed/27664824
50. Malcolm M, Frost H, Cowie J. Loneliness and social isolation causal association with health-related lifestyle risk in older adults: a systematic review and meta-analysis protocol. Syst Rev. 2019;8(1):48. PMCID: PMC6366024. http://www.ncbi.nlm.nih.gov/pubmed/30732659
51. Rico-Uribe LA, Caballero FF, Martín-María N, Cabello M, Ayuso-Mateos JL, Miret M. Association of loneliness with all-cause mortality: a meta-analysis. PLoS One. 2018;13(1):e0190033. PMCID: PMC5754055. http://www.ncbi.nlm.nih.gov/pubmed/29300743
52. Courtin E, Knapp M. Social isolation, loneliness and health in old age: a scoping review. Health Soc Care Community. 2017;25(3):799–812. PMID: 26712585. http://www.ncbi.nlm.nih.gov/pubmed/26712585
53. Hodgson S, Watts I, Fraser S, Roderick P, Dambha-Miller H. Loneliness, social isolation, cardiovascular disease and mortality: a synthesis of the literature and conceptual framework. J R Soc Med. 2020;113(5):185–92. PMCID: PMC7366328. http://www.ncbi.nlm.nih.gov/pubmed/32407646
54. Ho KHM, Yang C, Ng MSN, Tao A, Chan HYL. Loneliness at end-of-life: a scoping review. J Clin Nurs. 2023;32(17–18):6179–95. PMID: 37149735. http://www.ncbi.nlm.nih.gov/pubmed/37149735
55. Cacioppo JT, Cacioppo S. The growing problem of loneliness. Lancet. 2018;391(10119):426. PMCID: PMC6530780. http://www.ncbi.nlm.nih.gov/pubmed/29407030.
56. Wilson RS, Krueger KR, Arnold SE, Schneider JA, Kelly JF, Barnes LL, Tang Y, Bennett DA. Loneliness and risk of Alzheimer disease. Arch Gen Psychiatry. 2007;64(2):234–40. PMID: 17283291. http://www.ncbi.nlm.nih.gov/pubmed/17283291
57. van Roekel E, Verhagen M, Engels RCME, Scholte RHJ, Cacioppo S, Cacioppo JT. Trait and state levels of loneliness in early and late adolescents: examining the differential reactivity hypothesis. J Clin Child Adolesc Psychol. 2018;47(6):888–99. PMID: 27191708. http://www.ncbi.nlm.nih.gov/pubmed/27191708
58. Wang F, Gao Y, Han Z, Yu Y, Long Z, Jiang X, Wu Y, Pei B, Cao Y, Ye J, Wang M, Zhao Y. A systematic review and meta-analysis of 90 cohort studies of social isolation, loneliness and mortality. Nat Hum Behav. 2023;7(8):1307–19. PMID: 37337095. http://www.ncbi.nlm.nih.gov/pubmed/37337095
59. Zhou X, Yang F, Gao Y. A meta-analysis of the association between loneliness and all-cause mortality in older adults. Psychiatry Res. 2023;328:115430. PMID: 37647699. http://www.ncbi.nlm.nih.gov/pubmed/37647699
60. Long RM, Terracciano A, Sutin AR, Creaven AM, Gerstorf D, D'Arcy-Bewick S, O'Súilleabháin PS. Loneliness, Social isolation, and living alone associations with mortality risk in individuals living with cardiovascular disease: a systematic review, meta-analysis, and meta-regression. Psychosom Med. 2023;85(1):8–17. PMID: 36441849. http://www.ncbi.nlm.nih.gov/pubmed/36441849
61. Zhang X, Dong S. The relationships between social support and loneliness: a meta-analysis and review. Acta Psychol. 2022;227:103616. PMID: 35576818. http://www.ncbi.nlm.nih.gov/pubmed/35576818
62. Gabarrell-Pascuet A, García-Mieres H, Giné-Vázquez I, Moneta MV, Koyanagi A, Haro JM, Domènech-Abella J. The Association of Social Support and Loneliness with Symptoms of Depression, Anxiety, and Posttraumatic Stress during the COVID-19 Pandemic: a Meta-Analysis. Int J Environ Res Public Health. 2023;20(4):2765. PMCID: PMC9957328. http://www.ncbi.nlm.nih.gov/pubmed/36833463
63. Wen Z, Wang H, Liang Q, Liu L, Zhang W, Zhang X. Mediating effect of social support and resilience between loneliness and depression in older adults: a systematic review and meta-analytic structural equation modeling. J Affect Disord. 2024;365:246–57. PMID: 39147150. http://www.ncbi.nlm.nih.gov/pubmed/39147150
64. Machado N, Abreo L, Petkari E, Pinto da Costa M. The relationship of social contacts with prisoners' mental health: a systematic review. Public Health. 2024;234:199–216. PMID: 39053366. http://www.ncbi.nlm.nih.gov/pubmed/39053366
65. Freak-Poli R, Phyo AZZ, Hu J, Barker SF. Are social isolation, lack of social support or loneliness risk factors for cardiovascular disease in Australia and New Zealand? A systematic review and meta-analysis. Health Promot J Austr. 2022;33 Suppl 1(Suppl 1):278–315. PMCID: PMC9790538. http://www.ncbi.nlm.nih.gov/pubmed/35263481
66. Winterton A, Rødevand L, Westlye LT, Steen NE, Andreassen OA, Quintana DS. Associations of loneliness and social isolation with cardiovascular and metabolic health: a systematic review and meta-analysis protocol. Syst Rev. 2020;9(1):102. PMCID: PMC7199368. http://www.ncbi.nlm.nih.gov/pubmed/32366295
67. Meng M, Ma Z, Zhou H, Xie Y, Lan R, Zhu S, Miao D, Shen X. The impact of social relationships on the risk of stroke and post-stroke mortality: a systematic review and meta-analysis. BMC Public Health. 2024;24(1):2403. PMCID: PMC11373457. http://www.ncbi.nlm.nih.gov/pubmed/39232685
68. Chau AKC, Zhu C, So SHW. Loneliness and the psychosis continuum: a meta-analysis on positive psychotic experiences and a meta-analysis on negative psychotic experiences. Int Rev Psychiatry. 2019;31(5–6):471–90. PMID: 31331209. http://www.ncbi.nlm.nih.gov/pubmed/31331209
69. Cacioppo JT, Cacioppo S, Capitanio JP, Cole SW. The neuroendocrinology of social isolation. Annu Rev Psychol. 2015;66:733–67. PMCID: PMC5130104. http://www.ncbi.nlm.nih.gov/pubmed/25148851
70. Miller G. Social neuroscience. Why loneliness is hazardous to your health. Science. 2011;331(6014):138–40. PMID: 21233358. http://www.ncbi.nlm.nih.gov/pubmed/21233358
71. Cacioppo S, Capitanio JP, Cacioppo JT. Toward a neurology of loneliness. Psychol Bull. 2014;140(6):1464–504. PMCID: PMC5130107. http://www.ncbi.nlm.nih.gov/pubmed/25222636
72. Lim MH, Eres R, Vasan S. Understanding loneliness in the twenty-first century: an update on correlates, risk factors,

and potential solutions. Soc Psychiatry Psychiatr Epidemiol. 2020;55(7):793–810. PMID: 32524169. http://www.ncbi.nlm.nih.gov/pubmed/32524169

73. Abdellaoui A, Sanchez-Roige S, Sealock J, Treur JL, Dennis J, Fontanillas P, Elson S, 23andme Research Team, Nivard MG, Ip HF, van der Zee M, Baselmans BML, Hottenga JJ, Willemsen G, Mosing M, Lu Y, Pedersen NL, Denys D, Amin N, M van Duijn C, Szilagyi I, Tiemeier H, Neumann A, Verweij KJH, Cacioppo S, Cacioppo JT, Davis LK, Palmer AA, Boomsma DI. Phenome-wide investigation of health outcomes associated with genetic predisposition to loneliness. Hum Mol Genet 2019;28(22):3853–3865. PMCID: PMC6935385 PubMed entry [Internet]. [cited 2024 Dec 31]. Available from: http://www.ncbi.nlm.nih.gov/pubmed/31518406
74. Hartley S, McArthur M, Coenen M, Cabello M, Covelli V, Roszczynska-Michta J, Pitkänen T, Bickenbach J, Cieza A. Narratives reflecting the lived experiences of people with brain disorders: common psychosocial difficulties and determinants. PLoS One. 2014;9(5):e96890. PMCID: PMC4013080. http://www.ncbi.nlm.nih.gov/pubmed/24805128
75. Social Isolation and Loneliness in Older Adults: Opportunities for the Health Care System | The National Academies Press
76. Personal Autonomy (Stanford Encyclopedia of Philosophy)
77. Henning-Smith C, Moscovice I, Kozhimannil K. Differences in social isolation and its relationship to health by rurality. J Rural Health. 2019;35(4):540–9. PMID: 30609155. http://www.ncbi.nlm.nih.gov/pubmed/30609155
78. Naito R, Leong DP, Bangdiwala SI, McKee M, Subramanian SV, Rangarajan S, Islam S, Avezum A, Yeates KE, Lear SA, Gupta R, Yusufali A, Dans AL, Szuba A, Alhabib KF, Kaur M, Rahman O, Seron P, Diaz R, Puoane T, Liu W, Zhu Y, Sheng Y, Lopez-Jaramillo P, Chifamba J, Rosnah I, Karsidag K, Kelishadi R, Rosengren A, Khatib R, K R LIA, Azam SI, Teo K, Yusuf S. Impact of social isolation on mortality and morbidity in 20 high-income, middle-income and low-income countries in five continents. BMJ Glob Health. 2021;6(3):e004124. PMCID: PMC7986654. http://www.ncbi.nlm.nih.gov/pubmed/33753400
79. Au A, Murad-Kassam S, Mukanoheli V, Idrees S, Ben Mabrouk E, Abdi K, Kennedy M, Whitfield K, Salma J. Immigrant older adults' experiences of aging in place and their neighborhoods: a qualitative systematic review. Int J Environ Res Public Health. 2024;21(7):904. PMCID: PMC11277252. http://www.ncbi.nlm.nih.gov/pubmed/39063481
80. Gallardo-Peralta LP, Sánchez-Moreno E, Rodríguez Rodríguez V, García Martín M. Studying loneliness and social support networks among older people: a systematic review in Europe. Rev Esp Salud Publica. 2023;97:e202301006. PMCID: PMC10540907. http://www.ncbi.nlm.nih.gov/pubmed/36700292
81. Vieira MF, Méio MDBB, Reis ABR, Villela LD, de Rodrigues MCC, de Almeida Di Maio Ferreira FCP, de Paula Barros LB, Costa RP, Menezes ER, Campos CO, Moreira MEL, Gomes-Junior SCS. High-risk children and social isolation: the importance of family functioning. Front Psychol. 2023;14:1190438. PMCID: PMC10325665. http://www.ncbi.nlm.nih.gov/pubmed/37425187
82. Salmon C, Quesnel-Vallée A, Parent MÉ. Family structure and living arrangements as indicators of social isolation, and prostate cancer risk. Prev Med. 2023;172:107544. PMID: 37178831. http://www.ncbi.nlm.nih.gov/pubmed/37178831
83. Heshmati S, Blackard MB, Beckmann B, Chipidza W. Family relationships and adolescent loneliness: an application of social network analysis in family studies. J Fam Psychol. 2021;35(2):182–91. PMID: 33871279. http://www.ncbi.nlm.nih.gov/pubmed/33871279
84. Liang J, Aranda MP, Jang Y, Wilber K. The role of social isolation on mediating depression and anxiety among primary family caregivers of older adults: a two-wave mediation analysis. Int J Behav Med. 2024;31(3):445–58. PMCID: PMC11043211. http://www.ncbi.nlm.nih.gov/pubmed/37878186
85. Litchfield I, Shukla D, Greenfield S. Impact of COVID-19 on the digital divide: a rapid review. BMJ Open 2021;11(10):e053440. PMCID: PMC8520586. http://www.ncbi.nlm.nih.gov/pubmed/34642200
86. COVID-19 Mental Disorders Collaborators. Global prevalence and burden of depressive and anxiety disorders in 204 countries and territories in 2020 due to the COVID-19 pandemic. Lancet. 2021;398(10312):1700–12. PMCID: PMC8500697. http://www.ncbi.nlm.nih.gov/pubmed/34634250
87. GBD 2017 Disease and Injury Incidence and Prevalence Collaborators. Global, regional, and national incidence, prevalence, and years lived with disability for 354 diseases and injuries for 195 countries and territories, 1990–2017: a systematic analysis for the Global Burden of Disease Study 2017. Lancet. 2018;392(10159):1789–858. PMCID: PMC6227754. http://www.ncbi.nlm.nih.gov/pubmed/30496104
88. Depressive disorder (depression)
89. Silva C, Fonseca C, Ferreira R, Weidner A, Morgado B, Lopes MJ, Moritz S, Jelinek L, Schneider BC, Pinho LG. Depression in older adults during the COVID-19 pandemic: a systematic review. J Am Geriatr Soc. 2023;71(7):2308–25. PMID: 37029710. http://www.ncbi.nlm.nih.gov/pubmed/37029710
90. Azevedo LVDS, Calandri IL, Slachevsky A, Graviotto HG, Vieira MCS, de Andrade CB, Rossetti AP, Generoso AB, Carmona KC, Pinto LAC, Sorbara M, Pinto A, Guajardo T, Olavarria L, Thumala D, Crivelli L, Vivas L, Allegri RF, Barbosa MT, Serrano CM, Miranda-Castillo C, Caramelli P. Impact of social isolation on people with dementia and their family caregivers. J Alzheimers Dis. 2021;81(2):607–17. PMCID: PMC11185189. http://www.ncbi.nlm.nih.gov/pubmed/33814446
91. Barguilla A, Fernández-Lebrero A, Estragués-Gázquez I, García-Escobar G, Navalpotro-Gómez I, Manero RM, Puente-Periz V, Roquer J, Puig-Pijoan A. Effects of COVID-19 pandemic confinement in patients with cognitive impairment. Front Neurol. 2020;11:589901. PMCID: PMC7732426. http://www.ncbi.nlm.nih.gov/pubmed/33329337
92. Koszalinski RS, Olmos B. Communication challenges in social isolation, subjective cognitive decline, and mental health status in older adults: a scoping review (2019–2021). Perspect Psychiatr Care. 2022;58(4):2741–55. PMID: 35582750. http://www.ncbi.nlm.nih.gov/pubmed/35582750
93. Harrington KD, Vasan S, Kang JE, Sliwinski MJ, Lim MH. Loneliness and cognitive function in older adults without dementia: a systematic review and meta-analysis. J Alzheimers Dis. 2023;91(4):1243–59. PMCID: PMC9983432. http://www.ncbi.nlm.nih.gov/pubmed/36617781
94. Lara E, Martín-María N, De la Torre-Luque A, Koyanagi A, Vancampfort D, Izquierdo A, Miret M. Does loneliness contribute to mild cognitive impairment and dementia? A systematic review and meta-analysis of longitudinal studies. Ageing Res Rev. 2019;52:7–16. PMID: 30914351. http://www.ncbi.nlm.nih.gov/pubmed/30914351
95. Fan K, Seah B, Lu Z, Wang T, Zhou Y. Association between loneliness and mild cognitive impairment in older adults: a meta-analysis of longitudinal studies. Aging Ment Health. 2024;28(12):1650–8. PMID: 38825970. http://www.ncbi.nlm.nih.gov/pubmed/38825970
96. Cole SW, Cacioppo JT, Cacioppo S, Bone K, Del Rosso LA, Spinner A, Arevalo JMG, Dizon TP, Capitanio JP. The type I interferon antiviral gene program is impaired by lockdown and preserved by caregiving. Proc Natl Acad Sci USA.

2021;118(29):e2105803118. PMCID: PMC8307615. http://www.ncbi.nlm.nih.gov/pubmed/34272291
97. Capitanio JP, Cacioppo S, Cole SW. Loneliness in monkeys: Neuroimmune mechanisms. Curr Opin Behav Sci. 2019;28:51–7. PMCID: PMC6857932. http://www.ncbi.nlm.nih.gov/pubmed/31737750
98. Spithoven AWM, Cacioppo S, Goossens L, Cacioppo JT. Genetic contributions to loneliness and their relevance to the evolutionary theory of loneliness. Perspect Psychol Sci. 2019;14(3):376–96. PMID: 30844327. http://www.ncbi.nlm.nih.gov/pubmed/30844327
99. Cacioppo S, Bangee M, Balogh S, Cardenas-Iniguez C, Qualter P, Cacioppo JT. Loneliness and implicit attention to social threat: a high-performance electrical neuroimaging study. Cogn Neurosci. 2016;7(1–4):138–59. PMID: 26274315. http://www.ncbi.nlm.nih.gov/pubmed/26274315
100. Goossens L, van Roekel E, Verhagen M, Cacioppo JT, Cacioppo S, Maes M, Boomsma DI. The genetics of loneliness: linking evolutionary theory to genome-wide genetics, epigenetics, and social science. Perspect Psychol Sci. 2015;10(2):213–26. PMID: 25910391. http://www.ncbi.nlm.nih.gov/pubmed/25910391
101. Layden EA, Cacioppo JT, Cacioppo S. Loneliness predicts a preference for larger interpersonal distance within intimate space. PLoS One. 2018;13(9):e0203491. PMCID: PMC6126853. http://www.ncbi.nlm.nih.gov/pubmed/30188950
102. Cacioppo JT, Chen HY, Cacioppo S. Reciprocal influences between loneliness and self-centeredness: a cross-lagged panel analysis in a population-based sample of African American, Hispanic, and Caucasian adults. Pers Soc Psychol Bull. 2017;43(8):1125–35. PMID: 28903715. http://www.ncbi.nlm.nih.gov/pubmed/28903715
103. Loboprabhu S, Molinari V. Appreciating the 4 "Ts" of loneliness when providing psychiatric care for the lonely patient. J Psychiatr Pract. 2019;25(5):402–10. PMID: 31505529. http://www.ncbi.nlm.nih.gov/pubmed/31505529
104. King-Mullins E, Maccou E, Miller P. Intersectionality: understanding the interdependent systems of discrimination and disadvantage. Clin Colon Rectal Surg. 2023;36(5):356–64. PMCID: PMC10411112. http://www.ncbi.nlm.nih.gov/pubmed/37564344
105. Singh RS, Bhambhani Y, Skinta MD, Torres-Harding SR. Measurement of intersectional microaggressions: conceptual barriers and recommendations. Perspect Psychol Sci. 2021;16(5):956–71. PMID: 34498531. http://www.ncbi.nlm.nih.gov/pubmed/34498531
106. Ghavami N, Katsiaficas D, Rogers LO. Toward an intersectional approach in developmental science: the role of race, gender, sexual orientation, and immigrant status. Adv Child Dev Behav. 2016;50:31–73. PMID: 26956069. http://www.ncbi.nlm.nih.gov/pubmed/26956069
107. Evans CR, Erickson N. Intersectionality and depression in adolescence and early adulthood: a MAIHDA analysis of the national longitudinal study of adolescent to adult health, 1995–2008. Soc Sci Med. 2019;220:1–11. PMID: 30390469. http://www.ncbi.nlm.nih.gov/pubmed/30390469
108. Christian LM, Cole SW, McDade T, Pachankis JE, Morgan E, Strahm AM, Kamp Dush CM. A biopsychosocial framework for understanding sexual and gender minority health: a call for action. Neurosci Biobehav Rev. 2021;129:107–116. PMCID: PMC8429206. http://www.ncbi.nlm.nih.gov/pubmed/34097981
109. Balki E, Hayes N, Holland C. Effectiveness of technology interventions in addressing social isolation, connectedness, and loneliness in older adults: systematic umbrella review. JMIR Aging. 2022;5(4):e40125. PMCID: PMC9641519. http://www.ncbi.nlm.nih.gov/pubmed/36279155
110. Sen K, Prybutok G, Prybutok V. The use of digital technology for social wellbeing reduces social isolation in older adults: a systematic review. SSM Popul Health. 2022;17:101020. PMCID: PMC8733322. http://www.ncbi.nlm.nih.gov/pubmed/35024424
111. Hoge E, Bickham D, Cantor J. Digital media, anxiety, and depression in children. Pediatrics. 2017;140(Suppl 2):S76–80. PMID: 29093037. http://www.ncbi.nlm.nih.gov/pubmed/29093037
112. Sales-Filho GS, Bandeira ID, Argollo N, Lucena R. Hikikomori syndrome and digital technologies: a systematic review. Harv Rev Psychiatry. 2023;31(2):50–9. PMID: 36884037. http://www.ncbi.nlm.nih.gov/pubmed/36884037
113. Neoh MJY, Carollo A, Lim M, Esposito G. Hikikomori: a scientometric review of 20 years of research. Int J Environ Res Public Health. 2023;20(9):5657. PMCID: PMC10177810. http://www.ncbi.nlm.nih.gov/pubmed/37174175.
114. Ghaemi SN. Digital depression: a new disease of the millennium? Acta Psychiatr Scand. 2020;141(4):356–61. PMID: 31955405. http://www.ncbi.nlm.nih.gov/pubmed/31955405
115. Twenge JM. Why increases in adolescent depression may be linked to the technological environment. Curr Opin Psychol. 2020;32:89–94. PMID: 31415993. http://www.ncbi.nlm.nih.gov/pubmed/31415993
116. Twenge JM, Campbell WK. Media use is linked to lower psychological Well-being: evidence from three datasets. Psychiatr Q. 2019;90(2):311–31. PMID: 30859387. http://www.ncbi.nlm.nih.gov/pubmed/30859387
117. Twenge JM. Increases in depression, self-harm, and suicide among U.S. adolescents after 2012 and links to technology use: possible mechanisms. Psychiatr Res Clin Pract. 2020;2(1):19–25. PMCID: PMC9176070. http://www.ncbi.nlm.nih.gov/pubmed/36101887
118. Noone C, McSharry J, Smalle M, Burns A, Dwan K, Devane D, Morrissey EC. Video calls for reducing social isolation and loneliness in older people: a rapid review. Cochrane Database Syst Rev. 2020;5(5):CD013632. PMCID: PMC7387868. http://www.ncbi.nlm.nih.gov/pubmed/32441330
119. Odgers CL, Jensen MR. Annual research review: adolescent mental health in the digital age: facts, fears, and future directions. J Child Psychol Psychiatry. 2020;61(3):336–48. PMCID: PMC8221420. http://www.ncbi.nlm.nih.gov/pubmed/31951670
120. Hilty DM, Stubbe D, McKean AJ, Hoffman PE, Zalpuri I, Myint MT, Joshi SV, Pakyurek M, Li STT. A scoping review of social media in child, adolescents and young adults: research findings in depression, anxiety and other clinical challenges. BJPsych Open. 2023;9(5):e152. PMCID: PMC10594088. http://www.ncbi.nlm.nih.gov/pubmed/37563766
121. Masi CM, Chen HY, Hawkley LC, Cacioppo JT. A meta-analysis of interventions to reduce loneliness. Pers Soc Psychol Rev. 2011;15(3):219–66. PMCID: PMC3865701. http://www.ncbi.nlm.nih.gov/pubmed/20716644
122. "Demarginalizing the Intersection of Race and Sex: A Black Feminist Cri" by Kimberle Crenshaw
123. Cacioppo S, Grippo AJ, London S, Goossens L, Cacioppo JT. Loneliness: clinical import and interventions. Perspect Psychol Sci. 2015;10(2):238–49. PMCID: PMC4391342. http://www.ncbi.nlm.nih.gov/pubmed/25866548
124. Yu DSF, Li PWC, Lin RSY, Kee F, Chiu A, Wu W. Effects of non-pharmacological interventions on loneliness among community-dwelling older adults: a systematic review, network meta-analysis,

and meta-regression. Int J Nurs Stud. 2023;144:104524. PMID: 37295285. http://www.ncbi.nlm.nih.gov/pubmed/37295285
125. Hughes ME, Waite LJ, Hawkley LC, Cacioppo JT. A short scale for measuring loneliness in large surveys: results from two population-based studies. Res Aging. 2004;26(6):655–72. PMCID: PMC2394670. http://www.ncbi.nlm.nih.gov/pubmed/18504506
126. Della Longa L, Valori I, Farroni T. Interpersonal affective touch in a virtual world: feeling the social presence of others to overcome loneliness. Front Psychol. 2021;12:795283. PMCID: PMC8787079. http://www.ncbi.nlm.nih.gov/pubmed/35087455
127. von Mohr M, Kirsch LP, Fotopoulou A. The soothing function of touch: affective touch reduces feelings of social exclusion. Sci Rep. 2017;7(1):13516. PMCID: PMC5647341. http://www.ncbi.nlm.nih.gov/pubmed/29044137
128. von Mohr M, Kirsch LP, Fotopoulou A. Social touch deprivation during COVID-19: effects on psychological wellbeing and craving interpersonal touch. R Soc Open Sci. 2021;8(9):210287. PMCID: PMC8424338. http://www.ncbi.nlm.nih.gov/pubmed/34527270
129. Cauberghe V, Van Wesenbeeck I, De Jans S, Hudders L, Ponnet K. How adolescents use social Media to cope with feelings of loneliness and anxiety during COVID-19 lockdown. Cyberpsychol Behav Soc Netw. 2021;24(4):250–7. PMID: 33185488. http://www.ncbi.nlm.nih.gov/pubmed/33185488

Depression Associated with Other Medical Conditions

12

Franklin Sunzeri and Elizabeth Sunzeri

Introduction

A patient's history of disease is frequently associated with subsequent depression [1–6, 8], and depression is associated with future disease occurrence [1, 7–9].

To shed some light on this bidirectional interaction, a *scoping review*[1] of depression and multiple morbidity was published in 2019 [1]. *Multiple morbidity* is the occurrence of two or more chronic medical conditions [11]. Multiple morbidity has significantly increased since the late 1980s to the extent that almost 60% of adults meet the criteria [12]. The scoping review used two data sets. One was a large, randomly selected, population-based sample [10]. The second group included 25 systematic reviews and meta-analyses. The first study found that depression was most commonly related to hypertension and arthritis. The second study found that preexisting depression was related to all the common diseases, but with particular connections to ischemic heart disease, diabetes, and hypertension, and perhaps a sizable association with arthritis.

The researchers reached four primary conclusions: (1) depression serves as a highly central connector in multimorbidity; (2) it is associated with a greater burden of chronic diseases; (3) it correlates with unhealthy behaviors, including regular smoking, alcohol use, and physical inactivity; and (4) it predicts the subsequent incidence of some of the most prevalent diseases found in multimorbid clusters, diseases that commonly occur in multimorbid clusters.

According to data analyzed from the *National Health and Nutrition Examination Survey (NHANES)*, in 2014, 59.6% met the multiple morbidity criteria, 38.5% had 3 or more co-occurring chronic diseases, and 22.7% had 4 or more. In 1988, 45.7% had multiple morbidity. In 1988, 41.9% of these were obese. In 2014, 54.1% were obese. In adults, 65 years of age or more, multiple morbidity prevalence was 91.8% [13]. Women had more multiple morbidity than men did (58.4% vs. 55.9%, respectively). Whites and blacks had significantly higher prevalence than Hispanic or "other" race (59.2%, 60.1%, and 45.0%, respectively). See Fig. 12.1.

Analysis of data on 40 morbidities in 1,751,841 people registered with 314 medical practices in Scotland as of March 2007 found that multimorbidity began 10–15 years earlier in people living in the most deprived areas compared with the most affluent [14]. The prevalence of multimorbidity was 11.0% versus 5.9% in the most deprived versus the most affluent areas. Mental health disorders increased as the number of physical morbidities increased, and they were much greater in more impoverished areas: adjusted odds ratio (AOR) 2.2 versus 1.08 in more affluent areas.

In a German sample of more than 120,000 people 65 years of age or older, 62% were multimorbid [13]. A person was defined as multimorbid if she/he had at least three diagnoses out of a list of 46 chronic conditions in three or more quarters within the one-year observation period. Triads of the six most prevalent individual chronic conditions (hypertension, lipid metabolism disorders, chronic low back pain, diabetes mellitus, osteoarthritis, and chronic ischemic heart disease) accounted for 42% of the multimorbid sample. There were insignificant gender differences.

The single most common co-occurring disease in older adults is depression [15]. A systematic review in 2013 of twenty disease pairs found depression was the most commonly clustered and was paired with eight different diseases. Hypertension and diabetes mellitus were the second most

[1] *A scoping review* is a systematic review of literature that maps a field of knowledge in a particular area [10]. For example, "The scoping review has become an increasingly popular approach for synthesizing research evidence. It is a relatively new approach for which a universal study definition or definitive procedure has not been established. The purpose of this scoping review was to provide an overview of scoping reviews in the literature." [10].

F. Sunzeri (✉) · E. Sunzeri
Heather Hills Consulting, Coos Bay, OR, USA

J. Raber et al. (eds.), *Understanding and Treating Depressive Disorders*, https://doi.org/10.1007/978-3-032-14465-2_12

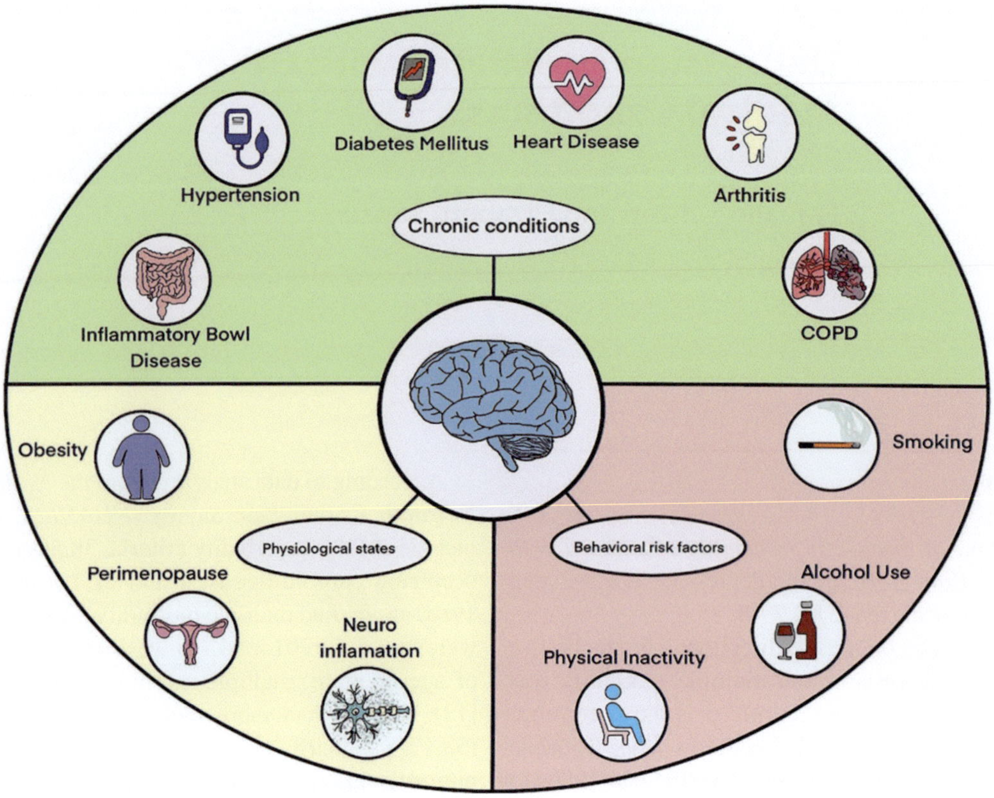

Fig. 12.1 Common comorbidities associated with depression. This illustration highlights a spectrum of physiological and behavioral conditions frequently comorbid with depression. Depicted are inflammatory bowel disease, obesity, and perimenopause, representing chronic inflammatory and hormonal disruptions. Neuroinflammation is shown as a central component linking brain-immune interactions with mood disorders. Lifestyle factors—including physical inactivity, alcohol use, and smoking—are included for their established roles in exacerbating depressive symptoms. Comorbid chronic diseases such as chronic obstructive pulmonary disease (COPD), arthritis, heart disease, diabetes mellitus, and hypertension underscore the bidirectional relationship between systemic health and mental well-being. Together, these interconnected conditions reflect the multifactorial nature of depression and its impact across biological systems

clustered diseases, both with six different diseases. Prevalence rates were highest in pairs that included hypertension, coronary artery disease, and diabetes mellitus.

Depression seems to be two to three times more common in patients who have multiple diseases compared to those who do not have multiple diseases [1]. A 2017 systematic review and meta-analysis found that depression is two to three times greater risk for people with multiple morbidity than it is for people who have no comorbidity or no chronic medical condition [16].

Depression can be triggered by substance abuse, alcohol, benzodiazepines, and, as discussed above, other medical conditions. Associations between depression and individual medical disorders were reviewed in 2017 [17]. The following are some of these associations.

Inflammatory bowel disorders and depression share activated immune-inflammatory, oxidative, and nitrosative stress pathways, including tryptophan catabolite, autoimmune, and gut-brain pathways [18]. *Oxidative and nitrosative stress* refers to an imbalance between increased levels of reactive oxygen species and reactive nitrogen species and antioxidants, where oxidants predominate.

Multiple sclerosis and MDD share abnormal conditions of chronic oxidative and nitrosative stress, neuroendocrine abnormalities, microglial pathology, mitochondrial dysfunction, gut dysbiosis, increased intestinal barrier permeability, and peripheral and neuro-inflammation [19].

More than one-half of patients who have autoimmune disorders show depression-like symptoms [23]. A comprehensive review found that more than one-third of COPD patients suffer from depression and anxiety [20].

Depression has been associated with endocrine disorders, including autoimmune thyroiditis, Hashimoto thyroiditis, and subclinical or overt hypothyroidism [21].

Twenty-five percent of people with type 2 diabetes have clinically significant depression [22]. The risk of metabolic syndrome is increased in patients who suffer from major depressive disorder (MDD), PTSD, ADHD, bipolar disorder, schizophrenia, or anxiety disorders [24]. There is a genetic overlap between cardio-metabolic diseases and depression [25].

Depression and cognitive decline of dementia are often associated [26, 27].

Patients with cirrhosis are likely to suffer from MDD [28]. One study found a prevalence of 18% [28].

Although the highest rates of depression are seen in the 25–45 age range, the elderly have the highest rates of systemic neuroinflammation [29, 30].

Women with perimenopausal depression are associated with more severe and frequent hot flashes than those without perimenopausal depression [31]. However, there is no increase in proinflammatory cytokines and decreased anti-inflammatory cytokines.

That is quite a list. Let us look at a couple of the diseases that have a strong association with depression.

Hypertension

There is another list of factors involved in both MDD and hypertension. These include the immune system, the cortisol response system, the sympathetic nervous system [32], shared genetics [33], unhealthy lifestyles [34], obstructive sleep apnea [35], sleep deprivation [36], metabolic syndrome [37], and the renin-angiotensin system [38]. Genome-wide studies have shown that calcium channel polymorphisms that are common to hypertension and blood pressure control [39] also add to the risk for MDD and bipolar disorder [40–42]. Regulation of adrenergic activity often fails in people who have MDD, and such alterations may be instrumental in sustaining elevated blood pressure [43–45].

There is disagreement as to whether depression increases blood pressure or lowers blood pressure [46]. However, depression has generally been found to be associated longitudinally with hypertension incidence [47, 48] and cross-sectionally with hypertension prevalence [49, 50].

In 2000, 26.4% of the adult population in the world had hypertension (26.6% of men and 26.1% of women) [51]. By 2025, it is projected that 29.2% will have hypertension (29.0% men and 29.5% of women). In 2001, worldwide, 13.5% of premature deaths and 6.0% of the global disability-adjusted life years (DALYs) total were attributed to high blood pressure [52]. Worldwide, about 54% of stroke and 47% of ischemic heart disease were attributable to high blood pressure [52]. The majority of those who have high blood pressure are in low- and middle-income countries and are middle aged with prehypertension. Prehypertension is a systolic pressure from 120 to 139 mm Hg or a diastolic pressure from 80 to 89 mm Hg. Pressures greater than or equal to 140/90 mm Hg are considered hypertension.

Some studies have shown MDD to be comorbid with hypertension in about 27% of patients [49, 53, 54]. It has been estimated that by the year 2030, MDD and cardiovascular disease (CVD) will be the two leading causes of disability worldwide [55]. When MDD is comorbid with CVD, the outcome is usually worse [56]. The more severe the depression, the worse the prognosis for CVD [57]. Data on hypertension comorbid with CVD suggest a possible additive connection to decreased survival [58].

However, even though depressive symptoms are associated with higher rates of cardiovascular disease, the association between depressive symptoms and hypertension is mixed, especially in young adults [48, 59–61]. MDD was associated with low blood pressure in some studies [62, 63]. Medications used to treat MDD can have an effect either beneficial or adverse on blood pressure, as can antihypertensives on MDD [64–66].

The deleterious effects of some antidepressant medications on blood pressure may contribute to the mixed findings [66]. For example, the 2009 *Netherlands Study of Depression and Anxiety* (n = 2981) showed that MDD was associated with low systolic blood pressure and less hypertension; in contrast, certain antidepressants (tricyclics, noradrenergics, and serotonergics) were associated with both high diastolic and systolic blood pressures and hypertension [65]. So, the culprit seems to be SSRIs and non-selective serotonin reuptake inhibitors, at least in young adults [66]. But maybe not. Results of a 2014 Croatian study suggested that antidepressant therapy in patients receiving antihypertensives and who were also depressed were associated with better control of blood pressure in addition to alleviating depressive symptoms [67].

A community-based sample of Australian men (N = 1195, aged 35–80 years; for 2002–2005) found that depression was significantly associated with previously diagnosed anxiety (12.0) and insomnia (4.4), not married (1.7), current smoker (1.7), low muscle strength tertile (1.7, P = 0.059), high triglycerides (1.6), high storage lower urinary tract symptoms tertile (1.8), past year general practitioner visits 5-9 (1.9), middle energy density tertile (0.4), and high systolic blood pressure (0.5) [68].

Low blood pressure and depression are quite common in elderly people [69]. For example, a 1994 community-based sample in California of men aged 60–89 years limited to 594 men not taking drugs for hypertension found association of relatively low diastolic blood pressure with higher depressive symptom scores [70].

The *Northern Finland 1966 Birth Cohort Study*, conducted in 1998 and reported in 2006, found no association between depression and metabolic syndrome (which includes hypertension) [71].

The population-based *Nord-Trøndelag Health Study* [72], *Norway*, of 60,799 men and women aged 20–89 years found an association of low blood pressure with anxiety and depression, which is not caused by cardiovascular disease [73]. When these same people were reassessed 11 years later, they found that change in symptom level of anxiety and depression between baseline and follow-up was inversely associated with change in systolic blood pressure but not diastolic pressure [73]. Similar results were seen 22 years after the first study [73]. A high symptom level of combined anxiety and depression present at all three examinations was associated with a stronger decrease in mean systolic and diastolic blood pressure and with a 20% ($p = 0.001$) lower risk of developing hypertension at year 22.

A cross-sectional community-based study in 9294 participants aged 65 years and over, living at home, in three French cities (Bordeaux, Dijon, and Montpellier) reported in 2008 that people with depression had lower systolic and diastolic blood pressure values compared with people who were not depressed [74]. In that study, 31% of participants were depressed, 77.5% had hypertension, and 49.5% were on antihypertensive drugs. They found that this association was independent of the use of antihypertensive or psychotropic medications.

A 2009 reported population-based study of 2723 Mexican Americans aged 65 or older not living in institutions found that independent of antihypertensive medications there was a significant relationship between depression and low blood pressure [75].

On the other hand, trajectories of depressive episodes and hypertension over 24 years in the *Whitehall II prospective cohort study* showed that the risk of hypertension increased with repeated experience of depressive episodes over time and became evident in later adulthood [76]. The study followed 6889 men and 3413 women (London-based civil servants aged 35–55 years at baseline) for 24 years between 1985 and 2009.

Some of the relationship studies relied on self-reporting of symptoms, which makes data difficult to interpret [60, 61, 77]. A 2010 report looked at insomnia and sleep duration as mediators of the relationship between depression and hypertension incidence [77]. They found that depression, sleep duration, and insomnia were significantly associated with hypertension incidence only in middle-aged subjects and not in the elderly.

A 2004 analysis of data from the *Baltimore Epidemiologic Catchment Area (ECA) Follow-up Study (n = 1920)*, a longitudinal population-based study of mental illness in East Baltimore, used self-reported data to suggest that depression may be an independent risk factor for hypertension, particularly for those with recurrent episodes or a long-term history of the disease [60].

The self-reporting *Canadian National Population Health Survey (NPHS)* of 12,270 respondents who did not report high blood pressure or the use of antihypertensive medications at a baseline interview conducted in 1994 were followed up for 10 years [61]. They found that after adjustment for age, the risk of developing high blood pressure increased in those with MDD. The hazard ratio was 1.6, indicating a 60% increase in risk.

Data from the *Multi-ethnic Study of Atherosclerosis*, a population-based prospective cohort study of 6814 US adults from four different racial/ethnic groups, found that there might be an association between depression symptoms and hypertension [59]. A 2002 quantitative review of prospective evidence linking psychological factors with hypertension development analyzed data from 15 prospective cohort studies (greater than 1-year follow-up) [78]. They concluded that there is moderate support for psychological factors as predictors of hypertension development. The strongest support was for anger, anxiety, and depression.

Possible explanations for divergent results include self-reporting, age effects, short duration of follow-up, ethnicity, and use of antidepressants or other medications [46].

Most of the studies referenced above use self-reported data, which is inherently not verifiable and subject to bias [79–82]. Some of the studies have looked at hypertension and depression interactions without consideration of the age of the participants [46]. For example, short sleep duration is more strongly associated with hypertension and obesity in middle-aged subjects than it is with older subjects [83, 84]. Elderly people have more difficulty in falling asleep and maintaining sleep [85]. So, sleep influences on depression will be less influenced in the older folks than in the younger ones. Middle-aged patients with hypertension are usually afflicted with combined systolic and diastolic hypertension, while the elderly are most frequently suffering from isolated systolic hypertension [86]. In addition, depression in older subjects is associated with systolic hypotension [75, 87]. So, studies that do not account for differences in age group responses may give an inaccurate picture of relationships between depression and blood pressure.

A prospective, multicenter, general community cohort of young adults (aged 23–35 years at study entry) who did not have hypertension was followed up for 5 years [48]. The sample included 3343 adults from four urban areas stratified by race from the *CARDIA (Coronary Artery Risk Development in Young Adults)* study. Those who had high and intermediate depressive symptoms were at risk of later hypertension incidence. Young blacks who had depressive symptoms were at high risk of developing hypertension.

Analysis of participants in the *National Health and Nutrition Examination Survey I Epidemiologic Follow-up Study* who were followed up for 7–16 showed significant increased risk of depression predicting hypertension for whites aged 45–64 years (RR[2]1.82) and a greater risk for blacks aged 25–64 years (RR 2.99) [47]. US blacks have the highest morbidity and mortality rates due to cardiovascular disease anywhere in the world, and it is highly related to hypertension [88].

Alteration of sleep duration has been associated with depression and with hypertension prevalence in cross-sectional studies and with hypertension incidence in longitudinal studies. A 2015 meta-analysis showed that short and long sleep durations were significantly associated with increased risk of depression in adults [89]. Compared with normal sleep duration, RR was 1.31 for the short sleep duration overall and the pooled RR was 1.42 for the long duration.

The Sleep Heart Health Study is a community-based prospective study of the cardiovascular consequences of sleep-disordered breathing in 2813 men and 3097 women, aged 40–100 years [90]. They found that typical sleep duration above or below the median of 7–8 h per night was associated with increased prevalence of hypertension. This was especially true for less than 6 h per night. These associations held even after self-reported adjustments for caffeine and alcohol consumption, current smoking, insomnia symptoms, depression symptoms, sleep efficiency, and prevalent diabetes mellitus or cardiovascular disease. The day after a lack of adequate sleep, SNS activity and blood pressure can increase [91].

Lack of sleep can also decrease insulin sensitivity [92], increase ghrelin, and decrease leptin, leading to increased appetite [93]. It has also been associated with increased obesity and diabetes [84, 94]. All of these are risk factors for hypertension [94].

During sleep, blood pressure usually drops 10–20% [95]. So, it has been suggested that with chronic sleep deprivation the average 24-h blood pressure and heart rate increase. It is reasoned that the increased hemodynamic load can result in a "structural upward" resetting of the whole cardiovascular system to function at a higher-pressure equilibrium.

Sleep deprivation and depression in adolescents seem to be reciprocally associated [96]. In young women but not in young men, sleep deprivation appears to increase the risk of MDD [97].

On the other hand, sleep deprivation may act as an antidepressant according to a meta-analysis [98]. A model of therapeutic sleep deprivation has shown that within hours, sleep deprivation can lead to a dramatic decrease in depressive symptoms in 50–60% of patients with MDD [99]. In another study, although there was antidepressant response with hours after sleep deprivation in 40–60% of depressed patients, more than 80% of the responded relapsed after the recovery night [100].

A meta-analysis of sleep duration and depression has indicated that short and long sleep durations are significantly associated with increased risk of adult depression [89]. In another study, depressed middle-aged people were 65% more likely to be hypertensive during follow-up [77]. Short, but not long, sleep duration appeared to be a significant moderator in that relationship. The study's authors suggested that chronic short duration of sleep could mean that a prolonged exposure to non-sleep levels of blood pressure and heart rate could entrain cardiovascular adaptations to operate at the higher pressures [95]. In addition, insomnia might increase HPA activation, and a through neuroendocrine dysregulation via the same processes leads to hypertension [101, 102].

Compounding the relationships between sleep, depression, and hypertension is the use of antidepressants [103]. In short-term treatment, many antidepressants have activating effects that can disrupt sleep (e.g., Imipramine, desipramine, fluoxetine, paroxetine, venlafaxine, reboxetine, and bupropion) [104]. Others that have sedative properties can improve sleep but may be over-sedating and adversely influencing sleep cycles (e.g., doxepin, mirtazapine, trazodone, trimipramine, and agomelatine) [104–107].

More on sleep and depression can be found in its own chapter in this monograph.

Cardiovascular Disease

In addition to being a risk factor for suicide, well-controlled studies have shown that symptoms of depression as well as the psychiatric illness of major depression are associated with increased risk of other serious illness such as of coronary heart disease (CHD) [108–110]. Several appropriately controlled studies have shown that depression increases the risk of CHD, the number one killer in the USA, and the number one killer of women over 40 [111–113]. Indeed, CHD has a worse prognosis in women [114].

The constellation of the so-called *type D distressed personality style* and social inhibition shows predictive value for 10-year cardiac morbidity and mortality [115, 116]. The tendency to experience negative emotions and suppress emotional expression of these emotions in social interactions is a hallmark of the type D [117]. It seems that type D personality is an independent predictor of negative cardiac events after controlling for current stress symptoms.

[2]*Relative risk (RR)* is perhaps the most common method of expressing the estimated risk of experiencing a result. RR compares the probability of a specific outcome in the treatment group with that of a control group. When an RR is greater than 1, there seems to be an increased risk of an event. When the RR is less than 1, there appears to be a decreased risk of experiencing an event. If the RR is 1, there is no apparent risk. If the RR = 5, it is 5 times more likely to occur than in the control group. If the RR = 0.5, it is half as likely to happen as in the control group. For more information, see Chap. 4 Evidence Basics.

One study [118] concluded that the risk of dying from heart disease among depressed elderly women was as great as the danger conferred by other cardiovascular risk factors, including smoking, hyperlipidemia, high blood pressure, diabetes, and obesity.

There is convincing evidence for a psychological and social impact on coronary artery disease (CAD) morbidity and mortality [119]. Five key variables have been identified as possible psychosocial risk factors: acute and chronic stress, hostility, depression, social support, and socioeconomic status. There is considerable evidence to suggest that the immune system has a role to play in the incidence and progression of CAD [120].

It appears that autonomic nervous system (ANS) dysfunction mediates effects of depression on the course and increased risks of mortality and cardiac morbidity of CHD [121]. Depressed patients with CHD frequently have ANS dysfunction that includes elevated heart rate, low heart rate variability, exaggerated heart rate responses to physical stressors, high variability in ventricular repolarization, and low baroreceptor sensitivity [121]. Depressed folks without CHD frequently exhibit increased plasma catecholamines.

The most common arrhythmia, atrial fibrillation (AF), has reached epidemic proportions in the USA and is associated with significant morbidity and mortality; as of 2010, it affected more than 3 million people [123–125]. And it is increasing rapidly [122]. In 2014, AF was estimated to affect 2–3% of Europeans and North Americans, whereas in the developing world about 0.6% of males and 0.4% of females were affected [122]. In Asia, 2018 estimates were 0.49%–1.9% [126]. In 2014, AF prevalence differed between the sexes (male-to-female ratio of 1.2:1) and by age [127]. AF prevalence in people less than 49 years of age in 2014 was 0.12%–0.16%. Between 60 and 70 years of age it was 3.7% to 4.2%, and over 80 years of age it was 10% to 17%.

Obesity, aging population, diabetes, congestive heart failure, hypertension, and being male are common risk factors for AF [128]. Significant decrement is seen with AF on health-related quality of life (HRQOL) [129]. Anxiety and depression have a complex and circular cause-and-effect relationship with AF [130].

Initiation and propagation of AF is hypothesized to be instigated by inflammation and oxidative stress [131]. It is common to find decreased anti-inflammatory molecules, increased acute phase reactants, including heat shock proteins, C-reactive proteins (CRP), and inflammatory cytokines [132]. Higher levels of circulating CRP have been associated with the incidence and recurrence of AF [133].

Increased activation of the sympathetic nervous system, which occurs in depression and anxiety, may be associated with inciting paroxysmal AF [134]. Post-surgical anxiety, depression, stress, and elevation of the sympathetic nervous system may also be associated with post-cardiac surgical AF [135].

Activation of the HPA axis and the renin-angiotensin-aldosterone system that occurs in depression may activate enzymes that may result in cardiac fibrosis formation and transforming growth factor (TGF)-$\beta 1$ production, which promotes atrial fibrosis, a dilated left atrium and aberrant conduction [136]. Moreover, angiotensin induces production of inflammatory cytokines, adhesion molecules, and free radical reactive oxygen molecules [137].

Analysis of data from 3682 patients in the Framingham offspring study who were followed for 10 years revealed that tension predicted coronary artery disease, mortality, and AF, and anxiety predicted total mortality in women and men, and was a risk factor for incident AF [138]. In another population of AF patients, unadjusted analysis but not multivariate analysis showed mild to moderate and severe depression was associated with increased inflammatory reaction as measured by high sensitivity (hs)–CRP [139, 140]. In 114 chronic AF patients, 32% had type D personality, and those who had type D personality had higher levels of hs-CRP measurements [141].

In addition, when folks are depressed or anxious, perception of AF can be maladaptive and decrease utilization of healthcare and decrease effectiveness of standard treatments [130]. SSRI use can be problematic—sometimes inhibiting the vasovagal reflex and stopping AF [142], sometimes apparently provoking AF [143], or dangerously prolonging QT intervals, especially in females or the elderly [144–147]. In addition, SSRI use can interact with anticoagulants and precipitate bleeding [145–148].

Cancer

A complex interaction occurs between depression and cancer [149]. Comprehensive reviews of stress and depression as they relate to cancer, by Reiche and her colleagues, are particularly well written and definitely are worth reading [150, 151]. Depression may follow cancer, or cancer may follow depression because they share common biobehavioral mechanisms [152, 153].

Depression in cancer can range through sadness, adjustment disorder, subclinical depression, and MDD [154, 155]. Emotional and psychosocial dimensions of cancer can include overwhelming stress from employment, family, finances, physical appearance, and independence. When a patient's capabilities to cope are overwhelmed, a feeling of low mood, anhedonia, despair, and hopelessness can emerge.

Depression can influence participation in cancer treatment, resulting in worse outcomes and higher mortality rates [156, 157]. Pretreatment depression can increase treatment levels of depression and decrease quality of life [158, 159]. Greater suicide risk and increased time of hospitalization are also associated with depression [160, 161]. Depression may contribute to decreased tumor suppression activity, increased cancer invasion, and increased mortality [156, 157, 162–166].

Anxiety and depression vary widely by cancer type, gender, and age [158]. In 2004, a review of depression prevalence in cancer studies found the prevalence of major depression to be 0%–38% and depression spectrum syndromes to be 0%–58% [167]. The differences varied based on the definitions used, methodological approaches, and study populations. They reported depression prevalence in oropharyngeal (22%–57%), pancreatic (33%–50%), breast (1.5%–46%), lung (11%–44%), colon (13%–25%), gynecological (12%–23%), and lymphoma (8%–19%) cancers. Depression symptoms in MDD patients who do not have cancer may be different from those arising from cancer patients [168, 681, 682]. For example, one study showed that a sense of guilt was higher among MDD patients (56.5%) and was lower among cancer patients (4%) [168].

In 2013, another study found that the pooled mean prevalence of depression in cancer patients ranged from 8% to 24% [169]. The prevalence of depression was highest during treatment: 14% to 27%. They found 3% prevalence in breast cancer and 31% in gastrointestinal tract cancer.

A study conducted on 10,153 consecutive cancer patients found that 19.0% of patients showed clinical levels of anxiety, 22.6% had subclinical symptoms, 12.9% had clinical symptoms of depression, and 16.5% had subclinical symptoms. Women showed two to three times greater rates of anxiety and depression than men for some cancers. An inverse relationship in emotional distress was seen with age. In more than ½ of the cases, patients younger than 50 and women had either subclinical levels or clinical levels of anxiety.

Mixed anxiety and depression in cancer is associated with less favorable psychosocial and treatment outcomes [156], worse quality of life, worse adherence to treatment [157], slower recovery, greater suicide risk, and higher cost-utilization [170, 171].

A meta-analysis found mortality rates independent of clinical prognosticators were up to 25% higher in patients who had depressive symptoms and up to 39% higher in patients diagnosed with major or minor depression [157]. There seems to be a higher rate of depression when there is greater pain and metastases [172].

One study found that household income, perceived subjective health status, and employment status were the main factors affecting depression and health-related quality of life in cancer survivors [173]. Otherwise, depression and health-related quality of life were similar to the general population. A study of bladder cancer patients undergoing adjuvant chemotherapy found that quality of life was retained while anxiety and depression increased [174]. Factors such as gender, age, BMI, hypertension, smoking, and diabetes increased the risk of depression.

Psychosocial stress in patients induces transcription factor nuclear factor-κ-β (NFκβ), which controls inflammatory gene expression [175]. In addition to the psychosocial contribution to depression in cancer patients, there is a strong correlation to biological contributors [176]. *Damage-associated molecular patterns (DAMPs)* on damaged tissue are produced by the cancer itself as well as treatments such as surgery or chemo and radio therapy [177]. DAMPs bind to *pattern recognition receptors (PRRs)* on macrophages and other white blood cells. This interaction triggers expression of many pro-inflammatory cytokines, such as interleukin-1 (IL-1), interferon-α (INF-α), IL-6, and TNF-α.

NFκβ regulates production of TNF, IL-1alpha, IL-1beta, IL-6, IL-8, IL-18, chemokines, MMP-9, VEGF, COX-2, and 5-LOX [178]. When chronically activated, these products may suppress apoptosis while encouraging proliferation, angiogenesis, invasion, and metastases; thereby contributing to cancer progression [179, 180]. It has been reported that approximately 15–20% of all malignancies are initiated or exacerbated by inflammation [181]. In addition, *cancer-related inflammation* is implicated in subversion of adaptive immunity, reduced response to hormones and chemotherapeutic agents, and induction of genetic instability, leading to accumulation of random genetic alterations in cancer cells [182].

TNF-α, IL-1, INF-α, and some of these other cytokines can decrease concentrations of serotonin and norepinephrine [183–186], and dopamine [187], and can contribute to depression symptoms. Additionally, these cytokines can increase corticotropin-releasing hormone (CRH) and decrease brain-derived neurotrophic factor (BDNF), which is vital for neurogenesis. Increased CRH [188] and decreased BDNF have been associated with producing depression [189].

Through mechanisms described above, some anticancer drugs, such as INF-α, and other cancer treatments have been reported to cause cognitive issues and depression in a significant number of patients receiving them [190–195].

Additional contributions to depression come from chronic stress during cancer. The *parasympathetic nervous system (PSNS) is inhibited, the sympathetic nervous system (SNS) is stimulated,* and the hypothalamic-pituitary-adrenal (HPA) axis is activated [183, 184, 196–198, 203]. Normally, increased activation of the HPA should increase the potent glucocorticoid anti-inflammatories, but DAMP activation of PRRs results in inactivation of glucocorticoid receptors and decreased effects of corticoids on leukocytes [177, 199]. The result is increased cytokines, which also may decrease the sensitivity of the rest of the activated glucocorticoid receptors and even more cytokine production [200].

Chronic SNS activation increases norepinephrine stimulation of macrophages, resulting in increased NFκβ activation and cytokine expression, followed by more reduction of serotonin and norepinephrine in the synapses [183, 184]. The PSNS would normally inhibit the production of the pro-inflammatory cytokines via acetylcholine binding to nicotinic receptors on leukocytes to inhibit NFκβ production [197, 198]. But, in chronic stress, the PSNS is inhibited, leading to more pro-inflammatory cytokines and less serotonin and norepinephrine in the synapses [197, 198].

Depression's contribution to cancer incidence and progression has been investigated by various researchers [152, 153, 201]. As mentioned above, clinical depression is frequently accompanied by significantly elevated systemic inflammation [150, 151] but dampened cellular immune response [202]. Depressed (or highly stressed) folks typically have a generalized leukocytosis and increased numbers of circulating neutrophils, but with decreased activity, decreased mitogen-stimulated lymphocyte proliferation, and a shift from *Th1 to Th2* predominance [207].

It is common to find decreased NK cell and cytotoxic T cell activity and associated tumor surveillance and increased genomic instability with elevations in somatic mutations. In chronically stressed or depressed persons, elevations are commonly seen of tumor-related factors, such as damaged DNA, tumor anxiogenic and growth factors, free radical production and reactive oxygen species, proteases, and metalloproteinases.

Increased risk of mortality in depressed cancer patients may be related to a reduced number of NK cells [164], cytotoxic T cells, T h1 cells, and INF-γ [165, 202]. Increased SNS activity may suppress the p53 tumor suppressor gene [166]. As mentioned above for cancer-related inflammation, depression may also be associated with increased expression of angiogenic factors that promote invasion [204] and anti-apoptotic factors that prevent cell death [205].

Penninx et al. [206] reported that chronically depressed mood is linked to a variety of cancers by a hazard ratio of 1.88. That is, after adjusting for demographics and risk factors, those persons with a depressed mood are 1.88 times more likely to have one of those cancers than someone who is not depressed.

On the other hand, some studies have looked for but have not found a linkage between negative emotions and malignancies [66, 118].

Obesity

Obesity[3] is growing worldwide [212, 213]. In 1990 being underweight was more prevalent than obesity but the global age-standardized prevalence of underweight began to decrease so that by 2022 obesity became more prevalent than underweight in many countries [214]. The global prevalence of obesity increased from less than 1% in 1975 to between 6% and 8% in 2016 among girls and boys, between 3% and 11% among men, and between 6% and 15% among women over the same time period [214].

In 2017, the *Global Burden of Disease Study* found that out of 84 risk factors, high body mass index (BMI) demonstrated the greatest relative increase in exposure since 1990 [211]. High BMI was in the top five risk factors for attributable deaths and disability-adjusted life-years.[4] As of 2020, almost 39% of the general population in the USA was overweight or obese [209]. In 2015, obesity had a mean prevalence of 19.5% in *Organization for Economic Co-operation and Development (OECD)* [210] countries [215]. During midlife, 50 to 71, the increased risk of death is 20% to 40% greater among overweight persons and by two to at least three times greater among obese persons [216, 217].

A 2024 analysis of self-reported and measured anthropometric data from 134 unique sources—including all major national surveillance survey datasets—found that nearly 75% of US adults over the age of 25 were overweight or obese as of 2021 [218] .[5] The southern states had the highest prevalence of overweight or obesity. For example, Texas showed the highest rate in male adolescents (15–24 years of age); they had a prevalence of 52.4%. Mississippi showed the highest rates in female adolescents at 63.0%. The highest rate for male adults was in North Dakota at 80.6%, and for female adults it was in Mississippi at 79.9%.

Projections are for increasing rates all around if there is not a population level intervention. The highest prevalence rates are forecast to continue to be concentrated in the southern states. The prevalence of overweight and obesity in ado-

[3]The *National Health and Nutrition Examination Survey (NHANES)* [208] defined obesity among adults aged 20 years and older as a body mass index (BMI: calculated as weight in kilograms divided by height in meters squared) of 30 or more and severe obesity as a BMI of 40 or more [209]. Among youth aged 2 to 19 years, obesity was defined as a BMI at or above the 95th percentile of sex-specific BMI-for-age, and severe obesity was defined as a BMI at or above 120% of the 95th percentile. Pregnant females were excluded.

[4]The five leading risks in 2017 were high systolic blood pressure, smoking, high fasting plasma glucose, high BMI and short gestation for birthweight [211]

[5]For individuals older than 18 years, overweight was defined as a BMI of 25 to less than 30 and obesity was defined as a BMI of 30 or higher, and for individuals younger than 18 years definitions were based on International Obesity Task Force criteria [219]

lescence and childhood has dramatically increased since 1990. For female adolescents, it has been a 95–99% increase.

Although population-wide obesity in the USA is a result of the socially acceptable imbalance between excessive energy intake and energy expenditure, mainly by lack of physical exercise, the triggers behind that imbalance are complex [220–222]. Overeating can be aroused or triggered by a multitude of factors, including environmental influences—such as marketing pressures that activate our reward systems and create or reinforce habits; emotional drivers, including attempts at stress reduction; family eating patterns, such as the influence of maternal malnutrition, which may engage epigenetic mechanisms in offspring; genetically predisposed eating or metabolic disorders; lack of information; and inadequate sleep.

The trigger for the energy imbalance that drives obesity is proposed to be a product of repeated exposure to intense and often profoundly increasing commercial, social, and structural forces across interacting systems, such as food supply systems, agriculture practices, urban design, land use, and transportation [214, 215, 223, 224]. Mixed drivers of these are economic, demographic, and technological changes, often supported by structural racism and gender inequities [214, 220, 225, 226]. Manipulations of consumer behaviors and the food environment by transnational food and beverage manufactures to drive commercial profits are a recognized force [224, 225, 227, 228].

A 2009 review of seventeen studies totaling 204,507 participants suggested a very significant association between depression and obesity [229]. Obese people are almost 55% more likely to have depressive symptoms than those who are not obese [230, 231]. A very significant association has been reported between depression and obesity, and this association appeared to be stronger for women [229]. Obesity is often associated with stigma that diminishes quality of life and increases premature mortality [232–234]. Societal stigma of obesity adversely affects screening services for breast, cervical, and colon cancer [235].

Maladaptive behaviors that may accompany and reinforce depression include high rates of co-morbid addictive behaviors such as overeating to obesity, smoking, alcohol, and drug abuse [236–243]. In attempting to self-medicate depression symptoms, it is frequent to find excessive eating leading to obesity [244–246], alcohol abuse [247], smoking [248–250], and use of recreational drugs [251, 252].

In addition to addiction risk, increased isolation, and poor work performance may be associated with obesity [253, 254].

Although many people with classic depression are obese, only atypical depression appears to be associated with an elevated risk of obesity compared to the overall population [255, 256]. The atypical subtype of depression is characterized by increased appetite and weight gain, whereas classic depression is characterized by decreased appetite and weight loss. Data from the 2001–2002 *National Epidemiologic Survey on Alcohol and Related Conditions (NESARC)* showed marked elevation of obesity in atypical depression compared to population controls and to other subtypes (OR[6] > 2.0: $p < 0.001$). Obesity rates in classic depression were not significantly different from non-depressed subjects.

Epidemiological transitions [257] and nutritional transitions [258] are at work in important population trends. *Nutritional transition* refers to how people's diets, physical activity, and health change as a result of economic, demographic, and technological changes [259]. As far back as 1993, it was observed that there is a worldwide shift toward a diet high in fat and processed foods low in fiber, with corresponding increases in degenerative disease [258]. Health parameters, underlying determinants, positive deviants, and future trends have been discussed as stages of obesity transitions [214]. Four stages are posited that relate to sex, socioeconomics, and age [214].[7] There is evidence that current food environments exploit people's biological, psychological, social, and economic vulnerabilities, which make it easier to eat unhealthy foods [260].

Between the 1960s and 2010, the per capita caloric intake in the USA increased by about 28% [268]. As detailed in other places in this text, a high-fat diet can lead to a variety of problems [269], including depression [255, 256, 271, 272], obesity [273], cardiovascular problems [274], and diabetes [275]. A 2013 study has shed some new light on the molecular bases of these connections. In mice, a high-fat diet appears to induce widespread alterations in the circadian clock [276, 277].[8] And, chronic consumption of high-fat foods and obesity can induce neuroplastic changes in the *mesolimbic reward circuitry* that is associated with depression, including behavioral despair [272].[9]

[6] Odds ratio (OR) is a way to represent the odds that an outcome will result when a given exposure to a variable of interest occurs compared to when the exposure does not occur. OR quantifies the strength of the association between two events. An OR greater than 1 indicates a positive association or that exposure to that variable increases the odds of that outcome. An OR less than one indicates a negative relationship between two events. An OR of 1 suggests no relationship between two events. An OR is frequently accompanied by a 95% confidence interval (CI). CI is a measure of precision of the OR. The smaller the CI the higher precision as long as it does not overlap OR = 1. For more information, see Chap. 4 on evidence basics in this text.

[7] The *NCD Risk Factor Collaboration* [212], the *WHO Global Health Observatory* [261], the *Global Burden of Disease Study* [262], and the *Global Nutrition Report* [267] monitor changes in age and sex-specific BMI, overweight and obesity.

[8] The *circadian clock* is the time keeper for metabolic processes and the circadian system [263]. Metabolites and nutrients regulate the circadian clock. Nuclear receptors can act as metabolic sensors and clock regulators. Clock modulation and feeding patterns influence the development of obesity

[9] A common tool for assessing dietary fat intake is *the Fat and Fiber-related Diet Behavior Questionnaire* [264, 265]. Physical Activity can be measured via the *Framingham Physical Activity Index* [266].

High intakes of fruit, vegetables, fish, and whole grains may be associated with a reduced depression risk [278]. Several current meta-analyses have shown that dietary interventions with high intakes of fruit, vegetables, whole grains, fish, olive oil, low-fat dairy, and antioxidants and low intakes of animal foods are associated with a decreased risk of depression [279–283].

The role of nutrients in obesity can be found in [270].

Deficiencies in maternal and early postnatal nutrition contribute to health-risk factors in adult life, including hypertension, insulin resistance, obesity, cardiovascular disease, diabetes, and the metabolic syndrome [284]. Molecular, cellular, metabolic, neuroendocrine, and physiological adaptations to changes in the early nutritional environment can permanently change developmental patterns of cellular proliferation and differentiation in tissues and organs that can have pathological effects later in life [284]. Inadequate nutrition during pregnancy (both over and under) is associated with increased incidence of several diseases in offspring [285–287]. These include diabetes and obesity [288].

The role of healthy diets in decreasing and poor diets in increasing the prevalence of depression in children has been seen in several adolescent populations [289–292]. For example, a brief 3-week dietary RCT intervention showed that young adults with elevated depression symptoms can engage in and adhere to a diet intervention resulting in significantly decreased symptoms of depression [283].

Obesity is significantly associated with reduced quality of life. Obesity is a powerful and independent risk factor for type 2 diabetes mellitus, coronary heart disease, stroke, cancers, dyslipidemia and other metabolic diseases, hypertension, and obstructive sleep apnea (OSA), and is highly associated with increased mortality [293–295]. Obesity can increase the risk of other conditions such as osteoarthritis and infertility [296–299], as well as mental health difficulties [300, 301]. Comorbidities include depression and anxiety [230, 254, 302, 303], poor physical functioning [304–307], gastroesophageal reflux disease [308], pelvic floor disorders [309], and sexual dysfunction [310].

Multifaceted relationships exist between many of the comorbidities. For example, anxiety and depression along with obesity have complex relationships with atrial fibrillation [130]. There is strong evidence that OSA is connected directly or indirectly to depression [311]. Possible bidirectional connections to OSA comediators include obesity, hypertension, and decreased quality of life [312]. In addition, depressed mood increases the risk of complications of obesity [313]. Major depressive disorder is associated with an advanced aging phenotype, including increased risk of mortality and age-related diseases such as cardiovascular disease, cancer, obesity, cognitive decline, and frailty [314, 315].

Obesity increases both the incidence of depression and its severity [316, 317]. Obesity, depression, and diabetes track with low socioeconomic status; the most socioeconomically disadvantaged have the greatest risk for poor mental and physical health [318–321]. Obesity and depression appear to be mutually dependent [322] and may be moderated by the effect of chronic systemic inflammation and the gut microbiota [323].

A variety of genetic associations between obesity and depression have been identified. There are key genes that are associated with MDD and obesity:

1. OLFM4 and NEGR1 are associated with obesity and body mass index [324–326]. These genes play a role in synaptic function, glutamate signaling, insulin secretion/action, energy metabolism, lipid biology, and adipogenesis.
2. Many of these peptides associated with depression play a hypothalamic role in regulating appetite and eating [327]. This relationship may tie into the comorbidity of obesity and psychiatric disorders [328, 329].
3. Alterations in the GI microbiota can have an impact on disorders ranging from obesity [330] to allergies [331], autoimmune disorders [332], inflammatory bowel disease [333] and irritable bowel syndrome [334] and to psychiatric disorders such as depression [335–338]. In addition to communicating with the CNS to influence host behavior, our microbiome functions include producing vitamins, metabolizing fatty acids, and educating the immune system [339–341].
4. Depression may interact with functional polymorphisms of the dopamine transporter (SLC6A3) to modify food intake. Such a relationship was investigated using the *National Longitudinal Study of Adolescent Health* [342]. The researchers examined interactions between symptoms of depression and functional polymorphisms of dopamine transporter (SLC6A3), monoamine oxidase A (MAOA), dopamine receptor D2 (DRD2), and dopamine receptor D4 (DRD4) on intake of high-calorie sweet, high-calorie non-sweet, and low-calorie foods. They found that females with high levels of depression and the SLC6A3 10/10 allele exhibited significantly greater intake of high-calorie sweet foods than women with similar levels of depression who had any SLC6A3 9 allele ($p < 0.05$).
5. It seems that relatively brief indulgence in diets rich in sugar, or rich in both sugar and fats, can compromise hippocampal-dependent place-recognition memory—but not perirhinal-dependent object recognition—even before weight increases [343]. A 2012 experiment in rats has suggested that oxidative stress and neuroinflammation may be involved in this decrement of memory [343]. Rats

fed sucrose had both increased hippocampal inflammation (increased TNF-α and IL-1β mRNA) and oxidative stress (increased NRF1 mRNA)

6. Alterations in glucocorticoids, adipose-derived hormones, insulin, and inflammatory signaling that are typical of central obesity may be directly or indirectly implicated in the increased incidence of depression in obesity [344, 345]. Premenopausal women with both major depression and the specific polymorphisms of the glucocorticoid receptor GG genotype Bcl1 polymorphism have shown greater abdominal obesity compared with non-GG carriers [346]. Elevated cortisol levels are associated with mood disorders, abdominal obesity, type 2 diabetes, osteoporosis, and cardiovascular disease [347].
7. Inverted sleep-wake schedules, obesity, smoking, alcoholism, and physical activity [348] can modify epigenetic patterns [349]. Interconnections exist between nutrition, epigenetics, lifestyle, disease, and metabolic stress pathways [350, 351].

Treatment of Obesity

Treating overeating is a great challenge to clinicians. The approaches usually begin with recommendations for lifestyle changes (diet, exercise, and behavioral changes) [352]. If these recommendations are not successful, the next step is adding medications to the regimen [353]. If those measures are not successful, the final step is invasive bariatric surgery. See Fig. 12.2.

The best obesity treatments are individually tailored combinations of behavioral interventions, nutrition, physical activity, pharmacotherapy, and metabolic/bariatric procedures, depending on the amount of weight loss desired and patient characteristics. The best treatments combine the elements from the major categories of evidence-based treatment: behavioral interventions, nutrition, physical activity, pharmacotherapy, and bariatric procedures [354–359].

A 2023 review of obesity management in adults concluded that behavioral interventions could result in about a 5% to 10% decrease in weight. GLP-1 agonists and combi-

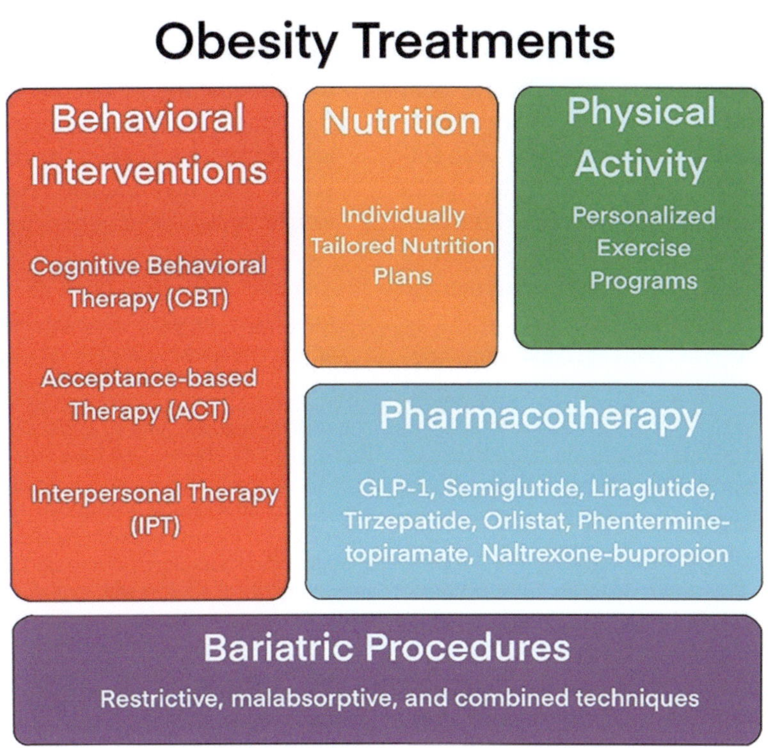

Fig. 12.2 Multimodal approaches to obesity treatment. This illustration presents key strategies employed in the management of obesity. Behavioral interventions form the foundation for sustainable lifestyle changes. Nutrition strategies emphasize balanced dietary patterns that support caloric regulation and metabolic health. Physical activity is depicted as a vital element for energy expenditure and cardiovascular fitness. Pharmacotherapy options are included to highlight the role of anti-obesity medications in complementing lifestyle efforts. Bariatric procedures demonstrate an option for severe obesity with associated comorbidities. Together, these modalities underscore a comprehensive, individualized approach to treatment

nation glucose-dependent insulinotropic polypeptide/GLP-1 receptor agonists may achieve 8% to 21% reduction in weight. Bariatric surgery may attain a 25% to 30% reduction in weight [360].

A systematic review and meta-analysis showed a statistically significant overall effect of both psychotherapeutic interventions and support groups on weight loss [361]. Effective treatment of obesity ranges from behavioral therapy to bariatric surgery [362]. CBT, as discussed in detail elsewhere in this text, may be useful for treating various disorders in adults [363], including depression [364], anxiety [365], obesity [229], and eating disorders [230, 364–367]. Bariatric surgery can be safe and very effective for weight loss in those who have been unsuccessful in multiple attempts at weight loss and have severe obesity [368]. Bariatric surgery can improve comorbidities although there can be some complications and adverse side effects [369, 370], and improvement of mental health status may be problematic [230, 369, 371, 372].

Treatment of Obesity: Behavioral Approach

Behavioral interventions may be an individualized group, in person, remote, or technology driven. They are multicomponent and can be conducted in primary care, evidence-based commercial programs, or community settings [233, 355, 373]. Typical interventions include 14 or more sessions in the first 6 months or at least 12 sessions in the first year, followed by follow-up maintenance sessions for up to 2 years [373, 374]. Evidence-based behavioral approaches for obesity treatment include cognitive-behavioral therapy (CBT), acceptance-based therapy (ACT), and interpersonal therapy (IPT) [375].

Treatment focuses on lifestyle changes, education, cognitive restructuring, goal setting, self-monitoring, peer support, and coaching [233, 353, 375]. Particular foci include chronic stress and sleep effects on appetite and metabolism [376]. Results of intense multicomponent behavioral interventions may produce 5% to 10% weight loss, most of which comes between 6 months and 1 year [234, 353–373]. Weight loss and weight maintenance appear to be improved by self-weighing [377]. When communicating with a patient-centered supportive and non-judgmental approach, it is likely that patients will lose more weight [378].

Perhaps the biggest challenge is the willingness to change. Elsewhere in this text, we have discussed the six stages of the *Transtheoretical Model of change* [379, 380]. Briefly, they are (1) pre-contemplation (I can't/won't), (2) contemplation (I might), (3) preparation (I will), (4) action (I am doing), (5) maintenance (I am still doing), and (6) following a sufficient maintenance period, either relapse to the undesirable behavior or termination of the behavior with no desire to return to that undesirable behavior.

The five A's (assess, advise, agree, assist, arrange) that have been used for smoking cessation [355, 381] are being used by clinicians to increase motivation and confidence in changing dietary intake [381, 382]. Medicare and other insurance policies cover this approach for treating obesity [383].

Culturally relevant interventions accounting for root causes and intersectional stressors are vital to achieving the best results [384–387].

Decisions as to when to discuss and pursue each of these steps depend upon the wishes and readiness of the patients [360, 381, 388, 389].

1. *Assessment* begins by asking permission from the patient to discuss their weight, nutrition, exercise, and their willingness to change. Screening for psychosocial risk factors are essential as is asking what the patient's goals are.
2. *Advice* regarding the health benefits of weight loss and lifestyle changes is presented strongly and clearly.
3. *Agreement* is necessary for specific measurable and achievable goals personalized to the patient. These usually include dietary, exercise, sleep, and stress management.
4. *Assistance* is provided by offering behavioral management counseling or referral to possible intensive multicomponent evidence-based nutritional programs, anti-obesity medication, or metabolic and bariatric surgery.[10] This may include referral to an evidence-based weight reduction program, obesity medicine clinic, or bariatric clinic.
5. *Arrange* for follow-up with an appropriate referral to maximize support accountability and feedback, and to adjust the treatment plan as required.

[10]A 2020 systematic review of 14 popular dietary programs can be found in [390]. Their conclusion was, "…*most* macronutrient diets, over six months, result in modest weight loss and substantial improvements in cardiovascular risk factors, particularly blood pressure. At 12 months the effects on weight reduction and improvements in cardiovascular risk factors largely disappear. Estimated effects at the 12-month follow-up for weight loss and cardiovascular risk factor improvements diminished for all popular named diets, except for the *Mediterranean Diet*" [233, 391].

Physical activity is suggested for all adults regardless of BMI [392]. A 2018 review found that approximately 80% of Americans are insufficiently active [393]. Physical activity guidelines are suggested in [234, 393]. Individualized to patient health and limitation, the general guidelines are moderate-intensity (50%–70% maximal heart rate) physical activity 150–300 min/wk. (e.g., 30 min 5 times per wk.), or vigorous-intensity physical activity 75–150 min/wk. And resistance training 2–3 times per wk. More than 200 min/wk. is associated with better maintenance of weight loss [234].

Anti-obesity medications are usually suggested if BMI is ≥30 and ≤35 or if BMI is ≥27 with an obesity related comorbidity. *Metabolic or bariatric surgery* is usually suggested if the BMI is ≥35, or ≥30 with a metabolic disorder such as diabetes, or if the patients is ethnically Asian and the BMI is ≥27.5.

Motivational interviewing (MI) is an essential bag of tools to help guide the patient with the process of change [394–396]. It works well as a standalone at times and particularly effectively when combined with CBT, ACT, and IPT. MI activities include engaging, focusing, evoking, and planning. Basic principles of MI are expressing empathy, supporting self-efficacy, avoiding arguments or rolling with resistance, and resolving ambivalence by revealing discrepancies [397].

Expressing empathy begins by asking the patient's motivation for change. It is collaborative and evocative, and it uses open-ended questions (affirmations, reflections, and summaries) that help to show that the clinician has understood the patient.

Supporting self-efficacy focuses on successes, strengths, and skills and provides affirmation, especially during the preparation, action, and maintenance stages of change.

Rolling with resistance is avoiding arguments by reflection, reframing, shifting focus, and siding with the negative. Resistance is frequently manifested as interrupting, arguing, denying, and ignoring during the counseling session.

Resolving ambivalence attempts to resolve the uncertainty for change by helping the patient to recognize how there is a discrepancy between their current behavior and their core values and desired behaviors [398].

Motivational interviewing is not sufficient for many people, especially for people with eating disorders [395]. So, more intensive interventions such as CBT or ACT are the next steps.

Cognitive behavioral therapy is the primary treatment for eating disorders and for depression, which are frequently comorbid with obesity [399, 400]. CBT also serves as an important adjunct to bariatric surgery for addressing depression and mood disorders, which are highly prevalent in individuals with severe obesity [229]. A CBT behavioral and cognitive approach to overeating frequently employs the following five major components of habit reversal [401].

1. *Awareness*:
   (a) Become aware that we have a choice.
   (b) Pay attention to the setting and our habitual response.
2. *Competing thoughts*:
   (a) Thinking about outcomes can change the way we feel about the stimulus and thereby change our behavior.
3. *Competing behavior*:
   (a) Break the pattern of stimulus and response by substituting a competing behavior.
   (b) Use executive brain functions to override primitive, hardwired responses.
   (c) Be ready to substitute another behavior as soon as possible when presented with the cues.
4. *Support:*
   (a) Helps us to recognize and avoid cues and acknowledge our success.
   (b) Helps to sustain and reinforce motivation not to succumb to conditioned overeating.
   (c) They need to be the right people.
   (d) Social engagement can be a competing behavior or a substitute reward, which can reduce anxiety.
   (e) Avoiding disapproval or disappointment of an ally can also be a strong motivator.
5. *Emotional learning:*
   (a) Learning is most effective when it is a combination of being drawn toward something we want while at the same time being repulsed by something we no longer view as desirable.
   (b) Conditioned overeating involves comforting stimuli. We can assign an emotional value (good or bad) to food. If we assign emotionally negative values to hyperfat, hypersugar, and hypersalty foods and positive values to eschewing these we can reverse the conditioning.

Cognitive functioning may be problematic in obese individuals, especially in the arena of executive functions [402–404]. ADHD and obesity are frequently comorbid, and executive functions such as impulse control, planning, and organization may present a challenge [405–409].

The personality trait of persistence has been a persistent predictor of weight loss success [410–412].

Acute and chronic stress can limit a patient's adherence to self-care, so it is important to make sure there is a good support system in place [413, 414]. Indeed, the quality of and extent of social support for behavioral weight management is often found to be a crucial factor in weight loss [361, 414–416].

There are several classes of medications that are associated with excess weight gain [417–419]. Of note are antidepressants such as mirtazapine and amitriptyline, antipsychotics, antiepileptics, antihyperglycemics including insulin, corticosteroids, beta-blockers, progesterone-based contraceptives, and antiretroviral therapeutics like protease inhibitors. If substitute medications that do not have the same risk of gaining weight are not available and an agent is not available to counteract the weight-gaining effects, it will be especially difficult to achieve good results even with lifestyle modifications [420–422].

Treatment of Obesity: Pharmacological Approach

Attempts at dropping excess weight have traditionally focused on increased energy use through exercise and decreased calorie consumption. However, due to environmental and genetic influences, this has often been an illusory goal. So, in modern times, weight loss medications have become a focus of attempts.

The early medications focused on increasing metabolic rates. These most commonly were thyroid extracts, sympathomimetics, and amphetamines. However, the dangerous cardiovascular effects were unacceptable. Next attempts focused on decreasing the excess drive for food. These included serotonergics, dopaminergics, and endocannabinoid antagonists. However, these were not very effective, and they too had adverse cardiovascular effects and unacceptable psychiatric effects.

More recent attempts have focused on the complex of reciprocal satiety and energy-seeking signals between CNS metabolic control areas and the rest of the body. Leptin was one of these tissue hormones that induced satiety and increased energy use and initially showed promise [423, 424]. Alas, pharmacological leptin did not produce the desired results [425, 426]. But it spurred interest in genetic studies that pursued other similar control system molecules, especially those that appear in the CNS [427]. Most of the results of the studies using these obesity molecules were not promising and were beset with adverse effects [428–432]. For example, the selective serotonin receptor agonist (lorcaserin) was originally approved by the FDA for use and then withdrawn due to cancer risk [433].

Nevertheless, some drugs have been approved by the FDA for weight management in nonpregnant patients. As of 2023, there are six drugs [360]. These include glucagon-like peptide receptor 1 (GLP-1) agonists (semaglutide and liraglutide only), tirzepatide (a combined glucose-dependent insulinotropic polypeptide/GLP-1 agonist), phentermine-topiramate, naltrexone-bupropion, and orlistat. The most promising of these molecules, which we will discuss, are analogs of the glucagon-like peptide 1 (GLP-1) [434].

These medications must be used with lifestyle changes and likely will need to be used throughout life, as it is very common for all the weight to be regained when the medication is discontinued [356–436]. Most common side effects of all of these are gastrointestinal (abdominal pain, diarrhea, constipation, nausea, vomiting).

Glucagon-like peptide-1 receptor agonists (GLP-1 agonists, GLP-1RA, GLP-1DAs, incretin mimetics, or GLP-1 analogs) have revolutionized the treatment of obesity and type 2 diabetes [437]. Agonists are chemicals that bind to a receptor to produce the same response as the substance that normally binds to the receptor. In this case, the normal substance is GLP-1.

In 2010, the FDA approved high subcutaneous daily doses of the GLP-1 agonist liraglutide for chronic weight management in patients aged 12 or older with a BMI of 30 or greater [356, 438]. In 2021, the FDA also approved a once-a-week 2.4 mg subcutaneous injection of the GLP-1 agonist semaglutide for the management of overweight or obesity [356, 439]. Semaglutide is more effective than liraglutide at producing weight loss [440–442]. In addition, semaglutide is better than liraglutide in improving-related comorbidities and are associated with fewer gastrointestinal side effects [443, 444].

Due to poor oral absorption, they are only used by injection. When combined with diet and exercise, they have been effective in managing weight.

Incretins are gastrointestinal tract-derived metabolic hormones that are produced from enteroendocrine cells [445] and released into the bloodstream as a response to nutrient ingestion, primarily glucose and fat [446]. The two principal incretins are *GIP (glucose-dependent insulinotropic polypeptide aka gastric inhibitory peptide)* and *GLP-1 (glucagon-like peptide-1)*. GIP is produced and secreted into the blood circulation by K cells, which are in the mucosa of the duodenum and upper jejunum [447]. GLP-1 is produced and secreted into the bloodstream by L cells located primarily in the ileum and colon, but also occasionally in the duodenum and jejunum [448]; a small amount is also found in the brainstem [449].

Some enteroendocrine cells, the K/L cells, secrete both GIP and GLP [450, 451].

GIP and GLP-1 stimulate insulin secretion. GLP-1 inhibits glucagon secretion and gastric emptying, resulting in reduced postprandial glycemia. GLP-1 has insulinomimetic, insulinotropic, and antiapoptotic properties [434, 461].[11] GIP

[11] So what do all these terms mean? First let's look at glucagon. *Glucagon* is short for glucose antagonist [452]. Briefly, glucagon is produced in the alpha cells of the pancreas and is released into the circulation where it acts on the liver to stimulate de novo glucose production and glycogenolysis: the main effect of which is to increase glucose in the circulation. However, glucagon is pleiotropic. Glucagon stimulates insulin secretion as a reaction to increased glycemia, decreases body weight by increasing energy expenditure and decreasing feeding. It slows gastric emptying, inhibits lipid synthesis and stimulates lipolysis, increases cardiac output, increases the natural process of breaking down cells and recycling their parts (apoptosis), and increases renal glomerular filtration.

Glucagon has been used to treat severe hypoglycemia and has been combined with GLP-1 to treat type-2 diabetes, obesity [453, 454] and nonalcoholic steatohepatitis. An interesting tidbit is that different types of fats and their sources have a variable effect on stimulating glucagon secretion [455]. Glucagon during fasting mobilizes lipids to provide energy [456]. Control of glucagon is a complex relationship orchestrated by multiple glycemic, paracrine, endocrine, and neural factors.

As mentioned above, *GLP-1* is a hormone produced and secreted by cells in the digestive tract and the brain stem as a response to food consumption. GLP-1 slows digestion and suppresses hunger and improves satiety GLP-1 receptor agonists are frequently used in treating type 2 diabetes and obesity [437, 456]. By their ability to inhibit secretion of insulin and zinc, GIP and GLP-1 indirectly inhibit secretion of glucagon [457, 458]. *GIP* actually has a bifunctional role in maintaining appropriate glucose levels as it stimulates glucagon secretion in hypoglycemia and insulin in hyperglycemic states [459]. Insulinomimetic means that it mimics insulin. Insulinotropic means that it can stimulate production or activity of insulin. GLP-1 prolongs the life of the beta cells of the pancreas while promoting their proliferation [460].

and GLP-1 also have a role to play in the health of the cardiovascular system, adipose cells, and bones [462].

In obese individuals, GLP-1 secretion may be impaired. Post-Roux-en-Y gastric bypass may deliver more nutrients to the lower small intestines, where the L cells are located.

GLP-1 agonists appear to produce an average weight loss of 2.9 kg compared to placebo and improve cardiovascular effects [463, 464].

GLP-1 agonists also increase satiety by interacting with the hypothalamus, slowing gastric emptying, and decreasing inappropriate glucagon secretion [465]. Added benefits include decreased hepatic gluconeogenesis, increased neuroprotection, decreased all-cause mortality, and improved A1C levels in folks with type 2 diabetes mellitus [466]. Combinations of GIP and GLP-1 agonists like tirzepatide have also found promise in diabetes therapy [467].

Although very useful, the use of GLP-1 agonists is not all goodness and light. The most frequent side effects are gastrointestinal. Because the GLP-1 agonists slow gastric emptying and produces early feelings of satiety, nausea and vomiting and other gastrointestinal side effects can occur if one attempts to overeat [468]. Diarrhea may lead to acute kidney injury due to volume contraction. Dyspepsia, mild tachycardia, headaches, dizziness, irritation at the injection sites, and increased infections are also reported [469, 470]. Discontinuation rates are about 10% [471, 472]. Additional cautions include increased risk of pancreatitis and thyroid disorders [473].

More distressing are reports of suicidal thoughts and adverse events following GLP-1 agonist use [474]. A 2024 pharmacovigilance analysis of individual case safety reports submitted to the *EudraVigilance* database found that out of all the adverse events reported only 1.2% were psychiatric [474, 475]. Of those, depression—followed by anxiety and suicidal ideation—was the most prevalent. Of these, 9 deaths were associated with depression and completed suicide. Investigations of associations between GLP-1 agonists and suicidality reports to the *Food and Drug Administration Adverse Event Reporting System (FAERS)* were conducted up to 2023 [476–479]. They found disproportionate reporting of suicidal ideation and "depression/suicidal" with semaglutide and liraglutide, but not disproportionate reporting of suicidal behavior, suicide attempts, and completed suicide with any of the FDA-approved GLP-1's. WHO data reported in 2024 showed significant disproportionality only for semaglutide-associated suicidal ideation, which remained significant in patients with co-reported use of antidepressants and benzodiazepines [480]. A replication study of the reports to the *WHO pharmacovigilance database (WHO VigiBase)* [481], unlike the first report with FEARS, found a mixed pattern of reporting odds ratios [680] with respect to suicidality and exposure to select GLP-1 agonists [482]. In 2024, a large cohort study using the *TrinetX database* [483] investigated the impact of liraglutide and semaglutide on the risk of developing depression, anxiety, and suicidal behaviors in obese patients [484]. They found that patients on GLP-1 RA's had a 195% higher risk of major depression, a 108% increased risk for anxiety, and a 106% elevated risk for suicidal behavior. Given the mixed reports available at this point in time (2024), assigning causation remains difficult.

For maximum benefit and lower risk, smaller meals, eating more slowly, avoiding fatty foods, and getting sufficient exercise are necessary. It is important that there are routine follow-ups to monitor blood counts, kidney function, and blood glucose levels.

In 2023, the FDA approved tirzepatide, a dual hormone agonist that interacts with the GLP-1 receptor—like semaglutide—and with the glucose-dependent insulinotropic polypeptide (GIP) receptor, regulating energy balance via signaling in the central nervous system and adipose tissue [357, 485]. Tirzepatide seems to be the most effective pharmacological agent with a mean weight loss of 21% at 6 years [360].

In 2012, the FDA approved phentermine-topiramate oral medication for obesity [356]. Phentermine is a noradrenergic that reduces appetite [486]. Topiramate mechanisms are largely unknown.

In 2014, FDA approved naltrexone-bupropion for obesity [356]. Naltrexone has been used to treat opioid and alcohol dependence [487]. Naltrexone blocks opioid-mediated proopiomelanocortin (PMOC) autoinhibition, which reduces reactivity to food cues and improves dysregulation of eating control in the hypothalamus mesolimbic dopamine reward pathways [488]. Bupropion is a weak dopamine and norepinephrine reuptake inhibitor that stimulates hypothalamic PMOC neurons [489]. Naltrexone-bupropion has been useful for obesity comorbid with depression [356].

Over-the-counter Orlistat, a pancreatic lipase inhibitor, was approved in 1999 for the treatment of obesity, but it is not very effective [356]. Gelesis 100, an orally administered superabsorbent gel capsule that increases bulk in the stomach, was approved in 2019 [356]. It has limited efficacy [490]. Short-term use of four oral sympathomimetics has been used [356]. Of these, phentermine is the most frequently prescribed [491, 492]. Although phentermine is a schedule IV controlled substance, it has not been associated with increased risk of abuse/dependency or cardiovascular events [492–494].

Off-label use of several medications that were approved to treat diabetes has been widely used for obesity. These include Metformin, Mounjaro (tirzepatide injection), Ozempic (semaglutide injection), Rybelsus (oral semaglutide), and Victoza (liraglutide injection). Tirzepatide, under the name Zepbound, has been approved by FDA (2024) for obesity in adults with a BMI of >30 [495].

Metformin increases insulin and leptin sensitivity and decreases ghrelin levels and hunger [496]. Metformin is inexpensive and although not FDA approved, it has been used in folks with prediabetes, polycystic ovarian syndrome, obesity, and those experiencing weight gain from antipsychotic medications.

The FDA, for a while in 2024, as a result of manufacturing shortages principally due to off-label demand, permitted the compounding of Tirzepatide injection, Dulaglutide injection, Semaglutide injection, and Liraglutide injection [497].

Discontinuation rates may be high for use of liraglutide due to out-of-pocket costs [498].

The anorectic gut peptide, Peptide YY3-36 (PYY3-36), is secreted from the same intestinal cells as GLP-1 and is being investigated as a possible dual agonist [499].

Antidepressants may diminish the weight loss effects of GLP-1 agonists [500].

GLP-1 receptor agonists may be useful in improving cognitive functions in adults with mood disorders [501].

GLP-1 in a rodent experiment has shown both acute anxiogenic and chronic antidepressant effects on amygdala serotonin signaling [502].

Treatment of Obesity: Bariatric Surgery

Bariatric surgical interventions for obesity quintupled worldwide from 2003 to 2018 [503]. Between 1997 and 2013, the number of bariatric surgeries worldwide increased tenfold [213, 293, 504].[12] The adjustable gastric band has fallen out of favor and has been replaced by the laparoscopic sleeve gastrectomy and the Roux-en-Y gastric bypass as the most common interventions [505].[13]

It has been asserted that the most effective method for losing substantial weight and managing diabetes is bariatric surgery [509]. A 2023 systematic review of outcomes and adverse events after bariatric surgery reported that Roux-en-Y-gastric bypass (RYGB) produced significantly better results for better short-term (1–2 years) and long-term (3–10 years) weight loss than medical treatment and gastric banding (GB) [215].[14] RYGB was the most effective in maintaining substantial weight loss, followed by sleeve gastrectomy (SG), GB, and medical treatment. Improvements were seen with diabetes but less so with hypertension and dyslipidemia.

Evidence suggests that weight loss from bariatric surgery is more attributable to caloric, glucose, and lipid metabolism and less from mechanical changes such as shrinking stomach size [453]. Most bariatric patients experience significant changes in GLP-1, GIP, glucagon, ghrelin, fibroblast growth factors, and peptide YY.

RYGB had higher rates of complications, including intestinal obstructions [215]. Reflux problems were greater in sleeve gastrectomy. Late complication rates were higher in the SG and GB groups than in the RYGB group. RYGB showed a rate of 35% (21–49%); SG, 44% (17–22%); and GB, 57% (4–111%). Increased prevalence of dumping syndrome associated with RYGB: GERD associated with SG. Abdominal pain was the most prevalent complication of bariatric surgery, presenting in 3-61% of subjects with healthcare contacts or readmissions 1–5 years after surgery. This could be explained by behavioral, anatomical, and/or functional disorders [510].

Among bariatric surgery patients prior to surgery, rates of lifetime mood disorders have been reported to range from 22.4% [511] to 45% [512], while rates of current mood disorders range from 11% to 33% [513]. Depression symptoms frequently improve following bariatric surgery [514–517]. However, when used alone, surgery is not likely to solve long-term psychological problems [515].

The effect of personality disorder on weight loss surgery is uncertain [519, 520]. Prevalence of personality disorders among patients seeking surgery has been estimated to be up to 30% [521, 522].

History of trauma, especially childhood abuse, while linked to obesity, may impact the result of surgery [523–526].

Among the most common preexisting conditions in bariatric candidates are depression, anxiety, substance abuse, and binge-eating disorder [512, 527]. Considerable variation in prevalence rates is reported, which may be dependent upon the population studied [528]. For example, in veterans, the prevalence for PTSD is higher compared to other groups [528].

[12] *Types of bariatric surgeries* include restrictive, malabsorptive and combined techniques. *Restrictive types* include *laparoscopic adjustable gastric banding* which creates an adjustable pouch of approximately 30 mL and a *laparoscopic sleeve gastrectomy* which removes part of the stomach and staples the rest to form a sleeve of 60 to 120 mL. Both of these limit food intake and induce early satiety. *Malabsorptive types* include *jejunoileal bypass* which joins the proximal part of the small intestine to the distal part of the small intestine such that only a small portion of the gastrointestinal tract is available for normal absorption. *Combined types* include the *Roux-en-Y-gastric bypass* which creates an approximately 30 mL gastric pouch which is then connected to a segment of the jejunum for passage of contents. The *biliopancreatic diversion* removes a small part of the stomach and creates an alternative route to the small intestine. One example is the *biliopancreatic diversion with a duodenal switch* that combines a vertical sleeve gastrectomy with a doudenoenterostomy.

[13] Two *bariatric endoscopic procedures* are FDA approved. They are intragastric balloons that take up space in the stomach, delay gastric emptying and increases satiety [506, 507] and endoscopic sleeve gastroplasty [508]. These procedures can result in 10% to 13% weight loss at 6 months [360].

[14] Heterogeneity in outcome was high. Subject populations varied between studies in terms of age, sex, race and preoperative weight. There was a variable number of studies assessing outcome of each surgical type. And follow-up periods were not the same.

Psychotic symptoms, severe depression, untreated eating disorders such as anorexia nervosa or bulimia nervosa, and active substance use disorders are considered relative—but not absolute—contraindications to bariatric surgery [529]. Patients with preexisting depression may have a more difficult time with weight loss, but not always [530, 531]. Preexisting binge eating studies generally support successful weight loss if the patient is receiving behavioral support [532]. There is some evidence that the prevalence of alcohol use disorder increases significantly after 2 years in patients undergoing gastric bypass surgery, but not in those undergoing gastric banding [533].

In addition to weight loss, bariatric surgery may also be associated with improved metabolic status and medical comorbidities, increased quality of life, and better psychosocial and behavioral functioning [534–537]. As discussed below, post-surgical psychosocial difficulties and challenges are very real and may benefit from presurgical psychosocial evaluation to identify risk factors and be ready for appropriate post-surgical intervention. These complications include body image dissatisfaction [538], interpersonal relationships [539], substance abuse [540], and suicide [541].

Some reports suggest that patients with *higher levels of preoperative depression have higher rates of postoperative complications* [518]. Others suggest that postoperative depressive rates are the most predictive of weight loss [513, 542]. For example, in one study, depressive symptoms of 15 or greater on the *Beck Depression Inventory* were seen in 45% of patients prior to surgery [543].[15] At a 6-month post-surgery follow-up, it was 12%; at a 12-month follow-up, it was 13%; and at a 24-month follow-up, it was 18%. The preoperative depressive symptoms did not predict postoperative weight loss. However, higher postoperative depressive symptoms at every point in time predicted a greater degree of concurrent and subsequent eating disorder psychopathology and lower quality of life. In another study in patients who were eligible for bariatric surgery, depression and bipolar were comorbid with obesity in 22.0% to 54.8% [547]. Postsurgical results of folks with mood disorders appeared to be the same as those without mood disorders.

Some studies find that patients who are depressed preoperatively lose less weight [519, 548] or have comparatively poor postoperative adherence [549–551]. Data from the *Michigan Bariatric Surgery Collaborative* showed that nearly one-third of patients undergoing bariatric surgery are depressed, and 10% are moderately or severely depressed [552]. Preoperative depressive symptoms and extended length of stay after bariatric surgery were significantly associated. And, there were higher rates of smoking and use of marijuana, prescription opiates, and alcohol.

A systematic review of preoperative depression effects on outcomes of bariatric surgery 6 months to 6 years post-surgery has found that results are mixed and are subject to a high risk of bias [553]. Different results between studies may reflect differences in cohort characteristics, outcome definitions, and instruments used to measure depression. However, there is evidence that pre-surgical depression may have negative impacts on a variety of post-surgical outcomes, such as decreased quality of life, worse acute pain, and complications. The reviewers suggested that factors that may have made the review challenging were a lack of accounting for variables such as sociodemographic factors, comorbidities, the perioperative use of medications causing weight loss or weight gain (e.g., serotonergic antidepressants and antipsychotics), psychological factors (e.g., motivation), and lifestyle factors (e.g., exercise and diet). A small number of studies reported that preoperative depression was associated with lower quality of life, worse acute pain, and more perioperative complications after surgery. The reviewers suggested that although there was no clear relationship between preoperative depression and weight loss outcome, postoperative motivation and mood may be the key to effective changes [554].

Most studies have found no difference in outcomes in patients depressed at baseline and those who were not [555–558]. On the other hand, postoperative depression is associated with a poorer outcome [513, 557, 559, 560].

Psychiatric complications from bariatric surgery are quite real [594]. Although bariatric surgery can improve mental health in patients suffering from chronic disease, there is a potential for depression, anxiety disorders, eating disorders, dissatisfaction due to unmet weight loss expectations, body image disturbances, and psychotic syndromes [561, 562]. Complications may depend upon the type of bariatric surgery. For example, one study found a 1.7 times increased risk for major depressive disorders after malabsorptive procedures compared to restrictive procedures [563]. At time points more than 4 years after surgery, major depressive disorders were significantly increased in both procedures after an initial improvement in the initial postoperative years [563].

Bariatric surgery may also increase the risk of alcohol use disorder (AUD) [540]. AUD was greater in the second postoperative year than in the first postoperative year and in the year preceding surgery. AUD was associated with male sex and younger age and preoperative factors including smoking, regular alcohol consumption, AUD, recreational drug use, and lower interpersonal support. AUD was more heavily associated with the Roux-en-Y gastric bypass procedure.

[15] Because there is some overlap between depression symptoms and consequences of obesity such as fatigue, increased appetite and poor quality sleep, it is important to differentiate between the primary disorder [544]. The Beck Depression Inventory must be used with care not to confuse depression symptoms with physical consequences of obesity such as sleep disturbance, chronic pain, or sexual dysfunction [545, 546].

Availability of postoperative psychosocial interventions and support is associated with better outcomes of bariatric surgery [361, 559, 564–566]. Adverse outcomes include insufficient weight loss [567], nonadherence to the postoperative program [549, 567–570], weight regain [571–573], eating disorders [573–576], substance abuse [540, 577], and suicide [541, 578].

The *National Institutes of Health Consensus Conference Development Panel* recommends a multidisciplinary team approach to the surgical treatment of morbid obesity [579].

Presurgical psychosocial evaluations of prospective bariatric patients are usually thought to be essential [580]. Psychosocial evaluations screen for risk factors or postoperative challenges that may produce less than optimal outcomes from bariatric surgery [580, 581]. In some cases, results of these evaluations may result in recommendations for behavioral or other management before or after surgery [582] or even militate against bariatric surgery.

However, preoperative psychological testing prior to surgery is not without controversy [583]. Critics suggest that abnormal psychological profiles identified preoperatively do not universally predict less favorable postoperative weight loss outcomes.

The most common elements of psychosocial evaluations for bariatric surgery are clinical interviews, symptom inventories, objective personality and psychopathology tests [584]. Some researchers have used the *Weight and Lifestyle Inventory* [585]. Whatever inventory is used, the common core of domains includes weight history, eating disorder symptoms, psychiatric history, psychosocial functioning, developmental and family history, current and past mental health treatment, cognitive functioning, personality traits and temperament, current stressors, social support, quality of life, health-related behaviors, and patient motivation and knowledge.

Eating disorders include binge eating and binge eating disorder [587], night eating syndrome [586], compensation behaviors such as purging [588, 589], and anorexia nervosa [574]. Various other eating behaviors include grazing [590], loss of control eating [587, 589, 590], and eating large portions or frequent fast food restaurant meals [591].

Patients who seek bariatric surgery appear to exhibit more psychopathology than community samples of obese patients [544, 592]. The more severe the obesity, the more likely the patient is to report current or lifetime depression, PTSD, social phobias, or panic disorder [521, 593].

Bipolar disorders, anxiety disorders [595], schizophrenia [596], and personality disorders [519, 597] associations with both obesity and weight loss surgery are not well characterized. Presurgical psychopathology has a complex relationship with weight loss surgery that is not well revealed for several reasons. These include exclusion of severely compromised patients from surgery [544, 597, 598], and variations in data collection and duration of studies [559, 599, 600].

It appears that the severity of the symptoms impact on the patient's life is most important, not just the presence of a psychiatric diagnosis. For example, if depression is stable and is being managed well, a better prognosis of weight loss surgery can be anticipated [564, 601]. If the symptoms are severe and/or there is no management in place, it is generally considered to be a contraindication for bariatric surgery [233, 565, 588, 601].

Cognitive behavioral therapy pre- and post-surgery has been effective in reducing disordered eating behaviors and promoting weight loss [602]. A key to success may be accessing adaptability to behavioral changes for patients with depression undergoing bariatric surgery.

Almost half of patients who are depressed before bariatric surgery may find some relief from depression after surgery [604] perhaps via a renewed sense of motivation [603] and feeling of autonomy over their health [605]. However, bariatric surgery is not a magic panacea. There are important postoperative reasons for caution.

Postoperative psychosocial concerns include maladaptive eating, substance use disorders, lack of social support, and suicide [371]. A meta-analysis and systematic review of post-bariatric surgery depression suggests a pooled prevalence of 15.3 [606]. Depression was associated with weight regain, eating disorders, and decreased quality of life.

The first year after surgery is the period when most weight loss occurs. But after that it is difficult to lose more weight without severe dietary restrictions and long-term behavioral modifications [607]. Stress of unreasonable expectations and body dissatisfaction increases the risk of depression [608–610] and suicide [606, 610]. *Potential risks of mental health disorders after bariatric surgery include substance abuse, self-harm, and suicide* [611–615]. An aggregate account from five healthcare systems between 2009 and 2017 found that *the relative risk of suicide was 64% higher in a cohort with bariatric surgery versus a nonsurgical cohort* [616].

The nonrandomized, prospective, controlled *Swedish Obese Subjects* study found that the risk for self-harm/suicide was 1.98 times as high in surgical patients compared to control patients [617]. They found that male sex, previous healthcare visits for self-harm or mental disorders, psychiatric drug use, and sleep difficulties predicted a higher risk. Reviews suggest that a variety of psychosocial, medical, biological, and genetic factors are involved in risk factors for suicide [618]. These include changes in ghrelin and GLP-1[16] mechanisms, disinhibition and impulsivity related to the dif-

[16] *Ghrelin* is known as the hunger hormone as it increase appetite. It is produced primarily in the stomach, duodenum and other parts of the gastrointestinal tract [619].

ference in alcohol absorption, and changes in absorption of antidepressants or other medications. Psychosocial factors might include low quality of life, continued or recurring physical disabilities, sexual and relationship dysfunctions, disappointment in amount of weight loss, low self-esteem, and lingering effects of childhood maltreatment.

Suicide rates are higher in bariatric patients than in control groups. One study estimated a suicide rate of 4.1/10,000 person-years (95% CI: 3.2 to 5.1/10,000 person-years) [611]. A large meta-analysis of data through January 2018 revealed the risk of non-fatal self-harm/suicide attempts was 1.9 times higher after bariatric surgery within the same population, and it was 3.8 times higher compared to age-, sex-, and BMI-matched controls [620]. Completed suicide in that post-bariatric population was 2.7/1000.

The *Longitudinal Assessment of Bariatric Surgery-2* is a cohort study with pre-surgery and annual post-surgery assessments conducted at ten US hospitals [621]. About 25% of the participants reported suicidal thoughts or behavior pre-surgery. Prevalence of self-harm/suicidal ideation was 5.3% pre-surgery, 3.8% at the first year, and increased post-surgery to 6.6% at year 5, but it was not significantly different from pre-surgery.

Another study found that compared to the general population a fourfold increase in risk of attempted suicide was seen [543, 622]. Data from the *Pennsylvania Health Care Cost and Containment Council* tracked mortality from suicides between September 1, 1996, and December 28, 2006 [541]. There were 31 suicides out of 16,683 operations, which yields an overall rate of 6.6/10,000. The rates were 13.7 per 10,000 among men and 5.2 per 10,000 among women. Over that same period, age and sex-matched controls in the USA, suicide rates for ages 35-64 were 2.4/10,000 (men) and 0.7/10,000 (women). Seventy percent of those suicides occurred in the first 3 years, and 30% occurred within the first 2 years post-surgery.

It is a challenge to identify risk factors that would allow targeting postoperative surgical monitoring and support [541]. A Nordic study identified risk factors for bariatric-associated suicide in their population [623]. They found an increased risk in men irrespective of age and comorbidity. Gastric bypass carried a higher risk than other forms of bariatric surgery (HR = 0.44, 95%CI: 0.27–0.99). Increased risk was seen with a history of depression or anxiety (HR = 6.87, 95%CI: 3.97–11.90); mania, bipolar disorder, psychosis, or schizophrenia (HR = 2.70, 95%CI: 1.1–6.37); and substance use (HR = 2.28, 95%CI: 1.08–4.80). Multiple diagnoses increased the suicide risk HR = 22.59, 95%CI: 12.96–39.38 for ≥ 2 compared to 0 diagnoses. Pre- and post-surgical psychosocial, pharmacokinetic, physiologic, and medical factors may be involved [620]. Postoperative psychosocial monitoring and support for high-risk patients are advisable based upon presurgical risk factors [623].

Some speculate that increased suicide or worsened post-surgical depression may relate to lack of psychological follow-up [618], increased and or chronic pain due to gastric ulcers [510], or guilty feelings of not adhering to the strict post-surgical regimen and relapsing [624].

Several factors may be at play in these psychiatric complications from bariatric surgery. These include preexisting psychiatric conditions, nutritional deficiencies, gut microbiome changes, and addiction transfer.

Neurohormonal mechanisms underlying changes in reward-related behaviors after bariatric surgery may be involved in increased risk for substance use disorders, especially alcohol use disorder (AUD) [625, 626]. Of interest is that, in rats, different types of weight loss surgical procedures—such as Roux-en-Y gastric bypass (RYGB) and sleeve gastrectomy (SG)—have differential effects on alcohol consumption. Alterations in alcohol metabolism and pharmacokinetics resulting from bariatric surgery have not been found to be the primary cause [626, 627].

Postsurgical nutritional deficiencies that are most commonly reported include vitamins B(12), B(1), C, folate, A, D, and K, along with the trace minerals iron, selenium, zinc, and copper [628, 629]. It has also been found that typical over-the-counter multivitamin and mineral supplements do not supply adequate amounts of such as vitamin B(12), iron, or fat-soluble vitamins which necessitate additional doses of prophylactic supplementation throughout life to achieve optimal nutrient status [630]. Metabolic and nutrient problems are more common in patients who undergo restrictive-malabsorptive or malabsorptive surgical procedures than those who have restrictive procedures [631]. For example, due to a decreased number of parietal cells and intrinsic factor, vitamin B12 deficiency has been found to occur more than three times more often in malabsorptive or combined procedures than in restrictive procedures [632]. Iron, calcium, and other mineral deficiencies are common when the main sites of absorption in the duodenum and proximal jejunum are bypassed in restrictive surgeries so that about 17% of these patients are anemic [633]. Antidepressant medications may need to be altered after surgery [634, 635].

Bone health is another concern [636, 637]. Fracture risk has been reported to increase 2 years post-surgery and is more problematic following malabsorptive procedures like RYGB and biliopancreatic diversion (BPD). Fractures were reported at axial, weight-bearing sites and at appendicular sites [638]. Monitoring and managing nutrient imbalances after bariatric surgery is very important, especially in the [639].

Pregnant women who have had bariatric surgery need supplementation of iron, vitamin A, vitamin B(12), vitamin K, and folate to prevent maternal and fetal complications, such as severe anemia, congenital abnormalities, low birth weight, and failure to thrive [640, 641]. Some nutritionists suggest that all bariatric surgery patients should receive regular monitoring of serum nutrient levels starting at 3 months after surgery and periodically afterwards [628, 642].

Preoperative deficiency of vitamin D, iron, and selenium seems to be common [644]. Vitamin D deficiency is strongly linked to depression [643]. Vitamin D deficiency in spite of post-surgical supplementation has been reported in 10% of post-surgical patients in one observational study [644]. Thiamine deficiency and B12 deficiency can contribute to postoperative psychosis [632].

Alterations of gastrointestinal microbiome-associated products, including ghrelin, glucagon-like peptide 1, peptide YY, and cholecystokinin, are associated with behavior as documented in a separate chapter in this text. Changes in their expression and effects on appetite and glycaemia regulation after bariatric surgery are being explored in the context of bariatric surgery effects on suicide risk, depression, and substance abuse [645, 646]. It has been suggested that post-surgical rewarding effects of alcohol increases may relate to these changes [647]. It is believed that after bariatric surgery, metabolic phenotypes change due to alterations in the gut-brain axis, resulting in changes in taste preferences and central reward reactivity toward palatable food, apparently via pathways in brain areas involved in sensorimotor, reward-motivational, emotional-arousal, and executive control components of food intake [646].

Addiction transfer involves replacing prior addictive eating habits with new or increased substance use [648]. The most frequently abused substance is alcohol. All too frequently, bariatric patients die during the postoperative period due to hepatic cirrhosis [649]. Undergoing Roux-en-Y gastric bypass versus laparoscopic adjustable gastric banding has been associated with twice the risk of incident alcohol use disorder [649]. In that study, one-fifth of the participants reported alcohol use disorder within a 5-year post-Roux-en-Y gastric bypass. Multiple studies report increased risk of suicide in the postoperative period [611]. A 2016 review found that postoperative prevalence of alcohol use ranged from 7.6% to 11.8% among patients who underwent bariatric surgery [650].

Binge eating (BE) or BE disorder (BED) and loss of control (LOC) are quite common among the severely obese before surgery [651]. Unfortunately, BE, BED, and LOC can develop post-surgically and are associated with less weight loss and more weight regain [587].

Psychoeducation prior to surgery to prepare the patient for possible complications will facilitate earlier support and intervention should it be needed. Experts in the field highly encourage the postoperative team to acknowledge potential psychiatric complications postoperatively, conduct screenings, and adopt an interdisciplinary, team-based approach to their management [652]. AUD education, screening, evaluation, and treatment referral should be incorporated in pre- and postoperative care [649]. Especially important is evaluation for signs of MDD or other mood disorders. Important are anhedonia, dysphoria, fatigue, appetite changes, guilt, and psychomotor symptoms that present for more than 2 weeks. Appearance or worsening symptoms of psychosis include delusions, hallucinations, or paranoia, and the emergence of any eating disorder such as binging and purging. Anxiety symptoms including palpitations should be evaluated for organic causes such as electrolyte imbalances, dumping syndrome, Wernicke encephalopathy,[17] thyroid conditions, and other endocrine and metabolic complications [653].

An especially useful tool is the *Patient Health Questionnaire (PHQ-9),* which is a brief self-administered tool [655]. The PHQ-9 targets important symptoms of depression, including anhedonia, dysphoria, fatigue, appetite irregularities, feelings of guilt, lack of motivation, difficulty concentrating, changes in motor activity (such as agitation and retardation), and suicide ideation, and scores them based on the frequency of these symptoms over the assessment period. The *US Substance Abuse and Mental Health Services Administration, Center for Substance Abuse Treatment (SAMHSA, CSAT) Screening, Brief Intervention, and Referral for Treatment (SBIRT)* tool [656] is useful for screening for substance abuse.

Pharmacotherapeutic treatment and management of depression and other disorders could be a challenge as absorption and metabolism of pharmaceuticals, as well as food, vitamins, and minerals, will have changed [657]. Antidepressant medications may need to be altered after surgery [634, 635, 658]. Noteworthy are the cytochrome CYP 450 3A enzymes subfamily in the small intestine, which is involved in the bioavailability of various psychiatric medications, including antidepressants and antipsychotics [659–661].

Most likely due to physiological processes, behavioral characteristics, and psychological factors, it appears that between 20% and 30% of patients experience suboptimal weight loss or significant weight regain within the first few postoperative years [622]. The *American Gastroenterological Association Best Practice Advice* for post-bariatric surgery states that: "Clinicians should screen and follow up on all patients undergoing endoscopic management of bariatric/metabolic surgical complications and dietary intolerance for comorbid medical (nutrient deficiencies, infection, pulmonary embolism) and psychological (depression, anxiety) conditions to minimize complications and improve results" [639].

[17] Wernicke encephalopathy is most often encountered in thiamine deficiency and is associated with severe alcohol use disorder and of concern in this context is impaired absorption from the intestines [654].

Diabetes

According to the International Diabetes Foundation [662] in 2019, worldwide, 1 in 11 adults aged 20–79 had diabetes; 10% of global health expenditure was on diabetes; and two-thirds of people with diabetes lived in rural areas. In developed countries, depression and anxiety are the fourth and diabetes is the eighth leading cause of disability adjusted life years [663]. Diabetes is an independent risk factor for depression, and the risk of depression is greater in subjects with diabetes compared to the general population [664].

People with diabetes mellitus have been said to be two to three times more likely to have depression [665]. However, a 2019 systematic review and meta-analysis found a lower but still substantial risk [664]. They found the pooled OR for all of the studies to be 1.33; 95% CI: 1.18–1.51. The ORs varied by study types. Prospective studies OR = 1.34; 95% CI: 1.14–1.57; retrospective OR = 1.30; 95% CI: 1.05–1.62; self-reported doctor's diagnosis OR = 1.37; 95% CI: 1.17–1.60) and blood test diagnosis OR = 1.25; 95% CI: 1.04–1.52.

A systematic review in 2012 showed that compared to those without diabetes, prevalence of depression was more than three-times higher in people with type 1 diabetes (12%, range 5.8–43.3% vs. 3.2%, range 2.7–11.4%) and nearly twice as high in people with type 2 diabetes (19.1%, range 6.5–33% vs. 10.7%, range 3.8–19.4%) [666]. Another systematic review showed that in patients who participated in clinical studies, generalized anxiety disorder was present in 14% and increased anxiety symptoms were present in 40% of the diabetic patients [667].

A 2008 meta-analysis revealed that depression imparted a 60% increase in risk (RR[18] 1.60 (1.37–1.88) of type 2 diabetes, while in the other direction diabetes showed a modest risk (RR 1.15 (1.02–1.30) of depression [668]. It has been suggested that associations between the comorbidities may be based upon nonspecific pathophysiological mechanisms, or that specific changes in brain structure or function in diabetics may dispose to depression, or antidepressant treatment in depression may adversely affect metabolic pathways leading to diabetes [669].

In terms of common etiology, genetic and environmental factors have been considered [669]. Investigations of genetic factors that both type 2 diabetes and depression might have in common have been few and non-revealing [670, 671]. There is a substantially higher prevalence rate of comorbid type 2 diabetes and depression in females compared with males [672–674].

A 2016 study has identified genetic overlap between type 2 diabetes and depression in large population-based Swedish and Danish twin registries [675]. Their findings also suggested that males and females might have different risk factors.

A 2019 review of shared and unique risk factors for depression and diabetes found the following [676].

- Shared risk factors were hypertension, daily smoking, lack of physical activity, and obesity.
- Unique associations with depression were being female, family stress, traumatic events, and having any chronic disease or heart disease.
- Unique associations with diabetes were increasing age and ethnicity (non-white).
- Risk factors for major depressive disorder in both sexes were being underweight, family stress, chronic disease, and heart disease.
- Risk factors for incident diabetes in both sexes were age, ethnicity (non-white), high blood pressure, daily smoking, physical inactivity, and body mass index.

When depression and anxiety are present in diabetic patients, the diabetic prognosis is worse; non-compliance is more pronounced [677]; all-cause mortality is increased [678]; and quality of life is diminished [679].

Summary

Depression is two to three times greater risk for people with multiple morbidity than it is for people who have no comorbidity or no chronic medical condition. Evidence has been accumulating for some of the specific characteristics that associate a variety of illnesses with depression. For example, depression is associated with engaging in unhealthy behaviors, including regular smoking, overeating, alcohol use, and lack of exercise.

Depression predicts the subsequent incidence of some of the most prevalent diseases that commonly occur in multimorbid clusters. An example of abnormal conditions shared by a disorder is MS and MDD. They have a common condition of chronic oxidative and nitrosative stress, neuroendocrine abnormalities, microglial pathology, mitochondrial dysfunction, gut dysbiosis, increased intestinal barrier permeability, and peripheral and neuro-inflammation.

Personality types and stressors are variously associated with depression. Twenty-five percent of people with type 2 diabetes have clinically significant depression. The risk of metabolic syndrome is increased in patients who suffer from

[18] *Relative risk (RR)* is perhaps the most common method of expressing the estimated risk of experiencing a result. RR compares the probability of a specific outcome in the treatment group with that of a control group. When an RR is greater than 1, there seems to be an increased risk of an event. When the RR is less than 1, there appears to be a decreased risk of experiencing an event. If the RR is 1, there is no apparent risk. If the RR = 5, it is 5 times more likely to occur than in the control group. If the RR = 0.5, it is half as likely to happen as in the control group. For more information, see Chap. 4 Evidence Basics.

major MDD, PTSD, ADHD, bipolar disorder, schizophrenia, or anxiety disorders. There is a genetic overlap between cardio-metabolic diseases and depression.

Hypertension, cardiovascular disease, obesity, and diabetes are prominently associated with depression. However, some of the relationship studies relied on self-reporting of symptoms, which makes data difficult to interpret. As a result, some studies report divergent results. Other possible explanations for divergent results include age effects, short duration of follow-up, ethnicity, and use of antidepressants or other medications.

References

1. Birk JL, Kronish IM, Moise N, Falzon L, Yoon S, Davidson KW. Depression and multimorbidity: considering temporal characteristics of the associations between depression and multiple chronic diseases. Health Psychol. 2019;38(9):802–11. PMCID: PMC6706317. http://www.ncbi.nlm.nih.gov/pubmed/31008648.
2. Köhler-Forsberg O, Petersen L, Ishtiak-Ahmed K, Østergaard SD, Gasse C. Medical diseases prior to first-time depression diagnosis and subsequent risk of admissions for depression: a nationwide study of 117,585 patients. J Affect Disord. 2020;276:1030–7. PMID: 32763587. http://www.ncbi.nlm.nih.gov/pubmed/32763587.
3. Huang CQ, Dong BR, Lu ZC, Yue JR, Liu QX. Chronic diseases and risk for depression in old age: a meta-analysis of published literature. Ageing Res Rev. 2010;9(2):131–41. PMID: 19524072. http://www.ncbi.nlm.nih.gov/pubmed/19524072.
4. Wu Q, Feng J, Pan CW. Risk factors for depression in the elderly: an umbrella review of published meta-analyses and systematic reviews. J Affect Disord. 2022;307:37–45. PMID: 35351490. http://www.ncbi.nlm.nih.gov/pubmed/35351490.
5. Cho Y, Mishiro I, Akaki T, Akimoto T, Fujikawa K. Diseases prevalent before major depressive disorder diagnosis: an exploratory nested case-control study using health insurance-based claims data. BMJ Open. 2022;12(2):e048233. PMCID: PMC8852671. http://www.ncbi.nlm.nih.gov/pubmed/35168961.
6. Thombs BD, Bass EB, Ford DE, Stewart KJ, Tsilidis KK, Patel U, Fauerbach JA, Bush DE, Ziegelstein RC. Prevalence of depression in survivors of acute myocardial infarction. J Gen Intern Med. 2006;21(1):30–8. PMCID: PMC1484630. http://www.ncbi.nlm.nih.gov/pubmed/16423120.
7. Polenick CA, Renn BN, Birditt KS. Dyadic effects of depressive symptoms on medical morbidity in middle-aged and older couples. Health Psychol. 2018;37(1):28–36. PMCID: PMC5764774. http://www.ncbi.nlm.nih.gov/pubmed/29154606.
8. Feng MY, Bi YH, Wang HX, Pei JJ. Influence of chronic diseases on the occurrence of depression: a 13-year follow-up study from the Survey of Health, Ageing and Retirement in Europe. Psychiatry Res. 2023;326:115268. PMID: 37270866. http://www.ncbi.nlm.nih.gov/pubmed/37270866.
9. Herrera PA, Campos-Romero S, Szabo W, Martínez P, Guajardo V, Rojas G. Understanding the relationship between depression and chronic diseases such as diabetes and hypertension: a grounded theory study. Int J Environ Res Public Health. 2021;18(22):12130. PMCID: PMC8618720. http://www.ncbi.nlm.nih.gov/pubmed/34831886.
10. Pham MT, Rajić A, Greig JD, Sargeant JM, Papadopoulos A, McEwen SA. A scoping review of scoping reviews: advancing the approach and enhancing the consistency. Res Synth Methods. 2014;5(4):371–85. PMCID: PMC4491356. http://www.ncbi.nlm.nih.gov/pubmed/26052958.
11. Tinetti ME, Fried TR, Boyd CM. Designing health care for the most common chronic condition—multimorbidity. JAMA. 2012;307(23):2493–4. PMCID: PMC4083627. http://www.ncbi.nlm.nih.gov/pubmed/22797447.
12. King DE, Xiang J, Pilkerton CS. Multimorbidity trends in United States adults, 1988-2014. J Am Board Fam Med. 2018;31(4):503–13. PMCID: PMC6368177. http://www.ncbi.nlm.nih.gov/pubmed/29986975.
13. van den Bussche H, Koller D, Kolonko T, Hansen H, Wegscheider K, Glaeske G, von Leitner EC, Schäfer I, Schön G. Which chronic diseases and disease combinations are specific to multimorbidity in the elderly? Results of a claims data based cross-sectional study in Germany. BMC Public Health. 2011;11:101. PMCID: PMC3050745. http://www.ncbi.nlm.nih.gov/pubmed/21320345.
14. Barnett K, Mercer SW, Norbury M, Watt G, Wyke S, Guthrie B. Epidemiology of multimorbidity and implications for health care, research, and medical education: a cross-sectional study. Lancet. 2012;380(9836):37–43. PMID: 22579043. http://www.ncbi.nlm.nih.gov/pubmed/22579043.
15. Sinnige J, Braspenning J, Schellevis F, Stirbu-Wagner I, Westert G, Korevaar J. The prevalence of disease clusters in older adults with multiple chronic diseases—a systematic literature review. PLoS One. 2013;8(11):e79641. PMCID: PMC3823581. http://www.ncbi.nlm.nih.gov/pubmed/24244534.
16. Read JR, Sharpe L, Modini M, Dear BF. Multimorbidity and depression: a systematic review and meta-analysis. J Affect Disord. 2017;221:36–46. PMID: 28628766. http://www.ncbi.nlm.nih.gov/pubmed/28628766.
17. Lang UE, Walter M. Depression in the context of medical disorders: new pharmacological pathways revisited. Neurosignals. 2017;25(1):54–73. PMID: 29041003. http://www.ncbi.nlm.nih.gov/pubmed/29041003.
18. Martin-Subero M, Anderson G, Kanchanatawan B, Berk M, Maes M. Comorbidity between depression and inflammatory bowel disease explained by immune-inflammatory, oxidative, and nitrosative stress; tryptophan catabolite; and gut-brain pathways. CNS Spectr. 2016;21(2):184–98. PMID: 26307347. http://www.ncbi.nlm.nih.gov/pubmed/26307347.
19. Morris G, Reiche EMV, Murru A, Carvalho AF, Maes M, Berk M, Puri BK. Multiple immune-inflammatory and oxidative and nitrosative stress pathways explain the frequent presence of depression in multiple sclerosis. Mol Neurobiol. 2018;55(8):6282–306. PMCID: PMC6061180. http://www.ncbi.nlm.nih.gov/pubmed/29294244.
20. Panagioti M, Scott C, Blakemore A, Coventry PA. Overview of the prevalence, impact, and management of depression and anxiety in chronic obstructive pulmonary disease. Int J Chron Obstruct Pulmon Dis. 2014;9:1289–306. PMCID: PMC4235478. http://www.ncbi.nlm.nih.gov/pubmed/25419126.
21. Siegmann EM, Müller HHO, Luecke C, Philipsen A, Kornhuber J, Grömer TW. Association of Depression and Anxiety Disorders with autoimmune thyroiditis: a systematic review and meta-analysis. JAMA Psychiatry. 2018;75(6):577–84. PMCID: PMC6137529. http://www.ncbi.nlm.nih.gov/pubmed/29800939.
22. Semenkovich K, Brown ME, Svrakic DM, Lustman PJ. Depression in type 2 diabetes mellitus: prevalence, impact, and treatment. Drugs. 2015;75(6):577–87. PMID: 25851098. http://www.ncbi.nlm.nih.gov/pubmed/25851098.
23. Pryce CR, Fontana A. Depression in autoimmune diseases. Curr Top Behav Neurosci. 2017;31:139–54. PMID: 27221625. http://www.ncbi.nlm.nih.gov/pubmed/27221625.
24. Penninx BWJH, Lange SMM. Metabolic syndrome in psychiatric patients: overview, mechanisms, and implications. Dialogues Clin

Neurosci. 2018;20(1):63–73. PMCID: PMC6016046. http://www.ncbi.nlm.nih.gov/pubmed/29946213.
25. Amare AT, Schubert KO, Klingler-Hoffmann M, Cohen-Woods S, Baune BT. The genetic overlap between mood disorders and cardiometabolic diseases: a systematic review of genome wide and candidate gene studies. Transl Psychiatry. 2017;7(1):e1007. PMCID: PMC5545727. http://www.ncbi.nlm.nih.gov/pubmed/28117839.
26. Bennett S, Thomas AJ. Depression and dementia: cause, consequence or coincidence? Maturitas. 2014;79(2):184–90. PMID: 24931304. http://www.ncbi.nlm.nih.gov/pubmed/24931304.
27. Helvik AS, Barca ML, Bergh S, Šaltytė-Benth J, Kirkevold Ø, Borza T. The course of depressive symptoms with decline in cognitive function - a longitudinal study of older adults receiving in-home care at baseline. BMC Geriatr. 2019;19(1):231. PMCID: PMC6708209. http://www.ncbi.nlm.nih.gov/pubmed/31443638.
28. Buganza-Torio E, Mitchell N, Abraldes JG, Thomas L, Ma M, Bailey RJ, Tandon P. Depression in cirrhosis - a prospective evaluation of the prevalence, predictors and development of a screening nomogram. Aliment Pharmacol Ther. 2019;49(2):194–201. PMID: 30485460. http://www.ncbi.nlm.nih.gov/pubmed/30485460.
29. Hein AM, O'Banion MK. Neuroinflammation and cognitive dysfunction in chronic disease and aging. J Neuroimmune Pharmacol. 2012;7(1):3–6. PMID: 22252623. http://www.ncbi.nlm.nih.gov/pubmed/22252623.
30. Kessler RC, Berglund P, Demler O, Jin R, Merikangas KR, Walters EE. Lifetime prevalence and age-of-onset distributions of DSM-IV disorders in the National Comorbidity Survey Replication. Arch Gen Psychiatry. 2005;62(6):593–602. PMID: 15939837. http://www.ncbi.nlm.nih.gov/pubmed/15939837.
31. Karaoulanis SE, Daponte A, Rizouli KA, Rizoulis AA, Lialios GA, Theodoridou CT, Christakopoulos C, Angelopoulos NV. The role of cytokines and hot flashes in perimenopausal depression. Ann General Psychiatry. 2012;11:9. PMCID: PMC3348044. http://www.ncbi.nlm.nih.gov/pubmed/22490187.
32. Barton DA, Dawood T, Lambert EA, Esler MD, Haikerwal D, Brenchley C, Socratous F, Kaye DM, Schlaich MP, Hickie I, Lambert GW. Sympathetic activity in major depressive disorder: identifying those at increased cardiac risk? J Hypertens. 2007;25(10):2117–24. PMID: 17885556. http://www.ncbi.nlm.nih.gov/pubmed/17885556.
33. Grewen KM, Girdler SS, Hinderliter A, Light KC. Depressive symptoms are related to higher ambulatory blood pressure in people with a family history of hypertension. Psychosom Med. 2004;66(1):9–16. PMID: 14747632. http://www.ncbi.nlm.nih.gov/pubmed/14747632.
34. Wu ZS. Importance must be attached to correcting unhealthy lifestyles in prevention and control of hypertension. J Geriatr Cardiol. 2019;16(3):176–7. PMCID: PMC6500572. http://www.ncbi.nlm.nih.gov/pubmed/31080463.
35. Aloia MS, Arnedt JT, Smith L, Skrekas J, Stanchina M, Millman RP. Examining the construct of depression in obstructive sleep apnea syndrome. Sleep Med. 2005;6(2):115–21. PMID: 15716215. http://www.ncbi.nlm.nih.gov/pubmed/15716215.
36. Kalmbach DA, Arnedt JT, Song PX, Guille C, Sen S. Sleep disturbance and short sleep as risk factors for depression and perceived medical errors in first-year residents. Sleep. 2017;40(3):zsw073. PMCID: PMC6084763. http://www.ncbi.nlm.nih.gov/pubmed/28369654.
37. Skilton MR, Moulin P, Terra JL, Bonnet F. Associations between anxiety, depression, and the metabolic syndrome. Biol Psychiatry. 2007;62(11):1251–7. PMID: 17553465. http://www.ncbi.nlm.nih.gov/pubmed/17553465.
38. Scalco AZ, Scalco MZ, Azul JBS, Lotufo NF. Hypertension and depression. Clinics (Sao Paulo). 2005;60(3):241–50. PMID: 15962086. http://www.ncbi.nlm.nih.gov/pubmed/15962086.
39. Johnson AD, Newton-Cheh C, Chasman DI, Ehret GB, Johnson T, Rose L, Rice K, Verwoert GC, Launer LJ, Gudnason V, Larson MG, Chakravarti A, Psaty BM, Caulfield M, van Duijn CM, Ridker PM, Munroe PB, Levy D. Cohorts for heart and aging research in Genomic Epidemiology Consortium, Global BPgen Consortium, Women's Genome Health Study. Association of hypertension drug target genes with blood pressure and hypertension in 86,588 individuals. Hypertension. 2011;57(5):903–10. PMCID: PMC3099407. http://www.ncbi.nlm.nih.gov/pubmed/21444836.
40. Casamassima F, Huang J, Fava M, Sachs GS, Smoller JW, Cassano GB, Lattanzi L, Fagerness J, Stange JP, Perlis RH. Phenotypic effects of a bipolar liability gene among individuals with major depressive disorder. Am J Med Genet B Neuropsychiatr Genet. 2010;153B(1):303–9. PMID: 19388002. http://www.ncbi.nlm.nih.gov/pubmed/19388002.
41. Green EK, Grozeva D, Jones I, Jones L, Kirov G, Caesar S, Gordon-Smith K, Fraser C, Forty L, Russell E, Hamshere ML, Moskvina V, Nikolov I, Farmer A, McGuffin P, Wellcome Trust Case Control Consortium, Holmans PA, Owen MJ, O'Donovan MC, Craddock N. The bipolar disorder risk allele at CACNA1C also confers risk of recurrent major depression and of schizophrenia. Mol Psychiatry. 2010;15(10):1016–22. PMCID: PMC3011210. http://www.ncbi.nlm.nih.gov/pubmed/19621016.
42. Ferreira MAR, O'Donovan MC, Meng YA, Jones IR, Ruderfer DM, Jones L, Fan J, Kirov G, Perlis RH, Green EK, Smoller JW, Grozeva D, Stone J, Nikolov I, Chambert K, Hamshere ML, Nimgaonkar VL, Moskvina V, Thase ME, Caesar S, Sachs GS, Franklin J, Gordon-Smith K, Ardlie KG, Gabriel SB, Fraser C, Blumenstiel B, Defelice M, Breen G, Gill M, Morris DW, Elkin A, Muir WJ, McGhee KA, Williamson R, MacIntyre DJ, MacLean AW, St CD, Robinson M, Van Beck M, Pereira ACP, Kandaswamy R, McQuillin A, Collier DA, Bass NJ, Young AH, Lawrence J, Ferrier IN, Anjorin A, Farmer A, Curtis D, Scolnick EM, McGuffin P, Daly MJ, Corvin AP, Holmans PA, Blackwood DH, Gurling HM, Owen MJ, Purcell SM, Sklar P, Craddock N. Wellcome Trust Case Control Consortium. Collaborative genome-wide association analysis supports a role for ANK3 and CACNA1C in bipolar disorder. Nat Genet. 2008;40(9):1056–8. PMCID: PMC2703780. http://www.ncbi.nlm.nih.gov/pubmed/18711365.
43. Siever LJ, Davis KL. Overview: toward a dysregulation hypothesis of depression. Am J Psychiatry. 1985;142(9):1017–31. PMID: 2862799. http://www.ncbi.nlm.nih.gov/pubmed/2862799.
44. Perez-Caballero L, Torres-Sanchez S, Romero-López-Alberca C, González-Saiz F, Mico JA, Berrocoso E. Monoaminergic system and depression. Cell Tissue Res. 2019;377(1):107–13. PMID: 30627806. http://www.ncbi.nlm.nih.gov/pubmed/30627806.
45. Hamon M, Blier P. Monoamine neurocircuitry in depression and strategies for new treatments. Prog Neuro-Psychopharmacol Biol Psychiatry. 2013;45:54–63. PMID: 23602950. http://www.ncbi.nlm.nih.gov/pubmed/23602950.
46. Hildrum B, Romild U, Holmen J. Anxiety and depression lowers blood pressure: 22-year follow-up of the population based HUNT study, Norway. BMC Public Health. 2011;11:601. PMCID: PMC3162525. http://www.ncbi.nlm.nih.gov/pubmed/21797992.
47. Jonas BS, Franks P, Ingram DD. Are symptoms of anxiety and depression risk factors for hypertension? Longitudinal evidence from the National Health and Nutrition Examination Survey I epidemiologic follow-up study. Arch Fam Med. 1997;6(1):43–9. PMID: 9003169. http://www.ncbi.nlm.nih.gov/pubmed/9003169.
48. Davidson K, Jonas BS, Dixon KE, Markovitz JH. Do depression symptoms predict early hypertension incidence in young adults in the CARDIA study? Coronary Artery Risk Development in

Young Adults. Arch Intern Med. 2000;160(10):1495–500. PMID: 10826464. http://www.ncbi.nlm.nih.gov/pubmed/10826464.
49. Li Z, Li Y, Chen L, Chen P, Hu Y. Prevalence of depression in patients with hypertension: a systematic review and meta-analysis. Medicine (Baltimore). 2015;94(31):e1317. PMCID: PMC4616591. http://www.ncbi.nlm.nih.gov/pubmed/26252317.
50. Maatouk I, Herzog W, Böhlen F, Quinzler R, Löwe B, Saum KU, Brenner H, Wild B. Association of hypertension with depression and generalized anxiety symptoms in a large population-based sample of older adults. J Hypertens. 2016;34(9):1711–20. PMID: 27341438. http://www.ncbi.nlm.nih.gov/pubmed/27341438.
51. Kearney PM, Whelton M, Reynolds K, Muntner P, Whelton PK, He J. Global burden of hypertension: analysis of worldwide data. Lancet. 2005;365(9455):217–23. PMID: 15652604. http://www.ncbi.nlm.nih.gov/pubmed/15652604.
52. Lawes CMM, Vander Hoorn S, Rodgers A. International Society of Hypertension. Global burden of blood-pressure-related disease, 2001. Lancet. 2008;371(9623):1513–8. PMID: 18456100. http://www.ncbi.nlm.nih.gov/pubmed/18456100.
53. Meng L, Chen D, Yang Y, Zheng Y, Hui R. Depression increases the risk of hypertension incidence: a meta-analysis of prospective cohort studies. J Hypertens. 2012;30(5):842–51. PMID: 22343537. http://www.ncbi.nlm.nih.gov/pubmed/22343537.
54. Wu EL, Chien IC, Lin CH, Chou YJ, Chou P. Increased risk of hypertension in patients with major depressive disorder: a population-based study. J Psychosom Res. 2012;73(3):169–74. PMID: 22850255. http://www.ncbi.nlm.nih.gov/pubmed/22850255.
55. 9789241563710_eng.pdf.
56. Hare DL, Toukhsati SR, Johansson P, Jaarsma T. Depression and cardiovascular disease: a clinical review. Eur Heart J. 2014;35(21):1365–72. PMID: 24282187. http://www.ncbi.nlm.nih.gov/pubmed/24282187.
57. Kuo PL, Pu C. The contribution of depression to mortality among elderly with self-reported hypertension: analysis using a national representative longitudinal survey. J Hypertens. 2011;29(11):2084–90. PMID: 21934532. http://www.ncbi.nlm.nih.gov/pubmed/21934532.
58. Graham N, Ward J, Mackay D, Pell JP, Cavanagh J, Padmanabhan S, Smith DJ. Impact of major depression on cardiovascular outcomes for individuals with hypertension: prospective survival analysis in UK Biobank. BMJ Open. 2019;9(9):e024433. PMCID: PMC6797415. http://www.ncbi.nlm.nih.gov/pubmed/31575565.
59. Delaney JAC, Oddson BE, Kramer H, Shea S, Psaty BM, McClelland RL. Baseline depressive symptoms are not associated with clinically important levels of incident hypertension during two years of follow-up: the multi-ethnic study of atherosclerosis. Hypertension. 2010;55(2):408–14. PMCID: PMC2821214. http://www.ncbi.nlm.nih.gov/pubmed/20065156.
60. Meyer CM, Armenian HK, Eaton WW, Ford DE. Incident hypertension associated with depression in the Baltimore Epidemiologic Catchment area follow-up study. J Affect Disord. 2004;83(2–3):127–33. PMID: 15555705. http://www.ncbi.nlm.nih.gov/pubmed/15555705.
61. Patten SB, Williams JVA, Lavorato DH, Modgill G, Jetté N, Eliasziw M. Major depression as a risk factor for chronic disease incidence: longitudinal analyses in a general population cohort. Gen Hosp Psychiatry. 2008;30(5):407–13. PMID: 18774423. http://www.ncbi.nlm.nih.gov/pubmed/18774423.
62. Hildrum B, Mykletun A, Holmen J, Dahl AA. Effect of anxiety and depression on blood pressure: 11-year longitudinal population study. Br J Psychiatry. 2008;193(2):108–13. PMID: 18669991. http://www.ncbi.nlm.nih.gov/pubmed/18669991.
63. Paterniti S, Verdier-Taillefer MH, Geneste C, Bisserbe JC, Alpérovitch A. Low blood pressure and risk of depression in the elderly. A prospective community-based study. Br J Psychiatry. 2000;176:464–7. PMID: 10912223. http://www.ncbi.nlm.nih.gov/pubmed/10912223.
64. Boal AH, Smith DJ, McCallum L, Muir S, Touyz RM, Dominiczak AF, Padmanabhan S. Monotherapy with major antihypertensive drug classes and risk of hospital admissions for mood disorders. Hypertension. 2016;68(5):1132–8. PMCID: PMC5058642. http://www.ncbi.nlm.nih.gov/pubmed/27733585.
65. Licht CMM, de Geus EJC, Seldenrijk A, van Hout HPJ, Zitman FG, van Dyck R, Penninx BWJH. Depression is associated with decreased blood pressure, but antidepressant use increases the risk for hypertension. Hypertension. 2009;53(4):631–8. PMID: 19237679. http://www.ncbi.nlm.nih.gov/pubmed/19237679.
66. Crookes DM, Demmer RT, Keyes KM, Koenen KC, Suglia SF. Depressive symptoms, antidepressant use, and hypertension in young adulthood. Epidemiology. 2018;29(4):547–55. PMCID: PMC5980764. http://www.ncbi.nlm.nih.gov/pubmed/29629939.
67. Diminic-Lisica I, Popovic B, Rebic J, Klaric M, Franciškovic T. Outcome of treatment with antidepressants in patients with hypertension and undetected depression. Int J Psychiatry Med. 2014;47(2):115–29. PMID: 25084798. http://www.ncbi.nlm.nih.gov/pubmed/25084798.
68. Atlantis E, Lange K, Goldney RD, Martin S, Haren MT, Taylor A, O'Loughlin PD, Marshall V, Tilley W, Wittert GA. Specific medical conditions associated with clinically significant depressive symptoms in men. Soc Psychiatry Psychiatr Epidemiol. 2011;46(12):1303–12. PMID: 20976591. http://www.ncbi.nlm.nih.gov/pubmed/20976591.
69. Gould CE, Beaudreau SA. Association between depression and anxiety on blood pressure dysregulation and pulse in the Health and Retirement Study. Int J Geriatr Psychiatry. 2013;28(10):1045–53. PMID: 23335009. http://www.ncbi.nlm.nih.gov/pubmed/23335009.
70. Barrett-Connor E, Palinkas LA. Low blood pressure and depression in older men: a population based study. BMJ. 1994;308(6926):446–9. PMCID: PMC2539519. http://www.ncbi.nlm.nih.gov/pubmed/8124175.
71. Herva A, Räsänen P, Miettunen J, Timonen M, Läksy K, Veijola J, Laitinen J, Ruokonen A, Joukamaa M. Co-occurrence of metabolic syndrome with depression and anxiety in young adults: the Northern Finland 1966 Birth Cohort Study. Psychosom Med. 2006;68(2):213–6. PMID: 16554385. http://www.ncbi.nlm.nih.gov/pubmed/16554385.
72. HUNT - The Trøndelag Health Study - NTNU.
73. Hildrum B, Mykletun A, Stordal E, Bjelland I, Dahl AA, Holmen J. Association of low blood pressure with anxiety and depression: the Nord-Trøndelag Health Study. J Epidemiol Community Health. 2007;61(1):53–8. PMCID: PMC2465598. http://www.ncbi.nlm.nih.gov/pubmed/17183016.
74. Lenoir H, Lacombe JM, Dufouil C, Ducimetière P, Hanon O, Ritchie K, Dartigues JF, Alpérovitch A, Tzourio C. Relationship between blood pressure and depression in the elderly. The Three-City Study. J Hypertens. 2008;26(9):1765–72. PMID: 18698210. http://www.ncbi.nlm.nih.gov/pubmed/18698210.
75. Stroup-Benham CA, Markides KS, Black SA, Goodwin JS. Relationship between low blood pressure and depressive symptomatology in older people. J Am Geriatr Soc. 2000;48(3):250–5. PMID: 10733049. http://www.ncbi.nlm.nih.gov/pubmed/10733049.
76. Nabi H, Chastang JF, Lefèvre T, Dugravot A, Melchior M, Marmot MG, Shipley MJ, Kivimäki M, Singh-Manoux A. Trajectories of depressive episodes and hypertension over 24 years: the Whitehall II prospective cohort study. Hypertension. 2011;57(4):710–6. PMCID: PMC3065997. http://www.ncbi.nlm.nih.gov/pubmed/21339474.

77. Gangwisch JE, Malaspina D, Posner K, Babiss LA, Heymsfield SB, Turner JB, Zammit GK, Pickering TG. Insomnia and sleep duration as mediators of the relationship between depression and hypertension incidence. Am J Hypertens. 2010;23(1):62–9. PMCID: PMC4415616. http://www.ncbi.nlm.nih.gov/pubmed/19893498.
78. Rutledge T, Hogan BE. A quantitative review of prospective evidence linking psychological factors with hypertension development. Psychosom Med. 2002;64(5):758–66. PMID: 12271106. http://www.ncbi.nlm.nih.gov/pubmed/12271106.
79. Knäuper B, Turner PA. Measuring health: improving the validity of health assessments. Qual Life Res. 2003;12(Suppl 1):81–9. PMID: 12803314. http://www.ncbi.nlm.nih.gov/pubmed/12803314.
80. Newell SA, Girgis A, Sanson-Fisher RW, Savolainen NJ. The accuracy of self-reported health behaviors and risk factors relating to cancer and cardiovascular disease in the general population: a critical review. Am J Prev Med. 1999;17(3):211–29. PMID: 10987638. http://www.ncbi.nlm.nih.gov/pubmed/10987638.
81. Kimberlin CL, Winterstein AG. Validity and reliability of measurement instruments used in research. Am J Health Syst Pharm. 2008;65(23):2276–84. PMID: 19020196. http://www.ncbi.nlm.nih.gov/pubmed/19020196.
82. Piper MA, Evans CV, Burda BU, Margolis KL, O'Connor E, Smith N, Webber E, Perdue LA, Bigler KD, Whitlock EP. Screening for high blood pressure in adults: a systematic evidence review for the U.S. Preventive Services Task Force [Internet]. Rockville: Agency for Healthcare Research and Quality (US); 2014 [cited 2025 Jan 1]. Available from: http://www.ncbi.nlm.nih.gov/books/NBK269495/ PMID: 25632496 http://www.ncbi.nlm.nih.gov/pubmed/25632496.
83. Gangwisch JE, Heymsfield SB, Boden-Albala B, Buijs RM, Kreier F, Pickering TG, Rundle AG, Zammit GK, Malaspina D. Short sleep duration as a risk factor for hypertension: analyses of the first National Health and Nutrition Examination Survey. Hypertension. 2006;47(5):833–9. PMID: 16585410. http://www.ncbi.nlm.nih.gov/pubmed/16585410.
84. Gangwisch JE, Heymsfield SB, Boden-Albala B, Buijs RM, Kreier F, Opler MG, Pickering TG, Rundle AG, Zammit GK, Malaspina D. Sleep duration associated with mortality in elderly, but not middle-aged, adults in a large US sample. Sleep. 2008;31(8):1087–96. PMCID: PMC2542954. http://www.ncbi.nlm.nih.gov/pubmed/18714780.
85. Prinz PN. Age impairments in sleep, metabolic and immune functions. Exp Gerontol. 2004;39(11–12):1739–43. PMID: 15582290. http://www.ncbi.nlm.nih.gov/pubmed/15582290.
86. Kannel WB. Blood pressure as a cardiovascular risk factor: prevention and treatment. JAMA. 1996;275(20):1571–6. PMID: 8622248. http://www.ncbi.nlm.nih.gov/pubmed/8622248.
87. Robbins MA, Elias PK, Elias MF. Low blood pressure and depression: comorbidity and competing outcomes. J Am Geriatr Soc. 2000;48(3):336–7. PMID: 10733064. http://www.ncbi.nlm.nih.gov/pubmed/10733064.
88. Qureshi AI, Suri MFK, Kirmani JF, Divani AA. Prevalence and trends of prehypertension and hypertension in United States: National Health and Nutrition Examination Surveys 1976 to 2000. Med Sci Monit. 2005;11(9):CR403-409. PMID: 16127357. http://www.ncbi.nlm.nih.gov/pubmed/16127357.
89. Zhai L, Zhang H, Zhang D. Sleep duration and depression among adults: a meta-analysis of prospective studies. Depress Anxiety. 2015;32(9):664–70. PMID: 26047492. http://www.ncbi.nlm.nih.gov/pubmed/26047492.
90. Gottlieb DJ, Redline S, Nieto FJ, Baldwin CM, Newman AB, Resnick HE, Punjabi NM. Association of usual sleep duration with hypertension: the Sleep Heart Health Study. Sleep. 2006;29(8):1009–14. PMID: 16944668. http://www.ncbi.nlm.nih.gov/pubmed/16944668.
91. Tochikubo O, Ikeda A, Miyajima E, Ishii M. Effects of insufficient sleep on blood pressure monitored by a new multibiomedical recorder. Hypertension. 1996;27(6):1318–24. PMID: 8641742. http://www.ncbi.nlm.nih.gov/pubmed/8641742.
92. Spiegel K, Leproult R, Van Cauter E. Impact of sleep debt on metabolic and endocrine function. Lancet. 1999;354(9188):1435–9. PMID: 10543671. http://www.ncbi.nlm.nih.gov/pubmed/10543671.
93. Spiegel K, Tasali E, Penev P, Van Cauter E. Brief communication: sleep curtailment in healthy young men is associated with decreased leptin levels, elevated ghrelin levels, and increased hunger and appetite. Ann Intern Med. 2004;141(11):846–50. PMID: 15583226. http://www.ncbi.nlm.nih.gov/pubmed/15583226.
94. Gangwisch JE, Malaspina D, Boden-Albala B, Heymsfield SB. Inadequate sleep as a risk factor for obesity: analyses of the NHANES I. Sleep. 2005;28(10):1289–96. PMID: 16295214. http://www.ncbi.nlm.nih.gov/pubmed/16295214.
95. Folkow B. "Structural factor" in primary and secondary hypertension. Hypertension. 1990;16(1):89–101. PMID: 2365448. http://www.ncbi.nlm.nih.gov/pubmed/2365448.
96. Roberts RE, Duong HT. The prospective association between sleep deprivation and depression among adolescents. Sleep. 2014;37(2):239–44. PMCID: PMC3900610. http://www.ncbi.nlm.nih.gov/pubmed/24497652.
97. Conklin AI, Yao CA, Richardson CG. Chronic sleep deprivation and gender-specific risk of depression in adolescents: a prospective population-based study. BMC Public Health. 2018;18(1):724. PMCID: PMC5996474. http://www.ncbi.nlm.nih.gov/pubmed/29890964.
98. Boland EM, Rao H, Dinges DF, Smith RV, Goel N, Detre JA, Basner M, Sheline YI, Thase ME, Gehrman PR. Meta-analysis of the antidepressant effects of acute sleep deprivation. J Clin Psychiatry. 2017;78(8):e1020–34. PMID: 28937707. http://www.ncbi.nlm.nih.gov/pubmed/28937707.
99. Wolf E, Kuhn M, Normann C, Mainberger F, Maier JG, Maywald S, Bredl A, Klöppel S, Biber K, van Calker D, Riemann D, Sterr A, Nissen C. Synaptic plasticity model of therapeutic sleep deprivation in major depression. Sleep Med Rev. 2016;30:53–62. PMID: 26803484. http://www.ncbi.nlm.nih.gov/pubmed/26803484.
100. Hemmeter UM, Hemmeter-Spernal J, Krieg JC. Sleep deprivation in depression. Expert Rev Neurother. 2010;10(7):1101–15. PMID: 20586691. http://www.ncbi.nlm.nih.gov/pubmed/20586691.
101. Rodenbeck A, Hajak G. Neuroendocrine dysregulation in primary insomnia. Rev Neurol (Paris). 2001;157(11 Pt 2):S57–61. PMID: 11924040. http://www.ncbi.nlm.nih.gov/pubmed/11924040.
102. Prejbisz A, Kabat M, Januszewicz A, Szelenberger W, Piotrowska AJ, Piotrowski W, Piwoński J, Makowiecka-Cieśla M, Widecka K, Patera B, Bieniaszewski L, Narkiewicz K, Tykarski A, Piejko A, Grodzicki T, Czerwieńska B, Wiecek A. Characterization of insomnia in patients with essential hypertension. Blood Press. 2006;15(4):213–9. PMID: 17078157. http://www.ncbi.nlm.nih.gov/pubmed/17078157.
103. Wichniak A, Wierzbicka A, Walęcka M, Jernajczyk W. Effects of antidepressants on sleep. Curr Psychiatry Rep. 2017;19(9):63. PMCID: PMC5548844. http://www.ncbi.nlm.nih.gov/pubmed/28791566.
104. Webb-Johnson DC, Andrews JL. Drug therapy: bronchodilator therapy (first of two parts). N Engl J Med. 1977;297(9):476–82. PMID: 6999. http://www.ncbi.nlm.nih.gov/pubmed/69991.
105. Everitt H, Baldwin DS, Stuart B, Lipinska G, Mayers A, Malizia AL, Manson CC, Wilson S. Antidepressants for insomnia in adults. Cochrane Database Syst Rev. 2018;5(5):CD010753. PMCID: PMC6494576. http://www.ncbi.nlm.nih.gov/pubmed/29761479.
106. Santos Moraes WA, dos, Burke PR, Coutinho PL, Guilleminault C, Bittencourt AG, Tufik S, Poyares D. Sedative antidepres-

sants and insomnia. Braz. J Psychiatry. 2011;33(1):91–5. PMID: 21537726. http://www.ncbi.nlm.nih.gov/pubmed/21537726.
107. Ostuzzi G, Matcham F, Dauchy S, Barbui C, Hotopf M. Antidepressants for the treatment of depression in people with cancer. Cochrane Database Syst Rev. 2018;4(4):CD011006. PMCID: PMC6494588. http://www.ncbi.nlm.nih.gov/pubmed/29683474.
108. Everson SA, Roberts RE, Goldberg DE, Kaplan GA. Depressive symptoms and increased risk of stroke mortality over a 29-year period. Arch Intern Med. 1998;158(10):1133–8. PMID: 9605786. http://www.ncbi.nlm.nih.gov/pubmed/9605786.
109. Pratt LA, Ford DE, Crum RM, Armenian HK, Gallo JJ, Eaton WW. Depression, psychotropic medication, and risk of myocardial infarction. Prospective data from the Baltimore ECA follow-up. Circulation. 1996;94(12):3123–9. PMID: 8989119. http://www.ncbi.nlm.nih.gov/pubmed/8989119.
110. Glassman AH, Shapiro PA. Depression and the course of coronary artery disease. Am J Psychiatry. 1998;155(1):4–11. PMID: 9433332. http://www.ncbi.nlm.nih.gov/pubmed/9433332.
111. Sansone RA, Sansone LA. Depression and cardiovascular disease: just an urban legend? Psychiatry (Edgmont). 2008;5(11):45–8. PMCID: PMC2695723. http://www.ncbi.nlm.nih.gov/pubmed/19724717.
112. Grippo AJ, Johnson AK. Stress, depression and cardiovascular dysregulation: a review of neurobiological mechanisms and the integration of research from preclinical disease models. Stress. 2009;12(1):1–21. PMCID: PMC2613299. http://www.ncbi.nlm.nih.gov/pubmed/19116888.
113. Grippo AJ. Mechanisms underlying altered mood and cardiovascular dysfunction: the value of neurobiological and behavioral research with animal models. Neurosci Biobehav Rev. 2009;33(2):171–80. PMCID: PMC2593749. http://www.ncbi.nlm.nih.gov/pubmed/18703084.
114. Bankier B, Littman AB. Psychiatric disorders and coronary heart disease in women — a still neglected topic: review of the literature from 1971 to 2000. Psychother Psychosom. 2002;71(3):133–40. PMID: 12021555. http://www.ncbi.nlm.nih.gov/pubmed/12021555.
115. Denollet J, Brutsaert DL. Personality, disease severity, and the risk of long-term cardiac events in patients with a decreased ejection fraction after myocardial infarction. Circulation. 1998;97(2):167–73. PMID: 9445169. http://www.ncbi.nlm.nih.gov/pubmed/9445169.
116. Denollet J, Sys SU, Stroobant N, Rombouts H, Gillebert TC, Brutsaert DL. Personality as independent predictor of long-term mortality in patients with coronary heart disease. Lancet. 1996;347(8999):417–21. PMID: 8618481. http://www.ncbi.nlm.nih.gov/pubmed/8618481.
117. Denollet J, Pedersen SS, Vrints CJ, Conraads VM. Usefulness of type D personality in predicting five-year cardiac events above and beyond concurrent symptoms of stress in patients with coronary heart disease. Am J Cardiol. 2006;97(7):970–3. PMID: 16563897. http://www.ncbi.nlm.nih.gov/pubmed/16563897.
118. Whooley MA, Browner WS. Association between depressive symptoms and mortality in older women. Study of Osteoporotic Fractures Research Group. Arch Intern Med. 1998;158(19):2129–35. PMID: 9801180. http://www.ncbi.nlm.nih.gov/pubmed/9801180.
119. Krantz DS, McCeney MK. Effects of psychological and social factors on organic disease: a critical assessment of research on coronary heart disease. Annu Rev Psychol. 2002;53:341–69. PMID: 11752489. http://www.ncbi.nlm.nih.gov/pubmed/11752489.
120. Kop WJ, Gottdiener JS. The role of immune system parameters in the relationship between depression and coronary artery disease. Psychosom Med. 2005;67(Suppl 1):S37–41. PMID: 15953799. http://www.ncbi.nlm.nih.gov/pubmed/15953799.
121. Carney RM, Freedland KE, Veith RC. Depression, the autonomic nervous system, and coronary heart disease. Psychosom Med. 2005;67(Suppl 1):S29–33. PMID: 15953797. http://www.ncbi.nlm.nih.gov/pubmed/15953797.
122. Munger TM, Wu LQ, Shen WK. Atrial fibrillation. J Biomed Res. 2014;28(1):1–17. PMCID: PMC3904170. http://www.ncbi.nlm.nih.gov/pubmed/24474959.
123. Coromilas J. Obesity and atrial fibrillation: is one epidemic feeding the other? JAMA. 2004;292(20):2519–20. PMID: 15562134. http://www.ncbi.nlm.nih.gov/pubmed/15562134.
124. Naccarelli GV, Varker H, Lin J, Schulman KL. Increasing prevalence of atrial fibrillation and flutter in the United States. Am J Cardiol. 2009;104(11):1534–9. PMID: 19932788. http://www.ncbi.nlm.nih.gov/pubmed/19932788.
125. Stroke Prevention in Patients With Atrial Fibrillation: A Systematic Review Update - NCBI Bookshelf
126. Zulkifly H, Lip GYH, Lane DA. Epidemiology of atrial fibrillation. Int J Clin Pract. 2018;72(3):e13070. PMID: 29493854. http://www.ncbi.nlm.nih.gov/pubmed/29493854.
127. Zoni-Berisso M, Lercari F, Carazza T, Domenicucci S. Epidemiology of atrial fibrillation: European perspective. Clin Epidemiol. 2014;6:213–20. PMCID: PMC4064952. http://www.ncbi.nlm.nih.gov/pubmed/24966695.
128. Lip GYH, Fauchier L, Freedman SB, Van Gelder I, Natale A, Gianni C, Nattel S, Potpara T, Rienstra M, Tse HF, Lane DA. Atrial fibrillation. Nat Rev Dis Primers. 2016;2:16016. PMID: 27159789. http://www.ncbi.nlm.nih.gov/pubmed/27159789.
129. Thrall G, Lane D, Carroll D, Lip GYH. Quality of life in patients with atrial fibrillation: a systematic review. Am J Med. 2006;119(5):448.e1–19. PMID: 16651058. http://www.ncbi.nlm.nih.gov/pubmed/16651058.
130. Patel D, Mc Conkey ND, Sohaney R, Mc Neil A, Jedrzejczyk A, Armaganijan L. A systematic review of depression and anxiety in patients with atrial fibrillation: the mind-heart link. Cardiovasc Psychiatry Neurol. 2013;2013:159850. PMCID: PMC3655604. http://www.ncbi.nlm.nih.gov/pubmed/23710335.
131. Aviles RJ, Martin DO, Apperson-Hansen C, Houghtaling PL, Rautaharju P, Kronmal RA, Tracy RP, Van Wagoner DR, Psaty BM, Lauer MS, Chung MK. Inflammation as a risk factor for atrial fibrillation. Circulation. 2003;108(24):3006–10. PMID: 14623805. http://www.ncbi.nlm.nih.gov/pubmed/14623805.
132. Pasic J, Levy WC, Sullivan MD. Cytokines in depression and heart failure. Psychosom Med. 2003;65(2):181–93. PMID: 12651985. http://www.ncbi.nlm.nih.gov/pubmed/12651985.
133. Chung MK, Martin DO, Sprecher D, Wazni O, Kanderian A, Carnes CA, Bauer JA, Tchou PJ, Niebauer MJ, Natale A, Van Wagoner DR. C-reactive protein elevation in patients with atrial arrhythmias: inflammatory mechanisms and persistence of atrial fibrillation. Circulation. 2001;104(24):2886–91. PMID: 11739301. http://www.ncbi.nlm.nih.gov/pubmed/11739301.
134. Hansson A, Madsen-Härdig B, Olsson SB. Arrhythmia-provoking factors and symptoms at the onset of paroxysmal atrial fibrillation: a study based on interviews with 100 patients seeking hospital assistance. BMC Cardiovasc Disord. 2004;4:13. PMCID: PMC514544. http://www.ncbi.nlm.nih.gov/pubmed/15291967.
135. Yamakami Y, Kojima Y, Tsuruoka M. Physiological identification and property of afferents from the masseter muscle to the caudal part of the trigeminal nucleus in rat. Showa Shigakkai Zasshi. 1989;9(2):122–9. PMID: 2561864. http://www.ncbi.nlm.nih.gov/pubmed/2561864.
136. Murck H, Held K, Ziegenbein M, Künzel H, Koch K, Steiger A. The renin-angiotensin-aldosterone system in patients with depression compared to controls—a sleep endocrine study. BMC Psychiatry. 2003;3:15. PMCID: PMC280657. http://www.ncbi.nlm.nih.gov/pubmed/14585110.

137. Takahashi N, Kume O, Wakisaka O, Fukunaga N, Teshima Y, Hara M, Saikawa T. Novel strategy to prevent atrial fibrosis and fibrillation. Circ J. 2012;76(10):2318–26. PMID: 22972366. http://www.ncbi.nlm.nih.gov/pubmed/22972366.
138. Eaker ED, Sullivan LM, Kelly-Hayes M, D'Agostino RB, Benjamin EJ. Tension and anxiety and the prediction of the 10-year incidence of coronary heart disease, atrial fibrillation, and total mortality: the Framingham Offspring Study. Psychosom Med. 2005;67(5):692–6. PMID: 16204425. http://www.ncbi.nlm.nih.gov/pubmed/16204425.
139. Rommel J, Simpson R, Mounsey JP, Chung E, Schwartz J, Pursell I, Gehi A. Effect of body mass index, physical activity, depression, and educational attainment on high-sensitivity C-reactive protein in patients with atrial fibrillation. Am J Cardiol. 2013;111(2):208–12. PMID: 23127689. http://www.ncbi.nlm.nih.gov/pubmed/23127689.
140. hs-CRP Test (C-Reactive Protein High-Sensitivity) - Testing.com.
141. Son YJ, Song EK. The impact of type D personality and high-sensitivity C-reactive protein on health-related quality of life in patients with atrial fibrillation. Eur J Cardiovasc Nurs. 2012;11(3):304–12. PMID: 21601531. http://www.ncbi.nlm.nih.gov/pubmed/21601531.
142. Shirayama T, Sakamoto T, Sakatani T, Mani H, Yamamoto T, Matsubara H. Usefulness of paroxetine in depressed men with paroxysmal atrial fibrillation. Am J Cardiol. 2006;97(12):1749–51. PMID: 16765127. http://www.ncbi.nlm.nih.gov/pubmed/16765127.
143. Buff DD, Brenner R, Kirtane SS, Gilboa R. Dysrhythmia associated with fluoxetine treatment in an elderly patient with cardiac disease. J Clin Psychiatry. 1991;52(4):174–6. PMID: 2016253. http://www.ncbi.nlm.nih.gov/pubmed/2016253.
144. Fayssoil A, Issi J, Guerbaa M, Raynaud JC, Heroguelle V. Torsade de pointes induced by citalopram and amiodarone. Ann Cardiol Angeiol (Paris). 2011;60(3):165–8. PMID: 21295285. http://www.ncbi.nlm.nih.gov/pubmed/21295285.
145. Castro VM, Clements CC, Murphy SN, Gainer VS, Fava M, Weilburg JB, Erb JL, Churchill SE, Kohane IS, Iosifescu DV, Smoller JW, Perlis RH. QT interval and antidepressant use: a cross sectional study of electronic health records. BMJ. 2013;346:f288. PMCID: PMC3558546. http://www.ncbi.nlm.nih.gov/pubmed/23360890.
146. Cochran KA, Cavallari LH, Shapiro NL, Bishop JR. Bleeding incidence with concomitant use of antidepressants and warfarin. Ther Drug Monit. 2011;33(4):433–8. PMCID: PMC3212440. http://www.ncbi.nlm.nih.gov/pubmed/21743381.
147. Roden DM. Drug-induced prolongation of the QT interval. N Engl J Med. 2004;350(10):1013–22. PMID: 14999113. http://www.ncbi.nlm.nih.gov/pubmed/14999113.
148. Dalton SO, Johansen C, Mellemkjaer L, Nørgård B, Sørensen HT, Olsen JH. Use of selective serotonin reuptake inhibitors and risk of upper gastrointestinal tract bleeding: a population-based cohort study. Arch Intern Med. 2003;163(1):59–64. PMID: 12523917. http://www.ncbi.nlm.nih.gov/pubmed/12523917.S
149. Niedzwiedz CL, Knifton L, Robb KA, Katikireddi SV, Smith DJ. Depression and anxiety among people living with and beyond cancer: a growing clinical and research priority. BMC Cancer. 2019;19(1):943. PMCID: PMC6788022. http://www.ncbi.nlm.nih.gov/pubmed/31604468.
150. Reiche EMV, Morimoto HK, Nunes SMV. Stress and depression-induced immune dysfunction: implications for the development and progression of cancer. Int Rev Psychiatry. 2005;17(6):515–27. PMID: 16401550. http://www.ncbi.nlm.nih.gov/pubmed/16401550.
151. Reiche EMV, Nunes SOV, Morimoto HK. Stress, depression, the immune system, and cancer. Lancet Oncol. 2004;5(10):617–25. PMID: 15465465. http://www.ncbi.nlm.nih.gov/pubmed/15465465.
152. Bortolato B, Hyphantis TN, Valpione S, Perini G, Maes M, Morris G, Kubera M, Köhler CA, Fernandes BS, Stubbs B, Pavlidis N, Carvalho AF. Depression in cancer: the many biobehavioral pathways driving tumor progression. Cancer Treat Rev. 2017;52:58–70. PMID: 27894012. http://www.ncbi.nlm.nih.gov/pubmed/27894012.
153. Sotelo JL, Musselman D, Nemeroff C. The biology of depression in cancer and the relationship between depression and cancer progression. Int Rev Psychiatry. 2014;26(1):16–30. PMID: 24716498. http://www.ncbi.nlm.nih.gov/pubmed/24716498.
154. Schwartz RM, Ornstein KA, Liu B, Alpert N, Bevilacqua KG, Taioli E. Change in quality of life after a cancer diagnosis among a nationally representative cohort of older adults in the US. Cancer Investig. 2019;37(7):299–310. PMCID: PMC6755900. http://www.ncbi.nlm.nih.gov/pubmed/31379217.
155. Yi JC, Syrjala KL. Anxiety and depression in cancer survivors. Med Clin North Am. 2017;101(6):1099–113. PMCID: PMC5915316. http://www.ncbi.nlm.nih.gov/pubmed/28992857.
156. Pinquart M, Duberstein PR. Depression and cancer mortality: a meta-analysis. Psychol Med. 2010;40(11):1797–810. PMCID: PMC2935927. http://www.ncbi.nlm.nih.gov/pubmed/20085667.
157. Satin JR, Linden W, Phillips MJ. Depression as a predictor of disease progression and mortality in cancer patients: a meta-analysis. Cancer. 2009;115(22):5349–61. PMID: 19753617. http://www.ncbi.nlm.nih.gov/pubmed/19753617.
158. Linden W, Vodermaier A, Mackenzie R, Greig D. Anxiety and depression after cancer diagnosis: prevalence rates by cancer type, gender, and age. J Affect Disord. 2012;141(2–3):343–51. PMID: 22727334. http://www.ncbi.nlm.nih.gov/pubmed/22727334.
159. Fann JR, Thomas-Rich AM, Katon WJ, Cowley D, Pepping M, McGregor BA, Gralow J. Major depression after breast cancer: a review of epidemiology and treatment. Gen Hosp Psychiatry. 2008;30(2):112–26. PMID: 18291293. http://www.ncbi.nlm.nih.gov/pubmed/18291293.
160. Koenig HG, Shelp F, Goli V, Cohen HJ, Blazer DG. Survival and health care utilization in elderly medical inpatients with major depression. J Am Geriatr Soc. 1989;37(7):599–606. PMID: 2738278. http://www.ncbi.nlm.nih.gov/pubmed/2738278.
161. Misono S, Weiss NS, Fann JR, Redman M, Yueh B. Incidence of suicide in persons with cancer. J Clin Oncol. 2008;26(29):4731–8. PMCID: PMC2653137. http://www.ncbi.nlm.nih.gov/pubmed/18695257.
162. Liu L, Fiorentino L, Natarajan L, Parker BA, Mills PJ, Sadler GR, Dimsdale JE, Rissling M, He F, Ancoli-Israel S. Pre-treatment symptom cluster in breast cancer patients is associated with worse sleep, fatigue and depression during chemotherapy. Psychooncology. 2009;18(2):187–94. PMCID: PMC2762479. http://www.ncbi.nlm.nih.gov/pubmed/18677716.
163. Giese-Davis J, Collie K, Rancourt KMS, Neri E, Kraemer HC, Spiegel D. Decrease in depression symptoms is associated with longer survival in patients with metastatic breast cancer: a secondary analysis. J Clin Oncol. 2011;29(4):413–20. PMCID: PMC3058287. http://www.ncbi.nlm.nih.gov/pubmed/21149651.
164. Maes M, Meltzer HY, Stevens W, Calabrese J, Cosyns P. Natural killer cell activity in major depression: relation to circulating natural killer cells, cellular indices of the immune response, and depressive phenomenology. Prog Neuro-Psychopharmacol Biol Psychiatry. 1994;18(4):717–30. PMID: 7938562. http://www.ncbi.nlm.nih.gov/pubmed/7938562.
165. Saul AN, Oberyszyn TM, Daugherty C, Kusewitt D, Jones S, Jewell S, Malarkey WB, Lehman A, Lemeshow S, Dhabhar FS. Chronic stress and susceptibility to skin cancer. J Natl Cancer Inst. 2005;97(23):1760–7. PMCID: PMC3422720. http://www.ncbi.nlm.nih.gov/pubmed/16333031.

166. Feng Z, Liu L, Zhang C, Zheng T, Wang J, Lin M, Zhao Y, Wang X, Levine AJ, Hu W. Chronic restraint stress attenuates p53 function and promotes tumorigenesis. Proc Natl Acad Sci USA. 2012;109(18):7013–8. PMCID: PMC3345015. http://www.ncbi.nlm.nih.gov/pubmed/22509031.
167. Massie MJ. Prevalence of depression in patients with cancer. J Natl Cancer Inst Monogr. 2004;(32):57–71. PMID: 15263042. http://www.ncbi.nlm.nih.gov/pubmed/15263042.
168. Pasquini M, Speca A, Mastroeni S, Delle Chiaie R, Sternberg CN, Biondi M. Differences in depressive thoughts between major depressive disorder, IFN-alpha-induced depression, and depressive disorders among cancer patients. J Psychosom Res. 2008;65(2):153–6. https://doi.org/10.1016/j.jpsychores.2008.01.009. PMID: 18655860. http://www.ncbi.nlm.nih.gov/pubmed/18655860.
169. Krebber AMH, Buffart LM, Kleijn G, Riepma IC, de Bree R, Leemans CR, Becker A, Brug J, van Straten A, Cuijpers P, Verdonck-de Leeuw IM. Prevalence of depression in cancer patients: a meta-analysis of diagnostic interviews and self-report instruments. Psychooncology. 2014;23(2):121–30. PMCID: PMC4282549. http://www.ncbi.nlm.nih.gov/pubmed/24105788.
170. Colleoni M, Mandala M, Peruzzotti G, Robertson C, Bredart A, Goldhirsch A. Depression and degree of acceptance of adjuvant cytotoxic drugs. Lancet. 2000;356(9238):1326–7. PMID: 11073026. http://www.ncbi.nlm.nih.gov/pubmed/11073026.
171. Brintzenhofe-Szoc KM, Levin TT, Li Y, Kissane DW, Zabora JR. Mixed anxiety/depression symptoms in a large cancer cohort: prevalence by cancer type. Psychosomatics. 2009;50(4):383–91. PMID: 19687179. http://www.ncbi.nlm.nih.gov/pubmed/19687179.
172. Ciaramella A, Poli P. Assessment of depression among cancer patients: the role of pain, cancer type and treatment. Psychooncology. 2001;10(2):156–65. PMID: 11268142. http://www.ncbi.nlm.nih.gov/pubmed/11268142.
173. Spiegel D, Sands S, Koopman C. Pain and depression in patients with cancer. Cancer. 1994;74(9):2570–8. PMID: 7923013. http://www.ncbi.nlm.nih.gov/pubmed/7923013.
174. Lee SJ, Cartmell KB. Self-reported depression in cancer survivors versus the general population: a population-based propensity score-matching analysis. Qual Life Res. 2020;29(2):483–94. PMID: 31707694. http://www.ncbi.nlm.nih.gov/pubmed/31707694.
175. Zhang Y, Wang Y, Song B, Li H. Patients' self-report anxiety, depression and quality of life and their predictive factors in muscle invasive bladder cancer patients receiving adjuvant chemotherapy. Psychol Health Med. 2020;25(2):190–200. PMID: 31698952. http://www.ncbi.nlm.nih.gov/pubmed/31698952.
176. Bierhaus A, Wolf J, Andrassy M, Rohleder N, Humpert PM, Petrov D, Ferstl R, von Eynatten M, Wendt T, Rudofsky G, Joswig M, Morcos M, Schwaninger M, McEwen B, Kirschbaum C, Nawroth PP. A mechanism converting psychosocial stress into mononuclear cell activation. Proc Natl Acad Sci USA. 2003;100(4):1920–5. PMCID: PMC149934. http://www.ncbi.nlm.nih.gov/pubmed/12578963.
177. Bianchi ME. DAMPs, PAMPs and alarmins: all we need to know about danger. J Leukoc Biol. 2007;81(1):1–5. PMID: 17032697. http://www.ncbi.nlm.nih.gov/pubmed/17032697.
178. Aggarwal BB, Shishodia S, Sandur SK, Pandey MK, Sethi G. Inflammation and cancer: how hot is the link? Biochem Pharmacol. 2006;72(11):1605–21. PMID: 16889756. http://www.ncbi.nlm.nih.gov/pubmed/16889756.
179. Sethi G, Shanmugam MK, Ramachandran L, Kumar AP, Tergaonkar V. Multifaceted link between cancer and inflammation. Biosci Rep. 2012;32(1):1–15. PMID: 21981137. http://www.ncbi.nlm.nih.gov/pubmed/21981137.
180. Lu H, Ouyang W, Huang C. Inflammation, a key event in cancer development. Mol Cancer Res. 2006;4(4):221–33. PMID: 16603636. http://www.ncbi.nlm.nih.gov/pubmed/16603636.
181. Ono M. Molecular links between tumor angiogenesis and inflammation: inflammatory stimuli of macrophages and cancer cells as targets for therapeutic strategy. Cancer Sci. 2008;99(8):1501–6. PMCID: PMC11158258. http://www.ncbi.nlm.nih.gov/pubmed/18754859.
182. Colotta F, Allavena P, Sica A, Garlanda C, Mantovani A. Cancer-related inflammation, the seventh hallmark of cancer: links to genetic instability. Carcinogenesis. 2009;30(7):1073–81. PMID: 19468060. http://www.ncbi.nlm.nih.gov/pubmed/19468060.
183. Raison CL, Capuron L, Miller AH. Cytokines sing the blues: inflammation and the pathogenesis of depression. Trends Immunol. 2006;27(1):24–31. PMCID: PMC3392963. http://www.ncbi.nlm.nih.gov/pubmed/16316783.
184. Zhu CB, Carneiro AM, Dostmann WR, Hewlett WA, Blakely RD. p38 MAPK activation elevates serotonin transport activity via a trafficking-independent, protein phosphatase 2A-dependent process. J Biol Chem. 2005;280(16):15649–58. PMID: 15728187. http://www.ncbi.nlm.nih.gov/pubmed/15728187.
185. DeMyer MK, Shea PA, Hendrie HC, Yoshimura NN. Plasma tryptophan and five other amino acids in depressed and normal subjects. Arch Gen Psychiatry. 1981;38(6):642–6. PMID: 7247626. http://www.ncbi.nlm.nih.gov/pubmed/7247626.
186. Myint AM, Kim YK. Cytokine-serotonin interaction through IDO: a neurodegeneration hypothesis of depression. Med Hypotheses. 2003;61(5–6):519–25. PMID: 14592780. http://www.ncbi.nlm.nih.gov/pubmed/14592780.
187. Felger JC, Li L, Marvar PJ, Woolwine BJ, Harrison DG, Raison CL, Miller AH. Tyrosine metabolism during interferon-alpha administration: association with fatigue and CSF dopamine concentrations. Brain Behav Immun. 2013;31:153–60. PMCID: PMC3578984. http://www.ncbi.nlm.nih.gov/pubmed/23072726.
188. Holsboer F, Ising M. Central CRH system in depression and anxiety—evidence from clinical studies with CRH1 receptor antagonists. Eur J Pharmacol. 2008;583(2–3):350–7. PMID: 18272149. http://www.ncbi.nlm.nih.gov/pubmed/18272149.
189. Duman RS, Monteggia LM. A neurotrophic model for stress-related mood disorders. Biol Psychiatry. 2006;59(12):1116–27. PMID: 16631126. http://www.ncbi.nlm.nih.gov/pubmed/16631126.
190. Bagnall-Moreau C, Chaudhry S, Salas-Ramirez K, Ahles T, Hubbard K. Chemotherapy-induced cognitive impairment is associated with increased inflammation and oxidative damage in the hippocampus. Mol Neurobiol. 2019;56(10):7159–72. PMCID: PMC6728167. http://www.ncbi.nlm.nih.gov/pubmed/30989632.
191. Gottschalk LA, Holcombe RF, Jackson D, Bechtel RJ. The effects of anticancer chemotherapeutic drugs on cognitive function and other neuropsychiatric dimensions in breast cancer patients. Methods Find Exp Clin Pharmacol. 2003;25(2):117–22. PMID: 12731457. http://www.ncbi.nlm.nih.gov/pubmed/12731457.
192. Wefel JS, Schagen SB. Chemotherapy-related cognitive dysfunction. Curr Neurol Neurosci Rep. 2012;12(3):267–75. PMID: 22453825. http://www.ncbi.nlm.nih.gov/pubmed/22453825.
193. Raffa RB. Imaging as a means of studying chemotherapy-related cognitive impairment. Adv Exp Med Biol. 2010;678:70–6. PMID: 20738008. http://www.ncbi.nlm.nih.gov/pubmed/20738008.
194. Scherling CS, Smith A. Opening up the window into "chemobrain": a neuroimaging review. Sensors (Basel). 2013;13(3):3169–203. PMCID: PMC3658739. http://www.ncbi.nlm.nih.gov/pubmed/23467031.
195. López Zunini RA, Scherling C, Wallis N, Collins B, MacKenzie J, Bielajew C, Smith AM. Differences in verbal memory retrieval in breast cancer chemotherapy patients compared to healthy controls: a prospective fMRI study. Brain Imaging Behav.

2013;7(4):460–77. PMID: 23242968. http://www.ncbi.nlm.nih.gov/pubmed/23242968.
196. Pace TWW, Hu F, Miller AH. Cytokine-effects on glucocorticoid receptor function: relevance to glucocorticoid resistance and the pathophysiology and treatment of major depression. Brain Behav Immun. 2007;21(1):9–19. PMCID: PMC1820632. http://www.ncbi.nlm.nih.gov/pubmed/17070667.
197. Pavlov VA, Tracey KJ. The cholinergic anti-inflammatory pathway. Brain Behav Immun. 2005;19(6):493–9. PMID: 15922555. http://www.ncbi.nlm.nih.gov/pubmed/15922555.
198. Besedovsky HO, del Rey A. Immune-neuro-endocrine interactions: facts and hypotheses. Endocr Rev. 1996;17(1):64–102. PMID: 8641224. http://www.ncbi.nlm.nih.gov/pubmed/8641224.
199. Wang X, Wu H, Miller AH. Interleukin 1alpha (IL-1alpha) induced activation of p38 mitogen-activated protein kinase inhibits glucocorticoid receptor function. Mol Psychiatry. 2004;9(1):65–75. PMID: 14699442. http://www.ncbi.nlm.nih.gov/pubmed/14699442.
200. Raison CL, Miller AH. When not enough is too much: the role of insufficient glucocorticoid signaling in the pathophysiology of stress-related disorders. Am J Psychiatry. 2003;160(9):1554–65. PMID: 12944327. http://www.ncbi.nlm.nih.gov/pubmed/12944327.
201. Huang T, Zhou F, Wang-Johanning F, Nan K, Wei Y. Depression accelerates the development of gastric cancer through reactive oxygen species-activated ABL1 (review). Oncol Rep. 2016;36(5):2435–43. PMID: 27666407. http://www.ncbi.nlm.nih.gov/pubmed/27666407.
202. Moynihan JA. Mechanisms of stress-induced modulation of immunity. Brain Behav Immun. 2003;17(Suppl 1):S11–6. PMID: 12615181. http://www.ncbi.nlm.nih.gov/pubmed/12615181.
203. Lutgendorf SK, Lamkin DM, DeGeest K, Anderson B, Dao M, McGinn S, Zimmerman B, Maiseri H, Sood AK, Lubaroff DM. Depressed and anxious mood and T-cell cytokine expressing populations in ovarian cancer patients. Brain Behav Immun. 2008;22(6):890–900. PMCID: PMC2605940. http://www.ncbi.nlm.nih.gov/pubmed/18276105.
204. Hassan S, Karpova Y, Baiz D, Yancey D, Pullikuth A, Flores A, Register T, Cline JM, D'Agostino R, Danial N, Datta SR, Kulik G. Behavioral stress accelerates prostate cancer development in mice. J Clin Invest. 2013;123(2):874–86. PMCID: PMC3561807. http://www.ncbi.nlm.nih.gov/pubmed/23348742.
205. Sun X, Bao J, Nelson KC, Li KC, Kulik G, Zhou X. Systems modeling of anti-apoptotic pathways in prostate cancer: psychological stress triggers a synergism pattern switch in drug combination therapy. PLoS Comput Biol. 2013;9(12):e1003358. PMCID: PMC3854132. http://www.ncbi.nlm.nih.gov/pubmed/24339759.
206. Penninx BW, Guralnik JM, Pahor M, Ferrucci L, Cerhan JR, Wallace RB, Havlik RJ. Chronically depressed mood and cancer risk in older persons. J Natl Cancer Inst. 1998;90(24):1888–93. PMID: 9862626. http://www.ncbi.nlm.nih.gov/pubmed/9862626.
207. Belizário JE, Brandão W, Rossato C, Peron JP. Thymic and post-thymic regulation of Naïve CD4(+) T-Cell lineage fates in humans and Mice Models. Mediators Inflamm. 2016;2016:9523628. PMCID: PMC4904118. http://www.ncbi.nlm.nih.gov/pubmed/27313405.
208. National Health and Nutrition Examination Survey | National Health and Nutrition Examination Survey | CDC.
209. Hales CM, Fryar CD, Carroll MD, Freedman DS, Ogden CL. Trends in obesity and severe obesity prevalence in US youth and adults by sex and age, 2007-2008 to 2015-2016. JAMA. 2018;319(16):1723–5. PMCID: PMC5876828. http://www.ncbi.nlm.nih.gov/pubmed/29570750.
210. Members and partners | OECD.
211. GBD 2017 Risk Factor Collaborators. Global, regional, and national comparative risk assessment of 84 behavioural, environmental and occupational, and metabolic risks or clusters of risks for 195 countries and territories, 1990–2017: a systematic analysis for the Global Burden of Disease Study 2017. Lancet. 2018;392(10159):1923–94. PMCID: PMC6227755. http://www.ncbi.nlm.nih.gov/pubmed/30496105.
212. NCD Risk Factor Collaboration (NCD-RisC). Worldwide trends in underweight and obesity from 1990 to 2022: a pooled analysis of 3663 population-representative studies with 222 million children, adolescents, and adults. Lancet. 2024;403(10431):1027–50. PMCID: PMC7615769. http://www.ncbi.nlm.nih.gov/pubmed/38432237.
213. Abelson P, Kennedy D. The obesity epidemic. Science. 2004;304(5676):1413. PMID: 15178768. http://www.ncbi.nlm.nih.gov/pubmed/15178768.
214. Jaacks LM, Vandevijvere S, Pan A, McGowan CJ, Wallace C, Imamura F, Mozaffarian D, Swinburn B, Ezzati M. The obesity transition: stages of the global epidemic. Lancet Diabetes Endocrinol. 2019;7(3):231–40. PMCID: PMC7360432. http://www.ncbi.nlm.nih.gov/pubmed/30704950.
215. Blüher M. Obesity: global epidemiology and pathogenesis. Nat Rev Endocrinol. 2019;15(5):288–98. PMID: 30814686. http://www.ncbi.nlm.nih.gov/pubmed/30814686.
216. Adams KF, Schatzkin A, Harris TB, Kipnis V, Mouw T, Ballard-Barbash R, Hollenbeck A, Leitzmann MF. Overweight, obesity, and mortality in a large prospective cohort of persons 50 to 71 years old. N Engl J Med. 2006;355(8):763–78. PMID: 16926275. http://www.ncbi.nlm.nih.gov/pubmed/16926275.
217. Flegal KM, Graubard BI, Williamson DF, Gail MH. Excess deaths associated with underweight, overweight, and obesity. JAMA. 2005;293(15):1861–7. PMID: 15840860. http://www.ncbi.nlm.nih.gov/pubmed/15840860.
218. GBD 2021 US Obesity Forecasting Collaborators. National-level and state-level prevalence of overweight and obesity among children, adolescents, and adults in the USA, 1990–2021 and forecasts up to 2050. Lancet. 2024;404(10469):2278–98. PMID: 39551059. http://www.ncbi.nlm.nih.gov/pubmed/39551059.
219. Cole TJ, Lobstein T. Extended international (IOTF) body mass index cut-offs for thinness, overweight and obesity. Pediatr Obes. 2012;7(4):284–94. PMID: 22715120. http://www.ncbi.nlm.nih.gov/pubmed/22715120.
220. Swinburn B, Sacks G, Ravussin E. Increased food energy supply is more than sufficient to explain the US epidemic of obesity. Am J Clin Nutr. 2009;90(6):1453–6. PMID: 19828708. http://www.ncbi.nlm.nih.gov/pubmed/19828708.
221. Bray GA, Kim KK, Wilding JPH, World Obesity Federation. Obesity: a chronic relapsing progressive disease process. A position statement of the World Obesity Federation. Obes Rev. 2017;18(7):715–23. PMID: 28489290. http://www.ncbi.nlm.nih.gov/pubmed/28489290.
222. Norris SA, Frongillo EA, Black MM, Dong Y, Fall C, Lampl M, Liese AD, Naguib M, Prentice A, Rochat T, Stephensen CB, Tinago CB, Ward KA, Wrottesley SV, Patton GC. Nutrition in adolescent growth and development. Lancet. 2022;399(10320):172–84. PMID: 34856190. http://www.ncbi.nlm.nih.gov/pubmed/34856190.
223. Swinburn BA, Sacks G, Hall KD, McPherson K, Finegood DT, Moodie ML, Gortmaker SL. The global obesity pandemic: shaped by global drivers and local environments. Lancet. 2011;378(9793):804–14. PMID: 21872749. http://www.ncbi.nlm.nih.gov/pubmed/21872749.
224. Buse K, Tanaka S, Hawkes S. Healthy people and healthy profits? Elaborating a conceptual framework for governing the commercial determinants of non-communicable diseases and identifying options for reducing risk exposure. Glob Health. 2017;13(1):34. PMCID: PMC5472958. http://www.ncbi.nlm.nih.gov/pubmed/28619031.

225. Bell CN, Kerr J, Young JL. Associations between obesity, obesogenic environments, and structural racism vary by county-level racial composition. Int J Environ Res Public Health. 2019;16(5):861. PMCID: PMC6427384. http://www.ncbi.nlm.nih.gov/pubmed/30857286.
226. Gartner DR, Taber DR, Hirsch JA, Robinson WR. The spatial distribution of gender differences in obesity prevalence differs from overall obesity prevalence among US adults. Ann Epidemiol. 2016;26(4):293–8. PMCID: PMC4901384. http://www.ncbi.nlm.nih.gov/pubmed/27039046.
227. Stuckler D, Nestle M. Big food, food systems, and global health. PLoS Med. 2012;9(6):e1001242. PMCID: PMC3378592. http://www.ncbi.nlm.nih.gov/pubmed/22723746.
228. Swinburn BA, Kraak VI, Allender S, Atkins VJ, Baker PI, Bogard JR, Brinsden H, Calvillo A, De Schutter O, Devarajan R, Ezzati M, Friel S, Goenka S, Hammond RA, Hastings G, Hawkes C, Herrero M, Hovmand PS, Howden M, Jaacks LM, Kapetanaki AB, Kasman M, Kuhnlein HV, Kumanyika SK, Larijani B, Lobstein T, Long MW, Matsudo VKR, Mills SDH, Morgan G, Morshed A, Nece PM, Pan A, Patterson DW, Sacks G, Shekar M, Simmons GL, Smit W, Tootee A, Vandevijvere S, Waterlander WE, Wolfenden L, Dietz WH. The global syndemic of obesity, undernutrition, and climate change: the Lancet Commission report. Lancet. 2019;393(10173):791–846. PMID: 30700377. http://www.ncbi.nlm.nih.gov/pubmed/30700377.
229. Symposium on Lipid Abnormalities in Renal Diseases. Sardinia, Italy, 1990. Kidney Int Suppl. 1991;31:S1–72. PMID: 2046264. http://www.ncbi.nlm.nih.gov/pubmed/2046264.
230. Dawes AJ, Maggard-Gibbons M, Maher AR, Booth MJ, Miake-Lye I, Beroes JM, Shekelle PG. Mental health conditions among patients seeking and undergoing bariatric surgery: a meta-analysis. JAMA. 2016;315(2):150–63. PMID: 26757464. http://www.ncbi.nlm.nih.gov/pubmed/26757464.
231. Osterhues A, von Lengerke T, Mall JW, de Zwaan M, Müller A. Health-related quality of life, anxiety, and depression in bariatric surgery candidates compared to patients from a psychosomatic inpatient hospital. Obes Surg. 2017;27(9):2378–87. PMID: 28285469. http://www.ncbi.nlm.nih.gov/pubmed/28285469.
232. Kost C, Jamie K, Mohr E. "Whatever I said didn't register with her": medical fatphobia and interactional and relational disconnect in healthcare encounters. Front Sociol. 2024;9:1303919. PMCID: PMC10996856. http://www.ncbi.nlm.nih.gov/pubmed/38586083.
233. Garvey WT, Mechanick JI, Brett EM, Garber AJ, Hurley DL, Jastreboff AM, Nadolsky K, Pessah-Pollack R, Plodkowski R. Reviewers of the AACE/ACE Obesity Clinical Practice Guidelines. American Association of Clinical Endocrinologists and American College of endocrinology comprehensive clinical practice guidelines for medical care of patients with obesity. Endocr Pract. 2016;22 Suppl 3:1–203. PMID: 27219496. http://www.ncbi.nlm.nih.gov/pubmed/27219496.
234. Jensen MD, Ryan DH, Apovian CM, Ard JD, Comuzzie AG, Donato KA, Hu FB, Hubbard VS, Jakicic JM, Kushner RF, Loria CM, Millen BE, Nonas CA, Pi-Sunyer FX, Stevens J, Stevens VJ, Wadden TA, Wolfe BM, Yanovski SZ, Jordan HS, Kendall KA, Lux LJ, Mentor-Marcel R, Morgan LC, Trisolini MG, Wnek J, Anderson JL, Halperin JL, Albert NM, Bozkurt B, Brindis RG, Curtis LH, DeMets D, Hochman JS, Kovacs RJ, Ohman EM, Pressler SJ, Sellke FW, Shen WK, Smith SC, Tomaselli GF. American College of Cardiology/American Heart Association Task Force on Practice Guidelines, Obesity Society. 2013 AHA/ACC/TOS guideline for the management of overweight and obesity in adults: a report of the American College of Cardiology/American Heart Association Task Force on Practice Guidelines and The Obesity Society. Circulation. 2014;129(25 Suppl 2):S102–38. PMCID: PMC5819889. http://www.ncbi.nlm.nih.gov/pubmed/24222017.
235. Graham Y, Hayes C, Cox J, Mahawar K, Fox A, Yemm H. A systematic review of obesity as a barrier to accessing cancer screening services. Obes Sci Pract. 2022;8(6):715–27. PMCID: PMC9722456. http://www.ncbi.nlm.nih.gov/pubmed/36483123.
236. Paterson NE, Markou A. Animal models and treatments for addiction and depression co-morbidity. Neurotox Res. 2007;11(1):1–32. PMID: 17449445. http://www.ncbi.nlm.nih.gov/pubmed/17449445.
237. Flórez KR, Dubowitz T, Ghosh-Dastidar MB, Beckman R, Collins RL. Associations between depressive symptomatology, diet, and body mass index among participants in the supplemental nutrition assistance program. J Acad Nutr Diet. 2015;115(7):1102–8. PMCID: PMC4484316. http://www.ncbi.nlm.nih.gov/pubmed/25769748.
238. Lalanne L, Ayranci G, Kieffer BL, Lutz PE. The kappa opioid receptor: from addiction to depression, and back. Front. Psychiatry. 2014;5:170. PMCID: PMC4258993. http://www.ncbi.nlm.nih.gov/pubmed/25538632.
239. Treadway MT, Zald DH. Reconsidering anhedonia in depression: lessons from translational neuroscience. Neurosci Biobehav Rev. 2011;35(3):537–55. PMCID: PMC3005986. http://www.ncbi.nlm.nih.gov/pubmed/20603146.
240. Mineur YS, Picciotto MR. Biological basis for the comorbidity between smoking and mood disorders. J Dual Diagn. 2009;5(2):122–30. PMCID: PMC2707026. http://www.ncbi.nlm.nih.gov/pubmed/20046987.
241. Filip M, Frankowska M, Jastrzębska J, Wydra K, Przegaliński E. Preclinical studies on comorbidity between depression and psychostimulant addiction. Pharmacol Rep. 2013;65(6):1529–34. PMID: 24553001. http://www.ncbi.nlm.nih.gov/pubmed/24553001.
242. Slavich GM, Irwin MR. From stress to inflammation and major depressive disorder: a social signal transduction theory of depression. Psychol Bull. 2014;140(3):774–815. PMCID: PMC4006295. http://www.ncbi.nlm.nih.gov/pubmed/24417575.
243. Preiss K, Brennan L, Clarke D. A systematic review of variables associated with the relationship between obesity and depression. Obes Rev. 2013;14(11):906–18. PMID: 23809142. http://www.ncbi.nlm.nih.gov/pubmed/23809142.
244. Arterburn D, Westbrook EO, Ludman EJ, Operskalski B, Linde JA, Rohde P, Jeffery RW, Simon GE. Relationship between obesity, depression, and disability in middle-aged women. Obes Res Clin Pract. 2012;6(3):e197–206. PMCID: PMC3418708. http://www.ncbi.nlm.nih.gov/pubmed/22905068.
245. Mazzeschi C, Pazzagli C, Buratta L, Reboldi GP, Battistini D, Piana N, Pippi R, Fatone C, De Feo P. Mutual interactions between depression/quality of life and adherence to a multidisciplinary lifestyle intervention in obesity. J Clin Endocrinol Metab. 2012;97(12):E2261–5. PMID: 23007686. http://www.ncbi.nlm.nih.gov/pubmed/23007686.
246. Dave DM, Tennant J, Colman G. Isolating the effect of major depression on obesity: role of selection bias. J Ment Health Policy Econ. 2011;14(4):165–86. PMID: 22345359. http://www.ncbi.nlm.nih.gov/pubmed/22345359.
247. Boden JM, Fergusson DM. Alcohol and depression. Addiction. 2011;106(5):906–14. PMID: 21382111. http://www.ncbi.nlm.nih.gov/pubmed/21382111.
248. Park S, Romer D. Associations between smoking and depression in adolescence: an integrative review. Taehan Kanho Hakhoe Chi. 2007;37(2):227–41. PMID: 17435408. http://www.ncbi.nlm.nih.gov/pubmed/17435408.
249. Chaiton MO, Cohen JE, O'Loughlin J, Rehm J. A systematic review of longitudinal studies on the association between depression and smoking in adolescents. BMC Public Health. 2009;9:356. PMCID: PMC2758872. http://www.ncbi.nlm.nih.gov/pubmed/19772635.

250. Paperwalla KN, Levin TT, Weiner J, Saravay SM. Smoking and depression. Med Clin North Am. 2004;88(6):1483–1494, x–xi. PMID: 15464109. http://www.ncbi.nlm.nih.gov/pubmed/15464109.
251. Simon NM. Generalized anxiety disorder and psychiatric comorbidities such as depression, bipolar disorder, and substance abuse. J Clin Psychiatry. 2009;70(Suppl 2):10–4. PMID: 19371501. http://www.ncbi.nlm.nih.gov/pubmed/19371501.
252. Gilman SE, Trinh NH, Smoller JW, Fava M, Murphy JM, Breslau J. Psychosocial stressors and the prognosis of major depression: a test of Axis IV. Psychol Med. 2013;43(2):303–16. PMCID: PMC3721739. http://www.ncbi.nlm.nih.gov/pubmed/22640506.
253. Sagar R, Gupta T. Psychological aspects of obesity in children and adolescents. Indian J Pediatr. 2018;85(7):554–9. PMID: 29150753. http://www.ncbi.nlm.nih.gov/pubmed/29150753.
254. Yazdani N, Hosseini SV, Amini M, Sobhani Z, Sharif F, Khazraei H. Relationship between body image and psychological well-being in patients with morbid obesity. Int J Commun Based Nurs Midwifery. 2018;6(2):175–84. PMCID: PMC5845121. http://www.ncbi.nlm.nih.gov/pubmed/29607346.
255. Levitan RD, Davis C, Kaplan AS, Arenovich T, Phillips DIW, Ravindran AV. Obesity comorbidity in unipolar major depressive disorder: refining the core phenotype. J Clin Psychiatry. 2012;73(8):1119–24. PMID: 22687640. http://www.ncbi.nlm.nih.gov/pubmed/22687640.
256. Chou KL, Yu KM. Atypical depressive symptoms and obesity in a national sample of older adults with major depressive disorder. Depress Anxiety. 2013;30(6):574–9. PMID: 23554014. http://www.ncbi.nlm.nih.gov/pubmed/23554014.
257. Omran AR. The epidemiologic transition. A theory of the epidemiology of population change. Milbank Mem Fund Q. 1971;49(4):509–38. PMID: 5155251. http://www.ncbi.nlm.nih.gov/pubmed/5155251.
258. Popkin BM. Nutritional patterns and transitions. Population and development review, 138–157, 1993. (PDF) Nutritional Patterns and Transitions.
259. Popkin BM, Ng SW. The nutrition transition to a stage of high obesity and noncommunicable disease prevalence dominated by ultra-processed foods is not inevitable. Obes Rev. 2022;23(1):e13366. PMCID: PMC8639733. http://www.ncbi.nlm.nih.gov/pubmed/34632692.
260. Roberto CA, Swinburn B, Hawkes C, Huang TTK, Costa SA, Ashe M, Zwicker L, Cawley JH, Brownell KD. Patchy progress on obesity prevention: emerging examples, entrenched barriers, and new thinking. Lancet. 2015;385(9985):2400–9. PMID: 25703111. http://www.ncbi.nlm.nih.gov/pubmed/25703111.
261. Noncommunicable diseases: Risk factors and conditions.
262. GBD 2015 Obesity Collaborators, Afshin A, Forouzanfar MH, Reitsma MB, Sur P, Estep K, Lee A, Marczak L, Mokdad AH, Moradi-Lakeh M, Naghavi M, Salama JS, Vos T, Abate KH, Abbafati C, Ahmed MB, Al-Aly Z, Alkerwi A, Al-Raddadi R, Amare AT, Amberbir A, Amegah AK, Amini E, Amrock SM, Anjana RM, Ärnlöv J, Asayesh H, Banerjee A, Barac A, Baye E, Bennett DA, Beyene AS, Biadgilign S, Biryukov S, Bjertness E, Boneya DJ, Campos-Nonato I, Carrero JJ, Cecilio P, Cercy K, Ciobanu LG, Cornaby L, Damtew SA, Dandona L, Dandona R, Dharmaratne SD, Duncan BB, Eshrati B, Esteghamati A, Feigin VL, Fernandes JC, Fürst T, Gebrehiwot TT, Gold A, Gona PN, Goto A, Habtewold TD, Hadush KT, Hafezi-Nejad N, Hay SI, Horino M, Islami F, Kamal R, Kasaeian A, Katikireddi SV, Kengne AP, Kesavachandran CN, Khader YS, Khang YH, Khubchandani J, Kim D, Kim YJ, Kinfu Y, Kosen S, Ku T, Defo BK, Kumar GA, Larson HJ, Leinsalu M, Liang X, Lim SS, Liu P, Lopez AD, Lozano R, Majeed A, Malekzadeh R, Malta DC, Mazidi M, McAlinden C, McGarvey ST, Mengistu DT, Mensah GA, Mensink GBM, Mezgebe HB, Mirrakhimov EM, Mueller UO, Noubiap JJ, Obermeyer CM, Ogbo FA, Owolabi MO, Patton GC, Pourmalek F, Qorbani M, Rafay A, Rai RK, Ranabhat CL, Reinig N, Safiri S, Salomon JA, Sanabria JR, Santos IS, Sartorius B, Sawhney M, Schmidhuber J, Schutte AE, Schmidt MI, Sepanlou SG, Shamsizadeh M, Sheikhbahaei S, Shin MJ, Shiri R, Shiue I, Roba HS, Silva DAS, Silverberg JI, Singh JA, Stranges S, Swaminathan S, Tabarés-Seisdedos R, Tadese F, Tedla BA, Tegegne BS, Terkawi AS, Thakur JS, Tonelli M, Topor-Madry R, Tyrovolas S, Ukwaja KN, Uthman OA, Vaezghasemi M, Vasankari T, Vlassov VV, Vollset SE, Weiderpass E, Werdecker A, Wesana J, Westerman R, Yano Y, Yonemoto N, Yonga G, Zaidi Z, Zenebe ZM, Zipkin B, Murray CJL. Health effects of overweight and obesity in 195 countries over 25 years. N Engl J Med. 2017;377(1):13–27. PMCID: PMC5477817. http://www.ncbi.nlm.nih.gov/pubmed/28604169.
263. Albrecht U. The circadian clock, metabolism and obesity. Obes Rev. 2017;18(Suppl 1):25–33. PMID: 28164453. http://www.ncbi.nlm.nih.gov/pubmed/28164453.
264. Shannon J, Kristal AR, Curry SJ, Beresford SA. Application of a behavioral approach to measuring dietary change: the fat- and fiber-related diet behavior questionnaire. Cancer Epidemiol Biomarkers Prev. 1997;6(5):355–61. PMID: 9149896. http://www.ncbi.nlm.nih.gov/pubmed/9149896.
265. Kristal AR, Shattuck AL, Henry HJ. Patterns of dietary behavior associated with selecting diets low in fat: reliability and validity of a behavioral approach to dietary assessment. J Am Diet Assoc. 1990;90(2):214–20. PMID: 2303658. http://www.ncbi.nlm.nih.gov/pubmed/2303658.
266. Kannel WB, Sorlie P. Some health benefits of physical activity. The Framingham study. Arch Intern Med. 1979;139(8):857–61. PMID: 464698. http://www.ncbi.nlm.nih.gov/pubmed/464698.
267. 2017 Global Nutrition Report - Global Nutrition Report.
268. (PDF) United States Dietary Trends Since 1800: Lack of Association Between Saturated Fatty Acid Consumption and Non-communicable Diseases.
269. Schmid A. The role of meat fat in the human diet. Crit Rev Food Sci Nutr. 2011;51(1):50–66. PMID: 21229418. http://www.ncbi.nlm.nih.gov/pubmed/21229418.
270. Ramos-Lopez O, Milagro FI, Allayee H, Chmurzynska A, Choi MS, Curi R, De Caterina R, Ferguson LR, Goni L, Kang JX, Kohlmeier M, Marti A, Moreno LA, Pérusse L, Prasad C, Qi L, Reifen R, Riezu-Boj JI, San-Cristobal R, Santos JL, Martínez JA. Guide for current nutrigenetic, nutrigenomic, and nutriepigenetic approaches for precision nutrition involving the prevention and management of chronic diseases associated with obesity. J Nutrigenet Nutrigenomics. 2017;10(1–2):43–62. PMID: 28689206. http://www.ncbi.nlm.nih.gov/pubmed/28689206.
271. Hammerton G, Thapar A, Thapar AK. Association between obesity and depressive disorder in adolescents at high risk for depression. Int J Obes. 2014;38(4):513–9. PMID: 23887062. http://www.ncbi.nlm.nih.gov/pubmed/23887062.
272. Sharma S, Fulton S. Diet-induced obesity promotes depressive-like behaviour that is associated with neural adaptations in brain reward circuitry. Int J Obes. 2013;37(3):382–9. PMID: 22508336. http://www.ncbi.nlm.nih.gov/pubmed/22508336.
273. Hariri N, Thibault L. High-fat diet-induced obesity in animal models. Nutr Res Rev. 2010;23(2):270–99. PMID: 20977819. http://www.ncbi.nlm.nih.gov/pubmed/20977819.
274. Dirkx E, Schwenk RW, Glatz JFC, Luiken JJFP, van Eys GJJM. High fat diet induced diabetic cardiomyopathy. Prostaglandins Leukot Essent Fatty Acids. 2011;85(5):219–25. PMID: 21571515. http://www.ncbi.nlm.nih.gov/pubmed/21571515.
275. Coelho DF, Pereira-Lancha LO, Chaves DS, Diwan D, Ferraz R, Campos-Ferraz PL, Poortmans JR, Lancha Junior AH. Effect of

high-fat diets on body composition, lipid metabolism and insulin sensitivity, and the role of exercise on these parameters. Braz J Med Biol Res. 2011;44(10):966–72. PMID: 21876873. http://www.ncbi.nlm.nih.gov/pubmed/21876873.
276. Eckel-Mahan KL, Patel VR, de Mateo S, Orozco-Solis R, Ceglia NJ, Sahar S, Dilag-Penilla SA, Dyar KA, Baldi P, Sassone-Corsi P. Reprogramming of the circadian clock by nutritional challenge. Cell. 2013;155(7):1464–78. PMCID: PMC4573395. http://www.ncbi.nlm.nih.gov/pubmed/24360271.
277. Sebti Y, Hebras A, Pourcet B, Staels B, Duez H. The Circadian clock and obesity. Handb Exp Pharmacol. 2022;274:29–56. PMID: 35112237. http://www.ncbi.nlm.nih.gov/pubmed/35112237.
278. Lai JS, Hiles S, Bisquera A, Hure AJ, McEvoy M, Attia J. A systematic review and meta-analysis of dietary patterns and depression in community-dwelling adults. Am J Clin Nutr. 2014;99(1):181–97. PMID: 24196402. http://www.ncbi.nlm.nih.gov/pubmed/24196402.
279. Jacka FN, O'Neil A, Opie R, Itsiopoulos C, Cotton S, Mohebbi M, Castle D, Dash S, Mihalopoulos C, Chatterton ML, Brazionis L, Dean OM, Hodge AM, Berk M. Correction to: a randomised controlled trial of dietary improvement for adults with major depression (the "SMILES" trial). BMC Med. 2018;16(1):236. PMCID: PMC6309070. http://www.ncbi.nlm.nih.gov/pubmed/30591046.
280. Li Y, Lv MR, Wei YJ, Sun L, Zhang JX, Zhang HG, Li B. Dietary patterns and depression risk: a meta-analysis. Psychiatry Res. 2017;253:373–82. PMID: 28431261. http://www.ncbi.nlm.nih.gov/pubmed/28431261.
281. Jacka FN, O'Neil A, Opie R, Itsiopoulos C, Cotton S, Mohebbi M, Castle D, Dash S, Mihalopoulos C, Chatterton ML, Brazionis L, Dean OM, Hodge AM, Berk M. A randomised controlled trial of dietary improvement for adults with major depression (the "SMILES" trial). BMC Med. 2017;15(1):23. PMCID: PMC5282719. http://www.ncbi.nlm.nih.gov/pubmed/28137247.
282. The effects of dietary improvement on symptoms of depression and anxiety: a meta-analysis of randomized controlled trials: erratum. Psychosom Med. 2020;82(5):536. PMCID: PMC7515462. http://www.ncbi.nlm.nih.gov/pubmed/32310838.
283. Francis HM, Stevenson RJ, Chambers JR, Gupta D, Newey B, Lim CK. A brief diet intervention can reduce symptoms of depression in young adults - a randomised controlled trial. PLoS One. 2019;14(10):e0222768. PMCID: PMC6784975. http://www.ncbi.nlm.nih.gov/pubmed/31596866.
284. McMillen IC, Robinson JS. Developmental origins of the metabolic syndrome: prediction, plasticity, and programming. Physiol Rev. 2005;85(2):571–633. PMID: 15788706. http://www.ncbi.nlm.nih.gov/pubmed/15788706.
285. Simmons R. Epigenetics and maternal nutrition: nature v. nurture. Proc Nutr Soc. 2011;70(1):73–81. PMID: 21110912. http://www.ncbi.nlm.nih.gov/pubmed/21110912.
286. Dominguez-Salas P, Cox SE, Prentice AM, Hennig BJ, Moore SE. Maternal nutritional status, C(1) metabolism and offspring DNA methylation: a review of current evidence in human subjects. Proc Nutr Soc. 2012;71(1):154–65. PMCID: PMC3491641. http://www.ncbi.nlm.nih.gov/pubmed/22124338.
287. Chmurzynska A. Fetal programming: link between early nutrition, DNA methylation, and complex diseases. Nutr Rev. 2010;68(2):87–98. PMID: 20137054. http://www.ncbi.nlm.nih.gov/pubmed/20137054.
288. Li M, Sloboda DM, Vickers MH. Maternal obesity and developmental programming of metabolic disorders in offspring: evidence from animal models. Exp Diabetes Res. 2011;2011:592408. PMCID: PMC3182397. http://www.ncbi.nlm.nih.gov/pubmed/21969822.
289. Weng TT, Hao JH, Qian QW, Cao H, Fu JL, Sun Y, Huang L, Tao FB. Is there any relationship between dietary patterns and depression and anxiety in Chinese adolescents? Public Health Nutr. 2012;15(4):673–82. PMID: 22115495. http://www.ncbi.nlm.nih.gov/pubmed/22115495.
290. Jacka FN, Kremer PJ, Berk M, de Silva-Sanigorski AM, Moodie M, Leslie ER, Pasco JA, Swinburn BA. A prospective study of diet quality and mental health in adolescents. PLoS One. 2011;6(9):e24805. PMCID: PMC3177848. http://www.ncbi.nlm.nih.gov/pubmed/21957462.
291. Oddy WH, Robinson M, Ambrosini GL, O'Sullivan TA, de Klerk NH, Beilin LJ, Silburn SR, Zubrick SR, Stanley FJ. The association between dietary patterns and mental health in early adolescence. Prev Med. 2009;49(1):39–44. PMID: 19467256. http://www.ncbi.nlm.nih.gov/pubmed/19467256.
292. Jacka FN, Kremer PJ, Leslie ER, Berk M, Patton GC, Toumbourou JW, Williams JW. Associations between diet quality and depressed mood in adolescents: results from the Australian Healthy Neighbourhoods Study. Aust N Z J Psychiatry. 2010;44(5):435–42. PMID: 20397785. http://www.ncbi.nlm.nih.gov/pubmed/20397785.
293. Hill JJ. Obesity: an emerging threat. J Natl Black Nurses Assoc. 2018;29(2):36–9. PMID: 31022338. http://www.ncbi.nlm.nih.gov/pubmed/31022338.
294. Smith BM, Criminisi A, Sorek N, Harari Y, Sood N, Heymsfield SB. Modeling health risks using neural network ensembles. PLoS One. 2024;19(10):e0308922. PMCID: PMC11463747. http://www.ncbi.nlm.nih.gov/pubmed/39383158.
295. Must A, Spadano J, Coakley EH, Field AE, Colditz G, Dietz WH. The disease burden associated with overweight and obesity. JAMA. 1999;282(16):1523–9. PMID: 10546691. http://www.ncbi.nlm.nih.gov/pubmed/10546691.
296. Safaei M, Sundararajan EA, Driss M, Boulila W, Shapi'i A. A systematic literature review on obesity: understanding the causes & consequences of obesity and reviewing various machine learning approaches used to predict obesity. Comput Biol Med. 2021;136:104754. PMID: 34426171. http://www.ncbi.nlm.nih.gov/pubmed/34426171.
297. Wu YK, Berry DC. Impact of weight stigma on physiological and psychological health outcomes for overweight and obese adults: a systematic review. J Adv Nurs. 2018;74(5):1030–42. PMID: 29171076. http://www.ncbi.nlm.nih.gov/pubmed/29171076.
298. Alfaris N, Alqahtani AM, Alamuddin N, Rigas G. Global impact of obesity. Gastroenterol Clin N Am. 2023;52(2):277–93. PMID: 37197873. http://www.ncbi.nlm.nih.gov/pubmed/37197873.
299. Merrell J, Lavery M, Ashton K, Heinberg L. Depression and infertility in women seeking bariatric surgery. Surg Obes Relat Dis. 2014;10(1):132–7. PMID: 24507079. http://www.ncbi.nlm.nih.gov/pubmed/24507079.
300. Avila C, Holloway AC, Hahn MK, Morrison KM, Restivo M, Anglin R, Taylor VH. An overview of links between obesity and mental health. Curr Obes Rep. 2015;4(3):303–10. PMID: 26627487. http://www.ncbi.nlm.nih.gov/pubmed/26627487.
301. Steptoe A, Frank P. Obesity and psychological distress. Philos Trans R Soc Lond Ser B Biol Sci. 1888;2023(378):20220225. PMCID: PMC10475872. http://www.ncbi.nlm.nih.gov/pubmed/37661745.
302. Lin HY, Huang CK, Tai CM, Lin HY, Kao YH, Tsai CC, Hsuan CF, Lee SL, Chi SC, Yen YC. Psychiatric disorders of patients seeking obesity treatment. BMC Psychiatry. 2013;13:1. PMCID: PMC3543713. http://www.ncbi.nlm.nih.gov/pubmed/23281653.
303. Riaz H, Khan MS, Siddiqi TJ, Usman MS, Shah N, Goyal A, Khan SS, Mookadam F, Krasuski RA, Ahmed H. Association between obesity and cardiovascular outcomes: a systematic review and meta-analysis of mendelian randomization studies. JAMA Netw Open. 2018;1(7):e183788. PMCID: PMC6324374. http://www.ncbi.nlm.nih.gov/pubmed/30646365.
304. Tompkins J, Bosch PR, Chenowith R, Tiede JL, Swain JM. Changes in functional walking distance and health-

related quality of life after gastric bypass surgery. Phys Ther. 2008;88(8):928–35. PMID: 18583427. http://www.ncbi.nlm.nih.gov/pubmed/18583427.
305. Josbeno DA, Jakicic JM, Hergenroeder A, Eid GM. Physical activity and physical function changes in obese individuals after gastric bypass surgery. Surg Obes Relat Dis. 2010;6(4):361–6. PMID: 18996771. http://www.ncbi.nlm.nih.gov/pubmed/18996771.
306. Vargas CB, Picolli F, Dani C, Padoin AV, Mottin CC. Functioning of obese individuals in pre- and postoperative periods of bariatric surgery. Obes Surg. 2013;23(10):1590–5. PMID: 23515976. http://www.ncbi.nlm.nih.gov/pubmed/23515976.
307. Vincent HK, Ben-David K, Conrad BP, Lamb KM, Seay AN, Vincent KR. Rapid changes in gait, musculoskeletal pain, and quality of life after bariatric surgery. Surg Obes Relat Dis. 2012;8(3):346–54. PMID: 22336495. http://www.ncbi.nlm.nih.gov/pubmed/14699442.
308. Woodman G, Cywes R, Billy H, Montgomery K, Cornell C, Okerson T, APEX Study Group. Effect of adjustable gastric banding on changes in gastroesophageal reflux disease (GERD) and quality of life. Curr Med Res Opin. 2012;28(4):581–9. PMID: 22356120. http://www.ncbi.nlm.nih.gov/pubmed/22356120.
309. Cuicchi D, Lombardi R, Cariani S, Leuratti L, Lecce F, Cola B. Clinical and instrumental evaluation of pelvic floor disorders before and after bariatric surgery in obese women. Surg Obes Relat Dis. 2013;9(1):69–75. PMID: 21978747. http://www.ncbi.nlm.nih.gov/pubmed/21978747.
310. Hernández Hernández JR, López-Tomassetti Fernández E, Caballero Díaz Y, Molina Cabrillana J, Morales García D, Núñez JV. Remission of female sexual dysfunction in morbidly obese female patients with the Scopinaro procedure. Surg Obes Relat Dis. 2013;9(6):987–90. PMID: 23561961. http://www.ncbi.nlm.nih.gov/pubmed/23561961.
311. Hobzova M, Prasko J, Vanek J, Ociskova M, Genzor S, Holubova M, Grambal A, Latalova K. Depression and obstructive sleep apnea. Neuro Endocrinol Lett. 2017;38(5):343–52. PMID: 29106789. http://www.ncbi.nlm.nih.gov/pubmed/29106789.
312. Pan ML, Tsao HM, Hsu CC, Wu KM, Hsu TS, Wu YT, Hu GC. Bidirectional association between obstructive sleep apnea and depression: a population-based longitudinal study. Medicine (Baltimore). 2016;95(37):e4833. PMCID: PMC5402579. http://www.ncbi.nlm.nih.gov/pubmed/27631236.
313. Shelton RC, Falola M, Li L, Zajecka J, Fava M, Papakostas GI. The pro-inflammatory profile of depressed patients is (partly) related to obesity. J Psychiatr Res. 2015;70:91–97. PMCID: PMC4734093. http://www.ncbi.nlm.nih.gov/pubmed/26424427.
314. Ben-Avraham D, Muzumdar RH, Atzmon G. Epigenetic genome-wide association methylation in aging and longevity. Epigenomics. 2012;4(5):503–9. PMCID: PMC4123813. http://www.ncbi.nlm.nih.gov/pubmed/23130832.
315. Buigues C, Padilla-Sánchez C, Garrido JF, Navarro-Martínez R, Ruiz-Ros V, Cauli O. The relationship between depression and frailty syndrome: a systematic review. Aging Ment Health. 2015;19(9):762–72. PMID: 25319638. http://www.ncbi.nlm.nih.gov/pubmed/25319638.
316. Salk RH, Hyde JS, Abramson LY. Gender differences in depression in representative national samples: meta-analyses of diagnoses and symptoms. Psychol Bull. 2017;143(8):783–822. PMCID: PMC5532074. http://www.ncbi.nlm.nih.gov/pubmed/28447828.
317. Freeman A, Tyrovolas S, Koyanagi A, Chatterji S, Leonardi M, Ayuso-Mateos JL, Tobiasz-Adamczyk B, Koskinen S, Rummel-Kluge C, Haro JM. The role of socio-economic status in depression: results from the COURAGE (aging survey in Europe). BMC Public Health. 2016;16(1):1098. PMCID: PMC5069819. http://www.ncbi.nlm.nih.gov/pubmed/27760538.
318. Fluharty M, Taylor AE, Grabski M, Munafò MR. The Association of Cigarette Smoking with depression and anxiety: a systematic review. Nicotine Tob Res. 2017;19(1):3–13. PMCID: PMC5157710. http://www.ncbi.nlm.nih.gov/pubmed/27199385.
319. Buka SL. Disparities in health status and substance use: ethnicity and socioeconomic factors. Public Health Rep. 2002;117 Suppl 1(Suppl 1):S118–25. PMCID: PMC1913692. http://www.ncbi.nlm.nih.gov/pubmed/12435835.
320. Adler NE, Newman K. Socioeconomic disparities in health: pathways and policies. Health Aff (Millwood). 2002;21(2):60–76. PMID: 11900187. http://www.ncbi.nlm.nih.gov/pubmed/11900187.
321. Adler NE, Ostrove JM. Socioeconomic status and health: what we know and what we don't. Ann NY Acad Sci. 1999;896:3–15. PMID: 10681884. http://www.ncbi.nlm.nih.gov/pubmed/10681884.
322. Luppino FS, de Wit LM, Bouvy PF, Stijnen T, Cuijpers P, Penninx BWJH, Zitman FG. Overweight, obesity, and depression: a systematic review and meta-analysis of longitudinal studies. Arch Gen Psychiatry. 2010;67(3):220–9. PMID: 20194822. http://www.ncbi.nlm.nih.gov/pubmed/20194822.
323. Schachter J, Martel J, Lin CS, Chang CJ, Wu TR, Lu CC, Ko YF, Lai HC, Ojcius DM, Young JD. Effects of obesity on depression: a role for inflammation and the gut microbiota. Brain Behav Immun. 2018;69:1–8. PMID: 28888668. http://www.ncbi.nlm.nih.gov/pubmed/28888668.
324. Locke AE, Kahali B, Berndt SI, Justice AE, Pers TH, Day FR, Powell C, Vedantam S, Buchkovich ML, Yang J, Croteau-Chonka DC, Esko T, Fall T, Ferreira T, Gustafsson S, Kutalik Z, Luan J, Mägi R, Randall JC, Winkler TW, Wood AR, Workalemahu T, Faul JD, Smith JA, Zhao JH, Zhao W, Chen J, Fehrmann R, Hedman ÅK, Karjalainen J, Schmidt EM, Absher D, Amin N, Anderson D, Beekman M, Bolton, Ingelsson E, Hirschhorn JN, Loos RJF, Speliotes EK, et al. Genetic studies of body mass index yield new insights for obesity biology. Nature. 2015;518(7538):197–206. PMCID: PMC4382211. http://www.ncbi.nlm.nih.gov/pubmed/25673413.
325. Berndt SI, Gustafsson S, Mägi R, Ganna A, Wheeler E, Feitosa MF, Justice AE, Monda KL, Croteau-Chonka DC, Day FR, Esko T, Fall T, Ferreira T, Gentilini D, Jackson AU, Luan J, Randall JC, Vedantam S, Willer CJ, Winkler TW, Wood AR, Workalemahu T, Hu YJ, Lee SH, Liang L, Lin DY, Min JL, Neale BM, Thorleifsson G, et al. EK, North KE, Loos RJF, Ingelsson E. Genome-wide meta-analysis identifies 11 new loci for anthropometric traits and provides insights into genetic architecture. Nat Genet. 2013;45(5):501–12. PMCID: PMC3973018. http://www.ncbi.nlm.nih.gov/pubmed/23563607.
326. Bradfield JP, Taal HR, Timpson NJ, Scherag A, Lecoeur C, Warrington NM, Hypponen E, Holst C, Valcarcel B, Thiering E, Salem RM, Schumacher FR, Cousminer et al. Jaddoe VWV, Smith GD, Hakonarson H, Grant SFA, Early Growth Genetics Consortium. A genome-wide association meta-analysis identifies new childhood obesity loci. Nat Genet. 2012;44(5):526–31. PMCID: PMC3370100. http://www.ncbi.nlm.nih.gov/pubmed/22484627.
327. Cummings DE, Overduin J. Gastrointestinal regulation of food intake. J Clin Invest. 2007;117(1):13–23. PMCID: PMC1716217. http://www.ncbi.nlm.nih.gov/pubmed/17200702.
328. Gariepy G, Wang J, Lesage A, Schmitz N. The interaction of obesity and psychological distress on disability. Soc Psychiatry Psychiatr Epidemiol. 2010;45(5):531–40. PMID: 19575138. http://www.ncbi.nlm.nih.gov/pubmed/19575138.
329. Kloiber S, Ising M, Reppermund S, Horstmann S, Dose T, Majer M, Zihl J, Pfister H, Unschuld PG, Holsboer F, Lucae S. Overweight and obesity affect treatment response in major depression. Biol Psychiatry. 2007;62(4):321–6. PMID: 17241618. http://www.ncbi.nlm.nih.gov/pubmed/17241618.
330. Patterson E, Ryan PM, Cryan JF, Dinan TG, Ross RP, Fitzgerald GF, Stanton C. Gut microbiota, obesity and diabetes. Postgrad

Med J. 2016;92(1087):286–300. PMID: 26912499. http://www.ncbi.nlm.nih.gov/pubmed/26912499.
331. Inoue Y, Shimojo N. Microbiome/microbiota and allergies. Semin Immunopathol. 2015;37(1):57–64. PMID: 25326106. http://www.ncbi.nlm.nih.gov/pubmed/25326106.
332. Shamriz O, Mizrahi H, Werbner M, Shoenfeld Y, Avni O, Koren O. Microbiota at the crossroads of autoimmunity. Autoimmun Rev. 2016;15(9):859–69. PMID: 27392501. http://www.ncbi.nlm.nih.gov/pubmed/27392501.
333. Rapozo DCM, Bernardazzi C, de Souza HSP. Diet and microbiota in inflammatory bowel disease: the gut in disharmony. World J Gastroenterol. 2017;23(12):2124–40. PMCID: PMC5374124. http://www.ncbi.nlm.nih.gov/pubmed/28405140.
334. De Palma G, Collins SM, Bercik P. The microbiota-gut-brain axis in functional gastrointestinal disorders. Gut Microbes. 2014;5(3):419–29. PMCID: PMC4153782. http://www.ncbi.nlm.nih.gov/pubmed/24921926.
335. Inserra A, Rogers GB, Licinio J, Wong ML. The microbiota-inflammasome hypothesis of major depression. BioEssays. 2018;40(9):e1800027. PMID: 30004130. http://www.ncbi.nlm.nih.gov/pubmed/30004130.
336. Dinan TG, Cryan JF. Melancholic microbes: a link between gut microbiota and depression? Neurogastroenterol Motil. 2013;25(9):713–9. PMID: 23910373. http://www.ncbi.nlm.nih.gov/pubmed/23910373.
337. Koopman M, El Aidy S, MIDtrauma consortium. Depressed gut? The microbiota-diet-inflammation trialogue in depression. Curr Opin Psychiatry. 2017;30(5):369–77. PMID: 28654462. http://www.ncbi.nlm.nih.gov/pubmed/28654462.
338. Neufeld KAM, Kang N, Bienenstock J, Foster JA. Effects of intestinal microbiota on anxiety-like behavior. Commun Integr Biol. 2011;4(4):492–4. PMCID: PMC3181531. http://www.ncbi.nlm.nih.gov/pubmed/21966581.
339. Bäckhed F, Ley RE, Sonnenburg JL, Peterson DA, Gordon JI. Host-bacterial mutualism in the human intestine. Science. 2005;307(5717):1915–20. PMID: 15790844. http://www.ncbi.nlm.nih.gov/pubmed/15790844.
340. Cryan JF, Dinan TG. Mind-altering microorganisms: the impact of the gut microbiota on brain and behaviour. Nat Rev Neurosci. 2012;13(10):701–12. PMID: 22968153. http://www.ncbi.nlm.nih.gov/pubmed/22968153.
341. Rajilić-Stojanović M. Function of the microbiota. Best Pract Res Clin Gastroenterol. 2013;27(1):5–16. PMID: 23768548. http://www.ncbi.nlm.nih.gov/pubmed/23768548.
342. Agurs-Collins T, Fuemmeler BF. Dopamine polymorphisms and depressive symptoms predict foods intake. Results from a nationally representative sample. Appetite. 2011;57(2):339–48. PMCID: PMC3156384. http://www.ncbi.nlm.nih.gov/pubmed/21672565.
343. Beilharz JE, Maniam J, Morris MJ. Short exposure to a diet rich in both fat and sugar or sugar alone impairs place, but not object recognition memory in rats. Brain Behav Immun. 2014;37:134–41. PMID: 24309633. http://www.ncbi.nlm.nih.gov/pubmed/24309633.
344. Hryhorczuk C, Sharma S, Fulton SE. Metabolic disturbances connecting obesity and depression. Front Neurosci. 2013;7:177. PMCID: PMC3791387. http://www.ncbi.nlm.nih.gov/pubmed/24109426.
345. Liu C, Lee S, Elmquist JK. Circuits controlling energy balance and mood: inherently intertwined or just complicated intersections? Cell Metab. 2014;19(6):902–9. PMCID: PMC4047152. http://www.ncbi.nlm.nih.gov/pubmed/24630814.
346. Krishnamurthy P, Romagni P, Torvik S, Gold PW, Charney DS, Detera-Wadleigh S, Cizza G, P.O.W.E.R. (Premenopausal, Osteoporosis Women, Alendronate, Depression) Study Group. Glucocorticoid receptor gene polymorphisms in premenopausal women with major depression. Horm Metab Res. 2008;40(3):194–8. PMID: 18246526. http://www.ncbi.nlm.nih.gov/pubmed/18246526.
347. Manenschijn L, Koper JW, Lamberts SWJ, van Rossum EFC. Evaluation of a method to measure long term cortisol levels. Steroids. 2011;76(10–11):1032–6. PMID: 21515299. http://www.ncbi.nlm.nih.gov/pubmed/21515299.
348. Archer T, Fredriksson A, Schütz E, Kostrzewa RM. Influence of physical exercise on neuroimmunological functioning and health: aging and stress. Neurotox Res. 2011;20(1):69–83. PMID: 20953749. http://www.ncbi.nlm.nih.gov/pubmed/20953749.
349. Vanden Berghe W, Haegeman G. Epigenetic remedies by dietary phytochemicals against inflammatory skin disorders: myth or reality? Curr Drug Metab. 2010;11(5):436–50. PMID: 20540697. http://www.ncbi.nlm.nih.gov/pubmed/20540697.
350. vel Szarc Szic K, Ndlovu MN, Haegeman G, Vanden Berghe W. Nature or nurture: let food be your epigenetic medicine in chronic inflammatory disorders. Biochem Pharmacol. 2010;80(12):1816–32. PMID: 20688047. http://www.ncbi.nlm.nih.gov/pubmed/20688047.
351. Keating ST, El-Osta A. Epigenetics and metabolism. Circ Res. 2015;116(4):715–36. PMID: 25677519. http://www.ncbi.nlm.nih.gov/pubmed/25677519.
352. Monteleone AM, Pellegrino F, Croatto G, Carfagno M, Hilbert A, Treasure J, Wade T, Bulik CM, Zipfel S, Hay P, Schmidt U, Castellini G, Favaro A, Fernandez-Aranda F, Il Shin J, Voderholzer U, Ricca V, Moretti D, Busatta D, Abbate-Daga G, Ciullini F, Cascino G, Monaco F, Correll CU, Solmi M. Treatment of eating disorders: a systematic meta-review of meta-analyses and network meta-analyses. Neurosci Biobehav Rev. 2022;142:104857. PMCID: PMC9813802. http://www.ncbi.nlm.nih.gov/pubmed/36084848.
353. LeBlanc EL, Patnode CD, Webber EM, Redmond N, Rushkin M, O'Connor EA. Behavioral and pharmacotherapy weight loss interventions to prevent obesity-related morbidity and mortality in adults: an updated systematic review for the U.S. Preventive Services Task Force [Internet]. Rockville: Agency for Healthcare Research and Quality (US); 2018 [cited 2025 Jan 2]. Available from: http://www.ncbi.nlm.nih.gov/books/NBK532379/ PMID: 30354042 http://www.ncbi.nlm.nih.gov/pubmed/30354042.
354. Eisenberg D, Shikora SA, Aarts E, Aminian A, Angrisani L, Cohen RV, De Luca M, Faria SL, Goodpaster KPS, Haddad A, Himpens JM, Kow L, Kurian M, Loi K, Mahawar K, Nimeri A, O'Kane M, Papasavas PK, Ponce J, Pratt JSA, Rogers AM, Steele KE, Suter M, Kothari SN. 2022 American Society for Metabolic and Bariatric Surgery (ASMBS) and International Federation for the Surgery of Obesity and Metabolic Disorders (IFSO): indications for metabolic and bariatric surgery. Surg Obes Relat Dis. 2022;18(12):1345–56. PMID: 36280539. http://www.ncbi.nlm.nih.gov/pubmed/36280539.
355. Wharton S, Lau DCW, Vallis M, Sharma AM, Biertho L, Campbell-Scherer D, Adamo K, Alberga A, Bell R, Boulé N, Boyling E, Brown J, Calam B, Clarke C, Crowshoe L, Divalentino D, Forhan M, Freedhoff Y, Gagner M, Glazer S, Grand C, Green M, Hahn M, Hawa R, Henderson R, Hong D, Hung P, Janssen I, Jacklin K, Johnson-Stoklossa C, Kemp A, Kirk S, Kuk J, Langlois MF, Lear S, McInnes A, Macklin D, Naji L, Manjoo P, Morin MP, Nerenberg K, Patton I, Pedersen S, Pereira L, Piccinini-Vallis H, Poddar M, Poirier P, Prud'homme D, Salas XR, Rueda-Clausen C, Russell-Mayhew S, Shiau J, Sherifali D, Sievenpiper J, Sockalingam S, Taylor V, Toth E, Twells L, Tytus R, Walji S, Walker L, Wicklum S. Obesity in adults: a clinical practice guideline. CMAJ. 2020;192(31):E875–91. PMCID: PMC7828878. http://www.ncbi.nlm.nih.gov/pubmed/32753461.
356. Grunvald E, Shah R, Hernaez R, Chandar AK, Pickett-Blakely O, Teigen LM, Harindhanavudhi T, Sultan S, Singh S, Davitkov P. AGA clinical guidelines committee. AGA clinical practice

guideline on pharmacological interventions for adults with obesity. Gastroenterology. 2022;163(5):1198–225. PMID: 36273831. http://www.ncbi.nlm.nih.gov/pubmed/36273831.
357. Jastreboff AM, Aronne LJ, Ahmad NN, Wharton S, Connery L, Alves B, Kiyosue A, Zhang S, Liu B, Bunck MC, Stefanski A. SURMOUNT-1 Investigators. Tirzepatide once weekly for the treatment of obesity. N Engl J Med. 2022;387(3):205–16. PMID: 35658024. http://www.ncbi.nlm.nih.gov/pubmed/35658024.
358. Chao AM, Quigley KM, Wadden TA. Dietary interventions for obesity: clinical and mechanistic findings. J Clin Invest. 2021;131(1):e140065, 140065. PMCID: PMC7773341. http://www.ncbi.nlm.nih.gov/pubmed/33393504.
359. Look AHEAD Research Group, Chao AM, Wadden TA, Berkowitz RI, Blackburn G, Bolin P, Clark JM, Coday M, Curtis JM, Delahanty LM, Dutton GR, Evans M, Ewing LJ, Foreyt JP, Gay LJ, Gregg EW, Hazuda HP, Hill JO, Horton ES, Houston DK, Jakicic JM, Jeffery RW, Johnson KC, Kahn SE, Knowler WC, Kure A, Michalski KL, Montez MG, Neiberg RH, Patricio J, Peters A, Pi-Sunyer X, Pownall H, Reboussin D, Redmon B, Rejeski WJ, Steinburg H, Walker M, Williamson DA, Wing RR, Wyatt H, Yanovski SZ, Zhang P. Weight change 2 years after termination of the intensive lifestyle intervention in the Look AHEAD Study. Obesity (Silver Spring). 2020;28(5):893–901. PMCID: PMC7437140. http://www.ncbi.nlm.nih.gov/pubmed/32320144.
360. Elmaleh-Sachs A, Schwartz JL, Bramante CT, Nicklas JM, Gudzune KA, Jay M. Obesity management in adults: a review. JAMA. 2023;330(20):2000–15. PMCID: PMC11325826. http://www.ncbi.nlm.nih.gov/pubmed/38015216.
361. Beck NN, Johannsen M, Støving RK, Mehlsen M, Zachariae R. Do postoperative psychotherapeutic interventions and support groups influence weight loss following bariatric surgery? A systematic review and meta-analysis of randomized and nonrandomized trials. Obes Surg. 2012;22(11):1790–7. PMID: 22930073. http://www.ncbi.nlm.nih.gov/pubmed/22930073.
362. Semlitsch T, Stigler FL, Jeitler K, Horvath K, Siebenhofer A. Management of overweight and obesity in primary care-a systematic overview of international evidence-based guidelines. Obes Rev. 2019;20(9):1218–30. PMCID: PMC6852048. http://www.ncbi.nlm.nih.gov/pubmed/31286668.
363. Hayes SC, Villatte M, Levin M, Hildebrandt M. Open, aware, and active: contextual approaches as an emerging trend in the behavioral and cognitive therapies. Annu Rev Clin Psychol. 2011;7:141–68. PMID: 21219193. http://www.ncbi.nlm.nih.gov/pubmed/21219193.
364. Foroushani PS, Schneider J, Assareh N. Meta-review of the effectiveness of computerised CBT in treating depression. BMC Psychiatry. 2011;11:131. PMCID: PMC3180363. http://www.ncbi.nlm.nih.gov/pubmed/21838902.
365. Keefe JR, Chambless DL, Barber JP, Milrod BL. Treatment of anxiety and mood comorbidities in cognitive-behavioral and psychodynamic therapies for panic disorder. J Psychiatr Res. 2019;114:34–40. PMID: 31015099. http://www.ncbi.nlm.nih.gov/pubmed/31015099.
366. Wilfley DE, Kolko RP, Kass AE. Cognitive-behavioral therapy for weight management and eating disorders in children and adolescents. Child Adolesc Psychiatr Clin N Am. 2011;20(2):271–85. PMCID: PMC3065663. http://www.ncbi.nlm.nih.gov/pubmed/21440855.
367. Murphy R, Straebler S, Cooper Z, Fairburn CG. Cognitive behavioral therapy for eating disorders. Psychiatr Clin North Am. 2010;33(3):611–27. PMCID: PMC2928448. http://www.ncbi.nlm.nih.gov/pubmed/20599136.
368. Chang SH, Stoll CRT, Song J, Varela JE, Eagon CJ, Colditz GA. The effectiveness and risks of bariatric surgery: an updated systematic review and meta-analysis, 2003-2012. JAMA Surg. 2014;149(3):275–87. PMCID: PMC3962512. http://www.ncbi.nlm.nih.gov/pubmed/24352617.
369. O'Brien PE, Hindle A, Brennan L, Skinner S, Burton P, Smith A, Crosthwaite G, Brown W. Long-term outcomes after bariatric surgery: a systematic review and meta-analysis of weight loss at 10 or more years for all bariatric procedures and a single-centre review of 20-year outcomes after adjustable gastric banding. Obes Surg. 2019;29(1):3–14. PMCID: PMC6320354. http://www.ncbi.nlm.nih.gov/pubmed/30293134.
370. Khosravi-Largani M, Nojomi M, Aghili R, Otaghvar HA, Tanha K, Seyedi SHS, Mottaghi A. Evaluation of all types of metabolic bariatric surgery and its consequences: a systematic review and meta-analysis. Obes Surg. 2019;29(2):651–90. PMID: 30443720. http://www.ncbi.nlm.nih.gov/pubmed/30443720.
371. Kalarchian MA, Marcus MD. Psychosocial concerns following bariatric surgery: current status. Curr Obes Rep. 2019;8(1):1–9. PMID: 30659459. http://www.ncbi.nlm.nih.gov/pubmed/30659459.
372. Golzarand M, Toolabi K, Farid R. The bariatric surgery and weight losing: a meta-analysis in the long- and very long-term effects of laparoscopic adjustable gastric banding, laparoscopic Roux-en-Y gastric bypass and laparoscopic sleeve gastrectomy on weight loss in adults. Surg Endosc. 2017;31(11):4331–45. PMID: 28378086. http://www.ncbi.nlm.nih.gov/pubmed/28378086.
373. US Preventive Services Task Force, Curry SJ, Krist AH, Owens DK, Barry MJ, Caughey AB, Davidson KW, Doubeni CA, Epling JW, Grossman DC, Kemper AR, Kubik M, Landefeld CS, Mangione CM, Phipps MG, Silverstein M, Simon MA, Tseng CW, Wong JB. Behavioral weight loss interventions to prevent obesity-related morbidity and mortality in adults: US Preventive Services Task Force recommendation statement. JAMA. 2018;320(11):1163–71. PMID: 30326502. http://www.ncbi.nlm.nih.gov/pubmed/30326502.
374. American Diabetes Association Professional Practice Committee. 8. Obesity and weight management for the prevention and treatment of type 2 diabetes: standards of medical care in diabetes-2022. Diabetes Care. 2022;45(Suppl 1):S113–24. PMID: 34964843. http://www.ncbi.nlm.nih.gov/pubmed/34964843.
375. Tronieri JS, Alamuddin N, Wadden TA. Behavioral approaches to obesity management. In: Feingold KR, Anawalt B, Blackman MR, Boyce A, Chrousos G, Corpas E, de Herder WW, Dhatariya K, Dungan K, Hofland J, Kalra S, Kaltsas G, Kapoor N, Koch C, Kopp P, Korbonits M, Kovacs CS, Kuohung W, Laferrère B, Levy M, McGee EA, McLachlan R, New M, Purnell J, Sahay R, Shah AS, Singer F, Sperling MA, Stratakis CA, Trence DL, Wilson DP, editors. Endotext [Internet]. South Dartmouth: MDText.com, Inc.; 2000 [cited 2025 Jan 2]. Available from: http://www.ncbi.nlm.nih.gov/books/NBK278952/ PMID: 25905187 http://www.ncbi.nlm.nih.gov/pubmed/25905187
376. Duan D, Kim LJ, Jun JC, Polotsky VY. Connecting insufficient sleep and insomnia with metabolic dysfunction. Ann N Y Acad Sci. 2023;1519(1):94–117. PMCID: PMC9839511. http://www.ncbi.nlm.nih.gov/pubmed/36373239.
377. Varkevisser RDM, van Stralen MM, Kroeze W, Ket JCF, Steenhuis IHM. Determinants of weight loss maintenance: a systematic review. Obes Rev. 2019;20(2):171–211. PMCID: PMC7416131. http://www.ncbi.nlm.nih.gov/pubmed/30324651.
378. Gudzune KA, Bennett WL, Cooper LA, Bleich SN. Perceived judgment about weight can negatively influence weight loss: a cross-sectional study of overweight and obese patients. Prev Med. 2014;62:103–7. PMCID: PMC4006987. http://www.ncbi.nlm.nih.gov/pubmed/24521530.
379. Carvalho MCR de, Menezes MC de, Toral N, Lopes ACS. Effect of a Transtheoretical Model-based intervention on fruit and vegetable intake according to perception of intake adequacy: a randomized

controlled community trial. Appetite. 2021;161:105159. PMID: 33577862. http://www.ncbi.nlm.nih.gov/pubmed/33577862.
380. Prochaska JO, Velicer WF. The transtheoretical model of health behavior change. Am J Health Promot. 1997;12(1):38–48. PMID: 10170434. http://www.ncbi.nlm.nih.gov/pubmed/10170434.
381. Serdula MK, Khan LK, Dietz WH. Weight loss counseling revisited. JAMA. 2003;289(14):1747–50. PMID: 1268433. http://www.ncbi.nlm.nih.gov/pubmed/12684339.
382. Pollak KI, Tulsky JA, Bravender T, Østbye T, Lyna P, Dolor RJ, Coffman CJ, Bilheimer A, Lin PH, Farrell D, Bodner ME, Alexander SC. Teaching primary care physicians the 5 A's for discussing weight with overweight and obese adolescents. Patient Educ Couns. 2016;99(10):1620–5. PMCID: PMC5964297. http://www.ncbi.nlm.nih.gov/pubmed/27228899.
383. Centers for Medicare & Medicaid Services. CMS Manual System publication 100–04: Medicare claims processing: transmittal 2421: intensive behavioral therapy for obesity. Published March 7, 2012. R2421CP.pdf.
384. Herbozo S, Brown KL, Burke NL, LaRose JG. A call to reconceptualize obesity treatment in service of health equity: review of evidence and future directions. Curr Obes Rep. 2023;12(1):24–35. PMCID: PMC9894524. http://www.ncbi.nlm.nih.gov/pubmed/36729299.
385. Lewis KH, Edwards-Hampton SA, Ard JD. Disparities in treatment uptake and outcomes of patients with obesity in the USA. Curr Obes Rep. 2016;5(2):282–90. PMID: 27023070. http://www.ncbi.nlm.nih.gov/pubmed/27023070.
386. Kane RM, Nicklas JM, Schwartz JL, Bramante CT, Yancy WS, Gudzune KA, Jay MR. Opportunities for general internal medicine to promote equity in obesity care. J Gen Intern Med. 2024; PMID: 39414737. http://www.ncbi.nlm.nih.gov/pubmed/39414737.
387. Ward ZJ, Bleich SN, Cradock AL, Barrett JL, Giles CM, Flax C, Long MW, Gortmaker SL. Projected U.S. state-level prevalence of adult obesity and severe obesity. N Engl J Med. 2019;381(25):2440–50. PMID: 31851800. http://www.ncbi.nlm.nih.gov/pubmed/31851800.
388. Jay M, Gillespie C, Schlair S, Sherman S, Kalet A. Physicians' use of the 5As in counseling obese patients: is the quality of counseling associated with patients' motivation and intention to lose weight? BMC Health Serv Res. 2010;10:159. PMCID: PMC2903583. http://www.ncbi.nlm.nih.gov/pubmed/20534160.
389. Welzel FD, Bär J, Stein J, Löbner M, Pabst A, Luppa M, Grochtdreis T, Kersting A, Blüher M, Luck-Sikorski C, König HH, Riedel-Heller SG. Using a brief web-based 5A intervention to improve weight management in primary care: results of a cluster-randomized controlled trial. BMC Fam Pract. 2021;22(1):61. PMCID: PMC8017625. http://www.ncbi.nlm.nih.gov/pubmed/33794781.
390. Ge L, Sadeghirad B, Ball GDC, da Costa BR, Hitchcock CL, Svendrovski A, Kiflen R, Quadri K, Kwon HY, Karamouzian M, Adams-Webber T, Ahmed W, Damanhoury S, Zeraatkar D, Nikolakopoulou A, Tsuyuki RT, Tian J, Yang K, Guyatt GH, Johnston BC. Comparison of dietary macronutrient patterns of 14 popular named dietary programmes for weight and cardiovascular risk factor reduction in adults: systematic review and network meta-analysis of randomised trials. BMJ. 2020;369:m696. PMCID: PMC7190064. http://www.ncbi.nlm.nih.gov/pubmed/32238384.
391. Salas-Salvadó J, Díaz-López A, Ruiz-Canela M, Basora J, Fitó M, Corella D, Serra-Majem L, Wärnberg J, Romaguera D, Estruch R, Vidal J, Martínez JA, Arós F, Vázquez C, Ros E, Vioque J, López-Miranda J, Bueno-Cavanillas A, Tur JA, Tinahones FJ, Martín V, Lapetra J, Pintó X, Daimiel L, Delgado-Rodríguez M, Matía P, Gómez-Gracia E, Díez-Espino J, Babio N, Castañer O, Sorlí JV, Fiol M, Zulet MÁ, Bulló M, Goday A, Martínez-González MÁ, PREDIMED-Plus investigators. Effect of a lifestyle intervention program with energy-restricted Mediterranean diet and exercise on weight loss and cardiovascular risk factors: one-year results of the PREDIMED-Plus trial. Diabetes Care. 2019;42(5):777–88. PMID: 30389673.
392. Piercy KL, Troiano RP, Ballard RM, Carlson SA, Fulton JE, Galuska DA, George SM, Olson RD. The physical activity guidelines for Americans. JAMA. 2018;320(19):2020–8. PMCID: PMC9582631. http://www.ncbi.nlm.nih.gov/pubmed/30418471.
393. Healthy People 2030 | odphp.health.gov.
394. Rodriguez-Cristobal JJ, Alonso-Villaverde C, Panisello JM, Travé-Mercade P, Rodriguez-Cortés F, Marsal JR, Peña E. Effectiveness of a motivational intervention on overweight/obese patients in the primary healthcare: a cluster randomized trial. BMC Fam Pract. 2017;18(1):74. PMCID: PMC5477747. http://www.ncbi.nlm.nih.gov/pubmed/28633627.
395. Lundahl B, Moleni T, Burke BL, Butters R, Tollefson D, Butler C, Rollnick S. Motivational interviewing in medical care settings: a systematic review and meta-analysis of randomized controlled trials. Patient Educ Couns. 2013;93(2):157–68. PMID: 24001658. http://www.ncbi.nlm.nih.gov/pubmed/24001658.
396. Rubak S, Sandbaek A, Lauritzen T, Christensen B. Motivational interviewing: a systematic review and meta-analysis. Br J Gen Pract. 2005;55(513):305–12. PMCID: PMC1463134. http://www.ncbi.nlm.nih.gov/pubmed/15826439.
397. Yearwood L, Masood W. Behavioral approaches to obesity treatmenT. StatPearls [Internet]. Treasure Island (FL): StatPearls Publishing; 2024 [cited 2025 Jan 2]. Available from: http://www.ncbi.nlm.nih.gov/books/NBK570565/ PMID: 34033327 http://www.ncbi.nlm.nih.gov/pubmed/34033327
398. Apodaca TR, Longabaugh R. Mechanisms of change in motivational interviewing: a review and preliminary evaluation of the evidence. Addiction. 2009;104(5):705–15. PMCID: PMC2756738. http://www.ncbi.nlm.nih.gov/pubmed/19413785.
399. Vocks S, Tuschen-Caffier B, Pietrowsky R, Rustenbach SJ, Kersting A, Herpertz S. Meta-analysis of the effectiveness of psychological and pharmacological treatments for binge eating disorder. Int J Eat Disord. 2010;43(3):205–17. PMID: 19402028. http://www.ncbi.nlm.nih.gov/pubmed/19402028.
400. Linardon J, Wade T, de la Piedad GX, Brennan L. Psychotherapy for bulimia nervosa on symptoms of depression: a meta-analysis of randomized controlled trials. Int J Eat Disord. 2017;50(10):1124–36. PMID: 28804915. http://www.ncbi.nlm.nih.gov/pubmed/28804915.
401. David A. Kessler: the end of overeating - taking control of the insatiable American Appetite.
402. Alosco ML, Galioto R, Spitznagel MB, Strain G, Devlin M, Cohen R, Crosby RD, Mitchell JE, Gunstad J. Cognitive function after bariatric surgery: evidence for improvement 3 years after surgery. Am J Surg. 2014;207(6):870–6. PMCID: PMC3983172. http://www.ncbi.nlm.nih.gov/pubmed/24119892.
403. Cserjési R, Luminet O, Poncelet AS, Lénárd L. Altered executive function in obesity. Exploration of the role of affective states on cognitive abilities. Appetite. 2009;52(2):535–9. PMID: 19260167. http://www.ncbi.nlm.nih.gov/pubmed/19260167.
404. Smith E, Hay P, Campbell L, Trollor JN. A review of the association between obesity and cognitive function across the lifespan: implications for novel approaches to prevention and treatment. Obes Rev. 2011;12(9):740–55. PMID: 21991597. http://www.ncbi.nlm.nih.gov/pubmed/21991597.
405. Davis C, Levitan RD, Smith M, Tweed S, Curtis C. Associations among overeating, overweight, and attention deficit/hyperactivity disorder: a structural equation modelling approach. Eat Behav. 2006;7(3):266–74. PMID: 16843230. http://www.ncbi.nlm.nih.gov/pubmed/16843230.
406. Pagoto SL, Curtin C, Lemon SC, Bandini LG, Schneider KL, Bodenlos JS, Ma Y. Association between adult attention deficit/

hyperactivity disorder and obesity in the US population. Obesity (Silver Spring). 2009;17(3):539–44. PMCID: PMC3221303. http://www.ncbi.nlm.nih.gov/pubmed/19131944.

407. Gruss B, Mueller A, Horbach T, Martin A, de Zwaan M. Attention-deficit/hyperactivity disorder in a prebariatric surgery sample. Eur Eat Disord Rev. 2012;20(1):e103–7. PMID: 21796736. http://www.ncbi.nlm.nih.gov/pubmed/21796736.

408. Schmidt F, Körber S, de Zwaan M, Müller A. Impulse control disorders in obese patients. Eur Eat Disord Rev. 2012;20(3):e144–7. PMID: 22367789. http://www.ncbi.nlm.nih.gov/pubmed/22367789.

409. Spitznagel MB, Galioto R, Limbach K, Gunstad J, Heinberg L. Cognitive function is linked to adherence to bariatric postoperative guidelines. Surg Obes Relat Dis. 2013;9(4):580–5. PMCID: PMC3737380. http://www.ncbi.nlm.nih.gov/pubmed/23791534.

410. Müller A, Claes L, Wilderjans TF, de Zwaan M. Temperament subtypes in treatment seeking obese individuals: a latent profile analysis. Eur Eat Disord Rev. 2014;22(4):260–6. PMID: 24809764. http://www.ncbi.nlm.nih.gov/pubmed/24809764.

411. De Panfilis C, Cero S, Torre M, Salvatore P, Dall'Aglio E, Adorni A, Maggini C. Utility of the temperament and character inventory (TCI) in outcome prediction of laparoscopic adjustable gastric banding: preliminary report. Obes Surg. 2006;16(7):842–7. PMID: 16839480. http://www.ncbi.nlm.nih.gov/pubmed/16839480.

412. Gordon PC, Sallet JA, Sallet PC. The impact of temperament and character inventory personality traits on long-term outcome of Roux-en-Y gastric bypass. Obes Surg. 2014;24(10):1647–55. PMID: 24682805. http://www.ncbi.nlm.nih.gov/pubmed/24682805.

413. Sarwer DB, Dilks RJ, West-Smith L. Dietary intake and eating behavior after bariatric surgery: threats to weight loss maintenance and strategies for success. Surg Obes Relat Dis. 2011;7(5):644–51. PMID: 21962227. http://www.ncbi.nlm.nih.gov/pubmed/21962227.

414. Phelan S, Wing RR, Loria CM, Kim Y, Lewis CE. Prevalence and predictors of weight-loss maintenance in a biracial cohort: results from the coronary artery risk development in young adults study. Am J Prev Med. 2010;39(6):546–54. PMCID: PMC3308341. http://www.ncbi.nlm.nih.gov/pubmed/21084075.

415. DiMatteo MR. Social support and patient adherence to medical treatment: a meta-analysis. Health Psychol. 2004;23(2):207–18. PMID: 15008666. http://www.ncbi.nlm.nih.gov/pubmed/15008666.

416. Livhits M, Mercado C, Yermilov I, Parikh JA, Dutson E, Mehran A, Ko CY, Shekelle PG, Gibbons MM. Is social support associated with greater weight loss after bariatric surgery?: a systematic review. Obes Rev. 2011;12(2):142–8. PMID: 20158617. http://www.ncbi.nlm.nih.gov/pubmed/20158617.

417. Apovian CM, Aronne LJ, Bessesen DH, McDonnell ME, Murad MH, Pagotto U, Ryan DH, Still CD, Endocrine Society. Pharmacological management of obesity: an endocrine Society clinical practice guideline. J Clin Endocrinol Metab. 2015;100(2):342–62. PMID: 25590212. http://www.ncbi.nlm.nih.gov/pubmed/25590212.

418. Wharton S, Raiber L, Serodio KJ, Lee J, Christensen RA. Medications that cause weight gain and alternatives in Canada: a narrative review. Diabetes Metab Syndr Obes. 2018;11:427–38. PMCID: PMC6109660. http://www.ncbi.nlm.nih.gov/pubmed/30174450.

419. Verhaegen AA, Van Gaal LF. Drugs affecting body weight, body fat distribution, and metabolic function-mechanisms and possible therapeutic or preventive measures: an update. Curr Obes Rep. 2021;10(1):1–13. PMID: 33400222. http://www.ncbi.nlm.nih.gov/pubmed/33400222.

420. Goh KK, Chen CH, Lu ML. Topiramate mitigates weight gain in antipsychotic-treated patients with schizophrenia: meta-analysis of randomised controlled trials. Int J Psychiatry Clin Pract. 2019;23(1):14–32. PMID: 29557263. http://www.ncbi.nlm.nih.gov/pubmed/29557263.

421. Yu O, Lu M, Lai TKY, Hahn M, Agarwal SM, O'Donoghue B, Ebdrup BH, Siskind D. Metformin co-commencement at time of antipsychotic initiation for attenuation of weight gain: a systematic review and meta-analysis. Ther Adv Psychopharmacol. 2024;14:20451253241255476. PMCID: PMC11141220. http://www.ncbi.nlm.nih.gov/pubmed/38827016.

422. Jensterle M, Ferjan S, Janez A. The maintenance of long-term weight loss after semaglutide withdrawal in obese women with PCOS treated with metformin: a 2-year observational study. Front Endocrinol (Lausanne). 2024;15:1366940. PMCID: PMC11043580. http://www.ncbi.nlm.nih.gov/pubmed/38665260.

423. Farooqi IS, Jebb SA, Langmack G, Lawrence E, Cheetham CH, Prentice AM, Hughes IA, McCamish MA, O'Rahilly S. Effects of recombinant leptin therapy in a child with congenital leptin deficiency. N Engl J Med. 1999;341(12):879–84. PMID: 10486419. http://www.ncbi.nlm.nih.gov/pubmed/10486419.

424. Halaas JL, Gajiwala KS, Maffei M, Cohen SL, Chait BT, Rabinowitz D, Lallone RL, Burley SK, Friedman JM. Weight-reducing effects of the plasma protein encoded by the obese gene. Science. 1995;269(5223):543–6. PMID: 7624777. http://www.ncbi.nlm.nih.gov/pubmed/7624777.

425. Bates SH, Stearns WH, Dundon TA, Schubert M, Tso AWK, Wang Y, Banks AS, Lavery HJ, Haq AK, Maratos-Flier E, Neel BG, Schwartz MW, Myers MG. STAT3 signalling is required for leptin regulation of energy balance but not reproduction. Nature. 2003;421(6925):856–9. PMID: 12594516. http://www.ncbi.nlm.nih.gov/pubmed/12594516.

426. Elias CF, Aschkenasi C, Lee C, Kelly J, Ahima RS, Bjorbaek C, Flier JS, Saper CB, Elmquist JK. Leptin differentially regulates NPY and POMC neurons projecting to the lateral hypothalamic area. Neuron. 1999;23(4):775–86. PMID: 10482243. http://www.ncbi.nlm.nih.gov/pubmed/10482243.

427. Locke AE, Kahali B, Berndt SI, Justice AE, Pers TH, Day FR, Powell C, Vedantam S, Buchkovich ML, Yang J, Croteau-Chonka DC, Esko T, Fall T, Ferreira T, Gustafsson S, Kutalik Z, Luan J, Mägi R, Randall JC, Winkler TW, Wood AR, Workalemahu T, Faul JD, Smith JA, Zhao JH, Zhao W, Chen J, Fehrmann R, Hedman ÅK, Karjalainen J, Schmidt EM, Absher D, Amin N, Anderson D, Beekman M, Bolton, Ingelsson E, Hirschhorn JN, Loos RJF, Speliotes EK, et al. Genetic studies of body mass index yield new insights for obesity biology. Nature. 2015;518(7538):197–206. PMCID: PMC4382211. http://www.ncbi.nlm.nih.gov/pubmed/25673413

428. Christensen R, Kristensen PK, Bartels EM, Bliddal H, Astrup A. Efficacy and safety of the weight-loss drug rimonabant: a meta-analysis of randomised trials. Lancet. 2007;370(9600):1706–13. PMID: 18022033. http://www.ncbi.nlm.nih.gov/pubmed/18022033.

429. Ettinger MP, Littlejohn TW, Schwartz SL, Weiss SR, McIlwain HH, Heymsfield SB, Bray GA, Roberts WG, Heyman ER, Stambler N, Heshka S, Vicary C, Guler HP. Recombinant variant of ciliary neurotrophic factor for weight loss in obese adults: a randomized, dose-ranging study. JAMA. 2003;289(14):1826–32. PMID: 12684362. http://www.ncbi.nlm.nih.gov/pubmed/12684362.

430. Allison DB, Gadde KM, Garvey WT, Peterson CA, Schwiers ML, Najarian T, Tam PY, Troupin B, Day WW. Controlled-release phentermine/topiramate in severely obese adults: a randomized controlled trial (EQUIP). Obesity (Silver Spring). 2012;20(2):330–42. PMCID: PMC3270297. http://www.ncbi.nlm.nih.gov/pubmed/22051941.

431. Davidson MH, Hauptman J, DiGirolamo M, Foreyt JP, Halsted CH, Heber D, Heimburger DC, Lucas CP, Robbins DC, Chung J, Heymsfield SB. Weight control and risk factor reduction in obese subjects treated for 2 years with orlistat: a randomized controlled

trial. JAMA. 1999;281(3):235–42. PMID: 9918478. http://www.ncbi.nlm.nih.gov/pubmed/9918478.
432. Plodkowski RA, Nguyen Q, Sundaram U, Nguyen L, Chau DL, St JS. Bupropion and naltrexone: a review of their use individually and in combination for the treatment of obesity. Expert Opin Pharmacother. 2009;10(6):1069–81. PMID: 19364254. http://www.ncbi.nlm.nih.gov/pubmed/19364254.
433. FDA requests the withdrawal of the weight-loss drug Belviq, Belviq XR (lorcaserin) from the market | FDA.
434. Vilsbøll T, Christensen M, Junker AE, Knop FK, Gluud LL. Effects of glucagon-like peptide-1 receptor agonists on weight loss: systematic review and meta-analyses of randomised controlled trials. BMJ. 2012;344:d7771. PMCID: PMC3256253. http://www.ncbi.nlm.nih.gov/pubmed/22236411.
435. Rubino D, Abrahamsson N, Davies M, Hesse D, Greenway FL, Jensen C, Lingvay I, Mosenzon O, Rosenstock J, Rubio MA, Rudofsky G, Tadayon S, Wadden TA, Dicker D, STEP 4 Investigators. Effect of continued weekly subcutaneous Semaglutide vs Placebo on weight loss maintenance in adults with overweight or obesity: the STEP 4 randomized clinical trial. JAMA. 2021;325(14):1414–25. PMCID: PMC7988425. http://www.ncbi.nlm.nih.gov/pubmed/33755728.
436. Wilding JPH, Batterham RL, Davies M, Van Gaal LF, Kandler K, Konakli K, Lingvay I, McGowan BM, Oral TK, Rosenstock J, Wadden TA, Wharton S, Yokote K, Kushner RF. STEP 1 Study Group. Weight regain and cardiometabolic effects after withdrawal of semaglutide: the STEP 1 trial extension. Diabetes Obes Metab. 2022;24(8):1553–64. PMCID: PMC9542252. http://www.ncbi.nlm.nih.gov/pubmed/35441470.
437. Latif W, Lambrinos KJ, Patel P, Rodriguez R. Compare and contrast the Glucagon-Like Peptide-1 Receptor Agonists (GLP1RAs). StatPearls [Internet]. Treasure Island (FL): StatPearls Publishing; 2024 [cited 2025 Jan 2]. Available from: http://www.ncbi.nlm.nih.gov/books/NBK572151/ PMID: 34283517 http://www.ncbi.nlm.nih.gov/pubmed/34283517.
438. Jensterle M, Rizzo M, Haluzík M, Janež A. Efficacy of GLP-1 RA approved for weight management in patients with or without diabetes: a narrative review. Adv Ther. 2022;39(6):2452–67. PMCID: PMC9063254. http://www.ncbi.nlm.nih.gov/pubmed/35503498.
439. Wilding JPH, Batterham RL, Calanna S, Davies M, Van Gaal LF, Lingvay I, McGowan BM, Rosenstock J, Tran MTD, Wadden TA, Wharton S, Yokote K, Zeuthen N, Kushner RF, STEP 1 Study Group. Once-weekly Semaglutide in adults with overweight or obesity. N Engl J Med. 2021;384(11):989–1002. PMID: 33567185. http://www.ncbi.nlm.nih.gov/pubmed/33567185.
440. Xie Z, Yang S, Deng W, Li J, Chen J. Efficacy and safety of Liraglutide and Semaglutide on weight loss in people with obesity or overweight: a systematic review. Clin Epidemiol. 2022;14:1463–76. PMCID: PMC9738168. http://www.ncbi.nlm.nih.gov/pubmed/36510488.
441. O'Neil PM, Birkenfeld AL, McGowan B, Mosenzon O, Pedersen SD, Wharton S, Carson CG, Jepsen CH, Kabisch M, Wilding JPH. Efficacy and safety of semaglutide compared with liraglutide and placebo for weight loss in patients with obesity: a randomised, double-blind, placebo and active controlled, dose-ranging, phase 2 trial. Lancet. 2018;392(10148):637–49. PMID: 30122305. http://www.ncbi.nlm.nih.gov/pubmed/30122305.
442. Shyangdan DS, Royle P, Clar C, Sharma P, Waugh N, Snaith A. Glucagon-like peptide analogues for type 2 diabetes mellitus. Cochrane Database Syst Rev. 2011;2011(10):CD006423. PMCID: PMC6486297. http://www.ncbi.nlm.nih.gov/pubmed/21975753.
443. Moore PW, Malone K, VanValkenburg D, Rando LL, Williams BC, Matejowsky HG, Ahmadzadeh S, Shekoohi S, Cornett EM, Kaye AD. GLP-1 agonists for weight loss: pharmacology and clinical implications. Adv Ther. 2023;40(3):723–42. PMID: 36566341. http://www.ncbi.nlm.nih.gov/pubmed/36566341.
444. Guo X, Zhou Z, Lyu X, Xu H, Zhu H, Pan H, Wang L, Yang H, Gong F. The Antiobesity effect and safety of GLP-1 receptor agonist in overweight/obese patients without diabetes: a systematic review and meta-analysis. Horm Metab Res. 2022;54(7):458–71. PMID: 35512849. http://www.ncbi.nlm.nih.gov/pubmed/35512849.
445. Moran GW, Leslie FC, Levison SE, Worthington J, McLaughlin JT. Enteroendocrine cells: neglected players in gastrointestinal disorders? Ther Adv Gastroenterol. 2008;1(1):51–60. PMCID: PMC3002486. http://www.ncbi.nlm.nih.gov/pubmed/21180514.
446. Nauck MA, Meier JJ. Incretin hormones: their role in health and disease. Diabetes Obes Metab. 2018;20(Suppl 1):5–21. PMID: 29364588. http://www.ncbi.nlm.nih.gov/pubmed/29364588.
447. Gutierrez-Aguilar R, Woods SC. Nutrition and L and K-enteroendocrine cells. Curr Opin Endocrinol Diabetes Obes. 2011;18(1):35–41. PMCID: PMC3884637. http://www.ncbi.nlm.nih.gov/pubmed/21124210.
448. Drucker DJ, Nauck MA. The incretin system: glucagon-like peptide-1 receptor agonists and dipeptidyl peptidase-4 inhibitors in type 2 diabetes. Lancet. 2006;368(9548):1696–705. PMID: 17098089. http://www.ncbi.nlm.nih.gov/pubmed/17098089.
449. Drucker DJ, Asa S. Glucagon gene expression in vertebrate brain. J Biol Chem. 1988;263(27):13475–8. PMID: 2901414. http://www.ncbi.nlm.nih.gov/pubmed/2901414.
450. Mortensen K, Christensen LL, Holst JJ, Orskov C. GLP-1 and GIP are colocalized in a subset of endocrine cells in the small intestine. Regul Pept. 2003;114(2–3):189–96. PMID: 12832109. http://www.ncbi.nlm.nih.gov/pubmed/12832109.
451. Theodorakis MJ, Carlson O, Michopoulos S, Doyle ME, Juhaszova M, Petraki K, Egan JM. Human duodenal enteroendocrine cells: source of both incretin peptides, GLP-1 and GIP. Am J Physiol Endocrinol Metab. 2006;290(3):E550–9. PMID: 16219666. http://www.ncbi.nlm.nih.gov/pubmed/16219666.
452. Zeigerer A, Sekar R, Kleinert M, Nason S, Habegger KM, Müller TD. Glucagon's metabolic action in health and disease. Compr Physiol. 2021;11(2):1759–83. PMCID: PMC8513137. http://www.ncbi.nlm.nih.gov/pubmed/33792899.
453. Tschöp MH, Finan B, Clemmensen C, Gelfanov V, Perez-Tilve D, Müller TD, DiMarchi RD. Unimolecular polypharmacy for treatment of diabetes and obesity. Cell Metab. 2016;24(1):51–62. PMID: 27411008. http://www.ncbi.nlm.nih.gov/pubmed/27411008.
454. Ambery PD, Klammt S, Posch MG, Petrone M, Pu W, Rondinone C, Jermutus L, Hirshberg B. MEDI0382, a GLP-1/glucagon receptor dual agonist, meets safety and tolerability endpoints in a single-dose, healthy-subject, randomized, Phase 1 study. Br J Clin Pharmacol. 2018;84(10):2325–35. PMCID: PMC6138475. http://www.ncbi.nlm.nih.gov/pubmed/29926478.
455. Hong J, Abudula R, Chen J, Jeppesen PB, Dyrskog SEU, Xiao J, Colombo M, Hermansen K. The short-term effect of fatty acids on glucagon secretion is influenced by their chain length, spatial configuration, and degree of unsaturation: studies in vitro. Metabolism. 2005;54(10):1329–36. PMID: 16154432. http://www.ncbi.nlm.nih.gov/pubmed/16154432.
456. Rui L. Energy metabolism in the liver. Compr Physiol. 2014;4(1):177–97. PMCID: PMC4050641. http://www.ncbi.nlm.nih.gov/pubmed/24692138.
457. Hare KJ, Vilsbøll T, Asmar M, Deacon CF, Knop FK, Holst JJ. The glucagonostatic and insulinotropic effects of glucagon-like peptide 1 contribute equally to its glucose-lowering action. Diabetes. 2010;59(7):1765–70. PMCID: PMC2889777. http://www.ncbi.nlm.nih.gov/pubmed/20150286.
458. Finan B, Müller TD, Clemmensen C, Perez-Tilve D, DiMarchi RD, Tschöp MH. Reappraisal of GIP pharmacology for metabolic diseases. Trends Mol Med. 2016;22(5):359–76. PMID: 27038883. http://www.ncbi.nlm.nih.gov/pubmed/27038883.

459. Christensen M, Vedtofte L, Holst JJ, Vilsbøll T, Knop FK. Glucose-dependent insulinotropic polypeptide: a bifunctional glucose-dependent regulator of glucagon and insulin secretion in humans. Diabetes. 2011;60(12):3103–9. PMCID: PMC3219957. http://www.ncbi.nlm.nih.gov/pubmed/21984584.
460. Garber AJ. Long-acting glucagon-like peptide 1 receptor agonists: a review of their efficacy and tolerability. Diabetes Care. 2011;34 Suppl 2(Suppl 2):S279–84. PMCID: PMC3632193. http://www.ncbi.nlm.nih.gov/pubmed/21525469.
461. Davidson MH. Cardiovascular effects of glucagonlike peptide-1 agonists. Am J Cardiol. 2011;108(3 Suppl):33B–41B. PMID: 21802579. http://www.ncbi.nlm.nih.gov/pubmed/21802579.
462. Ramos AC, Galvão Neto MP, de Souza YM, Galvão M, Murakami AH, Silva AC, Canseco EG, Santamaría R, Zambrano TA. Laparoscopic duodenal-jejunal exclusion in the treatment of type 2 diabetes mellitus in patients with BMI<30 kg/m2 (LBMI). Obes Surg. 2009;19(3):307–12. PMID: 18987919. http://www.ncbi.nlm.nih.gov/pubmed/18987919.
463. Zheng SL, Roddick AJ, Aghar-Jaffar R, Shun-Shin MJ, Francis D, Oliver N, Meeran K. Association between use of sodium-glucose Cotransporter 2 inhibitors, Glucagon-like Peptide 1 agonists, and dipeptidyl peptidase 4 inhibitors with all-cause mortality in patients with type 2 diabetes: a systematic review and meta-analysis. JAMA. 2018;319(15):1580–91. PMCID: PMC5933330. http://www.ncbi.nlm.nih.gov/pubmed/29677303.
464. Bethel MA, Patel RA, Merrill P, Lokhnygina Y, Buse JB, Mentz RJ, Pagidipati NJ, Chan JC, Gustavson SM, Iqbal N, Maggioni AP, Öhman P, Poulter NR, Ramachandran A, Zinman B, Hernandez AF, Holman RR, EXSCEL Study Group. Cardiovascular outcomes with glucagon-like peptide-1 receptor agonists in patients with type 2 diabetes: a meta-analysis. Lancet Diabetes Endocrinol. 2018;6(2):105–13. PMID: 29221659. http://www.ncbi.nlm.nih.gov/pubmed/29221659.
465. Nolen-Doerr E, Stockman MC, Rizo I. Mechanism of Glucagon-Like Peptide 1 improvements in type 2 diabetes mellitus and obesity. Curr Obes Rep. 2019;8(3):284–91. PMID: 31124035. http://www.ncbi.nlm.nih.gov/pubmed/31124035.
466. Tran S, Retnakaran R, Zinman B, Kramer CK. Efficacy of glucagon-like peptide-1 receptor agonists compared to dipeptidyl peptidase-4 inhibitors for the management of type 2 diabetes: a meta-analysis of randomized clinical trials. Diabetes Obes Metab. 2018;20(Suppl 1):68–76. PMID: 29364587. http://www.ncbi.nlm.nih.gov/pubmed/29364587.
467. ElSayed NA, Aleppo G, Aroda VR, Bannuru RR, Brown FM, Bruemmer D, Collins BS, Hilliard ME, Isaacs D, Johnson EL, Kahan S, Khunti K, Leon J, Lyons SK, Perry ML, Prahalad P, Pratley RE, Seley JJ, Stanton RC, Gabbay RA, on behalf of the American Diabetes Association null. 9. Pharmacologic approaches to Glycemic treatment: standards of care in diabetes-2023. Diabetes Care. 2023;46(Suppl 1):S140–57. PMCID: PMC9810476. http://www.ncbi.nlm.nih.gov/pubmed/36507650.
468. Htike ZZ, Zaccardi F, Papamargaritis D, Webb DR, Khunti K, Davies MJ. Efficacy and safety of glucagon-like peptide-1 receptor agonists in type 2 diabetes: a systematic review and mixed-treatment comparison analysis. Diabetes Obes Metab. 2017;19(4):524–36. PMID: 27981757. http://www.ncbi.nlm.nih.gov/pubmed/27981757.
469. Filippatos TD, Panagiotopoulou TV, Elisaf MS. Adverse effects of GLP-1 Receptor agonists. Rev Diabet Stud. 2014;11(3–4):202–30. PMCID: PMC5397288. http://www.ncbi.nlm.nih.gov/pubmed/26177483.
470. Trujillo JM, Nuffer W, Ellis SL. GLP-1 receptor agonists: a review of head-to-head clinical studies. Ther. Adv Endocrinol Metab. 2015;6(1):19–28. PMCID: PMC4321870. http://www.ncbi.nlm.nih.gov/pubmed/25678953.
471. Madsbad S. Review of head-to-head comparisons of glucagon-like peptide-1 receptor agonists. Diabetes Obes Metab. 2016;18(4):317–32. PMCID: PMC5064617. http://www.ncbi.nlm.nih.gov/pubmed/26511102.
472. Unger JR, Parkin CG. Glucagon-like peptide-1 (GLP-1) receptor agonists: differentiating the new medications. Diabet Ther. 2011;2(1):29–39. PMCID: PMC3124643. http://www.ncbi.nlm.nih.gov/pubmed/22127767.
473. Elashoff M, Matveyenko AV, Gier B, Elashoff R, Butler PC. Pancreatitis, pancreatic, and thyroid cancer with glucagon-like peptide-1-based therapies. Gastroenterology. 2011;141(1):150–6. PMCID: PMC4404515. http://www.ncbi.nlm.nih.gov/pubmed/21334333.
474. Tobaiqy M, Elkout H. Psychiatric adverse events associated with semaglutide, liraglutide and tirzepatide: a pharmacovigilance analysis of individual case safety reports submitted to the EudraVigilance database. Int. J Clin Pharm. 2024;46(2):488–95. PMCID: PMC10960895. http://www.ncbi.nlm.nih.gov/pubmed/38265519.
475. EudraVigilance | European Medicines Agency (EMA).
476. FDA Adverse Event Reporting System (FAERS) Database | FDA.
477. McIntyre RS, Mansur RB, Rosenblat JD, Kwan ATH. The association between glucagon-like peptide-1 receptor agonists (GLP-1 RAs) and suicidality: reports to the Food and Drug Administration Adverse Event Reporting System (FAERS). Expert Opin Drug Saf. 2024;23(1):47–55. PMID: 38087976. http://www.ncbi.nlm.nih.gov/pubmed/38087976.
478. Guirguis A, Chiappini S, Papanti PGD, Vickers-Smith R, Harris D, Corkery JM, Arillotta D, Floresta G, Martinotti G, Schifano F. Exploring the association between suicidal thoughts, self-injury, and GLP-1 receptor agonists in weight loss treatments: insights from pharmacovigilance measures and unmasking analysis. Eur Neuropsychopharmacol. 2024;82:82–91. PMID: 38508100
479. McIntyre RS. Glucagon-like peptide-1 receptor agonists (GLP-1 RAs) and suicidality: what do we know and future vistas. Expert Opin Drug Saf. 2024;23(5):539–42. PMID: 38520274. http://www.ncbi.nlm.nih.gov/pubmed/38520274.
480. Schoretsanitis G, Weiler S, Barbui C, Raschi E, Gastaldon C. Disproportionality analysis from World Health Organization data on Semaglutide, Liraglutide, and Suicidality. JAMA Netw Open. 2024;7(8):e2423385. PMCID: PMC11337067. http://www.ncbi.nlm.nih.gov/pubmed/39163046.
481. VigiBase, WHO's global database | UMC.
482. McIntyre RS, Mansur RB, Rosenblat JD, Rhee TG, Cao B, Teopiz KM, Wong S, Le GH, Ho R, Kwan ATH. Glucagon-like peptide-1 receptor agonists (GLP-1 RAs) and suicidality: a replication study using reports to the World Health Organization pharmacovigilance database (VigiBase®). J Affect Disord. 2025;369:922–7. PMID: 39433133. http://www.ncbi.nlm.nih.gov/pubmed/39433133.
483. Real-world data for the life sciences and healthcare | TriNetX
484. Kornelius E, Huang JY, Lo SC, Huang CN, Yang YS. The risk of depression, anxiety, and suicidal behavior in patients with obesity on glucagon like peptide-1 receptor agonist therapy. Sci Rep. 2024;14(1):24433. PMCID: PMC11489776. http://www.ncbi.nlm.nih.gov/pubmed/39424950.
485. Alkhezi OS, Alahmed AA, Alfayez OM, Alzuman OA, Almutairi AR, Almohammed OA. Comparative effectiveness of glucagon-like peptide-1 receptor agonists for the management of obesity in adults without diabetes: a network meta-analysis of randomized clinical trials. Obes Rev. 2023;24(3):e13543. PMID: 36579723. http://www.ncbi.nlm.nih.gov/pubmed/36579723.
486. Alfaris N, Minnick AM, Hopkins CM, Berkowitz RI, Wadden TA. Combination phentermine and topiramate extended release in the management of obesity. Expert Opin Pharmacother. 2015;16(8):1263–74. PMID: 25958964. http://www.ncbi.nlm.nih.gov/pubmed/25958964.

487. Billes SK, Greenway FL. Combination therapy with naltrexone and bupropion for obesity. Expert Opin Pharmacother. 2011;12(11):1813–26. PMID: 21689063. http://www.ncbi.nlm.nih.gov/pubmed/21689063.
488. Sherman MM, Ungureanu S, Rey JA. Naltrexone/Bupropion ER (Contrave): newly approved treatment option for chronic weight management in obese adults. P T. 2016;41(3):164–72. PMCID: PMC4771085. http://www.ncbi.nlm.nih.gov/pubmed/26957883.
489. Pennock RL, Hentges ST. Differential expression and sensitivity of presynaptic and postsynaptic opioid receptors regulating hypothalamic proopiomelanocortin neurons. J Neurosci. 2011;31(1):281–8. PMCID: PMC3061472. http://www.ncbi.nlm.nih.gov/pubmed/21209213/.
490. Greenway FL, Aronne LJ, Raben A, Astrup A, Apovian CM, Hill JO, Kaplan LM, Fujioka K, Matejkova E, Svacina S, Luzi L, Gnessi L, Navas-Carretero S, Martinez JA, Still CD, Sannino A, Saponaro C, Demitri C, Urban LE, Leider H, Chiquette E, Ron ES, Zohar Y, Heshmati HM. Erratum: a randomized, double-blind, placebo-controlled study of Gelesis100: A novel nonsystemic oral hydrogel for weight loss. Obesity (Silver Spring). 2019;27(7):1210. PMCID: PMC6885974. http://www.ncbi.nlm.nih.gov/pubmed/31231960.
491. LiverTox: Clinical and Research Information on Drug-Induced Liver Injury [Internet]. Bethesda (MD): National Institute of Diabetes and Digestive and Kidney Diseases; 2012 [cited 2025 Jan 2]. Available from: http://www.ncbi.nlm.nih.gov/books/NBK547852/ PMID: 31643176 http://www.ncbi.nlm.nih.gov/pubmed/31643176.
492. Yanovski SZ, Yanovski JA. Progress in pharmacotherapy for obesity. JAMA. 2021;326(2):129–30. PMCID: PMC8277731. http://www.ncbi.nlm.nih.gov/pubmed/34160571.
493. Pilitsi E, Farr OM, Polyzos SA, Perakakis N, Nolen-Doerr E, Papathanasiou AE, Mantzoros CS. Pharmacotherapy of obesity: available medications and drugs under investigation. Metabolism. 2019;92:170–92. PMID: 30391259. http://www.ncbi.nlm.nih.gov/pubmed/30391259.
494. Ahmad NN, Robinson S, Kennedy-Martin T, Poon JL, Kan H. Clinical outcomes associated with anti-obesity medications in real-world practice: a systematic literature review. Obes Rev. 2021;22(11):e13326. PMCID: PMC9285776. http://www.ncbi.nlm.nih.gov/pubmed/34423889.
495. Tirzepatide (Zepbound) for chronic weight management. Med Lett Drugs Ther. 2023;65(1692):205–7. PMID: 38133594. http://www.ncbi.nlm.nih.gov/pubmed/38133594.
496. Apolzan JW, Venditti EM, Edelstein SL, Knowler WC, Dabelea D, Boyko EJ, Pi-Sunyer X, Kalyani RR, Franks PW, Srikanthan P, Gadde KM, Diabetes Prevention Program Research Group. Long-term weight loss with metformin or lifestyle intervention in the diabetes prevention program outcomes study. Ann Intern Med. 2019;170(10):682–90. PMCID: PMC6829283. http://www.ncbi.nlm.nih.gov/pubmed/31009939.
497. FDA clarifies policies for compounders as national GLP-1 supply begins to stabilize | FDA.
498. Tempia Valenta S, Stecchi M, Perazza F, Nuccitelli C, Villanova N, Pironi L, Atti AR, Petroni ML. Liraglutide 3.0 mg and mental health: can psychiatric symptoms be associated to adherence to therapy? Insights from a clinical audit. Eat Weight Disord. 2023;28(1):99. PMCID: PMC10684642. http://www.ncbi.nlm.nih.gov/pubmed/38015342.
499. Dumiaty Y, Underwood BM, Phy-Lim J, Chee MJ. Neurocircuitry underlying the actions of glucagon-like peptide 1 and peptide YY3-36 in the suppression of food, drug-seeking, and anxiogenesis. Neuropeptides. 2024;105:102427. PMID: 38579490. http://www.ncbi.nlm.nih.gov/pubmed/38579490.
500. Durell N, Franks R, Coon S, Cowart K, Carris NW. Effect of antidepressants on Glucagon-Like Peptide-1 Receptor agonist-related weight loss. J Pharm Technol. 2022;38(5):283–8. PMCID: PMC9420918. http://www.ncbi.nlm.nih.gov/pubmed/36046348.
501. Mansur RB, Lee Y, Subramaniapillai M, Brietzke E, McIntyre RS. Cognitive dysfunction and metabolic comorbidities in mood disorders: a repurposing opportunity for glucagon-like peptide 1 receptor agonists? Neuropharmacology. 2018;136(Pt B):335–42. PMID: 29481915. http://www.ncbi.nlm.nih.gov/pubmed/29481915.
502. Anderberg RH, Richard JE, Hansson C, Nissbrandt H, Bergquist F, Skibicka KP. GLP-1 is both anxiogenic and antidepressant; divergent effects of acute and chronic GLP-1 on emotionality. Psychoneuroendocrinology. 2016;65:54–66. PMID: 26724568. http://www.ncbi.nlm.nih.gov/pubmed/26724568.
503. Lazzati A. Epidemiology of the surgical management of obesity. J Visc Surg. 2023;160(2S):S3–6. PMID: 36725453. http://www.ncbi.nlm.nih.gov/pubmed/36725453.
504. Lee WJ, Almalki O. Recent advancements in bariatric/metabolic surgery. Ann Gastroenterol Surg. 2017;1(3):171–9. PMCID: PMC5881368. http://www.ncbi.nlm.nih.gov/pubmed/29863165.
505. Peterli R, Wölnerhanssen BK, Peters T, Vetter D, Kröll D, Borbély Y, Schultes B, Beglinger C, Drewe J, Schiesser M, Nett P, Bueter M. Effect of laparoscopic sleeve gastrectomy vs laparoscopic Roux-en-Y gastric bypass on weight loss in patients with morbid obesity: the SM-BOSS randomized clinical trial. JAMA. 2018;319(3):255–65. PMCID: PMC5833546. http://www.ncbi.nlm.nih.gov/pubmed/29340679.
506. Courcoulas A, Abu Dayyeh BK, Eaton L, Robinson J, Woodman G, Fusco M, Shayani V, Billy H, Pambianco D, Gostout C. Intragastric balloon as an adjunct to lifestyle intervention: a randomized controlled trial. Int J Obes. 2017;41(3):427–33. PMID: 28017964. http://www.ncbi.nlm.nih.gov/pubmed/28017964.
507. Qureshi H, Saeed N, Jovani M. Updates in endoscopic bariatric and metabolic therapies. J Clin Med. 2023;12(3):1126. PMCID: PMC9917553. http://www.ncbi.nlm.nih.gov/pubmed/36769774.
508. Abu Dayyeh BK, Bazerbachi F, Vargas EJ, Sharaiha RZ, Thompson CC, Thaemert BC, Teixeira AF, Chapman CG, Kumbhari V, Ujiki MB, Ahrens J, Day C, MERIT Study Group, Galvao Neto M, Zundel N, Wilson EB. Endoscopic sleeve gastroplasty for treatment of class 1 and 2 obesity (MERIT): a prospective, multicentre, randomised trial. Lancet. 2022;400(10350):441–51. PMID: 35908555. http://www.ncbi.nlm.nih.gov/pubmed/35908555.
509. Arterburn DE, Telem DA, Kushner RF, Courcoulas AP. Benefits and risks of bariatric surgery in adults: a review. JAMA. 2020;324(9):879–87. PMID: 32870301. http://www.ncbi.nlm.nih.gov/pubmed/32870301.
510. Simoni AH, Ladebo L, Christrup LL, Drewes AM, Johnsen SP, Olesen AE. Chronic abdominal pain and persistent opioid use after bariatric surgery. Scand. J Pain. 2020;20(2):239–51. PMID: 31756166. http://www.ncbi.nlm.nih.gov/pubmed/31756166.
511. Rosenberger PH, Henderson KE, Grilo CM. Psychiatric disorder comorbidity and association with eating disorders in bariatric surgery patients: a cross-sectional study using structured interview-based diagnosis. J Clin Psychiatry. 2006;67(7):1080–5. PMID: 16889451. http://www.ncbi.nlm.nih.gov/pubmed/16889451.
512. Kalarchian MA, Marcus MD, Levine MD, Courcoulas AP, Pilkonis PA, Ringham RM, Soulakova JN, Weissfeld LA, Rofey DL. Psychiatric disorders among bariatric surgery candidates: relationship to obesity and functional health status. Am J Psychiatry. 2007;164(2):328–34. quiz 374. PMID: 17267797. http://www.ncbi.nlm.nih.gov/pubmed/17267797.
513. de Zwaan M, Enderle J, Wagner S, Mühlhans B, Ditzen B, Gefeller O, Mitchell JE, Müller A. Anxiety and depression in bariatric surgery patients: a prospective, follow-up study using structured clinical interviews. J Affect Disord. 2011;133(1–2):61–8. PMID: 21501874. http://www.ncbi.nlm.nih.gov/pubmed/21501874.

514. Hayden MJ, Dixon JB, Dixon ME, Shea TL, O'Brien PE. Characterization of the improvement in depressive symptoms following bariatric surgery. Obes Surg. 2011;21(3):328–35. PMID: 20559893. http://www.ncbi.nlm.nih.gov/pubmed/20559893.
515. Fu R, Zhang Y, Yu K, Mao D, Su H. Bariatric surgery alleviates depression in obese patients: a systematic review and meta-analysis. Obes Res Clin Pract. 2022;16(1):10–6. PMID: 34802982. http://www.ncbi.nlm.nih.gov/pubmed/34802982.
516. Rutledge T, Braden AL, Woods G, Herbst KL, Groesz LM, Savu M. Five-year changes in psychiatric treatment status and weight-related comorbidities following bariatric surgery in a veteran population. Obes Surg. 2012;22(11):1734–41. PMID: 23011461. http://www.ncbi.nlm.nih.gov/pubmed/23011461.
517. Lier HO, Biringer E, Hove O, Stubhaug B, Tangen T. Quality of life among patients undergoing bariatric surgery: associations with mental health- a 1 year follow-up study of bariatric surgery patients. Health Qual Life Outcomes. 2011;9:79. PMCID: PMC3192661. http://www.ncbi.nlm.nih.gov/pubmed/21943381.
518. Mitchell JE, King WC, Chen JY, Devlin MJ, Flum D, Garcia L, Inabet W, Pender JR, Kalarchian MA, Khandelwal S, Marcus MD, Schrope B, Strain G, Wolfe B, Yanovski S. Course of depressive symptoms and treatment in the longitudinal assessment of bariatric surgery (LABS-2) study. Obesity (Silver Spring). 2014;22(8):1799–806. PMCID: PMC4115026. http://www.ncbi.nlm.nih.gov/pubmed/24634371.
519. Livhits M, Mercado C, Yermilov I, Parikh JA, Dutson E, Mehran A, Ko CY, Gibbons MM. Preoperative predictors of weight loss following bariatric surgery: systematic review. Obes Surg. 2012;22(1):70–89. PMID: 21833817. http://www.ncbi.nlm.nih.gov/pubmed/21833817.
520. Pontiroli AE, Fossati A, Vedani P, Fiorilli M, Folli F, Paganelli M, Marchi M, Maffei C. Post-surgery adherence to scheduled visits and compliance, more than personality disorders, predict outcome of bariatric restrictive surgery in morbidly obese patients. Obes Surg. 2007;17(11):1492–7. PMID: 18219777. http://www.ncbi.nlm.nih.gov/pubmed/18219777.
521. Mauri M, Rucci P, Calderone A, Santini F, Oppo A, Romano A, Rinaldi S, Armani A, Polini M, Pinchera A, Cassano GB. Axis I and II disorders and quality of life in bariatric surgery candidates. J Clin Psychiatry. 2008;69(2):295–301. PMID: 18251626. http://www.ncbi.nlm.nih.gov/pubmed/18251626.
522. Martínez EP, González ST, Vicente MM, van-der Hofstadt Román CJ, Rodríguez-Marín J. Psychopathology in a sample of candidate patients for bariatric surgery. Int J Psychiatry Clin Pract. 2013;17(3):197–205. PMID: 22746988. http://www.ncbi.nlm.nih.gov/pubmed/22746988.
523. Alciati A, Gesuele F, Casazza G, Foschi D. The relationship between childhood parental loss and metabolic syndrome in obese subjects. Stress Health. 2013;29(1):5–13. PMID: 22190357. http://www.ncbi.nlm.nih.gov/pubmed/22190357.
524. Alciati A, Gesuele F, Rizzi A, Sarzi-Puttini P, Foschi D. Childhood parental loss and bipolar spectrum in obese bariatric surgery candidates. Int J Psychiatry Med. 2011;41(2):155–71. PMID: 21675347. http://www.ncbi.nlm.nih.gov/pubmed/21675347.
525. Salwen JK, Hymowitz GF, O'Leary KD, Pryor AD, Vivian D. Childhood verbal abuse: a risk factor for depression in pre-bariatric surgery psychological evaluations. Obes Surg. 2014;24(9):1572–5. PMID: 24858597. http://www.ncbi.nlm.nih.gov/pubmed/24858597.
526. Buser AT, Lam CS, Poplawski SC. A long-term cross-sectional study on gastric bypass surgery: impact of self-reported past sexual abuse. Obes Surg. 2009;19(4):422–6. PMID: 18516655. http://www.ncbi.nlm.nih.gov/pubmed/18516655.
527. Troisi A. Emergence of bariatric psychiatry as a new subspecialty. World. J Psychiatry. 2022;12(1):108–16. PMCID: PMC8783166. http://www.ncbi.nlm.nih.gov/pubmed/35111582.
528. Gibbons MM, Maher AR, Dawes AJ, Booth MS, Miake-Lye IM, Beroes JM, Shekelle PG. Mental health assessment and psychosocial interventions for bariatric surgery [Internet]. Washington (DC): Department of Veterans Affairs (US). 2014 [cited 2025 Jan 3]. Available from: http://www.ncbi.nlm.nih.gov/books/NBK343838/ PMID: 26889521 http://www.ncbi.nlm.nih.gov/pubmed/26889521.
529. Fried M, Yumuk V, Oppert JM, Scopinaro N, Torres AJ, Weiner R, Yashkov Y, Frühbeck G. European Association for the Study of Obesity, International Federation for the Surgery of Obesity - European Chapter. Interdisciplinary European guidelines on metabolic and bariatric surgery. Obes Facts. 2013;6(5):449–68. PMCID: PMC5644681. http://www.ncbi.nlm.nih.gov/pubmed/24135948.
530. Susmallian S, Nikiforova I, Azoulai S, Barnea R. Outcomes of bariatric surgery in patients with depression disorders. PLoS One. 2019;14(8):e0221576. PMCID: PMC6711535. http://www.ncbi.nlm.nih.gov/pubmed/31454382.
531. Alshammari SA, Alassiri MA, Allami HA, Almousa HM, Alobaid AS, Ismail DH, Bin Onayq AI. The prevalence of depression and anxiety in post-bariatric surgery patients at King Khalid University Hospital, Riyadh. Cureus. 2022;14(12):e32500. PMCID: PMC9837663. http://www.ncbi.nlm.nih.gov/pubmed/36644066.
532. Wadden TA, Faulconbridge LF, Jones-Corneille LR, Sarwer DB, Fabricatore AN, Thomas JG, Wilson GT, Alexander MG, Pulcini ME, Webb VL, Williams NN. Binge eating disorder and the outcome of bariatric surgery at one year: a prospective, observational study. Obesity (Silver Spring). 2011;19(6):1220–8. PMCID: PMC3085093. http://www.ncbi.nlm.nih.gov/pubmed/21253005.
533. Azam H, Shahrestani S, Phan K. Alcohol use disorders before and after bariatric surgery: a systematic review and meta-analysis. Ann Transl Med. 2018;6(8):148. PMCID: PMC5952017. http://www.ncbi.nlm.nih.gov/pubmed/29862237.
534. García Díaz E, Martín FT. Preoperative determinants of outcomes of laparoscopic gastric bypass in the treatment of morbid obesity. Nutr Hosp. 2011;26(4):851–5. PMID: 22470034. http://www.ncbi.nlm.nih.gov/pubmed/22470034.
535. Ortega J, Fernandez-Canet R, Alvarez-Valdeita S, Cassinello N, Baguena-Puigcerver MJ. Predictors of psychological symptoms in morbidly obese patients after gastric bypass surgery. Surg Obes Relat Dis. 2012;8(6):770–6. PMID: 21640667. http://www.ncbi.nlm.nih.gov/pubmed/21640667.
536. van Hout GCM, Boekestein P, Fortuin FAM, Pelle AJM, van Heck GL. Psychosocial functioning following bariatric surgery. Obes Surg. 2006;16(6):787–94. PMID: 16756745. http://www.ncbi.nlm.nih.gov/pubmed/16756745.
537. Aarts EO, Dogan K, Koehestanie P, Aufenacker TJ, Janssen IMC, Berends FJ. Long-term results after laparoscopic adjustable gastric banding: a mean fourteen year follow-up study. Surg Obes Relat Dis. 2014;10(4):633–40. PMID: 25066440. http://www.ncbi.nlm.nih.gov/pubmed/25066440.
538. Biörserud C, Olbers T, Fagevik OM. Patients' experience of surplus skin after laparoscopic gastric bypass. Obes Surg. 2011;21(3):273–7. PMID: 19455374. http://www.ncbi.nlm.nih.gov/pubmed/19455374.
539. Sogg S, Gorman MJ. Interpersonal changes and challenges after weight-loss surgery. Prim Psychiatry. 2008;15(8):61–6. (PDF) Interpersonal changes and challenges after weight-loss surgery.
540. King WC, Chen JY, Mitchell JE, Kalarchian MA, Steffen KJ, Engel SG, Courcoulas AP, Pories WJ, Yanovski SZ. Prevalence of alcohol use disorders before and after bariatric surgery. JAMA. 2012;307(23):2516–25. PMCID: PMC3682834. http://www.ncbi.nlm.nih.gov/pubmed/22710289.

541. Tindle HA, Omalu B, Courcoulas A, Marcus M, Hammers J, Kuller LH. Risk of suicide after long-term follow-up from bariatric surgery. Am J Med. 2010;123(11):1036–42. PMCID: PMC4296730. http://www.ncbi.nlm.nih.gov/pubmed/20843498.
542. Dixon JB, Dixon ME, O'Brien PE. Depression in association with severe obesity: changes with weight loss. Arch Intern Med. 2003;163(17):2058–65. PMID: 14504119. http://www.ncbi.nlm.nih.gov/pubmed/14504119.
543. White MA, Kalarchian MA, Levine MD, Masheb RM, Marcus MD, Grilo CM. Prognostic significance of depressive symptoms on weight loss and psychosocial outcomes following gastric bypass surgery: a prospective 24-month follow-up study. Obes Surg. 2015;25(10):1909–16. PMCID: PMC4551611. http://www.ncbi.nlm.nih.gov/pubmed/25720515.
544. Berkowitz RI, Fabricatore AN. Obesity, psychiatric status, and psychiatric medications. Psychiatr Clin North Am. 2011;34(4):747–64. PMID: 22098801. http://www.ncbi.nlm.nih.gov/pubmed/22098801.
545. Krukowski RA, Friedman KE, Applegate KL. The utility of the Beck Depression Inventory in a bariatric surgery population. Obes Surg. 2010;20(4):426–31. PMID: 18841428. http://www.ncbi.nlm.nih.gov/pubmed/18841428.
546. Munoz DJ, Chen E, Fischer S, Roehrig M, Sanchez-Johnson L, Alverdy J, Dymek-Valentine M, le Grange D. Considerations for the use of the Beck Depression Inventory in the assessment of weight-loss surgery seeking patients. Obes Surg. 2007;17(8):1097–101. PMID: 17953246. http://www.ncbi.nlm.nih.gov/pubmed/17953246.
547. Mowoh DPM, Cole R, Sarvepalli S, Grover K, Abbas M, Khaitan L. Bariatric surgery efficacy in patients with mood disorders. Surgery. 2024;175(4):943–6. PMID: 38171967. http://www.ncbi.nlm.nih.gov/pubmed/38171967.
548. Brunault P, Jacobi D, Miknius V, Bourbao-Tournois C, Huten N, Gaillard P, Couet C, Camus V, Ballon N. High preoperative depression, phobic anxiety, and binge eating scores and low medium-term weight loss in sleeve gastrectomy obese patients: a preliminary cohort study. Psychosomatics. 2012;53(4):363–70. PMID: 22458986. http://www.ncbi.nlm.nih.gov/pubmed/22458986.
549. Toussi R, Fujioka K, Coleman KJ. Pre- and postsurgery behavioral compliance, patient health, and postbariatric surgical weight loss. Obesity (Silver Spring). 2009;17(5):996–1002. PMID: 19165167. http://www.ncbi.nlm.nih.gov/pubmed/19165167.
550. Gorin AA, Raftopoulos I. Effect of mood and eating disorders on the short-term outcome of laparoscopic Roux-en-Y gastric bypass. Obes Surg. 2009;19(12):1685–90. PMID: 18810566. http://www.ncbi.nlm.nih.gov/pubmed/18810566.
551. Júnior WS, do Amaral JL, Nonino-Borges CB. Factors related to weight loss up to 4 years after bariatric surgery. Obes Surg. 2011;21(11):1724–30. PMID: 21509481. http://www.ncbi.nlm.nih.gov/pubmed/21509481.
552. Ramirez JL, Kim E, Fregenal AC, Vigran HJ, Hughes SE, Reynolds CW, Varban OA, Carlin AM, Ehlers AP, Bonham AJ, Finks JF. Depression as a risk factor for adverse outcomes and increased healthcare utilization in bariatric surgery patients. Surg Endosc. 2023;37(12):9582–90. PMID: 37735218. http://www.ncbi.nlm.nih.gov/pubmed/37735218.
553. Diep C, Lee S, Xue Y, Xiao M, Pivetta B, Daza JF, Jung JJ, Wijeysundera DN, Ladha KS. Preoperative depression and outcomes after metabolic and bariatric surgery: a systematic narrative review. Obes Rev. 2024;25(7):e13743. PMID: 38572605. http://www.ncbi.nlm.nih.gov/pubmed/38572605.
554. Wimmelmann CL, Dela F, Mortensen EL. Psychological predictors of weight loss after bariatric surgery: a review of the recent research. Obes Res Clin Pract. 2014;8(4):e299–313. PMID: 25091351. http://www.ncbi.nlm.nih.gov/pubmed/25091351.
555. Alger-Mayer S, Rosati C, Polimeni JM, Malone M. Preoperative binge eating status and gastric bypass surgery: a long-term outcome study. Obes Surg. 2009;19(2):139–45. PMID: 18478306. http://www.ncbi.nlm.nih.gov/pubmed/18478306.
556. Thonney B, Pataky Z, Badel S, Bobbioni-Harsch E, Golay A. The relationship between weight loss and psychosocial functioning among bariatric surgery patients. Am J Surg. 2010;199(2):183–8. PMID: 19362287. http://www.ncbi.nlm.nih.gov/pubmed/19362287.
557. Scholtz S, Bidlake L, Morgan J, Fiennes A, El-Etar A, Lacey JH, McCluskey S. Long-term outcomes following laparoscopic adjustable gastric banding: postoperative psychological sequelae predict outcome at 5-year follow-up. Obes Surg. 2007;17(9):1220–5. PMID: 18074498. http://www.ncbi.nlm.nih.gov/pubmed/18074498.
558. Masheb RM, White MA, Toth CM, Burke-Martindale CH, Rothschild B, Grilo CM. The prognostic significance of depressive symptoms for predicting quality of life 12 months after gastric bypass. Compr Psychiatry. 2007;48(3):231–6. PMID: 17445516. http://www.ncbi.nlm.nih.gov/pubmed/17445516.
559. Sheets CS, Peat CM, Berg KC, White EK, Bocchieri-Ricciardi L, Chen EY, Mitchell JE. Post-operative psychosocial predictors of outcome in bariatric surgery. Obes Surg. 2015;25(2):330–45. PMCID: PMC4538993. http://www.ncbi.nlm.nih.gov/pubmed/25381119.
560. Rutledge T, Groesz LM, Savu M. Psychiatric factors and weight loss patterns following gastric bypass surgery in a veteran population. Obes Surg. 2011;21(1):29–35. PMCID: PMC3008931. http://www.ncbi.nlm.nih.gov/pubmed/19847571.
561. Becerra AZ, Khalid SI, Morgenstern AS, Rembert EA, Carroll MM, Omotosho PA, Torquati A. The association between bariatric surgery and psychiatric disorders: a National Cohort Study. Obes Surg. 2022;32(4):1110–8. PMID: 35044598. http://www.ncbi.nlm.nih.gov/pubmed/35044598.
562. Thanos PK, Gold MS, Blum K, Badgaiyan RD, Avena NM. Bariatric surgery: potential post-operative heightened sensitivity to substances or behaviors. J Syst Integr Neurosci. 2021;8:1. PMCID: PMC9367099. http://www.ncbi.nlm.nih.gov/pubmed/35965990.
563. Lu CW, Chang YK, Lee YH, Kuo CS, Chang HH, Huang CT, Hsu CC, Huang KC. Increased risk for major depressive disorder in severely obese patients after bariatric surgery - a 12-year nationwide cohort study. Ann Med. 2018;50(7):605–12. PMID: 30101619. http://www.ncbi.nlm.nih.gov/pubmed/30101619.
564. Sauerland S, Angrisani L, Belachew M, Chevallier JM, Favretti F, Finer N, Fingerhut A, Garcia Caballero M, Guisado Macias JA, Mittermair R, Morino M, Msika S, Rubino F, Tacchino R, Weiner R, Neugebauer E, a. M, European Association for Endoscopic Surgery. Obesity surgery: evidence-based guidelines of the European Association for Endoscopic Surgery (EAES). Surg Endosc. 2005;19(2):200–21. PMID: 15580436. http://www.ncbi.nlm.nih.gov/pubmed/15580436.
565. Greenberg I, Sogg S, Perna MF. Behavioral and psychological care in weight loss surgery: best practice update. Obesity (Silver Spring). 2009;17(5):880–4. PMID: 19396066. http://www.ncbi.nlm.nih.gov/pubmed/19396066.
566. Mechanick JI, Kushner RF, Sugerman HJ, Gonzalez-Campoy JM, Collazo-Clavell ML, Spitz AF, Apovian CM, Livingston EH, Brolin R, Sarwer DB, Anderson WA, Dixon J, Guven S, American Association of Clinical Endocrinologists, Obesity Society, American Society for Metabolic & Bariatric Surgery. American Association of Clinical Endocrinologists, The Obesity Society, and American Society for Metabolic & Bariatric Surgery medical guidelines for clinical practice for the perioperative nutritional,

metabolic, and nonsurgical support of the bariatric surgery patient. Obesity (Silver Spring). 2009;17 Suppl 1:S1–70, v. PMID: 19319140. http://www.ncbi.nlm.nih.gov/pubmed/19319140.
567. Zijlstra H, Boeije HR, Larsen JK, van Ramshorst B, Geenen R. Patients' explanations for unsuccessful weight loss after laparoscopic adjustable gastric banding (LAGB). Patient Educ Couns. 2009;75(1):108–13. PMID: 19019618. http://www.ncbi.nlm.nih.gov/pubmed/19019618.
568. Wardé-Kamar J, Rogers M, Flancbaum L, Laferrère B. Calorie intake and meal patterns up to 4 years after Roux-en-Y gastric bypass surgery. Obes Surg. 2004;14(8):1070–9. PMID: 15479596. http://www.ncbi.nlm.nih.gov/pubmed/15479596.
569. Welch G, Wesolowski C, Zagarins S, Kuhn J, Romanelli J, Garb J, Allen N. Evaluation of clinical outcomes for gastric bypass surgery: results from a comprehensive follow-up study. Obes Surg. 2011;21(1):18–28. PMID: 20087678. http://www.ncbi.nlm.nih.gov/pubmed/20087678.
570. Sarwer DB, Wadden TA, Moore RH, Baker AW, Gibbons LM, Raper SE, Williams NN. Preoperative eating behavior, postoperative dietary adherence, and weight loss after gastric bypass surgery. Surg Obes Relat Dis. 2008;4(5):640–6. PMCID: PMC2610859. http://www.ncbi.nlm.nih.gov/pubmed/18586571.
571. Higa K, Ho T, Tercero F, Yunus T, Boone KB. Laparoscopic Roux-en-Y gastric bypass: 10-year follow-up. Surg Obes Relat Dis. 2011;7(4):516–25. PMID: 21333610. http://www.ncbi.nlm.nih.gov/pubmed/21333610.
572. Christou NV, Look D, Maclean LD. Weight gain after short- and long-limb gastric bypass in patients followed for longer than 10 years. Ann Surg. 2006;244(5):734–40. PMCID: PMC1856611. http://www.ncbi.nlm.nih.gov/pubmed/17060766.
573. Kofman MD, Lent MR, Swencionis C. Maladaptive eating patterns, quality of life, and weight outcomes following gastric bypass: results of an Internet survey. Obesity (Silver Spring). 2010;18(10):1938–43. PMID: 20168309. http://www.ncbi.nlm.nih.gov/pubmed/20168309.
574. Rusch MD, Andris D. Maladaptive eating patterns after weight-loss surgery. Nutr Clin Pract. 2007;22(1):41–9. PMID: 17242453. http://www.ncbi.nlm.nih.gov/pubmed/17242453.
575. de Zwaan M, Hilbert A, Swan-Kremeier L, Simonich H, Lancaster K, Howell LM, Monson T, Crosby RD, Mitchell JE. Comprehensive interview assessment of eating behavior 18-35 months after gastric bypass surgery for morbid obesity. Surg Obes Relat Dis. 2010;6(1):79–85. PMID: 19837012. http://www.ncbi.nlm.nih.gov/pubmed/19837012.
576. Colles SL, Dixon JB, O'Brien PE. Grazing and loss of control related to eating: two high-risk factors following bariatric surgery. Obesity (Silver Spring). 2008;16(3):615–22. PMID: 18239603. http://www.ncbi.nlm.nih.gov/pubmed/18239603.
577. Conason A, Teixeira J, Hsu CH, Puma L, Knafo D, Geliebter A. Substance use following bariatric weight loss surgery. JAMA Surg. 2013;148(2):145–50. PMID: 23560285. http://www.ncbi.nlm.nih.gov/pubmed/23560285.
578. Omalu BI, Luckasevic T, Shakir AM, Rozin L, Wecht CH, Kuller LH. Postbariatric surgery deaths, which fall under the jurisdiction of the coroner. Am J Forensic Med Pathol. 2004;25(3):237–42. PMID: 15322466. http://www.ncbi.nlm.nih.gov/pubmed/15322466.
579. NIH conference. Gastrointestinal surgery for severe obesity. Consensus development conference panel. Ann Intern Med. 1991;115(12):956–61. PMID: 1952493. http://www.ncbi.nlm.nih.gov/pubmed/1952493.
580. Sogg S, Lauretti J, West-Smith L. Recommendations for the presurgical psychosocial evaluation of bariatric surgery patients. Surg Obes Relat Dis. 2016;12(4):731–49. PMID: 27179400. http://www.ncbi.nlm.nih.gov/pubmed/27179400.
581. Lanyon RI, Maxwell BM. Predictors of outcome after gastric bypass surgery. Obes Surg. 2007;17(3):321–8. PMID: 17546839. http://www.ncbi.nlm.nih.gov/pubmed/17546839.
582. Wadden TA, Butryn ML, Sarwer DB, Fabricatore AN, Crerand CE, Lipschutz PE, Faulconbridge L, Raper SE, Williams NN. Comparison of psychosocial status in treatment-seeking women with class III vs. class I-II obesity. Obesity (Silver Spring). 2006;14(Suppl 2):90S–8S. PMID: 16648600. http://www.ncbi.nlm.nih.gov/pubmed/16648600.
583. Ashton D, Favretti F, Segato G. Preoperative psychological testing—another form of prejudice. Obes Surg. 2008;18(10):1330–7. PMID: 18335282. http://www.ncbi.nlm.nih.gov/pubmed/18335282.
584. Fabricatore AN, Crerand CE, Wadden TA, Sarwer DB, Krasucki JL. How do mental health professionals evaluate candidates for bariatric surgery? Survey results. Obes Surg. 2006;16(5):567–73. PMID: 16687023. http://www.ncbi.nlm.nih.gov/pubmed/16687023.
585. Wadden TA, Sarwer DB. Behavioral assessment of candidates for bariatric surgery: a patient-oriented approach. Obesity (Silver Spring). 2006;14(Suppl 2):53S–62S. PMID: 16648595. http://www.ncbi.nlm.nih.gov/pubmed/16648595.
586. Allison KC, Wadden TA, Sarwer DB, Fabricatore AN, Crerand CE, Gibbons LM, Stack RM, Stunkard AJ, Williams NN. Night eating syndrome and binge eating disorder among persons seeking bariatric surgery: prevalence and related features. Obesity (Silver Spring). 2006;14(Suppl 2):77S–82S. PMID: 16648598. http://www.ncbi.nlm.nih.gov/pubmed/16648598.
587. Meany G, Conceição E, Mitchell JE. Binge eating, binge eating disorder and loss of control eating: effects on weight outcomes after bariatric surgery. Eur Eat Disord Rev. 2014;22(2):87–91. PMCID: PMC4420157. http://www.ncbi.nlm.nih.gov/pubmed/24347539.
588. Mechanick JI, Youdim A, Jones DB, Timothy Garvey W, Hurley DL, Molly McMahon M, Heinberg LJ, Kushner R, Adams TD, Shikora S, Dixon JB, Brethauer S. Clinical practice guidelines for the perioperative nutritional, metabolic, and nonsurgical support of the bariatric surgery patient--2013 update: cosponsored by American Association of Clinical Endocrinologists, the Obesity Society, and American Society for Metabolic & Bariatric Surgery. Surg Obes Relat Dis. 2013;9(2):159–91. PMID: 23537696. http://www.ncbi.nlm.nih.gov/pubmed/23537696.
589. Marino JM, Ertelt TW, Lancaster K, Steffen K, Peterson L, de Zwaan M, Mitchell JE. The emergence of eating pathology after bariatric surgery: a rare outcome with important clinical implications. Int J Eat Disord. 2012;45(2):179–84. PMID: 21495051. http://www.ncbi.nlm.nih.gov/pubmed/21495051.
590. Conceição EM, Crosby R, Mitchell JE, Engel SG, Wonderlich SA, Simonich HK, Peterson CB, Crow SJ, Le Grange D. Picking or nibbling: frequency and associated clinical features in bulimia nervosa, anorexia nervosa, and binge eating disorder. Int J Eat Disord. 2013;46(8):815–8. PMCID: PMC4009470. http://www.ncbi.nlm.nih.gov/pubmed/23922133.
591. Mitchell JE, King WC, Courcoulas A, Dakin G, Elder K, Engel S, Flum D, Kalarchian M, Khandelwal S, Pender J, Pories W, Wolfe B. Eating behavior and eating disorders in adults before bariatric surgery. Int J Eat Disord. 2015;48(2):215–22. PMCID: PMC4192110. http://www.ncbi.nlm.nih.gov/pubmed/24719222.
592. Malik S, Mitchell JE, Engel S, Crosby R, Wonderlich S. Psychopathology in bariatric surgery candidates: a review of studies using structured diagnostic interviews. Compr Psychiatry. 2014;55(2):248–59. PMCID: PMC3985130. http://www.ncbi.nlm.nih.gov/pubmed/24290079.
593. Bonfà F, Marchetta L, Avanzi M, Baldini E, Raselli R, Uber E, Cabrini S. Exploratory evaluation of an obese population seeking bariatric surgery in an Italian public service. Eat Weight Disord.

2010;15(3):e119–26. PMID: 21150247. http://www.ncbi.nlm.nih.gov/pubmed/21150247.

594. Wadden TA, Sarwer DB, Fabricatore AN, Jones L, Stack R, Williams NS. Psychosocial and behavioral status of patients undergoing bariatric surgery: what to expect before and after surgery. Med Clin North Am. 2007;91(3):451–469, xi–xii. PMID: 17509389. http://www.ncbi.nlm.nih.gov/pubmed/17509389.
595. Hayden MJ, Murphy KD, Brown WA, O'Brien PE. Axis I disorders in adjustable gastric band patients: the relationship between psychopathology and weight loss. Obes Surg. 2014;24(9):1469–75. PMID: 24570091. http://www.ncbi.nlm.nih.gov/pubmed/24570091.
596. Hamoui N, Kingsbury S, Anthone GJ, Crookes PF. Surgical treatment of morbid obesity in schizophrenic patients. Obes Surg. 2004;14(3):349–52. PMID: 15072656. http://www.ncbi.nlm.nih.gov/pubmed/15072656.
597. Lier HØ, Biringer E, Stubhaug B, Eriksen HR, Tangen T. Psychiatric disorders and participation in pre- and postoperative counselling groups in bariatric surgery patients. Obes Surg. 2011;21(6):730–7. PMID: 20396993. http://www.ncbi.nlm.nih.gov/pubmed/20396993.
598. Miras AD, Al-Najim W, Jackson SN, McGirr J, Cotter L, Tharakan G, Vusirikala A, le Roux CW, Prechtl CG, Scholtz S. Psychological characteristics, eating behavior, and quality of life assessment of obese patients undergoing weight loss interventions. Scand J Surg. 2015;104(1):10–7. PMID: 25053582. http://www.ncbi.nlm.nih.gov/pubmed/25053582.
599. Rutledge T, Adler S, Friedman R. A prospective assessment of psychosocial factors among bariatric versus non-bariatric surgery candidates. Obes Surg. 2011;21(10):1570–9. PMCID: PMC3179584. http://www.ncbi.nlm.nih.gov/pubmed/20872090.
600. Legenbauer T, De Zwaan M, Benecke A, Muhlhans B, Petrak F, Herpertz S. Depression and anxiety: their predictive function for weight loss in obese individuals. Obes Facts. 2009;2(4):227–34. PMCID: PMC6515937. http://www.ncbi.nlm.nih.gov/pubmed/20054228.
601. Sogg S, Mori DL. Psychosocial evaluation for bariatric surgery: the Boston interview and opportunities for intervention. Obes Surg. 2009;19(3):369–77. PMID: 18795379. http://www.ncbi.nlm.nih.gov/pubmed/18795379.
602. Paul L, van der Heiden C, Hoek HW. Cognitive behavioral therapy and predictors of weight loss in bariatric surgery patients. Curr Opin Psychiatry. 2017;30(6):474–9. PMID: 28795980. http://www.ncbi.nlm.nih.gov/pubmed/28795980.
603. Gill H, Kang S, Lee Y, Rosenblat JD, Brietzke E, Zuckerman H, McIntyre RS. The long-term effect of bariatric surgery on depression and anxiety. J Affect Disord. 2019;246:886–894. PMID: 30795495. http://www.ncbi.nlm.nih.gov/pubmed/30795495.
604. By-Band-Sleeve Collaborating Group. Prevalence and short-term change in symptoms of anxiety and depression following bariatric surgery: a prospective cohort study. BMJ Open. 2024;14(1):e071231. PMCID: PMC10773381. http://www.ncbi.nlm.nih.gov/pubmed/38171620.
605. Teixeira PJ, Silva MN, Mata J, Palmeira AL, Markland D. Motivation, self-determination, and long-term weight control. Int J Behav Nutr Phys Act. 2012;9:22. PMCID: PMC3312817. http://www.ncbi.nlm.nih.gov/pubmed/22385818.
606. Alyahya RA, Alnujaidi MA. Prevalence and outcomes of depression after bariatric surgery: a systematic review and meta-analysis. Cureus. 2022;14(6):e25651. PMCID: PMC9249077. http://www.ncbi.nlm.nih.gov/pubmed/35784972.
607. Sockalingam S, Leung SE, Wnuk S, Cassin SE, Yanofsky R, Hawa R. Psychiatric management of bariatric surgery patients: a review of psychopharmacological and psychological treatments and their impact on postoperative mental health and weight outcomes. Psychosomatics. 2020;61(5):498–507. PMID: 32451127. http://www.ncbi.nlm.nih.gov/pubmed/32451127.
608. Baillot A, Brais-Dussault E, Bastin A, Cyr C, Brunet J, Aimé A, Romain AJ, Langlois MF, Bouchard S, Tchernof A, Rabasa-Lhoret R, Garneau PY, Bernard P. What is known about the correlates and impact of excess skin after bariatric surgery: a scoping review. Obes Surg. 2017;27(9):2488–98. PMID: 28681262. http://www.ncbi.nlm.nih.gov/pubmed/28681262.
609. The Impact of Bariatric Surgery on Depression: a Review | Current Cardiovascular Risk Reports
610. Risk of Depression and Suicide in Patients with Extreme Obesity Who Seek Bariatric Surgery | Obesity Management
611. Peterhänsel C, Petroff D, Klinitzke G, Kersting A, Wagner B. Risk of completed suicide after bariatric surgery: a systematic review. Obes Rev. 2013;14(5):369–82. PMID: 23297762. http://www.ncbi.nlm.nih.gov/pubmed/23297762.
612. Neovius M, Bruze G, Jacobson P, Sjöholm K, Johansson K, Granath F, Sundström J, Näslund I, Marcus C, Ottosson J, Peltonen M, Carlsson LMS. Risk of suicide and non-fatal self-harm after bariatric surgery: results from two matched cohort studies. Lancet Diabetes Endocrinol. 2018;6(3):197–207. PMCID: PMC5932484. http://www.ncbi.nlm.nih.gov/pubmed/29329975.
613. Lagerros YT, Brandt L, Hedberg J, Sundbom M, Bodén R. Suicide, self-harm, and depression after gastric bypass surgery: a Nationwide Cohort Study. Ann Surg. 2017;265(2):235–43. PMID: 27387654. http://www.ncbi.nlm.nih.gov/pubmed/27387654.
614. Morgan DJR, Ho KM. Incidence and risk factors for deliberate self-harm, mental illness, and suicide following bariatric surgery: a state-wide population-based linked-data Cohort Study. Ann Surg. 2017;265(2):244–52. PMID: 27433913. http://www.ncbi.nlm.nih.gov/pubmed/27433913.
615. Bhatti JA, Nathens AB, Thiruchelvam D, Grantcharov T, Goldstein BI, Redelmeier DA. Self-harm emergencies after bariatric surgery: a population-based Cohort Study. JAMA Surg. 2016;151(3):226–32. PMID: 26444444. http://www.ncbi.nlm.nih.gov/pubmed/26444444.
616. Miller-Matero LR, Yeh HH, Ahmedani BK, Rossom RC, Harry ML, Daida YG, Coleman KJ. Suicide attempts after bariatric surgery: comparison to a nonsurgical cohort of individuals with severe obesity. Surg Obes Relat Dis. 2023;19(12):1458–66. PMCID: PMC10843496. http://www.ncbi.nlm.nih.gov/pubmed/37758538.
617. Konttinen H, Sjöholm K, Jacobson P, Svensson PA, Carlsson LMS, Peltonen M. Prediction of suicide and nonfatal self-harm after bariatric surgery: a risk score based on sociodemographic factors, lifestyle behavior, and mental health: a nonrandomized controlled trial. Ann Surg. 2021;274(2):339–45. PMCID: PMC7283001 PubMed entry [Internet]. [cited 2025 Jan 3]. Available from: http://www.ncbi.nlm.nih.gov/pubmed/31850987.
618. Mitchell JE, Crosby R, de Zwaan M, Engel S, Roerig J, Steffen K, Gordon KH, Karr T, Lavender J, Wonderlich S. Possible risk factors for increased suicide following bariatric surgery. Obesity (Silver Spring). 2013;21(4):665–72. PMCID: PMC4372842. http://www.ncbi.nlm.nih.gov/pubmed/23404774.
619. Biochemistry, Ghrelin - StatPearls - NCBI Bookshelf.
620. Castaneda D, Popov VB, Wander P, Thompson CC. Risk of suicide and self-harm is increased after bariatric surgery-a systematic review and meta-analysis. Obes Surg. 2019;29(1):322–33. PMID: 30343409. http://www.ncbi.nlm.nih.gov/pubmed/30343409.
621. Gordon KH, King WC, White GE, Belle SH, Courcoulas AP, Ebel FE, Engel SG, Flum DR, Hinojosa MW, Pomp A, Pories WJ, Spaniolas D, Wolfe BM, Yanovski SZ, Mitchell JE. A longitudinal examination of suicide-related thoughts and behaviors among bariatric surgery patients. Surg Obes Relat Dis. 2019;15(2):269–78. PMCID: PMC6481310. http://www.ncbi.nlm.nih.gov/pubmed/31010651.

622. Sarwer DB, Allison KC, Wadden TA, Ashare R, Spitzer JC, McCuen-Wurst C, LaGrotte C, Williams NN, Edwards M, Tewksbury C, Wu J. Psychopathology, disordered eating, and impulsivity as predictors of outcomes of bariatric surgery. Surg Obes Relat Dis. 2019;15(4):650–5. PMCID: PMC6538470. http://www.ncbi.nlm.nih.gov/pubmed/30858009.
623. Courcoulas A. Who, why, and how? Suicide and harmful behaviors after bariatric surgery. Ann Surg. 2017;265(2):253–4. PMID: 27735820. http://www.ncbi.nlm.nih.gov/pubmed/27735820.
624. Jumbe S, Hamlet C, Meyrick J. Psychological aspects of bariatric surgery as a treatment for obesity. Curr Obes Rep. 2017;6(1):71–8. PMCID: PMC5359375. http://www.ncbi.nlm.nih.gov/pubmed/28243838.
625. Orellana ER, Covasa M, Hajnal A. Neuro-hormonal mechanisms underlying changes in reward related behaviors following weight loss surgery: potential pharmacological targets. Biochem Pharmacol. 2019;164:106–114. PMID: 30954487. http://www.ncbi.nlm.nih.gov/pubmed/30954487.
626. Blackburn AN, Hajnal A, Leggio L. The gut in the brain: the effects of bariatric surgery on alcohol consumption. Addict Biol. 2017;22(6):1540–53. PMCID: PMC5332539. http://www.ncbi.nlm.nih.gov/pubmed/27578259.
627. Ivezaj V, Benoit SC, Davis J, Engel S, Lloret-Linares C, Mitchell JE, Pepino MY, Rogers AM, Steffen K, Sogg S. Changes in alcohol use after metabolic and bariatric surgery: predictors and mechanisms. Curr Psychiatry Rep. 2019;21(9):85. PMCID: PMC7057935. http://www.ncbi.nlm.nih.gov/pubmed/31410716.
628. Shankar P, Boylan M, Sriram K. Micronutrient deficiencies after bariatric surgery. Nutrition. 2010;26(11–12):1031–7. PMID: 20363593. http://www.ncbi.nlm.nih.gov/pubmed/20363593.
629. Valentino D, Sriram K, Shankar P. Update on micronutrients in bariatric surgery. Curr Opin Clin Nutr Metab Care. 2011;14(6):635–41. PMID: 21892077. http://www.ncbi.nlm.nih.gov/pubmed/21892077.
630. Bal BS, Finelli FC, Shope TR, Koch TR. Nutritional deficiencies after bariatric surgery. Nat Rev Endocrinol. 2012;8(9):544–56. PMID: 22525731. http://www.ncbi.nlm.nih.gov/pubmed/22525731.
631. Lupoli R, Lembo E, Saldalamacchia G, Avola CK, Angrisani L, Capaldo B. Bariatric surgery and long-term nutritional issues. World J Diabetes. 2017;8(11):464–74. PMCID: PMC5700383. http://www.ncbi.nlm.nih.gov/pubmed/29204255.
632. Al Mansoori A, Shakoor H, Ali HI, Feehan J, Al Dhaheri AS, Cheikh Ismail L, Bosevski M, Apostolopoulos V, Stojanovska L. The effects of bariatric surgery on vitamin B status and mental health. Nutrients. 2021;13(4):1383. PMCID: PMC8073305. http://www.ncbi.nlm.nih.gov/pubmed/33923999.
633. Miedziaszczyk M, Ciabach P, Szałek E. The effects of bariatric surgery and gastrectomy on the absorption of drugs, vitamins, and mineral elements. Pharmaceutics. 2021;13(12):2111. PMCID: PMC8708306. http://www.ncbi.nlm.nih.gov/pubmed/34959391.
634. Roerig JL, Steffen K, Zimmerman C, Mitchell JE, Crosby RD, Cao L. Preliminary comparison of sertraline levels in postbariatric surgery patients versus matched nonsurgical cohort. Surg Obes Relat Dis. 2012;8(1):62–6. PMID: 21256091. http://www.ncbi.nlm.nih.gov/pubmed/21256091.
635. Miller AD, Smith KM. Medication and nutrient administration considerations after bariatric surgery. Am J Health Syst Pharm. 2006;63(19):1852–7. PMID: 16990631. http://www.ncbi.nlm.nih.gov/pubmed/16990631.
636. Saad R, Habli D, El Sabbagh R, Chakhtoura M. Bone health following bariatric surgery: an update. J Clin Densitom. 2020;23(2):165–81. PMID: 31519474. http://www.ncbi.nlm.nih.gov/pubmed/31519474.
637. Wasserman H, Jenkins T, Inge T, Ryder J, Michalsky M, Sisley S, Xie C, Kalkwarf HJ. Bone mineral density in young adults 5 to 11 years after adolescent metabolic and bariatric surgery for severe obesity compared to peers. Int J Obes. 2024;48(4):575–83. PMID: 38177697. http://www.ncbi.nlm.nih.gov/pubmed/38177697.
638. Paccou J, Tsourdi E, Meier C, Palermo A, Pepe J, Body JJ, Zillikens MC. Bariatric surgery and skeletal health: a narrative review and position statement for management by the European Calcified Tissue Society (ECTS). Bone. 2022;154:116236. PMID: 34688942. http://www.ncbi.nlm.nih.gov/pubmed/34688942.
639. Kumbhari V, Cummings DE, Kalloo AN, Schauer PR. AGA clinical practice update on evaluation and management of early complications after bariatric/metabolic surgery: expert review. Clin Gastroenterol Hepatol. 2021;19(8):1531–7. PMID: 33741500. http://www.ncbi.nlm.nih.gov/pubmed/33741500.
640. Jans G, Matthys C, Bogaerts A, Lannoo M, Verhaeghe J, Van der Schueren B, Devlieger R. Maternal micronutrient deficiencies and related adverse neonatal outcomes after bariatric surgery: a systematic review. Adv Nutr. 2015;6(4):420–9. PMCID: PMC4496736. http://www.ncbi.nlm.nih.gov/pubmed/26178026.
641. Via MA, Mechanick JI. Nutritional and micronutrient care of bariatric surgery patients: current evidence update. Curr Obes Rep. 2017;6(3):286–96. PMID: 28718091. http://www.ncbi.nlm.nih.gov/pubmed/28718091.
642. Devlieger R, Guelinckx I, Jans G, Voets W, Vanholsbeke C, Vansant G. Micronutrient levels and supplement intake in pregnancy after bariatric surgery: a prospective cohort study. PLoS One. 2014;9(12):e114192. PMCID: PMC4254913. http://www.ncbi.nlm.nih.gov/pubmed/25470614.
643. Menon V, Kar SK, Suthar N, Nebhinani N. Vitamin D and depression: a critical appraisal of the evidence and future directions. Indian J Psychol Med. 2020;42(1):11–21. PMCID: PMC6970300. http://www.ncbi.nlm.nih.gov/pubmed/31997861.
644. Lewis CA, Osland EJ, de Jersey S, Hopkins G, Seymour M, Webb L, Chatfield MD, Hickman IJ. Monitoring for micronutrient deficiency after bariatric surgery-what is the risk? Eur J Clin Nutr. 2023;77(11):1071–83. PMCID: PMC10630125. http://www.ncbi.nlm.nih.gov/pubmed/37550536.
645. Martinou E, Stefanova I, Iosif E, Angelidi AM. Neurohormonal changes in the gut-brain axis and underlying neuroendocrine mechanisms following bariatric surgery. Int J Mol Sci. 2022;23(6):3339. PMCID: PMC8954280. http://www.ncbi.nlm.nih.gov/pubmed/35328759.
646. Guerrero-Hreins E, Foldi CJ, Oldfield BJ, Stefanidis A, Sumithran P, Brown RM. Gut-brain mechanisms underlying changes in disordered eating behaviour after bariatric surgery: a review. Rev Endocr Metab Disord. 2022;23(4):733–51. PMID: 34851508. http://www.ncbi.nlm.nih.gov/pubmed/34851508.
647. Brown RM, Guerrero-Hreins E, Brown WA, le Roux CW, Sumithran P. Potential gut-brain mechanisms behind adverse mental health outcomes of bariatric surgery. Nat Rev Endocrinol. 2021;17(9):549–59. PMID: 34262156. http://www.ncbi.nlm.nih.gov/pubmed/34262156.
648. Meule A. The relation between body mass index and substance use: a true can of worms. Innov Clin Neurosci. 2014;11(3–4):11–2. PMCID: PMC4008295. http://www.ncbi.nlm.nih.gov/pubmed/24800127.
649. King WC, Chen JY, Courcoulas AP, Dakin GF, Engel SG, Flum DR, Hinojosa MW, Kalarchian MA, Mattar SG, Mitchell JE, Pomp A, Pories WJ, Steffen KJ, White GE, Wolfe BM, Yanovski SZ. Alcohol and other substance use after bariatric surgery: prospective evidence from a U.S. multicenter cohort study. Surg Obes Relat Dis. 2017;13(8):1392–402. PMCID: PMC5568472. http://www.ncbi.nlm.nih.gov/pubmed/28528115.
650. Li L, Wu LT. Substance use after bariatric surgery: a review. J Psychiatr Res. 2016;76:16–29. PMCID: PMC4789154. http://www.ncbi.nlm.nih.gov/pubmed/26871733.

651. Brode CS, Mitchell JE. Problematic eating behaviors and eating disorders associated with bariatric surgery. Psychiatr Clin North Am. 2019;42(2):287–97. PMCID: PMC6501797. http://www.ncbi.nlm.nih.gov/pubmed/31046930.
652. Francois Z, Rizvi A. Psychiatric complications of bariatric surgery. In: StatPearls [Internet]. Treasure Island (FL): StatPearls Publishing. 2024 [cited 2025 Jan 3]. Available from: http://www.ncbi.nlm.nih.gov/books/NBK604208/ PMID: 38861640 http://www.ncbi.nlm.nih.gov/pubmed/38861640.
653. Jammah AA. Endocrine and metabolic complications after bariatric surgery. Saudi. J Gastroenterol. 2015;21(5):269–77. PMCID: PMC4632250. http://www.ncbi.nlm.nih.gov/pubmed/26458852.
654. Wernicke Encephalopathy - StatPearls - NCBI Bookshelf.
655. Kroenke K, Spitzer RL, Williams JB. The PHQ-9: validity of a brief depression severity measure. J Gen Intern Med. 2001;16(9):606–13. PMCID: PMC1495268. http://www.ncbi.nlm.nih.gov/pubmed/11556941.
656. Bray JW, Del Boca FK, McRee BG, Hayashi SW, Babor TF. Screening, Brief Intervention and Referral to Treatment (SBIRT): rationale, program overview and cross-site evaluation. Addiction. 2017;112(Suppl 2):3–11. PMID: 28074566. http://www.ncbi.nlm.nih.gov/pubmed/28074566.
657. Lorico S, Colton B. Medication management and pharmacokinetic changes after bariatric surgery. Can Fam Physician. 2020;66(6):409–16. PMCID: PMC7292522. http://www.ncbi.nlm.nih.gov/pubmed/32532720.
658. Padwal R, Brocks D, Sharma AM. A systematic review of drug absorption following bariatric surgery and its theoretical implications. Obes Rev. 2010;11(1):41–50. PMID: 19493300. http://www.ncbi.nlm.nih.gov/pubmed/19493300.
659. Angeles PC, Robertsen I, Seeberg LT, Krogstad V, Skattebu J, Sandbu R, Åsberg A, Hjelmesaeth J. The influence of bariatric surgery on oral drug bioavailability in patients with obesity: a systematic review. Obes Rev. 2019;20(9):1299–311. PMCID: PMC6852510. http://www.ncbi.nlm.nih.gov/pubmed/31232513.
660. Bernhardt R. Cytochromes P450 as versatile biocatalysts. J Biotechnol. 2006;124(1):128–45. PMID: 16516322. http://www.ncbi.nlm.nih.gov/pubmed/16516322.
661. Biochemistry, Cytochrome P450 - StatPearls - NCBI Bookshelf.
662. IDF Diabetes Atlas.
663. VizHub - GBD Compare.
664. Chireh B, Li M, D'Arcy C. Diabetes increases the risk of depression: a systematic review, meta-analysis and estimates of population attributable fractions based on prospective studies. Prev Med Rep. 2019;14:100822. PMCID: PMC6378921. http://www.ncbi.nlm.nih.gov/pubmed/30815337.
665. Bădescu SV, Tătaru C, Kobylinska L, Georgescu EL, Zahiu DM, Zăgrean AM, Zăgrean L. The association between diabetes mellitus and depression. J Med Life. 2016;9(2):120–5. PMCID: PMC4863499. http://www.ncbi.nlm.nih.gov/pubmed/27453739.
666. Roy T, Lloyd CE. Epidemiology of depression and diabetes: a systematic review. J Affect Disord. 2012;142(Suppl):S8–21. PMID: 23062861. http://www.ncbi.nlm.nih.gov/pubmed/23062861.
667. Grigsby AB, Anderson RJ, Freedland KE, Clouse RE, Lustman PJ. Prevalence of anxiety in adults with diabetes: a systematic review. J Psychosom Res. 2002;53(6):1053–60. PMID: 12479986. http://www.ncbi.nlm.nih.gov/pubmed/12479986.
668. Mezuk B, Eaton WW, Albrecht S, Golden SH. Depression and type 2 diabetes over the lifespan: a meta-analysis. Diabetes Care. 2008;31(12):2383–90. PMCID: PMC2584200. http://www.ncbi.nlm.nih.gov/pubmed/19033418.
669. Berge LI, Riise T. Comorbidity between type 2 diabetes and depression in the adult population: directions of the association and its possible pathophysiological mechanisms. Int J Endocrinol. 2015;2015:164760. PMCID: PMC4589629. http://www.ncbi.nlm.nih.gov/pubmed/26457080.
670. Clarke TK, Obsteter J, Hall LS, Hayward C, Thomson PA, Smith BH, Padmanabhan S, Hocking LJ, Deary IJ, Porteous DJ, McIntosh AM. Investigating shared aetiology between type 2 diabetes and major depressive disorder in a population based cohort. Am J Med Genet B Neuropsychiatr Genet. 2017;174(3):227–34. PMCID: PMC5363226. http://www.ncbi.nlm.nih.gov/pubmed/27480393.
671. Alzoubi A, Abunaser R, Khassawneh A, Alfaqih M, Khasawneh A, Abdo N. The bidirectional relationship between diabetes and depression: a literature review. Korean J Fam Med. 2018;39(3):137–46. PMCID: PMC5975983. http://www.ncbi.nlm.nih.gov/pubmed/29788701.
672. Alonso-Morán E, Satylganova A, Orueta JF, Nuño-Solinis R. Prevalence of depression in adults with type 2 diabetes in the Basque Country: relationship with glycaemic control and health care costs. BMC Public Health. 2014;14:769. PMCID: PMC4129099. http://www.ncbi.nlm.nih.gov/pubmed/25073532.
673. Anderson RJ, Freedland KE, Clouse RE, Lustman PJ. The prevalence of comorbid depression in adults with diabetes: a meta-analysis. Diabetes Care. 2001;24(6):1069–78. PMID: 11375373. http://www.ncbi.nlm.nih.gov/pubmed/11375373.
674. Ali S, Stone MA, Peters JL, Davies MJ, Khunti K. The prevalence of co-morbid depression in adults with Type 2 diabetes: a systematic review and meta-analysis. Diabet Med. 2006;23(11):1165–73. PMID: 17054590. http://www.ncbi.nlm.nih.gov/pubmed/17054590.
675. Kan C, Pedersen NL, Christensen K, Bornstein SR, Licinio J, MacCabe JH, Ismail K, Rijsdijk F. Genetic overlap between type 2 diabetes and depression in Swedish and Danish twin registries. Mol Psychiatry. 2016;21(7):903–9. PMCID: PMC5414070. http://www.ncbi.nlm.nih.gov/pubmed/27021822.
676. Chireh B, D'Arcy C. Shared and unique risk factors for depression and diabetes mellitus in a longitudinal study, implications for prevention: an analysis of a longitudinal population sample aged ⩾45 years. Ther Adv Endocrinol Metab. 2019;10:2042018819865828. PMCID: PMC6659182. http://www.ncbi.nlm.nih.gov/pubmed/31384422.
677. Gonzalez JS, Peyrot M, McCarl LA, Collins EM, Serpa L, Mimiaga MJ, Safren SA. Depression and diabetes treatment nonadherence: a meta-analysis. Diabetes Care. 2008;31(12):2398–403. PMCID: PMC2584202. http://www.ncbi.nlm.nih.gov/pubmed/19033420.
678. Egede LE, Nietert PJ, Zheng D. Depression and all-cause and coronary heart disease mortality among adults with and without diabetes. Diabetes Care. 2005;28(6):1339–45. PMID: 15920049. http://www.ncbi.nlm.nih.gov/pubmed/15920049.
679. Baumeister H, Hutter N, Bengel J, Härter M. Quality of life in medically ill persons with comorbid mental disorders: a systematic review and meta-analysis. Psychother Psychosom. 2011;80(5):275–86. PMID: 21646822. http://www.ncbi.nlm.nih.gov/pubmed/21646822.
680. Szumilas M. Explaining odds ratios. J Can Acad Child Adolesc Psychiatry. 2010;19(3):227–9. Erratum in: J Can Acad Child Adolesc Psychiatry. 2015 Winter;24(1):58. PMID: 20842279; PMCID: PMC2938757. Explaining odds ratios - PubMed.
681. Akechi T, Nakano T, Akizuki N, Okamura M, Sakuma K, Nakanishi T, Yoshikawa E, Uchitomi Y. Somatic symptoms for diagnosing major depression in cancer patients. Psychosomatics. 2003;44(3):244–8. https://doi.org/10.1176/appi.psy.44.3.244. PMID: 12724506.
682. Musselman DL, Miller AH, Porter MR, Manatunga A, Gao F, Penna S, Pearce BD, Landry J, Glover S, McDaniel JS, Nemeroff CB. Higher than normal plasma interleukin-6 concentrations in cancer patients with depression: preliminary findings. Am J Psychiatry. 2001;158(8):1252–7. https://doi.org/10.1176/appi.ajp.158.8.1252. PMID: 11481159.

Depression and Sleep

13

Franklin Sunzeri

Introduction

Sleep is defined by electrophysiologists as *synchronous* activity detected on an *electroencephalogram (EEG)*. When we are awake, our EEGs show a *desynchronous* pattern. Depolarizations in the brain are recorded on the scalp by electrodes. The average of all the electrical changes in the brain when someone is awake is not synchronized, so it shows no obvious pattern and not much amplitude. This low-amplitude high-frequency wave pattern is the average of many simultaneous electrical vectors that seem to attenuate each other. When we fall asleep, our brain activity begins to synchronize, and the pattern shows a higher amplitude and lower frequency than when we are awake.

Types of *brain waves* that are shown on EEGs are from fastest to slowest: beta, alpha, theta, and delta [1]. See Fig. 13.1.

Beta is seen with eyes open and at attention. Beta brain waves are associated with normal waking consciousness and a heightened state of alertness, logic, and critical reasoning. It is also increased by some medications such as benzodiazepines.

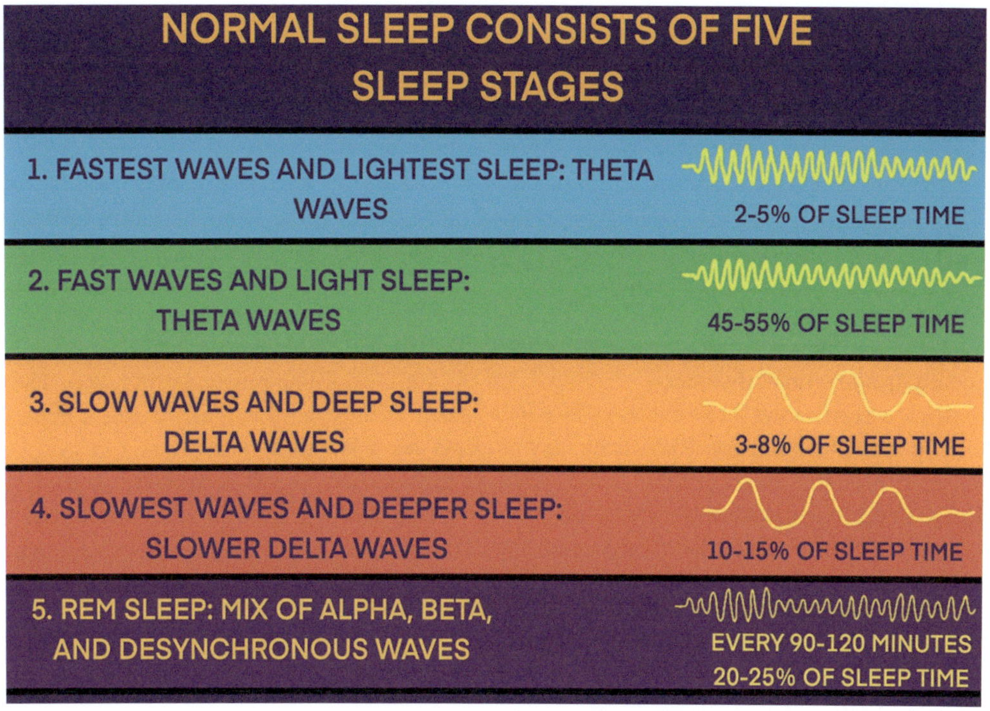

Fig. 13.1 This figure depicts the progression of sleep through five distinct stages: N1, N2, and N3 non-REM phases, followed by REM sleep and wakefulness. Each stage is characterized by unique brain activity patterns, physiological changes, and roles in rest and restoration. The cycle repeats throughout the night, supporting cognitive, emotional, and physical health

F. Sunzeri (✉)
Heather Hills Consulting, Coos Bay, OR, USA

J. Raber et al. (eds.), *Understanding and Treating Depressive Disorders*, https://doi.org/10.1007/978-3-032-14465-2_13

Alpha is seen in relaxed states with eyes closed and decreased attentiveness. When we begin to relax, our brain waves become more synchronous, slower, and higher in amplitude. Alpha waves are often seen in meditation and biofeedback when we are relaxed and peaceful.

Theta waves are slower frequency and lower in amplitude than alpha waves. The first and second stages of sleep demonstrate theta waves. There are very subtle and there are gradual differences between relaxation and stage 1 sleep. Stage 2 sleep adds two defining characteristic waves that occur periodically every minute or so. These waves are sleep spindles (a sudden increase in frequency) and K complexes (a sudden increase in amplitude). Stages 1 and 2 sleep are so light that if someone is awakened during these stages, often they will say that they have not been sleeping.

Delta waves (the slowest frequency and the highest amplitude waves) are shown in the deep sleep of stages 3 and 4. The primary difference between stages 3 and 4 is the percentage of waves that are delta: less than 50% in stage 3 and more than 50% in stage 4. Sleepwalking and sleep-talking are most frequent in stages 3 and 4. If someone is awakened during delta sleep, they are most likely to be disoriented and groggy.

Normal sleep consists of five stages [1]:

1. The fastest waves and lightest sleep: theta waves, 2–5% of total adult sleep time.
2. Fast waves and light sleep: theta waves, 45–55% of adult sleep time.
3. Slow waves and deep sleep: delta waves, 3–8% of adult sleep time.
4. Slowest waves and deeper sleep: slower delta waves, 10–15% of adult sleep time.
5. Rapid eye movement (REM) sleep: a mix of alpha, beta, and desynchronous waves, every 90–120 minutes, 20–25% of total adult sleep time.

Theta and delta are also seen diffusely in delirium and focally in some brain disorders.

REM sleep follows 4 to 6 cycles of non-REM sleep. In the early part of the night, non-REM sleep may progress through stages 1 through 4 and back up to 2 or 3 before giving way to REM sleep. Later during the night, stages 3 or 4 may not occur. REM sleep is a well-characterized stage of sleep and is associated with many sleep activities. It lasts for a few minutes initially during the night, and 20–40 minutes later in the evening. REM sleep is accompanied by elevated blood pressure, heart rate, increased deep and rapid breathing, decreased skeletal muscle tone with the exception of the eyes, the muscles of the middle ear (which twitch), and penile and clitoral erection. See Fig. 13.2.

REM sleep occurs when cholinergic activity increases and noradrenergic and serotonergic activity decreases [2]. REM sleep is also called *paradoxical sleep* because although the body appears deeper asleep than in other stages, the EEGs are very similar to the awake brain (alpha, beta, and desynchronous waves). Possibly, this is due to dreaming.

Dreaming is often considered to be a nighttime continuation of conscious processing of daytime thoughts or reprogramming for the next day's events [3, 4]. Learning and memory processing and adaptation to emotional stress may be some of the important events of dreaming [5].

Dreams arise in all stages of sleep. Dreams are reported by 80% of those awakened from stages 1, 2, and REM sleep, and from 40% of those awakened from stages 3 and 4 deep sleep [6]. Stage 1 and 2 dreams are simple and with few associations. REM sleep dreams tend to be bizarre and are often reported in detail. Dreams in deep sleep tend to be more diffuse, often relating to colors or emotions [7]. Dream recall is greater in those stages that are more like the waking state [8].

Although sleep appears to serve important functions, it is still unclear what they are beyond the classic rest and recuperation [9]. Poor sleep almost always accompanies systemic illness and acute psychiatric disorders. Folks who get less than 4 hours or more than 10 hours of sleep per night are statistically more likely to live a shorter life [9]. Linked to circadian endocrine rhythms, independent of a good night's sleep or a noon meal, people normally tend to become drowsy in mid-afternoon.

When we sleep, we are not aware of our sensory world until something of sufficient stimulation arouses us. One of the intriguing phenomena of sleep is: How can we be "dead to the world" and yet be aroused? The answer is the thalamus, the gatekeeper for Morpheus. Activity in an acetylcholine system, the reticular nucleus, and the sensory thalamus are the principal factors. Ascending acetylcholinergic neurons from the fourth ventricle near the midbrain in the rostral pons contact the sensory areas of the thalamus and the *reticular nucleus*. The reticular nucleus acts as a brake on the sensory processing of the thalamus. The reticular neurons and the sensory neurons have different acetylcholine receptors and respond differently. The acetylcholine acting on the sensory neurons closes a hyperpolarizing potassium channel in these neurons and in so doing sensitizes them to sensations, i.e., they become primed to receive sensory input. At the same time, the acetylcholine inhibits the reticular nucleus, i.e., the inhibitor becomes inhibited. So, the thalamus is active and alert, the thalamocortical path is open, the cortex is humming along, and we are awake. When we are asleep, the ascending acetylcholine pathway is silent. The reticular nucleus is not inhibited, so it inhibits the sensory nuclei that are not sensitized. The result is that the gate is closed; the thalamus is coasting along in a hyperpolarized state but can still respond if the sensory input is sufficiently strong. In this resting state, the thalamocortical neurons are still firing but slowly, so the cortex still has some degree of activity.

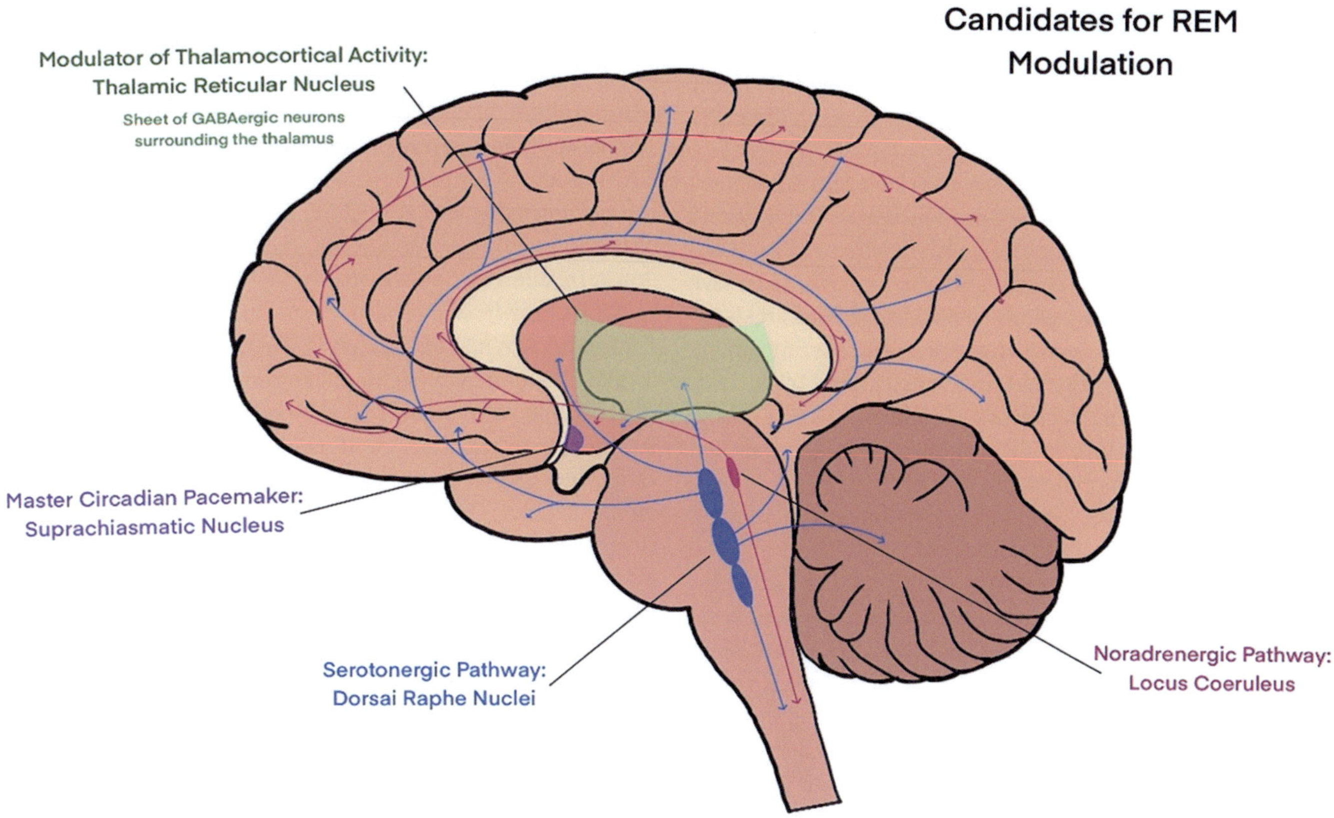

Fig. 13.2 Brain regions implicated in REM sleep modulation. This illustration depicts key neural structures involved in regulating rapid eye movement (REM) sleep. The thalamic reticular nucleus facilitates sensory gating and oscillatory rhythms during sleep transitions. The suprachiasmatic nucleus, the brain's master circadian clock, orchestrates temporal cues essential for REM onset and duration. Serotonergic projections from the dorsal raphe nuclei and noradrenergic input from the locus coeruleus modulate cortical arousal and REM suppression, reflecting complex monoaminergic control of sleep architecture. Collectively, these regions represent a dynamic network influencing REM sleep expression and homeostasis

Curiously, in REM sleep, the ascending acetylcholine system turns back on, but paradoxically we are still without consciousness. This phenomenon reflects the complexity of the multilayers of control that are characteristic of the nervous system. It is likely that other neurotransmitters from cells in other nuclei are involved. Candidates include a group of noradrenergic neurons in the *locus ceruleus* and a group of serotonergic neurons in the *dorsal raphe nuclei*, both in the rostral pons. Lack of movement when we are in REM sleep, versus tossing and turning in most other stages, may be the result of a *descending inhibition system* that originates in the medulla. A very rare occurrence of *violent sleeping* has been documented when damage to this system results in the dreamer acting out the dream.

Two interacting processes regulate the sleep-wake cycle [10–13]. These are the circadian process and the homeostatic or recovery process. The *circadian process* is regulated by oscillations within the *suprachiasmatic nucleus of the hypothalamus* that controls basic circadian, ultradian, and infradian phenomena such as hormones and metabolism. This circadian function is susceptible to environmental and psychosocial cues and not dependent upon time awake or tiredness [10, 11, 14, 15]. The *homeostatic or recovery process* on the other hand is dependent upon time awake and regulates the urge to sleep.

When we get less sleep than usual, we incur a sleep debt that results in a drive to longer hours of deeper sleep. Both of these processes are altered in someone experiencing depression [15]. The sleep disorders that are most often encountered in depression are insomnia, hypersomnia, nightmares, and pavor nocturnus.

Independent of other factors, sleep patterns change with age [16]. Most of these patterns occur between young and middle age and become stable in older age. These include advanced sleep timing, shortened nocturnal sleep duration, increased frequency of daytime naps, increased number of nighttime awakenings, duration of being awake during the night, and decreased slow-wave sleep. Circadian sleep-related hormones and homeostatic mechanisms change with normal aging.

Sleep Disturbances

The International Classification of Sleep Disorders is the authoritative clinical text for the diagnosis of sleep disorders [17].

Endogenously depressed individuals have less slow-wave sleep, reach REM sleep sooner, have increased REM earlier in the evening and less later in the night: the reverse of the normal pattern [9, 18]. They also have more frequent eye movement in REM. Only people with narcolepsy start sleeping with REM. REM is associated with intense, recallable dreams and occurs in neonates, individuals blind from birth, and animals reared in the absence of light.

Nightmares also lurk in the shadows of REM sleep and are more common in children. They are most often associated with fatigue, fever, or alcohol consumption. A number of pharmaceuticals interfere with REM sleep. These include alcohol, tricyclic antidepressants, barbiturates, phenothiazines, benzodiazepines, and monoamine oxidase inhibitors. When these inhibitors (except for benzodiazepines) are withdrawn, REM sleep begins earlier and lasts longer (*REM rebound*). Excess alcohol consumed in the evening can also lead to withdrawal effects in the early morning, so restlessness on awakening or even tremulousness and fear can occur in severely dependent people. Sleep attacks, but not narcolepsy, are episodes of REM sleep.

Stage 4 sleep and sometimes stage 3 sleep are associated with several sleep disorders. *Night terrors*, or *pavor nocturnus*, are most common in children. They wake from sleep screaming and inconsolable until they fall back to sleep in a few minutes and only recall vague, ill-formed images. When night terrors occur in adults, they are most often associated with alcoholism or psychological disturbances.

Benzodiazepines decrease stage-4 sleep, so they have been used for treating night terrors. *Enuresis* (bedwetting) often but not always occurs in stage 4 sleep. It has a high incidence of about 20% of all children between 3 and 15. *Somnambulism* (sleep walking, sitting, or performing other complex activities) usually occurs with eyes wide open, is not recalled upon awakening; it lasts several minutes, and is accompanied by *visual agnosia* (non-recognition of familiar objects). The somnambulists may injure themselves, perhaps because of the agnosia. There is no accompanying dream. They often mumble incessantly. It is most common in childhood and early adolescence.

A chronic desire for increased sleep can result from depression, lesions in the hypothalamus or the upper-brain stem, or other unusual disorders such as narcolepsy. Acute *hypersomnia* often is a component of acute infections such as influenza or may be associated with systemic problems such as hypothyroidism, hypo-or hyperglycemia, anemia, and liver problems [19].

Narcolepsy is a rare syndrome that may have four components. Hypersomnia, sleep paralysis, cataplexy, and hypnagogic phenomena. Hypersomnia is the most common manifestation. Sleep can occur at any time and lasts from minutes to hours, several to many times per day. The onset of REM sleep is almost instantaneous. The afflicted can be roused normally, feel refreshed, and then fall asleep again. Total sleep time may be normal, but nighttime sleep may be non-refreshing and punctuated by wild, scary dreams.

Sleep paralysis can also occur in normal children and some adults. When the sleeper is just falling asleep, or is just awakening, there is a frightening moment when movement is not possible. *Hypnagogic phenomena* are intense visual or auditory hallucinations or illusions at the onset of sleep. *Hypnopompic phenomena* are similar phenomena sometimes on awakening. They can occur in young children and occasionally in adults who do not have narcolepsy. *Cataplexy* is a brief episode of paralysis, most often in the limbs, without loss of consciousness. The episodes are provoked by intense emotions such as surprise, fear, anger, or laughter.

Complaints of poor sleep are quite common in the general population [20]. They are often accompanied by significant social, psychological, and medical problems. Disturbances include breathing difficulties while asleep, snoring, frequent awakenings, diurnal sleepiness, fatigue, moodiness, and compromised quality of life [21, 22]. Increased complaints are seen in veterans [23, 24] and the elderly [25]. In the USA, sleep disordered breathing is more common in African Americans [26] and Asian-Americans [27] than in Caucasians.

Significant *insomnia* afflicts about 50% of the population at some time [28]. Approximately 10% have chronic insomnia. As we age, total sleep time tends to decrease; sleep may become more fragmented, and stage 4 sleep may disappear. The ability to sleep is decreased by intense feelings, caffeinated foods and beverages, cocaine, amphetamines, monoamine oxidase inhibitors, and a few tricyclic antidepressants. Difficulty in initially falling asleep is most often associated with an emotional disturbance, but other common causes are a variable sleep schedule, pain, breathing difficulties, restless legs syndrome, withdrawal from sedatives, sleep apnea, or circadian rhythm disturbances [28]. Early morning awakening or drifting into restless sleep is common in aging, but it is also commonly associated with self-reproachful thinking, anxiety, and self-punishment.

Trouble sleeping, trouble falling asleep, and trouble staying asleep, independent of sleep apnea, may be associated with increased risk of coronary heart disease [29]. Some reviewers believe these sleep problems may be part of a larger syndrome that includes depression and poor health, or autonomic dysfunctions, reduced slow-wave sleep, or continual stressors. Ten studies between January 1976 and

August 1997 were analyzed [12]. The highest quality studies showed a combined effect of 1.7, with risk ratios of 1.47 to 3.90, $p < 0.0001$ for trouble falling asleep and coronary events when age and various risk factors were adjusted.

One night's partial sleep loss will elevate cortisol levels the next night [30]. Deep sleep is the normal stimulus for a considerable amount of growth hormone release. So, when sleep is disturbed, there is less growth hormone released. And, as growth hormone enhances several facets of immune function there may be resultant dysregulation of immune functions [31].

Decreased *sleep efficiency* under episodes of stress is frequently associated with increases in phases 1 and 2 sleep, intermittent awakenings, anxiety, social inhibition, increased sleep latency, and impulsiveness [32–34]. Abnormal *sleep architecture* (decreased slow wave sleep, reduced latency to first episode of REM, and increased eye movements during REM) is frequent and associated with intense dreams and nightmares [35].

Sleep and Depression

As many as 70% of people with depression have sleep disturbances [36]. Primary disturbances include problems falling asleep, frequently awakening, waking sooner than desired, lack of restorative sleep, pavor nocturnus, nightmares, and hypersomnia [12, 35–39]. Insomnia may be present in 60–80% of depressed patients [12]. Some pharmacotherapeutics prescribed for depression increase insomnia [12]. Epidemiological and biologic findings about insomnia as a clinical predictor of subsequent depression are discussed in reference [40].

Even during remissions, patients with major depression, and those with higher anxiety scores or who are divorced, continue to experience increased frequency of sleep disturbances [41–43].

Circadian sleep disturbances are common [12]. There are increased REM sleep and decreased slow-wave sleep [44]. Hyperactivation occurs in the HPA axis and in the habenula [45], and CLOCK gene polymorphisms are associated [45].

In depressed patients, cortisol and ACTH are usually elevated at night and may indicate an acute episode of MDD [46].

In sufferers with MDD compared to healthy folks, in transitioning from waking to non-REM sleep, there may be less of a decrease in metabolic activity in frontal, temporal and parietal cortices, and anterior cingulate cortex, amygdala, and thalamus [44]. In addition, these areas may show increased activity in REM sleep [47]. This may be related to imbalances in monoaminergic-cholinergic systems in depression [47]. The habenula, which is adjacent to the thalamus, may be implicated in these disturbances [48, 49].

During adolescence, depression and sleep disturbances increase together in a gender-specific fashion [50]. However, inconsistencies in these disturbances occur, probably reflecting lifestyle changes, the highly dynamic changes in the brain's genetic expressions, and neurotransmitter and hormone metabolism.

Many studies indicate a high incidence of insomnia and other sleep disturbances preceding depression [37, 51]. Chronically disturbed sleep has the potential to provoke neurobiological changes very much like those found in depression. Hypotheses suggest there is an upset in the regulation of neural plasticity and neurogenesis.

Sleep-related breathing disorders may be associated in a dose-response relationship with depression [52].

Depression is the most common cause of *insomnia* [53]. The suprachiasmatic nucleus (SQN) in the anterior hypothalamus synchronizes sleep with the help of the CLOCK genes [54]. The C alleles of the CLOCK appear to be implicated in patients with MDD and insomnia [54–56]. The C allele is also associated with increased early insomnia in those patients treated with antidepressants [56]. Polymorphisms of the monoamine-oxidase A gene and the promoter of the serotonin transporter gene are also associated with citalopram side effects and greater severity of insomnia [57, 58]. An additional association with late insomnia has been seen with the T allele of the polymorphism *rs76481776* of the micro-RNA gene (*pre-miR-182*) that endogenously modulates the circadian cycle [59].

Insomnia and nightmares, along with other sleep disturbances, are significantly associated with suicidal thoughts and behaviors [60]. Repetitive and frightening dreams may be a link to increased suicide attempts [61, 62].

Nightmares are the most common parasomnias in depression [63]. Poor self-image, threats to self-esteem, survival, and masochism are frequent themes. Emotions expressed in nightmares include despair, anxiety, and overwhelming sadness (DSM-5). For most children, and in some creative adults [64], frequent nightmares are unrelated to any underlying psychopathology [6, 65–67]. Recurrent nightmares, however, are one of the most defining symptoms of PTSD [6].

It is frequently difficult to fall back to sleep after a nightmare. Depression and insomnia can be significant predictors of frequent nightmares [68]. Nightmare frequency seems to be strongly connected to sleep and mood difficulties and a variety of factors related to physical and psychological health [68]. Residual sleep disturbances after depression symptoms have subsided appear to be related to comorbid anxiety, baseline sleep difficulties, and a host of personality and psychosocial factors [41].

Various hypotheses have been suggested for the etiopathogenesis of nightmares. These include neurobiological models [69–71], neopsychoanalytical hypotheses [72], and evolutionary models [4]. For example, in a neurocognitive explanation, the underlying belief is that dreaming is an emotionally adaptive function of intensifying the expression of an emotion or a dysfunction in the fear extinction function of dreaming [73].

Distinctions between bad dreams and nightmares often suggest that in nightmares the dreams frequently awaken the dreamer [74]. One study found that 51% of bad dreams and 30% of nightmares had primary emotions besides fear [74]. Data from the *National FINRISK Study* found that sex, age, impairment in the ability to work, low life satisfaction, use of antidepressants or hypnotics, and heavy alcohol use were strongly associated with frequent nightmares ($p < 0.001$ for all) [68]. The strongest risk factors were insomnia (OR[1] 6.90), exhaustion and fatigue (OR 6.86), and a negative attitude toward the self-associated with depression (OR 1.32 per 1-point increase) ($p < 0.001$ for all).

In contradistinction to night terrors upon awakening from a nightmare, orientation is quickly recovered, and the individual often retains a detailed memory of the nightmarish plot [75]. Prevalence of nightmares in the general population is reported to be 1–8% [17, 75]. Between 20% and 39% of children between 5 and 12 years of age have nightmares [5].

Increased nocturnal awakenings, sleep onset insomnia, anxiety about poor sleep, and memory difficulties in the daytime are commonly associated with nightmares [76]. Women are more likely to have nightmares, and as we age, we are all more likely to have nightmares [75].

Frequency of nightmares related to depression in adults as well as in children may be associated with a trait-like augmenting of negative emotions relating to maternal separation [77]. Medications such as antidepressants, barbiturates, beta-blockers, amphetamines, and narcotics may increase the frequency and onset of nightmares [78–80]. Rebounding of REM sleep upon withdrawal from drugs such as benzodiazepines, ethanol, and barbiturates may produce intense, frightening dreams [7, 81].

Night terrors (pavor nocturnus) occur during sudden arousal from usually the first cycle of stage 4 non-REM sleep, where there is limited awareness of surroundings [82–84]. Manifestations include a strong autonomic discharge resulting in feelings of panic, sometimes accompanied by a terrified scream, and sometimes stereotyped motor discharge [85]. People who experience night terrors have a higher incidence of depression, OCD, anxiety, and phobias [86]. Genetics, developmental, and psychological factors are involved. Night terrors show a prevalence of 1–6% among children [87] and less than 1% among adults (DSM-5). In children, they are most common in ages 3 to 12 and usually disappear in adolescence. In adults, their highest incidence is between 20 and 30 years of age [83]. Substance abuse, affective disorders [88], and sleep apnea [89] are the most common adult associations with night terrors. Night terrors and sleepwalking may be closely related parasomnias [84].

Sleep apnea, while highly associated with night terrors, appears to have an inverse relationship with nightmares [90, 91]. It has been suggested that this association is secondary to REM suppression in patients with significant obstructive sleep apnea. Nightmares decrease in patients treated with continuous positive airway pressure therapy [91].

There is strong evidence that *obstructive sleep apnea (OSA)* is connected directly or indirectly to depression [92, 93]. Possible connections to OSA comediators include obesity, hypertension, and decreased quality of life. OSA patients that had comorbid depression may have more severe and longer periods of depression [92]. There is an increased risk of developing depression among people with OSA, and an association between OSA severity and the likelihood of developing depression [93]. The relationship of OSA with depression appears to be bidirectional [94].

OSA and restless legs syndrome that occur during sleep are more frequent in people with MDD than those without MDD [95]. The association with MDD is greater in women (5.2) than in men (2.4). Associations for OSA might be with hypoxemia or metabolic syndrome [96].

In a Swiss sleep clinic, the prevalence of clinical depression was 21.5% [97]. A 2015 systematic review found evidence (albeit with considerable heterogeneity and high risk for bias) for the prevalence of OSA with MDD and PTSD but not with schizophrenia and psychotic disorders, bipolar and related disorders, and anxiety disorders other than PTSD [98].

Men with co-morbid OSA and insomnia appear to have a greater risk for depression and for greater severity of depression than men with only OSA or insomnia have [99].

In one study, *Restless Legs Syndrome* (RLS) was found in 26% of patients with MDD [100]. Connections between RLS and MDD and chronic insomnia may be the low functioning of dopamine pathways [101–103].

Narcolepsy may be 3 times more prevalent in patients with MDD than in the general population [104]. Narcolepsy is caused by hypocretin deficiency and is more frequent in inactive and obese people. Hypersomnia that is frequently associated with depression may also relate to hypocretin deficiency [105].

[1]Odds ratio (OR) is a way to represent the odds that an outcome will result when a given exposure to a variable of interest occurs compared to when the exposure does not occur. OR quantifies the strength of the association between two events. An OR greater than 1 indicates a positive association or that exposure to that variable increases the odds of that outcome. An OR less than one indicates a negative relationship between two events. An OR of 1 suggests no relationship between two events. An OR is frequently accompanied by a 95% confidence interval (CI). CI is a measure of precision of the OR. The smaller the CI the higher precision as long as it does not overlap OR = 1. For more information, see Chap. 4.

Treatment of Sleep Disorders

Because of the activating properties of many antidepressants, they can make sleep worse [106, 107]. These drugs include imipramine, desipramine, fluoxetine, paroxetine, venlafaxine, and reboxetine. Clomipramine and phenelzine completely suppress REM sleep [33]. Because of their perturbations of sleep, patients are frequently co-prescribed other drugs to help them sleep. As many as 30–40% of these patients still experience insomnia even with these sleep medications. Sedative antidepressants, including doxepin, mirtazapine, trazodone, trimipramine, and agomelatine, appear to help regulate circadian sleep rhythms and increase REM sleep [33]. Bupropion may improve latency to REM sleep but still is associated with increased insomnia [108–110].

There is little evidence to support long-term usage of sedative antidepressants for MDD and insomnia [111]. Studies have suggested that zolpidem that agonizes benzodiazepine receptors improves SSRI-associated sleep disturbances [112]. However, zolpidem has been linked to rebound insomnia, residual next-day effects on psychomotor performance, including driving and memory, and complex sleep-related behaviors [112]. Trazodone may afford some help but may have considerable side effects [113]. Agomelatine may improve sleep perhaps through its melatonin agonist activity [114, 115] but has serious potential toxicity [116].

A *2016 Agency for Healthcare Research and Quality (AHRQ) comprehensive assessment* of the efficacy, comparative effectiveness, and harms of treatments for insomnia disorder in the general adult population and older adults [117] has stated, "Low- to moderate-strength evidence indicated that the nonbenzodiazepine hypnotics eszopiclone and zolpidem, and the orexin receptor antagonist suvorexant, improved short-term global and sleep outcomes in general adult populations. Doxepin improved sleep outcomes. The absolute mean effect was small. Evidence for benzodiazepine hypnotics, melatonin agonists, and antidepressants in general populations and for most pharmacologic interventions in older adults was generally insufficient. Evidence on adverse effects from RCT data was generally insufficient or of low strength. Observational studies suggest that hypnotics may be associated with dementia, fractures, and major injury. Food and Drug Administration (FDA) labels warn about cognitive and behavioral changes, including driving impairment, and other harms, and advise lower doses for females and older/debilitated adults." [118].

CBT has found success in treating both MDD and associated insomnia [112, 119–121]. A systematic review and meta-analysis of CBT for insomnia in cancer survivors has shown large effect sizes for insomnia severity ($d = 0.77$) with effects lasting up to 5 months [122]. *The 2016 AHRQ review mentioned earlier* also stated, "*Cognitive behavioral therapy for insomnia (CBT-I)* [123] improved global outcomes and nearly all sleep parameters in the general adult population, older adults, and adults with pain. We found insufficient evidence of adverse effects of these interventions. Evidence was less robust for psychological interventions other than CBT-I, but low-strength evidence shows that some interventions improve some sleep outcomes." [118]. The 2016 AHRQ review also stated, "Evidence on complementary and alternative medicine was insufficient. Evidence was insufficient to compare hypnotic medications within or across classes or versus CBT-I." [118]. A protocol for youth-oriented CBT therapy for insomnia is presented in [124].

American College of Physicians recommends CBT-I as the *first-line treatment for insomnia*, due to its efficacy and safety, whether the underlying cause has been identified or not [125–129]. Some pharmacologicals may have similar acute effects, but only CBT-I has shown durable long-term effects after treatment has stopped [127, 128].

We will discuss more about therapies for sleep in Chap. 16 and in Chap. 17.

Summary

A wide variety of factors mediate sleep and depression. Sleep problems may be the cause and/or effect of depression.

Although sleep appears to serve important functions, it is still unclear what they are beyond the classic rest and recuperation. Poor sleep almost always accompanies systemic illness and acute psychiatric disorders.

Two interacting processes regulate the sleep-wake cycle. The circadian process is regulated by oscillations within the suprachiasmatic nucleus of the hypothalamus that controls basic circadian, ultradian, and infradian phenomena such as hormones and metabolism. This circadian function is susceptible to environmental and psychosocial cues and is not dependent upon time awake or tiredness. On the other hand, the homeostatic or recovery process is dependent upon time awake and regulates the urge to sleep.

There are a number of depression related changes in sleep cycles. For example, in individuals afflicted with MDD, the transition from waking to non-REM sleep may involve a smaller decrease in metabolic activity in the frontal, temporal, and parietal cortices, as well as the anterior cingulate cortex, amygdala, and thalamus. These areas may show increased activity in REM sleep and may be related to imbalances in monoaminergic-cholinergic systems in depression.

Depression is the most common cause of insomnia. The suprachiasmatic nucleus in the anterior hypothalamus synchronizes sleep with the help of the CLOCK genes. The C alleles of the CLOCK appear to be implicated in patients with MDD and insomnia. Insomnia and nightmares, along with other sleep disturbances, are significantly associated with suicidal thoughts and behaviors. Repetitive and frightening dreams may be a link to increased suicidal attempts.

When we get less sleep than usual, we incur a sleep debt that results in a drive to longer hours of deeper sleep. Both of these processes are altered in someone experiencing depression. The sleep disorders that are most often encountered in depression are insomnia, hypersomnia, nightmares, and pavor nocturnus.

Even during remissions, patients with major depression, higher anxiety scores, or a history of divorce continue to experience increased frequency of sleep disturbances.

References

1. Kryger MH, Roth T, Dement WC, editors. Principles and practice of sleep medicine. 4th ed. Saunders; 2005.
2. Pace-Schott EF, Hobson JA. The neurobiology of sleep: genetics, cellular physiology and subcortical networks. Nat Rev Neurosci. 2002;3(8):591–605. PMID: 12154361. http://www.ncbi.nlm.nih.gov/pubmed/12154361
3. Hobson JA. Dreaming as delirium: a mental status analysis of our nightly madness. Semin Neurol. 1997;17(2):121–8. PMID: 9195654. http://www.ncbi.nlm.nih.gov/pubmed/9195654
4. Schredl M, Hofmann F. Continuity between waking activities and dream activities. Conscious Cogn. 2003;12(2):298–308. PMID: 12763010. http://www.ncbi.nlm.nih.gov/pubmed/12763010
5. Moffitt A, Kramer M, Hoffmann R, editors. The functions of dreaming. Albany: State University of New York Press; 1993.
6. Pagel JF. Nightmares and disorders of dreaming. Am Fam Physician. 2000;61(7):2037–42. 2044. PMID: 10779247. http://www.ncbi.nlm.nih.gov/pubmed/10779247
7. Gieselmann A, Ait Aoudia M, Carr M, Germain A, Gorzka R, Holzinger B, Kleim B, Krakow B, Kunze AE, Lancee J, Nadorff MR, Nielsen T, Riemann D, Sandahl H, Schlarb AA, Schmid C, Schredl M, Spoormaker VI, Steil R, van Schagen AM, Wittmann L, Zschoche M, Pietrowsky R. Aetiology and treatment of nightmare disorder: State of the art and future perspectives. J Sleep Res. 2019;28(4):e12820. https://doi.org/10.1111/jsr.12820. Epub 2019 Jan 29. PMID: 30697860; PMCID: PMC6850667. Aetiology and treatment of nightmare disorder: State of the art and future perspectives – PubMed
8. Malcolm-Smith S, Solms M. Incidence of threat in dreams: a response to Revonsuo's threat simulation theory. Dreaming. 2004;14:220–9.
9. Roehrs T. Sleep physiology and pathophysiology. Clin Cornerstone. 2000;2(5):1–15. PMID: 10875042. http://www.ncbi.nlm.nih.gov/pubmed/10875042
10. Borbély AA. A two process model of sleep regulation. Hum Neurobiol. 1982;1(3):195–204. PMID: 7185792. http://www.ncbi.nlm.nih.gov/pubmed/7185792
11. Golombek DA, Rosenstein RE. Physiology of circadian entrainment. Physiol Rev. 2010;90(3):1063–102. PMID: 20664079. http://www.ncbi.nlm.nih.gov/pubmed/20664079
12. Luca A, Luca M, Calandra C. Sleep disorders and depression: brief review of the literature, case report, and nonpharmacologic interventions for depression. Clin Interv Aging. 2013;8:1033–9. PMCID: PMC3760296. http://www.ncbi.nlm.nih.gov/pubmed/24019746
13. Cermakian N, Boivin DB. The regulation of central and peripheral circadian clocks in humans. Obes Rev. 2009;10(Suppl 2):25–36. PMID: 19849799. http://www.ncbi.nlm.nih.gov/pubmed/19849799
14. Zee PC, Attarian H, Videnovic A. Circadian rhythm abnormalities. Continuum (Minneap Minn). 2013;19(1 Sleep Disorders):132–47. PMCID: PMC3654533. http://www.ncbi.nlm.nih.gov/pubmed/23385698
15. Lu BS, Zee PC. Circadian rhythm sleep disorders. Chest. 2006;130(6):1915–23. PMID: 17167016. http://www.ncbi.nlm.nih.gov/pubmed/17167016
16. Li J, Vitiello MV, Gooneratne NS. Sleep in normal aging. Sleep Med Clin. 2018;13(1):1–11. PMCID: PMC5841578. http://www.ncbi.nlm.nih.gov/pubmed/29412976
17. The International Classification of Sleep Disorders – Third Edition (ICSD-3) About AASM – Board of Directors, Mission, History & More.
18. Steiger A, Pawlowski M. Depression and Sleep. Int J Mol Sci. 2019;20(3):607. PMCID: PMC6386825. http://www.ncbi.nlm.nih.gov/pubmed/30708948
19. Trotti LM, Arnulf I. Idiopathic hypersomnia and other hypersomnia syndromes. Neurotherapeutics. 2021;18(1):20–31. PMCID: PMC8116415. http://www.ncbi.nlm.nih.gov/pubmed/32901432
20. Redline S, Strohl KP. Recognition and consequences of obstructive sleep apnea hypopnea syndrome. Otolaryngol Clin N Am. 1999;32(2):303–31. PMID: 10385539. http://www.ncbi.nlm.nih.gov/pubmed/10385539
21. Vgontzas AN, Zoumakis E, Bixler EO, Lin HM, Follett H, Kales A, Chrousos GP. Adverse effects of modest sleep restriction on sleepiness, performance, and inflammatory cytokines. J Clin Endocrinol Metab. 2004;89(5):2119–26. PMID: 15126529. http://www.ncbi.nlm.nih.gov/pubmed/15126529
22. Bixler EO, Vgontzas AN, Lin HM, Calhoun SL, Vela-Bueno A, Kales A. Excessive daytime sleepiness in a general population sample: the role of sleep apnea, age, obesity, diabetes, and depression. J Clin Endocrinol Metab. 2005;90(8):4510–5. PMID: 15941867. http://www.ncbi.nlm.nih.gov/pubmed/15941867
23. Mustafa M, Erokwu N, Ebose I, Strohl K. Sleep problems and the risk for sleep disorders in an outpatient veteran population. Sleep Breath. 2005;9(2):57–63. PMID: 15875229. http://www.ncbi.nlm.nih.gov/pubmed/15875229
24. Ocasio-Tascón ME, Alicea-Colón E, Torres-Palacios A, Rodríguez-Cintrón W. The veteran population: one at high risk for sleep-disordered breathing. Sleep Breath. 2006;10(2):70–5. PMID: 16496117. http://www.ncbi.nlm.nih.gov/pubmed/16496117
25. Piani A, Brotini S, Dolso P, Budai R, Gigli GL. Sleep disturbances in elderly: a subjective evaluation over 65. Arch Gerontol Geriatr Suppl. 2004;9:325–31. PMID: 15207430. http://www.ncbi.nlm.nih.gov/pubmed/15207430
26. Redline S, Tishler PV, Hans MG, Tosteson TD, Strohl KP, Spry K. Racial differences in sleep-disordered breathing in African-Americans and Caucasians. Am J Respir Crit Care Med. 1997;155(1):186–92. PMID: 9001310. http://www.ncbi.nlm.nih.gov/pubmed/9001310
27. Ong KC, Clerk AA. Comparison of the severity of sleep-disordered breathing in Asian and Caucasian patients seen at a sleep disorders center. Respir Med. 1998;92(6):843–8. PMID: 9850368. http://www.ncbi.nlm.nih.gov/pubmed/9850368
28. The Merck manual of diagnosis and therapy 17. Merck, 1999.
29. Schwartz S, McDowell Anderson W, Cole SR, Cornoni-Huntley J, Hays JC, Blazer D. Insomnia and heart disease: a review of epidemiologic studies. J Psychosom Res. 1999;47(4):313–33. PMID: 10616226. http://www.ncbi.nlm.nih.gov/pubmed/10616226
30. Leproult R, Copinschi G, Buxton O, Van Cauter E. Sleep loss results in an elevation of cortisol levels the next evening. Sleep.

1997;20(10):865–70. PMID: 9415946. http://www.ncbi.nlm.nih.gov/pubmed/9415946
31. Veldhuis JD, Iranmanesh A. Physiological regulation of the human growth hormone (GH)-insulin-like growth factor type I (IGF-I) axis: predominant impact of age, obesity, gonadal function, and sleep. Sleep. 1996;19(10 Suppl):S221–4. PMID: 9085516. http://www.ncbi.nlm.nih.gov/pubmed/9085516
32. Hatzinger M, Brand S, Perren S, Stadelmann S, von Wyl A, von Klitzing K, Holsboer-Trachsler E. Electroencephalographic sleep profiles and hypothalamic-pituitary-adrenocortical (HPA)-activity in kindergarten children: early indication of poor sleep quality associated with increased cortisol secretion. J Psychiatr Res. 2008;42(7):532–43. PMID: 17645894. http://www.ncbi.nlm.nih.gov/pubmed/17645894
33. Steiger A, Kimura M. Wake and sleep EEG provide biomarkers in depression. J Psychiatr Res. 2010;44(4):242–52. PMID: 19762038. http://www.ncbi.nlm.nih.gov/pubmed/19762038
34. Lam RW. Sleep disturbances and depression: a challenge for antidepressants. Int Clin Psychopharmacol. 2006;21(Suppl 1):S25–9. PMID: 16436937. http://www.ncbi.nlm.nih.gov/pubmed/16436937
35. Peterson M, Benca R. Sleep in Mood Disorders. Sleep Med Clin. 2008;3:231–49.
36. Medina AB, Lechuga DA, Escandón OS, Moctezuma JV. Update of sleep alterations in depression. Sleep Sci. 2014;7(3):165–9. PMCID: PMC4559588. http://www.ncbi.nlm.nih.gov/pubmed/26483922
37. Benca RM, Peterson MJ. Insomnia and depression. Sleep Med. 2008;9(Suppl 1):S3–9. PMID: 18929317. http://www.ncbi.nlm.nih.gov/pubmed/18929317
38. Ohayon MM. Epidemiology of insomnia: what we know and what we still need to learn. Sleep Med Rev. 2002;6(2):97–111. PMID: 12531146. http://www.ncbi.nlm.nih.gov/pubmed/12531146
39. Ohayon MM. Prevalence and correlates of nonrestorative sleep complaints. Arch Intern Med. 2005;165(1):35–41. PMID: 15642872. http://www.ncbi.nlm.nih.gov/pubmed/15642872
40. Baglioni C, Riemann D. Is chronic insomnia a precursor to major depression? Epidemiological and biological findings. Curr Psychiatry Rep. 2012;14(5):511–8. PMID: 22865155. http://www.ncbi.nlm.nih.gov/pubmed/22865155
41. Li SX, Lam SP, Chan JWY, Yu MWM, Wing YK. Residual sleep disturbances in patients remitted from major depressive disorder: a 4-year naturalistic follow-up study. Sleep. 2012;35(8):1153–61. PMCID: PMC3397819. http://www.ncbi.nlm.nih.gov/pubmed/22851811
42. Rush AJ, Erman MK, Giles DE, Schlesser MA, Carpenter G, Vasavada N, Roffwarg HP. Polysomnographic findings in recently drug-free and clinically remitted depressed patients. Arch Gen Psychiatry. 1986;43(9):878–84. PMID: 3753165. http://www.ncbi.nlm.nih.gov/pubmed/3753165
43. Kupfer DJ, Spiker DG, Coble PA, Neil JF, Ulrich R, Shaw DH. Sleep and treatment prediction in endogenous depression. Am J Psychiatry. 1981;138(4):429–34. PMID: 7212100. http://www.ncbi.nlm.nih.gov/pubmed/7212100
44. Peterson MJ, Benca RM. Sleep in mood disorders. Psychiatr Clin North Am. 2006;29(4):1009–32. abstract ix. PMID: 17118279. http://www.ncbi.nlm.nih.gov/pubmed/17118279
45. Ehlers CL, Kupfer DJ. Hypothalamic peptide modulation of EEG sleep in depression: a further application of the S-process hypothesis. Biol Psychiatry. 1987;22(4):513–7. PMID: 3032289. http://www.ncbi.nlm.nih.gov/pubmed/3032289
46. Linkowski P, Mendlewicz J, Kerkhofs M, Leclercq R, Golstein J, Brasseur M, Copinschi G, Van Cauter E. 24-hour profiles of adrenocorticotropin, cortisol, and growth hormone in major depressive illness: effect of antidepressant treatment. J Clin Endocrinol Metab. 1987;65(1):141–52. PMID: 3034952. http://www.ncbi.nlm.nih.gov/pubmed/3034952
47. Riemann D. Insomnia and comorbid psychiatric disorders. Sleep Med. 2007;8(Suppl 4):S15–20. PMID: 18346672. http://www.ncbi.nlm.nih.gov/pubmed/18346672
48. Lawson RP, Drevets WC, Roiser JP. Defining the habenula in human neuroimaging studies. Neuroimage. 2013;64:722–7. PMCID: PMC3650642. http://www.ncbi.nlm.nih.gov/pubmed/22986224
49. Grant P, Kuepper Y, Mueller EA, Wielpuetz C, Mason O, Hennig J. Dopaminergic foundations of schizotypy as measured by the German version of the Oxford-Liverpool Inventory of Feelings and Experiences (O-LIFE)-a suitable endophenotype of schizophrenia. Front Hum Neurosci. 2013;7:1. PMCID: PMC3553421. http://www.ncbi.nlm.nih.gov/pubmed/23355817
50. Urrila AS, Paunio T, Palomäki E, Marttunen M. Sleep in adolescent depression: physiological perspectives. Acta Physiol (Oxf). 2015;213(4):758–77. PMID: 25561272. http://www.ncbi.nlm.nih.gov/pubmed/25561272
51. Meerlo P, Havekes R, Steiger A. Chronically restricted or disrupted sleep as a causal factor in the development of depression. Curr Top Behav Neurosci. 2015;25:459–81. PMID: 25646723. http://www.ncbi.nlm.nih.gov/pubmed/25646723
52. Peppard PE, Szklo-Coxe M, Hla KM, Young T. Longitudinal association of sleep-related breathing disorder and depression. Arch Intern Med. 2006;166(16):1709–15. PMID: 16983048. http://www.ncbi.nlm.nih.gov/pubmed/16983048
53. Berk M. Sleep and depression - theory and practice. Aust Fam Physician. 2009;38(5):302–4. PMID: 19458799. http://www.ncbi.nlm.nih.gov/pubmed/19458799
54. Bunney JN, Potkin SG. Circadian abnormalities, molecular clock genes and chronobiological treatments in depression. Br Med Bull. 2008;86:23–32. PMID: 18487629. http://www.ncbi.nlm.nih.gov/pubmed/18487629
55. Serretti A, Cusin C, Benedetti F, Mandelli L, Pirovano A, Zanardi R, Colombo C, Smeraldi E. Insomnia improvement during antidepressant treatment and CLOCK gene polymorphism. Am J Med Genet B Neuropsychiatr Genet. 2005;137B(1):36–9. PMID: 15952199. http://www.ncbi.nlm.nih.gov/pubmed/15952199
56. Serretti A, Benedetti F, Mandelli L, Lorenzi C, Pirovano A, Colombo C, Smeraldi E. Genetic dissection of psychopathological symptoms: insomnia in mood disorders and CLOCK gene polymorphism. Am J Med Genet B Neuropsychiatr Genet. 2003;121B(1):35–8. PMID: 12898572. http://www.ncbi.nlm.nih.gov/pubmed/12898572
57. Benedetti F, Colombo C, Serretti A, Lorenzi C, Pontiggia A, Barbini B, Smeraldi E. Antidepressant effects of light therapy combined with sleep deprivation are influenced by a functional polymorphism within the promoter of the serotonin transporter gene. Biol Psychiatry. 2003;54(7):687–92. PMID: 14512208. http://www.ncbi.nlm.nih.gov/pubmed/14512208
58. Hu XZ, Rush AJ, Charney D, Wilson AF, Sorant AJM, Papanicolaou GJ, Fava M, Trivedi MH, Wisniewski SR, Laje G, Paddock S, McMahon FJ, Manji H, Lipsky RH. Association between a functional serotonin transporter promoter polymorphism and citalopram treatment in adult outpatients with major depression. Arch Gen Psychiatry. 2007;64(7):783–92. PMID: 17606812. http://www.ncbi.nlm.nih.gov/pubmed/17606812
59. Saus E, Soria V, Escaramís G, Vivarelli F, Crespo JM, Kagerbauer B, Menchón JM, Urretavizcaya M, Gratacòs M, Estivill X. Genetic variants and abnormal processing of pre-miR-182, a circadian clock modulator, in major depression patients with late insomnia. Hum Mol Genet. 2010;19(20):4017–25. PMID: 20656788. http://www.ncbi.nlm.nih.gov/pubmed/20656788
60. Pigeon WR, Pinquart M, Conner K. Meta-analysis of sleep disturbance and suicidal thoughts and behaviors. J Clin Psychiatry.

2012;73(9):e1160–7. PMID: 23059158. http://www.ncbi.nlm.nih.gov/pubmed/23059158
61. Agargun MY, Besiroglu L, Cilli AS, Gulec M, Aydin A, Inci R, Selvi Y. Nightmares, suicide attempts, and melancholic features in patients with unipolar major depression. J Affect Disord. 2007;98(3):267–70. PMID: 16938351. http://www.ncbi.nlm.nih.gov/pubmed/16938351
62. Littlewood DL, Gooding PA, Panagioti M, Kyle SD. Nightmares and suicide in posttraumatic stress disorder: the mediating role of defeat, entrapment, and hopelessness. J Clin Sleep Med. 2016;12(3):393–9. PMCID: PMC4773636. http://www.ncbi.nlm.nih.gov/pubmed/26564386
63. Beauchemin KM, Hays P. Dreaming away depression: the role of REM sleep and dreaming in affective disorders. J Affect Disord. 1996;41(2):125–33. PMID: 8961040. http://www.ncbi.nlm.nih.gov/pubmed/8961040
64. Hartmann E, Elkin R, Garg M. Personality and dreaming: the dreams of people with very thick or very thin boundaries. Dreaming. 1991;1:311–24.
65. Terr LC. Nightmares in children. In: Guilleminault C, editor. Sleep and its disorders in children. New York: Raven; 1987.
66. Hartmann E. The nightmare: the psychology and biology of terrifying dreams. New York: Basic Books; 1984.
67. Hawkins C, Williams TI. Nightmares, life events and behaviour problems in preschool children. Child Care Health Dev. 1992;18(2):117–28. PMID: 1587010. http://www.ncbi.nlm.nih.gov/pubmed/1587010
68. Sandman N, Valli K, Kronholm E, Revonsuo A, Laatikainen T, Paunio T. Nightmares: risk factors among the Finnish general adult population. Sleep. 2015;38(4):507–14. PMCID: PMC4355890. http://www.ncbi.nlm.nih.gov/pubmed/25325474
69. Nielsen T, Paquette T, Solomonova E, Lara-Carrasco J, Colombo R, Lanfranchi P. Changes in cardiac variability after REM sleep deprivation in recurrent nightmares. Sleep. 2010;33(1):113–22. PMCID: PMC2802238. http://www.ncbi.nlm.nih.gov/pubmed/20120628
70. Simor P, Bódizs R, Horváth K, Ferri R. Disturbed dreaming and the instability of sleep: altered nonrapid eye movement sleep microstructure in individuals with frequent nightmares as revealed by the cyclic alternating pattern. Sleep. 2013;36(3):413–9. PMCID: PMC3571751. http://www.ncbi.nlm.nih.gov/pubmed/23449753
71. Hobson JA, Pace-Schott EF, Stickgold R. Dreaming and the brain: toward a cognitive neuroscience of conscious states. Behav Brain Sci. 2000;23(6):793–842. discussion 904–1121. PMID: 11515143. http://www.ncbi.nlm.nih.gov/pubmed/11515143
72. Solms M. Dreaming and REM sleep are controlled by different brain mechanisms. Behav Brain Sci. 2000;23(6):843–50. discussion 904–1121. PMID: 11515144 http://www.ncbi.nlm.nih.gov/pubmed/11515144
73. Nielsen T, Levin R. Nightmares: a new neurocognitive model. Sleep Med Rev. 2007;11(4):295–310. PMID: 17498981. http://www.ncbi.nlm.nih.gov/pubmed/17498981
74. Zadra A, Pilon M, Donderi DC. Variety and intensity of emotions in nightmares and bad dreams. J Nerv Ment Dis. 2006;194(4):249–54. PMID: 16614545. http://www.ncbi.nlm.nih.gov/pubmed/16614545
75. Klink M, Quan SF. Prevalence of reported sleep disturbances in a general adult population and their relationship to obstructive airways diseases. Chest. 1987;91(4):540–6. PMID: 3829746. http://www.ncbi.nlm.nih.gov/pubmed/3829746
76. Ohayon MM, Morselli PL, Guilleminault C. Prevalence of nightmares and their relationship to psychopathology and daytime functioning in insomnia subjects. Sleep. 1997;20(5):340–8. PMID: 9381055. http://www.ncbi.nlm.nih.gov/pubmed/9381055
77. Csóka S, Simor P, Szabó G, Kopp MS, Bódizs R. Early maternal separation, nightmares, and bad dreams: results from the Hungarostudy epidemiological panel. Attach Hum Dev. 2011;13(2):125–40. PMID: 21390906. http://www.ncbi.nlm.nih.gov/pubmed/21390906
78. Pagel JF. Nightmares. Am Fam Physician. 1989;39(3):145–8. PMID: 2646879. http://www.ncbi.nlm.nih.gov/pubmed/2646879
79. Thompson DF, Pierce DR. Drug-induced nightmares. Ann Pharmacother. 1999;33(1):93–8. PMID: 9972389. http://www.ncbi.nlm.nih.gov/pubmed/9972389
80. Pagel JF, Helfter P. Drug induced nightmares–an etiology based review. Hum Psychopharmacol. 2003;18(1):59–67. PMID: 12532316. http://www.ncbi.nlm.nih.gov/pubmed/12532316
81. Winokur A, Gary KA, Rodner S, Rae-Red C, Fernando AT, Szuba MP. Depression, sleep physiology, and antidepressant drugs. Depress Anxiety. 2001;14(1):19–28. PMID: 11568979. http://www.ncbi.nlm.nih.gov/pubmed/11568979
82. Hartman D, Crisp AH, Sedgwick P, Borrow S. Is there a dissociative process in sleepwalking and night terrors? Postgrad Med J. 2001;77(906):244–9. PMCID: PMC1741968. http://www.ncbi.nlm.nih.gov/pubmed/11264487.
83. Haupt M, Sheldon SH, Loghmanee D. Just a scary dream? A brief review of sleep terrors, nightmares, and rapid eye movement sleep behavior disorder. Pediatr Ann. 2013;42(10):211–6. PMID: 24126984. http://www.ncbi.nlm.nih.gov/pubmed/24126984
84. Szelenberger W, Niemcewicz S, Dabrowska AJ. Sleepwalking and night terrors: psychopathological and psychophysiological correlates. Int Rev Psychiatry. 2005;17(4):263–70. PMID: 16194798. http://www.ncbi.nlm.nih.gov/pubmed/16194798
85. Crisp AH, Matthews BM, Oakey M, Crutchfield M. Sleepwalking, night terrors, and consciousness. BMJ. 1990;300(6721):360–2. PMCID: PMC1662124. http://www.ncbi.nlm.nih.gov/pubmed/2106985
86. Kales JD, Kales A, Soldatos CR, Caldwell AB, Charney DS, Martin ED. Night terrors. Clinical characteristics and personality patterns. Arch Gen Psychiatry. 1980;37(12):1413–7. PMID: 7447622. http://www.ncbi.nlm.nih.gov/pubmed/7447622
87. Stores G. Aspects of parasomnias in childhood and adolescence. Arch Dis Child. 2009;94(1):63–9. PMID: 18499772. http://www.ncbi.nlm.nih.gov/pubmed/18499772
88. Llorente MD, Currier MB, Norman SE, Mellman TA. Night terrors in adults: phenomenology and relationship to psychopathology. J Clin Psychiatry. 1992;53(11):392–4. PMID: 1459969. http://www.ncbi.nlm.nih.gov/pubmed/1459969
89. Pressman MR, Meyer TJ, Kendrick-Mohamed J, Figueroa WG, Greenspon LW, Peterson DD. Night terrors in an adult precipitated by sleep apnea. Sleep. 1995;18(9):773–5. PMID: 8638070. http://www.ncbi.nlm.nih.gov/pubmed/8638070
90. Pagel JF, Kwiatkowski C. The nightmares of sleep apnea: nightmare frequency declines with increasing apnea hypopnea index. J Clin Sleep Med. 2010;6(1):69–73. PMCID: PMC2823279. http://www.ncbi.nlm.nih.gov/pubmed/20191941
91. BaHammam AS, Al-Shimemeri SA, Salama RI, Sharif MM. Clinical and polysomnographic characteristics and response to continuous positive airway pressure therapy in obstructive sleep apnea patients with nightmares. Sleep Med. 2013;14(2):149–54. PMID: 22959148. http://www.ncbi.nlm.nih.gov/pubmed/22959148
92. Hobzova M, Prasko J, Vanek J, Ociskova M, Genzor S, Holubova M, Grambal A, Latalova K. Depression and obstructive sleep apnea. Neuro Endocrinol Lett. 2017;38(5):343–52. PMID: 29106789. http://www.ncbi.nlm.nih.gov/pubmed/29106789
93. BaHammam AS, Kendzerska T, Gupta R, Ramasubramanian C, Neubauer DN, Narasimhan M, Pandi-Perumal SR, Moscovitch A. Comorbid depression in obstructive sleep apnea: an under-recognized association. Sleep Breath. 2016;20(2):447–56. PMID: 26156890. http://www.ncbi.nlm.nih.gov/pubmed/26156890

94. Pan ML, Tsao HM, Hsu CC, Wu KM, Hsu TS, Wu YT, Hu GC. Bidirectional association between obstructive sleep apnea and depression: a population-based longitudinal study. Medicine (Baltimore). 2016;95(37):e4833. PMCID: PMC5402579. http://www.ncbi.nlm.nih.gov/pubmed/27631236
95. Wheaton AG, Perry GS, Chapman DP, Croft JB. Sleep disordered breathing and depression among U.S. adults: National Health and Nutrition Examination Survey, 2005–2008. Sleep. 2012;35(4):461–7. PMCID: PMC3296787. http://www.ncbi.nlm.nih.gov/pubmed/22467983
96. Sala M, Vicentini A, Brambilla P, Montomoli C, Jogia JR, Caverzasi E, Bonzano A, Piccinelli M, Barale F, De Ferrari GM. QT interval prolongation related to psychoactive drug treatment: a comparison of monotherapy versus polytherapy. Ann Gen Psychiatry. 2005;4(1):1. PMCID: PMC1088007. http://www.ncbi.nlm.nih.gov/pubmed/15845138
97. Acker J, Richter K, Piehl A, Herold J, Ficker JH, Niklewski G. Obstructive sleep apnea (OSA) and clinical depression-prevalence in a sleep center. Sleep Breath. 2017;21(2):311–8. PMID: 27704327. http://www.ncbi.nlm.nih.gov/pubmed/27704327
98. Gupta MA, Simpson FC. Obstructive sleep apnea and psychiatric disorders: a systematic review. J Clin Sleep Med. 2015;11(2):165–75. PMCID: PMC4298774. http://www.ncbi.nlm.nih.gov/pubmed/25406268
99. Lang CJ, Appleton SL, Vakulin A, McEvoy RD, Wittert GA, Martin SA, Catcheside PG, Antic NA, Lack L, Adams RJ. Co-morbid OSA and insomnia increases depression prevalence and severity in men. Respirology. 2017;22(7):1407–15. PMID: 28589663. http://www.ncbi.nlm.nih.gov/pubmed/28589663
100. Numthavaj P, Thakkinstian A, Dejthevaporn C, Attia J. Corticosteroid and antiviral therapy for bell's palsy: a network meta-analysis. BMC Neurol. 2011;11:1. PMCID: PMC3025847. http://www.ncbi.nlm.nih.gov/pubmed/21208452
101. Picchietti D, Winkelman JW. Restless legs syndrome, periodic limb movements in sleep, and depression. Sleep. 2005;28(7):891–8. PMID: 16124671. http://www.ncbi.nlm.nih.gov/pubmed/16124671
102. Ohayon MM, Roth T. Prevalence of restless legs syndrome and periodic limb movement disorder in the general population. J Psychosom Res. 2002;53(1):547–54. PMID: 12127170. http://www.ncbi.nlm.nih.gov/pubmed/12127170
103. Kim KW, Yoon IY, Chung S, Shin YK, Lee SB, Choi EA, Park JH, Kim JM. Prevalence, comorbidities and risk factors of restless legs syndrome in the Korean elderly population – results from the Korean longitudinal study on health and aging. J Sleep Res. 2010;19(1 Pt 1):87–92. PMID: 19686313. http://www.ncbi.nlm.nih.gov/pubmed/19686313
104. Ohayon MM. Narcolepsy is complicated by high medical and psychiatric comorbidities: a comparison with the general population. Sleep Med. 2013;14(6):488–92. PMID: 23643648. http://www.ncbi.nlm.nih.gov/pubmed/23643648
105. Dauvilliers Y, Lopez R, Ohayon M, Bayard S. Hypersomnia and depressive symptoms: methodological and clinical aspects. BMC Med. 2013;11:78. PMCID: PMC3621400. http://www.ncbi.nlm.nih.gov/pubmed/23514569
106. Wichniak A, Wierzbicka A, Jernajczyk W. Sleep and antidepressant treatment. Curr Pharm Des. 2012;18(36):5802–17. PMID: 22681161. http://www.ncbi.nlm.nih.gov/pubmed/22681161
107. Postuma RB, Gagnon JF, Tuineaig M, Bertrand JA, Latreille V, Desjardins C, Montplaisir JY. Antidepressants and REM sleep behavior disorder: isolated side effect or neurodegenerative signal? Sleep. 2013;36(11):1579–85. PMCID: PMC3792373. http://www.ncbi.nlm.nih.gov/pubmed/24179289
108. Schramm PJ, Poland RE, Rao U. Bupropion response on sleep quality in patients with depression: implications for increased cardiovascular disease risk. Eur Neuropsychopharmacol. 2014;24(2):207–14. PMCID: PMC3948318. http://www.ncbi.nlm.nih.gov/pubmed/24239431
109. Wilkes S. Bupropion. Drugs Today (Barc). 2006;42(10):671–81. PMID: 17136226. http://www.ncbi.nlm.nih.gov/pubmed/17136226
110. Thase ME. Depression, sleep, and antidepressants. J Clin Psychiatry. 1998;59(Suppl 4):55–65. PMID: 9554322. http://www.ncbi.nlm.nih.gov/pubmed/9554322
111. Kurian BT, Greer TL, Trivedi MH. Strategies to enhance the therapeutic efficacy of antidepressants: targeting residual symptoms. Expert Rev Neurother. 2009;9(7):975–84. PMCID: PMC2720783. http://www.ncbi.nlm.nih.gov/pubmed/19589048
112. Franzen PL, Buysse DJ. Sleep disturbances and depression: risk relationships for subsequent depression and therapeutic implications. Dialogues Clin Neurosci. 2008;10(4):473–81. PMCID: PMC3108260. http://www.ncbi.nlm.nih.gov/pubmed/19170404
113. Fagiolini A, Comandini A, Catena Dell'Osso M, Kasper S. Rediscovering trazodone for the treatment of major depressive disorder. CNS Drugs. 2012;26(12):1033–49. PMCID: PMC3693429. http://www.ncbi.nlm.nih.gov/pubmed/23192413
114. De Berardis D, Marini S, Fornaro M, Srinivasan V, Iasevoli F, Tomasetti C, Valchera A, Perna G, Quera-Salva MA, Martinotti G, di Giannantonio M. The melatonergic system in mood and anxiety disorders and the role of agomelatine: implications for clinical practice. Int J Mol Sci. 2013;14(6):12458–83. PMCID: PMC3709794. http://www.ncbi.nlm.nih.gov/pubmed/23765220
115. Komaram RB, Nukala S, Palla J, Nambaru LR, Kasturi SM. A comparative study of efficacy and safety of Agomelatine and escitalopram in major depressive disorder. J Clin Diagn Res. 2015;9(6):VC05–8. PMCID: PMC4525586. http://www.ncbi.nlm.nih.gov/pubmed/26266196
116. Gahr M, Kratzer W, Fuchs M, Connemann BJ. Safety and tolerability of agomelatine: focus on hepatotoxicity. Curr Drug Metab. 2014;15(7):694–702. PMID: 25255870. http://www.ncbi.nlm.nih.gov/pubmed/25255870
117. AHRQ Comparative Effectiveness Reviews – NCBI Bookshelf.
118. Brasure M, MacDonald R, Fuchs E, Olson CM, Carlyle M, Diem S, Koffel E, Khawaja IS, Ouellette J, Butler M, Kane RL, Wilt TJ. Management of Insomnia Disorder [Internet]. Rockville (MD): Agency for Healthcare Research and Quality (US); 2015 [cited 2025 Jan 4]. Available from: http://www.ncbi.nlm.nih.gov/books/NBK343503/. PMID: 26844312 http://www.ncbi.nlm.nih.gov/pubmed/26844312
119. Haynes P. Application of cognitive behavioral therapies for comorbid insomnia and depression. Sleep Med Clin. 2015;10(1):77–84. PMID: 26055675. http://www.ncbi.nlm.nih.gov/pubmed/26055675
120. Manber R, Bernert RA, Suh S, Nowakowski S, Siebern AT, Ong JC. CBT for insomnia in patients with high and low depressive symptom severity: adherence and clinical outcomes. J Clin Sleep Med. 2011;7(6):645–52. PMCID: PMC3227711. http://www.ncbi.nlm.nih.gov/pubmed/22171204
121. Matthews EE, Arnedt JT, McCarthy MS, Cuddihy LJ, Aloia MS. Adherence to cognitive behavioral therapy for insomnia: a systematic review. Sleep Med Rev. 2013;17(6):453–64. PMCID: PMC3720832. http://www.ncbi.nlm.nih.gov/pubmed/23602124
122. Johnson JA, Rash JA, Campbell TS, Savard J, Gehrman PR, Perlis M, Carlson LE, Garland SN. A systematic review and meta-analysis of randomized controlled trials of cognitive behavior therapy for insomnia (CBT-I) in cancer survivors. Sleep Med Rev. 2016;27:20–8. PMID: 26434673. http://www.ncbi.nlm.nih.gov/pubmed/26434673
123. Cognitive Behavioral Therapy for Insomnia (CBT-I): An Overview
124. Clarke G, Harvey AG. The complex role of sleep in adolescent depression. Child Adolesc Psychiatr Clin N Am.

2012;21(2):385–400. PMCID: PMC3605974. http://www.ncbi.nlm.nih.gov/pubmed/22537732.
125. Qaseem A, Kansagara D, Forciea MA, Cooke M, Denberg TD, Clinical guidelines Committee of the American College of physicians. Management of Chronic Insomnia Disorder in adults: a clinical practice guideline from the American College of Physicians. Ann Intern Med. 2016;165(2):125–33. PMID: 27136449. http://www.ncbi.nlm.nih.gov/pubmed/27136449
126. Riemann D, Baglioni C, Bassetti C, Bjorvatn B, Dolenc Groselj L, Ellis JG, Espie CA, Garcia-Borreguero D, Gjerstad M, Gonçalves M, Hertenstein E, Jansson-Fröjmark M, Jennum PJ, Leger D, Nissen C, Parrino L, Paunio T, Pevernagie D, Verbraecken J, Weeß HG, Wichniak A, Zavalko I, Arnardottir ES, Deleanu OC, Strazisar B, Zoetmulder M, Spiegelhalder K. European guideline for the diagnosis and treatment of insomnia. J Sleep Res. 2017;26(6):675–700. PMID: 28875581. http://www.ncbi.nlm.nih.gov/pubmed/28875581
127. Perlis ML, Posner D, Riemann D, Bastien CH, Teel J, Thase M. Insomnia. Lancet. 2022;400(10357):1047–60. PMID: 36115372. http://www.ncbi.nlm.nih.gov/pubmed/36115372
128. Trauer JM, Qian MY, Doyle JS, Rajaratnam SMW, Cunnington D. Cognitive behavioral therapy for chronic insomnia: a systematic review and meta-analysis. Ann Intern Med. 2015;163(3):191–204. PMID: 26054060. http://www.ncbi.nlm.nih.gov/pubmed/26054060
129. Vitiello MV. Cognitive-behavioural therapy for insomnia: effective, long-lasting and safe. Evid Based Ment Health 2016;19(1):e2. PMCID: PMC10699350. http://www.ncbi.nlm.nih.gov/pubmed/26674632

What Can We Change and How?

14

Franklin Sunzeri

Introduction

Expression of many genes is controlled by experience that can modify their transcription [107]. Some genetic patterns are age- or developmental-stage-related changes, and others are plasticity-related changes [108]. These changes are perhaps best understood in terms of epigenetics. And it appears that learning, synaptic plasticity [109], and consolidating and stabilizing cognitive-behavioral memories are dependent upon epigenetic processes [110, 111].

In many, if not most, mental disorders, genetic factors are involved [112]. However, discordance rates in identical twin studies, especially in stress-related illnesses such as depression, suggest that other processes are implicated [112–115]. Maladaptation in gene expression, neural network functions, and behavior may be induced by environmental exposure [116]. These changes appear to be sustained and are distinct depending upon exposure at critical developmental times or in adulthood [117]. These changes are highly correlated with mental disorders such as depression, schizophrenia, and bipolar disorder [116]. Comprehensive reviews of epigenetic mechanisms in depression can be found in these references [118–124].

Epigenetics

Epigenetics (epi = in addition to, above, or upon) is usually taken to mean the relationship between genotype and phenotype [the discernible characteristics that are a product of genes and the environment], or the global mechanisms of gene regulation involved in growth and development [125–127]. On one level, this relates to inheritable expression or repression of genes during development, and it probably obeys different rules than Mendelian inheritance [128]. The underlying assumption is that characteristics may be passed from one cell, tissue, or organism generation to the next generation via mechanisms that do not involve changes to the DNA sequences themselves.

Phenotypes are dependent upon which genes become transcribed and upon the level at which these genes are expressed. Expression of genes can be controlled at several levels. We will discuss changes to DNA that modify transcription and small RNA functions that have effects on both transcription and post-transcription processes. And, as we shall see later, various experiments have shown that the environment can play an important role in modifying genetic expression. This expression is stable, but is capable of being changed [129, 130].

In 2010, *the International Human Epigenome Consortium* (IHEC) began [131–133]. In 2013, the NIH *Roadmap Epigenomics Project* began as part of the IHEC [134]. These projects support reference epigenome production centers that develop reference epigenomes of a variety of human cells.

The goal is to identify potential therapeutic targets, enhance understanding of disease mechanisms, provide additional insights into genetic susceptibility of disease, pursue therapeutic opportunities in stem cell-based and tissue regeneration strategies, and understand normal differentiation, development, and aging/senescence. One of the multiple initiatives is to identify fundamental epigenomic changes or mechanisms underlying specific diseases, conditions of development or aging, or response to exposures (physical, chemical, behavioral, and social factors).

They define epigenetics as both heritable changes in gene activity and expression (in the progeny of cells or of individuals) and stable, long-term alterations in the transcriptional potential of a cell that are not necessarily heritable.

There is a consensus that *multiple mechanistic steps are required* for the stable inheritance of a phenotype resulting from changes in a chromosome without alterations in the DNA sequence [135, 136]. These changes operate on the basis of methylation and other modifications of DNA, post-translational modifications of histones [137], maneuvering

F. Sunzeri (✉)
Heather Hills Consulting, Coos Bay, OR, USA

J. Raber et al. (eds.), *Understanding and Treating Depressive Disorders*, https://doi.org/10.1007/978-3-032-14465-2_14

of small RNAs [138], and 3D conformations of chromosomes [139]. Epigenetic changes have been linked to autoimmune diseases, aging, cancer, and psychiatric disorders, such as depression [140, 141]. Because epigenetic aberrations can, in some instances, be reversed, they represent a topic worth investigating from a behavioral medicine standpoint [137].

An *epigenator* from the extracellular environment begins the process (e.g., temperature changes, differentiation signals).[1] These transient signals are relayed (via various pathways) through the cytoplasm to the nucleus, where the *epigenetic initiators* are found. These initiators include noncoding RNAs and DNA-binding factors that have specific sequence recognition ability. These initiators determine the exact chromatin and DNA environment that are appropriate for the epigenetic pathway. Positive feedback appears to be a general requirement to maintain self-renewal and self-reinforcement.

To maintain those epigenetic changes in the present and subsequent generations, *epigenetic maintainers* are stimulated. These include DNA and histone modifiers, nucleosome positioning, and histone variants. However, not all post-translational modifications of histones are epigenetic. The maintainers do not need sequence specificity. The initiators and the maintainers appear to work in consort to maintain the chromatin modifications.

It has become clear that hundreds of proteins are associated with the activation and repression of genes in an immensely complicated epigenetic network in stress-related depression disorders [142, 143].

Inherited cis-linked (on the same DNA strand) chromatin structures are called *epitypes* or *epigenotypes* [144–146]. Somatic epitypes appear to be dynamic and alterable both before and after birth by such things as maternal care, exercise, nutritional, or behavioral stress. Gene expressions but not amino acid sequences are altered by somatic epitypes. Reprogramming of epitypes appears to be more susceptible at particular times in development and in particular tissues.

There is an *extremely complex cause-and-effect relationship* among genotype, epitype, and phenotype. However, it appears that genotypes predispose epitypes. That is, methylation of CpG is determined by gene sequence and the influence of paired sequence-specific complementary small RNAs that direct their transgenerational remethylation [146]. Epitypes modify gene expression and risk phenotype. Therefore, DNA and RNA sequences heavily influence epigenetic controls. So, a revised definition of epigenetics could be that presented by David Nanney in 1958: "*epigenetic systems regulate the expression of the genetically determined potentialities*" [147].

[1]The terms epigenator, epigenetic initiators, and epigenetic maintainers are not widely used but are suitable descriptors [149].

Our 6 billion nucleotides are wrapped into 23 pairs of chromosomes. Each chromosome is composed of two chromatins. The *chromatins* are the packaged form of an individual strand of DNA plus proteins. The principal proteins are the *histones*. The fundamental unit of the chromatins is the *nucleosome*, which is a 146 bp segment of DNA wound ~1.65 times around a cluster of eight histone proteins. Each histone octamer is composed of two copies each of the histones H2A, H2B, H3, and H4 [148, 150]. Each nucleosome is bound to the next one via one *linker histone* (H1) from the linker histone family [151, 152]. This group of one nucleosome plus a linker histone is called a *chromatosome* [153]. The chromatosome is composed of 146 bp of DNA from the nucleosome, the nucleosome histone octamer, plus 20–80 bp of DNA of the H1 plus the linker H1 itself [154].

The conformational relationships of histones and DNA change the access of transcription factors to the DNA [155]. These 3D chromatin changes are controlled by various epigenetic factors. A family of *nucleosome remodeling ATPases* is in charge of keeping the chromatin flexible enough to respond to developmental, metabolic, and environmental signals [156, 157]. Upon binding and hydrolyzing ATP, the ATPases change their conformation while simultaneously interacting with the nucleosomes [157, 158]. This interaction may result in various degrees of assembly or disassembly of nucleosomes and/or movement or exchanges of histones [159, 160].

Remodeling of nucleosomes allows DNA access or denies DNA access by proteins. In so doing, they integrate with other processes, including RNA metabolism and histone modifications, to affect a stable epigenetic state [148, 150]. The state of chromatin that is open for transcription is called *euchromatin*. The inactivated closed state that represses transcription is called *heterochromatin*.

One of the most studied ways in which transcription can be suppressed is through covalently attaching a methyl group to the C5 position of cytosine *(5mC)* most frequently at cytosine-guanine dyads (*CpG*) sites [161]. However, methylation can occur at non-CpG sites and methylation of DNA can also produce enhanced expression of DNA depending upon the context [162].

CpG's tend to be in or around promoter regions and are usually not extensively methylated in normal somatic cells [161, 163]. When methylation of these promoter islands occurs, it can repress expression of DNA in one of two ways. It can bind to methyl-CpG-binding proteins to recruit transcriptional corepressors to affect a heterochromatin state. Alternatively, it can block the start site from binding transcriptional activators and RNA polymerase II [161, 163, 164].

Critically, *methylation is reversible* [165–167]. *Methylcytosine oxidase ten-eleven translocation (TET) proteins* catalyze the sequential oxidation of 5-methylcytosine

(5mC) to oxidized methylcytosines, including 5-hydroxymethylcytosine (*5hmC*), 5-formylcytosine, and 5-carboxylcytosine. In so doing, TETs contribute to the regulation of lineage-specific gene expression by modulating DNA *5mC/5hmC balance*. As such, TET participates in ensuring neuronal plasticity by establishing and/or maintaining hypomethylated 5mC/5hmC domains at multiple differentiation-associated genes.

Approximately 40% of the modified cytosine in the brain is 5hmC and compared to 5mC is more correlated to plasticity instead of repression [168, 169]. The 5-hmC-regulated regions show stable and dynamically modified loci during postnatal neurodevelopment and aging. These methylation-related plasticity-regulating processes in the CNS [170] influence neuronal activity-dependent gene regulation [171, 172], learning, and memory [173, 174].

During fetal to young adult development and corresponding with synaptogenesis, there is widespread *methylome*[2] reconfiguration [162]. At that time, highly conserved *non-CG methylation* becomes the principal methylation form in human neurons but not in glial cells.

Methyl groups come from nutrients such as methionine, choline, and folic acid. The *DNA methyltransferase 3 (DNMT3)* catalyzes DNA methylation, and DNMT1 maintains methylation during mitosis and DNA repair [175].

Along with the DNA modifications, *post-translational modifications to histones* are important parts of the epigenome [176, 177]. It has been estimated that the histone code has a far greater potential for different combinations than gene transcription does [148].

Most frequently, N-terminal histone tails protruding from the nucleosome are dynamically modified. The most common modifications are acetylation, ubiquitination or *SUMOylation* at lysine (K)[3] residues, methylation at lysine or arginine residues, and phosphorylation at serine or threonine residues.

Acetylation of histones is usually associated with euchromatin and increased transcription. *Histone acetyltransferases (HATs)* add acetyl, and *histone deacetylases (HDACs)* remove the acetyl [178].

Experiments in yeast have shown that reversal of targeted deacetylation occurs within 5–8 min, while reversal of targeted acetylation is more rapid, taking 1.5 min [179].

Location and valence (mono-, di-, or tri-methylation) of histone methylation will determine whether there will be a euchromatin or heterochromatin state. *Histone methyltransferases (HMTs)* methylate the tails and *histone demethylases (HDMs)* demethylate the tails [178]. In some instances, there seems to be a rather speedy removal of histone methyl. An experiment in yeast noted that methylation patterns induced by high temperature were erased within one cell cycle, during S phase [180].

A large family of *chromatin remodeling proteins* binds to specifically modified histones and produces the transcriptional changes in an ATP-dependent manner [181–183]. These epigenetic changes are associated with stress and depression.

In addition to epigenetic DNA and histone modifications, *supranucleosomal 3D looping of chromosomes* in neurons and glial cells may affect transcription [139].

Prenatal epigenetic programming is influenced by maternal metabolic and nutritional environment [184–186]. Indeed, the interrelationship is so strong that maternal plasma DNA sequencing can reveal the genome-wide genetic and mutational profile of the fetus [187]. Postnatal epigenetic programming depends upon nutrition via the alimentary tract [184].

Contrary to earlier beliefs, mammalian sperm transmits a highly complex set of epigenetic information [188–190]. These include combinations of histone variants, transcription factors, chromatin-associated and chromatin-modifying proteins [199].

Adverse early life stressors may result in epigenetic modification of gene expression, some of which have been associated with MDD [123, 191–196]. Prenatal stressors also influence gene expression that may predispose to depression [197].

A 2018 review of imaging genetic studies on childhood adversity analyzed complex pathways of genetic factors, early psychosocial environments, and the accompanying morphologic changes in emotion-processing neural circuitry [191]. The major findings were that childhood adversity is associated with the following:

- Structural changes in the hippocampus, amygdala, anterior cingulate cortex (ACC), and prefrontal cortex (PFC).
- Changes in white matter tracts, including the corpus callosum, cingulum, and uncinate fasciculus.
- Interaction with the brain-derived neurotrophic factor (BDNF) gene Val66Met polymorphism, serotonin transporter-linked promoter region (5-HTTLPR), and FK506 binding protein 51 (FKBP5) gene rs1360780 in brain morphologic changes in patients with depression and in a non-clinical population.
- A reduced volume in the hippocampus and its subfields, amygdala, and PFC and thinner rostral ACC in people with the met allele of BDNF (Val66Met).
- A smaller hippocampal volume and subsequent onset of depression when combined with the S allele of 5-HTTLPR.

[2] The methylome is the set of nucleic acid methylation modifications in an organism's genome or in a particular cell.

[3] Lysine (K) residue in the Walker A protein sequence motif (that has a highly conserved 3-D structure), along with the main chain NH atoms, are vital for nucleotide-binding [196].

- Diminished white matter integrity of brain regions involved in emotion processing when interacting with the FKBP5 gene rs160780.

Combinations of genetic and epigenetic factors have been proposed as underlying mechanisms for major psychiatric disorders [117, 200]. Moreover, integration of chromatin structure and epigenetic control of the immune system might be the link between environmental and differentiation influences on stress responses [201–204].

Individual differences in behavior and susceptibility to different psychopathologies may be influenced by differences in neuroendocrine responses to stress [205–210]. Experiments with rats have shown differences in base level and stress-induced expression of some stress-related molecules [206, 211, 212]. Individual differences in expression of stress-related genes have been documented in rats [211, 212] and humans [213].

Psychosocial influences on individual human stress responses are extremely difficult to ferret out of studies that do not control those variables [214, 215]. For example, happiness throughout the workday has been highly correlated with decreased cortisol on both working and nonworking days, and increased health in both middle-aged men and women [216]. Loss of job control may have the inverse effect [217].

Socioeconomic status can influence hemodynamic recovery from mental stress [218], and lower status may increase risk for cardiovascular disease [219]. It appears that inflammatory cytokines may have an individualized delayed response to acute mental stress, and individual differences in cytokine responses may be related to sympathetic reactivity [220].

Fetal and early-life stress has been associated with epigenetic modifications of key developmental or stress-related genes that may determine lifetime susceptibility to chronic disease states [117, 221–223]. Nutritional, endocrine, and placental cues may influence cell-specific and developmentally specific gene expression and modulate behavioral responses to social or environmental cues [224, 225].

Relevant genes include the familiar glucocorticoid receptor (NR3C1*)* [226] and brain-derived neurotrophic factor (BDNF) [227, 228]. The role of BDNF in neurodevelopment puts it as a logical focus for a molecular correlate of developmental stress. BDNF contributes to neuronal activity-dependent processes for memory formation, contextual and spatial learning [229].

Associations studies of MDD with DNA methylation of BDNF, SLC6A4, NR3C1, 5-HTR (1A, 2A, and 3A), FKBP5, MAO-A, and OXTR have been reviewed in 2017 [230]. They found that most studies showed BDNF, and NR3C1 gene methylation levels were correlated with MDD and that SLC6A4 correlations were inconsistent.

A systematic review of stress, epigenetics, and depression in humans looked at data up to February 2018 [120]. They found correlations with depression with genes for NRC31, SLCA4, BDNF, FKBP5, SKA2, OXTR, LINGO3, POU3F1, and ITGB1. The most promising therapeutic targets were epigenetic changes in glucocorticoid signaling (e.g., NR3C1, FKBP5), serotonergic signaling (e.g., SLC6A4), and neurotrophins (e.g., BDNF) genes. They did find inconsistencies with the directions of effects ascribed to epigenetic changes. They also suggested that widespread use of psychotropics and their effects on epigenes are important to factor into study results.

A comprehensive 2018 review of *genetic and epigenetic mechanisms that regulate BDNF* expression and function with relevance to MDD is presented in [231]. Altered levels of BDNF have been seen in animal models of maltreatment [232] and in subjects with bipolar disorder [228, 233]. Chronic defeat in mice, a model of depression, can induce downregulation of BDNF promoter/exon IV and can be associated with increases in histone H3 lysine 27 methylation (H3K27) at the corresponding promoter [234]. Post-translational modifications of histones are also important correlates of environmental epigenetic modifications.

In an adult rat model of PTSD, psychosocial stress significantly increased BDNF DNA methylation in the dorsal hippocampus (especially in the dorsal CA1 subregion) and decreased BDNF mRNA in the dorsal and ventral CA1 [235]. In addition, it significantly decreased DNA methylation in the ventral hippocampus (CA3) but produced no changes in BDNF DNA methylation in the medial prefrontal cortex or basolateral amygdala. These results suggest an epigenetic relationship in the association of PTSD with hippocampal-related symptoms.

Differential regulation of exon-specific BDNF mRNAs associated with BDNF DNA methylation and altered local chromatin structure has been induced by contextual fear in rats [236].

Transgenerational and lifelong perpetuation of changes in gene expression and behavior may result from early life neglect and abuse. Early maltreatment of rats can induce persistent changes in methylation of BDNF DNA and altered BDNF gene expression in adult prefrontal cortex [237]. Offspring of females who had previously experienced the maltreatment also showed altered methylation of BDNF DNA.

Post-mortem tissue from suicide victims has shown hypermethylation of BDNF promoter/exon IV in the Wernicke area irrespective of genome-wide methylation levels [238].

In humans, early-life stress is associated with alterations in BDNF expression and DNA methylation in depression, schizophrenia, bipolar disorder, and autism [239].

One of the neuropsychiatric disorders that have been highly associated with early life conditions is borderline personality disorder. It may serve to illustrate the relationship between adverse environments and epigenetics. Aberrant epigenetic regulation of neuropsychiatric-associated genes may contribute to the pathogenesis of borderline personality disorder (BPD) [240]. Significantly increased methylation has been seen in promoter regions of HTR2A, NR3C1, MAOA, MAOB and soluble COMT (S-COMT). In addition, significantly increased average methylation (1.7%) has been seen in the blood of BPD patients ($p < 0.0001$).

Experiments with borderline personality disorder have also shown that epigenetic marks may be changed via psychotherapy and that these changes are associated with cognitive improvements [241].

In people suffering from major depressive disorder (MDD), serum BDNF levels are frequently low and can be increased by some antidepressants [242, 243] and cognitive behavioral therapy [241, 244].

According to one study, increases in serum level of BDNF, however, do not parallel clinical characteristics such as symptom severity [245]. Other studies disagree. For example, 2 months of treatment with citalopram decreased H3K27 methylation levels at promoter/exon IV of the BDNF gene in the prefrontal cortex and was associated with symptom relief [246].

The polymorphisms of BDNF by themselves do not appear to associate with treatment response in MDD [247].

Glial cell-derived neurotrophic factor (GDNF) promotes the development, differentiation, and protection of CNS neurons [248]. A 2015 published meta-analysis showed that compared to controls, blood GDNF levels were significantly decreased in patients with depression. They concluded that blood GDNF levels could be a biomarker of depression as a whole, but the results were modulated by psychiatric diagnosis, age of included subjects, and sampling sources [248].

GDNF is important for the maintenance of dopamine neurons [249]. GDNF also appears to modulate the serotonin system in the brain [250]. In mice, histone modification and DNA methylation of GDNF in the ventral striatum, along with genetic and environmental factors, determine adaptability and susceptibility to daily stressors [251].

A 2017 review of the role of GDNF in the pathogenesis and treatment of mood disorders came to two conclusions. Brain GDNF contributes to the mechanism underlying depressive disorders and the effects of antidepressants and mood stabilizers. There is a crosstalk between GDNF and neurotransmitters representing a feedback system [252].

There is some indication that low serum BDNF and GDNF levels may be involved in the pathophysiology of first-episode depression and differences in serum BDNF levels may occur at different ages [253].

There is a positive association between *serotonin transporter (SLC6A4)*-linked polymorphic region methylation and depression in humans [254, 255]. SLC6A4 performs an important role in brain development, mood, cognition, and psychopathology [256].

Twin studies have shown that higher SLC6A4 methylation levels associate with greater orbitofrontal cortical (OFC) activity and left amygdala-anterior cingulate cortex (ACC) and left amygdala-right OFC connectivity in response to sadness as well as greater ACC-left amygdala and ACC-left insula connectivity in response to fearful stimuli [257]. Increased activation of the amygdala is associated with an increased response to threat and regulates a positive family history for depression and the later manifestation of depressive symptoms [258].

Peripheral blood SLC6A4 methylation can be used as a surrogate to assay for frontal-limbic SLC6A4 methylation processes in humans and may be a useful biomarker [257].

Some studies have found that some antidepressants can reverse SLC6A4 methylation [230].

Resilience to social stress occurs with functional DNA methylation of corticotropin-releasing hormone (CRH) in the paraventricular nucleus (PVN) of the hypothalamus [259]. Chronic social stress in adult mice induced a long-term decrease in methylation of the CRH gene at that location. On the other hand, chronic *unpredictable* stress can increase methylation of the CRH promoter in the PVN of female rats [260]. In humans and rats, early life adversity is associated with increased DNA methylation of hippocampal glucocorticoid receptor (*NR3C1*), which is also associated with depression [261].

Maltreatment of children that is associated with epigenetic changes in ID3, GRIN1, and TPPP genes appears to be a risk factor for depression [262].

Rapid behavioral adaptation is linked to *neocortical Tet3-mediated accumulation of 5-hydroxymethylcytosine (5-hmc)* [263]. The ten-eleven translocation (Tet) family of enzymes is essential for converting methylated DNA to 5-hmC. The 5-hmC is a DNA modification that is highly enriched in the adult brain. It accumulates over a lifetime, and it is dynamically regulated by neural activity. Extinction of fear can lead to a dramatic genome-wide redistribution of 5-hmC within the infralimbic prefrontal cortex. Experiments in mice have shown that extinction-learning-induced, Tet3-mediated accumulation of 5-hmC is associated with establishing epigenetic states that promote gene expression and rapid behavioral adaptation.

As mentioned above, but worth repeating here, *more than 90% of the human genome is actively transcribed, but only about 2% codes for functional protein* [264]. Those RNAs not translating to proteins, the *non-coding RNAs (ncRNAs)*, are critical regulators of transcription, epigenetic processes, and gene silencing [264, 265]. It is likely that they evolved to control genomic functions that coordinate tissue- and developmental stage-specific regulation of gene expression [266]. As such, they have a role in neural plasticity and cognition. They are highly expressed in the brain. They contribute to neuropsychiatric disorders, for example, fear [267], addiction, anxiety, schizophrenia, and depression [268–270].

There are several *classifications of ncRNAs*, most of which seem to be capable of directing epigenetic processes [271]. The simplest current classification is that of *small ncRNAs*, between 20 and 200 nucleotides, and *long ncRNAs*, defined as any ncRNA over 200 nucleotides. For example, a class of endogenous small ncRNAs, *microRNAs*, is thought to affect up to 60% of protein-coding transcripts [272]. Familiar ncRNAs include transfer RNA (tRNA) and ribosomal RNA (rRNA).

A myriad of noncoding RNAs have been identified; however, few functions have been demonstrated [273, 274]. Transcription into non-protein-coding RNA is actually widespread [275]. Studies have estimated that there are thousands [276]. Many of these are associated with known genes [277]. It has also been speculated that many of these may be just junk transcripts [274].

Many ncRNAs remain silent until the appropriate developmental age or environmental trigger occurs [278]. In addition, different classes of ncRNAs are expressed either in the oocytes (*siRNA*) [279] or in the sperm (*piRNA*) [280], which makes them interesting candidates for transgenerational epigenetic controls [265].

There may be an intimate relationship between retrotransposons like LINES and SINES, microRNAs and other ncRNAs [281].

Epigenetic structural and functional activity in the brain is highly complex and entwined [282]. Interactive phenotypes and genotypes provide the myriad individual manifestations of reactions to environmental cues [223, 283].

Lifestyles can modify epigenetic patterns [284]. These include inverted sleep-wake schedules, obesity, smoking, alcoholism, and physical activity [285]. Interconnections exist between nutrition, epigenetics, lifestyle, disease, and metabolic stress pathways [186, 286]. Some bioactive food components (e.g., fatty acids, folate, polyphenols, isothiocyanates, selenium, retinoids, and allyl compounds) impact DNA and histone epigenetic processes involved in cell differentiation, proliferation, and senescence [284, 287–289].

The *epigenetic clock* is an interesting concept that relates to the aging of individual cells and possibly the onset of diseases that increase with age [290].[4] MDD is associated with an advanced aging phenotype, including increased risk of mortality and age-related diseases such as cardiovascular disease, cancer, obesity, cognitive decline, and frailty [292, 293]. Chronological age can be gauged by using DNA methylation age (*DNAmAge*) data to produce an epigenetic clock [294–296].

Various studies have shown that MDD is associated with accelerated brain aging [297] and shorter telomere length [298, 299]. Patients with MDD have higher epigenetic aging in blood and brain tissue, suggesting that they are biologically older than their corresponding chronological age. When childhood trauma is present, the effect is even more pronounced [141].

Depression and epigenetics related to the brain-gut axis have been reviewed in 2022 and 2023 [300–302]. A 2000–2022 systematic scoping review in rodents has found limited but suggestive evidence for a role of brain epigenetics on diet-induced protective or detrimental effects, specifically on anxiety and depressive-like behavior [303]. Diet induced changes in the epigenome most often through the action of DNA methylation, histone acetylation, and microRNAs associated with behavioral changes. Changes in the epigenome also paralleled inadequate maternal diets and susceptibility of offspring to later development of anxiety and depressive-like behavior.

Neurogenesis and Plasticity

Brain-based learning and memory (change) is the result of alterations in neuronal transmission in response to experience and use [304]. These alterations are known as *neuronal plasticity*. If the efficacy of transmission is increased, it is called *potentiation*. If the efficacy is decreased, it is called *depression*. Both excitatory and inhibitory circuits are influenced by experience [305]. See Fig. 14.1.

These changes may be physiological or structural. Physiological changes may be due to functional modification of existing synapses, neurons [304] or glial cells [306]. Structural changes may be physical alterations in neuronal networks, such as synapse morphological modifications, growth, or elimination.

One of the core concepts of neuroplasticity is put forth in the *Hebbian Theory* formulated by Donald Hebb in 1949 [1, 2]. It states that:

> Let us assume that the persistence or repetition of a reverberatory activity (or 'trace') tends to induce lasting cellular changes that add to its stability… When an axon of cell *A* is near enough to excite a cell *B* and repeatedly or persistently takes part in firing it, some growth process or metabolic change takes place in one or both cells such that *A*'s efficiency, as one of the cells firing *B*, is increased.

Short-term plasticity may be due to *synaptic fatigue* [307], *synaptic augmentation* [308, 309] or *neuronal facilitation* [310]. Short-term changes in the order of a few seconds or less may be due to a change in the size of the easily releasable pool of neurotransmitters or to the amount of

[4] The epigenetic clock is discussed in [289].

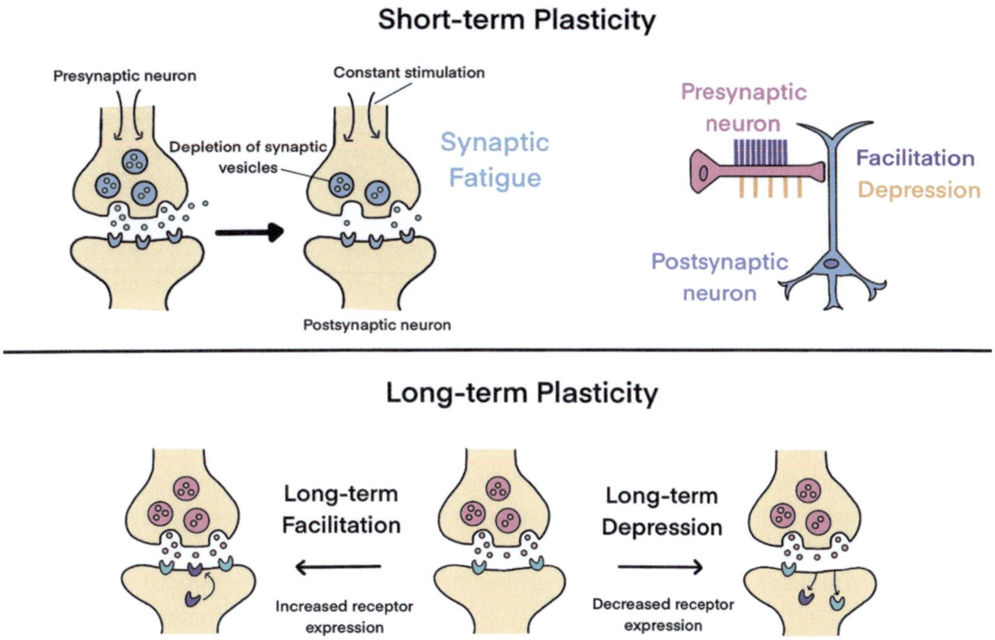

Fig. 14.1 Cartoon representation of neural plasticity. This illustration highlights short-term and long-term synaptic plasticity mechanisms. Short-term plasticity includes synaptic fatigue, facilitation, and depression, reflecting rapid changes in synaptic strength due to prior activity. Long-term plasticity features sustained modifications, including long-term facilitation and long-term depression, essential for learning and memory formation

transmitter released as the result of an action potential [311]. *Synaptic fatigue* is a temporary inhibition of neuronal transmission because of constant stimulation and is related to depletion of synaptic vesicles that house the neurotransmitters [307]. *Synaptic augmentation* is a temporary (a few seconds) increase in the efficiency of neurotransmission [309]. *Neuronal facilitation* is a phenomenon wherein postsynaptic potentials elicited by an impulse increase when that impulse is closely preceded by a prior impulse [310, 312].

Long-term plasticity [313] that lasts minutes to hours at excitatory synapses includes *long-term potentiation (LTP)* and *long-term depression (LTD)*. LTP and LTD also occur at inhibitory synapses but are not as well studied [314]. Neurotransmitter receptors are transiently stabilized at synapses by scaffolding molecules, which affect extracellular and intramembrane diffusion [315]. LTP is a facilitation of synaptic responses or strength for several hours in vitro or weeks to months in vivo following synchronous neuronal stimulation [316–318]. LTP is rapid, usually brief, and strongly correlated with pre- and post-synaptic activity [305]. LTP is specific to the pathway that was stimulated and involves coincident activity of presynaptic, postsynaptic, and glial cells [319]. Based upon experiments in the hippocampus and elsewhere, it is widely thought that LTP is involved in learning and memory [320, 321]. LTP and LDP are often discussed as part of the Hebbian Theory.

LTD is an activity-dependent decrease in efficacy of neuronal transmission that can last hours or longer [314, 322–324]. LTD is probably widespread if not ubiquitous and varies in response to weak or strong stimuli depending upon their location and neuronal development stage. Mechanisms may be pre- or post-synaptic. LTD may be necessary to prepare specific synapses for new LTP [325]. In contrast to LTP, LTD is usually sustained and weakly correlated with pre- and post-synaptic activity [323, 326].

Metaplasticity is a persistent change in the ability to induce subsequent synaptic plasticity and is induced by former cellular activity [327, 328]. *Homeostatic plasticity* is the counterbalancing of destabilizing influences and restores or maintains the set point of cellular or network activity [329]. *Heterosynaptic plasticity* is activity on one set of synapses that drives activity on another set of synapses on the same postsynaptic cell [330].

Glial cells modulate synaptic plasticity by modifying their synaptic coverage, release of chemokines and cytokines, and glial transmitters [306, 331, 332]. In this way, they can influence LTP, LDP, homeostatic plasticity, and metaplasticity.

A pervasive theme underlying molecular research into depression is that symptoms result from deregulation and destabilization of *synaptic plasticity* [333–336]. In prefrontal and hippocampal areas, chronic or repeated stress triggers reduced dendritic complexity [337–339], selective alterations in makers of excitatory synapses [340–342], and depressive-like symptoms in rodents. In humans with MDD, similar changes such as decreased genetic expression and decreased number of synaptic contacts are seen in prefrontal and limbic areas [341–347]. When therapeutic interventions alleviate depressive-like symptoms in rodents, these aberrant changes reverse [348–350]. It is well known that synaptic plasticity is affected by varying levels of a variety of neurotransmitters [351], biogenic amines [352], BDNF [353], and, of course, glucocorticoids [338] under stress.

It has been hypothesized that psychological and immune stressors can interact (via trophic factors) with a susceptible genetic background to promote depression by disrupting BDNF and neuroplastic processes and that relapses in depression may be related to aberrant hippocampal and cortical neuroplasticity resulting in faulty wiring of emotional circuits [354].

Feldman has pointed out that even basic sensory perception is influenced by prior experience and learning [305]. A variety of plastic mechanisms for learning and adaptive behavior has been proposed [8, 355, 356]. Indeed, the Internet phenomenon #theDress of 2015 may be an example of such experienced-based sensory perception [357]. Another such example is #theshoe [358].

A mild to moderate amount of stress provokes the release of neurogenic growth hormones that are conducive to new learning [359]. Influence of stress via maternal-offspring interactions on neurodevelopmental programming begins prior to birth [360]. Adult cortical plasticity depends upon early postnatal critical periods [361].

The relevance of these concepts will be discussed when we visit the sections on critical periods and arousal in psychotherapy.

Therapygenetics

Just as there is considerable variation in interindividual responses to antidepressants, which seem to have a genetic component [362, 363], so there are differences in individual responses to psychotherapy that appear to have a genetic component [364]. *Pharmacogenetics* as applied to depression is the study of the genetic variants that are associated with the response to antidepressants [365]. *Therapygenetics* is a term of recent vintage that is the study of genetic determinants of response to psychological therapies [364, 366–370]. The underlying goal is to explore the possibility that genotype and epigenotype-associated traits can be brought to bear on developing personalized therapeutic interventions [371].

It has been widely suggested that within the framework of the *diathesis-stress model of behavior-gene-environment (G x E) interactions*, some individuals are more susceptible to adversity [372, 373]. It is widely held that personal characteristics modify the influence of negative environmental stressors such as poor parenting or poverty [374–376]. It is believed that behavioral characteristics such as temperament or intermediate traits called *endophenotype* are at play along with genetics and epigenetics [377, 378]. Endophenotypes are traits that are not directly seen. They may be neurophysiological, biochemical, endocrinological, neuroanatomical, cognitive, or neuropsychological [379, 380].

It is suggested that a child who has an endophenotype that may include, for example, a difficult temperament or vulnerability genes/risky alleles may be more susceptible to developmental stressors and may manifest psychopathologies such as depression when they are exposed to certain stressors. *The Early Growth and Development Study*: a prospective adoption study from birth through middle childhood [381] has begun to shed light on the relationships between temperament, parenting, genes, and environmental influences. Ongoing results are being published beginning in 2007 [381–386].

A corollary to the diathesis-stress model has been proposed that the same genes that produce the vulnerability may also increase the probability that there will be greater benefit from supportive therapy. In other words, these may be "*plasticity genes*" that may render folks more amenable to environmental influences, which may be harmful or beneficial. The *differential susceptibility hypothesis* proposes that the exact individuals who may be the most adversely impacted by stressors may also be the ones who can profit the most from enriching environments [387–392]. For example, in the *SPOKES trial* (ISRCTN 77566446), a randomized controlled trial of 112 schoolchildren 5- to 6-years-old, children who showed emotionally dysregulated behavior before receiving parenting treatment were more responsive to improvements in parental care [393].

Ellis, Boyce, Belsky, and their collaborators have taken an *evolutionary-neurodevelopmental* approach to evaluating neurobiological susceptibility to environmental influences [388, 394]. Two evolutionary models have emerged that have in common the hypothesis that some individuals are more sensitive than others to both risk-promoting (negative) and development-enhancing (positive) environmental factors [395–398]. These two theories are the *biological sensitivity to context theory (BSCT)* and *the differential susceptibility theory (DST)*. BSCT and DST are in opposition to the diathesis stress/dual risk perspective that is more commonly used to describe individual interactions with the environment during development [399–401].

Ellis et al. propose that individual susceptibility to the environment has the following characteristics [394]:

1. Individuals who are highly susceptible to the environment are sensitive to both positive and negative environments.
2. This sensitivity increases developmental receptivity to the environment.
3. This susceptibility is grounded on neurobiological susceptibility.
4. Individual differences in susceptibility are a product of at least heritable polygenic variation and developmental experience.

5. All individuals vary in their neurobiological susceptibility and do so in an age-dependent fashion.
6. During the course of human evolution, this differential neurobiological susceptibility has been adaptive and conserved. This may be due to fluctuating environmental pressures that produce different fitness depending upon social, physical, and historical contexts.
7. Differential susceptibility moderates the effect of the environment on developmental and life outcomes. The result is that some individuals will be more influenced by their environment than others will be.

Such *conditional adaptation* has been comprehensively discussed in the following references [10, 394, 402–404]. One especially salient example of conditional adaptation can be seen in the work of Michael Meaney and his colleagues at McGill University [405–407]. Low levels of maternal care in the rat make a significant difference in the offspring's brain morphology and stress biochemistry. These changes, such as lower spine density and dendritic lengths in areas such as the hippocampus, and increased corticosterone levels, increased fearful and defensive behaviors. However, learning and memory processes are actually enhanced when encountering stressors [405]. Indeed, the low levels of maternal nurturing may prove to be adaptive in high-threat environments, perhaps enhancing contextual (hippocampal) but not fear-cued (amygdala) learning [408]. It has been suggested that these behaviors in the face of adversity may be evolutionarily highly adaptive [409–411].

Maternally enhanced defensive capacity in her offspring appears to act via programming cognitive, emotional, and endocrine sensitivity to harsh conditions, which may have an immediate adaptive benefit [412]. The downside of increased flexibility appears to be a heightened risk for multiple pathologies later [413, 414].

Indeed, human childhood trauma can lead to physical illnesses such as PTSD, phobias, eating problems, substance abuse, irritable bowel syndrome, multiple personality disorders, and autoimmune disorders [413–415].

So, what are the putative genes that may be involved in adaptive neurodevelopment? Three of these candidate plastic genes are *monoamine oxidase-A (MAOA), 5-HTTLPR (5-hydroxytryptamine-linked polymorphic region), and dopamine receptor D4 (DRD4)*. Do these sound familiar? We discussed them in the chapter on molecular underpinnings of depression.

A functional polymorphism of the neurotransmitter-metabolizing enzyme MAOA (MAOA-uVNTR) appears to relate to contextual childhood adversity and antisocial behavior [416–418]. Alleles that result in low MAOA activity are associated with vulnerability to environmental stressors [417]. In addition, the vulnerability may manifest as a vulnerability to become antisocial when experiencing a variety of adversity, especially in childhood. Several experiments with the MAOA genes have shown that children with the low activity gene have more behavior problems than controls when they experience poor-quality parenting but more-social skills and fewer problems than controls when they get high-quality parenting [375, 417, 419–422].

As detailed above, the short allele of the 5-HTTLPR is associated with increased depression when experiencing high stress, whereas the long allele seems to offer some protection [423, 424]. However, there are apparent cognitive advantages to the short allele. Frequently, the carriers of the short alleles outperformed the long allele carriers when they were not subjected to as many stressors [425–428].

A 7-repeat allele of the DRD4 has been associated with ADHD [376]. However, the most externalizing behavior followed the quality of parenting. For example, when mothers were the most insensitive, the externalizing behavior was most prominent and with the most sensitive mothers, externalizing behavior was less prominent; but this was only in the 7-repeat allele carriers [398, 429–433].

Some interesting therapygenetics observations have been seen. Here are a few examples. A sample of 374 white, anxiety-disordered children received cognitive behavioral therapy (CBT) and had their buccal DNA examined for single-nucleotide polymorphisms in nerve growth factor (NGF) [rs6330) and brain-derived neurotrophic factor (BDNF) (rs6265) genes [364]. These genes are good candidates as they are widely involved in mood and cognition and neuroplastically respond to stress. Anxiety-associated phenotypes have been associated with alleles in these genes. Results indicated that children who had the T allele of NGF rs6330 were significantly more likely to be rid of anxiety at the end of CBT (OR[5] = 0.60; 95% CI: 0.42 to 0.85, $p = 0.005$). There was no significant association between CBT and BDNF rs6265.

In children diagnosed with anxiety disorder, CBT produced a better response 6 months after treatment if they were homozygous for the S-allele of 5-HTTLPR [367].

[5] Odds ratio (OR) is a way to represent the odds that an outcome will result when a given exposure to a variable of interest occurs compared to when the exposure does not occur. OR quantifies the strength of the association between two events. An OR greater than 1 indicates a positive association or that exposure to that variable increases the odds of that outcome. An OR less than one indicates a negative relationship between two events. An OR of 1 suggests no relationship between two events. An OR is frequently accompanied by a 95% confidence interval (CI). CI is a measure of precision of the OR. The smaller the CI the higher precision as long as it does not overlap OR = 1. For more information, see the Chap. 4 on evidence basics in this text.

Neuronal Plasticity and Epigenetic Memory

As Catherine Dulac has suggested, even though the mechanisms behind the formation of memories and plasticity of neuron functions are unknown, they are likely to involve a combination of alterations in gene expression, protein synthesis, and cellular and anatomical structure [434]. Dulac points out that there is a similarity between epigenetic events that are self-perpetuating in the absence of the original stimulus that caused them and the long-lasting effects apparently involved in memory.

Plasticity Implications for Human Health

Pre- and early post-natal maternal environment has been shown in mice to have a significant impact on the behavior of the progeny [435]. Two different inbred genetically identical mouse strains (C57BL/6J and BALB/cj C57BL/6J) were used in the experiment. A C57BL/6J embryo was cross-transferred into a BALB/cj uterus and cross-fostered by a BALB/cj mother. The fostered offspring demonstrated three out of four tested behaviors that were distinctly different from their non-fostered siblings and identical to those of the foster mother. These included anxiety-associated behaviors, sensory motor gating,[6] and water maze performances.[7] All of these behaviors were previously thought to be genetically determined.

Deficiencies in maternal and early postnatal nutrition contribute to health risk factors in adult life. These include hypertension, insulin resistance, obesity, cardiovascular disease, diabetes, and the metabolic syndrome [436]. Molecular, cellular, metabolic, neuroendocrine, and physiological adaptations to changes in the early nutritional environment can permanently change developmental patterns of cellular proliferation and differentiation in tissues and organs that can have pathological effects later in life [436].

Chromatin remodeling may be the target for these pathological changes. One level of influence may be the effects of early life nutrition on methylation of cytosine including in imprinted genes [445] and retrotransposons[8] [446] and in histones [447]. There are some questions about the unintended consequences of nutritional supplementation, however [446]. Supplementing a mouse mother's nutritionally adequate diet with extra folic acid, vitamin B12, choline, and betaine was shown to permanently affect the offspring's DNA methylation at epigenetically susceptible loci, e.g., in transposable elements [446].

Genomic imprinting is an epigenetic process that results in some genes being expressed in a parental-origin-specific manner [448]. It is essential for normal mammalian growth and development [449]. The establishment, maintenance, and erasing of epigenetic marks is extremely complex and timing dependent [450, 451]. In humans, dozens of imprinted genes have been described [452–454]. Many of these imprinted genes are found in the brain. Some of these genes are involved in brain homeostasis, social behaviors including maternal and mating behaviors, risk taking and food sharing and circadian rhythms [455–458]. The monoallelic expression makes these genes vulnerable to the effects of dysregulation and mutations that could have a radiating effect [459, 460]. This effect may be transgenerational [461, 462].

As mentioned before, many ncRNAs remain silent until the appropriate developmental age or environmental trigger occurs [278]. In addition, different classes of ncRNAs are expressed either in the oocytes [279] or in the sperm [280], which makes them interesting candidates for transgenerational epigenetic controls [265]. There may be an intimate relationship between retrotransposons—such as LINEs and SINEs—and microRNAs and other ncRNAs [281].

It is still unknown how these chromatin modifications are carried through. For example, as mentioned above, histone marks are rather quickly erased, so involvement in long-term epigenetic memory seems to be unlikely [179, 180].

Conditioning

Changing responses to external or internal cues can be accomplished in various ways involving different levels of awareness. *Conditioning* is the procedure whereby new responses are acquired, developed, trained, educated, established, or learned in or by an individual. A stimulus that unconditionally elicits a physiological response is repeatedly paired with a neutral stimulus that does not originally elicit the same response. After sufficient repetition, the neutral stimulus becomes a conditioned stimulus that elicits the

[6] Sensory gating is the neurological process of filtering out unnecessary stimuli in the brain from all possible environmental stimuli to prevent information overload in the higher cortical areas [435]. Sensory-motor gating is related but not the same. It refers to gating that influences the startle response. Both of these phenomena have been investigated in relationship to schizophrenia [436, 437].

[7] The Morris water maze assesses hippocampal-dependent spatial learning and memory in transgenic mouse models of disease, including neurocognitive disorders such as Alzheimer's disease [438]. The strain of mice used in these tests has significant effects on the behavioral phenotype, with some strains exhibiting superior learning ability relative to other strains.

[8] *Transposable elements* may be found in many human genes [439] and comprise about 17% of the human genome [440]. Many human genes are transcribed from the antisense promoter of the L1 retrotransposon, which is analogous to the transposons in the mouse experiment [441, 442].

physiological response in the absence of the unconditioned stimulus. A parallel reasoning follows for the unconditioned response, i.e., the response normally associated with the unconditioned stimulus. It can become associated with the conditioned stimulus when the conditioned stimulus is properly presented in time and space with the unconditioned stimulus. The broadest categories of conditioning are classical and operant.

Classical conditioning (*respondent* or *Pavlovian conditioning*) with sufficient repetition and close enough timing, pairs a previously neutral stimulus with an unconditioned stimulus such that the neutral stimulus becomes the conditioned stimulus and can evoke the unconditioned response without the unconditioned stimulus. A second-order and higher-order conditioning pairs a conditioned stimulus with a new neutral stimulus to further produce conditioned stimuli. Many of our life experiences that are paired become associated and conditioned.

Operant conditioning (*Skinnerian* or *instrumental conditioning*) waits for an individual to spontaneously, voluntarily, perform an operation (an activity) that is to be conditioned, and then a positive reward is immediately given to reinforce that behavior. With sufficient repetitions, the targeted response will increase in frequency to a higher level than it was before. Escape and avoidance responses are ways that an individual has learned to avoid aversive stimuli by making a new response or terminating a response, respectively. Therefore, it can be seen that the consequences of a behavior may alter the frequency of its occurrence.

Consequences, stimuli, or objects given after the performance of a targeted behavior may be either a reinforcer if the behavior is increased in frequency or a punishment if the behavior decreases in frequency.

Deconditioning of responses may take place passively or naturally if there is a lack of association over time with the conditioned stimuli. Deconditioning can also take place actively if cognitive processes can intercede in the trigger response cycle.

In a classical learned maladaptive response, it may be possible to apply classical conditioning to designing treatments. Additionally, as we shall discuss within the context of cognitive behavioral therapy, it may be possible to decondition or extinguish maladaptive conditioned responses.

In real life, conditioning may be operant or classical. When the immune system or endocrine system is involved, conditioning is a result of multidirectional central nervous-endocrine-immune system communication. It is well to remember that just as CNS changes affect the immune system, such as are revealed in classical conditioning and stress experiments, so does the immune system affect behavior by way of interactions on the CNS [463–466].

The mesolimbic dopamine reward system, composed of the ventral tegmental area (VTA) and ventral striatum aka nucleus accumbens (NAc) (VTA-NAc), is the most important brain reward pathway [467]. It is evolutionarily ancient. The dopamine neurotransmitters that mediate behavioral responses are found in flies and worms. See Fig. 14.2.

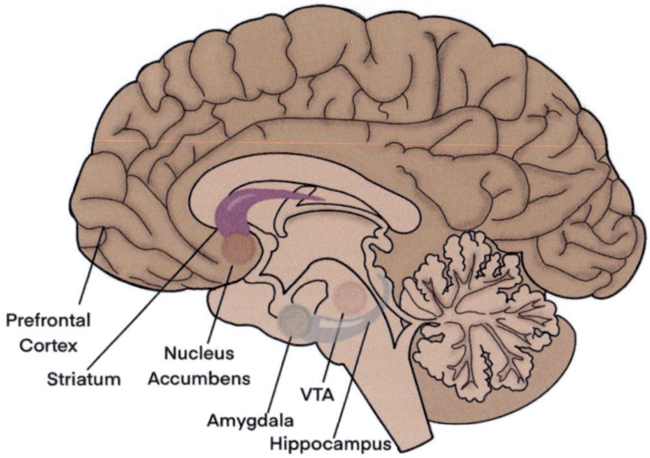

Fig. 14.2 Neural circuitry of the mesolimbic dopamine reward system. This figure highlights key brain regions involved in reward processing and motivational behavior. Dopaminergic projections from the ventral tegmental area (VTA) innervate the nucleus accumbens within the striatum, facilitating reward signaling. The prefrontal cortex modulates executive function and decision-making in response to incentive cues. The amygdala contributes to emotional valence, while the hippocampus encodes contextual and memory-based associations. Together, these regions form an interconnected network underlying reinforcement, goal-directed behavior, and addiction-related neuroplasticity

VTA-NAc is the primary reward-detecting circuit that is tuned to respond to natural rewards, including food, sex, and positive social interactions. It also responds to rewards from drugs of abuse. When the VTA-NAc is activated, it motivates and incentivizes an individual to repeat the behavior that elicited the reward. In so doing, the VTA-NAc prompts memory of the details of the process and features of the reward.

The VTA-NAc communicates with and integrates with several areas of the brain. These include the amygdala, hippocampus, and hypothalamus, prefrontal regions of the cerebral cortex, locus coeruleus, and the dorsal raphe.

The amygdala helps establish connections between environmental cues and the rewarding or aversive nature of the experience. The amygdala is highly associated with conditioned learning.

The hippocampus, in collaboration with the amygdala, is vital for remembering persons, places, or things that are associated with the rewards.

The hypothalamus integrates an interest in rewards with an individual's physiological needs.

The prefrontal regions (including the medial prefrontal cortex, anterior cingulate cortex, and orbitofrontal cortex) control the actual executive decision to seek a particular reward.

The locus coeruleus with its noradrenergic neurons regulates activation state and mood. The dorsal raphe is the principal location for serotonergic innervation in the brain, which also regulates activation state and mood. Acetylcholine from the pons modulates the motivation to seek the reward [468].

Sensitization is a conditioning response where facilitator interneurons increase cyclic AMP in sensory neurons as a response to stimuli. *Habituation* is another phenomenon of neural chemistry conditioning wherein the nervous system reduces or inhibits responses to repeated stimulation.

It appears that amygdala activity is closely related to behavioral output, not just threats or rewards [469]. Pavlovian and operant conditioning studies have implicated the *basolateral amygdaloid complex* [470] in rewarding approach conditions [470–472] and aversive defensive conditions [473–475]. Many of these neurons strongly respond after these conditioning experiments in a way that reflects the intensity of the unconditioned stimulus and somatic requirements of the tasks [476–480].

However, it has become clearer that the design in conditioning experiments has been an artificial construct in a non-natural setting [469]. When rats have been placed in a condition to replicate natural foraging, it has been found that the amygdala regulates risky foraging decisions based on risk assessments for rewards versus risks [481]. Amygdala activity in those situations may be high or low depending upon the decisions in any given trial [469]. Opposing processes balance actual threats against potential rewards (including threat reduction) [469].

Complex functions of the basolateral amygdaloid complex are precisely controlled and exquisitely plastic, especially during *critical stages of maturation and development* when emotional memory and learning are at play [3, 4, 470, 482, 483]. Difficulties at these times have been highly associated with later psychiatric problems. These include unconscious fear, phobias, panic attacks, and various neuroses.

Critical Periods

While stress certainly influences the brain throughout the life span, the developing brain is most vulnerable to stress during several critical periods [484–488]. These periods include prenatal, perinatal, infancy, childhood, and adolescence. During prenatal and early postnatal periods, the brain is developing rapidly, making and breaking neuronal connections at a fast clip. During later childhood and adolescence, the processes slow down. By adulthood, plasticity still exists but the pace has slowed considerably [484].

Exposure of the developing brain to high levels of stress or persistent stress at these critical times may have potent effects [485] that may persist for life. These may include hyperactivity of the amygdala, resulting in prominent fear reactions; hyperreactivity or hypersensitivity of the stress system, leading to excessive cortisol production; hypoactivity of the reproductive, immune, growth, and thyroid systems; and disturbed pain perception [484, 489]. Brain remodeling in areas such as the hippocampus, amygdala, and prefrontal cortex occurs in response to both acute and chronic stress.

One way that environmental effects generate such potent and long-term effects is via epigenetic modifications of DNA expression without altering the genotype. Epigenetic processes are more active during times when rates of DNA synthesis are high during prenatal, infancy, and early childhood periods, when growth rates are highest [490]. This cellular and molecular remodeling can change cognitive, behavioral, and physiological responses to stress. The underlying epigenetic changes appear to be dependent upon many factors, such as maturational stage (e.g., pre- or post-puberty) and gender [492]. *Whether or not malfunctioning epigenetic affects can be therapeutically modified is an open question* [493]. *However, evidence is accumulating that many of these marks have the potential to be reset.*

Early life experiences at critical times can have lasting epigenetic effects on high-affinity type I mineralocorticoid receptors (MRs) or low-affinity type II glucocorticoid receptors (GRs) [129, 405, 494, 495]. For example,

1. Epigenetic factors have been shown to modulate promoter actions in the MR and GR genes [494–497]. For example, in classical maternal grooming experiments in rats, maternal licking increased GR expression in offspring by way of increased hippocampal serotonergic tone and increased histone acetylase transferase activity, histone acetylation, and DNA demethylation mediated by the nerve growth factor-inducible protein A (NGFI-A) transcription factor binding to the exon (7) GR promoter [496, 497].
2. Epigenetic changes in promoter regions of the GR (NR3C1) gene in human newborns are sensitive to prenatal maternal mood [498].
3. A litany of early-life distresses has been identified as risk factors for diseases [499–502]. These stressful situations include maternal diseases during pregnancy, maternal distress, loss of a parent, addicted or depressed parents, neglect and abuse, family conflict or violence. Many of these are associated with changes in glucocorticoid levels [503].
4. Stress responses and cognitive performance in rats appear to be programmed through different levels of maternal interactions [504].
5. Matching early life stressors with later life stressors may be the difference between predicting adaptive responses [405]. Exposure to trauma in early life is not invariably linked to increased risks of psychological or

physiological problems later on. If early-life adversity epigenetically prepares the stress response system to handle later-life stress, then there may be less chance of disease. So, context seems to determine at least to some extent if synaptic plasticity has become maladaptive or adaptive.

The first critical period begins in gestation [360]. It is likely that the environmental effects of the maternal-fetal interface may have a profound epigenetic effect on the offspring and determine vulnerabilities throughout life.

Interactions between mother and fetus during gestation are mostly via hormones. It is suggested that progestogens (pro-gestational hormones) such as progesterone (P_4) and its 5α-reduced/3α-hydroxylated metabolite, allopregnanolone (AlloP), may be especially important in that communication [360].

Even though the fetus is protected by the placenta and uterine environment from many influences, maternal strain may have an impact on neurodevelopment [505]. Childhood cognitive functioning and behavioral problems (e.g., inattention and hyperactivity) have been linked inversely to fetal growth. Fetal growth reflects the fetal environment and can be assessed by size at birth. Evidence is mixed for fetal growth, adversity, schizophrenia, and personality disorders. Mood disorders have an unclear association. However, prenatal stress as reflected in fetal growth appears to be associated with childhood problems of temperament, distress, and reaction to stress.

Considerable research has associated prenatal exposure to maternal alcohol consumption, nutritional deficits, smoking, drugs, toxins, infections, and psychosocial stressors with mental health problems in their offspring [506, 507].

Inadequate nutrition during pregnancy (both over and under) is associated with increased incidence of several diseases in offspring [145, 508, 509]. These include diabetes and obesity [510]. For example, fetal demands are high for folate and choline needed for neural tube closure and normal development. Deficiencies of methylation may arise if the maternal diet is low in methyl groups that are supplied via *C1 metabolism*[9] by way of choline, betaine, methionine, or folate, using riboflavin and vitamins B6 and B12 as cofactors [509].

Mechanisms for this influence appear to be based upon epigenetic gene regulation of chromatin remodeling and histone modifications that maintain a stable propagation of gene expression in succeeding generations of cells. Reduction in cell numbers and changes in organ structure and function may be the result of altered gene expression [145].

[9]C1 metabolism is the metabolic process of providing methyl groups for vital functions [509, 510].

SLC6A4 encodes the transmembrane serotonin transporter. Prenatal exposure to maternal depressed mood and the methylenetetrahydrofolate reductase (MTHFR) C677T variant affects SLC6A4 methylation in infants at birth [513]. MTHFR is important in generating methyl groups for DNA methylation. C677T, a common variant of MTHFR, is associated with depression in men and non-pregnant women, greater depressed mood in pregnant women, and with global changes in DNA methylation.

Synaptic density peaks in the human frontal cortex during childhood and early adolescence and then declines by about 30% to 40% during late adolescence and teenage [514]. Programmed cell death (apoptosis), synapse disassembly, and process elimination are involved [515]. The dying cells and their processes are removed by glial cells. Developmental processes appear to be precisely regulated by the interaction between neurons and glial cells [516, 517].

During early brain development, cortical axon and dendritic branches and dendritic spines can disappear and regrow in just a few minutes. In adults, reorganization is restricted mainly to dendritic spines and occurs at a much slower rate [518]. These neuroplastic changes are driven by experience [519, 520]. In the adult brain, dendritic spines are not as dynamic and are lost, retracted, or sprouted after a few days [520, 521]. Increased sensory stimulation or deprivation at all stages tends to make a significant impact on plasticity in the neocortex [522–524].

Social, emotional, and neurological changes that occur during adolescence may put vulnerable individuals in a susceptible state to psychopathology [525]. It has been suggested that stress associated with adolescent changes may be a diathesis for mental psychopathology [516, 526].

Willingness to Change: Motivation and More

Now that we have looked at evidence for those things that we need to change, let us look at how we can encourage our patients to make what changes that they can.

For our purposes, what we can change can be separated into the direct constellation of symptoms that define depression and those maladaptive behaviors that may accompany and reinforce depression. This latter category includes the high rates of comorbid addictive behaviors such as obesity, smoking, alcohol, and drug abuse [526–534].

A 2009 review of seventeen studies totaling 204,507 participants suggested a very significant association between depression and obesity [535]. In addition, this association appeared to be stronger for women.

First, a few clarifications. The subject of changing health behavior often uses the term volition. *Volition,* in psychological terms, is an individual's internally generated, self-initiated cognitive process that is used to commit to a specific action [536–540].

Brain networks that are involved in the series of decisions that underpin voluntary behavior include the pre-supplementary motor area, the anterior prefrontal cortex, and the parietal cortex [541, 542]. Although it is pretty straightforward to feel that we are in control of our behavior when we willfully intend to move and that *self-agency* is at work (i.e., that our actions are a consequence of this intention), the pathways and degrees of consciousness are nuanced [543].

Although the term "*habit*" is widely used in the context of health-related behavior, definitions in the literature are often implicit and not coherently linked to an underlying theoretical framework [544]. A scoping review of 136 empirical studies and 8 literature reviews regarding habits suggests that habit is a process by which a stimulus generates an impulse to act as a result of a learned stimulus-response association [544]. Those reviewers also emphasized that habit does not need to generate behavior. Instead, habits combine with impulses and inhibitions coming from other sources, including conscious decisions to elicit responses.

Research on health-related behavior has been dominated by one theory since 1985. However, there is surprisingly little evidence for its utility [5–7]. This theory is the *Theory of Planned Behavior* (TPB) [8–10, 108, 545], which is an extension of the *Theory of Reasoned Action* (TRA) [11].

The main tenets of the TPB are as follows [2]. TPB states that *intention* to perform the behavior and the perceived *behavioral control* are the foundations for the volitional behavior. Intentions are believed to be based upon the level of perceived control over the behavior, attitudes about the behavior, and subjective norms. Perceived behavioral control is based upon actual control. Strength and evaluation of accessible behavioral, normative, and control beliefs form the foundation upon which perceived behavioral control, attitudes, and subjective norms are built.

TPB postulates that intention fully mediates the effects of attitude and subjective norm and partially mediates perceived behavioral control. Furthermore, TPB hypothesizes that (i) perceived behavioral control mediates control beliefs on intention and behavior; (ii) subjective norm mediates normative beliefs on intention and behavior; and (iii) attitude mediates behavioral beliefs on intention and behavior. The *sufficiency assumption* suggests that TPB mediates all other biological, medical, social, cultural, economic, and environmental influences [12].

A 2011 meta-analysis of 237 tests from 206 prospective studies of TPB analyzed moderating relationships of behavior type, length of follow-up, sample age, and behavioral measure, controlling for past behavior where possible [13]. Behavior type significantly influenced the predictions. Risk, detection, safer sex, and abstinence from drugs poorly predicted between 13.8% and 15.3% of the variance. The variance of physical activity and diet behaviors was better explained (23.9% and 21.2%, respectively). The age of the sample population moderated the relationships: Student samples more accurately predicted physical activity, whereas adolescent samples more strongly predicted abstinence behaviors. Better predictions were seen for self-reports versus objective measurements and for short-term assessments.

A 2002 systematic review of studies that used TPB to analyze results of behavioral interventions identified 30 papers covering 24 studies [14]. Very rarely was TPB used to develop the intervention. Instead, these studies used TPB to measure process and outcome variables and to predict intention and behavior. The behavior change methods used in these studies were mainly persuasion and information. Increasing skills, goal setting, and rehearsal of skills were less common interventions. Although effect sizes, where calculable, were small, two-thirds of the studies successfully changed behavior, and half successfully changed intention. No relationship was seen between effectiveness and the theory used to produce the interventions.

The TPB seems to suffer from having a focus on rational reasoning and ignoring subconscious influences [14, 106], not considering the role of emotions [15], not accounting for the dynamic nature of behavioral changes on cognition [12, 13], and being of questionable validity and utility [16].

Reviews of the Theory of Planned Behavior (TPB) have challenged its validity [16, 27]. One particularly vexing issue is the phenomenon of inclined abstainers—individuals who intend to act but fail to follow through. Questions surrounding validity focus on several key points [16, 27], including the sufficiency hypothesis, which assumes that all theory-external processes are mediated through the TPB. This assumption is contradicted by evidence showing that, even when TPB predictors are controlled for, moderators such as age, socioeconomic status, physical health, mental health, and environment still forecast objectively measured physical activity [17]. TPB demonstrates stronger predictive power among individuals who are younger, more affluent, and healthier—and when behavior is measured over shorter time spans [13, 22].

A quality appraisal of TPB-based questionnaires between 2002 and 2012 revealed problem areas that include sample size estimation, direct and indirect measures, and questions on demographics [545].

Health behavior seems to be better predicted than TPB by habit strength [18], self-regulatory factors including planning [20], and motivational factors including identity, self-determination, and anticipated regret [19].

Changes in health behavior can occur without affecting perceived behavioral control or intention. These changes in health behavior can result from subtle changes below the awareness of an individual by varying salience, cost, and reinforcement [21].

The utility of the TPB has come into question due to its failure to incorporate the considerable progress that has been made in human behavioral research since its introduction in 1985 [23–26, 546].

Alternative approaches to explaining and changing health-related behaviors have been advanced [27]. These include theories based on self-regulation [560], temporal dynamics, e.g., PRIME [28], cost versus benefit in temporal context, e.g., temporal self-regulation theory [29], integrating planned behavior and self-determination [547, 548], self-determination and autonomy [549–551], integrating multiple goals [552], dual processes of impulse versus reflection [553–557], and sequential models suggesting different processes in motivation and implementation, e.g., HAPA [558].

Another way to categorize attempts at changing health behaviors is in terms of *motivation versus no motivation for change*.

The first group of approaches focuses on converting motivation into action. These include implementation intentions [30, 561], self-monitoring [31], goal setting [32, 33], and action planning [26].

The second group of approaches focuses on motivating the non-motivated [559]. A significant number of people who are at high risk of the consequences of non-healthy behavior are not motivated to change. These include studies showing that about one-third of individuals who could most benefit from exercise have no intention of exercising [562, 563]; more than 90% of smokers reportedly do not want to quit [564]; and in any given year, about 60% of smokers make no attempt to quit [565, 566]. *The two most common theories about non-motivated individuals are the self-determination theory* [34–37] *and the transtheoretical model of behavioral change* [567, 568].

Underpinning *self-determination theory* is the idea that there are different types of motivation or reasons for engaging in behavior. *Amotivation* is defined as the state in which an individual does not intend to act [38]. When individuals are amotivated relative to health behaviors, they do not identify reasons why they act and generally lack sufficient intentions, have poor uptake, and do not stick to health behaviors. It has been suggested that amotivation stems from low levels of self-efficacy, outcome expectancies, effort beliefs, and value beliefs [39, 569].

Transtheoretical Model of Behavioral Change

The *transtheoretical model of behavioral change (TTM)* (so called because it encompasses many theories of behavior change) is probably the most accepted model of health behavior change [225, 570–573]. Instead of recommending one particular approach, the TTM makes use of strategies from various psychotherapeutic approaches and provides an organizing and integrating biopsychosocial matrix for understanding and assisting behavioral changes [574]. It is used by the Centers for Disease Control and Prevention as a foundation for health care research and intervention [575–577]. TTM has been used across a spectrum of health behaviors, including addiction, HIV [578, 579], STD protection [580], exercise [581, 582], tobacco [583–585], nutrition [586], and cancer [587].

TTM suggests that to change a health behavior there is a continuum of change [40, 588, 589]. The model identifies six stages of change: *precontemplation, contemplation, preparation, action, maintenance, and termination* [590, 591]. The amount of time spent in each change varies, and it is possible to move backwards at any time. A variety of processes of change based upon various experiences and self-regulatory strategies facilitate movement from stage to stage [585]. *The whole process of change is influenced by self-efficacy.* Precontemplation, contemplation, and preparation deal with introspective intentions to change and no overt change. Action and maintenance stages are manifest as observable behavior [22]. It has been suggested that, as a general rule, at-risk populations have 40% in precontemplation, 40% in contemplation, and 20% in preparation [590].

Precontemplation is characterized by no apparent interest in changing health behavior, very similar to the amotivation states. This state encompasses those who are aware of the reasons for changing their behavior but do not want to change and those who are unaware of the reasons for changing or their ability to change. Both of these groups tend to avoid thinking, reading, or talking about their high-risk behavior. Frequently, the aware group has tried to change, failed, is disheartened, and has given up. They are frequently considered by other theories to be amotivated, resistant, or not ready to be helped. Cons outweigh the pros.

Contemplation is the stage where an individual is actively considering the pluses and minuses of changing. Ambivalence is the primary characteristic [592]. This stage may take quite a while and is akin to chronic procrastination in making a decision. It has been suggested that during this stage the procrastinator is hoping that the problem will go away by itself, or that in the process of contemplation a solution will be found that does not require action [572]. This process of contemplation is also referred to as *decisional balance* [41, 572, 593]. When ambivalence is resolved, the balance is tipped to action when activity is seen to be vital to obtaining a life goal.

Preparation is the stage during which an individual becomes committed to acting, often within the "next month." In this stage, a plan has been produced. Some small steps toward acting have often been taken. Commitment is frequently vocalized. The pros outweigh the cons.

Action is where an individual fully engages and is actively making changes. Incremental changes may not be fully engaged. For example, cutting down the number of cigarettes instead of quitting totally. It is a stage where it is important to be ready to head off recidivism.

Maintenance occurs when the new behavior is fully integrated into daily living. Relapse prevention is very important at this stage [592, 594].

Termination is the stage where there is no further temptation to relapse into maladaptive behavior.

The TTM also suggests that there are *ten processes of change* for producing progress, along with *decisional balance, self-efficacy* [595–600], and *temptations* [601].

The ten self-regulatory strategies known as the *processes of change* that have been identified in the TTM [573, 590] are independent variables that function between the stages [602, 603]. These broad processes of change categories can be used as the basis for formulating specific therapeutic interventions. Although each of the processes can be used in any stage, they have found their best utility in either the *experiential* pre-action preparation stages or in the *behavioral* processes action stages. Experiential strategies help raise awareness about the need for change and prompt a resolution of procrastination. Behavioral strategies are practical reinforcers of the manifest behavioral changes.

Those strategies most commonly used in the pre-action stages are as follows:

1. *Consciousness raising* is becoming aware of the nature of the unhealthy behavior and the benefit of changing it. Education, discussions, and personal feedback are learning tools.
2. *Emotional arousal or dramatic relief* is feeling negative emotions such as fear or anxiety about the unhealthy behavior and feeling relief when learning about how others were able to change away from the unhealthy behavior.
3. *Self-reevaluation* is realizing that changing behavior is in tune with one's personal values and identity.
4. *Social liberation* occurs with the realization that social norms are supporting the change in behavior. This may sometimes be due to a shifting of social norms.
5. *Self-liberation or commitment* occurs when one realizes that they are capable of changing, and one makes a commitment to change.

Those strategies most commonly used in the action and maintenance stages are as follows:

1. *Counter conditioning* is the process of substituting healthy alternative cognitions and behaviors for the maladaptive behavior.
2. *Stimulus control* is engaging cues and reminders to use the healthy behavior and to disengage the cues and reminders that trigger unhealthy behavior.
3. *Contingency or reinforcement management* increases the rewards for healthy behavior and decreases the rewards for unhealthy behavior.
4. *Helping relationships* is finding and using appropriate social interactions for support to help with facilitating behavioral changes.
5. *Environmental reevaluation* is the realization that the unhealthy behavior has a negative effect on others. Also, how the new behavior may have a beneficial effect on their social environment.

Self-Efficacy

Self-efficacy or *task-specific confidence* affects the process of movement from stage to stage [227, 604–608]. Self-efficacy is the confidence that an individual has about his or her own ability to accomplish a specific task in a specific situation [227–229]. It is the situation-specific confidence that one can handle high-risk situations without falling back upon their maladaptive behavior. Self-efficacy will also determine how long someone will attempt a task without giving up [229]. Self-efficacy perceptions can be changed [609, 610]. There are four principal theories that address self-efficacy. These are Social Cognitive Theory, Social Learning Theory, Self-Concept Theory, and Attribution Theory.

Social Cognitive Theory postulates that there are four bases of beliefs of self-efficacy [42, 611]. The four are mastery, vicarious experience, verbal persuasion, and emotional-physiological state. Self-efficacy determines action via motivational, cognitive, and affective intervention [43, 44].

1. *Mastery experience* is the successful accomplishment of a task. It lays a firm foundation for the belief in self-efficacy. However, if someone fails at a task it may be discouraging. Mastery of simple tasks encourages tackling more complex ones.
2. *Vicarious experience* observing a social model helps provide a model demonstrating processes that accomplish a behavior. This is considered to be the essential component of learning. Modeling can also be written or oral in addition to active. Identifying with the person modeling the behavior is more conducive to adopting the behavior. Outcome expectancies should be perceived. Reproduction of a modeled behavior is thought to be dependent upon three factors: (i) Perceived personal ability [self-efficacy). (ii) Behavioral factors which refer to the response received after correctly performing the behavior. (iii) Environmental factors that are the provision of suitable materials and a setting to accomplish the goal.
3. *Verbal persuasion* provides encouragement to continue to pursue the goal [45].

4. *Emotional physiological state* is the importance of the subject being in a rested or relaxed physical state when attempting to make a change.

Social Learning Theory proposes that learning is cognitive in a social context [46]. Learning may be a result of observing, direct instruction, or motor reinforcement. The following are the main principles of social learning theory [48]:

1. *Learning is cognitive* in a social context. It is not purely behavioral.
2. *Modeling* or observational learning with extraction of information and thinking about the behavior is frequent. Modeling may be live wherein an actual person demonstrates the targeted behavior. The stimuli may be verbal in which detailed instructions are given. Or modeling may be symbolic via real or fictional characters who are seen performing the behavior in the media (e.g., TV, Internet, literature, movies).
3. *Reinforcement* is important but not essential for learning.
4. *Vicarious reinforcement*: Observation of rewards and punishments can be sufficient to produce learning [47].
5. *Reciprocal determinism* is the mutual influence of cognition, environment, and behavior. Learning is active even if not overt.

Cognitive, behavioral, and model processes of learning are said to modify what is learned by observation [49, 50]. Attributes include attention, retention, reproduction, and motivation.

1. *Attention* is determined by features of the behavior observed (e.g., affective valence, novelty, relevance, complexity) and aspects of the observer (e.g., arousal, past experiences, perception, and cognitive ability).
2. *Retention* is the capability of remembering what has been observed. It is also influenced by aspects of the observer and the object being observed.
3. *Reproduction* is the ability to organize and reproduce a behavior. This is also dependent upon the characteristics of the observer.
4. *Motivation* and expectations of the observer to reproduce or not the observed behavior is also based upon characteristics of the observer.

Social learning, social cognition, observational learning, and motor cognition may involve *mirror neurons* [51, 52]. Mirror neurons fire when an individual observes the same action performed by another individual and when one performs the same act [612]. Mirror neurons have been found in the human premotor cortex, the supplementary motor area, the primary somatosensory cortex, and the inferior parietal cortex [54]. They have also been found in other primates and in birds.

Self-Concept Theory may be described as an organized, developmental, stable, hierarchical perception of oneself [55]. Self-concept is created by experience with one's environment and with significant others [57]. Carl Rogers believed that self-concept is composed of self-image (how you see yourself), self-esteem (how much you value yourself), and ideal self (how you would like to be) [56]. Others have argued that self-concept differs from self-esteem, which is opinionated and evaluative, and from self-awareness, which refers to introspection or how self-knowledge relates to one's attitudes and dispositions [58].

Attribution Theory is the study of models to explain the causes of behavior and events [59]. It has been suggested that attributing negative events to factors over which a person has no control leads to a lack of attempts to make conditions better [60]. This may, in turn, lead to negative moods and possibly to depression and other mental illnesses.

Acting in a way to produce a successful health behavior outcome can be problematic [570, 603, 613–615]. Three *primary reasons for problems with adherence* have been suggested to be strategy-to-stage mismatch, neglect of self-efficacy, and poor maintenance support [616]. A strategy that is not matched to a patient's stage of change may result in patient resistance and fail to achieve results [573, 592, 614, 617]. When a patient fails to change, the reasons for change are not important to the individual and that the patient lacks sufficient self-efficacy. Continued support after the action stage is completed may be necessary to boost the chances of long-term adherence to change. Degrees of self-reward and automaticity of the new behavior vary, so some degree of social support may be needed.

A meta-analysis of which psychological interventions are most effective in increasing self-efficacy for physical exercise showed that self-efficacy for physical activity seems to be enhanced by feedback on past performances by an individual or vicariously by feedback on performance by others [618]. Lower levels of self-efficacy were associated with persuasion, graded mastery, and barrier identification. Another meta-analysis showed that action planning, providing instruction, and reinforcing effort toward behavior were associated with significantly higher self-efficacy and greater physical activity [619]. Setting graded tasks and relapse prevention strategies are associated with significantly lower self-efficacy and less physical activity.

Self-efficacy to perform osteopathic psychomotor skills by medical students can be significantly modified by different instructional approaches [620]. A comparison was made between the instructor's demonstration, paired practice in the laboratory, independent self-paced practice outside class using an instructional handout and videotape, and after receiving individualized feedback on skill performance from an instructor acting as the patient. All students mastered the skills. However, the first two methods produced self-efficacy scores of 18% and 30%, respectively, whereas in the other two groups the self-efficacy scores were 75% and 85%, respectively.

Results of a study of the relationship between personal resources of self-mastery, optimism, and abstinence self-efficacy suggest that optimism and abstinence self-efficacy are effective personal resources for recovering substance abusers in 12-step programs [621].

The broad processes of change outlined above can be used as the basis for formulating specific therapeutic interventions. Indeed, Van Leer et al. [616] suggest that different psychotherapeutic approaches generally focus on a subset of these processes of change. They give the example of Gestalt therapy versus behavioral modification. Gestalt therapy tends to focus on experiential processes to develop awareness and resolve ambivalence, but not the outward manifestations of the behavior [61]. Behavioral modification reinforces overt behavior but does not address experiential or cognitive processes [62].

The role of the psychotherapist changes with the patient's needs. In the motivational stages, the therapist is a client-oriented counselor who directs the conversation about change but does not try to control the decision to commit to change [63–65, 622]. During the early action stages, the therapist becomes a coach and later becomes a consultant [65]. Matching processes of change to stages and providing ongoing support for self-efficacy is a dynamic process [616]. Reframing previous failures and restructuring treatment plans may be necessary to overcome poor self-efficacy.

A randomized trial of a computer-tailored intervention based upon the TTM for patients with depression showed significant improvements in depression [623]. The largest effect was seen in participants who had moderate or severe depression and who were in the precontemplation or contemplation stage at baseline.

Criticisms of the TTM have rested upon the assertion that stages are not really linear; rather, over time, individuals may cycle in or out of various stages [66, 624–626]. The rebuttal is that it may be better to think of the stages as cognitive benchmarks for the therapist while understanding the fluidity of the process [63, 622].

Other Processes for Change

Another set of theories to understand the lack of action in changing behavior posits a *dual process*. One is conscious and the other is non-conscious [67–71, 627]. The conscious process is reflective, concerned with knowledge about facts and values. The non-conscious process is an impulsive and spontaneous behavior that acts via associative motivational orientations.

Unhealthy behaviors are frequently conditioned by environmental cues coupled with rewards via the mesolimbic dopamine reward system that reinforces the cue-urge-reward cycle [72]. A powerful marshalling of cognitive forces may be necessary to override and change the connections in these pathways [72, 73, 628]. When an individual is low in internal resources and motivation, they are unlikely to be able to summon enough effort to overcome the automated cue-urge-reward system. In this case, introducing environmental modifiers may be useful [74].

Motivational Interviewing

Motivational interviewing is a counseling approach [68]. It is another way of looking at change as a balance between perceived importance to change and confidence to be able to make that change (self-efficacy) [64, 65]. This concept segregates individuals into four categories based upon the balance. Those with high confidence and high importance are ready to change. Those others need to have interventions tailored to their position in the matrix relative to importance and self-efficacy.

Strategies to reduce amotivation might use confidence-building plans, target decisional balance approaches, focus on changing effort, and value beliefs [67, 68, 629].

Therapeutic relational styles used in motivational interviewing include *reframing, overshooting, coming alongside, shifting focus, and emphasizing autonomy* [630].

Hardcastle et al. suggest the following *content-related techniques to overcome the lack of motivation* [559, 630]. Their techniques include *running head start, looking forward, and values exploration.* The goal of these three is to encourage arguments for change and decrease the person's own arguments for not changing.

Running head start is based upon the therapist asking open-ended questions to explore the advantages of changing versus the disadvantages of staying the same.

Looking forward prompts the client to imagine two possible scenarios: they continue the same behavior or make a change to a healthier way.

Value exploration is the exploration of what the client describes as their most important life goals and values and how the present behavior fits with those goals and values. Focus away from bad behaviors onto a more deeply satisfying lifestyle.

Rating of importance and self-efficacy on a readiness ruler or a visual analog scale may be a point of departure for asking why they rated themselves as they had. The follow-up questions would then focus on what it would take to move them to a higher level on the scale.

An RCT assessed the initial efficacy of *Motivational Interviewing* (MI), *Online Transtheoretical Model (*TTM)-tailored communications, and a brief *Health Risk Intervention* (HRI) on four health risk factors of inactivity, BMI, stress, and smoking in a worksite sample [75]. Over 6 months, everyone received an HRI session, but one group only got the MI, another group got three TTM sessions online, and the third group got three MI sessions in person or via telephone sessions. There were significantly more participants in the action stage for exercise and effective stress management and significantly fewer risk behaviors at 6 months in the MI and TTM groups than in the HRI only group.

The Health Action Process Approach (HAPA)

It has been suggested that health change models are either nonlinear sequential stage-based or continuum-based [76]. Stage-based models assume that stages of change are based upon dynamic qualitative steps as a manifestation of diverse mindsets of an individual as they approach the concept of change. Continuum models posit that change is a linear and continuous beginning with lack of motivation and progressing through readiness for action into implementation of change or disengagement.

On the other hand, *the health action process approach (HAPA)* combines both linear and nonlinear elements [77].

Ralf Schwarzer developed the HAPA as an open matrix of motivational and volitional concepts to attempt to explain and predict individual health behavior changes [78, 84, 631].

The HAPA posits two distinct self-regulating processes or phases (stages). These phases or stages are not fixed, and individuals may move in and out of these stages. The first is *pre-intentional motivation*, leading to a goal-setting intention to change a behavior. Individuals in this stage are referred to as *pre-intenders*. The second process is the *post-intentional volition* goal pursuit leading to the targeted behavior [78]. The volitional stage is subdivided into *pre-action and action phases*. The pre-action subdivision is characterized by the mindset of intention. Those individuals in this mindset are called *intenders*. Those in the action subdivision are called *actors*. These stages can be viewed as moderators on the continuum of change [83, 84].

The motivational and volitional variables specified in the HAPA are motivational self-efficacy, outcome expectancies, risk perception, intention, maintenance self-efficacy, action planning, coping planning, recovery self-efficacy, and social support [632]. These concepts are suggested to underlie adoption, initiation, and persistence of health change behaviors [79–81].

Post-intentional planning mediates the relationship between intentions and behavioral changes [82]. That is, when individuals plan how, when, and where to change, good intentions can be implemented as productive activity [82, 83]. There are two types of planning: action planning and coping planning [83, 85]. *Action planning* is important for the initiation of the planned behavior. *Coping planning* is developing a plan to manage prospective challenges to planned behavioral change. Coping planning is important for both initiation and maintenance of the behavioral changes [83].

In recognition of different challenges during different phases, self-efficacy in the concept of HAPA appears to vary with the phase [86]. *Pre-actional or task self-efficacy, coping or maintenance self-efficacy, and recovery self-efficacy* are recognized.

Interventions based upon the HAPA begin by recognizing the phase that an individual is in and then using a specific treatment targeted to that phase [87, 88, 633].

Non-intenders need to learn the benefits of the new behavior and the negative consequences of the current behavior [89]. Intenders have already set a goal; they now need plans to turn their intentions into action [90].

Actors only need relapse prevention skills based upon acquiring essential perceived recovery self-efficacy [86].

Phase-matched interventions based on the HAPA have been analyzed through randomized controlled trials across several health behaviors, including diet [88], dental hygiene [92], vaccination [634, 635], smoking [636, 637], condom use [638], and physical exercise [91]. These interventions have also been applied to various populations, such as patients with multiple sclerosis [639], sedentary middle-aged women [640], the elderly [641], individuals with chronic illness or disability [642], patients with schizophrenia [643], those undergoing physiotherapy [644], and participants in cardiac rehabilitation programs [645].

The following are some of the studies that looked at aspects of HAPA principles.

Deficits in motivation and in volition (especially negative expectations, self-efficacy, and planning) seem to be at work to partly explain the lower levels of exercise in people with depression [646]. The role of volitional mediators has been examined for physical exercise, breast self-examination, seat belt use, dietary behaviors, and dental flossing [78].

HAPA appears to be generalizable with regard to dietary behavior among cardiovascular disorder patients [647]. It seems that the process of change is the same for people at high risk of a coronary event and those who have already had the event.

Cross-behavior cognitions are related to a healthy lifestyle and may underlie the ability of an individual to regulate more than one health behavior [648]. Compensatory health beliefs are negatively related to intentions and hinder the adoption of a healthy lifestyle. Transfer cognitions are positively associated with intentions, action planning, and control (self-regulatory strategies) and encourage healthy lifestyles.

HAPA has been found to be relevant to engagement in physical activity by African American breast cancer survivors [649].

The HAPA model has been used in cardiac rehabilitation exercises to produce effective education curricula for increasing knowledge, enhancing intentions, self-efficacy, and action planning [650].

In China, HAPA online mindfulness has been successfully used to enhance mental health and well-being [651].

HAPA constructs showed that patients with acquired physical disabilities rate their health behavior constructs differently based upon their "sport intentions" [652].

In a population of obese men and women, HAPA assumptions were partly confirmed relative to exercise [632]. No relationships were seen between risk perception and intention and between planning and physical activity. Intention was related to motivational self-efficacy, outcome expectancies, and social support. Social support and self-efficacy were associated with physical activity. Maintenance self-efficacy and coping planning were associated.

An intervention based upon HAPA was able to predict health outcomes in patients with type 2 diabetes but was not successful in changing healthy eating [653].

Investigation of HAPA variables relating to binge eating in patients undergoing laparoscopic adjustable gastric banding for severe obesity showed that preoperative intentions but not planning and volitional self-efficacy were able to predict reduced binge eating following surgery [654].

The value of integrating social support into the HAPA for dietary support in overweight and obese patients has shown that instrumental support was more beneficial for men than for women in addition to self-regulation in achieving maintenance of a low-fat diet a year later [655].

More Constraints on Changing

Velleity is the lowest degree of inclination that has not led to action. It is often considered the lowest level of volition [655]. Velleity may work in two different directions at the same time. The existence of conflicting values may make the transition to activity or full-blown volition difficult. In making the decision to action, it has been suggested that there is a conflict between doing a particular activity and not doing it. Resolution of this conflict may hang in the balance between velleity and volition for the opposites.

Conation may be the link between cognitive ability and performance capabilities in everyday life [656]. Conation is the ability to focus and maintain intellectual energy over time to successfully complete a task [656–659].

Conation is considered the frequently ignored member of the mental trilogy of cognition, affect, and conation [656, 660, 661]. Conativity is the drive to act on the thoughts and feelings.

Relationships among conation and cognition, emotion, motivation, vigilance, and malingering are discussed in [657]. Conation is highly associated with determining differential performances on neuropsychological tests [657]. Conation may be equivalent to the *Power Factor* postulated by Halstead to be at the basis of intellectual energy: the energy source for production of intelligent behavior [94, 104 Conation has been called purposeful striving by early authors [94–99]. Conation has been thought to be related to temperament, educational attainment, and performance on intelligence tests [100, 102]. Connation may be the missing factor between intellectual capacity and achievement in many practical tasks [102]. Some researchers have suggested that the prefrontal cortex is the likely source of conation [101].

The *strength model of self-control* suggests that effortful control over dominant responses is limited by the capacity for self-control [662–665]. When the capacity is depleted, and performance is impaired, it is known as *ego depletion* [665]. Meta-analysis demonstrated significant effects (a medium-sized effect (d = 0.62) across 198 tests) of ego-depletion on effort, perceived difficulty, negative affect, subjective fatigue, and blood glucose levels [560]. In ego-depleted subjects, better self-control was seen by offering motivational incentives, training on self-control tasks, and glucose supplementation.

The strength model of self-control says that self-control is the volitional overriding of predominant impulses to attain a specific goal. It is the ability to resist immediate gratification when a more desirable outcome is possible [665]. Some researchers have suggested that every act of self-control is based upon a resource with finite capacity [666–669]. These acts include controlling impulses, overriding habitual responses, making choices [664], emotional regulation [104], attention regulation [105], and persistence [665].

However, some researchers have questioned if ego depletion really exists [670, 671]. They believe that small study effects and publication bias may have made suspect the meta-analysis presented in [560]. The authors of that meta-analysis reject that criticism [672]. Data from the meta-analysis may be found here [673].

Attentional control theory (ACT) suggests that anxiety negatively influences the efficient functioning of the goal-directed attentional system and increases the influence of the stimulus-driven attentional system, especially as related to threat-associated stimuli [674]. This increased vulnerability to threats may lead to emotional reactivity and decreased performance [675].

Integration of the strength model of self-control with the central tenets of the ACT suggests that anxiety will lead to attention disruption and distraction from subsequent cognitive or perceptual-motor tasks only if an individual does not have sufficient self-control [676].

An exploration of the role of *affective attitudes* versus *cognitive attitudes* for 14 health-promoting or health-risk behaviors suggested that affective attitude was significantly more powerful in predicting behavior than was cognitive attitude for nine behaviors [677]. There was especially higher divergence between affective and cognitive attitudes for illegal drug use, binge drinking, and smoking. However, intentions to change behaviors that are most strongly based on anticipated affective reactions may be a stronger predictor of health behaviors [678]. Performance on 20 health-related behaviors showed anticipated affective reactions, but not affective attitude, instrumental attitude, injunctive norms, descriptive norms, moral norms, self-efficacy, or past behavior was the only underlying cognition (motivator) that influenced the health behavior.

Higher socioeconomic status (SES) is generally associated with more health protection and fewer health-risking behaviors [679, 680]. This relationship was tested in smoking initiation in adolescents, breastfeeding in primiparous women, and physical activity in working adults [681]. Significant interactions between intentions and behavior were seen such that lower SES associated with lower interactions. No relationship between SES and self-efficacy was seen.

A comparison between *collaborative implementation intentions,* partner-only, implementation intentions, and a control group in promoting physical activity has suggested that participants in the collaborative implementation-intention group were more physically active and lost more weight than each of the other groups at 1-, 3-, and 6-months [682]. Collaborative implementation intentions involve planning and enacting behavior with a partner.

An inductive approach to identifying health behavior characteristics and exploring the differences in health behaviors identified *three key dimensions of perception* [683]. The three dimensions are "easy immediate pay-offs" versus "effortful long-term pay-offs," "private unproblematic" versus "public and problematic," and "important routines" versus "unimportant one-offs." Risk behaviors were characterized by "easy immediate pay-offs" and "public-problematic." Physical activity was perceived as "effortful long-term pay-offs."

A questionnaire-based study of *planned behavior and exercise* showed that intention certainty, past behavior, self-schema, anticipated regret, and attitudinal versus normative control associated with significant improvements in consistency between intention and behavior [684]. In addition, they found that temporal stability moderated the effects of the other moderators.

Meta-analysis has revealed that the benefits of *printed tailored health interventions for change* depend upon (1) type of comparison condition, (2) health behavior, (3) type of subject population (both type of recruitment and country of sample), (4) type of print material, (5) number of intervention contacts, (6) length of follow-up, (7) number and type-of theoretical concepts tailored on, and (8) whether or not demographics and/or behavior were tailored on [106, 107].

Self-help preferences and attitudes for treatment of depression versus psychotherapy and antidepressants were assessed by the random assignment of 536 people to read about one of five treatment options before rating how successful they thought the treatment would be and ranking them in their order of preference [685]. The treatments were bibliotherapy, Internet-based self-help, guided self-help, antidepressants, or psychotherapy. The most acceptable and preferred treatments were psychotherapy and guided self-help. The least acceptable were antidepressants and bibliotherapy. Antidepressants were rated as having the highest risk of side effects.

Self-affirmation inductions coupled with persuasive health information can enhance message acceptance, intentions to change, and resulting health behavior change [686]. Effect sizes are small but comparable to other health behavior interventions.

The reward-processing and valuation [687, 688], interval-timing [689], and decision-making sub-systems interact and integrate to form the *reward system* [690]. Motivation and the valuation system influence the reward system via direct connections to the timing system [691]. The amount of attention placed on an event influences our perception of time and the salience of the reward in the system [692, 693].

The *striatum embodies multiple learning signals and functions* across many cognitive domains and contexts, including learning and motivation [694]. Genes such as COMT, DARPP-32, DAT1, DRD2, and DRD4 controlling dopaminergic processes in frontostriatal areas may be involved in motivation, learning, and cognition [695, 696].

It appears that *placebo effects in therapeutic environments* are mediated by affective consequences of performing a motivated ritual (aka *motivational concordance*) [697]. Motivational concordance is the concept that the placebo response is the consequence of concordance between the placebo ritual and significant intrinsic motives [698]. In a controlled exercise experiment, the behavioral and affective consequences of pursuing a positively valued goal demonstrated that satisfaction mediated expectancy [697]. Expectancy, adherence, and effort correlated with perceived benefit [697]. Alternatively, response expectancy, conditioning, and goal activation may account for short-term placebo effects [698]. However, goal satisfaction and affect influences on the hypothalamic-pituitary-adrenal axis and inflammatory responses may be responsible for long-term therapeutic changes [698].

It appears that the lower amount of exercise that is common in people with depression is due to negative outcome expectations, self-efficacy deficits, and planning deficits, i.e., *deficits in motivation and volition,* respectively [646, 699]. Motivation can be successfully targeted to enhance exercise adherence [700].

Addictive disorders and experiments with addictive substances most frequently begin in adolescence and young adults [701, 702]. *Differential maturational changes* in frontal cortical and subcortical monoaminergic systems may explain adolescent impulsivity and novelty seeking as a transitional behavior [703–707]. It appears there is faster development in areas promoting novelty seeking and slower development in inhibitory areas. Vulnerability to drugs at those times may lead to changes in neurochemistry that enhance progression to neural changes fundamental to addiction.

Advantages and limitations of *Internet-based interventions* for mental disorders are discussed in reference [708].

A systematic review and meta-analysis of using the Internet to promote health behavior change was conducted on interventions that were published between 2000 and 2008 [709]. Results showed that more extensive use of theory, incorporation of more behavioral change techniques, and use of additional communications methods, especially the use of short message service or text messages, produced greater results.

Summary

This chapter considers what we can change to decrease the likelihood and impact of depression. Mechanisms involve epigenetics, neuroplasticity, and conditioning. Our targets for change are direct symptoms that define depression and those maladaptive behaviors that may accompany and reinforce depression.

Expression of many genes is controlled by experience that can modify their transcription. Some genetic patterns are age or developmental stage-related changes, and others are plasticity-related changes. These changes are perhaps best understood in terms of epigenetics. In many if not most mental disorders, genetic factors are involved. However, discordance rates in identical twin studies, especially in stress-related illnesses such as depression, suggest other processes are implicated. One way that environmental effects generate such potent and long-term effects is via epigenetic modifications of DNA expression without altering the genotype.

Epigenetic processes are more active during times when rates of DNA synthesis are high, e.g., during prenatal, infancy, and early childhood periods when growth rates are highest. This cellular and molecular remodeling can change cognitive, behavioral, and physiological responses to stress. The underlying epigenetic changes appear to be dependent upon many factors, such as maturational stage (e.g., pre- or post-puberty) and gender. There is an extremely complex cause-and-effect relationship among genotype, epitype, and phenotype. However, it appears that genotypes predispose epitypes.

Maladaptations in gene expression, neural network functions, and behavior may be induced by environmental exposure. These changes appear to be sustained and are distinct depending upon exposure at critical developmental times or in adulthood. These changes are highly correlated with mental disorders such as depression, schizophrenia, and bipolar disorder. Combinations of genetic and epigenetic factors have been proposed as underlying mechanisms for major psychiatric disorders. Integration of chromatin structure and epigenetic control of the immune system might be the link between environmental and differentiation influences on stress responses.

Maltreatment of children that is associated with epigenetic changes in ID3, GRIN1, and TPPP genes appears to be a risk factor for depression. Deficiencies in maternal and early postnatal nutrition contribute to health risk factors in adult life.

Conditioning may be operant or classical. When the immune system or endocrine system is involved, conditioning is a result of multidirectional central nervous-endocrine-immune system communication. Just as CNS changes affect the immune system, such as are revealed in classical conditioning and stress experiments, so does the immune system affect behavior by way of interactions on the CNS.

While stress influences the brain throughout the life span, the developing brain is most vulnerable to stress during several critical periods. These periods include prenatal, perinatal, infancy, childhood, and adolescence.

Social, emotional, and neurological changes that occur during adolescence may put vulnerable individuals in a susceptible state to psychopathology. It has been suggested that stress associated with adolescent changes may be a diathesis for mental psychopathology.

Whether or not malfunctioning epigenetic affects can be therapeutically modified is an open question. However, evidence is accumulating that many of these marks have the potential to be reset.

Just as there is considerable variation in interindividual responses to antidepressants, which seem to have a genetic component, so there are differences in individual responses to psychotherapy that appear to have a genetic component.

What we can change may be separated into two categories: the direct constellation of symptoms that define depression, and the maladaptive behaviors that often accompany and reinforce it. The latter includes high rates of comorbid addictive behaviors such as obesity, smoking, alcohol use, and drug abuse. Willingness to change, along with the motivation and ability to enact those changes, are matters of considerable importance.

Various theories have attempted to explain the range of this willingness and ability. One prominent example is the Theory of Planned Behavior (TPB), which posits that behavioral intention and perceived behavioral control—along with attitudes and subjective norms—jointly influence whether individuals act on their intentions. Other theories have more evidence behind them.

The Transtheoretical Model of Behavioral Change (TTM) encompasses many theories of behavior change and is probably the most accepted model of health behavior change. It is used by the Centers for Disease Control and Prevention as a foundation for health care research and intervention. Instead of recommending one particular approach, the TTM makes use of strategies from various psychotherapeutic approaches and provides an organizing and integrating biopsychosocial matrix for understanding and assisting behavioral changes.

It has been suggested that health change models are either nonlinear sequential stage-based or continuum-based. Stage-based models assume that stages of change are based upon dynamic qualitative steps as a manifestation of diverse mindsets of an individual as they approach the concept of change. Continuum models posit that change is a linear and continuous beginning with a lack of motivation and progressing through readiness for action into implementation of change or disengagement.

On the other hand, the Health Action Process Approach (HAPA) combines both linear and nonlinear elements. HAPA is an open matrix of motivational and volitional concepts to attempt to explain and predict individual health behavior changes. The HAPA posits two distinct self-regulating processes or phases (stages). These phases or stages are not fixed, and individuals may move in and out of these stages.

References

1. Hebb DO. The organization of behavior. New York: Wiley; 1949.
2. Hebb DO. Distinctive features of learning in the higher animal. In: Delafresnaye JF, editor. Brain mechanisms and learning. London: Oxford University Press; 1961.
3. Amaral DG, Price JL, Pitkänen A, Carmichael ST. Anatomical organisation of the primate amygdaloid complex. In: Aggleton JP, editor. The Amygdala: neurobiological aspects of emotion, memory, and mental dysfunction. New York: Wiley-Liss; 1992. p. 1–66.
4. McGaugh JL. Amygdala: role in modulation of memory storage. In: Aggleton JP, editor. The Amygdala: a functional analysis. New York: Oxford Univ. Press; 2000. p. 391–424.
5. Schwarzer R. Life and death of health behaviour theories. Health. Psychol Rev. 2014;8(1):53–6. PMID: 25053007. http://www.ncbi.nlm.nih.gov/pubmed/25053007.
6. Sniehotta FF, Presseau J, Araújo-Soares V. Time to retire the theory of planned behaviour. Health Psychol Rev. 2014;8(1):1–7. PMID: 25053004. http://www.ncbi.nlm.nih.gov/pubmed/25053004.
7. Schwarzer R. Modeling health behavior change: how to predict and modify the adoption and maintenance of health behaviors. Appl Psychol Int Rev. 2008;57:1–29. Modeling health behavior change: how to predict and modify the adoption and maintenance of health behaviors.
8. Ajzen I. The theory of planned behavior. Organ Behav Hum Decis Process. 1991;50:179–211. The theory of planned behavior.
9. Ajzen I. From intentions to actions: a theory of planned behavior. In: Kuhl J, Beckman J, editors. Action-control: from cognition to behavior. Heidelberg: Springer; 1985. p. 11–39.
10. Michie S, Wood CE, Johnston M, Abraham C, Francis JJ, Hardeman W. Behaviour change techniques: the development and evaluation of a taxonomic method for reporting and describing behaviour change interventions (a suite of five studies involving consensus methods, randomised controlled trials and analysis of qualitative data). Health Technol Assess. 2015;19(99):1–188. PMCID: PMC4781650. http://www.ncbi.nlm.nih.gov/pubmed/26616119.
11. Fishbein M, Ajzen I. Belief, attitude, intention, and behavior: an introduction to theory and research. Reading: Addison-Wesley; 1975.
12. Sutton S. The past predicts the future: interpreting behaviour-behaviour relationships in social psychological models of health behaviour. In: Rutter DR, Quine L, editors. Social psychology and health: European perspectives. Aldershot: Avebury; 1994. p. 71–88.
13. McEachan RRC, Conner M, Taylor N, Lawton RJ. Prospective prediction of health-related behaviors with the theory of planned behavior: a meta-analysis. Health Psychol Rev. 2011;5:97. Prospective prediction of health-related behaviours with the Theory of Planned Behaviour: a meta-analysis: Health Psychology Review: Vol 5 , No 2 - Get Access
14. Sheeran P, Gollwitzer PM, Bargh JA. Nonconscious processes and health. Health Psychol. 2013;32(5):460–73. PMID: http://www.ncbi.nlm.nih.gov/pubmed/22888816.
15. Conner M, Godin G, Sheeran P, Germain M. Some feelings are more important: cognitive attitudes, affective attitudes, anticipated affect, and blood donation. Health Psychol. 2013;32(3):264–72. PMID: 22612559. http://www.ncbi.nlm.nih.gov/pubmed/22612559.
16. Orbell S, Sheeran P. "Inclined abstainers": a problem for predicting health-related behaviour. Br J Soc Psychol. 1998;37(Pt 2):151–65. PMID: 9639861. http://www.ncbi.nlm.nih.gov/pubmed/9639861.
17. Sniehotta FF, Gellert P, Witham MD, Donnan PT, Crombie IK, McMurdo MET. Psychological theory in an interdisciplinary context: how do social cognitions predict physical activity in older adults alongside demographic, health-related, social, and environmental factors? Int J Behav Nutr Phys Act. 2013;10(1):106. Psychological theory in an interdisciplinary context: Psychological, demographic, health-related, social, and environmental correlates of physical activity in a representative cohort of community-dwelling older adults.
18. Gardner B, de Bruijn GJ, Lally P. A systematic review and meta-analysis of applications of the Self-Report Habit Index to nutrition and physical activity behaviours. Ann Behav Med. 2011;42(2):174–87. PMID: 21626256. http://www.ncbi.nlm.nih.gov/pubmed/21626256.
19. Conner M, Armitage CR. Extending the theory of planned behavior: a review and avenues for further research. J Appl Soc Psychol. 1998;28:1429–64. Extending the theory of planned behavior: A review and avenues for further research.

20. Carraro N, Gaudreau P. Spontaneous and experimentally induced action planning and coping planning for physical activity: a meta-analysis. Psychol Sport Exerc. 2013;14:228–48. Spontaneous and experimentally induced action planning and coping planning for physical activity: A meta-analysis - ScienceDirect
21. Marteau TM, Ogilvie D, Roland M, Suhrcke M, Kelly MP. Judging nudging: can nudging improve population health? BMJ. 2011;342:d228. PMID: 21266441. http://www.ncbi.nlm.nih.gov/pubmed/21266441.
22. Rhodes RE, Dickau L. Moderators of the intention-behaviour relationship in the physical activity domain: a systematic review. Br J Sports Med. 2013;47(4):215–25. PMID: 22278998. http://www.ncbi.nlm.nih.gov/pubmed/22278998.
23. Noar SM, Head KJ. Mind the gap: bringing our theories in line with the empirical data - a response to commentaries. Health. Psychol Rev. 2014;8(1):65–9. PMID: 25053009. http://www.ncbi.nlm.nih.gov/pubmed/25053009.
24. Head KJ, Noar SM. Facilitating progress in health behaviour theory development and modification: the reasoned action approach as a case study. Health. Psychol Rev. 2014;8(1):34–52. PMID: 25053006. http://www.ncbi.nlm.nih.gov/pubmed/25053006.
25. Kok G, Ruiter RAC. Who has the authority to change a theory? Everyone! A commentary on Head and Noar. Health. Psychol Rev. 2014;8(1):61–4. PMCID: PMC3919259. http://www.ncbi.nlm.nih.gov/pubmed/24575147.
26. Barley E, Lawson V. Using health psychology to help patients: theories of behaviour change. Br J Nurs. 2016;25(16):924–7. PMID: 27615529. http://www.ncbi.nlm.nih.gov/pubmed/27615529.
27. Ogden J. Time to retire the theory of planned behaviour?: one of us will have to go! A commentary on Sniehotta, Presseau and Araújo-Soares. Health. Psychol Rev. 2015;9(2):165–7. PMID: 26209205. http://www.ncbi.nlm.nih.gov/pubmed/26209205.
28. West R, Brown J. Theory of addiction. 2nd ed. Oxford: Wiley-Blackwell; 2013.
29. Hall PA, Fong GT. Temporal self-regulation theory: a neurobiologically informed model for physical activity behavior. Front Hum Neurosci. 2015;9:117. PMCID: PMC4373277. http://www.ncbi.nlm.nih.gov/pubmed/25859196.
30. Gollwitzer PM. Implementation intentions: strong effects of simple plans. Am Psychol. 1999;54:493–503. https://doi.org/10.1037/0003-066X.54.7.493. Implementation intentions: Strong effects of simple plans.
31. Miller ML, Thayer JF. On the nature of self-monitoring: relationships with adjustment and identity. Personal Soc Psychol Bull. 1988;14:544–53. https://doi.org/10.1177/0146167288143013. On the nature of self-monitoring: Relationships with adjustment and identity.
32. Locke EA. Motivation through conscious goal setting. Appl Prev Psychol. 1996;5:117–24. https://doi.org/10.1016/S0962--1849[96)80005-9. Motivation through conscious goal setting.
33. Fenner AA, Straker LM, Davis MC, Hagger MS. Theoretical underpinnings of a need-supportive intervention to address sustained healthy lifestyle changes in overweight and obese adolescents. Psychol Sport Exerc. 2013;14:819–29. https://doi.org/10.1016/j.psychsport.2013.06.005. Theoretical underpinnings of a need-supportive intervention to address sustained healthy lifestyle changes in overweight and obese adolescents - ScienceDirect
34. Deci EL, Ryan RM. Intrinsic motivation and self-determination in human behavior. New York: Plenum; 1985.
35. Deci EL, Ryan RM. The "what" and "why" of goal pursuits: human needs and the self-determination of behavior. Psychol Inq. 2000;11:227–68. https://doi.org/10.1207/S15327965PLI1104_01. The "what" and "why" of goal pursuits: Human needs and the self-determination of behavior.
36. Chatzisarantis NLD, Hagger MS, Brickell T. Using the construct of perceived autonomy support to understand social influence within the theory of planned behavior. Psychol Sport Exerc. 2008;9:27–44. https://doi.org/10.1016/j.psychsport.2006.12.003. Using the construct of perceived autonomy support to understand social influence within the theory of planned behavior - ScienceDirect
37. Chatzisarantis NLD, Hagger MS, Smith B. Influences of perceived autonomy support on physical activity within the theory of planned behavior. Eur J Soc Psychol. 2007;37:934–54. https://doi.org/10.1002/ejsp.407. Using the construct of perceived autonomy support to understand social influence within the theory of planned behavior - ScienceDirect
38. Vallerand RJ. A hierarchical model of intrinsic and extrinsic motivation in sport and exercise. In: Roberts GC, editor. Advances in motivation in sport and exercise. 2nd ed. Champaign: Human Kinetics; 2001. p. 263–319. A hierarchical model of intrinsic and extrinsic motivation for sport and physical activity.
39. Shen B, Wingert RK, Li W, Sun H, Rukavina PB. An amotivation model in physical education. J Teach Phys Educ. 2010;29:72–84. An amotivation model in physical education.
40. Glanz K, Rimer BK, Marcus LF. In: Glanz K, Rimer BK, Marcus Lewis F, editors. Health behavior and health education: theory, research, and practice. San Francisco: Jossey-Bass; 1990. p. 460.
41. Hall KL, Rossi JS. Meta-analytic examination of the strong and weak principles across 48 health behaviors. Prev Med. 2008;46(3):266–74. PMID: 18242667. http://www.ncbi.nlm.nih.gov/pubmed/18242667.
42. Luszczynska A, Schwarzer R. Social cognitive theory. In: Conner M, Norman P, editors. Predicting health behaviour. 2nd rev ed. Buckingham, UK: Open University Press; 2005. p. 127–69.
43. Bandura A. Human agency in social cognitive theory. Am Psychol. 1989;44:1175–84.
44. Bandura A. Self-efficacy in changing societies. Cambridge/New York: Cambridge University Press.
45. McAlister AL, Perry CL, Parcel GS. How individuals, environments, and health behaviors interact: social cognitive theory. In: Health behavior and health education: theory, research, and practice. 4th ed. San Francisco: Wiley; 2008. p. 169–88.
46. Bandura A. Social learning and personality development. New York: Holt, Rinehart, and Winston; 1963.
47. Bandura A. Social learning theory [PDF]. General Learning Corporation; 1971.
48. Grusec J. Social learning theory and developmental psychology: the legacies of Robert Sears and Albert Bandura. Dev Psychol. 1992;28(5):776–86. https://doi.org/10.1037/0012-1649.28.5.776. Social learning theory and developmental psychology: The legacies of Robert Sears and Albert Bandura.
49. Bandura A, Parke RD. Recent trends in social learning theory. New York: Academic Press, Inc; 1972.
50. Bandura A. Social learning theory. Oxford, UK: Prentice-Hall; 1977.
51. Fuhrmann D, Ravignani A, Marshall-Pescini S, Whiten A. Synchrony and motor mimicking in chimpanzee observational learning. Sci Rep. 2014;4
52. Reardon S. Monkey brains wired to share. Nature. 2014;506(7489):416–7. PMID: 24572401. http://www.ncbi.nlm.nih.gov/pubmed/24572401.
53. Uddin LQ, Iacoboni M, Lange C, Keenan JP. The self and social cognition: the role of cortical midline structures and mirror neurons. Trends Cogn Sci. 2007;11(4):153–7. PMID: 17300981. http://www.ncbi.nlm.nih.gov/pubmed/17300981.
54. Molenberghs P, Cunnington R, Mattingley JB. Is the mirror neuron system involved in imitation? A short review and meta-analysis. Neurosci Biobehav Rev. 2009;33(7):975–80. PMID: 19580913. http://www.ncbi.nlm.nih.gov/pubmed/19580913.
55. Shavelson RJ, Hubner JJ, Stanton GC. Self-concept: validation of construct interpretations. Rev Educ Res. 1976;46:407–41.

56. Rogers C. A theory of therapy, personality and interpersonal relationships as developed in the client-centered framework. In: Koch S, editor. Psychology: a study of science. Vol. 3: formulations of the person and the social context. New York: McGraw Hill; 1959.
57. Myers DG. Social psychology. 10th ed. New York: McGraw-Hill Higher Education; 2009.
58. Ayduk O, Gyurak A, Luerssen A. Rejection sensitivity moderates the impact of rejection on self-concept clarity. Personal Soc Psychol Bull. 2009;35(11):1467–78. PMCID: PMC4184908. http://www.ncbi.nlm.nih.gov/pubmed/19713567.
59. Kassin, Fein, Markus. Social psychology. 8th international ed. Wadsworth: C Engage Learning; 2010.
60. Seligman M. Helplessness: on depression, development, and death. Freeman/Times Books/Henry Holt & Co.; 1975.
61. Perls FS. The Gestalt approach & eyewitness to therapy. Palo Alto: Science & Behavior Books; 1973.
62. Skinner BF. Science and human behavior. New York: Macmillan; 1953.
63. Rollnick S, Mason P, Butler C. Health behavior change: a guide for practitioners. Edinburgh/New York: Churchill Livingstone; 1999. p. 225.
64. Miller WR, Rollnick S. Motivational interviewing: preparing people for change. New York: Guilford Press; 2002. p. 428.
65. Rogers CR. 'Client-centered' psychotherapy. Sci Am. 1952;187:66–74.
66. West R. The transtheoretical model of behaviour change and the scientific method. Addiction. 2006;101:774–8. The transtheoretical model of behaviour change and the scientific method.
67. Miller WR, Rollnick S. Motivational interviewing: preparing people for change. 3rd ed. New York: Guildford Press; 2013.
68. Hardcastle SJ, Taylor AH, Bailey MP, Harley RA, Hagger MS. Effectiveness of a motivational interviewing intervention on weight loss, physical activity and cardiovascular disease risk factors: a randomised controlled trial with a 12-month post-intervention follow-up. Int J Behav Nutr Phys Act. 2013;10:40. PMCID: PMC3639183. http://www.ncbi.nlm.nih.gov/pubmed/23537492.
69. Hagger MS, Chatzisarantis NLD. An integrated behavior change model for physical activity. Exerc Sport Sci Rev. 2014;42(2):62–9. PMID: 24508739. http://www.ncbi.nlm.nih.gov/pubmed/24508739.
70. Hagger MS, Chatzisarantis NLD. The trans-contextual model of autonomous motivation in education: conceptual and empirical issues and meta-analysis. Rev Educ Res. 2016;86(2):360–407. PMCID: PMC4873731. http://www.ncbi.nlm.nih.gov/pubmed/27274585.
71. Hagger MS, Rebar AL, Mullan B, Lipp OV, Chatzisarantis NLD. The subjective experience of habit captured by self-report indexes may lead to inaccuracies in the measurement of habitual action. Health. Psychol Rev. 2015;9(3):296–302. PMID: 25189762. http://www.ncbi.nlm.nih.gov/pubmed/25189762.
72. Rebar AL, Loftus AM, Hagger MS. Cognitive control and the non-conscious regulation of health behavior. Front Hum Neurosci. 2015;9:122. PMCID: PMC4350404. http://www.ncbi.nlm.nih.gov/pubmed/25798101.
73. Loftus AM, Yalcin O, Baughman FD, Vanman EJ, Hagger MS. The impact of transcranial direct current stimulation on inhibitory control in young adults. Brain Behav. 2015;5(5):e00332. PMCID: PMC4389055. http://www.ncbi.nlm.nih.gov/pubmed/25874165.
74. Sallis JF, Floyd MF, Rodríguez DA, Saelens BE. Role of built environments in physical activity, obesity, and cardiovascular disease. Circulation. 2012;125(5):729–37. PMCID: PMC3315587. http://www.ncbi.nlm.nih.gov/pubmed/22311885.
75. Prochaska JO, Butterworth S, Redding CA, Burden V, Perrin N, Leo M, Flaherty-Robb M, Prochaska JM. Initial efficacy of MI, TTM tailoring and HRI's with multiple behaviors for employee health promotion. Prev Med. 2008;46(3):226–31. PMCID: PMC3384542. http://www.ncbi.nlm.nih.gov/pubmed/18155287.
76. Lippke S, Ziegelmann JP. Theory-based health behavior change: developing, testing and applying theories for evidence-based interventions. Appl Psychol Int Rev. 2008;57:698–716. Theory-Based Health Behavior Change: Developing, Testing, and Applying Theories for Evidence-Based Interventions - Lippke - 2008 - Applied Psychology - Wiley Online Library
77. Schwarzer R. Modeling health behavior change: how to predict and modify the adoption and maintenance of health behaviors. Appl Psychol Int Rev. 2008;57:1–29. https://doi.org/10.1111/j.1464-0597.2007.00325. Modeling Health Behavior Change: How to Predict and Modify the Adoption and Maintenance of Health Behaviors - Schwarzer - 2008 - Applied Psychology - Wiley Online Library
78. Litt MD, Kleppinger A, Judge JO. Initiation and maintenance of exercise behavior in older women: predictors from the social learning model. J Behav Med. 2002;25(1):83–97. PMID: 11845560. http://www.ncbi.nlm.nih.gov/pubmed/11845560.
79. Sniehotta FF. Towards a theory of intentional behaviour change: plans, planning, and self-regulation. Br J Health Psychol. 2009;14(Pt 2):261–73. PMID: 19102817. http://www.ncbi.nlm.nih.gov/pubmed/19102817.
80. Conner M, Norman P, editors. Predicting health behavior: research and practice with social cognition models. 2nd ed. Buckingham, UK: Open University Press; 2005.
81. Sutton S. Stage models of health behaviour. In: Conner M, Norman P, editors. Predicting health behaviour: research and practice with social cognition models. 2nd ed. Maidenhead, UK: Open University Press; 2005. p. 223–75.
82. Gollwitzer PM, Sheeran P. Implementation intentions and goal achievement: a meta-analysis of effects and processes. Adv Exp Soc Psychol. 2006;38:69–119. Implementation intentions and goal achievement: A meta-analysis of effects and processes.
83. Sniehotta FF, Scholz U, Schwarzer R. Action plans and coping plans for physical exercise: a longitudinal intervention study in cardiac rehabilitation. Br J Health Psychol. 2006;11(Pt 1):23–37. PMID: 16480553. http://www.ncbi.nlm.nih.gov/pubmed/16480553.
84. Lippke S, Ziegelmann JP, Schwarzer R, Velicer WF. Validity of stage assessment in the adoption and maintenance of physical activity and fruit and vegetable consumption. Health Psychol. 2009;28(2):183–93. PMCID: PMC2939463. http://www.ncbi.nlm.nih.gov/pubmed/19290710.
85. Sniehotta FF, Schwarzer R, Scholz U, Schüz B. Action planning and coping planning for long-term lifestyle change: theory and assessment. Eur J Soc Psychol. 2005;35:565–76. Action Planning and Coping Planning for Long-Term Lifestyle Change: Theory and Assessment.
86. Luszczynska A, Mazurkiewicz M, Ziegelmann JP, Schwarzer R. Recovery self-efficacy and intention as predictors of running or jogging behavior: A cross-lagged panel analysis over a two-year period. Psychol Sport Exerc. 2007;8:247–60. Recovery self-efficacy and intention as predictors of running or jogging behavior: A cross-lagged panel analysis over a two-year period.
87. Schüz B, Sniehotta FF, Schwarzer R. Stage-specific effects of an action control intervention on dental flossing. Health Educ Res. 2007;22(3):332–41. PMID: 16945985. http://www.ncbi.nlm.nih.gov/pubmed/16945985.
88. Luszczynska A, Tryburcy M, Schwarzer R. Improving fruit and vegetable consumption: a self-efficacy intervention compared with a combined self-efficacy and planning intervention. Health Educ Res. 2007;22(5):630–8. PMID: 17060349. http://www.ncbi.nlm.nih.gov/pubmed/17060349.
89. Schwarzer R, Cao DS, Lippke S. Stage-matched minimal interventions to enhance physical activity in Chinese adolescents. J

Adolesc Health. 2010;47(6):533–9. PMID: 21094429. http://www.ncbi.nlm.nih.gov/pubmed/21094429.
90. Wiedemann AU, Schüz B, Sniehotta F, Scholz U, Schwarzer R. Disentangling the relation between intentions, planning, and behaviour: a moderated mediation analysis. Psychol Health. 2009;24(1):67–79. PMID: 20186640. http://www.ncbi.nlm.nih.gov/pubmed/20186640.
91. Lippke S, Schwarzer R, Ziegelmann JP, Scholz U, Schüz B. Testing stage-specific effects of a stage-matched intervention: a randomized controlled trial targeting physical exercise and its predictors. Health Educ Behav. 2010;37(4):533–46. PMID: 20547760. http://www.ncbi.nlm.nih.gov/pubmed/20547760.
92. Schüz B, Sniehotta FF, Mallach N, Wiedemann AU, Schwarzer R. Predicting transitions from preintentional, intentional and actional stages of change. Health Educ Res. 2009;24(1):64–75. PMID: 18245046. http://www.ncbi.nlm.nih.gov/pubmed/18245046.
93. Halstead WC. Brain and intelligence: a quantitative study of the frontal lobes. Chicago; 1947.
94. Boring EG. A history of experimental psychology. New York: D. Appleton-Century Co; 1929.
95. Anderson J. Mind as feeling. Aust J Psychol Philos. 1934;12:81–94.
96. Warren HC. In defense of some discarded concepts. Psychol Rev. 1931;38:392–405.
97. Burt C. The concept of mind. J Psychol Res. 1960;4:54–64.
98. Wild EH. Influences of conation on cognition. Br J Psychol. 1927;18:147–67.
99. Wild EH. Influence of conation on cognition. II. Br J Psychol. 1928;18:332–55.
100. Richardson CA. The measurement of conative factors in children and their influence. Br J Psychol. 1929;19:405–12.
101. Low MD, Borda RP, Kellaway P. "Contingent negative variation" in rhesus monkeys. An EEG sign of a specific mental process. Percept Mot Skills. 1966;22:443–6.
102. Sbordone RJ, Long CJ. Ecological validity of neuropsychological testing. Delray Beach: G. R. Press/St. Lucie Press; 1996.
103. Halstead WC. A power factor (P) in general intelligence: the effect of brain injuries. J Psychol. 1945;20:57–64.
104. Baumeister RF, Muraven M, Tice DM. Ego depletion: a resource model of volition, self-regulation, and controlled processing. Soc Cogn. 2000;18:130–50. https://doi.org/10.1521/soco.2000.18.2.130. Ego depletion: A resource model of volition, self-regulation, and controlled processing.
105. Schmeichel BJ, Baumeister RF. Effortful attention control. In: Bruya B, editor. Effortless attention: a new perspective in the cognitive science of attention and action. Cambridge, MA: MIT Press; 2010. p. 29–49.
106. Anagaw TF, Tiruneh MG, Fenta ET. Application of behavioral change theory and models on COVID-19 preventive behaviors, worldwide: a systematic review. SAGE Open Med. 2023;11:20503121231159750. PMCID: PMC10067469. http://www.ncbi.nlm.nih.gov/pubmed/37026109.
107. Dick DM. Gene-environment interaction in psychological traits and disorders. Annu Rev Clin Psychol. 2011;7:383–409. PMCID: PMC3647367. http://www.ncbi.nlm.nih.gov/pubmed/21219196.
108. Prasad SS, Kojic LZ, Li P, Mitchell DE, Hachisuka A, Sawada J, Gu Q, Cynader MS. Gene expression patterns during enhanced periods of visual cortex plasticity. Neuroscience. 2002;111(1):35–45. PMID: 11955710. http://www.ncbi.nlm.nih.gov/pubmed/11955710.
109. Puckett RE, Lubin FD. Epigenetic mechanisms in experience-driven memory formation and behavior. Epigenomics. 2011;3(5):649–64. PMCID: PMC3235677. http://www.ncbi.nlm.nih.gov/pubmed/22126252.
110. Sultan FA, Day JJ. Epigenetic mechanisms in memory and synaptic function. Epigenomics. 2011;3(2):157–81. PMCID: PMC3350307. http://www.ncbi.nlm.nih.gov/pubmed/22122279.
111. Day JJ, Sweatt JD. Epigenetic mechanisms in cognition. Neuron. 2011;70(5):813–29. PMCID: PMC3118503. http://www.ncbi.nlm.nih.gov/pubmed/21658577.
112. Adachi M, Monteggia LM. Decoding transcriptional repressor complexes in the adult central nervous system. Neuropharmacology. 2014;80:45–52. PMCID: PMC3984594. http://www.ncbi.nlm.nih.gov/pubmed/24418103.
113. Fullard JF, Halene TB, Giambartolomei C, Haroutunian V, Akbarian S, Roussos P. Understanding the genetic liability to schizophrenia through the neuroepigenome. Schizophr Res. 2016;177(1–3):115–24. PMCID: PMC4963306. http://www.ncbi.nlm.nih.gov/pubmed/26827128.
114. Guidotti A, Grayson DR. DNA methylation and demethylation as targets for antipsychotic therapy. Dialogues Clin Neurosci. 2014;16(3):419–29. PMCID: PMC4214182. http://www.ncbi.nlm.nih.gov/pubmed/25364290.
115. Bagot RC, Labonté B, Peña CJ, Nestler EJ. Epigenetic signaling in psychiatric disorders: stress and depression. Dialogues Clin Neurosci. 2014;16(3):281–95. PMCID: PMC4214172. http://www.ncbi.nlm.nih.gov/pubmed/25364280.
116. Peña CJ, Bagot RC, Labonté B, Nestler EJ. Epigenetic signaling in psychiatric disorders. J Mol Biol. 2014;426(20):3389–412. PMCID: PMC4177298. http://www.ncbi.nlm.nih.gov/pubmed/24709417.
117. Nestler EJ, Peña CJ, Kundakovic M, Mitchell A, Akbarian S. Epigenetic basis of mental illness. Neuroscientist. 2016;22(5):447–63. PMCID: PMC4826318. http://www.ncbi.nlm.nih.gov/pubmed/26450593.
118. Alshaya DS. Genetic and epigenetic factors associated with depression: an updated overview. Saudi. J Biol Sci. 2022;29(8):103311. PMCID: PMC9232544. http://www.ncbi.nlm.nih.gov/pubmed/35762011.
119. Penner-Goeke S, Binder EB. Epigenetics and depression. Dialogues Clin Neurosci. 2019;21(4):397–405. PMCID: PMC6952745. http://www.ncbi.nlm.nih.gov/pubmed/31949407.
120. Park C, Rosenblat JD, Brietzke E, Pan Z, Lee Y, Cao B, Zuckerman H, Kalantarova A, McIntyre RS. Stress, epigenetics and depression: a systematic review. Neurosci Biobehav Rev. 2019;102:139–52. PMID: 31005627. http://www.ncbi.nlm.nih.gov/pubmed/31005627.
121. Chmielewska N, Szyndler J, Maciejak P, Płaźnik A. Epigenetic mechanisms of stress and depression. Psychiatr Pol. 2019;53(6):1413–28. PMID: 32017826. http://www.ncbi.nlm.nih.gov/pubmed/32017826.
122. Talarowska M. Epigenetic mechanisms in the neurodevelopmental theory of depression. Depress Res Treat. 2020;2020:6357873. PMCID: PMC7196148. http://www.ncbi.nlm.nih.gov/pubmed/32373361.
123. Ochi S, Dwivedi Y. Dissecting early life stress-induced adolescent depression through epigenomic approach. Mol Psychiatry. 2023;28(1):141–53. PMCID: PMC9812796. http://www.ncbi.nlm.nih.gov/pubmed/36517640.
124. Zhang X, Qiao Y, Wang M, Liang X, Zhang M, Li C, Cairang J, Wang J, Bi H, Gao T. The influence of genetic and acquired factors on the vulnerability to develop depression: a review. Biosci Rep. 2023;43(5):BSR20222644. PMCID: PMC10214102. http://www.ncbi.nlm.nih.gov/pubmed/37140907.
125. Morange M. How to localize epigenetics in the landscape of biological research? Med Sci (Paris). 2005;21(4):367–9. PMID: 15811300. http://www.ncbi.nlm.nih.gov/pubmed/15811300.
126. Suzuki T, Miyata N. Epigenetic control using natural products and synthetic molecules. Curr Med Chem. 2006;13(8):935–58. PMID: 16611076. http://www.ncbi.nlm.nih.gov/pubmed/16611076.
127. Kleivi K. Advances in the genetics and epigenetics of gene regulation and human disease. Genome Biol. 2006;7(8):325. PMCID: PMC1779594. http://www.ncbi.nlm.nih.gov/pubmed/16934107.

128. Martin DIK, Ward R, Suter CM. Germline epimutation: a basis for epigenetic disease in humans. Ann N Y Acad Sci. 2005;1054:68–77. PMID: 16339653. http://www.ncbi.nlm.nih.gov/pubmed/16339653.
129. Szyf M, McGowan P, Meaney MJ. The social environment and the epigenome. Environ Mol Mutagen. 2008;49(1):46–60. PMID: 18095330. http://www.ncbi.nlm.nih.gov/pubmed/18095330.
130. Crews D. Epigenetics, brain, behavior, and the environment. Hormones (Athens). 2010;9(1):41–50. PMID: 20363720. http://www.ncbi.nlm.nih.gov/pubmed/20363720.
131. Bae JB. Perspectives of international human epigenome consortium. Genomics Inform. 2013;11(1):7–14. PMCID: PMC3630389. http://www.ncbi.nlm.nih.gov/pubmed/23613677.
132. Stunnenberg HG, International Human Epigenome Consortium, Hirst M. The International Human Epigenome Consortium: a blueprint for scientific collaboration and discovery. Cell. 2016;167(5):1145–9. PMID: 27863232. http://www.ncbi.nlm.nih.gov/pubmed/27863232.
133. Welcome to IHEC · IHEC
134. United States of America · IHEC
135. Berger SL, Kouzarides T, Shiekhattar R, Shilatifard A. An operational definition of epigenetics. Genes Dev. 2009;23(7):781–3. PMCID: PMC3959995. http://www.ncbi.nlm.nih.gov/pubmed/19339683.
136. Ptashne M. On the use of the word "epigenetic". Curr Biol. 2007;17(7):R233–6. PMID: 17407749. http://www.ncbi.nlm.nih.gov/pubmed/17407749.
137. Lu Q, Qiu X, Hu N, Wen H, Su Y, Richardson BC. Epigenetics, disease, and therapeutic interventions. Ageing Res Rev. 2006;5(4):449–67. PMID: 16965942. http://www.ncbi.nlm.nih.gov/pubmed/16965942.
138. Kim VN. Small RNAs: classification, biogenesis, and function. Mol Cells. 2005;19(1):1–15. PMID: 15750334. http://www.ncbi.nlm.nih.gov/pubmed/15750334.
139. Mitchell AC, Bharadwaj R, Whittle C, Krueger W, Mirnics K, Hurd Y, Rasmussen T, Akbarian S. The genome in three dimensions: a new frontier in human brain research. Biol Psychiatry. 2014;75(12):961–9. PMCID: PMC3925763. http://www.ncbi.nlm.nih.gov/pubmed/23958183.
140. Klengel T, Binder EB. Epigenetics of stress-related psychiatric disorders and gene × environment interactions. Neuron. 2015;86(6):1343–57. PMID: 26087162. http://www.ncbi.nlm.nih.gov/pubmed/26087162.
141. Han LKM, Aghajani M, Clark SL, Chan RF, Hattab MW, Shabalin AA, Zhao M, Kumar G, Xie LY, Jansen R, Milaneschi Y, Dean B, Aberg KA, van den Oord EJCG, Penninx BWJH. Epigenetic aging in major depressive disorder. Am J Psychiatry. 2018;175(8):774–82. PMCID: PMC6094380. http://www.ncbi.nlm.nih.gov/pubmed/29656664.
142. Sun H, Damez-Werno DM, Scobie KN, Shao NY, Dias C, Rabkin J, Koo JW, Korb E, Bagot RC, Ahn FH, Cahill ME, Labonté B, Mouzon E, Heller EA, Cates H, Golden SA, Gleason K, Russo SJ, Andrews S, Neve R, Kennedy PJ, Maze I, Dietz DM, Allis CD, Turecki G, Varga-Weisz P, Tamminga C, Shen L, Nestler EJ. ACF chromatin-remodeling complex mediates stress-induced depressive-like behavior. Nat Med. 2015;21(10):1146–53. PMCID: PMC4598281. http://www.ncbi.nlm.nih.gov/pubmed/26390241.
143. Vogel-Ciernia A, Wood MA. Neuron-specific chromatin remodeling: a missing link in epigenetic mechanisms underlying synaptic plasticity, memory, and intellectual disability disorders. Neuropharmacology. 2014;80:18–27. PMCID: PMC3984593. http://www.ncbi.nlm.nih.gov/pubmed/24140580.
144. Lahiri DK, Maloney B. Gene × environment interaction by a longitudinal epigenome-wide association study (LEWAS) overcomes limitations of genome-wide association study (GWAS). Epigenomics. 2012;4(6):685–99. PMCID: PMC4195244. http://www.ncbi.nlm.nih.gov/pubmed/23244313.
145. Chmurzynska A. Fetal programming: link between early nutrition, DNA methylation, and complex diseases. Nutr Rev. 2010;68(2):87–98. PMID: 20137054. http://www.ncbi.nlm.nih.gov/pubmed/20137054.
146. Meagher RB, Müssar KJ. The influence of DNA sequence on epigenome-induced pathologies. Epigenetics Chromatin. 2012;5(1):11. PMCID: PMC3439399. http://www.ncbi.nlm.nih.gov/pubmed/22818522.
147. Nanney DL. Epigenetic control systems. Proc Natl Acad Sci USA. 1958;44(7):712–7. PMCID: PMC528649. http://www.ncbi.nlm.nih.gov/pubmed/16590265.
148. Jenuwein T, Allis CD. Translating the histone code. Science. 2001;293(5532):1074–80. PMID: 11498575. http://www.ncbi.nlm.nih.gov/pubmed/11498575.
149. An operational definition of epigenetics.
150. Koyama M, Kurumizaka H. Structural diversity of the nucleosome. J Biochem. 2018;163(2):85–95. PMID: 29161414. http://www.ncbi.nlm.nih.gov/pubmed/29161414.
151. Zhou BR, Bai Y. Chromatin structures condensed by linker histones. Essays Biochem. 2019;63(1):75–87. PMID: 31015384. http://www.ncbi.nlm.nih.gov/pubmed/31015384.
152. Millán-Zambrano G, Burton A, Bannister AJ, Schneider R. Histone post-translational modifications - cause and consequence of genome function. Nat Rev Genet. 2022;23(9):563–80. PMID: 35338361. http://www.ncbi.nlm.nih.gov/pubmed/35338361.
153. Bharath MMS, Chandra NR, Rao MRS. Molecular modeling of the chromatosome particle. Nucleic Acids Res. 2003;31(14):4264–74. PMCID: PMC167642. http://www.ncbi.nlm.nih.gov/pubmed/12853645.
154. Yang J, Yin Y. PTEN in chromatin remodeling. Cold Spring Harb Perspect Med. 2020;10(2):a036160. PMCID: PMC6996446. http://www.ncbi.nlm.nih.gov/pubmed/31570373.
155. Workman JL, Kingston RE. Alteration of nucleosome structure as a mechanism of transcriptional regulation. Annu Rev Biochem. 1998;67:545–79. PMID: 9759497. http://www.ncbi.nlm.nih.gov/pubmed/9759497.
156. Chioda M, Becker PB. Soft skills turned into hard facts: nucleosome remodelling at developmental switches. Heredity (Edinb). 2010;105(1):71–9. PMID: 20372184. http://www.ncbi.nlm.nih.gov/pubmed/20372184.
157. Ho L, Crabtree GR. Chromatin remodelling during development. Nature. 2010;463(7280):474–84. PMCID: PMC3060774. http://www.ncbi.nlm.nih.gov/pubmed/20110991.
158. Becker PB, Hörz W. ATP-dependent nucleosome remodeling. Annu Rev Biochem. 2002;71:247–73. PMID: 12045097. http://www.ncbi.nlm.nih.gov/pubmed/12045097.
159. Clapier CR, Cairns BR. The biology of chromatin remodeling complexes. Annu Rev Biochem. 2009;78:273–304. PMID: 19355820. http://www.ncbi.nlm.nih.gov/pubmed/19355820.
160. Hargreaves DC, Crabtree GR. ATP-dependent chromatin remodeling: genetics, genomics and mechanisms. Cell Res. 2011;21(3):396–420. PMCID: PMC3110148. http://www.ncbi.nlm.nih.gov/pubmed/21358755.
161. Bird AP, Wolffe AP. Methylation-induced repression--belts, braces, and chromatin. Cell. 1999;99(5):451–4. PMID: 10589672. http://www.ncbi.nlm.nih.gov/pubmed/10589672.
162. Lister R, Mukamel EA, Nery JR, Urich M, Puddifoot CA, Johnson ND, Lucero J, Huang Y, Dwork AJ, Schultz MD, Yu M, Tonti-Filippini J, Heyn H, Hu S, Wu JC, Rao A, Esteller M, He C, Haghighi FG, Sejnowski TJ, Behrens MM, Ecker JR. Global epigenomic reconfiguration during mammalian brain development. Science. 2013;341(6146):1237905. PMCID: PMC3785061. http://www.ncbi.nlm.nih.gov/pubmed/23828890.

163. Razin A. CpG methylation, chromatin structure and gene silencing-a three-way connection. EMBO J. 1998;17(17):4905–8. PMCID: PMC1170819. http://www.ncbi.nlm.nih.gov/pubmed/9724627.
164. Fuks F. DNA methylation and histone modifications: teaming up to silence genes. Curr Opin Genet Dev. 2005;15(5):490–5. PMID: 16098738. http://www.ncbi.nlm.nih.gov/pubmed/16098738.
165. Wu X, Li G, Xie R. Decoding the role of TET family dioxygenases in lineage specification. Epigenetics Chromatin. 2018;11(1):58. PMCID: PMC6172806. http://www.ncbi.nlm.nih.gov/pubmed/30290828.
166. Li D, Guo B, Wu H, Tan L, Lu Q. TET family of dioxygenases: crucial roles and underlying mechanisms. Cytogenet Genome Res. 2015;146(3):171–80. PMID: 26302812. http://www.ncbi.nlm.nih.gov/pubmed/26302812.
167. Guo JU, Ma DK, Mo H, Ball MP, Jang MH, Bonaguidi MA, Balazer JA, Eaves HL, Xie B, Ford E, Zhang K, Ming G, Li, Gao Y, Song H. Neuronal activity modifies the DNA methylation landscape in the adult brain. Nat Neurosci. 2011;14(10):1345–51. PMCID: PMC3183401. http://www.ncbi.nlm.nih.gov/pubmed/21874013.
168. Szulwach KE, Li X, Li Y, Song CX, Wu H, Dai Q, Irier H, Upadhyay AK, Gearing M, Levey AI, Vasanthakumar A, Godley LA, Chang Q, Cheng X, He C, Jin P. 5-hmC-mediated epigenetic dynamics during postnatal neurodevelopment and aging. Nat Neurosci. 2011;14(12):1607–16. PMCID: PMC3292193. http://www.ncbi.nlm.nih.gov/pubmed/22037496.
169. Wu H, D'Alessio AC, Ito S, Wang Z, Cui K, Zhao K, Sun YE, Zhang Y. Genome-wide analysis of 5-hydroxymethylcytosine distribution reveals its dual function in transcriptional regulation in mouse embryonic stem cells. Genes Dev. 2011;25(7):679–84. PMCID: PMC3070931. http://www.ncbi.nlm.nih.gov/pubmed/21460036.
170. Riccio A. Dynamic epigenetic regulation in neurons: enzymes, stimuli and signaling pathways. Nat Neurosci. 2010;13(11):1330–7. PMID: 20975757. http://www.ncbi.nlm.nih.gov/pubmed/20975757.
171. Chen WG, Chang Q, Lin Y, Meissner A, West AE, Griffith EC, Jaenisch R, Greenberg ME. Derepression of BDNF transcription involves calcium-dependent phosphorylation of MeCP2. Science. 2003;302(5646):885–9. https://doi.org/10.1126/science.1086446. PMID: 14593183. http://www.ncbi.nlm.nih.gov/pubmed/14593183
172. Ma DK, Jang MH, Guo JU, Kitabatake Y, Chang ML, Pow-Anpongkul N, Flavell RA, Lu B, Ming GL, Song H. Neuronal activity-induced Gadd45b promotes epigenetic DNA demethylation and adult neurogenesis. Science. 2009;323(5917):1074–7. https://doi.org/10.1126/science.1166859. Epub 2009 Jan 1. PMID: 19119186; PMCID: PMC2726986. http://www.ncbi.nlm.nih.gov/pubmed/19119186
173. Day JJ, Sweatt JD. DNA methylation and memory formation. Nat Neurosci. 2010;13(11):1319–23. PMCID: PMC3130618. http://www.ncbi.nlm.nih.gov/pubmed/20975755.
174. Miller CA, Sweatt JD. Covalent modification of DNA regulates memory formation. Neuron. 2007;53(6):857–69. PMID: 17359920. http://www.ncbi.nlm.nih.gov/pubmed/17359920.
175. Lyko F. The DNA methyltransferase family: a versatile toolkit for epigenetic regulation. Nat Rev Genet. 2018;19(2):81–92. PMID: 29033456. http://www.ncbi.nlm.nih.gov/pubmed/29033456.
176. Khorasanizadeh S. The nucleosome: from genomic organization to genomic regulation. Cell. 2004;116(2):259–72. PMID: 14744436. http://www.ncbi.nlm.nih.gov/pubmed/14744436.
177. Ha M, Ng DWK, Li WH, Chen ZJ. Coordinated histone modifications are associated with gene expression variation within and between species. Genome Res. 2011;21(4):590–8. PMCID: PMC3065706. http://www.ncbi.nlm.nih.gov/pubmed/21324879.
178. Sun H, Kennedy PJ, Nestler EJ. Epigenetics of the depressed brain: role of histone acetylation and methylation. Neuropsychopharmacology. 2013;38(1):124–37. PMCID: PMC3521990. http://www.ncbi.nlm.nih.gov/pubmed/22692567.
179. Katan-Khaykovich Y, Struhl K. Dynamics of global histone acetylation and deacetylation in vivo: rapid restoration of normal histone acetylation status upon removal of activators and repressors. Genes Dev. 2002;16(6):743–52. PMCID: PMC155357. http://www.ncbi.nlm.nih.gov/pubmed/11914279.
180. Radman-Livaja M, Liu CL, Friedman N, Schreiber SL, Rando OJ. Replication and active demethylation represent partially overlapping mechanisms for erasure of H3K4me3 in budding yeast. PLoS Genet. 2010;6(2):e1000837. PMCID: PMC2816684. http://www.ncbi.nlm.nih.gov/pubmed/20140185.
181. Masliah-Planchon J, Bièche I, Guinebretière JM, Bourdeaut F, Delattre O. SWI/SNF chromatin remodeling and human malignancies. Annu Rev Pathol. 2015;10:145–171. PMID: 25387058. http://www.ncbi.nlm.nih.gov/pubmed/25387058.
182. Goodwin LR, Picketts DJ. The role of ISWI chromatin remodeling complexes in brain development and neurodevelopmental disorders. Mol Cell Neurosci. 2018;87:55–64. PMID: 29249292. http://www.ncbi.nlm.nih.gov/pubmed/29249292.
183. Wigley DB, Bowman GD. A glimpse into chromatin remodeling. Nat Struct Mol Biol. 2017;24(6):498–500. PMID: 28586327. http://www.ncbi.nlm.nih.gov/pubmed/28586327.
184. Waly MI, Hornig M, Trivedi M, Hodgson N, Kini R, Ohta A, Deth R. Prenatal and postnatal epigenetic programming: implications for GI, immune, and neuronal function in autism. Autism Res Treat. 2012;2012:190930. PMCID: PMC3420412. http://www.ncbi.nlm.nih.gov/pubmed/22934169.
185. Mazzio EA, Soliman KFA. Epigenetics and nutritional environmental signals. Integr Comp Biol. 2014;54(1):21–30. PMCID: PMC4072902. http://www.ncbi.nlm.nih.gov/pubmed/24861811.
186. Keating ST, El-Osta A. Epigenetics and metabolism. Circ Res. 2015;116(4):715–36. PMID: 25677519. http://www.ncbi.nlm.nih.gov/pubmed/25677519.
187. Lo YMD, Chan KCA, Sun H, Chen EZ, Jiang P, Lun FMF, Zheng YW, Leung TY, Lau TK, Cantor CR, Chiu RWK. Maternal plasma DNA sequencing reveals the genome-wide genetic and mutational profile of the fetus. Sci Transl Med. 2010;2(61):61ra91. PMID: 21148127. http://www.ncbi.nlm.nih.gov/pubmed/21148127.
188. Castillo J, Amaral A, Oliva R. Sperm nuclear proteome and its epigenetic potential. Andrology. 2014;2(3):326–38. PMID: 24327354. http://www.ncbi.nlm.nih.gov/pubmed/24327354.
189. Castillo J, Estanyol JM, Ballescá JL, Oliva R. Human sperm chromatin epigenetic potential: genomics, proteomics, and male infertility. Asian J Androl. 2015;17(4):601–9. PMCID: PMC4492051. http://www.ncbi.nlm.nih.gov/pubmed/25926607.
190. Castillo J, Amaral A, Azpiazu R, Vavouri T, Estanyol JM, Ballescà JL, Oliva R. Genomic and proteomic dissection and characterization of the human sperm chromatin. Mol Hum Reprod. 2014;20(11):1041–53. PMID: 25193639. http://www.ncbi.nlm.nih.gov/pubmed/25193639.
191. Kim YK, Ham BJ, Han KM. Interactive effects of genetic polymorphisms and childhood adversity on brain morphologic changes in depression. Prog Neuro-Psychopharmacol Biol Psychiatry. 2019;91:4–13. PMID: 29535036. http://www.ncbi.nlm.nih.gov/pubmed/29535036.
192. Booij L, Szyf M, Carballedo A, Frey EM, Morris D, Dymov S, Vaisheva F, Ly V, Fahey C, Meaney J, Gill M, Frodl T. DNA methylation of the serotonin transporter gene in peripheral cells and stress-related changes in hippocampal volume: a study in depressed patients and healthy controls. PLoS One. 2015;10(3):e0119061. PMCID: PMC4363605. http://www.ncbi.nlm.nih.gov/pubmed/25781010.

193. Cassiers LLM, Sabbe BGC, Schmaal L, Veltman DJ, Penninx BWJH, Van Den Eede F. Structural and functional brain abnormalities associated with exposure to different childhood trauma subtypes: a systematic review of neuroimaging findings. Front Psych. 2018;9:329. PMCID: PMC6086138. http://www.ncbi.nlm.nih.gov/pubmed/30123142.
194. Dalton VS, Kolshus E, McLoughlin DM. Epigenetics and depression: return of the repressed. J Affect Disord. 2014;155:1–12. PMID: 24238955. http://www.ncbi.nlm.nih.gov/pubmed/24238955.
195. Menke A, Binder EB. Epigenetic alterations in depression and antidepressant treatment. Dialogues Clin Neurosci. 2014;16(3):395–404. PMCID: PMC4214180. http://www.ncbi.nlm.nih.gov/pubmed/25364288.
196. Lewis CR, Olive MF. Early-life stress interactions with the epigenome: potential mechanisms driving vulnerability toward psychiatric illness. Behav Pharmacol. 2014;25(5–6):341–51. PMCID: PMC4119485. http://www.ncbi.nlm.nih.gov/pubmed/25003947.
197. Lo CL, Zhou FC. Environmental alterations of epigenetics prior to the birth. Int Rev Neurobiol. 2014;115:1–49. PMCID: PMC4158947. http://www.ncbi.nlm.nih.gov/pubmed/25131541.
198. Hanson PI, Whiteheart SW. AAA+ proteins: have engine, will work. Nat Rev Mol Cell Biol. 2005;6(7):519–29. PMID: 16072036. http://www.ncbi.nlm.nih.gov/pubmed/16072036.
199. Lismer A, Kimmins S. Emerging evidence that the mammalian sperm epigenome serves as a template for embryo development. Nat Commun. 2023;14(1):2142. PMCID: PMC10104880. http://www.ncbi.nlm.nih.gov/pubmed/37059740.
200. Abdolmaleky HM, Thiagalingam S, Wilcox M. Genetics and epigenetics in major psychiatric disorders: dilemmas, achievements, applications, and future scope. Am J Pharmacogenomics. 2005;5(3):149–60. PMID: 15952869. http://www.ncbi.nlm.nih.gov/pubmed/15952869.
201. Quina AS, Buschbeck M, Di Croce L. Chromatin structure and epigenetics. Biochem Pharmacol. 2006;72(11):1563–9. PMID: 16836980. http://www.ncbi.nlm.nih.gov/pubmed/16836980.
202. Vanden Berghe W, Ndlovu MN, Hoya-Arias R, Dijsselbloem N, Gerlo S, Haegeman G. Keeping up NF-kappaB appearances: epigenetic control of immunity or inflammation-triggered epigenetics. Biochem Pharmacol. 2006;72(9):1114–31. PMID: 16934762. http://www.ncbi.nlm.nih.gov/pubmed/16934762.
203. Pearce EL, Shen H. Making sense of inflammation, epigenetics, and memory CD8+ T-cell differentiation in the context of infection. Immunol Rev. 2006;211:197–202. PMID: 16824128. http://www.ncbi.nlm.nih.gov/pubmed/16824128.
204. Lee GR, Kim ST, Spilianakis CG, Fields PE, Flavell RA. T helper cell differentiation: regulation by cis elements and epigenetics. Immunity. 2006;24(4):369–79. PMID: 16618596. http://www.ncbi.nlm.nih.gov/pubmed/16618596.
205. Isgor C, Kabbaj M, Akil H, Watson SJ. Delayed effects of chronic variable stress during peripubertal-juvenile period on hippocampal morphology and on cognitive and stress axis functions in rats. Hippocampus. 2004;14(5):636–48. PMID: 15301440. http://www.ncbi.nlm.nih.gov/pubmed/15301440.
206. Kabbaj M. Neurobiological bases of individual differences in emotional and stress responsiveness: high responders-low responders model. Arch Neurol. 2004;61(7):1009–12. PMID: 15262729. http://www.ncbi.nlm.nih.gov/pubmed/15262729.
207. Holsboer F, Lauer CJ, Schreiber W, Krieg JC. Altered hypothalamic-pituitary-adrenocortical regulation in healthy subjects at high familial risk for affective disorders. Neuroendocrinology. 1995;62(4):340–7. PMID: 8544947. http://www.ncbi.nlm.nih.gov/pubmed/8544947.
208. Anisman H, Zacharko RM. Depression as a consequence of inadequate neurochemical adaptation in response to stressors. Br J Psychiatry Suppl. 1992;(15):36–43. PMID: 1356356. http://www.ncbi.nlm.nih.gov/pubmed/1356356.
209. Zuckerman M, Neeb M. Sensation seeking and psychopathology. Psychiatry Res. 1979;1(3):255–64. PMID: 298353. http://www.ncbi.nlm.nih.gov/pubmed/298353.
210. Zuckerman M. The psychophysiology of sensation seeking. J Pers. 1990;58(1):313–45. PMID: 2198341. http://www.ncbi.nlm.nih.gov/pubmed/2198341.
211. Kabbaj M, Akil H. Individual differences in novelty-seeking behavior in rats: a c-fos study. Neuroscience. 2001;106(3):535–45. PMID: 11591454. http://www.ncbi.nlm.nih.gov/pubmed/11591454.
212. Emmert MH, Herman JP. Differential forebrain c-fos mRNA induction by ether inhalation and novelty: evidence for distinctive stress pathways. Brain Res. 1999;845(1):60–7. PMID: 10529444. http://www.ncbi.nlm.nih.gov/pubmed/10529444.
213. Whitney AR, Diehn M, Popper SJ, Alizadeh AA, Boldrick JC, Relman DA, Brown PO. Individuality and variation in gene expression patterns in human blood. Proc Natl Acad Sci USA. 2003;100(4):1896–901. PMCID: PMC149930. http://www.ncbi.nlm.nih.gov/pubmed/12578971.
214. McEwen BS, Seeman T. Protective and damaging effects of mediators of stress. Elaborating and testing the concepts of allostasis and allostatic load. Ann N Y Acad Sci. 1999;896:30–47. PMID: 10681886. http://www.ncbi.nlm.nih.gov/pubmed/10681886.
215. Goodman E, McEwen BS, Dolan LM, Schafer-Kalkhoff T, Adler NE. Social disadvantage and adolescent stress. J Adolesc Health. 2005;37(6):484–92. PMID: 16310126. http://www.ncbi.nlm.nih.gov/pubmed/16310126.
216. Steptoe A, Wardle J. Positive affect and biological function in everyday life. Neurobiol Aging. 2005;26(Suppl 1):108–12. PMID: 16213629. http://www.ncbi.nlm.nih.gov/pubmed/16213629.
217. Steptoe A, Willemsen G. The influence of low job control on ambulatory blood pressure and perceived stress over the working day in men and women from the Whitehall II cohort. J Hypertens. 2004;22(5):915–20. PMID: 15097230. http://www.ncbi.nlm.nih.gov/pubmed/15097230.
218. Steptoe A, Willemsen G, Kunz-Ebrecht SR, Owen N. Socioeconomic status and hemodynamic recovery from mental stress. Psychophysiology. 2003;40(2):184–91. PMID: 12820859. http://www.ncbi.nlm.nih.gov/pubmed/12820859.
219. Steptoe A, Kunz-Ebrecht S, Owen N, Feldman PJ, Willemsen G, Kirschbaum C, Marmot M. Socioeconomic status and stress-related biological responses over the working day. Psychosom Med. 2003;65(3):461–70. PMID: 12764220. http://www.ncbi.nlm.nih.gov/pubmed/12764220.
220. Steptoe A, Willemsen G, Owen N, Flower L, Mohamed-Ali V. Acute mental stress elicits delayed increases in circulating inflammatory cytokine levels. Clin Sci (Lond). 2001;101(2):185–92. PMID: 11473494. http://www.ncbi.nlm.nih.gov/pubmed/11473494.
221. Leichsenring F, Leibing E, Kruse J, New AS, Leweke F. Borderline personality disorder. Lancet. 2011;377(9759):74–84. PMID: 21195251. http://www.ncbi.nlm.nih.gov/pubmed/21195251.
222. Archer T, Oscar-Berman M, Blum K, Gold M. Epigenetic modulation of mood disorders. J Genet Syndr Gene Ther. 2013;4(120):1000120. PMCID: PMC3615441. http://www.ncbi.nlm.nih.gov/pubmed/23565345.
223. Dudley KJ, Li X, Kobor MS, Kippin TE, Bredy TW. Epigenetic mechanisms mediating vulnerability and resilience to psychiatric disorders. Neurosci Biobehav Rev. 2011;35(7):1544–51. PMID: 21251925. http://www.ncbi.nlm.nih.gov/pubmed/21251925.
224. Hochberg Z, Feil R, Constancia M, Fraga M, Junien C, Carel JC, Boileau P, Le Bouc Y, Deal CL, Lillycrop K, Scharfmann R, Sheppard A, Skinner M, Szyf M, Waterland RA, Waxman DJ, Whitelaw E, Ong K, Albertsson-Wikland K. Child health, devel-

opmental plasticity, and epigenetic programming. Endocr Rev. 2011;32(2):159–224. PMCID: PMC3365792. http://www.ncbi.nlm.nih.gov/pubmed/20971919.
225. Uher R. Genes, environment, and individual differences in responding to treatment for depression. Harv Rev Psychiatry. 2011;19(3):109–24. PMID: 21631158. http://www.ncbi.nlm.nih.gov/pubmed/21631158.
226. Perroud N, Paoloni-Giacobino A, Prada P, Olié E, Salzmann A, Nicastro R, Guillaume S, Mouthon D, Stouder C, Dieben K, Huguelet P, Courtet P, Malafosse A. Increased methylation of glucocorticoid receptor gene (NR3C1) in adults with a history of childhood maltreatment: a link with the severity and type of trauma. Transl. Psychiatry. 2011;1(12):e59. PMCID: PMC3309499. http://www.ncbi.nlm.nih.gov/pubmed/22832351.
227. Mondal AC, Fatima M. Direct and indirect evidences of BDNF and NGF as key modulators in depression: role of antidepressants treatment. Int J Neurosci. 2019;129(3):283–96. PMID: 30235967. http://www.ncbi.nlm.nih.gov/pubmed/30235967.
228. Koenigsberg HW, Yuan P, Diaz GA, Guerreri S, Dorantes C, Mayson S, Zamfirescu C, New AS, Goodman M, Manji HK, Siever LJ. Platelet protein kinase C and brain-derived neurotrophic factor levels in borderline personality disorder patients. Psychiatry Res. 2012;199(2):92–7. PMCID: PMC4128317. http://www.ncbi.nlm.nih.gov/pubmed/22633012.
229. Martínez-Levy GA, Cruz-Fuentes CS. Genetic and epigenetic regulation of the brain-derived neurotrophic factor in the central nervous system. Yale J Biol Med. 2014;87(2):173–86. PMCID: PMC4031791. http://www.ncbi.nlm.nih.gov/pubmed/24910563.
230. Chen D, Meng L, Pei F, Zheng Y, Leng J. A review of DNA methylation in depression. J Clin Neurosci. 2017;43:39–46. PMID: 28645747. http://www.ncbi.nlm.nih.gov/pubmed/28645747.
231. Hing B, Sathyaputri L, Potash JB. A comprehensive review of genetic and epigenetic mechanisms that regulate BDNF expression and function with relevance to major depressive disorder. Am J Med Genet B Neuropsychiatr Genet. 2018;177(2):143–67. PMID: 29243873. http://www.ncbi.nlm.nih.gov/pubmed/29243873.
232. Kozlovsky N, Matar MA, Kaplan Z, Kotler M, Zohar J, Cohen H. Long-term down-regulation of BDNF mRNA in rat hippocampal CA1 subregion correlates with PTSD-like behavioural stress response. Int J Neuropsychopharmacol. 2007;10(6):741–58. PMID: 17291374. http://www.ncbi.nlm.nih.gov/pubmed/17291374.
233. Elzinga BM, Molendijk ML, Oude Voshaar RC, Bus BAA, Prickaerts J, Spinhoven P, Penninx BJWH. The impact of childhood abuse and recent stress on serum brain-derived neurotrophic factor and the moderating role of BDNF Val66Met. Psychopharmacology. 2011;214(1):319–28. PMCID: PMC3045516. http://www.ncbi.nlm.nih.gov/pubmed/20703451.
234. Tsankova NM, Berton O, Renthal W, Kumar A, Neve RL, Nestler EJ. Sustained hippocampal chromatin regulation in a mouse model of depression and antidepressant action. Nat Neurosci. 2006;9(4):519–25. PMID: 16501568. http://www.ncbi.nlm.nih.gov/pubmed/16501568.
235. Roth TL, Zoladz PR, Sweatt JD, Diamond DM. Epigenetic modification of hippocampal Bdnf DNA in adult rats in an animal model of post-traumatic stress disorder. J Psychiatr Res. 2011;45(7):919–26. PMCID: PMC3335738. http://www.ncbi.nlm.nih.gov/pubmed/21306736.
236. Lubin FD, Roth TL, Sweatt JD. Epigenetic regulation of BDNF gene transcription in the consolidation of fear memory. J Neurosci. 2008;28(42):10576–86. PMCID: PMC3312036. http://www.ncbi.nlm.nih.gov/pubmed/18923034.
237. Roth TL, Lubin FD, Funk AJ, Sweatt JD. Lasting epigenetic influence of early-life adversity on the BDNF gene. Biol Psychiatry. 2009;65(9):760–9. PMCID: PMC3056389. http://www.ncbi.nlm.nih.gov/pubmed/19150054.
238. Keller S, Sarchiapone M, Zarrilli F, Videtic A, Ferraro A, Carli V, Sacchetti S, Lembo F, Angiolillo A, Jovanovic N, Pisanti F, Tomaiuolo R, Monticelli A, Balazic J, Roy A, Marusic A, Cocozza S, Fusco A, Bruni CB, Castaldo G, Chiariotti L. Increased BDNF promoter methylation in the Wernicke area of suicide subjects. Arch Gen Psychiatry. 2010;67(3):258–67. PMID: 20194826. http://www.ncbi.nlm.nih.gov/pubmed/20194826.
239. Kundakovic M, Gudsnuk K, Herbstman JB, Tang D, Perera FP, Champagne FA. DNA methylation of BDNF as a biomarker of early-life adversity. Proc Natl Acad Sci USA. 2015;112(22):6807–13. PMCID: PMC4460453. http://www.ncbi.nlm.nih.gov/pubmed/25385582.
240. Dammann G, Teschler S, Haag T, Altmüller F, Tuczek F, Dammann RH. Increased DNA methylation of neuropsychiatric genes occurs in borderline personality disorder. Epigenetics. 2011;6(12):1454–62. PMID: 22139575. http://www.ncbi.nlm.nih.gov/pubmed/22139575.
241. Perroud N, Salzmann A, Prada P, Nicastro R, Hoeppli ME, Furrer S, Ardu S, Krejci I, Karege F, Malafosse A. Response to psychotherapy in borderline personality disorder and methylation status of the BDNF gene. Transl Psychiatry. 2013;3(1):e207. PMCID: PMC3566720. http://www.ncbi.nlm.nih.gov/pubmed/23422958.
242. Sen S, Duman R, Sanacora G. Serum brain-derived neurotrophic factor, depression, and antidepressant medications: meta-analyses and implications. Biol Psychiatry. 2008;64(6):527–32. PMCID: PMC2597158. http://www.ncbi.nlm.nih.gov/pubmed/18571629.
243. Polyakova M, Stuke K, Schuemberg K, Mueller K, Schoenknecht P, Schroeter ML. BDNF as a biomarker for successful treatment of mood disorders: a systematic & quantitative meta-analysis. J Affect Disord. 2015;174:432–40. PMID: 25553404. http://www.ncbi.nlm.nih.gov/pubmed/25553404.
244. Bakker JM, Lieverse R, Menne-Lothmann C, Viechtbauer W, Pishva E, Kenis G, Geschwind N, Peeters F, van Os J, Wichers M. Therapygenetics in mindfulness-based cognitive therapy: do genes have an impact on therapy-induced change in real-life positive affective experiences? Transl Psychiatry. 2014;4(4):e384. PMCID: PMC4012287. http://www.ncbi.nlm.nih.gov/pubmed/24755993.
245. Molendijk ML, Bus BA, Spinhoven P, Penninx BWJH, Kenis G, Prickaerts J, Voshaar RCO, Elzinga BM. Serum levels of brain-derived neurotrophic factor in major depressive disorder: state-trait issues, clinical features and pharmacological treatment. Mol Psychiatry. 2011;16(11):1088–95. PMCID: PMC3220395. http://www.ncbi.nlm.nih.gov/pubmed/20856249.
246. Lopez JP, Mamdani F, Labonte B, Beaulieu MM, Yang JP, Berlim MT, Ernst C, Turecki G. Epigenetic regulation of BDNF expression according to antidepressant response. Mol Psychiatry. 2013;18(4):398–9. PMCID: PMC5319860. http://www.ncbi.nlm.nih.gov/pubmed/22547115.
247. Musil R, Zill P, Seemüller F, Bondy B, Obermeier M, Spellmann I, Bender W, Adli M, Heuser I, Zeiler J, Gaebel W, Maier W, Rietschel M, Rujescu D, Schennach R, Möller HJ, Riedel M. No influence of brain-derived neurotrophic factor (BDNF) polymorphisms on treatment response in a naturalistic sample of patients with major depression. Eur Arch Psychiatry Clin Neurosci. 2013;263(5):405–12. PMID: 22965830. http://www.ncbi.nlm.nih.gov/pubmed/22965830.
248. Lin PY, Tseng PT. Decreased glial cell line-derived neurotrophic factor levels in patients with depression: a meta-analytic study. J Psychiatr Res. 2015;63:20–7. PMID: 25726496. http://www.ncbi.nlm.nih.gov/pubmed/25726496.
249. Ayanlaja AA, Zhang B, Ji G, Gao Y, Wang J, Kanwore K, Gao D. The reversible effects of glial cell line-derived neurotrophic factor (GDNF) in the human brain. Semin Cancer Biol. 2018;53:212–22. PMID: 30059726. http://www.ncbi.nlm.nih.gov/pubmed/30059726.

250. Naumenko VS, Bazovkina DV, Semenova AA, Tsybko AS, Il'chibaeva TV, Kondaurova EM, Popova NK. Effect of glial cell line-derived neurotrophic factor on behavior and key members of the brain serotonin system in mouse strains genetically predisposed to behavioral disorders. J Neurosci Res. 2013;91(12):1628–38. PMID: 24105724. http://www.ncbi.nlm.nih.gov/pubmed/24105724.
251. Uchida S, Hara K, Kobayashi A, Otsuki K, Yamagata H, Hobara T, Suzuki T, Miyata N, Watanabe Y. Epigenetic status of Gdnf in the ventral striatum determines susceptibility and adaptation to daily stressful events. Neuron. 2011;69(2):359–72. PMID: 21262472. http://www.ncbi.nlm.nih.gov/pubmed/21262472.
252. Tsybko AS, Ilchibaeva TV, Popova NK. Role of glial cell line-derived neurotrophic factor in the pathogenesis and treatment of mood disorders. Rev Neurosci. 2017;28(3):219–33. PMID: 28099138. http://www.ncbi.nlm.nih.gov/pubmed/28099138.
253. He X, Song J, Gao H, Li Z, Wang X, Zeng Q, Xiao Y, Feng J, Zhou D, Wang G. Serum brain-derived neurotrophic factor and glial cell-derived neurotrophic factor in patients with first-episode depression at different ages. Int J Psychiatry Clin Pract. 2023;27(2):118–26. PMID: 35980319. http://www.ncbi.nlm.nih.gov/pubmed/35980319.
254. Philibert R, Madan A, Andersen A, Cadoret R, Packer H, Sandhu H. Serotonin transporter mRNA levels are associated with the methylation of an upstream CpG Island. Am J Med Genet B Neuropsychiatr Genet. 2007;144B(1):101–5. PMID: 16958039. http://www.ncbi.nlm.nih.gov/pubmed/16958039.
255. Philibert RA, Sandhu H, Hollenbeck N, Gunter T, Adams W, Madan A. The relationship of 5HTT (SLC6A4) methylation and genotype on mRNA expression and liability to major depression and alcohol dependence in subjects from the Iowa Adoption Studies. Am J Med Genet B Neuropsychiatr Genet. 2008;147B(5):543–9. PMCID: PMC3643119. http://www.ncbi.nlm.nih.gov/pubmed/17987668.
256. Booij L, Tremblay RE, Szyf M, Benkelfat C. Genetic and early environmental influences on the serotonin system: consequences for brain development and risk for psychopathology. J Psychiatry Neurosci. 2015;40(1):5–18. PMCID: PMC4275332. http://www.ncbi.nlm.nih.gov/pubmed/25285876.
257. Ismaylova E, Lévesque ML, Pomares FB, Szyf M, Nemoda Z, Fahim C, Vitaro F, Brendgen M, Dionne G, Boivin M, Tremblay RE, Booij L. Serotonin transporter promoter methylation in peripheral cells and neural responses to negative stimuli: a study of adolescent monozygotic twins. Transl. Psychiatry. 2018;8(1):147. PMCID: PMC6082838. http://www.ncbi.nlm.nih.gov/pubmed/30089832.
258. Swartz JR, Hariri AR, Williamson DE. An epigenetic mechanism links socioeconomic status to changes in depression-related brain function in high-risk adolescents. Mol Psychiatry. 2017;22(2):209–14. PMCID: PMC5122474. http://www.ncbi.nlm.nih.gov/pubmed/27217150.
259. Elliott E, Ezra-Nevo G, Regev L, Neufeld-Cohen A, Chen A. Resilience to social stress coincides with functional DNA methylation of the Crf gene in adult mice. Nat Neurosci. 2010;13(11):1351–3. PMID: 20890295. http://www.ncbi.nlm.nih.gov/pubmed/20890295.
260. Sterrenburg L, Gaszner B, Boerrigter J, Santbergen L, Bramini M, Elliott E, Chen A, Peeters BWMM, Roubos EW, Kozicz T. Chronic stress induces sex-specific alterations in methylation and expression of corticotropin-releasing factor gene in the rat. PLoS One. 2011;6(11):e28128. PMCID: PMC3223222. http://www.ncbi.nlm.nih.gov/pubmed/22132228.
261. McGowan PO, Sasaki A, D'Alessio AC, Dymov S, Labonté B, Szyf M, Turecki G, Meaney MJ. Epigenetic regulation of the glucocorticoid receptor in human brain associates with childhood abuse. Nat Neurosci. 2009;12(3):342–8. PMCID: PMC2944040. http://www.ncbi.nlm.nih.gov/pubmed/19234457.
262. Weder N, Zhang H, Jensen K, Yang BZ, Simen A, Jackowski A, Lipschitz D, Douglas-Palumberi H, Ge M, Perepletchikova F, O'Loughlin K, Hudziak JJ, Gelernter J, Kaufman J. Child abuse, depression, and methylation in genes involved with stress, neural plasticity, and brain circuitry. J Am Acad Child Adolesc Psychiatry. 2014;53(4):417–424.e5. PMCID: PMC4126411. http://www.ncbi.nlm.nih.gov/pubmed/24655651.
263. Li X, Wei W, Zhao QY, Widagdo J, Baker-Andresen D, Flavell CR, D'Alessio A, Zhang Y, Bredy TW. Neocortical Tet3-mediated accumulation of 5-hydroxymethylcytosine promotes rapid behavioral adaptation. Proc Natl Acad Sci USA. 2014;111(19):7120–5. PMCID: PMC4024925. http://www.ncbi.nlm.nih.gov/pubmed/24757058.
264. Derrien T, Guigó R, Johnson R. The long non-coding RNAs: a New (P)layer in the "Dark Matter". Front Genet. 2011;2:107. PMCID: PMC3266617. http://www.ncbi.nlm.nih.gov/pubmed/22303401.
265. Spadaro PA, Bredy TW. Emerging role of non-coding RNA in neural plasticity, cognitive function, and neuropsychiatric disorders. Front Genet. 2012;3:132. PMCID: PMC3395882. http://www.ncbi.nlm.nih.gov/pubmed/22811697.
266. Mattick JS. The double life of RNA. Biochimie. 2011;93(11):viii–ix. PMID: 21963144. http://www.ncbi.nlm.nih.gov/pubmed/21963144.
267. Lin Q, Wei W, Coelho CM, Li X, Baker-Andresen D, Dudley K, Ratnu VS, Boskovic Z, Kobor MS, Sun YE, Bredy TW. The brain-specific microRNA miR-128b regulates the formation of fear-extinction memory. Nat Neurosci. 2011;14(9):1115–7. PMID: 21841775. http://www.ncbi.nlm.nih.gov/pubmed/21841775.
268. Dwivedi Y. MicroRNAs in depression and suicide: recent insights and future perspectives. J Affect Disord. 2018;240:146–54. PMCID: PMC6108934. http://www.ncbi.nlm.nih.gov/pubmed/30071418.
269. Tavakolizadeh J, Roshanaei K, Salmaninejad A, Yari R, Nahand JS, Sarkarizi HK, Mousavi SM, Salarinia R, Rahmati M, Mousavi SF, Mokhtari R, Mirzaei H. MicroRNAs and exosomes in depression: potential diagnostic biomarkers. J Cell Biochem. 2018;119(5):3783–97. PMID: 29236313. http://www.ncbi.nlm.nih.gov/pubmed/29236313.
270. Hu Z, Jiang Y, Huo X, Yang Y, Davies H, Botchway BOA, Fang M. Prospective role of MicroRNAs in depression. Curr Med Chem. 2017;24(32):3508–21. PMID: 28714388. http://www.ncbi.nlm.nih.gov/pubmed/28714388.
271. Mattick JS, Makunin IV. Non-coding RNA. Hum Mol Genet. 2006;15 Spec No 1:R17–29. PMID: 16651366. http://www.ncbi.nlm.nih.gov/pubmed/16651366.
272. Friedman RC, Farh KKH, Burge CB, Bartel DP. Most mammalian mRNAs are conserved targets of microRNAs. Genome Res. 2009;19(1):92–105. PMCID: PMC2612969. http://www.ncbi.nlm.nih.gov/pubmed/18955434.
273. Lee H, Zhang Z, Krause HM. Long noncoding RNAs and repetitive elements: junk or intimate evolutionary partners? Trends Genet. 2019;35(12):892–902. PMID: 31662190. http://www.ncbi.nlm.nih.gov/pubmed/31662190.
274. Palazzo AF, Lee ES. Non-coding RNA: what is functional and what is junk? Front Genet. 2015;6:2. PMCID: PMC4306305. http://www.ncbi.nlm.nih.gov/pubmed/25674102.
275. Backofen R, Gorodkin J, Hofacker IL, Stadler PF. Comparative RNA genomics. Methods Mol Biol. 2024;2802:347–93. PMID: 38819565. http://www.ncbi.nlm.nih.gov/pubmed/38819565.
276. Thind AS, Monga I, Thakur PK, Kumari P, Dindhoria K, Krzak M, Ranson M, Ashford B. Demystifying emerging bulk RNA-Seq applications: the application and utility of bioinformatic methodology. Brief Bioinform. 2021;22(6):bbab259. PMID: 34329375. http://www.ncbi.nlm.nih.gov/pubmed/34329375.

277. van Bakel H, Nislow C, Blencowe BJ, Hughes TR. Most "dark matter" transcripts are associated with known genes. PLoS Biol. 2010;8(5):e1000371. PMCID: PMC2872640. http://www.ncbi.nlm.nih.gov/pubmed/20502517.
278. Kretz M, Webster DE, Flockhart RJ, Lee CS, Zehnder A, Lopez-Pajares V, Qu K, Zheng GXY, Chow J, Kim GE, Rinn JL, Chang HY, Siprashvili Z, Khavari PA. Suppression of progenitor differentiation requires the long noncoding RNA ANCR. Genes Dev. 2012;26(4):338–43. PMCID: PMC3289881. http://www.ncbi.nlm.nih.gov/pubmed/22302877.
279. Nejepinska J, Malik R, Filkowski J, Flemr M, Filipowicz W, Svoboda P. dsRNA expression in the mouse elicits RNAi in oocytes and low adenosine deamination in somatic cells. Nucleic Acids Res. 2012;40(1):399–413. PMCID: PMC3245926. http://www.ncbi.nlm.nih.gov/pubmed/21908396.
280. Rajasethupathy P, Antonov I, Sheridan R, Frey S, Sander C, Tuschl T, Kandel ER. A role for neuronal piRNAs in the epigenetic control of memory-related synaptic plasticity. Cell. 2012;149(3):693–707. PMCID: PMC3442366. http://www.ncbi.nlm.nih.gov/pubmed/22541438.
281. Borchert GM, Holton NW, Williams JD, Hernan WL, Bishop IP, Dembosky JA, Elste JE, Gregoire NS, Kim JA, Koehler WW, Lengerich JC, Medema AA, Nguyen MA, Ower GD, Rarick MA, Strong BN, Tardi NJ, Tasker NM, Wozniak DJ, Gatto C, Larson ED. Comprehensive analysis of microRNA genomic loci identifies pervasive repetitive-element origins. Mob Genet Elements. 2011;1(1):8–17. PMCID: PMC3190270. http://www.ncbi.nlm.nih.gov/pubmed/22016841.
282. Gräff J, Kim D, Dobbin MM, Tsai LH. Epigenetic regulation of gene expression in physiological and pathological brain processes. Physiol Rev. 2011;91(2):603–49. PMID: 21527733. http://www.ncbi.nlm.nih.gov/pubmed/21527733.
283. Peerbooms OLJ, van Os J, Drukker M, Kenis G, Hoogveld L, MTHFR in Psychiatry Group, de Hert M, Delespaul P, van Winkel R, Rutten BPF. Meta-analysis of MTHFR gene variants in schizophrenia, bipolar disorder and unipolar depressive disorder: evidence for a common genetic vulnerability? Brain Behav Immun. 2011;25(8):1530–43. PMID: 21185933. http://www.ncbi.nlm.nih.gov/pubmed/21185933.
284. Vanden Berghe W, Haegeman G. Epigenetic remedies by dietary phytochemicals against inflammatory skin disorders: myth or reality? Curr Drug Metab. 2010;11(5):436–50. PMID: 20540697. http://www.ncbi.nlm.nih.gov/pubmed/20540697.
285. Archer T, Fredriksson A, Schütz E, Kostrzewa RM. Influence of physical exercise on neuroimmunological functioning and health: aging and stress. Neurotox Res. 2011;20(1):69–83. PMID: 20953749. http://www.ncbi.nlm.nih.gov/pubmed/20953749.
286. Szarc vel Szic K, Ndlovu MN, Haegeman G, Vanden Berghe W. Nature or nurture: let food be your epigenetic medicine in chronic inflammatory disorders. Biochem Pharmacol. 2010;80(12):1816–32. PMID: 20688047. http://www.ncbi.nlm.nih.gov/pubmed/20688047.
287. Szarc vel Szic K, Declerck K, Vidaković M, Vanden Berghe W. From inflammaging to healthy aging by dietary lifestyle choices: is epigenetics the key to personalized nutrition? Clin. Epigenetics. 2015;7(1):33. PMCID: PMC4389409. http://www.ncbi.nlm.nih.gov/pubmed/25861393.
288. Ong TP, Moreno FS, Ross SA. Targeting the epigenome with bioactive food components for cancer prevention. J Nutrigenet Nutrigenomics. 2011;4(5):275–92. PMCID: PMC3388269. http://www.ncbi.nlm.nih.gov/pubmed/22353664.
289. Hardy TM, Tollefsbol TO. Epigenetic diet: impact on the epigenome and cancer. Epigenomics. 2011;3(4):503–18. PMCID: PMC3197720. http://www.ncbi.nlm.nih.gov/pubmed/22022340.
290. Horvath S, Raj K. DNA methylation-based biomarkers and the epigenetic clock theory of ageing. Nat Rev Genet. 2018;19(6):371–84. PMID: 29643443. http://www.ncbi.nlm.nih.gov/pubmed/29643443.
291. Gibbs WW. Biomarkers and ageing: the clock-watcher. Nature. 2014;508(7495):168–70. PMID: 24717494. http://www.ncbi.nlm.nih.gov/pubmed/24717494.
292. Ben-Avraham D, Muzumdar RH, Atzmon G. Epigenetic genome-wide association methylation in aging and longevity. Epigenomics. 2012;4(5):503–9. PMCID: PMC4123813. http://www.ncbi.nlm.nih.gov/pubmed/23130832.
293. Buigues C, Padilla-Sánchez C, Garrido JF, Navarro-Martínez R, Ruiz-Ros V, Cauli O. The relationship between depression and frailty syndrome: a systematic review. Aging Ment Health. 2015;19(9):762–72. PMID: 25319638. http://www.ncbi.nlm.nih.gov/pubmed/25319638.
294. Horvath S. DNA methylation age of human tissues and cell types. Genome Biol. 2013;14(10):R115. PMCID: PMC4015143. http://www.ncbi.nlm.nih.gov/pubmed/24138928.
295. Hannum G, Guinney J, Zhao L, Zhang L, Hughes G, Sadda S, Klotzle B, Bibikova M, Fan JB, Gao Y, Deconde R, Chen M, Rajapakse I, Friend S, Ideker T, Zhang K. Genome-wide methylation profiles reveal quantitative views of human aging rates. Mol Cell. 2013;49(2):359–67. PMCID: PMC3780611. http://www.ncbi.nlm.nih.gov/pubmed/23177740.
296. Lim U, Song MA. DNA methylation as a biomarker of aging in epidemiologic studies. Methods Mol Biol. 2018;1856:219–31. PMID: 30178254. http://www.ncbi.nlm.nih.gov/pubmed/30178254.
297. Koutsouleris N, Davatzikos C, Borgwardt S, Gaser C, Bottlender R, Frodl T, Falkai P, Riecher-Rössler A, Möller HJ, Reiser M, Pantelis C, Meisenzahl E. Accelerated brain aging in schizophrenia and beyond: a neuroanatomical marker of psychiatric disorders. Schizophr Bull. 2014;40(5):1140–53. PMCID: PMC4133663. http://www.ncbi.nlm.nih.gov/pubmed/24126515.
298. Ridout KK, Ridout SJ, Price LH, Sen S, Tyrka AR. Depression and telomere length: a meta-analysis. J Affect Disord. 2016;191:237–47. PMCID: PMC4760624. http://www.ncbi.nlm.nih.gov/pubmed/26688493.
299. Schutte NS, Malouff JM. The association between depression and leukocyte telomere length: a meta-analysis. Depress Anxiety. 2015;32(4):229–38. PMID: 25709105. http://www.ncbi.nlm.nih.gov/pubmed/25709105.
300. Begum N, Mandhare A, Tryphena KP, Srivastava S, Shaikh MF, Singh SB, Khatri DK. Epigenetics in depression and gut-brain axis: a molecular crosstalk. Front Aging Neurosci. 2022;14:1048333. PMCID: PMC9794020. http://www.ncbi.nlm.nih.gov/pubmed/36583185.
301. Vitetta L, Bambling M, Strodl E. Probiotics and commensal bacteria metabolites trigger epigenetic changes in the gut and influence beneficial mood dispositions. Microorganisms. 2023;11(5):1334. PMCID: PMC10221035. http://www.ncbi.nlm.nih.gov/pubmed/37317308.
302. Wang J, Zhou T, Liu F, Huang Y, Xiao Z, Qian Y, Zhou W. Influence of gut microbiota on resilience and its possible mechanisms. Int J Biol Sci. 2023;19(8):2588–98. PMCID: PMC10197883. http://www.ncbi.nlm.nih.gov/pubmed/37215996.
303. Sánchez-Lafuente CL, Reive BS, Kalynchuk LE, Caruncho HJ. A scoping review of Rodent studies investigating the epigenetic mechanisms in the brain underlying the effects of diet on depressive-like behaviour. Biomedicine. 2022;10(12):3213. PMCID: PMC9775686. http://www.ncbi.nlm.nih.gov/pubmed/36551970.
304. Cline H, Haas K. The regulation of dendritic arbor development and plasticity by glutamatergic synaptic input: a review of the synaptotrophic hypothesis. J Physiol. 2008;586(6):1509–17. PMCID: PMC2375708. http://www.ncbi.nlm.nih.gov/pubmed/18202093.

305. Feldman DE. Synaptic mechanisms for plasticity in neocortex. Annu Rev Neurosci. 2009;32:33–55. PMCID: PMC3071739. http://www.ncbi.nlm.nih.gov/pubmed/19400721.
306. Ben Achour S, Pascual O. Glia: the many ways to modulate synaptic plasticity. Neurochem Int. 2010;57(4):440–5. PMID: 20193723. http://www.ncbi.nlm.nih.gov/pubmed/20193723.
307. Simons-Weidenmaier NS, Weber M, Plappert CF, Pilz PKD, Schmid S. Synaptic depression and short-term habituation are located in the sensory part of the mammalian startle pathway. BMC Neurosci. 2006;7:38. PMCID: PMC1479352. http://www.ncbi.nlm.nih.gov/pubmed/16684348.
308. Magleby KL, Zengel JE. Long term changes in augmentation, potentiation, and depression of transmitter release as a function of repeated synaptic activity at the frog neuromuscular junction. J Physiol. 1976;257(2):471–94. PMCID: PMC1309370. http://www.ncbi.nlm.nih.gov/pubmed/820855.
309. Schlösser B, ten Bruggencate G, Sutor B. Local disinhibition of neocortical neuronal circuits causes augmentation of glutamatergic and GABAergic synaptic transmission in the rat neostriatum in vitro. Exp Neurol. 1999;157(1):180–93. PMID: 10222121. http://www.ncbi.nlm.nih.gov/pubmed/10222121.
310. Zucker RS, Regehr WG. Short-term synaptic plasticity. Annu Rev Physiol. 2002;64:355–405. PMID: 11826273. http://www.ncbi.nlm.nih.gov/pubmed/11826273.
311. Stevens CF, Wesseling JF. Augmentation is a potentiation of the exocytotic process. Neuron. 1999;22(1):139–46. PMID: 10027296. http://www.ncbi.nlm.nih.gov/pubmed/10027296.
312. Abbott LF, Regehr WG. Synaptic computation. Nature. 2004;431(7010):796–803. PMID: 15483601. http://www.ncbi.nlm.nih.gov/pubmed/15483601.
313. Gerrow K, Triller A. Synaptic stability and plasticity in a floating world. Curr Opin Neurobiol. 2010;20(5):631–9. PMID: 20655734. http://www.ncbi.nlm.nih.gov/pubmed/20655734.
314. Gaiarsa JL, Ben-Ari Y. Long-term plasticity at inhibitory synapses: a phenomenon that has been overlooked. In: Kittler JT, Moss SJ, editors. The dynamic synapse: molecular methods in ionotropic receptor biology [Internet]. Boca Raton: CRC Press/Taylor & Francis; 2006 [cited 2025 Jan 6]. Available from: http://www.ncbi.nlm.nih.gov/books/NBK2553/ PMID: 21204478. http://www.ncbi.nlm.nih.gov/pubmed/21204478.
315. Rusakov DA, Savtchenko LP, Zheng K, Henley JM. Shaping the synaptic signal: molecular mobility inside and outside the cleft. Trends Neurosci. 2011;34(7):359–69. PMCID: PMC3133640. http://www.ncbi.nlm.nih.gov/pubmed/21470699.
316. Blundon JA, Zakharenko SS. Dissecting the components of long-term potentiation. Neuroscientist. 2008;14(6):598–608. PMCID: PMC2655119. http://www.ncbi.nlm.nih.gov/pubmed/18940785.
317. Bliss TV, Gardner-Medwin AR. Long-lasting potentiation of synaptic transmission in the dentate area of the unanaestetized rabbit following stimulation of the perforant path. J Physiol. 1973;232(2):357–74. PMCID: PMC1350459. http://www.ncbi.nlm.nih.gov/pubmed/4727085.
318. Abraham WC, Logan B, Greenwood JM, Dragunow M. Induction and experience-dependent consolidation of stable long-term potentiation lasting months in the hippocampus. J Neurosci. 2002;22(21):9626–34. PMCID: PMC6758050. http://www.ncbi.nlm.nih.gov/pubmed/12417688.
319. Cooke SF, Bliss TVP. Plasticity in the human central nervous system. Brain. 2006;129(Pt 7):1659–73. PMID: 16672292. http://www.ncbi.nlm.nih.gov/pubmed/16672292.
320. Bliss TV, Collingridge GL. A synaptic model of memory: long-term potentiation in the hippocampus. Nature. 1993;361(6407):31–9. PMID: 8421494. http://www.ncbi.nlm.nih.gov/pubmed/8421494.
321. Malenka RC, Nicoll RA. Long-term potentiation—a decade of progress? Science. 1999;285(5435):1870–4. PMID: 10489359. http://www.ncbi.nlm.nih.gov/pubmed/10489359.
322. Massey PV, Bashir ZI. Long-term depression: multiple forms and implications for brain function. Trends Neurosci. 2007;30(4):176–84. PMID: 17335914. http://www.ncbi.nlm.nih.gov/pubmed/17335914.
323. Malenka RC, Bear MF. LTP and LTD: an embarrassment of riches. Neuron. 2004;44(1):5–21. PMID: 15450156. http://www.ncbi.nlm.nih.gov/pubmed/15450156.
324. Zhuo M, Hawkins RD. Long-term depression: a learning-related type of synaptic plasticity in the mammalian central nervous system. Rev Neurosci. 1995;6(3):259–77. PMID: 8717637. http://www.ncbi.nlm.nih.gov/pubmed/8717637.
325. Malleret G, Alarcon JM, Martel G, Takizawa S, Vronskaya S, Yin D, Chen IZ, Kandel ER, Shumyatsky GP. Bidirectional regulation of hippocampal long-term synaptic plasticity and its influence on opposing forms of memory. J Neurosci. 2010;30(10):3813–25. PMCID: PMC6632240. http://www.ncbi.nlm.nih.gov/pubmed/20220016.
326. Kandel ER. The molecular biology of memory storage: a dialogue between genes and synapses. Science. 2001;294(5544):1030–8. PMID: 11691980. http://www.ncbi.nlm.nih.gov/pubmed/11691980.
327. Abraham WC, Bear MF. Metaplasticity: the plasticity of synaptic plasticity. Trends Neurosci. 1996;19(4):126–30. PMID: 8658594. http://www.ncbi.nlm.nih.gov/pubmed/8658594.
328. Vose LR, Stanton PK. Synaptic plasticity, metaplasticity and depression. Curr Neuropharmacol. 2017;15(1):71–86. PMCID: PMC5327460. http://www.ncbi.nlm.nih.gov/pubmed/26830964.
329. Turrigiano G. Homeostatic synaptic plasticity: local and global mechanisms for stabilizing neuronal function. Cold Spring Harb Perspect Biol. 2012;4(1):a005736. PMCID: PMC3249629. http://www.ncbi.nlm.nih.gov/pubmed/22086977.
330. Zhou JQ, Gafni A. Exposure of rat muscle phosphoglycerate kinase to a nonenzymatic MFO system generates the old form of the enzyme. J Gerontol. 1991;46(6):B217–21. PMID: 1940072. http://www.ncbi.nlm.nih.gov/pubmed/1940072.
331. Paixão S, Klein R. Neuron-astrocyte communication and synaptic plasticity. Curr Opin Neurobiol. 2010;20(4):466–73. PMID: 20471242. http://www.ncbi.nlm.nih.gov/pubmed/20471242.
332. Bernardinelli Y, Muller D, Nikonenko I. Astrocyte-synapse structural plasticity. Neural Plast. 2014;2014:232105. PMCID: PMC3910461. http://www.ncbi.nlm.nih.gov/pubmed/24511394..
333. Duman RS, Aghajanian GK. Synaptic dysfunction in depression: potential therapeutic targets. Science. 2012;338(6103):68–72. PMCID: PMC4424898. http://www.ncbi.nlm.nih.gov/pubmed/23042884.
334. Kraus C, Castrén E, Kasper S, Lanzenberger R. Serotonin and neuroplasticity - links between molecular, functional and structural pathophysiology in depression. Neurosci Biobehav Rev. 2017;77:317–26. PMID: 28342763. http://www.ncbi.nlm.nih.gov/pubmed/28342763.
335. Duman RS, Aghajanian GK, Sanacora G, Krystal JH. Synaptic plasticity and depression: new insights from stress and rapid-acting antidepressants. Nat Med. 2016;22(3):238–49. PMCID: PMC5405628. http://www.ncbi.nlm.nih.gov/pubmed/26937618.
336. Price JB, Bronars C, Erhardt S, Cullen KR, Schwieler L, Berk M, Walder K, McGee SL, Frye MA, Tye SJ. Bioenergetics and synaptic plasticity as potential targets for individualizing treatment for depression. Neurosci Biobehav Rev. 2018;90:212–20. PMID: 29656032. http://www.ncbi.nlm.nih.gov/pubmed/29656032.
337. Magariños AM, Verdugo JM, McEwen BS. Chronic stress alters synaptic terminal structure in hippocampus. Proc Natl Acad Sci U S A. 1997;94(25):14002–14008. PMCID: PMC28422. http://www.ncbi.nlm.nih.gov/pubmed/9391142.

338. Sousa N, Lukoyanov NV, Madeira MD, Almeida OF, Paula-Barbosa MM. Reorganization of the morphology of hippocampal neurites and synapses after stress-induced damage correlates with behavioral improvement. Neuroscience. 2000;97(2):253–66. PMID: 10799757. http://www.ncbi.nlm.nih.gov/pubmed/10799757.
339. Radley JJ, Rocher AB, Miller M, Janssen WGM, Liston C, Hof PR, McEwen BS, Morrison JH. Repeated stress induces dendritic spine loss in the rat medial prefrontal cortex. Cereb Cortex. 2006;16(3):313–20. PMID: 15901656. http://www.ncbi.nlm.nih.gov/pubmed/15901656.
340. Tzanoulinou S, Riccio O, de Boer MW, Sandi C. Peripubertal stress-induced behavioral changes are associated with altered expression of genes involved in excitation and inhibition in the amygdala. Transl Psychiatry. 2014;4(7):e410. PMCID: PMC4119221. http://www.ncbi.nlm.nih.gov/pubmed/25004390.
341. Kaster MP, Machado NJ, Silva HB, Nunes A, Ardais AP, Santana M, Baqi Y, Müller CE, Rodrigues ALS, Porciúncula LO, Chen JF, Tomé ÂR, Agostinho P, Canas PM, Cunha RA. Caffeine acts through neuronal adenosine A2A receptors to prevent mood and memory dysfunction triggered by chronic stress. Proc Natl Acad Sci USA. 2015;112(25):7833–8. PMCID: PMC4485143. http://www.ncbi.nlm.nih.gov/pubmed/26056314.
342. Gilabert-Juan J, Varea E, Guirado R, Blasco-Ibáñez JM, Crespo C, Nácher J. Alterations in the expression of PSA-NCAM and synaptic proteins in the dorsolateral prefrontal cortex of psychiatric disorder patients. Neurosci Lett. 2012;530(1):97–102. PMID: 23022470. http://www.ncbi.nlm.nih.gov/pubmed/23022470.
343. Feyissa AM, Chandran A, Stockmeier CA, Karolewicz B. Reduced levels of NR2A and NR2B subunits of NMDA receptor and PSD-95 in the prefrontal cortex in major depression. Prog Neuro-Psychopharmacol Biol Psychiatry. 2009;33(1):70–5. PMCID: PMC2655629. http://www.ncbi.nlm.nih.gov/pubmed/18992785.
344. Zhao J, Bao AM, Qi XR, Kamphuis W, Luchetti S, Lou JS, Swaab DF. Gene expression of GABA and glutamate pathway markers in the prefrontal cortex of non-suicidal elderly depressed patients. J Affect Disord. 2012;138(3):494–502. PMID: 22357337. http://www.ncbi.nlm.nih.gov/pubmed/22357337.
345. Duric V, Banasr M, Stockmeier CA, Simen AA, Newton SS, Overholser JC, Jurjus GJ, Dieter L, Duman RS. Altered expression of synapse and glutamate related genes in post-mortem hippocampus of depressed subjects. Int J Neuropsychopharmacol. 2013;16(1):69–82. PMCID: PMC3414647. http://www.ncbi.nlm.nih.gov/pubmed/22339950.
346. Rajkowska G, Miguel-Hidalgo JJ, Wei J, Dilley G, Pittman SD, Meltzer HY, Overholser JC, Roth BL, Stockmeier CA. Morphometric evidence for neuronal and glial prefrontal cell pathology in major depression. Biol Psychiatry. 1999;45(9):1085–98. PMID: 10331101. http://www.ncbi.nlm.nih.gov/pubmed/10331101.
347. Kang HJ, Voleti B, Hajszan T, Rajkowska G, Stockmeier CA, Licznerski P, Lepack A, Majik MS, Jeong LS, Banasr M, Son H, Duman RS. Decreased expression of synapse-related genes and loss of synapses in major depressive disorder. Nat Med. 2012;18(9):1413–7. PMCID: PMC3491115. http://www.ncbi.nlm.nih.gov/pubmed/22885997.
348. Li N, Lee B, Liu RJ, Banasr M, Dwyer JM, Iwata M, Li XY, Aghajanian G, Duman RS. mTOR-dependent synapse formation underlies the rapid antidepressant effects of NMDA antagonists. Science. 2010;329(5994):959–64. PMCID: PMC3116441. http://www.ncbi.nlm.nih.gov/pubmed/20724638.
349. Li N, Liu RJ, Dwyer JM, Banasr M, Lee B, Son H, Li XY, Aghajanian G, Duman RS. Glutamate N-methyl-D-aspartate receptor antagonists rapidly reverse behavioral and synaptic deficits caused by chronic stress exposure. Biol Psychiatry. 2011;69(8):754–61. PMCID: PMC3068225. http://www.ncbi.nlm.nih.gov/pubmed/21292242.
350. McEwen BS, Eiland L, Hunter RG, Miller MM. Stress and anxiety: structural plasticity and epigenetic regulation as a consequence of stress. Neuropharmacology. 2012;62(1):3–12. PMCID: PMC3196296. http://www.ncbi.nlm.nih.gov/pubmed/21807003.
351. Lesch KP, Waider J. Serotonin in the modulation of neural plasticity and networks: implications for neurodevelopmental disorders. Neuron. 2012;76(1):175–91. PMID: 23040814. http://www.ncbi.nlm.nih.gov/pubmed/23040814.
352. Marzo A, Bai J, Otani S. Neuroplasticity regulation by noradrenaline in mammalian brain. Curr Neuropharmacol. 2009;7(4):286–95. PMCID: PMC2811862. http://www.ncbi.nlm.nih.gov/pubmed/20514208.
353. Gray JD, Milner TA, McEwen BS. Dynamic plasticity: the role of glucocorticoids, brain-derived neurotrophic factor and other trophic factors. Neuroscience. 2013;239:214–27. PMCID: PMC3743657. http://www.ncbi.nlm.nih.gov/pubmed/22922121.
354. Hayley S, Litteljohn D. Neuroplasticity and the next wave of antidepressant strategies. Front Cell Neurosci. 2013;7:218. PMCID: PMC3834236. http://www.ncbi.nlm.nih.gov/pubmed/24312008.
355. Maren S. Synaptic mechanisms of associative memory in the amygdala. Neuron. 2005;47(6):783–6. PMID: 16157273. http://www.ncbi.nlm.nih.gov/pubmed/16157273.
356. Weinberger NM. Associative representational plasticity in the auditory cortex: a synthesis of two disciplines. Learn Mem. 2007;14(1–2):1–16. PMCID: PMC3601844. http://www.ncbi.nlm.nih.gov/pubmed/17202426.
357. Aston S, Hurlbert A. What #theDress reveals about the role of illumination priors in color perception and color constancy. J Vis. 2017;17(9):4. PMCID: PMC5812438. http://www.ncbi.nlm.nih.gov/pubmed/28793353.
358. Morimoto T, Fukuda K, Uchikawa K. Explaining #theShoe based on the optimal color hypothesis: the role of chromaticity vs. luminance distribution in an ambiguous image. Vis Res. 2021;178:117–23. PMCID: PMC7116573. http://www.ncbi.nlm.nih.gov/pubmed/33278815.
359. Schoenfeld TJ, Gould E. Stress, stress hormones, and adult neurogenesis. Exp Neurol. 2012;233(1):12–21. PMCID: PMC3715962. http://www.ncbi.nlm.nih.gov/pubmed/21281629.
360. Frye CA, Paris JJ, Osborne DM, Campbell JC, Kippin TE. Prenatal stress alters progestogens to mediate susceptibility to sex-typical, stress-sensitive disorders, such as drug abuse: a review. Front Psychiatry. 2011;2:52. PMCID: PMC3195272. http://www.ncbi.nlm.nih.gov/pubmed/22022315.
361. Greenhill SD, Juczewski K, de Haan AM, Seaton G, Fox K, Hardingham NR. NEURODEVELOPMENT. Adult cortical plasticity depends on an early postnatal critical period. Science. 2015;349(6246):424–7. PMID: 26206934. http://www.ncbi.nlm.nih.gov/pubmed/26206934.
362. Pitychoutis PM, Zisaki A, Dalla C, Papadopoulou-Daifoti Z. Pharmacogenetic insights into depression and antidepressant response: does sex matter? Curr Pharm Des. 2010;16(20):2214–23. PMID: 20459391. http://www.ncbi.nlm.nih.gov/pubmed/20459391.
363. Serretti A, Artioli P, Quartesan R. Pharmacogenetics in the treatment of depression: pharmacodynamic studies. Pharmacogenet Genomics. 2005;15(2):61–7. PMID: 15861029. http://www.ncbi.nlm.nih.gov/pubmed/15861029.
364. Lester KJ, Hudson JL, Tropeano M, Creswell C, Collier DA, Farmer A, Lyneham HJ, Rapee RM, Eley TC. Neurotrophic gene polymorphisms and response to psychological therapy. Transl Psychiatry. 2012;2(5):e108. PMCID: PMC3365252. http://www.ncbi.nlm.nih.gov/pubmed/22832952.

365. Keers R, Aitchison KJ. Pharmacogenetics of antidepressant response. Expert Rev Neurother. 2011;11(1):101–25. PMID: 21158559. http://www.ncbi.nlm.nih.gov/pubmed/21158559.
366. Rayner C, Coleman JRI, Purves KL, Hodsoll J, Goldsmith K, Alpers GW, Andersson E, Arolt V, Boberg J, Bögels S, Creswell C, Cooper P, Curtis C, Deckert J, Domschke K, El Alaoui S, Fehm L, Fydrich T, Gerlach AL, Grocholewski A, Hahlweg K, Hamm A, Hedman E, Heiervang ER, Hudson JL, Jöhren P, Keers R, Kircher T, Lang T, Lavebratt C, Lee SH, Lester KJ, Lindefors N, Margraf J, Nauta M, Pané-Farré CA, Pauli P, Rapee RM, Reif A, Rief W, Roberts S, Schalling M, Schneider S, Silverman WK, Ströhle A, Teismann T, Thastum M, Wannemüller A, Weber H, Wittchen HU, Wolf C, Rück C, Breen G, Eley TC. A genome-wide association meta-analysis of prognostic outcomes following cognitive behavioural therapy in individuals with anxiety and depressive disorders. Transl Psychiatry. 2019;9(1):150. PMCID: PMC6533285. http://www.ncbi.nlm.nih.gov/pubmed/31123309.
367. Eley TC, Hudson JL, Creswell C, Tropeano M, Lester KJ, Cooper P, Farmer A, Lewis CM, Lyneham HJ, Rapee RM, Uher R, Zavos HMS, Collier DA. Therapygenetics: the 5HTTLPR and response to psychological therapy. Mol Psychiatry. 2012;17(3):236–7. PMCID: PMC3272476. http://www.ncbi.nlm.nih.gov/pubmed/22024766.
368. Bockting CLH, Mocking RJ, Lok A, Koeter MWJ, Schene AH. Therapygenetics: the 5HTTLPR as a biomarker for response to psychological therapy? Mol Psychiatry. 2013;18(7):744–5. PMID: 22751490. http://www.ncbi.nlm.nih.gov/pubmed/22751490.
369. Beevers CG, McGeary JE. Therapygenetics: moving towards personalized psychotherapy treatment. Trends Cogn Sci. 2012;16(1):11–2. PMCID: PMC3253222. http://www.ncbi.nlm.nih.gov/pubmed/22104133.
370. Schosser A, Fischer-Hansal D, Swoboda MM, Ludwig B, Carlberg L, Swoboda P, Kienesberger K, Bernegger A, Fuxjäger M, Zotter M, Schmelzle N, Inaner M, Koller R, Kapusta ND, Haslacher H, Aigner M, Kasper S, Senft B. BDNF gene polymorphisms predicting treatment response to CBT-based rehabilitation of depression: to be submitted to: European Neuropsychopharmacology. Eur Neuropsychopharmacol. 2022;58:103–8. PMID: 35453068. http://www.ncbi.nlm.nih.gov/pubmed/35453068.
371. Uher R. The implications of gene-environment interactions in depression: will cause inform cure? Mol Psychiatry. 2008;13(12):1070–8. PMID: 18679406. http://www.ncbi.nlm.nih.gov/pubmed/18679406.
372. Belsky J, Jonassaint C, Pluess M, Stanton M, Brummett B, Williams R. Vulnerability genes or plasticity genes? Mol Psychiatry. 2009;14(8):746–54. PMCID: PMC2834322. http://www.ncbi.nlm.nih.gov/pubmed/19455150.
373. Rutter M, Moffitt TE, Caspi A. Gene-environment interplay and psychopathology: multiple varieties but real effects. J Child Psychol Psychiatry. 2006;47(3–4):226–61. PMID: 16492258. http://www.ncbi.nlm.nih.gov/pubmed/16492258.
374. Roisman GI, Newman DA, Fraley RC, Haltigan JD, Groh AM, Haydon KC. Distinguishing differential susceptibility from diathesis-stress: recommendations for evaluating interaction effects. Dev Psychopathol. 2012;24(2):389–409. PMID: 22559121. http://www.ncbi.nlm.nih.gov/pubmed/22559121.
375. Pluess M, Belsky J. Differential susceptibility to parenting and quality child care. Dev Psychol. 2010;46(2):379–90. PMID: 20210497. http://www.ncbi.nlm.nih.gov/pubmed/20210497.
376. Burmeister M, McInnis MG, Zöllner S. Psychiatric genetics: progress amid controversy. Nat Rev Genet. 2008;9(7):527–40. PMID: 18560438. http://www.ncbi.nlm.nih.gov/pubmed/18560438.
377. Radley JJ, Kabbaj M, Jacobson L, Heydendael W, Yehuda R, Herman JP. Stress risk factors and stress-related pathology: neuroplasticity, epigenetics and endophenotypes. Stress. 2011;14(5):481–97. PMCID: PMC3641164. http://www.ncbi.nlm.nih.gov/pubmed/21848436.
378. Hasler G, Northoff G. Discovering imaging endophenotypes for major depression. Mol Psychiatry. 2011;16(6):604–19. PMID: 21602829. http://www.ncbi.nlm.nih.gov/pubmed/21602829.
379. Gottesman II, Gould TD. The endophenotype concept in psychiatry: etymology and strategic intentions. Am J Psychiatry. 2003;160(4):636–45. PMID: 12668349. http://www.ncbi.nlm.nih.gov/pubmed/12668349.
380. Hasler G, Drevets WC, Manji HK, Charney DS. Discovering endophenotypes for major depression. Neuropsychopharmacology. 2004;29(10):1765–81. PMID: 15213704. http://www.ncbi.nlm.nih.gov/pubmed/15213704.
381. Leve LD, Neiderhiser JM, Ganiban JM, Natsuaki MN, Shaw DS, Reiss D. The early growth and development study: a dual-family adoption study from birth through adolescence. Twin Res Hum Genet. 2019;22(6):716–27. PMCID: PMC7056588. http://www.ncbi.nlm.nih.gov/pubmed/31526412.
382. Leve LD, Neiderhiser JM, Scaramella LV, Reiss D. The early growth and development study: using the prospective adoption design to examine genotype-environment interplay. Xin Li Xue Bao. 2008;40(10):1106–15. PMCID: PMC2674795. http://www.ncbi.nlm.nih.gov/pubmed/19458782.
383. Leve LD, Neiderhiser JM, Ge X, Scaramella LV, Conger RD, Reid JB, Shaw DS, Reiss D. The early growth and development study: a prospective adoption design. Twin Res Hum Genet. 2007;10(1):84–95. PMCID: PMC4169207. http://www.ncbi.nlm.nih.gov/pubmed/17539368.
384. Leve LD, Neiderhiser JM, Scaramella LV, Reiss D. The early growth and development study: using the prospective adoption design to examine genotype-environment interplay. 2008. Behav Genet. 2010;40(3):306–14. PMCID: PMC5575997. http://www.ncbi.nlm.nih.gov/pubmed/20358398.
385. Leve LD, Neiderhiser JM, Shaw DS, Ganiban J, Natsuaki MN, Reiss D. The early growth and development study: a prospective adoption study from birth through middle childhood. Twin Res Hum Genet. 2013;16(1):412–23. PMCID: PMC3572752. http://www.ncbi.nlm.nih.gov/pubmed/23218244.
386. Early Growth and Development Study: Phase II—Oregon Social Learning Center.
387. Grazioplene RG, Deyoung CG, Rogosch FA, Cicchetti D. A novel differential susceptibility gene: CHRNA4 and moderation of the effect of maltreatment on child personality. J Child Psychol Psychiatry. 2013;54(8):872–80. PMCID: PMC3608843. http://www.ncbi.nlm.nih.gov/pubmed/23240931.
388. Belsky J, Pluess M. Beyond diathesis stress: differential susceptibility to environmental influences. Psychol Bull. 2009;135(6):885–908. PMID: 19883141. http://www.ncbi.nlm.nih.gov/pubmed/19883141.
389. Sturge-Apple ML, Cicchetti D, Davies PT, Suor JH. Differential susceptibility in spillover between interparental conflict and maternal parenting practices: evidence for OXTR and 5-HTT genes. J Fam Psychol. 2012;26(3):431–42. PMCID: PMC3368084. http://www.ncbi.nlm.nih.gov/pubmed/22563705.
390. Ramchandani PG, Jzendoorn M van I, Bakermans-Kranenburg MJ. Differential susceptibility to fathers' care and involvement: the moderating effect of infant reactivity. Fam Sci. 2010;1(2):93–101. PMCID: PMC3208580. http://www.ncbi.nlm.nih.gov/pubmed/22073318.
391. Fortuna K, van Ijzendoorn MH, Mankuta D, Kaitz M, Avinun R, Ebstein RP, Knafo A. Differential genetic susceptibility to child risk at birth in predicting observed maternal behavior. PLoS One. 2011;6(5):e19765. PMCID: PMC3095622. http://www.ncbi.nlm.nih.gov/pubmed/21603618.
392. Boyce WT. Differential susceptibility of the developing brain to contextual adversity and stress. Neuropsychopharmacology.

2016;41(1):142–62. PMCID: PMC4677150. http://www.ncbi.nlm.nih.gov/pubmed/26391599.
393. Scott S, O'Connor TG. An experimental test of differential susceptibility to parenting among emotionally-dysregulated children in a randomized controlled trial for oppositional behavior. J Child Psychol Psychiatry. 2012;53(11):1184–93. PMID: 22881827. http://www.ncbi.nlm.nih.gov/pubmed/22881827.
394. Ellis BJ, Boyce WT, Belsky J, Bakermans-Kranenburg MJ, van Ijzendoorn MH. Differential susceptibility to the environment: an evolutionary--neurodevelopmental theory. Dev Psychopathol. 2011;23(1):7–28. PMID: 21262036. http://www.ncbi.nlm.nih.gov/pubmed/21262036.
395. Ellis BJ, Boyce WT. Differential susceptibility to the environment: toward an understanding of sensitivity to developmental experiences and context. Dev Psychopathol. 2011;23(1):1–5. PMID: 21262035. http://www.ncbi.nlm.nih.gov/pubmed/21262035.
396. Ellis BJ, Del Giudice M, Dishion TJ, Figueredo AJ, Gray P, Griskevicius V, Hawley PH, Jacobs WJ, James J, Volk AA, Wilson DS. The evolutionary basis of risky adolescent behavior: implications for science, policy, and practice. Dev Psychol. 2012;48(3):598–623. PMID: 22122473. http://www.ncbi.nlm.nih.gov/pubmed/22122473.
397. Bakermans-Kranenburg MJ, van Ijzendoorn MH. Differential susceptibility to rearing environment depending on dopamine-related genes: new evidence and a meta-analysis. Dev Psychopathol. 2011;23(1):39–52. PMID: 21262038. http://www.ncbi.nlm.nih.gov/pubmed/21262038.
398. Bakermans-Kranenburg MJ, Van IJzendoorn MH, Pijlman FTA, Mesman J, Juffer F. Experimental evidence for differential susceptibility: dopamine D4 receptor polymorphism (DRD4 VNTR) moderates intervention effects on toddlers' externalizing behavior in a randomized controlled trial. Dev Psychol. 2008;44(1):293–300. PMID: 18194028. http://www.ncbi.nlm.nih.gov/pubmed/18194028.
399. Boyce WT, Ellis BJ. Biological sensitivity to context: I. An evolutionary-developmental theory of the origins and functions of stress reactivity. Dev Psychopathol. 2005;17(2):271–301. PMID: 16761546. http://www.ncbi.nlm.nih.gov/pubmed/16761546.
400. Ellis BJ, Essex MJ, Boyce WT. Biological sensitivity to context: II. Empirical explorations of an evolutionary-developmental theory. Dev Psychopathol. 2005;17(2):303–28. PMID: 16761547. http://www.ncbi.nlm.nih.gov/pubmed/16761547.
401. Ellis BJ, Shirtcliff EA, Boyce WT, Deardorff J, Essex MJ. Quality of early family relationships and the timing and tempo of puberty: effects depend on biological sensitivity to context. Dev Psychopathol. 2011;23(1):85–99. PMCID: PMC3033698. http://www.ncbi.nlm.nih.gov/pubmed/21262041.
402. Gluckman PD, Hanson MA, Bateson P, Beedle AS, Law CM, Bhutta ZA, Anokhin KV, Bougnères P, Chandak GR, Dasgupta P, Smith GD, Ellison PT, Forrester TE, Gilbert SF, Jablonka E, Kaplan H, Prentice AM, Simpson SJ, Uauy R, West-Eberhard MJ. Towards a new developmental synthesis: adaptive developmental plasticity and human disease. Lancet. 2009;373(9675):1654–7. PMID: 19427960. http://www.ncbi.nlm.nih.gov/pubmed/19427960.
403. Belsky J, Steinberg L, Draper P. Childhood experience, interpersonal development, and reproductive strategy: and evolutionary theory of socialization. Child Dev. 1991;62(4):647–70. PMID: 1935336. http://www.ncbi.nlm.nih.gov/pubmed/1935336.
404. Ellis BJ. Timing of pubertal maturation in girls: an integrated life history approach. Psychol Bull. 2004;130(6):920–58. PMID: 15535743. http://www.ncbi.nlm.nih.gov/pubmed/15535743.
405. Champagne DL, Bagot RC, van Hasselt F, Ramakers G, Meaney MJ, de Kloet ER, Joëls M, Krugers H. Maternal care and hippocampal plasticity: evidence for experience-dependent structural plasticity, altered synaptic functioning, and differential responsiveness to glucocorticoids and stress. J Neurosci. 2008;28(23):6037–45. PMCID: PMC6670331. http://www.ncbi.nlm.nih.gov/pubmed/18524909.
406. Kaffman A, Meaney MJ. Neurodevelopmental sequelae of postnatal maternal care in rodents: clinical and research implications of molecular insights. J Child Psychol Psychiatry. 2007;48(3–4):224–44. PMID: 17355397. http://www.ncbi.nlm.nih.gov/pubmed/17355397.
407. Meaney MJ, Szyf M. Maternal care as a model for experience-dependent chromatin plasticity? Trends Neurosci. 2005;28(9):456–63. PMID: 16054244. http://www.ncbi.nlm.nih.gov/pubmed/16054244.
408. Bagot RC, van Hasselt FN, Champagne DL, Meaney MJ, Krugers HJ, Joëls M. Maternal care determines rapid effects of stress mediators on synaptic plasticity in adult rat hippocampal dentate gyrus. Neurobiol Learn Mem. 2009;92(3):292–300. PMID: 19292996. http://www.ncbi.nlm.nih.gov/pubmed/19292996.
409. Cameron NM, Shahrokh D, Del Corpo A, Dhir SK, Szyf M, Champagne FA, Meaney MJ. Epigenetic programming of phenotypic variations in reproductive strategies in the rat through maternal care. J Neuroendocrinol. 2008;20(6):795–801. PMID: 18513204. http://www.ncbi.nlm.nih.gov/pubmed/18513204.
410. Cameron NM, Fish EW, Meaney MJ. Maternal influences on the sexual behavior and reproductive success of the female rat. Horm Behav. 2008;54(1):178–84. PMID: 18417127. http://www.ncbi.nlm.nih.gov/pubmed/18417127.
411. Cameron NM, Champagne FA, Parent C, Fish EW, Ozaki-Kuroda K, Meaney MJ. The programming of individual differences in defensive responses and reproductive strategies in the rat through variations in maternal care. Neurosci Biobehav Rev. 2005;29(4–5):843–65. PMID: 15893378. http://www.ncbi.nlm.nih.gov/pubmed/15893378.
412. Diorio J, Meaney MJ. Maternal programming of defensive responses through sustained effects on gene expression. J Psychiatry Neurosci. 2007;32(4):275–84. PMCID: PMC1911190. http://www.ncbi.nlm.nih.gov/pubmed/17653296.
413. Mulvihill D. The health impact of childhood trauma: an interdisciplinary review, 1997-2003. Issues Compr Pediatr Nurs. 2005;28(2):115–36. PMID: 16006380 http://www.ncbi.nlm.nih.gov/pubmed/16006380.
414. Shonkoff JP, Boyce WT, McEwen BS. Neuroscience, molecular biology, and the childhood roots of health disparities: building a new framework for health promotion and disease prevention. JAMA. 2009;301(21):2252–9. PMID: 19491187. http://www.ncbi.nlm.nih.gov/pubmed/19491187.
415. Mock SE, Arai SM. Childhood trauma and chronic illness in adulthood: mental health and socioeconomic status as explanatory factors and buffers. Front Psychol. 2010;1:246. PMCID: PMC3153850. http://www.ncbi.nlm.nih.gov/pubmed/21833299.
416. Caspi A, McClay J, Moffitt TE, Mill J, Martin J, Craig IW, Taylor A, Poulton R. Role of genotype in the cycle of violence in maltreated children. Science. 2002;297(5582):851–4. PMID: 12161658. http://www.ncbi.nlm.nih.gov/pubmed/12161658.
417. Verhoeven FEA, Booij L, Kruijt AW, Cerit H, Antypa N, Does W. The effects of MAOA genotype, childhood trauma, and sex on trait and state-dependent aggression. Brain Behav. 2012;2(6):806–13. PMCID: PMC3500467. http://www.ncbi.nlm.nih.gov/pubmed/23170243.
418. Kim-Cohen J, Caspi A, Taylor A, Williams B, Newcombe R, Craig IW, Moffitt TE. MAOA, maltreatment, and gene-environment interaction predicting children's mental health: new evidence and a meta-analysis. Mol Psychiatry. 2006;11(10):903–13. PMID: 16801953. http://www.ncbi.nlm.nih.gov/pubmed/16801953.
419. Foley DL, Eaves LJ, Wormley B, Silberg JL, Maes HH, Kuhn J, Riley B. Childhood adversity, monoamine oxidase a geno-

type, and risk for conduct disorder. Arch Gen Psychiatry. 2004;61(7):738–44. PMID: 15237086. http://www.ncbi.nlm.nih.gov/pubmed/15237086.
420. Boeldt DL, Rhee SH, Dilalla LF, Mullineaux PY, Schulz-Heik RJ, Corley RP, Young SE, Hewitt JK. The association between positive parenting and externalizing behavior. Infant Child Dev. 2012;21(1):85–106. PMCID: PMC3347769. http://www.ncbi.nlm.nih.gov/pubmed/22577341.
421. Nilsson KW, Sjöberg RL, Damberg M, Leppert J, Ohrvik J, Alm PO, Lindström L, Oreland L. Role of monoamine oxidase A genotype and psychosocial factors in male adolescent criminal activity. Biol Psychiatry. 2006;59(2):121–7. PMID: 16125147. http://www.ncbi.nlm.nih.gov/pubmed/16125147.
422. Fergusson DM, Boden JM, Horwood LJ, Miller AL, Kennedy MA. MAOA, abuse exposure and antisocial behaviour: 30-year longitudinal study. Br J Psychiatry. 2011;198(6):457–63. PMCID: PMC3105117. http://www.ncbi.nlm.nih.gov/pubmed/21628708.
423. Zammit S, Owen MJ. Stressful life events, 5-HTT genotype and risk of depression. Br J Psychiatry. 2006;188:199–201. PMID: 16507957. http://www.ncbi.nlm.nih.gov/pubmed/16507957.
424. Owens M, Goodyer IM, Wilkinson P, Bhardwaj A, Abbott R, Croudace T, Dunn V, Jones PB, Walsh ND, Ban M, Sahakian BJ. 5-HTTLPR and early childhood adversities moderate cognitive and emotional processing in adolescence. PLoS One. 2012;7(11):e48482. PMCID: PMC3509124. http://www.ncbi.nlm.nih.gov/pubmed/23209555.
425. Taylor SE, Way BM, Welch WT, Hilmert CJ, Lehman BJ, Eisenberger NI. Early family environment, current adversity, the serotonin transporter promoter polymorphism, and depressive symptomatology. Biol Psychiatry. 2006;60(7):671–6. PMID: 16934775. http://www.ncbi.nlm.nih.gov/pubmed/16934775.
426. Zalsman G, Huang YY, Oquendo MA, Burke AK, Hu XZ, Brent DA, Ellis SP, Goldman D, Mann JJ. Association of a triallelic serotonin transporter gene promoter region (5-HTTLPR) polymorphism with stressful life events and severity of depression. Am J Psychiatry. 2006;163(9):1588–93. PMID: 16946185. http://www.ncbi.nlm.nih.gov/pubmed/16946185.
427. Wilhelm K, Mitchell PB, Niven H, Finch A, Wedgwood L, Scimone A, Blair IP, Parker G, Schofield PR. Life events, first depression onset and the serotonin transporter gene. Br J Psychiatry. 2006;188:210–5. PMID: 16507960. http://www.ncbi.nlm.nih.gov/pubmed/16507960.
428. Retz W, Freitag CM, Retz-Junginger P, Wenzler D, Schneider M, Kissling C, Thome J, Rösler M. A functional serotonin transporter promoter gene polymorphism increases ADHD symptoms in delinquents: interaction with adverse childhood environment. Psychiatry Res. 2008;158(2):123–31. PMID: 18155777. http://www.ncbi.nlm.nih.gov/pubmed/18155777.
429. Propper C, Willoughby M, Halpern CT, Carbone MA, Cox M. Parenting quality, DRD4, and the prediction of externalizing and internalizing behaviors in early childhood. Dev Psychobiol. 2007;49(6):619–32. PMID: 17680609. http://www.ncbi.nlm.nih.gov/pubmed/17680609.
430. Sheese BE, Voelker PM, Rothbart MK, Posner MI. Parenting quality interacts with genetic variation in dopamine receptor D4 to influence temperament in early childhood. Dev Psychopathol. 2007;19(4):1039–46. PMID: 17931433. http://www.ncbi.nlm.nih.gov/pubmed/17931433.
431. Bakermans-Kranenburg MJ, van IJzendoorn MH, Caspers K, Philibert R. DRD4 genotype moderates the impact of parental problems on unresolved loss or trauma. Attach Hum Dev. 2011;13(3):253–69. PMCID: PMC3098559. http://www.ncbi.nlm.nih.gov/pubmed/21506030.
432. Van Ijzendoorn MH, Bakermans-Kranenburg MJ. DRD4 7-repeat polymorphism moderates the association between maternal unresolved loss or trauma and infant disorganization. Attach Hum Dev. 2006;8(4):291–307. PMID: 17178609. http://www.ncbi.nlm.nih.gov/pubmed/17178609.
433. Seeger G, Schloss P, Schmidt MH, Rüter-Jungfleisch A, Henn FA. Gene-environment interaction in hyperkinetic conduct disorder (HD + CD) as indicated by season of birth variations in dopamine receptor (DRD4) gene polymorphism. Neurosci Lett. 2004;366(3):282–6. PMID: 15288435. http://www.ncbi.nlm.nih.gov/pubmed/15288435.
434. Dulac C. Brain function and chromatin plasticity. Nature. 2010;465(7299):728–35. PMCID: PMC3075582. http://www.ncbi.nlm.nih.gov/pubmed/20535202.
435. Francis DD, Szegda K, Campbell G, Martin WD, Insel TR. Epigenetic sources of behavioral differences in mice. Nat Neurosci. 2003;6(5):445–6. PMID: 12665797. http://www.ncbi.nlm.nih.gov/pubmed/12665797.
436. McMillen IC, Robinson JS. Developmental origins of the metabolic syndrome: prediction, plasticity, and programming. Physiol Rev. 2005;85(2):571–633. PMID: 15788706. http://www.ncbi.nlm.nih.gov/pubmed/15788706.
437. Geyer MA, Braff DL. Startle habituation and sensorimotor gating in schizophrenia and related animal models. Schizophr Bull. 1987;13(4):643–68. PMID: 3438708. http://www.ncbi.nlm.nih.gov/pubmed/3438708.
438. Kobayashi Y, Isa T. Sensory-motor gating and cognitive control by the brainstem cholinergic system. Neural Netw. 2002;15(4–6):731–41. PMID: 12371523. http://www.ncbi.nlm.nih.gov/pubmed/12371523.
439. Graham FK. Presidential address, 1974. The more or less startling effects of weak prestimulation. Psychophysiology. 1975;12(3):238–48. PMID: 1153628. http://www.ncbi.nlm.nih.gov/pubmed/1153628.
440. Weitzner DS, Engler-Chiurazzi EB, Kotilinek LA, Ashe KH, Reed MN. Morris water Maze test: optimization for mouse strain and testing environment. J Vis Exp. 2015;100:e52706. PMCID: PMC4545046. http://www.ncbi.nlm.nih.gov/pubmed/26132096.
441. Nekrutenko A, Li WH. Transposable elements are found in a large number of human protein-coding genes. Trends Genet. 2001;17(11):619–21. PMID: 11672845. http://www.ncbi.nlm.nih.gov/pubmed/11672845.
442. Singer T, McConnell MJ, Marchetto MCN, Coufal NG, Gage FH. LINE-1 retrotransposons: mediators of somatic variation in neuronal genomes? Trends Neurosci. 2010;33(8):345–54. PMCID: PMC2916067. http://www.ncbi.nlm.nih.gov/pubmed/20471112.
443. Nigumann P, Redik K, Mätlik K, Speek M. Many human genes are transcribed from the antisense promoter of L1 retrotransposon. Genomics. 2002;79(5):628–34. PMID: 11991712. http://www.ncbi.nlm.nih.gov/pubmed/11991712.
444. Whitelaw E, Martin DI. Retrotransposons as epigenetic mediators of phenotypic variation in mammals. Nat Genet. 2001;27(4):361–5. PMID: 11279513. http://www.ncbi.nlm.nih.gov/pubmed/11279513.
445. Waterland RA, Jirtle RL. Early nutrition, epigenetic changes at transposons and imprinted genes, and enhanced susceptibility to adult chronic diseases. Nutrition. 2004;20(1):63–8. PMID: 14698016. http://www.ncbi.nlm.nih.gov/pubmed/14698016.
446. Waterland RA, Jirtle RL. Transposable elements: targets for early nutritional effects on epigenetic gene regulation. Mol Cell Biol. 2003;23(15):5293–300. PMCID: PMC165709. http://www.ncbi.nlm.nih.gov/pubmed/12861015.
447. Huang D, Cui L, Ahmed S, Zainab F, Wu Q, Wang X, Yuan Z. An overview of epigenetic agents and natural nutrition products targeting DNA methyltransferase, histone deacetylases and microR-

NAs. Food Chem Toxicol. 2019;123:574–94. PMID: 30408543. http://www.ncbi.nlm.nih.gov/pubmed/30408543.
448. Ferguson-Smith AC. Genomic imprinting: the emergence of an epigenetic paradigm. Nat Rev Genet. 2011;12(8):565–75. PMID: 21765458. http://www.ncbi.nlm.nih.gov/pubmed/21765458.
449. Bartolomei MS. Genomic imprinting: employing and avoiding epigenetic processes. Genes Dev. 2009;23(18):2124–33. PMCID: PMC2751984. http://www.ncbi.nlm.nih.gov/pubmed/19759261.
450. Patten MM, Ross L, Curley JP, Queller DC, Bonduriansky R, Wolf JB. The evolution of genomic imprinting: theories, predictions and empirical tests. Heredity (Edinb). 2014;113(2):119–28. PMCID: PMC4105453. http://www.ncbi.nlm.nih.gov/pubmed/24755983.
451. Vasconcelos S, Ramalho C, Marques CJ, Doria S. Altered expression of epigenetic regulators and imprinted genes in human placenta and fetal tissues from second trimester spontaneous pregnancy losses. Epigenetics. 2019;14(12):1234–44. PMCID: PMC6791697. http://www.ncbi.nlm.nih.gov/pubmed/31221015.
452. Peters J. The role of genomic imprinting in biology and disease: an expanding view. Nat Rev Genet. 2014;15(8):517–30. PMID: 24958438. http://www.ncbi.nlm.nih.gov/pubmed/24958438.
453. Babak T, DeVeale B, Tsang EK, Zhou Y, Li X, Smith KS, Kukurba KR, Zhang R, Li JB, van der Kooy D, Montgomery SB, Fraser HB. Genetic conflict reflected in tissue-specific maps of genomic imprinting in human and mouse. Nat Genet. 2015;47(5):544–9. PMCID: PMC4414907. http://www.ncbi.nlm.nih.gov/pubmed/25848752.
454. Baran Y, Subramaniam M, Biton A, Tukiainen T, Tsang EK, Rivas MA, Pirinen M, Gutierrez-Arcelus M, Smith KS, Kukurba KR, Zhang R, Eng C, Torgerson DG, Urbanek C, GTEx Consortium, Li JB, Rodriguez-Santana JR, Burchard EG, Seibold MA, MacArthur DG, Montgomery SB, Zaitlen NA, Lappalainen T. The landscape of genomic imprinting across diverse adult human tissues. Genome Res. 2015;25(7):927–36. PMCID: PMC4484390. http://www.ncbi.nlm.nih.gov/pubmed/25953952.
455. Wilkinson LS, Davies W, Isles AR. Genomic imprinting effects on brain development and function. Nat Rev Neurosci. 2007;8(11):832–43. PMID: 17925812. http://www.ncbi.nlm.nih.gov/pubmed/17925812.
456. Crespi B. Genomic imprinting in the development and evolution of psychotic spectrum conditions. Biol Rev Camb Philos Soc. 2008;83(4):441–93. PMID: 18783362. http://www.ncbi.nlm.nih.gov/pubmed/18783362.
457. Kozlov SV, Bogenpohl JW, Howell MP, Wevrick R, Panda S, Hogenesch JB, Muglia LJ, Van Gelder RN, Herzog ED, Stewart CL. The imprinted gene Magel2 regulates normal circadian output. Nat Genet. 2007;39(10):1266–72. PMID: 17893678. http://www.ncbi.nlm.nih.gov/pubmed/17893678.
458. Jirtle RL, Skinner MK. Environmental epigenomics and disease susceptibility. Nat Rev Genet. 2007;8(4):253–62. PMCID: PMC5940010. http://www.ncbi.nlm.nih.gov/pubmed/17363974.
459. McCarrey JR. Distinctions between transgenerational and non-transgenerational epimutations. Mol Cell Endocrinol. 2014;398(1–2):13–23. PMID: 25079508. http://www.ncbi.nlm.nih.gov/pubmed/25079508.
460. Richards EJ. Inherited epigenetic variation--revisiting soft inheritance. Nat Rev Genet. 2006;7(5):395–401. PMID: 16534512. http://www.ncbi.nlm.nih.gov/pubmed/16534512.
461. Patisaul HB, Adewale HB. Long-term effects of environmental endocrine disruptors on reproductive physiology and behavior. Front. Behav Neurosci. 2009;3:10. PMCID: PMC2706654. http://www.ncbi.nlm.nih.gov/pubmed/19587848.
462. Whitelaw NC, Whitelaw E. Transgenerational epigenetic inheritance in health and disease. Curr Opin Genet Dev. 2008;18(3):273–9. PMID: 18662779. http://www.ncbi.nlm.nih.gov/pubmed/18662779.
463. Maier SF, Watkins LR, Fleshner M. Psychoneuroimmunology. The interface between behavior, brain, and immunity. Am Psychol. 1994;49(12):1004–17. PMID: 7818221. http://www.ncbi.nlm.nih.gov/pubmed/7818221.
464. Cohen N, Moynihan JA, Ader R. Pavlovian conditioning of the immune system. Int Arch Allergy Immunol. 1994;105(2):101–6. PMID: 7920010. http://www.ncbi.nlm.nih.gov/pubmed/7920010.
465. Yirmiya R, Pollak Y, Morag M, Reichenberg A, Barak O, Avitsur R, Shavit Y, Ovadia H, Weidenfeld J, Morag A, Newman ME, Pollmächer T. Illness, cytokines, and depression. Ann N Y Acad Sci. 2000;917:478–87. PMID: 11268375. http://www.ncbi.nlm.nih.gov/pubmed/11268375.
466. Capuron L, Hauser P, Hinze-Selch D, Miller AH, Neveu PJ. Treatment of cytokine-induced depression. Brain Behav Immun. 2002;16(5):575–80. PMID: 12401471. http://www.ncbi.nlm.nih.gov/pubmed/12401471.
467. Baik JH. Dopamine signaling in reward-related behaviors. Front Neural Circuits. 2013;7:152. PMCID: PMC3795306. http://www.ncbi.nlm.nih.gov/pubmed/24130517.
468. Mark GP, Shabani S, Dobbs LK, Hansen ST. Cholinergic modulation of mesolimbic dopamine function and reward. Physiol Behav. 2011;104(1):76–81. PMCID: PMC4495915. http://www.ncbi.nlm.nih.gov/pubmed/21549724.
469. Amir A, Lee SC, Headley DB, Herzallah MM, Pare D. Amygdala signaling during foraging in a hazardous environment. J Neurosci. 2015;35(38):12994–3005. PMCID: PMC4579372. http://www.ncbi.nlm.nih.gov/pubmed/26400931.
470. Moryś J, Berdel B, Jagalska-Majewska H, Luczyńska A. The basolateral amygdaloid complex--its development, morphology and functions. Folia Morphol (Warsz). 1999;58(3 Suppl 2):29–46. PMID: 10959259. http://www.ncbi.nlm.nih.gov/pubmed/10959259.
471. Everitt BJ, Cardinal RN, Parkinson JA, Robbins TW. Appetitive behavior: impact of amygdala-dependent mechanisms of emotional learning. Ann N Y Acad Sci. 2003;985:233–50. PMID: 12724162. http://www.ncbi.nlm.nih.gov/pubmed/12724162.
472. Ambroggi F, Ishikawa A, Fields HL, Nicola SM. Basolateral amygdala neurons facilitate reward-seeking behavior by exciting nucleus accumbens neurons. Neuron. 2008;59(4):648–61. PMCID: PMC2603341. http://www.ncbi.nlm.nih.gov/pubmed/18760700.
473. Maren S, Quirk GJ. Neuronal signalling of fear memory. Nat Rev Neurosci. 2004;5(11):844–52. PMID: 15496862. http://www.ncbi.nlm.nih.gov/pubmed/15496862.
474. Anglada-Figueroa D, Quirk GJ. Lesions of the basal amygdala block expression of conditioned fear but not extinction. J Neurosci. 2005;25(42):9680–5. PMCID: PMC6725741. http://www.ncbi.nlm.nih.gov/pubmed/16237172.
475. Duvarci S, Pare D. Amygdala microcircuits controlling learned fear. Neuron. 2014;82(5):966–80. PMCID: PMC4103014. http://www.ncbi.nlm.nih.gov/pubmed/24908482.
476. Rorick-Kehn LM, Steinmetz JE. Amygdalar unit activity during three learning tasks: eyeblink classical conditioning, Pavlovian fear conditioning, and signaled avoidance conditioning. Behav Neurosci. 2005;119(5):1254–76. PMID: 16300433. http://www.ncbi.nlm.nih.gov/pubmed/16300433.
477. Belova MA, Paton JJ, Salzman CD. Moment-to-moment tracking of state value in the amygdala. J Neurosci. 2008;28(40):10023–30. PMCID: PMC2610542. http://www.ncbi.nlm.nih.gov/pubmed/18829960.
478. Schønning K, Jansson B, Olofsson S, Nielsen JO, Hansen JS. Resistance to V3-directed neutralization caused by an N-linked oligosaccharide depends on the quaternary structure

of the HIV-1 envelope oligomer. Virology. 1996;218(1):134–40. PMID: 8615015. http://www.ncbi.nlm.nih.gov/pubmed/8615015.
479. Amano T, Duvarci S, Popa D, Paré D. The fear circuit revisited: contributions of the basal amygdala nuclei to conditioned fear. J Neurosci. 2011;31(43):15481–9. PMCID: PMC3221940. http://www.ncbi.nlm.nih.gov/pubmed/22031894.
480. Shabel SJ, Janak PH. Substantial similarity in amygdala neuronal activity during conditioned appetitive and aversive emotional arousal. Proc Natl Acad Sci U S A. 2009;106(35):15031–15036. PMCID: PMC2736461. http://www.ncbi.nlm.nih.gov/pubmed/19706473..
481. Choi JS, Kim JJ. Amygdala regulates risk of predation in rats foraging in a dynamic fear environment. Proc Natl Acad Sci USA. 2010;107(50):21773–7. PMCID: PMC3003044. http://www.ncbi.nlm.nih.gov/pubmed/21115817.
482. McKernan MG, Shinnick-Gallagher P. Fear conditioning induces a lasting potentiation of synaptic currents in vitro. Nature. 1997;390(6660):607–11. PMID: 9403689. http://www.ncbi.nlm.nih.gov/pubmed/9403689.
483. McGaugh JL. Memory consolidation and the amygdala: a systems perspective. Trends Neurosci. 2002;25(9):456. PMID: 12183206. http://www.ncbi.nlm.nih.gov/pubmed/12183206.
484. Charmandari E, Kino T, Souvatzoglou E, Chrousos GP. Pediatric stress: hormonal mediators and human development. Horm Res. 2003;59(4):161–79. PMID: 12649570. http://www.ncbi.nlm.nih.gov/pubmed/12649570.
485. Charmandari E, Tsigos C, Chrousos G. Endocrinology of the stress response. Annu Rev Physiol. 2005;67:259–84. PMID: 15709959. http://www.ncbi.nlm.nih.gov/pubmed/15709959.
486. Vaiserman AM, Koliada AK. Early-life adversity and long-term neurobehavioral outcomes: epigenome as a bridge? Hum Genomics. 2017;11(1):34. PMCID: PMC5732459. http://www.ncbi.nlm.nih.gov/pubmed/29246185.
487. Doherty TS, Roth TL. Epigenetic landscapes of the adversity-exposed brain. Prog Mol Biol Transl Sci. 2018;157:1–19. PMCID: PMC6056018. http://www.ncbi.nlm.nih.gov/pubmed/29933946.
488. Jiang S, Kamei N, Bolton JL, Ma X, Stern HS, Baram TZ, Mortazavi A. Intra-individual methylomics detects the impact of early-life adversity. Life Sci Alliance. 2019;2(2):e201800204. PMCID: PMC6445397. http://www.ncbi.nlm.nih.gov/pubmed/30936186.
489. Chrousos GP. The role of stress and the hypothalamic-pituitary-adrenal axis in the pathogenesis of the metabolic syndrome: neuro-endocrine and target tissue-related causes. Int J Obes Relat Metab Disord. 2000;24(Suppl 2):S50–5. PMID: 10997609. http://www.ncbi.nlm.nih.gov/pubmed/10997609.
490. Waterland RA, Dolinoy DC, Lin JR, Smith CA, Shi X, Tahiliani KG. Maternal methyl supplements increase offspring DNA methylation at Axin Fused. Genesis. 2006;44(9):401–6. PMID: 16868943. http://www.ncbi.nlm.nih.gov/pubmed/16868943.
491. Romeo RD, Ali FS, Karatsoreos IN, Bellani R, Chhua N, Vernov M, McEwen BS. Glucocorticoid receptor mRNA expression in the hippocampal formation of male rats before and after pubertal development in response to acute or repeated stress. Neuroendocrinology. 2008;87(3):160–7. PMID: 17923777. http://www.ncbi.nlm.nih.gov/pubmed/17923777.
492. McEwen BS. Central effects of stress hormones in health and disease: understanding the protective and damaging effects of stress and stress mediators. Eur J Pharmacol. 2008;583(2–3):174–85. PMCID: PMC2474765. http://www.ncbi.nlm.nih.gov/pubmed/18282566.
493. Meaney MJ, Szyf M. Environmental programming of stress responses through DNA methylation: life at the interface between a dynamic environment and a fixed genome. Dialogues Clin Neurosci. 2005;7(2):103–23. PMCID: PMC3181727. http://www.ncbi.nlm.nih.gov/pubmed/16262207.
494. Weaver ICG. Epigenetic effects of glucocorticoids. Semin Fetal Neonatal Med. 2009;14(3):143–50. PMID: 19217839. http://www.ncbi.nlm.nih.gov/pubmed/19217839.
495. Szyf M. The early life environment and the epigenome. Biochim Biophys Acta. 2009;1790(9):878–85. PMID: 19364482. http://www.ncbi.nlm.nih.gov/pubmed/19364482.
496. Weaver ICG. Epigenetic programming by maternal behavior and pharmacological intervention. Nature versus nurture: let's call the whole thing off. Epigenetics. 2007;2(1):22–8. PMID: 17965624. http://www.ncbi.nlm.nih.gov/pubmed/17965624.
497. Weaver ICG, D'Alessio AC, Brown SE, Hellstrom IC, Dymov S, Sharma S, Szyf M, Meaney MJ. The transcription factor nerve growth factor-inducible protein a mediates epigenetic programming: altering epigenetic marks by immediate-early genes. J Neurosci. 2007;27(7):1756–68. PMCID: PMC2951014. http://www.ncbi.nlm.nih.gov/pubmed/17301183.
498. Oberlander TF, Weinberg J, Papsdorf M, Grunau R, Misri S, Devlin AM. Prenatal exposure to maternal depression, neonatal methylation of human glucocorticoid receptor gene (NR3C1) and infant cortisol stress responses. Epigenetics. 2008;3(2):97–106. PMID: 18536531. http://www.ncbi.nlm.nih.gov/pubmed/18536531.
499. MacMillan HL, Georgiades K, Duku EK, Shea A, Steiner M, Niec A, Tanaka M, Gensey S, Spree S, Vella E, Walsh CA, De Bellis MD, Van der Meulen J, Boyle MH, Schmidt LA. Cortisol response to stress in female youths exposed to childhood maltreatment: results of the youth mood project. Biol Psychiatry. 2009;66(1):62–8. PMCID: PMC3816014. http://www.ncbi.nlm.nih.gov/pubmed/19217075.
500. De Bellis MD. Developmental traumatology: a contributory mechanism for alcohol and substance use disorders. Psychoneuroendocrinology. 2002;27(1–2):155–70. PMID: 11750776. http://www.ncbi.nlm.nih.gov/pubmed/11750776.
501. Heim C, Plotsky PM, Nemeroff CB. Importance of studying the contributions of early adverse experience to neurobiological findings in depression. Neuropsychopharmacology. 2004;29(4):641–8. PMID: 15034558. http://www.ncbi.nlm.nih.gov/pubmed/15034558.
502. King S, Laplante D, Joober R. Understanding putative risk factors for schizophrenia: retrospective and prospective studies. J Psychiatry Neurosci. 2005;30(5):342–8. PMCID: PMC1197279. http://www.ncbi.nlm.nih.gov/pubmed/16151539.
503. Lupien SJ, McEwen BS, Gunnar MR, Heim C. Effects of stress throughout the lifespan on the brain, behaviour and cognition. Nat Rev Neurosci. 2009;10(6):434–45. PMID: 19401723. http://www.ncbi.nlm.nih.gov/pubmed/19401723.
504. Liu D, Diorio J, Tannenbaum B, Caldji C, Francis D, Freedman A, Sharma S, Pearson D, Plotsky PM, Meaney MJ. Maternal care, hippocampal glucocorticoid receptors, and hypothalamic-pituitary-adrenal responses to stress. Science. 1997;277(5332):1659–62. PMID: 9287218. http://www.ncbi.nlm.nih.gov/pubmed/9287218.
505. Schlotz W, Phillips DIW. Fetal origins of mental health: evidence and mechanisms. Brain Behav Immun. 2009;23(7):905–16. PMID: 19217937. http://www.ncbi.nlm.nih.gov/pubmed/19217937.
506. Hackman DA, Farah MJ, Meaney MJ. Socioeconomic status and the brain: mechanistic insights from human and animal research. Nat Rev Neurosci. 2010;11(9):651–9. PMCID: PMC2950073. http://www.ncbi.nlm.nih.gov/pubmed/20725096.
507. Mathews HL, Janusek LW. Epigenetics and psychoneuroimmunology: mechanisms and models. Brain Behav Immun. 2011;25(1):25–39. PMCID: PMC2991515. http://www.ncbi.nlm.nih.gov/pubmed/20832468.
508. Simmons R. Epigenetics and maternal nutrition: nature v. nurture. Proc Nutr Soc. 2011;70(1):73–81. PMID: 21110912. http://www.ncbi.nlm.nih.gov/pubmed/21110912.

509. Dominguez-Salas P, Cox SE, Prentice AM, Hennig BJ, Moore SE. Maternal nutritional status, C(1) metabolism and offspring DNA methylation: a review of current evidence in human subjects. Proc Nutr Soc. 2012;71(1):154–65. PMCID: PMC3491641. http://www.ncbi.nlm.nih.gov/pubmed/22124338.
510. Li M, Sloboda DM, Vickers MH. Maternal obesity and developmental programming of metabolic disorders in offspring: evidence from animal models. Exp Diabetes Res. 2011;2011:592408. PMCID: PMC3182397. http://www.ncbi.nlm.nih.gov/pubmed/21969822.
511. Zeisel SH. Choline, homocysteine, and pregnancy. Am J Clin Nutr. 2005;82(4):719–20. PMID: 16210698. http://www.ncbi.nlm.nih.gov/pubmed/16210698.
512. Zeisel SH. Genetic polymorphisms in methyl-group metabolism and epigenetics: lessons from humans and mouse models. Brain Res. 2008;1237:5–11. PMCID: PMC2587491. http://www.ncbi.nlm.nih.gov/pubmed/18789905.
513. Devlin AM, Brain U, Austin J, Oberlander TF. Prenatal exposure to maternal depressed mood and the MTHFR C677T variant affect SLC6A4 methylation in infants at birth. PLoS One. 2010;5(8):e12201. PMCID: PMC2922376. http://www.ncbi.nlm.nih.gov/pubmed/20808944.
514. Hoffman RE, McGlashan TH. Synaptic elimination, neurodevelopment, and the mechanism of hallucinated "voices" in schizophrenia. Am J Psychiatry. 1997;154(12):1683–9. PMID: 9396946. http://www.ncbi.nlm.nih.gov/pubmed/9396946.
515. Purves D, Lichtman JW. Elimination of synapses in the developing nervous system. Science. 1980;210(4466):153–7. PMID: 7414326. http://www.ncbi.nlm.nih.gov/pubmed/7414326.
516. Riccomagno MM, Kolodkin AL. Sculpting neural circuits by axon and dendrite pruning. Annu Rev Cell Dev Biol. 2015;31:779–805. PMCID: PMC4668927. http://www.ncbi.nlm.nih.gov/pubmed/26436703.
517. Low LK, Cheng HJ. Axon pruning: an essential step underlying the developmental plasticity of neuronal connections. Philos Trans R Soc Lond Ser B Biol Sci. 2006;361(1473):1531–44. PMCID: PMC1664669. http://www.ncbi.nlm.nih.gov/pubmed/16939973.
518. Lendvai B, Stern EA, Chen B, Svoboda K. Experience-dependent plasticity of dendritic spines in the developing rat barrel cortex in vivo. Nature. 2000;404(6780):876–81. PMID: 10786794. http://www.ncbi.nlm.nih.gov/pubmed/10786794.
519. Trachtenberg JT, Chen BE, Knott GW, Feng G, Sanes JR, Welker E, Svoboda K. Long-term in vivo imaging of experience-dependent synaptic plasticity in adult cortex. Nature. 2002;420(6917):788–94. PMID: 12490942. http://www.ncbi.nlm.nih.gov/pubmed/12490942.
520. Zuo Y, Lin A, Chang P, Gan WB. Development of long-term dendritic spine stability in diverse regions of cerebral cortex. Neuron. 2005;46(2):181–9. PMID: 15848798. http://www.ncbi.nlm.nih.gov/pubmed/15848798.
521. Ortega F, Costa MR. Live imaging of adult neural stem cells in rodents. Front Neurosci. 2016;10:78. PMCID: PMC4779908. http://www.ncbi.nlm.nih.gov/pubmed/27013941.
522. Winkle CC, Gupton SL. Membrane trafficking in neuronal development: ins and outs of neural connectivity. Int Rev Cell Mol Biol. 2016;322:247–80. PMCID: PMC4797321. http://www.ncbi.nlm.nih.gov/pubmed/26940520.
523. Miner D, Triesch J. Plasticity-driven self-organization under topological constraints accounts for non-random features of cortical synaptic wiring. PLoS Comput Biol. 2016;12(2):e1004759. PMCID: PMC4750861. http://www.ncbi.nlm.nih.gov/pubmed/26866369.
524. Jasinska M, Siucinska E, Jasek E, Litwin JA, Pyza E, Kossut M. Effect of associative learning on memory spine formation in Mouse Barrel Cortex. Neural Plast. 2016;2016:9828517. PMCID: PMC4706958. http://www.ncbi.nlm.nih.gov/pubmed/26819780.
525. Hoffman RE, Hampson M. Functional connectivity studies of patients with auditory verbal hallucinations. Front Hum Neurosci. 2011;6:6. PMCID: PMC3269039. http://www.ncbi.nlm.nih.gov/pubmed/22375109.
526. Ihara K, Morgan C, Fearon P, Dazzan P, Demjaha A, Lloyd T, Kirkbride JB, Hayhurst H, Murray RM, Jones PB. The prevalence, diagnostic significance and demographic characteristics of Schneiderian first-rank symptoms in an epidemiological sample of first-episode psychoses. Psychopathology. 2009;42(2):81–91. PMID: 19225242. http://www.ncbi.nlm.nih.gov/pubmed/19225242.
527. Paterson NE, Markou A. Animal models and treatments for addiction and depression co-morbidity. Neurotox Res. 2007;11(1):1–32. PMID: 17449445. http://www.ncbi.nlm.nih.gov/pubmed/17449445.
528. Flórez KR, Dubowitz T, Ghosh-Dastidar MB, Beckman R, Collins RL. Associations between depressive symptomatology, diet, and body mass index among participants in the supplemental nutrition assistance program. J Acad Nutr Diet. 2015;115(7):1102–8. PMCID: PMC4484316. http://www.ncbi.nlm.nih.gov/pubmed/25769748.
529. Lalanne L, Ayranci G, Kieffer BL, Lutz PE. The kappa opioid receptor: from addiction to depression, and back. Front Psych. 2014;5:170. PMCID: PMC4258993. http://www.ncbi.nlm.nih.gov/pubmed/25538632.
530. Treadway MT, Zald DH. Reconsidering anhedonia in depression: lessons from translational neuroscience. Neurosci Biobehav Rev. 2011;35(3):537–55. PMCID: PMC3005986. http://www.ncbi.nlm.nih.gov/pubmed/20603146.
531. Mineur YS, Picciotto MR. Biological basis for the co-morbidity between smoking and mood disorders. J Dual Diagn. 2009;5(2):122–30. PMCID: PMC2707026. http://www.ncbi.nlm.nih.gov/pubmed/20046987.
532. Filip M, Frankowska M, Jastrzębska J, Wydra K, Przegaliński E. Preclinical studies on comorbidity between depression and psychostimulant addiction. Pharmacol Rep. 2013;65(6):1529–34. PMID: 24553001. http://www.ncbi.nlm.nih.gov/pubmed/24553001.
533. Slavich GM, Irwin MR. From stress to inflammation and major depressive disorder: a social signal transduction theory of depression. Psychol Bull. 2014;140(3):774–815. PMCID: PMC4006295. http://www.ncbi.nlm.nih.gov/pubmed/24417575.
534. Preiss K, Brennan L, Clarke D. A systematic review of variables associated with the relationship between obesity and depression. Obes Rev. 2013;14(11):906–18. PMID: 23809142. http://www.ncbi.nlm.nih.gov/pubmed/23809142.
535. Symposium on Lipid Abnormalities in Renal Diseases. Sardinia, Italy, 1990. Kidney Int Suppl. 1991;31:S1–72. PMID: 2046264. http://www.ncbi.nlm.nih.gov/pubmed/2046264.
536. Frith C. The psychology of volition. Exp Brain Res. 2013;229(3):289–99. PMCID: PMC3745827. http://www.ncbi.nlm.nih.gov/pubmed/23354664.
537. Brembs B. Towards a scientific concept of free will as a biological trait: spontaneous actions and decision-making in invertebrates. Proc Biol Sci. 2011;278(1707):930–9. PMCID: PMC3049057. http://www.ncbi.nlm.nih.gov/pubmed/21159679.
538. Zhu J. Locating volition. Conscious Cogn. 2004;13(2):302–22. PMID: 15134762. http://www.ncbi.nlm.nih.gov/pubmed/15134762.
539. What is VOLITION? definition of VOLITION (Psychology Dictionary).
540. Fried I, Mukamel R, Kreiman G. Internally generated preactivation of single neurons in human medial frontal cortex predicts

volition. Neuron. 2011;69(3):548–62. PMCID: PMC3052770. http://www.ncbi.nlm.nih.gov/pubmed/21315264.
541. Haggard P. Human volition: towards a neuroscience of will. Nat Rev Neurosci. 2008;9(12):934–46. PMID: 19020512. http://www.ncbi.nlm.nih.gov/pubmed/19020512.
542. Nachev P, Rees G, Parton A, Kennard C, Husain M. Volition and conflict in human medial frontal cortex. Curr Biol. 2005;15(2):122–8. PMCID: PMC2648721. http://www.ncbi.nlm.nih.gov/pubmed/15668167.
543. Kranick SM, Hallett M. Neurology of volition. Exp Brain Res. 2013;229(3):313–27. PMCID: PMC4744643. http://www.ncbi.nlm.nih.gov/pubmed/23329204.
544. Gardner B. A review and analysis of the use of "habit" in understanding, predicting and influencing health-related behaviour. Health. Psychol Rev. 2015;9(3):277–95. PMCID: PMC4566897. http://www.ncbi.nlm.nih.gov/pubmed/25207647.
545. Oluka OC, Nie S, Sun Y. Quality assessment of TPB-based questionnaires: a systematic review. PLoS One. 2014;9(4):e94419. PMCID: PMC3983195. http://www.ncbi.nlm.nih.gov/pubmed/24722323.
546. Ajzen I. The theory of planned behaviour: reactions and reflections. Psychol Health. 2011;26(9):1113–27. PMID: 21929476. http://www.ncbi.nlm.nih.gov/pubmed/21929476.
547. Chatzisarantis NLD, Hagger MS, Kamarova S, Kawabata M. When effects of the universal psychological need for autonomy on health behaviour extend to a large proportion of individuals: a field experiment. Br J Health Psychol. 2012;17(4):785–97. PMID: 22515432. http://www.ncbi.nlm.nih.gov/pubmed/22515432.
548. Hagger MS, Chatzisarantis NLD. Integrating the theory of planned behaviour and self-determination theory in health behaviour: a meta-analysis. Br J Health Psychol. 2009;14(Pt 2):275–302. PMID: 18926008. http://www.ncbi.nlm.nih.gov/pubmed/18926008.
549. Moustaka FC, Vlachopoulos SP, Kabitsis C, Theodorakis Y. Effects of an autonomy-supportive exercise instructing style on exercise motivation, psychological well-being, and exercise attendance in middle-age women. J Phys Act Health. 2012;9(1):138–50. PMID: 22232500. http://www.ncbi.nlm.nih.gov/pubmed/22232500.
550. Silva MN, Vieira PN, Coutinho SR, Minderico CS, Matos MG, Sardinha LB, Teixeira PJ. Using self-determination theory to promote physical activity and weight control: a randomized controlled trial in women. J Behav Med. 2010;33(2):110–22. PMID: 20012179. http://www.ncbi.nlm.nih.gov/pubmed/20012179.
551. Pavey LJ, Sparks P. Autonomy and reactions to health-risk information. Psychol Health. 2010;25(7):885–72. PMID: 20204958. http://www.ncbi.nlm.nih.gov/pubmed/20204958.
552. Presseau J, Tait RI, Johnston DW, Francis JJ, Sniehotta FF. Goal conflict and goal facilitation as predictors of daily accelerometer-assessed physical activity. Health Psychol. 2013;32(12):1179–87. PMID: 22888818. http://www.ncbi.nlm.nih.gov/pubmed/22888818.
553. Hofmann W, Friese M, Strack F. Impulse and self-control from a dual-systems perspective. Perspect Psychol Sci. 2009;4(2):162–76. PMID: 26158943. http://www.ncbi.nlm.nih.gov/pubmed/26158943.
554. Hofmann W, Friese M. Impulses got the better of me: alcohol moderates the influence of implicit attitudes toward food cues on eating behavior. J Abnorm Psychol. 2008;117(2):420–7. PMID: 18489218. http://www.ncbi.nlm.nih.gov/pubmed/18489218.
555. Hofmann W, Gschwendner T, Friese M, Wiers RW, Schmitt M. Working memory capacity and self-regulatory behavior: toward an individual differences perspective on behavior determination by automatic versus controlled processes. J Pers Soc Psychol. 2008;95(4):962–77. PMID: 18808271. http://www.ncbi.nlm.nih.gov/pubmed/18808271.
556. Sheeran P, Webb TL, Gollwitzer PM. The interplay between goal intentions and implementation intentions. Personal Soc Psychol Bull. 2005;31(1):87–98. PMID: 15574664. http://www.ncbi.nlm.nih.gov/pubmed/15574664.
557. Sheeran P, Harris P, Vaughan J, Oettingen G, Gollwitzer PM. Gone exercising: mental contrasting promotes physical activity among overweight, middle-aged, low-SES fishermen. Health Psychol. 2013;32(7):802–9. PMID: 22888817. http://www.ncbi.nlm.nih.gov/pubmed/22888817.
558. Lippke S, Fleig L, Wiedemann AU, Schwarzer R. A computerized lifestyle application to promote multiple health behaviors at the workplace: testing its behavioral and psychological effects. J Med Internet Res. 2015;17(10):e225. PMCID: PMC4642394. http://www.ncbi.nlm.nih.gov/pubmed/26429115.
559. Hardcastle SJ, Hancox J, Hattar A, Maxwell-Smith C, Thøgersen-Ntoumani C, Hagger MS. Motivating the unmotivated: how can health behavior be changed in those unwilling to change? Front Psychol. 2015;6:835. PMCID: PMC446835. http://www.ncbi.nlm.nih.gov/pubmed/26136716.
560. Hagger MS, Wood C, Stiff C, Chatzisarantis NLD. Ego depletion and the strength model of self-control: a meta-analysis. Psychol Bull. 2010;136(4):495–525. PMID: 20565167. http://www.ncbi.nlm.nih.gov/pubmed/20565167.
561. Hagger MS, Luszczynska A. Implementation intention and action planning interventions in health contexts: state of the research and proposals for the way forward. Appl Psychol Health Well Being. 2014;6(1):1–47. PMID: 24591064. http://www.ncbi.nlm.nih.gov/pubmed/24591064.
562. Ronda G, Van Assema P, Brug J. Stages of change, psychological factors and awareness of physical activity levels in The Netherlands. Health Promot Int. 2001;16(4):305–14. PMID: 11733449. http://www.ncbi.nlm.nih.gov/pubmed/11733449.
563. Rhodes RE, de Bruijn GJ. How big is the physical activity intention-behaviour gap? A meta-analysis using the action control framework. Br J Health Psychol. 2013;18(2):296–309. PMID: 23480428. http://www.ncbi.nlm.nih.gov/pubmed/23480428.
564. Wewers ME, Stillman FA, Hartman AM, Shopland DR. Distribution of daily smokers by stage of change: current population survey results. Prev Med. 2003;36(6):710–20. PMID: 12744915. http://www.ncbi.nlm.nih.gov/pubmed/12744915.
565. Centers for Disease Control and Prevention (CDC). Cigarette smoking among adults--United States, 2006. MMWR Morb Mortal Wkly Rep. 2007;56(44):1157–1161. PMID: 17989644. http://www.ncbi.nlm.nih.gov/pubmed/17989644.
566. Daoud N, Hayek S, Sheikh Muhammad A, Abu-Saad K, Osman A, Thrasher JF, Kalter-Leibovici O. Stages of change of the readiness to quit smoking among a random sample of minority Arab male smokers in Israel. BMC Public Health. 2015;15:672. PMCID: PMC4607270. http://www.ncbi.nlm.nih.gov/pubmed/26178347.
567. Prochaska JO, Velicer WF, Redding C, Rossi JS, Goldstein M, DePue J, Greene GW, Rossi SR, Sun X, Fava JL, Laforge R, Rakowski W, Plummer BA. Stage-based expert systems to guide a population of primary care patients to quit smoking, eat healthier, prevent skin cancer, and receive regular mammograms. Prev Med. 2005;41(2):406–16. PMID: 15896835. http://www.ncbi.nlm.nih.gov/pubmed/15896835.
568. Thøgersen-Ntoumani C, Ntoumanis N. The role of self-determined motivation in the understanding of exercise-related behaviours, cognitions and physical self-evaluations. J Sports Sci. 2006;24(4):393–404. PMID: 16492603. http://www.ncbi.nlm.nih.gov/pubmed/16492603.
569. Vlachopoulos SP, Gigoudi MA. Why don't you exercise? Development of the amotivation toward exercise scale among older

inactive individuals. J Aging Phys Act. 2008;16(3):316–41. PMID: 18660553. http://www.ncbi.nlm.nih.gov/pubmed/18660553.
570. Prochaska JO, DiClemente CC, Norcross JC. In search of how people change. Applications to addictive behaviors. Am Psychol. 1992;47(9):1102–14. PMID: 1329589. http://www.ncbi.nlm.nih.gov/pubmed/1329589.
571. Burbank PM, Padula CA, Nigg CR. Changing health behaviors of older adults. J Gerontol Nurs. 2000;26(3):26–33; quiz 52–53. PMID: 11111628. http://www.ncbi.nlm.nih.gov/pubmed/11111628.
572. Prochaska JO, Velicer WF, Rossi JS, Goldstein MG, Marcus BH, Rakowski W, Fiore C, Harlow LL, Redding CA, Rosenbloom D. Stages of change and decisional balance for 12 problem behaviors. Health Psychol. 1994;13(1):39–46. PMID: 8168470. http://www.ncbi.nlm.nih.gov/pubmed/8168470.
573. Prochaska JO, DiClemente CC. Stages and processes of self-change of smoking: toward an integrative model of change. J Consult Clin Psychol. 1983;51(3):390–5. PMID: 6863699. http://www.ncbi.nlm.nih.gov/pubmed/6863699.
574. Nigg CR, Burbank PM, Padula C, Dufresne R, Rossi JS, Velicer WF, Laforge RG, Prochaska JO. Stages of change across ten health risk behaviors for older adults. Gerontologist. 1999;39(4):473–82. PMID: 10495586. http://www.ncbi.nlm.nih.gov/pubmed/10495586.
575. Community-level HIV intervention in 5 cities: final outcome data from the CDC AIDS Community Demonstration Projects. Am J Public Health. 1999;89(3):336–45. PMCID: PMC1508588. http://www.ncbi.nlm.nih.gov/pubmed/10076482.
576. Blaney CL, Robbins ML, Paiva AL, Redding CA, Rossi JS, Blissmer B, Burditt C, Oatley K. Validation of the measures of the transtheoretical model for exercise in an adult African-American sample. Am J Health Promot. 2012;26(5):317–26. PMID: 22548428. http://www.ncbi.nlm.nih.gov/pubmed/22548428.
577. Ott U, Stanford JB, Greenwood JLJ, Murtaugh MA, Gren LH, Thiese MS, Hegmann KT. Stages of weight change among an occupational cohort. J Occup Environ Med. 2015;57(3):270–6. PMID: 25742533. http://www.ncbi.nlm.nih.gov/pubmed/25742533.
578. Prochaska JO, Redding CA, Harlow LL, Rossi JS, Velicer WF. The transtheoretical model of change and HIV prevention: a review. Health Educ Q. 1994;21(4):471–86. PMID: 7843978. http://www.ncbi.nlm.nih.gov/pubmed/7843978.
579. Plummer BA, Velicer WF, Redding CA, Prochaska JO, Rossi JS, Pallonen UE, Meier KS. Stage of change, decisional balance, and temptations for smoking: measurement and validation in a large, school-based population of adolescents. Addict Behav. 2001;26(4):551–71. PMID: 11456077. http://www.ncbi.nlm.nih.gov/pubmed/11456077.
580. Horowitz SM. Applying the transtheoretical model to pregnancy and STD prevention: a review of the literature. Am J Health Promot. 2003;17(5):304–28. PMID: 12769045. http://www.ncbi.nlm.nih.gov/pubmed/12769045.
581. Adams J, White M. Are activity promotion interventions based on the transtheoretical model effective? A critical review. Br J Sports Med. 2003;37(2):106–14. PMCID: PMC1724627. http://www.ncbi.nlm.nih.gov/pubmed/12663350.
582. Burbank PM, Reibe D, Padula CA, Nigg C. Exercise and older adults: changing behavior with the transtheoretical model. Orthop Nurs. 2002;21(4):51–61; quiz 61–63. PMID: 12224187. http://www.ncbi.nlm.nih.gov/pubmed/12224187.
583. A clinical practice guideline for treating tobacco use and dependence: a US Public Health service report. The tobacco use and dependence clinical practice guideline panel, staff, and consortium representatives. JAMA. 2000;283(24):3244–54. PMID: 10866874. http://www.ncbi.nlm.nih.gov/pubmed/10866874.
584. Gökbayrak NS, Paiva AL, Blissmer BJ, Prochaska JO. Predictors of relapse among smokers: transtheoretical effort variables, demographics, and smoking severity. Addict Behav. 2015;42:176–9. PMCID: PMC4272892. http://www.ncbi.nlm.nih.gov/pubmed/25481450.
585. Velicer WF, Norman GJ, Fava JL, Prochaska JO. Testing 40 predictions from the transtheoretical model. Addict Behav. 1999;24(4):455–69. PMID: 10466842. http://www.ncbi.nlm.nih.gov/pubmed/10466842.
586. Finckenor M, Byrd-Bredbenner C. Nutrition intervention group program based on preaction-stage-oriented change processes of the Transtheoretical Model promotes long-term reduction in dietary fat intake. J Am Diet Assoc. 2000;100(3):335–42. PMID: 10719408. http://www.ncbi.nlm.nih.gov/pubmed/10719408.
587. Comprehensive Cancer Information - NCI.
588. Daniels J, Farquhar C, Nathanson N, Mashalla Y, Petracca F, Desmond M, Green W, Davies L, O'Malley G. Afya Bora Consortium Working Group Members, Afya Bora Consortium Working Group Members. Training tomorrow's global health leaders: applying a transtheoretical model to identify behavior change stages within an intervention for health leadership development. Glob. Health Promot. 2014;21(4):24–34. PMID: 24763665. http://www.ncbi.nlm.nih.gov/pubmed/24763665.
589. Werch CE, Ames S, Moore MJ, Thombs D, Hart A. Health behavior insights: the transtheoretical/stages of change model: Carlo C. DiClemente, PhD. Health Promot Pract. 2009;10(1):41–8. PMID: 19116432. http://www.ncbi.nlm.nih.gov/pubmed/19116432.
590. Prochaska JO, Velicer WF. The transtheoretical model of health behavior change. Am J Health Promot. 1997;12(1):38–48. PMID: 10170434. http://www.ncbi.nlm.nih.gov/pubmed/10170434.
591. Bandura A. The anatomy of stages of change. Am J Health Promot. 1997;12(1):8–10. PMID: 10170438. http://www.ncbi.nlm.nih.gov/pubmed/10170438.
592. Levinson W, Cohen MS, Brady D, Duffy FD. To change or not to change: "Sounds like you have a dilemma". Ann Intern Med. 2001;135(5):386–91. PMID: 11529714. http://www.ncbi.nlm.nih.gov/pubmed/11529714.
593. Son HM. Differences in processes of change, decisional balance, and temptation across the stages of change for smoking cessation. Taehan Kanho Hakhoe Chi. 2005;35(5):904–13. PMID: 16208086. http://www.ncbi.nlm.nih.gov/pubmed/16208086.
594. Fiore MC. US public health service clinical practice guideline: treating tobacco use and dependence. Respir Care. 2000;45(10):1200–62. PMID: 11054899. http://www.ncbi.nlm.nih.gov/pubmed/11054899.
595. Bandura A. The assessment and predictive generality of self-percepts of efficacy. J Behav Ther Exp Psychiatry. 1982;13(3):195–9. PMID: 7142408. http://www.ncbi.nlm.nih.gov/pubmed/7142408.
596. Bandura A. Self-efficacy: toward a unifying theory of behavioral change. Psychol Rev. 1977;84(2):191–215. PMID: 847061. http://www.ncbi.nlm.nih.gov/pubmed/847061.
597. Bandura A, Caprara GV, Barbaranelli C, Gerbino M, Pastorelli C. Role of affective self-regulatory efficacy in diverse spheres of psychosocial functioning. Child Dev. 2003;74(3):769–82. PMID: 12795389. http://www.ncbi.nlm.nih.gov/pubmed/12795389.
598. Bandura A, Pastorelli C, Barbaranelli C, Caprara GV. Self-efficacy pathways to childhood depression. J Pers Soc Psychol. 1999;76(2):258–69. PMID: 10074708. http://www.ncbi.nlm.nih.gov/pubmed/10074708.
599. Bandura A, O'Leary A, Taylor CB, Gauthier J, Gossard D. Perceived self-efficacy and pain control: opioid and nonopioid mechanisms. J Pers Soc Psychol. 1987;53(3):563–71. PMID: 2821217. http://www.ncbi.nlm.nih.gov/pubmed/2821217.
600. Hawkins RM. Self-efficacy: a predictor but not a cause of behavior. J Behav Ther Exp Psychiatry. 1992;23(4):251–6. PMID: 1302251. http://www.ncbi.nlm.nih.gov/pubmed/1302251.

601. Cassidy CA. Facilitating behavior change. Use of the transtheoretical model in the occupational health setting. AAOHN J. 1997;45(5):239–46. PMID: 9171529. http://www.ncbi.nlm.nih.gov/pubmed/9171529.
602. Callaghan RC, Herzog TA. The relation between processes-of-change and stage-transition in smoking behavior: a two-year longitudinal test of the Transtheoretical Model. Addict Behav. 2006;31(8):1331–45. PMID: 16337342. http://www.ncbi.nlm.nih.gov/pubmed/16337342.
603. DiClemente CC, Prochaska JO. Self-change and therapy change of smoking behavior: a comparison of processes of change in cessation and maintenance. Addict Behav. 1982;7(2):133–42. PMID: 7102444. http://www.ncbi.nlm.nih.gov/pubmed/7102444.
604. Strecher VJ, DeVellis BM, Becker MH, Rosenstock IM. The role of self-efficacy in achieving health behavior change. Health Educ Q. 1986;13(1):73–92. PMID: 3957687. http://www.ncbi.nlm.nih.gov/pubmed/3957687.
605. Song KJ. The effects of self-efficacy promoting cardiac rehabilitation program on self-efficacy, health behavior, and quality of life. Taehan Kanho Hakhoe Chi. 2003;33(4):510–8. PMID: 15314427. http://www.ncbi.nlm.nih.gov/pubmed/15314427.
606. O'Hea EL, Boudreaux ED, Jeffries SK, Carmack Taylor CL, Scarinci IC, Brantley PJ. Stage of change movement across three health behaviors: the role of self-efficacy. Am J Health Promot. 2004;19(2):94–102. PMID: 15559709. http://www.ncbi.nlm.nih.gov/pubmed/15559709.
607. Andrew S. Self-efficacy as a predictor of academic performance in science. J Adv Nurs. 1998;27(3):596–603. PMID: 9543047. http://www.ncbi.nlm.nih.gov/pubmed/9543047.
608. Bandura A, Barbaranelli C, Caprara GV, Pastorelli C. Multifaceted impact of self-efficacy beliefs on academic functioning. Child Dev. 1996;67(3):1206–22. PMID: 8706518. http://www.ncbi.nlm.nih.gov/pubmed/8706518.
609. Marks R, Allegrante JP, Lorig K. A review and synthesis of research evidence for self-efficacy-enhancing interventions for reducing chronic disability: implications for health education practice (part II). Health Promot Pract. 2005;6(2):148–56. PMID: 15855284. http://www.ncbi.nlm.nih.gov/pubmed/15855284.
610. Bandura A, Adams NE, Beyer J. Cognitive processes mediating behavioral change. J Pers Soc Psychol. 1977;35(3):125–39. PMID: 15093. http://www.ncbi.nlm.nih.gov/pubmed/15093.
611. Islam KF, Awal A, Mazumder H, Munni UR, Majumder K, Afroz K, Tabassum MN, Hossain MM. Social cognitive theory-based health promotion in primary care practice: a scoping review. Heliyon. 2023;9(4):e14889. PMCID: PMC10070720. http://www.ncbi.nlm.nih.gov/pubmed/37025832.
612. Why the Mirror Neurons Cannot Support Action Understanding | Neurophysiology.
613. DiClemente CC, Schlundt D, Gemmell L. Readiness and stages of change in addiction treatment. Am J Addict. 2004;13(2):103–19. PMID: 15204662. http://www.ncbi.nlm.nih.gov/pubmed/15204662.
614. Prochaska JO, DiClemente CC, Velicer WF, Ginpil S, Norcross JC. Predicting change in smoking status for self-changers. Addict Behav. 1985;10(4):395–406. PMID: 4091072. http://www.ncbi.nlm.nih.gov/pubmed/4091072.
615. Ceccarini M, Borrello M, Pietrabissa G, Manzoni GM, Castelnuovo G. Assessing motivation and readiness to change for weight management and control: an in-depth evaluation of three sets of instruments. Front Psychol. 2015;6:511. PMCID: PMC4426708. http://www.ncbi.nlm.nih.gov/pubmed/26029126.
616. van Leer E, Hapner ER, Connor NP. Transtheoretical model of health behavior change applied to voice therapy. J Voice. 2008;22(6):688–98. PMCID: PMC2904548. http://www.ncbi.nlm.nih.gov/pubmed/18082367.
617. Dijkstra A, Conijn B, De Vries H. A match-mismatch test of a stage model of behaviour change in tobacco smoking. Addiction. 2006;101(7):1035–43. PMID: 16771895. http://www.ncbi.nlm.nih.gov/pubmed/16771895.
618. Ashford S, Edmunds J, French DP. What is the best way to change self-efficacy to promote lifestyle and recreational physical activity? A systematic review with meta-analysis. Br J Health Psychol. 2010;15(Pt 2):265–88. PMID: 19586583. http://www.ncbi.nlm.nih.gov/pubmed/19586583.
619. Williams SL, French DP. What are the most effective intervention techniques for changing physical activity self-efficacy and physical activity behaviour--and are they the same? Health Educ Res. 2011;26(2):308–22. PMID: 21321008. http://www.ncbi.nlm.nih.gov/pubmed/21321008.
620. Mann DD, Eland DC. Self-efficacy in mastery learning to apply a therapeutic psychomotor skill. Percept Mot Skills. 2005;100(1):77–84. PMID: 15773696. http://www.ncbi.nlm.nih.gov/pubmed/15773696.
621. Majer JM, Jason LA, Ferrari JR, Olson BD, North CS. Is self-mastery always a helpful resource? Coping wiith paradoxical findings in relation to optimism and abstinence self-efficacy. Am J Drug Alcohol Abuse. 2003;29(2):385–99. PMID: 12765212. http://www.ncbi.nlm.nih.gov/pubmed/12765212.
622. Behrman A. Facilitating behavioral change in voice therapy: the relevance of motivational interviewing. Am J Speech Lang Pathol. 2006;15(3):215–25. PMID: 16896171. http://www.ncbi.nlm.nih.gov/pubmed/16896171.
623. Levesque DA, Van Marter DF, Schneider RJ, Bauer MR, Goldberg DN, Prochaska JO, Prochaska JM. Randomized trial of a computer-tailored intervention for patients with depression. Am J Health Promot. 2011;26(2):77–89. PMID: 22040388. http://www.ncbi.nlm.nih.gov/pubmed/22040388.
624. Sutton S. Back to the drawing board? A review of applications of the transtheoretical model to substance use. Addiction. 2001;96(1):175–86. PMID: 11177528 http://www.ncbi.nlm.nih.gov/pubmed/11177528
625. Sutton S. Another nail in the coffin of the transtheoretical model? A comment on West (2005). Addiction. 2005;100(8):1043–6. author reply 1048-1050. PMID: 16042628. http://www.ncbi.nlm.nih.gov/pubmed/16042628.
626. Diclemente CC. A premature obituary for the transtheoretical model: a response to West (2005). Addiction. 2005;100(8):1046–8. author reply 1048-1050. PMID: 16042629. http://www.ncbi.nlm.nih.gov/pubmed/16042629.
627. Strack F, Deutsch R. Reflective and impulsive determinants of social behavior. Personal Soc Psychol Rev. 2004;8(3):220–47. PMID: 15454347. http://www.ncbi.nlm.nih.gov/pubmed/15454347.
628. Miller CK, Gutschall MD, Lawrence F. The development of self-efficacy and outcome expectation measures regarding glycaemic load and the nutritional management of type 2 diabetes. Public Health Nutr. 2007;10(6):628–34. PMID: 17381918. http://www.ncbi.nlm.nih.gov/pubmed/17381918.
629. Hardcastle S, Taylor A, Bailey M, Castle R. A randomised controlled trial on the effectiveness of a primary health care based counselling intervention on physical activity, diet and CHD risk factors. Patient Educ Couns. 2008;70(1):31–9. PMID: 17997263. http://www.ncbi.nlm.nih.gov/pubmed/17997263.
630. Hagger MS, Hardcastle SJ. Interpersonal style should be included in taxonomies of behavior change techniques. Front Psychol. 2014;5:254. PMCID: PMC3971167. http://www.ncbi.nlm.nih.gov/pubmed/24723904.
631. Health Action Process Approach.
632. Parschau L, Barz M, Richert J, Knoll N, Lippke S, Schwarzer R. Physical activity among adults with obesity: testing the Health Action Process Approach. Rehabil Psychol.

2014;59(1):42–9. PMID: 24446673. http://www.ncbi.nlm.nih.gov/pubmed/24446673.
633. Lippke S, Plotnikoff RC. Testing two principles of the Health Action Process Approach in individuals with type 2 diabetes. Health Psychol. 2014;33(1):77–84. PMID: 23088172. http://www.ncbi.nlm.nih.gov/pubmed/23088172.
634. Ernsting A, Gellert P, Schneider M, Lippke S. A mediator model to predict workplace influenza vaccination behaviour--an application of the health action process approach. Psychol Health. 2013;28(5):579–92. PMID: 23259583. http://www.ncbi.nlm.nih.gov/pubmed/23259583.
635. Payaprom Y, Bennett P, Alabaster E, Tantipong H. Using the Health Action Process Approach and implementation intentions to increase flu vaccine uptake in high risk Thai individuals: a controlled before-after trial. Health Psychol. 2011;30(4):492–500. PMID: 21534678. http://www.ncbi.nlm.nih.gov/pubmed/21534678.
636. Radtke T, Scholz U, Keller R, Hornung R. Smoking is ok as long as I eat healthily: compensatory health beliefs and their role for intentions and smoking within the Health Action Process Approach. Psychol Health. 2012;27(Suppl 2):91–107. PMID: 21812704. http://www.ncbi.nlm.nih.gov/pubmed/21812704.
637. Williams RJ, Herzog TA, Simmons VN. Risk perception and motivation to quit smoking: a partial test of the Health Action Process Approach. Addict Behav. 2011;36(7):789–91. PMCID: PMC3081897. http://www.ncbi.nlm.nih.gov/pubmed/21463920.
638. Teng Y, Mak WWS. The role of planning and self-efficacy in condom use among men who have sex with men: an application of the Health Action Process Approach model. Health Psychol. 2011;30(1):119–28. PMID: 21299300. http://www.ncbi.nlm.nih.gov/pubmed/21299300.
639. Chiu CY, Lynch RT, Chan F, Berven NL. The Health Action Process Approach as a motivational model for physical activity self-management for people with multiple sclerosis: a path analysis. Rehabil Psychol. 2011;56(3):171–81. PMID: 21767037. http://www.ncbi.nlm.nih.gov/pubmed/21767037.
640. Barg CJ, Latimer AE, Pomery EA, Rivers SE, Rench TA, Prapavessis H, Salovey P. Examining predictors of physical activity among inactive middle-aged women: an application of the health action process approach. Psychol Health. 2012;27(7):829–45. PMCID: PMC3288881. http://www.ncbi.nlm.nih.gov/pubmed/21867395.
641. Caudroit J, Stephan Y, Le Scanff C. Social cognitive determinants of physical activity among retired older individuals: an application of the health action process approach. Br J Health Psychol. 2011;16(Pt 2):404–17. PMID: 21489066. http://www.ncbi.nlm.nih.gov/pubmed/21489066.
642. Schwarzer R, Lippke S, Luszczynska A. Mechanisms of health behavior change in persons with chronic illness or disability: the Health Action Process Approach (HAPA). Rehabil Psychol. 2011;56(3):161–70. PMID: 21767036. http://www.ncbi.nlm.nih.gov/pubmed/21767036.
643. Arbour-Nicitopoulos KP, Duncan M, Remington G, Cairney J, Faulkner GE. Development and reliability testing of a Health Action Process Approach Inventory for physical activity participation among individuals with Schizophrenia. Front. Psychiatry. 2014;5:68. PMCID: PMC4051131. http://www.ncbi.nlm.nih.gov/pubmed/24959152.
644. Clark H, Bassett S. An application of the health action process approach to physiotherapy rehabilitation adherence. Physiother. Theory Pract. 2014;30(8):527–33. PMID: 24779488. http://www.ncbi.nlm.nih.gov/pubmed/24779488.
645. Dohnke B, Nowossadeck E, Müller-Fahrnow W. Motivation and participation in a phase III cardiac rehabilitation programme: an application of the health action process approach. Res. Sports Med. 2010;18(4):219–35. PMID: 21058208. http://www.ncbi.nlm.nih.gov/pubmed/21058208.
646. Krämer LV, Helmes AW, Seelig H, Fuchs R, Bengel J. Correlates of reduced exercise behaviour in depression: the role of motivational and volitional deficits. Psychol Health. 2014;29(10):1206–25. PMID: 24785393. http://www.ncbi.nlm.nih.gov/pubmed/24785393.
647. Steca P, Pancani L, Greco A, D'Addario M, Magrin ME, Miglioretti M, Sarini M, Scrignaro M, Vecchio L, Cesana F, Giannattasio C, Fattirolli F, Zanettini R. Changes in dietary behavior among coronary and hypertensive patients: a longitudinal investigation using the health action process approach. Appl Psychol Health Well Being. 2015;7(3):316–39. PMID: 26218746. http://www.ncbi.nlm.nih.gov/pubmed/26218746.
648. Fleig L, Ngo J, Roman B, Ntzani E, Satta P, Warner LM, Schwarzer R, Brandi ML. Beyond single behaviour theory: adding cross-behaviour cognitions to the health action process approach. Br J Health Psychol. 2015;20(4):824–41. PMID: 26112344. http://www.ncbi.nlm.nih.gov/pubmed/26112344.
649. Paxton RJ. The health action process approach applied to African American breast cancer survivors. Psychooncology. 2016;25(6):648–55. PMCID: PMC6581516. http://www.ncbi.nlm.nih.gov/pubmed/26058382.
650. de Ghisi GLM, Grace SL, Thomas S, Oh P. Behavior determinants among cardiac rehabilitation patients receiving educational interventions: an application of the health action process approach. Patient Educ Couns. 2015;98(5):612–21. PMID: 25638305. http://www.ncbi.nlm.nih.gov/pubmed/25638305.
651. Mak WWS, Chan ATY, Cheung EYL, Lin CLY, Ngai KCS. Enhancing web-based mindfulness training for mental health promotion with the health action process approach: randomized controlled trial. J Med Internet Res. 2015;17(1):e8. PMCID: PMC4319090. http://www.ncbi.nlm.nih.gov/pubmed/25599904.
652. Perrier MJ, Shirazipour CH, Latimer-Cheung AE. Sport participation among individuals with acquired physical disabilities: group differences on demographic, disability, and Health Action Process Approach constructs. Disabil Health J. 2015;8(2):216–22. PMID: 25458978. http://www.ncbi.nlm.nih.gov/pubmed/25458978.
653. MacPhail M, Mullan B, Sharpe L, MacCann C, Todd J. Using the health action process approach to predict and improve health outcomes in individuals with type 2 diabetes mellitus. Diabetes Metab Syndr Obes. 2014;7:469–79. PMCID: PMC4206248. http://www.ncbi.nlm.nih.gov/pubmed/25342914.
654. Wood KV, Ogden J. Predictors of decreased binge eating following laparoscopic adjustable gastric banding using the Health Action Process Approach model. Psychol Health Med. 2014;19(6):641–9. PMID: 24344688. http://www.ncbi.nlm.nih.gov/pubmed/24344688.
655. Velleity Definition & Meaning - Merriam-Webster.
656. Reitan RM, Wolfson D. Conation: a neglected aspect of neuropsychological functioning. Arch Clin Neuropsychol. 2000;15(5):443–53. PMID: 14590220. http://www.ncbi.nlm.nih.gov/pubmed/14590220.
657. Reitan RM, Wolfson D. The differential effect of conation on intelligence test scores among brain-damaged and control subjects. Arch Clin Neuropsychol. 2004;19(1):29–35. PMID: 14670377. http://www.ncbi.nlm.nih.gov/pubmed/14670377.
658. Silk-Eglit GM, Stenclik JH, Miele AS, Lynch JK, McCaffrey RJ. The degree of conation on neuropsychological tests does not account for performance invalidity among litigants. Arch Clin Neuropsychol. 2013;28(3):213–21. PMID: 23507448. http://www.ncbi.nlm.nih.gov/pubmed/23507448.

659. Gerdes KE, Stromwall LK. Conation: a missing link in the strengths perspective. Soc Work. 2008;53(3):233–42. PMID: 19275119. http://www.ncbi.nlm.nih.gov/pubmed/19275119.
660. Reitan RM, Wolfson D. The effect of conation in determining the differential variance among brain-damaged and nonbrain-damaged persons across a broad range of neuropsychological tests. Arch Clin Neuropsychol. 2005;20(8):957–66. PMID: 16297595. http://www.ncbi.nlm.nih.gov/pubmed/16297595.
661. Hilgard ER. The trilogy of mind: cognition, affection, and conation. J Hist Behav Sci. 1980;16(2):107–17. PMID: 11608381. http://www.ncbi.nlm.nih.gov/pubmed/11608381.
662. Wang L, Tao T, Fan C, Gao W, Wei C. The influence of chronic ego depletion on goal adherence: an experience sampling study. PLoS One. 2015;10(11):e0142220. PMCID: PMC4642976. http://www.ncbi.nlm.nih.gov/pubmed/26562839.
663. Baumeister RF, Gailliot M, DeWall CN, Oaten M. Self-regulation and personality: how interventions increase regulatory success, and how depletion moderates the effects of traits on behavior. J Pers. 2006;74(6):1773–801. PMID: 17083666. http://www.ncbi.nlm.nih.gov/pubmed/17083666.
664. Muraven M, Tice DM, Baumeister RF. Self-control as limited resource: regulatory depletion patterns. J Pers Soc Psychol. 1998;74(3):774–89. PMID: 9523419. http://www.ncbi.nlm.nih.gov/pubmed/9523419.
665. Baumeister RF, Bratslavsky E, Muraven M, Tice DM. Ego depletion: is the active self a limited resource? J Pers Soc Psychol. 1998;74(5):1252–65. PMID: 9599441. http://www.ncbi.nlm.nih.gov/pubmed/9599441.
666. Bertrams A, Baumeister RF, Englert C, Furley P. Ego depletion in color priming research: self-control strength moderates the detrimental effect of red on cognitive test performance. Personal Soc Psychol Bull. 2015;41(3):311–22. PMID: 25567999. http://www.ncbi.nlm.nih.gov/pubmed/25567999.
667. Baumeister RF. Self-regulation, ego depletion, and inhibition. Neuropsychologia. 2014;65:313–9. PMID: 25149821. http://www.ncbi.nlm.nih.gov/pubmed/25149821.
668. Daly M, Baumeister RF, Delaney L, MacLachlan M. Self-control and its relation to emotions and psychobiology: evidence from a Day Reconstruction Method study. J Behav Med. 2014;37(1):81–93. PMID: 23160950. http://www.ncbi.nlm.nih.gov/pubmed/23160950.
669. Hofmann W, Schmeichel BJ, Baddeley AD. Executive functions and self-regulation. Trends Cogn Sci. 2012;16(3):174–80. PMID: 22336729. http://www.ncbi.nlm.nih.gov/pubmed/22336729.
670. Carter EC, McCullough ME. Is ego depletion too incredible? Evidence for the overestimation of the depletion effect. Behav Brain Sci. 2013;36(6):683–4; discussion 707–726. PMID: 24304780. http://www.ncbi.nlm.nih.gov/pubmed/24304780.
671. Carter EC, McCullough ME. Publication bias and the limited strength model of self-control: has the evidence for ego depletion been overestimated? Front Psychol. 2014;5:823. PMCID: PMC4115664. http://www.ncbi.nlm.nih.gov/pubmed/25126083.
672. Hagger MS, Chatzisarantis NLD. It is premature to regard the ego-depletion effect as "Too Incredible". Front Psychol. 2014;5:298. PMCID: PMC3989757. http://www.ncbi.nlm.nih.gov/pubmed/24782802.
673. Dryad | Data -- It is premature to regard the ego-depletion effect as 'too incredible'.
674. Eysenck MW, Derakshan N, Santos R, Calvo MG. Anxiety and cognitive performance: attentional control theory. Emotion. 2007;7(2):336–53. PMID: 17516812. http://www.ncbi.nlm.nih.gov/pubmed/17516812.
675. Derakshan N, Smyth S, Eysenck MW. Effects of state anxiety on performance using a task-switching paradigm: an investigation of attentional control theory. Psychon Bull Rev. 2009;16(6):1112–7. PMID: 19966264. http://www.ncbi.nlm.nih.gov/pubmed/19966264.
676. Englert C, Bertrams A. Integrating attentional control theory and the strength model of self-control. Front Psychol. 2015;6:824. PMCID: PMC4468374. http://www.ncbi.nlm.nih.gov/pubmed/26136712.
677. Lawton R, Conner M, McEachan R. Desire or reason: predicting health behaviors from affective and cognitive attitudes. Health Psychol. 2009;28(1):56–65. PMID: 19210018. http://www.ncbi.nlm.nih.gov/pubmed/19210018.
678. Conner M, McEachan R, Lawton R, Gardner P. Basis of intentions as a moderator of the intention-health behavior relationship. Health Psychol. 2016;35(3):219–27. PMID: 26348498. http://www.ncbi.nlm.nih.gov/pubmed/26348498.
679. Adler NE, Stewart J. Using team science to address health disparities: MacArthur network as case example. Ann N Y Acad Sci. 2010;1186:252–60. PMID: 20201877. http://www.ncbi.nlm.nih.gov/pubmed/20201877.
680. Godin G. Does socioeconomic status moderate the relationship between health cognitions and behaviors?: a comment on Conner et al. Ann Behav Med. 2013;46(1):3–4. PMID: 23536122. http://www.ncbi.nlm.nih.gov/pubmed/23536122.
681. Conner M, McEachan R, Jackson C, McMillan B, Woolridge M, Lawton R. Moderating effect of socioeconomic status on the relationship between health cognitions and behaviors. Ann Behav Med. 2013;46(1):19–30. PMID: 23436276. http://www.ncbi.nlm.nih.gov/pubmed/23436276.
682. Prestwich A, Conner MT, Lawton RJ, Ward JK, Ayres K, McEachan RRC. Randomized controlled trial of collaborative implementation intentions targeting working adults' physical activity. Health Psychol. 2012;31(4):486–95. PMID: 22468716. http://www.ncbi.nlm.nih.gov/pubmed/22468716.
683. McEachan RRC, Lawton RJ, Conner M. Classifying health-related behaviours: exploring similarities and differences amongst behaviours. Br J Health Psychol. 2010;15(Pt 2):347–66. PMID: 19646330. http://www.ncbi.nlm.nih.gov/pubmed/19646330.
684. Sheeran P, Abraham C. Mediator of moderators: temporal stability of intention and the intention-behavior relation. Personal Soc Psychol Bull. 2003;29(2):205–15. PMID: 15272948. http://www.ncbi.nlm.nih.gov/pubmed/15272948.
685. Hanson K, Webb TL, Sheeran P, Turpin G. Attitudes and preferences towards self-help treatments for depression in comparison to psychotherapy and antidepressant medication. Behav Cogn Psychother. 2016;44(2):129–39. PMID: 25697236. http://www.ncbi.nlm.nih.gov/pubmed/25697236.
686. Epton T, Harris PR, Kane R, van Koningsbruggen GM, Sheeran P. The impact of self-affirmation on health-behavior change: a meta-analysis. Health Psychol. 2015;34(3):187–96. PMID: 25133846. http://www.ncbi.nlm.nih.gov/pubmed/25133846.
687. Peters J, Büchel C. Neural representations of subjective reward value. Behav Brain Res. 2010;213(2):135–41. PMID: 20420859. http://www.ncbi.nlm.nih.gov/pubmed/20420859.
688. Peters J, Büchel C. The neural mechanisms of inter-temporal decision-making: understanding variability. Trends Cogn Sci. 2011;15(5):227–39. PMID: 21497544. http://www.ncbi.nlm.nih.gov/pubmed/21497544.
689. Coull JT, Cheng RK, Meck WH. Neuroanatomical and neurochemical substrates of timing. Neuropsychopharmacology. 2011;36(1):3–25. PMCID: PMC3055517. http://www.ncbi.nlm.nih.gov/pubmed/20668434.
690. Doya K. Modulators of decision making. Nat Neurosci. 2008;11(4):410–6. PMID: 18368048. http://www.ncbi.nlm.nih.gov/pubmed/18368048.
691. Galtress T, Marshall AT, Kirkpatrick K. Motivation and timing: clues for modeling the reward system. Behav Process.

2012;90(1):142–53. PMCID: PMC3335954. http://www.ncbi.nlm.nih.gov/pubmed/22421220.
692. Coull JT, Vidal F, Nazarian B, Macar F. Functional anatomy of the attentional modulation of time estimation. Science. 2004;303(5663):1506–8. PMID: 15001776. http://www.ncbi.nlm.nih.gov/pubmed/15001776.
693. Frank MJ, Claus ED. Anatomy of a decision: striato-orbitofrontal interactions in reinforcement learning, decision making, and reversal. Psychol Rev. 2006;113(2):300–26. PMID: 16637763. http://www.ncbi.nlm.nih.gov/pubmed/16637763.
694. Shohamy D. Learning and motivation in the human striatum. Curr Opin Neurobiol. 2011;21(3):408–14. PMID: 21658933. http://www.ncbi.nlm.nih.gov/pubmed/21658933.
695. Frank MJ, Fossella JA. Neurogenetics and pharmacology of learning, motivation, and cognition. Neuropsychopharmacology. 2011;36(1):133–52. PMCID: PMC3055524. http://www.ncbi.nlm.nih.gov/pubmed/20631684.
696. Saez I, Set E, Hsu M. From genes to behavior: placing cognitive models in the context of biological pathways. Front Neurosci. 2014;8:336. PMCID: PMC4220121. http://www.ncbi.nlm.nih.gov/pubmed/25414628.
697. Gaitan-Sierra C, Hyland ME. Nonspecific mechanisms that enhance well-being in health-promoting behaviors. Health Psychol. 2011;30(6):793–6. PMID: 21942748. http://www.ncbi.nlm.nih.gov/pubmed/21942748.
698. Hyland ME. Motivation and placebos: do different mechanisms occur in different contexts? Philos Trans R Soc Lond B Biol Sci. 2011;366(1572):1828–37. PMCID: PMC3130400. http://www.ncbi.nlm.nih.gov/pubmed/21576140.
699. Broonen JP, Marty M, Legout V, Cedraschi C, Henrotin Y. Section Rachis de la SFR et de la Belgian Back Society. Is volition the missing link in the management of low back pain? Joint Bone Spine. 2011;78(4):364–7. PMID: 21159537. http://www.ncbi.nlm.nih.gov/pubmed/21159537.
700. McGrane N, Galvin R, Cusack T, Stokes E. Addition of motivational interventions to exercise and traditional physiotherapy: a review and meta-analysis. Physiotherapy. 2015;101(1):1–12. PMID: 25239472. http://www.ncbi.nlm.nih.gov/pubmed/25239472.
701. Kandel DB, Yamaguchi K, Chen K. Stages of progression in drug involvement from adolescence to adulthood: further evidence for the gateway theory. J Stud Alcohol. 1992;53(5):447–57. PMID: 1405637. http://www.ncbi.nlm.nih.gov/pubmed/1405637.
702. Wagner FA, Anthony JC. From first drug use to drug dependence; developmental periods of risk for dependence upon marijuana, cocaine, and alcohol. Neuropsychopharmacology. 2002;26(4):479–88. PMID: 11927172. http://www.ncbi.nlm.nih.gov/pubmed/11927172.
703. Chambers RA, Taylor JR, Potenza MN. Developmental neurocircuitry of motivation in adolescence: a critical period of addiction vulnerability. Am J Psychiatry. 2003;160(6):1041–52. PMCID: PMC2919168. http://www.ncbi.nlm.nih.gov/pubmed/12777258.
704. Jentsch JD, Ashenhurst JR, Cervantes MC, Groman SM, James AS, Pennington ZT. Dissecting impulsivity and its relationships to drug addictions. Ann N Y Acad Sci. 2014;1327:1–26. PMCID: PMC4360991. http://www.ncbi.nlm.nih.gov/pubmed/24654857.
705. Hammond CJ, Mayes LC, Potenza MN. Neurobiology of adolescent substance use and addictive behaviors: treatment implications. Adolesc Med State Art Rev. 2014;25(1):15–32. PMCID: PMC4446977. http://www.ncbi.nlm.nih.gov/pubmed/25022184.
706. Wetherill R, Tapert SF. Adolescent brain development, substance use, and psychotherapeutic change. Psychol Addict Behav. 2013;27(2):393–402. PMCID: PMC3700608. http://www.ncbi.nlm.nih.gov/pubmed/22732057.
707. Geier CF. Adolescent cognitive control and reward processing: implications for risk taking and substance use. Horm Behav. 2013;64(2):333–42. PMID: 23998676. http://www.ncbi.nlm.nih.gov/pubmed/23998676.
708. Andersson G, Titov N. Advantages and limitations of Internet-based interventions for common mental disorders. World Psychiatry. 2014;13(1):4–11. PMCID: PMC3918007. http://www.ncbi.nlm.nih.gov/pubmed/24497236.
709. Webb TL, Joseph J, Yardley L, Michie S. Using the internet to promote health behavior change: a systematic review and meta-analysis of the impact of theoretical basis, use of behavior change techniques, and mode of delivery on efficacy. J Med Internet Res. 2010;12(1):e4. PMCID: PMC2836773. http://www.ncbi.nlm.nih.gov/pubmed/20164043.

15 Perspective on Treatment of Depression

Franklin Sunzeri

Perspective

What are the best evidence-based treatments for depressive disorders? Alas, the answers to that question are not clear.

In 2012, a meta-analysis was published examining the effects of antidepressants, psychotherapy, and alternative therapies for depression—both individually and in combination [1]. Their results conclude that antidepressants or psychotherapy alone are not significantly different from alternative therapies or active ingredient controls. But there might be a slight advantage of the combination of antidepressants and psychotherapy. It should be noted that considerable evidence for publication bias was uncovered. For example, for antidepressants, there was significantly more reduction in symptoms reported in unblinded and published trials compared to those that were blinded or were unpublished FDA data.

The authors of the study suggest that the type of treatment for depression is less important than getting patients involved in an active therapeutic treatment program. They also believe treatment options might be best chosen based upon patient characteristics such as clinical presentations, risks, preferences, and acceptance.

A 2013 meta-analysis of RCTs on treatment of chronic major depression comparing antidepressants and psychotherapy or the combination of both indicated that the best treatment for chronic major depression is a combination of both [2]. However, the reviewers believed that these conclusions are preliminary because there was a lack of well-performed RCTs.

Similar results were seen in analyses of studies focusing on the treatment of MDD from 1970 to 2012 [3].

While the use of psychotherapy compared to pharmacotherapy declined between 1998 and 2007, outpatient treatment for depression increased from 2.37 per 100 persons in 1998 to 2.88 per 100 persons in 2007 [4]. The percentage of patients treated with antidepressants was 73.8% in 1998 and 75.2% in 2007. The percentage of patients receiving psychotherapy declined from 53.6% in 1998 to 43.1% in 2007. Outpatient costs for treating depression went from $10.05 billion to $12.45 billion in 2007. It appears to relate to the increase in medication costs from $4.59 billion in 1998 to $6.60 billion in 2007, which parallels the increase in Medicare spending from $0.52 billion in 1998 to $2.25 billion in 2007.

The declining use of psychotherapy was underscored by another study which found that, in the USA, the use of outpatient psychotherapy was 3.37% in 1998 and 3.18% in 2007 [5]. Use of only psychotherapy was 15.9% in 1998 and 10.5% in 2007; the combination of psychotherapy and psychotropic medication was 40.0% in 1998 and 32.1% in 2007. Meanwhile use of only psychotropics went from 44.1% in 1998 to 57.4% in 2007. Annual psychotherapy visits per patient went from 9.7 to 7.9; mean expense per psychotherapy visit went from $122.80 to $94.59, while total national psychotherapy expense went from $10.94 to $7.17 billion.

Depression treatment in the United States increased considerably from 1987 to 1997 and modestly from 1998 to 2007 [6]. Since that time, treatment appears to be influenced by changes in insurance coverage. Data that were analyzed came from *Medical Expenditure Panel Surveys* of 1998, 2007, and 2015. The data reviewers' principal conclusions are as follows:

- Outpatient treatment rates increased from 2.36 (95% CI, 2.12–2.61) per 100 population in 1998 to 3.47 (95% CI, 3.16–3.79) per 100 population in 2015.
- The proportion treated for depression using psychotherapy decreased from 53.7% (95% CI, 48.3%–59.1%) in 1998 to 43.2% (95% CI, 39.0%–47.4%) in 2007 and then increased to 50.4% (95% CI, 46.0%–54.9%) in 2015.
- The proportion receiving pharmacotherapy remained steady at 81.9% (95% CI, 77.9%–85.9%) in 1998, 82.4% (95% CI, 79.3%–85.4%) in 2007, and 80.8% (95% CI, 77.9%–83.7%) in 2015.

F. Sunzeri (✉)
Heather Hills Consulting, Coos Bay, OR, USA

J. Raber et al. (eds.), *Understanding and Treating Depressive Disorders*, https://doi.org/10.1007/978-3-032-14465-2_15

- Prescription expenditures after inflation adjustment decreased from $848 (95% CI, $713–$984) per year in 1998 to $603 (95% CI, $484–$722) per year in 2015, whereas the mean number of prescriptions decreased from 7.64 (95% CI, 6.61–8.67) in 1998 to 7.03 (95% CI, 6.51–7.56) in 2015.
- National costs for outpatient treatment of depression increased from $12,430,000 in 1997 to $15,554,000 in 2007 and then to $17,404,000 in 2015.
- The percentage of the cost that came from uninsured patients decreased from 32% in 1998 to 29% in 2007 and then to 20% in 2015.
- This decrease was largely associated with increasing Medicaid coverage: the percentage of this spending that was covered was 19% in 1998, 15% in 2007, and 36% in 2015.

Frequently, symptoms of depression will remit spontaneously. However, depression frequently recurs and may require long-term therapy.

The following recommendations for treatment of depression come from the American Psychiatric Association (APA) practice guidelines [7]. They purport to provide evidence-based recommendations for the assessment and treatment of psychiatric disorders. However, we cannot verify the sources of their evidence.

1. Most people with depression are treated as outpatients. Hospitalization is required for those who have psychotic symptoms or physical debilitation, or significant suicidal ideation, especially if there is no family support.
2. When substance abuse is involved, antidepressant treatment is likely to be far less effective as long as substance abuse continues. Within a few months of stopping substance abuse, depression symptoms usually resolve.
3. Treatment is directed first at any underlying physical disorder or drug toxicity. But if the diagnosis is uncertain or there are disabling symptoms, suicidal ideation, or feelings of hopelessness, treatment with an antidepressant or mood-stabilizing drug may help.
4. Initial support should include weekly or biweekly support and education to monitor progress. Telephone contact may supplement office visits.
5. Explanations that depression has a biological base and is not a character flaw may help to dispel worry or embarrassment about having a mental disorder. Perspective and adherence may be encouraged by conveying that this is a serious medical disorder requiring specific treatment and that it has a good prognosis with appropriate therapy. This may help to dispel feelings of helplessness when recovery fluctuates.
6. Suggestions are appropriate that self-blame should be avoided, and that dark thoughts that are part of being depressed will go away.
7. While acknowledging and balancing that patients may have a desire to avoid activities, it is good to encourage engaging in social interactions and gradually increasing simple activities such as walking or regular exercise.

A systematic review and network meta-analysis of pharmacological and non-pharmacological treatments for adult MDD was published in 2019 [8]. They found that all treatments studied (acupuncture, mirtazapine, herbal medicine, venlafaxine, physical exercise, cognitive-behavioral therapy (CBT), bupropion, fluoxetine, and vortioxetine) except for probiotics were significantly more effective than placebo.

As for safety, bupropion, fluoxetine, venlafaxine, and vortioxetine were significantly less safe than placebo. Herbal medicine and mirtazapine were not significantly different in overall risk of adverse events compared with placebo. Acupuncture, CBT, physical exercise, and probiotics did not have enough available safety data to evaluate their risk.

References

1. Khan A, Faucett J, Lichtenberg P, Kirsch I, Brown WA. A systematic review of comparative efficacy of treatments and controls for depression. PLoS One. 2012;7(7):e41778. PMCID: PMC3408478. http://www.ncbi.nlm.nih.gov/pubmed/22860015.
2. Spijker J, van Straten A, Bockting CLH, Meeuwissen JAC, van Balkom AJLM. Psychotherapy, antidepressants, and their combination for chronic major depressive disorder: a systematic review. Can J Psychiatr. 2013;58(7):386–92. PMID: 23870720. http://www.ncbi.nlm.nih.gov/pubmed/23870720.
3. van Hees ML, Rotter T, Ellermann T, Evers SM. The effectiveness of individual interpersonal psychotherapy as a treatment for major depressive disorder in adult outpatients: a systematic review. BMC Psychiatry. 2013;13:22. https://doi.org/10.1186/1471-244X-13-22. PMID: 23312024; PMCID: PMC3558333. http://www.ncbi.nlm.nih.gov/pubmed/23312024.
4. Marcus SC, Olfson M. National trends in the treatment for depression from 1998 to 2007. Arch Gen Psychiatry. 2010;67(12):1265–73. PMID: 21135326. http://www.ncbi.nlm.nih.gov/pubmed/21135326.
5. Olfson M, Marcus SC. National trends in outpatient psychotherapy. Am J Psychiatry. 2010;167(12):1456–63. PMID: 20686187. http://www.ncbi.nlm.nih.gov/pubmed/20686187.
6. Hockenberry JM, Joski P, Yarbrough C, Druss BG. Trends in treatment and spending for patients receiving outpatient treatment of depression in the United States, 1998–2015. JAMA Psychiatry. 2019;76(8):810–17. https://doi.org/10.1001/jamapsychiatry.2019.0633. Erratum in: JAMA Psychiatry. 2019;76(8):871–72. https://doi.org/10.1001/jamapsychiatry.2019.1393. PMID: 31017627; PMCID: PMC6487900. http://www.ncbi.nlm.nih.gov/pubmed/31017627.
7. Guidelines | Psychiatry Online.
8. Chen C, Shan W. Pharmacological and non-pharmacological treatments for major depressive disorder in adults: a systematic review and network meta-analysis. Psychiatry Res. 2019;281:112595. PMID: 31627074. http://www.ncbi.nlm.nih.gov/pubmed/31627074.

Pharmacotherapy

16

Franklin Sunzeri

Introduction

A 2017 review of systematic reviews summarized evidence of more than 140 pharmacological and nonpharmacological treatment options for MDD and evaluated the confidence that clinicians can have in their usefulness [15]. Their review did not consider the effects of the combination or augmentation of antidepressants with nonpharmacological interventions, which are common treatment strategies. They concluded that for general efficacy, only *second-generation antidepressants*[1] had high-strength evidence for successful treatment. They had "small beneficial treatment effects (SMD[2] = −0.35; 95% CI: −0.31 to −0.38), and a statistically significantly higher rate of discontinuation because of adverse events than patients on placebo (RR,[3] 1.88; 95% CI: 1.0–3.28)."

As for nonpharmacological interventions, they concluded "only CBT has reliable evidence (moderate strength of evidence) to produce responses to treatment similar to those of second-generation antidepressants (45.5% vs 44.2%; RR 1.10; 95% CI: 0.93–1.30)" [15]. They also concluded that the majority of nonpharmacological interventions for treating patients with MDD are not evidence-based.

As reviewed in 2008, the most frequently used and recommended treatments as a first step for acute MDD are selective serotonin reuptake inhibitors (SSRIs) or selective serotonin norepinephrine reuptake inhibitors (SNRIs) [17–19]. Almost 63% of patients taking these SSRIs or SNRIs have adverse effects, and 7–15% discontinue taking them due to the adverse effects [16]. Worry about possible addiction to antidepressants prevents many patients, especially women and minorities, from using the pharmacological approach to treatment [20, 21]. Also, stigma is higher for antidepressant drugs [22]. In such cases, nonpharmacological treatments have become the first choice [23, 24].

Since 1998, several respected studies have failed to find consistent evidence that antidepressant medication is any better than a placebo in treating depression [25–29].

For example, one of the studies [25] concluded that multiple and selective publication, and selective reporting in research sponsored by the pharmaceutical industry made it impossible to recommend a specific selective serotonin reuptake inhibitor. Selective publication of RCTs that are used in meta-analyses may result in serious inflation of reported treatment effects due to that publication bias [26, 30].

A 2008 NEJM analysis reviewed Food and Drug Administration (FDA) studies of 12 antidepressant agents involving 12,564 patients [26]. They found that in the published literature, it appeared that 94% of the trials conducted were positive, whereas the FDA analysis showed that 51% were positive. The reviewers stated that bias might have

[1] *Second-generation antidepressants* generally refer to antidepressants other than tricyclics and monoamine oxidase inhibitors used to treat major depressive disorder. The second generation refers to the era (1970s and 1980s) in which they were developed not any chemical property. The most familiar are the selective serotonin reuptake inhibitors (SSIRs) and selective serotonin norepinephrine reuptake inhibitors (SNRIs).

[2] *Standardized mean difference [SMD]* is a measure of effect size in meta-analyses when the studies all assess the same outcome but measure it in a variety of ways. In systematic reviews, the SMD is the mean difference in depression score between the intervention and control groups divided by the pooled SD at follow-up. This gives a unit-free effect size. The conventional SMD effects sizes of 0.2 (small), 0.5 (medium), and 0.8 (large) are used. Dichotomous variables are usually expressed as risk ratio with a 95% CI. For more information, see Chap. 4 Evidence Basics.

[3] *Relative risk (RR)* is perhaps the most common method of expressing the estimated risk of experiencing a result. RR compares the probability of a specific outcome in the treatment group with that of a control group. When an RR is greater than 1, there seems to be an increased risk of an event. When the RR is less than 1, there appears to be a decreased risk of experiencing an event. If the RR is 1, there is no apparent risk. If the RR = 5, it is 5 times more likely to occur than in the control group. If the RR = 0.5, it is half as likely to happen as in the control group. For more information, see Chap. 4 Evidence Basics.

F. Sunzeri (✉)
Heather Hills Consulting, Coos Bay, OR, USA

J. Raber et al. (eds.), *Understanding and Treating Depressive Disorders*, https://doi.org/10.1007/978-3-032-14465-2_16

come from failure to submit manuscripts or from decisions by journal editors and reviewers not to publish, or both.

A 2010 study published in JAMA [27] concluded that, "The magnitude of benefit of antidepressant medication compared with placebo increases with severity of depression symptoms and may be minimal or nonexistent, on average, in patients with mild or moderate symptoms. For patients with very severe depression, the benefit of medications over placebo is substantial."

About half of patients with major depression will respond to antidepressant treatment, and about one-third will achieve full symptom remission [31, 32]. According to a European Psychiatric Association position paper, antidepressants for depression have a number needed to treat of 5–7 for treatment of acute episodes and 4 for maintenance [33]. Moreover, these effects are achieved most often after the use of a variety of antidepressants, comedications, or augmentation therapies.

Studies have found that most patients taking antidepressants will not achieve symptom remission after initial treatment [34], and approximately one-third will not achieve remission even after several antidepressants are tried, and those who do remit have a higher relapse rate [32, 35, 36]. For example, after unsuccessful remission using the SSRI citalopram, the addition of bupropion-SR, sertraline, or venlafaxine-XR succeeded in producing a remission in approximately one out of four patients [36].

Sometimes, a combination of drugs is used if symptoms do not improve within 1–4 weeks. Drugs are frequently used as a bridge while psychotherapy is taking effect [37]. However, according to a 2019 systematic review, there is very low-quality evidence that augmenting current antidepressant therapy with other pharmacological interventions for treatment-resistant depression in adults has any benefits [38].

A 2018 Cochrane systematically reviewed psychological therapies for *treatment-resistant depression (TRD)* in adults [39]. They found moderate-quality evidence that psychotherapy added to usual care with antidepressants is beneficial for depressive symptoms and for response and remission rates over the short term and possibly for medium and long-term effects for patients with TRD. It was unclear which types of psychotherapy were most effective. There was no evidence to suggest that switching from antidepressants to psychotherapy was more beneficial.

To discover *relapse rates of antidepressant medications*, MDD patients who have responded to the antidepressant medication (ADM) are entered into *placebo substitution trials* (randomized, double-blind, placebo-controlled (RDBPC) effectiveness trials) to measure the rate of MDD relapse over time [40]. A 2017 systematic review of ADM randomized maintenance trials found that the placebo-substitution trials for patients who were abruptly switched to placebo resulted in unusually high (46%) rates of relapse over 6–12 months, twice the continuing ADM rate. However, these switch studies showed selective screening, high attrition, anxious anticipation of a switch to placebo, and risk of drug withdrawal symptoms. In nonindustry-sponsored RCTs of adults with multiple prior MDD episodes who were treated with ADM maintenance for 1–2 years, relapse rates averaging 40%. The reviewers suggest that industry sponsorship, attrition, the impact of the switch to placebo, and major relapse differences in MDD subpopulations are important considerations in evaluating ADM efficacy results.

According to a 2010 analysis, placebo responses in MDD trials appear to have increased until approximately 1997 but appear to have been stable since then and are not the cause of smaller reported treatment effects [41]. A 2016 systematic review of published and unpublished double-blind RCTs of placebo response rates in antidepressant trials found that the average placebo response rates in antidepressant trials have been stable for more than 25 years [42]. Average placebo response rates remained constant in the range between 35% and 40% (RR, 1.00, 95% CI: 0.97–1.03, $p = 0{\cdot}99$, for every 5-year increase).

A 2010 meta-analysis of RCTs of antidepressants found that the degree of benefit of antidepressant medications compared to placebo increases with the depression severity [42]. On average, the benefit of antidepressant medication may be minimal or nonexistent in patients with mild or moderate symptoms.

In 2019, data were used from 122 MDD trials conducted between the years 1983 and 2010 to determine if data support the implicit assumption of placebo additivity in placebo-controlled trials [41]. *Placebo additivity* means that effects not attributable to the active drug are equal in both the treatment and placebo arms. Several papers suggested that the mechanism of action in some drug classes can interact with placebo mechanisms and result in nonadditive effects [43–48].

Placebo effects in RCTs of antidepressant treatment of MDD have been reported to be approximately 82 per cent of the drug response, and about half of those RCTs with approved antidepressants fail [41, 49–51]. Various solutions to minimize the placebo response have been proposed [52–56]. One of those approaches that are being discussed is the *Sequential Parallel Comparison Design* [52, 56–59]. It is an interesting discussion that sheds light on the placebo in clinical trials. It aims to reduce the overall placebo response rate and the sample size required for these RCTs.

An interesting perspective on SSRIs is provided by Irving Kirsch in the 2014 book *Placebo* [60]. He asserts that the serotonin theory of depression may be wrong. He says that all antidepressants, whether they increase, decrease, or have no effect on serotonin levels, show the same therapeutic effect. And the little statistical difference between antidepressants and placebo may be, "due to the fact that most patients and doctors in clinical trials successfully break blind" [49].

Fava et al. suggest the following may be contributing to the problems with placebo response in clinical trials for psychiatric disorders [52]. "Diagnostic misclassification, issues concerning inclusion/exclusion criteria, outcome measures' lack of sensitivity to change, measurement errors, poor quality of data entry and verification, waxing and waning of the natural course of illness, regression toward the mean phenomenon, patient and clinician expectations about the trial, study design issues, nonspecific therapeutic effects, and high attrition." In addition, they suggest that some benefit may be realized from, "standardizing diagnostic procedures, managing clinicians' overestimation of change, simplification of study visits and assessments, minimizing nonspecific, therapeutic effects, extending trial duration, reducing number of sites, increasing the sensitivity of outcome measures, and reducing the number of treatment arms."

A review of symptom severity and the generalizability of *antidepressant efficacy trials* (AETs) from 1995 to 2014 found that a significantly higher percentage of patients in clinical practice would be excluded based on the severity thresholds used from 2010 to 2014 (59.3 ± 13.5 vs 49.0 ± 15.1; $t121 = 3.1$; $p < 0.005$). The study's authors suggest that results of AETs may not be applicable to less severely depressed patients who make up at least half of the patients that are treated in general practice [61].

Data from the *National Comorbidity Survey Replication (February 2001-April 2003)* were used to compare the characteristics of the presenting problem, the antidepressant type and dose, and continuity of treatment of adults prescribed antidepressants by psychiatrists or other medical providers [17]. About 10.5% of the participants received antidepressants in the past year, and most of them received the drugs from a general medical provider (73.6%), not from a psychiatrist. Those who were treated by a general provider were usually from a nonurban area and were over 65 years of age. These patients were less likely to meet the criteria for mood or anxiety disorders or to continue medication beyond the first month. Those who received medications from psychiatrists were more likely to have serious mood or anxiety symptoms and meet the corresponding diagnostic criteria for mood or anxiety disorders. Unlike those treated by general practitioners, most of them were male. They typically got higher doses of drugs, were likely to continue medications for at least 30 days, and were more likely to use them for a longer time [17].

Studies have found that a large proportion of psychotropics are given to patients who have not been diagnosed with any psychiatric disorder, or even if that drug is not appropriate for a putative diagnosis [62]. Especially in primary care visits, new psychotropic medications are commonly given without any psychiatric diagnosis, and the use of psychotropics has steadily increased since around the year 1998 [62–66]. About 16% of adults in the USA have taken psychotropics at least once [66]. Data from the *2006-2015 National Ambulatory Medical Care Survey (NAMCS)*, a nationally representative sample of office-based US outpatient care, found that visits to nonpsychiatric specialists showed 1.69 times greater odds of not having a psychiatric diagnosis when compared to primary care visits. Overall, 60.4% of the visits at which a new psychotropic prescription was initiated, no psychiatric diagnosis was given.

The proportion of the overall health expenditure on pharmaceuticals for the cost of psychotropics was about 3% per year in 2012 [67]. Between 2010 and 2018, the FDA approved at least 15 new or existing psychotropic medications for psychiatric purposes [68]. By 2011, psychotropic medicines in the USA were the third most prescribed class of drugs [69]. With annual sales of about 10 billion dollars, they were one of the most expensive classes of drugs [71, 72]. In 2009, chances of being prescribed psychotropics without a psychiatric diagnosis were 2.9 times greater among patients aged 50–64 than among younger patients [73]. In 2010, of those *Veterans Health Administration* (VHA) patients who were prescribed a psychotropic medication, 30% had no psychiatric diagnosis, with the highest proportions being among veterans ages 65–85 [74]. Reasons for this lack of documented diagnoses may include unnecessary use, underdiagnosis of mental illness, or incomplete documentation.

Little has changed by 2024 [70, 71]. As of 2024, psychotropic medications were the third most prescribed medications in the USA [70]. The top of the list for the most money spent on pharmaceuticals was semaglutide for diabetes and weight loss [71].

A significant increase in *polypharmacy*[4] involving antidepressant and antipsychotic medications has been seen [75]. Data from the 1996–2006 cross-sectional *National Ambulatory Medical Care Surveys*[5] found that in visits to office-based psychiatrists, prescriptions for 2 or more antidepressants, antipsychotics, sedative-hypnotics, and antidepressant-antipsychotic combinations, but not other combinations, significantly increased across survey years. The odds of receiving 2 or more antidepressants were significantly associated with a diagnosis of major depression (OR[6]= 3.44; 99% CI: 2.58–4.58); 2 or more antipsychotics, with schizophrenia (OR = 6.75; 99% CI: 3.52–12.92); 2 or more

[4]Polypharmacy is the concurrent use of multiple medications by a patient [79–81]. Polypharmacy is quite common in the elderly and may or may not present problems [82–85].

[5]The National Center for Health Statistics collects and publishes the National Ambulatory Medical Care Survey [576–578].

[6]Odds ratio (OR) is a way to represent the odds that an outcome will result when a given exposure to a variable of interest occurs compared to when the exposure does not occur. OR quantifies the strength of the association between two events. An OR greater than 1 indicates a positive association or that exposure to that variable increases the odds of that outcome. An OR less than one indicates a negative relationship between two events. An OR of 1 suggests no relationship between two events. An OR is frequently accompanied by a 95% confidence interval (CI). CI is a measure of precision of the OR. The smaller the CI, the higher precision as long as it does not overlap OR = 1. For more information, see Chap. 4 on evidence basics in this text.

mood stabilizers, with bipolar disorder (OR = 15.46; 99% CI: 6.77–35.31); and 2 or more sedative-hypnotics, with anxiety disorders (OR = 2.13; 99% CI: 1.41–3.22).

Polypharmacy, multiple side effects, and poor adherence to treatment regimens in older folks are real-world considerations. It is especially important to realize that, as with many prescriptions, metabolism of mood-altering chemotherapeutics changes with age. In this vein, the *Beers Criteria for Potentially Inappropriate Medication Use in Older Adults* is a professional reference that has been developed to identify medications that pose potential risks that may outweigh the potential benefits in folks older than 65 [76].

A copy of the Beers list can be found here [77]. For example, older folks may have decreased metabolism of long-acting antidepressants and increased sensitivity to benzodiazepines. Benzodiazepines appear to be prone to cause cognitive impairment, motor vehicle accidents, falls, and delirium [78].

Persistent forms of depression have a lifetime prevalence ranging from 3% to 6% in the Western world [87]. *Persistent depressive disorders* can include dysthymia, chronic major depression, recurrent major depression with incomplete remission between episodes, and double depression[7] that have lasted at least 2 years.

A Cochrane systematic review comparing the effectiveness of continuation and maintenance treatments for persistent depressive disorder (PDD) in adults was published in 2019 [86]. They concluded that due to moderate or high risk of bias as well as clinical heterogeneity in the analyzed studies, it was not possible to determine if continued or maintained pharmacotherapy (or both) with the reviewed antidepressants is an effective treatment for preventing relapse and recurrence of PDD. Continued or maintained psychotherapy might have been effective compared to no treatment, but for all other comparisons, there was not enough evidence to make any final conclusions. And, there is a need for more high-quality studies on psychological interventions.

An RCT published in 2019 evaluated the effects of psychoanalytic and CBT long-term therapy with chronically depressed patients [88]. They found that both long-term treatments produced significant and sustained improvements in depressive symptoms in chronically depressed patients. Their results exceeded the effect sizes of other international outcome studies.

A psychopharmacology review of studies from 1987 through 2017 found that continuing SSRIs for 1 year reduces the risk of MDD and relapse and that a combination of SSRIs and CBT may also reduce relapse [89]. They concluded that escitalopram appeared to have produced better results with fewer side effects than did other SSRIs or SNRIs. Tricyclic antidepressants and atypical antidepressants appeared to give similar results.

Crisafulli et al. in 2011 reviewed the data on *pharmacogenetics of antidepressants* and found that almost 60% of depressed patients do not show a complete response to antidepressants and up to 30% show no response [90]. Approximately half of the response is contributed by genetic factors. The genetic candidates that have been investigated seem to influence behavior, susceptibility to psychological disorders, and treatment response. Those *genes include* the cytochrome P-450 (aka CYP)[8] superfamily, the P-glycoprotein (ABCB1), the tryptophan hydroxylase, the catechol-O-methyltransferase, the monoamine oxidase A, the serotonin transporter (5-HTTLPR), the norepinephrine transporter, the dopamine transporter, variants in the 5-hydroxytryptamine receptors (5-HT1A, 5-HT2A, 5-HT3A, 5-HT3B, and 5-HT6), adrenoreceptor beta-1 and alpha-2, the dopamine receptors (D2), the G protein beta 3 subunit, the corticotropin releasing hormone receptors (CRHR1 and CRHR2), the glucocorticoid receptors, the c-AMP response-element binding, and the brain-derived neurotrophic factor [90]. In addition, some associations have been seen for angiotensin I converting enzyme, circadian locomotor output cycles kaput protein, glutamatergic system, nitric oxide synthase, and interleukin 1-beta gene. Many of these effects seem to be modulated by *gene x environment interactions.*

Some companies provide pharmacogenetics (PGx) testing to help determine which antidepressants may work the best for an individual [91]. The most common test is for genetic polymorphisms in the cytochrome P-450 (CYP) genes that mediate oxidative metabolism [92]. For instance, the *CYP2D6 enzyme* metabolizes at least 30 SSRI, SNRI, and tricyclic antidepressants. Alterations of the CYP2D6 enzyme may produce a wide variety of metabolic speeds, ranging from poor to very rapid metabolism of SSRIs. The actual utility of these tests for an individual is still open for discussion [91, 98–101]. Results are promising for the use of

[7] There is some ambiguity of terms in the literature. *Double depression* is defined as the coexistence of major depressive disorder (MDD) and *persistent depressive disorder (PDD)*. PDD subsumes several chronic depressive variations, including dysthymia with or without superimposed major depressive episodes, chronic major depression, and recurrent major depression without recovery between episodes [93]. Double depression tends to be more severe than either MDD or PDD and may have a greater relapse rate. However, some experts question if double depression is a separate entity from MDD or PDD [94, 95].

[8] *Cytochrome P-450 (CYP)* CYPs are a family of isoenzymes present in the endoplasmic reticulum. CYPs are central to oxidizing various compounds (e.g., fatty acids, steroids, and xenobiotics such as drugs). They are vital for synthesizing, breaking down, and clearing compounds [96].

Most chemical carcinogens are metabolically activated by CYPs through converting to highly reactive electrophiles that bind covalently to DNA [97].

pharmacogenetics in psychiatry [102–105]. In 2018, a systematic review identified available PGx tests, compared the genes they include with clinical guidelines and drug labels, and assessed the quality of published clinical studies [106].

Depression afflicts 1%–2% of children (6–12 years old) and 2%–5% of adolescents (13–18 years old). Peak incidence is around puberty [107, 108]. The course of pediatric disease is characterized by protracted episodes, frequent recurrence, and comorbid psychiatric disorders [109]. Due to undifferentiated signs and symptoms and atypical presentations, identification and diagnosis of depression in these age groups is problematic [110].

Serious problems in psychosocial relationships and school achievement can occur [111]. Increased risk of suicide and suicidal ideation can occur. The *American Academy of Child and Adolescent Psychiatry (AACAP)* suggests that depression contributes to more than 500,000 pediatric suicide attempts in a year [112, 113].

A systematic review and *network meta-analysis* of the comparative efficacy and acceptability of psychotherapies for depression in children and adolescents found that at post-treatment, only interpersonal therapy (IPT) and cognitive-behavioral therapy (CBT) were significantly more effective than most control conditions [114, 115]. Several alternative psychotherapies were understudied in this age group.

Psychotherapy is considered to be the first-line intervention for the management of depressive disorder in children and adolescents [116]. If psychotherapy does not work or the depression is quite severe, antidepressants are sometimes suggested. Side effects of psychotherapy include dependency on the therapist and potential distress for the family of the patients; however, there is little data systematically measuring safety and tolerance [117, 118].

Studies of pharmacological therapies of children and adolescent depression indicate that most antidepressants do not seem to afford a clear benefit for these patients [119–121]. Fluoxetine has been stated as an option if pharmacological therapy is indicated [119]. The potential risk of suicidality in children and adolescents who take antidepressants has not been completely resolved [122].

One study suggested that fluoxetine may be more effective than CBT in adolescents ages 12–17 with MDD and that the combination might be better than either one alone [123]. As discussed elsewhere in this text, some data in adults suggest that the combination is also better than either alone [124, 125].

A 2014 Cochrane meta-analysis concluded there is very limited evidence upon which to base conclusions about the relative effectiveness of psychological interventions, antidepressant medication, and a combination of these interventions in children and adolescents [126].

Antidepressants

Even if clinicians are not licensed to prescribe medications, it behooves them to be acquainted with these psychiatric medications. When reading the behavioral medicine literature relative to depression and anxiety, they will often encounter comparisons to standard treatments. In addition, it is common in dealing with patient symptoms to find symptoms that are associated with their medications. Keeping these admonitions in mind, psychotherapists as well as psychiatrists and general medical practitioners need to be aware of the abundant use of antidepressants. Especially, as their *side effects can provoke symptoms of comorbid disorders* and can even worsen the symptoms of the diseases for which they were originally prescribed [127–131].

In some instances, these include clinically important cardiac as well as vascular effects [127, 132], sexual dysfunctions [128], weight gain [133], extrapyramidal[9] side effects [134, 135], and psychological side effects such as emotional numbing [136, 137].

Sexual dysfunction is already present in a significant number of folks with depression [138, 139]. Moreover, antidepressants of many classes, with the notable exception of bupropion and nefazodone, may cause 30% to 40% of patients who take them to experience some degree of sexual dysfunction [138, 140, 141].

Most antidepressants after 6–12 months of therapy seem to produce a 3- to 4-kg weight gain. Mirtazapine is associated with significant *weight gain early in therapy* [133]. Fluvoxamine, nefazodone, and fluoxetine are most commonly associated with side effects because they are more likely to affect the metabolism of commonly prescribed medications [133].

The *prosuicidal effects* of antidepressants are well known for both monoamine reuptake inhibitors and tricyclics [142]. Neurological and somatic-metabolic as well as consecutive psychological activity of reuptake inhibitors may be prosuicidal in patients by increasing the intensity of existing suicidal predictors, including dysphoria, anxiety, impulsiveness, and agitation [142].

In addition, although suicide rates appear to decrease in those taking antidepressants, in some children, adolescents,

[9] *Extrapyramidal* functions are not an anatomically meaningful term. The *pyramidal (corticospinal)* tract is one of several tracts that subserve voluntary motor activity [159]. So, extrapyramidal refers to motor systems other than the pyramidal tract. Extrapyramidal refers to control of motor tone, the amount and velocity of movement, and the suppression of undesirable motor activity [160]. Extrapyramidal side effects imply impaired motor control usually associated with dysfunction of the forebrain basal ganglia. Other nonpyramidal motor functions of coordination, planning, sequencing, and inhibition also involve the cerebellum and neocortex. Hypotonicity can be found in short-term exposure to dopamine-blocking drugs, whereas hypertonicity may be an accompaniment to chronic exposure to dopamine-blocking drugs.

and young adults, suicidal thinking, feeling, and behavior may increase [143–146]. It may be that there is an increase in suicidal attempts but not completed suicide in those who have previously attempted suicide [145, 146].

The FDA requires all antidepressants to carry a warning on package inserts. This warning advises precautions about the risk for suicidal thoughts, hostility, and agitation in children and adults [147–149]. Controversy, however, exists as to the real and relative risks [150–155]. Information on the *Center for Drug Evaluation and Research (CDER)* process for ensuring safe and effective drugs are available to improve the health of people in the United States [156]. CDER is the part of the FDA that regulates over-the-counter and prescription drugs, including biological therapeutics and generic drugs. Their work covers more than just medicines (e.g., dandruff shampoos and fluoride-containing toothpaste) [157].

For insight into the process of developing drugs to treat major depression, the following FDA publication is available. *Major Depressive Disorder: Developing Drugs for Treatment Guidance for Industry* [158]. The introduction reads, "The purpose of this guidance is to assist sponsors in the clinical development of drugs for the monotherapeutic, combination, and adjunctive treatment of major depressive disorder (MDD). Specifically, this guidance addresses the FDA's current thinking regarding the overall development program and clinical trial designs for antidepressant drug products. This draft guidance is intended to serve as a focus for continued discussions among the Division of Psychiatry Products (the Division), pharmaceutical sponsors, the academic community, and the public."

The *National Ambulatory Medical Care Survey (NAMCS)* is an annual nationally representative sample survey of visits to nonfederal office-based patient care physicians, excluding anesthesiologists, radiologists, and pathologists [161]. In 2016, the top five chronic conditions documented during office visits were, in order: diabetes mellitus, hypertension, hyperlipidemia, arthritis, and depression. The most frequently mentioned drugs—by therapeutic category—were, in order: analgesics, antihyperlipidemics, dermatological agents, vitamins, and antidepressants.[10] In 2019, depressive disorders were the primary diagnosis in over 14 million visits to primary care physicians [162]. Depressive disorders were the fourth most common chronic conditions at office visits in 2019 and the top chronic conditions for patients under 45 [162].

Indeed, a glance at the most frequently prescribed and the top money-making pharmaceuticals in the USA shows the prominent place occupied by the antidepressants. According to a 2020 list of the most frequently prescribed medications, sertraline (Zoloft) ranked 14th; escitalopram (Lexapro), 20th; alprazolam (Xanax), a benzodiazepine used for anxiety, 21st; bupropion (Wellbutrin), 23rd; citalopram (Celexa), 26th; trazodone (Desyrel), 30th; fluoxetine (Prozac), 31st; and paroxetine (Paxil), 68th [163].

Of the 25 most frequently prescribed psychiatric medications in 2018, 14 were antidepressants [164]. Ranked among the top were Zoloft (sertraline) at number one; Lexapro (escitalopram), third; Wellbutrin (bupropion), fifth; Prozac (fluoxetine), seventh; Celexa (citalopram), eighth; and Cymbalta (duloxetine), ninth.

The antidepressant that made the most money for the manufacturer is Wellbutrin (for depression) —$1.024 billion. It came in 5th after three attention-deficit hyperactivity disorder (ADHD) medications and Abilify that is prescribed for bipolar disorder, depression, and schizophrenia. In 2016, there were more than 338 million prescriptions for antidepressant medications. In 2018, it decreased to 318 million, perhaps a slight decline in prescriptions for antidepressants. In 2023, sertraline was still number one, followed closely by trazodone and then fluoxetine [163]. Sertraline was number 11 on the most prescribed list with over 9 million patients receiving prescriptions [163].

There are abundant *Internet sites with detailed information on any drug*. These sites are often geared to the background of the researcher (e.g., for a health consumer or practitioner). One of our favorite consumer-oriented sites with many links is provided by USA tax dollars. It is *MedlinePlus*. Its depression information can be found at [165].

Another fine source of comparative benefits and side effects of the array of second-generation antidepressants is [166]. Again, this is our USA tax dollars at work. There are detailed consumer-oriented pamphlets also available that can be particularly useful for those who are taking or intending to take antidepressants.

For the more biochemically oriented, the widely available classic reference is *Martindale: Complete drug reference* [1].

The use of *antidepressants during cancer chemotherapy* may be problematic. Treatment of depression in cancer patients has been said to significantly improve quality of life and survival time [167, 168]. In one sample, decreasing depression symptoms in the first year of breast cancer diagnosis improved the mean survival time by 28.5 months [169]. Psychosocial therapy and pharmacotherapy can be effective, but they need to be tailored to the individual patient [170–172].

Antidepressants may improve depression and anxiety as well as provide analgesic, hypnotic, and pro-cognitive actions [173]. Some antidepressants may ameliorate specific symptoms, including insomnia (mirtazapine and trazodone), decreased appetite, nausea, and/or vomiting (mirtazapine),

[10] Rui P, Okeyode T. National Ambulatory Medical Care Survey: 2016 National Summary Tables. Available from [161].

fatigue (bupropion and methylphenidate), neuropathic pain (duloxetine and amitriptyline), and hot flashes (venlafaxine and SSRIs) [170]. Several antidepressants, perhaps related to influence on glial cells, may be immunomodulatory, cyto/neuroprotective, and antiinflammatory [173].

However, a 2019 Cochrane Systematic Review of antidepressants for the treatment of depression in people with cancer concluded, "Despite the impact of depression on people with cancer, available studies were very few and of low quality. This review found very low-quality evidence for the effects of these drugs compared with placebo. On the basis of these results, clear implications for practice cannot be made" [174].

Antidepressants for the treatment of depression in cancer patients need to be administered with caution [115, 171, 173]. Of course, there are possible side effects of second-generation SSRIs. Some of these are transient, and others may persist [175]. These include hypersensitivity reactions, hepatotoxicity, gastrointestinal, cardiovascular, or genitourinary symptoms, hyponatremia, metabolic disorders, and increased risk of bleeding [176]. In addition, risk of malignancies, overdose possibilities, suicidality, withdrawal syndromes, and adverse reactions during pregnancy are considerations. And there is the risk of drug-drug interactions. A 2019 JAMA published study analyzed data from published meta-analyses of observational studies that assessed the association between antidepressant use or exposure and adverse health outcomes [177]. They concluded that there are no absolute contraindications for using antidepressants, and they are safe for treating psychiatric disorders. But more work is needed to sort out matching antidepressants to underlying diseases.

SSRIs can also decrease the cytotoxic efficacy of some cytotoxic drugs [170, 178]. SSRIs are susceptible to metabolically based drug interactions with anticancer drugs principally through cytochrome P-450 isoenzymes [178, 179]. For example, it has been reported that women who have breast cancer who get paroxetine while taking tamoxifen have an increased risk of death [178, 180–183]. Although a 2019 review has disputed an increased risk of recurrence or contralateral breast cancer in early-stage breast cancer patients [181].

Paroxetine and fluoxetine potently inhibit *CYP2D6 (an enzyme system that metabolizes tamoxifen into its active form) and reduce the clinical efficacy of some cancer drugs* [184, 185]. On the other hand, citalopram and escitalopram are weak or negligible inhibitors of CYP2D6. Sertraline causes significant inhibition of CYP2D6 only at high doses. *Hypericum perforatum* extract induces CYP3A4 and the membrane transporter P-glycoprotein and can interfere with different antineoplastic agents, including imatinib, irinotecan, and docetaxel. One study found imipramine and tranylcypromine but not fluoxetine reduced the cytotoxic efficacy of temozolomide, under some oxygen conditions [173].

Various SSRIs used after colon cancer diagnosis did not seem to increase the risk of recurrence [186].

It should be mentioned that cancer patients are at a very high risk of potential drug-drug interactions, not just with antidepressants. It has been estimated that approximately 30% have been exposed to potentially dangerous combinations [187]. A 2019 review has produced a list of drugs for treating common comorbid conditions that can be safely administered concomitantly with palbociclib and/or ribociclib [188]. Similar lists are available for other drug-drug interactions.

Useful resources to check for drug interactions can be found on the Internet. For example, [189–191].

Databases from 1990 to 2009 were reviewed for the relevance of *sleep to vigilance* [192]. It was seen that neither the SSRIs nor the SNRIs have particularly beneficial effects on sleep. Among the medications that are the most reliable for improving sleep efficiency (e.g., mirtazapine and tricyclic antidepressants), side effects of daytime sedation may offset therapeutic benefits. When patients are taking other antidepressants, trazodone, which is frequently prescribed, does not appear to be a safe and effective hypnotic. There is no convincing evidence that benzodiazepines have any long-term efficacy. Agomelatine seems promising but may be hepatotoxic [193, 194].

A 2015 systematic review and network analysis on *efficacy and acceptability of pharmacological treatments* for depressive disorders in primary care found that tricyclic and tetracyclic antidepressants (TCAs), selective serotonin reuptake inhibitors (SSRIs), a serotonin-noradrenaline reuptake inhibitor (SNRI; venlafaxine), a low-dose serotonin antagonist and reuptake inhibitor (SARI; trazodone) and hypericum extracts (St. John's wort) were significantly superior to placebo, with estimated odds ratios between 1.69 and 2.03 [195]. No significant differences were seen between these drugs. There were fewer dropouts due to adverse effects in reversible inhibitors of monoaminoxidase A (rMAO-As) and hypericum extracts than in the rest of the drugs. Although effect sizes were small, TCAs and SSRIs had the most evidence for utility in primary care. There was little evidence for hypericum, rMAO-As, SNRI, NRI, NaSSAs (noradrenergic and specific serotonergic antidepressive agent (mianserin, mirtazapine), and SARI, even though there were a few positive results. With that admonition, TCAs, SSRIs, and hypericum extracts were significantly superior to NaSSAs and rMAO-As. Hypericum extracts were also more effective than NRI. SNRI and low-dose SARI were superior to NaSSAs.

On the Other Hand

Antidepressant treatment may be costly in time and money and have adverse effects. Dropout rates in clinical trials have been said to be between 12 and 40% in the first 6–8 weeks of treatment [30, 119].

A 2008 meta-analysis of data submitted to the Food and Drug Administration showed that differences between placebo and antidepressant drugs are minimal [30]. Any differences in effectiveness as the severity of depression increases appear to be due to decreased responsiveness to placebo among very severely depressed patients, rather than to increased responsiveness to medication.

Selective publication of clinical trials and outcomes within those trials can lead to unrealistic estimates of drug effectiveness and change the apparent risk-benefit ratio. In 2008, reviews were analyzed from the Food and Drug Administration (FDA) for studies of 12 antidepressant agents involving 12,564 patients [26]. The following is a direct quote,

> Among 74 FDA-registered studies, 31%, accounting for 3449 study participants, were not published. Whether and how the studies were published was associated with the study outcome. A total of 37 studies viewed by the FDA as having positive results were published; 1 study viewed as positive was not published. Studies viewed by the FDA as having negative or questionable results were, with 3 exceptions, either not published (22 studies) or published in a way that, in our opinion, conveyed a positive outcome (11 studies). According to the published literature, it appeared that 94% of the trials conducted were positive. By contrast, the FDA analysis showed that 51% were positive. Separate meta-analyses of the FDA and journal data sets showed that the increase in effect size ranged from 11 to 69% for individual drugs and was 32% overall. We cannot determine whether the bias observed resulted from a failure to submit manuscripts on the part of authors and sponsors, from decisions by journal editors and reviewers not to publish, or both. Selective reporting of clinical trial results may have adverse consequences for researchers, study participants, health care professionals, and patients.

A 2017 systematic review was conducted with meta-analysis and *Trial Sequential Analysis*[11] of selective serotonin reuptake inhibitors versus placebo in patients with MDD [196]. Direct quote, “A total of 131 randomised placebo-controlled trials enrolling a total of 27,422 participants were included. None of the trials used ‘active’ placebo or no intervention as control intervention.” They concluded, “SSRIs might have statistically significant effects on depressive symptoms, but all trials were at high risk of bias and the clinical significance seems questionable. SSRIs significantly increase the risk of both serious and nonserious adverse events. The potential small beneficial effects seem to be outweighed by harmful effects.”

A 2019 systematic review and meta-analysis of second-generation antidepressants for the treatment of older adults with depression concluded, “Second-generation antidepressants have uncertain benefit for older adults with depression and cause more adverse events compared to placebo. Until further research clarifies benefit, careful consideration of antidepressant prescribing with frailty is warranted” [198].

A 2016 systematic review and network meta-analysis compared *efficacy and acceptability of 21 antidepressant drugs for the acute treatment of adults* with major depressive disorder [199]. All 21 antidepressants were more effective than placebo, and the summary effect sizes were mostly modest. Escitalopram, mirtazapine, paroxetine, agomelatine, and sertraline, and a few others, achieved a relatively higher response and lower dropout rate than others. Reboxetine, trazodone, and fluvoxamine had generally comparatively inferior efficacy and acceptability profiles. More variability in efficacy and acceptability was seen in head-to-head trials than in placebo-controlled trials.

- ORs ranged between 2.13 (95% credible interval (CrI)[12]: 1.89–2.41) for amitriptyline and OR = 1.37; CrI: 1.16–1.63) for reboxetine.
- For acceptability, only agomelatine (OR = 0.84; 95% CrI: 0.72–0.97) and fluoxetine (OR = 0.88; CrI: 0.80–0.96) were associated with fewer dropouts than placebo; clomipramine was worse than placebo (OR 1.30, CrI: 1.01–1.68).
- When all trials were considered, differences in ORs between antidepressants ranged from 1.15 to 1.55 for efficacy and from 0.64 to 0.83 for acceptability; wide CrIs were seen in most of the comparative analyses.
- In head-to-head studies, agomelatine, amitriptyline, escitalopram, mirtazapine, paroxetine, venlafaxine, and vortioxetine were more effective than other antidepressants (range of ORs 1.19–1.96); fluoxetine, fluvoxamine, reboxetine, and trazodone were the least efficacious drugs (Ors 0.51–0.84).
- For acceptability, agomelatine, citalopram, escitalopram, fluoxetine, sertraline, and vortioxetine were more tolerable than other antidepressants (range of ORs 0.43–0.77); amitriptyline, clomipramine, duloxetine, fluvoxamine, reboxetine, trazodone, and venlafaxine had the highest dropout rates (1.30–2.32).

[11] *Trial Sequential Analysis* (TSA) combines an information size for a meta-analysis with the threshold of statistical significance. TSA is an advanced software technique for quantifying statistical reliability of data in the cumulative meta-analysis taking into account significance levels for sparse data and repetitive testing on accumulating data [197].

[12] A *credible interval (CrI)* characterizes a probability distribution wherein a particular unobserved event has the probability of occurring within that interval. The intervals may be predictive probabilities or posterior probabilities. A *credible set* is a generalization. For more details, please see Chap. 4.

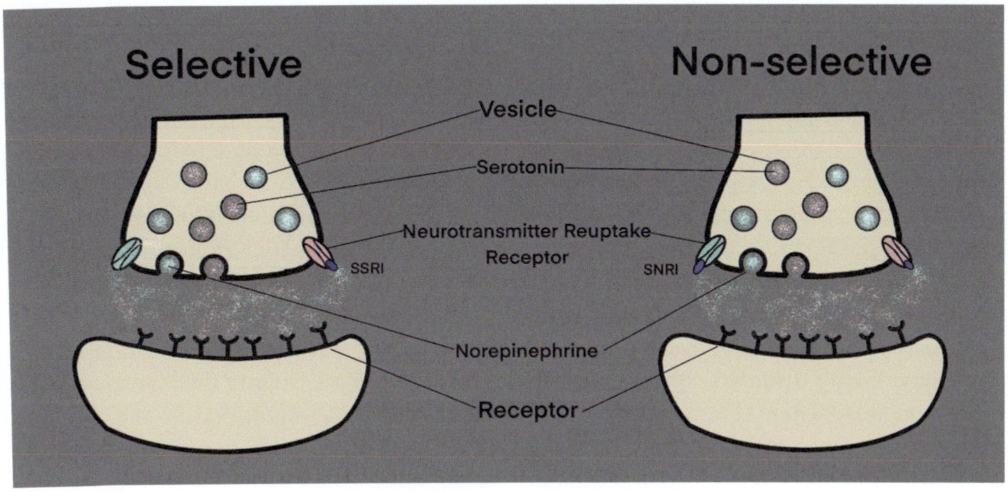

Fig. 16.1 Classification of selective and nonselective reuptake inhibitors. This illustration categorizes antidepressant reuptake inhibitors based on neurotransmitter targets. Selective agents include serotonin reuptake inhibitors (SRIs), dopamine reuptake inhibitors (DRIs), and norepinephrine reuptake inhibitors (NRIs), each modulating a single neurotransmitter system. Nonselective agents span combinations such as SNRIs, SDRIs, NDRIs, and SNDRIs, affecting multiple neurotransmitter pathways to alter mood and cognitive function

- For risk of bias, 46 (9%) of 522 trials were rated as high, 380 (73%) trials as moderate, and 96 (18%) as low; and the certainty of evidence was moderate to very low.

Effects of antidepressants on children and adolescents appear to be quite different than those on adults [109, 119]. It has been suggested that these differences may be due to underlying heterogeneous mechanisms of depression, fewer studies, or different methodological considerations involved in RCTs of adult versus pediatric populations [200]. A 2016 network meta-analysis of the comparative efficacy and tolerability of antidepressants for MDD in children and adolescents found that only fluoxetine was statistically significantly more effective than placebo (standardized mean difference −0.51, 95% credible interval CrI: −0.99 to −0.03) [119].

In 2024, results from a systematic review and network meta-analysis—covering studies conducted up to 2020—were published. The review evaluated psychological, psychosocial, pharmacological, physical, and combined treatments for adults experiencing a new episode of depression [201].

They concluded that in less severe depression, group cognitive/cognitive behavioral therapy (CT/CBT) and possibly group yoga and self-help may be efficacious; however, antidepressants did not show evidence of effect. In cases of more severe depression, the following treatments appeared efficacious: combined antidepressants with individual cognitive therapy (CT) or cognitive behavioral therapy (CBT); acupuncture and, possibly, group exercise; individual psychological therapies (CT/CBT) alone; and antidepressants alone. The quality of evidence for the effectiveness of these interventions on less severe depression was low, and for more severe depression was low to moderate.

Now, let us look at the characteristics of the major classes of antidepressants. *The three principal classifications* of antidepressants are the reuptake inhibitors, tricyclic antidepressants, and the monoamine oxidase inhibitors. The most commonly used antidepressants have varying degrees of effect on monoamine transporters and receptors. Antidepressants have been used to treat depression and anxiety, but there are also anxiety-specific pharmaceuticals.

Reuptake Inhibitors

According to the *monoamine hypothesis of depression*, norepinephrine may be associated with alertness, energy, anxiety, attention, and interest in life; serotonin with anxiety, obsessions, and compulsions; and dopamine with attention, motivation, pleasure, reward, and interest in life [202]. See Fig. 16.1.

Monoamine reuptake inhibitors (MRIs) are pharmaceuticals that inhibit the reuptake of at least one of the principal monoamine transmitters (i.e., serotonin, dopamine, or norepinephrine). Generally, they are classified as selective (binding to one monoamine transporter) or nonselective (binding to two or more monoamine transporters).

Selectives are serotonin reuptake inhibitors (SRIs), dopamine reuptake inhibitors (DRIs), or norepinephrine reuptake inhibitors (NRIs).

Nonselectives include serotonin-norepinephrine reuptake inhibitors (SNRI), serotonin-dopamine reuptake inhibitors (SDRI), norepinephrine-dopamine reuptake inhibitors (NDRI), and serotonin-norepinephrine-dopamine reuptake inhibitors (SNDRI).

In addition to prescribed MRIs, many of the abused or recreational psychoactive stimulants, such as cocaine and methylphenidate, are DRIs [203].

Selective Reuptake Inhibitors

SRIs are used principally as an antidepressant but are also used for treating anxiety, eating disorders, obesity, neuropathic pain, and premature ejaculation. For a description of the most common SRIs, a convenient source is [204, 205]. The most common subtype of SRIs is the selective serotonin reuptake inhibitors *(SSRIs)* [206].[13]

After neurotransmission, most of the neurotransmitters are removed from the postsynaptic receptors in the synaptic cleft and are recycled by monoamine or other transporters, which take them back into the presynaptic neuron [207]. After neurotransmission of serotonin, SSRIs inhibit the reuptake of serotonin by the presynaptic neuron, thereby increasing the amount of serotonin available to the postsynaptic cell. They are relatively specific for inhibiting serotonin and have little influence on inhibiting the reuptake of other monoamines such as dopamine or norepinephrine.

The underlying premise for reuptake inhibitors is that various conditions, such as depression, are due to a relative deficiency of neurotransmitters: more specifically, that the postsynaptic cells are not sufficiently stimulated. So, by inhibiting the reuptake of serotonin (5-HT), SSRIs increase the amount of time that serotonin hangs around the postsynaptic cell. In this way, it has been thought that the amount of serotonin has the potential to have a greater space/time effect and may fully activate the postsynaptic cell. However, the actual mechanisms for producing neuronal benefits are more complex than that. We will mention these in a few paragraphs later.

Now, as may have already occurred to the astute reader, the neuroendocrine system is dynamically auto-correcting. That is, there are usually feedback loops, sometimes redundant and multilayered, that do not ignore excess products. Such is the case here. Excess synaptic serotonin inhibits presynaptic production of serotonin and decreases the postsynaptic serotonin 5-HT receptors. The result is that the serotonin deficiency persists for a while after starting the SSRIs. But the brain gradually decreases its sensitivity to "excess" serotonin, and beneficial effects can be seen in many cases.

In those folks for whom antidepressants are useful, *it is common for 3–6 weeks of pharmacotherapy to be undertaken before full effects are seen* [37]. It appears that this delayed effect is due to modifications of gene expression resulting in changes in synaptic architecture and signaling, neurogenesis, receptor desensitization, and intracellular transduction cascades.

Due to this slow adaptation, SSRIs may take one to several weeks of continuous use until the beneficial effects are fully realized [210]. In the meantime, anxiety and depression can actually increase during the adjustment period.

Why does it take time for the effects of serotonin to be felt? One of the first things is a decrease in the density of postsynaptic receptors as a result of having more serotonin available in the synapse. The next thing is an increase in second messengers in the postsynaptic cells [211]. This includes cAMP. The culmination of these increased second messengers is an increase in trophic or protective molecules such as brain-derived neurotrophic factor (BDNF). Increased BDNF nourishes the neuron, making it more active and connecting it to other cells. Without BDNF and related trophic factors, cells decrease activity and connections.[14]

More specifically, mood stabilizers, antidepressants, and antipsychotics appear to produce their neurotrophic and neu-

---

[13] *Serotonin (5-hydroxytryptamine (5-HT))* is produced from the decarboxylation of 5-hydroxytryptophan, which is produced from the hydrolysis of tryptophan. Concentrations are controlled by tryptophan uptake and intraneuronal monoamine oxidase. High concentrations are found in the basal ganglia and the hypothalamus. The group of median raphe nuclei surrounding the midbrain aqueduct and midline neurons of the pons varolii and upper brain stem produce most of 5-HT that is produced in the brain. Those 5-HT neurons connected to the cerebral cortex and hypothalamus are associated with REM sleep; those connected to the limbic system relate to aggression; and those connected to the spinal column are associated with sensitivity to pain. About 90% of the serotonin is produced in the cells lining the gastrointestinal tract. Only about 10% is produced in the brain. Serotonin occurs in quite a few peripheral tissues and in some carcinoid tumors. It is also a vasoconstrictor stored in platelets, which actively concentrates it from plasma; it inhibits gastric secretions and stimulates the contraction of smooth muscle. Serotonin may also function as a neuromodulator or fine-tuner in the CNS by release from swellings (varicosities) along the axon. Fascinating reviews of serotonin can be found in [208, 209]. Serotonin does not cross the blood-brain barrier, and its production and, therefore, some behaviors can be moderated by dietary intake of tryptophan (for more, see the chapter on nutrition). However, it is important to realize that dietary sources of tryptophan are also usually high in other amino acids that compete for transport across the blood-brain barrier. Suppression of 5-HT reuptake and disruption of the serotonin system may result from the recreational use of methamphetamines, MDMA (ecstasy), and cocaine.

[14] *BDNF is also increased (as monitored by serum levels* [219] *and postmortem assays* [220]*) by other activities.* These include CBT [221, 222], exercise [223, 224], repetitive transcranial magnetic stimulation (rTMS) [225], and electroconvulsive shock [226]. In mice, an enriched environment may also increase BDNF in the hippocampus [227]. Estrogen is a neurotrophe/ neuroprotective too [228, 229]. There is some evidence that BDNF appears to be lowered by diets high in fat or sugar [230–234].

roprotective effects by stimulating the mitogen-activated protein kinase/extracellular signal-related kinase, PI3-kinase, and wingless/glycogen synthase kinase (GSK) 3 signaling pathways [211], and VEGF [212]. This results in increasing expression of neurotrophic and neuroprotective molecules such as BDNF, B-cell lymphoma 2 (Bcl-2), serine-threonine kinase, and Bcl-2-associated athanogene 1. At the same time, they inactivate neurodegenerative molecules [211, 212].

SSRIs have been used to treat clinical depression, anxiety disorders (such as panic disorders, social anxiety, posttraumatic stress syndrome, and obsessive-compulsive disorders), eating disorders, and some personality disorders [213–215]. They have also been used to treat premature ejaculation [216] and irritable bowel syndrome [217]. They are often the first-line treatment for depression [209]. It has been suggested that improvement in comorbidity of anxiety might be a consequence of interactions with GABA rather than with serotonin systems [245, 246].

Because of vast amounts of advertising, the trade names of several of these SSRIs have become familiar household names. These include Prozac (fluoxetine), Paxil (paroxetine), Celexa (citalopram), Zoloft (sertraline), and Lexapro (escitalopram oxalate).

Here is a list of the most common SSRIs:

1. Citalopram (Celexa) [235, 236]
2. Dapoxetine (Priligy) [237]
3. Escitalopram (Lexapro, Cipralex) [238]
4. Fluoxetine (Prozac) [239]
5. Fluvoxamine (Luvox) [240]
6. Paroxetine (Paxil, Seroxat) [241]
7. Sertraline (Zoloft, Lustral) [242]

The Merck Manual suggests the following [243]. For most types of antidepressants, therapeutic response takes about 2–3 weeks but may be as fast as 4 days or may take as much time as 8 weeks. They also suggest that for the first bout of mild to moderate depression, a 6-month course followed by gradual tapering (for SSRIs, about 25% per week) over the next 2 months should be instituted. For recurrent or severe depression, or when there is the risk of suicide, a dose that produces a full remission should be maintained. Antidepressant treatment for 6 months to 1 year and up to 2 years in folks older than 50 years of age may be necessary to prevent relapse.

Withdrawal likelihood and severity of symptoms (such as nausea, chills, muscle aches, dizziness, anxiety, irritability, insomnia, and fatigue) appear to be inversely related to the half-life of the SSRI.

Because serotonin is involved in many different functions in the central nervous system and in the gastrointestinal tract, there are *multiple side effects in inhibiting its reuptake*.[15] These side effects are quite variable in both duration and intensity. It has been said that most of the side effects disappear with time (1–4 weeks) as the body adapts to the changing levels; however, in some instances, they may persist [247, 248]. Side effects include blurred vision, drowsiness or insomnia, nausea, diarrhea, constipation, headache, changes in appetite and weight, increased depression or anxiety, tremors, sexual dysfunction, and sweating [133, 218]. It would appear that physicians tend to underestimate the frequency of side effects and how bothersome they are to their patients [218, 244].

There is debatable evidence that *suicide* is a side effect [151, 177, 249–259]. However, in the USA, the FDA mandates a prominent, black-boxed suicide warning label on SSRIs used for the treatment of children but not adults [256–259]. Early evidence had suggested that the critical periods appear to be the first few months after beginning the SSRIs, where suicidal ideations, gestures, or attempts may occur, especially in children and young adults [177].

Sexual dysfunctions have been reported to occur in 17% [218] to 41% [244] of folks taking SSRIs. These side effects include diminished libido, anorgasmia, and erectile dysfunction, and often persist after treatment with SSRIs is discontinued. Sexual dysfunction appears to correlate with duration of depression, but does not correlate with any measurement of depression, age, duration of treatment, dose, or plasma level of SSRI [244]. Genital anesthesia has been reported to persist for six or more years after discontinuing SSRIs [260]. SSRIs can cause an array of sexual side effects that may persist for months or years or be permanent even after the drugs have been discontinued [282]. This persistent condition is called *Post SSRI Sexual Dysfunction* [268].

Two alternatives to SSRIs that have sexual side effects are mirtazapine and bupropion [269].

Serotonin syndrome (aka *serotonergic syndrome* or *serotonin toxicity)* caused by excess serotonin activity produces cognitive, autonomic, and somatic symptoms that can range from barely noticeable to fatal [11, 270, 271]. The syndrome can result from several different types of drugs and combinations of drugs. Symptoms may begin within minutes to hours and include [272].

- Agitation or restlessness
- Diarrhea

[15]The 5-HT system has at least 15 different serotonin receptors [261, 262], some of which have opposing effects. SSRIs stimulate 5-HT1 receptors, which have anxiolytic and antidepressant effects [263–265]. However, SSRIs may also stimulate 5-HT2 receptors, which frequently cause anxiety, sexual dysfunction, and insomnia [15, 266]. Moreover, they stimulate 5-HT3 receptors, which may result in headaches and nausea [267]. In balance, therefore, SSRIs can cause anxiety or lessen anxiety and may do so in relation to the duration of treatment.

- Fast heartbeat and high blood pressure
- Mental status changes such as confusion, hypomania, or hallucinations
- Increased body temperature (e.g., manifested as fever or heavy sweating not due to activity)
- Loss of coordination
- Nausea
- Muscle spasms (myoclonus)
- Tremor, overactive reflexes
- Rapid changes in blood pressure
- Vomiting

Drug interactions can occur with some of the SSRIs, such as Prozac and Luvox, which interfere with cytochrome P-450 (CY P-450) isoenzymes [96]. Some of these side effects can be serious; for example, when they decrease the metabolism of some of the β-blockers, which can lead to hypotension and bradycardia. Another example is ethanol interactions that can also be serious with some SSRIs via pharmacodynamic synergism in producing CNS depression. There are several fine online databases to check for multidrug interactions. For example, [189–191].

When *nursing mothers* take antidepressants, it is unclear if they pose a risk to nursing infants [273]. Infant doses from breast milk of less than 10% of the maternal weight-adjusted dose are generally considered safe [143]. Paroxetine (Paxil) and sertraline (Zoloft) reach 0.5% to 3% in infants' sera; however, fluoxetine (Prozac), citalopram (Celexa), and desvenlafaxine [274] appear in levels close to or above 10% [275–280]. A 2013 review states, "Newer antidepressants transfer into breast milk in low amounts and have not been associated with serious adverse events" [281].

Norepinephrine reuptake inhibitors (NRIs), due to their psychostimulant properties, are most frequently used as treatments for schizophrenia, ADHD [283], and narcolepsy [284], and are also controversially used in major depression [285–288].

Dopamine reuptake inhibitors (DRIs) are used for similar conditions as NRIs, but due to their addiction properties by feeding into the reward system, they are seldom used for mood disorder treatments [289].

Reuptake Inhibitors Targeting Multiple Receptors

Norepinephrine-dopamine reuptake inhibitors (NDRIs) have been used for ADHD [291], social anxiety disorder [290], Parkinson's disease [292, 293], and narcolepsy [294, 295], and clinical depression [296–298].

Bupropion (Wellbutrin, Zyban, Voxra, Budeprion, Buproban, or Aplenzin), the most well-known of the NDRIs, has also been used to treat cocaine dependence and those who are attempting to stop smoking [299]. It has found popular use as an add-on medication to SSRIs [300].

Bupropion may not cause sexual dysfunctions or weight gain to the same extent as other antidepressants [269].

Bupropion, as a substituted amphetamine, is a mild psychostimulant. It can cause agitation, seizures (especially in bulimics), and can interact with other medications, inhibit CYP2D6 hepatic enzyme, but it appears to have little adverse sexual effects [300].

Primary behavioral effects appear to be related to inhibition of norepinephrine reuptake [301]. Its efficacy in smoking cessation appears to be related to its nicotinic acetylcholine receptor antagonism [302, 303].

Nicotine replacement therapies (patches and gum), bupropion, and varenicline (Chantix: a nicotine receptor partial agonist) may provide therapeutic effects in assisting with smoking cessation. Partial agonists reduce cravings and the pleasurable effects of nicotine-containing products. As an agonist, they maintain a moderate level of dopamine to moderate withdrawal, and as an antagonist, they decrease the satisfaction of smoking [304].

Comparative levels of effectiveness in smoking cessation are detailed in the following comprehensive reviews and meta-analyses [305, 306]. It appears that more folks quit successfully with varenicline than with bupropion.

Serotonin-norepinephrine reuptake inhibitors (SNRIs) are among the most commonly prescribed medications in the USA [307]. Some common SNRIs include Effexor (venlafaxine) [308], Cymbalta (duloxetine) [309], and Pristiq (desvenlafaxine) [310]. They are used to treat *Mood disorders* (major depression) [311–313]; postpartum depression [314]; and during pregnancy [315].[16] *Anxiety disorders* (panic disorders, phobias, and social anxiety) [316]. *ADHD* [317, 318]. *OCD* [319, 320]. *Pain* (fibromyalgia, chronic neuropathic pain) [321, 322]. *Menopausal symptoms* [323, 324].

Serotonin-dopamine reuptake inhibitors use is rare [325]. Some work has been done on the potential use of SDRIs for stimulant and alcohol addiction [326].

Serotonin-norepinephrine-dopamine reuptake inhibitors (SNDRIs) also known as triple uptake inhibitors are used for major depression [329, 330], alcoholism [331, 332], psychostimulant addiction [333], ADHD [334, 335], obesity [336], Parkinson's disease [337], and chronic pain [329, 338]. Nefazodone is currently the only SNDRI approved for major depression treatment [339]. Nontherapeutic SNDRIs include cocaine [340] and St. John's wort [341].

[16] Studies of risks of SNRI use during pregnancy include [315, 318, 327, 328].

Tricyclics

Tricyclic antidepressants were first used to treat depression starting in the 1950s and were the first line until the mid-1970s when the SSRIs were introduced. The tricyclics (their core structure is three rings) are believed to work by blocking the reuptake of norepinephrine, dopamine, and serotonin. The tricyclics also block α_1-adrenergic, H1 histaminergic, and muscarinic receptors.

Because of their wide range of receptors affected, many more side effects are experienced with tricyclics than with SSRIs. The tricyclics' most common side effects relate to their anticholinergic activity. These include dry mouth, constipation, ocular side effects, and urinary hesitancy [342].

Their *therapeutic index* is quite narrow [343]. That is, the toxic dose is very close to the therapeutic dose. *Serious toxic effects* include CNS perturbations and cardiac problems. Indeed, they are one of the most common causes of poisoning seen in emergency rooms [344]. Tricyclics may be second only to analgesics as a cause of fatal poisonings [345–347]. And as with all antidepressants, the FDA of the USA requires a suicide-warning label on the packaging insert [148, 348].

Nevertheless, tricyclics are still used for certain disorders. These most commonly include clinical depression that is refractory to the SSRIs [349]. They are also used in attention deficit disorder (ADHD) when psychostimulants are not effective [350]. They have minimal effect on attention and cognitive functions but seem to diminish hyperactivity and impulsivity. They can be useful for treating certain types of pain (e.g., neuropathic), possibly by indirectly modifying the CNS opioid systems [351].

Some common tricyclics are imipramine (Tofranil, et al.), amitriptyline (Elavil, et al.), and doxepin (Adapin, et al.).

Monoamine Oxidase Inhibitors

The oldest type of antidepressants is the monoamine oxidase inhibitors (MAOIs). Unlike the uptake inhibitors, MAOIs slow the activity of monoamine oxidase (MAO) in its role of oxidatively deaminating and hence deactivating both dietary and biogenic amines such as the monoamine neurotransmitters. MAO has two isoforms, which are found in the outer membranes of mitochondria in most cells, including neurons and glial cells. MAO-A isoform preferentially deaminates norepinephrine, epinephrine, serotonin, dopamine, and melatonin. MAO-B deaminates dopamine, phenylethylamine, and trace amines [352].

Oral MAOIs inhibit the catabolism of dietary amines. This is extremely important when the diet is high in tyramines [353]. Apparently, excessive *tyramine* may displace norepinephrine from storage depots; or as a building block for catecholamines, tyramine can trigger increased synthesis of catecholamines. The result may be an increased heart rate and increased vasoconstriction, causing a hypertensive crisis. Tyramine may be produced from any food high in aromatic amino acids when aging, fermenting, contamination, prolonged storage, or spoilage occurs [353]. These foods include various aged cheeses, such as those used in gourmet pizzas, tofu and soy sauce, aged wines such as Chianti, tap beer, chocolate; aged or cured meat such as air-dried sausage, bologna, and pepperoni; some meat extracts, liver, yeast extracts, overripe fruit; and sauerkraut [354–356]. Caffeinated foods may also present a problem.

Foods that have high *tryptophan* content, such as fava (broad) beans, may cause hyperserotonemia. Additionally, some birth-control pills, cold and allergy medications, pain relievers such as Advil, Motrin, and Tylenol, and some herbal supplements (such as St. John's Wort) may react with MAOIs to dangerously increase blood pressure [357]. The amount of any of the interacting substances that are dangerous seems to vary individually, and with the dose and selectivity of the MAOI.

Because they have serious and potentially deadly dietary and drug interactions, MAOIs are generally used as *a last resort* when other antidepressants have been tried and failed.

Anxiolytics

As mentioned above, mood disorders are frequently accompanied by comorbid conditions such as anxiety [358] and panic attacks [359–361]. Comorbidity prevalence between anxiety disorder and major depressive disorder has been reported to be as high as 60% in the USA and may be even higher if subsyndromal symptoms are included [362–364]. As such, it would be wise here to include information on drugs used for treating anxiety.

Anxiolytics are drugs used to treat the symptoms of anxiety. They are generally classified as benzodiazepines or nonbenzodiazepines.

Benzodiazepines

Benzodiazepines are often referred to as the minor tranquilizers. As a group, they share varying degrees of hypnotic, sedative, anxiolytic, muscle relaxation, amnestic (memory interfering) [365], and anticonvulsant features [366]. Benzodiazepines began to be used in the 1960s for stress-related illnesses.

Benzodiazepines decrease the high degree of physical arousal associated with panic attacks or anxiety, and some are used for insomnia. They are often used in tandem with

SSRIs. Popularity of anxiolytics such as Xanax, Valium, and Ativan is quite high due to speedy action and short half-life.

Benzodiazepine pharmacological action is *mediated by enhancing the action of GABA*. As mentioned above and discussed in more detail below, GABA is the major inhibitory neurotransmitter in the brain. About 40% of all the neurons in the CNS respond to GABA, so it has a natural soothing or tranquilizing effect [14]. After its interaction with the postsynaptic GABA-A cell receptor, GABA is actively pumped back up by the presynaptic cell and metabolized. Inhibition is due to increased permeability of chloride ions in the postsynaptic cell. This increased negative charge makes the postsynaptic neuron less responsive to excitation. Benzodiazepines interact with an area on the GABA receptors to further the inhibition. It apparently does this by changing the conformation of the GABA-A receptor in such a way that it has a much greater affinity for GABA. This results in a higher rate of opening the chloride channels and increasing the negative polarity [367–370].

GABA-A receptors are a family of various subtypes. Each of these is composed of 5 out of 19 possible subunits. Each of these subtypes has different properties, and they are found in different locations in the brain. In addition, they all have different interactions with benzodiazepines. For interaction with benzodiazepines, the GABA-A receptors need to have an α and a γ subunit. It appears that the $\alpha 2$ and $\alpha 3$ subtypes mediate the anxiolytic properties of benzodiazepines and $\alpha 1$ mediates the sedative properties [372].

Adverse effects of benzodiazepine interactions are common. Due to the increased inhibitory action, the postsynaptic cell releases less of the generally excitatory neurotransmitters such as norepinephrine, dopamine, serotonin, and acetylcholine. As a result of decreased excitatory transmitters, normal alertness, memory, emotional responses, heart rate, blood pressure, endocrine functions, muscle tone, and coordination take a hit [2]. In addition, non-GABA benzodiazepine receptors in the adrenal cortex, kidneys, colon, and blood cells may be perturbed by some benzodiazepines [2].

The various benzodiazepines differ in their *primary effects:* anxiolysis, hypnosis, sedation, anticonvulsant, and muscle relaxation. Taken as needed, some act in 20–30 min. Elimination rates vary widely among individuals. In addition, they vary in the length of their activity. Short-acting compounds last less than 6 h and have relatively few residual effects. They are more often used for treating insomnia. Intermediates last 6–10 h and may have some residual effects. Long-lasting ones have strong, persistent sedative effects. High-potency benzodiazepines are considered to be alprazolam, clonazepam, and lorazepam [371]. Benzodiazepines are usually taken daily for several weeks, but not any longer.

Potentially addictive, they should not be used by folks who have been addicted to alcohol, and they should *never be taken with alcohol*. Alcohol is synergistic with benzodiazepines and may produce intoxication, behavioral changes, and severe sedation [373, 374].

Some common benzodiazepines are:

1. Xanax (alprazolam): treating GAD and panic disorder; peak levels 1–2 h; ½ life about 6–27 h; most effects last 6–12 h.
2. Ativan (lorazepam): the intermediate-acting, has been used to treat panic disorder; peak concentration is about 2 h, ½ life about 12–16 h; most CNS effects last about 6 h.
3. Klonopin (clonazepam): treating generalized anxiety disorder (GAD) and social phobia; onset 1–2 h; long-acting: 19–60 h half-life.
4. Valium (diazepam): long acting; has anxiolytic, hypnotic, muscle relaxant, and anticonvulsant properties.
5. Librium (chlordiazepoxide): the original benzodiazepine is primarily an anxiolytic.
6. Dalmane (flurazepam): very long-acting hypnotic.

Tolerance to sedative and hypnotic effects usually occurs within days. But, tolerance to anxiolytic effects happens very slowly, if at all [2]. Dependence can also occur in up to 50 percent of patients within 6 months with therapeutic doses of diazepam [2].

One of the most *controversial negative effects* of benzodiazepines is on cognition [375–377]. A meta-analysis published in 2004 showed moderate-to-large weighted effect sizes for all cognitive domains assessed in people with long-term benzodiazepine use compared to controls. Another meta-analysis, published in 2005, found that cognitive dysfunction did occur with long-term treatment with benzodiazepines, and even though cognitive dysfunction improved after withdrawal, the patients did not return to levels of cognitive function that matched their benzodiazepine controls [376]. Neuroimages showed transient changes during benzodiazepine use, but no apparent long-term effects during prolonged use. The researchers state that the cognitive impairments may be insignificant in ordinary functioning.

The *Ashton Manual,* aka *Benzodiazepines: How they work and how to withdraw,* is remarkably comprehensive and well written. It is available on the Internet [378]. Dr. Heather Ashton is a world-renowned expert in the field.

Benzodiazepines can *dramatically suppress the HPA-axis*, probably mediated at the hypothalamic and/or suprahypothalamic level via suppression of CRH. [379]. Through apparent effects on the hypothalamus or pituitary, other pituitary hormones, such as gonadotropins and prolactin, are also affected.

Psychological dependence, physical dependence, and tolerance may result from prolonged use of benzodiazepines [380, 381]. Withdrawal symptoms may or may not reflect a true dependence and be due to a rebound effect that is a recurrence of anxiety symptoms that the medication was masking [383]. Typical withdrawal symptoms include insomnia, malaise, weakness, dizziness, lightheadedness, rebound anxiety, and tachycardia [382].

Withdrawal symptoms relate to the benzodiazepine used, how long it is used, dose frequency and amount, personality factors of the user, current and previous use, or cross-tolerant/dependent drugs such as other hypno-sedatives and alcohol [384–386].

Withdrawal symptoms are generally less common with diazepam (Valium) and oxazepam (Serepax) than with alprazolam (Xanax), temazepam (Restoril/Normison), or lorazepam (Temesta/Ativan) [387].

Major depressive disorder may be associated with the use of benzodiazepines or with the benzodiazepine withdrawal syndrome [12–14, 388, 389]. Decreased levels of norepinephrine and serotonin may be responsible for increased depression [390–392]. It may take up to 6–12 months for depression reacting to benzodiazepine withdrawal to subside [2, 3].

Nonbenzodiazepines

Barbiturates are basically obsolete for treating anxiety [393, 394]. *Buspirone* (Buspar et al.), a serotonin 5-HT_{1A} receptor agonist and a mixed dopamine postsynaptic receptor agonist/antagonist, has been used to treat anxiety [395]. It appears to be nonsedating, noncognition impairing, and less dependence-inducing than benzodiazepines. Beta-adrenergic blockers like propranolol (Inderal et al.) have been used to block physical symptoms of anxiety such as for public speaking [396].

Novel Pharmacotherapy Treatments

A solid 2022 review has categorized and expounded upon the novel pharmacological targets that may have the potential to fill in the gap (lack of efficacy, adverse effects, and risks) left by currently available antidepressants [397]. The following descriptions begin with their categories. The reader is encouraged to peruse their review for more and different details than what we present here.

Ketamine

Phencyclidine (*aka PCP, angel dust, whack, etc.*) is a hallucinogen well known for its ability to induce the fantasy of euphoria, omnipotence, superhuman strength, and social and sexual prowess [4, 398, 400].[17] Designer analogs were common for street use and PCP is still found laced into marijuana [400].

Phencyclidine has the greatest affinity for *NMDA*[18] *receptor complexes* in the hippocampus, neocortex, basal ganglia, and limbic system [401]. NMDA receptors are one of three subgroups of ionotropic glutamate receptors. Glutamate receptors include ionotropic and metabotropic receptors. They are critical for neuroplasticity and mediate most of the excitatory neurotransmission in the mammalian CNS [402].

The NMDA receptor (NMDAR) is a heteromeric ionotropic glutamatergic receptor. It is activated through glycine binding to an NR1 subunit or by glutamate binding to an NR2 subunit. Magnesium ions binding will block its activity [398, 403].

In decreasing order, PCP has affinity to NMDA receptors, to neuronal norepinephrine, dopamine, and serotonin reuptake systems, and to the σ opioid receptors [5]. PCP inhibits dopamine, norepinephrine, and serotonin reuptake, and increases dopamine and norepinephrine production by stimulating tyrosine hydroxylase, resulting in dopaminergic and sympathomimetic effects [6].

PCP intoxication is characterized by violent behavior, nystagmus, tachycardia, hypertension, anesthesia, and analgesia [398]. So, what does PCP have to do with depression treatment? The answer is ketamine.

NMDA receptor antagonists, particularly those targeting the GluN2B subunit, have been used for the treatment of severe mood disorders [404]. Ketamine is one of these [405].

Ketamine is a phencyclidine derivative that is a noncompetitive NMDAR antagonist that blocks the receptor pores [403, 404]. However, there is debate about whether monoamine reuptake inhibition is part of ketamine's effects on depressive disorders [406, 407]. Furthermore, dopamine agony is also debatable [408]. The mechanisms of action of ketamine in alleviating depression are unclear [405]. One hypothesis for ketamine antidepressant activity is inhibiting the *NMDA receptor-dependent bursting activity* in the "*anti-reward center*," the lateral habenula, in its role of modulating the mesolimbic reward pathway [409]. Another possibility is downstream effects on regulators like BDNF [410]. Other mechanisms with varying degrees of evidence have been suggested [411–414].

Ketamine has *two enantiomers* with antidepressant activity. These are R-ketamine (arketamine) and S-ketamine (esketamine). Although arketamine has lower affinity for the NMDA receptor, it has longer antidepressant effects [415, 416].

Ketamine *acts fast, but its effectiveness is not long-lasting* [417, 418]. Used as an IV infusion in treating treatment-resistant patients with BD and MDD, symptoms may be reduced within 4 h and achieve maximal benefit within 24 h

[17] PCP is the abbreviation of its organic name 1-(1-phenylcyclohexyl) piperidine.

[18] NMDA is the abbreviation for N-Methyl-DL-aspartic acid [399].

[419, 420]. Effects are variable, but for most patients, the antidepressant effects greatly diminish within 7 days, and most patients relapse within 10 days [421]. A 2021 Cochrane systematic review finds that ketamine and esketamine may be more efficacious than placebo at 24 h and are associated with improved symptoms that last 1–7 days [422].

Some folks may continue to have positive effects up to 30 days [420, 423]. Single dose and repeated doses *may produce antisuicidal effects* within 4.5 h in more than half of patients, and effects may be sustained over several weeks with 2 or 3 doses a week [420]. Significant reduction in suicidal ideation may be achieved from a single dose for up to 3 days [136].

Use of ketamine has been impractical due to the need for intravenous administration. A nasal spray form of esketamine has been approved for use in treatment-resistant depression (TRD) and MDD [424–426]. Esketamine has been used alone or in combination with standard antidepressants, and the results have been somewhat promising for use in patients with suicidal ideations and severe illness [427]. However, there are safety concerns over adverse events, including suicidal ideation [428–431].

Esketamine has been recommended by the Canadian Network for Mood and Anxiety Treatments (CANMAT) as a *third-line depression treatment* [432]. However, the cost of esketamine (sold under the brand name Spravato) is very steep for its modest efficacy.[19] There are *serious side effects* such as sedation, dissociation, respiratory depression, abuse, misuse, and suicidal thoughts and behaviors [7].

A 2022 review of human and clinical research has summarized data showing that ketamine can induce neurotoxicity and apoptosis, and changes in locomotor activity, social behaviors, anxiety- and depression-like behaviors, and memory [433]. Ketamine appeared to improve mood and reduce anxiety and depression symptoms in adolescents. But most of the data did not include females, and outcomes were dependent on dose and length of exposure. Harmful effects on various brain functions were notable.

γ-Aminobutyric Acid (GABA)

γ-Aminobutyric acid (GABA) is the *primary inhibitory neurotransmitter* in the brain and a major inhibitor in the spinal column (but in early stages of life, until the first postnatal week, it was exciting instead) [434, 435]. GABAergic neurons are mainly found in the GABAergic neurons located in the hippocampus, thalamus, basal ganglia, hypothalamus, and brainstem [436, 437]. See Fig. 16.2.

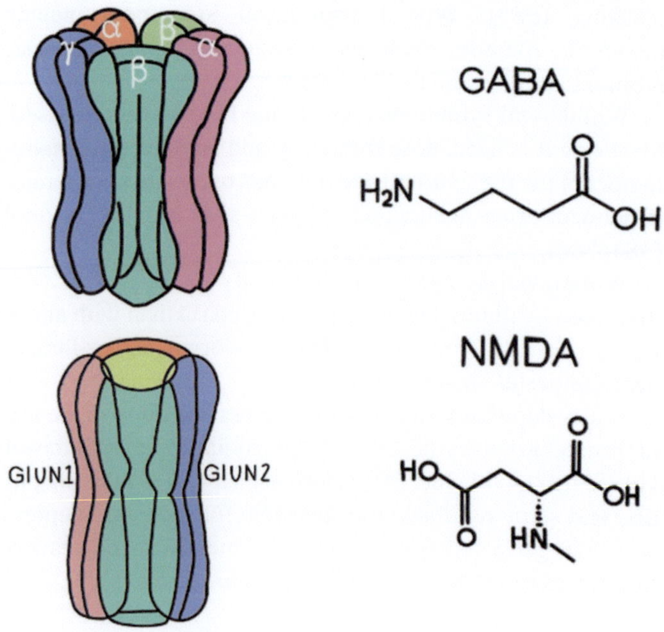

Fig. 16.2 Structural Representation of GABA and NMDA Receptor Proteins. This illustration depicts the distinct architectures of two major neurotransmitter receptors: the GABA receptor and the NMDA receptor. The GABA receptor is shown as a pentameric chloride channel composed of multiple subunits, facilitating inhibitory signaling via GABA binding. The NMDA receptor appears as a heterotetrameric glutamate-gated ion channel, requiring both glutamate and glycine for activation, and is critical for excitatory neurotransmission and synaptic plasticity

GABA is also *produced in a variety of peripheral tissues,* including the pancreas [438], intestines, stomach, fallopian tubes, uterus, ovaries, testicles, kidneys, urinary bladder, lungs, and liver [439]. Immune system cells have GABA receptors [441] astrocytes can synthesize and release GABA [440].

GABA activates GABA-A, an ionotropic receptor [442], and GABA-B, a metabotropic receptor [8, 443]. GABA is converted from glutamate by the action of glutamate decarboxylase and vitamin B [444, 445]. *Balances between glutamate excitatory transmission and GABA-mediated inhibitory functions* are vital for appropriate functioning in the brain [437, 446]. There are several GABA-A receptor subtypes [447, 448] as well as GABA-B subtypes [449, 450]. A second GABA ionotropic receptor has been identified: it is called GABA-C [451].

GABA function is determined by the neural circuit that it is inhibiting. It participates in complex circuits throughout the central nervous system [437, 452]. GABA-A receptor subtypes [453] are involved in specific brain circuits controlling fear, anxiety, learning, memory, reward, addiction, and stress-related behaviors [454, 455].

[19] Spravato is available for treatment of depression only from certified providers through a restricted program under a *Risk Evaluation and Mitigation Strategy (REMS)* [461]. REMS can provide safe access for patients to certain drugs with serious risks that may otherwise not be approved and available on the market.

Dysregulation of the GABAergic system is found in depression [456–458]. Astrocytes have a crucial role in regulating GABA homeostasis and synaptic neurotransmission [459, 460], and astrocyte GABA dysregulation is found in MDD and alcohol use disorders [440, 460]. Down-or dysregulation of GABA in MDD patients is seen in the orbitofrontal cortex [462], in treatment-resistant depression [463], and in postpartum depression [464, 465].

Several GABAergic drugs have shown preclinical evidence of antidepressant activity. These include valproate [466], amino-oxyacetic acid [467], beta-phenyl-GABA [468], diazepam [469], carbamazepine, and oxcarbazepine [470]. *GABA-As are targets of benzodiazepines and barbiturates in treating anxiety* [471]. Ethanol exerts effects on the GABA-A receptor, and benzodiazepines are cross-tolerant and are used for facilitating alcohol withdrawal [472, 473].

Using GABA-A receptor antagonists is not considered for first-line therapy because of the *high potential for addiction and possible fatality* [474].

GABA, when used as a dietary supplement, may or may not cross the blood-brain barrier or may exert some influence via the enteric nervous system [475].

Receptor Families as Potential Antidepressants

Preclinical and clinical data have shown glimpses of the usefulness of focusing on specific types of receptors rather than transmitters for the treatment of MDD. These include agonists, antagonists and regulators targeting opioid receptors, N-methyl-D-aspartate receptors (NMDARs), peroxisome proliferator-activated receptors (PPARs), G-protein-coupled receptor 39 (GPR39), metabotropic glutamate receptors (mGluRs) and galanin receptors (GALRs).

Epidrugs

Epidrugs are pharmacological interventions using drugs that selectively influence the epigenetic realm while having the potential to influence a wide range of genetic and environmental mechanisms of central nervous system disorders [476].

Biological Processes as Targets

Novel therapeutics show promise in targeting biological processes known to be involved in depression [397]. These include the hypothalamic–pituitary–adrenal axis (HPA) [477, 478], enteric microbiome [479–484], inflammation [485–489], brain plasticity [490], miRNAs [491], and cholesterol biosynthesis [492, 493].

Natural Products

Using natural products that target molecular pathways involved in depression has also shown promise in relieving depression symptoms [494]. These natural products include plant derivatives [495–498], N-3 polyunsaturated fatty acids (PUFAs) [487, 499–501], and resolvins [502, 503].

Stratified Treatment

The Depression Task Force sponsored by the *Hope for Depression Research Foundation* [504] was created in 2015 to develop novel strategies in antidepressant drug discovery to treat the significant number of patients with treatment-resistant depression. They use a systems biology approach to take advantage of advances in genomics and neural circuitry, and to integrate discoveries in animal models with results from MDD patients and high-risk cohorts. In that way, they hope to *identify biomarkers* that will allow patient subtyping and treatment stratification of those distinct depression subtypes [505].

A multistage multicenter prospective study was begun in China in 2013 to define subtypes of MDD [506]. Their goal is to develop a multidimensional diagnostic test and combine predictors to improve diagnostic accuracy and promote *personalized antidepressant drug interventions* in MDD patients.

Pharmacological Treatment of Sleep Disturbances in Depressed Patients

There are at least 40 recognized sleep disorders [507, 508]. Top-level categories include insomnia, hypersomnia, parasomnias, sleep-related breathing disorders, and sleep-related movement disorders. A good description of each of these and resources for management can be found on the *American Academy of Sleep Medicine* (AASM) website.[20]

Insomnia is the most common sleep disturbance and the one most associated with depression [510]. As a result,

[20]The AASM has both professional and patient resources [509]. "The American Academy of Sleep Medicine launched the Sleep Education website in 2005. The site has reliable information about sleep, sleep disorders, and treatment options. It is a valuable resource for patients who have sleep disorders. The site provides accurate medical and scientific insight in a concise manner that is easy to understand. It also provides facts that will be useful to anyone who wants to learn more about sleep."

insomnia is the sleep disorder most frequently treated with pharmaceuticals. So, we will focus our discussion on insomnia. More information on insomnia occurring with depression and nonpharmaceutical treatments can be found in Chap. 13 in this text. Briefly, insomnia is difficulty in either initiating sleep, maintaining sleep continuity, or poor sleep quality [14]. AASM 2017 clinical practice guidelines for the pharmacologic treatment of chronic insomnia in adults can be found in [511].

Compromised sleep quality, sleep deprivation, or restriction can lead to negative physiological and behavioral effects and increased mortality [512–515]. These include metabolic dysfunction, hypertension, vascular disorders, neurocognitive, and cardiovascular diseases.

Because of the activating properties of many antidepressants, they can make sleep worse [516, 517]. These drugs include imipramine, desipramine, fluoxetine, paroxetine, venlafaxine, and reboxetine. Clomipramine and phenelzine completely suppress REM sleep [518]. Because of their perturbations of sleep, patients are frequently coprescribed other drugs to help them sleep. As many as 30–40% of these patients still experience insomnia even with these sleep medications. Sedative antidepressants include doxepin, mirtazapine, trazodone, trimipramine, and agomelatine appear to help regulate circadian sleep rhythms and increase REM sleep [518]. Bupropion may improve latency to REM sleep, but it is still associated with increased insomnia [519–521].

There is little evidence to support long-term usage of sedative antidepressants for MDD and insomnia [522]. Studies have suggested that zolpidem that agonizes benzodiazepine receptors, improves SSRI-associated sleep disturbances [523]. However, zolpidem has been linked to rebound insomnia, residual next-day effects on psychomotor performance, including driving and memory, and complex sleep-related behaviors [524]. Trazodone may afford some help but may have considerable side effects [525]. Agomelatine may improve sleep, perhaps through its melatonin agonist activity [526, 527], but has serious potential toxicity [528].

A *2016 Agency for Healthcare Research and Quality (AHRQ) comprehensive assessment* of the efficacy, comparative effectiveness, and harms of treatments for insomnia disorder in the general adult population and older adults [529] has stated, "Low- to moderate-strength evidence indicated that the nonbenzodiazepine hypnotics eszopiclone and zolpidem, and the orexin receptor antagonist suvorexant, improved short-term global and sleep outcomes in general adult populations. Doxepin improved sleep outcomes. The absolute mean effect was small. Evidence for benzodiazepine hypnotics, melatonin agonists, and antidepressants in general populations and for most pharmacologic interventions in older adults was generally insufficient. Evidence on adverse effects from RCT data was generally insufficient or of low strength. Observational studies suggest that hypnotics may be associated with dementia, fractures, and major injury. Food and Drug Administration (FDA) labels warn about cognitive and behavioral changes, including driving impairment, and other harms, and advise lower doses for females and older/debilitated adults" [530].

Caution should be used when considering *sleep aids*. Older adults are susceptible to cognitive difficulties that may make some sleep aids dangerous. Children may be more susceptible to adverse effects than adults are. Pregnant or breast-feeding women may have health risks to themselves or their developing infant. It is convenient to think of medications used for sleep as either prescriptions, over-the-counter drugs, or dietary supplements [531].

Prescription Sleep Medications

The *prescription sleep medications* include sedative-hypnotic drugs, orexin receptor antagonists, melatonin receptor agonists, benzodiazepines, antidepressants, antipsychotics, and anticonvulsants.

Sedative-hypnotics are also known as the *Z drugs* (so called due to the Z in the trade names reflecting the vernacular of Z for sleep) [532]. Three of the Z drugs have received FDA approval. These are zolpidem [533], eszopiclone [534], and zaleplon [535]. Common treatments associated with adverse effects include next morning impairment, such as lingering drowsiness, impaired alertness even if feeling fully awake, impaired cognition, odd and dangerous behavior, including sleepwalking and sleep driving [536]. Additional negative effects include dependence, withdrawal, increased depression, and allergic reactions. Due to a slower rate of elimination, women seem to be more at risk than men for some of these side effects [9]. Respiratory depression can occur when combined with other sedatives.[21]

Orexin receptor antagonists decrease the production of orexin. Orexins (aka hypocretin) are neuropeptides that bind orexin receptor types 1 and 2 to regulate several physiologic processes involved in reacting to stressful stimuli, including feeding behavior, sleep-wake rhythm, reward and addiction, and energy balance [538]. In addition, orexin/receptor pathways are involved in the pathology of neurological diseases, including narcolepsy, depression, ischemic stroke, drug addiction, and Alzheimer's disease. A review of orexins in acute and chronic stress and how they contribute to sex differences in mental health can be found here [539].

As of 2024, the FDA has approved two orexin antagonists. They are suvorexant [540] and Lemborexant [541, 542]. Common adverse effects are similar to sedative hyp-

[21] The FDA has more than 100 entries listed under sleep medicines that detail risks of drugs used for sleep disorders listed on their Drug Safety and Availability web site [537].

notics [543]. But, in addition, they include narcolepsy, sleep paralysis, and hallucinations [544].

Melatonin receptor agonists activate melatonin receptors in the body [545]. Melatonin is produced from dietary tryptophan via serotonin. Melatonin helps to synchronize circadian rhythms in the body, including the sleep-wake cycle. Other activities include antioxidant, anti-inflammatory, and immune modulatory effects, memory improvement, neuroprotection, cardiovascular system modulation, bone homeostasis, lipid and glucose metabolism, and tumor inhibition [10]. The highest level of melatonin produced from the pineal gland via control of the suprachiasmatic nucleus is around 1–4 am when we are in the dark [546]. However, it is not essential for sleep. Endogenous levels of melatonin decrease with age [547].

The only FDA-approved melatonin receptor agonist as of 2024 is ramelteon [548]. Possible adverse effects are not as prominent as in the other prescribed sleep medications. They include daytime drowsiness, slowed thinking, decreased coordination, sleepwalking and sleep driving, and increased depression.

Benzodiazepines are well described above. They are recommended for maximum use of 7–10 days. The FDA has approved several benzodiazepines to treat insomnia. These are temazepam [549], triazolam [550], estazolam [551], quazepam [552], and flurazepam [553]. Treatment associated with adverse effects is similar to the sedative hypnotics, with the additional warning that benzodiazepines may increase the risk of serious or life-threatening breathing problems, sedation, or coma if used along with certain medications.

Antidepressants, as detailed above, treat depression and have been used for the treatment of depression associated insomnia [554, 555]. Two antidepressants have been approved for insomnia. These are doxepin [556] and trazodone [557]. A particular concern about the use of antidepressants includes the familiar association with increased suicidal ideation in patients less than 24 years of age. Additional concerns are blurred vision by altering pupil diameter and glaucoma risk; compromised cognitive thinking, including balance problems; and risky behavior when partially asleep.

Some *antipsychotics and anticonvulsants* have sedative properties, but none of them have been approved by the FDA for treating sleeping disorders.

Over-the-Counter (OTC) Sleep Aids

Over-the-counter (OTC) sleep aids are not FDA-approved or regulated but must comply with FDA standards [558].[22] Most OTC sleeping pills contain antihistamines. These medicines are commonly used to treat allergies. Those products that are used for allergies but are sedating are often labeled PM.

Two antihistamines that are specifically labeled for sleep aids are diphenhydramine [560] and doxylamine [561]. Within 30 min after taking one of these OTCs, sleep is likely to occur and last 7–8 h.

The FDA warns that nonprescription cough and cold combination products, including products that can cause serious side effects or death in young children.

Side effects include feeling tired or groggy the next day and impaired ability to drive. In elderly folks, their anticholinergic properties may result in dry mouth, nose, and throat, and confusion and memory problems. Dependency may be a problem because, although not addictive, our bodies quickly adapt to them, and their efficacy is fleeting.

Systematic reviews of RCTs have found that the most used OTC sleep-aid agents, especially diphenhydramine and valerian, do not have robust clinical evidence that supports their efficacy and safety [562].

Dietary Supplements

Dietary supplements are a diverse lot. Studies of effects on sleep are plagued by experimental difficulties, including adequate placebo controls, variability of active ingredients, and heterogeneity [563, 564]. For example, a 2020 review found that amino acids, vitamin D, and melatonin supplements were significantly beneficial to improve sleep quality [565]. However, high heterogeneity and wide confidence levels were observed in vitamin D and melatonin. Research was insufficient to analyze the effects of magnesium, zinc, resveratrol, and nitrate supplementation on improving sleep quality.

Melatonin again: There are a variety of dietary sources of melatonin. For example, melatonin is found in a variety of plants, including coffee beans, nuts, seeds, fruits, cereals, oils, beer, and wine [11, 12, 566]. Wheat, oats, and barley have relatively high levels. Of the fruit's grapes and their derivatives (wine and juice), cherries, strawberries, and kiwis have the highest. Of the vegetables, peppers, tomatoes, and mushrooms are the highest.

In foods of animal origin, the highest levels of melatonin are found in eggs, animal milk, human milk,[23] fish, and meat [569, 570].

Dietary intake of food sources of melatonin has been shown to significantly increase blood levels in humans and has produced positive effects on insomnia [571–574]. Oral intake of melatonin is well absorbed, distributed widely, and

[22] The difference between prescription drugs and over-the-counter drugs, as described by the FDA, can be found here [559].

[23] Milking cattle at night produces significantly higher melatonin values in cows' milk [567, 568].

completely metabolized and can pass the brain barrier [12, 572, 575]. A potential reciprocal association between sleep and fruit and vegetable consumption has been reported [13].

Summary

We have presented evidence for various antidepressants, their benefits, and drawbacks. Adverse effects and questionable efficacy have driven a shift to nonpharmacological treatments. Nevertheless, pharmacogenetic insights have suggested the possibility of matching antidepressant therapy to individual patient profiles to minimize variability in patient responses and associated risks with antidepressant medications. New pharmacotherapeutic approaches have begun to investigate alternative targets such as receptor families, biological processes, and the use of natural products.

References

1. Martindale: The Complete Drug Reference | Pharmaceutical Press.
2. Ashton CH. benzo.org.uk : Protracted Withdrawal From Benzodiazepines : Professor CH Ashton, DM, FRCP 1995.
3. Heather Ashton. benzo.org.uk : Protracted Withdrawal Symptoms from Benzodiazepines, Professor C H Ashton, 2004.
4. NIDA PCP (Phencyclidine). NIDA InfoFacts, Washington (DC), USA: U.S. Department of Health and Human Services20061–3. Commonly Used Drugs Charts | National Institute on Drug Abuse (NIDA).
5. Nelson LS, Goldfrank LR. Goldfrank's toxicologic emergencies, 2019.
6. Williams LC, Keyes C. Psychoactive drugs. In: Clinical toxicology, vol. 200. Philadelphia: WB Saunders; 2001. p. 640–9.
7. DailyMed - SPRAVATO- esketamine hydrochloride solution (nih.gov).
8. Structure and pharmacology of gamma-aminobutyric acidA receptor subtypes. | Pharmacological Reviews (aspetjournals.org).
9. Questions and Answers: Risk of next-morning impairment after use of insomnia drugs; FDA requires lower recommended doses for certain drugs containing zolpidem (Ambien, Ambien CR, Edluar, and Zolpimist) | FDA.
10. Kim HJ, Kim HJ, Bae MK, Kim YD. Suppression of Osteoclastogenesis by Melatonin: a melatonin receptor-independent action. Int J Mol Sci. 2017;18(6):1142. PMCID: PMC5485966. http://www.ncbi.nlm.nih.gov/pubmed/28587149.
11. Meng X, Li Y, Li S, Zhou Y, Gan RY, Xu DP, Li HB. Dietary sources and bioactivities of melatonin. Nutrients. 2017;9(4):367. PMCID: PMC5409706. http://www.ncbi.nlm.nih.gov/pubmed/28387721.
12. Circadin A. Australian public assessment report for melatonin. Commercial Eyes Pty Ltd; 2009. p. 1–57.
13. Noorwali E, Hardie L, Cade J. Bridging the reciprocal gap between sleep and fruit and vegetable consumption: a review of the evidence, potential mechanisms, implications, and directions for future work. Nutrients. 2019;11(6):1382. PMCID: PMC6627504. http://www.ncbi.nlm.nih.gov/pubmed/31248175.
14. http https://www.merckmanuals.com/professional/psychiatric-disorders/mood-disorders/medications-for-treatment-of-depressions://aasm.org/clinical-resources/international-classification-sleep-disorders/.
15. Gartlehner G, Wagner G, Matyas N, Titscher V, Greimel J, Lux L, Gaynes BN, Viswanathan M, Patel S, Lohr KN. Pharmacological and non-pharmacological treatments for major depressive disorder: review of systematic reviews. BMJ Open. 2017;7(6):e014912. PMCID: PMC5623437. http://www.ncbi.nlm.nih.gov/pubmed/28615268.
16. Gartlehner G, Thieda P, Hansen RA, Gaynes BN, Deveaugh-Geiss A, Krebs EE, Lohr KN. Comparative risk for harms of second-generation antidepressants : a systematic review and meta-analysis. Drug Saf. 2008;31(10):851–65. PMID: 18759509. http://www.ncbi.nlm.nih.gov/pubmed/18759509.
17. Mojtabai R, Olfson M. National patterns in antidepressant treatment by psychiatrists and general medical providers: results from the national comorbidity survey replication. J Clin Psychiatry. 2008;69(7):1064–74. PMID: 18399725. http://www.ncbi.nlm.nih.gov/pubmed/18399725.
18. Qaseem A, Barry MJ, Kansagara D. Clinical guidelines Committee of the American College of Physicians. Nonpharmacologic versus pharmacologic treatment of adult patients with major depressive disorder: a clinical practice guideline from the American College of Physicians. Ann Intern Med. 2016;164(5):350–9. PMID: 26857948. http://www.ncbi.nlm.nih.gov/pubmed/26857948.
19. Jobst A, Brakemeier EL, Buchheim A, Caspar F, Cuijpers P, Ebmeier KP, Falkai P, Jan van der Gaag R, Gaebel W, Herpertz S, Kurimay T, Sabaß L, Schnell K, Schramm E, Torrent C, Wasserman D, Wiersma J, Padberg F. European Psychiatric Association Guidance on psychotherapy in chronic depression across Europe. Eur Psychiatry. 2016;33:18–36. PMID: 26854984. http://www.ncbi.nlm.nih.gov/pubmed/26854984.
20. Churchill R, Khaira M, Gretton V, Chilvers C, Dewey M, Duggan C, Lee A. Nottingham Counselling and Antidepressants in Primary Care (CAPC) Study Group. Treating depression in general practice: factors affecting patients' treatment preferences. Br J Gen Pract. 2000;50(460):905–6. PMCID: PMC1313855. http://www.ncbi.nlm.nih.gov/pubmed/11141877.
21. van Schaik DJF, Klijn AFJ, van Hout HPJ, van Marwijk HWJ, Beekman ATF, de Haan M, van Dyck R. Patients' preferences in the treatment of depressive disorder in primary care. Gen Hosp Psychiatry. 2004;26(3):184–9. PMID: 15121346. http://www.ncbi.nlm.nih.gov/pubmed/15121346.
22. Givens JL, Katz IR, Bellamy S, Holmes WC. Stigma and the acceptability of depression treatments among african americans and whites. J Gen Intern Med. 2007;22(9):1292–7. PMCID: PMC2219769. http://www.ncbi.nlm.nih.gov/pubmed/17610120.
23. Cooper LA, Gonzales JJ, Gallo JJ, Rost KM, Meredith LS, Rubenstein LV, Wang NY, Ford DE. The acceptability of treatment for depression among African-American, Hispanic, and white primary care patients. Med Care. 2003;41(4):479–89. PMID: 12665712. http://www.ncbi.nlm.nih.gov/pubmed/12665712.
24. Givens JL, Houston TK, Van Voorhees BW, Ford DE, Cooper LA. Ethnicity and preferences for depression treatment. Gen Hosp Psychiatry. 2007;29(3):182–91. PMID: 17484934. http://www.ncbi.nlm.nih.gov/pubmed/17484934.
25. Melander H, Ahlqvist-Rastad J, Meijer G, Beermann B. Evidence b(i)ased medicine—selective reporting from studies sponsored by pharmaceutical industry: review of studies in new drug applications. BMJ. 2003;326(7400):1171–3. PMCID: PMC156459. http://www.ncbi.nlm.nih.gov/pubmed/12775615.
26. Turner EH, Matthews AM, Linardatos E, Tell RA, Rosenthal R. Selective publication of antidepressant trials and its influence on apparent efficacy. N Engl J Med. 2008;358(3):252–60. PMID: 18199864. http://www.ncbi.nlm.nih.gov/pubmed/18199864.
27. Fournier JC, DeRubeis RJ, Hollon SD, Dimidjian S, Amsterdam JD, Shelton RC, Fawcett J. Antidepressant drug effects and depression severity: a patient-level meta-analysis. JAMA.

2010;303(1):47–53. PMCID: PMC3712503. http://www.ncbi.nlm.nih.gov/pubmed/20051569.
28. Khan A, Leventhal RM, Khan SR, Brown WA. Severity of depression and response to antidepressants and placebo: an analysis of the Food and Drug Administration database. J Clin Psychopharmacol. 2002;22(1):40–5. PMID: 11799341. http://www.ncbi.nlm.nih.gov/pubmed/11799341.
29. Khan A, Faucett J, Lichtenberg P, Kirsch I, Brown WA. A systematic review of comparative efficacy of treatments and controls for depression. PLoS One. 2012;7(7):e41778. PMCID: PMC3408478. http://www.ncbi.nlm.nih.gov/pubmed/22860015.
30. Kirsch I, Deacon BJ, Huedo-Medina TB, Scoboria A, Moore TJ, Johnson BT. Initial severity and antidepressant benefits: a meta-analysis of data submitted to the Food and Drug Administration. PLoS Med. 2008;5(2):e45. PMCID: PMC2253608. http://www.ncbi.nlm.nih.gov/pubmed/18303940.
31. Narasimhan S, Lohoff FW. Pharmacogenetics of antidepressant drugs: current clinical practice and future directions. Pharmacogenomics. 2012;13(4):441–64. PMID: 22380000. http://www.ncbi.nlm.nih.gov/pubmed/22380000.
32. El-Hage W, Leman S, Camus V, Belzung C. Mechanisms of antidepressant resistance. Front Pharmacol. 2013;4:146. PMCID: PMC3837246. http://www.ncbi.nlm.nih.gov/pubmed/24319431.
33. Möller HJ, Bitter I, Bobes J, Fountoulakis K, Höschl C, Kasper S, European Psychiatric Association. Position statement of the European Psychiatric Association (EPA) on the value of antidepressants in the treatment of unipolar depression. Eur Psychiatry. 2012;27(2):114–28. PMID: 22119161. http://www.ncbi.nlm.nih.gov/pubmed/22119161.
34. Trivedi MH, Rush AJ, Wisniewski SR, Nierenberg AA, Warden D, Ritz L, Norquist G, Howland RH, Lebowitz B, McGrath PJ, Shores-Wilson K, Biggs MM, Balasubramani GK, Fava M, STAR*D Study Team. Evaluation of outcomes with citalopram for depression using measurement-based care in STAR*D: implications for clinical practice. Am J Psychiatry. 2006;163(1):28–40. PMID: 16390886. http://www.ncbi.nlm.nih.gov/pubmed/16390886.
35. Rush AJ, Trivedi MH, Wisniewski SR, Nierenberg AA, Stewart JW, Warden D, Niederehe G, Thase ME, Lavori PW, Lebowitz BD, McGrath PJ, Rosenbaum JF, Sackeim HA, Kupfer DJ, Luther J, Fava M. Acute and longer-term outcomes in depressed outpatients requiring one or several treatment steps: a STAR*D report. Am J Psychiatry. 2006;163(11):1905–17. PMID: 17074942. http://www.ncbi.nlm.nih.gov/pubmed/17074942.
36. Rush AJ, Trivedi MH, Wisniewski SR, Stewart JW, Nierenberg AA, Thase ME, Ritz L, Biggs MM, Warden D, Luther JF, Shores-Wilson K, Niederehe G, Fava M, STAR*D Study Team. Bupropion-SR, sertraline, or venlafaxine-XR after failure of SSRIs for depression. N Engl J Med. 2006;354(12):1231–42. PMID: 16554525. http://www.ncbi.nlm.nih.gov/pubmed/16554525.
37. Millan MJ. Multi-target strategies for the improved treatment of depressive states: conceptual foundations and neuronal substrates, drug discovery and therapeutic application. Pharmacol Ther. 2006;110(2):135–370. PMID: 16522330. http://www.ncbi.nlm.nih.gov/pubmed/16522330.
38. Davies P, Ijaz S, Williams CJ, Kessler D, Lewis G, Wiles N. Pharmacological interventions for treatment-resistant depression in adults. Cochrane Database Syst Rev. 2019;12(12):CD010557. PMCID: PMC6916711. http://www.ncbi.nlm.nih.gov/pubmed/31846068.
39. Ijaz S, Davies P, Williams CJ, Kessler D, Lewis G, Wiles N. Psychological therapies for treatment-resistant depression in adults. Cochrane Database Syst Rev. 2018;5(5):CD010558. PMCID: PMC6494651. http://www.ncbi.nlm.nih.gov/pubmed/29761488.
40. Safer DJ. Differing antidepressant maintenance methodologies. Contemp Clin Trials. 2017;61:87–95. PMID: 28739537. http://www.ncbi.nlm.nih.gov/pubmed/28739537.
41. Whitlock ME, Woodward PW, Alexander RC. Is high placebo response really a problem in depression trials? A critical re-analysis of depression studies. Innov Clin Neurosci. 2019;16(7–08):12–7. PMCID: PMC6850502. http://www.ncbi.nlm.nih.gov/pubmed/31832258.
42. Furukawa TA, Cipriani A, Atkinson LZ, Leucht S, Ogawa Y, Takeshima N, Hayasaka Y, Chaimani A, Salanti G. Placebo response rates in antidepressant trials: a systematic review of published and unpublished double-blind randomised controlled studies. Lancet Psychiatry. 2016;3(11):1059–66. PMID: 27726982. http://www.ncbi.nlm.nih.gov/pubmed/27726982.
43. Kirsch I. Are drug and placebo effects in depression additive? Biol Psychiatry. 2000;47(8):733–5. PMID: 10773181. http://www.ncbi.nlm.nih.gov/pubmed/10773181.
44. Fountoulakis KN, Möller HJ. Antidepressant drugs and the response in the placebo group: the real problem lies in our understanding of the issue. J Psychopharmacol. 2012;26(5):744–50. PMID: 21926425. http://www.ncbi.nlm.nih.gov/pubmed/21926425.
45. Enck P, Klosterhalfen S. The placebo response in clinical trials-the current state of play. Complement Ther Med. 2013;21(2):98–101. PMID: 23497810. http://www.ncbi.nlm.nih.gov/pubmed/23497810.
46. Eippert F, Bingel U, Schoell ED, Yacubian J, Klinger R, Lorenz J, Büchel C. Activation of the opioidergic descending pain control system underlies placebo analgesia. Neuron. 2009;63(4):533–43. PMID: 19709634. http://www.ncbi.nlm.nih.gov/pubmed/19709634.
47. Petrovic P, Kalso E, Petersson KM, Andersson J, Fransson P, Ingvar M. A prefrontal non-opioid mechanism in placebo analgesia. Pain. 2010;150(1):59–65. PMID: 20399560. http://www.ncbi.nlm.nih.gov/pubmed/20399560.
48. Homma G, Daimon T. A simple test for the treatment effect in clinical trials with a sequential parallel comparison design and negative binomial outcomes. Pharm Stat. 2019;18(2):184–97. PMID: 30411482. http://www.ncbi.nlm.nih.gov/pubmed/30411482.
49. Kirsch I. The emperor's new drugs: medication and placebo in the treatment of depression. Handb Exp Pharmacol. 2014;225:291–303. PMID: 25304538. http://www.ncbi.nlm.nih.gov/pubmed/25304538.
50. Laughren TP. The scientific and ethical basis for placebo-controlled trials in depression and schizophrenia: an FDA perspective. Eur Psychiatry. 2001;16(7):418–23. PMID: 11728855. http://www.ncbi.nlm.nih.gov/pubmed/11728855.
51. Khan A, Khan S, Brown WA. Are placebo controls necessary to test new antidepressants and anxiolytics? Int J Neuropsychopharmacol. 2002;5(3):193–7. PMID: 12366872. http://www.ncbi.nlm.nih.gov/pubmed/12366872.
52. Fava M, Evins AE, Dorer DJ, Schoenfeld DA. The problem of the placebo response in clinical trials for psychiatric disorders: culprits, possible remedies, and a novel study design approach. Psychother Psychosom. 2003;72(3):115–27. PMID: 12707478. http://www.ncbi.nlm.nih.gov/pubmed/12707478.
53. Merlo-Pich E, Alexander RC, Fava M, Gomeni R. A new population-enrichment strategy to improve efficiency of placebo-controlled clinical trials of antidepressant drugs. Clin Pharmacol Ther. 2010;88(5):634–42. PMID: 20861834. http://www.ncbi.nlm.nih.gov/pubmed/20861834.
54. Iovieno N, Papakostas GI. Correlation between different levels of placebo response rate and clinical trial outcome in major depressive disorder: a meta-analysis. J Clin Psychiatry. 2012;73(10):1300–6. PMID: 23140647. http://www.ncbi.nlm.nih.gov/pubmed/23140647.

55. Papakostas GI, Østergaard SD, Iovieno N. The nature of placebo response in clinical studies of major depressive disorder. J Clin Psychiatry. 2015;76(4):456–66. PMID: 25700292. http://www.ncbi.nlm.nih.gov/pubmed/25700292.
56. Schoenfeld DA, Doros G, Fava M. A commentary on: statistical inference problems in sequential parallel comparison designs. J Biopharm Stat. 2019;29(6):1130–3. PMID: 30794042. http://www.ncbi.nlm.nih.gov/pubmed/30794042.
57. Lui KJ. Estimation of the relative difference (or relative risk reduction) under the sequential parallel comparison design. Stat Methods Med Res. 2019;28(7):2125–36. PMID: 29284368. http://www.ncbi.nlm.nih.gov/pubmed/29284368.
58. Homma G, Daimon T. Sequential parallel comparison design for "gold standard" noninferiority trials with a prespecified margin. Biom J. 2019;61(6):1493–506. PMID: 31456230. http://www.ncbi.nlm.nih.gov/pubmed/31456230.
59. Cui Y, Ogbagaber S, Hung HMJ. Statistical inference problems in sequential parallel comparison design. J Biopharm Stat. 2019;29(6):1116–29. PMID: 31035859. http://www.ncbi.nlm.nih.gov/pubmed/31035859.
60. Placebo | SpringerLink.
61. Zimmerman M, Clark HL, Multach MD, Walsh E, Rosenstein LK, Gazarian D. Symptom severity and the generalizability of antidepressant efficacy trials: changes during the past 20 years. J Clin Psychopharmacol. 2016;36(2):153–6. PMID: 26848791. http://www.ncbi.nlm.nih.gov/pubmed/26848791.
62. Mojtabai R, Olfson M. Proportion of antidepressants prescribed without a psychiatric diagnosis is growing. Health Aff (Millwood). 2011;30(8):1434–42. PMID: 21821561. http://www.ncbi.nlm.nih.gov/pubmed/21821561.
63. Rhee TG, Rosenheck RA. Initiation of new psychotropic prescriptions without a psychiatric diagnosis among US adults: rates, correlates, and national trends from 2006 to 2015. Health Serv Res. 2019;54(1):139–48. PMCID: PMC6338322. http://www.ncbi.nlm.nih.gov/pubmed/30334247.
64. Mark TL, Levit KR, Buck JA. Datapoints: psychotropic drug prescriptions by medical specialty. Psychiatr Serv. 2009;60(9):1167. PMID: 19723729. http://www.ncbi.nlm.nih.gov/pubmed/19723729.
65. Rhee TG, Schommer JC, Capistrant BD, Hadsall RL, Uden DL. Potentially inappropriate antidepressant prescriptions among older adults in office-based outpatient settings: National Trends from 2002 to 2012. Admin Pol Ment Health. 2018;45(2):224–35. PMID: 28730279. http://www.ncbi.nlm.nih.gov/pubmed/28730279.
66. Moore TJ, Mattison DR. Adult utilization of psychiatric drugs and differences by sex, age, and race. JAMA Intern Med. 2017;177(2):274–5. PMID: 27942726. http://www.ncbi.nlm.nih.gov/pubmed/27942726.
67. Hodgkin D, Thomas CP, O'Brien PL, Levit K, Richardson J, Mark TL, Malone K. Projected spending on psychotropic medications 2013-2020. Admin Pol Ment Health. 2016;43(4):497–505. PMID: 26041078. http://www.ncbi.nlm.nih.gov/pubmed/26041078.
68. Depression Medicines | FDA.
69. The Top Prescription Drugs of 2011 in the United States: Antipsychotics and Antidepressants Once Again Lead CNS Therapeutics | ACS Chemical Neuroscience.
70. 2024 FDA-approved psychotropic medications: A conspectus - ScienceDirect.
71. Prescription drug expenditure U.S. 1960-2024 | Statista.
72. 2024 Pharmacy Forecast: A Focus on Mental Health.
73. Wiechers IR, Leslie DL, Rosenheck RA. Prescribing of psychotropic medications to patients without a psychiatric diagnosis. Psychiatr Serv. 2013;64(12):1243–8. PMID: 23999894. http://www.ncbi.nlm.nih.gov/pubmed/23999894.
74. Wiechers IR, Kirwin PD, Rosenheck RA. Increased risk among older veterans of prescribing psychotropic medication in the absence of psychiatric diagnoses. Am J Geriatr Psychiatry. 2014;22(6):531–9. PMID: 24211029. http://www.ncbi.nlm.nih.gov/pubmed/24211029.
75. Mojtabai R, Olfson M. National trends in psychotropic medication polypharmacy in office-based psychiatry. Arch Gen Psychiatry. 2010;67(1):26–36. PMID: 20048220. http://www.ncbi.nlm.nih.gov/pubmed/20048220.
76. By the 2023 American Geriatrics Society Beers Criteria® Update Expert Panel. American Geriatrics Society 2023 updated AGS Beers Criteria® for potentially inappropriate medication use in older adults. J Am Geriatr Soc. 2023;71(7):2052–81. PMID: 37139824. http://www.ncbi.nlm.nih.gov/pubmed/37139824.
77. American Geriatrics Society 2023 updated AGS Beers Criteria® for potentially inappropriate medication use in older adults.
78. Geriatrics Care | Geriatric Resources | Online events | Updates - Geriatrics Care Online.
79. Munger MA. Polypharmacy and combination therapy in the management of hypertension in elderly patients with co-morbid diabetes mellitus. Drugs Aging. 2010;27(11):871–83. PMID: 20964461. http://www.ncbi.nlm.nih.gov/pubmed/20964461.
80. Haider SI, Johnell K, Weitoft GR, Thorslund M, Fastbom J. The influence of educational level on polypharmacy and inappropriate drug use: a register-based study of more than 600,000 older people. J Am Geriatr Soc. 2009;57(1):62–9. PMID: 19054196. http://www.ncbi.nlm.nih.gov/pubmed/19054196.
81. Ong GJ, Page A, Caughey G, Johns S, Reeve E, Shakib S. Clinician agreement and influence of medication-related characteristics on assessment of polypharmacy. Pharmacol Res Perspect. 2017;5(3):e00321. PMCID: PMC5464348. http://www.ncbi.nlm.nih.gov/pubmed/28603638.
82. Ersoy S, Engin VS. Risk factors for polypharmacy in older adults in a primary care setting: a cross-sectional study. Clin Interv Aging. 2018;13:2003–11. PMCID: PMC6197244. http://www.ncbi.nlm.nih.gov/pubmed/30410317.
83. Holvast F, van Hattem BA, Sinnige J, Schellevis F, Taxis K, Burger H, Verhaak PFM. Late-life depression and the association with multimorbidity and polypharmacy: a cross-sectional study. Fam Pract. 2017;34(5):539–45. PMID: 28369380. http://www.ncbi.nlm.nih.gov/pubmed/28369380.
84. Masnoon N, Shakib S, Kalisch-Ellett L, Caughey GE. What is polypharmacy? A systematic review of definitions. BMC Geriatr. 2017;17(1):230. PMCID: PMC5635569. http://www.ncbi.nlm.nih.gov/pubmed/29017448.
85. Lee GB, Etherton-Beer C, Hosking SM, Pasco JA, Page AT. The patterns and implications of potentially suboptimal medicine regimens among older adults: a narrative review. Ther Adv Drug Saf. 2022;13:20420986221100117. PMCID: PMC9260603. http://www.ncbi.nlm.nih.gov/pubmed/35814333.
86. Machmutow K, Meister R, Jansen A, Kriston L, Watzke B, Härter MC, Liebherz S. Comparative effectiveness of continuation and maintenance treatments for persistent depressive disorder in adults. Cochrane Database Syst Rev. 2019;5(5):CD012855. PMCID: PMC6526465. http://www.ncbi.nlm.nih.gov/pubmed/31106850.
87. Patel RK, Aslam SP, Rose GM. Persistent depressive disorder. StatPearls [Internet]. Treasure Island: StatPearls Publishing; 2025 [cited 2025 Jan 10]. Available from: http://www.ncbi.nlm.nih.gov/books/NBK541052/ PMID: 31082096. http://www.ncbi.nlm.nih.gov/pubmed/31082096.
88. Leuzinger-Bohleber M, Hautzinger M, Fiedler G, Keller W, Bahrke U, Kallenbach L, Kaufhold J, Ernst M, Negele A, Schoett M, Küchenhoff H, Günther F, Rüger B, Beutel M. Outcome of psychoanalytic and cognitive-behavioural long-term therapy with chronically depressed patients: a controlled trial with preferential and randomized allocation. Can J Psychiatr. 2019;64(1):47–58.

PMCID: PMC6364135. http://www.ncbi.nlm.nih.gov/pubmed/30384775.
89. Clevenger SS, Malhotra D, Dang J, Vanle B, IsHak WW. The role of selective serotonin reuptake inhibitors in preventing relapse of major depressive disorder. Ther Adv Psychopharmacol. 2018;8(1):49–58. PMCID: PMC5761909. http://www.ncbi.nlm.nih.gov/pubmed/29344343.
90. Crisafulli C, Fabbri C, Porcelli S, Drago A, Spina E, De Ronchi D, Serretti A. Pharmacogenetics of antidepressants. Front Pharmacol. 2011;2:6. PMCID: PMC3108562. http://www.ncbi.nlm.nih.gov/pubmed/21687501.
91. Dubovsky SL. The usefulness of genotyping cytochrome P450 enzymes in the treatment of depression. Expert Opin Drug Metab Toxicol. 2015;11(3):369–79. PMID: 25554071. http://www.ncbi.nlm.nih.gov/pubmed/25554071.
92. Samer CF, Lorenzini KI, Rollason V, Daali Y, Desmeules JA. Applications of CYP450 testing in the clinical setting. Mol Diagn Ther. 2013;17(3):165–84. PMCID: PMC3663206. http://www.ncbi.nlm.nih.gov/pubmed/23588782.
93. Schramm E, Klein DN, Elsaesser M, Furukawa TA, Domschke K. Review of dysthymia and persistent depressive disorder: history, correlates, and clinical implications. Lancet Psychiatry. 2020;7(9):801–12. PMID: 32828168. http://www.ncbi.nlm.nih.gov/pubmed/32828168.
94. McCullough JP, Klein DN, Keller MB, Holzer CE, Davis SM, Kornstein SG, Howland RH, Thase ME, Harrison WM. Comparison of DSM-III-R chronic major depression and major depression superimposed on dysthymia (double depression): validity of the distinction. J Abnorm Psychol. 2000;109(3):419–27. PMID: 11016111. http://www.ncbi.nlm.nih.gov/pubmed/11016111.
95. Case SM, Sawhney M, Stewart JC. Atypical depression and double depression predict new-onset cardiovascular disease in U.S. adults. Depress Anxiety. 2018;35(1):10–7. PMCID: PMC5741545. http://www.ncbi.nlm.nih.gov/pubmed/28640965.
96. Biochemistry, Cytochrome P450 - StatPearls - NCBI Bookshelf.
97. Gonzalez FJ, Gelboin HV. Human cytochromes P450: evolution and cDNA-directed expression. Environ Health Perspect. 1992;98:81–5. PMCID: PMC1519618. http://www.ncbi.nlm.nih.gov/pubmed/1486867.
98. Bishop JR. Pharmacogenetics. Handb Clin Neurol. 2018;147:59–73. PMID: 29325628. http://www.ncbi.nlm.nih.gov/pubmed/29325628.
99. Drozda K, Müller DJ, Bishop JR. Pharmacogenomic testing for neuropsychiatric drugs: current status of drug labeling, guidelines for using genetic information, and test options. Pharmacotherapy. 2014;34(2):166–84. PMCID: PMC3939793. http://www.ncbi.nlm.nih.gov/pubmed/24523097.
100. Perlis RH. Pharmacogenomic testing and personalized treatment of depression. Clin Chem. 2014;60(1):53–9. PMID: 24281779. http://www.ncbi.nlm.nih.gov/pubmed/24281779.
101. Frieling H, Tadić A. Value of genetic and epigenetic testing as biomarkers of response to antidepressant treatment. Int Rev Psychiatry. 2013;25(5):572–8. PMID: 24151802. http://www.ncbi.nlm.nih.gov/pubmed/24151802.
102. Rosenblat JD, Lee Y, McIntyre RS. The effect of pharmacogenomic testing on response and remission rates in the acute treatment of major depressive disorder: a meta-analysis. J Affect Disord. 2018;241:484–91. PMID: 30149336. http://www.ncbi.nlm.nih.gov/pubmed/30149336.
103. Corponi F, Fabbri C, Serretti A. Pharmacogenetics in psychiatry. Adv Pharmacol. 2018;83:297–331. PMID: 29801579. http://www.ncbi.nlm.nih.gov/pubmed/29801579.
104. Ampong DN. Depression and Pharmacogenetics. Arch Psychiatr Nurs. 2018;32(1):71–4. PMID: 29413077. http://www.ncbi.nlm.nih.gov/pubmed/29413077.
105. Chang DD, Eyreeuro HA, Abbott R, Coudreaut M, Baune BT, Shaman JA, Lavretsky H, Lenze EJ, Merrill DA, Singh AB, Mulsant BH, Reynolds CF, Müller DJ, Bousman C. Pharmacogenetic guidelines and decision support tools for depression treatment: application to late-life. Pharmacogenomics. 2018;19(16):1269–84. PMID: 30422065. http://www.ncbi.nlm.nih.gov/pubmed/30422065.
106. Fabbri C, Zohar J, Serretti A. Pharmacogenetic tests to guide drug treatment in depression: comparison of the available testing kits and clinical trials. Prog Neuro-Psychopharmacol Biol Psychiatry. 2018;86:36–44. PMID: 29777729. http://www.ncbi.nlm.nih.gov/pubmed/29777729.
107. Costello EJ, Mustillo S, Erkanli A, Keeler G, Angold A. Prevalence and development of psychiatric disorders in childhood and adolescence. Arch Gen Psychiatry. 2003;60(8):837–44. PMID: 12912767. http://www.ncbi.nlm.nih.gov/pubmed/12912767.
108. Kessler RC, Berglund P, Demler O, Jin R, Merikangas KR, Walters EE. Lifetime prevalence and age-of-onset distributions of DSM-IV disorders in the National Comorbidity Survey Replication. Arch Gen Psychiatry. 2005;62(6):593–602. PMID: 15939837. http://www.ncbi.nlm.nih.gov/pubmed/15939837.
109. Thapar A, Collishaw S, Pine DS, Thapar AK. Depression in adolescence. Lancet. 2012;379(9820):1056–67. PMCID: PMC3488279. http://www.ncbi.nlm.nih.gov/pubmed/22305766.
110. Hazell P. Depression in children. BMJ. 2002;325(7358):229–30. PMCID: PMC1123757. http://www.ncbi.nlm.nih.gov/pubmed/12153903.
111. Puig-Antich J, Lukens E, Davies M, Goetz D, Brennan-Quattrock J, Todak G. Psychosocial functioning in prepubertal major depressive disorders. II. Interpersonal relationships after sustained recovery from affective episode. Arch Gen Psychiatry. 1985;42(5):511–7. PMID: 3985761. http://www.ncbi.nlm.nih.gov/pubmed/3985761.
112. Gould MS, King R, Greenwald S, Fisher P, Schwab-Stone M, Kramer R, Flisher AJ, Goodman S, Canino G, Shaffer D. Psychopathology associated with suicidal ideation and attempts among children and adolescents. J Am Acad Child Adolesc Psychiatry. 1998;37(9):915–23. PMID: 9735611. http://www.ncbi.nlm.nih.gov/pubmed/9735611.
113. Centers for Disease Control and Prevention (CDC). Suicide trends among youths and young adults aged 10-24 years—United States, 1990-2004. MMWR Morb Mortal Wkly Rep. 2007;56(35):905–8. PMID: 17805220. http://www.ncbi.nlm.nih.gov/pubmed/17805220.
114. Zhou X, Hetrick SE, Cuijpers P, Qin B, Barth J, Whittington CJ, Cohen D, Del Giovane C, Liu Y, Michael KD, Zhang Y, Weisz JR, Xie P. Comparative efficacy and acceptability of psychotherapies for depression in children and adolescents: a systematic review and network meta-analysis. World Psychiatry. 2015;14(2):207–22. PMCID: PMC4471978. http://www.ncbi.nlm.nih.gov/pubmed/26043339.
115. Weisz JR, McCarty CA, Valeri SM. Effects of psychotherapy for depression in children and adolescents: a meta-analysis. Psychol Bull. 2006;132(1):132–49. PMCID: PMC2150594. http://www.ncbi.nlm.nih.gov/pubmed/16435960.
116. Depression in Children and Young People - NCBI Bookshelf.
117. Nutt DJ, Sharpe M. Uncritical positive regard? Issues in the efficacy and safety of psychotherapy. J Psychopharmacol. 2008;22(1):3–6. PMID: 18187527. http://www.ncbi.nlm.nih.gov/pubmed/18187527.
118. Linden M, Schermuly-Haupt ML. Definition, assessment and rate of psychotherapy side effects. World Psychiatry. 2014;13(3):306–9. PMCID: PMC4219072. http://www.ncbi.nlm.nih.gov/pubmed/25273304.
119. Cipriani A, Zhou X, Del Giovane C, Hetrick SE, Qin B, Whittington C, Coghill D, Zhang Y, Hazell P, Leucht S, Cuijpers

P, Pu J, Cohen D, Ravindran AV, Liu Y, Michael KD, Yang L, Liu L, Xie P. Comparative efficacy and tolerability of antidepressants for major depressive disorder in children and adolescents: a network meta-analysis. Lancet. 2016;388(10047):881–90. PMID: 27289172. http://www.ncbi.nlm.nih.gov/pubmed/27289172.

120. Hetrick SE, McKenzie JE, Cox GR, Simmons MB, Merry SN. Newer generation antidepressants for depressive disorders in children and adolescents. Cochrane Database Syst Rev. 2012;11(11):CD004851. PMCID: PMC8786271. http://www.ncbi.nlm.nih.gov/pubmed/23152227.
121. Hazell P, Mirzaie M. Tricyclic drugs for depression in children and adolescents. Cochrane Database Syst Rev. 2013;2013(6):CD002317. PMCID: PMC7093893. http://www.ncbi.nlm.nih.gov/pubmed/23780719.
122. Suicidality in Children and Adolescents Being Treated With Antidepressant Medications | FDA.
123. March J, Silva S, Petrycki S, Curry J, Wells K, Fairbank J, Burns B, Domino M, McNulty S, Vitiello B, Severe J. Treatment for Adolescents With Depression Study (TADS) Team. Fluoxetine, cognitive-behavioral therapy, and their combination for adolescents with depression: Treatment for Adolescents With Depression Study (TADS) randomized controlled trial. JAMA. 2004;292(7):807–20. PMID: 15315995. http://www.ncbi.nlm.nih.gov/pubmed/15315995.
124. Pampallona S, Bollini P, Tibaldi G, Kupelnick B, Munizza C. Combined pharmacotherapy and psychological treatment for depression: a systematic review. Arch Gen Psychiatry. 2004;61(7):714–9. PMID: 15237083. http://www.ncbi.nlm.nih.gov/pubmed/15237083.
125. de Maat SM, Dekker J, Schoevers RA, de Jonghe F. Relative efficacy of psychotherapy and combined therapy in the treatment of depression: a meta-analysis. Eur Psychiatry. 2007;22(1):1–8. PMID: 17194571. http://www.ncbi.nlm.nih.gov/pubmed/17194571.
126. Cox GR, Callahan P, Churchill R, Hunot V, Merry SN, Parker AG, Hetrick SE. Psychological therapies versus antidepressant medication, alone and in combination for depression in children and adolescents. Cochrane Database Syst Rev. 2014;2014(11):CD008324. PMCID: PMC8556660. http://www.ncbi.nlm.nih.gov/pubmed/25433518.
127. Pacher P, Kecskemeti V. Cardiovascular side effects of new antidepressants and antipsychotics: new drugs, old concerns? Curr Pharm Des. 2004;10(20):2463–75. PMCID: PMC2493295. http://www.ncbi.nlm.nih.gov/pubmed/15320756.
128. Schweitzer I, Maguire K, Ng C. Sexual side-effects of contemporary antidepressants: review. Aust N Z J Psychiatry. 2009;43(9):795–808. PMID: 19670052. http://www.ncbi.nlm.nih.gov/pubmed/19670052.
129. Hert DE, Correll CU, Bobes J, Cetkovich-Bakmas M, Cohen D, Asai I, Detraux J, Gautam S, Möller HJ, Ndetei DM, Newcomer JW, Uwakwe R, Leucht S. Physical illness in patients with severe mental disorders. I. Prevalence, impact of medications and disparities in health care. World Psychiatry. 2011;10(1):52–77. PMCID: PMC3048500. http://www.ncbi.nlm.nih.gov/pubmed/21379357.
130. De Hert M, Cohen D, Bobes J, Cetkovich-Bakmas M, Leucht S, Ndetei DM, Newcomer JW, Uwakwe R, Asai I, Möller HJ, Gautam S, Detraux J, Correll CU. Physical illness in patients with severe mental disorders. II. Barriers to care, monitoring and treatment guidelines, plus recommendations at the system and individual level. World Psychiatry. 2011;10(2):138–51. PMCID: PMC3104888. http://www.ncbi.nlm.nih.gov/pubmed/21633691.
131. Uzun S, Kozumplik O. Management of side effects of antidepressants - brief review of recommendations from guidelines for treatment of major depressive disorder. Psychiatr Danub. 2009;21(1):91–4. PMID: 19270629. http://www.ncbi.nlm.nih.gov/pubmed/19270629.
132. Marano G, Traversi G, Romagnoli E, Catalano V, Lotrionte M, Abbate A, Biondi-Zoccai G, Mazza M. Cardiologic side effects of psychotropic drugs. J Geriatr Cardiol. 2011;8(4):243–53. PMCID: PMC3390089. http://www.ncbi.nlm.nih.gov/pubmed/22783311.
133. Masand PS, Gupta S. Long-term side effects of newer-generation antidepressants: SSRIS, venlafaxine, nefazodone, bupropion, and mirtazapine. Ann Clin Psychiatry. 2002;14(3):175–82. PMID: 12585567. http://www.ncbi.nlm.nih.gov/pubmed/12585567.
134. Bet PM, Hugtenburg JG, Penninx BWJH, Hoogendijk WJG. Side effects of antidepressants during long-term use in a naturalistic setting. Eur Neuropsychopharmacol. 2013;23(11):1443–51. PMID: 23726508. http://www.ncbi.nlm.nih.gov/pubmed/23726508.
135. Allsbrook M, Fries BE, Szafara KL, Regal RE. Do SSRI antidepressants increase The risk of extrapyramidal side effects in patients taking antipsychotics? P T. 2016;41(2):115–9. PMCID: PMC4745639. http://www.ncbi.nlm.nih.gov/pubmed/26909002.
136. Widespread psychological side effects of antidepressants. Researchers say side effects such as "emotional numbness" are more common than you might think. Duke Med Health News. 2014;20(5):3–4. PMID: 24960845. http://www.ncbi.nlm.nih.gov/pubmed/24960845.
137. Price J, Cole V, Doll H, Goodwin GM. The Oxford Questionnaire on the Emotional Side-effects of Antidepressants (OQuESA): development, validity, reliability and sensitivity to change. J Affect Disord. 2012;140(1):66–74. PMID: 22387055. http://www.ncbi.nlm.nih.gov/pubmed/22387055.
138. Ferguson JM. The effects of antidepressants on sexual functioning in depressed patients: a review. J Clin Psychiatry. 2001;62(Suppl 3):22–34. PMID: 11229450. http://www.ncbi.nlm.nih.gov/pubmed/11229450.
139. Kennedy SH, Rizvi S. Sexual dysfunction, depression, and the impact of antidepressants. J Clin Psychopharmacol. 2009;29(2):157–64. PMID: 19512977. http://www.ncbi.nlm.nih.gov/pubmed/19512977.
140. Rothschild AJ. Sexual side effects of antidepressants. J Clin Psychiatry. 2000;61(Suppl 11):28–36. PMID: 10926052. http://www.ncbi.nlm.nih.gov/pubmed/10926052.
141. Hsu JH, Shen WW. Male sexual side effects associated with antidepressants: a descriptive clinical study of 32 patients. Int J Psychiatry Med. 1995;25(2):191–201. PMID: 7591493. http://www.ncbi.nlm.nih.gov/pubmed/7591493.
142. Mihanović M, Restek-Petrović B, Bodor D, Molnar S, Oresković A, Presecki P. Suicidality and side effects of antidepressants and antipsychotics. Psychiatr Danub. 2010;22(1):79–84. PMID: 20305596. http://www.ncbi.nlm.nih.gov/pubmed/20305596.
143. Mulder RT. Antidepressants and suicide: population benefit vs. individual risk. Acta Psychiatr Scand. 2010;122(6):442–3. PMID: 21054281. http://www.ncbi.nlm.nih.gov/pubmed/21054281.
144. Mandour RA. Antidepressants medications and the relative risk of suicide attempt. Toxicol Int. 2012;19(1):42–6. PMCID: PMC3339244. http://www.ncbi.nlm.nih.gov/pubmed/22736902.
145. Nischal A, Tripathi A, Nischal A, Trivedi JK. Suicide and antidepressants: what current evidence indicates. Mens Sana Monogr. 2012;10(1):33–44. PMCID: PMC3353604. http://www.ncbi.nlm.nih.gov/pubmed/22654381.
146. Friedman RA, Leon AC. Expanding the black box - depression, antidepressants, and the risk of suicide. N Engl J Med. 2007;356(23):2343–6. PMID: 17485726. http://www.ncbi.nlm.nih.gov/pubmed/17485726.
147. Kafali N, Progovac A, Hou SSY, Cook BL. Long-run trends in antidepressant use among youths after the FDA Black Box warning. Psychiatr Serv. 2018;69(4):389–95. PMCID: PMC5942898. http://www.ncbi.nlm.nih.gov/pubmed/29241433.
148. Kaizar EE, Greenhouse JB, Seltman H, Kelleher K. Do antidepressants cause suicidality in children? A Bayesian meta-analysis.

Clin Trials. 2006;3(2):73–90; discussion 91-98. PMID: 16773951. http://www.ncbi.nlm.nih.gov/pubmed/16773951.
149. Simon GE, Savarino J, Operskalski B, Wang PS. Suicide risk during antidepressant treatment. Am J Psychiatry. 2006;163(1):41–7. PMID: 16390887. http://www.ncbi.nlm.nih.gov/pubmed/16390887.
150. Klein DF. The flawed basis for FDA post-marketing safety decisions: the example of anti-depressants and children. Neuropsychopharmacology. 2006;31(4):689–99. PMID: 16395296. http://www.ncbi.nlm.nih.gov/pubmed/16395296.
151. Khan A, Khan S, Kolts R, Brown WA. Suicide rates in clinical trials of SSRIs, other antidepressants, and placebo: analysis of FDA reports. Am J Psychiatry. 2003;160(4):790–2. PMID: 12668373. http://www.ncbi.nlm.nih.gov/pubmed/12668373.
152. Miller M, Pate V, Swanson SA, Azrael D, White A, Stürmer T. Antidepressant class, age, and the risk of deliberate self-harm: a propensity score matched cohort study of SSRI and SNRI users in the USA. CNS Drugs. 2014;28(1):79–88. https://doi.org/10.1007/s40263-013-0120-8. PMID: 24146116; PMCID: PMC3947090.
153. Hammad TA, Laughren T, Racoosin J. Suicidality in pediatric patients treated with antidepressant drugs. Arch Gen Psychiatry. 2006;63(3):332–9. PMID: 16520440. http://www.ncbi.nlm.nih.gov/pubmed/16520440.
154. Richmond TK, Rosen DS. The treatment of adolescent depression in the era of the black box warning. Curr Opin Pediatr. 2005;17(4):466–72. PMID: 16012257. http://www.ncbi.nlm.nih.gov/pubmed/16012257.
155. Giner L, Nichols CM, Zalsman G, Oquendo MA. Selective serotonin reuptake inhibitors and the risk for suicidality in adolescents: an update. Int J Adolesc Med Health. 2005;17(3):211–20. PMID: 16231472. http://www.ncbi.nlm.nih.gov/pubmed/16231472.
156. Center for Drug Evaluation and Research (CDER) | FDA.
157. FDA's Labeling Resources for Human Prescription Drugs | FDA.
158. Major Depressive Disorder: Developing Drugs for Treatment Guidance for Industry.
159. Sander RD. Motor examinations in psychiatry. Psychiatry (Edgmont). 2010;7(11):37–41. PMCID: PMC3010968. http://www.ncbi.nlm.nih.gov/pubmed/21191532.
160. Sanders RD, Gillig PM. Extrapyramidal examinations in psychiatry. Innov Clin Neurosci. 2012;9(7–8):10–6. PMCID: PMC3442750. http://www.ncbi.nlm.nih.gov/pubmed/22984647.
161. National Ambulatory Medical Care Survey | NAMCS | CDC.
162. National Ambulatory Medical Care Survey: 2019 National Summary.
163. ClinCalc DrugStats Database.
164. Products - Data Briefs - Number 377 - September 2020.
165. Antidepressants: MedlinePlus.
166. Depression Treatment | Effective Health Care (EHC) Program.
167. Colleoni M, Mandala M, Peruzzotti G, Robertson C, Bredart A, Goldhirsch A. Depression and degree of acceptance of adjuvant cytotoxic drugs. Lancet. 2000;356(9238):1326–7. PMID: 11073026. http://www.ncbi.nlm.nih.gov/pubmed/11073026.
168. Pinquart M, Duberstein PR. Depression and cancer mortality: a meta-analysis. Psychol Med. 2010;40(11):1797–810. PMCID: PMC2935927. http://www.ncbi.nlm.nih.gov/pubmed/20085667.
169. Giese-Davis J, Collie K, Rancourt KMS, Neri E, Kraemer HC, Spiegel D. Decrease in depression symptoms is associated with longer survival in patients with metastatic breast cancer: a secondary analysis. J Clin Oncol. 2011;29(4):413–20. PMCID: PMC3058287. http://www.ncbi.nlm.nih.gov/pubmed/21149651.
170. Grassi L, Nanni MG, Rodin G, Li M, Caruso R. The use of antidepressants in oncology: a review and practical tips for oncologists. Ann Oncol. 2018;29(1):101–11. PMID: 29272358. http://www.ncbi.nlm.nih.gov/pubmed/29272358.
171. Li M, Fitzgerald P, Rodin G. Evidence-based treatment of depression in patients with cancer. J Clin Oncol. 2012;30(11):1187–96. PMID: 22412144. http://www.ncbi.nlm.nih.gov/pubmed/22412144.
172. Jacobsen PB, Jim HS. Psychosocial interventions for anxiety and depression in adult cancer patients: achievements and challenges. CA Cancer J Clin. 2008;58(4):214–30. PMID: 18558664. http://www.ncbi.nlm.nih.gov/pubmed/18558664.
173. Bielecka AM, Obuchowicz E. Antidepressant drugs can modify cytotoxic action of temozolomide. Eur J Cancer Care (Engl). 2017;26(5). PMID: 27480195. http://www.ncbi.nlm.nih.gov/pubmed/27480195.
174. Bielecka AM, Obuchowicz E. Antidepressant drugs as a complementary therapeutic strategy in cancer. Exp Biol Med (Maywood). 2013;238(8):849–58. PMID: 23970405. http://www.ncbi.nlm.nih.gov/pubmed/23970405.
175. Bull SA, Hunkeler EM, Lee JY, Rowland CR, Williamson TE, Schwab JR, Hurt SW. Discontinuing or switching selective serotonin-reuptake inhibitors. Ann Pharmacother. 2002;36(4):578–84. PMID: 11918502. http://www.ncbi.nlm.nih.gov/pubmed/11918502.
176. Carvalho AF, Sharma MS, Brunoni AR, Vieta E, Fava GA. The safety, tolerability and risks associated with the use of newer generation antidepressant drugs: a critical review of the literature. Psychother Psychosom. 2016;85(5):270–88. PMID: 27508501. http://www.ncbi.nlm.nih.gov/pubmed/27508501.
177. Dragioti E, Solmi M, Favaro A, Fusar-Poli P, Dazzan P, Thompson T, Stubbs B, Firth J, Fornaro M, Tsartsalis D, Carvalho AF, Vieta E, McGuire P, Young AH, Shin JI, Correll CU, Evangelou E. Association of Antidepressant use with adverse health outcomes: a systematic umbrella review. JAMA Psychiatry. 2019;76(12):1241–55. PMCID: PMC6777224. http://www.ncbi.nlm.nih.gov/pubmed/31577342.
178. Caraci F, Crupi R, Drago F, Spina E. Metabolic drug interactions between antidepressants and anticancer drugs: focus on selective serotonin reuptake inhibitors and hypericum extract. Curr Drug Metab. 2011;12(6):570–7. PMID: 21395523. http://www.ncbi.nlm.nih.gov/pubmed/21395523.
179. Wedret JJ, Tu TG, Paul D, Rousseau C, Bonta A, Bota RG. Interactions between antidepressants, sleep aids and selected breast cancer therapy. Ment Illn. 2019;11(1):8115. PMCID: PMC6589536. http://www.ncbi.nlm.nih.gov/pubmed/31281608.
180. Kelly CM, Juurlink DN, Gomes T, Duong-Hua M, Pritchard KI, Austin PC, Paszat LF. Selective serotonin reuptake inhibitors and breast cancer mortality in women receiving tamoxifen: a population based cohort study. BMJ. 2010;340:c693. PMCID: PMC2817754. http://www.ncbi.nlm.nih.gov/pubmed/20142325.
181. Haque R, Shi J, Schottinger JE, Ahmed SA, Cheetham TC, Chung J, Avila C, Kleinman K, Habel LA, Fletcher SW, Kwan ML. Tamoxifen and antidepressant drug interaction in a Cohort of 16,887 breast cancer survivors. J Natl Cancer Inst. 2016;108(3):djv337. PMCID: PMC5072369. http://www.ncbi.nlm.nih.gov/pubmed/26631176.
182. Baker H. Use of antidepressants and breast cancer recurrence. Lancet Oncol. 2016;17(1):e11. PMID: 26687592. http://www.ncbi.nlm.nih.gov/pubmed/26687592.
183. Mayer SE, Weiss NS, Chubak J, Doody DR, Carlson CS, Makar KW, Wurscher MA, Malone KE. CYP2D6-inhibiting medication use and inherited CYP2D6 variation in relation to adverse breast cancer outcomes after tamoxifen therapy. Cancer Causes Control. 2019;30(1):103–12. PMCID: PMC6353670. http://www.ncbi.nlm.nih.gov/pubmed/30542984.
184. Alfaro CL, Lam YW, Simpson J, Ereshefsky L. CYP2D6 inhibition by fluoxetine, paroxetine, sertraline, and venlafaxine in a crossover study: intraindividual variability and plasma concentration correlations. J Clin Pharmacol. 2000;40(1):58–66. PMID: 10631623. http://www.ncbi.nlm.nih.gov/pubmed/10631623.

185. Binkhorst L, Mathijssen RHJ, van Herk-Sukel MPP, Bannink M, Jager A, Wiemer EAC, van Gelder T. Unjustified prescribing of CYP2D6 inhibiting SSRIs in women treated with tamoxifen. Breast Cancer Res Treat. 2013;139(3):923–9. PMID: 23760858. http://www.ncbi.nlm.nih.gov/pubmed/23760858.
186. Pocobelli G, Yu O, Ziebell RA, Aiello Bowles EJ, Fujii MM, Sterrett AT, Boggs JM, Chen L, Boudreau DM, Ritzwoller DP, Hubbard RA, Chubak J. Use of antidepressants after colon cancer diagnosis and risk of recurrence. Psychooncology. 2019;28(4):750–8. PMCID: PMC6445707. http://www.ncbi.nlm.nih.gov/pubmed/30703275.
187. Riechelmann RP, Krzyzanowska MK. Drug interactions and oncological outcomes: a hidden adversary. Ecancermedicalscience. 2019;13:ed88. PMCID: PMC6467454. http://www.ncbi.nlm.nih.gov/pubmed/31123502.
188. Bellet M, Ahmad F, Villanueva R, Valdivia C, Palomino-Doza J, Ruiz A, Gonzàlez X, Adrover E, Azaro A, Valls-Margarit M, Parra JL, Aguilar J, Vidal M, Martín A, Gavilá J, Escrivá-de-Romaní S, Perelló A, Hernando C, Lahuerta A, Zamora P, Reyes V, Alcalde M, Masanas H, Céliz P, Ruíz I, Gil M, Seguí MÀ, de la Peña L. Palbociclib and ribociclib in breast cancer: consensus workshop on the management of concomitant medication. Ther Adv Med Oncol. 2019;11:1758835919833867. PMCID: PMC6535716. http://www.ncbi.nlm.nih.gov/pubmed/31205497.
189. Drug Interaction Checker - Find Interactions Between Medications.
190. Drug Interactions Checker - Check Your Brand and Generic Drugs - RxList.
191. Drug Interaction Checker ← Quickly Check Your Meds.
192. Thase ME, Murck H, Post A. Clinical relevance of disturbances of sleep and vigilance in major depressive disorder: a review. Prim Care Companion J Clin Psychiatry. 2010;12(6):PCC.08m00676. PMCID: PMC3067979. http://www.ncbi.nlm.nih.gov/pubmed/21494354.
193. Guo YH, Zhou L, Cui ZA, Wang J, Zhang L, Xu T, Xie YD, Chen H. Efficacy and safety of agomelatine in the treatment of patients with depressive disorder: a meta-analysis. Medicine (Baltimore). 2023;102(45):e35871. PMCID: PMC10637518. http://www.ncbi.nlm.nih.gov/pubmed/37960759.
194. Fahri Aydın E, Güleç M, Oral E, Gökhan DA. The effects of fluoxetine and Agomelatine on neurocognitive functions and sleep in patients with major depressive disorder. Psychiatry Clin Psychopharmacol. 2024;34(1):9–18. PMCID: PMC11177640. http://www.ncbi.nlm.nih.gov/pubmed/38883888.
195. Linde K, Kriston L, Rücker G, Jamil S, Schumann I, Meissner K, Sigterman K, Schneider A. Efficacy and acceptability of pharmacological treatments for depressive disorders in primary care: systematic review and network meta-analysis. Ann Fam Med. 2015;13(1):69–79. PMCID: PMC4291268. http://www.ncbi.nlm.nih.gov/pubmed/25583895.
196. Jakobsen JC, Katakam KK, Schou A, Hellmuth SG, Stallknecht SE, Leth-Møller K, Iversen M, Banke MB, Petersen IJ, Klingenberg SL, Krogh J, Ebert SE, Timm A, Lindschou J, Gluud C. Selective serotonin reuptake inhibitors versus placebo in patients with major depressive disorder. A systematic review with meta-analysis and Trial Sequential Analysis. BMC Psychiatry. 2017;17(1):58. PMCID: PMC5299662. http://www.ncbi.nlm.nih.gov/pubmed/28178949.
197. TSA – ctu.dk.
198. Mallery L, MacLeod T, Allen M, McLean-Veysey P, Rodney-Cail N, Bezanson E, Steeves B, LeBlanc C, Moorhouse P. Systematic review and meta-analysis of second-generation antidepressants for the treatment of older adults with depression: questionable benefit and considerations for frailty. BMC Geriatr. 2019;19(1):306. PMCID: PMC6852920. http://www.ncbi.nlm.nih.gov/pubmed/31718566.
199. Cipriani A, Furukawa TA, Salanti G, Chaimani A, Atkinson LZ, Ogawa Y, Leucht S, Ruhe HG, Turner EH, Higgins JPT, Egger M, Takeshima N, Hayasaka Y, Imai H, Shinohara K, Tajika A, Ioannidis JPA, Geddes JR. Comparative efficacy and acceptability of 21 antidepressant drugs for the acute treatment of adults with major depressive disorder: a systematic review and network meta-analysis. Lancet. 2018;391(10128):1357–66. PMCID: PMC5889788. http://www.ncbi.nlm.nih.gov/pubmed/29477251.
200. Walkup JT. Antidepressant efficacy for depression in children and adolescents: industry- and NIMH-funded studies. Am J Psychiatry. 2017;174(5):430–7. PMID: 28253735. http://www.ncbi.nlm.nih.gov/pubmed/28253735.
201. Mavranezouli I, Megnin-Viggars O, Pedder H, Welton NJ, Dias S, Watkins E, Nixon N, Daly CH, Keeney E, Eadon H, Caldwell DM, O'Donoghue KJM, Stockton S, Arnold S, Thomas J, Kapur N, Pilling S. A systematic review and network meta-analysis of psychological, psychosocial, pharmacological, physical and combined treatments for adults with a new episode of depression. EClinicalMedicine. 2024;75:102780. PMCID: PMC11377144. http://www.ncbi.nlm.nih.gov/pubmed/39246718.
202. Nutt DJ. Relationship of neurotransmitters to the symptoms of major depressive disorder. J Clin Psychiatry. 2008;69 Suppl E1:4–7. PMID: 18494537. http://www.ncbi.nlm.nih.gov/pubmed/18494537.
203. Hadlock GC, Webb KM, McFadden LM, Chu PW, Ellis JD, Allen SC, Andrenyak DM, Vieira-Brock PL, German CL, Conrad KM, Hoonakker AJ, Gibb JW, Wilkins DG, Hanson GR, Fleckenstein AE. 4-Methylmethcathinone (mephedrone): neuropharmacological effects of a designer stimulant of abuse. J Pharmacol Exp Ther. 2011;339(2):530–6. PMCID: PMC3200001. http://www.ncbi.nlm.nih.gov/pubmed/21810934.
204. Tatsumi M, Groshan K, Blakely RD, Richelson E. Pharmacological profile of antidepressants and related compounds at human monoamine transporters. Eur J Pharmacol. 1997;340(2–3):249–58. PMID: 9537821. http://www.ncbi.nlm.nih.gov/pubmed/9537821.
205. Owens MJ, Knight DL, Nemeroff CB. Second-generation SSRIs: human monoamine transporter binding profile of escitalopram and R-fluoxetine. Biol Psychiatry. 2001;50(5):345–50. PMID: 11543737. http://www.ncbi.nlm.nih.gov/pubmed/11543737.
206. Chu A, Wadhwa R. Selective Serotonin reuptake inhibitors. StatPearls [Internet]. Treasure Island: StatPearls Publishing; 2025 [cited 2025 Jan 10]. Available from: http://www.ncbi.nlm.nih.gov/books/NBK554406/ PMID: 32119293. http://www.ncbi.nlm.nih.gov/pubmed/32119293.
207. Melikian HE. Neurotransmitter transporter trafficking: endocytosis, recycling, and regulation. Pharmacol Ther. 2004;104(1):17–27. PMID: 15500906. http://www.ncbi.nlm.nih.gov/pubmed/15500906.
208. Törk I. Anatomy of the serotonergic system. Ann N Y Acad Sci. 1990;600:9–34; discussion 34-35. PMID: 2252340. http://www.ncbi.nlm.nih.gov/pubmed/2252340.
209. Jacobs BL, Azmitia EC. Structure and function of the brain serotonin system. Physiol Rev. 1992;72(1):165–229. PMID: 1731370. http://www.ncbi.nlm.nih.gov/pubmed/1731370.
210. Taylor MJ, Freemantle N, Geddes JR, Bhagwagar Z. Early onset of selective serotonin reuptake inhibitor antidepressant action: systematic review and meta-analysis. Arch Gen Psychiatry. 2006;63(11):1217–23. PMCID: PMC2211759. http://www.ncbi.nlm.nih.gov/pubmed/17088502.
211. Hunsberger J, Austin DR, Henter ID, Chen G. The neurotrophic and neuroprotective effects of psychotropic agents. Dialogues Clin Neurosci. 2009;11(3):333–48. PMCID: PMC2804881. http://www.ncbi.nlm.nih.gov/pubmed/19877500.
212. Nowacka MM, Obuchowicz E. Vascular endothelial growth factor (VEGF) and its role in the central nervous system: a new element in the neurotrophic hypothesis of antidepressant drug action.

Neuropeptides. 2012;46(1):1–10. PMID: 21719103. http://www.ncbi.nlm.nih.gov/pubmed/21719103.
213. Weilburg JB. An overview of SSRI and SNRI therapies for depression. Manag Care. 2004;13(6 Suppl Depression):25–33. PMID: 15293768. http://www.ncbi.nlm.nih.gov/pubmed/15293768.
214. Labellarte MJ, Walkup JT, Riddle MA. The new antidepressants. Selective serotonin reuptake inhibitors. Pediatr Clin N Am. 1998;45(5):1137–55. ix. PMID: 9884679. http://www.ncbi.nlm.nih.gov/pubmed/9884679.
215. Vaswani M, Linda FK, Ramesh S. Role of selective serotonin reuptake inhibitors in psychiatric disorders: a comprehensive review. Prog Neuro-Psychopharmacol Biol Psychiatry. 2003;27(1):85–102. PMID: 12551730. http://www.ncbi.nlm.nih.gov/pubmed/12551730.
216. Giuliano F, Clément P. Serotonin and premature ejaculation: from physiology to patient management. Eur Urol. 2006;50(3):454–66. PMID: 16844284. http://www.ncbi.nlm.nih.gov/pubmed/16844284.
217. Tack J, Broekaert D, Fischler B, Van Oudenhove L, Gevers AM, Janssens J. A controlled crossover study of the selective serotonin reuptake inhibitor citalopram in irritable bowel syndrome. Gut. 2006;55(8):1095–103. PMCID: PMC1856276. http://www.ncbi.nlm.nih.gov/pubmed/16401691.
218. Hu XH, Bull SA, Hunkeler EM, Ming E, Lee JY, Fireman B, Markson LE. Incidence and duration of side effects and those rated as bothersome with selective serotonin reuptake inhibitor treatment for depression: patient report versus physician estimate. J Clin Psychiatry. 2004;65(7):959–65. PMID: 15291685. http://www.ncbi.nlm.nih.gov/pubmed/15291685.
219. Shimizu E, Hashimoto K, Okamura N, Koike K, Komatsu N, Kumakiri C, Nakazato M, Watanabe H, Shinoda N, Okada S, ichi, Iyo M. Alterations of serum levels of brain-derived neurotrophic factor (BDNF) in depressed patients with or without antidepressants. Biol Psychiatry. 2003;54(1):70–5. PMID: 12842310. http://www.ncbi.nlm.nih.gov/pubmed/12842310.
220. Chen B, Dowlatshahi D, MacQueen GM, Wang JF, Young LT. Increased hippocampal BDNF immunoreactivity in subjects treated with antidepressant medication. Biol Psychiatry. 2001;50(4):260–5. PMID: 11522260. http://www.ncbi.nlm.nih.gov/pubmed/11522260.
221. Lester KJ, Hudson JL, Tropeano M, Creswell C, Collier DA, Farmer A, Lyneham HJ, Rapee RM, Eley TC. Neurotrophic gene polymorphisms and response to psychological therapy. Transl Psychiatry. 2012;2(5):e108. PMCID: PMC3365252. http://www.ncbi.nlm.nih.gov/pubmed/22832952.
222. Kobayashi K, Shimizu E, Hashimoto K, Mitsumori M, Koike K, Okamura N, Koizumi H, Ohgake S, Matsuzawa D, Zhang L, Nakazato M, Iyo M. Serum brain-derived neurotrophic factor (BDNF) levels in patients with panic disorder: as a biological predictor of response to group cognitive behavioral therapy. Prog Neuro-Psychopharmacol Biol Psychiatry. 2005;29(5):658–63. PMID: 15905010. http://www.ncbi.nlm.nih.gov/pubmed/15905010.
223. Oliff HS, Berchtold NC, Isackson P, Cotman CW. Exercise-induced regulation of brain-derived neurotrophic factor (BDNF) transcripts in the rat hippocampus. Brain Res Mol Brain Res. 1998;61(1–2):147–53. PMID: 9795193. http://www.ncbi.nlm.nih.gov/pubmed/9795193.
224. Zoladz JA, Pilc A. The effect of physical activity on the brain derived neurotrophic factor: from animal to human studies. J Physiol Pharmacol. 2010;61(5):533–41. PMID: 21081796. http://www.ncbi.nlm.nih.gov/pubmed/21081796.
225. Müller MB, Toschi N, Kresse AE, Post A, Keck ME. Long-term repetitive transcranial magnetic stimulation increases the expression of brain-derived neurotrophic factor and cholecystokinin mRNA, but not neuropeptide tyrosine mRNA in specific areas of rat brain. Neuropsychopharmacology. 2000;23(2):205–15. PMID: 10882847. http://www.ncbi.nlm.nih.gov/pubmed/10882847.
226. Duman RS, Vaidya VA. Molecular and cellular actions of chronic electroconvulsive seizures. J ECT. 1998;14(3):181–93. PMID: 9773357. http://www.ncbi.nlm.nih.gov/pubmed/9773357.
227. Jha S, Dong B, Sakata K. Enriched environment treatment reverses depression-like behavior and restores reduced hippocampal neurogenesis and protein levels of brain-derived neurotrophic factor in mice lacking its expression through promoter IV. Transl. Psychiatry. 2011;1(9):e40. PMCID: PMC3309483. http://www.ncbi.nlm.nih.gov/pubmed/22832656.
228. Shao B, Cheng Y, Jin K. Estrogen, neuroprotection and neurogenesis after ischemic stroke. Curr Drug Targets. 2012;13(2):188–98. PMID: 22204318. http://www.ncbi.nlm.nih.gov/pubmed/22204318.
229. Scott E, Guang ZQ, Wang R, Vadlamudi R, Brann D. Estrogen neuroprotection and the critical period hypothesis. Front Neuroendocrinol. 2012;33(1):85–104. PMCID: PMC3288697. http://www.ncbi.nlm.nih.gov/pubmed/22079780.
230. Molteni R, Barnard RJ, Ying Z, Roberts CK, Gómez-Pinilla F. A high-fat, refined sugar diet reduces hippocampal brain-derived neurotrophic factor, neuronal plasticity, and learning. Neuroscience. 2002;112(4):803–14. PMID: 12088740. http://www.ncbi.nlm.nih.gov/pubmed/12088740.
231. Grillo CA, Piroli GG, Junor L, Wilson SP, Mott DD, Wilson MA, Reagan LP. Obesity/hyperleptinemic phenotype impairs structural and functional plasticity in the rat hippocampus. Physiol Behav. 2011;105(1):138–44. PMCID: PMC3129487. http://www.ncbi.nlm.nih.gov/pubmed/21354191.
232. Noble EE, Billington CJ, Kotz CM, Wang C. The lighter side of BDNF. Am J Physiol Regul Integr Comp Physiol. 2011;300(5):R1053–69. PMCID: PMC3293512. http://www.ncbi.nlm.nih.gov/pubmed/21346243.
233. Stranahan AM, Mattson MP. Bidirectional metabolic regulation of neurocognitive function. Neurobiol Learn Mem. 2011;96(4):507–16. PMCID: PMC3084367. http://www.ncbi.nlm.nih.gov/pubmed/21236352.
234. Kanoski SE, Davidson TL. Western diet consumption and cognitive impairment: links to hippocampal dysfunction and obesity. Physiol Behav. 2011;103(1):59–68. PMCID: PMC3056912. http://www.ncbi.nlm.nih.gov/pubmed/21167850.
235. Citalopram Monograph for Professionals - Drugs.com.
236. DailyMed - CELEXA- citalopram tablet, film coated.
237. Barrett EL, Clark MA. Tetrathionate reduction and production of hydrogen sulfide from thiosulfate. Microbiol Rev. 1987;51(2):192–205. PMCID: PMC373103. http://www.ncbi.nlm.nih.gov/pubmed/3299028.
238. Escitalopram Monograph for Professionals - Drugs.com.
239. FLUoxetine Monograph for Professionals - Drugs.com.
240. FluvoxaMINE Monograph for Professionals - Drugs.com.
241. PARoxetine Monograph for Professionals - Drugs.com.
242. Sertraline Monograph for Professionals - Drugs.com.
243. Medications for Treatment of Depression - Psychiatric Disorders - Merck Manual Professional Edition.
244. Landén M, Högberg P, Thase ME. Incidence of sexual side effects in refractory depression during treatment with citalopram or paroxetine. J Clin Psychiatry. 2005;66(1):100–6. PMID: 15669895. http://www.ncbi.nlm.nih.gov/pubmed/15669895.
245. Bhagwagar Z, Wylezinska M, Taylor M, Jezzard P, Matthews PM, Cowen PJ. Increased brain GABA concentrations following acute administration of a selective serotonin reuptake inhibitor. Am J Psychiatry. 2004;161(2):368–70. PMID: 14754790. http://www.ncbi.nlm.nih.gov/pubmed/14754790.
246. Vollenweider I, Smith KS, Keist R, Rudolph U. Antidepressant-like properties of α2-containing GABA(A) receptors. Behav Brain

Res. 2011;217(1):77–80. PMCID: PMC3023881. http://www.ncbi.nlm.nih.gov/pubmed/20965216.
247. Dording CM, Mischoulon D, Petersen TJ, Kornbluh R, Gordon J, Nierenberg AA, Rosenbaum JE, Fava M. The pharmacologic management of SSRI-induced side effects: a survey of psychiatrists. Ann Clin Psychiatry. 2002;14(3):143–7. PMID: 12585563. http://www.ncbi.nlm.nih.gov/pubmed/12585563.
248. Lane RM. SSRI-induced extrapyramidal side-effects and akathisia: implications for treatment. J Psychopharmacol. 1998;12(2):192–214. PMID: 9694033. http://www.ncbi.nlm.nih.gov/pubmed/9694033.
249. Fergusson D, Doucette S, Glass KC, Shapiro S, Healy D, Hebert P, Hutton B. Association between suicide attempts and selective serotonin reuptake inhibitors: systematic review of randomised controlled trials. BMJ. 2005;330(7488):396. PMCID: PMC549110. http://www.ncbi.nlm.nih.gov/pubmed/15718539.
250. Hall WD. How have the SSRI antidepressants affected suicide risk? Lancet. 2006;367(9527):1959–62. PMID: 16782468. http://www.ncbi.nlm.nih.gov/pubmed/16782468.
251. Painuly N, Basu D. SSRI and suicide? Psychother Psychosom. 2004;73(4):261–2. author reply 262. PMID: 15184724. http://www.ncbi.nlm.nih.gov/pubmed/15184724.
252. Casey P. SSRI and suicide. Psychother Psychosom. 2004;73(4):259–60. author reply 260-261. PMID: 15184722. http://www.ncbi.nlm.nih.gov/pubmed/15184722.
253. Regan J, Hamer G, Wright A, White C. SSRI and suicide in adolescents. Tenn Med. 2004;97(3):121–2. PMID: 15054945. http://www.ncbi.nlm.nih.gov/pubmed/15054945.
254. Ham P. Suicide risk not increased with SSRI antidepressants. J Fam Pract. 2003;52(8):587–8. PMID: 12899805. http://www.ncbi.nlm.nih.gov/pubmed/12899805.
255. Gibbons RD, Hur K, Bhaumik DK, Mann JJ. The relationship between antidepressant prescription rates and rate of early adolescent suicide. Am J Psychiatry. 2006;163(11):1898–904. PMID: 17074941. http://www.ncbi.nlm.nih.gov/pubmed/17074941.
256. Fornaro M, Anastasia A, Valchera A, Carano A, Orsolini L, Vellante F, Rapini G, Olivieri L, Di Natale S, Perna G, Martinotti G, Di Giannantonio M, De Berardis D. The FDA "Black Box" warning on antidepressant suicide risk in young adults: more harm than benefits?. Front Psychiatry. 2019;10:294. PMCID: PMC6510161. http://www.ncbi.nlm.nih.gov/pubmed/31130881.
257. Solmi M, Fornaro M, Ostinelli EG, Zangani C, Croatto G, Monaco F, Krinitski D, Fusar-Poli P, Correll CU. Safety of 80 antidepressants, antipsychotics, anti-attention-deficit/hyperactivity medications and mood stabilizers in children and adolescents with psychiatric disorders: a large scale systematic meta-review of 78 adverse effects. World Psychiatry. 2020;19(2):214–32. PMCID: PMC7215080.
258. Plöderl M, Hengartner MP. Effect of the FDA Black Box suicidality warnings for antidepressants on suicide rates in the USA. Crisis. 2023;44(2):128–34. PMID: 34915730. http://www.ncbi.nlm.nih.gov/pubmed/34915730.
259. Soumerai SB, Koppel R, Naci H, Madden JM, Fry A, Halbisen A, Angeles J, Koppel J, Rubin R, Lu CY. Intended and unintended outcomes after FDA pediatric antidepressant warnings: a systematic review. Health Aff (Millwood). 2024;43(10):1360–9. PMID: 39374452. http://www.ncbi.nlm.nih.gov/pubmed/39374452.
260. Bolton JM, Sareen J, Reiss JP. Genital anaesthesia persisting six years after sertraline discontinuation. J Sex Marital Ther. 2006;32(4):327–30. PMID: 16709553. http://www.ncbi.nlm.nih.gov/pubmed/16709553.
261. Yohn CN, Gergues MM, Samuels BA. The role of 5-HT receptors in depression. Mol. Brain. 2017;10(1):28. PMCID: PMC5483313. http://www.ncbi.nlm.nih.gov/pubmed/28646910.
262. Mechanisms of signal transduction by hormones and growth factors. Proceedings of the second international symposium on cellular endocrinology. Lake Placid, New York, September 8–11, 1986. Prog Clin Biol Res. 1987;249:1–321. PMID: 2823287. http://www.ncbi.nlm.nih.gov/pubmed/2823287.
263. Haddjeri N, Blier P, de Montigny C. Long-term antidepressant treatments result in a tonic activation of forebrain 5-HT1A receptors. J Neurosci. 1998;18(23):10150–6. PMCID: PMC6793307. http://www.ncbi.nlm.nih.gov/pubmed/9822768.
264. Celada P, Puig M, Amargós-Bosch M, Adell A, Artigas F. The therapeutic role of 5-HT1A and 5-HT2A receptors in depression. J Psychiatry Neurosci. 2004;29(4):252–65. PMCID: PMC446220. http://www.ncbi.nlm.nih.gov/pubmed/15309042.
265. Ślifirski G, Król M, Turło J. 5-HT receptors and the development of new antidepressants. Int J Mol Sci. 2021;22(16):9015. PMCID: PMC8396477. http://www.ncbi.nlm.nih.gov/pubmed/34445721.
266. Millan MJ. Serotonin 5-HT2C receptors as a target for the treatment of depressive and anxious states: focus on novel therapeutic strategies. Therapie. 2005;60(5):441–60. PMID: 16433010. http://www.ncbi.nlm.nih.gov/pubmed/16433010.
267. Boyarsky BK, Haque W, Rouleau MR, Hirschfeld RM. Sexual functioning in depressed outpatients taking mirtazapine. Depress Anxiety. 1999;9(4):175–9. PMID: 10431683. http://www.ncbi.nlm.nih.gov/pubmed/10431683.
268. Farnsworth KD, Dinsmore WW. Persistent sexual dysfunction in genitourinary medicine clinic attendees induced by selective serotonin reuptake inhibitors. Int J STD AIDS. 2009;20(1):68–9. PMID: 19103903. http://www.ncbi.nlm.nih.gov/pubmed/19103903.
269. Pereira VM, Arias-Carrión O, Machado S, Nardi AE, Silva AC. Bupropion in the depression-related sexual dysfunction: a systematic review. CNS Neurol Disord Drug Targets. 2014;13(6):1079–88. PMID: 24923342. http://www.ncbi.nlm.nih.gov/pubmed/24923342.
270. Boyer EW, Shannon M. The serotonin syndrome. N Engl J Med. 2005;352(11):1112–20. PMID: 15784664. http://www.ncbi.nlm.nih.gov/pubmed/15784664.
271. Arora B, Kannikeswaran N. The serotonin syndrome-the need for physician's awareness. Int J Emerg Med. 2010;3(4):373–7. PMCID: PMC3047867. http://www.ncbi.nlm.nih.gov/pubmed/21373307.
272. Serotonin syndrome: MedlinePlus Medical Encyclopedia.
273. Weissman AM, Levy BT, Hartz AJ, Bentler S, Donohue M, Ellingrod VL, Wisner KL. Pooled analysis of antidepressant levels in lactating mothers, breast milk, and nursing infants. Am J Psychiatry. 2004;161(6):1066–78. PMID: 15169695. http://www.ncbi.nlm.nih.gov/pubmed/15169695.
274. Ito S. Drug therapy for breast-feeding women. N Engl J Med. 2000;343(2):118–26. PMID: 10891521. http://www.ncbi.nlm.nih.gov/pubmed/10891521.
275. Rampono J, Teoh S, Hackett LP, Kohan R, Ilett KF. Estimation of desvenlafaxine transfer into milk and infant exposure during its use in lactating women with postnatal depression. Arch Womens Ment Health. 2011;14(1):49–53. PMID: 20960017. http://www.ncbi.nlm.nih.gov/pubmed/20960017.
276. Berle JØ, Spigset O. Antidepressant use during breastfeeding. Curr Womens Health Rev. 2011;7(1):28–34. PMCID: PMC3267169. http://www.ncbi.nlm.nih.gov/pubmed/22299006.
277. Ilett KF, Watt F, Hackett LP, Kohan R, Teoh S. Assessment of infant dose through milk in a lactating woman taking amisulpride and desvenlafaxine for treatment-resistant depression. Ther Drug Monit. 2010;32(6):704–7. PMID: 20926994. http://www.ncbi.nlm.nih.gov/pubmed/20926994.
278. Moretti M. Breastfeeding and the use of antidepressants. J Popul Ther Clin Pharmacol. 2012;19(3):e387–90. PMID: 23075497. http://www.ncbi.nlm.nih.gov/pubmed/23075497.

279. Fitelson E, Kim S, Baker AS, Leight K. Treatment of postpartum depression: clinical, psychological and pharmacological options. Int J Women's Health. 2010;3:1–14. PMCID: PMC3039003. http://www.ncbi.nlm.nih.gov/pubmed/21339932.
280. O'Hara MW, McCabe JE. Postpartum depression: current status and future directions. Annu Rev Clin Psychol. 2013;9:379–407. PMID: 23394227. http://www.ncbi.nlm.nih.gov/pubmed/23394227.
281. Chad L, Pupco A, Bozzo P, Koren G. Update on antidepressant use during breastfeeding. Can Fam Physician. 2013;59(6):633–4. PMCID: PMC3681447. http://www.ncbi.nlm.nih.gov/pubmed/23766044.
282. Csoka AB, Bahrick A, Mehtonen OP. Persistent sexual dysfunction after discontinuation of selective serotonin reuptake inhibitors. J Sex Med. 2008;5(1):227–33. PMID: 18173768. http://www.ncbi.nlm.nih.gov/pubmed/18173768.
283. Hu X, Pan L, Li W. Meta-analysis on the efficacy of the norepinephrine reuptake inhibitors reboxetine and atomoxetine for the treatment of schizophrenia and attention deficit hyperactivity disorder. Adv. Clin Exp Med. 2023;32(5):511–22. PMID: 36449401. http://www.ncbi.nlm.nih.gov/pubmed/36449401.
284. Wang J, Ye Y, Shang Z, Zheng Q, Zhang S, Li L, Liu W. Effect of norepinephrine reuptake inhibitors combined with antimuscarinic agents vs monotherapy for OSA: a systematic review and meta-analysis. J Clin Sleep Med. 2024;20(8):1363–72. PMCID: PMC11294128. http://www.ncbi.nlm.nih.gov/pubmed/38494994.
285. Cipriani A, Furukawa TA, Salanti G, Geddes JR, Higgins JP, Churchill R, Watanabe N, Nakagawa A, Omori IM, McGuire H, Tansella M, Barbui C. Comparative efficacy and acceptability of 12 new-generation antidepressants: a multiple-treatments meta-analysis. Lancet. 2009;373(9665):746–58. PMID: 19185342. http://www.ncbi.nlm.nih.gov/pubmed/19185342.
286. Eyding D, Lelgemann M, Grouven U, Härter M, Kromp M, Kaiser T, Kerekes MF, Gerken M, Wieseler B. Reboxetine for acute treatment of major depression: systematic review and meta-analysis of published and unpublished placebo and selective serotonin reuptake inhibitor controlled trials. BMJ. 2010;341:c4737. PMCID: PMC2954275. http://www.ncbi.nlm.nih.gov/pubmed/20940209.
287. Hajós M, Fleishaker JC, Filipiak-Reisner JK, Brown MT, Wong EHF. The selective norepinephrine reuptake inhibitor antidepressant reboxetine: pharmacological and clinical profile. CNS Drug Rev. 2004;10(1):23–44. PMCID: PMC6741733. http://www.ncbi.nlm.nih.gov/pubmed/14978512.
288. Preskorn SH. Reboxetine: a norepinephrine selective reuptake pump inhibitor. J Psychiatr Pract. 2004;10(1):57–63. PMID: 15334987. http://www.ncbi.nlm.nih.gov/pubmed/15334987.
289. DOPamine Monograph for Professionals - Drugs.com.
290. Fink M, Akimova E, Spindelegger C, Hahn A, Lanzenberger R, Kasper S. Social anxiety disorder: epidemiology, biology and treatment. Psychiatr Danub. 2009;21(4):533–42. PMID: 19935490. http://www.ncbi.nlm.nih.gov/pubmed/19935490.
291. Perugi G, De Rosa U, Barbuti M. What value do norepinephrine/dopamine dual reuptake inhibitors have to the current treatment of adult attention deficit hyperactivity disorder (ADHD) treatment armamentarium? Expert Opin Pharmacother. 2022;23(18):1975–8. PMID: 36384367. http://www.ncbi.nlm.nih.gov/pubmed/36384367.
292. Lin CH, Lane HY. Bupropion interferes with the image diagnosis of Parkinson's disease. Neuropsychiatr Dis Treat. 2017;13:2637–9. PMCID: PMC5656353. http://www.ncbi.nlm.nih.gov/pubmed/29089770.
293. Gebhardt S, Röttgers H, Bäcker A, Schu U, Krieg JC. Treatment of panic disorder with bupropion in a patient with Parkinson's disease. J Clin Pharm Ther. 2008;33(5):575–7. PMID: 18834374. http://www.ncbi.nlm.nih.gov/pubmed/18834374.
294. Subedi R, Singh R, Thakur RK, Jha D, Ray BK. Efficacy and safety of solriamfetol for excessive daytime sleepiness in narcolepsy and obstructive sleep apnea: a systematic review and meta-analysis of clinical trials. Sleep Med. 2020;75:510–21. PMID: 33032062. http://www.ncbi.nlm.nih.gov/pubmed/33032062.
295. Abad VC, Guilleminault C. Solriamfetol for the treatment of daytime sleepiness in obstructive sleep apnea. Expert Rev Respir Med. 2018;12(12):1007–19. PMID: 30365900. http://www.ncbi.nlm.nih.gov/pubmed/30365900.
296. Stahl SM, Pradko JF, Haight BR, Modell JG, Rockett CB, Learned-Coughlin S. A review of the neuropharmacology of Bupropion, a dual Norepinephrine and Dopamine Reuptake inhibitor. Prim Care Companion J Clin Psychiatry. 2004;6(4):159–66. PMCID: PMC514842. http://www.ncbi.nlm.nih.gov/pubmed/15361919.
297. Wang P, Yan F, Dong J, Wang S, Shi Y, Zhu M, Zuo Y, Ma H, Xue R, Zhai D, Song X. A multiple-step screening protocol to identify norepinephrine and dopamine reuptake inhibitors for depression. Phys Chem Chem Phys. 2023;25(12):8341–54. PMID: 36880666. http://www.ncbi.nlm.nih.gov/pubmed/36880666.
298. Hetrick SE, McKenzie JE, Bailey AP, Sharma V, Moller CI, Badcock PB, Cox GR, Merry SN, Meader N. New generation antidepressants for depression in children and adolescents: a network meta-analysis. Cochrane Database Syst Rev. 2021;5(5):CD013674. PMCID: PMC8143444. http://www.ncbi.nlm.nih.gov/pubmed/34029378.
299. Hughes JR, Stead LF, Hartmann-Boyce J, Cahill K, Lancaster T. Antidepressants for smoking cessation. Cochrane Database Syst Rev. 2014;2014(1):CD000031. PMCID: PMC7027688. http://www.ncbi.nlm.nih.gov/pubmed/24402784.
300. Huecker MR, Smiley A, Saadabadi A. Bupropion. StatPearls [Internet]. Treasure Island: StatPearls Publishing; 2025 [cited 2025 Jan 11]. Available from: http://www.ncbi.nlm.nih.gov/books/NBK470212/ PMID: 29262173. http://www.ncbi.nlm.nih.gov/pubmed/29262173.
301. Learned-Coughlin SM, Bergström M, Savitcheva I, Ascher J, Schmith VD, Långstrom B. In vivo activity of bupropion at the human dopamine transporter as measured by positron emission tomography. Biol Psychiatry. 2003;54(8):800–5. PMID: 14550679. http://www.ncbi.nlm.nih.gov/pubmed/14550679.
302. Slemmer JE, Martin BR, Damaj MI. Bupropion is a nicotinic antagonist. J Pharmacol Exp Ther. 2000;295(1):321–7. PMID: 10991997. http://www.ncbi.nlm.nih.gov/pubmed/10991997.
303. Bailey SR, Crew EE, Riske EC, Ammerman S, Robinson TN, Killen JD. Efficacy and tolerability of pharmacotherapies to aid smoking cessation in adolescents. Paediatr Drugs. 2012;14(2):91–108. PMCID: PMC3319092. http://www.ncbi.nlm.nih.gov/pubmed/22248234.
304. Gómez-Coronado N, Walker AJ, Berk M, Dodd S. Current and emerging pharmacotherapies for Cessation of tobacco smoking. Pharmacotherapy. 2018;38(2):235–58. PMID: 29250815. http://www.ncbi.nlm.nih.gov/pubmed/29250815.
305. Cahill K, Stead LF, Lancaster T. Nicotine receptor partial agonists for smoking cessation. Cochrane Database Syst Rev. 2012;(4):CD006103. PMID: 22513936. http://www.ncbi.nlm.nih.gov/pubmed/22513936.
306. Wu P, Wilson K, Dimoulas P, Mills EJ. Effectiveness of smoking cessation therapies: a systematic review and meta-analysis. BMC Public Health. 2006;6:300. PMCID: PMC1764891. http://www.ncbi.nlm.nih.gov/pubmed/17156479.
307. Fuentes AV, Pineda MD, Venkata KCN. Comprehension of top 200 prescribed drugs in the US as a resource for pharmacy teaching, training and practice. Pharmacy (Basel). 2018;6(2):43. PMCID: PMC6025009. http://www.ncbi.nlm.nih.gov/pubmed/29757930.
308. Effexor: Package Insert / Prescribing Information.
309. Cymbalta: Package Insert - Drugs.com.
310. Pristiq: Package Insert - Drugs.com.

311. SNRIs (Serotonin and Norepinephrine Reuptake Inhibitors): Uses [clevelandclinic.org).
312. Cashman JR, Ghirmai S. Inhibition of serotonin and norepinephrine reuptake and inhibition of phosphodiesterase by multi-target inhibitors as potential agents for depression. Bioorg Med Chem. 2009;17(19):6890–7. PMID: 19740668. http://www.ncbi.nlm.nih.gov/pubmed/19740668.
313. Spina E, Santoro V, D'Arrigo C. Clinically relevant pharmacokinetic drug interactions with second-generation antidepressants: an update. Clin Ther. 2008;30(7):1206–27. PMID: 18691982. http://www.ncbi.nlm.nih.gov/pubmed/18691982.
314. Suryawanshi O, Pajai S. A comprehensive review on postpartum depression. Cureus. 2022;14(12):e32745. PMCID: PMC9851410. http://www.ncbi.nlm.nih.gov/pubmed/36686097.
315. Leshem R, Bar-Oz B, Diav-Citrin O, Gbaly S, Soliman J, Renoux C, Matok I. Selective Serotonin Reuptake Inhibitors (SSRIs) and Serotonin Norepinephrine Reuptake Inhibitors (SNRIs) during pregnancy and the risk for autism spectrum disorder (ASD) and attention deficit hyperactivity disorder (ADHD) in the offspring: a true effect or a bias? a systematic review & meta-analysis. Curr Neuropharmacol. 2021;19(6):896–906. PMCID: PMC8686301. http://www.ncbi.nlm.nih.gov/pubmed/33655866.
316. Guaiana G, Meader N, Barbui C, Davies SJ, Furukawa TA, Imai H, Dias S, Caldwell DM, Koesters M, Tajika A, Bighelli I, Pompoli A, Cipriani A, Dawson S, Robertson L. Pharmacological treatments in panic disorder in adults: a network meta-analysis. Cochrane Database Syst Rev. 2023;11(11):CD012729. PMCID: PMC10683020. http://www.ncbi.nlm.nih.gov/pubmed/38014714.
317. Strawn JR, Dobson ET, Giles LL. Primary pediatric care psychopharmacology: focus on medications for ADHD, depression, and anxiety. Curr Probl Pediatr Adolesc Health Care. 2017;47(1):3–14. PMCID: PMC5340601. http://www.ncbi.nlm.nih.gov/pubmed/28043839.
318. Locher C, Koechlin H, Zion SR, Werner C, Pine DS, Kirsch I, Kessler RC, Kossowsky J. Efficacy and safety of selective serotonin reuptake inhibitors, serotonin-norepinephrine reuptake inhibitors, and placebo for common psychiatric disorders among children and adolescents: a systematic review and meta-analysis. JAMA Psychiatry. 2017;74(10):1011–20. PMCID: PMC5667359. http://www.ncbi.nlm.nih.gov/pubmed/28854296.
319. Elsouri KN, Heiser SE, Cabrera D, Alqurneh S, Hawat J, Demory ML. Management and treatment of obsessive-compulsive disorder (OCD): a literature review. Cureus. 2024;16(5):e60496. PMCID: PMC11180522. http://www.ncbi.nlm.nih.gov/pubmed/38883111.
320. Albert U, Marazziti D, Di Salvo G, Solia F, Rosso G, Maina G. A systematic review of evidence-based treatment strategies for obsessive- compulsive disorder resistant to first-line pharmacotherapy. Curr Med Chem. 2018;25(41):5647–61. PMID: 29278206. http://www.ncbi.nlm.nih.gov/pubmed/29278206.
321. Fanelli D, Weller G, Liu H. New Serotonin-Norepinephrine Reuptake inhibitors and their anesthetic and analgesic considerations. Neurol Int. 2021;13(4):497–509. PMCID: PMC8544373. http://www.ncbi.nlm.nih.gov/pubmed/34698218.
322. Wright ME, Rizzolo D. An update on the pharmacologic management and treatment of neuropathic pain. JAAPA. 2017;30(3):13–7. PMID: 28151738. http://www.ncbi.nlm.nih.gov/pubmed/28151738.
323. Newhouser LM, Maneval M, Rayalam K, Sabeeh G, Varela L. SSRIs vs. SNRIs for vasomotor symptoms of Menopause. Am Fam Physician. 2022;105(4):430–1. PMID: 35426647. http://www.ncbi.nlm.nih.gov/pubmed/35426647.
324. Hemachandra C, Taylor S, Islam RM, Fooladi E, Davis SR. A systematic review and critical appraisal of menopause guidelines. BMJ Sex Reprod Health. 2024;50(2):122–38. PMID: 38336466. http://www.ncbi.nlm.nih.gov/pubmed/38336466.
325. Kitaichi Y, Inoue T, Nakagawa S, Boku S, Kakuta A, Izumi T, Koyama T. Sertraline increases extracellular levels not only of serotonin, but also of dopamine in the nucleus accumbens and striatum of rats. Eur J Pharmacol. 2010;647(1–3):90–6. PMID: 20816814. http://www.ncbi.nlm.nih.gov/pubmed/20816814.
326. Rothman RB, Blough BE, Baumann MH. Dual dopamine/serotonin releasers as potential medications for stimulant and alcohol addictions. AAPS J. 2007;9(1):E1–10. PMCID: PMC2751297. http://www.ncbi.nlm.nih.gov/pubmed/17408232.
327. Hendson L, Shah V, Trkulja S. Selective serotonin reuptake inhibitors or serotonin-norepinephrine reuptake inhibitors in pregnancy: infant and childhood outcomes. Paediatr Child Health. 2021;26(5):321–2. PMCID: PMC8318525. http://www.ncbi.nlm.nih.gov/pubmed/34336063.
328. Uguz F. Neonatal and childhood outcomes in offspring of pregnant women using antidepressant medications: a critical review of current meta-analyses. J Clin Pharmacol. 2021;61(2):146–58. PMID: 32840005. http://www.ncbi.nlm.nih.gov/pubmed/32840005.
329. Marks DM, Pae CU, Patkar AA. Triple reuptake inhibitors: a premise and promise. Psychiatry Investig. 2008;5(3):142–7. PMCID: PMC2796030. http://www.ncbi.nlm.nih.gov/pubmed/20046357.
330. Marks DM, Pae CU, Patkar AA. Triple reuptake inhibitors: the next generation of antidepressants. Curr Neuropharmacol. 2008;6(4):338–43. PMCID: PMC2701280. http://www.ncbi.nlm.nih.gov/pubmed/19587855.
331. Yang ARST, Yi HS, Warnock KT, Mamczarz J, June HL, Mallick N, Krieter PA, Tonelli L, Skolnick P, Basile AS, June HL. Effects of the triple monoamine uptake inhibitor DOV 102,677 on alcohol-motivated responding and antidepressant activity in alcohol-preferring (P) rats. Alcohol Clin Exp Res. 2012;36(5):863–73. PMCID: PMC3464941. http://www.ncbi.nlm.nih.gov/pubmed/22150508.
332. McMillen BA, Shank JE, Jordan KB, Williams HL, Basile AS. Effect of DOV 102,677 on the volitional consumption of ethanol by Myers' high ethanol-preferring rat. Alcohol Clin Exp Res. 2007;31(11):1866–71. PMID: 17908267. http://www.ncbi.nlm.nih.gov/pubmed/17908267.
333. Gardner EL, Liu X, Paredes W, Giordano A, Spector J, Lepore M, Wu KM, Froimowitz M. A slow-onset, long-duration indanamine monoamine reuptake inhibitor as a potential maintenance pharmacotherapy for psychostimulant abuse: effects in laboratory rat models relating to addiction. Neuropharmacology. 2006;51(5):993–1003. PMID: 16901516. http://www.ncbi.nlm.nih.gov/pubmed/16901516.
334. Wilens TE, Klint T, Adler L, West S, Wesnes K, Graff O, Mikkelsen B. A randomized controlled trial of a novel mixed monoamine reuptake inhibitor in adults with ADHD. Behav Brain Funct. 2008;4:24. PMCID: PMC2442604. http://www.ncbi.nlm.nih.gov/pubmed/18554401.
335. Wilens TE, Morrison NR, Prince J. An update on the pharmacotherapy of attention-deficit/hyperactivity disorder in adults. Expert Rev Neurother. 2011;11(10):1443–65. PMCID: PMC3229037. http://www.ncbi.nlm.nih.gov/pubmed/21955201.
336. Tizzano JP, Stribling DS, Perez-Tilve D, Strack A, Frassetto A, Chen RZ, Fong TM, Shearman L, Krieter PA, Tschöp MH, Skolnick P, Basile AS. The triple uptake inhibitor (1R,5S)-(+)-1-(3,4-dichlorophenyl)-3-azabicyclo[3.1.0] hexane hydrochloride (DOV 21947) reduces body weight and plasma triglycerides in rodent models of diet-induced obesity. J Pharmacol Exp Ther. 2008;324(3):1111–26. PMID: 18089843. http://www.ncbi.nlm.nih.gov/pubmed/18089843.
337. Hauser RA, Salin L, Juhel N, Konyago VL. Randomized trial of the triple monoamine reuptake inhibitor NS 2330 (tesofensine) in early Parkinson's disease. Mov Disord. 2007;22(3):359–65. PMID: 17149725. http://www.ncbi.nlm.nih.gov/pubmed/17149725.

338. Basile AS, Janowsky A, Golembiowska K, Kowalska M, Tam E, Benveniste M, Popik P, Nikiforuk A, Krawczyk M, Nowak G, Krieter PA, Lippa AS, Skolnick P, Koustova E. Characterization of the antinociceptive actions of bicifadine in models of acute, persistent, and chronic pain. J Pharmacol Exp Ther. 2007;321(3):1208–25. PMID: 17325229. http://www.ncbi.nlm.nih.gov/pubmed/17325229.
339. Nefazodone Uses, Side Effects & Warnings.
340. Roque Bravo R, Faria AC, Brito-da-Costa AM, Carmo H, Mladěnka P, Dias da Silva D, Remião F. On Behalf Of The Oemonom Researchers null. Cocaine: an updated overview on chemistry, detection, biokinetics, and pharmacotoxicological aspects including abuse pattern. Toxins (Basel). 2022;14(4):278. PMCID: PMC9032145. http://www.ncbi.nlm.nih.gov/pubmed/35448887.
341. Ng QX, Venkatanarayanan N, Ho CYX. Clinical use of Hypericum perforatum (St John's wort) in depression: a meta-analysis. J Affect Disord. 2017;210:211–21. PMID: 28064110. http://www.ncbi.nlm.nih.gov/pubmed/28064110.
342. Remick RA. Anticholinergic side effects of tricyclic antidepressants and their management. Prog Neuro-Psychopharmacol Biol Psychiatry. 1988;12(2–3):225–31. PMID: 3290996. http://www.ncbi.nlm.nih.gov/pubmed/3290996.
343. McFee RB, Mofenson HC, Caraccio TR. A nationwide survey of the management of unintentional-low dose tricyclic antidepressant ingestions involving asymptomatic children: implications for the development of an evidence-based clinical guideline. J Toxicol Clin Toxicol. 2000;38(1):15–9. PMID: 10696919. http://www.ncbi.nlm.nih.gov/pubmed/10696919.
344. Kerr GW, McGuffie AC, Wilkie S. Tricyclic antidepressant overdose: a review. Emerg Med J. 2001;18(4):236–41. PMCID: PMC1725608. http://www.ncbi.nlm.nih.gov/pubmed/11435353.
345. Thomas SH, Bevan L, Bhattacharyya S, Bramble MG, Chew K, Connolly J, Dorani B, Han KH, Horner JE, Rodgers A, Sen B, Tesfayohannes B, Wynne H, Bateman DN. Presentation of poisoned patients to accident and emergency departments in the north of England. Hum Exp Toxicol. 1996;15(6):466–70. PMID: 8793528. http://www.ncbi.nlm.nih.gov/pubmed/8793528.
346. Kposowa AJ, McElvain JP. Gender, place, and method of suicide. Soc Psychiatry Psychiatr Epidemiol. 2006;41(6):435–43. PMID: 16565913. http://www.ncbi.nlm.nih.gov/pubmed/16565913.
347. Vieweg WVR, Pandurangi AK, Anum EA, Lanier JO, Fierro MF, Fernandez A. Toxicology findings in child and adolescent suicides in Virginia: 1987-2003. Prim Care Companion J Clin Psychiatry. 2006;8(3):142–6. PMCID: PMC1540399. http://www.ncbi.nlm.nih.gov/pubmed/16912816.
348. Hatzinger M. Antidepressants and suicidality: a contradiction? Praxis (Bern 1994). 2019;108(7):487–94. PMID: 31136275. http://www.ncbi.nlm.nih.gov/pubmed/31136275.
349. Broquet KE. Status of treatment of depression. South Med J. 1999;92(9):846–56. PMID: 10498158. http://www.ncbi.nlm.nih.gov/pubmed/10498158.
350. Biederman J, Spencer T. Attention-deficit/hyperactivity disorder (ADHD) as a noradrenergic disorder. Biol Psychiatry. 1999;46(9):1234–42. PMID: 10560028. http://www.ncbi.nlm.nih.gov/pubmed/10560028.
351. Micó JA, Ardid D, Berrocoso E, Eschalier A. Antidepressants and pain. Trends Pharmacol Sci. 2006;27(7):348–54. PMID: 16762426. http://www.ncbi.nlm.nih.gov/pubmed/16762426.
352. Shih JC, Chen K, Ridd MJ. Role of MAO A and B in neurotransmitter metabolism and behavior. Pol J Pharmacol. 1999;51(1):25–9. PMID: 10389141. http://www.ncbi.nlm.nih.gov/pubmed/10389141.
353. McCabe BJ. Dietary tyramine and other pressor amines in MAOI regimens: a review. J Am Diet Assoc. 1986;86(8):1059–64. PMID: 3525654. http://www.ncbi.nlm.nih.gov/pubmed/3525654.
354. Walker SE, Shulman KI, Tailor SA, Gardner D. Tyramine content of previously restricted foods in monoamine oxidase inhibitor diets. J Clin Psychopharmacol. 1996;16(5):383–8. PMID: 8889911. http://www.ncbi.nlm.nih.gov/pubmed/8889911.
355. Sweet RA, Brown EJ, Heimberg RG, Ciafre L, Scanga DM, Cornelius JR, Dube S, Forsyth KM, Holt CS. Monoamine oxidase inhibitor dietary restrictions: what are we asking patients to give up? J Clin Psychiatry. 1995;56(5):196–201. PMID: 7737959. http://www.ncbi.nlm.nih.gov/pubmed/7737959.
356. Gardner DM, Shulman KI, Walker SE, Tailor SA. The making of a user friendly MAOI diet. J Clin Psychiatry. 1996;57(3):99–104. PMID: 8617704. http://www.ncbi.nlm.nih.gov/pubmed/8617704.
357. Nieuwstraten C, Labiris NR, Holbrook A. Systematic overview of drug interactions with antidepressant medications. Can J Psychiatr. 2006;51(5):300–16. PMID: 16986820. http://www.ncbi.nlm.nih.gov/pubmed/16986820.
358. Simon NM. Generalized anxiety disorder and psychiatric comorbidities such as depression, bipolar disorder, and substance abuse. J Clin Psychiatry. 2009;70(Suppl 2):10–4. PMID: 19371501. http://www.ncbi.nlm.nih.gov/pubmed/19371501.
359. Batelaan NM, Spijker J, de Graaf R, Cuijpers P. Mixed anxiety depression should not be included in DSM-5. J Nerv Ment Dis. 2012;200(6):495–8. PMID: 22652614. http://www.ncbi.nlm.nih.gov/pubmed/22652614.
360. Johnson MR, Lydiard RB. Comorbidity of major depression and panic disorder. J Clin Psychol. 1998;54(2):201–10. PMID: 9467764. http://www.ncbi.nlm.nih.gov/pubmed/9467764.
361. Srinivasa K, Neerakal I. A study of panic patients with and without depression. Indian J Psychiatry. 2002;44(3):246–52. PMCID: PMC2954395. http://www.ncbi.nlm.nih.gov/pubmed/21206579.
362. Kessler RC, Chiu WT, Demler O, Merikangas KR, Walters EE. Prevalence, severity, and comorbidity of 12-month DSM-IV disorders in the National Comorbidity Survey Replication. Arch Gen Psychiatry. 2005;62(6):617–27. PMCID: PMC2847357. http://www.ncbi.nlm.nih.gov/pubmed/15939839.
363. Kaufman J, Charney D. Comorbidity of mood and anxiety disorders. Depress Anxiety. 2000;12(Suppl 1):69–76. PMID: 11098417. http://www.ncbi.nlm.nih.gov/pubmed/11098417.
364. Allen LB, White KS, Barlow DH, Shear MK, Gorman JM, Woods SW. Cognitive-Behavior Therapy (CBT) for panic disorder: relationship of anxiety and depression comorbidity with treatment outcome. J Psychopathol Behav Assess. 2010;32(2):185–92. PMCID: PMC2855025. http://www.ncbi.nlm.nih.gov/pubmed/20421906.
365. Beracochea D. Anterograde and retrograde effects of benzodiazepines on memory. ScientificWorldJournal. 2006;6:1460–5. PMCID: PMC5917174. http://www.ncbi.nlm.nih.gov/pubmed/17115086.
366. Utilizing benzodiazepines in clinical practice: an evidence-based discussion. J Clin Psychiatry. 2004;65(11):1565–74. PMID: 15554774. http://www.ncbi.nlm.nih.gov/pubmed/15554774.
367. Wilson MA. GABA physiology: modulation by benzodiazepines and hormones. Crit Rev Neurobiol. 1996;10(1):1–37. PMID: 8853952. http://www.ncbi.nlm.nih.gov/pubmed/8853952.
368. Atack JR. The benzodiazepine binding site of GABA(A) receptors as a target for the development of novel anxiolytics. Expert Opin Investig Drugs. 2005;14(5):601–18. PMID: 15926867. http://www.ncbi.nlm.nih.gov/pubmed/15926867.
369. Malcolm RJ. GABA systems, benzodiazepines, and substance dependence. J Clin Psychiatry. 2003;64(Suppl 3):36–40. PMID: 12662132. http://www.ncbi.nlm.nih.gov/pubmed/12662132.
370. Nemeroff CB. The role of GABA in the pathophysiology and treatment of anxiety disorders. Psychopharmacol Bull. 2003;37(4):133–46. PMID: 15131523. http://www.ncbi.nlm.nih.gov/pubmed/15131523.
371. Chouinard G. Issues in the clinical use of benzodiazepines: potency, withdrawal, and rebound. J Clin Psychiatry.

2004;65(Suppl 5):7–12. PMID: 15078112. http://www.ncbi.nlm.nih.gov/pubmed/15078112.
372. Morris HV, Dawson GR, Reynolds DS, Atack JR, Stephens DN. Both alpha2 and alpha3 GABAA receptor subtypes mediate the anxiolytic properties of benzodiazepine site ligands in the conditioned emotional response paradigm. Eur J Neurosci. 2006;23(9):2495–504. PMID: 16706856. http://www.ncbi.nlm.nih.gov/pubmed/16706856.
373. Dassanayake T, Michie P, Carter G, Jones A. Effects of benzodiazepines, antidepressants and opioids on driving: a systematic review and meta-analysis of epidemiological and experimental evidence. Drug Saf. 2011;34(2):125–56. PMID: 21247221. http://www.ncbi.nlm.nih.gov/pubmed/21247221.
374. Tanaka E. Toxicological interactions between alcohol and benzodiazepines. J Toxicol Clin Toxicol. 2002;40(1):69–75. PMID: 11990206. http://www.ncbi.nlm.nih.gov/pubmed/11990206.
375. Barker MJ, Greenwood KM, Jackson M, Crowe SF. Persistence of cognitive effects after withdrawal from long-term benzodiazepine use: a meta-analysis. Arch Clin Neuropsychol. 2004;19(3):437–54. PMID: 15033227. http://www.ncbi.nlm.nih.gov/pubmed/15033227.
376. Stewart SA. The effects of benzodiazepines on cognition. J Clin Psychiatry. 2005;66(Suppl 2):9–13. PMID: 15762814. http://www.ncbi.nlm.nih.gov/pubmed/15762814.
377. Barker MJ, Greenwood KM, Jackson M, Crowe SF. Cognitive effects of long-term benzodiazepine use: a meta-analysis. CNS Drugs. 2004;18(1):37–48. PMID: 14731058. http://www.ncbi.nlm.nih.gov/pubmed/14731058.
378. benzo.org.uk : Benzodiazepines: How They Work & How to Withdraw, Prof C H Ashton DM, FRCP, 2002.
379. Arvat E, Giordano R, Grottoli S, Ghigo E. Benzodiazepines and anterior pituitary function. J Endocrinol Investig. 2002;25(8):735–47. PMID: 12240908. http://www.ncbi.nlm.nih.gov/pubmed/12240908.
380. Klein E. The role of extended-release benzodiazepines in the treatment of anxiety: a risk-benefit evaluation with a focus on extended-release alprazolam. J Clin Psychiatry. 2002;63(Suppl 14):27–33. PMID: 12562116. http://www.ncbi.nlm.nih.gov/pubmed/12562116.
381. Susman J, Klee B. The role of high-potency Benzodiazepines in the treatment of panic disorder. Prim Care Companion J Clin Psychiatry. 2005;7(1):5–11. PMCID: PMC1076453. http://www.ncbi.nlm.nih.gov/pubmed/15841187.
382. benzo.org.uk: Toxicity and Adverse Consequences of Benzodiazepine Use, Professor Ashton, 1995.
383. Isbister GK, O'Regan L, Sibbritt D, Whyte IM. Alprazolam is relatively more toxic than other benzodiazepines in overdose. Br J Clin Pharmacol. 2004;58(1):88–95. PMCID: PMC1884537. http://www.ncbi.nlm.nih.gov/pubmed/15206998.
384. Uzun S, Kozumplik O, Jakovljević M, Sedić B. Side effects of treatment with benzodiazepines. Psychiatr Danub. 2010;22(1):90–3. PMID: 20305598. http://www.ncbi.nlm.nih.gov/pubmed/20305598.
385. Authier N, Balayssac D, Sautereau M, Zangarelli A, Courty P, Somogyi AA, Vennat B, Llorca PM, Eschalier A. Benzodiazepine dependence: focus on withdrawal syndrome. Ann Pharm Fr. 2009;67(6):408–13. PMID: 19900604. http://www.ncbi.nlm.nih.gov/pubmed/19900604.
386. O'brien CP. Benzodiazepine use, abuse, and dependence. J Clin Psychiatry. 2005;66(Suppl 2):28–33. PMID: 15762817. http://www.ncbi.nlm.nih.gov/pubmed/15762817.
387. Wolf B, Griffiths RR. Physical dependence on benzodiazepines: differences within the class. Drug Alcohol Depend. 1991;29(2):153–6. PMID: 1686752. http://www.ncbi.nlm.nih.gov/pubmed/1686752.
388. Modell JG. Protracted benzodiazepine withdrawal syndrome mimicking psychotic depression. Psychosomatics. 1997;38(2):160–1. PMID: 9063050. http://www.ncbi.nlm.nih.gov/pubmed/9063050.
389. Lader M. Anxiety or depression during withdrawal of hypnotic treatments. J Psychosom Res. 1994;38(Suppl 1):113–23; discussion 118-123. PMID: 7799243. http://www.ncbi.nlm.nih.gov/pubmed/7799243.
390. Lydiard RB, Laraia MT, Ballenger JC, Howell EF. Emergence of depressive symptoms in patients receiving alprazolam for panic disorder. Am J Psychiatry. 1987;144(5):664–5. PMID: 3578580. http://www.ncbi.nlm.nih.gov/pubmed/3578580.
391. Holt RL, Lydiard RB. Management of treatment-resistant panic disorder. Psychiatry (Edgmont). 2007;4(10):48–59. PMCID: PMC2860526. http://www.ncbi.nlm.nih.gov/pubmed/20428311.
392. Nathan RG, Robinson D, Cherek DR, Davison S, Sebastian S, Hack M. Long-term benzodiazepine use and depression. Am J Psychiatry. 1985;142(1):144–5. PMID: 2857068. http://www.ncbi.nlm.nih.gov/pubmed/2857068.
393. Ator NA, Griffiths RR. Selectivity in the generalization profile in baboons trained to discriminate lorazepam: benzodiazepines, barbiturates and other sedative/anxiolytics. J Pharmacol Exp Ther. 1997;282(3):1442–57. PMID: 9316858. http://www.ncbi.nlm.nih.gov/pubmed/9316858.
394. Griffiths RR, Lamb RJ, Sannerud CA, Ator NA, Brady JV. Self-injection of barbiturates, benzodiazepines and other sedative-anxiolytics in baboons. Psychopharmacology. 1991;103(2):154–61. PMID: 1674158. http://www.ncbi.nlm.nih.gov/pubmed/1674158.
395. Strawn JR, Mills JA, Cornwall GJ, Mossman SA, Varney ST, Keeshin BR, Croarkin PE. Buspirone in children and adolescents with anxiety: a review and Bayesian analysis of abandoned randomized controlled trials. J Child Adolesc Psychopharmacol. 2018;28(1):2–9. PMCID: PMC5771537. http://www.ncbi.nlm.nih.gov/pubmed/28846022.
396. Archer C, Wiles N, Kessler D, Turner K, Caldwell DM. Beta-blockers for the treatment of anxiety disorders: a systematic review and meta-analysis. J Affect Disord. 2025;368:90–9. PMID: 39271062. http://www.ncbi.nlm.nih.gov/pubmed/39271062.
397. Elias E, Zhang AY, Manners MT. Novel pharmacological approaches to the treatment of depression. Life (Basel). 2022;12(2):196. PMCID: PMC8879976. http://www.ncbi.nlm.nih.gov/pubmed/35207483.
398. Bey T, Patel A. Phencyclidine intoxication and adverse effects: a clinical and pharmacological review of an illicit drug. Cal. J Emerg Med. 2007;8(1):9–14. PMCID: PMC2859735. http://www.ncbi.nlm.nih.gov/pubmed/20440387.
399. N-Methyl-DL-aspartic acid | C5H9NO4 | CID 4376 - PubChem.
400. O'Shea B. Phencyclidine, ketamine, and khat phencyclidine (PCP, DOA, "angel dust," "crystal," 'hog'). Ir Med J. 2000;93(6):185. PMID: 11105446. http://www.ncbi.nlm.nih.gov/pubmed/11105446.
401. Javitt DC, Zukin SR. Recent advances in the phencyclidine model of schizophrenia. Am J Psychiatry. 1991;148(10):1301–8. PMID: 1654746. http://www.ncbi.nlm.nih.gov/pubmed/1654746.
402. Ozawa S, Kamiya H, Tsuzuki K. Glutamate receptors in the mammalian central nervous system. Prog Neurobiol. 1998;54(5):581–618. PMID: 9550192. http://www.ncbi.nlm.nih.gov/pubmed/9550192.
403. Lord B, Wintmolders C, Langlois X, Nguyen L, Lovenberg T, Bonaventure P. Comparison of the ex vivo receptor occupancy profile of ketamine to several NMDA receptor antagonists in mouse hippocampus. Eur J Pharmacol. 2013;715(1–3):21–5. PMID: 23872376. http://www.ncbi.nlm.nih.gov/pubmed/23872376.
404. Tyler MW, Yourish HB, Ionescu DF, Haggarty SJ. Classics in chemical neuroscience: Ketamine. ACS Chem Neurosci.

2017;8(6):1122–34. PMID: 28418641. http://www.ncbi.nlm.nih.gov/pubmed/28418641.

405. Hashimoto K. Rapid-acting antidepressant ketamine, its metabolites and other candidates: a historical overview and future perspective. Psychiatry Clin Neurosci. 2019;73(10):613–27. PMCID: PMC6851782. http://www.ncbi.nlm.nih.gov/pubmed/31215725.
406. Kraus C, Rabl U, Vanicek T, Carlberg L, Popovic A, Spies M, Bartova L, Gryglewski G, Papageorgiou K, Lanzenberger R, Willeit M, Winkler D, Rybakowski JK, Kasper S. Administration of ketamine for unipolar and bipolar depression. Int J Psychiatry Clin Pract. 2017;21(1):2–12. PMID: 28097909. http://www.ncbi.nlm.nih.gov/pubmed/28097909.
407. Can A, Zanos P, Moaddel R, Kang HJ, Dossou KSS, Wainer IW, Cheer JF, Frost DO, Huang XP, Gould TD. Effects of Ketamine and Ketamine metabolites on evoked striatal dopamine release, dopamine receptors, and monoamine transporters. J Pharmacol Exp Ther. 2016;359(1):159–70. PMCID: PMC5034706. http://www.ncbi.nlm.nih.gov/pubmed/27469513.
408. Kapur S, Seeman P. NMDA receptor antagonists ketamine and PCP have direct effects on the dopamine D(2) and serotonin 5-HT(2)receptors-implications for models of schizophrenia. Mol Psychiatry. 2002;7(8):837–44. PMID: 12232776. http://www.ncbi.nlm.nih.gov/pubmed/12232776.
409. Yang Y, Cui Y, Sang K, Dong Y, Ni Z, Ma S, Hu H. Ketamine blocks bursting in the lateral habenula to rapidly relieve depression. Nature. 2018;554(7692):317–22. PMID: 29446381. http://www.ncbi.nlm.nih.gov/pubmed/29446381.
410. Zanos P, Gould TD. Mechanisms of ketamine action as an antidepressant. Mol Psychiatry. 2018;23(4):801–11. PMCID: PMC5999402. http://www.ncbi.nlm.nih.gov/pubmed/29532791.
411. Jiang C, Lin WJ, Labonté B, Tamminga CA, Turecki G, Nestler EJ, Russo SJ, Salton SR. VGF and its C-terminal peptide TLQP-62 in ventromedial prefrontal cortex regulate depression-related behaviors and the response to ketamine. Neuropsychopharmacology. 2019;44(5):971–81. PMCID: PMC6462025. http://www.ncbi.nlm.nih.gov/pubmed/30504797.
412. Fukumoto K, Iijima M, Funakoshi T, Chaki S. Role of 5-HT1A receptor stimulation in the medial prefrontal cortex in the sustained antidepressant effects of Ketamine. Int J Neuropsychopharmacol. 2018;21(4):371–81. PMCID: PMC5888010. http://www.ncbi.nlm.nih.gov/pubmed/29309585.
413. Pałucha-Poniewiera A, Podkowa K, Pilc A. Role of AMPA receptor stimulation and TrkB signaling in the antidepressant-like effect of ketamine co-administered with a group II mGlu receptor antagonist, LY341495, in the forced swim test in rats. Behav Pharmacol. 2019;30(6):471–7. PMID: 30724804. http://www.ncbi.nlm.nih.gov/pubmed/30724804.
414. Mastrodonato A, Martinez R, Pavlova IP, LaGamma CT, Brachman RA, Robison AJ, Denny CA. Ventral CA3 activation mediates prophylactic Ketamine efficacy against stress-induced depressive-like behavior. Biol Psychiatry. 2018;84(11):846–56. PMCID: PMC6107435. http://www.ncbi.nlm.nih.gov/pubmed/29615190.
415. Leal GC, Bandeira ID, Correia-Melo FS, Telles M, Mello RP, Vieira F, Lima CS, Jesus-Nunes AP, Guerreiro-Costa LNF, Marback RF, Caliman-Fontes AT, Marques BLS, Bezerra MLO, Dias-Neto AL, Silva SS, Sampaio AS, Sanacora G, Turecki G, Loo C, Lacerda ALT, Quarantini LC. Intravenous arketamine for treatment-resistant depression: open-label pilot study. Eur Arch Psychiatry Clin Neurosci. 2021;271(3):577–82. PMID: 32078034. http://www.ncbi.nlm.nih.gov/pubmed/32078034.
416. Fukumoto K, Toki H, Iijima M, Hashihayata T, Yamaguchi JI, Hashimoto K, Chaki S. Antidepressant potential of (R)-Ketamine in Rodent models: comparison with (S)-Ketamine. J Pharmacol Exp Ther. 2017;361(1):9–16. PMID: 28115553. http://www.ncbi.nlm.nih.gov/pubmed/28115553.
417. Sachdeva B, Sachdeva P, Ghosh S, Ahmad F, Sinha JK. Ketamine as a therapeutic agent in major depressive disorder and posttraumatic stress disorder: potential medicinal and deleterious effects. Ibrain. 2023;9(1):90–101. PMCID: PMC10528797. http://www.ncbi.nlm.nih.gov/pubmed/37786516.
418. Sanacora G, Frye MA, McDonald W, Mathew SJ, Turner MS, Schatzberg AF, Summergrad P, Nemeroff CB. American Psychiatric Association (APA) Council of Research Task Force on novel biomarkers and treatments. A consensus statement on the use of Ketamine in the treatment of mood disorders. JAMA Psychiatry. 2017;74(4):399–405. PMID: 28249076. http://www.ncbi.nlm.nih.gov/pubmed/28249076.
419. Zhang K, Hashimoto K. An update on ketamine and its two enantiomers as rapid-acting antidepressants. Expert Rev Neurother. 2019;19(1):83–92. PMID: 30513009. http://www.ncbi.nlm.nih.gov/pubmed/30513009.
420. Molero P, Ramos-Quiroga JA, Martin-Santos R, Calvo-Sánchez E, Gutiérrez-Rojas L, Meana JJ. Antidepressant efficacy and tolerability of Ketamine and Esketamine: a critical review. CNS Drugs. 2018;32(5):411–20. PMID: 29736744. http://www.ncbi.nlm.nih.gov/pubmed/29736744.
421. Marcantoni WS, Akoumba BS, Wassef M, Mayrand J, Lai H, Richard-Devantoy S, Beauchamp S. A systematic review and meta-analysis of the efficacy of intravenous ketamine infusion for treatment resistant depression: January 2009 - January 2019. J Affect Disord. 2020;277:831–41. PMID: 33065824. http://www.ncbi.nlm.nih.gov/pubmed/33065824.
422. Dean RL, Hurducas C, Hawton K, Spyridi S, Cowen PJ, Hollingsworth S, Marquardt T, Barnes A, Smith R, McShane R, Turner EH, Cipriani A. Ketamine and other glutamate receptor modulators for depression in adults with unipolar major depressive disorder. Cochrane Database Syst Rev. 2021;9(9):CD011612. PMCID: PMC8434915. http://www.ncbi.nlm.nih.gov/pubmed/34510411.
423. Singh I, Morgan C, Curran V, Nutt D, Schlag A, McShane R. Ketamine treatment for depression: opportunities for clinical innovation and ethical foresight. Lancet. Psychiatry. 2017;4(5):419–26. PMID: 28395988. http://www.ncbi.nlm.nih.gov/pubmed/28395988.
424. Ionescu DF, Fu DJ, Qiu X, Lane R, Lim P, Kasper S, Hough D, Drevets WC, Manji H, Canuso CM. Esketamine nasal spray for rapid reduction of depressive symptoms in patients with major depressive disorder who have active suicide ideation with intent: results of a phase 3, double-blind, randomized study (ASPIRE II). Int J Neuropsychopharmacol. 2021;24(1):22–31. PMCID: PMC7816667. http://www.ncbi.nlm.nih.gov/pubmed/32861217.
425. Wajs E, Aluisio L, Holder R, Daly EJ, Lane R, Lim P, George JE, Morrison RL, Sanacora G, Young AH, Kasper S, Sulaiman AH, Li CT, Paik JW, Manji H, Hough D, Grunfeld J, Jeon HJ, Wilkinson ST, Drevets WC, Singh JB. Esketamine nasal spray plus oral antidepressant in patients with treatment-resistant depression: assessment of long-term safety in a phase 3, open-label study (SUSTAIN-2). J Clin Psychiatry. 2020;81(3):19m12891. PMID: 32316080. http://www.ncbi.nlm.nih.gov/pubmed/32316080.
426. Fu DJ, Ionescu DF, Li X, Lane R, Lim P, Sanacora G, Hough D, Manji H, Drevets WC, Canuso CM. Esketamine nasal spray for rapid reduction of major depressive disorder symptoms in patients who have active suicidal ideation with intent: double-blind, randomized study (ASPIRE I). J Clin Psychiatry. 2020;81(3):19m13191. PMID: 32412700. http://www.ncbi.nlm.nih.gov/pubmed/32412700.
427. McIntyre RS, Rosenblat JD, Nemeroff CB, Sanacora G, Murrough JW, Berk M, Brietzke E, Dodd S, Gorwood P, Ho R, Iosifescu DV, Lopez Jaramillo C, Kasper S, Kratiuk K, Lee JG, Lee Y, Lui

LMW, Mansur RB, Papakostas GI, Subramaniapillai M, Thase M, Vieta E, Young AH, Zarate CA, Stahl S. Synthesizing the evidence for Ketamine and Esketamine in treatment-resistant depression: an International Expert Opinion on the available evidence and implementation. Am J Psychiatry. 2021;178(5):383–99. PMCID: PMC9635017. http://www.ncbi.nlm.nih.gov/pubmed/33726522.

428. Wang YT, Wang XL, Lei L, Guo ZY, Kan FF, Hu D, Gai C, Zhang Y. A systematic review and meta-analysis of the efficacy of ketamine and esketamine on suicidal ideation in treatment-resistant depression. Eur J Clin Pharmacol. 2024;80(2):287–96. PMID: 38117332. http://www.ncbi.nlm.nih.gov/pubmed/38117332.
429. Turner EH. Esketamine for treatment-resistant depression: seven concerns about efficacy and FDA approval. Lancet Psychiatry. 2019;6(12):977–9. PMID: 31680014. http://www.ncbi.nlm.nih.gov/pubmed/31680014.
430. Zimmermann KS, Richardson R, Baker KD. Esketamine as a treatment for paediatric depression: questions of safety and efficacy. Lancet Psychiatry. 2020;7(10):827–9. PMID: 31952957. http://www.ncbi.nlm.nih.gov/pubmed/31952957.
431. Kaur U, Pathak BK, Singh A, Chakrabarti SS. Esketamine: a glimmer of hope in treatment-resistant depression. Eur Arch Psychiatry Clin Neurosci. 2021;271(3):417–29. PMID: 31745646. http://www.ncbi.nlm.nih.gov/pubmed/31745646.
432. Swainson J, McGirr A, Blier P, Brietzke E, Richard-Devantoy S, Ravindran N, Blier J, Beaulieu S, Frey BN, Kennedy SH, McIntyre RS, Milev RV, Parikh SV, Schaffer A, Taylor VH, Tourjman V, van Ameringen M, Yatham LN, Ravindran AV, Lam RW. The Canadian Network for Mood and Anxiety Treatments (CANMAT) Task Force Recommendations for the Use of Racemic Ketamine in Adults with Major Depressive Disorder: Recommandations Du Groupe De Travail Du Réseau Canadien Pour Les Traitements De L'humeur Et De L'anxiété (Canmat) Concernant L'utilisation De La Kétamine Racémique Chez Les Adultes Souffrant De Trouble Dépressif Majeur. Can J Psychiatry. 2021;66(2):113–25. PMCID: PMC7918868. http://www.ncbi.nlm.nih.gov/pubmed/33174760.
433. Acevedo J, Siegel JA. Neurobiological, behavioral, and cognitive effects of ketamine in adolescents: a review of human and pre-clinical research. Behav Brain Res. 2022;435:114049. PMID: 35952776. http://www.ncbi.nlm.nih.gov/pubmed/35952776.
434. Leinekugel X, Khalilov I, McLean H, Caillard O, Gaiarsa JL, Ben-Ari Y, Khazipov R. GABA is the principal fast-acting excitatory transmitter in the neonatal brain. Adv Neurol. 1999;79:189–201. PMID: 10514814. http://www.ncbi.nlm.nih.gov/pubmed/10514814.
435. Li K, Xu E. The role and the mechanism of gamma-aminobutyric acid during central nervous system development. Neurosci Bull. 2008;24(3):195–200. PMCID: PMC5552538. http://www.ncbi.nlm.nih.gov/pubmed/18500393.
436. Pelkey KA, Chittajallu R, Craig MT, Tricoire L, Wester JC, McBain CJ. Hippocampal GABAergic inhibitory interneurons. Physiol Rev. 2017;97(4):1619–747. PMCID: PMC6151493. http://www.ncbi.nlm.nih.gov/pubmed/28954853.
437. Marín O, Müller U. Lineage origins of GABAergic versus glutamatergic neurons in the neocortex. Curr Opin Neurobiol. 2014;26:132–41. PMCID: PMC4159607. http://www.ncbi.nlm.nih.gov/pubmed/24549207.
438. Rorsman P, Berggren PO, Bokvist K, Ericson H, Möhler H, Ostenson CG, Smith PA. Glucose-inhibition of glucagon secretion involves activation of GABAA-receptor chloride channels. Nature. 1989;341(6239):233–6. PMID: 2550826. http://www.ncbi.nlm.nih.gov/pubmed/2550826.
439. Erdö SL, Wolff JR. gamma-Aminobutyric acid outside the mammalian brain. J Neurochem. 1990;54(2):363–72. PMID: 2405103. http://www.ncbi.nlm.nih.gov/pubmed/2405103.
440. Ali DN, Ali HM, Lopez MR, Kang S, Choi DS. Astrocytic GABAergic regulation in alcohol use and major depressive disorders. Cells. 2024;13(4):318. PMCID: PMC10887002. http://www.ncbi.nlm.nih.gov/pubmed/38391931.
441. Mendu SK, Bhandage A, Jin Z, Birnir B. Different subtypes of GABA-A receptors are expressed in human, mouse and rat T lymphocytes. PLoS One. 2012;7(8):e42959. PMCID: PMC3424250. http://www.ncbi.nlm.nih.gov/pubmed/22927941.
442. Phulera S, Zhu H, Yu J, Claxton DP, Yoder N, Yoshioka C, Gouaux E. Cryo-EM structure of the benzodiazepine-sensitive α1β1γ2S tri-heteromeric GABAA receptor in complex with GABA. elife. 2018;7:e39383. PMCID: PMC6086659. http://www.ncbi.nlm.nih.gov/pubmed/30044221.
443. Allen MJ, Sabir S, Sharma S. GABA Receptor. StatPearls [Internet]. Treasure Island: StatPearls Publishing; 2025 [cited 2025 Jan 11]. Available from: http://www.ncbi.nlm.nih.gov/books/NBK526124/ PMID: 30252380. http://www.ncbi.nlm.nih.gov/pubmed/30252380.
444. Petroff OAC. GABA and glutamate in the human brain. Neuroscientist. 2002;8(6):562–73. PMID: 12467378. http://www.ncbi.nlm.nih.gov/pubmed/12467378.
445. Schousboe A, Waagepetersen HS. GABA: homeostatic and pharmacological aspects. Prog Brain Res. 2007;160:9–19. PMID: 17499106. http://www.ncbi.nlm.nih.gov/pubmed/17499106.
446. Wong CGT, Bottiglieri T, Snead OC. GABA, gamma-hydroxybutyric acid, and neurological disease. Ann Neurol. 2003;54(Suppl 6):S3–12. PMID: 12891648. http://www.ncbi.nlm.nih.gov/pubmed/12891648.
447. Engin E. GABAA receptor subtypes and benzodiazepine use, misuse, and abuse. Front Psych. 2022;13:1060949. PMCID: PMC9879605. http://www.ncbi.nlm.nih.gov/pubmed/36713896.
448. Maillard PY, Baer S, Schaefer É, Desnous B, Villeneuve N, Lépine A, Fabre A, Lacoste C, El Chehadeh S, Piton A, Porter LF, Perriard C, Wardé MTA, Spitz MA, Laugel V, Lesca G, Putoux A, Ville D, Mignot C, Héron D, Nabbout R, Barcia G, Rio M, Roubertie A, Meyer P, Paquis-Flucklinger V, Patat O, Lefranc J, Gerard M, Epigen Consortium, de Bellescize J, Villard L, De Saint Martin A, Milh M. Molecular and clinical descriptions of patients with GABAA receptor gene variants (GABRA1, GABRB2, GABRB3, GABRG2): a cohort study, review of literature, and genotype-phenotype correlation. Epilepsia. 2022;63(10):2519–33. PMCID: PMC9804453. http://www.ncbi.nlm.nih.gov/pubmed/35718920.
449. Nieto A, Bailey T, Kaczanowska K, McDonald P. GABAB receptor chemistry and pharmacology: agonists, antagonists, and allosteric modulators. Curr Top Behav Neurosci. 2022;52:81–118. PMID: 34036555. http://www.ncbi.nlm.nih.gov/pubmed/34036555.
450. Fritzius T, Stawarski M, Isogai S, Bettler B. Structural basis of GABAB receptor regulation and signaling. Curr Top Behav Neurosci. 2022;52:19–37. PMID: 32812202. http://www.ncbi.nlm.nih.gov/pubmed/32812202.
451. Wong LW, Tae HS, Cromer BA. Role of the ρ1 GABA(C) receptor N-terminus in assembly, trafficking and function. ACS Chem Neurosci. 2014;5(12):1266–77. PMID: 25347026. http://www.ncbi.nlm.nih.gov/pubmed/25347026.
452. Engin E, Benham RS, Rudolph U. An emerging circuit pharmacology of GABAA receptors. Trends Pharmacol Sci. 2018;39(8):710–32. PMCID: PMC6056379. http://www.ncbi.nlm.nih.gov/pubmed/29903580.
453. Qian X, Zhao X, Yu L, Yin Y, Zhang XD, Wang L, Li JX, Zhu Q, Luo JL. Current status of GABA receptor subtypes in analgesia. Biomed Pharmacother. 2023;168:115800. PMID: 37935070. http://www.ncbi.nlm.nih.gov/pubmed/37935070.
454. Menzikov SA, Zaichenko DM, Moskovtsev AA, Morozov SG, Kubatiev AA. Phenols and GABAA receptors: from structure and molecular mechanisms action to neuropsychiatric sequelae. Front

Pharmacol. 2024;15:1272534. PMCID: PMC10831359. http://www.ncbi.nlm.nih.gov/pubmed/38303988.

455. Ghit A, Assal D, Al-Shami AS, Hussein DEE. GABAA receptors: structure, function, pharmacology, and related disorders. J Genet Eng Biotechnol. 2021;19(1):123. PMCID: PMC8380214. http://www.ncbi.nlm.nih.gov/pubmed/34417930.
456. Cutler AJ, Mattingly GW, Maletic V. Understanding the mechanism of action and clinical effects of neuroactive steroids and GABAergic compounds in major depressive disorder. Transl Psychiatry. 2023;13(1):228. PMCID: PMC10293235. http://www.ncbi.nlm.nih.gov/pubmed/37365161.
457. Jellinger KA. The heterogeneity of late-life depression and its pathobiology: a brain network dysfunction disorder. J Neural Transm (Vienna). 2023;130(8):1057–76. PMCID: PMC10162005. http://www.ncbi.nlm.nih.gov/pubmed/37145167.
458. Della Vecchia A, Arone A, Piccinni A, Mucci F, Marazziti D. GABA system in depression: impact on pathophysiology and psychopharmacology. Curr Med Chem. 2022;29(36):5710–30. PMID: 34781862. http://www.ncbi.nlm.nih.gov/pubmed/34781862.
459. Andersen JV, Schousboe A, Wellendorph P. Astrocytes regulate inhibitory neurotransmission through GABA uptake, metabolism, and recycling. Essays Biochem. 2023;67(1):77–91. PMID: 36806927. http://www.ncbi.nlm.nih.gov/pubmed/36806927.
460. Ishibashi M, Egawa K, Fukuda A. Diverse actions of astrocytes in GABAergic Signaling. Int J Mol Sci. 2019;20(12):2964. PMCID: PMC6628243. http://www.ncbi.nlm.nih.gov/pubmed/31216630.
461. Frequently Asked Questions (FAQs) about REMS | FDA.
462. Sundman-Eriksson I, Allard P. [(3)H]Tiagabine binding to GABA transporter-1 (GAT-1) in suicidal depression. J Affect Disord. 2002;71(1–3):29–33. PMID: 12167498. http://www.ncbi.nlm.nih.gov/pubmed/12167498.
463. Kosel M, Rudolph U, Wielepp P, Luginbühl M, Schmitt W, Fisch HU, Schlaepfer TE. Diminished GABA(A) receptor-binding capacity and a DNA base substitution in a patient with treatment-resistant depression and anxiety. Neuropsychopharmacology. 2004;29(2):347–50. PMID: 14628001. http://www.ncbi.nlm.nih.gov/pubmed/14628001.
464. Epperson CN, Gueorguieva R, Czarkowski KA, Stiklus S, Sellers E, Krystal JH, Rothman DL, Mason GF. Preliminary evidence of reduced occipital GABA concentrations in puerperal women: a 1H-MRS study. Psychopharmacology. 2006;186(3):425–33. PMID: 16724188. http://www.ncbi.nlm.nih.gov/pubmed/16724188.
465. Feng YF, Zhou YY, Duan KM. The role of Extrasynaptic GABA receptors in postpartum depression. Mol Neurobiol. 2024;61(1):385–96. PMID: 37612480. http://www.ncbi.nlm.nih.gov/pubmed/37612480.
466. Fernández Teruel A, Boix F, Escorihuela RM, Yáñez P, Tobeña A. Sodium valproate reduces immobility in the behavioral "despair" test in rats. Eur J Pharmacol. 1988;152(1–2):1–7. PMID: 3145207. http://www.ncbi.nlm.nih.gov/pubmed/3145207.
467. Borsini F, Mancinelli A, D'Aranno V, Evangelista S, Meli A. On the role of endogenous GABA in the forced swimming test in rats. Pharmacol Biochem Behav. 1988;29(2):275–9. PMID: 3362921. http://www.ncbi.nlm.nih.gov/pubmed/3362921.
468. Rägo L, Kiivet RA, Adojaan A, Harro J, Allikmets L. Stress-protection action of beta-phenyl(GABA): involvement of central and peripheral type benzodiazepine binding sites. Pharmacol Toxicol. 1990;66(1):41–4. PMID: 2155416. http://www.ncbi.nlm.nih.gov/pubmed/2155416.
469. Nishimura H, Ida Y, Tsuda A, Tanaka M. Opposite effects of diazepam and beta-CCE on immobility and straw-climbing behavior of rats in a modified forced-swim test. Pharmacol Biochem Behav. 1989;33(1):227–31. PMID: 2506583. http://www.ncbi.nlm.nih.gov/pubmed/2506583.
470. Joca SR, Skalisz LL, Beijamini V, Vital MA, Andreatini R. The antidepressive-like effect of oxcarbazepine: possible role of dopaminergic neurotransmission. Eur Neuropsychopharmacol. 2000;10(4):223–8. PMID: 10871703. http://www.ncbi.nlm.nih.gov/pubmed/10871703.
471. Olsen RW, Sapp DW. Neuroactive steroid modulation of GABAA receptors. Adv Biochem Psychopharmacol. 1995;48:57–74. PMID: 7653326. http://www.ncbi.nlm.nih.gov/pubmed/7653326.
472. Liang J, Olsen RW. Alcohol use disorders and current pharmacological therapies: the role of GABA(A) receptors. Acta Pharmacol Sin. 2014;35(8):981–93. PMCID: PMC4125717. http://www.ncbi.nlm.nih.gov/pubmed/25066321.
473. Olsen RW, Liang J. Role of GABAA receptors in alcohol use disorders suggested by chronic intermittent ethanol (CIE) rodent model. Mol Brain. 2017;10(1):45. PMCID: PMC5605989. http://www.ncbi.nlm.nih.gov/pubmed/28931433.
474. Edinoff AN, Nix CA, Hollier J, Sagrera CE, Delacroix BM, Abubakar T, Cornett EM, Kaye AM, Kaye AD. Benzodiazepines: uses, dangers, and clinical considerations. Neurol Int. 2021;13(4):594–607. PMCID: PMC8629021. http://www.ncbi.nlm.nih.gov/pubmed/34842811.
475. Boonstra E, de Kleijn R, Colzato LS, Alkemade A, Forstmann BU, Nieuwenhuis S. Neurotransmitters as food supplements: the effects of GABA on brain and behavior. Front Psychol. 2015;6:1520. PMCID: PMC4594160. http://www.ncbi.nlm.nih.gov/pubmed/26500584.
476. Gladkova MG, Leidmaa E, Anderzhanova EA. Epidrugs in the therapy of central nervous system disorders: a way to drive on? Cells. 2023;12(11):1464. PMCID: PMC10253154. http://www.ncbi.nlm.nih.gov/pubmed/37296584.
477. Menke A, The HPA. Axis as target for depression. Curr Neuropharmacol. 2024;22(5):904–15. PMCID: PMC10845091. http://www.ncbi.nlm.nih.gov/pubmed/37581323.
478. Liu J, Meng T, Wang C, Cheng W, Zhang Q, Cheng G. Natural products for the treatment of depression: insights into signal pathways influencing the hypothalamic-pituitary-adrenal axis. Medicine (Baltimore). 2023;102(44):e35862. PMCID: PMC10627670. http://www.ncbi.nlm.nih.gov/pubmed/37932977.
479. Potter K, Gayle EJ, Deb S. Effect of gut microbiome on serotonin metabolism: a personalized treatment approach. Naunyn Schmiedeberg's Arch Pharmacol. 2024;397(5):2589–602. PMID: 37922012. http://www.ncbi.nlm.nih.gov/pubmed/37922012.
480. Matin S, Dadkhah M. BDNF/CREB signaling pathway contribution in depression pathogenesis: a survey on the non-pharmacological therapeutic opportunities for gut microbiota dysbiosis. Brain Res Bull. 2024;207:110882. PMID: 38244808. http://www.ncbi.nlm.nih.gov/pubmed/38244808.
481. Makris AP, Karianaki M, Tsamis KI, Paschou SA. The role of the gut-brain axis in depression: endocrine, neural, and immune pathways. Hormones (Athens). 2021;20(1):1–12. PMID: 32827123. http://www.ncbi.nlm.nih.gov/pubmed/32827123.
482. Liu L, Wang H, Chen X, Zhang Y, Zhang H, Xie P. Gut microbiota and its metabolites in depression: from pathogenesis to treatment. EBioMedicine. 2023;90:104527. PMCID: PMC10051028. http://www.ncbi.nlm.nih.gov/pubmed/36963238.
483. Li B, Xu M, Wang Y, Feng L, Xing H, Zhang K. Gut microbiota: a new target for traditional Chinese medicine in the treatment of depression. J Ethnopharmacol. 2023;303:116038. PMID: 36529248. http://www.ncbi.nlm.nih.gov/pubmed/36529248.
484. Pascale A, Marchesi N, Govoni S, Barbieri A. Targeting the microbiota in pharmacology of psychiatric disorders. Pharmacol Res. 2020;157:104856. PMID: 32389857. http://www.ncbi.nlm.nih.gov/pubmed/32389857.
485. Bhatt S, Devadoss T, Jha NK, Baidya M, Gupta G, Chellappan DK, Singh SK, Dua K. Targeting inflammation: a potential

approach for the treatment of depression. Metab Brain Dis. 2023;38(1):45–59. PMID: 36239867. http://www.ncbi.nlm.nih.gov/pubmed/36239867.
486. Miller AH, Raison CL. The role of inflammation in depression: from evolutionary imperative to modern treatment target. Nat Rev Immunol. 2016;16(1):22–34. PMCID: PMC5542678. http://www.ncbi.nlm.nih.gov/pubmed/26711676.
487. Borsini A, Nicolaou A, Camacho-Muñoz D, Kendall AC, Di Benedetto MG, Giacobbe J, Su KP, Pariante CM. Omega-3 polyunsaturated fatty acids protect against inflammation through production of LOX and CYP450 lipid mediators: relevance for major depression and for human hippocampal neurogenesis. Mol Psychiatry. 2021;26(11):6773–88. PMCID: PMC8760043. http://www.ncbi.nlm.nih.gov/pubmed/34131267.
488. Xia CY, Guo YX, Lian WW, Yan Y, Ma BZ, Cheng YC, Xu JK, He J, Zhang WK. The NLRP3 inflammasome in depression: potential mechanisms and therapies. Pharmacol Res. 2023;187:106625. PMID: 36563870. http://www.ncbi.nlm.nih.gov/pubmed/36563870.
489. Hassamal S. Chronic stress, neuroinflammation, and depression: an overview of pathophysiological mechanisms and emerging anti-inflammatories. Front Psych. 2023;14:1130989. PMCID: PMC10213648. http://www.ncbi.nlm.nih.gov/pubmed/37252156.
490. Li G, Forero MG, Wentzell JS, Durmus I, Wolf R, Anthoney NC, Parker M, Jiang R, Hasenauer J, Strausfeld NJ, Heisenberg M, Hidalgo A. A Toll-receptor map underlies structural brain plasticity. elife. 2020;9:e52743. PMCID: PMC7077983. http://www.ncbi.nlm.nih.gov/pubmed/32066523.
491. Lopizzo N, Zonca V, Cattane N, Pariante CM, Cattaneo A. miRNAs in depression vulnerability and resilience: novel targets for preventive strategies. J Neural Transm (Vienna). 2019;126(9):1241–58. PMCID: PMC6746676. http://www.ncbi.nlm.nih.gov/pubmed/31350592.
492. Sarkar P, Chattopadhyay A. Interplay of cholesterol and actin in neurotransmitter GPCR Signaling: insights from chronic cholesterol depletion using statin. ACS Chem Neurosci. 2023;14(20):3855–68. PMID: 37804226. http://www.ncbi.nlm.nih.gov/pubmed/37804226.
493. Yang W, Yin H, Wang Y, Wang Y, Li X, Wang C, Liu P, Hu Y. New insights into effects of Kaixin Powder on depression via lipid metabolism related adiponectin signaling pathway. Chin Herb Med. 2023;15(2):240–50. PMCID: PMC10230638. http://www.ncbi.nlm.nih.gov/pubmed/37265759.
494. Pannu A, Sharma PC, Thakur VK, Goyal RK. Emerging role of flavonoids as the treatment of depression. Biomolecules. 2021;11(12):1825. PMCID: PMC8698856. http://www.ncbi.nlm.nih.gov/pubmed/34944471.
495. Kou Y, Li Z, Yang T, Shen X, Wang X, Li H, Zhou K, Li L, Xia Z, Zheng X, Zhao Y. Therapeutic potential of plant iridoids in depression: a review. Pharm Biol. 2022;60(1):2167–81. PMCID: PMC9621214. http://www.ncbi.nlm.nih.gov/pubmed/36300881.
496. German-Ponciano LJ, Rosas-Sánchez GU, Cueto-Escobedo J, Fernández-Demeneghi R, Guillén-Ruiz G, Soria-Fregozo C, Herrera-Huerta EV, Rodríguez-Landa JF. Participation of the serotonergic system and brain-derived neurotrophic factor in the antidepressant-like effect of flavonoids. Int J Mol Sci. 2022;23(18):10896. PMCID: PMC9505567. http://www.ncbi.nlm.nih.gov/pubmed/36142808.
497. Hong H, Lu X, Lu Q, Huang C, Cui Z. Potential therapeutic effects and pharmacological evidence of sinomenine in central nervous system disorders. Front Pharmacol. 2022;13:1015035. PMCID: PMC9523510. http://www.ncbi.nlm.nih.gov/pubmed/36188580.
498. Akwu NA, Lekhooa M, Deqiang D, Aremu AO. Antidepressant effects of coumarins and their derivatives: a critical analysis of research advances. Eur J Pharmacol. 2023;956:175958. PMID: 37543158. http://www.ncbi.nlm.nih.gov/pubmed/37543158.
499. Bazinet RP, Metherel AH, Chen CT, Shaikh SR, Nadjar A, Joffre C, Layé S. Brain eicosapentaenoic acid metabolism as a lead for novel therapeutics in major depression. Brain Behav Immun. 2020;85:21–8. PMID: 31278982. http://www.ncbi.nlm.nih.gov/pubmed/31278982.
500. Chang JPC, Su KP. Nutritional neuroscience as mainstream of psychiatry: The evidence- based treatment guidelines for using Omega-3 fatty acids as a new treatment for psychiatric disorders in children and adolescents. Clin Psychopharmacol Neurosci. 2020;18(4):469–83. PMCID: PMC7609218. http://www.ncbi.nlm.nih.gov/pubmed/33124582.
501. Kalkman HO, Hersberger M, Walitza S, Berger GE. Disentangling the molecular mechanisms of the antidepressant activity of Omega-3 polyunsaturated fatty acid: a comprehensive review of the literature. Int J Mol Sci. 2021;22(9):4393. PMCID: PMC8122828. http://www.ncbi.nlm.nih.gov/pubmed/33922396.
502. Deyama S, Minami M, Kaneda K. Resolvins as potential candidates for the treatment of major depressive disorder. J Pharmacol Sci. 2021;147(1):33–9. PMID: 34294370. http://www.ncbi.nlm.nih.gov/pubmed/34294370.
503. Deyama S, Kaneda K, Minami M. Resolution of depression: antidepressant actions of resolvins. Neurosci Res. 2022;S0168-0102(22):00266–8. PMID: 36272561. http://www.ncbi.nlm.nih.gov/pubmed/36272561.
504. Hope for Depression | Hope for Depression Research Foundation.
505. Akil H, Gordon J, Hen R, Javitch J, Mayberg H, McEwen B, Meaney MJ, Nestler EJ. Treatment resistant depression: a multi-scale, systems biology approach. Neurosci Biobehav Rev. 2018;84:272–88. PMCID: PMC5729118. http://www.ncbi.nlm.nih.gov/pubmed/28859997.
506. Lv X, Si T, Wang G, Wang H, Liu Q, Hu C, Wang J, Su Y, Huang Y, Jiang H, Yu X. The establishment of the objective diagnostic markers and personalized medical intervention in patients with major depressive disorder: rationale and protocol. BMC Psychiatry. 2016;16:240. PMCID: PMC4946102. http://www.ncbi.nlm.nih.gov/pubmed/27422150.
507. Learn about Sleep Disorders - Sleep Education by AASM.
508. AASM | International Classification of Sleep Disorders.
509. Home Page - Sleep Education - American Academy of Sleep Medicine.
510. Insomnia: Symptoms, Causes, and Treatments.
511. Sateia MJ, Buysse DJ, Krystal AD, Neubauer DN, Heald JL. Clinical practice guideline for the pharmacologic treatment of chronic insomnia in adults: an American Academy of sleep medicine clinical practice guideline. J Clin Sleep Med. 2017;13(2):307–49. PMCID: PMC5263087. http://www.ncbi.nlm.nih.gov/pubmed/27998379.
512. Cappuccio FP, Taggart FM, Kandala NB, Currie A, Peile E, Stranges S, Miller MA. Meta-analysis of short sleep duration and obesity in children and adults. Sleep. 2008;31(5):619–26. PMCID: PMC2398753. http://www.ncbi.nlm.nih.gov/pubmed/18517032.
513. Cappuccio FP, D'Elia L, Strazzullo P, Miller MA. Quantity and quality of sleep and incidence of type 2 diabetes: a systematic review and meta-analysis. Diabetes Care. 2010;33(2):414–20. PMCID: PMC2809295. http://www.ncbi.nlm.nih.gov/pubmed/19910503.
514. Kripke DF, Garfinkel L, Wingard DL, Klauber MR, Marler MR. Mortality associated with sleep duration and insomnia. Arch Gen Psychiatry. 2002;59(2):131–6. PMID: 11825133. http://www.ncbi.nlm.nih.gov/pubmed/11825133.
515. Hoevenaar-Blom MP, Spijkerman AMW, Kromhout D, van den Berg JF, Verschuren WMM. Sleep duration and sleep quality in relation to 12-year cardiovascular disease incidence: the MORGEN study. Sleep. 2011;34(11):1487–92. PMCID: PMC3198203. http://www.ncbi.nlm.nih.gov/pubmed/22043119.

516. Wichniak A, Wierzbicka A, Jernajczyk W. Sleep and antidepressant treatment. Curr Pharm Des. 2012;18(36):5802–17. PMID: 22681161. http://www.ncbi.nlm.nih.gov/pubmed/22681161.
517. Postuma RB, Gagnon JF, Tuineaig M, Bertrand JA, Latreille V, Desjardins C, Montplaisir JY. Antidepressants and REM sleep behavior disorder: isolated side effect or neurodegenerative signal? Sleep. 2013;36(11):1579–85. PMCID: PMC3792373. http://www.ncbi.nlm.nih.gov/pubmed/24179289.
518. Steiger A, Kimura M. Wake and sleep EEG provide biomarkers in depression. J Psychiatr Res. 2010;44(4):242–52. PMID: 19762038. http://www.ncbi.nlm.nih.gov/pubmed/19762038.
519. Schramm PJ, Poland RE, Rao U. Bupropion response on sleep quality in patients with depression: implications for increased cardiovascular disease risk. Eur Neuropsychopharmacol. 2014;24(2):207–14. PMCID: PMC3948318. http://www.ncbi.nlm.nih.gov/pubmed/24239431.
520. Wilkes S. Bupropion. Drugs Today (Barc). 2006;42(10):671–81. PMID: 17136226. http://www.ncbi.nlm.nih.gov/pubmed/17136226.
521. Thase ME. Depression, sleep, and antidepressants. J Clin Psychiatry. 1998;59(Suppl 4):55–65. PMID: 9554322. http://www.ncbi.nlm.nih.gov/pubmed/9554322.
522. Kurian BT, Greer TL, Trivedi MH. Strategies to enhance the therapeutic efficacy of antidepressants: targeting residual symptoms. Expert Rev Neurother. 2009;9(7):975–84. PMCID: PMC2720783. http://www.ncbi.nlm.nih.gov/pubmed/19589048.
523. Franzen PL, Buysse DJ. Sleep disturbances and depression: risk relationships for subsequent depression and therapeutic implications. Dialogues Clin Neurosci. 2008;10(4):473–81. PMCID: PMC3108260. http://www.ncbi.nlm.nih.gov/pubmed/19170404.
524. Westermeyer J, Carr TM. Zolpidem-associated consequences: an updated literature review with case reports. J Nerv Ment Dis. 2020;208(1):28–32. PMID: 31834190. http://www.ncbi.nlm.nih.gov/pubmed/31834190.
525. Fagiolini A, Comandini A, Catena Dell'Osso M, Kasper S. Rediscovering trazodone for the treatment of major depressive disorder. CNS Drugs. 2012;26(12):1033–49. PMCID: PMC3693429. http://www.ncbi.nlm.nih.gov/pubmed/23192413.
526. De Berardis D, Marini S, Fornaro M, Srinivasan V, Iasevoli F, Tomasetti C, Valchera A, Perna G, Quera-Salva MA, Martinotti G, di Giannantonio M. The melatonergic system in mood and anxiety disorders and the role of agomelatine: implications for clinical practice. Int J Mol Sci. 2013;14(6):12458–83. PMCID: PMC3709794. http://www.ncbi.nlm.nih.gov/pubmed/23765220.
527. Komaram RB, Nukala S, Palla J, Nambaru LR, Kasturi SM. A comparative study of efficacy and safety of Agomelatine and Escitalopram in major depressive disorder. J Clin Diagn Res. 2015;9(6):VC05–8. PMCID: PMC4525586. http://www.ncbi.nlm.nih.gov/pubmed/26266196.
528. Gahr M, Kratzer W, Fuchs M, Connemann BJ. Safety and tolerability of agomelatine: focus on hepatotoxicity. Curr Drug Metab. 2014;15(7):694–702. PMID: 25255870. http://www.ncbi.nlm.nih.gov/pubmed/25255870.
529. AHRQ Comparative Effectiveness Reviews - NCBI Bookshelf.
530. Brasure M, MacDonald R, Fuchs E, Olson CM, Carlyle M, Diem S, Koffel E, Khawaja IS, Ouellette J, Butler M, Kane RL, Wilt TJ. Management of insomnia disorder [Internet]. Rockville: Agency for Healthcare Research and Quality (US); 2015 [cited 2025 Jan 11]. Available from: http://www.ncbi.nlm.nih.gov/books/NBK343503/ PMID: 26844312. http://www.ncbi.nlm.nih.gov/pubmed/26844312.
531. Compare Sleep Aids: Understanding the Differences.
532. Sleep Disorder (Sedative-Hypnotic) Drug Information | FDA.
533. Zolpidem: MedlinePlus Drug Information.
534. Eszopiclone: MedlinePlus Drug Information.
535. Zaleplon: MedlinePlus Drug Information.
536. Certain Prescription Insomnia Medicines: New Boxed Warning - Due to Risk of Serious Injuries Caused by Sleepwalking, Sleep Driving and Engaging in Other Activities While Not Fully Awake | FDA.
537. Search | FDA.
538. Wang C, Wang Q, Ji B, Pan Y, Xu C, Cheng B, Bai B, Chen J. The Orexin/Receptor system: molecular mechanism and therapeutic potential for neurological diseases. Front Mol Neurosci. 2018;11:220. PMCID: PMC6031739. http://www.ncbi.nlm.nih.gov/pubmed/30002617.
539. Grafe LA, Bhatnagar S. Orexins and stress. Front Neuroendocrinol. 2018;51:132–45. PMCID: PMC6345253. http://www.ncbi.nlm.nih.gov/pubmed/29932958\.
540. Suvorexant: MedlinePlus Drug Information.
541. Lemborexant: MedlinePlus Drug Information.
542. Kärppä M, Yardley J, Pinner K, Filippov G, Zammit G, Moline M, Perdomo C, Inoue Y, Ishikawa K, Kubota N. Long-term efficacy and tolerability of lemborexant compared with placebo in adults with insomnia disorder: results from the phase 3 randomized clinical trial SUNRISE 2. Sleep. 2020;43(9):zsaa123. PMCID: PMC7487867. http://www.ncbi.nlm.nih.gov/pubmed/32585700.
543. Xue T, Wu X, Chen S, Yang Y, Yan Z, Song Z, Zhang W, Zhang J, Chen Z, Wang Z. The efficacy and safety of dual orexin receptor antagonists in primary insomnia: a systematic review and network meta-analysis. Sleep Med Rev. 2022;61:101573. PMID: 34902823. http://www.ncbi.nlm.nih.gov/pubmed/34902823.
544. Na HJ, Jeon N, Staatz CE, Han N, Baek IH. Clinical safety and narcolepsy-like symptoms of dual orexin receptor antagonists in patients with insomnia: a systematic review and meta-analysis. Sleep. 2024;47(2):zsad293. PMID: 37950346. http://www.ncbi.nlm.nih.gov/pubmed/37950346.
545. Maruani J, Reynaud E, Chambe J, Palagini L, Bourgin P, Geoffroy PA. Efficacy of melatonin and ramelteon for the acute and long-term management of insomnia disorder in adults: a systematic review and meta-analysis. J Sleep Res. 2023;32(6):e13939. PMID: 37434463. http://www.ncbi.nlm.nih.gov/pubmed/37434463.
546. Daugaard S, Garde AH, Bonde JPE, Christoffersen J, Hansen ÄM, Markvart J, Schlünssen V, Skene DJ, Vistisen HT, Kolstad HA. Night work, light exposure and melatonin on work days and days off. Chronobiol Int. 2017;34(7):942–55. PMID: 28613972. http://www.ncbi.nlm.nih.gov/pubmed/28613972.
547. Wu DZ, Zhu GZ, Zhao K, Gao JW, Cai GX, Li HZ, Huang YS, Tu C, Zhuang JS, Huang ZW, Zhong ZM. Age-related decline in melatonin contributes to enhanced osteoclastogenesis via disruption of redox homeostasis. Mol Med. 2024;30(1):10. PMCID: PMC10785421. http://www.ncbi.nlm.nih.gov/pubmed/38216878.
548. Ramelteon: MedlinePlus Drug Information.
549. Temazepam: MedlinePlus Drug Information.
550. Triazolam: MedlinePlus Drug Information.
551. Estazolam: MedlinePlus Drug Information.
552. DailyMed - QUAZEPAM tablet.
553. Flurazepam: MedlinePlus Drug Information.
554. De Crescenzo F, D'Alò GL, Ostinelli EG, Ciabattini M, Di Franco V, Watanabe N, Kurtulmus A, Tomlinson A, Mitrova Z, Foti F, Del Giovane C, Quested DJ, Cowen PJ, Barbui C, Amato L, Efthimiou O, Cipriani A. Comparative effects of pharmacological interventions for the acute and long-term management of insomnia disorder in adults: a systematic review and network meta-analysis. Lancet. 2022;400(10347):170–84. PMID: 35843245. http://www.ncbi.nlm.nih.gov/pubmed/35843245.
555. Everitt H, Baldwin DS, Stuart B, Lipinska G, Mayers A, Malizia AL, Manson CC, Wilson S. Antidepressants for insomnia in adults. Cochrane Database Syst Rev. 2018;5(5):CD010753. PMCID: PMC6494576. http://www.ncbi.nlm.nih.gov/pubmed/29761479.
556. Doxepin (Insomnia): MedlinePlus Drug Information.
557. Trazodone: MedlinePlus Drug Information.

558. Medicines for sleep: MedlinePlus Medical Encyclopedia.
559. Prescription Drugs and Over-the-Counter (OTC) Drugs: Questions and Answers | FDA.
560. Diphenhydramine: MedlinePlus Drug Information.
561. Doxylamine: MedlinePlus Drug Information.
562. Culpepper L, Wingertzahn MA. Over-the-counter agents for the treatment of occasional disturbed sleep or transient insomnia: a systematic review of efficacy and safety. Prim Care Companion CNS Disord. 2015;17(6). PMCID: PMC4805417. http://www.ncbi.nlm.nih.gov/pubmed/27057416.
563. Abboud M, Vitamin D. Supplementation and sleep: a systematic review and meta-analysis of intervention studies. Nutrients. 2022;14(5):1076. PMCID: PMC8912284. http://www.ncbi.nlm.nih.gov/pubmed/35268051.
564. Wu Y, Huang X, Zhong C, Wu T, Sun D, Wang R, Zhan Q, Luo H. Efficacy of dietary supplements on sleep quality and daytime function of shift workers: a systematic review and meta-analysis. Front Nutr. 2022;9:850417. PMCID: PMC9097162. http://www.ncbi.nlm.nih.gov/pubmed/35571888.
565. Chan V, Lo K. Efficacy of dietary supplements on improving sleep quality: a systematic review and meta-analysis. Postgrad Med J. 2022;98(1158):285–93. PMID: 33441476. http://www.ncbi.nlm.nih.gov/pubmed/33441476.
566. Tan DX, Hardeland R, Manchester LC, Korkmaz A, Ma S, Rosales-Corral S, Reiter RJ. Functional roles of melatonin in plants, and perspectives in nutritional and agricultural science. J Exp Bot. 2012;63(2):577–97. PMID: 22016420. http://www.ncbi.nlm.nih.gov/pubmed/22016420.
567. Milagres MP, Minim VPR, Minim LA, Simiqueli AA, Moraes LES, Martino HSD. Night milking adds value to cow's milk. J Sci Food Agric. 2014;94(8):1688–92. PMID: 24243550. http://www.ncbi.nlm.nih.gov/pubmed/24243550.
568. Valtonen M, Niskanen L, Kangas AP, Koskinen T. Effect of melatonin-rich night-time milk on sleep and activity in elderly institutionalized subjects. Nord J Psychiatry. 2005;59(3):217–21. PMID: 16195124. http://www.ncbi.nlm.nih.gov/pubmed/16195124.
569. Karunanithi D, Radhakrishna A, Sivaraman KP, Biju VMN. Quantitative determination of melatonin in milk by LC-MS/MS. J Food Sci Technol. 2014;51(4):805–12. PMCID: PMC3981994. http://www.ncbi.nlm.nih.gov/pubmed/24741180.
570. Hansen AL, Dahl L, Olson G, Thornton D, Graff IE, Frøyland L, Thayer JF, Pallesen S. Fish consumption, sleep, daily functioning, and heart rate variability. J Clin Sleep Med. 2014;10(5):567–75. PMCID: PMC4013386. http://www.ncbi.nlm.nih.gov/pubmed/24812543.
571. González-Flores D, Gamero E, Garrido M, Ramírez R, Moreno D, Delgado J, Valdés E, Barriga C, Rodríguez AB, Paredes SD. Urinary 6-sulfatoxymelatonin and total antioxidant capacity increase after the intake of a grape juice cv. Tempranillo stabilized with HHP. Food Funct. 2012;3(1):34–9. PMID: 22033761. http://www.ncbi.nlm.nih.gov/pubmed/22033761.
572. Oba S, Nakamura K, Sahashi Y, Hattori A, Nagata C. Consumption of vegetables alters morning urinary 6-sulfatoxymelatonin concentration. J Pineal Res. 2008;45(1):17–23. PMID: 18205730. http://www.ncbi.nlm.nih.gov/pubmed/18205730.
573. Reiter RJ, Manchester LC, Tan D, xian. Melatonin in walnuts: influence on levels of melatonin and total antioxidant capacity of blood. Nutrition. 2005;21(9):920–4. PMID: 15979282. http://www.ncbi.nlm.nih.gov/pubmed/15979282.
574. Salehi B, Sharopov F, Fokou PVT, Kobylinska A, Jonge L de, Tadio K, Sharifi-Rad J, Posmyk MM, Martorell M, Martins N, Iriti M. Melatonin in medicinal and food plants: occurrence, bioavailability, and health potential for humans. Cells. 2019;8(7):681. PMCID: PMC6678868. http://www.ncbi.nlm.nih.gov/pubmed/31284489.
575. Ng KY, Leong MK, Liang H, Paxinos G. Melatonin receptors: distribution in mammalian brain and their respective putative functions. Brain Struct Funct. 2017;222(7):2921–39. PMID: 28478550. http://www.ncbi.nlm.nih.gov/pubmed/28478550.
576. Goodson JD, Shahbazi S. The national ambulatory medical care survey (NAMCS) at fifty: past and future. Healthc (Amst). 2024;12(4):100754. https://doi.org/10.1016/j.hjdsi.2024.100754. Epub 2024 Nov 11. PMID: 39531953. The national ambulatory medical care survey (NAMCS) at fifty: Past and future - PubMed.
577. NAMCS Questionnaires, Datasets, and Documentation | NAMCS | CDC.
578. NAMCS 2025.

Psychotherapy

17

Elizabeth Sunzeri and Franklin Sunzeri

Introduction

A meta-analytic database of randomized trials (Metapsy) on psychological interventions for mental health issues, including depression, anxiety, PTSD, suicide prevention, psychosis, and gambling, among other mental health issues, is an especially valuable resource [59]. Its depression database contains controlled and comparative studies examining the effects of psychotherapy for depression for different populations, ages, and sexes [60]. It has been collected and analyzed by a group of researchers from VU University Amsterdam, The Netherlands and Linköping University, Sweden. The goal of Metapsy is to be a central hub for meta-analytical research domains that facilitate the total fields of psychotherapy research in a manner that is consistent, transparent, and accessible to the research community. Metapsy is a *WHO Collaborating Center for Research and Dissemination of Psychological Interventions* [61].

Under the auspices of Pim Cuijpers, the data have been used in a series of freely accessible meta-analyses. In 2019, Cuijpers and colleagues published a meta-analytic review examining the effects of 15 evidence-supported therapies for adult depression [62]. These therapies include: acceptance and commitment therapy; mindfulness-based cognitive behavioral therapy (CBT); guided self-help using a book by David Burns; Beck's CBT; the "Coping with Depression" course; two subtypes of behavioral activation; extended and brief problem-solving therapy; self-examination therapy; brief psychodynamic therapy; nondirective counseling; full and brief interpersonal psychotherapy; and life review therapy.

They found high levels of heterogeneity, publication bias, and the risk of bias in most studies, which made the evidence nonconclusive. The overall pooled effect size for all psychotherapies was g = 0.72 (95% CI: 0.67 ~ 0.78), which corresponds with an NNT of 4.04. Heterogeneity was high ($I^2 = 81$; 95% CI: 79 ~ 81), and the prediction interval ranged from −0.17 to 1.61. However, despite these difficulties, they concluded that the 15 types of therapy that were examined in this meta-analysis may be effective in the treatment of depression.

A 2019 overview of recent developments in psychological treatments of depression in primary care found that psychotherapies can effectively be delivered through *e-health applications* and that lay counselors can be effective in delivering that care [63]. For example, behavioral activation therapy, which is less complex than CBT, can be equally as effective as CBT [64]. When subthreshold depression is treated, it may reduce symptoms and prevent the onset of major depressive disorder (MDD). In addition, the review indicated that use of psychotherapy in primary care can have longer-lasting effects than pharmacological treatment, is preferred by most of the patients, and can be presented effectively with different formats to a variety of targets.

Emerging understanding of interactions between critical periods and genetics has suggested the existence of core *cognitive endophenotypes* [65]. Recognition of the commonality of cognitive dysfunctions that underlie more than just a single mental disorder has opened the doors to more effective personalized treatments that do more than just treat symptoms. Knowledge of developmental neuroscience may help to individualize treatment that homes in on precise mediators and moderators that can be harnessed for effective treatment.

In this section, we will discuss the best current evidence for various psychotherapeutic approaches to treating depression. We will peek at what nondirective supportive therapy (NDST) can teach us. Then we will first look at the major psychotherapies: cognitive behavioral therapy, psychodynamic psychotherapy, psychoeducation, interpersonal psychotherapy, problem-solving therapy, nondirective supportive therapy, and behavioral activation therapy.

Then, evidence will be discussed for nondirective supportive therapy (NDST), time-limited cognitive behavioral

E. Sunzeri (✉) · F. Sunzeri
Heather Hills Consulting, Coos Bay, OR, USA

J. Raber et al. (eds.), *Understanding and Treating Depressive Disorders*, https://doi.org/10.1007/978-3-032-14465-2_17

intervention (Competitive Memory Training, or COMET for depressive rumination), bibliotherapy, mindfulness-based stress reduction (MBSR), guided self-help, and stepped-care approaches to deliver accessible and efficient services for depression.

Innovative e-based delivery of psychotherapy holds a promising position to begin and maintain therapy in a cost-effective and efficient manner [66]. Therefore, we will see what evidence exists for e-health delivered Internet-based therapies. These include Guided Internet-based cognitive behavior therapy (ICBT), Mobile Cognitive Therapy (M-CT), GET.ON-Mood Enhancer-WL, transdiagnostic Internet-based maintenance treatment, psychodynamic psychotherapy via the Internet (IPDT), Interpersonal Psychotherapy (IPT), Do not Panic Online, Master Your Mood (MYM), and Internet-based problem-solving therapy (IPST).

Because the comorbidity of depressive disorders with anxiety and panic disorders is so high [67–69] and similar treatments are used, we will also mention psychotherapeutic approaches to treating anxiety disorders. As such, we will give a nod to a couple of evidence-based special CBT interventions. One of these is the Barlow approach to managing panic and anxiety [1, 70–72]. Another is the scientifically based approach of James Phelps and his colleagues in treating bipolar disorders [73].

We will also take a brief look at evidence for adjunctive therapies that have at least some evidence to support them. These include music therapy, art therapy, animal-assisted therapy, and systematic emotion regulation training (ERT). We will also look at the evidence for exercise in the management of depression and anxiety. See Fig. 17.1.

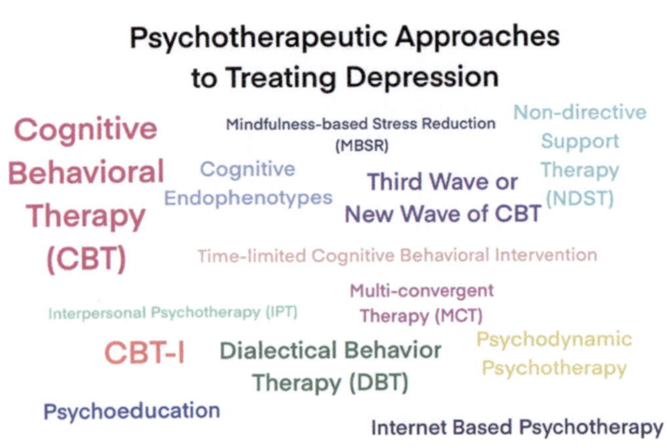

Fig. 17.1 Word cloud of psychotherapeutic approaches for depression. This figure displays a word cloud highlighting the diversity of psychotherapeutic modalities used in the treatment of depression, illustrating the expansive landscape of psychological treatments tailored to individual needs

Nondirective Supportive Therapy

Back in 1992, Lambert suggested that 40% of the improvement in patients was caused by extra-therapeutic change, 30% by the therapeutic relationship, 15% by client expectations, and the remaining 15% by specific techniques [80]. To investigate Lambert's original assertion, a meta-analysis of *nondirective supportive therapy (NDST)* was conducted in 2012 [74].

NDST is defined as "A psychological treatment in which therapists do not engage in any therapeutic strategies other than active listening and offering support, focusing on participants' problems and concerns" [74].

Unfortunately, there was not a lot of useful data to be analyzed. Out of 280 RCTs using psychotherapy for depression, only 31 targeted supportive therapy. Of those, the majority, 23 out of 31, did not meet sufficient study criteria to include in the meta-analysis. Nevertheless, meta-analysis of NDST for depression has shown effectiveness in adults ($g = 0.58$; 95% CI: 0.45–0.72) [74]. NDST appeared to be less effective than other psychological treatments (differential effect size $g = -0.20$; 95% CI: −0.32 to −0.08, $p < 0.010$), but this difference disappeared when research allegiance was considered.

The study's authors calculated that those processes functioning in waiting-list and care-as-usual controls accounted for 33.3% of the overall improvement, the effects of NDST compared with control groups contributed 49.6%, and the effects of NDST compared with other therapies accounted for 17.1%. The implication is that considerable, if not most, of the effect of psychotherapy for adult depression is contributed by nonspecific factors.

Armed with these admonitions, we will look at evidence for psychotherapeutic interventions for depression.

Cognitive Behavioral Therapy

The mainstay and at the heart of many evidence-based psychotherapies is cognitive behavioral therapy. There are many excellent references on cognitive behavioral therapy (CBT).[1]

Probably the most investigated form of psychotherapy is cognitive behavioral therapy (CBT). Evidence has been accumulating over the past several decades that suggests CBT may be useful for treating various disorders in adults [78–80]. These disorders include depression [81, 82], anxiety [82–85], obesity [86], eating disorders [87, 88], sub-

[1]One succinct (~5 pages) overview of CBT can be found at [75]. The *StatPearls* Knowledge Base is available in Apps, eBooks, and online CME/CE Learning Management System covering over 470 medical specialties. Their goal is to provide health professionals with the educational tools needed to identify weaknesses and stay current.

stance abuse [89], personality disorders [90], psychotic disorders [91, 92], chronic fatigue syndrome [93], hoarding disorders [94], insomnia [95], and schizophrenia [96]. In addition, CBT has been used to treat psychological distress of cancer [97], spinal cord injuries [98], fibromyalgia [99, 100], and lower back pain [79].

CBT is also efficacious in specific subsets, including in older adults, women with postpartum depression, patients with general medical disorders, in inpatients, in primary care patients, patients with chronic depression, and in subthreshold depression [101]. *Alexithymia*[2] does not appear to impede CBT [474]. One study asserts that there is strong evidence that CBT interventions are effective for treating and preventing depression during the perinatal period [102].

Various systematic goal-oriented, problem-focused approaches are used to investigate maladaptive behaviors, dysfunctional emotions, and cognitive processes and to help the individual replace the troubled parameters with more adaptive ones [2, 3]. The client and therapist fashion homework assignments to attain therapeutically measurable goals [4].

The central issues in CBT revolve around relationships among cognition, emotion, and behavior. The core issues of cognition are automatic thoughts, cognitive distortions, and underlying beliefs or schemas.

Traditional CBT Has 6 Phases Assessment, reconceptualization, acquisition of skills, consolidation of skills and application training, generalization and maintenance, and posttreatment follow-up [79]. There are a variety of protocols for delivering CBT, some of which are specific to individual disorders [103]. CBT can be delivered in groups [104] or to individuals; approaches can be predominantly cognitively oriented (such as in cognitive restructuring) or behaviorally oriented (such as in vivo exposure therapy) [105].

Typically, there are about 6–18 sessions, an hour long every 1–3 weeks, with booster sessions after 1–3 months [106]. Computerized CBT can also be successfully delivered for depression and anxiety via the Internet [82, 107–110].

CBT, when used for the treatment of depression in contrast to antidepressant medications, may produce a longer-lasting effect and protection against relapse after the end of active treatment [81].

As mentioned above, even though there was a dearth of good RCTs, a 2013 meta-analysis of RCTs on the treatment of chronic major depression compared antidepressants and psychotherapy or the combination of both and indicated that the best treatment for chronic major depression is a combination of both [111]. Similar results were seen in analyses of studies focusing on the treatment of MDD from 1970 to 2012 [112].

CBT appears effective for treating adolescents who are depressed [113, 114] and suicidal [115]. It appears that CBT improves suicidal ideation and depressed mood, generally comparable to active comparison treatments [115]. However, Spirito et al. point out that a significant percentage of adolescents reattempt suicide (5–40%) during any active interventions [115]. Core cognitive, affective, and behavioral techniques used in CBT treatments of suicidal ideation and behavior in depressed adolescents can be found in the following treatment manuals [116]. Cognitive restructuring, problem solving, and affect regulation are the key concepts.

CBT has also been shown to be useful for treating children and adolescents who have eating disorders [88], anxiety [117], PTSD [118], body dysmorphic disorder [119], OCD [120], and repetitive behavior disorders [121].

A 2019 meta-analysis examined CBT for adult depression delivered in individual, group, telephone-administered, guided self-help, and unguided self-help formats [122]. They found that for acute depression, the effectiveness of individual, group, telephone, and guided self-help CBT did not differ statistically significantly from each other and were significantly more effective than waiting list, care as usual, unguided self-help, or placebo. In terms of dropout for any reason, individual and group CBT were significantly better than guided self-help. Guided self-help was also less acceptable than being on a waiting list and care as usual.

A 12-week clinical trial of CBT for depressed adolescent females ($N = 33$; ages 13–18 years; 69.7% White) examined the role of cognitive versus behavioral skills in predicting symptom improvement in depressed youth [123]. Therapist and patient measures of CBT skills obtained at Sessions 1, 3, 6, 9, and 12 showed small to moderate associations ($rs = 0.20$–0.38). Acquisition of behavioral skills vs. cognitive skills predicted subsequent symptom changes.

A multicenter RCT compared the addition of eight weekly sessions of preventive cognitive therapy (PCT) to care as usual (CAU) versus CAU alone in patients with a history of depression in remission following treatment with CBT [124]. Over the 15-month follow-up, the addition of PCT significantly delayed time to relapse/recurrence relative to CAU alone, hazard ratio = 1.807 (number needed to treat = 8.1), $p = 0.02$, 95% CI: 1.029 to 3.174).

A 2016 meta-analytical update reviewed the effects of CBT in the treatment of MDD, generalized anxiety disorder (GAD), panic disorder (PAD), and social anxiety disorder (SAD) [125]. They concluded that CBT is probably effective in the treatment of MDD, GAD, PAD, and SAD; that the effects are large when the control condition is waiting list, but small to moderate when it is care-as-usual or pill pla-

[2]*Alexithymia (emotional blindness)* is a personality trait characterized by the subclinical inability to identify and describe emotions experienced by one's self or others [76, 77].

cebo. The reviewers state that because of the small number of high-quality trials, these effects are still uncertain.

A 2013 meta-analysis was conducted on studies of psychotherapy for depression in which outcomes on *suicidality* and the strongly associated *hopelessness* were reported [126]. Results indicated only a nonsignificant small effect on suicidal ideation and suicide risk. However, the effects on hopelessness were large and significant ($g = 1.10$; 95% CI: 0.72 to 1.48). But there was significant heterogeneity and publication bias. After adjustment, the effect size became 0.60. It would seem that there was no evidence that psychotherapy for depression is sufficient for suicide prevention.

A 2011 meta-analysis and trial sequential analyses of randomized trials compared the effects of cognitive therapy versus "no intervention" for MDD [127]. They found that cognitive therapy significantly reduced depressive symptoms (four trials; mean difference − 3.05 (95% confidence interval (CI: −5.23 to −0.87; $p < 0.006$)) compared with "no intervention." However, trial sequential analysis could not confirm that result. Cognitive therapy significantly reduced depressive symptoms (eight trials; mean difference − 4.86 (95% CI: −6.44 to 3.28; $p = 0.00001$)). Trial sequential analysis on these data confirmed the result. They summarized that cognitive therapy might be an effective treatment for depression, but outcomes may be overestimated due to risks of systematic errors (bias) and random errors (play of chance). And effects on remission, suicidality, adverse events, and quality of life were unclear.

Overestimation effects can influence the effect size of psychotherapy RCTs [128]. *The experimenter's allegiance* is the probable reason for the overestimation. Experimenter's allegiance (EA) is a personal confidence in the superiority of a specific psychotherapy treatment. It is an optimism, nonfinancial bias. But the pattern of treatment effects attributable to EA is not straightforward.

A 2019 study conducted a systematic review and meta-analysis of primary care-based CBT for depression and anxiety [129]. The secondary meta-analysis covered 57 eligible RCTs, which included 10,701 participants and 221 effect sizes. They found an overall significant treatment effect of $d = 0.400$ (95% CI: 0.235 to 0.566), $p < 0.001$, of CBT for depression and anxiety in primary care. There were significant moderators, including the percentage of White participants, treatment composition (CBT only versus CBT + other approaches), and treatment duration. Significant treatment effects for subgroups were (1) depressive ($d = 0.425$, $p < 0.001$) and anxiety ($d = 0.393$, $p < 0.01$) outcomes, (2) studies conducted inside primary care ($d = 0.412$, $p < 0.001$), (3) studies using individual-based CBT ($d = 0.412$, $p < 0.001$), (4) studies without primary care physician involvement ($d = 0.395$, $p < 0.001$), and (5) studies using both tele-health ($d = 0.563$, $p < 0.001$) and in-person CBT ($d = 0.363$, $p < 0.001$).

A comprehensive meta-analysis published in 2023 concludes that CBT for depression has a moderate to large effect size across different delivery formats, ages, and target groups [130]. Furthermore, CBT's effect is still significant up to 12 months and appears to be as effective as pharmacotherapies in the short term, but more effective in the longer term. Combined treatment appears to be superior to pharmacotherapy alone but not to CBT alone. It was not clear if CBT was more effective than other psychotherapies.

Cognitive Behavioral Therapy for Insomnia (CBT-I)

CBT has found good success in treating both MDD and associated insomnia [131–134]. *The 2016 AHRQ review*[3] stated, "*Cognitive behavioral therapy for insomnia (CBT-I)* improved global outcomes and nearly all sleep parameters in the general adult population, older adults, and adults with pain." They found insufficient evidence for any adverse effects of psychotherapeutic interventions [135]. A protocol for youth-oriented CBT therapy for insomnia is presented in [136]. A systematic review and meta-analysis of CBT for insomnia in cancer survivors has shown large effect sizes for insomnia severity ($d = 0.77$) with effects lasting up to 5 months [26434673].

As with all forms of CBT, CBT-I focuses on identifying thoughts, feelings, and behaviors that contribute to insomnia symptoms [54, 55]. Once maladaptive thoughts and misconceptions have been identified and examined, the therapist helps the patient reframe them to promote more relaxing and restorative sleep [139]. The American College of Physicians recommends CBT-I as the first-line treatment for insomnia due to its safety and proven efficacy, regardless of whether an underlying cause has been identified [140–142]. Although some pharmacological treatments may offer similar acute benefits, only CBT-I has demonstrated durable long-term effects following the cessation of therapy [142, 143].

Cognitive components focus on changing misconceptions and unhelpful thinking about sleep. Behavioral interventions focus on incorporating healthy sleep habits, including relaxation, sleep restriction, stimulus control, and compression. Psychoeducation looms large in connecting thoughts, feelings, behavior, and sleep.

Therapists who provide CBT-I can be found through contacts with the *American Board of Sleep Medicine* [144], the *Association of Behavioral and Cognitive Therapists* [145],

[3] A *2016 Agency for Healthcare Research and Quality (AHRQ) comprehensive assessment* of the efficacy, comparative effectiveness, and harms of treatments for insomnia disorder in the general adult population and older adults [137, 138].

the *Society of Behavioral Sleep Medicine* [146], and *the American Psychological Association* [147].

Classic stimulus control aims to restructure the bedroom environment to associate it exclusively with sleep and sex, to encourage getting out of bed when falling asleep becomes difficult, to maintain a consistent sleep–wake cycle, and to discourage daytime napping. Sleep restriction limits the time in bed without sleeping. It begins by keeping track of the amount of time usually spent sleeping, for example, 6 out of 8 desired hours. Next, add 30 min to that time and go to bedtime 30 min later than normal. The idea is to slightly increase fatigue. If successful in inducing more sleep time, the process might be repeated, adding more latent time. Alternatively, sleep compression would reduce the time in bed to equal the number of hours that are typically slept. The relaxation training [56] that is most frequently used with CBT-I includes breathing exercises, autogenics, progressive muscle relaxation exercises, guided imagery, self-hypnosis, meditation, and biofeedback.

Several systematic reviews and meta-analyses have shown CBT-I to be an effective treatment for insomnia and other sleep problems [148–151]. Clinically meaningful effect sizes are seen, and changes seem to be sustainable with no apparent adverse effects.

A 2024 *systematic review and component network meta-analysis (cNMA)*[4] suggests that the most *successful CBT-I packages may include* cognitive restructuring,[5] third-wave components,[6] sleep restriction,[7] stimulus control,[8] and in-person delivery [150]. However, they point out that potential undetected interactions could undermine these conclusions. Sleep hygiene education[9] was not essential, and relaxation procedures[10] were found to be potentially counterproductive. They concluded that a) sleep restriction was associated with improved subjective sleep quality, sleep efficiency, and waking after sleep onset; and b) stimulus control was associated with improved subjective sleep quality, sleep efficiency, and sleep latency.

They did not find evidence of superiority of the in-person format over the self-help format with human encouragement.

Their findings for *relaxation therapy* are similar to those found for cNMAs of potential harm in *panic disorder* [155], and in *Internet CBT for depression* [156]. The reviewers suggested that relaxation might lead to lying down longer, which might run counter to sleep restrictions or stimulus control.

Third Wave or New Wave of CBT

A number of CBT variants, often called the *third wave or new wave of CBT,* have become popular [103, 157]. These include mindfulness-based treatments (e.g., mindfulness-based stress reduction (MBSR), mindfulness-based cognitive therapy (MBCT), acceptance and commitment therapy (ACT), and dialectical behavior therapy (DBT) [25–28], exposure therapy [158, 159], cognitive processing therapy [160], and lesser-known cognitive behavioral analysis system of psychotherapy (CBASP) [161], functional analytic psychotherapy (FAP) [476], and integrative behavioral couple therapy (IBCT) [49, 162].

A 2008 meta-analysis of third wave treatment RCTs found that there were 13 RCTs both in Acceptance and Commitment Therapy (ACT) and dialectical behavior therapy (DBT), one in cognitive behavioral analysis system of psychotherapy (CBASP), two in integrative behavioral couple therapy (IBCT, and none in functional analytic psychotherapy (FAP) [163]. The reviewers concluded that the third wave treatment RCTs were significantly less stringent than CBT studies. ACT and DBT had moderate effect sizes, whereas the others had no empirical support.

Since that time, a 2009 RCT of CBASP for depression indicated that CBASP plus medication was approximately equal to brief supportive psychotherapy plus medication and both were better than medication alone [164].

A 2013 meta-analysis of behavioral therapies compared to other psychological therapies for acute depression in adults found low to moderate quality evidence of equal effectiveness [165]. The behavioral therapies were behavioral therapy, behavioral activation, social skills training, and relaxation training. The psychotherapies were CBT, third

[4] *Component network meta-analysis (cNMA)* is an extension of standard network meta-analysis [152] that can be used to examine complex associations of different components that might contribute to the outcomes in multicomponent interventions [153, 154].

[5] Cognitive restructuring was defined as "Skills to identify, challenge, and change unhelpful beliefs about sleep that may disturb sleep. Sometimes simply called cognitive therapy. This may include behavioral experiments."

[6] The third-wave components that were assessed were mindfulness and acceptance and commitment therapy.

[7] Sleep restriction they defined as "Skills to improve sleep by limiting time in bed. First, time in bed is restricted to the average sleep duration plus 30 minutes, and then it is increased or decreased depending on sleep efficiency."

[8] Stimulus control was defined as "Skills to reassociate the bed with sleep. Patients are instructed to wake up at the same time every morning, refrain from daytime napping, go to bed only when sleepy, get out of bed when unable to sleep, and use the bed and bedroom for sleep and sex only."

[9] The researchers defined sleep hygiene education as "general explanation about sleep (e.g., sleep biology, characteristics of healthy sleep, and changes in sleep patterns with aging) and general recommendations about lifestyle (e.g., diet, exercise, and substance use) and environmental factors (e.g., light, noise, and temperature) to improve sleep."

[10] Relaxation was defined as "Structured exercises to reduce somatic tension (e.g., abdominal breathing, progressive muscle relaxation, autogenic training) and cognitive arousal (e.g., guided imagery training)."

wave CBT, psychodynamic, humanistic, and integrative psychological therapies.

Another 2013 Cochrane database meta-analysis concluded that although there is very low-quality evidence, there are suggestions that third wave CBT and standard CBT approaches are equally effective and acceptable in the treatment of acute depression [166, 167]. The paucity of evidence is such that they could not draw any conclusions as to their short- or long-term equivalences. There was substantial heterogeneity. The RCTs suffered from several deficiencies, including small sample sizes, lack of follow-up, and researcher allegiance.

A 2016 Cochrane review examined CBT, third-wave CBT, and interpersonal therapy (IPT) based interventions for preventing depression in children and adolescents [168]. The target population was ages 5–19 years, who did not currently meet diagnostic criteria for depression but who had a history of depression. The evidence was low to moderate, and the results were heterogeneous. However, small positive benefits were seen for decreased depressive symptoms postintervention and depression diagnosis up to 12 months. The number needed to treat to benefit was 11, which is similar to other public health interventions. *Attention placebo* comparison groups (a control intervention that controls for non-specific factors such as involvement in a trial and attention from researchers) were seldom present, and when they were, the effect sizes diminished significantly. They concluded that there is not enough evidence to support the implementation of depression prevention programs.

Mindfulness-Based Therapies

Mindfulness-based therapies (MBT) are clinical applications of spiritual practices based upon nonjudgmental acceptance of distress with the goal of reducing catastrophizing or the tendency to ruminate [5, 6, 169].

The concept of *mindfulness* was introduced to the West from Buddhist philosophy in the 1970s by Jon Kabat-Zinn [5]. Mindfulness can be defined as purposefully bringing one's complete attention nonjudgmentally to the present experience on a moment-to-moment basis [91]. In this present-centered awareness, each thought, feeling, or sensation that arises in the attentional field is acknowledged and accepted as it is [5–7, 170]. In that experience, a practitioner can identify habitual thought patterns about which they were unaware and, in so doing, may allow them to engage in a new way with curiosity, openness, and acceptance. Gaining *metacognitive* skills[11] involves accepting one's *mind stream* and developing a *Beginner's Mind* [56–58].

One of the goals of practicing mindfulness is to create an interval of time in which to make conscious life choices based upon possible responses to life events such as stressors [173]. Through this process, it is possible to reveal self-inflicted stress caused by the interpretation of events.

Some scholars have objected to the Western attempts to define mindfulness that they believe is different in some important ways from the Buddhist tradition [174–177].

Mindfulness scales are used in RCTs to establish an evidence base in investigating the effects of mindfulness [178].

Four mechanisms have been proposed for the effects of mindfulness [7, 179]. These are attention regulation, body awareness, emotion regulation, and changes in perspective on the self.

A 2011 clinical review concluded that mindfulness brings about various positive psychological effects, including increased subjective well-being, reduced psychological symptoms and emotional reactivity, and improved behavioral regulation [169]. Mindfulness is in opposition to suppression and avoidance and is associated with greater activation in the prefrontal cortex and greater deactivation of the amygdala during affect labeling [180]. Mindfulness appears to improve emotional regulation by enhancing cortical regulation of limbic circuits and attentional control [181].

Changes in amygdala activity seem to be correlated both with depression and with mindfulness-based treatment. A study of relationships of mindfulness and depression in young normal adults found that depressive symptomatology was positively correlated with resting activity in self-referential processing areas, while dispositional mindfulness was negatively correlated with resting activity in these areas [182]. Depressive symptoms were positively correlated with activity in the right amygdala, whereas dispositional mindfulness was negatively correlated with resting activity bilaterally in the amygdala. When reviewing emotional faces, depressive symptoms were positively correlated with amygdala reactivity, whereas dispositional mindfulness was negatively correlated with amygdala reactivity.

Mindfulness association with intrinsic neural activity and alterations in resting amygdala activity has been suggested to underpin positive results from mindfulness-based depression treatment [182]. Individual disposition to mindfulness seems to be associated with extensive activation of the prefrontal cortex and decreased bilateral amygdala activity [183]. Strong negative associations have been seen between areas of the prefrontal cortex and right amygdala responses in people who are highly proficient in mindfulness, but not in those who are low in mindfulness. These characteristics are associated with tighter control of immune responses [184].

Mindfulness practice in one study increased left-sided anterior activation and significantly increased antibody titers to the influenza vaccine in an association where the increase

[11] Metacognition is thinking about thinking [171, 172].

in left-sided activation predicted the magnitude of antibody titer response to the vaccine [185].

Specific facets of mindfulness and dimensions of anxiety and depression symptoms have been associated in a study of treatment-seeking adults [186]. Results indicated that all facets of mindfulness were significantly related to all dimensions of anxiety and depression except for describing and observing. In particular, nonreactivity was significantly inversely associated with general distress anxiety symptoms; describing was significantly inversely associated with anxious arousal, and observing was significantly positively associated with anxious arousal; general distress-depression and anhedonic depression symptomatology were significantly inversely related to nonjudging and nonreactivity. There was no significant association between acting with awareness and any dimensions of anxiety or depression.

Mindfulness-based therapies have been seen in some relatively high-quality RCTs to be useful for cancer patients and survivors with symptoms of anxiety and depression [187]. Mindfulness training can result in verifiable improvements in measurements of disability such as depression and anxiety [173], diabetes [188], pain [189, 190], and psoriasis [191, 192].

Since its introduction in the West, mindfulness has been incorporated into several therapeutic applications, including *Mindfulness-Based Stress Reduction (MBSR), Mindfulness-Based Cognitive Therapy (MBCT), Acceptance and Commitment Therapy (ACT), Dialectical Behavioral Therapy,* and the lesser-known *Mindfulness-based relapse prevention (MBRP), Mindfulness-Based Intervention (MBI-ld), and Multiconvergent therapy (MCT).* These emotion regulation-training interventions focus on emotional reactivity to stress in a variety of clinical and nonclinical populations.

A 2018 systematic review and meta-analysis analyzed mindfulness-based interventions for psychiatric disorders [193]. They included 142 nonoverlapping samples with 12,005 participants. They suggested that mindfulness-based interventions are promising as evidence-based treatments.

1. At posttreatment, mindfulness-based interventions were superior to no treatment (d = 0.55), minimal treatment (d = 0.37), nonspecific active controls (d = 0.35), and specific active controls (d = 0.23). Mindfulness conditions did not differ from evidence-based treatments (d = −0.004).
2. At follow-up, mindfulness-based interventions were superior to no treatment conditions (d = 0.50), nonspecific active controls (d = 0.52), and specific active controls (d = 0.29). Mindfulness conditions did not differ from minimal treatment conditions (d = 0.38) and evidence-based treatments (d = 0.09).
3. The most consistent evidence in support of mindfulness was for depression, pain conditions, smoking, and addictive disorders.

A 2016 study suggested that mindfulness-based interventions suffered from several difficulties [194]. These included the use of nonactive control conditions in RCTs and the lack of outcome specificity.

Another 2016 review of mindfulness-based RCTs raised questions of overstating the efficacy of mindfulness-based interventions that might introduce systematic bias into the relevant literature [195]. An effect size of d = 0.55 was seen based upon 109 out of 124 published trials concluding that mindfulness-based therapy was effective. This was 1.6 times greater number of reported positive RCTs than the expected number of positive trials based on effect size d = 0.55 (the expected number of positive trials is 65.7). Of registered RCTs, 13 out of 21 were still unpublished 30 months after RCT completion. Nevertheless, the current investigators found that not one of 36 systematic reviews and meta-analyses concluded that effect estimates were overestimated due to reporting biases.

A 2014 systematic review and meta-analysis of meditation programs for psychological stress and well-being found moderate evidence of improved anxiety (effect size, 0.38 [95% CI, 0.12–0.64] at 8 weeks and 0.22 [0.02–0.43] at 3–6 months), depression (0.30 [0.00–0.59] at 8 weeks and 0.23 [0.05–0.42] at 3–6 months), and pain (0.33 [0.03–0.62]) and low evidence of improved stress/distress and mental health-related quality of life. They found low evidence or no effect or insufficient evidence of any effect of meditation programs on positive mood, attention, substance use, eating habits, sleep, and weight. They found no evidence that meditation programs were better than any active treatment (drugs, exercise, and other behavioral therapies). [196].

A 2013 meta-analysis has concluded that mindfulness-based therapies are an effective treatment for a variety of psychological problems, and are especially effective for reducing anxiety, depression, and stress [23796855]. They found moderate effect sizes in pre-post comparisons (n = 72; Hedge's g = 0.55), in comparison to other active treatments (n = 68; Hedge's g = 0.33), and other psychological treatments (n = 35; Hedge's g = 0.22). They found no difference compared to traditional CBT or behavioral therapies (n = 9; Hedge's g = −0.07) or pharmacological treatments (n = 3; Hedge's g = 0.13).

Mindfulness-based stress reduction (MBSR) is a structured program using mindfulness meditation to help with a diversity of health issues [173]. A variety of meditation techniques are used in MBSR, including focusing on sitting meditation (breath awareness, focused attention), body scanning (awareness of sensations in the body), mindful movement, walking meditation, and insight meditation.

The standard MBSR format consists of 26 h of session time, including 8 classes of 2–1/2 h and an all-day class [197]. It was thought that this length of time was necessary for participants to understand the principles of self-regulation using mindfulness and gain the ability and independence in mindfulness. However, a review of class contact hours and effect sizes for psychological distress has found that the correlation between mean effect size and number of in-class hours was not significant for both clinical and nonclinical samples [197]. At home, practice is essential and is typically 45 min a day, 6 days a week, during the 8-day training.

Modifications to the MBSR while maintaining the core principles of the 8-week program and inclusion of a retreat have reduced the time committed to meetings, and formal practice has still produced good results [197–202]. For example, a 6-week shortened work-site MBSR intervention reduced perceived stress ($p = 0.0025$) and increased mindfulness ($p = 0.0149$) [203]. Global measures of sleep improved ($p = 0.0018$) as well as for the control group ($p = 0.0072$). Five days of *Integrative Body-Mind Training (IBMT)* improved self-regulation of the autonomic nervous system via a subgenual and adjacent ventral anterior cingulate cortex brain system, the executive attention network [204]. Compared to a relaxation control, IBMT is associated with better physiological reactions in heart rate, respiratory amplitude and rate, and skin conductance. IBMT has also been associated with higher salivary IgA levels and lower salivary cortisol levels following an acute stressor [205].

A *low-dose Mindfulness-Based Intervention (MBI-ld)* that reduced the time devoted to meetings and formal mindfulness practice while conducting the sessions during the workday significantly increased mindfulness while decreasing some markers of inflammation [202]. A 2011 meta-analytical review of 72 MBSR articles found that there was a medium effect size overall, supporting the conclusion that it is a useful method for improving mental health and reducing symptoms of stress, anxiety, and depression [206]. They also suggested that the experience of the MBSR teachers makes a significant impact on the effectiveness of MBSR.

Reviews of MBSR for chronic diseases such as fibromyalgia, chronic pain, rheumatoid arthritis, type 2 diabetes, chronic fatigue syndrome, multiple chemical sensitivity, and cardiovascular diagnoses disease have been difficult to compare, but it seems that overall positive changes in psychological and physical measurements seem to occur [207].

A meta-analysis of MBSR covering a wide range of clinical populations (including pain, cancer, heart disease, depression, and anxiety) and stressed nonclinical groups showed an effect size of approximately 0.5 ($p < 0.0001$) homogeneously distributed [208].

Acceptance-based interventions such as *mindfulness-based stress reduction* programs and *acceptance and commitment therapy* have small to medium effects on physical and mental health in chronic pain patients comparable to those of cognitive behavioral therapy [209].

Eight weekly 2.5-h sessions of MBSR for patients afflicted with fibromyalgia have resulted in significant improvements in depression symptoms [210].

However, a review of several studies of MBSR for chronic low back pain found short-term improvements in pain acceptance, whereas some other studies found no short-term or long-term improvements in pain or disability for chronic specific or nonspecific low back pain [211].

A 2011 comprehensive overview and meta-analysis of MBSR in cancer showed an improvement in quality of life with an effect size of 0.29 (95% CI: 0.17–0.40; $p \leq 0.00005$), mood with an effect size of 0.42 (95% CI: 0.26–0.58; $p < 0.0001$), and reduction in distress with an effect size of 0.58 (95% CI: 0.45–0.72; $p < 0.0001$) [212].

Postsurgical women with early-stage breast cancer who received group MBSR were able to reestablish their natural killer cell activity and IFN-γ production levels and lower their IL-4, IL-6, and IL-10 production [213]. They were also able to reduce cortisol levels, improve quality of life, and increase coping effectiveness.

A review of articles on MBSR among breast cancer survivors published from 1987 to 2009 showed large effect sizes on perceived stress and state anxiety and medium effect sizes on symptoms of stress and mood disturbance [214]. Biological influences showed small effect sizes, except for cytokine production, which had a large effect size at 6- and 12-month follow-ups.

MBSR has been shown to reduce ruminative thinking and trait anxiety and increase empathy and self-compassion [215]. *Mindfulness-based relapse prevention (MBRP)* can be effective for reducing craving in substance use that is part of the conditioned response in depression [216]. A 9-week *Web-based program, Deprexis*, which integrates behavioral activation, cognitive restructuring, mindfulness/acceptance exercises, and social skills training, has been shown to significantly reduce depression symptoms [217].

A 2011 review of 39 studies conducted in ten countries found that mindfulness-based therapies were superior to standard care in reducing depressive symptoms and preventing relapse, with effect sizes ranging from 0.11 to 1.65 [218]. The most effective therapy was exposure-based cognitive therapy ($d = 2.09$), followed by MBSR ($d = 1.92$), acceptance-based behavior therapy ($d = 1.33$), and mindfulness ($d = 1.31$). Effect sizes correlated with the length of intervention sessions.

A 2019 RCT of the effects of Modified MBSR on the psychological health of adolescents in China with subthreshold depression showed positive effects on psychological health among adolescents, including decreased depression and rumination, and increased mindfulness [223]. In another study of adolescents in China, MBSR had moderate effects

(Hedges' $g = -0.45$) in reducing depression at the end of the intervention [219]. However, on follow-up, there was no evidence of the effect persisting: the effect size was Hedges' $g = -0.24$.

MBSR appears to be capable of alleviating depression, anxiety, and pain in patients with postherpetic neuralgia [220]. MBSR and CBT appear to be equally effective in reducing comorbid anxiety and depression in adults with autism spectrum disorder [221]. MBSR training can reduce mean depression, anxiety, and stress scores in women with multiple sclerosis [222]. MBSR may be effective in treating depression in veterans [223].

The effects of an MBSR intervention on depression, anxiety, and stress symptoms of older adults showed that MBSR is more effective than a wait-list-control group in reducing depression in older adults with clinically significant symptoms immediately following the intervention. However, there was no evidence that MBSR reduced the perception of stress and anxiety, or for how long those positive effects are maintained [225].

In 1995, Zindel Segal, Mark Williams, and John Teasdale presented an information processing analysis of mindfulness and mindlessness and their relevance to preventing depression relapse [226]. They proposed integrating cognitive behavioral therapy (CBT) with mindfulness training in a new approach that they called *Attentional Control Training*.

This was the foundation for *Mindfulness-Based Cognitive Therapy (MBCT)*, which was developed by Segal, Williams, and Teasdale based on Jon Kabat-Zinn's *Mindfulness-Based Stress Reduction* program [227, 228]. As they put it, they designed MBCT as a group intervention to train recovered recurrently depressed patients to disengage from dysphoria-activated depression generating thinking that may mediate relapse or recurrence [228]. They believed that in those individuals who were predisposed to depression, life stressors could lead to dysphoria that activates automatic negative thinking patterns, which escalate negative affect cycling into full-blown depression [229].

MBCT is an 8-week group intervention, 2 h at a time, with 1 day-long class following the fifth week [230]. Homework is a key concept wherein the participants practice guided meditations and attempt to incorporate mindfulness into their everyday lives. It seems that the number of minutes of practice a week may not correlate with depression outcomes [231]. The regularity of practice may be more important. Self-help versions seem to be promising [232].

MDD is frequently chronic. Relapse and recurrence occur despite successful treatments that induce remission [231]. As mentioned above, it is this recurrence that was the original target of MBCT.

MBCT targets the *cognitive reactivity* of the cognition-affect cycle [233]. Cognitive reactivity is the magnitude of change in response to negative mood provocation [234]. MBCT teaches depressed individuals to step away from negative ruminations and self-evaluations, thereby breaking the positive feedback loop between negative thinking and negative affect [8, 226]. Little emphasis is placed on challenging specific cognitions [181]. Greater cognitive reactivity in patients who recovered through antidepressant medication or CBT, had a higher 18-month relapse rate [233]. In addition, those who recovered via antidepressants had a higher relapse rate and significantly more cognitive reactivity than those who recovered via CBT.

However, MBCT, in contradistinction to CBT, helps patients to hold negative thoughts in awareness instead of diminishing them [235–237]. An RCT found that patients who received MBCT were more highly cognitive reacting than those who took antidepressants while in a dysphoric mood, but this reactivity did not produce affective deterioration [235]. At 15-month follow-up, cognitive reactivity and relapse were decoupled for MBCT but not for antidepressants. It was further substantiated that, in addition to the decoupling between reactivity of depressive thinking and a poor outcome, the treatment effect is associated with both developing augmented self-compassion toward one's own feelings and thoughts and mindfulness [235].

In addition, affective or *emotional reactivity*, the intensity and duration of negative affect in response to a stressor, is also modified by MBCT [9, 237]. The goal in emotional reactivity is to acknowledge the negative thoughts and emotions, hold them in awareness, and compassionately accept them without self-referential negative judgment that can make them worse [236, 237]. This compassionate acceptance seems to mediate the successful regulation of emotions in response to stressors that would tend to provoke a negative response [238, 239].

Indeed, it has been suggested that reduced emotional reactivity to stress, instead of depression specific cognitive reactivity, may be the target of MBCT [240–242].

Greater prefrontal inhibition of the amygdala [182, 238, 241] and decreased sympathetic nervous system hyperarousal [243–245] have been seen to occur as a result of better emotional regulation in people who meditate.

MBCT has expanded its scope to include acute and residual depression treatment [246–250]. Moreover, MBCT has been seen to be useful in treating a variety of emotional difficulties [251–254], including anxiety disorders [255–258], sleep disturbance [247], and bipolar disorder [259]. The role of meditation in substance use disorders is reviewed in [260]. Attentional factors and mood response are discussed in [261].

There is some evidence that MBCT may be superior to psychoeducation for some people who did not fully achieve remission from MDD after antidepressant treatment [262]. A meta-analysis of six RCTs (n = 593 participants) found that MBCT reduced the risk of MDD relapse/recurrence 34%

[21802618]. For those who had three or more previous episodes, the risk was reduced by 43%, and no risk reduction was seen for those who had only two relapses. Two studies indicated that MBCT was at least as effective as maintenance antidepressant medication.

In a 14-month follow-up study, MBCT plus treatment as usual produced a significantly longer time to relapse than treatment as usual (median 204 and 69 days, respectively); however, both groups relapsed at a similar rate [263]. In that study, brief and informal mindfulness practice, but longer formal meditation, decreased over the 14 months.

A 2012 meta-analysis of MBCT in MDD showed significantly reduced risk for relapse [264]. Positive results were more likely to occur when there had been three or more MDD episodes. However, MBCT can reduce residual depressive symptoms regardless of the number of previous episodes of MDD [265]. Results of an RCT indicated that MBCT was superior to the control condition across subgroups ($\beta = -0.56$, $P < 0.001$).

Long-term success of MBCT as a relapse prevention for MDD appears to be significant at least in an observational study of 39 participants [20374671]. Gains were maintained for Group 1, 1–12 months, $p = 0.002$; Group 2, 13–24 months, $p = 0.001$; and Group 3, 25–34 months, $p = 0.04$. Better depression scores correlated with booster sessions ($p = 0.003$) and ongoing mindfulness practice ($p = 0.03$). Rumination and mindful attention were significantly negatively associated ($p < 0.001$).

MBCT appears to be as effective for patients with recurrent depression who are currently depressed as for patients who are not currently depressed [266]. MBCT also appears to be equally effective in protecting against MDD relapse as maintenance antidepressants [267]. An RCT found that metacognitive skills of decentering and curiosity were significantly increased by MBCT but not by medication treatments for prevention of depressive relapse [268]. Pharmacological treatment was associated with decreased rumination and increased Wider Experiences subscales of the Experiences Questionnaire and the Toronto Mindfulness Scale.

MBCT has achieved good results for men with advanced prostate cancer [10, 269]. Improvements were seen in anxiety ($p = 0.027$), avoidance ($p = 0.032$), and mindfulness skills ($p = 0.019$). There was a trend for a reduction in fear of cancer recurrence ($p = 0.062$), and effect sizes were moderate to large.

A mindfulness-based intervention for patients with multiple sclerosis, compared to usual care, improved psychological symptoms postintervention and at follow-up ($p < 0.002$) [270]. Overall effect sizes posttreatment were 0.4–0.9, and at follow-up, it was 0.3–0.5. Those participants who had clinically relevant levels of preintervention depression, fatigue, or anxiety showed larger effect sizes.

In a review of eight published randomized controlled outcome studies for folks with chronic somatic diseases, MBCT appeared to have small effects on depression (0.32) and anxiety (0.24) [271].

American Lung Association's Freedom from Smoking (FFS) treatment and a mindfulness-based treatment (MBT) were compared for smoking cessation [272]. Both treatments were delivered twice weekly over 4 weeks in a group format. Participants who received the MBT demonstrated a greater reduction in cigarette use during treatment and maintained their improvement during follow-up ($F = 11.11$, $p = 0.001$). At 17-week follow-up, there was a significant difference in abstinence rate (31% MBT vs. 6% FFS, $p = 0.012$).

MBCT is associated with increases in self-reported and objectively measured polysomnographic sleep profiles in antidepressant medications users [273].

Acceptance and Commitment Therapy

Acceptance and Commitment Therapy (ACT) is a type of clinical behavior analysis [11, 274–277] philosophically based in *Functional Contextualism* [104, 105] and grounded in *Relational Frame Theory* [12, 20]. ACT uses mindfulness and acceptance approaches along with commitment and behavior-changing methods designed to increase psychological flexibility [13]. Relational Frame Theory is a comprehensive active basic research program on the nature of human language and cognition [278].

ACT was developed in the late 1980s by Steven Hayes, Kelly Wilson, and Kirk Strosahl and was originally called *Comprehensive Distancing* [14, 15, 18, 19]. ACT was designed as a treatment for *Experiential Avoidance Disorder* [21].

A goal of ACT is to help an individual get in touch with a transcendent sense of self that is called *self-as-context* [13]. This self is distinct from one's thoughts, memories, sensations, and feelings, but is always present, experiencing and observing. It is thought that this will enhance psychological flexibility and permit an individual to clarify their personal values and act upon them. In contrast to CBT, which teaches how to better control their thoughts, memories, sensations, and feelings, ACT teaches just noticing and accepting these.

ACT posits that psychological processing in the normal human is frequently destructive [16] and psychological difficulties arise from experiential avoidance and cognitive rigidity that prevents the flexibility needed to change behavior in a way that is commensurate with core values [17, 279]. The reference summarizes the view of ACT that the core issues of many problems are due to FEAR [280]

1. *F*usion with your thoughts
2. *E*valuation of experience

3. *A*voidance of your experience
4. *R*eason-giving for your behavior

And the healthy alternative is to *ACT*:

5. *A*ccept your reactions and be present
6. *C*hoose a valued direction
7. *T*ake action

The six core principles that ACT uses to foster psychological flexibility are [16, 281][12]:

1. *Acceptance*: Active and aware embracing of thoughts without struggling against them. It is a method of increasing value-based action.
2. Observing the self: Self as context for relationships within time and space. A transcendent side to experience without becoming attached to them.
3. *Cognitive defusion*: Leaning methods that attempt to change the undesirable functions of thoughts, images, memories, and emotions [283].
4. *Being in contact with the present:* Nonjudgmental awareness of psychological and environmental events as they happen. A defused description of processes observed with openness, receptiveness, and interest. Being fully engaged in the moment.
5. *Values:* Discovering and choosing what qualities of life are the most important to one's own true self. The goal is not to lead to choices based on avoidance, fusion, or compliance.
6. *Committed action:* Selecting goals that are behaviorally coherent with stated values and responsibly carrying them through with an appropriate action plan.

Three previous meta-analyses of ACT were published in 2006, 2008, and 2009. The 2009 meta-analysis found 18 suitable quality RCTs [280]. Hedges' g effect sizes were interpreted with Cohen's convention of small (0.2), medium (0.5), and large (0.8) effects. Overall, ACT, compared to controls, had an effect size of 0.42 for several problem domains. ACT was not significantly better than established treatments (effect size = 0.18, $p = 0.13$). ACT was better than waiting lists and psychological placebos (effect size = 0.68) and treatment as usual (effect size = 0.42). However, ACT was not superior to control conditions for treating anxiety and depression (effect size = 0.03, $p = 0.84$).

A 2012 RCT showed ACT and CBT were equally effective at posttreatment in terms of depression, anxiety, overall (social/occupational/symptom-related) functioning, and quality of life [281, 284]. However, at the 1 ½ year follow-up, one-third more CBT patients were in the normative range of depressive symptoms, and more than twice as many CBT patients were in the normative range of functioning.

[12]The Veterans Health Administration provides a video series about ACT that addresses the six core processes [282].

Further comparisons between CBT and ACT are presented in [285]. It appears that ACT and CBT produce their results through different mechanisms [286, 287].

Five sessions over 15 weeks of ACT or relaxation training for multiple sclerosis showed a 3-month follow-up for significantly reduced anxiety for the relaxation treatment and acceptance, while living an active, valued life for the ACT group [288].

Internet-based ACT may be a viable alternative to CBT for managing tinnitus [284, 289]. ACT may be worth exploring for OCD [289]. An ACT self-help program with minimal email support for people with mild to moderate depression produced a 3-month sustainable significant improvement in depression, anxiety, fatigue, experiential avoidance, and improvements in positive mental health and mindfulness [290]. Effect sizes were Cohen's $d = 0.51–1.00$.

ACT has been seen to be a good alternative to CBT for chronic pain [291, 292]. A large series of RCTs showed ACT had an effect size on pain of 0.37 and on depression of 0.32 [209]. ACT and CBT appeared to be equally effective. Manual-based self-help ACT with weekly therapist support can help in the treatment of chronic pain [293, 294]. ACT has moderated the influence of pain on the quality of life in pediatric longstanding pain syndromes [295].

Twelve weeks of ACT for women with fibromyalgia showed significant improvements in pain-related functioning, fibromyalgia impact, mental health-related quality of life, self-efficacy, depression, anxiety, and psychological inflexibility [296].

Before and after 12 weekly sessions of ACT or wait-list control in groups of six women suffering from fibromyalgia, fMRI was assessed during pressure-evoked pain [297]. Women treated with ACT reported better improvement of fibromyalgia, depression, and anxiety, but there were no effects on clinical pain or pain sensitivity. ACT led to increased activity in the ventrolateral prefrontal/lateral orbitofrontal cortex, the executive cognitive control regions. It is hypothesized that reappraisal of pain is derived from an altered cerebral loop between pain signals, emotions, and cognitions.

ACT may decrease depression and crisis contacts in psychosis [298]. Patients with MDD with psychotic features received up to 6 months of *Acceptance-Based Depression and Psychosis Therapy (ADAPT)* combined with pharmacotherapy [299]. Improvement was seen in depression and psychotic symptoms, psychosocial functioning, and processes such as acceptance, mindfulness, and living a value-based life. Psychological flexibility seems to account for a larger proportion of variance in depression and anxiety in people with psychosis [300].

Self-help ACT workbooks can have significant effects on the prevention and amelioration of depression, anxiety, and stress [301].

Early intervention by ACT increased acceptance and reduced depression symptoms in adults with mild to moderate depression [302]. The effect size was Cohen's d of 0.60.

ACT appears to be similar to CBT in overall benefit in treating anxiety disorders [303].

Dialectical Behavior Therapy

Dialectical Behavior Therapy (DBT), which was developed by Marsha Linehan in the late 1970s, combines CBT techniques of reality testing and emotional regulation with acceptance, distress tolerance, and mindfulness [304]. She originally created DBT to deal with chronically suicidal individuals, many of whom were suffering from borderline personality disorder (BPD). DBT has been successful in reducing interpersonal problems, anger, suicidal behavior, substance abuse [305], treatment dropout, eating disorders [306], traumatic brain injuries, ADHD [307, 308], and mood disorders [29]. In addition to BPD [309], DBT has also been successful in treating bipolar disorders [310], PTSD [311], and major depressive disorders [312].

Linehan discovered that her patients needed loving kindness, validation of the patient's feelings, and somewhat unconditional metaphysical acceptance from the therapist while informing the patient that some of the behaviors and feelings are maladaptive and showing them that there are better alternatives [22–24]. In essence, an *intersubjective* tough love [314].[13] In addition, patients needed to commit and be willing to accept their emotional dysfunction [22–24].

As a basis for acceptance and change, Linehan and her followers embraced the Hegelian *dialectical* process of reasoning to resolve a disagreement through rational discussion in the search for truth [30, 31]. The *Socratic Method* is the classically familiar dialectical process, which begins with accepting a hypothesis that leads to contradictions and rejecting that hypothesis in the search for truth [32]. *Reductio ad absurdum* is a common technique. Another dialectical approach is that of denying a presupposition of a thesis and antithesis to achieve a third possible thesis that is the synthesis [30, 31].

Skills for emotional self-regulation were based upon CBT, IPCBT, assertiveness training, and mindfulness meditation. Skills in processing emotions are based upon adaptive awareness, expression, regulation, tolerance, and acceptance of emotions [313].

For a cogent discussion of DBT, we suggest Behavioral Tech [304] and which was started by Marsha Linehan. A periodically updated database of DBT studies can be found here. The following are a few highlights of the evidence-based articles on DBT.

A 12-month outpatient DBT program for patients with BPD in an unselected, comorbid population of female patients (mean age, 32.65 years) produced a significant reduction ($p < 0.05$) of depressive symptoms, suicidal thoughts, anxiety, and anger [309].

A DBT-informed group therapy intensive outpatient program for a sample of participants with mood disorder (80%) and/or anxiety (~50%) showed significant improvement in depression, anxiety, and hope [312]. Over half of the participants had more than one diagnosis, and 20% had comorbid substance abuse or dependence. Treatment duration ranged from 2 to 16 weeks (average was 6 weeks) based on the individual's needs. Although mindfulness did not significantly increase, the amount of increase from baseline of hope and mindfulness predicted the final depression and anxiety levels.

Twelve weekly 90-min sessions of training for euthymic, depressed, or hypomanic Bipolar I or II patients in DBT skills, mindfulness techniques, and psychoeducation of bipolar disorders showed a trend toward reduced depressive symptoms, significant improvement in mindful awareness, and less fear toward and more control of emotional states [310]. In addition, during the following 6 months, there were fewer emergency room visits and mental health admissions.

A 2013 pilot study evaluating the efficacy of integrating PTSD treatment (*Prolonged Exposure (PE))* into DBT for women with BPD, PTSD, and intentional self-injury showed promising results [311]. DBT PE, compared to DBT alone, produced larger and more stable improvements in PTSD and doubled the remission rate among those who completed the protocol (80% vs. 40%). Those who completed the DBT PE protocol vs. the DBT only protocol were 2.4 times less likely to attempt suicide and 1.5 times less likely to perform self-injury. There were moderate to large effect sizes for dissociation, trauma-related guilt cognitions, shame, anxiety, depression, and global functioning in those who completed DBT PE vs. DBT alone.

A gold standard Cochrane Systematic Review by two independent review authors to assess the effects of psychological interventions for BPD was published in 2012 [315]. They concluded that, "none of the treatments has a very robust evidence base, and there are some concerns regarding the quality of individual studies. Overall, the findings support a substantial role for psychotherapy in the treatment of people with BPD but clearly indicate a need for replicatory studies."

A systematic review of randomized clinical trials with meta-analysis and trial sequential analysis published in 2021 concluded that 10 trials on adolescents with BPD had a high risk of bias and very low quality of evidence [473]. As a result, they found that it was very difficult to derive any con-

[13] Intersubjectivity is the variety of possible relations between perspectives.

clusions on the efficacy of psychological therapies for BPD in adolescence.

Cognitive Processing Therapy

Cognitive processing therapy (CPT) was started by Patricia Resick in 1988 and followed up by Candice Monson to treat rape victims who had PTSD [316]. CPT has been extended to treat combat veterans, young adults, refugees, and others who suffer from PTSD [317]. CPT is based upon an *information processing hypothesis of PTSD*. CPT postulates that an individual's beliefs about traumatic events produce strong emotions that prevent appropriate processing of the memory of the trauma. The individual gets stuck and does not adequately recover. In order to unstick the maladaptive behavior, CPT includes elements of education, exposure, and especially cognitive processing [318]. It is a manualized approach, usually of 12 sessions, 90 min each, and can be conducted in individual or group sessions. [319].

In the VA setting, studies have shown consistent improvement in PTSD, depressive symptoms, and other mood disorders [320, 321]. Another study included 50 women diagnosed with PTSD secondary to rape who participated in an RCT of CPT for PTSD [322]. After CPT, changes in rape survivors' trauma-related beliefs were shown to relate to significant improvement in PTSD and depression symptoms 5–10 years after treatment. Reduction in symptoms was linked to increased accommodated (realistic) thinking and decreased over-accommodated or assimilated (distorted) thinking.

Interpersonal Psychotherapy

Interpersonal psychotherapy (IPT) is a structured and time-limited therapy taking 12–16 weeks and is frequently used for unipolar depression [52, 53, 323, 324]. IPT takes its structure from psychodynamic psychotherapy and its time limits, homework, structured interviews, and assessment tools from CBT. IPT has one of the strongest evidence bases for treatment of major depression [325].

Interpersonal problems are the main therapeutic targets of IPT [325]. Whatever the cause of depression, it occurs in an interpersonal context and most often is associated with disruption of significant attachments and social roles [323]. It is believed that reciprocations between interpersonal problems and depression are at the heart of the onset and maintenance of depressive disorders. Consequently, the focus is on the relationship between mood and social circumstances. IPT improves social functioning and builds social support while improving symptoms [323].

Four main areas of interpersonal problems are (1) interpersonal role disputes (antagonistic relationships), (2) role transitions (life disruptions or losses), (3) complicated bereavement (the death of a significant other), and (4) interpersonal deficits (isolative lack of social support). To sever the interactions between problems and depressive symptoms, therapy is based upon improving communication, expressing affect in an effective way to improve social situations, and proactively engaging with their current interpersonal network [324].

Quality of social relationships appears to be a significant risk factor for MDD [326]. In a cohort of 4642 American adults aged 25–75 who completed surveys at baseline in 1995–1996 and at 10-year follow-up, the depression risk was significantly greater in those who had baseline social strain (OR = 1.99; 95% CI: 1.47 to 2.70), lack of social support (OR[14] =1.79; 95% CI: 1.37 to 2.35), and poor overall relationship quality (OR = 2.60; 95% CI: 1.84 to 3.69). Social isolation did not influence future depression or relationship quality. There was more than twice the risk of depression in those who had the lowest overall quality of social relationships (OR = 14.0; 95% CI: 12.0 to 16.0; $p < 0.001$) compared to those who had the highest quality (OR = 6.7; 95% CI: 5.3 to 8.1; $p < 0.001$).

Early work on IPT indicated that when the patient and therapist can maintain a high degree of interpersonal focus, monthly sessions of IPT could have a considerable effect on preventing relapse of depression [327].

IPT has been used for a variety of depressive subtypes, including adolescent [85], geriatric [328], medically ill with MDD [329], postpartum [330], dysthymic disorder [86, 331], and subthreshold depression [332, 333], and as adjunctive therapy to pharmacotherapy for bipolar disorder [334, 335].

Information on obtaining training and certification in IPT can be found at *the International Society of Interpersonal Psychotherapy (ISIPT)* [475].

A 2011 meta-analysis compared IPT with no treatment, usual care, other psychological treatments, and pharmacotherapy [325]. They also analyzed studies that compared combination treatment with pharmacotherapy and IPT. Overall, Cohen's d effect size of 16 studies comparing IPT with a control group was 0.63 (95% CI: 0.36 to 0.90), with a number needed to treat of 2.91. Comparisons of IPT and other psychotherapies ($n = 10$) revealed a nonsignificant

[14]Odds ratio (OR) is a way to represent the odds that an outcome will result when a given exposure to a variable of interest occurs compared to when the exposure does not occur. OR quantifies the strength of the association between two events. An OR greater than 1 indicates a positive association or that exposure to that variable increases the odds of that outcome. An OR less than one indicates a negative relationship between two events. An OR of 1 suggests no relationship between two events. An OR is frequently accompanied by a 95% confidence interval (CI). CI is a measure of precision of the OR. The smaller the CI, the higher precision as long as it does not overlap OR = 1. For more information, see Chap. 4 on evidence basics in this text.

effect size, in favor of IPT, of 0.04 (95% CI: −0.14 to 0.21; number needed to treat = 45.45). After discarding one outlier, IPT was less effective than pharmacotherapy ($d = -0.19$, 95% CI: −0.38 to −0.01; number needed to treat = 9.43). The combination of pharmacotherapy and IPT was not more effective than IPT alone in treating depression. However, maintenance of remission was more effective with pharmacotherapy and IPT than with pharmacotherapy alone (OR = 0.37; 95% CI: 0.19 to 0.73; number needed to treat =7.63).

A systematic review was conducted of RCTs of IPT for MDD in adult outpatients from January 1970 through August 2012 [112]. Unipolar, nonpsychotic MDD was the primary diagnosis. Contradictory results were seen in studies comparing IPT with pharmacotherapy. IPT plus nefazodone improved depressive symptoms significantly better than nefazodone by itself. Nondefined pharmacotherapy plus clinical management improved symptoms better than IPT by itself. Imipramine or IPT plus clinical management was better than placebo plus clinical management. The cognitive behavioral analysis system of psychotherapy did better than IPT, which did better than wait-list control or usual care. The mean difference between CBT and IPT was 1.01 (95% CI: −0.34, 2.37), favoring CBT over IPT, but was not significant. The researchers concluded that the differences between CBT, IPT, and pharmacotherapy are small, and any of these can be recommended for first-line treatment. The study's authors suggest that the results of this review had several limitations, including the small number of studies that met the inclusion criteria. Their bottom line is that patient preferences should be a primary consideration when choosing one of these therapies.

A 2012 meta-analysis comparing CBT and IPT for depression found 7 appropriate trials, all of which carried a high risk of bias [336]. Their analysis showed comparable results in reducing the symptoms of depression.

A Cochrane systematic review published in 2011analyzed the effect of interpersonal psychotherapy and other psychodynamic therapies versus "treatment as usual" in patients with MDD [337]. They found a high risk of bias in the six trials that they analyzed. Results of these studies did show that psychodynamic interventions significantly reduced depressive symptoms on the 17-item Hamilton Rating Scale for Depression (mean difference − 3.12 (95% CI: −4.39 to −1.86; $p < 0.00001$), with no heterogeneity compared with "treatment as usual."

In order to test relative efficacy for depression, 4 weeks of face-to-face cognitive behavioral therapy (CBT) and *Internet-delivered interpersonal psychotherapy* (IPT) were compared to an active control intervention (*MoodGYM*:[339]) [338]. A significant reduction in symptoms was seen in all groups. No differences in clinically significant changes were seen between the groups. Medium to large effect sizes were seen within all groups. Consistently higher rates of reliable change were seen in CBT. IPT participants were less satisfied than were those who took part in CBT or MoodGYM. The dropout rate overall was 70% [1294/1843], with the highest rate for MoodGYM.

A 2013 study found that adolescent interpersonal problems relating to interpersonal stress and loss, poor interpersonal relationships, insecure attachment style, and poor social skills appear more often in depressed adolescents compared to their nondepressed peers [340]. It was uncertain if these problems were causes or effects. The study's authors suggest that IPT would be helpful by focusing on handling interpersonal conflicts, role transitions, and interpersonal losses, and building social support and social skills.

A mixed methods evaluation of the implementation of IPT in the first fully-powered trial of any treatment for MDD in an incarcerated population found that IPT was a good fit for prisoners, and that prisoners and providers were enthusiastic about IPT [341]. An RCT targeting American Indians combined *Historical Trauma and Unresolved Grief Intervention (HTUG)* with Group IPT, to reduce symptoms of depression and related trauma and grief [342, 345].

A 2019 scoping review and historical perspective of IPT can be seen in [343].

According to a meta-analysis, *prevention* of depression symptoms based on interpersonal psychotherapy may be more effective than prevention based on cognitive-behavioral therapy [344].

Psychoeducation

Psychoeducation does not have a consensus definition: this has made it difficult for meta-analyses to evaluate its efficacy [346]. However, it can be said that it is an applied educational intervention usually in a behavioral context [347].

According to Casañas et al., the various interventions that share a didactic and psychoeducational group structure are usually composed of behavioral elements (behavior changes and pleasant activities), cognition (cognitive restructuring and counseling), education (direct instruction and lectures), and enhancing competence (broad skill training); and homework is frequently employed [346]. Pleasant activities are considered quite important as decreased frequency and quality of pleasant activities and increased aversive activities appear to covary with depression [36]. Mood tends to increase with pleasurable activities and decrease with aversive ones.

A central tenet of psychoeducation is that *clearly understanding cause and effects* increases the awareness of resources and potentials within the context of the etiology of the mental disorder and plays an important role in personally changing emotions and behavior. Family members are often included in the psychoeducation process. The ultimate goal is to empower the patient.

Critical analyses have shown that psychoeducation can be effective in managing depression symptoms [346–349]. However, the effects (ranging from 0.21 to 0.80] depend at least upon the type of psychoeducation [346], and the intensity of depression symptoms upon initiation of treatment [350–352]. In addition, the time to possible relapse or symptom recurrence appears to be variable based upon yet not clearly understood factors [346].

Psychoeducational interventions include the *Coping with Depression Course (CWD)* [348, 351, 353]. CWD is a stepped care multicomponent approach [349] of CBT interventions with a psychoeducational format [354], and drug treatment [347]. That is, CWD is a cognitive behavioral intervention delivered by a psychoeducational method [355]. CWD is based upon a classical behavioral model of depression that suggests that depression may be provoked by a stressor that perturbs normal behavior patterns that causing a low rate of response-contingent positive reinforcement [33, 34]. This rate of reinforcement is functionally associated with access to reinforcing events, the impact of certain types of events, and the personal capacity (skills) to act on the environment. If the individual cannot reverse the low rate of reinforcement, increased self-awareness leading to self-criticism and withdrawal behavior may result [35]. It is also suggested that when family and social networks are mobilized to support the depressed person, a negative reinforcing feedback loop can be produced.

CWD can be used with both adolescents and adults [37–40]. It has also been adapted for elderly individuals [41, 42]; frail or cognitively impaired older adults and their caregivers [43, 44]; the prevention of depression in high-risk, low-income, minority medical outpatients [45]; American Indian populations [46]; and individuals attempting smoking cessation [47].

The typical CWD course for adults is highly structured and uses a text and instructional materials [68, 69]. The intervention spans 12 two-hour sessions conducted over 8 weeks. Groups of 6 to 10 are usual. Twice-weekly sessions are held for the first 4 weeks. Follow-up sessions at 1 and 6 months are used to maintain and monitor treatment.

In addition to the skills included in the adult course, the adolescent CWD course [39] adds teaching basic communication, negotiation, and conflict-resolution skills [356]. CWD also has a parallel course for the parents of depressed youths [71].

Sixteen weeks of CWD were delivered for a group of patients, many of whom had experienced multiple episodes of depression and about half of whom were only partially remitted [357, 358]. Two-thirds of the patients showed clinically significant improvements by the end of the intervention. However, the relapse rates after the active intervention were 13.6% at 6 months, 30% at 12 months, 37% at 17 months, and 44.9% at 23 months.

A 2009 meta-analysis of CWD found that CWD resulted in a 38% reduction (incidence rate ratio = 0.62) in the risk of getting MDD and a Cohen's d of 0.28 in treating depression [359].

According to a 2008 meta-analysis, *brief passive psychoeducational interventions (BPPE)* for depression and psychological distress can be effective in reducing symptoms [360]. It was suggested that BPPE is quick and easy to use and inexpensive. And it could be used as the initial step in stepped interventions.

An interesting study of anxiety and depression in an elderly population aged 75 or older combined a *sequential stepped protocol* of watchful waiting, CBT-based bibliotherapy, CBT-based problem-solving, and referral to primary care for medication as needed [361]. The 12-month incidence of anxiety and depression was about half (RR[15] 0.49; 95% CI: 0.24 to 0.98) in the stepped group compared to the usual care group.

The effectiveness of 12 weeks of 1.5 h sessions led by two nurses providing psychoeducational personal care and a healthy lifestyle program for patients with mild/moderate depression symptoms showed good results for patients with mild depression but not for moderate depression [346]. Among individuals with mild depression, 59% of the intervention group showed improvement at the 6-month follow-up, compared to 42% in the usual care group. At the 9-month follow-up, 65% improved in the intervention group versus 38% in the control group, representing a significant between-group difference of 27% (p = 0.006). The moderately depressed group showed significant improvement at the end of the intervention, but the results were not sustained.

Psychodynamic Psychotherapy

A meta-analytical comparison of CBT and psychodynamic psychotherapy has found CBT to be superior in treating anxiety and depression [362]. However, another meta-analysis published in 2008 has found that all the major psychotherapies (cognitive-behavior therapy, nondirective supportive treatment, behavioral activation treatment, psychodynamic treatment, problem-solving therapy, interpersonal psycho-

[15] *Relative risk (RR)* is perhaps the most common method of expressing the estimated risk of experiencing a result. RR compares the probability of a specific outcome in the treatment group with that of a control group. When an RR is greater than 1, there seems to be an increased risk of an event. When the RR is less than 1, there appears to be a decreased risk of experiencing an event. If the RR is 1, there is no apparent risk. If the RR = 5, it is 5 times more likely to occur than in the control group. If the RR = 0.5, it is half as likely to happen as in the control group. For more information, see Chap. 4 Evidence Basics.

therapy, and social skills training) used for treating mild to moderate depression are about equal in efficacy [48].

Short-term psychodynamic psychotherapy (STPP) may be effective in treating adults who have depressive symptoms [363]. Meta-analysis published in 2010 found STPP was significantly more effective than control at posttreatment ($d = 0.69$). Depression level changes during treatment were large ($d = 1.34$) and persisted at least through 1 year follow-up. Other psychotherapies appeared to be better immediately after treatment ($d = -0.30$), but there were no significant differences at 3 months ($d = -0.05$) and 1-year follow-up. Group formats showed significantly lower effect sizes ($d = 0.83$) than individual treatment ($d = 1.48$). Expressive ($d = 1.30$) and supportive ($d = 1.36$) modes were equally effective.

A 2011Cochrane systematic review was conducted with meta-analysis and trial sequential analysis of randomized trials comparing the effect of psychodynamic therapies versus "treatment as usual" for major depressive disorder [337]. They found that psychodynamic interventions significantly reduced depressive symptoms on the 17-item Hamilton Rating Scale for Depression (mean difference − 3.12 (95% CI: −4.39 to −1.86; $p < 0.00001$), no heterogeneity) compared with "treatment as usual." Trial sequential analysis confirmed the result. However, they concluded, "We did not find convincing evidence supporting or refuting the effect of interpersonal psychotherapy or psychodynamic therapy compared with 'treatment as usual' for patients with major depressive disorder. The potential beneficial effect seems small, and effects on major outcomes are unknown."

A 2012 systematic review of RCTs with meta-analyses and trial sequential analyses measured the effect of adding psychodynamic therapy to antidepressants in patients with major depressive disorder [364]. They found psychodynamic therapy significantly reduced depressive symptoms on the 17-item Hamilton Rating Scale for Depression (mean difference − 3.01 (95% CI: −3.98 to −2.03; $p < 0.00001$), no significant heterogeneity between trials) compared with "no intervention." Trial sequential analysis confirmed this result. However, they concluded that the results are based on a few trials with a high risk of bias and a limited number of participants. Adding psychodynamic therapy to antidepressants might be helpful, but the treatment effect is small.

Internet-Based Psychotherapy

Prevalence, severity, and comorbidity of 12-month DSM-IV disorders in the National Comorbidity Survey Replication conducted between February 2001 and April 2003 indicated that about 7% of the population in the USA suffered from depression [67]. Published in 2019, MDD global prevalence and incidence were meta-analyzed to quantify the burden in the *Global Burden of Disease (GBD) 2017 Study* [366]. Results from 1990 were compared to those in 2017 [365]. During that time, incident cases of depression increased worldwide from 172 million to 258 million: an increase of almost 50%. People who have major depressive disorder have almost twice the mortality of nondepressed persons [367]. They also have higher medical costs [368] and exacerbations of other medical conditions [369].

In 2016–2017, data were analyzed that were collected from April 2012 to June 2013, from the *National Epidemiologic Survey on Alcohol and Related Conditions III (NESARC-III)* [370]. Using DSM-5 criteria, they found 12-month and lifetime prevalence of MDD were 10.4% and 20.6%, respectively.

Symptoms of depression and depressive disorders appear to affect between one-quarter to more than one-third of primary care patients, many of whom do not receive or do not complete treatment [371, 372]. Psychotherapy is effective in treating depression [373], and most patients prefer psychotherapy instead of medications [374–376]. Most primary care patients considered antidepressants to be addictive and psychotherapy to cure the cause of depression. However, when referred for psychotherapy, most patients do not follow through [377]. Furthermore, rates of dropping out of clinical psychotherapy are quite high, often 50% or more [378]. In addition, in clinical trials, it is frequently 30% [48].

One of the possible explanations for low usage of psychotherapy is access barriers [379–381]. Some studies have reported that up to 75% of depressed primary care patients describe barriers that make it very difficult or impossible to take part in regular sessions. These include a dearth of available and accessible services, time constraints, cost, and transportation difficulties.

Some Internet-based interventions for depression are showing promising results in changing that situation. Delivery of CBT in primary care, including computer- or Internet-based self-help programs, can be successful [382]. According to the *Interapy* research group of the University of Amsterdam [383], which has been examining the effects of online cognitive behavioral treatment since 1996, online CBT is a viable and effective alternative to face-to-face treatment [384, 385]. They have found that overall treatment adherence was 82%, and reductions in psychopathology have a large between-group effect size of SMD[16] = 0.9 (95%

[16]*Standardized mean difference [SMD]* is a measure of effect size in meta-analyses when the studies all assess the same outcome but measure it in a variety of ways [122]. In systematic reviews, the SMD is the mean difference in depression score between the intervention and control groups divided by the pooled SD at follow-up. This gives a unit-free effect size. The conventional SMD effect sizes of 0.2 (small), 0.5 (medium), and 0.8 (large) are used. Dichotomous variables are usually expressed as risk ratio with a 95% CI. For more information, see Chap. 4 Evidence Basics.

CI: 0.7 to 1.1), with a strong postintervention continuation of positive results.

A systematic review and meta-analysis of *online CBT (oCBT) for MDD* showed that therapist-supported oCBT was equivalent to face-to-face CBT at improving depressive symptoms and was better than treatment-as-usual, waitlist control, and attention control [386]. There was some evidence that oCBT was more costly but produced greater benefits in the short term.

In 2019, a systematic review was conducted of prevention programs targeting depression, anxiety, and stress in college, graduate, or professional students across 15 countries [387]. Programs were delivered in a group-based, online/computer-delivered, or self-administered format and at the universal, selective, or indicated prevention level. Moderate average effect sizes (overall $g = 0.65$) were achieved irrespective of prevention level or delivery format. Overall, and for programs generating large effects, the most common programs were psychoeducation (72%), relaxation (69%), and cognitive monitoring/restructuring (47%).

The *International Society for Research on Internet Interventions (ISRII)* was formed in 2004 to encourage eHealth researchers to collaborate in their efforts to further the science behind developing, testing, and disseminating Web-based treatment programs [388, 389].

A 2018 meta-analysis and systematic review of third-wave behavioral and cognitive eHealth treatment can be found in [157]. The reviewers concluded that *third-wave eHealth* significantly outperformed inactive control conditions in improving anxiety, depression, and quality-of-life outcomes. In addition, third-wave eHealth significantly outperformed active control conditions in alleviating anxiety and depression. There were small to medium effect sizes. They did not find significant differences compared to other interventions.

The following are some examples of Internet-based interventions for treating depression.

A web-based guided self-help intervention *(GET. ON-Mood Enhancer-WL)* was developed for patients waiting to begin inpatient therapy for MDD [390]. The idea is that patients may reduce the wait for admission and get a jump-start on the reduction of their symptoms before starting inpatient treatment. The hope is that this might decrease inpatient time, reduce cost, and possibly increase remission rates.

A *transdiagnostic Internet-based maintenance treatment (TIMT)* has been designed for a wide range of patients who have different clinical, motivational, and demographic characteristics [391, 392]. The designers of the program hope that it will be particularly effective for participants who are not well educated. TIMT involves an online self-management module, asynchronous patient–therapist communication, a peer support group, and online-based progress monitoring. Results of an RCT indicated that TIMT vs. the control was most effective among participants with a low (vs. high) education, participants with high (vs. low) positive outcome expectations, and participants with anxiety disorder (vs. mood disorder). However, all subgroups still benefited significantly.

A *culturally sensitive, guided, self-help, problem-solving* intervention through the Internet for reducing depressive symptoms in Turkish migrants did not show a significant effect [393]. However, the effect size was high, but the sample may not have been large enough to accurately measure the possible effectiveness.

Evidence suggests that different online mental health programs may offer greater benefits to patients with specific characteristics [394]. A fully automated, self-guided randomized controlled intervention incorporating Interpersonal Psychotherapy (IPT) and Cognitive Behavioral Therapy (CBT) was delivered over a 4-week period to spontaneous visitors of an Internet-based therapy website. This intervention was compared to an active control condition, MoodGYM [339, 395]. Results indicated that regardless of the intervention, being female, lower mastery, and lower dysfunctional attitudes predicted better outcomes at posttest and/or follow-up. It seems that for older folks, CBT may be most beneficial, whereas for younger folks, IPT may be preferable. Despite a large sample size, there was not sufficient power to detect moderator effects.

In order to test relative efficacy for depression, 4 weeks of face-to-face *cognitive behavioral therapy (CBT)* and *Internet-delivered interpersonal psychotherapy (IPT)* were compared to an active control intervention (*MoodGYM*: [339]) [338]. A significant reduction in symptoms was seen in all groups. No differences in clinically significant changes were seen between the groups. Medium to large effect sizes were seen within all groups. Consistently higher rates of reliable change were seen in CBT. IPT participants were less satisfied than were those who took part in CBT or MoodGYM. The dropout rate overall was 70% [1294/1843], with the highest rate for MoodGYM.

Master Your Mood (MYM) is a cognitive-based, online intervention for young adults who have depressive symptoms [396, 397]. To determine if circularity between anxiety and depression was associated with mastery symptoms, 244 participants with depressive symptoms were examined. Results indicated that comorbidity of depression and anxiety was high (69.2%) and the association between depression and changing anxiety was strong ($r = 0.677$, $p < 0.01$); changes in depression mediated changes in anxiety (79%) and mastery (75%). Changes in anxiety and mastery mediated change in depression (mediation proportion 44%). They did not find that an early change in anxiety predicted a late change in depression, and vice versa.

The onset of depression is usually in adolescence, an age group wherein services are readily used [398]. ICBT for adults shows good results in treating depression, so an RCT investigated the effect of MYM, which was designed for people aged 16–25 years, compared to a wait-listed control group [22677437]. The MYM group demonstrated significantly greater improvement than the control group in depressive symptoms at 3 months ($p < 0.001$), with a large between-group effect size of $d = 0.94$ (95% CI: 0.64–1.23). The MYM group also had greater improvement in anxiety $p < 0.001$, $d = 0.49$, (95% CI: 0.24 to 0.75) and mastery $p = 0.001$, $d = 0.44$, (95% CI: 0.19 to 0.70). At 12 weeks, 56% (68/121) of the participants in the MYM group and 20% (24/123) in the control group demonstrated reliable and clinically significant change ($p < 0.001$) with a number needed to treat of 2.7. MYM group improvements were maintained at 6 months.

A 45-min, eight-session interactive computer software program called *Stressbusters* is based upon a clinically effective in-person CBT protocol for teenagers who have mild to moderate depression [399]. In a small trial of Stressbusters, 95% of the participants met the criteria for depression with a group score of 35.48, while postintervention, 22% met the criteria for depression with a group mean score of 20.32. These significant gains were maintained at the 3-month follow-up. Significant improvements were seen in global functioning, self-reported anxiety, depressive cognitions, and attributions, and in self- and parent-reported emotional and behavioral problems.

It has been suggested that for Internet-based cognitive therapies to work well, it is important to make a proper diagnosis before the treatment starts, and to use a comprehensive treatment that is user-friendly and not too technically advanced support. And it is vital to provide adequate support and a clear deadline throughout the treatment [400].

Internet cognitive behavioral therapy (ICBT) is delivered via a diverse amount of contact with the therapist, and it consists of a variety of treatment content [401, 402]. Contact ranges from nonexistent to a complete pretreatment assessment and continuous support during treatment. A review of RCTs has shown a strong correlation between the degree of support and outcome. Treatment content may also modify results.

ICBT for MDD appears to be most effective when therapist support is through email or telephone calls [403]. Text-based treatments are less sensitive to therapist effects, and nontargeted treatment effects seem to be more sensitive to the way therapy is presented and by whom.

ICBT can be as effective as face-to-face CBT [404]. However, there has been some concern that poor patient compliance with homework and other adherence issues are frequent, along with psychotherapists drifting away from best evidence-based CBT [405]. To overcome these deficiencies, a novel approach blended ICBT with conventional CBT was devised [405]. They designed an online support system of basic CBT components and a library of interventions from ICBT manuals that could be used by both patients and therapists. Patients with mild to moderate anxiety and/or depression participated in the 9-week intervention and were followed up at 12 months. Symptoms across all measures were significantly reduced: 60 to 87% reliability changes were observed for both anxiety and depression. Large effect sizes were seen: Cohen's d ranged from 1.62 (95% CI: 0.59 to 2.66) to 2.43 (95% CI: 1.12 to 3.74). Patients felt that the interventions were helpful. No problems with compliance, and no dropouts were seen, and results were maintained for at least 12 months.

American Psychological Association criteria for empirically supported treatments [406] were used to determine efficacy and cost-effectiveness in a meta-analysis of RCTs for ICBT [404]. Although 25 different clinical disorders had been examined, most ICBT RCTs examined depression, anxiety, and chronic pain. The highest level of evidence was well established for depression, social phobia, and panic disorder. RCTs of depression, anxiety disorders, severe health anxiety, irritable bowel syndrome, female sexual dysfunction, eating disorders, cannabis use, and pathological gambling all yielded large effect sizes. Effect sizes were small to moderate for other clinical disorders. Conventional CBT and ICBT showed equivalent results. The large effect sizes and the limited therapist time appear to make ICBT highly cost-effective.

An additional study has indicated that the return on investment of using preventive telemedicine for depressive disorders seems to be a better value than a healthcare system that does not use Internet-based prevention [407].

An eight lesson Internet based diabetes specific CBT for depression with minimal therapist support showed that MDD, anxiety disorder, and elevated diabetes distress were not significant effect modifiers in the treatment of self-assessed depressive symptoms [408]. Results suggested that this approach was suitable for patients who have a range of mental health problems.

Guided ICBT for insomnia has resulted in good acceptance by patients and improved sleep [409].

Both ICBT and *Internet psychodynamic therapy (IPDT)* for depression treatment can be delivered successfully via the Internet [410]. In a head-to-head comparison, both performed equally well in decreasing depression symptoms. Strength of preference was associated with following the treatment regimen and completing the program, and for the ICBT, for the long-term outcome. Greater completion rates were seen with IPDT, but at follow-up, those who chose ICBT showed greater improvements in quality of life. ICBT participants also showed a significant increase in those who recovered from depression between posttreatment to follow-up.

Guided *Internet-based cognitive behavior therapy (ICBT)* has been effectively used to treat depression and anxiety, including *generalized anxiety disorder (GAD)* [404]. The efficacy of *Internet-based psychodynamic therapy (IPDT)* to treat GAD has been compared to ICBT and a wait-list control [411]. Both ICBT and IPDT showed a modest reduction in symptoms compared to controls. Immediately posttreatment, there were no significant differences between the groups; however, ICBT and IPDT at 3- and 18-month follow-up showed moderate to large within-group effect sizes.

Adult MDD participants who had 10 weeks of *Internet psychodynamic psychotherapy (IPDT)* made large and better improvements compared to an active control group (a structured support intervention that contained psychoeducation and scheduled weekly contacts online) [410]. The Beck Depression Inventory-II (BDI-II) showed a between-group Cohen's d effect size of 1.11. Treatment effects were maintained at a 10-month follow-up.

Comparisons of *Internet cognitive behavioral therapy (ICBT), Internet problem-solving therapy (IPST),* and a waiting list control group found ICBT and IPST were more effective than controls in improving depression symptoms [412, 413]. Dysfunctional attitudes, worrying, negative problem orientation, and perceived control were all important in ICBT as well as in IPST. Both ICBT and IPST appear to have a high probability of being cost-effective as well as useful for treating depression [414].

IPST has shown good results in treating the commonly associated depression of patients who have multiple sclerosis [415]. The compliance rate was 52%. Depression symptoms significantly decreased, $p = 0.01$, $d = 0.51$ in intention-to-treat analysis and $p < 0.001$, $d = 1.50$ in completers analysis. The intervention was rated as good or excellent by 85% of the patients.

In further attempts to determine for whom Internet therapy is best for depression treatment, 8 weeks of *ICBT* was compared to 8 weeks of *Internet-based problem-solving therapy (IPST)* [416]. Improvement was predicted by higher baseline depression and higher education. Clinically significant change across all participants was associated with higher education, less avoidance behavior, and decreased rational problem-solving skills. They did not find any variables that predicted differences in outcomes between ICBT and PST.

However, reported in 2012, a 5-week IPST for adolescents compared to a waiting-list control did not show greater efficacy in reducing mild to moderate symptoms of depression or anxiety [417]. Both groups did show improvements in symptoms.

Attempts have been made to develop a clear theoretical model based on relevant empirical research that can guide the development of human support components, *manualization* of *eHealth* interventions [418]. One of the attempts has been developing a model called *Supportive Accountability* in which human support increases patient adherence by being accountable to a coach who is perceived to be a trustworthy, benevolent expert [418]. Important issues include patient participation in determining clear, process-oriented expectations and explicit reciprocity with clear benefits. The more intrinsically motivated a patient is, the less support they are likely to need. The type of medium used for communication (such as e-mail, texting, or telephone) has its benefits and deficiencies.

However, poor adherence results were obtained when a comparison was made between a 12-week manualized telephone coaching intervention (*TeleCoach*) designed to increase adherence to a web-based intervention (*moodManager*) and 12 weeks of moodManager without coaching [419,420]. Compared to a wait list control, *TeleCoach + moodManager*, compared to self-directed moodManager, achieved significantly more login days ($p = 0.01$), more time until last use ($p = 0.007$), more lessons ($p = 0.03$), greater variety of interactive tools used ($p = 0.02$), but not significantly more tool use ($p = 0.07$). Greater adherence was seen with TeleCoach+moodManager. However, most users had stopped treatment by week 12. Significantly greater reductions in depression scores at any time and with respect to self-directed moodManager were only seen for TeleCoach+moodManager relative to wait list control at week 6 ($p = 0.04$). Baseline depression scores were not related to adherence issues.

A Web-based intervention, *Living to the Full*, for the prevention of depression using both a fully automated and human-supported format was used in an attempt to determine characteristics that would modify adherence to the protocol, elements of the program that would make a difference to adherence, and what patterns of usage might be different between adherers and nonadherers [421]. Being female (OR = 2.02; 95% CI: 1.01–4.04; $p = 0.046$) and having a higher need for cognition (OR = 1.02; 95% CI: 1.00 to 1.05; $p = 0.02$) increased the odds of adhering to the intervention. Adherers logged in significantly more times per lesson than nonadherers ($p < 0.001$). Overall, they found that characteristics of users are significantly associated with adherence, but their predictive values are small.

An 8-week ICBT for depression targeted registered university students to specifically address engagement issues, especially by integrating online therapist support and communication within the interactive platform [422]. Results showed a high level of engagement and statistically significant ($p < 0.001$) decrease in self-reported depressive symptomatology with a large effect size ($d = 1.17$).

A six-session interactive guided Web-based intervention for postpartum depression, *MomMoodBooster* (MMB), has shown promising results [426]. Results indicated that 87%

(46/53) of participants completed all sessions with a high degree of usage. At pretest, 55% (29/53) of participants met criteria for minor or major depression. Three months after enrolling in the program, 90% (26/29) no longer met the criteria.

To better understand motivators to encourage use of a primary care support portal focused on an *Internet-based peer support group* (*Psycho-Babble*) for depression, an RCT was set up [372]. The portal connected primary care patients to fact-based information and Psycho-Babble. Psycho-Babble permitted visitors to view messages and then to decide if they wanted to register there. After randomization, three groups were populated. The control was a simple generic referral card. The external motivator was a physician's letter of recommendation. The internal motivator was a patient-oriented brochure with examples of online postings and experience. Out of 50 participants, 62% visited the portal and 54% visited Psycho-Babble. The internally motivated group showed significantly greater participation than the control group, whereas the externally motivated group spent significantly less time in the portal than the control group. The internals demonstrated significantly greater participation than the externals. So, it would seem that the internally motivated folks were more inclined to use the peer support group.

Providing *telephone-administered CBT* for 18 weeks to primary care patients compared to in-person CBT decreased the attrition rate and close to the same improvement in depression at the end of the intervention and at 6-month follow-up compared to baseline ($p < 0.001$) [423]. However, at 6-month follow-up, those who had face-to-face CBT were significantly less depressed than the group who had the telephone CBT: Ham-D (difference, 2.91; 95% CI: 1.20–4.63; $P < 0.001$) and the PHQ-9 (difference, 2.12; 95% CI: 0.68–3.56; $P = 0.004$).

Another telephone-administered CBT (TCBT) showed that TCBT was not inferior to face-to-face CBT except for people with more severe depression [424].

Evaluation of an 11-week *computerized cognitive-bias modification (CBM)* protocol for MDD targeting imagery and interpretation bias (CBM-I) independently and combined with Internet-based cognitive behavioral therapy (ICBT) has shown promising results [425]. The combined protocol was 1 week of CBM-I + 10 weeks of ICBT. Significantly decreased primary symptoms compared to a wait list control were seen with a medium to large effect sizes (Cohen's $d = 0.62–2.40$) with both CBM-I and the combined protocol. Following the combined treatment, significant reductions were also seen in disability, anxiety, and repetitive negative thinking (Cohen's $d = 1.51–2.23$). Following CBM-I, 27% of the patients demonstrated clinically significant improvement. With combined treatment, the percentage improved to 65%.

Studies have suggested that guided self-help based on cognitive-behavioral principles for eating disorders is a brief, cost-effective treatment that can be implemented by a wide range of mental health providers, including nonspecialists, by either personal contact or Internet-based technology [428]. It appears that such an approach can be an effective treatment for binge eating disorder and bulimia nervosa, but it is contraindicated for anorexia nervosa.

Computer-aided (including stand-alone or Internet-linked computers, palmtop computers, phone-interactive voice response, DVDs, and cell phones) psychotherapies for anxiety disorders have also shown promise [429]. A 2009 meta-analysis found an overall mean effect size of a computer-aided compared with a noncomputer-aided aided to be 1.08 (95% CI: 0.84–1.32). Comparison of computer-aided and face-to-face psychotherapy showed no significant difference (13 comparisons, $d = -0.06$).

Mobilyze!, a mobile phone- and Internet-based intervention including ecological momentary intervention and context sensing, has been undergoing preliminary investigations into its feasibility to assist in treating MDD [430]. To use the researchers' own description: "machine learning predicted patients' mood, emotions, cognitive/motivational states, activities, environmental context, and social context based on at least 38 concurrent phone sensor values (e.g., global positioning system, ambient light, recent calls)." Their website included "feedback graphs illustrating correlations between patients' self-reported states, as well as didactics and tools teaching patients behavioral activation concepts. Brief telephone calls and emails with a clinician were used to promote adherence." The concept was evaluated on 8 MDD patients. Based upon categorical contextual states, accuracy was 60 to 91%, but predictive accuracy based upon scales was poor. Participants reported significant improvement in depression symptoms ($p < 0.001$, per-protocol Cohen $d = 3.43–3.55$). Per protocol remission rate was 85.71% ($p = 0.03$), and comorbid anxiety symptoms significantly improved ($p < 0.001$, per-protocol Cohen $d = 2.58$).

Self-management supported by online CBT with therapist support, accompanied by *Short Message Service (SMS) based tele-monitoring of depressive symptomatology (Mobile Cognitive Therapy)*, has been proposed as an approach to prevent relapse in remitted recurrent MDD [431].

A comprehensive literature search (2008–2013) in MEDLINE, Embase, the Cochrane Central Register of Controlled Trials, PsycINFO, PsycTESTS, Compendex, and Inspec reviewed the evidence for the efficacy of *mental health apps* for mobile devices (such as smartphones and tablets) [432]. They examined apps for depression, anxiety, substance use, sleep disturbances, suicidal behavior, self-harm, psychotic disorders, eating disorders, stress, and gambling. They identified 5464 abstracts. Of those, 5 apps that targeted depression, anxiety, and substance abuse met the criteria for further evidence-based evaluation. Two of these were available commercially. Four of the apps provided support from a professional mental health worker. Significant reductions in depression, stress, and substance use were seen. Within-group and between-group intention-to-treat effect sizes ranged from 0.29 to 2.28 at posttest and 0.01–0.48 at follow-up. Most apps that are currently available do not have scientific evidence for their efficacy.

In 2016, a systematic review identified self-help apps available exclusively for people with depression and evaluated those that offer CBT or behavioral activation (BA) [433]. They found 117 apps of those 12 (10.26%) offer support that seems to be consistent with evidence-based principles of CBT or BA. The reviewers question the utility of these apps due to the nonexistence of effectiveness/efficacy studies, and the low level of adherence to the core ingredients of the CBT/BA models. They found usability to be highly variable and rarely accompanied by explicit privacy or safety policies.

A 2017 systematic review studied the efficacy, usability, and feasibility of mobile apps and short message service as mHealth interventions for self-guided care [434]. *Short message service (SMS)* messages involve psychoeducation, medication reminders, and links to useful, informative Web pages. RCTs showed improvement in physical health and significant reductions in anxiety, stress, and depression. Within-group and between-group effect sizes ranged from 0.05 to 3.37 (immediately posttest), 0.05–3.25 (1-month follow-up), 0.08–3.08 (2-month follow-up), 0.00–3.10 (3-month follow-up), and 0.02–0.27 (6-month follow-up). Promising, significant results of usability and feasibility of mHealth interventions were also seen. A 2018 systematic review produced the same conclusions [435].

A systematic review of mental health mobile apps for preadolescents and adolescents was published in 2017 in *The Journal of Medical Internet Research* [436, 437]. They concluded that there is currently insufficient research evidence to support the effectiveness of apps for children, preadolescents, and adolescents with mental health problems. New mHealth apps are being released at a rapid pace with very little done to evaluate their safety, efficacy, and effectiveness.

Patient Interest and barriers to engagement on the adoption of mobile apps for depression and anxiety were examined in a cross-sectional survey study of veterans [438]. At a single Veterans Health Administration facility, 149 veterans who attended an appointment in early 2016 that was associated with either unipolar depression, any anxiety disorder, or posttraumatic stress disorder were studied. High-interest ratings were for context-sensitive apps (85.2%, 127/149), and apps focused on increasing exercise (75.8%, 113/149), improving sleep (73.2%, 109/149), changing negative thinking (70.5%, 105/149), and increasing involvement in activities (67.1%, 100/149). The study suggested that improved adoption of apps might be achieved by including provider endorsement, greater publicity of efficacious apps, and clear messaging about efficacy and privacy of information. In addition, they suggest multifaceted apps that address a range of concerns, from sleep to negative thought patterns, may be the best received.

Health professionals' perspective on the promotion of e-mental health apps in the context of maternal depression was gathered from the USA, Spain, and Swiss health professionals in the field of pregnancy and maternal health by means of an online survey [439]. Health professionals would, in general, intend to recommend and use e-mental health applications. But attitudes about e-mental health applications vary regarding their respective use (positive psychology intervention, assessment and diagnosis, prevention program, and treatment program) and among health professions. For most of the uses, psychologists and psychiatrists see the value in e-mental health apps, but they are skeptical about the assessment, diagnosis, and treatment of depression. The literature suggests that at least part of the reasons for the skepticism is the lack of technology usage and the fear of being replaced by technology [440, 441].

In 2018, mobile mental health apps were analyzed to determine whether the app had been developed with mental health expert input; if they had been developed in association with a government body, academic institution, or medical facility; and if they were free to download [442]. Apple App Store and Google Play Store revealed a total of 293 apps that claimed to have an evidence base. Overall, only 3.41% of apps cited published research to justify their claims of effectiveness. The majority of that research was done by those involved in developing the app. Only 1.02% of the 293 apps had support shown in independent research. Of these apps, 30.38% claimed to have expert development input; 20.48% were affiliated with a government body, academic institution, or medical facility; and 74.06% were free to download.

More Psychotherapies

Trials of adding *psychosocial mood management* to a standard smoking cessation program have indicated that long-term cessation rates in smokers with both current and past depression are enhanced compared with the standard intervention alone without necessarily preventing the recurrence of depression [443, 444].

A study in the Netherlands has indicated that in psychiatric patients, the symptoms of depression, general anxiety, and agoraphobia were more severe in nicotine-dependent smokers than in never-smokers, former smokers, and nondependent smokers [445].

Results of a meta-analysis suggest that *mindfulness-based stress reduction (MBSR)* appears to have a small effect on depression, anxiety, and psychological distress in people with chronic somatic diseases [271].

Hypnotherapy may be a useful adjunct to CBT for depression [446–449].

Integrating *systematic emotion regulation training (ERT)* may enhance the efficacy of routine inpatient cognitive behavioral therapy (CBT) for MDD [450]. An RCT showed significantly greater reduction in depression (response rates—CBT: 75.5%, CBT-ERT: 84.9%; remission rates—CBT: 51.1%, CBT-ERT: 65.1%). CBT-ERT participants had a significantly greater reduction of negative affect, and a greater increase of well-being and emotion regulation skills.

One proposal for delivering accessible, effective, and efficient services to treat depression is *Stepped Care* [451–453]. Stepped care results are carefully monitored by a care manager. It begins with low-cost self-management and proceeds to higher-cost treatments only if necessary. All treatments are evidence-based. The first step is watchful waiting. Spontaneous recovery of half of all patients is likely to occur within 3 months. The second step is guided self-help, a central tenet of stepped care. It is frequently delivered through the Internet or CBT-based bibliotherapy. The third step is brief face-to-face psychotherapy, usually CBT-based, and problem-solving. The fourth step is continued face-to-face psychotherapy with the possibility of adding an antidepressant.

Stepped care in the elderly has shown promising results [453, 454]. One study found that stepped care decreased by 50% the incidence of depression and anxiety after 1 year and sustained these effects for 24 months [453, 454]. Another RCT examined the stepped effects on individuals 75 years and older who had subthreshold symptom levels of depression or anxiety who did not meet the full diagnostic criteria for the disorders [361]. In the elderly, subthreshold symptom levels of depression or anxiety carry a high prevalence and an unfavorable prognosis, predicting significant pathology. Twelve-month incidence of depressive and anxiety disorders decreased from 0.24 (20 of 84) in the usual care group to 0.12 (10 of 86) in the stepped-care group (relative risk, 0.49; 95% CI: 0.24 to 0.98).

Rumination is an important component of anxiety and depression. Rumination is compulsively focused attention on one's own symptoms of distress, their possible causes and consequences, rather than their solutions. As opposed to worry, which focuses on potential bad events, rumination focuses on past bad feelings and events [455]. A time-limited cognitive behavioral intervention (*Competitive Memory Training,* or *COMET* for depressive rumination) has been investigated for its effect on depression and rumination in older adult depressed outpatients [456]. The RCT used two treatment conditions: 7 weeks of COMET + treatment-as-usual (TAU) versus TAU only. COMET + TAU yielded significant improvements in depression and rumination compared with TAU alone.

One of the self-guided sole or supplementary therapies for mild to moderate depression or subthreshold symptoms is bibliotherapy. *Bibliotherapy* is a home-based therapy in which a patient more or less independently works through a standardized treatment in the form of a structured book [457]. There is no traditional relationship with a therapist: therapist support is facilitative or supportive in answering any questions or concerns that the patient may have.

It is generally believed that patients need to have a reading ability above 12 years of age and a positive disposition about self-help. A typical approach begins with an intake in which the patient learns about the options and chooses a book. This is followed in 2 weeks by a 30-min consultation to answer any questions and provide empathetic support. Depending upon the patient's progress, ongoing contact is arranged, which is generally once a week. This may be face-to-face, email, or telephone. The therapist and the patient determine the duration of therapy.

Frequently, used books that may be available from a library or purchased, and may be available as e-books, include the following [50, 51].

1. *Feeling good: the new mood therapy*, by David D. Burns. New York: HarperCollins Publishers, 1999.
2. *Beating the blues: a self-help approach to overcoming depression*, by Susan Tanner and Jillian Ball. Sydney: Susan Tanner and Jillian Ball, 1998.
3. *Change your thinking: overcome stress, anxiety, and depression, and improve your life with CBT*, by Sarah Edelman. San Francisco: Marlow and Company, 2007.
4. *Mind over mood: change how you feel by changing the way you think*, by Dennis Greenberger and Christine Padesky. New York: The Guilford Press, 1995.
5. *Control your depression*, by Peter Lewinsohn, Ricardo Muñoz, Mary Ann Youngren, and Antoinette Zeiss. New York: Fireside, 1992.
6. *Dealing with depression*, by Gordon Parker. Sydney: Allen & Unwin, 2004.

A meta-analysis published in 2010 compared *guided self-help* for depression and anxiety to face-to-face psychotherapies for depression and anxiety [458]. Results indicated that the overall effect size of the difference between self-help and face-to-face was $d = -0.02$ in favor of guided self-help. There was no difference in dropout rates. At 1-year follow-up, there were no significant differences.

Bibliotherapy was not more successful than usual care in reducing depression in folks 75 years and older [459]. Guidelines for bibliotherapy for older adults have been presented in reference [460].

Brief CBT for adolescent MDD significantly reduced MDD onset compared to brochure control and bibliotherapy [461]. CBT risk was 0.8% vs. CB bibliotherapy (6.3%) and brochure control (6.5%); hazard ratios = 8.1 and 8.3, respectively. However, the 6-month follow-up showed no significant difference among any of the interventions. Four weeks of cognitive bibliotherapy for depressive symptoms may be useful for jail and prison inmates [462].

At least with panic disorder, pacing of the bibliotherapy material does not seem to be important [463]. Bibliotherapy was seen to decrease the psychological distress of a group of folks in Thailand who were suffering from moderate depression [464]. A small study where patients were assigned to read Burns' book Feeling Good (q.s.) or usual care often involving antidepressants, showed equal effects in significantly decreasing depression symptoms and dysfunctional attitudes, and increasing quality of life [465].

For a group of patients 60 years of age or older, 16 sessions of CBT and reading Feeling Good showed individualized CBT to be superior at posttreatment in terms of self-rated depression, but not to be any different on clinician-rated depression; both were superior to delayed treatment control [466]. However, those who had participated in bibliotherapy continued to improve to the extent that 3 months after treatment, there were no differences between the groups. Similar maintenance of results has been seen in to be maintained for at least 2 years [467], or 3 years after bibliotherapy for folks with mild to moderate depression [468].

Estimates of the prevalence of depression in *cancer* vary between 8 and 24% depending largely upon the type of cancer and methods used for evaluation [469].

Meaning-centered interventions for cancer have suggested that relationships and experiences are the predominant themes [470]. Some cancer survivors find enhanced meaning through relationships, experiences, resilience, goal-orientation, and leaving a legacy. Other survivors suffer a loss of meaning through experiences, social roles, relationships, and uncertainties about their future.

A review of psychological and pharmacological approaches has found that therapy can be successfully targeted to deal with depression arising from cancer [97].

Multiconvergent therapy (MCT), a type of psychotherapy that combines mindfulness meditation with CBT, has been used in the management of irritable bowel syndrome (IBS) [472].

To test the effects of Internet-based CBT, callers to Australia's 24 h telephone counseling service received either 6 weeks of Internet CBT plus weekly telephone follow-up; Internet CBT only; weekly telephone follow-up only, or a wait-list treatment as usual control group [471]. All participants showed significant reductions in suicidal ideation over 12 months ($p < 0.001$). Those patients who had higher baseline suicidal behavior had less chance of postintervention remission of suicidal ideation (OR = 0.409, $p < 0.001$). Decreased depression during treatment was associated with decreased suicidal ideation (OR = 1.165, $p < 0.001$).

Summary

A variety of psychotherapies have been examined, and many of them offer hope for those who suffer from depression. Unfortunately, many of these analyses and studies have been beset with heterogeneity and bias of various kinds. Nevertheless, glimpses have been seen of the human variables that increase the likelihood of successful treatment and prevention of depression. Awareness of these mediators may allow for a more individually targeted psychotherapy.

CBT is the mainstay of psychotherapy for depression. Comprehensive meta-analyses have found CBT for depression has a moderate to large effect size across different delivery formats, ages, and target groups. CBT's effect is as effective as pharmacotherapies in the short term, but more effective in the long term. Combined treatment appears to be superior to pharmacotherapy alone but not to CBT alone. CBT may or may not be more effective than other psychotherapies.

A number of CBT variants, often called the third wave or new wave of CBT, have become popular. These include mindfulness-based treatments (e.g., mindfulness-based stress reduction (MBSR), mindfulness-based cognitive therapy (MBCT), acceptance and commitment therapy (ACT), and dialectical behavior therapy (DBT), exposure therapy, cognitive processing therapy, and lesser-known cognitive behavioral analysis system of psychotherapy (CBASP), functional analytic psychotherapy (FAP), and integrative behavioral couple therapy (IBCT).

Systematic reviews have shown that RCTs of these therapies have substantial heterogeneity. Many of the RCTs suffer from several deficiencies, including small sample sizes, lack of follow-up, and researcher allegiance bias. Some studies have shown small to medium effect sizes. Of these, mindfulness-based therapies are popular, and some reviewers believe they present promising evidence-based treatments. Some RCTs of ACT, DBT, and CPT also show promise.

Psychoeducation can be effective in managing depression symptoms. However, the effects depend at least upon the type of psychoeducation and the intensity of depression symptoms upon initiation of treatment. Adding psychodynamic therapy to antidepressants might be helpful, but the treatment effect is small.

Bibliotherapy has variable effects, which seem to depend mostly upon the characteristics of the study population. Among appealing therapies are innovative Internet-based delivery of psychotherapy that may begin and maintain therapy cost-effectively and efficiently.

References

1. Barlow DH, Craske MG. Mastery of your anxiety and panic: workbook. 5th ed. Oxford University Press; 2022. ISBN-13 9780197584095
2. Schacter DL, Gilbert DT, Wegner DM. Psychology. 2nd ed. New York: Worth Pub; 2010. p. 600.
3. Rachman, S The evolution of cognitive behaviour therapy. In Clark, D, Fairburn, CG & Gelder, MG. Science and practice of cognitive behaviour therapy. Oxford: Oxford University Press. 1997. pp. 1–26. ISBN 0-19-262726-0.
4. Hofmann SG. An introduction to modern CBT. In: Psychological solutions to mental health problems. Chichester: Wiley-Blackwell; 2011. ISBN 0-470-97175-4.
5. Kabat-Zinn J. Mindfulness-based interventions in context: past, present, and future. Clin Psychol Sci Pract. 2003;10:144–56.
6. Kabat-Zinn J. Full catastrophe living: using the wisdom of your body and mind to face stress, pain, and illness: Delta; 1990.
7. Hölzel BK, Lazar SW, Gard T, Schuman-Olivier Z, Vago DR, Ott U. How Does mindfulness meditation work? Proposing mechanisms of action from a conceptual and neural perspective. Perspect Psychol Sci. 2011;6(6):537–59. PMID: 26168376. http://www.ncbi.nlm.nih.gov/pubmed/26168376.
8. Teasdale JD. Cognitive vulnerability to persistent depression. Cognit Emot. 1988;2:247–74.
9. Segal ZV, Teasdale JD, Williams JM, Gemar M. The mindfulness-based cognitive therapy adherence scale: inter-rater reliability, adherence to and treatment distinctiveness. Clin Psychol Psychother. 2002;9:131–8.
10. Segal ZV, Williams JMG, Teasdale JD. Mindfulness-based cognitive therapy for depression: a new approach to preventing relapse. New York: Guilford Press; 2002.
11. Kohlenberg RJ, Bolling MY, Kanter JW, Parker CR. Clinical behavior analysis: where it went wrong, how it was made good again, and why its future is so bright (PDF). Behav Anal Today. 2002;3:248–53. ISSN 1539-4352
12. Blackledge JT. An introduction to relational frame theory: basics and applications. Behav Anal Today. 2003;3(4):421–42. BAO
13. Hayes S. Acceptance & Commitment Therapy (ACT). ContextualPsychology.org.
14. Murdock NL. Theories of counseling and psychotherapy: a case approach. Upper Saddle River: Merrill/Pearson; 2009.
15. Jump up ^ "Getting in on the act – The Irish Times – Tue, Jun 07, 2011". The Irish Times 2011-06-07. Retrieved March 16, 2012.
16. Harris R. Embracing your demons: an overview of Acceptance and Commitment Therapy. 2006.
17. Robb H. Values as leading principles in acceptance and commitment therapy. Int J Behav Consult Ther. 2007;3(1):118–23.
18. Hayes SC. Analytic goals and the varieties of scientific contextualism. In: Hayes SC, Hayes LJ, Reese HW, Sarbin TR, editors. Varieties of scientific contextualism. Reno: Context Press; 1993. p. 11–27.
19. Hayes SC, Hayes LJ, Reese HW. Finding the philosophical core: a review of Stephen C. Pepper's world hypotheses. J Exp Anal Behav. 1988;50:91–111.
20. Hayes SC, Barnes-Holmes D, Roche B. Relational frame theory. A post-skinnerian account of human language and cognition. New York: Kluwer Academic; 2001.
21. Hayes SC, Wilson KG, Gifford EV, Follette VM, Strosahl K. Experimental avoidance and behavioral disorders: a functional dimensional approach to diagnosis and treatment. J Consult Clin Psychol. 1996;64(6):1152–68. PMID: 8991302. http://www.ncbi.nlm.nih.gov/pubmed/8991302.
22. Linehan MM. Cognitive behavioral therapy for borderline personality disorder. New York: Guilford Press; 1993a.
23. Linehan MM. Skills training manual for treating borderline personality disorder. New York: Guilford Press; 1993b.
24. Mindfulness and acceptance expanding the cognitive-behavioral tradition Edited by Hayes, Follette, and Linehan New York: Guilford Press; 2011.
25. Linehan MM, Armstrong HE, Suarez A, Allmon D, Heard HL. Cognitive-behavioral treatment of chronically parasuicidal borderline patients. Arch Gen Psychiatry. 1991;48(12):1060–4. PMID: 1845222. http://www.ncbi.nlm.nih.gov/pubmed/1845222.
26. Koons CR, Robins CJ, Tweed JL, Lynch TR, Gonzalez AM, Morse JQ, Bishop GK, Butterfield MI, Bastian LA. Efficacy of dialectical behavior therapy in women veterans with borderline personality disorder. Behav Ther. 2001;32:371–90.
27. Linehan MM, Schmidt H, Dimeff LA, Craft JC, Kanter J, Comtois KA. Dialectical behavior therapy for patients with borderline personality disorder and drug-dependence. Am J Addict. 1999;8(4):279–92. PMID: 10598211. http://www.ncbi.nlm.nih.gov/pubmed/10598211.
28. Verheul R, Van Den Bosch LMC, Koeter MWJ, De Ridder MAJ, Stijnen T, Van Den Brink W. Dialectical behaviour therapy for women with borderline personality disorder: 12-month, randomised clinical trial in The Netherlands. Br J Psychiatry. 2003;182:135–40. PMID: 12562741. http://www.ncbi.nlm.nih.gov/pubmed/12562741.
29. Linehan MM, Dimeff L. Dialectical behavior therapy in a nutshell. Calif Psychol. 2001;34:10–3.
30. Pinto RC. Argument, inference, and dialectic: collected papers on informal logic, Argumentation library, vol. 4. Dordrecht: Kluwer Academic; 2001. p. 138–9.
31. Eemeren FH v. Anyone who has a view: theoretical contributions to the study of argumentation, Argumentation library, vol. 8. Dordrecht: Kluwer Academic; 2003. p. 92.
32. Frede M. "Plato's arguments and the dialogue form", Oxford studies in ancient philosophy, supplementary volume 1992. Oxford; 1992. p. 201–19.
33. Lewinsohn PM, Youngren MA, Grosscup SJ. Reinforcement and depression. In: Dupue RA, editor. The psychobiology of depressive disorders: implications for the effects of stress. New York: Academic; 1979. p. 291–316.
34. Teri L, Lewinsohn PM. Individual treatment of unipolar depression: comparison of treatment outcome and identification of predictors of successful treatment outcome. Behav Ther. 1986;17:215–28.
35. Lewinsohn PM, Hoberman HM, Teri L, Hautzinger M. An integrated theory of depression. In: Reiss S, Bootzin R, editors. Theoretical issues in behavior therapy. New York: Academic; 1985. p. 331–59.
36. Lewinsohn PM, Sullivan JM, Grosscup SJ. Changing reinforcing events: an approach to the treatment of depression. Psychother Theory Res Pract. 1980;47:322–34.
37. Lewinsohn PM, Munoz RF, Youngren MA, Zeiss AM. Control your depression. 2nd ed. Englewood Cliffs: Prentice-Hall; 1986.
38. Lewinsohn PM, Antonuccio DO, Steinmetz-Breckenridge JL, Teri L. The coping with depression course: a psychoeducational intervention for unipolar depression. Eugene: Castalia Publishing; 1984.
39. Clarke GN, Lewinsohn PM, Hops H. Adolescent coping with depression course. Eugene: Castalia Publishing; 1990.
40. Lewinsohn PM, Rhode P, Hops H, Clarke GN. Leader's manual for parent groups: adolescent coping with depression course. Unpublished manuscript; 1991.
41. Breckenridge JS, Zeiss AM, Breckenridge J, Thompson L. Behavioral group therapy with the elderly: a psychoeducational model. In: Upper D, Ross S, editors. Handbook of behavioral group therapy; 1985. p. 275–302.

42. Gallagher D, Thompson LW. Depression in the elderly: a behavioral treatment manual. Los Angeles: University of Southern California Press 1981.
43. Lovett S, Gallagher D. Psychoeducational interventions for family caregivers: preliminary efficacy data. Behav Ther. 1988;19:321–30.
44. Teri L, Gallagher-Thompson D. Cognitive-behavioral interventions for treatment of depression in Alzheimer's patients. Gerontologist. 1991;31(3):413–6. PMID: 1879719. http://www.ncbi.nlm.nih.gov/pubmed/1879719.
45. Munoz RF, Ying YW, editors. The prevention of depression: research and practice. Baltimore: The Johns Hopkins University Press; 1993.
46. Manson SM. American Indian and Alaska native mental health research. J Natl Center. 1988;1:1–64.
47. Hall SM, Muñoz RF, Reus VI. Cognitive-behavioral intervention increases abstinence rates for depressive-history smokers. J Consult Clin Psychol. 1994;62(1):141–6. PMID: 8034816. http://www.ncbi.nlm.nih.gov/pubmed/8034816.
48. Cuijpers P, van Straten A, Andersson G, van Oppen P. Psychotherapy for depression in adults: a meta-analysis of comparative outcome studies. J Consult Clin Psychol. 2008;76(6):909–22. PMID: 19045960. http://www.ncbi.nlm.nih.gov/pubmed/19045960.
49. Lambert MJ. Psychotherapy outcome research: implications for integrative and eclectic therapists. In: Norcross JC, Goldfield MR, editors. Handbook of psychotherapy integration. New York: Basic Books; 1992. p. 94–129.
50. Anderson L, Lewis G, Araya R, Elgie R, Harrison G, Proudfoot J, Schmidt U, Sharp D, Weightman A, Williams C. Self-help books for depression: how can practitioners and patients make the right choice? Br J Gen Pract. 2005;55(514):387–92. PMCID: PMC1463163. http://www.ncbi.nlm.nih.gov/pubmed/15904559.
51. Gregory RJ, Canning SS, Lee TW, Wise JC. Cognitive bibliotherapy for depression: a meta-analysis. Prof Psychol Res Pr. 2004;35:275–80.
52. Markowitz JC, Weissman MM, editors. Casebook of interpersonal psychotherapy. New York: Oxford University Press; 2012.
53. Weissman MM, Markowitz JC, Klerman GL. Clinician's quick guide to interpersonal psychotherapy. New York: Oxford University Press; 2007.
54. Clinical Management of Insomnia Using Cognitive Therapy. Behav Sleep Med. 4(3) (tandfonline.com)
55. Understanding and Treating Insomnia | Annual Reviews.
56. Keown D. A dictionary of Buddhism. Oxford: Oxford University Press; 2003.
57. Nandini D. Karunamuni The five-aggregate model of the mind 2015.
58. Panjvani C. Buddhism: a philosophical approach. Broadview Press; 2013.
59. Databases.
60. Depression Psychotherapy | Metapsy Online Meta-Analysis Tool.
61. WHOCC – WHO Collaborating Centres.
62. Cuijpers P, Karyotaki E, de Wit L, Ebert DD. The effects of fifteen evidence-supported therapies for adult depression: a meta-analytic review. Psychother Res. 2020;30(3):279–93. PMID: 31394976. http://www.ncbi.nlm.nih.gov/pubmed/31394976.
63. Cuijpers P, Quero S, Dowrick C, Arroll B. Psychological treatment of depression in primary care: recent developments. Curr Psychiatry Rep. 2019;21(12):129. PMCID: PMC6875158. http://www.ncbi.nlm.nih.gov/pubmed/31760505
64. Richards DA, Ekers D, McMillan D, Taylor RS, Byford S, Warren FC, Barrett B, Farrand PA, Gilbody S, Kuyken W, O'Mahen H, Watkins ER, Wright KA, Hollon SD, Reed N, Rhodes S, Fletcher E, Finning K. Cost and outcome of behavioural activation versus cognitive behavioural therapy for depression (COBRA): a randomised, controlled, non-inferiority trial. Lancet. 2016;388(10047):871–80. PMCID: PMC5007415. http://www.ncbi.nlm.nih.gov/pubmed/27461440.
65. Riper H, Andersson G, Hunter SB, de Wit J, Berking M, Cuijpers P. Treatment of comorbid alcohol use disorders and depression with cognitive-behavioural therapy and motivational interviewing: a meta-analysis. Addiction. 2014;109(3):394–406. PMCID: PMC4227588. http://www.ncbi.nlm.nih.gov/pubmed/24304463.
66. Emmelkamp PMG, David D, Beckers T, Muris P, Cuijpers P, Lutz W, Andersson G, Araya R, Banos Rivera RM, Barkham M, Berking M, Berger T, Botella C, Carlbring P, Colom F, Essau C, Hermans D, Hofmann SG, Knappe S, Ollendick TH, Raes F, Rief W, Riper H, Van Der Oord S, Vervliet B. Advancing psychotherapy and evidence-based psychological interventions. Int J Methods Psychiatr Res. 2014;23((Suppl 1)):58–91. PMCID: PMC6878277. http://www.ncbi.nlm.nih.gov/pubmed/24375536.
67. Kessler RC, Chiu WT, Demler O, Merikangas KR, Walters EE. Prevalence, severity, and comorbidity of 12-month DSM-IV disorders in the National Comorbidity Survey Replication. Arch Gen Psychiatry. 2005;62(6):617–27. PMCID: PMC2847357. http://www.ncbi.nlm.nih.gov/pubmed/15939839.
68. Kaufman J, Charney D. Comorbidity of mood and anxiety disorders. Depress Anxiety. 2000;12(Suppl 1):69–76. PMID: 11098417. http://www.ncbi.nlm.nih.gov/pubmed/11098417.
69. Allen LB, White KS, Barlow DH, Shear MK, Gorman JM, Woods SW. Cognitive-Behavior Therapy (CBT) for panic disorder: relationship of anxiety and depression comorbidity with treatment outcome. J Psychopathol Behav Assess. 2010;32(2):185–92. PMCID: PMC2855025. http://www.ncbi.nlm.nih.gov/pubmed/20421906.
70. Barlow DH, Gorman JM, Shear MK, Woods SW. Cognitive-behavioral therapy, imipramine, or their combination for panic disorder: a randomized controlled trial. JAMA. 2000;283(19):2529–36. PMID: 10815116. http://www.ncbi.nlm.nih.gov/pubmed/10815116.
71. Hofmann SG, Smits JAJ. Cognitive-behavioral therapy for adult anxiety disorders: a meta-analysis of randomized placebo-controlled trials. J Clin Psychiatry. 2008;69(4):621–32. PMCID: PMC2409267. http://www.ncbi.nlm.nih.gov/pubmed/18363421.
72. Ley R. Blood, breath, fears redux, and panic attacks: comment on Roth, Wilhelm, and Pettit (2005). Psychol Bull. 2005;131(2):193–8. Author reply 199–201. PMID: 15740415. http://www.ncbi.nlm.nih.gov/pubmed/15740415.
73. Psych Education – Mental health education you can trust.
74. Cuijpers P, Driessen E, Hollon SD, van Oppen P, Barth J, Andersson G. The efficacy of non-directive supportive therapy for adult depression: a meta-analysis. Clin Psychol Rev. 2012;32(4):280–91. PMID: 22466509. http://www.ncbi.nlm.nih.gov/pubmed/22466509.
75. Cognitive behavior therapy – StatPearls – NCBI Bookshelf.
76. Sifneos PE. The prevalence of "alexithymic" characteristics in psychosomatic patients. Psychother Psychosom. 1973;22(2):255–62. PMID: 4770536. http://www.ncbi.nlm.nih.gov/pubmed/4770536.
77. ≡ Alexithymia Online – Emotional Blindness.
78. Hayes SC, Villatte M, Levin M, Hildebrandt M. Open, aware, and active: contextual approaches as an emerging trend in the behavioral and cognitive therapies. Annu Rev Clin Psychol. 2011;7:141–68. PMID: 21219193. http://www.ncbi.nlm.nih.gov/pubmed/21219193.
79. Gatchel RJ, Rollings KH. Evidence-informed management of chronic low back pain with cognitive behavioral therapy. Spine J. 2008;8(1):40–4. PMCID: PMC3237294. http://www.ncbi.nlm.nih.gov/pubmed/18164452.
80. Longmore RJ, Worrell M. Do we need to challenge thoughts in cognitive behavior therapy? Clin Psychol Rev.

2007;27(2):173–87. PMID: 17157970. http://www.ncbi.nlm.nih.gov/pubmed/17157970.
81. Driessen E, Hollon SD. Cognitive behavioral therapy for mood disorders: efficacy, moderators and mediators. Psychiatr Clin North Am. 2010;33(3):537–55. PMCID: PMC2933381. http://www.ncbi.nlm.nih.gov/pubmed/20599132.
82. Foroushani PS, Schneider J, Assareh N. Meta-review of the effectiveness of computerised CBT in treating depression. BMC Psychiatry. 2011;11:131. PMCID: PMC3180363. http://www.ncbi.nlm.nih.gov/pubmed/21838902.
83. Keefe JR, Chambless DL, Barber JP, Milrod BL. Treatment of anxiety and mood comorbidities in cognitive-behavioral and psychodynamic therapies for panic disorder. J Psychiatr Res. 2019;114:34–40. PMID: 31015099. http://www.ncbi.nlm.nih.gov/pubmed/31015099.
84. Sahranavard S, Esmaeili A, Salehiniya H, Behdani S. The effectiveness of group training of cognitive behavioral therapy-based stress management on anxiety, hardiness and self-efficacy in female medical students. J Educ Health Promot. 2019;8:49. PMCID: PMC6432834. http://www.ncbi.nlm.nih.gov/pubmed/30993142.
85. Robinson E, Titov N, Andrews G, McIntyre K, Schwencke G, Solley K. Internet treatment for generalized anxiety disorder: a randomized controlled trial comparing clinician vs. technician assistance. PLoS One. 2010;5(6):e10942. PMCID: PMC2880592. http://www.ncbi.nlm.nih.gov/pubmed/20532167.
86. Symposium on Lipid Abnormalities in Renal Diseases. Sardinia, Italy, 1990. Kidney Int Suppl. 1991;31:S1–72. PMID: 2046264. http://www.ncbi.nlm.nih.gov/pubmed/2046264.
87. Murphy R, Straebler S, Cooper Z, Fairburn CG. Cognitive behavioral therapy for eating disorders. Psychiatr Clin North Am. 2010;33(3):611–27. PMCID: PMC2928448. http://www.ncbi.nlm.nih.gov/pubmed/20599136.
88. Wilfley DE, Kolko RP, Kass AE. Cognitive-behavioral therapy for weight management and eating disorders in children and adolescents. Child Adolesc Psychiatr Clin N Am. 2011;20(2):271–85. PMCID: PMC3065663. http://www.ncbi.nlm.nih.gov/pubmed/21440855.
89. McHugh RK, Hearon BA, Otto MW. Cognitive behavioral therapy for substance use disorders. Psychiatr Clin North Am. 2010;33(3):511–25. PMCID: PMC2897895. http://www.ncbi.nlm.nih.gov/pubmed/20599130.
90. Matusiewicz AK, Hopwood CJ, Banducci AN, Lejuez CW. The effectiveness of cognitive behavioral therapy for personality disorders. Psychiatr Clin North Am. 2010;33(3):657–85. PMCID: PMC3138327. http://www.ncbi.nlm.nih.gov/pubmed/20599139.
91. Gutiérrez M, Sánchez M, Trujillo A, Sánchez L. Cognitive-behavioral therapy for chronic psychosis. Actas Esp Psiquiatr. 2009;37(2):106–14. PMID: 19401859. http://www.ncbi.nlm.nih.gov/pubmed/19401859.
92. Kumari V, Fannon D, Peters ER, Ffytche DH, Sumich AL, Premkumar P, Anilkumar AP, Andrew C, Phillips ML, Williams SCR, Kuipers E. Neural changes following cognitive behaviour therapy for psychosis: a longitudinal study. Brain. 2011;134(Pt 8):2396–407. PMCID: PMC3155705. http://www.ncbi.nlm.nih.gov/pubmed/21772062.
93. Janse A, Bleijenberg G, Knoop H. Prediction of long-term outcome after cognitive behavioral therapy for chronic fatigue syndrome. J Psychosom Res. 2019;121:93–9. PMID: 31006534. http://www.ncbi.nlm.nih.gov/pubmed/31006534.
94. Tolin DF, Wootton BM, Levy HC, Hallion LS, Worden BL, Diefenbach GJ, Jaccard J, Stevens MC. Efficacy and mediators of a group cognitive-behavioral therapy for hoarding disorder: a randomized trial. J Consult Clin Psychol. 2019;87(7):590–602. PMID: 31008633. http://www.ncbi.nlm.nih.gov/pubmed/31008633.
95. Heenan A, Pipe A, Lemay K, Davidson JR, Tulloch H. Cognitive-behavioral therapy for insomnia tailored to patients with cardiovascular disease: a pre-post study. Behav Sleep Med. 2020;18(3):372–85. PMID: 31007057. http://www.ncbi.nlm.nih.gov/pubmed/31007057.
96. Rathod S, Phiri P, Kingdon D. Cognitive behavioral therapy for schizophrenia. Psychiatr Clin North Am. 2010;33(3):527–36. PMID: 20599131. http://www.ncbi.nlm.nih.gov/pubmed/20599131.
97. Hart SL, Hoyt MA, Diefenbach M, Anderson DR, Kilbourn KM, Craft LL, Steel JL, Cuijpers P, Mohr DC, Berendsen M, Spring B, Stanton AL. Meta-analysis of efficacy of interventions for elevated depressive symptoms in adults diagnosed with cancer. J Natl Cancer Inst. 2012;104(13):990–1004. PMCID: PMC3634552. http://www.ncbi.nlm.nih.gov/pubmed/22767203.
98. Mehta S, Orenczuk S, Hansen KT, Aubut JAL, Hitzig SL, Legassic M, Teasell RW, Spinal Cord Injury Rehabilitation Evidence Research Team. An evidence-based review of the effectiveness of cognitive behavioral therapy for psychosocial issues post-spinal cord injury. Rehabil Psychol. 2011;56(1):15–25. PMCID: PMC3206089. http://www.ncbi.nlm.nih.gov/pubmed/21401282.
99. Hassett AL, Gevirtz RN. Nonpharmacologic treatment for fibromyalgia: patient education, cognitive-behavioral therapy, relaxation techniques, and complementary and alternative medicine. Rheum Dis Clin North Am. 2009;35(2):393–407. PMCID: PMC2743408. http://www.ncbi.nlm.nih.gov/pubmed/19647150.
100. Friedberg F, Williams DA, Collinge W. Lifestyle-oriented non-pharmacological treatments for fibromyalgia: a clinical overview and applications with home-based technologies. J Pain Res. 2012;5:425–35. PMCID: PMC3500923. http://www.ncbi.nlm.nih.gov/pubmed/23166446.
101. Cuijpers P, Andersson G, Donker T, van Straten A. Psychological treatment of depression: results of a series of meta-analyses. Nord J Psychiatry. 2011;65(6):354–64. PMID: 21770842. http://www.ncbi.nlm.nih.gov/pubmed/21770842.
102. Sockol LE. A systematic review of the efficacy of cognitive behavioral therapy for treating and preventing perinatal depression. J Affect Disord. 2015;177:7–21. PMID: 25743368. http://www.ncbi.nlm.nih.gov/pubmed/25743368.
103. Hofmann SG, Sawyer AT, Fang A. The empirical status of the "new wave" of cognitive behavioral therapy. Psychiatr Clin North Am. 2010;33(3):701–10. PMCID: PMC2898899. http://www.ncbi.nlm.nih.gov/pubmed/20599141.
104. Houghton S, Saxon D. An evaluation of large group CBT psycho-education for anxiety disorders delivered in routine practice. Patient Educ Couns. 2007;68(1):107–10. PMID: 17582724. http://www.ncbi.nlm.nih.gov/pubmed/17582724.
105. Butler AC, Chapman JE, Forman EM, Beck AT. The empirical status of cognitive-behavioral therapy: a review of meta-analyses. Clin Psychol Rev. 2006;26(1):17–31. PMID: 16199119. http://www.ncbi.nlm.nih.gov/pubmed/16199119.
106. Overview | Depression in adults: treatment and management | Guidance | NICE.
107. Kirkpatrick T, Manoukian L, Dear BF, Johnston L, Titov N. A feasibility open trial of internet-delivered cognitive-behavioural therapy (iCBT) among consumers of a non-governmental mental health organisation with anxiety. PeerJ. 2013;1:e210. PMCID: PMC3845869. http://www.ncbi.nlm.nih.gov/pubmed/24349897.
108. Dear BF, Zou J, Titov N, Lorian C, Johnston L, Spence J, Anderson T, Sachdev P, Brodaty H, Knight RG. Internet-delivered cognitive behavioural therapy for depression: a feasibility open trial for older adults. Aust N Z J Psychiatry. 2013;47(2):169–76. PMID: 23152358. http://www.ncbi.nlm.nih.gov/pubmed/23152358.
109. Gega L, Swift L, Barton G, Todd G, Reeve N, Bird K, Holland R, Howe A, Wilson J, Molle J. Computerised therapy for depression with clinician vs. assistant and brief vs. extended phone

support: study protocol for a randomised controlled trial. Trials. 2012;13:151. PMCID: PMC3495903. http://www.ncbi.nlm.nih.gov/pubmed/22925596.
110. Titov N, Andrews G, Sachdev P. Computer-delivered cognitive behavioural therapy: effective and getting ready for dissemination. F1000 Med Rep. 2010;2:49. PMCID: PMC2950044. http://www.ncbi.nlm.nih.gov/pubmed/20948835.
111. Spijker J, van Straten A, Bockting CLH, Meeuwissen JAC, van Balkom AJLM. Psychotherapy, antidepressants, and their combination for chronic major depressive disorder: a systematic review. Can J Psychiatr. 2013;58(7):386–92. PMID: 23870720. http://www.ncbi.nlm.nih.gov/pubmed/23870720.
112. van Hees MLJM, Rotter T, Ellermann T, Evers SMAA. The effectiveness of individual interpersonal psychotherapy as a treatment for major depressive disorder in adult outpatients: a systematic review. BMC Psychiatry. 2013;13:22. PMCID: PMC3558333. http://www.ncbi.nlm.nih.gov/pubmed/23312024.
113. Brent D, Emslie G, Clarke G, Wagner KD, Asarnow JR, Keller M, Vitiello B, Ritz L, Iyengar S, Abebe K, Birmaher B, Ryan N, Kennard B, Hughes C, DeBar L, McCracken J, Strober M, Suddath R, Spirito A, Leonard H, Melhem N, Porta G, Onorato M, Zelazny J. Switching to another SSRI or to venlafaxine with or without cognitive behavioral therapy for adolescents with SSRI-resistant depression: the TORDIA randomized controlled trial. JAMA. 2008;299(8):901–13. PMCID: PMC2277341. http://www.ncbi.nlm.nih.gov/pubmed/18314433.
114. David-Ferdon C, Kaslow NJ. Evidence-based psychosocial treatments for child and adolescent depression. J Clin Child Adolesc Psychol. 2008;37(1):62–104. PMID: 18444054. http://www.ncbi.nlm.nih.gov/pubmed/18444054.
115. Spirito A, Esposito-Smythers C, Wolff J, Uhl K. Cognitive-behavioral therapy for adolescent depression and suicidality. Child Adolesc Psychiatr Clin N Am. 2011;20(2):191–204. PMCID: PMC3073681. http://www.ncbi.nlm.nih.gov/pubmed/21440850.
116. Donaldson D, Spirito A, Esposito-Smythers C. Treatment for adolescents following a suicide attempt: results of a pilot trial. J Am Acad Child Adolesc Psychiatry. 2005;44(2):113–20. PMID: 15689724. http://www.ncbi.nlm.nih.gov/pubmed/15689724.
117. Seligman LD, Ollendick TH. Cognitive-behavioral therapy for anxiety disorders in youth. Child Adolesc Psychiatr Clin N Am. 2011;20(2):217–38. PMCID: PMC3091167. http://www.ncbi.nlm.nih.gov/pubmed/21440852.
118. Kowalik J, Weller J, Venter J, Drachman D. Cognitive behavioral therapy for the treatment of pediatric posttraumatic stress disorder: a review and meta-analysis. J Behav Ther Exp Psychiatry. 2011;42(3):405–13. PMID: 21458405. http://www.ncbi.nlm.nih.gov/pubmed/21458405.
119. Phillips KA, Rogers J. Cognitive-behavioral therapy for youth with body dysmorphic disorder: current status and future directions. Child Adolesc Psychiatr Clin N Am. 2011;20(2):287–304. PMCID: PMC3070293. http://www.ncbi.nlm.nih.gov/pubmed/21440856.
120. Boileau B. A review of obsessive-compulsive disorder in children and adolescents. Dialogues Clin Neurosci. 2011;13(4):401–11. PMCID: PMC3263388. http://www.ncbi.nlm.nih.gov/pubmed/22275846.
121. Flessner CA. Cognitive-behavioral therapy for childhood repetitive behavior disorders: tic disorders and trichotillomania. Child Adolesc Psychiatr Clin N Am. 2011;20(2):319–28. PMCID: PMC3074180. http://www.ncbi.nlm.nih.gov/pubmed/21440858.
122. Cuijpers P, Noma H, Karyotaki E, Cipriani A, Furukawa TA. Effectiveness and acceptability of cognitive behavior therapy delivery formats in adults with depression: a network meta-analysis. JAMA Psychiat. 2019;76(7):700–7. PMCID: PMC6583673. http://www.ncbi.nlm.nih.gov/pubmed/30994877.
123. Webb CA, Stanton CH, Bondy E, Singleton P, Pizzagalli DA, Auerbach RP. Cognitive versus behavioral skills in CBT for depressed adolescents: disaggregating within-patient versus between-patient effects on symptom change. J Consult Clin Psychol. 2019;87(5):484–90. PMCID: PMC6506214. http://www.ncbi.nlm.nih.gov/pubmed/30998049.
124. de Jonge M, Bockting CLH, Kikkert MJ, van Dijk MK, van Schaik DJF, Peen J, Hollon SD, Dekker JJM. Preventive cognitive therapy versus care as usual in cognitive behavioral therapy responders: a randomized controlled trial. J Consult Clin Psychol. 2019;87(6):521–9. PMID: 31008635. http://www.ncbi.nlm.nih.gov/pubmed/31008635.
125. Cuijpers P, Cristea IA, Karyotaki E, Reijnders M, Huibers MJH. How effective are cognitive behavior therapies for major depression and anxiety disorders? A meta-analytic update of the evidence. World Psychiatry. 2016;15(3):245–58. PMCID: PMC5032489. http://www.ncbi.nlm.nih.gov/pubmed/27717254.
126. Cuijpers P, de Beurs DP, van Spijker BAJ, Berking M, Andersson G, Kerkhof AJFM. The effects of psychotherapy for adult depression on suicidality and hopelessness: a systematic review and meta-analysis. J Affect Disord. 2013;144(3):183–90. PMID: 22832172. http://www.ncbi.nlm.nih.gov/pubmed/22832172.
127. Jakobsen JC, Hansen JL, Storebø OJ, Simonsen E, Gluud C. The effects of cognitive therapy versus "no intervention" for major depressive disorder. PLoS One. 2011;6(12):e28299. PMCID: PMC3235113. http://www.ncbi.nlm.nih.gov/pubmed/22174786.
128. Dragioti E, Dimoliatis I, Fountoulakis KN, Evangelou E. A systematic appraisal of allegiance effect in randomized controlled trials of psychotherapy. Ann Gen Psychiatry. 2015;14:25. PMCID: PMC4570291. http://www.ncbi.nlm.nih.gov/pubmed/26379758.
129. Zhang A, Borhneimer LA, Weaver A, Franklin C, Hai AH, Guz S, Shen L. Cognitive behavioral therapy for primary care depression and anxiety: a secondary meta-analytic review using robust variance estimation in meta-regression. J Behav Med. 2019;42(6):1117–41. PMID: 31004323. http://www.ncbi.nlm.nih.gov/pubmed/31004323.
130. Cuijpers P, Miguel C, Harrer M, Plessen CY, Ciharova M, Ebert D, Karyotaki E. Cognitive behavior therapy vs. control conditions, other psychotherapies, pharmacotherapies and combined treatment for depression: a comprehensive meta-analysis including 409 trials with 52,702 patients. World Psychiatry. 2023;22(1):105–15. PMCID: PMC9840507. http://www.ncbi.nlm.nih.gov/pubmed/36640411.
131. Haynes P. Application of cognitive behavioral therapies for comorbid insomnia and depression. Sleep Med Clin. 2015;10(1):77–84. PMID: 26055675. http://www.ncbi.nlm.nih.gov/pubmed/26055675.
132. Franzen PL, Buysse DJ. Sleep disturbances and depression: risk relationships for subsequent depression and therapeutic implications. Dialogues Clin Neurosci. 2008;10(4):473–81. PMCID: PMC3108260. http://www.ncbi.nlm.nih.gov/pubmed/19170404.
133. Manber R, Bernert RA, Suh S, Nowakowski S, Siebern AT, Ong JC. CBT for insomnia in patients with high and low depressive symptom severity: adherence and clinical outcomes. J Clin Sleep Med. 2011;7(6):645–52. PMCID: PMC3227711. http://www.ncbi.nlm.nih.gov/pubmed/22171204.
134. Matthews EE, Arnedt JT, MS MC, Cuddihy LJ, Aloia MS. Adherence to cognitive behavioral therapy for insomnia: a systematic review. Sleep Med Rev. 2013;17(6):453–64. PMCID: PMC3720832. http://www.ncbi.nlm.nih.gov/pubmed/23602124.
135. Brasure M, MacDonald R, Fuchs E, Olson CM, Carlyle M, Diem S, Koffel E, Khawaja IS, Ouellette J, Butler M, Kane RL, Wilt TJ. Management of insomnia disorder [Internet]. Rockville: Agency for Healthcare Research and Quality (US); 2015. [cited 2025 Jan 12]. Available from:. http://www.ncbi.nlm.nih.gov/

books/NBK343503/ PMID: 26844312. http://www.ncbi.nlm.nih.gov/pubmed/26844312.
136. Clarke G, Harvey AG. The complex role of sleep in adolescent depression. Child Adolesc Psychiatr Clin N Am. 2012;21(2):385–400. PMCID: PMC3605974. http://www.ncbi.nlm.nih.gov/pubmed/22537732.
137. AHRQ Comparative Effectiveness Reviews – NCBI Bookshelf.
138. Cognitive Behavioral Therapy for Insomnia (CBT-I): An Overview.
139. Mitchell MD, Gehrman P, Perlis M, Umscheid CA. Comparative effectiveness of cognitive behavioral therapy for insomnia: a systematic review. BMC Fam Pract. 2012;13:40. PMCID: PMC3481424. http://www.ncbi.nlm.nih.gov/pubmed/22631616.
140. Qaseem A, Kansagara D, Forciea MA, Cooke M, Denberg TD. Clinical guidelines committee of the American College of physicians. Management of chronic insomnia disorder in adults: a clinical practice guideline from the American College of Physicians. Ann Intern Med. 2016;165(2):125–33. PMID: 27136449. http://www.ncbi.nlm.nih.gov/pubmed/27136449.
141. Riemann D, Baglioni C, Bassetti C, Bjorvatn B, Dolenc Groselj L, Ellis JG, Espie CA, Garcia-Borreguero D, Gjerstad M, Gonçalves M, Hertenstein E, Jansson-Fröjmark M, Jennum PJ, Leger D, Nissen C, Parrino L, Paunio T, Pevernagie D, Verbraecken J, Weeß HG, Wichniak A, Zavalko I, Arnardottir ES, Deleanu OC, Strazisar B, Zoetmulder M, Spiegelhalder K. European guideline for the diagnosis and treatment of insomnia. J Sleep Res. 2017;26(6):675–700. PMID: 28875581. http://www.ncbi.nlm.nih.gov/pubmed/28875581.
142. Perlis ML, Posner D, Riemann D, Bastien CH, Teel J, Thase M. Insomnia. Lancet. 2022;400(10357):1047–60. PMID: 36115372. http://www.ncbi.nlm.nih.gov/pubmed/36115372.
143. Trauer JM, Qian MY, Doyle JS, Rajaratnam SMW, Cunnington D. Cognitive behavioral therapy for chronic insomnia: a systematic review and meta-analysis. Ann Intern Med. 2015;163(3):191–204. PMID: 26054060. http://www.ncbi.nlm.nih.gov/pubmed/26054060.
144. American Board of Sleep Medicine (ABSM).
145. Find a CBT Therapist | Association for Behavioral and Cognitive Therapies.
146. Society of Behavioral Sleep Medicine.
147. APA Psychologist Locator—American Psychological Association.
148. Hertenstein E, Trinca E, Wunderlin M, Schneider CL, Züst MA, Fehér KD, Su T, Straten AV, Berger T, Baglioni C, Johann A, Spiegelhalder K, Riemann D, Feige B, Nissen C. Cognitive behavioral therapy for insomnia in patients with mental disorders and comorbid insomnia: a systematic review and meta-analysis. Sleep Med Rev. 2022;62:101597. PMID: 35240417. http://www.ncbi.nlm.nih.gov/pubmed/35240417.
149. Alimoradi Z, Jafari E, Broström A, Ohayon MM, Lin CY, Griffiths MD, Blom K, Jernelöv S, Kaldo V, Pakpour AH. Effects of cognitive behavioral therapy for insomnia (CBT-I) on quality of life: a systematic review and meta-analysis. Sleep Med Rev. 2022;64:101646. PMID: 35653951. http://www.ncbi.nlm.nih.gov/pubmed/35653951.
150. Furukawa Y, Sakata M, Yamamoto R, Nakajima S, Kikuchi S, Inoue M, Ito M, Noma H, Takashina HN, Funada S, Ostinelli EG, Furukawa TA, Efthimiou O, Perlis M. Components and delivery formats of cognitive behavioral therapy for chronic insomnia in adults: a systematic review and component network meta-analysis. JAMA Psychiatr. 2024;81(4):357–65. PMCID: PMC10794978. http://www.ncbi.nlm.nih.gov/pubmed/38231522.
151. Yu DJ, Recchia F, Bernal JDK, Yu AP, Fong DY, Li SX, Chan RNY, Hu X, Siu PM. Effectiveness of exercise, cognitive behavioral therapy, and pharmacotherapy on improving sleep in adults with chronic insomnia: a systematic review and network meta-analysis of randomized controlled trials. Healthcare (Basel). 2023;11(15):2207. PMCID: PMC10418444. http://www.ncbi.nlm.nih.gov/pubmed/37570447.
152. Efthimiou O, Debray TPA, van Valkenhoef G, Trelle S, Panayidou K, Moons KGM, Reitsma JB, Shang A, Salanti G, GetReal Methods Review Group. GetReal in network meta-analysis: a review of the methodology. Res Synth Methods. 2016;7(3):236–63. PMID: 26754852. http://www.ncbi.nlm.nih.gov/pubmed/26754852.
153. Welton NJ, Caldwell DM, Adamopoulos E, Vedhara K. Mixed treatment comparison meta-analysis of complex interventions: psychological interventions in coronary heart disease. Am J Epidemiol. 2009;169(9):1158–65. PMID: 19258485. http://www.ncbi.nlm.nih.gov/pubmed/19258485.
154. Petropoulou M, Efthimiou O, Rücker G, Schwarzer G, Furukawa TA, Pompoli A, Koek HL, Del Giovane C, Rodondi N, Mavridis D. A review of methods for addressing components of interventions in meta-analysis. PLoS One. 2021;16(2):e0246631. PMCID: PMC7870082. http://www.ncbi.nlm.nih.gov/pubmed/33556155.
155. Pompoli A, Furukawa TA, Efthimiou O, Imai H, Tajika A, Salanti G. Dismantling cognitive-behaviour therapy for panic disorder: a systematic review and component network meta-analysis. Psychol Med. 2018;48(12):1945–53. PMCID: PMC6137372. http://www.ncbi.nlm.nih.gov/pubmed/29368665.
156. Furukawa TA, Suganuma A, Ostinelli EG, Andersson G, Beevers CG, Shumake J, Berger T, Boele FW, Buntrock C, Carlbring P, Choi I, Christensen H, Mackinnon A, Dahne J, Huibers MJH, Ebert DD, Farrer L, Forand NR, Strunk DR, Ezawa ID, Forsell E, Kaldo V, Geraedts A, Gilbody S, Littlewood E, Brabyn S, Hadjistavropoulos HD, Schneider LH, Johansson R, Kenter R, Kivi M, Björkelund C, Kleiboer A, Riper H, Klein JP, Schröder J, Meyer B, Moritz S, Bücker L, Lintvedt O, Johansson P, Lundgren J, Milgrom J, Gemmill AW, Mohr DC, Montero-Marin J, Garcia-Campayo J, Nobis S, Zarski AC, O'Moore K, Williams AD, Newby JM, Perini S, Phillips R, Schneider J, Pots W, Pugh NE, Richards D, Rosso IM, Rauch SL, Sheeber LB, Smith J, Spek V, Pop VJ, Ünlü B, van Bastelaar KMP, van Luenen S, Garnefski N, Kraaij V, Vernmark K, Warmerdam L, van Straten A, Zagorscak P, Knaevelsrud C, Heinrich M, Miguel C, Cipriani A, Efthimiou O, Karyotaki E, Cuijpers P. Dismantling, optimising, and personalising internet cognitive behavioural therapy for depression: a systematic review and component network meta-analysis using individual participant data. Lancet. Psychiatry. 2021;8(6):500–11. PMCID: PMC8838916. http://www.ncbi.nlm.nih.gov/pubmed/33957075.
157. O'Connor M, Munnelly A, Whelan R, McHugh L. The efficacy and acceptability of third-wave behavioral and cognitive eHealth treatments: a systematic review and meta-analysis of randomized controlled trials. Behav Ther. 2018;49(3):459–75. PMID: 29704973. http://www.ncbi.nlm.nih.gov/pubmed/29704973.
158. Pull CB. Current empirical status of acceptance and commitment therapy. Curr Opin Psychiatry. 2009;22(1):55–60. PMID: 19122536. http://www.ncbi.nlm.nih.gov/pubmed/19122536.
159. Hofmann SG, Asmundson GJG. Acceptance and mindfulness-based therapy: new wave or old hat? Clin Psychol Rev. 2008;28(1):1–16. PMID: 17904260. http://www.ncbi.nlm.nih.gov/pubmed/17904260.
160. Hunot V, Moore THM, Caldwell DM, Furukawa TA, Davies P, Jones H, Honyashiki M, Chen P, Lewis G, Churchill R. "Third wave" cognitive and behavioural therapies versus other psychological therapies for depression. Cochrane Database Syst Rev. 2013;18(10):CD008704. PMID: 24142844. http://www.ncbi.nlm.nih.gov/pubmed/24142844.
161. Vivian D, Salwen J. Key process issues in cognitive behavioral analysis system of psychotherapy (CBASP): translation of an evidence-based model into clinical practice and training.

Psychotherapy (Chic). 2013;50(3):398–403. PMID: 24000859. http://www.ncbi.nlm.nih.gov/pubmed/24000859.
162. Sevier M, Atkins DC, Doss BD, Christensen A. Up and down or down and up? The process of change in constructive couple behavior during traditional and integrative behavioral couple therapy. J Marital Fam Ther. 2015;41(1):113–27. PMID: 24303810. http://www.ncbi.nlm.nih.gov/pubmed/24303810.
163. Ost LG. Efficacy of the third wave of behavioral therapies: a systematic review and meta-analysis. Behav Res Ther. 2008;46(3):296–321. PMID: 18258216. http://www.ncbi.nlm.nih.gov/pubmed/18258216.
164. Klein DN, Leon AC, Li C, D'Zurilla TJ, Black SR, Vivian D, Dowling F, Arnow BA, Manber R, Markowitz JC, Kocsis JH. Social problem solving and depressive symptoms over time: a randomized clinical trial of cognitive-behavioral analysis system of psychotherapy, brief supportive psychotherapy, and pharmacotherapy. J Consult Clin Psychol. 2011;79(3):342–52. PMCID: PMC3109172. http://www.ncbi.nlm.nih.gov/pubmed/21500885.
165. Shinohara K, Honyashiki M, Imai H, Hunot V, Caldwell DM, Davies P, Moore THM, Furukawa TA, Churchill R. Behavioural therapies versus other psychological therapies for depression. Cochrane Database Syst Rev. 2013;2013(10):CD008696. PMCID: PMC7433301. http://www.ncbi.nlm.nih.gov/pubmed/24129886.
166. Hunot V, Moore THM, Caldwell DM, Furukawa TA, Davies P, Jones H, Honyashiki M, Chen P, Lewis G, Churchill R. "Third wave" cognitive and behavioural therapies versus other psychological therapies for depression. Cochrane Database Syst Rev. 2013;2013(10):CD008704. PMID: 24142844. http://www.ncbi.nlm.nih.gov/pubmed/24142844.
167. Churchill R, Moore THM, Furukawa TA, Caldwell DM, Davies P, Jones H, Shinohara K, Imai H, Lewis G, Hunot V. "Third wave" cognitive and behavioural therapies versus treatment as usual for depression. Cochrane Database Syst Rev. 2013;10:CD008705. PMID: 24142810. http://www.ncbi.nlm.nih.gov/pubmed/24142810.
168. Hetrick SE, Cox GR, Witt KG, Bir JJ, Merry SN. Cognitive behavioural therapy (CBT), third-wave CBT and interpersonal therapy (IPT) based interventions for preventing depression in children and adolescents. Cochrane Database Syst Rev. 2016;2016(8):CD003380. PMCID: PMC8407360. http://www.ncbi.nlm.nih.gov/pubmed/27501438.
169. Keng SL, Smoski MJ, Robins CJ. Effects of mindfulness on psychological health: a review of empirical studies. Clin Psychol Rev. 2011;31(6):1041–56. PMCID: PMC3679190. http://www.ncbi.nlm.nih.gov/pubmed/21802619.
170. Chiesa A, Calati R, Serretti A. Does mindfulness training improve cognitive abilities? A systematic review of neuropsychological findings. Clin Psychol Rev. 2011;31(3):449–64. PMID: 21183265. http://www.ncbi.nlm.nih.gov/pubmed/21183265.
171. Borkowski JG. Metacognitive theory: a framework for teaching literacy, writing, and math skills. J Learn Disabil. 1992;25(4):253–7. PMID: 1573335. http://www.ncbi.nlm.nih.gov/pubmed/1573335.
172. Molenberghs P, Trautwein FM, Böckler A, Singer T, Kanske P. Neural correlates of metacognitive ability and of feeling confident: a large-scale fMRI study. Soc Cogn Affect Neurosci. 2016;11(12):1942–51. PMCID: PMC5141950. http://www.ncbi.nlm.nih.gov/pubmed/27445213.
173. Ludwig DS, Kabat-Zinn J. Mindfulness in medicine. JAMA. 2008;300(11):1350–2. PMID: 18799450. http://www.ncbi.nlm.nih.gov/pubmed/18799450.
174. Chiesa A. The difficulty of defining mindfulness: current thought and critical issues. Mindfulness. 2013;4:255–68.
175. Rosch E. More than mindfulness: when you have a tiger by the tail, let it eat you. Psychol Inq. 18(4):258–64.
176. Wallace BA, Shapiro SL. Mental balance and Well-being: building bridges between Buddhism and Western psychology. Am Psychol. 2006;61(7):690–701. PMID: 17032069. http://www.ncbi.nlm.nih.gov/pubmed/17032069.
177. Walsh R, Shapiro SL. The meeting of meditative disciplines and Western psychology: a mutually enriching dialogue. Am Psychol. 2006;61(3):227–39. PMID: 16594839. http://www.ncbi.nlm.nih.gov/pubmed/16594839.
178. Dunning DL, Griffiths K, Kuyken W, Crane C, Foulkes L, Parker J, Dalgleish T. Research review: the effects of mindfulness-based interventions on cognition and mental health in children and adolescents – a meta-analysis of randomized controlled trials. J Child Psychol Psychiatry. 2019;60(3):244–58. PMCID: PMC6546608. http://www.ncbi.nlm.nih.gov/pubmed/30345511.
179. Rapgay L, Bystrisky A. Classical mindfulness: an introduction to its theory and practice for clinical application. Ann N Y Acad Sci. 2009;1172:148–62. PMID: 19735247. http://www.ncbi.nlm.nih.gov/pubmed/19735247.
180. Stein DJ, Ives-Deliperi V, Thomas KGF. Psychobiology of mindfulness. CNS Spectr. 2008;13(9):752–6. PMID: 18849893. http://www.ncbi.nlm.nih.gov/pubmed/18849893.
181. Sipe WEB, Eisendrath SJ. Mindfulness-based cognitive therapy: theory and practice. Can J Psychiatr. 2012;57(2):63–9. PMID: 22340145. http://www.ncbi.nlm.nih.gov/pubmed/22340145.
182. Way BM, Creswell JD, Eisenberger NI, Lieberman MD. Dispositional mindfulness and depressive symptomatology: correlations with limbic and self-referential neural activity during rest. Emotion. 2010;10(1):12–24. PMCID: PMC2868367. http://www.ncbi.nlm.nih.gov/pubmed/20141298.
183. Creswell JD, Way BM, Eisenberger NI, Lieberman MD. Neural correlates of dispositional mindfulness during affect labeling. Psychosom Med. 2007;69(6):560–5. PMID: 17634566. http://www.ncbi.nlm.nih.gov/pubmed/17634566.
184. Cerqueira JJ, Almeida OFX, Sousa N. The stressed prefrontal cortex. Left? Right! Brain Behav Immun. 2008;22(5):630–8. PMID: 18281193. http://www.ncbi.nlm.nih.gov/pubmed/18281193.
185. Davidson RJ, Kabat-Zinn J, Schumacher J, Rosenkranz M, Muller D, Santorelli SF, Urbanowski F, Harrington A, Bonus K, Sheridan JF. Alterations in brain and immune function produced by mindfulness meditation. Psychosom Med. 2003;65(4):564–70. PMID: 12883106. http://www.ncbi.nlm.nih.gov/pubmed/12883106.
186. Desrosiers A, Klemanski DH, Nolen-Hoeksema S. Mapping mindfulness facets onto dimensions of anxiety and depression. Behav Ther. 2013;44(3):373–84. PMCID: PMC4012250. http://www.ncbi.nlm.nih.gov/pubmed/23768665.
187. Piet J, Würtzen H, Zachariae R. The effect of mindfulness-based therapy on symptoms of anxiety and depression in adult cancer patients and survivors: a systematic review and meta-analysis. J Consult Clin Psychol. 2012;80(6):1007–20. PMID: 22563637. http://www.ncbi.nlm.nih.gov/pubmed/22563637.
188. Hartmann M, Kopf S, Kircher C, Faude-Lang V, Djuric Z, Augstein F, Friederich HC, Kieser M, Bierhaus A, Humpert PM, Herzog W, Nawroth PP. Sustained effects of a mindfulness-based stress-reduction intervention in type 2 diabetic patients: design and first results of a randomized controlled trial (the Heidelberger diabetes and stress-study). Diabetes Care. 2012;35(5):945–7. PMCID: PMC3329807. http://www.ncbi.nlm.nih.gov/pubmed/22338101.
189. Morone NE, Greco CM, Weiner DK. Mindfulness meditation for the treatment of chronic low back pain in older adults: a randomized controlled pilot study. Pain. 2008;134(3):310–9. PMCID: PMC2254507. http://www.ncbi.nlm.nih.gov/pubmed/17544212.
190. Zautra AJ, Davis MC, Reich JW, Nicassario P, Tennen H, Finan P, Kratz A, Parrish B, Irwin MR. Comparison of cognitive behavioral and mindfulness meditation interventions on adaptation to rheumatoid arthritis for patients with and without history of recurrent

depression. J Consult Clin Psychol. 2008;76(3):408–21. PMID: 18540734. http://www.ncbi.nlm.nih.gov/pubmed/18540734.
191. Kabat-Zinn J, Wheeler E, Light T, Skillings A, Scharf MJ, Cropley TG, Hosmer D, Bernhard JD. Influence of a mindfulness meditation-based stress reduction intervention on rates of skin clearing in patients with moderate to severe psoriasis undergoing phototherapy (UVB) and photochemotherapy (PUVA). Psychosom Med. 1998;60(5):625–32. PMID: 9773769. http://www.ncbi.nlm.nih.gov/pubmed/9773769.
192. Moon HS, Mizara A, McBride SR. Psoriasis and psycho-dermatology. Dermatol Ther (Heidelb). 2013;3(2):117–30. PMCID: PMC3889305. http://www.ncbi.nlm.nih.gov/pubmed/24318414.
193. Stuart LD, James LF, Panter KE, Call JW, Short RE. Pine needle abortion in cattle: pathological observations. Cornell Vet. 1989;79(1):61–9. PMID: 2912674. http://www.ncbi.nlm.nih.gov/pubmed/2912674.
194. Farias M, Wikholm C, Delmonte R. What is mindfulness-based therapy good for? Lancet Psychiatry. 2016;3(11):1012–3. PMID: 27794365. http://www.ncbi.nlm.nih.gov/pubmed/27794365.
195. Coronado-Montoya S, Levis AW, Kwakkenbos L, Steele RJ, Turner EH, Thombs BD. Reporting of positive results in randomized controlled trials of mindfulness-based mental health interventions. PLoS One. 2016;11(4):e0153220. PMCID: PMC4825994. http://www.ncbi.nlm.nih.gov/pubmed/27058355.
196. Goyal M, Singh S, Sibinga EMS, Gould NF, Rowland-Seymour A, Sharma R, Berger Z, Sleicher D, Maron DD, Shihab HM, Ranasinghe PD, Linn S, Saha S, Bass EB, Haythornthwaite JA. Meditation programs for psychological stress and Well-being: a systematic review and meta-analysis. JAMA Intern Med. 2014;174(3):357–68. PMCID: PMC4142584. http://www.ncbi.nlm.nih.gov/pubmed/24395196.
197. Carmody J, Baer RA. How long does a mindfulness-based stress reduction program need to be? A review of class contact hours and effect sizes for psychological distress. J Clin Psychol. 2009;65(6):627–38. PMID: 19309694. http://www.ncbi.nlm.nih.gov/pubmed/19309694.
198. Ott MJ, Norris RL, Bauer-Wu SM. Mindfulness meditation for oncology patients: a discussion and critical review. Integr Cancer Ther. 2006;5(2):98–108. PMID: 16685074. http://www.ncbi.nlm.nih.gov/pubmed/16685074.
199. Olivo EL, Dodson-Lavelle B, Wren A, Fang Y, Oz MC. Feasibility and effectiveness of a brief meditation-based stress management intervention for patients diagnosed with or at risk for coronary heart disease: a pilot study. Psychol Health Med. 2009;14(5):513–23. PMID: 19844830. http://www.ncbi.nlm.nih.gov/pubmed/19844830.
200. Nakamura Y, Lipschitz DL, Kuhn R, Kinney AY, Donaldson GW. Investigating efficacy of two brief mind-body intervention programs for managing sleep disturbance in cancer survivors: a pilot randomized controlled trial. J Cancer Surviv. 2013;7(2):165–82. PMCID: PMC3622018. http://www.ncbi.nlm.nih.gov/pubmed/23338490.
201. Pace TWW, Negi LT, Sivilli TI, Issa MJ, Cole SP, Adame DD, Raison CL. Innate immune, neuroendocrine and behavioral responses to psychosocial stress do not predict subsequent compassion meditation practice time. Psychoneuroendocrinology. 2010;35(2):310–5. PMCID: PMC3083925. http://www.ncbi.nlm.nih.gov/pubmed/19615827.
202. Malarkey WB, Jarjoura D, Klatt M. Workplace based mindfulness practice and inflammation: a randomized trial. Brain Behav Immun. 2013;27(1):145–54. PMCID: PMC3528077. http://www.ncbi.nlm.nih.gov/pubmed/23078984.
203. Klatt MD, Buckworth J, Malarkey WB. Effects of low-dose mindfulness-based stress reduction (MBSR-ld) on working adults. Health Educ Behav. 2009;36(3):601–14. PMID: 18469160. http://www.ncbi.nlm.nih.gov/pubmed/18469160.
204. Tang YY, Ma Y, Fan Y, Feng H, Wang J, Feng S, Lu Q, Hu B, Lin Y, Li J, Zhang Y, Wang Y, Zhou L, Fan M. Central and autonomic nervous system interaction is altered by short-term meditation. Proc Natl Acad Sci USA. 2009;106(22):8865–70. PMCID: PMC2690030. http://www.ncbi.nlm.nih.gov/pubmed/19451642.
205. Tang YY, Ma Y, Wang J, Fan Y, Feng S, Lu Q, Yu Q, Sui D, Rothbart MK, Fan M, Posner MI. Short-term meditation training improves attention and self-regulation. Proc Natl Acad Sci U S A. 2007;104(43):17152–6. PMCID: PMC2040428. http://www.ncbi.nlm.nih.gov/pubmed/17940025.
206. Fjorback LO, Arendt M, Ornbøl E, Fink P, Walach H. Mindfulness-based stress reduction and mindfulness-based cognitive therapy: a systematic review of randomized controlled trials. Acta Psychiatr Scand. 2011;124(2):102–19. PMID: 21534932. http://www.ncbi.nlm.nih.gov/pubmed/21534932.
207. Merkes M. Mindfulness-based stress reduction for people with chronic diseases. Aust J Prim Health. 2010;16(3):200–10. PMID: 20815988. http://www.ncbi.nlm.nih.gov/pubmed/20815988.
208. Grossman P, Niemann L, Schmidt S, Walach H. Mindfulness-based stress reduction and health benefits. A meta-analysis. J Psychosom Res. 2004;57(1):35–43. PMID: 15256293. http://www.ncbi.nlm.nih.gov/pubmed/15256293.
209. Veehof MM, Oskam MJ, Schreurs KMG, Bohlmeijer ET. Acceptance-based interventions for the treatment of chronic pain: a systematic review and meta-analysis. Pain. 2011;152(3):533–42. PMID: 21251756. http://www.ncbi.nlm.nih.gov/pubmed/21251756.
210. Sephton SE, Salmon P, Weissbecker I, Ulmer C, Floyd A, Hoover K, Studts JL. Mindfulness meditation alleviates depressive symptoms in women with fibromyalgia: results of a randomized clinical trial. Arthritis Rheum. 2007;57(1):77–85. PMID: 17266067. http://www.ncbi.nlm.nih.gov/pubmed/17266067.
211. Cramer H, Haller H, Lauche R, Dobos G. Mindfulness-based stress reduction for low back pain. A systematic review. BMC Complement Altern Med. 2012;12:162. PMCID: PMC3520871. http://www.ncbi.nlm.nih.gov/pubmed/23009599.
212. Musial F, Büssing A, Heusser P, Choi KE, Ostermann T. Mindfulness-based stress reduction for integrative cancer care: a summary of evidence. Forsch Komplementmed. 2011;18(4):192–202. PMID: 21934319. http://www.ncbi.nlm.nih.gov/pubmed/21934319.
213. Witek-Janusek L, Albuquerque K, Chroniak KR, Chroniak C, Durazo-Arvizu R, Mathews HL. Effect of mindfulness based stress reduction on immune function, quality of life and coping in women newly diagnosed with early stage breast cancer. Brain Behav Immun. 2008;22(6):969–81. PMCID: PMC2586059. http://www.ncbi.nlm.nih.gov/pubmed/18359186.
214. Matchim Y, Armer JM, Stewart BR. Mindfulness-based stress reduction among breast cancer survivors: a literature review and discussion. Oncol Nurs Forum. 2011;38(2):E61–71. PMID: 21356643. http://www.ncbi.nlm.nih.gov/pubmed/21356643.
215. Chiesa A, Serretti A. Mindfulness-based stress reduction for stress management in healthy people: a review and meta-analysis. J Altern Complement Med. 2009;15(5):593–600. PMID: 19432513. http://www.ncbi.nlm.nih.gov/pubmed/19432513.
216. Witkiewitz K, Bowen S. Depression, craving, and substance use following a randomized trial of mindfulness-based relapse prevention. J Consult Clin Psychol. 2010;78(3):362–74. PMCID: PMC3280693. http://www.ncbi.nlm.nih.gov/pubmed/20515211.
217. Meyer B, Berger T, Caspar F, Beevers CG, Andersson G, Weiss M. Effectiveness of a novel integrative online treatment for depression (Deprexis): randomized controlled trial. J Med Internet Res. 2009;11(2):e15. PMCID: PMC2762808. http://www.ncbi.nlm.nih.gov/pubmed/19632969.

218. Klainin-Yobas P, Cho MAA, Creedy D. Efficacy of mindfulness-based interventions on depressive symptoms among people with mental disorders: a meta-analysis. Int J Nurs Stud. 2012;49(1):109–21. PMID: 21963234. http://www.ncbi.nlm.nih.gov/pubmed/21963234.
219. Chi X, Bo A, Liu T, Zhang P, Chi I. Effects of mindfulness-based stress reduction on depression in adolescents and Young adults: a systematic review and meta-analysis. Front Psychol. 2018;9:1034. PMCID: PMC6021542. http://www.ncbi.nlm.nih.gov/pubmed/29977221.
220. Zhu X, Hu P, Fan Z, Zhan W, Wang H, Yang Y, Zhou Z, Ma L, Gao H. Effects of mindfulness-based stress reduction on depression, anxiety, and pain in patients with Postherpetic neuralgia. J Nerv Ment Dis. 2019;207(6):482–6. PMID: 31045954. http://www.ncbi.nlm.nih.gov/pubmed/31045954.
221. Sizoo BB, Kuiper E. Cognitive behavioural therapy and mindfulness based stress reduction may be equally effective in reducing anxiety and depression in adults with autism spectrum disorders. Res Dev Disabil. 2017;64:47–55. PMID: 28342404. http://www.ncbi.nlm.nih.gov/pubmed/28342404.
222. Kolahkaj B, Zargar F. Effect of mindfulness-based stress reduction on anxiety, depression and stress in women with multiple sclerosis. Nurs Midwifery Stud. 2015;4(4):e29655. PMCID: PMC4733502. http://www.ncbi.nlm.nih.gov/pubmed/26835467.
223. Serpa JG, Taylor SL, Tillisch K. Mindfulness-based stress reduction (MBSR) reduces anxiety, depression, and suicidal ideation in veterans. Med Care. 2014;52(12 Suppl 5):S19–24. PMID: 25397818. http://www.ncbi.nlm.nih.gov/pubmed/25397818.
224. Zhang JY, Ji XZ, Meng LN, Cai YJ. Effects of modified mindfulness-based stress reduction (MBSR) on the psychological health of adolescents with subthreshold depression: a randomized controlled trial. Neuropsychiatr Dis Treat. 2019;15:2695–704. PMCID: PMC6758632. http://www.ncbi.nlm.nih.gov/pubmed/31571885.
225. Li SYH, Bressington D. The effects of mindfulness-based stress reduction on depression, anxiety, and stress in older adults: a systematic review and meta-analysis. Int J Ment Health Nurs. 2019;28(3):635–56. PMID: 30656813. http://www.ncbi.nlm.nih.gov/pubmed/30656813.
226. Teasdale JD, Segal Z, Williams JM. How does cognitive therapy prevent depressive relapse and why should attentional control (mindfulness) training help? Behav Res Ther. 1995;33(1):25–39. PMID: 7872934. http://www.ncbi.nlm.nih.gov/pubmed/7872934.
227. Home – MBCT.com.
228. Teasdale JD, Segal ZV, Williams JM, Ridgeway VA, Soulsby JM, Lau MA. Prevention of relapse/recurrence in major depression by mindfulness-based cognitive therapy. J Consult Clin Psychol. 2000;68(4):615–23. PMID: 10965637. http://www.ncbi.nlm.nih.gov/pubmed/10965637.
229. Segal ZV, Williams JM, Teasdale JD, Gemar M. A cognitive science perspective on kindling and episode sensitization in recurrent affective disorder. Psychol Med. 1996;26(2):371–80. PMID: 8685293. http://www.ncbi.nlm.nih.gov/pubmed/8685293.
230. A Head for Work | learning and development | Cambridge.
231. Munshi K, Eisendrath S, Delucchi K. Preliminary long-term follow-up of Mindfulness-based cognitive therapy-induced remission of depression. Mindfulness (N Y). 2013;4(4):354–61. PMCID: PMC3891780. http://www.ncbi.nlm.nih.gov/pubmed/24443660.
232. MacKenzie MB, Abbott KA, Kocovski NL. Mindfulness-based cognitive therapy in patients with depression: current perspectives. Neuropsychiatr Dis Treat. 2018;14:1599–605. PMCID: PMC6018485. http://www.ncbi.nlm.nih.gov/pubmed/29950842.
233. Segal ZV, Kennedy S, Gemar M, Hood K, Pedersen R, Buis T. Cognitive reactivity to sad mood provocation and the prediction of depressive relapse. Arch Gen Psychiatry. 2006;63(7):749–55. PMID: 16818864. http://www.ncbi.nlm.nih.gov/pubmed/16818864.
234. Segal ZV, Gemar M, Williams S. Differential cognitive response to a mood challenge following successful cognitive therapy or pharmacotherapy for unipolar depression. J Abnorm Psychol. 1999;108(1):3–10. PMID: 10066988. http://www.ncbi.nlm.nih.gov/pubmed/10066988.
235. Kuyken W, Watkins E, Holden E, White K, Taylor RS, Byford S, Evans A, Radford S, Teasdale JD, Dalgleish T. How does mindfulness-based cognitive therapy work? Behav Res Ther. 2010;48(11):1105–12. PMID: 20810101. http://www.ncbi.nlm.nih.gov/pubmed/20810101.
236. Arch JJ, Craske MG. Mechanisms of mindfulness: emotion regulation following a focused breathing induction. Behav Res Ther. 2006;44(12):1849–58. PMID: 16460668. http://www.ncbi.nlm.nih.gov/pubmed/16460668.
237. Britton WB, Shahar B, Szepsenwol O, Jacobs WJ. Mindfulness-based cognitive therapy improves emotional reactivity to social stress: results from a randomized controlled trial. Behav Ther. 2012;43(2):365–80. PMCID: PMC3495556. http://www.ncbi.nlm.nih.gov/pubmed/22440072.
238. Farb NAS, Segal ZV, Mayberg H, Bean J, McKeon D, Fatima Z, Anderson AK. Attending to the present: mindfulness meditation reveals distinct neural modes of self-reference. Soc Cogn Affect Neurosci. 2007;2(4):313–22. PMCID: PMC2566754. http://www.ncbi.nlm.nih.gov/pubmed/18985137.
239. Grant JA, Courtemanche J, Rainville P. A non-elaborative mental stance and decoupling of executive and pain-related cortices predicts low pain sensitivity in Zen meditators. Pain. 2011;152(1):150–6. PMID: 21055874. http://www.ncbi.nlm.nih.gov/pubmed/21055874.
240. Chambers R, Gullone E, Allen NB. Mindful emotion regulation: an integrative review. Clin Psychol Rev. 2009;29(6):560–72. PMID: 19632752. http://www.ncbi.nlm.nih.gov/pubmed/19632752.
241. Taylor VA, Grant J, Daneault V, Scavone G, Breton E, Roffe-Vidal S, Courtemanche J, Lavarenne AS, Beauregard M. Impact of mindfulness on the neural responses to emotional pictures in experienced and beginner meditators. Neuroimage. 2011;57(4):1524–33. PMID: 21679770. http://www.ncbi.nlm.nih.gov/pubmed/21679770.
242. Arch JJ, Craske MG. Laboratory stressors in clinically anxious and non-anxious individuals: the moderating role of mindfulness. Behav Res Ther. 2010;48(6):495–505. PMID: 20303471. http://www.ncbi.nlm.nih.gov/pubmed/20303471.
243. Barnes VA, Treiber FA, Davis H. Impact of transcendental meditation on cardiovascular function at rest and during acute stress in adolescents with high normal blood pressure. J Psychosom Res. 2001;51(4):597–605. PMCID: PMC3216051. http://www.ncbi.nlm.nih.gov/pubmed/11595248.
244. Sudsuang R, Chentanez V, Veluvan K. Effect of Buddhist meditation on serum cortisol and total protein levels, blood pressure, pulse rate, lung volume and reaction time. Physiol Behav. 1991;50(3):543–8. PMID: 1801007. http://www.ncbi.nlm.nih.gov/pubmed/1801007.
245. Carlson LE, Speca M, Faris P, Patel KD. One year pre-post intervention follow-up of psychological, immune, endocrine and blood pressure outcomes of mindfulness-based stress reduction (MBSR) in breast and prostate cancer outpatients. Brain Behav Immun. 2007;21(8):1038–49. PMID: 17521871. http://www.ncbi.nlm.nih.gov/pubmed/17521871.
246. Manicavasgar V, Parker G, Perich T. Mindfulness-based cognitive therapy vs cognitive behaviour therapy as a treatment for non-melancholic depression. J Affect Disord. 2011;130(1–2):138–44. PMID: 21093925. http://www.ncbi.nlm.nih.gov/pubmed/21093925.

247. Britton WB, Haynes PL, Fridel KW, Bootzin RR. Polysomnographic and subjective profiles of sleep continuity before and after mindfulness-based cognitive therapy in partially remitted depression. Psychosom Med. 2010;72(6):539–48. PMID: 20467003. http://www.ncbi.nlm.nih.gov/pubmed/20467003.
248. Schroevers MJ, Brandsma R. Is learning mindfulness associated with improved affect after mindfulness-based cognitive therapy? Br J Psychol. 2010;101(Pt 1):95–107. PMID: 19327220. http://www.ncbi.nlm.nih.gov/pubmed/19327220.
249. Kuyken W, Byford S, Taylor RS, Watkins E, Holden E, White K, Barrett B, Byng R, Evans A, Mullan E, Teasdale JD. Mindfulness-based cognitive therapy to prevent relapse in recurrent depression. J Consult Clin Psychol. 2008;76(6):966–78. PMID: 19045965. http://www.ncbi.nlm.nih.gov/pubmed/19045965.
250. Barnhofer T, Crane C, Hargus E, Amarasinghe M, Winder R, Williams JMG. Mindfulness-based cognitive therapy as a treatment for chronic depression: a preliminary study. Behav Res Ther. 2009;47(5):366–73. PMCID: PMC2866254. http://www.ncbi.nlm.nih.gov/pubmed/19249017.
251. van der Lee ML, Garssen B. Mindfulness-based cognitive therapy reduces chronic cancer-related fatigue: a treatment study. Psychooncology. 2012;21(3):264–72. PMID: 22383268. http://www.ncbi.nlm.nih.gov/pubmed/22383268.
252. Sachse S, Keville S, Feigenbaum J. A feasibility study of mindfulness-based cognitive therapy for individuals with borderline personality disorder. Psychol Psychother. 2011;84(2):184–200. PMID: 22903856. http://www.ncbi.nlm.nih.gov/pubmed/22903856.
253. Rimes KA, Wingrove J. Pilot study of mindfulness-based cognitive therapy for trainee clinical psychologists. Behav Cogn Psychother. 2011;39(2):235–41. PMID: 21144122. http://www.ncbi.nlm.nih.gov/pubmed/21144122.
254. Oken BS, Fonareva I, Haas M, Wahbeh H, Lane JB, Zajdel D, Amen A. Pilot controlled trial of mindfulness meditation and education for dementia caregivers. J Altern Complement Med. 2010;16(10):1031–8. PMCID: PMC3110802. http://www.ncbi.nlm.nih.gov/pubmed/20929380.
255. Vøllestad J, Nielsen MB, Nielsen GH. Mindfulness- and acceptance-based interventions for anxiety disorders: a systematic review and meta-analysis. Br J Clin Psychol. 2012;51(3):239–60. PMID: 22803933. http://www.ncbi.nlm.nih.gov/pubmed/22803933.
256. Piet J, Hougaard E, Hecksher MS, Rosenberg NK. A randomized pilot study of mindfulness-based cognitive therapy and group cognitive-behavioral therapy for young adults with social phobia. Scand J Psychol. 2010;51(5):403–10. PMID: 20210911. http://www.ncbi.nlm.nih.gov/pubmed/20210911.
257. Kim YW, Lee SH, Choi TK, Suh SY, Kim B, Kim CM, Cho SJ, Kim MJ, Yook K, Ryu M, Song SK, Yook KH. Effectiveness of mindfulness-based cognitive therapy as an adjuvant to pharmacotherapy in patients with panic disorder or generalized anxiety disorder. Depress Anxiety. 2009;26(7):601–6. PMID: 19242985. http://www.ncbi.nlm.nih.gov/pubmed/19242985.
258. Lovas DA, Barsky AJ. Mindfulness-based cognitive therapy for hypochondriasis, or severe health anxiety: a pilot study. J Anxiety Disord. 2010;24(8):931–5. PMID: 20650601. http://www.ncbi.nlm.nih.gov/pubmed/20650601.
259. Williams JMG, Alatiq Y, Crane C, Barnhofer T, Fennell MJV, Duggan DS, Hepburn S, Goodwin GM. Mindfulness-based cognitive therapy (MBCT) in bipolar disorder: preliminary evaluation of immediate effects on between-episode functioning. J Affect Disord. 2008;107(1–3):275–9. PMCID: PMC2881943. http://www.ncbi.nlm.nih.gov/pubmed/17884176.
260. Dakwar E, Levin FR. The emerging role of meditation in addressing psychiatric illness, with a focus on substance use disorders. Harv Rev Psychiatry. 2009;17(4):254–67. PMCID: PMC3109319. http://www.ncbi.nlm.nih.gov/pubmed/19637074.
261. De Raedt R, Koster EHW. Understanding vulnerability for depression from a cognitive neuroscience perspective: a reappraisal of attentional factors and a new conceptual framework. Cogn Affect Behav Neurosci. 2010;10(1):50–70. PMID: 20233955. http://www.ncbi.nlm.nih.gov/pubmed/20233955.
262. Chiesa A, Mandelli L, Serretti A. Mindfulness-based cognitive therapy versus psycho-education for patients with major depression who did not achieve remission following antidepressant treatment: a preliminary analysis. J Altern Complement Med. 2012;18(8):756–60. PMID: 22794787. http://www.ncbi.nlm.nih.gov/pubmed/22794787.
263. Bondolfi G, Jermann F, der Linden MV, Gex-Fabry M, Bizzini L, Rouget BW, Myers-Arrazola L, Gonzalez C, Segal Z, Aubry JM, Bertschy G. Depression relapse prophylaxis with mindfulness-based cognitive therapy: replication and extension in the Swiss health care system. J Affect Disord. 2010;122(3):224–31. PMCID: PMC2866251. http://www.ncbi.nlm.nih.gov/pubmed/19666195.
264. Piet J, Hougaard E. The effect of mindfulness-based cognitive therapy for prevention of relapse in recurrent major depressive disorder: a systematic review and meta-analysis. Clin Psychol Rev. 2011;31(6):1032–40. PMID: 21802618. http://www.ncbi.nlm.nih.gov/pubmed/21802618.
265. Geschwind N, Peeters F, Huibers M, van Os J, Wichers M. Efficacy of mindfulness-based cognitive therapy in relation to prior history of depression: randomised controlled trial. Br J Psychiatry. 2012;201(4):320–5. PMID: 22878133. http://www.ncbi.nlm.nih.gov/pubmed/22878133.
266. van Aalderen JR, Donders ART, Giommi F, Spinhoven P, Barendregt HP, Speckens AEM. The efficacy of mindfulness-based cognitive therapy in recurrent depressed patients with and without a current depressive episode: a randomized controlled trial. Psychol Med. 2012;42(5):989–1001. PMID: 22017808. http://www.ncbi.nlm.nih.gov/pubmed/22017808.
267. Segal ZV, Bieling P, Young T, MacQueen G, Cooke R, Martin L, Bloch R, Levitan RD. Antidepressant monotherapy vs sequential pharmacotherapy and mindfulness-based cognitive therapy, or placebo, for relapse prophylaxis in recurrent depression. Arch Gen Psychiatry. 2010;67(12):1256–64. PMCID: PMC3311113. http://www.ncbi.nlm.nih.gov/pubmed/21135325.
268. Bieling PJ, Hawley LL, Bloch RT, Corcoran KM, Levitan RD, Young LT, Macqueen GM, Segal ZV. Treatment-specific changes in decentering following mindfulness-based cognitive therapy versus antidepressant medication or placebo for prevention of depressive relapse. J Consult Clin Psychol. 2012;80(3):365–72. PMCID: PMC3365628. http://www.ncbi.nlm.nih.gov/pubmed/22409641.
269. Chambers SK, Foley E, Galt E, Ferguson M, Clutton S. Mindfulness groups for men with advanced prostate cancer: a pilot study to assess feasibility and effectiveness and the role of peer support. Support Care Cancer. 2012;20(6):1183–92. PMID: 21625914. http://www.ncbi.nlm.nih.gov/pubmed/21625914.
270. Grossman P, Kappos L, Gensicke H, D'Souza M, Mohr DC, Penner IK, Steiner C. MS quality of life, depression, and fatigue improve after mindfulness training: a randomized trial. Neurology. 2010;75(13):1141–9. PMCID: PMC3463050. http://www.ncbi.nlm.nih.gov/pubmed/20876468.
271. Bohlmeijer E, Prenger R, Taal E, Cuijpers P. The effects of mindfulness-based stress reduction therapy on mental health of adults with a chronic medical disease: a meta-analysis. J Psychosom Res. 2010;68(6):539–44. PMID: 20488270. http://www.ncbi.nlm.nih.gov/pubmed/20488270.
272. Brewer JA, Mallik S, Babuscio TA, Nich C, Johnson HE, Deleone CM, Minnix-Cotton CA, Byrne SA, Kober H, Weinstein AJ, Carroll KM, Rounsaville BJ. Mindfulness training for smoking cessation: results from a randomized controlled trial. Drug Alcohol Depend. 2011;119(1–2):72–80. PMCID: PMC3191261. http://www.ncbi.nlm.nih.gov/pubmed/21723049.

273. Britton WB, Haynes PL, Fridel KW, Bootzin RR. Mindfulness-based cognitive therapy improves polysomnographic and subjective sleep profiles in antidepressant users with sleep complaints. Psychother Psychosom. 2012;81(5):296–304. PMCID: PMC3495555. http://www.ncbi.nlm.nih.gov/pubmed/22832540.
274. Coto-Lesmes R, Fernández-Rodríguez C, González-Fernández S. Acceptance and commitment therapy in group format for anxiety and depression. A systematic review. J Affect Disord. 2020;263:107–20. PMID: 31818766. http://www.ncbi.nlm.nih.gov/pubmed/31818766.
275. Bai Z, Luo S, Zhang L, Wu S, Chi I. Acceptance and commitment therapy (ACT) to reduce depression: a systematic review and meta-analysis. J Affect Disord. 2020;260:728–37. PMID: 31563072. http://www.ncbi.nlm.nih.gov/pubmed/31563072.
276. Pohar R, Argáez C. Acceptance and commitment therapy for post-traumatic stress disorder, anxiety, and depression: a review of clinical effectiveness [Internet]. Ottawa: Canadian Agency for Drugs and Technologies in Health; 2017. [cited 2025 Jan 13]. Available from:. http://www.ncbi.nlm.nih.gov/books/NBK525684/. PMID: 30226695. http://www.ncbi.nlm.nih.gov/pubmed/30226695.
277. Twohig MP, Levin ME. Acceptance and commitment therapy as a treatment for anxiety and depression: a review. Psychiatr Clin North Am. 2017;40(4):751–70. PMID: 29080598. http://www.ncbi.nlm.nih.gov/pubmed/29080598.
278. Hayes SC, Luoma JB, Bond FW, Masuda A, Lillis J. Acceptance and commitment therapy: model, processes and outcomes. Behav Res Ther. 2006;44(1):1–25. PMID: 16300724. http://www.ncbi.nlm.nih.gov/pubmed/16300724.
279. Fledderus M, Bohlmeijer ET, Fox JP, Schreurs KMG, Spinhoven P. The role of psychological flexibility in a self-help acceptance and commitment therapy intervention for psychological distress in a randomized controlled trial. Behav Res Ther. 2013;51(3):142–51. PMID: 23337183. http://www.ncbi.nlm.nih.gov/pubmed/23337183.
280. Powers MB, Zum Vorde Sive Vording MB, Emmelkamp PMG. Acceptance and commitment therapy: a meta-analytic review. Psychother Psychosom. 2009;78(2):73–80. PMID: 19142046. http://www.ncbi.nlm.nih.gov/pubmed/19142046.
281. The Six Core Processes of ACT | Association for Contextual Behavioral Science.
282. Acceptance and Commitment Therapy – YouTube.
283. Arch JJ, Wolitzky-Taylor KB, Eifert GH, Craske MG. Longitudinal treatment mediation of traditional cognitive behavioral therapy and acceptance and commitment therapy for anxiety disorders. Behav Res Ther. 2012;50(7–8):469–78. PMID: 22659156. http://www.ncbi.nlm.nih.gov/pubmed/22659156.
284. Forman EM, Shaw JA, Goetter EM, Herbert JD, Park JA, Yuen EK. Long-term follow-up of a randomized controlled trial comparing acceptance and commitment therapy and standard cognitive behavior therapy for anxiety and depression. Behav Ther. 2012;43(4):801–11. PMID: 23046782. http://www.ncbi.nlm.nih.gov/pubmed/23046782.
285. Forman EM, Chapman JE, Herbert JD, Goetter EM, Yuen EK, Moitra E. Using session-by-session measurement to compare mechanisms of action for acceptance and commitment therapy and cognitive therapy. Behav Ther. 2012;43(2):341–54. PMID: 22440070. http://www.ncbi.nlm.nih.gov/pubmed/22440070.
286. Zettle RD, Rains JC, Hayes SC. Processes of change in acceptance and commitment therapy and cognitive therapy for depression: a mediation reanalysis of Zettle and Rains. Behav Modif. 2011;35(3):265–83. PMID: 21362745. http://www.ncbi.nlm.nih.gov/pubmed/21362745.
287. Forman EM, Herbert JD, Moitra E, Yeomans PD, Geller PA. A randomized controlled effectiveness trial of acceptance and commitment therapy and cognitive therapy for anxiety and depression. Behav Modif. 2007;31(6):772–99. PMID: 17932235. http://www.ncbi.nlm.nih.gov/pubmed/17932235.
288. Nordin L, Rorsman I. Cognitive behavioural therapy in multiple sclerosis: a randomized controlled pilot study of acceptance and commitment therapy. J Rehabil Med. 2012;44(1):87–90. PMID: 22234322. http://www.ncbi.nlm.nih.gov/pubmed/22234322.
289. Hesser H, Gustafsson T, Lundén C, Henrikson O, Fattahi K, Johnsson E, Zetterqvist Westin V, Carlbring P, Mäki-Torkko E, Kaldo V, Andersson G. A randomized controlled trial of internet-delivered cognitive behavior therapy and acceptance and commitment therapy in the treatment of tinnitus. J Consult Clin Psychol. 2012;80(4):649–61. PMID: 22250855. http://www.ncbi.nlm.nih.gov/pubmed/22250855.
290. Fledderus M, Bohlmeijer ET, Pieterse ME, Schreurs KMG. Acceptance and commitment therapy as guided self-help for psychological distress and positive mental health: a randomized controlled trial. Psychol Med. 2012;42(3):485–95. PMID: 21740624. http://www.ncbi.nlm.nih.gov/pubmed/21740624.
291. Wetherell JL, Afari N, Rutledge T, Sorrell JT, Stoddard JA, Petkus AJ, Solomon BC, Lehman DH, Liu L, Lang AJ, Atkinson HJ. A randomized, controlled trial of acceptance and commitment therapy and cognitive-behavioral therapy for chronic pain. Pain. 2011;152(9):2098–107. PMID: 21683527. http://www.ncbi.nlm.nih.gov/pubmed/21683527.
292. Wicksell RK, Olsson GL, Hayes SC. Psychological flexibility as a mediator of improvement in acceptance and commitment therapy for patients with chronic pain following whiplash. Eur J Pain. 2010;14(10):1059.e1–1059.e11. PMID: 20538493. http://www.ncbi.nlm.nih.gov/pubmed/20538493.
293. Thorsell J, Finnes A, Dahl J, Lundgren T, Gybrant M, Gordh T, Buhrman M. A comparative study of 2 manual-based self-help interventions, acceptance and commitment therapy and applied relaxation, for persons with chronic pain. Clin J Pain. 2011;27(8):716–23. PMID: 21540740. http://www.ncbi.nlm.nih.gov/pubmed/21540740.
294. Johnston M, Foster M, Shennan J, Starkey NJ, Johnson A. The effectiveness of an acceptance and commitment therapy self-help intervention for chronic pain. Clin J Pain. 2010;26(5):393–402. PMID: 20473046. http://www.ncbi.nlm.nih.gov/pubmed/20473046.
295. Wicksell RK, Melin L, Lekander M, Olsson GL. Evaluating the effectiveness of exposure and acceptance strategies to improve functioning and quality of life in longstanding pediatric pain--a randomized controlled trial. Pain. 2009;141(3):248–57. PMID: 19108951. http://www.ncbi.nlm.nih.gov/pubmed/19108951.
296. Wicksell RK, Kemani M, Jensen K, Kosek E, Kadetoff D, Sorjonen K, Ingvar M, Olsson GL. Acceptance and commitment therapy for fibromyalgia: a randomized controlled trial. Eur J Pain. 2013;17(4):599–611. PMID: 23090719. http://www.ncbi.nlm.nih.gov/pubmed/23090719.
297. Jensen KB, Kosek E, Wicksell R, Kemani M, Olsson G, Merle JV, Kadetoff D, Ingvar M. Cognitive behavioral therapy increases pain-evoked activation of the prefrontal cortex in patients with fibromyalgia. Pain. 2012;153(7):1495–503. PMID: 22617632. http://www.ncbi.nlm.nih.gov/pubmed/22617632.
298. White R, Gumley A, McTaggart J, Rattrie L, McConville D, Cleare S, Mitchell G. A feasibility study of acceptance and commitment therapy for emotional dysfunction following psychosis. Behav Res Ther. 2011;49(12):901–7. PMID: 21975193. http://www.ncbi.nlm.nih.gov/pubmed/21975193.
299. Gaudiano BA, Nowlan K, Brown LA, Epstein-Lubow G, Miller IW. An open trial of a new acceptance-based behavioral treatment for major depression with psychotic features. Behav Modif. 2013;37(3):324–55. PMCID: PMC4049629. http://www.ncbi.nlm.nih.gov/pubmed/23223385.
300. White RG, Gumley AI, McTaggart J, Rattrie L, McConville D, Cleare S, Mitchell G. Depression and anxiety following psycho-

sis: associations with mindfulness and psychological flexibility. Behav Cogn Psychother. 2013;41(1):34–51. PMID: 22578715. http://www.ncbi.nlm.nih.gov/pubmed/22578715.
301. Jeffcoat T, Hayes SC. A randomized trial of ACT bibliotherapy on the mental health of K-12 teachers and staff. Behav Res Ther. 2012;50(9):571–9. PMID: 22750188. http://www.ncbi.nlm.nih.gov/pubmed/22750188.
302. Bohlmeijer ET, Fledderus M, Rokx TAJJ, Pieterse ME. Efficacy of an early intervention based on acceptance and commitment therapy for adults with depressive symptomatology: evaluation in a randomized controlled trial. Behav Res Ther. 2011;49(1):62–7. PMID: 21074752. http://www.ncbi.nlm.nih.gov/pubmed/21074752.
303. Arch JJ, Eifert GH, Davies C, Plumb Vilardaga JC, Rose RD, Craske MG. Randomized clinical trial of cognitive behavioral therapy (CBT) versus acceptance and commitment therapy (ACT) for mixed anxiety disorders. J Consult Clin Psychol. 2012;80(5):750–65. PMCID: PMC4718567. http://www.ncbi.nlm.nih.gov/pubmed/22563639.
304. General DBT – Behavioral Tech Institute.
305. Bornovalova MA, Daughters SB. How does dialectical behavior therapy facilitate treatment retention among individuals with comorbid borderline personality disorder and substance use disorders? Clin Psychol Rev. 2007;27(8):923–43. PMID: 17376574. http://www.ncbi.nlm.nih.gov/pubmed/17376574.
306. Bankoff SM, Karpel MG, Forbes HE, Pantalone DW. A systematic review of dialectical behavior therapy for the treatment of eating disorders. Eat Disord. 2012;20(3):196–215. PMID: 22519897. http://www.ncbi.nlm.nih.gov/pubmed/22519897.
307. Robins CJ, Chapman AL. Dialectical behavior therapy: current status, recent developments, and future directions. J Personal Disord. 2004;18(1):73–89. PMID: 15061345. http://www.ncbi.nlm.nih.gov/pubmed/15061345.
308. Vidal-Estrada R, Bosch-Munso R, Nogueira-Morais M, Casas-Brugue M, Ramos-Quiroga JA. Psychological treatment of attention deficit hyperactivity disorder in adults: a systematic review. Actas Esp Psiquiatr. 2012;40(3):147–54. PMID: 22723133. http://www.ncbi.nlm.nih.gov/pubmed/22723133.
309. Gutteling BM, Montagne B, Nijs M, van den Bosch LMCW. Dialectical behavior therapy: is outpatient group psychotherapy an effective alternative to individual psychotherapy?: Preliminary conclusions. Compr Psychiatry. 2012;53(8):1161–8. PMID: 22560774. http://www.ncbi.nlm.nih.gov/pubmed/22560774.
310. Van Dijk S, Jeffrey J, Katz MR. A randomized, controlled, pilot study of dialectical behavior therapy skills in a psychoeducational group for individuals with bipolar disorder. J Affect Disord. 2013;145(3):386–93. PMID: 22858264. http://www.ncbi.nlm.nih.gov/pubmed/22858264.
311. Harned MS, Korslund KE, Linehan MM. A pilot randomized controlled trial of dialectical behavior therapy with and without the dialectical behavior therapy prolonged exposure protocol for suicidal and self-injuring women with borderline personality disorder and PTSD. Behav Res Ther. 2014;55:7–17. PMCID: PMC3987949. http://www.ncbi.nlm.nih.gov/pubmed/24562087.
312. Ritschel LA, Cheavens JS, Nelson J. Dialectical behavior therapy in an intensive outpatient program with a mixed-diagnostic sample. J Clin Psychol. 2012;68(3):221–35. PMID: 22422561. http://www.ncbi.nlm.nih.gov/pubmed/22422561.
313. Feldman G, Harley R, Kerrigan M, Jacobo M, Fava M. Change in emotional processing during a dialectical behavior therapy-based skills group for major depressive disorder. Behav Res Ther. 2009;47(4):316–21. PMID: 19232571. http://www.ncbi.nlm.nih.gov/pubmed/19232571.
314. STORRE: Intersubjectivity: Towards a Dialogical Analysis.
315. Stoffers JM, Völlm BA, Rücker G, Timmer A, Huband N, Lieb K. Psychological therapies for people with borderline personality disorder. Cochrane Database Syst Rev. 2012;2012(8):CD005652. PMCID: PMC6481907. http://www.ncbi.nlm.nih.gov/pubmed/22895952.
316. About Us | Cognitive Processing Therapy.
317. Cognitive Processing Therapy for PTSD: Second Edition: A Comprehensive Therapist Manual.
318. Resick PA, Schnicke MK. Cognitive processing therapy for sexual assault victims. J Consult Clin Psychol. 1992;60(5):748–56. PMID: 1401390. http://www.ncbi.nlm.nih.gov/pubmed/1401390.
319. Cognitive Processing Therapy (CPT).
320. Chard KM, Ricksecker EG, Healy ET, Karlin BE, Resick PA. Dissemination and experience with cognitive processing therapy. J Rehabil Res Dev. 2012;49(5):667–78. PMID: 23015578. http://www.ncbi.nlm.nih.gov/pubmed/23015578.
321. Tran K, Moulton K, Santesso N, Rabb D. Cognitive processing therapy for post-traumatic stress disorder: a systematic review and meta-analysis [Internet]. Ottawa: Canadian Agency for Drugs and Technologies in Health; 2016. [cited 2025 Jan 13]. Available from: http://www.ncbi.nlm.nih.gov/books/NBK362346/ PMID: 27227199 http://www.ncbi.nlm.nih.gov/pubmed/27227199.
322. Iverson KM, King MW, Cunningham KC, Resick PA. Rape survivors' trauma-related beliefs before and after cognitive processing therapy: associations with PTSD and depression symptoms. Behav Res Ther. 2015;66:49–55. PMID: 25698164. http://www.ncbi.nlm.nih.gov/pubmed/25698164.
323. Markowitz JC, Weissman MM. Interpersonal psychotherapy: past, present and future. Clin Psychol Psychother. 2012;19(2):99–105. PMCID: PMC3427027. http://www.ncbi.nlm.nih.gov/pubmed/22331561.
324. Brakemeier EL, Frase L. Interpersonal psychotherapy (IPT) in major depressive disorder. Eur Arch Psychiatry Clin Neurosci. 2012;262(Suppl 2):S117–21. PMID: 22955493. http://www.ncbi.nlm.nih.gov/pubmed/22955493.
325. Cuijpers P, Geraedts AS, van Oppen P, Andersson G, Markowitz JC, van Straten A. Interpersonal psychotherapy for depression: a meta-analysis. Am J Psychiatry. 2011;168(6):581–92. PMCID: PMC3646065. http://www.ncbi.nlm.nih.gov/pubmed/21362740.
326. Teo AR, Choi H, Valenstein M. Social relationships and depression: ten-year follow-up from a nationally representative study. PLoS One. 2013;8(4):e62396. PMCID: PMC3640036. http://www.ncbi.nlm.nih.gov/pubmed/23646128.
327. Frank E, Kupfer DJ, Wagner EF, McEachran AB, Cornes C. Efficacy of interpersonal psychotherapy as a maintenance treatment of recurrent depression. Contributing factors. Arch Gen Psychiatry. 1991;48(12):1053–9. PMID: 1845438. http://www.ncbi.nlm.nih.gov/pubmed/1845438.
328. Reynolds CF, Frank E, Perel JM, Imber SD, Cornes C, Miller MD, Mazumdar S, Houck PR, Dew MA, Stack JA, Pollock BG, Kupfer DJ. Nortriptyline and interpersonal psychotherapy as maintenance therapies for recurrent major depression: a randomized controlled trial in patients older than 59 years. JAMA. 1999;281(1):39–45. PMID: 9892449. http://www.ncbi.nlm.nih.gov/pubmed/9892449.
329. Schulberg HC, Block MR, Madonia MJ, Scott CP, Rodriguez E, Imber SD, Perel J, Lave J, Houck PR, Coulehan JL. Treating major depression in primary care practice. Eight-month clinical outcomes. Arch Gen Psychiatry. 1996;53(10):913–9. PMID: 8857868. http://www.ncbi.nlm.nih.gov/pubmed/8857868.
330. O'Hara MW, Stuart S, Gorman LL, Wenzel A. Efficacy of interpersonal psychotherapy for postpartum depression. Arch Gen Psychiatry. 2000;57(11):1039–45. PMID: 11074869. http://www.ncbi.nlm.nih.gov/pubmed/11074869.
331. Browne G, Steiner M, Roberts J, Gafni A, Byrne C, Dunn E, Bell B, Mills M, Chalklin L, Wallik D, Kraemer J. Sertraline and/or interpersonal psychotherapy for patients with dysthymic

disorder in primary care: 6-month comparison with longitudinal 2-year follow-up of effectiveness and costs. J Affect Disord. 2002;68(2–3):317–30. PMID: 12063159. http://www.ncbi.nlm.nih.gov/pubmed/12063159.

332. Klerman GL, Budman S, Berwick D, Weissman MM, Damico-White J, Demby A, Feldstein M. Efficacy of a brief psychosocial intervention for symptoms of stress and distress among patients in primary care. Med Care. 1987;25(11):1078–88. PMID: 3695638. http://www.ncbi.nlm.nih.gov/pubmed/3695638.
333. Mossey JM, Knott KA, Higgins M, Talerico K. Effectiveness of a psychosocial intervention, interpersonal counseling, for subdysthymic depression in medically ill elderly. J Gerontol A Biol Sci Med Sci. 1996;51(4):M172–8. PMID: 8681000. http://www.ncbi.nlm.nih.gov/pubmed/8681000.
334. Frank E, Kupfer DJ, Thase ME, Mallinger AG, Swartz HA, Fagiolini AM, Grochocinski V, Houck P, Scott J, Thompson W, Monk T. Two-year outcomes for interpersonal and social rhythm therapy in individuals with bipolar I disorder. Arch Gen Psychiatry. 2005;62(9):996–1004. PMID: 16143731. http://www.ncbi.nlm.nih.gov/pubmed/16143731.
335. Swartz HA, Frank E, Frankel DR, Novick D, Houck P. Psychotherapy as monotherapy for the treatment of bipolar II depression: a proof of concept study. Bipolar Disord. 2009;11(1):89–94. PMCID: PMC3394543. http://www.ncbi.nlm.nih.gov/pubmed/19133971.
336. Jakobsen JC, Hansen JL, Simonsen S, Simonsen E, Gluud C. Effects of cognitive therapy versus interpersonal psychotherapy in patients with major depressive disorder: a systematic review of randomized clinical trials with meta-analyses and trial sequential analyses. Psychol Med. 2012;42(7):1343–57. PMID: 22051174. http://www.ncbi.nlm.nih.gov/pubmed/22051174.
337. Jakobsen JC, Hansen JL, Simonsen E, Gluud C. The effect of interpersonal psychotherapy and other psychodynamic therapies versus "treatment as usual" in patients with major depressive disorder. PLoS One. 2011;6(4):e19044. PMCID: PMC3083428. http://www.ncbi.nlm.nih.gov/pubmed/21556370.
338. Donker T, Bennett K, Bennett A, Mackinnon A, van Straten A, Cuijpers P, Christensen H, Griffiths KM. Internet-delivered interpersonal psychotherapy versus internet-delivered cognitive behavioral therapy for adults with depressive symptoms: randomized controlled noninferiority trial. J Med Internet Res. 2013;15(5):e82. PMCID: PMC3668608. http://www.ncbi.nlm.nih.gov/pubmed/23669884.
339. Moodgym – Interactive skills training for depression and anxiety.
340. O'Shea G, Spence SH, Donovan CL. Interpersonal factors associated with depression in adolescents: are these consistent with theories underpinning interpersonal psychotherapy? Clin Psychol Psychother. 2014;21(6):548–58. PMID: 23801523. http://www.ncbi.nlm.nih.gov/pubmed/23801523.
341. Johnson JE, Hailemariam M, Zlotnick C, Richie F, Sinclair J, Chuong A, Stirman SW. Mixed methods analysis of implementation of interpersonal psychotherapy (IPT) for major depressive disorder in prisons in a hybrid type I randomized trial. Adm Policy Ment Health. 2020;47(3):410–26. PMCID: PMC9187220. http://www.ncbi.nlm.nih.gov/pubmed/31797190.
342. Brave Heart MYH, Chase J, Myers O, Elkins J, Skipper B, Schmitt C, Mootz J, Waldorf VA. Iwankapiya American Indian pilot clinical trial: historical trauma and group interpersonal psychotherapy. Psychotherapy (Chic). 2020;57(2):184–96. PMCID: PMC8216771. http://www.ncbi.nlm.nih.gov/pubmed/31789541.
343. Ravitz P, Watson P, Lawson A, Constantino MJ, Bernecker S, Park J, Swartz HA. Interpersonal psychotherapy: a scoping review and historical perspective (1974–2017). Harv Rev Psychiatry. 2019;27(3):165–80. PMID: 30883446. http://www.ncbi.nlm.nih.gov/pubmed/30883446.
344. Cuijpers P, van Straten A, Smit F, Mihalopoulos C, Beekman A. Preventing the onset of depressive disorders: a meta-analytic review of psychological interventions. Am J Psychiatry. 2008;165(10):1272–80. PMID: 18765483. http://www.ncbi.nlm.nih.gov/pubmed/18765483.
345. Historical Trauma and Unresolved Grief.
346. Casañas R, Catalán R, del Val JL, Real J, Valero S, Casas M. Effectiveness of a psycho-educational group program for major depression in primary care: a randomized controlled trial. BMC Psychiatry. 2012;12:230. PMCID: PMC3551665. http://www.ncbi.nlm.nih.gov/pubmed/23249399.
347. Peveler R, George C, Kinmonth AL, Campbell M, Thompson C. Effect of antidepressant drug counselling and information leaflets on adherence to drug treatment in primary care: randomised controlled trial. BMJ. 1999;319(7210):612–5. PMCID: PMC28214. http://www.ncbi.nlm.nih.gov/pubmed/10473477.
348. Dalgard OS. A randomized controlled trial of a psychoeducational group program for unipolar depression in adults in Norway (NCT00319540). Clin Pract Epidemiol Ment Health. 2006;2:15. PMCID: PMC1538590. http://www.ncbi.nlm.nih.gov/pubmed/16805912.
349. Araya R, Rojas G, Fritsch R, Gaete J, Rojas M, Simon G, Peters TJ. Treating depression in primary care in low-income women in Santiago, Chile: a randomised controlled trial. Lancet. 2003;361(9362):995–1000. PMID: 12660056. http://www.ncbi.nlm.nih.gov/pubmed/12660056.
350. Rodríguez MR, Nuevo R, Chatterji S, Ayuso-Mateos JL. Definitions and factors associated with subthreshold depressive conditions: a systematic review. BMC Psychiatry. 2012;12:181. PMCID: PMC3539957. http://www.ncbi.nlm.nih.gov/pubmed/23110575.
351. Allart-van Dam E, Hosman CMH, Hoogduin CAL, Schaap CPDR. Prevention of depression in subclinically depressed adults: follow-up effects on the "coping with depression" course. J Affect Disord. 2007;97(1–3):219–28. PMID: 16860874. http://www.ncbi.nlm.nih.gov/pubmed/16860874.
352. Cuijpers P, Smit F, van Straten A. Psychological treatments of subthreshold depression: a meta-analytic review. Acta Psychiatr Scand. 2007;115(6):434–41. PMID: 17498154. http://www.ncbi.nlm.nih.gov/pubmed/17498154.
353. Dowrick C, Dunn G, Ayuso-Mateos JL, Dalgard OS, Page H, Lehtinen V, Casey P, Wilkinson C, Vazquez-Barquero JL, Wilkinson G. Problem solving treatment and group psychoeducation for depression: multicentre randomised controlled trial. Outcomes of Depression International Network (ODIN) Group. BMJ. 2000;321(7274):1450–4. PMCID: PMC27549. http://www.ncbi.nlm.nih.gov/pubmed/11110739.
354. Bright JI, Baker KD, Neimeyer RA. Professional and paraprofessional group treatments for depression: a comparison of cognitive-behavioral and mutual support interventions. J Consult Clin Psychol. 1999;67(4):491–501. PMID: 10450619. http://www.ncbi.nlm.nih.gov/pubmed/10450619.
355. Adolescent Coping with Depression Course — Saavsus, Inc.
356. Adolescent Coping With Depression.
357. APA Clinical Practice Guideline for the Treatment of Depression Across Three Age Cohorts.
358. Kuehner C. An evaluation of the "coping with depression course" for relapse prevention with unipolar depressed patients. Psychother Psychosom. 2005;74(4):254–9. PMID: 15947516. http://www.ncbi.nlm.nih.gov/pubmed/15947516.
359. Cuijpers P, Muñoz RF, Clarke GN, Lewinsohn PM. Psychoeducational treatment and prevention of depression: the "coping with depression" course thirty years later. Clin Psychol Rev. 2009;29(5):449–58. PMID: 19450912. http://www.ncbi.nlm.nih.gov/pubmed/19450912.

360. Donker T, Griffiths KM, Cuijpers P, Christensen H. Psychoeducation for depression, anxiety and psychological distress: a meta-analysis. BMC Med. 2009;7:79. PMCID: PMC2805686. http://www.ncbi.nlm.nih.gov/pubmed/20015347.
361. van't Veer-Tazelaar PJ, van Marwijk HWJ, van Oppen P, van Hout HPJ, van der Horst HE, Cuijpers P, Smit F, Beekman ATF. Stepped-care prevention of anxiety and depression in late life: a randomized controlled trial. Arch Gen Psychiatry. 2009;66(3):297–304. PMID: 19255379. http://www.ncbi.nlm.nih.gov/pubmed/19255379.
362. Tolin DF. Is cognitive-behavioral therapy more effective than other therapies? A meta-analytic review. Clin Psychol Rev. 2010;30(6):710–20. PMID: 20547435. http://www.ncbi.nlm.nih.gov/pubmed/20547435.
363. Driessen E, Cuijpers P, de Maat SCM, Abbass AA, de Jonghe F, Dekker JJM. The efficacy of short-term psychodynamic psychotherapy for depression: a meta-analysis. Clin Psychol Rev. 2010;30(1):25–36. PMID: 19766369. http://www.ncbi.nlm.nih.gov/pubmed/19766369.
364. Jakobsen JC, Hansen JL, Simonsen E, Gluud C. The effect of adding psychodynamic therapy to antidepressants in patients with major depressive disorder. A systematic review of randomized clinical trials with meta-analyses and trial sequential analyses. J Affect Disord. 2012;137(1–3):4–14. PMID: 21501877. http://www.ncbi.nlm.nih.gov/pubmed/21501877.
365. Global Health Data Exchange | GHDx.
366. Liu Q, He H, Yang J, Feng X, Zhao F, Lyu J. Changes in the global burden of depression from 1990 to 2017: findings from the global burden of disease study. J Psychiatr Res. 2020;126:134–40. PMID: 31439359. http://www.ncbi.nlm.nih.gov/pubmed/31439359.
367. Cuijpers P, Smit F. Excess mortality in depression: a meta-analysis of community studies. J Affect Disord. 2002;72(3):227–36. PMID: 12450639. http://www.ncbi.nlm.nih.gov/pubmed/12450639.
368. Simon GE. Social and economic burden of mood disorders. Biol Psychiatry. 2003;54(3):208–15. PMID: 12893097. http://www.ncbi.nlm.nih.gov/pubmed/12893097.
369. Katon W, Ciechanowski P. Impact of major depression on chronic medical illness. J Psychosom Res. 2002;53(4):859–63. PMID: 12377294. http://www.ncbi.nlm.nih.gov/pubmed/12377294.
370. Hasin DS, Sarvet AL, Meyers JL, Saha TD, Ruan WJ, Stohl M, Grant BF. Epidemiology of adult DSM-5 major depressive disorder and its specifiers in the United States. JAMA Psychiatry. 2018;75(4):336–46. PMCID: PMC5875313. http://www.ncbi.nlm.nih.gov/pubmed/29450462.
371. Herrman H, Patrick DL, Diehr P, Martin ML, Fleck M, Simon GE, Buesching DP. Longitudinal investigation of depression outcomes in primary care in six countries: the LIDO study. Functional status, health service use and treatment of people with depressive symptoms. Psychol Med. 2002;32(5):889–902. PMID: 12171383. http://www.ncbi.nlm.nih.gov/pubmed/12171383.
372. Van Voorhees BW, Hsiung RC, Marko-Holguin M, Houston TK, Fogel J, Lee R, Ford DE. Internal versus external motivation in referral of primary care patients with depression to an internet support group: randomized controlled trial. J Med Internet Res. 2013;15(3):e42. PMCID: PMC3636270. http://www.ncbi.nlm.nih.gov/pubmed/23482332.
373. Cuijpers P, van Straten A, Bohlmeijer E, Hollon SD, Andersson G. The effects of psychotherapy for adult depression are overestimated: a meta-analysis of study quality and effect size. Psychol Med. 2010;40(2):211–23. PMID: 19490745. http://www.ncbi.nlm.nih.gov/pubmed/19490745.
374. Winter SE, Barber JP. Should treatment for depression be based more on patient preference? Patient Prefer Adherence. 2013;7:1047–57. PMCID: PMC3797653. http://www.ncbi.nlm.nih.gov/pubmed/24143080.
375. Dwight-Johnson M, Sherbourne CD, Liao D, Wells KB. Treatment preferences among depressed primary care patients. J Gen Intern Med. 2000;15(8):527–34. PMCID: PMC1495573. http://www.ncbi.nlm.nih.gov/pubmed/10940143.
376. van Schaik DJF, Klijn AFJ, van Hout HPJ, van Marwijk HWJ, Beekman ATF, de Haan M, van Dyck R. Patients' preferences in the treatment of depressive disorder in primary care. Gen Hosp Psychiatry. 2004;26(3):184–9. PMID: 15121346. http://www.ncbi.nlm.nih.gov/pubmed/15121346.
377. Jaycox LH, Miranda J, Meredith LS, Duan N, Benjamin B, Wells K. Impact of a primary care quality improvement intervention on use of psychotherapy for depression. Ment Health Serv Res. 2003;5(2):109–20. PMID: 12801074. http://www.ncbi.nlm.nih.gov/pubmed/12801074.
378. Mohr DC, Vella L, Hart S, Heckman T, Simon G. The effect of telephone-administered psychotherapy on symptoms of depression and attrition: a meta-analysis. Clin Psychol (New York). 2008;15(3):243–53. PMCID: PMC3045729. http://www.ncbi.nlm.nih.gov/pubmed/21369344.
379. Mohr DC, Ho J, Duffecy J, Baron KG, Lehman KA, Jin L, Reifler D. Perceived barriers to psychological treatments and their relationship to depression. J Clin Psychol. 2010;66(4):394–409. PMCID: PMC2907887. http://www.ncbi.nlm.nih.gov/pubmed/20127795.
380. Mohr DC, Hart SL, Howard I, Julian L, Vella L, Catledge C, Feldman MD. Barriers to psychotherapy among depressed and nondepressed primary care patients. Ann Behav Med. 2006;32(3):254–8. PMID: 17107299. http://www.ncbi.nlm.nih.gov/pubmed/17107299.
381. Simon GE, Fleck M, Lucas R, Bushnell DM, LIDO Group. Prevalence and predictors of depression treatment in an international primary care study. Am J Psychiatry. 2004;161(9):1626–34. PMID: 15337653. http://www.ncbi.nlm.nih.gov/pubmed/15337653.
382. Høifødt RS, Strøm C, Kolstrup N, Eisemann M, Waterloo K. Effectiveness of cognitive behavioural therapy in primary health care: a review. Fam Pract. 2011;28(5):489–504. PMID: 21555339. http://www.ncbi.nlm.nih.gov/pubmed/21555339.
383. Online psychologische hulp nodig – Interapy.
384. Ruwaard J, Lange A, Schrieken B, Emmelkamp P. Efficacy and effectiveness of online cognitive behavioral treatment: a decade of interapy research. Stud Health Technol Inform. 2011;167:9–14. PMID: 21685634. http://www.ncbi.nlm.nih.gov/pubmed/21685634.
385. A Decade of Interapy Research | PPT.
386. Ahern E, Kinsella S, Semkovska M. Clinical efficacy and economic evaluation of online cognitive behavioral therapy for major depressive disorder: a systematic review and meta-analysis. Expert Rev Pharmacoecon Outcomes Res. 2018;18(1):25–41. PMID: 29145746. http://www.ncbi.nlm.nih.gov/pubmed/29145746.
387. Rith-Najarian LR, Boustani MM, Chorpita BF. A systematic review of prevention programs targeting depression, anxiety, and stress in university students. J Affect Disord. 2019;257:568–84. PMID: 31326690. http://www.ncbi.nlm.nih.gov/pubmed/31326690.
388. Ritterband LM, Andersson G, Christensen HM, Carlbring P, Cuijpers P. Directions for the International Society for Research on internet interventions (ISRII). J Med Internet Res. 2006;8(3):e23. PMCID: PMC2018834. http://www.ncbi.nlm.nih.gov/pubmed/17032639.
389. ISRII – International Society for Research on Internet Interventions.
390. Reins JA, Ebert DD, Lehr D, Riper H, Cuijpers P, Berking M. Internet-based treatment of major depression for patients on a waiting list for inpatient psychotherapy: protocol for a multi-Centre randomised controlled trial. BMC Psychiatry. 2013;13:318. PMCID: PMC4222859. http://www.ncbi.nlm.nih.gov/pubmed/24279841.

391. Ebert DD, Gollwitzer M, Riper H, Cuijpers P, Baumeister H, Berking M. For whom does it work? Moderators of outcome on the effect of a transdiagnostic internet-based maintenance treatment after inpatient psychotherapy: randomized controlled trial. J Med Internet Res. 2013;15(10):e191. PMCID: PMC3849694. http://www.ncbi.nlm.nih.gov/pubmed/24113764.
392. González-Robles A, García-Palacios A, Baños R, Riera A, Llorca G, Traver F, Haro G, Palop V, Lera G, Romeu JE, Botella C. Effectiveness of a transdiagnostic internet-based protocol for the treatment of emotional disorders versus treatment as usual in specialized care: study protocol for a randomized controlled trial. Trials. 2015;16:488. PMCID: PMC4628388. http://www.ncbi.nlm.nih.gov/pubmed/26519046.
393. Ünlü Ince B, Cuijpers P, van 't Hof E, van Ballegooijen W, Christensen H, Riper H. Internet-based, culturally sensitive, problem-solving therapy for Turkish migrants with depression: randomized controlled trial. J Med Internet Res. 2013;15(10):e227. PMCID: PMC3849840. http://www.ncbi.nlm.nih.gov/pubmed/24121307.
394. Donker T, Batterham PJ, Warmerdam L, Bennett K, Bennett A, Cuijpers P, Griffiths KM, Christensen H. Predictors and moderators of response to internet-delivered interpersonal psychotherapy and cognitive behavior therapy for depression. J Affect Disord. 2013;151(1):343–51. PMID: 23953024. http://www.ncbi.nlm.nih.gov/pubmed/23953024.
395. Updated program e-couch – self-help and information for common mental health issues.
396. Home – Master Your Moods.
397. van der Zanden R, Galindo-Garre F, Curie K, Kramer J, Cuijpers P. Online cognitive-based intervention for depression: exploring possible circularity in mechanisms of change. Psychol Med. 2014;44(6):1159–70. PMID: 23866103. http://www.ncbi.nlm.nih.gov/pubmed/23866103.
398. van der Zanden R, Kramer J, Gerrits R, Cuijpers P. Effectiveness of an online group course for depression in adolescents and young adults: a randomized trial. J Med Internet Res. 2012;14(3):e86. PMCID: PMC3414873. http://www.ncbi.nlm.nih.gov/pubmed/22677437.
399. Abeles P, Verduyn C, Robinson A, Smith P, Yule W, Proudfoot J. Computerized CBT for adolescent depression ("Stressbusters") and its initial evaluation through an extended case series. Behav Cogn Psychother. 2009;37(2):151–65. PMID: 19364416. http://www.ncbi.nlm.nih.gov/pubmed/19364416.
400. Andersson G, Carlbring P, Berger T, Almlöv J, Cuijpers P. What makes internet therapy work? Cogn Behav Ther. 2009;38(Suppl 1):55–60. PMID: 19675956. http://www.ncbi.nlm.nih.gov/pubmed/19675956.
401. Johansson R, Andersson G. Internet-based psychological treatments for depression. Expert Rev Neurother 2012;12(7):861–869; quiz 870. PMID: 22853793. http://www.ncbi.nlm.nih.gov/pubmed/22853793.
402. Andersson G. The promise and pitfalls of the internet for cognitive behavioral therapy. BMC Med. 2010;8:82. PMCID: PMC3004806. http://www.ncbi.nlm.nih.gov/pubmed/21138574.
403. Almlöv J, Carlbring P, Berger T, Cuijpers P, Andersson G. Therapist factors in internet-delivered cognitive behavioural therapy for major depressive disorder. Cogn Behav Ther. 2009;38(4):247–54. PMID: 19802751. http://www.ncbi.nlm.nih.gov/pubmed/19802751.
404. Hedman E, Ljótsson B, Lindefors N. Cognitive behavior therapy via the internet: a systematic review of applications, clinical efficacy and cost-effectiveness. Expert Rev Pharmacoecon Outcomes Res. 2012;12(6):745–64. PMID: 23252357. http://www.ncbi.nlm.nih.gov/pubmed/23252357.
405. Månsson KNT, Skagius Ruiz E, Gervind E, Dahlin M, Andersson G. Development and initial evaluation of an internet-based support system for face-to-face cognitive behavior therapy: a proof of concept study. J Med Internet Res. 2013;15(12):e280. PMCID: PMC3868964. http://www.ncbi.nlm.nih.gov/pubmed/24326065.
406. APA Publications and Communications Board Working Group on Journal Article Reporting Standards. Reporting standards for research in psychology: why do we need them? What might they be? Am Psychol. 2008;63(9):839–51. PMCID: PMC2957094. http://www.ncbi.nlm.nih.gov/pubmed/19086746.
407. Lokkerbol J, Adema D, Cuijpers P, Reynolds CF, Schulz R, Weehuizen R, Smit F. Improving the cost-effectiveness of a healthcare system for depressive disorders by implementing telemedicine: a health economic modeling study. Am J Geriatr Psychiatry. 2014;22(3):253–62. PMCID: PMC4096928. http://www.ncbi.nlm.nih.gov/pubmed/23759290.
408. van Bastelaar KMP, Pouwer F, Cuijpers P, Riper H, Twisk JWR, Snoek FJ. Is a severe clinical profile an effect modifier in a web-based depression treatment for adults with type 1 or type 2 diabetes? Secondary analyses from a randomized controlled trial. J Med Internet Res. 2012;14(1):e2. PMCID: PMC3846344. http://www.ncbi.nlm.nih.gov/pubmed/22262728.
409. van Straten A, Emmelkamp J, de Wit J, Lancee J, Andersson G, van Someren EJW, Cuijpers P. Guided internet-delivered cognitive behavioural treatment for insomnia: a randomized trial. Psychol Med. 2014;44(7):1521–32. PMID: 24001364. http://www.ncbi.nlm.nih.gov/pubmed/24001364.
410. Johansson R, Nyblom A, Carlbring P, Cuijpers P, Andersson G. Choosing between internet-based psychodynamic versus cognitive behavioral therapy for depression: a pilot preference study. BMC Psychiatry. 2013;13:268. PMCID: PMC3852703. http://www.ncbi.nlm.nih.gov/pubmed/24139066.
411. Andersson G, Paxling B, Roch-Norlund P, Östman G, Norgren A, Almlöv J, Georén L, Breitholtz E, Dahlin M, Cuijpers P, Carlbring P, Silverberg F. Internet-based psychodynamic versus cognitive behavioral guided self-help for generalized anxiety disorder: a randomized controlled trial. Psychother Psychosom. 2012;81(6):344–55. PMID: 22964540. http://www.ncbi.nlm.nih.gov/pubmed/22964540.
412. Warmerdam L, van Straten A, Jongsma J, Twisk J, Cuijpers P. Online cognitive behavioral therapy and problem-solving therapy for depressive symptoms: exploring mechanisms of change. J Behav Ther Exp Psychiatry. 2010;41(1):64–70. PMID: 19913781. http://www.ncbi.nlm.nih.gov/pubmed/19913781.
413. Warmerdam L, van Straten A, Twisk J, Riper H, Cuijpers P. Internet-based treatment for adults with depressive symptoms: randomized controlled trial. J Med Internet Res. 2008;10(4):e44. PMCID: PMC2629364. http://www.ncbi.nlm.nih.gov/pubmed/19033149.
414. Warmerdam L, Smit F, van Straten A, Riper H, Cuijpers P. Cost-utility and cost-effectiveness of internet-based treatment for adults with depressive symptoms: randomized trial. J Med Internet Res. 2010;12(5):e53. PMCID: PMC3057305. http://www.ncbi.nlm.nih.gov/pubmed/21169166.
415. Pedowitz RA, Rydevik BL, Gershuni DH, Hargens AR. An animal model for the study of neuromuscular injury induced beneath and distal to a pneumatic tourniquet. J Orthop Res. 1990;8(6):899–908. PMID: 2213347. http://www.ncbi.nlm.nih.gov/pubmed/2213347.
416. Warmerdam L, Van Straten A, Twisk J, Cuijpers P. Predicting outcome of internet-based treatment for depressive symptoms. Psychother Res. 2013;23(5):559–67. PMID: 23848944. http://www.ncbi.nlm.nih.gov/pubmed/23848944.
417. Hoek W, Schuurmans J, Koot HM, Cuijpers P. Effects of internet-based guided self-help problem-solving therapy for adolescents with depression and anxiety: a randomized controlled trial. PLoS One. 2012;7(8):e43485. PMCID: PMC3432036. http://www.ncbi.nlm.nih.gov/pubmed/22952691.
418. Mohr DC, Cuijpers P, Lehman K. Supportive accountability: a model for providing human support to enhance adherence to eHealth interventions. J Med Internet Res. 2011;13(1):e30.

PMCID: PMC3221353. http://www.ncbi.nlm.nih.gov/pubmed/21393123.
419. Mohr DC, Duffecy J, Ho J, Kwasny M, Cai X, Burns MN, Begale M. A randomized controlled trial evaluating a manualized TeleCoaching protocol for improving adherence to a web-based intervention for the treatment of depression. PLoS One. 2013;8(8):e70086. PMCID: PMC3749146. http://www.ncbi.nlm.nih.gov/pubmed/23990896.
420. Mohr DC, Duffecy J, Jin L, Ludman EJ, Lewis A, Begale M, McCarthy M. Multimodal e-mental health treatment for depression: a feasibility trial. J Med Internet Res. 2010;12(5):e48. PMCID: PMC3057313. http://www.ncbi.nlm.nih.gov/pubmed/21169164.
421. Kelders SM, Bohlmeijer ET, Van Gemert-Pijnen JE. Participants, usage, and use patterns of a web-based intervention for the prevention of depression within a randomized controlled trial. J Med Internet Res. 2013;15(8):e172. PMCID: PMC3757912. http://www.ncbi.nlm.nih.gov/pubmed/23963284.
422. Sharry J, Davidson R, McLoughlin O, Doherty G. A service-based evaluation of a therapist-supported online cognitive behavioral therapy program for depression. J Med Internet Res. 2013;15(6):e121. PMCID: PMC3713925. http://www.ncbi.nlm.nih.gov/pubmed/23807565.
423. Mohr DC, Ho J, Duffecy J, Reifler D, Sokol L, Burns MN, Jin L, Siddique J. Effect of telephone-administered vs face-to-face cognitive behavioral therapy on adherence to therapy and depression outcomes among primary care patients: a randomized trial. JAMA. 2012;307(21):2278–85. PMCID: PMC3697075. http://www.ncbi.nlm.nih.gov/pubmed/22706833.
424. Hammond GC, Croudace TJ, Radhakrishnan M, Lafortune L, Watson A, McMillan-Shields F, Jones PB. Comparative effectiveness of cognitive therapies delivered face-to-face or over the telephone: an observational study using propensity methods. PLoS One. 2012;7(9):e42916. PMCID: PMC3460939. http://www.ncbi.nlm.nih.gov/pubmed/23028436.
425. Williams AD, Blackwell SE, Mackenzie A, Holmes EA, Andrews G. Combining imagination and reason in the treatment of depression: a randomized controlled trial of internet-based cognitive-bias modification and internet-CBT for depression. J Consult Clin Psychol. 2013;81(5):793–9. PMCID: PMC3780629. http://www.ncbi.nlm.nih.gov/pubmed/23750459.
426. MomMoodBooster | Helping women with perinatal depression.
427. Danaher BG, Milgrom J, Seeley JR, Stuart S, Schembri C, Tyler MS, Ericksen J, Lester W, Gemmill AW, Kosty DB, Lewinsohn P. MomMoodBooster web-based intervention for postpartum depression: feasibility trial results. J Med Internet Res. 2013;15(11):e242. PMCID: PMC3841354. http://www.ncbi.nlm.nih.gov/pubmed/24191345.
428. Wilson GT, Zandberg LJ. Cognitive-behavioral guided self-help for eating disorders: effectiveness and scalability. Clin Psychol Rev. 2012;32(4):343–57. PMID: 22504491. http://www.ncbi.nlm.nih.gov/pubmed/22504491.
429. Cuijpers P, Marks IM, van Straten A, Cavanagh K, Gega L, Andersson G. Computer-aided psychotherapy for anxiety disorders: a meta-analytic review. Cogn Behav Ther. 2009;38(2):66–82. PMID: 20183688. http://www.ncbi.nlm.nih.gov/pubmed/20183688.
430. Burns MN, Begale M, Duffecy J, Gergle D, Karr CJ, Giangrande E, Mohr DC. Harnessing context sensing to develop a mobile intervention for depression. J Med Internet Res. 2011;13(3):e55. PMCID: PMC3222181. http://www.ncbi.nlm.nih.gov/pubmed/21840837.
431. Bockting CLH, Kok GD, van der Kamp L, Smit F, van Valen E, Schoevers R, van Marwijk H, Cuijpers P, Riper H, Dekker J, Beck AT. Disrupting the rhythm of depression using Mobile cognitive therapy for recurrent depression: randomized controlled trial design and protocol. BMC Psychiatry. 2011;11:12. PMCID: PMC3036590. http://www.ncbi.nlm.nih.gov/pubmed/21235774.
432. Donker T, Petrie K, Proudfoot J, Clarke J, Birch MR, Christensen H. Smartphones for smarter delivery of mental health programs: a systematic review. J Med Internet Res. 2013;15(11):e247. PMCID: PMC3841358. http://www.ncbi.nlm.nih.gov/pubmed/24240579.
433. Huguet A, Rao S, McGrath PJ, Wozney L, Wheaton M, Conrod J, Rozario S. A systematic review of cognitive behavioral therapy and behavioral activation apps for depression. PLoS One. 2016;11(5):e0154248. PMCID: PMC4852920. http://www.ncbi.nlm.nih.gov/pubmed/27135410.
434. Rathbone AL, Prescott J. The use of Mobile apps and SMS messaging as physical and mental health interventions: systematic review. J Med Internet Res. 2017;19(8):e295. PMCID: PMC5590007. http://www.ncbi.nlm.nih.gov/pubmed/28838887.
435. Wang K, Varma DS, Prosperi M. A systematic review of the effectiveness of mobile apps for monitoring and management of mental health symptoms or disorders. J Psychiatr Res. 2018;107:73–8. PMID: 30347316. http://www.ncbi.nlm.nih.gov/pubmed/30347316.
436. Grist R, Porter J, Stallard P. Mental health Mobile apps for preadolescents and adolescents: a systematic review. J Med Internet Res. 2017;19(5):e176. PMCID: PMC5465380. http://www.ncbi.nlm.nih.gov/pubmed/28546138.
437. Journal of Medical Internet Research.
438. Lipschitz J, Miller CJ, Hogan TP, Burdick KE, Lippin-Foster R, Simon SR, Burgess J. Adoption of Mobile apps for depression and anxiety: cross-sectional survey study on patient interest and barriers to engagement. JMIR Ment Health. 2019;6(1):e11334. PMCID: PMC6367667. http://www.ncbi.nlm.nih.gov/pubmed/30681968.
439. Sprenger M, Mettler T, Osma J. Health professionals' perspective on the promotion of e-mental health apps in the context of maternal depression. PLoS One. 2017;12(7):e0180867. PMCID: PMC5507525. http://www.ncbi.nlm.nih.gov/pubmed/28704442.
440. Lal S, Adair CE. E-mental health: a rapid review of the literature. Psychiatr Serv. 2014;65(1):24–32. PMID: 24081188. http://www.ncbi.nlm.nih.gov/pubmed/24081188.
441. Emmelkamp PMG. Technological innovations in clinical assessment and psychotherapy. Psychother Psychosom. 2005;74(6):336–43. PMID: 16244509. http://www.ncbi.nlm.nih.gov/pubmed/16244509.
442. Marshall JM, Dunstan DA, Bartik W. The digital psychiatrist: in search of evidence-based apps for anxiety and depression. Front Psychiatry. 2019;10:831. PMCID: PMC6872533. http://www.ncbi.nlm.nih.gov/pubmed/31803083.
443. van der Meer RM, Willemsen MC, Smit F, Cuijpers P. Smoking cessation interventions for smokers with current or past depression. Cochrane Database Syst Rev. 2013;8:CD006102. PMID: 23963776. http://www.ncbi.nlm.nih.gov/pubmed/23963776.
444. van der Meer RM, Willemsen MC, Smit F, Cuijpers P, Schippers GM. Effectiveness of a mood management component as an adjunct to a telephone counselling smoking cessation intervention for smokers with a past major depression: a pragmatic randomized controlled trial. Addiction. 2010;105(11):1991–9. PMID: 20735366. http://www.ncbi.nlm.nih.gov/pubmed/20735366.
445. Jamal M, Willem Van der Does AJ, Cuijpers P, Penninx BWJH. Association of smoking and nicotine dependence with severity and course of symptoms in patients with depressive or anxiety disorder. Drug Alcohol Depend. 2012;126(1–2):138–46. PMID: 22633368. http://www.ncbi.nlm.nih.gov/pubmed/22633368.
446. Kirsch I, Montgomery G, Sapirstein G. Hypnosis as an adjunct to cognitive-behavioral psychotherapy: a meta-analysis. J Consult Clin Psychol. 1995;63(2):214–20. PMID: 7751482. http://www.ncbi.nlm.nih.gov/pubmed/7751482.

447. McCann BS, Landes SJ. Hypnosis in the treatment of depression: considerations in research design and methods. Int J Clin Exp Hypn. 2010;58(2):147–64. PMCID: PMC2856099. http://www.ncbi.nlm.nih.gov/pubmed/20390688.
448. Schnur JB, David D, Kangas M, Green S, Bovbjerg DH, Montgomery GH. A randomized trial of a cognitive-behavioral therapy and hypnosis intervention on positive and negative affect during breast cancer radiotherapy. J Clin Psychol. 2009;65(4):443–55. PMCID: PMC2756503. http://www.ncbi.nlm.nih.gov/pubmed/19226611.
449. Alladin A, Alibhai A. Cognitive hypnotherapy for depression: an empirical investigation. Int J Clin Exp Hypn. 2007;55(2):147–66. PMID: 17365072. http://www.ncbi.nlm.nih.gov/pubmed/17365072.
450. Berking M, Ebert D, Cuijpers P, Hofmann SG. Emotion regulation skills training enhances the efficacy of inpatient cognitive behavioral therapy for major depressive disorder: a randomized controlled trial. Psychother Psychosom. 2013;82(4):234–45. PMID: 23712210. http://www.ncbi.nlm.nih.gov/pubmed/23712210.
451. Krebber AMH, Leemans CR, de Bree R, van Straten A, Smit F, Smit EF, Becker A, Eeckhout GM, Beekman ATF, Cuijpers P, Verdonck-de Leeuw IM. Stepped care targeting psychological distress in head and neck and lung cancer patients: a randomized clinical trial. BMC Cancer. 2012;12:173. PMCID: PMC3502336. http://www.ncbi.nlm.nih.gov/pubmed/22574757.
452. van Straten A, Seekles W, van 't Veer-Tazelaar NJ, Beekman ATF, Cuijpers P. Stepped care for depression in primary care: what should be offered and how? Med J Aust. 2010;192(S11):S36–9. PMID: 20528706. http://www.ncbi.nlm.nih.gov/pubmed/20528706.
453. van't Veer-Tazelaar PJ, van Marwijk HWJ, van Oppen P, van der Horst HE, Smit F, Cuijpers P, Beekman ATF. Prevention of late-life anxiety and depression has sustained effects over 24 months: a pragmatic randomized trial. Am J Geriatr Psychiatry. 2011;19(3):230–9. PMID: 21425519. http://www.ncbi.nlm.nih.gov/pubmed/21425519.
454. van 't Veer-Tazelaar PJ, Cuijpers P, Beekman AJ. Prevention of depression and anxiety in older people. Tijdschr Psychiatr. 2011;53(9):579–84. PMID: 21898310.
455. Nolen-Hoeksema S, Wisco BE, Lyubomirsky S. Rethinking Rumination. Perspect Psychol Sci. 2008;3(5):400–24. PMID: 26158958. http://www.ncbi.nlm.nih.gov/pubmed/26158958.
456. Ekkers W, Korrelboom K, Huijbrechts I, Smits N, Cuijpers P, van der Gaag M. Competitive memory training for treating depression and rumination in depressed older adults: a randomized controlled trial. Behav Res Ther. 2011;49(10):588–96. PMID: 21784413. http://www.ncbi.nlm.nih.gov/pubmed/21784413.
457. HANDI Project Team, Usher T. Bibliotherapy for depression. Aust Fam Physician. 2013;42(4):199–200. PMID: 23550243. http://www.ncbi.nlm.nih.gov/pubmed/23550243.
458. Cuijpers P, Donker T, van Straten A, Li J, Andersson G. Is guided self-help as effective as face-to-face psychotherapy for depression and anxiety disorders? A systematic review and meta-analysis of comparative outcome studies. Psychol Med. 2010;40(12):1943–57. PMID: 20406528. http://www.ncbi.nlm.nih.gov/pubmed/20406528.
459. Joling KJ, van Hout HPJ, van't Veer-Tazelaar PJ, van der Horst HE, Cuijpers P, van de Ven PM, van Marwijk HWJ. How effective is bibliotherapy for very old adults with subthreshold depression? A randomized controlled trial. Am J Geriatr Psychiatry. 2011;19(3):256–65. PMID: 20808151. http://www.ncbi.nlm.nih.gov/pubmed/20808151.
460. Floyd M. Bibliotherapy as an adjunct to psychotherapy for depression in older adults. J Clin Psychol. 2003;59(2):187–95. PMID: 12552627. http://www.ncbi.nlm.nih.gov/pubmed/12552627
461. Rohde P, Stice E, Shaw H, Brière FN. Indicated cognitive behavioral group depression prevention compared to bibliotherapy and brochure control: acute effects of an effectiveness trial with adolescents. J Consult Clin Psychol. 2014;82(1):65–74. PMCID: PMC3932106. http://www.ncbi.nlm.nih.gov/pubmed/24099432.
462. Pardini J, Scogin F, Schriver J, Domino M, Wilson D, LaRocca M. Efficacy and process of cognitive bibliotherapy for the treatment of depression in jail and prison inmates. Psychol Serv. 2014;11(2):141–52. PMID: 23834667. http://www.ncbi.nlm.nih.gov/pubmed/23834667.
463. Carlbring P, Maurin T, Sjömark J, Maurin L, Westling BE, Ekselius L, Cuijpers P, Andersson G. All at once or one at a time? A randomized controlled trial comparing two ways to deliver bibliotherapy for panic disorder. Cogn Behav Ther. 2011;40(3):228–35. PMID: 21660778. http://www.ncbi.nlm.nih.gov/pubmed/21660778.
464. Songprakun W, McCann TV. Evaluation of a bibliotherapy manual for reducing psychological distress in people with depression: a randomized controlled trial. J Adv Nurs. 2012;68(12):2674–84. PMID: 22381065. http://www.ncbi.nlm.nih.gov/pubmed/22381065.
465. Naylor EV, Antonuccio DO, Litt M, Johnson GE, Spogen DR, Williams R, McCarthy C, Lu MM, Fiore DC, Higgins DL. Bibliotherapy as a treatment for depression in primary care. J Clin Psychol Med Settings. 2010;17(3):258–71. PMID: 20803165. http://www.ncbi.nlm.nih.gov/pubmed/20803165.
466. Floyd M, Scogin F, McKendree-Smith NL, Floyd DL, Rokke PD. Cognitive therapy for depression: a comparison of individual psychotherapy and bibliotherapy for depressed older adults. Behav Modif. 2004;28(2):297–318. PMID: 14997954. http://www.ncbi.nlm.nih.gov/pubmed/14997954.
467. Scogin F, Jamison C, Davis N. Two-year follow-up of bibliotherapy for depression in older adults. J Consult Clin Psychol. 1990;58(5):665–7. PMID: 2254516. http://www.ncbi.nlm.nih.gov/pubmed/2254516.
468. Smith NM, Floyd MR, Scogin F, Jamison CS. Three-year follow-up of bibliotherapy for depression. J Consult Clin Psychol. 1997;65(2):324–7. PMID: 9086697. http://www.ncbi.nlm.nih.gov/pubmed/9086697.
469. Krebber AMH, Buffart LM, Kleijn G, Riepma IC, de Bree R, Leemans CR, Becker A, Brug J, van Straten A, Cuijpers P, Verdonck-de Leeuw IM. Prevalence of depression in cancer patients: a meta-analysis of diagnostic interviews and self-report instruments. Psychooncology. 2014;23(2):121–30. PMCID: PMC4282549. http://www.ncbi.nlm.nih.gov/pubmed/24105788.
470. van der Spek N, Vos J, van Uden-Kraan CF, Breitbart W, Tollenaar RAEM, Cuijpers P, Verdonck-de Leeuw IM. Meaning making in cancer survivors: a focus group study. PLoS One. 2013;8(9):e76089. PMCID: PMC3784408. http://www.ncbi.nlm.nih.gov/pubmed/24086695.
471. Christensen H, Farrer L, Batterham PJ, Mackinnon A, Griffiths KM, Donker T. The effect of a web-based depression intervention on suicide ideation: secondary outcome from a randomised controlled trial in a helpline. BMJ Open. 2013;3(6):e002886. PMCID: PMC3696875. http://www.ncbi.nlm.nih.gov/pubmed/23811172.
472. Berrill JW, Sadlier M, Hood K, Green JT. Mindfulness-based therapy for inflammatory bowel disease patients with functional abdominal symptoms or high perceived stress levels. J Crohns Colitis. 2014;8(9):945–55. PMID: 24529603. http://www.ncbi.nlm.nih.gov/pubmed/24529603.
473. Jørgensen MS, Storebø OJ, Stoffers-Winterling JM, Faltinsen E, Todorovac A, Simonsen E. Psychological therapies for adolescents with borderline personality disorder (BPD) or BPD features-a systematic review of randomized clinical trials with meta-analysis and Trial sequential analysis. PLoS One. 2021;16(1):e0245331. https://doi.org/10.1371/journal.pone.0245331. PMID: 33444397; PMCID: PMC7808579. Psychological therapies for adolescents with borderline personality disorder (BPD) or BPD features-A

systematic review of randomized clinical trials with meta-analysis and Trial Sequential Analysis – PubMed.
474. Spek V, Nyklícek I, Cuijpers P, Pop V. Alexithymia and cognitive behaviour therapy outcome for subthreshold depression. Acta Psychiatr Scand. 2008;118(2):164–7. https://doi.org/10.1111/j.1600-0447.2008.01199.x. Epub 2008 May 22. PMID: 18498434. Alexithymia and cognitive behaviour therapy outcome for subthreshold depression – PubMed
475. International Society of Interpersonal Psychotherapy – ISIPT.
476. Tsai M, Callaghan GM, Kohlenberg RJ. The use of awareness, courage, therapeutic love, and behavioral interpretation in Functional Analytic Psychotherapy. Psychotherapy (Chic). 2013;50(3):366–70. https://doi.org/10.1037/a0031942. PMID: 24000853.

Psychotherapy Compared to Pharmacotherapy

18

Franklin Sunzeri

Introduction

A common problem in making pharmacotherapy versus psychotherapy comparisons is the use of different types of antidepressants with their own characteristics and idiosyncrasies [1]. In addition, there is a variety of psychotherapeutic techniques that have been brought to bear upon depression [2].

Psychotherapy can be defined as the informed and intentional application of clinical methods and interpersonal stances derived from established psychological principles for the purpose of assisting people to modify their behaviors, cognitions, emotions, and/or other personal characteristics in directions that the participants deem desirable [3].

Pharmacotherapy is the treatment or prevention of health conditions by using pharmaceutical products as medication [4].

Current thoughts on responses to psychotherapy and antidepressants consider both neurovegetative symptoms and cognitive and emotional dysregulation [5].

It is a common finding in PET scans and fMRI studies that depressed individuals have less prefrontal activity than healthy subjects do [6–9] and have more problems working on tasks that require executive control and working memory [10–13].

An imbalance between limbic and prefrontal control seems to be at the base of sustained emotional reactivity present in depression and anxiety disorders [14, 15]. A cognitive model of depression suggests that deficits in automatic prefrontal mechanisms and in upper-level areas, perhaps in the *dorsolateral prefrontal cortex (DLPFC)*, result in decreased executive control over amygdala activity [16–19]. Beck has suggested that a hypersensitive amygdala and hypofunctional prefrontal areas are associated with genetic polymorphisms, dysfunctional beliefs, and cognitive biases, leading to automatic negative thoughts, diminishing cognitive appraisals, and depression [19].

Alternative emphasis has been placed upon neurochemical systems rather than brain regions [20–24]. Neural mechanisms underlying cognitive bias in depression have been summarized by Jiang in 2024 [25].

Several regions of the orbital prefrontal cortex and ventromedial regions, including the rostral and subgenual cingulate gyri, are known to have inhibitory connections with the limbic system, especially with the amygdala. These include Brodmann areas 24 and 25, in which altered activity has been associated with depressive symptoms [26–28]. Farther upstream, the DLPFC might operate through the orbital prefrontal cortex to inhibit the amygdala [29, 30].

A systematic meta-analysis suggests that distinct differences exist between reactions to antidepressants in healthy volunteers and depressed patients [31]. In patients, during both positive and negative emotions, antidepressants increase activity in the DLPFC,[1] a key region mediating emotion regulation. Essentially, engaging the DLPFC regulatory network, normalizing responses by increasing brain responses to positive stimuli and decreasing brain responses to negative stimuli in the emotions involved network. In healthy volunteers, repeated administration of antidepressants decreases responses to positive emotions in the nucleus accumbens, putamen, medial prefrontal cortex, and midbrain.

Longitudinal fMRI has been used to examine changes in the DLPFC associated with CBT in treating depression [33–36].

Most recent studies suggest that CBT appears to have the potential to correct inaccurate beliefs and maladaptive processing of emotion-relevant information that are the baes of

[1] *Functional MRI and PET neuroimaging studies of placebo effects* have shown that a common set of brain regions, the left dorsolateral prefrontal cortex (DLPFC) and the left subgenual anterior cingulate cortex (sgACC)/ventral striatum are involved in placebo effects in healthy individuals and patients and appear to overlap with depression treatment targets [32].

F. Sunzeri (✉)
Heather Hills Consulting, Coos Bay, OR, USA

J. Raber et al. (eds.), *Understanding and Treating Depressive Disorders*, https://doi.org/10.1007/978-3-032-14465-2_18

negative thinking, causal in relapsing and recurrence of depression [37, 38]. Repetitive negative thinking characteristic of depression is associated with decreased prefrontal cortex activity and increased limbic activity [39, 40]. Increased and relatively non-modulated limbic activity, especially in the amygdalas, is associated with cognitive processes that underlie the expression of depressive symptoms [6, 16, 41–43]. The amygdala modulates mood-congruent memory in individuals who are vulnerable to depression relapse [44].

Psychotherapies based on cognitive approaches such as CBT focus on developing more controlled processing to replace automatic emotional reactions [26, 45–53]. PET scans have verified changes in the DLPFC and amygdalas in response to CBT that have tracked with improvement in depression symptoms [49, 54].

Antidepressants appear to be symptom-suppressive rather than curative [55]. There is little evidence that shows antidepressants reduce the risk of future depressive episodes once the antidepressants are no longer used [56, 57]. Early work indicated that CBT was as effective as antidepressants and their effects were more enduring [58–65]. However, later studies suggested that antidepressants might be more effective than CBT for patients with severe depression, that CBT was not more effective than placebo [66], and the effects were not more enduring [65]. It was noted that the outcome of CBT in those studies varied among the treatment sites and might have reflected therapist experience [37, 67]. Other studies indicated that CBT can be equally effective as antidepressants in treating moderate to severe depression, but the degree of effectiveness depends on the level of therapist expertise [5, 38]. Other work has indicated the time course for effects is important to recognize [68].

Antidepressants such as SSRIs can directly inhibit the amygdala, whereas there appears to be less evidence for increasing activity in the prefrontal cortex [69–75]. It has been suggested that when antidepressants are ceased, the prefrontal cortex cognitive functions have not been developed enough and the patient is more at risk in responding aversely to future environmental assault [5]. Cognitive therapies, on the other hand, have helped patients build stronger prefrontal cortex functions, skills that with practice the patient can continue to use on their own. Consequently, when psychotherapy has ended, the therapeutic effects may be longer lasting, and the patient may be capable of handling further environmental insults.

Indeed, RCTs have found that changes in negative expectations change depression symptoms and mitigate against relapse in those patients treated with cognitive therapy but not in those treated with antidepressant therapy [76, 77]. Post-intervention differences in resting states of brain functioning can be seen in patients treated with cognitive therapy versus antidepressants [23, 78]. The brain after CBT intervention has a top-down cortical pattern with a decreased resting-state activity in the prefrontal cortex, and with increased resting-state activity in the hippocampus and the dorsal cingulate [69]. Antidepressants show a resting state bottom-up subcortical control with prefrontal increases and hippocampal and subgenual cingulate decreases [79]. Further differences between metabolic changes were seen in several prefrontal regions [80]. CBT and venlafaxine were both associated with bilateral decreased glucose metabolism in the orbitofrontal cortex and left medial prefrontal cortex, along with increased metabolism in the right occipital-temporal cortex. However, CBT was associated with reciprocal modulation of cortical and limbic connections, whereas venlafaxine recruited previously unreported cortical and striatal regions.

Response to CBT further suggests effects start with the cortex as improvement in hopelessness and self-worth occur before motivational and vegetative symptoms improve [46, 81], a time course that does not occur with antidepressants.

Increased amygdala hyperarousal even outside of consciousness awareness can be normalized by some antidepressants [82].

Antidepressant medications mediate their activity via aminergic reuptake inhibition and associated presynaptic autoregulatory desensitization, up- and downregulation of multiple postsynaptic receptor sites, and receptor-mediated second messenger and neurotrophic intracellular signaling effects [54, 83–87]. Brain regions involved in these effects include dorsal raphe, locus coeruleus, hippocampus, and frontal cortex [88–91]. Frontal cortex changes that are associated with treatment are normalizing over- and underactivity [69, 70, 79, 92]. Subcortical and limbic changes frequently include a reduction in the activity of the hippocampus, subgenual cingulate, posterior cingulate, and insula [69, 79].

To compare brain changes, 15–20 CBT sessions were compared to paroxetine treated controls [54]. Significant clinical responses were seen with both regimens. With CBT, significant metabolic changes were seen as increases in hippocampus and dorsal cingulate (Brodmann area [BA] 24) and decreases in dorsal (BA 9/46), ventral (BA 47/11), and medial (BA 9/10/11) frontal cortex. In contrast, paroxetine treated patients demonstrated prefrontal increases and hippocampal and subgenual cingulate decreases. Many of the same sites for both treatments were affected but they were in the opposite direction. This may seem paradoxical, as one might have expected the reverse changes. The study's authors suggest the following explanation. The hippocampal, mid and anterior cingulate increases along with decreases in medial frontal, dorsolateral, and ventrolateral prefrontal activity with CBT treatment, they believe, "increases in attention to personally relevant emotional and environmental stimuli associated with a learned ability to reduce online cortical processes at the level of encoding and retrieval of maladaptive associative memories, as well as a reduction in both ruminations and the overprocessing of irrelevant information." The authors point out that other studies that target social phobias and OCD show other patterns that are different from those induced by cognitive therapies for depression. They believe this may be due to differences in underlying psychopathologies and CBT variations in treatment for those disorders.

Involvement of these areas was anticipated because they are involved in a depressive state [93–95]. (1) The anterior cingulate and orbital frontal cortex is involved in directed attention, reward-based decision making, and monitoring of emotional salience [94, 96–98]. (2) The hippocampus is involved in memory encoding, retrieval, and consolidation [99–101]. (3) The medial frontal and ventral prefrontal cortex are involved in working memory, self-referential processing, and cognitive ruminations [102–104].

In 2013, a meta-analysis *comparing CBT to other treatments* reaffirmed that CBT is an effective treatment for adult depression [105]. The analyzers found 115 suitable studies. Analysis showed an effect size as Hedges $g^2 = 0.71$ (95% CI: 0.62–0.79) based on 94 comparisons from 75 studies of CBT and control groups. This yielded a number needed to treat of 2.6. They believe that this effect size is inflated due to publication bias and inclusion of lower-quality studies. Problems with publication bias have been suggested in other meta-analyses [107]. After adjustment, the effect size was $g = 0.53$. A combination of CBT and pharmacotherapy was more effective than CBT alone ($g = 0.49$). This superiority of combined effect is born out in other studies [108, 109].

About 50%–60% of patients being treated with CBT or psychotherapy compared to 40% receiving placebo have been reported to have a favorable response and do so on the average of a level of about 0.3 SD below placebo pills [110–113].

A 2011 comparison of cognitive behavior therapy, interpersonal psychotherapy, problem-solving therapy, non-directive supportive therapy, and behavioral activation therapy has shown very small if any differences among them [105, 109]. For mild to moderate depression, the efficacy of psychotherapy appears to be equal to that of pharmacotherapy [109, 114]. For severe depression, there was no evidence found that psychotherapy is any less effective than pharmacotherapy, but there was a smaller effect size in chronic depression [109].

Contrary to conventional wisdom, CBT may be more effective for high-severity rather than for low-severity patients. In one meta-analysis conducted in 2010, psychotherapy was shown to be consistently superior to control conditions ($d = 0.40$–0.88), and post-treatment effect sizes were higher for high-severity patients ($d = 0.63$) than for low-severity patients ($d = 0.22$) [115].

A 2011 meta-analysis of psychological treatments for inpatients showed a small ($g = 0.29$) effect on depression compared to usual care and structured pharmacological treatments only [116]. The numbers-needed-to-be-treated were 6.17, heterogeneity was insignificant, and there was no evidence of publication bias. Population characteristics, interventions, and study designs did not associate with the effects.

A 2018 Cochrane systematically reviewed psychological therapies for the treatment of mental disorders in low- and middle-income countries affected by humanitarian crises [117]. They found that there is low-quality evidence that psychological therapies have large or moderate effects in reducing PTSD, depressive, and anxiety symptoms in adults living in humanitarian settings in low- and middle-income countries. Treatment effects were smaller at 4–6-month follow-ups. There were very few RCTs that analyzed children and adolescents. The risk of bias was present, and substantial amounts of heterogeneity were seen.

Integration of direct and indirect evidence from randomized clinical trials up to November 2012 using network meta-analysis compared the efficacy of seven psychotherapeutic interventions for adult depression [118]. They found that each of the seven psychotherapeutic interventions was better than waitlist controls and exhibited moderate to large effects (range $d = -0.62$ to -0.92). There were a range of effects from absent to small differences among the seven (range $d = 0.01$ to -0.30). For several of the therapies, there was limited empirical evidence. Nevertheless, considering sample size, there were strong effects for cognitive-behavioral therapy, interpersonal therapy, and problem-solving therapy (all $d > 0.46$) compared to waitlist controls. Interpersonal therapy appeared more effective than supportive therapy ($d = -0.30$).

A meta-analysis conducted of psychotherapy for depression studies prior to 2010 showed that the standardized mean effect size found for the high-quality studies ($d = 0.22$) was significantly smaller than in the other studies ($d = 0.74$, $p < 0.001$) [119]. There was zero heterogeneity in the high-quality studies, with numbers needed to treat of 8, versus 2 in the lower-quality studies.

Psychological treatments of depression in general appear to be safe and effective in older adults [120]. One review

[2] *Conventional values for the effect size expressed as d or g are*: Small: $d = 0.20$, Medium: $d = 0.50$, Large: $d = 0.80$ [106, 107]. Effects size values are perhaps the easiest to comprehend in terms of the average percentile ranking of the experimental group compared to that of the control group. If the sample has a normal distribution, an effect size of $d = 0.0$ says that the mean of the experimental group is comparable to the 50th percentile of the control group. If $d = 0.5$, the mean of the experimental group is comparable to the 69th percentile of the control. If $d = 0.8$, it is comparable to the 79th percentile. If $d = 1.3$ it is comparable to the 90th percentile. If $d = 2.0$ it is equivalent to the 97.7th percentile. If $d = 3.0$, it is equivalent to the 99.9th percentile.

found an effect size of $g = 0.64$ (95% CI: 0.47–0.80) corresponding to a number needed to treat of 3 [120].

A 2008 study analyzed which characteristics of thc intervention, target population, and study design are related to the effects of psychotherapies on depression [121]. The mean effect size of all comparisons was 0.69 (95% CI: 0.60–0.79). Results showed that problem-solving interventions and those targeting women with postpartum depression or specific populations had higher effect sizes. When studies used students as therapists, or participants were recruited from clinical populations and through systematic screening, and those that used care-as-usual or placebo control groups there were lower effect sizes.

A 2013 direct comparison of all types of psychotherapy and antidepressant medication in the treatment of adult depression and anxiety disorders demonstrated an insignificant effect size in favor of psychotherapy versus pharmacotherapy after treatment of major depression, panic disorder, and social anxiety disorder ($g = 0.02$; 95% CI: −0.07 to 0.10) [122]. There was moderate to high heterogeneity. Unfortunately, there were not enough studies available that examined PTSD and GAD.

Of the 78 psychotherapy studies, 49 were CBT; 11 were interpersonal psychotherapy (IPT), 5 were problem-solving therapy, 6 were non-directive counseling, 4 were psychodynamic therapies, and three were other therapies. Most therapies ($n = 62$) were individual treatment, and the number of treatment sessions ranged from 6 to 20, most of which ($n = 45$) ranging between 12 and 18 sessions. The antidepressants included SSRIs ($n = 37$), TCAs ($n = 20$), SNRIs ($n = 2$), MAOIs ($n = 7$), and different types of antidepressant medication ($n = 12$).

For dysthymia, antidepressants were significantly more effective than psychotherapy ($g = -0.30$) until other characteristics were analyzed. At which time the significance disappeared. For obsessive-compulsive disorder, psychotherapy was significantly more efficacious than pharmacotherapy ($g = 0.64$). Psychotherapy was significantly more efficacious than pharmacotherapy with tricyclic antidepressants ($g = 0.21$). Pharmacotherapy was significantly more efficacious than non-directive counseling ($g = 0.33$). Other characteristics of the studies did not change the significance of the results. It is interesting that all types of psychotherapies were more effective than all pharmacotherapies for treating OCD, which is generally considered to be the most severe anxiety disorder.

Even though overall results between psychotherapies and pharmacotherapies are as recounted earlier, there were differences in the relative effects of different treatments and drugs. For example, psychodynamic psychotherapy [123] and non-directive supportive counseling [124] do not appear as efficacious as other approaches. In addition, there is some evidence from other studies that interpersonal psychotherapy (IPT) may be a bit better than other therapies for treating depression [118, 125]. However, another meta-analysis suggests that while IPT is effective, this may not be the case that it is better than others [126].

Negative psychotherapeutic effects that are well known for pharmacotherapy [127] were not possible to determine and compare. In addition, patient preference and costs were not addressed in the analyzed studies. There were insufficient data available to examine the long-term post-treatment effects.

A 2008 meta-analysis revealed that *psychotherapy had a significant advantage at follow-ups compared to antidepressants* [128]. This effect was positively associated with the length of follow-ups. Additionally, discontinued acute phase psychotherapy did not differ from continued medication use at follow-ups. This effect has also been analyzed in a 2013 meta-analysis. That 2013 meta-analysis showed that patients who received acute phase CBT with no continued treatment were significantly less likely to relapse than patients who withdrew from pharmacotherapy (OR[3] = 2.61; 95% CI: 1.58–4.31, $p < 0.001$; numbers-needed-to-be-treated = 5) [129]. Moreover, there was a trend ($p < 0.1$) suggesting that patients who had acute phase CBT may be less likely to relapse following termination of acute treatment than patients who continued with pharmacotherapy (OR = 1.62; 95% CI: 0.97–2.72; NNT = 10). There were significantly fewer dropouts with CBT than with pharmacotherapy. Short-term therapeutic effects seemed comparable.

A 2010 meta-analysis of the effects of psychotherapy on chronic depression and dysthymia showed a small but significant effect ($d = 0.23$) compared to controls [130]. In this meta-analysis, for dysthymic patients, psychotherapy was significantly less effective than pharmacotherapy, especially with SSRIs ($d = -0.31$). Combined psychotherapy and pharmacotherapy was better than pharmacotherapy alone ($d = 0.23$) and psychotherapy alone ($d = 0.45$). That study's authors believe this difference may be related to a larger number of dysthymics in the psychotherapy alone group. There was no evidence of significant dropout rate differences, and at least 18 treatments were necessary to achieve optimal effects.

An earlier analysis (2008) suggested that pharmacologic treatments may be more effective than psychological inter-

[3]Odds ratio (OR) is a way to represent the odds that an outcome will result when a given exposure to a variable of interest occurs compared to when the exposure does not occur. OR quantifies the strength of the association between two events. An OR greater than 1 indicates a positive association or that exposure to that variable increases the odds of that outcome. An OR less than one indicates a negative relationship between two events. An OR of 1 suggests no relationship between two events. An OR is frequently accompanied by a 95% confidence interval (CI). CI is a measure of precision of the OR. The smaller the CI the higher precision as long as it does not overlap OR = 1. For more information, see Chap. 4 on evidence basics in this text.

ventions in treating dysthymia, and SSRIs may be more effective in the treatment of MDD [131]. However, a reanalysis of the data, including high-quality psychotherapies, showed that psychotherapy and SSRIs were equally effective in treating MDD [132]. In fact, the examination suggested that high-quality psychotherapy appears equally effective as second-generation antidepressants in short-term treatment of depression and is probably a bit more effective in long-term management of depression.

Meta-analysis (2013) of psychotherapy compared to pill placebo has shown an effect size comparable to that of pharmacotherapy [112]. Although the role of placebo in psychotherapy is difficult to interpret, post-test effects of psychotherapy compared to pill placebo was $g = 0.25$ (95% CI: 0.14–0.36). This effect size gives a number needed to treat of 7.14 (95% CI: 5.00–12.82). The Beck Depression Inventory score was 3.20 points lower, and the Hamilton Depression Rating Scale score was 2.66 points lower than placebo.

Primary care rather than specialized care may be the site for treatment of most cases of depression [133]. It appears that most patients tend to prefer psychological instead of pharmacological treatment [134]. Depression treatment in primary care has been shown by meta-analysis to be effective, especially when PCPs refer patients for depression treatment [135].

In Spanish-speaking patients, negative perceptions about medications, patient noncompliance, and a lack of sufficient bilingual behavioral healthcare providers make treatment difficult [136].

The prevalence of MDD is said to be 20%–25% in patients who have non-dialysis chronic kidney disease and end-stage kidney disease [137] and is associated with increased harmful consequences [138–141]. Studies examining the use of CBT versus pharmacological interventions appear to be underpowered or undercontrolled [137]. However, A Trial of Sertraline versus Cognitive Behavioral Therapy (CBT) for End-stage Renal Disease Patients with Depression (*ASCEND*) has suggested that SSRIs might be useful if carefully monitored for side effects [142]. CBT was judged to be low risk and possibly effective.

A retrospective, cross-sectional analysis of data obtained from the *Medical Expenditure Panel Surveys (MEPS)*, for the years 2011, 2013, and 2015, examined depression treatment among stroke patients [143]. The data were categorized into either antidepressant only, a combination of antidepressants and psychotherapy, and no treatment. Approximately 51.2% of the stroke patients received only antidepressants and 12.6% received a combination. The majority of not treated patients were males 40–64 years of age and African Americans. Treatment adherence was higher for combination therapy than for antidepressants alone. Additional factors in receiving treatment included gender, age, race, marital status, and comorbidity burden.

A cross-lagged study showed that *patient outcome expectancy* can lead to therapeutically favorable outcomes in treating MDD with either CBT or pharmacotherapy [144]. For pharmacotherapy, higher optimism and lower pessimism in the middle of the treatment predicted a favorable response. For CBT, higher optimism expectancy before treatment and less pessimism at mid-treatment predicted a more favorable response. Active ingredients might be expected to be shared between CBT and pharmacotherapies. These include expectations by both the patient and the clinician and regular support [145].

As with pharmacotherapy, negative outcomes of psychotherapy are possible [146, 147], It is possible for symptom severity to increase during or after therapy [127, 147, 148] and extreme nonresponse [149]. Extreme nonresponders are patients who demonstrated an extremely poor response to CBT [150]. It has been suggested that deterioration of symptoms in psychotherapy happens at a higher rate in children than in adults [148, 149, 151, 152] and is probably at a comparable level to pharmacotherapy [153].

Negative outcomes in practice are not as easily recognized in psychotherapy as they are in pharmacotherapy [154]. It has been suggested that there are five reasons for this lack of awareness [152]: (1) perceptual bias by the therapist looking for the positive and not the negative effects [155]; (2) treatment exists in a social context which is not as easily assessed [156]; (3) ambiguities of what is negative; (4) the difficulty of differentiating between therapy side effects and deterioration of the disease; and (5) there are no guidelines or acceptable means of assessing psychotherapy side effects [157].

The prediction of CBT or pharmacotherapy responses is inconsistent [158]. Relationships between depression severity and outcome are complex [159]. Comorbidity, suicidality, unemployment, prior hospitalizations, and other pretreatment indicators of greater pathology predict less improvement in pharmacotherapy [160, 161] and in CBT [158, 162]. Extreme nonresponse in CBT has been associated with pretreatment conditions of being severely depressed, having higher anxiety, being functionally impaired, and having primary support group problems [149, 150]. Lower baseline scores are significantly related to being a better responder [163].

It is difficult to know if improvement or deterioration of depression is due to treatment or the natural course of the disease. This is especially true with unipolar depression, which is often reactive and episodic.

Unusual positive and negative outcomes from therapy for unipolar depression were tested in RCTs comparing CBT versus pharmacotherapy [164]. Using the Hamilton Depression Rating Scale (HAM-D) and/or Beck Depression

Inventory (BDI) [145], 5%–7% of patients showed any deterioration, 1% reliable deterioration, 4%–5% extreme nonresponse, 6%–10% superior improvement, and 4%–5% superior response. Lower pretreatment levels are associated with deterioration or superior response. Higher levels of pretreatment symptoms are associated with extreme nonresponse and superior improvement. Attrition and superior improvement, as demonstrated on the HAM-D only, were more frequent in the pharmacotherapy individuals (OR = 1.67).

Data from the *2017–2019 Medical Expenditure Panel Survey (MEPS)*[4] were used to probe rates and associations of psychotherapy and psychiatry visits by age/sex and antidepressant/antipsychotic use [166]. In an individual year, about 5.2% used psychotherapy and no psychiatry and 3.2% used psychiatry visits. Males were less likely than females over the age of 15 to use psychotherapy. The highest rate for psychotherapy visits ranged between 10 and 25 years of age for males and between 15 and 30 years of age for females. Psychiatry visits did not vary by age as psychotherapy did. Females had lower rates than males during preteen years, similar rates through teen years, higher rates though adulthood, and similar rates after 60 years of age. Younger antidepressant or antipsychotic users were more likely to visit a psychotherapist or psychiatrist.

A 2023 rapid review assessed evidence on the *cost-effectiveness* of pharmacologic and nonpharmacologic interventions as first- and second-step treatments in patients with MDD [167]. They found that there is low certainty evidence that CBT may be a cost-effective first-step treatment compared to second-generation antidepressants at least in the first 4 years, and there is no evidence for cost-effectiveness of second-step treatment.

A significant number of studies indicate that *the effectiveness of antidepressants may be greatly overestimated* due to methodological issues with the antidepressant efficacy studies, which include publication bias, unintentional unblinding, and confusion between withdrawal symptoms and relapse [168].

The beneficial short-term use of antidepressants for severe depression has been well substantiated [169–171]. Prescribing antidepressants has been increasing since the introduction of SSRIs, and the median length of use seems to be about 2 years in the United Kingdom and 5 years in the USA [172, 173]. This is problematic, as such medications should be prescribed only for a limited duration. Without psychological support following cessation, patients may experience withdrawal symptoms and relapse.

Long-term use of antidepressants may be appropriate for some patients to prevent relapse [174, 175]. However, well-controlled RCTs of maintenance antidepressants do not extend very far beyond 2 years [176]. Long-term maintenance studies of preventing relapse have mainly been conducted on patients in secondary care who are at higher risk of relapse [175, 176], and it is hard to generalize to patients who are in primary care and at potentially lower relapse risk [177, 178].

Surveys of long-term antidepressant use have found that 30–50% of users in the UK and the Netherlands have no evidence to suggest they need to continue taking them [178–180].

Critical reviews of antidepressant use suggest that consideration for their use should include harmful side effects [181], discontinuation reactions and rebound effects that encourage prolonged use [182, 183], and overestimation of therapeutic benefit [169, 184, 185]. It has even been suggested that the use of antidepressants may exacerbate the prognosis of depression [186–188].

Side effects can be more severe with age. For folks over 65 years of age, a retrospective study found absolute risks over 1 year of exposure to SSRIs (after adjusting for comorbidities and other potential confounding variables) of 5.7% for falls, 2.6% for stroke/TIA, 0.5% for upper gastrointestinal bleeding, 0.38% for seizures, and 0.44% for hyponatremia [189]. For patients not taking antidepressants, the absolute risk over 1 year for all-cause mortality was 7.04%; for those taking TCAs it was 8.12%; for those taking SSRIs it was 10.61%; and for those taking other antidepressants it was 11.43%. The study's authors note that some of the associations might be explained by differences in patient characteristics [189]. In addition, side effects of SSRIs include sexual dysfunction, sleep disturbance, and significant weight gain [190]. Almost half of patients who take monoaminergic antidepressants long term may experience blunting of emotions and may have an associated poorer quality of remission [191].

Supervised tapering off antidepressants over several weeks is routine but that supervision is most often cursory [192–194] and is even more infrequent after prolonged use.[5] Frequently, patients after repeat doses of antidepressants believe that they are expected to continue taking these medications for life [199, 200]. A belief reinforced by the lack of follow-up counseling and recurrence of depression symp-

[4]The *Agency for Healthcare Research and Quality*, a division of the *US Department of Health and Human Services* produces the Medical Expenditure Panel Survey (MEPS). The MEPS is a "set of large-scale surveys of families and individuals, their medical providers, and employers across the United States. MEPS is the most complete source of data on the cost and use of health care and health insurance coverage" [165]. "Researchers in government, the health care industry, think tanks, advocacy groups, and universities use MEPS data for policy-related and behavioral research on the determinants of health care use, spending, and insurance coverage, as well as microsimulation models analyzing alternative health care delivery proposals."

[5]Strategies to reduce long-term antidepressant use can be found in the following resources [195–198].

toms upon withdrawal. Sometimes, anxiety about withdrawing results in mood swings and other symptoms that feel like depression have returned.

Withdrawal symptoms such as insomnia, sensory changes, anxiety, depression, and suicidal ideations appear to occur in up to 50% of patients after they quit the antidepressants [201, 202]. That figure may be somewhat high due to reliance on Internet surveys.

It is important to remember that a significant number of patients will improve on their own within a few weeks of active monitoring without antidepressants [203, 204]. Standard recommendations are for initial limited treatment for 3–6 months and then for up to another 6 months after improvement to limit the risk of relapse [203]. Guidance also says that continued prescription should only be if there have been two or more previous bouts of depression, a significant risk due to ongoing symptoms, or continuing significant life difficulties.

Psychotherapy Combined with Pharmacotherapy

Combination treatments of psychotherapy and pharmacotherapy may be more effective for adult depression than each of the treatments by themselves [205, 206]. A 2009 meta-analysis found that the mean effect size of the difference between psychological and combined treatment was 0.35 (95% CI: 0.24–0.45; $p < 0.001$), with low heterogeneity [207]. Significantly less difference was seen when just CBT was compared to combined treatment. At follow-ups, no difference between psychological and combined treatments was seen.

Meta-analysis (2010) has shown that the active medication contributes a small but significant amount to the efficacy of the combined treatment [208]. Mean differences between the combination of psychotherapy and pharmacotherapy and the combination of psychotherapy and placebo were 0.25 (95% CI: 0.03–0.46), which yields a number needed to treat of 7.14.

However, it has been suggested that increased effects of combined treatment may not be clinically relevant [131, 207]. A longitudinal study of CBT versus CBT plus antidepressants found very good efficacy for both and no improvement in efficacy when antidepressants were added to CBT [168].

In addition to allegiance effects, clinical trials that compare pharmaceutical and psychotherapies or evaluate combination therapy have special methodological problems due to differing structures of behavior and drug therapy, and confounding variables, differential expectations, preferences, and adherence for pharmaceutical or behavioral therapy [209].

Patient preference may be a powerful moderator of treatment response for people who have chronic MDD [210]. A randomized (but not blinded and without a placebo) multicenter trial of nefazodone, *Cognitive Behavioral Analysis System of Psychotherapy (CBASP)*, or combination therapy for chronic MDD, tested patients who indicated their preference for a type of treatment at study entry. Patients who preferred psychotherapy achieved a higher remission rate (50.0%) and lower depression scores if they received psychotherapy than if they received medication (remission rate 7.7%). Those who preferred medication showed a higher remission rate (45.5%) and lower depression scores at the end of the study if they received medication than if they received psychotherapy (remission rate, 22.2%).

A network meta-analysis of the effects of psychotherapies, pharmacotherapies, and their combination in the treatment of adult depression was published in 2020 [211, 212]. A total of 101 studies with 11,910 patients were analyzed, and in most studies, depression was moderate to severe. In achieving response at the end of treatment, combined treatment was more effective than psychotherapy alone (RR = 1.27; 95% CI: 1.14–1.39) and pharmacotherapy alone (RR[6] = 1.25; 95% CI: 1.14–1.37). There was no significant difference between psychotherapy alone and pharmacotherapy alone (RR = 0.99; 95% CI: 0.92–1.08). There was more acceptance for combined treatment (RR = 1.23; 95% CI: 1.05–1.45) and psychotherapy alone (RR = 1.17; 95% CI: 1.02–1.32) than there was for pharmacotherapy. Results for remission, chronic, and treatment-resistant depression were similar.

A Cochrane review of *treatment-resistant depression (TRD)* of adults 18–74 years of age concluded that moderate quality evidence shows that psychotherapy added to usual care with antidepressants is beneficial for depressive symptoms and for response and remission rates over the short term and probably over the medium and long term [213]. At the time of that collation (2018), there was no evidence that switching to psychotherapy in TRD was better than staying with antidepressants.

A 2020 systematic review compared and ranked all available treatment interventions for the acute treatment of depressive disorders in children and adolescents [214]. They concluded that even though there is a lack of high-quality

[6] *Relative risk (RR)* is perhaps the most common method of expressing the estimated risk of experiencing a result. RR compares the probability of a specific outcome in the treatment group with that of a control group. When an RR is greater than 1, there seems to be an increased risk of an event. When the RR is less than 1, there appears to be a decreased risk of experiencing an event. If the RR is 1, there is no apparent risk. If the RR = 5, it is 5 times more likely to occur than in the control group. If the RR = 0.5, it is half as likely to happen as in the control group. For more information, see Chap. 4.

evidence fluoxetine alone or combined with CBT seems to be the best choice for that group.

A 2023 comprehensive meta-analysis was conducted on CBT versus control conditions, other psychotherapies, pharmacotherapies, and combined treatment for depression [215]. They found that (1) efficacy of CBT in depression is documented across different formats, ages, target groups, and settings. (2) CBT appears to be as effective as pharmacotherapies in the short term, but more effective in the longer term. (3) It is not clear if CBT is superior to other psychotherapies. (4) Combined treatments were more effective than pharmacotherapy alone, but not more effective than CBT alone. (5) CBT was effective as an unguided self-help in children and adolescents and in institutions.

Changes of functional connectivity have been seen in the subgenual anterior cingulate cortex and precuneus after CBT only and combined with fluoxetine in young, depressed patients who had attempted suicide [216].

A systematic search of RCTs through 2020 found limited evidence that CBT plus fluoxetine or CBT with non-SSRIs were superior to other active treatment options for depression in children and adolescents [217]. They did have concerns with the risks of bias in the 14 RCTs that they analyzed.

Summary

Psychotherapy and pharmacotherapy seem to engage both similar neural mechanisms and dissimilar mechanisms to influence depression. There is conflicting information, but CBT and antidepressant medications appear to be equally effective in treating some patients with depression. But individual responses are based upon the precise pairing of the treatment selected with the characteristics of the patient. CBT seems to reduce the risk of relapse even after its discontinuation, which seems to be less likely to be the case for antidepressants. A comprehensive meta-analysis has shown that CBT is likely to be equally effective in the short term and more effective than pharmacotherapy in the long term.

References

1. Higgins JPT, Green S, editors. Cochrane handbook for systematic reviews of interventions. Version 5.1.0 [updated March 2011]. The Cochrane Collaboration; 2011. Available from http://www.cochrane-handbook.org.
2. Cuijpers P, Karyotaki E, de Wit L, Ebert DD. The effects of fifteen evidence-supported therapies for adult depression: a meta-analytic review. Psychother Res. 2020;30(3):279–93. PMID: 31394976. http://www.ncbi.nlm.nih.gov/pubmed/31394976.
3. Campbell LF, Norcross JC, Vasquez MJT, Kaslow NJ. Recognition of psychotherapy effectiveness: the APA resolution. Psychotherapy (Chic). 2013;50(1):98–101. PMID: 23505985. http://www.ncbi.nlm.nih.gov/pubmed/23505985.
4. Pharmacotherapeutics, pharmacokinetics, and pharmacodynamics – Johns Hopkins University.
5. DeRubeis RJ, Siegle GJ, Hollon SD. Cognitive therapy versus medication for depression: treatment outcomes and neural mechanisms. Nat Rev Neurosci. 2008;9(10):788–96. PMCID: PMC2748674. http://www.ncbi.nlm.nih.gov/pubmed/18784657.
6. Siegle GJ, Thompson W, Carter CS, Steinhauer SR, Thase ME. Increased amygdala and decreased dorsolateral prefrontal BOLD responses in unipolar depression: related and independent features. Biol Psychiatry. 2007;61(2):198–209. PMID: 17027931. http://www.ncbi.nlm.nih.gov/pubmed/17027931.
7. Mayberg HS, Liotti M, Brannan SK, McGinnis S, Mahurin RK, Jerabek PA, Silva JA, Tekell JL, Martin CC, Lancaster JL, Fox PT. Reciprocal limbic-cortical function and negative mood: converging PET findings in depression and normal sadness. Am J Psychiatry. 1999;156(5):675–82. PMID: 10327898. http://www.ncbi.nlm.nih.gov/pubmed/10327898.
8. Baxter LR, Schwartz JM, Phelps ME, Mazziotta JC, Guze BH, Selin CE, Gerner RH, Sumida RM. Reduction of prefrontal cortex glucose metabolism common to three types of depression. Arch Gen Psychiatry. 1989;46(3):243–50. PMID: 2784046. http://www.ncbi.nlm.nih.gov/pubmed/2784046.
9. Bench CJ, Friston KJ, Brown RG, Frackowiak RS, Dolan RJ. Regional cerebral blood flow in depression measured by positron emission tomography: the relationship with clinical dimensions. Psychol Med. 1993;23(3):579–90. PMID: 7901863. http://www.ncbi.nlm.nih.gov/pubmed/7901863.
10. Ottowitz WE, Dougherty DD, Savage CR. The neural network basis for abnormalities of attention and executive function in major depressive disorder: implications for application of the medical disease model to psychiatric disorders. Harv Rev Psychiatry. 2002;10(2):86–99. PMID: 11897749. http://www.ncbi.nlm.nih.gov/pubmed/11897749.
11. Liotti M, Mayberg HS. The role of functional neuroimaging in the neuropsychology of depression. J Clin Exp Neuropsychol. 2001;23(1):121–36. PMID: 11320448. http://www.ncbi.nlm.nih.gov/pubmed/11320448.
12. Cohen JD, Perlstein WM, Braver TS, Nystrom LE, Noll DC, Jonides J, Smith EE. Temporal dynamics of brain activation during a working memory task. Nature. 1997;386(6625):604–8. PMID: 9121583. http://www.ncbi.nlm.nih.gov/pubmed/9121583.
13. Harvey PO, Le Bastard G, Pochon JB, Levy R, Allilaire JF, Dubois B, Fossati P. Executive functions and updating of the contents of working memory in unipolar depression. J Psychiatr Res. 2004;38(6):567–76. PMID: 15458852. http://www.ncbi.nlm.nih.gov/pubmed/15458852.
14. Ray JP, Price JL. The organization of projections from the mediodorsal nucleus of the thalamus to orbital and medial prefrontal cortex in macaque monkeys. J Comp Neurol. 1993;337(1):1–31. PMID: 7506270. http://www.ncbi.nlm.nih.gov/pubmed/7506270.
15. Ghashghaei HT, Barbas H. Pathways for emotion: interactions of prefrontal and anterior temporal pathways in the amygdala of the rhesus monkey. Neuroscience. 2002;115(4):1261–79. PMID: 12453496. http://www.ncbi.nlm.nih.gov/pubmed/12453496.
16. Siegle GJ, Steinhauer SR, Thase ME, Stenger VA, Carter CS. Can't shake that feeling: event-related fMRI assessment of sustained amygdala activity in response to emotional information in depressed individuals. Biol Psychiatry. 2002;51(9):693–707. PMID: 11983183. http://www.ncbi.nlm.nih.gov/pubmed/11983183.
17. Davidson RJ. Affective style, psychopathology, and resilience: brain mechanisms and plasticity. Am Psychol. 2000;55(11):1196–214. PMID: 11280935. http://www.ncbi.nlm.nih.gov/pubmed/11280935.

18. Phillips ML, Ladouceur CD, Drevets WC. A neural model of voluntary and automatic emotion regulation: implications for understanding the pathophysiology and neurodevelopment of bipolar disorder. Mol Psychiatry. 2008;13(9):829, 833–57. PMCID: PMC2745893. https://pmc.ncbi.nlm.nih.gov/articles/PMC2745893/pdf/nihms105442.pdf.
19. Beck AT. The evolution of the cognitive model of depression and its neurobiological correlates. Am J Psychiatry. 2008;165(8):969–77. PMID: 18628348. http://www.ncbi.nlm.nih.gov/pubmed/18628348.
20. Mayberg HS. Positron emission tomography imaging in depression: a neural systems perspective. Neuroimaging Clin N Am. 2003;13(4):805–15. PMID: 15024963. http://www.ncbi.nlm.nih.gov/pubmed/15024963.
21. Mayberg HS. Modulating dysfunctional limbic-cortical circuits in depression: towards development of brain-based algorithms for diagnosis and optimised treatment. Br Med Bull. 2003;65:193–207. PMID: 12697626. http://www.ncbi.nlm.nih.gov/pubmed/12697626.
22. Seminowicz DA, Mayberg HS, AR MI, Goldapple K, Kennedy S, Segal Z, Rafi-Tari S. Limbic-frontal circuitry in major depression: a path modeling metanalysis. Neuroimage. 2004;22(1):409–18. PMID: 15110034. http://www.ncbi.nlm.nih.gov/pubmed/15110034.
23. Ohira H, Nomura M, Ichikawa N, Isowa T, Iidaka T, Sato A, Fukuyama S, Nakajima T, Yamada J. Association of neural and physiological responses during voluntary emotion suppression. Neuroimage. 2006;29(3):721–33. PMID: 16249100. http://www.ncbi.nlm.nih.gov/pubmed/16249100.
24. Ray RD, Ochsner KN, Cooper JC, Robertson ER, Gabrieli JDE, Gross JJ. Individual differences in trait rumination and the neural systems supporting cognitive reappraisal. Cogn Affect Behav Neurosci. 2005;5(2):156–68. PMID: 16180622. http://www.ncbi.nlm.nih.gov/pubmed/16180622.
25. Jiang Y. A theory of the neural mechanisms underlying negative cognitive bias in major depression. Front Psychiatry. 2024;15:1348474. PMCID: PMC10963437. http://www.ncbi.nlm.nih.gov/pubmed/38532986.
26. Ochsner KN, Bunge SA, Gross JJ, Gabrieli JDE. Rethinking feelings: an FMRI study of the cognitive regulation of emotion. J Cogn Neurosci. 2002;14(8):1215–29. PMID: 12495527. http://www.ncbi.nlm.nih.gov/pubmed/12495527.
27. Drevets WC. Neuroimaging studies of mood disorders. Biol Psychiatry. 2000;48(8):813–29. PMID: 11063977. http://www.ncbi.nlm.nih.gov/pubmed/11063977.
28. Mayberg HS. Limbic-cortical dysregulation: a proposed model of depression. J Neuropsychiatry Clin Neurosci. 1997;9(3):471–81. PMID: 9276848. http://www.ncbi.nlm.nih.gov/pubmed/9276848.
29. Carter CS, Macdonald AM, Botvinick M, Ross LL, Stenger VA, Noll D, Cohen JD. Parsing executive processes: strategic vs. evaluative functions of the anterior cingulate cortex. Proc Natl Acad Sci USA. 2000;97(4):1944–8. PMCID: PMC26541. http://www.ncbi.nlm.nih.gov/pubmed/10677559.
30. Davidson RJ. Affective neuroscience and psychophysiology: toward a synthesis. Psychophysiology. 2003;40(5):655–65. PMID: 14696720. http://www.ncbi.nlm.nih.gov/pubmed/14696720.
31. Ma Y. Neuropsychological mechanism underlying antidepressant effect: a systematic meta-analysis. Mol Psychiatry. 2015;20(3):311–9. PMID: 24662929. http://www.ncbi.nlm.nih.gov/pubmed/24662929.
32. Burke MJ, Romanella SM, Mencarelli L, Greben R, Fox MD, Kaptchuk TJ, Pascual-Leone A, Santarnecchi E. Placebo effects and neuromodulation for depression: a meta-analysis and evaluation of shared mechanisms. Mol Psychiatry. 2022;27(3):1658–66. PMID: 34903861. http://www.ncbi.nlm.nih.gov/pubmed/34903861.
33. Schrammen E, Roesmann K, Rosenbaum D, Redlich R, Harenbrock J, Dannlowski U, Leehr EJ. Functional neural changes associated with psychotherapy in anxiety disorders – a meta-analysis of longitudinal fMRI studies. Neurosci Biobehav Rev. 2022;142:104895. PMID: 36179918. http://www.ncbi.nlm.nih.gov/pubmed/36179918.
34. Pantazatos SP, Yttredahl A, Rubin-Falcone H, Kishon R, Oquendo MA, John Mann J, Miller JM. Depression-related anterior cingulate prefrontal resting state connectivity normalizes following cognitive behavioral therapy. Eur Psychiatry. 2020;63(1):e37. PMCID: PMC7355178. http://www.ncbi.nlm.nih.gov/pubmed/32284075.
35. Bajbouj M, Aust S, Spies J, Herrera-Melendez AL, Mayer SV, Peters M, Plewnia C, Fallgatter AJ, Frase L, Normann C, Behler N, Wulf L, Brakemeier EL, Padberg F. PsychotherapyPlus: augmentation of cognitive behavioral therapy (CBT) with prefrontal transcranial direct current stimulation (tDCS) in major depressive disorder-study design and methodology of a multicenter double-blind randomized placebo-controlled trial. Eur Arch Psychiatry Clin Neurosci. 2018;268(8):797–808. PMID: 29214483. http://www.ncbi.nlm.nih.gov/pubmed/29214483.
36. Yang Z, Oathes DJ, Linn KA, Bruce SE, Satterthwaite TD, Cook PA, Satchell EK, Shou H, Sheline YI. Cognitive behavioral therapy is associated with enhanced cognitive control network activity in major depression and posttraumatic stress disorder. Biol Psychiatry Cogn Neurosci Neuroimaging. 2018;3(4):311–9. PMCID: PMC5908226. http://www.ncbi.nlm.nih.gov/pubmed/29628063.
37. Jacobson NS, Hollon SD. Prospects for future comparisons between drugs and psychotherapy: lessons from the CBT-versus-pharmacotherapy exchange. J Consult Clin Psychol. 1996;64(1):104–8. PMID: 8907089. http://www.ncbi.nlm.nih.gov/pubmed/8907089.
38. Bhar SS, Gelfand LA, Schmid SP, Gallop R, DeRubeis RJ, Hollon SD, Amsterdam JD, Shelton RC, Beck AT. Sequence of improvement in depressive symptoms across cognitive therapy and pharmacotherapy. J Affect Disord. 2008;110(1–2):161–6. PMCID: PMC2566850. http://www.ncbi.nlm.nih.gov/pubmed/18276017.
39. Abercrombie HC, Schaefer SM, Larson CL, Oakes TR, Lindgren KA, Holden JE, Perlman SB, Turski PA, Krahn DD, Benca RM, Davidson RJ. Metabolic rate in the right amygdala predicts negative affect in depressed patients. Neuroreport. 1998;9(14):3301–7. PMID: 9831467. http://www.ncbi.nlm.nih.gov/pubmed/9831467.
40. Sheline YI, Sanghavi M, Mintun MA, Gado MH. Depression duration but not age predicts hippocampal volume loss in medically healthy women with recurrent major depression. J Neurosci. 1999;19(12):5034–43. PMCID: PMC6782668. http://www.ncbi.nlm.nih.gov/pubmed/10366636.
41. Drevets WC. Prefrontal cortical-amygdalar metabolism in major depression. Ann N Y Acad Sci. 1999;877:614–37. PMID: 10415674. http://www.ncbi.nlm.nih.gov/pubmed/10415674.
42. Dougherty D, Rauch SL. Neuroimaging and neurobiological models of depression. Harv Rev Psychiatry. 1997;5(3):138–59. PMID: 9385033. http://www.ncbi.nlm.nih.gov/pubmed/9385033.
43. Evans KC, Wright CI, Wedig MM, Gold AL, Pollack MH, Rauch SL. A functional MRI study of amygdala responses to angry schematic faces in social anxiety disorder. Depress Anxiety. 2008;25(6):496–505. PMID: 17595018. http://www.ncbi.nlm.nih.gov/pubmed/17595018.
44. Ramel W, Goldin PR, Eyler LT, Brown GG, Gotlib IH, McQuaid JR. Amygdala reactivity and mood-congruent memory in individuals at risk for depressive relapse. Biol Psychiatry. 2007;61(2):231–9. PMID: 16950223. http://www.ncbi.nlm.nih.gov/pubmed/16950223.
45. Siegle GJ, Ghinassi F, Thase ME. Neurobehavioral therapies in the 21st century: summary of an emerging field and an extended

example of cognitive control training for depression. Cogn Ther Res. 2007;31:235–62.
46. Rush AJ, Beck AT, Kovacs M, Weissenburger J, Hollon SD. Comparison of the effects of cognitive therapy and pharmacotherapy on hopelessness and self-concept. Am J Psychiatry. 1982;139(7):862–6. PMID: 7091401. http://www.ncbi.nlm.nih.gov/pubmed/7091401.
47. Straube T, Glauer M, Dilger S, Mentzel HJ, Miltner WHR. Effects of cognitive-behavioral therapy on brain activation in specific phobia. Neuroimage. 2006;29(1):125–35. PMID: 16087353. http://www.ncbi.nlm.nih.gov/pubmed/16087353.
48. Paquette V, Lévesque J, Mensour B, Leroux JM, Beaudoin G, Bourgouin P, Beauregard M. "Change the mind and you change the brain": effects of cognitive-behavioral therapy on the neural correlates of spider phobia. Neuroimage. 2003;18(2):401–9. PMID: 12595193. http://www.ncbi.nlm.nih.gov/pubmed/12595193.
49. Brody AL, Saxena S, Mandelkern MA, Fairbanks LA, Ho ML, Baxter LR. Brain metabolic changes associated with symptom factor improvement in major depressive disorder. Biol Psychiatry. 2001;50(3):171–8. PMID: 11513815. http://www.ncbi.nlm.nih.gov/pubmed/11513815.
50. Blackburn IM, Bishop S. Changes in cognition with pharmacotherapy and cognitive therapy. Br J Psychiatry. 1983;143:609–17. PMID: 6661604. http://www.ncbi.nlm.nih.gov/pubmed/6661604.
51. DeRubeis RJ, Evans MD, Hollon SD, Garvey MJ, Grove WM, Tuason VB. How does cognitive therapy work? Cognitive change and symptom change in cognitive therapy and pharmacotherapy for depression. J Consult Clin Psychol. 1990;58(6):862–9. PMID: 2292637. http://www.ncbi.nlm.nih.gov/pubmed/2292637.
52. Simons AD, Garfield SL, Murphy GE. The process of change in cognitive therapy and pharmacotherapy for depression. Changes in mood and cognition. Arch Gen Psychiatry. 1984;41(1):45–51. PMID: 6691784. http://www.ncbi.nlm.nih.gov/pubmed/6691784.
53. Garamoni GL, Reynolds CF, Thase ME, Frank E, Fasiczka AL. Shifts in affective balance during cognitive therapy of major depression. J Consult Clin Psychol. 1992;60(2):260–6. PMID: 1592956. http://www.ncbi.nlm.nih.gov/pubmed/1592956.
54. Goldapple K, Segal Z, Garson C, Lau M, Bieling P, Kennedy S, Mayberg H. Modulation of cortical-limbic pathways in major depression: treatment-specific effects of cognitive behavior therapy. Arch Gen Psychiatry. 2004;61(1):34–41. PMID: 14706942. http://www.ncbi.nlm.nih.gov/pubmed/14706942.
55. Hollon SD, Thase ME, Markowitz JC. Treatment and prevention of depression. Psychol Sci Public Interest. 2002;3(2):39–77. PMID: 26151569. http://www.ncbi.nlm.nih.gov/pubmed/26151569.
56. American Psychiatric Association. Practice guideline for the treatment of patients with major depressive disorder (revision). Am J Psychiatry. 2000;157(4 Suppl):1–45. PMID: 10767867. http://www.ncbi.nlm.nih.gov/pubmed/10767867.
57. Drahota A, Revell-Smith Y. Continuation and maintenance treatments for depression in older people. Issues Ment Health Nurs. 2019;40(4):369–70. PMID: 30759038. http://www.ncbi.nlm.nih.gov/pubmed/30759038.
58. Blackburn IM, Bishop S, Glen AI, Whalley LJ, Christie JE. The efficacy of cognitive therapy in depression: a treatment trial using cognitive therapy and pharmacotherapy, each alone and in combination. Br J Psychiatry. 1981;139:181–9. PMID: 7317698. http://www.ncbi.nlm.nih.gov/pubmed/7317698.
59. Murphy GE, Simons AD, Wetzel RD, Lustman PJ. Cognitive therapy and pharmacotherapy. Singly and together in the treatment of depression. Arch Gen Psychiatry. 1984;41(1):33–41. PMID: 6691783. http://www.ncbi.nlm.nih.gov/pubmed/6691783.
60. Hollon SD, DeRubeis RJ, Evans MD, Wiemer MJ, Garvey MJ, Grove WM, Tuason VB. Cognitive therapy and pharmacotherapy for depression. Singly and in combination. Arch Gen Psychiatry. 1992;49(10):774–81. PMID: 1417429. http://www.ncbi.nlm.nih.gov/pubmed/1417429.
61. Kovacs M, Rush AJ, Beck AT, Hollon SD. Depressed outpatients treated with cognitive therapy or pharmacotherapy. A one-year follow-up. Arch Gen Psychiatry. 1981;38(1):33–9. PMID: 7006557. http://www.ncbi.nlm.nih.gov/pubmed/7006557.
62. Blackburn IM, Eunson KM, Bishop S. A two-year naturalistic follow-up of depressed patients treated with cognitive therapy, pharmacotherapy and a combination of both. J Affect Disord. 1986;10(1):67–75. PMID: 2939125. http://www.ncbi.nlm.nih.gov/pubmed/2939125.
63. Simons AD, Murphy GE, Levine JL, Wetzel RD. Cognitive therapy and pharmacotherapy for depression. Sustained improvement over one year. Arch Gen Psychiatry. 1986;43(1):43–8. PMID: 3942473. http://www.ncbi.nlm.nih.gov/pubmed/3942473.
64. Evans MD, Hollon SD, DeRubeis RJ, Piasecki JM, Grove WM, Garvey MJ, Tuason VB. Differential relapse following cognitive therapy and pharmacotherapy for depression. Arch Gen Psychiatry. 1992;49(10):802–8. PMID: 1417433. http://www.ncbi.nlm.nih.gov/pubmed/1417433.
65. Shea MT, Elkin I, Imber SD, Sotsky SM, Watkins JT, Collins JF, Pilkonis PA, Beckham E, Glass DR, Dolan RT. Course of depressive symptoms over follow-up. Findings from the National Institute of Mental Health Treatment of Depression Collaborative Research Program. Arch Gen Psychiatry. 1992;49(10):782–7. PMID: 1417430. http://www.ncbi.nlm.nih.gov/pubmed/1417430.
66. Elkin I, Gibbons RD, Shea MT, Sotsky SM, Watkins JT, Pilkonis PA, Hedeker D. Initial severity and differential treatment outcome in the National Institute of Mental Health Treatment of Depression Collaborative Research Program. J Consult Clin Psychol. 1995;63(5):841–7. PMID: 7593878. http://www.ncbi.nlm.nih.gov/pubmed/7593878.
67. DeRubeis RJ, Gelfand LA, Tang TZ, Simons AD. Medications versus cognitive behavior therapy for severely depressed outpatients: mega-analysis of four randomized comparisons. Am J Psychiatry. 1999;156(7):1007–13. PMID: 10401443. http://www.ncbi.nlm.nih.gov/pubmed/10401443.
68. DiMascio A, Weissman MM, Prusoff BA, Neu C, Zwilling M, Klerman GL. Differential symptom reduction by drugs and psychotherapy in acute depression. Arch Gen Psychiatry. 1979;36(13):1450–6. PMID: 518245. http://www.ncbi.nlm.nih.gov/pubmed/518245.
69. Mayberg HS, Brannan SK, Tekell JL, Silva JA, Mahurin RK, McGinnis S, Jerabek PA. Regional metabolic effects of fluoxetine in major depression: serial changes and relationship to clinical response. Biol Psychiatry. 2000;48(8):830–43. PMID: 11063978. http://www.ncbi.nlm.nih.gov/pubmed/11063978.
70. Buchsbaum MS, Wu J, Siegel BV, Hackett E, Trenary M, Abel L, Reynolds C. Effect of sertraline on regional metabolic rate in patients with affective disorder. Biol Psychiatry. 1997;41(1):15–22. PMID: 8988791. http://www.ncbi.nlm.nih.gov/pubmed/8988791.
71. Nobler MS, Olvet KR, Sackeim HA. Effects of medications on cerebral blood flow in late-life depression. Curr Psychiatry Rep. 2002;4(1):51–8. PMID: 11814396. http://www.ncbi.nlm.nih.gov/pubmed/11814396.
72. Fu CHY, Williams SCR, Cleare AJ, Brammer MJ, Walsh ND, Kim J, Andrew CM, Pich EM, Williams PM, Reed LJ, Mitterschiffthaler MT, Suckling J, Bullmore ET. Attenuation of the neural response to sad faces in major depression by antidepressant treatment: a prospective, event-related functional magnetic resonance imaging study. Arch Gen Psychiatry. 2004;61(9):877–89. PMID: 15351766. http://www.ncbi.nlm.nih.gov/pubmed/15351766.
73. Davidson RJ, Irwin W, Anderle MJ, Kalin NH. The neural substrates of affective processing in depressed patients treated

with venlafaxine. Am J Psychiatry. 2003;160(1):64–75. PMID: 12505803. http://www.ncbi.nlm.nih.gov/pubmed/12505803.
74. Anand A, Li Y, Wang Y, Wu J, Gao S, Bukhari L, Mathews VP, Kalnin A, Lowe MJ. Antidepressant effect on connectivity of the mood-regulating circuit: an FMRI study. Neuropsychopharmacology. 2005;30(7):1334–44. PMID: 15856081. http://www.ncbi.nlm.nih.gov/pubmed/15856081.
75. Canli T, Cooney RE, Goldin P, Shah M, Sivers H, Thomason ME, Whitfield-Gabrieli S, Gabrieli JDE, Gotlib IH. Amygdala reactivity to emotional faces predicts improvement in major depression. Neuroreport. 2005;16(12):1267–70. PMID: 16056122. http://www.ncbi.nlm.nih.gov/pubmed/16056122.
76. De Jesús-Romero R, Holder-Dixon AR, Buss JF, Lorenzo-Luaces L. Race, ethnicity, and other cultural background factors in trials of internet-based cognitive behavioral therapy for depression: systematic review. J Med Internet Res. 2024;26:e50780. PMCID: PMC10870215. http://www.ncbi.nlm.nih.gov/pubmed/38300699.
77. McClure EB, Adler A, Monk CS, Cameron J, Smith S, Nelson EE, Leibenluft E, Ernst M, Pine DS. fMRI predictors of treatment outcome in pediatric anxiety disorders. Psychopharmacology (Berl). 2007;191(1):97–105. PMID: 16972100. http://www.ncbi.nlm.nih.gov/pubmed/16972100.
78. Fu CHY, Williams SCR, Cleare AJ, Scott J, Mitterschiffthaler MT, Walsh ND, Donaldson C, Suckling J, Andrew C, Steiner H, Murray RM. Neural responses to sad facial expressions in major depression following cognitive behavioral therapy. Biol Psychiatry. 2008;64(6):505–12. PMID: 18550030. http://www.ncbi.nlm.nih.gov/pubmed/18550030.
79. Kennedy SH, Evans KR, Krüger S, Mayberg HS, Meyer JH, McCann S, Arifuzzman AI, Houle S, Vaccarino FJ. Changes in regional brain glucose metabolism measured with positron emission tomography after paroxetine treatment of major depression. Am J Psychiatry. 2001;158(6):899–905. PMID: 11384897. http://www.ncbi.nlm.nih.gov/pubmed/11384897.
80. Kennedy SH, Konarski JZ, Segal ZV, Lau MA, Bieling PJ, McIntyre RS, Mayberg HS. Differences in brain glucose metabolism between responders to CBT and venlafaxine in a 16-week randomized controlled trial. Am J Psychiatry. 2007;164(5):778–88. PMID: 17475737. http://www.ncbi.nlm.nih.gov/pubmed/17475737.
81. Rush AJ, Kovacs M, Beck AT, Weissenburger J, Hollon SD. Differential effects of cognitive therapy and pharmacotherapy on depressive symptoms. J Affect Disord. 1981;3(3):221–9. PMID: 6456289. http://www.ncbi.nlm.nih.gov/pubmed/6456289.
82. Sheline YI, Barch DM, Donnelly JM, Ollinger JM, Snyder AZ, Mintun MA. Increased amygdala response to masked emotional faces in depressed subjects resolves with antidepressant treatment: an fMRI study. Biol Psychiatry. 2001;50(9):651–8. PMID: 11704071. http://www.ncbi.nlm.nih.gov/pubmed/11704071.
83. Frazer A, Hensler JG. 5-HT1A receptors and 5-HT1A-mediated responses: effect of treatments that modify serotonergic neurotransmission. Ann N Y Acad Sci. 1990;600:460–74; discussion 474–475. PMID: 2174665. http://www.ncbi.nlm.nih.gov/pubmed/2174665.
84. Chaput Y, de Montigny C, Blier P. Presynaptic and postsynaptic modifications of the serotonin system by long-term administration of antidepressant treatments. An in vivo electrophysiologic study in the rat. Neuropsychopharmacology. 1991;5(4):219–29. PMID: 1839498. http://www.ncbi.nlm.nih.gov/pubmed/1839498.
85. Haddjeri N, Blier P, de Montigny C. Long-term antidepressant treatments result in a tonic activation of forebrain 5-HT1A receptors. J Neurosci. 1998;18(23):10150–6. PMCID: PMC6793307. http://www.ncbi.nlm.nih.gov/pubmed/9822768.
86. Hyman SE, Nestler EJ. Initiation and adaptation: a paradigm for understanding psychotropic drug action. Am J Psychiatry. 1996;153(2):151–62. PMID: 8561194. http://www.ncbi.nlm.nih.gov/pubmed/8561194.
87. Duman RS, Malberg J, Thome J. Neural plasticity to stress and antidepressant treatment. Biol Psychiatry. 1999;46(9):1181–91. PMID: 10560024. http://www.ncbi.nlm.nih.gov/pubmed/10560024.
88. Vaidya VA, Marek GJ, Aghajanian GK, Duman RS. 5-HT2A receptor-mediated regulation of brain-derived neurotrophic factor mRNA in the hippocampus and the neocortex. J Neurosci. 1997;17(8):2785–95. PMCID: PMC6573109. http://www.ncbi.nlm.nih.gov/pubmed/9092600.
89. Chen B, Dowlatshahi D, MacQueen GM, Wang JF, Young LT. Increased hippocampal BDNF immunoreactivity in subjects treated with antidepressant medication. Biol Psychiatry. 2001;50(4):260–5. PMID: 11522260. http://www.ncbi.nlm.nih.gov/pubmed/11522260.
90. Blier P, de Montigny C. Serotonin and drug-induced therapeutic responses in major depression, obsessive-compulsive and panic disorders. Neuropsychopharmacology. 1999;21(2 Suppl):91S–8S. PMID: 10432494. http://www.ncbi.nlm.nih.gov/pubmed/10432494.
91. Freo U, Ori C, Dam M, Merico A, Pizzolato G. Effects of acute and chronic treatment with fluoxetine on regional glucose cerebral metabolism in rats: implications for clinical therapies. Brain Res. 2000;854(1–2):35–41. PMID: 10784104. http://www.ncbi.nlm.nih.gov/pubmed/10784104.
92. Passero S, Nardini M, Battistini N. Regional cerebral blood flow changes following chronic administration of antidepressant drugs. Prog Neuro-Psychopharmacol Biol Psychiatry. 1995;19(4):627–36. PMID: 8588061. http://www.ncbi.nlm.nih.gov/pubmed/8588061.
93. Elliott R, Rubinsztein JS, Sahakian BJ, Dolan RJ. The neural basis of mood-congruent processing biases in depression. Arch Gen Psychiatry. 2002;59(7):597–604. PMID: 12090812. http://www.ncbi.nlm.nih.gov/pubmed/12090812.
94. Murphy FC, Sahakian BJ, Rubinsztein JS, Michael A, Rogers RD, Robbins TW, Paykel ES. Emotional bias and inhibitory control processes in mania and depression. Psychol Med. 1999;29(6):1307–21. PMID: 10616937. http://www.ncbi.nlm.nih.gov/pubmed/10616937.
95. Zhang B, Rolls ET, Wang X, Xie C, Cheng W, Feng J. Roles of the medial and lateral orbitofrontal cortex in major depression and its treatment. Mol Psychiatry. 2024;29(4):914–28. PMID: 38212376. http://www.ncbi.nlm.nih.gov/pubmed/38212376.
96. Rolls ET. The orbitofrontal cortex. Philos Trans R Soc Lond Ser B Biol Sci. 1996;351(1346):1433–43; discussion 1443–1444. PMID: 8941955. http://www.ncbi.nlm.nih.gov/pubmed/8941955.
97. Tremblay L, Schultz W. Relative reward preference in primate orbitofrontal cortex. Nature. 1999;398(6729):704–8. PMID: 10227292. http://www.ncbi.nlm.nih.gov/pubmed/10227292.
98. Elliott R, Rubinsztein JS, Sahakian BJ, Dolan RJ. Selective attention to emotional stimuli in a verbal go/no-go task: an fMRI study. Neuroreport. 2000;11(8):1739–44. PMID: 10852235. http://www.ncbi.nlm.nih.gov/pubmed/10852235.
99. McIntosh AR. Mapping cognition to the brain through neural interactions. Memory. 1999;7(5–6):523–48. PMID: 10659085. http://www.ncbi.nlm.nih.gov/pubmed/10659085.
100. Strange BA, Fletcher PC, Henson RN, Friston KJ, Dolan RJ. Segregating the functions of human hippocampus. Proc Natl Acad Sci USA. 1999;96(7):4034–9. PMCID: PMC22415. http://www.ncbi.nlm.nih.gov/pubmed/10097158.
101. Grön G, Bittner D, Schmitz B, Wunderlich AP, Tomczak R, Riepe MW. Hippocampal activations during repetitive learning and recall of geometric patterns. Learn Mem. 2001;8(6):336–45. PMCID: PMC311390. http://www.ncbi.nlm.nih.gov/pubmed/11773433.

102. Grady C. Neuroimaging & activation of the frontal lobes. In: Miller BL, Cummings JL, editors. The human frontal lobes, functions and disorders. Baltimore: Guilford; 1999. p. 196–230.
103. Fossati P, Hevenor SJ, Graham SJ, Grady C, Keightley ML, Craik F, Mayberg H. In search of the emotional self: an fMRI study using positive and negative emotional words. Am J Psychiatry. 2003;160(11):1938–45. PMID: 14594739. http://www.ncbi.nlm.nih.gov/pubmed/14594739.
104. Kelley WM, Macrae CN, Wyland CL, Caglar S, Inati S, Heatherton TF. Finding the self? An event-related fMRI study. J Cogn Neurosci. 2002;14(5):785–94. PMID: 12167262. http://www.ncbi.nlm.nih.gov/pubmed/12167262.
105. Cuijpers P, Berking M, Andersson G, Quigley L, Kleiboer A, Dobson KS. A meta-analysis of cognitive-behavioural therapy for adult depression, alone and in comparison with other treatments. Can J Psychiatr. 2013;58(7):376–85. PMID: 23870719. http://www.ncbi.nlm.nih.gov/pubmed/23870719.
106. Cohen J. Statistical power analysis for the behavioral sciences. 1st ed. Hillsdale: Lawrence Erlbaum Associates; 1969 (2nd ed.; 1988). https://books.google.com/books?id=2v9zDAsLvA0C&pg=PP1#v=onepage&q&f=false.
107. Kelley K, Preacher KJ. On effect size. Psychol Methods. 2012;17(2):137–52. PMID: 22545595. http://www.ncbi.nlm.nih.gov/pubmed/22545595.
108. Cuijpers P, Smit F, Bohlmeijer E, Hollon SD, Andersson G. Efficacy of cognitive-behavioural therapy and other psychological treatments for adult depression: meta-analytic study of publication bias. Br J Psychiatry. 2010;196(3):173–8. PMID: 20194536. http://www.ncbi.nlm.nih.gov/pubmed/20194536.
109. Cuijpers P, Andersson G, Donker T, van Straten A. Psychological treatment of depression: results of a series of meta-analyses. Nord J Psychiatry. 2011;65(6):354–64. PMID: 21770842. http://www.ncbi.nlm.nih.gov/pubmed/21770842.
110. Iovieno N, Tedeschini E, Ameral VE, Rigatelli M, Papakostas GI. Antidepressants for major depressive disorder in patients with a co-morbid axis-III disorder: a meta-analysis of patient characteristics and placebo response rates in randomized controlled trials. Int Clin Psychopharmacol. 2011;26(2):69–74. PMID: 20962663. http://www.ncbi.nlm.nih.gov/pubmed/20962663.
111. Cuijpers P, Karyotaki E, Weitz E, Andersson G, Hollon SD, van Straten A. The effects of psychotherapies for major depression in adults on remission, recovery and improvement: a meta-analysis. J Affect Disord. 2014;159:118–26. PMID: 24679399. http://www.ncbi.nlm.nih.gov/pubmed/24679399.
112. Cuijpers P, Turner EH, Mohr DC, Hofmann SG, Andersson G, Berking M, Coyne J. Comparison of psychotherapies for adult depression to pill placebo control groups: a meta-analysis. Psychol Med. 2014;44(4):685–95. PMID: 23552610. http://www.ncbi.nlm.nih.gov/pubmed/23552610.
113. Dunlop BW, Thase ME, Wun CC, Fayyad R, Guico-Pabia CJ, Musgnung J, Ninan PT. A meta-analysis of factors impacting detection of antidepressant efficacy in clinical trials: the importance of academic sites. Neuropsychopharmacology. 2012;37(13):2830–6. PMCID: PMC3499718. http://www.ncbi.nlm.nih.gov/pubmed/22910458.
114. Li X, Wang Q. Psychological treatment for depressive disorder. Adv Exp Med Biol. 2019;1180:233–65. PMID: 31784967. http://www.ncbi.nlm.nih.gov/pubmed/31784967.
115. Driessen E, Cuijpers P, Hollon SD, Dekker JJM. Does pretreatment severity moderate the efficacy of psychological treatment of adult outpatient depression? A meta-analysis. J Consult Clin Psychol. 2010;78(5):668–80. PMID: 20873902. http://www.ncbi.nlm.nih.gov/pubmed/20873902.
116. Cuijpers P, Clignet F, van Meijel B, van Straten A, Li J, Andersson G. Psychological treatment of depression in inpatients: a systematic review and meta-analysis. Clin Psychol Rev. 2011;31(3):353–60. PMID: 21382540. http://www.ncbi.nlm.nih.gov/pubmed/21382540.
117. Purgato M, Gastaldon C, Papola D, van Ommeren M, Barbui C, Tol WA. Psychological therapies for the treatment of mental disorders in low- and middle-income countries affected by humanitarian crises. Cochrane Database Syst Rev. 2018;7(7):CD011849. PMCID: PMC6513488. http://www.ncbi.nlm.nih.gov/pubmed/29975811.
118. Barth J, Munder T, Gerger H, Nüesch E, Trelle S, Znoj H, Jüni P, Cuijpers P. Comparative efficacy of seven psychotherapeutic interventions for patients with depression: a network meta-analysis. PLoS Med. 2013;10(5):e1001454. PMCID: PMC3665892. http://www.ncbi.nlm.nih.gov/pubmed/23723742.
119. Cuijpers P, van Straten A, Bohlmeijer E, Hollon SD, Andersson G. The effects of psychotherapy for adult depression are overestimated: a meta-analysis of study quality and effect size. Psychol Med. 2010;40(2):211–23. PMID: 19490745. http://www.ncbi.nlm.nih.gov/pubmed/19490745.
120. Cuijpers P, Karyotaki E, Pot AM, Park M, Reynolds CF. Managing depression in older age: psychological interventions. Maturitas. 2014;79(2):160–9. PMCID: PMC4537161. http://www.ncbi.nlm.nih.gov/pubmed/24973043.
121. Cuijpers P, Van Straten A, Warmerdam L, Smits N. Characteristics of effective psychological treatments of depression: a metaregression analysis. Psychother Res. 2008;18(2):225–36. PMID: 18815968. http://www.ncbi.nlm.nih.gov/pubmed/18815968.
122. Cuijpers P, Sijbrandij M, Koole SL, Andersson G, Beekman AT, Reynolds CF. The efficacy of psychotherapy and pharmacotherapy in treating depressive and anxiety disorders: a meta-analysis of direct comparisons. World Psychiatry. 2013;12(2):137–48. PMCID: PMC3683266. http://www.ncbi.nlm.nih.gov/pubmed/23737423.
123. Driessen E, Cuijpers P, de Maat SCM, Abbass AA, de Jonghe F, Dekker JJM. The efficacy of short-term psychodynamic psychotherapy for depression: a meta-analysis. Clin Psychol Rev. 2010;30(1):25–36. PMID: 19766369. http://www.ncbi.nlm.nih.gov/pubmed/19766369.
124. Cuijpers P, Driessen E, Hollon SD, van Oppen P, Barth J, Andersson G. The efficacy of non-directive supportive therapy for adult depression: a meta-analysis. Clin Psychol Rev. 2012;32(4):280–91. PMID: 22466509. http://www.ncbi.nlm.nih.gov/pubmed/22466509.
125. Cuijpers P, van Straten A, Andersson G, van Oppen P. Psychotherapy for depression in adults: a meta-analysis of comparative outcome studies. J Consult Clin Psychol. 2008;76(6):909–22. PMID: 19045960. http://www.ncbi.nlm.nih.gov/pubmed/19045960.
126. Cuijpers P, Geraedts AS, van Oppen P, Andersson G, Markowitz JC, van Straten A. Interpersonal psychotherapy for depression: a meta-analysis. Am J Psychiatry. 2011;168(6):581–92. PMCID: PMC3646065. http://www.ncbi.nlm.nih.gov/pubmed/21362740.
127. Barlow DH. Negative effects from psychological treatments: a perspective. Am Psychol. 2010;65(1):13–20. PMID: 20063906. http://www.ncbi.nlm.nih.gov/pubmed/20063906.
128. Imel ZE, Malterer MB, McKay KM, Wampold BE. A meta-analysis of psychotherapy and medication in unipolar depression and dysthymia. J Affect Disord. 2008;110(3):197–206. PMID: 18456340. http://www.ncbi.nlm.nih.gov/pubmed/18456340.
129. Cuijpers P, Hollon SD, van Straten A, Bockting C, Berking M, Andersson G. Does cognitive behaviour therapy have an enduring effect that is superior to keeping patients on continuation pharmacotherapy? A meta-analysis. BMJ Open. 2013;3(4):e002542. PMCID: PMC3641456. http://www.ncbi.nlm.nih.gov/pubmed/23624992.
130. Cuijpers P, van Straten A, Schuurmans J, van Oppen P, Hollon SD, Andersson G. Psychotherapy for chronic major depression and dysthymia: a meta-analysis. Clin Psychol Rev.

2010;30(1):51–62. PMID: 19781837. http://www.ncbi.nlm.nih.gov/pubmed/19781837.

131. Cuijpers P, van Straten A, van Oppen P, Andersson G. Are psychological and pharmacologic interventions equally effective in the treatment of adult depressive disorders? A meta-analysis of comparative studies. J Clin Psychiatry. 2008;69(11):1675–85; quiz 1839–1841. PMID: 18945396. http://www.ncbi.nlm.nih.gov/pubmed/18945396.
132. Spielmans GI, Berman MI, Usitalo AN. Psychotherapy versus second-generation antidepressants in the treatment of depression: a meta-analysis. J Nerv Ment Dis. 2011;199(3):142–9. PMID: 21346483. http://www.ncbi.nlm.nih.gov/pubmed/21346483.
133. Bijl RV, Ravelli A. Psychiatric morbidity, service use, and need for care in the general population: results of The Netherlands Mental Health Survey and Incidence Study. Am J Public Health. 2000;90(4):602–7. PMCID: PMC1446190. http://www.ncbi.nlm.nih.gov/pubmed/10754976.
134. van Schaik DJF, Klijn AFJ, van Hout HPJ, van Marwijk HWJ, Beekman ATF, de Haan M, van Dyck R. Patients' preferences in the treatment of depressive disorder in primary care. Gen Hosp Psychiatry. 2004;26(3):184–9. PMID: 15121346. http://www.ncbi.nlm.nih.gov/pubmed/15121346.
135. Cuijpers P, van Straten A, van Schaik A, Andersson G. Psychological treatment of depression in primary care: a meta-analysis. Br J Gen Pract. 2009;59(559):e51–60. PMCID: PMC2629842. http://www.ncbi.nlm.nih.gov/pubmed/19192368.
136. Stephenson J, Distelberg B, Morton KR, Ortiz L, Montgomery SB. Different depression treatment recommendations and adherence for Spanish- and English-speaking patients. J Am Board Fam Med. 2019;32(6):904–12. PMID: 31704759. http://www.ncbi.nlm.nih.gov/pubmed/31704759.
137. Gregg LP, Hedayati SS. Pharmacologic and psychological interventions for depression treatment in patients with kidney disease. Curr Opin Nephrol Hypertens. 2020;29(5):457–64. PMCID: PMC7735461. http://www.ncbi.nlm.nih.gov/pubmed/32701597.
138. Hedayati SS, Minhajuddin AT, Toto RD, Morris DW, Rush AJ. Prevalence of major depressive episode in CKD. Am J Kidney Dis. 2009;54(3):424–32. PMCID: PMC3210064. http://www.ncbi.nlm.nih.gov/pubmed/19493599.
139. Palmer S, Vecchio M, Craig JC, Tonelli M, Johnson DW, Nicolucci A, Pellegrini F, Saglimbene V, Logroscino G, Fishbane S, Strippoli GFM. Prevalence of depression in chronic kidney disease: systematic review and meta-analysis of observational studies. Kidney Int. 2013;84(1):179–91. PMID: 23486521. http://www.ncbi.nlm.nih.gov/pubmed/23486521.
140. Hedayati SS, Jiang W, O'Connor CM, Kuchibhatla M, Krishnan KR, Cuffe MS, Blazing MA, Szczech LA. The association between depression and chronic kidney disease and mortality among patients hospitalized with congestive heart failure. Am J Kidney Dis. 2004;44(2):207–15. PMID: 15264178. http://www.ncbi.nlm.nih.gov/pubmed/15264178.
141. Hedayati SS, Bosworth HB, Briley LP, Sloane RJ, Pieper CF, Kimmel PL, Szczech LA. Death or hospitalization of patients on chronic hemodialysis is associated with a physician-based diagnosis of depression. Kidney Int. 2008;74(7):930–6. PMID: 18580856. http://www.ncbi.nlm.nih.gov/pubmed/18580856.
142. Hedayati SS, Daniel DM, Cohen S, Comstock B, Cukor D, Diaz-Linhart Y, Dember LM, Dubovsky A, Greene T, Grote N, Heagerty P, Katon W, Kimmel PL, Kutner N, Linke L, Quinn D, Rue T, Trivedi MH, Unruh M, Weisbord S, Young BA, Mehrotra R. Rationale and design of a trial of sertraline vs. cognitive behavioral therapy for end-stage renal disease patients with depression (ASCEND). Contemp Clin Trials. 2016;47:1–11. PMCID: PMC4818161. http://www.ncbi.nlm.nih.gov/pubmed/26621218.
143. Desai R, Sonawane K. Depression treatment use among stroke individuals with depression: a cross-sectional analysis of the Medical Expenditure Panel Survey. Res Social Adm Pharm. 2019;15(11):1338–43. PMID: 30473397. http://www.ncbi.nlm.nih.gov/pubmed/30473397.
144. Thiruchselvam T, Dozois DJA, Bagby RM, Lobo DSS, Ravindran LN, Quilty LC. The role of outcome expectancy in therapeutic change across psychotherapy versus pharmacotherapy for depression. J Affect Disord. 2019;251:121–9. PMID: 30921595. http://www.ncbi.nlm.nih.gov/pubmed/30921595.
145. Vittengl JR, Jarrett RB, Weitz E, Hollon SD, Twisk J, Cristea I, David D, DeRubeis RJ, Dimidjian S, Dunlop BW, Faramarzi M, Hegerl U, Kennedy SH, Kheirkhah F, Mergl R, Miranda J, Mohr DC, Rush AJ, Segal ZV, Siddique J, Simons AD, Cuijpers P. Divergent outcomes in cognitive-behavioral therapy and pharmacotherapy for adult depression. Am J Psychiatry. 2016;173(5):481–90. PMCID: PMC4934129. http://www.ncbi.nlm.nih.gov/pubmed/26869246.
146. Lilienfeld SO. Psychological treatments that cause harm. Perspect Psychol Sci. 2007;2(1):53–70. PMID: 26151919. http://www.ncbi.nlm.nih.gov/pubmed/26151919.
147. Berk M, Parker G. The elephant on the couch: side-effects of psychotherapy. Aust N Z J Psychiatry. 2009;43(9):787–94. PMID: 19670051. http://www.ncbi.nlm.nih.gov/pubmed/19670051.
148. Ogles BM, Lambert MJ, Sawyer JD. Clinical significance of the National Institute of Mental Health Treatment of Depression Collaborative Research Program data. J Consult Clin Psychol. 1995;63(2):321–6. PMID: 7751495. http://www.ncbi.nlm.nih.gov/pubmed/7751495.
149. Coffman SJ, Martell CR, Dimidjian S, Gallop R, Hollon SD. Extreme nonresponse in cognitive therapy: can behavioral activation succeed where cognitive therapy fails? J Consult Clin Psychol. 2007;75(4):531–41. PMID: 17663608. http://www.ncbi.nlm.nih.gov/pubmed/17663608.
150. Koenig AM, Jarrett RB, Gallop R, Barrett MS, Thase ME. Extreme nonresponse to acute phase cognitive therapy for depression: an attempt to replicate and extend. Behav Ther. 2014;45(3):300–13. PMCID: PMC4221276. http://www.ncbi.nlm.nih.gov/pubmed/24680227.
151. Lambert MJ. Bergin and Garfield's handbook of psychotherapy and behavior change. Wiley; 2013.
152. Linden M, Schermuly-Haupt ML. Definition, assessment and rate of psychotherapy side effects. World Psychiatry. 2014;13(3):306–9. PMCID: PMC4219072. http://www.ncbi.nlm.nih.gov/pubmed/25273304.
153. Blais MA, Malone JC, Stein MB, Slavin-Mulford J, O'Keefe SM, Renna M, Sinclair SJ. Treatment as usual (TAU) for depression: a comparison of psychotherapy, pharmacotherapy, and combined treatment at a large academic medical center. Psychotherapy (Chic). 2013;50(1):110–8. PMID: 23505987. http://www.ncbi.nlm.nih.gov/pubmed/23505987.
154. Dimidjian S, Hollon SD. How would we know if psychotherapy were harmful? Am Psychol. 2010;65(1):21–33. PMID: 20063907. http://www.ncbi.nlm.nih.gov/pubmed/20063907.
155. Hatfield D, McCullough L, Frantz SHB, Krieger K. Do we know when our clients get worse? An investigation of therapists' ability to detect negative client change. Clin Psychol Psychother. 2010;17(1):25–32. PMID: 19916162. http://www.ncbi.nlm.nih.gov/pubmed/19916162.
156. Szapocznik J, Prado G. Negative effects on family functioning from psychosocial treatments: a recommendation for expanded safety monitoring. J Fam Psychol. 2007;21(3):468–78. PMID: 17874932. http://www.ncbi.nlm.nih.gov/pubmed/17874932.
157. Horigian VE, Robbins MS, Dominguez R, Ucha J, Rosa CL. Principles for defining adverse events in behavioral intervention research: lessons from a family-focused adolescent drug abuse trial. Clin Trials. 2010;7(1):58–68. PMCID: PMC3163837. http://www.ncbi.nlm.nih.gov/pubmed/20156957.
158. Driessen E, Hollon SD. Cognitive behavioral therapy for mood disorders: efficacy, moderators and mediators. Psychiatr Clin

North Am. 2010;33(3):537–55. PMCID: PMC2933381. http://www.ncbi.nlm.nih.gov/pubmed/20599132.
159. Van HL, Schoevers RA, Dekker J. Predicting the outcome of antidepressants and psychotherapy for depression: a qualitative, systematic review. Harv Rev Psychiatry. 2008;16(4):225–34. PMID: 18661365. http://www.ncbi.nlm.nih.gov/pubmed/18661365.
160. Rush AJ, Wisniewski SR, Warden D, Luther JF, Davis LL, Fava M, Nierenberg AA, Trivedi MH. Selecting among second-step antidepressant medication monotherapies: predictive value of clinical, demographic, or first-step treatment features. Arch Gen Psychiatry. 2008;65(8):870–80. PMID: 18678792. http://www.ncbi.nlm.nih.gov/pubmed/18678792.
161. Souery D, Oswald P, Massat I, Bailer U, Bollen J, Demyttenaere K, Kasper S, Lecrubier Y, Montgomery S, Serretti A, Zohar J, Mendlewicz J, Group for the Study of Resistant Depression. Clinical factors associated with treatment resistance in major depressive disorder: results from a European multicenter study. J Clin Psychiatry. 2007;68(7):1062–70. PMID: 17685743. http://www.ncbi.nlm.nih.gov/pubmed/17685743.
162. Jarrett RB, Minhajuddin A, Kangas JL, Friedman ES, Callan JA, Thase ME. Acute phase cognitive therapy for recurrent major depressive disorder: who drops out and how much do patient skills influence response? Behav Res Ther. 2013;51(4–5):221–30. PMCID: PMC3685278. http://www.ncbi.nlm.nih.gov/pubmed/23485420.
163. Tedlow J, Fava M, Uebelacker L, Nierenberg AA, Alpert JE, Rosenbaum J. Outcome definitions and predictors in depression. Psychother Psychosom. 1998;67(4–5):266–70. PMID: 9693355. http://www.ncbi.nlm.nih.gov/pubmed/9693355.
164. Fairbairn N, Wood E. Commentary on Enns et al. (2016): Supervised injection facilities as a cost-effective intervention. Addiction. 2016;111(3):490–1. PMCID: PMC5279864. http://www.ncbi.nlm.nih.gov/pubmed/26860246.
165. Medical Expenditure Panel Survey Background.
166. Johansen ME, Sicker K. Psychotherapy and psychiatry visits in the United States: a study of MEPS, 2017–2019. J Am Board Fam Med. 2022:jabfm.2022.AP.210503. PMID: 36096657. http://www.ncbi.nlm.nih.gov/pubmed/36096657.
167. Dobrescu A, Chapman A, Affengruber L, Persad E, Toromanova A, Wagner G, Klerings I, Emprechtinger R, Gartlehner G. Cost-effectiveness of first- and second-step treatment strategies for major depressive disorder: a rapid review. Ann Intern Med. 2023;176(2):212–6. PMID: 36689742. http://www.ncbi.nlm.nih.gov/pubmed/36689742.
168. Maß R, Backhaus K, Lohrer K, Szelies M, Unkelbach BK. No benefit of antidepressants in inpatient treatment of depression. A longitudinal, quasi-experimental field study. Psychopharmacology (Berl). 2023;240(9):1963–71. PMCID: PMC10471650. http://www.ncbi.nlm.nih.gov/pubmed/37526699.
169. Stone MB, Yaseen ZS, Miller BJ, Richardville K, Kalaria SN, Kirsch I. Response to acute monotherapy for major depressive disorder in randomized, placebo controlled trials submitted to the US Food and Drug Administration: individual participant data analysis. BMJ. 2022;378:e067606. PMCID: PMC9344377. http://www.ncbi.nlm.nih.gov/pubmed/35918097.
170. Cipriani A, Furukawa TA, Salanti G, Chaimani A, Atkinson LZ, Ogawa Y, Leucht S, Ruhe HG, Turner EH, Higgins JPT, Egger M, Takeshima N, Hayasaka Y, Imai H, Shinohara K, Tajika A, Ioannidis JPA, Geddes JR. Comparative efficacy and acceptability of 21 antidepressant drugs for the acute treatment of adults with major depressive disorder: a systematic review and network meta-analysis. Lancet. 2018;391(10128):1357–66. PMCID: PMC5889788. http://www.ncbi.nlm.nih.gov/pubmed/29477251.
171. Tondo L, Baldessarini RJ, Vázquez G, Lepri B, Visioli C. Clinical responses to antidepressants among 1036 acutely depressed patients with bipolar or unipolar major affective disorders. Acta Psychiatr Scand. 2013;127(5):355–64. PMID: 23121222. http://www.ncbi.nlm.nih.gov/pubmed/23121222.
172. Mojtabai R, Olfson M. National trends in long-term use of antidepressant medications: results from the U.S. National Health and Nutrition Examination Survey. J Clin Psychiatry. 2014;75(2):169–77. PMID: 24345349. http://www.ncbi.nlm.nih.gov/pubmed/24345349.
173. Kendrick T. Strategies to reduce use of antidepressants. Br J Clin Pharmacol. 2021;87(1):23–33. PMID: 32656861. http://www.ncbi.nlm.nih.gov/pubmed/32656861.
174. Reid I, Cameron I, MacGillivray S. Increased prescription of antidepressants shows correction of inadequate duration of treatment of depression. BMJ. 2014;348:g228. PMID: 24448343. http://www.ncbi.nlm.nih.gov/pubmed/24448343.
175. Geddes JR, Carney SM, Davies C, Furukawa TA, Kupfer DJ, Frank E, Goodwin GM. Relapse prevention with antidepressant drug treatment in depressive disorders: a systematic review. Lancet. 2003;361(9358):653–61. PMID: 12606176. http://www.ncbi.nlm.nih.gov/pubmed/12606176.
176. Sim K, Lau WK, Sim J, Sum MY, Baldessarini RJ. Prevention of relapse and recurrence in adults with major depressive disorder: systematic review and meta-analyses of controlled trials. Int J Neuropsychopharmacol. 2015;19(2):pyv076. PMCID: PMC4772815. http://www.ncbi.nlm.nih.gov/pubmed/26152228.
177. Mangin D, Dowson C, Mulder R, Wells E, Toop L, Dowel T. The effectiveness of maintenance SSRI treatment in primary care depression to prevent recurrence: multicentre double blinded placebo-controlled RCT. In: North American Primary Care Research Group annual meeting, October; 2015.
178. Ambresin G, Palmer V, Densley K, Dowrick C, Gilchrist G, Gunn JM. What factors influence long-term antidepressant use in primary care? Findings from the Australian diamond cohort study. J Affect Disord. 2015;176:125–32. PMID: 25704565. http://www.ncbi.nlm.nih.gov/pubmed/25704565.
179. Cruickshank G, Macgillivray S, Bruce D, Mather A, Matthews K, Williams B. Cross-sectional survey of patients in receipt of long-term repeat prescriptions for antidepressant drugs in primary care. Ment Health Fam Med. 2008;5(2):105–9. PMCID: PMC2777559. http://www.ncbi.nlm.nih.gov/pubmed/22477855.
180. Eveleigh R, Grutters J, Muskens E, Oude Voshaar R, van Weel C, Speckens A, Lucassen P. Cost-utility analysis of a treatment advice to discontinue inappropriate long-term antidepressant use in primary care. Fam Pract. 2014;31(5):578–84. PMID: 25121977. http://www.ncbi.nlm.nih.gov/pubmed/25121977.
181. Hengartner MP, Plöderl M. Newer-generation antidepressants and suicide risk in randomized controlled trials: a re-analysis of the FDA database. Psychother Psychosom. 2019;88(4):247–8. PMID: 31234169. http://www.ncbi.nlm.nih.gov/pubmed/31234169.
182. Davies J, Read J, Hengartner MP, Cosci F, Fava G, Chouinard G, van Os J, Nardi A, Gøtzsche P, Groot P, Offidani E, Timimi S, Moncrieff J, Spada M, Guy A. Clinical guidelines on antidepressant withdrawal urgently need updating. BMJ. 2019;365:l2238. PMID: 31109968. http://www.ncbi.nlm.nih.gov/pubmed/31109968.
183. Amrein MA, Hengartner MP, Näpflin M, Farcher R, Huber CA. Prevalence, trends, and individual patterns of long-term antidepressant medication use in the adult Swiss general population. Eur J Clin Pharmacol. 2023;79(11):1505–13. PMCID: PMC10618304. http://www.ncbi.nlm.nih.gov/pubmed/37668659.
184. Turner EH, Cipriani A, Furukawa TA, Salanti G, de Vries YA. Selective publication of antidepressant trials and its influence on apparent efficacy: updated comparisons and meta-analyses of newer versus older trials. PLoS Med. 2022;19(1):e1003886. PMCID: PMC8769343. http://www.ncbi.nlm.nih.gov/pubmed/35045113.

185. Holper L, Hengartner MP. Comparative efficacy of placebos in short-term antidepressant trials for major depression: a secondary meta-analysis of placebo-controlled trials. BMC Psychiatry. 2020;20(1):437. PMCID: PMC7487933. http://www.ncbi.nlm.nih.gov/pubmed/32894088.
186. Hengartner MP, Passalacqua S, Andreae A, Heinsius T, Hepp U, Rössler W, von Wyl A. Antidepressant use during acute inpatient care is associated with an increased risk of psychiatric rehospitalisation over a 12-month follow-up after discharge. Front Psychiatry. 2019;10:79. PMCID: PMC6396716. http://www.ncbi.nlm.nih.gov/pubmed/30853919.
187. Hengartner MP, Angst J, Rössler W. Antidepressant use prospectively relates to a poorer long-term outcome of depression: results from a prospective community cohort study over 30 years. Psychother Psychosom. 2018;87(3):181–3. PMID: 29680831. http://www.ncbi.nlm.nih.gov/pubmed/29680831.
188. Hengartner MP. How effective are antidepressants for depression over the long term? A critical review of relapse prevention trials and the issue of withdrawal confounding. Ther Adv Psychopharmacol. 2020;10:2045125320921694. PMCID: PMC7225779. http://www.ncbi.nlm.nih.gov/pubmed/32435449.
189. Coupland C, Dhiman P, Morriss R, Arthur A, Barton G, Hippisley-Cox J. Antidepressant use and risk of adverse outcomes in older people: population based cohort study. BMJ. 2011;343:d4551. PMCID: PMC3149102. http://www.ncbi.nlm.nih.gov/pubmed/21810886.
190. Ferguson JM. SSRI antidepressant medications: adverse effects and tolerability. Prim Care Companion J Clin Psychiatry. 2001;3(1):22–7. PMCID: PMC181155. http://www.ncbi.nlm.nih.gov/pubmed/15014625.
191. Goodwin GM, Price J, De Bodinat C, Laredo J. Emotional blunting with antidepressant treatments: a survey among depressed patients. J Affect Disord. 2017;221:31–5. PMID: 28628765. http://www.ncbi.nlm.nih.gov/pubmed/28628765.
192. Haddad PM, Anderson IM. Recognising and managing antidepressant discontinuation symptoms. Adv Psychiatr Treat. 2007;13(6):447–57.
193. Middleton DJ, Cameron IM, Reid IC. Continuity and monitoring of antidepressant therapy in a primary care setting. Qual Prim Care. 2011;19(2):109–13. PMID: 21575333. http://www.ncbi.nlm.nih.gov/pubmed/21575333.
194. Sinclair JE, Aucott LS, Lawton K, Reid IC, Cameron IM. The monitoring of longer term prescriptions of antidepressants: observational study in a primary care setting. Fam Pract. 2014;31(4):419–26. PMID: 24850795. http://www.ncbi.nlm.nih.gov/pubmed/24850795.
195. Kendrick T. Strategies to reduce use of antidepressants. Br J Clin Pharmacol. 2021. Wiley Online Library.
196. Kendrick T, Geraghty AWA, Bowers H, Stuart B, Leydon G, May C, Yao G, O'Brien W, Glowacka M, Holley S, Williams S, Zhu S, Dewar-Haggart R, Palmer B, Bell M, Collinson S, Fry I, Lewis G, Griffiths G, Gilbody S, Moncrieff J, Moore M, Macleod U, Little P, Dowrick C. REDUCE (Reviewing long-term antidepressant use by careful monitoring in everyday practice) internet and telephone support to people coming off long-term antidepressants: protocol for a randomised controlled trial. Trials. 2020;21(1):419. PMCID: PMC7245840. http://www.ncbi.nlm.nih.gov/pubmed/32448374.
197. WiserAD: A randomised trial of a structured online intervention to promote and support antidepressant de-prescribing in primary care (previously STOPS).
198. Ruhe HG, Horikx A, van Avendonk MJP, Groeneweg BF, Woutersen-Koch H, Discontinuation of Antidepressants Taskforce. Tapering of SSRI treatment to mitigate withdrawal symptoms. Lancet Psychiatry. 2019;6(7):561–2. PMID: 31230677. http://www.ncbi.nlm.nih.gov/pubmed/31230677.
199. Leydon GM, Rodgers L, Kendrick T. A qualitative study of patient views on discontinuing long-term selective serotonin reuptake inhibitors. Fam Pract. 2007;24(6):570–5. PMID: 18032401. http://www.ncbi.nlm.nih.gov/pubmed/18032401.
200. Dickinson R, Knapp P, House AO, Dimri V, Zermansky A, Petty D, Holmes J, Raynor DK. Long-term prescribing of antidepressants in the older population: a qualitative study. Br J Gen Pract. 2010;60(573):e144–55. PMCID: PMC2845505. http://www.ncbi.nlm.nih.gov/pubmed/20353660.
201. Taylor S, Annand F, Burkinshaw P, Greaves F, Kelleher M, Knight J. Dependence and withdrawal associated with some prescribed medicines. London: Public Health England; 2019.
202. Davies J, Read J. A systematic review into the incidence, severity and duration of antidepressant withdrawal effects: are guidelines evidence-based? Addict Behav. 2019;97:111–21. PMID: 30292574. http://www.ncbi.nlm.nih.gov/pubmed/30292574.
203. Ganasan S. Managing depression in the primary care setting. J Prescr Pract. 2019;1(8):388–92.
204. Arroll B, Chin WY, Moir F, Dowrick C. An evidence-based first consultation for depression: nine key messages. Br J Gen Pract. 2018;68(669):200–1. PMCID: PMC5863674. http://www.ncbi.nlm.nih.gov/pubmed/29592945.
205. Cuijpers P, Reynolds CF, Donker T, Li J, Andersson G, Beekman A. Personalized treatment of adult depression: medication, psychotherapy, or both? A systematic review. Depress Anxiety. 2012;29(10):855–64. PMID: 22815247. http://www.ncbi.nlm.nih.gov/pubmed/22815247.
206. Cuijpers P, Dekker J, Hollon SD, Andersson G. Adding psychotherapy to pharmacotherapy in the treatment of depressive disorders in adults: a meta-analysis. J Clin Psychiatry. 2009;70(9):1219–29. PMID: 19818243. http://www.ncbi.nlm.nih.gov/pubmed/19818243.
207. Cuijpers P, van Straten A, Warmerdam L, Andersson G. Psychotherapy versus the combination of psychotherapy and pharmacotherapy in the treatment of depression: a meta-analysis. Depress Anxiety. 2009;26(3):279–88. PMID: 19031487. http://www.ncbi.nlm.nih.gov/pubmed/19031487.
208. Cuijpers P, van Straten A, Hollon SD, Andersson G. The contribution of active medication to combined treatments of psychotherapy and pharmacotherapy for adult depression: a meta-analysis. Acta Psychiatr Scand. 2010;121(6):415–23. PMID: 19922522. http://www.ncbi.nlm.nih.gov/pubmed/19922522.
209. Holroyd KA, Powers SW, Andrasik F. Methodological issues in clinical trials of drug and behavior therapies. Headache. 2005;45(5):487–92. PMID: 15953265. http://www.ncbi.nlm.nih.gov/pubmed/15953265.
210. Kocsis JH, Leon AC, Markowitz JC, Manber R, Arnow B, Klein DN, Thase ME. Patient preference as a moderator of outcome for chronic forms of major depressive disorder treated with nefazodone, cognitive behavioral analysis system of psychotherapy, or their combination. J Clin Psychiatry. 2009;70(3):354–61. PMID: 19192474. http://www.ncbi.nlm.nih.gov/pubmed/19192474.
211. Cuijpers P, Noma H, Karyotaki E, Vinkers CH, Cipriani A, Furukawa TA. A network meta-analysis of the effects of psychotherapies, pharmacotherapies and their combination in the treatment of adult depression. World Psychiatry. 2020;19(1):92–107. PMCID: PMC6953550. http://www.ncbi.nlm.nih.gov/pubmed/31922679.
212. Cuijpers P, Noma H, Karyotaki E, Cipriani A, Furukawa TA. Effectiveness and acceptability of cognitive behavior therapy delivery formats in adults with depression: a network meta-analysis. JAMA Psychiatr. 2019;76(7):700–7. PMCID: PMC6583673. http://www.ncbi.nlm.nih.gov/pubmed/30994877.
213. Ijaz S, Davies P, Williams CJ, Kessler D, Lewis G, Wiles N. Psychological therapies for treatment-resistant depression in adults. Cochrane Database Syst Rev. 2018;5(5):CD010558.

PMCID: PMC6494651. http://www.ncbi.nlm.nih.gov/pubmed/29761488.

214. Zhou X, Teng T, Zhang Y, Del Giovane C, Furukawa TA, Weisz JR, Li X, Cuijpers P, Coghill D, Xiang Y, Hetrick SE, Leucht S, Qin M, Barth J, Ravindran AV, Yang L, Curry J, Fan L, Silva SG, Cipriani A, Xie P. Comparative efficacy and acceptability of antidepressants, psychotherapies, and their combination for acute treatment of children and adolescents with depressive disorder: a systematic review and network meta-analysis. Lancet Psychiatry. 2020;7(7):581–601. PMCID: PMC7303954. http://www.ncbi.nlm.nih.gov/pubmed/32563306.

215. Cuijpers P, Miguel C, Harrer M, Plessen CY, Ciharova M, Ebert D, Karyotaki E. Cognitive behavior therapy vs. control conditions, other psychotherapies, pharmacotherapies and combined treatment for depression: a comprehensive meta-analysis including 409 trials with 52,702 patients. World Psychiatry. 2023;22(1):105–15. PMCID: PMC9840507. http://www.ncbi.nlm.nih.gov/pubmed/36640411.

216. Shu Y, Wu G, Bi B, Liu J, Xiong J, Kuang L. Changes of functional connectivity of the subgenual anterior cingulate cortex and precuneus after cognitive behavioral therapy combined with fluoxetine in young depressed patients with suicide attempt. Behav Brain Res. 2022;417:113612. PMID: 34600960. http://www.ncbi.nlm.nih.gov/pubmed/34600960.

217. Xiang Y, Cuijpers P, Teng T, Li X, Fan L, Liu X, Jiang Y, Du K, Lin J, Zhou X, Xie P. Comparative short-term efficacy and acceptability of a combination of pharmacotherapy and psychotherapy for depressive disorder in children and adolescents: a systematic review and meta-analysis. BMC Psychiatry. 2022;22(1):139. PMCID: PMC8862472. http://www.ncbi.nlm.nih.gov/pubmed/35193522.

Cognitive Dysfunction and Suicide

19

Franklin Sunzeri

Introduction to Cognitive Dysfunctions

Cognitive dysfunction (diminished ability to think or concentrate or indecisiveness) is a diagnostic criterion for major depressive disorder (MDD) [12]. This dysfunction includes deficiencies in concentration and attention, executive functions, learning and memory (working, episodic, and/or visuospatial), and processing speed [50].

Cognitive dysfunctions have particularly negative effects on function and clinical outcome in MDD [51–53]. They may contribute to other symptoms of MDD, such as anhedonia and psychomotor retardation, and may influence and be influenced by poor quality sleep and fatigue. When cognitive dysfunction occurs, it is frequently observable at the onset of depression [54], and for some people, it may persist when MDD is in remission [55].

Cognitive heterogeneity exists in patients with acute depressive episodes [60]. Some patients never suffer from cognitive impairment during episodes, while others range from mild to severe deficits [56–59]. Cognitive performance may improve for some patients upon remission, but for others, cognitive impairments can persist.

Cognitive dysfunction is associated with worse work performance and social relationships [61–63].

Cognitive dysfunction can be associated with early/late illness onset and severity [55, 64], higher levels of resistance to antidepressant strategies [65–67], and the number of previous depressive episodes [55]. Cognitive dysfunctions are also linked to age [68, 69], poor intellectual ability [70], and years of school [71, 72].

Inflammation association with cognitive decrements is not unique to depression. Inflammation has been linked to cognitive dysfunction in folks who are otherwise healthy [73–77] and to a variety of medical conditions [78–81]. Common risk factors of substance use, sedentary behavior, inflammation, obesity, and life stress are linked to cognitive dysfunction and depression beginning in youth [73, 75, 76].

The intersection of immune responses and neurocircuits, especially in the brain in response to stressors, has probably endowed humans with a survival advantage [82]. However, modern stressors may have pushed this relationship into the development of depression. This may be seen in sickness responses that share behavioral symptoms with depression [83].

Some investigators have suggested different types of cognitive symptoms and deficits, such as being either hot or cold and being trait- and state-like cognitive alterations [23]. These dysfunctions can alter the course of depression, including remission, residual symptoms, functioning, and treatment responses. *Hot dysfunctions* are ones that lead to cognitive distortions. *Cold dysfunctions* lead to cognitive deficits. Hot dysfunctions can be recognized by patient interviews, whereas cold dysfunctions are revealed through neuropsychological tests or neurophysiological examinations [13].

Patients' *hot cognitive distortions* result in errors in information processing by focusing on negative information and denying positive aspects of the world and the patient themselves. The distorted view of reality enhances and perpetuates depressive symptoms [14]. *Executive functions* aim to (1) make plans to achieve targets by deliberate, intentional, and volitional actions; and (2) control reactions that are inimical to achieving those targets. Deficits in executive functions often block patients from achieving even the most pedestrian goals and result in withdrawal from social activities.

Attention relates to the selection of information and controls memory functions [84]. Deficits in *short-term memory*, especially sensory memory and working memory, are common in MDD. The *sensory memory deficits* include those of visuospatial and auditory-verbal memory, that is, the ability to receive, process, and store visual and auditory experiences [15]. *Working (operational) memory* is the temporary storage necessary for language processing, learning, and reasoning.

F. Sunzeri (✉)
Heather Hills Consulting, Coos Bay, OR, USA

J. Raber et al. (eds.), *Understanding and Treating Depressive Disorders*, https://doi.org/10.1007/978-3-032-14465-2_19

Psychomotor retardation includes both physical symptoms and cognitive processing problems [85, 86]. Physical symptoms may include diminished coordination, slower speed of response, slowing down of gait, stooping, low voice timbre, and poorly modulated affect.

Czerwińska and Pawłowski have proposed pathological mechanisms of cognitive impairments in MDD [87]. In MDD patients with cognitive impairments, the *amygdala* requires stronger and longer activation to process information. This activation often is accompanied by increased cortisol and norepinephrine [16]. It is proposed that this increase may predispose to focusing on negative memories. There is some evidence that the *dorsolateral prefrontal cortex (dlPFC)*, which normally acts as a brake to the amygdala, may be malfunctioning [17].

Malfunctions in some other areas of the cerebral cortex may also be involved. The *anterior cingulate cortex (ACC)* integrates neuronal circuits responsible for emotion processing and affect regulation [19, 20]. There are two parts to the ACC. The *dorsal anterior cingulate cortex (dACC)* roles in regulating cognitive functions are performing executive functions, processing stimuli, decision-making, detecting errors, monitoring performance, and assessing risk. The *ventral anterior cingulate cortex (vACC)* role is regulating emotions, motivation, and tasks with high emotional loads. Patients with MDD have reduced activity of the vACC and, consequently, less stimulation of dopamine in the limbic system [18].

Disruptions in *neurotransmitters*, especially serotonin, norepinephrine, and dopamine in these areas may lead to problems with attention, operational memory, and cognitive flexibility [21, 22].

In MDD patients, areas of the brain that show reduced gray matter have also shown increased glucose levels reflecting *increased glutaminergic* transmission and overstimulation of the *N-methyl-D-aspartate (NMDA) receptors* and an excessive secretion of glutamine [23, 24, 88–92]. An increase in glutaminergic transmission in pyramidal neurons of the PFC leads to a decrement of operational memory in patients with MDD. It has been suggested that glial cell malfunction may be involved because one of the roles of glial cells is to protect neurons against excessive glutamine that could send the neurons into apoptosis. Glial cells are particularly active in the hippocampus, cerebral cortex, and amygdala, areas of the brain that are sensitive to stress.

In response to stress, the immune system becomes highly active, and microglia—the primary immune cells of the central nervous system—release factors such as IL-1β, IL-6, TNF-α, and BDNF [24, 93, 94]. One trigger for microglial activation is a decline in CX3CL1, a neurochemokine that regulates synaptic plasticity and cognitive functions [25]. CX3CL1 levels decrease when neurons are damaged.

The *hippocampus* is particularly vulnerable to increased levels of IL-1β and has been associated with impaired learning, associative, and spatial motor skills. Immune system activation seems to increase amygdala and dACC reactivity to psychosocial skills [26, 27]. The increased hypothalamic-pituitary adrenal (HPA) axis activity of chronic stress increases glutaminergic transmission and apoptosis of neurons in the corticolimbic system [28]. Increased microglia and decreased dendritic connections result in decreased hippocampal volume in MDD, which is associated with poorer prognosis and relapse [28, 29]. A decreased number of neurons is associated with cognitive function deficits [95]. The longer MDD persists, the greater the deficit is in gray matter volume of the hippocampus [96] and the more difficult it is to achieve a response to antidepressants [30].

Pharmacological or psychological treatment does not seem to be sufficiently capable of altering cognitive dysfunctions [23]. Cognitive dysfunctions may persist after the mood symptoms have improved [11]. Through the use of some medications, a limited number of people may find some relief from cognitive deficits [31]. A general improvement of cognitive processes may be achieved with the SSRIs fluoxetine [32, 97, 98], paroxetine [33–35], and escitalopram [36–38]. Sertraline may improve executive functions and attention and may improve psychomotor retardation [39]. Bupropion may improve verbal and spatial memory and information processing [36–41]. Improved attention and executive functions may be seen with the SNRIs venlafaxine and duloxetine, which may also improve memory [37, 39, 41].

For some people, operational memory, information processing, and executive functions may be improved by mirtazapine, a noradrenergic and 5-HT1A receptor-specific serotonergic antidepressant [42]. The selective noradrenergic reuptake inhibitor reboxetine may also have a positive effect on cognitive functions [42].

The multimodal serotonin modulator vortioxetine may have positive effects on cognitive functions by increasing neuroplasticity [43, 44] and boosting immune system functions [46]. Clinical trials suggest that vortioxetine may be the best antidepressant for improving cognitive functions in MDD. However, meta-analyses show only weak evidence for improved depression compared to other SRIs [46, 28677828, 38863483].

Repetitive transcranial magnetic stimulation (rTMS) may improve cognitive functions [47–49].

Physical exercise can enhance memory function, executive function, and reward processing in depression patients by increasing functional brain regions [101]. Mechanisms appear to relate to increased neurogenesis, synaptic plasticity, and the release of brain-derived neurotrophic factor (BDNF) and other neurotrophic factors [99, 100]. An RCT testing receptive music therapy in older adults showed significant improvement in cognitive function and reduced depression [102].

Cognitive behavioral treatments typically show cognitive improvement along with functional and/or clinical recovery, but it appears that the long-term benefits on cognition are not certain [103].

Cerebral small vessel disease is a common disease in older folks and plays a central role in dementia and stroke [104–106]. Symptoms include cognitive decline, gait disturbance, and psychiatric disorders [107, 108]. There is evidence that cerebral microbleeds, as hallmarks of cerebral small vessel disease, may underlie depression and cognitive dysfunction [107, 109, 110].

A small study showed that there are moderate decrements in cognitive functioning in depressed older U.S. military veterans compared to nondepressed veterans [111]. Depressed carriers of single nucleotide *BDNF polymorphism* (Val66Met; rs6265) vs. Val/Val homozygotes exercisers scored better than nonexercisers on subjective cognitive, and objective measures of visual learning and working memory.[1] Those who got physical exercise scored better on a subjective measure of reasoning, and objective measures of processing speed, attention, and visual learning.

It appears that treatment-resistant depression patients may have higher verbal memory deficits compared to nonresistant patients, irrespective of symptom severity or pharmacological treatment [114].

Attention

Concentration problems are common in MDD; however, this problem with attention is rarely addressed by therapeutic interventions [115]. A 2019 comprehensive review of neural mechanisms supporting goal-directed attention can be found in Keller et al. [115]. Just as MDD is heterogeneous, attention impairment does not afflict all depressed individuals [116]. See Fig. 19.1.

Katsuki and Constantinidis have defined *attention as two distinct activities* [84]. They are *bottom-up* attention, referring to attentional guidance purely by externally driven factors to stimuli that are salient because of their inherent properties relative to the background; and *top-down* attention, referring to internal guidance of attention based on prior knowledge, willful plans, and current goals. *The fronto-parietal network* is the critical element in both.

Top-down attention has been discussed in three subdomains: selective, sustained, and divided attention [115]. *Selective attention* is the ability to attend to important (task-relevant) information while ignoring distracting (task-irrelevant) information. Task relevance is either related to spatial location or feature-based [84, 116–120]. There is some evidence that selective attention impairments in MDD are specific to feature-based selective attention while spatial selective attention remains intact [121–125].

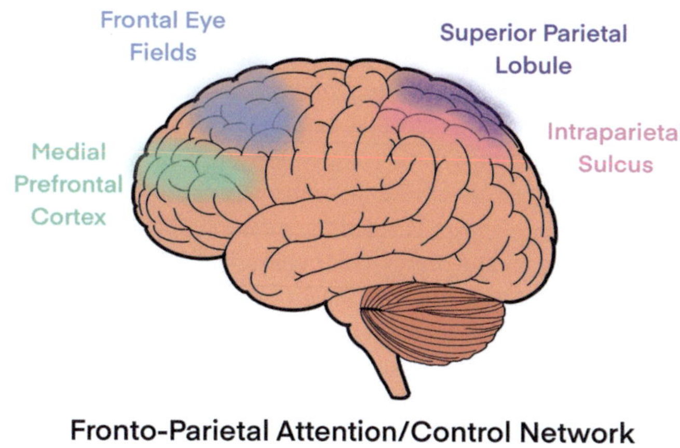

Fig. 19.1 This illustration highlights key regions of the fronto-parietal network involved in attentional regulation and executive control, including the medial prefrontal cortex, frontal eye fields, superior parietal lobule, and intraparietal sulcus. Together, these regions support top-down modulation of attention, visual orientation, and goal-directed behavior

Sustained attention is the ability to continuously attend to, or monitor, task-relevant information, in the relative absence of distractions. It is frequently manifested by an inability to maintain focus at work or school. The speed of detection of intermittent eccentric stimuli, such as in the Continuous Performance Task, is used to measure the degree of sustained attention. Impaired detection has sometimes been seen in MDD patients [128–130] and sometimes not [126, 127]. Rumination and worry may underlie decrements in sustained attention [131, 132].

Divided attention encompasses the functions of multitasking and of simultaneously attending to multiple sources of task-relevant information [133]. The prefrontal cortex is the vital element in paying simultaneous attention to multiple sensory modalities [134], performing more than one task at a time [8442936], and switching attention between multiple tasks [135]. Having better divided attention seems to be associated with better treatment outcome [136]. Poor divided attention is associated with higher suicidality [137] and relapse risk [53].

Symptoms of depression are often ameliorated with no improvement in attention, and selective attention does not correlate with insomnia or excessive worry [130, 138, 139]. Interactions between selective, sustained, and divided attention are complex [140].

Goal-directed, selective, sustained, and divided attention are necessary for cognitive control, perception, and decision-

[1] BDNF Val66Met polymorphism is more important in the development of MDD in men than in women [112, 113].

making. *Cognitive control functions* are discussed in references [141–144]. Cognitive control encompasses executive subfunctions, including selection and updating goal representations, response selection and suppression, and performance monitoring. Top-down attention and cognitive control processes appear to involve the same neurocircuitry.

Sensory perception is gated by attention [145]. Attention helps us to form and organize our conscious experience from the large amount of sensory information that surrounds us. Automatic and voluntary attention can alter the overall appearance of sensory information, hence impacting perception [146–149]. Higher-level perceptions, including attractiveness and emotional intensity of facial expressions, are also influenced by attention [148, 149]. *Retinal contrast* is significantly lower in both medicated and nonmedicated MDD patients. As a marker for depression, one study showed a specificity of 92.5% and a sensitivity of 77.5% [150, 151]. There was a strong correlation between increased severity and decreased contrast gain.

Decision-making is also dependent upon attention [152]. Krajbich summarizes that in making a decision, evidence for a given alternative is collected over time in proportion to its subjective value amplified by attention. And attention is drawn to noisier and more salient stimuli in a two-alternative choice, and to higher-value options in a multialternative choice. *Gaze bias* influences and reflects preferences [153]. Gaze-bias effect is a fundamental aspect of visual decision-making [153, 154]. When confronted with multiple options, we tend to fixate longer on stimuli that are ultimately chosen than on those that are not. *Reward bias* affects the attention that we place on the reward-associated locations [155]. Attention influences the choices we make and is associated with rewards [156]. Reinforcement in multidimensional reinforcement learning relies upon selective attention [157]. In depression, there are dysfunctions in model-based decision-making [158].

Negative Valence Systems are primarily responsible for responses to aversive situations or contexts, such as fear, anxiety, and loss [159]. *Negative attentional biases* in depressed patients are manifested as a tendency to spend more time paying attention to negative information rather than neutral or positive information [160]. It has been suggested that negative attentional biases come into play in depressed persons when their attention is initially arrested by salient negative information, but there is a lack of ability to redirect attention from the negative information toward goal-relevant information [161]. The result is a perpetual sad mood [162].

This *persistent mood state*, in turn, influences in a circular fashion the conscious or unconscious allocation of attention [163, 164]. *Affect-as-information* framework suggests that emotional/mood states can influence attention and overall cognitive styles [25067943]. The *mood-as-input* theory suggests that positive mood improves attention or makes tasks more pleasurable and therefore more acceptable even if performance is low [163]. The *broaden-and-build theory* postulates that positive moods improve cognition by increasing the scope of attention, enhancing creativity and flexibility [165–167].

Critical for control of goal-directed attention is the *fronto-parietal attention/control network*, which includes the frontal eye fields, intraparietal sulcus, medial prefrontal cortex (mPFC), and superior parietal lobule, among other regions [168–172]. Hypo-conductivity in the fronto-parietal attention/control network is associated with problems in goal-directed attention in MDD [122]. Evidence has increasingly pointed to the role of the fronto-parietal network in depression [173–177]. Varying results in exploring structures and functions in this network imply a dynamic and complex system [115]. The electrophysiology of the attention network is reviewed in reference [115].

It has been proposed that stress hyperreactivity associated with depression might interfere with the fronto-parietal attention/control network [115]. The mPFC part of the fronto-parietal attention/control network [178] interacts with the HPA-axis, which is dysregulated in depression [179]. In prolonged depression, there is elevation of cortisol, and neuronal atrophy of the hippocampus and the mPFC [180–182]. It has been suggested that stress hyperreactivity disruption of hippocampal-mPFC communication that is important for cognitive functions [183–185] may be the basis for MDD-associated problems with top–down attention [186]. In addition, the mPFC may be an integration site for cognition and emotions such that emotions may guide attention and vice versa [187].

Treatment of MDD does not appear to have adequately addressed attention problems. A 2019 review of potential pharmacological, brain stimulation, and behavioral interventions and their effects on subdomains of goal-directed attention (selective, sustained, and divided) is presented in reference [115].

Despite improvements in mood symptoms, *SSRI pharmacological* interventions show no change in sustained attention [130, 188], selective attention [138], or divided attention [53, 189]. Moreover, in healthy individuals, there is some evidence of decreased divided and sustained attention with SSRIs [190]. There appears to be one exception, and that is an SRI Vortioxetine that has mixed agonist/antagonist/partial-agonist effects [191]. Vortioxetine appears to have sustained and selective attention benefits.

Catecholaminergics such as those used to treat ADHD as well as MDD do seem to improve attention and other cognitive functions [192, 193].

In some but not all studies [194], *selective noradrenergic agonists*, including serotonin and norepinephrine reuptake inhibitors (SNRIs), atomoxetine, and the alpha2 agonists, may improve selective [195] and sustained attention [191, 196]. Guanfacine, an alpha2 agonist, may have positive effects on selective attention [197]. The SSNRI venlafaxine did not appear to improve cognitive functions in healthy volunteers [198], but results have been mixed in improving selective attention in MDD patients [138, 188, 196].

Dopaminergics appear to improve sustained attention, and possibly selective and divided attention. Amphetamines [199–201] and methylphenidate [202–205] can improve sustained attention and selective attention. Methylphenidate can also improve divided attention [204].

The *norepinephrine and dopamine reuptake inhibitor bupropion* can improve sustained attention [206, 207]. Modafinil as an adjunctive treatment can improve sustained and selective attention in some patients [193, 208–211]. Pramipexole, a D3 agonist used to treat restless legs syndrome, can improve sustained attention in low performers [212].

Noninvasive brain stimulation, including transcranial magnetic stimulation (TMS) and transcranial direct-current stimulation (tDCS), has the potential to target specific brain areas more precisely than chemical neuromodulators [213]. Selective and sustained attention has been improved in healthy subjects when the left dorsolateral prefrontal cortex (DLPFC) has been stimulated [214]. In depressed patients, sustained attention has been improved when the DLPFC has been stimulated [215–218]. However, systematic reviews have shown no improvements in selective, sustained, and divided attention in depressed subjects [219]. Other reviews found significant improvements only in working memory [220] and verbal memory [221].

Behavioral interventions can enhance attention; however, MDD is not typically their primary therapeutic target. Mindfulness meditation, which involves directing attention to a single sensation—such as breathing—while deliberately disengaging from distracting thoughts, has been shown to improve selective attention [222–225]. Neurofeedback-assisted technology-supported mindfulness training (N-tsMT) has been able to improve selective attention [226]. Exercise, in addition to improving mood, may improve selective attention [227–229]. However, some systematic reviews have yielded mixed results [230, 231]. Some computerized cognitive training apps using immersive video games or cognitive exercises have shown promising effects on both attentional and mood-related symptoms in some [232–234] but not in all studies [235].

Neurochemistry of Suicide

Suicide is a vicious act against the self [236–241], associated with violent and impulsive-aggressive behavior [242–244], and depression [245–249].[2]

Suicide is generally considered to result from an interplay of trait-like susceptibility to suicidal behaviors and environmental stressors: a stress diathesis model [254–257]. Suicidal behavior is heritable [258, 259]. Twin studies suggest a role of genetic factors contributing to a heritability of 30 to 55% [259, 260], which is in the range of heritability of psychiatric illnesses [261, 262]. Monozygotes vs. dizygotes are reported to have a 175 times greater risk of suicide behaviors, including attempts and completions [263]. In relatives of those who completed suicide, there are indications of a ten-fold greater risk [264]. Suicide attempts are up to 30 times more common in some populations compared to suicides and are important predictors of repeated attempts and completed suicides [265].

Adverse childhood experience (aka early life stress or childhood maltreatment) includes physical, sexual, or emotional abuse or neglect, violence within the home, or a hostile social environment (bullying)[3] [266, 267]. Early traumatic experiences are associated with deficits in brain development, psychiatric disorders, addiction disorders, and suicide [268–272]. Risks are also increased for negative physical health outcomes such as cancer, chronic pain, and metabolic syndromes [273–276].

These experiences and their consequences may also be passed along to succeeding generations [277–279].

Suicidal behavior may be the result of genetic factors predisposing to overreaction to negative social stressors, compromised higher-order cognitive control of mood, self-criticism, internalizing problems, overwhelming emotional pain, pessimism, impulsivity, anger, and reactive aggression, leading to suicidal ideation [255, 256, 280–284]. Epigenetics may be the link between neurochemical abnor-

[2]An early review back in 1995 found that 23 of 37 risk factors for violence were shared with suicide [250]. They also found that 17 variables that are protective factors for violence are also protective of suicide. In some European countries, the incidence of suicide among murderers is 30% [251, 252].

[3]According to the World Health Organization (2006), Preventing child maltreatment: a guide to taking action and generating evidence [253]. Childhood maltreatment is all forms of physical and/or emotional ill-treatment, sexual abuse, neglect, or negligent treatment or commercial or other exploitation, resulting in actual or potential harm to the child's health, survival, development, or dignity in the context of a relationship of responsibility, trust, or power.

Another restating of that definition is that childhood maltreatment is "abuse and neglect of children less than 18 years of age including all types of physical, sexual, and psychological/emotional violence, and the neglect of infants, children, and adolescents by parents, caregivers, and other authority figures, at home and in settings such as schools and orphanages" [268].

malities and environmental stressors [285]. Exposure in childhood to domestic violence may increase the rate of impulsive and suicidal behavior by two to seven times [286–289].

Various studies, both in vivo and postmortem, have revealed associations with problems in the hypothalamic-pituitary adrenal (HPA) system and with serotonin (5-hydroxytryptamine; 5-HT) responses in the brain [290]. State-of-the-art genetic studies have identified a variety of genes and proteins that associate with suicide in different populations [258]. Immunological studies have shown relationships between inflammatory system states and risk of suicide [291]. Nutritional factors have also been associated with suicide [292].

Genetic Interactions and Suicide

The *serotonin theory of depression*—namely, the hypothesis that depression is associated with lower levels of serotonin in the brain—has received considerable attention. Much of this focus has centered on the serotonin transporter gene and various serotonin receptor genes.

One of the genes that was first investigated for its relationship with depression and suicide is the gene *SLC6A4*[4] coding for the *serotonin transporter* [293, 294]. Early observations had found low *5-Hydroxyindoleacetic acid (5-HIAA)* concentrations in the cortical spinal fluid of depressed suicidal patients [299, 300]. 5-HIAA is the main metabolite of serotonin.[5] A particular focus of investigation was insertions and deletions in the *5-HTTLPR.* The 5-HTTLPR (*serotonin-transporter-linked promoter region*) is a polymorphic region in *SLC6A4,* the gene encoding the serotonin transporter, a type of monoamine transporter protein that transports the neurotransmitter serotonin from the synaptic cleft back to the presynaptic neuron, in the serotonin reuptake [4].

The 5-HTTLPR contains variations of repeat sequence containing GC-rich, 20–23-bp-long repeat elements [301]. The first two alleles to be identified were called the short (S) allele and the long (L) allele (14- and 16-copy repeats, respectively). Since that time, other alleles have been identified [302]. Each of the 14-copy repeat alleles has 4 variants (14-A, 14-B, 14-C,14-D). Each of the 16-copy repeats has six variants (16-A, 16-B, 16-C, 16-D, 16-E, 16-F). In addition, 15, 18, 19, 20, and 22 copy repeats have been described. One study found significant ethnic differences in the distribution of alleles and genotypes between a Japanese and a Caucasian population [302].

Considerable research has gone into investigating possible links of the serotonin transporter gene polymorphisms to affective disorders. Here are a few of those papers [303–306]. However, results from early studies have not always been replicated [307–310]. After a few words about serotonin receptors, we will summarize below the results of a 2022 comprehensive review on the role of these receptors in depression [316] and a 2023 umbrella review about the serotonin theory of depression [311].

There are at least 15 different *serotonin receptors* [312, 313]. Most of these have been associated with depression and depressive-like behavior. Serotonin 1A (5-HT 1A) and 1B (5-HT 1B) are the most well studied in relationship to MDD [314]. The 5-HT 1A receptors are autoreceptors that inhibit presynaptic serotonin release [315].

In 2022, a comprehensive review was published on the role of 5-HT_{1A}, 5-HT_{1B}, 5-HT_{2A}, 5-HT_{2B}, 5-HT_{2C}, 5-HT_3, and 5-HT_7 receptors in the mechanisms underlying the predisposition to aggression, depression, and suicidal behavior [316]. They concluded that: 1) depression-related 5-HT receptors include those receptors with pro-depressive properties (5-HT_{2A}, 5-HT_3, and 5-HT_7) as well as those providing an antidepressant effect (5-HT_{1A}, 5-HT_{1B}, and 5-HT_{2C} subtypes). 2) Aggression-related 5-HT receptors are identical to depression-related 5-HT receptors except for 5-HT_7 receptors. 3) Activation of 5-HT_{1A}, 5-HT_{1B}, 5-HT_{2A}, 5-HT_{2C} receptors attenuate aggressiveness, whereas agonists of 5-HT_3 intensify aggressive behavior. SSRIs operate by being agonists at the 5-HT1A, 5-HT1B, 5-HT2C, 5-HT4, and 5-HT6 receptors and antagonists at the 5-HT1A, 5-HT2A, 5-HT2C,

[4]Human *SLC6A4* (solute carrier family 6 member 4) is also known as HTT; 5HTT; OCD1; SERT; 5-HTT; SERT1; and hSERT. It is found on chromosome 17q11.2 and is composed of 14 exons that span ~40 kb. The sequence of the transcript predicts a protein of 630 amino acids with 12 transmembrane domains [7, 295]. Complexity is provided by alternative promoters, differential splicing, and 3′-untranslated-region variability, resulting in the transcription of multiple mRNA species. Several single nucleotide polymorphisms (SNPs), especially rs25531 and rs25532, and a variable number of tandem repeats (VNTRs) can change the structure or function of the protein. The rs25531 polymorphism has a minor-allele frequency of 9–15% in Caucasians and 24% in African Americans. Some of the polymorphisms appear to be associated with behavioral phenotypes.

The following description about *SLC6A4* is quoted from the *National Library of Medicine National Center for Biotechnology Information and updated on 11-Apr-2024* [327].

> This gene encodes an integral membrane protein that transports the neurotransmitter serotonin from synaptic spaces into presynaptic neurons. The encoded protein terminates the action of serotonin and recycles it in a sodium-dependent manner. This protein is a target of psychomotor stimulants, such as amphetamines and cocaine, and is a member of the sodium: neurotransmitter symporter family. A repeat length polymorphism in the promoter of this gene has been shown to affect the rate of serotonin uptake. There have been conflicting results in the literature about the possible effect, if any, that this polymorphism may play in behavior and depression.

[5]Serotonin is produced principally by enterochromaffin cells in the gut and also, importantly for the discussion of suicide and depression, by neurons [296–298].

5-HT3, 5- HT6, and 5-HT7 receptors [317]. Paradoxical antidepressant effects of both agonists and antagonists at specific 5-HT receptors are common [317].

Indeed, the use of SSRIs as antidepressants has been predicated on the serotonin theory of depression [312, 318, 319]. Surveys of the general population showed that most people believe that depression is caused by an imbalance of brain chemicals [320–322], a view also shared by many general practitioners [323]. Nevertheless, that hypothesis has been questioned [5, 6, 324–326].

A 2023 systematic umbrella review of the evidence offers insight into the prevailing state of the serotonin theory of depression—namely, whether depression is associated with reduced serotonin levels in the brain [311].[6] The following is a summary of their major points. (1) 5-HIAA concentrations showed no association with depression; (2) cohort studies of plasma serotonin showed no relationship with depression, and showed no evidence that lowered serotonin concentration was associated with antidepressant use; (3) 5-HT_{1A} receptor and SERT binding showed weak and inconsistent evidence of reduced binding in some areas, which would have been consistent with increased synaptic availability of serotonin in people with depression, if this was the original, causal abnormality, but prior antidepressant use was not reliably excluded; (4) tryptophan depletion studies found no effect in most healthy volunteers, but weak evidence of an effect in those with a family history of depression; but no systematic review had been conducted after 2007; (5) there was no evidence that the SERT gene had an association with depression, or of an interaction between genotype, stress and depression; (6) there was no consistent evidence of there being an association between serotonin and depression, and no support for the hypothesis that depression is caused by lowered serotonin activity or concentrations: and (7) some evidence might exist that long-term antidepressant use reduces serotonin concentration.

Reconciling the above 2022 review [316] *with the 2023 review* [311] *is a daunting task.* There may be a nuanced interpretation of conflicting data. For example, a recent study *5-HTTLPR* impacts only certain types of suicide risk-related behaviors and that it interacts with only distinct types of recent stressors [328]. That study found that even though *5-HTTLPR* did not influence previous suicide attempts or interact with childhood adversities, it did influence current suicidal ideation in an interaction with recent relationship problems. Significant associations have been seen in genetic variants of serotonin transportation (*5HTTLPR SLC6A4* intron 2) and of the serotonin receptor gene (*5HTR2AT102C*) in individuals who died of suicide [329]. The LL genotype of 5HTTLPR was associated with a higher risk. The heterozygous 12/10 genotype of SLC6A4 intron 2 polymorphisms increased among those who committed suicide, and serum serotonin levels were lower.

Genetic liability for MDD increases the risk for suicide attempts [330]. Genome-wide association studies (GWASs) results suggest that polygenic risk and specific genetic loci that overlap with MDD associate with a higher risk of attempting suicide [331]. An example is genes involved in anaerobic energy production (LDHB), circadian clock regulation (ARNTL2), and catabolism of tyrosine (FAH).

Novel suicide research has revealed three proteins that might be significantly associated with prospective suicide attempts (SCGB1A1, ANXA10, and CETN2) [332]. Tryptophan degradation via the *kynurenine pathway* produces several neuroactive metabolites, including kynurenic acid (KYNA), quinolinic acid (QUIN), and picolinic acid (PIC), that might be active in the pathophysiology of psychosis, major depression, and suicidal behavior [333].

The results of two large-scale GWASs validated loci for suicide attempts in multiancestry and European subjects [258]. Significant enrichment was seen in brain tissue gene expression, most notably in the pituitary. Twelve mostly intergenic risk loci with $p < 5 \times 10–8$ were identified. These loci were *DRD2, SLC6A9, FURIN, NLGN1, SOX5, PDE4B, and CACNG2*. The multiancestry single nucleotide polymorphisms (SNP)-based heritability estimate of suicide attempts was 5.7% on the liability scale ($SE = 0.003, p = 5.7 \times 10–80$). Genetic variation in these loci was shared between MDD, PTSD, smoking, and risk tolerance. Significant overlap was seen with previously identified regions implicated in suicide attempts. In these GWASs, the locus most strongly associated with suicide attempts was in an intergenic region on chromosome 7. Drug target enrichment results suggested that suicide attempts risk is most associated with the targets of antipsychotic and antidepressant drug classes. Pathways associated with epigenetics, gene regulation, and transcription were enriched but only in European ancestry.

Another GWAS found two loci with genome-wide significance [334]. These loci were the same intergenic area on chromosome 7 and the major histocompatibility locus. The chromosome 7 locus has been associated with risk-taking behavior, smoking, pain, sleep disturbances, lower educational attainment, reproductive traits, lower socioeconomic status, and poorer general health. The reviewers suggested that this locus is not mediated by psychiatric disorders but shows a strong association with those other factors. Strong correlations were seen with MDD but independent of the above-mentioned nonpsychiatric characteristics.

P2X7 is an ATP-sensitive ligand-gated nonselective cation channel, expressed in the brain primarily by microglia

[6] The review included 17 studies through December 2020. There were 12 systematic reviews and meta-analyses, 1 collaborative meta-analysis, 1 meta-analysis of large cohort studies, 1 systematic review and narrative synthesis, 1 genetic association study, and 1 umbrella review. They stated that the quality of reviews was variable with some genetic studies of high quality.

[335]. Activation can lead to *NLRP3* inflammasome complex-mediated release of proinflammatory cytokines and neurotransmitters (including IL-1 β, IL-18, and glutamate) into the extracellular space [336, 337]. Variations in *P2RX7* have been associated with mediating effects of stressors on the severity of depressive and anxiety symptoms [338, 339]. Variations of the *P2RX7* gene encoding the purinergic receptor P2X7R may interact with and mediate effects of early childhood adversities and traumas, as well as current stress, on lifetime emergence of suicide attempts and current suicide risk markers [288]. Current suicidal ideation was associated with clumps of top SNPs *rs641940* and *rs1653613*. Childhood trauma was associated with a clump with top SNP *psy_rs11615992* and another clump on hopelessness containing *rs78473339* as the index SNP.

Acute stress-associated epigenetic changes to genes associated with regulating vitamin D levels, tumor suppressors, structural framework, immune response, oxytocin, and possible relationships to suicide have been reviewed in [279].

Neuroinflammation and Suicide

A comprehensive model focusing on immune system influence on the pathophysiology of suicide behavior suggests that childhood abuse, sleep disturbance, infections, and other stressors induce a chronic inflammatory condition, causing dysregulation of the hypothalamic–pituitary–adrenal axis [340]. This leads to cortisol and *indolamine 2,3-dioxygenase* activation, which influences serotonin metabolism and increases in *N-methyl-d-aspartate (NMDA)* agonist [341–343].

In depressed patients, bidirectional dysregulation of both the innate and adaptive immune system is common [344]. There is another chapter in this focus volume that provides more detail on those relationships. Another chapter speaks about the role of the microbiota-immune-brain axis in neurodevelopment, wherein microbiota influences communication between the immune system and the brain is essential to neuronal development, neuronal excitability, neuroplasticity, and neurotransmission [345, 346]. Investigations for relationships between the microbiome and suicidality are in their infancy [347]. For example, preliminary evidence suggests that individuals who have attempted suicide exhibit differences in beta diversity compared to control subjects [348]. In addition, increased gut permeability may allow lipopolysaccharides (LPS) from gram-negative bacteria to enter the circulation, triggering low-grade systemic inflammation [349, 350]. Indeed, gut permeability markers zonulin and intestinal fatty acid binding protein were altered along with the elevation of IL-6 in patients with a recent suicide attempt [351].

According to a 2020 systematic review, the exact and specific immune pathways involved in suicidal behavior are not clear [352]. Most studies did show a link between abnormally higher *interleukin (IL)-1β, IL-6, tumor necrosis factor (TNF)-α, transforming growth factor (TGF)-β1, vascular endothelial growth factor (VEGF), kynurenic acid (KYN), and lower IL-2, IL-4, and interferon (IFN)-γ* levels in specific brain regions and suicidal behavior.

During chronic stress, low-level inflammation, especially neuroinflammation,[7] may be present [353]. Manifestations include activation of *microglia*, the resident immune system cells in the CNS, which produce proinflammatory cytokines such as TNF-alpha and IL-1 and neuroactive molecules including BDNF, glutamate, nitrous oxide, and ATP [354, 355]. Activation of microglia has been associated with increased depression and suicide [356–358]. An especially compelling 2022 narrative review of the role of microglia in neuropsychiatric disorders and suicide is quite revealing and well worth the read by anyone interested in the role of the immune system in depression and suicide [355].

Microglia in the dorsal raphe nucleus may have a role in both suicide facilitation and prevention in affective disorders [359]. Disruption of serotonergic transmission in the *dorsal raphe nucleus* (DRN) [360–362] has been implicated in the pathophysiology of schizophrenia, MDD, and suicidal behavior [363–367]. The serotonin system has been the frequent target of discussions that link depression and suicide [368–371]. Serotonin deficiency appears to contribute to MDD and suicidal behavior [372–375].

Suicide appears to involve neuroinflammation activation of the kynurenine pathway causing serotonin depletion and stimulation of glutamate neurotransmission [376]. Associated decreased BDNF (brain-derived neurotrophic factor) is linked to impaired neuroplasticity and cognitive deficits. Hyperactivity of the HPA is a frequent finding. Epigenetic control is exerted on these changes. Stanek et al. explore the mechanisms of action of antisuicidal treatments considering such an etiopathogenesis [376].

A large meta-analysis of immune biomarkers found that higher blood levels of C-reactive protein (CRP) have been associated with suicidal behavior independent of any psychiatric disorders [382]. Dysregulation of sex hormones in MDD may also be associated with suicide [383].

An exploratory analysis of cytokine and chemokine levels compared after controlling for age, gender, body mass index, race, ethnicity, and *C-reactive protein (CRP)* levels showed that adolescent and young adult patients with recent suicide behavior had lower IL-4 levels [384].

[7]Neuroinflammation is inflammation of nervous system tissue [377]. Neuroinflammation can be triggered by a diverse array including infections, psychosocial stress [378, 379], autoimmune disorders, neurodegenerative disorders, and traumatic brain injury. Microglia appear to be the critical mediator between stress and neuroimmune consequences. For more on neuroinflammation in the CNS, the following resources are available [378, 380, 381].

A meta-analysis of postmortem brain gene expression in relation to suicide underscored involvement of astrocytes, stress response, immune system, and microglia in suicide [385]. They found reduced expression of the *KCNJ2 (Potassium Inwardly Rectifying Channel Subfamily J Member 2), A2M (Alpha-2-Macroglobulin), AGT (Angiotensinogen), PMP2 (Peripheral Myelin Protein 2), and VEZF1 (Vascular Endothelial Zinc Finger 1) genes* (FDR $p < 0.05$).

A large cohort of MDD patients was assessed for percentages of circulating peripheral blood mononuclear cells focused on T helper cell subsets (memory T helper cells, Th1, Th2, Th17, and T regulatory cells) [386]. They found (1) there is a greater abundance of memory T helper in MDD patients including in young adults, which may signal premature aging of the immune system; (2) reduced percentages of NK cells, and higher percentages of B and T cells in MDD patients; and (3) the highest risk group showed the highest number of memory T helper cells and showed a robust increase of Th17 cells compared to other suicide risk groups.

Neutrophil-to-lymphocyte ratio (NLR), monocyte-to-lymphocyte ratio (MLR), and platelet-to-lymphocyte ratio (PLR) are important peripheral inflammatory biomarkers [387–390]. There is some evidence that NLR may be significantly higher in depressed suicidal patients [391–393].

A combination of cytokines and kynurenine metabolites in the second trimester may have a >99% probability of accurately predicting third trimester depression [394]. Blood samples in pregnant women were analyzed for plasma IL-1β, IL-2, IL-6, IL-8, IL-10, TNF, kynurenine, tryptophan, serotonin, kynurenic, quinolinic, and picolinic acids, and used mixed-effects models to assess the association between biomarkers and depression severity [394]. Results showed that IL-1β and IL-6 levels associated positively with the severity of depressive symptoms throughout pregnancy and postpartum, and that the odds of experiencing significant depressive symptoms increased by >30% per median absolute deviation for both IL-1β and IL-6 (both $P = 0.01$).

Depression, suicidal ideation, and behavior are frequently seen in patients being treated with monoclonal antibodies (mAbs); this is especially seen with mAbs for treating autoimmune diseases that suppress the immune system [395].

Nutrition and Suicide

A comprehensive narrative review suggests that links between the one-carbon cycle, folate-homocysteine balance, immune system function, glutamate excitation via NMDA (N-methyl-D-aspartate) receptors, and gut microbiome eubiosis play a role in mood regulation and suicidality [292]. Low levels of serum and red blood cell folate are often found in depressed people [396–398]. Mixed reviews suggest that folic acid and its derivative, L-methylfolate, could be used to supplement depression treatment [399–401].

Epigenetics and Suicide

Epigenetic processes can influence depressive symptoms by regulating genes associated with depression [279, 402–409]. For example, activation of the tryptophan-kynurenine metabolic pathway results in bioactive molecules with oxidant, antioxidant, neurotoxic, neuroprotective, and/or immunomodulatory properties [410–412]. Epigenetic changes in these bioactive amines, glucocorticoid, and serotonin regulatory pathways are highly involved in suicide, depression, and anxiety [279].

A 2023 comprehensive narrative review of the literature investigated the epigenetic changes that occur with acute stress, chronic stress, early childhood stress, and traumatic stress exposures [279]. In addition, they examined epigenetic changes in postmortem brains or blood samples of suicide completers and attempters. Powerfully, they also looked at the transgenerational effects of these changes. They found that for all types of stress studies examined, the genes *Nr3c1*, *OXTR*, *SLC6A4*, and *BDNF* reproducibly showed epigenetic change, and some modifications were passed down to subsequent generations following stress exposures. *Nr3c1*,[8] *OXTR*,[9] *SLC6A4*,[10] and *BDNF*[11] participate in neuronal development and hormonal regulation, and all are associated with susceptibility to mental health disorders, including depression, anxiety, personality disorders, and PTSD. Those four genes demonstrated region-and site-specific methylation patterns in response to various stressors. These patterns for each of these genes were different for acute stress, chronic stress, early childhood stress, traumatic stress, and in suicide completers and noncompleters. Those changes are well illustrated in [279]. There are tables that are summaries of epigenetic changes to these and other genes associated with acute stress, chronic stress, early childhood stress, traumatic stress, and suicide.[12]

[8] *Nr3c1* glucocorticoid receptor gene [413].

[9] *OXTR* oxytocin receptor gene [414].

[10] *SLC6A4* serotonin transporter gene [415].

[11] *BDNF* brain-derived neurotropic factor [416].

[12] A partial list of genes that have been shown as of 2023 to be epigenetically associated with suicide includes [279]:

1. *GRIK2, BEGAIN, BDNF,* and *TrkB,* involved in neuron survival, cell-to-cell communication, and development [417, 418].
2. *Elovl5, ARHGEF38, PSORS1C3, OXTR,* and *CYP2D6* are involved in the elongation of long-chain fatty acids, the regulation of catalytic activity, and a gene involved in psoriasis, respectively [419].
3. *ZNF714, NRIP3, Nr3c1, 5-HT1A, SKA2, MAOA, GABRA1,* and CERC2 [279].
4. *ZNF714* was hypomethylated and *NRIP3* showed mixed methylation in 9 male hanging suicides [420].

Epigenetics-targeted treatment for stress-related disorders suggests that some psychotherapies can reverse adverse methylation changes [421–423]. For example, in response to narrative exposure therapy for PTSD, protective effects in *Nr3c1* may occur [424].

Exercise may beneficially change methylation profiles in inflammation, cancer, neurodegenerative diseases, and aging [425–427].

MDMA treatment-responsive PTSD patients appear to undergo favorable methylation changes in the *NR3C1* gene [428].

Assorted Associations with Suicide

Sunlight has profound and complex influences on physiology and human behavior, such as depression [3, 429–432]. Besides vision, sunlight modulates circadian rhythms of a variety of physiological functions, including autonomic, neuroendocrine, immunological, mood, thermal regulation, alertness, and performance [433–436]. Suicide rates in the circumpolar communities are quite high [437].

A large international study has revealed that the risk of suicide attempts by folks with bipolar 1 disorder appears to increase when there is a large change in solar insolation, both between winter and summer and between the minimum and maximum monthly values [438]. The lowest odds of a suicide attempt are at the equator and the highest at the poles. Results also indicated that living in a country with a state-sponsored religion decreased the odds by 65%. Being male increased the odds by 54%. Being in the youngest cohort increased the odds by 127%. Substance abuse or alcohol abuse increased the odds by 58%. Adult depression is associated with low and decreasing self esteem in adolescence [443].

A complex relation exists between the psychological and behavioral indicators of impulsivity and anger [439]. A 2021 study revealed a correlation between psychological and blood biochemical indicators in suicide attempters among adolescents who have MDD and have engaged in nonsuicidal self-injury (NSSI). In suicide attempters, an inverse relation was seen between impulsivity scores[13] and lower serum C-reactive protein and cortisol levels than those having MDD who participated in NSSI. An increased frequency of NSSI is a potential risk factor for suicide.

Impulsivity can be dangerously risky for self-injury. For example, emotional instability and impulsive behavior in borderline personality disorder (BPD), bulimia nervosa (BN), and anorexia nervosa (AN) contribute to high rates of suicidal ideation and behavior [440]. More than 60% of people with BPD, and 25–33% of individuals with AN or BN attempt suicide [441].

A 2023 study has identified transdiagnostic inflammatory/oxidative biomarkers relevant to suicidal behavior in impulsive and unstable disorders [442]. They sampled patients with BPD, patients with restrictive eating disorder (rED), and patients with purging eating disorder (pED). They found that more *JNK and ERK*, and *less GPx, SOD, and Keap1*, predicted nonsuicidal self-injury, and three components with higher *JNK, TBARS, and TNF-α* levels, and lower *GPx, SOD, and iNOS* levels, predicted suicide attempts.

Significantly higher levels of proinflammatory cytokines IL-8 and TNF-α have been associated with low self-esteem [45, 444][14] in Native Hawaiians and other Pacific Islanders [516]. Metagenomics showed relative abundance of specific gut bacteria differed between groups with different self-esteem scores. In addition, differences between groups were seen in epigenetic changes in genes involved with immunometabolism. The *Horvath clock* [445, 446][15] indicated genetic acceleration in those who had normal self-esteem and deceleration in those who had low self-esteem.

Tools for Predicting Suicide

Ecological momentary assessments (EMA) are a type of e-mental health intensive time sampling that relies on repeated measurements of self-reported daily experiences [461]. EMA consists of asking patients questions in real time in their usual habitat [462]. EMA can use smartphone sensing technology to collect data, machine learning, and mobile apps to relay that information to a remote practitioner [463, 464]. Typically, self-report assessments are triggered by a daily event or at a fixed or random time.

Machine learning has been proposed to widen understanding of neurobiology, depression, and suicide [465].

EMA studies focus on identifying the proximal relationship between individual risk factors and suicidal ideations [462, 466, 467]. Associations have been seen between daily negative affect and positive affect, rumination, interpersonal

[13] Inventories that were used in this study were the following: Ottawa Self-Injury Inventory (OSI) [447], Beck Depression Inventory-II (BDI-II) [448], State-Trait Anxiety Inventory (STAI) [449], Barratt Impulsiveness Scale (BIS-11) [450], Difficulties in Emotion Regulation Scale (DERS) [451], State-Trait Anger Expression Inventory (STAXI-2), Borderline Symptom List (BSL-23) [452], Childhood Trauma Questionnaire (CTQ) [453], Eysenck personality Questionnaire (EPQ) [1, 453, 454], Defense Style Questionnaire (DSQ) [455], and Coping Style Questionnaire (CSQ) [2].

[14] The Rosenberg Self-Esteem Scale is the most widely used measure of global self-esteem with evidence of generalizability across ethnic groups [456, 457].

[15] Many changes that happen with age are epigenetic [458, 459]. According to Steve Horvath, the Horvath Clock focuses on one type of epigenetic control: cytosine-5 methylation within CpG dinucleotides (also known as DNA methylation). Genes or genomic regions either get hypermethylated or hypomethylated with age [460]. Many CpGs are subject to age-related hypermethylation [445].

interactions, daily nonsuicidal self-injury, social support, sleep, and emotions, and a history of suicide and self-harm. The goal is to monitor behaviors of people who are at high risk for suicide, especially in patients who have depressive disorders who may be prone to quick changes in intensity of risk factors [463, 468, 469]. Mobile-based ecological momentary assessments, but not passive sensing alone, have the potential to identify short-term, immediate, suicide risk [470].

A deep-learning model has shown promise in predicting the risk of suicide-related events (SREs) in PTSD sufferers [471]. The *DeepBiomarker* analyzed electronic medical records of 38,807 PTSD patients and found that it could predict SRE within the following 3 months with an area under the ROC curve score of 0.93.[16] They identified important abnormal laboratory tests, medication use, and other factors that implied that regulation of the immune system, respiratory system, cardiovascular system, and gut microbiome participated in shaping the pathophysiological pathways promoting depression and suicidal risks in those PTSD patients.

Suicide Prevention

Suicide frequently coincides with depressive episodes [8, 9, 477, 478]. For each completed suicide, worldwide, there may be 10–30 times more attempts made [479]. The highest mortality rate worldwide in suicide is due to depression. Depression is the most prevalent psychiatric disorder associated with suicide [334]. A spectrum exists from suicidal ideation through the pain of helplessness and hopelessness; if coping skills, both innate and learned, are exceeded, then planning begins, and suicide attempts seem the way out [480].

Globally, suicide was the fourth leading cause of death in 2023 among 15–29-year-olds [481]. It is the second leading cause worldwide of death of adolescents [482]. Prevalence of suicidal ideation, suicidal behavior, and completed suicide all increase dramatically during adolescence, the exceptional time of developmental vulnerability for suicidal ideation and behaviors [483–485].

Traumatic stress that occurs in response to catastrophes of the rapid loss of important resources, such as during natural disasters, tragic deaths, sexual assault, and war, increases the likelihood of suicide in vulnerable individuals [10, 486–488].

The cumulative burden of chronic stress and life events (allostatic load), which depends upon the nature of the stressor, severity, and duration, may interact with epigenetic factors to reach the tipping point [489]. That is, if personalized intervention resources are insufficient.

Suicide is an increasing public health problem. In the USA, the national rate increased by 30% from 2000 to 2016 [473]. The *Centers for Disease Control and Prevention* reports that the national suicide rate increased from 10.4 to 13.5 per 100,000 persons, with average annual increases of 1% from 2000 to 2006 and 2% from 2006 to 2016 [474].

Substance Abuse and Mental Health Services Administration (SAMHSA) in 2017 reports that suicidal ideation, suicide planning, and suicide attempts have especially increased from 2006 to 2017 among people 18 to 25 years of age [475]. These increases have co-occurred with an increase in the prevalence of mental health conditions that cause significant impairment in daily functioning, especially major depressive episodes, and chronic substance abuse. At least one study has found that anxiety symptoms, high rates of depressive symptoms, ongoing substance use issues, sleeping difficulties, and fatigue were common in the final week before suicide [490]. One bit of good news is that the suicide rates fell age-adjusted rate of deaths by suicide declining between 2018 and 2020. Nevertheless, suicide was the second leading cause of death among people aged 10 to 34 and the fifth leading cause among people aged 35 to 54 [476].

Prediction and prevention of suicidal behavior usually rely on scales that consider clinical factors such as depression, previous suicide attempts, and stressful events [491–493]. However, these suicide predictor models do not perform as well as hoped [492, 493]. This makes attempts very attractive for finding a sensitive and specific *biomarker*[17] that can differentiate between diagnostic subgroups and predict worsening symptoms [492, 498, 499]. A 2022 comprehensive review concludes that the serotonergic system, inflammation, hypothalamic-pituitary-adrenal axis, lipids, and endocannabinoids emerged as the most promising diagnostic, predictive, and therapeutic indicators [500].

Machine learning and artificial intelligence approaches to suicide prediction using healthcare data are currently being explored and show promise [501–505].

CDC's Preventing Suicide: A Technical Package of Policies, Programs, and Practices highlights strategies based on the best available evidence to help states and communities prevent suicide.[18]

[16]Quoted from [472]: "The **receiver operating characteristic (ROC) curve** is a well-known graphical tool routinely used for evaluating the discriminatory ability of continuous markers, referring to a binary characteristic. The **area under the curve (AUC)** has been proposed as a summarized accuracy index. Higher values of the marker are usually associated with higher probabilities of having the characteristic under study." The value of 0.93 is better than other traditional machine learning models.

[17]A biomarker is defined as "any substance, structure, or process that can be measured in the body," which can "influence or predict the incidence of outcome or disease" [494] as well as the treatment response [495, 496].

[18]Contact the *National Suicide Prevention Lifeline Call 1-800-273-TALK (1-800–273-8255)* [497].

A 2019 systematic review assessed the benefits and harms of nonpharmacological and pharmacological interventions to prevent suicide and reduce suicide behaviors in at-risk adults [506]. Nonpharmacological interventions included psychotherapies, crisis response planning (CRP), and community support programs. CBT reduced suicide attempts, suicidal ideation, and hopelessness compared with treatment as usual. Limited evidence suggested that DBT reduced suicidal ideation compared with wait-list control or crisis planning. They saw low-strength evidence for the *World Health Organization's Brief Intervention and Contact method (WHO-BIC)* to reduce suicide, CRP to reduce suicide attempts, and *Window to Hope* to reduce suicidal ideation and hopelessness.

Pharmacologic interventions were antidepressants and anxiety medications, lithium, antipsychotics, ketamine, and naloxone. Ketamine reduced suicidal ideation with negligible adverse events compared with placebo or midazolam. Lithium reduced suicide rates among patients with unipolar or bipolar mood disorders compared with placebo. However, no differences were observed between lithium and other medications in reducing suicide. There was limited information on potential harm. There are some suggestions that some pharmaceuticals may exert some anti suicidal effects through their anti-inflammatory properties [376, 507].

The procedures used in cognitive behavioral therapy for suicide prevention (*CBT-SP*) as an empirically supported treatment approach for suicidal patients are presented in [508].

On the other hand, a meta-analysis of RCTs up until December of 2015 of strategies to prevent death by suicide reported that the WHO-BIC was associated with significantly lower odds of suicide (OR[19] = 0.20; 95% CI: 0.09 to 0.42) [509]. Whereas CBT (OR = 0.34; 95% CI: 0.12 to 1.03) and lithium (OR = 0.23; 95% CI: 0.05 to 1.02) gave nonsignificant results.

A systematic review and meta-analysis of studies between 2011 and 2017 found a significant effect for suicide prevention interventions on completed suicides (d = −0.535, 95% CI: −0.898 to −0.171, p = 0.0040 and on suicide attempts (d = −0.449, 95% CI: −0.618 to −0.280, $p < 0.001$) [515]. In addition, there was a significantly higher synergistic effect related to the number of levels of the intervention ($p = 0.032$).

[19] Odds ratio (OR) is a way to represent the odds that an outcome will result when a given exposure to a variable of interest occurs compared to when the exposure does not occur. OR quantifies the strength of the association between two events. An OR greater than 1 indicates a positive association or that exposure to that variable increases the odds of that outcome. An OR less than one indicates a negative relationship between two events. An OR of 1 suggests no relationship between two events. An OR is frequently accompanied by a 95% confidence interval (CI). CI is a measure of the precision of the OR. The smaller the CI, the higher the precision as long as it does not overlap OR = 1. For more information, see Chap. 4 on evidence basics in this text.

According to a Swedish study, females compared to males tend to use healthcare more frequently in the 2 years before suicide [510]. In that study, younger people sought psychiatric services, whereas older adults used predominantly non-psychiatric services.

Suicidal ideation in acute suicidal episodes may be in the form of verbal thoughts or mental imagery [6]. Mental imagery is perception in the absence of external sensory input [511, 512]. It is multisensory, ranging from fleeting sensory impressions and static scenes to detailed pre- or re-play of events in a specific time and space [6]. Mental imagery may have a stronger impact on affective responses and influence on behavior than verbal processing [513]. Interestingly, in previously depressed and never depressed individuals, higher levels of image processing were significantly associated with more positive affect and better momentary mood irrespective of positive or negative valence [514]. One study identified two themes. They were 1) Suicide-approaching imagery: intrusive looming images that contributed to loss of control, flashforwards that clarified the suicidal solution, or desirable but unattainable images. 2) Suicide preventive imagery: death-alienating, life-affirming, or potentially helpful images [6].

If you or someone you know is struggling with loneliness, or is feeling helpless and suicidal, there are many resources available. If you are in the USA, support can be found at Find a support group | AFSP . *If suicide is a possibility and you need assistance, immediately call 988 or the National Suicide Prevention Helpline on 1–800-273-TALK (8255). The Helpline is a free, confidential crisis hotline that is available to everyone 24 hours a day, seven days a week.* National Hotline for Mental Health Crises and Suicide Prevention | NAMI

If you are in another country, you can go to www.befrienders.org *to find a helpline near you.*

Summary

This chapter introduced some of the complexities of cognitive dysfunction as it relates to many of the symptoms of depressive disorders. Just as MDD is heterogeneous, attention impairment does not afflict all depressed individuals. When cognitive deficiencies occur in concentration and attention, executive functions, learning and memory, and processing speed can have profound effects on function and clinical outcome in MDD.

Cognitive dysfunction is associated with worse work performance and social relationships and can occur early or late in illness. The dysfunction may also relate to higher levels of resistance to antidepressant strategies and the number of previous depressive episodes. Cognitive dysfunctions are also linked to age, poor intellectual ability, and years of schooling.

Common risk factors of substance use, sedentary behavior, inflammation, obesity, and life stress are linked to cognitive dysfunction and depression. Therapeutic attempts to improve cognitive functions, including attention-related problems, have achieved only mixed results.

Genetics and epigenetics may alter both the occurrence of cognitive dysfunctions and their resistance to treatment. A complex relationship exists among stress, inflammation, cognition, and mood. Symptoms of depression and suicide are frequently associated with gross neuroanatomical changes and allostatic changes in control circuits.

Immune and neurocircuits response to stressors has probably given us a survival advantage. But modern stressors may have predisposed us to the development of depression.

Pharmacological or psychological treatment does not seem to be sufficiently capable of altering cognitive dysfunctions, which may persist after the mood symptoms have improved. However, exercise and rTMS have shown some promising effects for some patients.

Suicide is discussed in terms of psychosocial and biochemical interactions responsible for self-harm. Emphasis has been focused on research dealing with genetics, neuroinflammation, and epigenetics. Detection of suicidal behavior and prevention based upon current evidence is discussed. It has become clear that predisposition to suicide is heritable in a stress diathesis model. Successful prevention will need to embrace personal medicine.

References

1. Barrett PT, Petrides KV, Eysenck SBG, Eysenck HJ. "The Eysenck personality questionnaire: an examination of the factorial similarity of P, E, N, and L across 34 countries" (PDF). Personal Individ Differ. 1998;25(5):805–19. https://doi.org/10.1016/S0191-8869(98)00026-9.
2. Xiao JH, Xu XF. Study on validity and reliability of coping style questionnaire. Chin Ment Health J. 1996;4:164–8.
3. Münch M, Brøndsted AE, Brown SA, Gjedde A, Kantermann T, Martiny K, et al. The effect of light on humans. In: Changing perspectives on daylight: science, technology, and culture. Washington, DC: Sponsored supplement to Science/AAS; Science/AAAS Custom Publishing Office; 2017. p. 16–23.
4. SLC6A4 – Sodium-dependent serotonin transporter – Homo sapiens (Human) | UniProtKB | UniProt.
5. Psychiatry's New Brain-Mind and the Legend of the "Chemical Imbalance"
6. Nilsson AM, Waern M, Ehnvall A, Skärsäter I. The meaning of mental imagery in acute suicidal episodes: A qualitative exploration of lived experiences. Omega (Westport). 2023:302228231218562. PMID: 38006244. http://www.ncbi.nlm.nih.gov/pubmed/38006244
7. Murphy DL, Lesch KP. Targeting the murine serotonin transporter: insights into human neurobiology. Nat Rev Neurosci 9: 85–96.
8. Suicidal Ideation – StatPearls – NCBI Bookshelf
9. Depressive disorder (depression)
10. Traumatic stress in overview: Definition, context, scope, and long-term outcomes.
11. Murrough JW, Iacoviello B, Neumeister A, Charney DS, Iosifescu DV. Cognitive dysfunction in depression: neurocircuitry and new therapeutic strategies. Neurobiol Learn Mem. 2011;96(4):553–63. PMID: 21704176. http://www.ncbi.nlm.nih.gov/pubmed/21704176
12. Psychiatry.org – DSM
13. Wojcik GM, Masiak J, Kawiak A, Schneider P, Kwasniewicz L, Polak N, Gajos-Balinska A. New protocol for quantitative analysis of brain cortex electroencephalographic activity in patients with psychiatric disorders. Front Neuroinform. 2018;12:27. PMCID: PMC5976787. http://www.ncbi.nlm.nih.gov/pubmed/29881339
14. Hammer-Helmich L, Haro JM, Jönsson B, Tanguy Melac A, Di Nicola S, Chollet J, Milea D, Rive B, Saragoussi D. Functional impairment in patients with major depressive disorder: the 2-year PERFORM study. Neuropsychiatr Dis Treat. 2018;14:239–49. PMCID: PMC5767094. http://www.ncbi.nlm.nih.gov/pubmed/29386897
15. Talarowska M, Zajączkowska M, Gałecki P. Cognitive functions in first-episode depression and recurrent depressive disorder. Psychiatr Danub. 2015;27(1):38–43. PMID: 25751430. http://www.ncbi.nlm.nih.gov/pubmed/25751430
16. Stuhrmann A, Dohm K, Kugel H, Zwanzger P, Redlich R, Grotegerd D, Rauch AV, Arolt V, Heindel W, Suslow T, Zwitserlood P, Dannlowski U. Mood-congruent amygdala responses to subliminally presented facial expressions in major depression: associations with anhedonia. J Psychiatry Neurosci. 2013;38(4):249–58. PMCID: PMC3692722. http://www.ncbi.nlm.nih.gov/pubmed/23171695
17. Disner SG, Beevers CG, Haigh EAP, Beck AT. Neural mechanisms of the cognitive model of depression. Nat Rev Neurosci. 2011;12(8):467–77. http://www.ncbi.nlm.nih.gov/pubmed/21731066
18. Drevets WC, Savitz J, Trimble M. The subgenual anterior cingulate cortex in mood disorders. CNS Spectr. 2008;13(8):663–81. PMCID: PMC2729429. http://www.ncbi.nlm.nih.gov/pubmed/18704022
19. Etkin A, Egner T, Kalisch R. Emotional processing in anterior cingulate and medial prefrontal cortex. Trends Cogn Sci. 2011;15(2):85–93. PMCID: PMC3035157. http://www.ncbi.nlm.nih.gov/pubmed/21167765
20. Stevens FL, Hurley RA, Taber KH. Anterior cingulate cortex: unique role in cognition and emotion. J Neuropsychiatry Clin Neurosci. 2011;23(2):121–5. http://www.ncbi.nlm.nih.gov/pubmed/21677237
21. Pehrson AL, Leiser SC, Gulinello M, Dale E, Li Y, Waller JA, Sanchez C. Treatment of cognitive dysfunction in major depressive disorder—a review of the preclinical evidence for efficacy of selective serotonin reuptake inhibitors, serotonin-norepinephrine reuptake inhibitors and the multimodal-acting antidepressant vortioxetine. Eur J Pharmacol. 2015;753:19–31. PMID: 25107284. http://www.ncbi.nlm.nih.gov/pubmed/25107284
22. Li Y, Waller JA, et al. Treatment of cognitive dysfunction in major depressive disorder—a review of the preclinical evidence for efficacy of selective serotonin reuptake inhibitors, serotonin-norepinephrine reuptake inhibitors and the multimodal-acting antidepressant vortioxetine. Eur J Pharmacol. 2015;753:19–31.
23. Gonda X, Pompili M, Serafini G, Carvalho AF, Rihmer Z, Dome P. The role of cognitive dysfunction in the symptoms and remission from depression. Ann General Psychiatry. 2015;14:27. PMCID: PMC4578787. http://www.ncbi.nlm.nih.gov/pubmed/26396586
24. Yuen EY, Liu W, Karatsoreos IN, Ren Y, Feng J, McEwen BS, Yan Z. Mechanisms for acute stress-induced enhancement of glutamatergic transmission and working memory. Mol Psychiatry.

2011;16(2):156–70. PMCID: PMC3108461. http://www.ncbi.nlm.nih.gov/pubmed/20458323
25. Reus GZ, de Moura AB, Silva RH, Resende WR, Quevedo J. Resilience dysregulation in major depressive disorder: focus on glutamatergic imbalance and microglial activation. Curr Neuropharmacol. 2018;16(3):297–307. PMCID: PMC5843981. http://www.ncbi.nlm.nih.gov/pubmed/28676011
26. Rogers JT, Morganti JM, Bachstetter AD, Hudson CE, Peters MM, Grimmig BA, Weeber EJ, Bickford PC, Gemma C. CX3CR1 deficiency leads to impairment of hippocampal cognitive function and synaptic plasticity. J Neurosci. 2011;31(45):16241–50. PMCID: PMC3236509. http://www.ncbi.nlm.nih.gov/pubmed/22072675
27. Muscatell KA, Moieni M, Inagaki TK, Dutcher JM, Jevtic I, Breen EC, Irwin MR, Eisenberger NI. Exposure to an inflammatory challenge enhances neural sensitivity to negative and positive social feedback. Brain Behav Immun. 2016;57:21–9. PMCID: PMC5011017. http://www.ncbi.nlm.nih.gov/pubmed/27032568
28. Ménard C, Pfau ML, Hodes GE, Russo SJ. Immune and neuroendocrine mechanisms of stress vulnerability and resilience. Neuropsychopharmacology. 2017;42(1):62–80. PMCID: PMC5143517. http://www.ncbi.nlm.nih.gov/pubmed/27291462
29. Drevets WC, Price JL, Furey ML. Brain structural and functional abnormalities in mood disorders: implications for neurocircuitry models of depression. Brain Struct Funct. 2008;213(1–2):93–118. PMCID: PMC2522333. http://www.ncbi.nlm.nih.gov/pubmed/18704495
30. Sheline YI, Pieper CF, Barch DM, Welsh-Bohmer K, McKinstry RC, MacFall JR, D'Angelo G, Garcia KS, Gersing K, Wilkins C, Taylor W, Steffens DC, Krishnan RR, Doraiswamy PM. Support for the vascular depression hypothesis in late-life depression: results of a 2-site, prospective, antidepressant treatment trial. Arch Gen Psychiatry. 2010;67(3):277–85. PMCID: PMC2838210. http://www.ncbi.nlm.nih.gov/pubmed/20194828
31. Bukh JD, Bock C, Vinberg M, Kessing LV. The effect of prolonged duration of untreated depression on antidepressant treatment outcome. J Affect Disord. 2013;145(1):42–8. PMID: 22854096. http://www.ncbi.nlm.nih.gov/pubmed/22854096
32. Rosenblat JD, Kakar R, McIntyre RS. The cognitive effects of antidepressants in major depressive disorder: a systematic review and meta-analysis of randomized clinical trials. Int J Neuropsychopharmacol. 2015;19(2):pyv082. PMCID: PMC4772818. http://www.ncbi.nlm.nih.gov/pubmed/26209859
33. Levkovitz Y, Caftori R, Avital A, Richter-Levin G. The SSRIs drug fluoxetine, but not the noradrenergic tricyclic drug Desipramine, improves memory performance during acute major depression. Brain Res Bull. 2002;58(4):345–50. PMID: 12183009. http://www.ncbi.nlm.nih.gov/pubmed/12183009
34. Ferguson JM, Wesnes KA, Schwartz GE. Reboxetine versus paroxetine versus placebo: effects on cognitive functioning in depressed patients. Int Clin Psychopharmacol. 2003;18(1):9–14. PMID: 12490769. http://www.ncbi.nlm.nih.gov/pubmed/12490769
35. Deuschle M, Kniest A, Niemann H, Erb-Bies M, Colla N, Hamann B, Heuser I. Impaired declarative memory in depressed patients is slow to recover: clinical experience. Pharmacopsychiatry. 2004;37(4):147–51. PMID: 15467969. http://www.ncbi.nlm.nih.gov/pubmed/15467969
36. Gorlyn M, Keilp J, Burke A, Oquendo M, Mann JJ, Grunebaum M. Treatment-related improvement in neuropsychological functioning in suicidal depressed patients: paroxetine vs. bupropion. Psychiatry Res. 2015;225(3):407–12. PMCID: PMC4314330. http://www.ncbi.nlm.nih.gov/pubmed/25555415
37. Soczynska JK, Ravindran LN, Styra R, McIntyre RS, Cyriac A, Manierka MS, Kennedy SH. The effect of bupropion XL and escitalopram on memory and functional outcomes in adults with major depressive disorder: results from a randomized controlled trial. Psychiatry Res. 2014;220(1–2):245–50. PMID: 25124683. http://www.ncbi.nlm.nih.gov/pubmed/25124683
38. Herrera-Guzmán I, Herrera-Abarca JE, Gudayol-Ferré E, Herrera-Guzmán D, Gómez-Carbajal L, Peña-Olvira M, Villuendas-González E, Joan GO. Effects of selective serotonin reuptake and dual serotonergic-noradrenergic reuptake treatments on attention and executive functions in patients with major depressive disorder. Psychiatry Res. 2010;177(3):323–9. PMID: 20385412. http://www.ncbi.nlm.nih.gov/pubmed/20385412
39. Herrera-Guzmán I, Gudayol-Ferré E, Herrera-Guzmán D, Guàrdia-Olmos J, Hinojosa-Calvo E, Herrera-Abarca JE. Effects of selective serotonin reuptake and dual serotonergic-noradrenergic reuptake treatments on memory and mental processing speed in patients with major depressive disorder. J Psychiatr Res. 2009;43(9):855–63. PMID: 19128810. http://www.ncbi.nlm.nih.gov/pubmed/19128810
40. Constant EL, Adam S, Gillain B, Seron X, Bruyer R, Seghers A. Effects of sertraline on depressive symptoms and attentional and executive functions in major depression. Depress Anxiety. 2005;21(2):78–89. PMID: 15884090. http://www.ncbi.nlm.nih.gov/pubmed/15884090
41. Herrera-Guzmán I, Gudayol-Ferré E, Lira-Mandujano J, Herrera-Abarca J, Herrera-Guzmán D, Montoya-Pérez K, Guardia-Olmos J. Cognitive predictors of treatment response to bupropion and cognitive effects of bupropion in patients with major depressive disorder. Psychiatry Res. 2008;160(1):72–82. PMID: 18501971. http://www.ncbi.nlm.nih.gov/pubmed/18501971
42. Borkowska A, Drozdz W, Ziółkowska-Kochan M, Rybakowski J. Enhancing effect of mirtazapine on cognitive functions associated with prefrontal cortex in patients with recurrent depression. Neuropsychopharmacol Hung. 2007;9(3):131–6. PMID: 18399031. http://www.ncbi.nlm.nih.gov/pubmed/18399031
43. Connolly KR, Thase ME. Vortioxetine: a new treatment for major depressive disorder. Expert Opin Pharmacother. 2016;17(3):421–31. PMID: 26679430. http://www.ncbi.nlm.nih.gov/pubmed/26679430
44. Baune BT, Brignone M, Larsen KG. A network meta-analysis comparing effects of various antidepressant classes on the digit symbol substitution test (DSST) as a measure of cognitive dysfunction in patients with major depressive disorder. Int J Neuropsychopharmacol. 2018;21(2):97–107. PMCID: PMC5793828. http://www.ncbi.nlm.nih.gov/pubmed/29053849
45. Talmon M, Rossi S, Pastore A, Cattaneo CI, Brunelleschi S, Fresu LG. Vortioxetine exerts anti-inflammatory and immunomodulatory effects on human monocytes/macrophages. Br J Pharmacol. 2018;175(1):113–24. PMCID: PMC5740236. http://www.ncbi.nlm.nih.gov/pubmed/29057467
46. McIntyre RS, Harrison J, Loft H, Jacobson W, Olsen CK. The effects of Vortioxetine on cognitive function in patients with major depressive disorder: a meta-analysis of three randomized controlled trials. Int J Neuropsychopharmacol. 2016;19(10):pyw055. PMCID: PMC5091829. http://www.ncbi.nlm.nih.gov/pubmed/27312740
47. George MS, Lisanby SH, Avery D, McDonald WM, Durkalski V, Pavlicova M, Anderson B, Nahas Z, Bulow P, Zarkowski P, Holtzheimer PE, Schwartz T, Sackeim HA. Daily left prefrontal transcranial magnetic stimulation therapy for major depressive disorder: a sham-controlled randomized trial. Arch Gen Psychiatry. 2010;67(5):507–16. PMID: 20439832. http://www.ncbi.nlm.nih.gov/pubmed/20439832
48. George MS, Taylor JJ, Short EB. The expanding evidence base for rTMS treatment of depression. Curr Opin Psychiatry. 2013;26(1):13–8. PMCID: PMC4214363. http://www.ncbi.nlm.nih.gov/pubmed/23154644
49. Serafini G, Pompili M, Belvederi Murri M, Respino M, Ghio L, Girardi P, Fitzgerald PB, Amore M. The effects of repeti-

tive transcranial magnetic stimulation on cognitive performance in treatment-resistant depression. A systematic review. Neuropsychobiology. 2015;71(3):125–39. PMID: 25925699. http://www.ncbi.nlm.nih.gov/pubmed/25925699

50. Zuckerman H, Pan Z, Park C, Brietzke E, Musial N, Shariq AS, Iacobucci M, Yim SJ, Lui LMW, Rong C, McIntyre RS. Recognition and treatment of cognitive dysfunction in major depressive disorder. Front Psychiatry. 2018;9:655. PMCID: PMC6288549. http://www.ncbi.nlm.nih.gov/pubmed/30564155
51. Fehnel SE, Forsyth BH, DiBenedetti DB, Danchenko N, François C, Brevig T. Patient-centered assessment of cognitive symptoms of depression. CNS Spectr. 2016;21(1):43–52. PMID: 24067243. http://www.ncbi.nlm.nih.gov/pubmed/24067243
52. Cotrena C, Branco LD, Shansis FM, Fonseca RP. Executive function impairments in depression and bipolar disorder: association with functional impairment and quality of life. J Affect Disord. 2016;190:744–53. PMID: 26606718. http://www.ncbi.nlm.nih.gov/pubmed/26606718
53. Majer M, Ising M, Künzel H, Binder EB, Holsboer F, Modell S, Zihl J. Impaired divided attention predicts delayed response and risk to relapse in subjects with depressive disorders. Psychol Med. 2004;34(8):1453–63. PMID: 15724876. http://www.ncbi.nlm.nih.gov/pubmed/15724876
54. Ahern E, Semkovska M. Cognitive functioning in the first-episode of major depressive disorder: a systematic review and meta-analysis. Neuropsychology. 2017;31(1):52–72. PMID: 27732039. http://www.ncbi.nlm.nih.gov/pubmed/27732039
55. Semkovska M, Quinlivan L, O'Grady T, Johnson R, Collins A, O'Connor J, Knittle H, Ahern E, Gload T. Cognitive function following a major depressive episode: a systematic review and meta-analysis. Lancet Psychiatry. 2019;6(10):851–61. PMID: 31422920. http://www.ncbi.nlm.nih.gov/pubmed/31422920
56. Biringer E, Mykletun A, Sundet K, Kroken R, Stordal KI, Lund A. A longitudinal analysis of neurocognitive function in unipolar depression. J Clin Exp Neuropsychol. 2007;29(8):879–91. PMID: 17852600. http://www.ncbi.nlm.nih.gov/pubmed/17852600
57. Burdick KE, Russo M, Frangou S, Mahon K, Braga RJ, Shanahan M, Malhotra AK. Empirical evidence for discrete neurocognitive subgroups in bipolar disorder: clinical implications. Psychol Med. 2014;44(14):3083–96. PMCID: PMC4797987. http://www.ncbi.nlm.nih.gov/pubmed/25065409
58. Hasselbalch BJ, Knorr U, Kessing LV. Cognitive impairment in the remitted state of unipolar depressive disorder: a systematic review. J Affect Disord. 2011;134(1–3):20–31. PMID: 21163534. http://www.ncbi.nlm.nih.gov/pubmed/21163534
59. Vicent-Gil M, Keymer-Gausset A, Serra-Blasco M, Carceller-Sindreu M, de Diego-Adeliño J, Trujols J, Mur M, Pérez V, Alvarez E, Cardoner N, Portella MJ. Cognitive predictors of illness course at 12 months after first-episode of depression. Eur Neuropsychopharmacol. 2018;28(4):529–37. PMID: 29482974. http://www.ncbi.nlm.nih.gov/pubmed/29482974
60. Vicent-Gil M, Portella MJ, Serra-Blasco M, Navarra-Ventura G, Crivillés S, Aguilar E, Palao D, Cardoner N. Dealing with heterogeneity of cognitive dysfunction in acute depression: a clustering approach. Psychol Med. 2021;51(16):2886–94. PMCID: PMC8640365. http://www.ncbi.nlm.nih.gov/pubmed/32476636
61. Evans VC, Iverson GL, Yatham LN, Lam RW. The relationship between neurocognitive and psychosocial functioning in major depressive disorder: a systematic review. J Clin Psychiatry. 2014;75(12):1359–70. PMID: 25551235. http://www.ncbi.nlm.nih.gov/pubmed/25551235
62. Cotrena C, Branco LD, Kochhann R, Shansis FM, Fonseca RP. Quality of life, functioning and cognition in bipolar disorder and major depression: a latent profile analysis. Psychiatry Res. 2016;241:289–96. PMID: 27209359. http://www.ncbi.nlm.nih.gov/pubmed/27209359
63. Clark M, DiBenedetti D, Perez V. Cognitive dysfunction and work productivity in major depressive disorder. Expert Rev Pharmacoecon Outcomes Res. 2016;16(4):455–63. PMID: 27268275. http://www.ncbi.nlm.nih.gov/pubmed/27268275
64. McDermott LM, Ebmeier KP. A meta-analysis of depression severity and cognitive function. J Affect Disord. 2009;119(1–3):1–8. PMID: 19428120. http://www.ncbi.nlm.nih.gov/pubmed/19428120
65. Pimontel MA, Rindskopf D, Rutherford BR, Brown PJ, Roose SP, Sneed JR. A meta-analysis of executive dysfunction and antidepressant treatment response in late-life depression. Am J Geriatr Psychiatry. 2016;24(1):31–41. PMCID: PMC4928373. http://www.ncbi.nlm.nih.gov/pubmed/26282222
66. Serra-Blasco M, de Vita S, Rodríguez MR, de Diego-Adeliño J, Puigdemont D, Martín-Blanco A, Pérez-Egea R, Molet J, Álvarez E, Pérez V, Portella MJ. Cognitive functioning after deep brain stimulation in subcallosal cingulate gyrus for treatment-resistant depression: an exploratory study. Psychiatry Res. 2015;225(3):341–6. PMID: 25592978. http://www.ncbi.nlm.nih.gov/pubmed/25592978
67. Murrough JW, Burdick KE, Levitch CF, Perez AM, Brallier JW, Chang LC, Foulkes A, Charney DS, Mathew SJ, Iosifescu DV. Neurocognitive effects of ketamine and association with antidepressant response in individuals with treatment-resistant depression: a randomized controlled trial. Neuropsychopharmacology. 2015;40(5):1084–90. PMCID: PMC4367458. http://www.ncbi.nlm.nih.gov/pubmed/25374095
68. Wei J, Ying M, Xie L, Chandrasekar EK, Lu H, Wang T, Li C. Late-life depression and cognitive function among older adults in the U.S.: the National Health and nutrition examination survey, 2011–2014. J Psychiatr Res. 2019;111:30–5. PMID: 30660811. http://www.ncbi.nlm.nih.gov/pubmed/30660811
69. Dotson VM, Resnick SM, Zonderman AB. Differential association of concurrent, baseline, and average depressive symptoms with cognitive decline in older adults. Am J Geriatr Psychiatry. 2008;16(4):318–30. PMCID: PMC2405887. http://www.ncbi.nlm.nih.gov/pubmed/18378557
70. Pu S, Noda T, Setoyama S, Nakagome K. Empirical evidence for discrete neurocognitive subgroups in patients with non-psychotic major depressive disorder: clinical implications. Psychol Med. 2018;48(16):2717–29. PMID: 29679991. http://www.ncbi.nlm.nih.gov/pubmed/29679991
71. Venezia RG, Gorlyn M, Burke AK, Oquendo MA, Mann JJ, Keilp JG. The impact of cognitive reserve on neurocognitive performance in major depressive disorder. Psychiatry Res. 2018;270:211–8. PMID: 30267985. http://www.ncbi.nlm.nih.gov/pubmed/30267985
72. McLaren ME, Szymkowicz SM, Kirton JW, Dotson VM. Impact of education on memory deficits in subclinical depression. Arch Clin Neuropsychol. 2015;30(5):387–93. PMCID: PMC4542750. http://www.ncbi.nlm.nih.gov/pubmed/26109434
73. Mac Giollabhui N, Kautz MM, Moriarity DP, Chat IKY, Murray S, Ellman LM, Alloy LB. Chronic inflammation is associated with worsening working memory performance: preliminary evidence from a diverse, longitudinal cohort of adolescents and young adults. Psychoneuroendocrinology. 2024;164:106992. PMCID: PMC11031287. http://www.ncbi.nlm.nih.gov/pubmed/38422797
74. Singh-Manoux A, Dugravot A, Brunner E, Kumari M, Shipley M, Elbaz A, Kivimaki M. Interleukin-6 and C-reactive protein as predictors of cognitive decline in late midlife. Neurology. 2014;83(6):486–93. PMCID: PMC4141998. http://www.ncbi.nlm.nih.gov/pubmed/24991031
75. Mac Giollabhui N, Alloy LB, Hartman CA. Investigating whether depressed youth exhibiting elevated C reactive protein perform worse on measures of executive functioning, verbal fluency and episodic memory in a large, population based sample of Dutch

adolescents. Brain Behav Immun. 2021;94:369–80. PMCID: PMC7921209. http://www.ncbi.nlm.nih.gov/pubmed/32889083
76. Mac Giollabhui N, Hartman CA. Examining inflammation, health, stress and lifestyle variables linking low socioeconomic status with poorer cognitive functioning during adolescence. Brain Behav Immun. 2022;104:1–5. PMID: 35491005. http://www.ncbi.nlm.nih.gov/pubmed/35491005
77. Giollabhui NM, Slaney C, Hemani G, Foley ÉM, van der Most PJ, Nolte IM, Snieder H, Smith GD, Khandaker G, Hartman CA. Role of Inflammation in Depressive and Anxiety Disorders, Affect, and Cognition: Genetic and Non-Genetic Findings in the Lifelines Cohort Study. medRxiv. 2024;2024.04.17.24305950. PMCID: PMC11065023. http://www.ncbi.nlm.nih.gov/pubmed/38699368
78. Slaney C, Sallis HM, Jones HJ, Dardani C, Charge Inflammation Working Group, Tilling K, Munafò MR, Davey Smith G, Mahedy L, Khandaker GM. Association between inflammation and cognition: triangulation of evidence using a population-based cohort and Mendelian randomization analyses. Brain Behav Immun 2023;110:30–42. PMCID: PMC10728829. http://www.ncbi.nlm.nih.gov/pubmed/36791891
79. Crişan AF, Oancea C, Timar B, Fira-Mladinescu O, Crişan A, Tudorache V. Cognitive impairment in chronic obstructive pulmonary disease. PLoS One. 2014;9(7):e102468. PMCID: PMC4102489. http://www.ncbi.nlm.nih.gov/pubmed/25033379
80. Li X, Robertson CMT, Yu X, Cheypesh A, Dinu IA, Li J. Early postoperative systemic inflammatory response is an important determinant for adverse 2-year neurodevelopment-associated outcomes after the Norwood procedure. J Thorac Cardiovasc Surg. 2014;148(1):202–6. PMID: 24060363. http://www.ncbi.nlm.nih.gov/pubmed/24060363
81. Huang YS, Guilleminault C, Hwang FM, Cheng C, Lin CH, Li HY, Lee LA. Inflammatory cytokines in pediatric obstructive sleep apnea. Medicine (Baltimore). 2016;95(41):e4944. PMCID: PMC5072934. http://www.ncbi.nlm.nih.gov/pubmed/27741107.
82. Miller AH, Raison CL. The role of inflammation in depression: from evolutionary imperative to modern treatment target. Nat Rev Immunol. 2016;16(1):22–34. PMCID: PMC5542678. http://www.ncbi.nlm.nih.gov/pubmed/26711676
83. Dantzer R, O'Connor JC, Freund GG, Johnson RW, Kelley KW. From inflammation to sickness and depression: when the immune system subjugates the brain. Nat Rev Neurosci. 2008;9(1):46–56. PMCID: PMC2919277. https://pmc.ncbi.nlm.nih.gov/articles/PMC2919277/pdf/nihms213147.pdf
84. Katsuki F, Constantinidis C. Bottom-up and top-down attention: different processes and overlapping neural systems. Neuroscientist. 2014;20(5):509–21. PMID: 24362813. http://www.ncbi.nlm.nih.gov/pubmed/24362813
85. Bennabi D, Vandel P, Papaxanthis C, Pozzo T, Haffen E. Psychomotor retardation in depression: a systematic review of diagnostic, pathophysiologic, and therapeutic implications. Biomed Res Int. 2013;2013:158746. PMCID: PMC3830759. http://www.ncbi.nlm.nih.gov/pubmed/24286073
86. Buyukdura JS, McClintock SM, Croarkin PE. Psychomotor retardation in depression: biological underpinnings, measurement, and treatment. Prog Neuro-Psychopharmacol Biol Psychiatry. 2011;35(2):395–409. PMCID: PMC3646325. http://www.ncbi.nlm.nih.gov/pubmed/21044654
87. Czerwińska A, Pawłowski T. Cognitive dysfunctions in depression – significance, description and treatment prospects. Psychiatr Pol. 2020;54(3):453–66. PMID: 33038880. http://www.ncbi.nlm.nih.gov/pubmed/33038880
88. Mamelak M. Depression and the glutamate/GABA-glutamine cycle. Curr Neuropharmacol. 2024;23(1):75–84. PMCID: PMC11519819. http://www.ncbi.nlm.nih.gov/pubmed/39150032
89. Price RB, Duman R. Neuroplasticity in cognitive and psychological mechanisms of depression: an integrative model. Mol Psychiatry. 2020;25(3):530–43. PMCID: PMC7047599. http://www.ncbi.nlm.nih.gov/pubmed/31801966
90. Tartt AN, Mariani MB, Hen R, Mann JJ, Boldrini M. Dysregulation of adult hippocampal neuroplasticity in major depression: pathogenesis and therapeutic implications. Mol Psychiatry. 2022;27(6):2689–99. PMCID: PMC9167750. http://www.ncbi.nlm.nih.gov/pubmed/35354926
91. Niciu MJ, Ionescu DF, Richards EM, Zarate CA. Glutamate and its receptors in the pathophysiology and treatment of major depressive disorder. J Neural Transm (Vienna). 2014;121(8):907–24. PMCID: PMC4048804. http://www.ncbi.nlm.nih.gov/pubmed/24318540
92. Steiner J, Walter M, Gos T, Guillemin GJ, Bernstein HG, Sarnyai Z, Mawrin C, Brisch R, Bielau H, Meyer zu Schwabedissen L, Bogerts B, Myint AM. Severe depression is associated with increased microglial quinolinic acid in subregions of the anterior cingulate gyrus: evidence for an immune-modulated glutamatergic neurotransmission? J Neuroinflammation. 2011;8:94. PMCID: PMC3177898. http://www.ncbi.nlm.nih.gov/pubmed/21831269
93. Delpech JC, Valdearcos M, Nadjar A. Stress and microglia: a double-edged relationship. Adv Neurobiol. 2024;37:333–42. PMID: 39207700. http://www.ncbi.nlm.nih.gov/pubmed/39207700
94. González Ibáñez F, VanderZwaag J, Deslauriers J, Tremblay MÈ. Ultrastructural features of psychological stress resilience in the brain: a microglial perspective. Open Biol. 2024;14(11):240079. PMCID: PMC11576122. http://www.ncbi.nlm.nih.gov/pubmed/39561812
95. Du R, Yang K, Li W, Wang Z, Cai H. Research status and global trends of late-life depression from 2004 to 2023: bibliometric analysis. Front Aging Neurosci. 2024;16:1393110. PMCID: PMC11095109. http://www.ncbi.nlm.nih.gov/pubmed/38752209
96. Szymkowicz SM, Gerlach AR, Homiack D, Taylor WD. Biological factors influencing depression in later life: role of aging processes and treatment implications. Transl Psychiatry. 2023;13(1):160. PMCID: PMC10169845. http://www.ncbi.nlm.nih.gov/pubmed/37160884
97. Bougea A, Angelopoulou E, Vasilopoulos E, Gourzis P, Papageorgiou S. Emerging therapeutic potential of fluoxetine on cognitive decline in Alzheimer's disease: systematic review. Int J Mol Sci. 2024;25(12):6542. PMCID: PMC11203451. http://www.ncbi.nlm.nih.gov/pubmed/38928248
98. Talaee N, Azadvar S, Khodadadi S, Abbasi N, Asli-Pashaki ZN, Mirabzadeh Y, Kholghi G, Akhondzadeh S, Vaseghi S. Comparing the effect of fluoxetine, escitalopram, and sertraline, on the level of BDNF and depression in preclinical and clinical studies: a systematic review. Eur J Clin Pharmacol. 2024;80(7):983–1016. PMID: 38558317. http://www.ncbi.nlm.nih.gov/pubmed/38558317
99. Hird EJ, Slanina-Davies A, Lewis G, Hamer M, Roiser JP. From movement to motivation: a proposed framework to understand the antidepressant effect of exercise. Transl Psychiatry. 2024;14(1):273. PMCID: PMC11222551. http://www.ncbi.nlm.nih.gov/pubmed/38961071
100. Sanaeifar F, Pourranjbar S, Pourranjbar M, Ramezani S, Mehr SR, Wadan AHS, Khazeifard F. Beneficial effects of physical exercise on cognitive-behavioral impairments and brain-derived neurotrophic factor alteration in the limbic system induced by neurodegeneration. Exp Gerontol. 2024;195:112539. PMID: 39116955. http://www.ncbi.nlm.nih.gov/pubmed/39116955
101. Tian H, Wang Z, Meng Y, Geng L, Lian H, Shi Z, Zhuang Z, Cai W, He M. Neural mechanisms underlying cognitive impairment in depression and cognitive benefits of exercise intervention. Behav Brain Res. 2025;476:115218. PMID: 39182624. http://www.ncbi.nlm.nih.gov/pubmed/39182624
102. Xue B, Meng X, Liu Q, Luo X. The effect of receptive music therapy on older adults with mild cognitive impairment and depres-

sion: a randomized controlled trial. Sci Rep. 2023;13(1):22159. PMCID: PMC10719334. http://www.ncbi.nlm.nih.gov/pubmed/38092791
103. Knight MJ, Mills NT, Baune BT. Contemporary methods of improving cognitive dysfunction in clinical depression. Expert Rev Neurother. 2019;19(5):431–43. PMID: 31020872. http://www.ncbi.nlm.nih.gov/pubmed/31020872
104. Cannistraro RJ, Badi M, Eidelman BH, Dickson DW, Middlebrooks EH, Meschia JF. CNS small vessel disease: a clinical review. Neurology. 2019;92(24):1146–56. PMCID: PMC6598791. http://www.ncbi.nlm.nih.gov/pubmed/31142635
105. Li Q, Yang Y, Reis C, Tao T, Li W, Li X, Zhang JH. Cerebral small vessel disease. Cell Transplant. 2018;27(12):1711–22. PMCID: PMC6300773. http://www.ncbi.nlm.nih.gov/pubmed/30251566
106. Wardlaw JM, Smith C, Dichgans M. Small vessel disease: mechanisms and clinical implications. Lancet Neurol. 2019;18(7):684–96. PMID: 31097385. http://www.ncbi.nlm.nih.gov/pubmed/31097385
107. Feng M, Wen H, Xin H, Wang S, Gao Y, Sui C, Liang C, Guo L. Decreased local specialization of brain structural networks associated with cognitive Dysfuntion revealed by probabilistic diffusion Tractography for different cerebral small vessel disease burdens. Mol Neurobiol. 2024;61(1):326–39. PMCID: PMC10791730. http://www.ncbi.nlm.nih.gov/pubmed/37606718
108. Zhang X, Liang C, Feng M, Xin H, Fu Y, Gao Y, Sui C, Wang N, Wang Y, Zhang N, Guo L, Wen H. Aberrant brain structural-functional connectivity coupling associated with cognitive dysfunction in different cerebral small vessel disease burdens. CNS Neurosci Ther. 2024;30(9):e70005. PMCID: PMC11371661. http://www.ncbi.nlm.nih.gov/pubmed/39228091
109. Xin H, Liang C, Fu Y, Feng M, Wang S, Gao Y, Sui C, Zhang N, Guo L, Wen H. Disrupted brain structural networks associated with depression and cognitive dysfunction in cerebral small vessel disease with microbleeds. Prog Neuro-Psychopharmacol Biol Psychiatry. 2024;131:110944. PMID: 38246218. http://www.ncbi.nlm.nih.gov/pubmed/38246218
110. Gao Y, Wang S, Xin H, Feng M, Zhang Q, Sui C, Guo L, Liang C, Wen H. Disrupted gray matter networks associated with cognitive dysfunction in cerebral small vessel disease. Brain Sci. 2023;13(10):1359. PMCID: PMC10605932. http://www.ncbi.nlm.nih.gov/pubmed/37891728
111. Pitts BL, Wen V, Whealin JM, Fogle BM, Southwick SM, Esterlis I, Pietrzak RH. Depression and cognitive dysfunction in older U.S. Military Veterans: Moderating effects of BDNF Val66Met polymorphism and physical exercise. Am J Geriatr Psychiatry. 2020;28(9):959–67. PMID: 32122804. http://www.ncbi.nlm.nih.gov/pubmed/32122804
112. Verhagen M, van der Meij A, van Deurzen P a M, Janzing JGE, Arias-Vásquez A, Buitelaar JK, Franke B. Meta-analysis of the BDNF Val66Met polymorphism in major depressive disorder: effects of gender and ethnicity. Mol Psychiatry. 2010;15(3):260–71. PMID: 18852698. http://www.ncbi.nlm.nih.gov/pubmed/18852698
113. Suktas A, Ekalaksananan T, Aromseree S, Bumrungthai S, Songserm N, Pientong C. Genetic polymorphism involved in major depressive disorder: a systemic review and meta-analysis. BMC Psychiatry. 2024;24(1):716. PMCID: PMC11515766. http://www.ncbi.nlm.nih.gov/pubmed/39438912
114. López-Solà C, Subirà M, Serra-Blasco M, Vicent-Gil M, Navarra-Ventura G, Aguilar E, Acebillo S, Palao DJ, Cardoner N. Is cognitive dysfunction involved in difficult-to-treat depression? Characterizing resistance from a cognitive perspective. Eur Psychiatry. 2020;63(1):e74. PMCID: PMC7443785. http://www.ncbi.nlm.nih.gov/pubmed/32571441
115. Keller AS, Leikauf JE, Holt-Gosselin B, Staveland BR, Williams LM. Paying attention to attention in depression. Transl Psychiatry. 2019;9(1):279. PMCID: PMC6838308. http://www.ncbi.nlm.nih.gov/pubmed/31699968
116. Fried EI, Nesse RM. Depression is not a consistent syndrome: an investigation of unique symptom patterns in the STAR*D study. J Affect Disord. 2015;(172):96–102. PMCID: PMC4397113. http://www.ncbi.nlm.nih.gov/pubmed/25451401
117. Ibos G, Freedman DJ. Interaction between spatial and feature attention in posterior parietal cortex. Neuron. 2016;91(4):931–43. PMCID: PMC5015486. http://www.ncbi.nlm.nih.gov/pubmed/27499082
118. Patzwahl DR, Treue S. Combining spatial and feature-based attention within the receptive field of MT neurons. Vis Res. 2009;49(10):1188–93. PMID: 19362573. http://www.ncbi.nlm.nih.gov/pubmed/19362573
119. Giesbrecht B, Woldorff MG, Song AW, Mangun GR. Neural mechanisms of top-down control during spatial and feature attention. NeuroImage. 2003;19(3):496–512. PMID: 12880783. http://www.ncbi.nlm.nih.gov/pubmed/12880783
120. Galashan D, Siemann J. Differences and similarities for spatial and feature-based selective attentional orienting. Front Neurosci. 2017;11:283. PMCID: PMC5435748. http://www.ncbi.nlm.nih.gov/pubmed/28572756
121. Holmes AJ, Pizzagalli DA. Response conflict and frontocingulate dysfunction in unmedicated participants with major depression. Neuropsychologia. 2008;46(12):2904–13. PMCID: PMC2538441. http://www.ncbi.nlm.nih.gov/pubmed/18577391
122. Keller AS, Ball TM, Williams LM. Deep phenotyping of attention impairments and the “inattention biotype” in major depressive disorder. Psychol Med. 2020;50(13):2203–12. PMCID: PMC8022888. http://www.ncbi.nlm.nih.gov/pubmed/31477195
123. Degl’Innocenti A, Agren H, Bäckman L. Executive deficits in major depression. Acta Psychiatr Scand. 1998;97(3):182–8. PMID: 9543305. http://www.ncbi.nlm.nih.gov/pubmed/9543305
124. Ladouceur CD, Slifka JS, Dahl RE, Birmaher B, Axelson DA, Ryan ND. Altered error-related brain activity in youth with major depression. Dev Cogn Neurosci. 2012;2(3):351–62. PMCID: PMC3369189. http://www.ncbi.nlm.nih.gov/pubmed/22669036
125. Olvet DM, Klein DN, Hajcak G. Depression symptom severity and error-related brain activity. Psychiatry Res. 2010;179(1):30–7. PMID: 20630603. http://www.ncbi.nlm.nih.gov/pubmed/20630603
126. Li X, Wu H, Lou C, Xing B, Yu E. Study on the executive function of attention in depression patients based on SPECT technology. Int J Clin Exp Med. 2014;7(4):1110–5. PMCID: PMC4057870. http://www.ncbi.nlm.nih.gov/pubmed/24955191
127. Li Y, Kang C, Qu X, Zhou Y, Wang W, Hu Y. Depression-related brain connectivity analyzed by EEG event-related phase synchrony measure. Front Hum Neurosci. 2016;10:477. PMCID: PMC5035751. http://www.ncbi.nlm.nih.gov/pubmed/27725797
128. Kemp AH, Hopkinson PJ, Hermens DF, Rowe DL, Sumich AL, Clark CR, Drinkenburg W, Abdi N, Penrose R, McFarlane A, Boyce P, Gordon E, Williams LM. Fronto-temporal alterations within the first 200 ms during an attentional task distinguish major depression, non-clinical participants with depressed mood and healthy controls: a potential biomarker? Hum Brain Mapp. 2009;30(2):602–14. PMCID: PMC6870851. http://www.ncbi.nlm.nih.gov/pubmed/18181154
129. Tenke CE, Kayser J, Shankman SA, Griggs CB, Leite P, Stewart JW, Bruder GE. Hemispatial PCA dissociates temporal from parietal ERP generator patterns: CSD components in healthy adults and depressed patients during a dichotic oddball task. Int J Psychophysiol. 2008;67(1):1–16. PMCID: PMC2271144. http://www.ncbi.nlm.nih.gov/pubmed/17963912

130. Gyurak A, Patenaude B, Korgaonkar MS, Grieve SM, Williams LM, Etkin A. Frontoparietal activation during response inhibition predicts remission to antidepressants in patients with major depression. Biol Psychiatry. 2016;79(4):274–81. PMID: 25891220. http://www.ncbi.nlm.nih.gov/pubmed/25891220
131. van Vugt MK, van der Velde M, ESM-MERGE Investigators. How does rumination impact cognition? A first mechanistic model. Top Cogn Sci. 2018;10(1):175–91. PMID: 29383884. http://www.ncbi.nlm.nih.gov/pubmed/29383884
132. Keller AS, Jagadeesh AV, Bugatus L, Williams LM, Grill-Spector K. Attention enhances category representations across the brain with strengthened residual correlations to ventral temporal cortex. Neuroimage. 2022;249:118900. PMCID: PMC8947761 http://www.ncbi.nlm.nih.gov/pubmed/35021039
133. McMains SA, Somers DC. Processing efficiency of divided spatial attention mechanisms in human visual cortex. J Neurosci. 2005;25(41):9444–8. PMCID: PMC6725695. http://www.ncbi.nlm.nih.gov/pubmed/16221854
134. Godefroy O, Rousseaux M. Divided and focused attention in patients with lesion of the prefrontal cortex. Brain Cogn. 1996;30(2):155–74. PMID: 8811992. http://www.ncbi.nlm.nih.gov/pubmed/8811992
135. Owen AM, Roberts AC, Polkey CE, Sahakian BJ, Robbins TW. Extra-dimensional versus intra-dimensional set shifting performance following frontal lobe excisions, temporal lobe excisions or amygdalo-hippocampectomy in man. Neuropsychologia. 1991;29(10):993–1006. PMID: 1762678. http://www.ncbi.nlm.nih.gov/pubmed/1762678
136. Mikoteit T, Hemmeter U, Eckert A, Brand S, Bischof R, Delini-Stula A, Holsboer-Trachsler E, Beck J. Improved alertness is associated with early increase in serum brain-derived neurotrophic factor and antidepressant treatment outcome in major depression. Neuropsychobiology. 2015;72(1):16–28. PMID: 26337518. http://www.ncbi.nlm.nih.gov/pubmed/26337518
137. Kim SJ, Kang SG, Cho IH, Lee YJG, Hong JP, Park J, Lee YJ. The relationship between poor performance on attention tasks and increased suicidal ideation in adolescents. Eur Child Adolesc Psychiatry. 2015;24(11):1361–8. PMID: 25663429. http://www.ncbi.nlm.nih.gov/pubmed/25663429
138. Luo LL, Chen X, Chai Y, Li JH, Zhang M, Zhang JN. A distinct pattern of memory and attention deficiency in patients with depression. Chin Med J. 2013;126(6):1144–9. PMID: 23506595. http://www.ncbi.nlm.nih.gov/pubmed/23506595
139. Pines A, Keller AS, Larsen B, Bertolero M, Ashourvan A, Bassett DS, Cieslak M, Covitz S, Fan Y, Feczko E, Houghton A, Rueter AR, Saggar M, Shafiei G, Tapera TM, Vogel J, Weinstein SM, Shinohara RT, Williams LM, Fair DA, Satterthwaite TD. Development of top-down cortical propagations in youth. Neuron. 2023;111(8):1316–1330.e5. PMCID: PMC10121821. http://www.ncbi.nlm.nih.gov/pubmed/36803653
140. Giollabhui NM, Olino TM, Nielsen J, Abramson LY, Alloy LB. Is worse attention a risk factor for or a consequence of depression, or are worse attention and depression better accounted for by stress? A prospective test of three hypotheses. Clin Psychol Sci. 2019;7(1):93–109. PMCID: PMC6425724. http://www.ncbi.nlm.nih.gov/pubmed/30906675
141. LeMoult J, Gotlib IH. Depression: a cognitive perspective. Clin Psychol Rev. 2019;69:51–66. PMID: 29961601. http://www.ncbi.nlm.nih.gov/pubmed/29961601
142. Snyder HR. Major depressive disorder is associated with broad impairments on neuropsychological measures of executive function: a meta-analysis and review. Psychol Bull. 2013;139(1):81–132. PMCID: PMC3436964. http://www.ncbi.nlm.nih.gov/pubmed/22642228
143. Gratton G, Cooper P, Fabiani M, Carter CS, Karayanidis F. Dynamics of cognitive control: theoretical bases, paradigms, and a view for the future. Psychophysiology. 2018;55(3). PMID: 29044552 http://www.ncbi.nlm.nih.gov/pubmed/29044552
144. Cognitive Systems: Workshop Proceedings – National Institute of Mental Health (NIMH)
145. Carrasco M, Barbot A. Spatial attention alters visual appearance. Curr Opin Psychol. 2019;29:56–64. PMCID: PMC7661009. http://www.ncbi.nlm.nih.gov/pubmed/30572280
146. Liu T, Abrams J, Carrasco M. Voluntary attention enhances contrast appearance. Psychol Sci. 2009;20(3):354–62. PMCID: PMC2657200. http://www.ncbi.nlm.nih.gov/pubmed/19254239
147. Fuller S, Carrasco M. Exogenous attention and color perception: performance and appearance of saturation and hue. Vis Res. 2006;46(23):4032–47. PMID: 16979690. http://www.ncbi.nlm.nih.gov/pubmed/16979690
148. Störmer VS, Alvarez GA. Attention alters perceived attractiveness. Psychol Sci. 2016;27(4):563–71. PMID: 26966228. http://www.ncbi.nlm.nih.gov/pubmed/26966228
149. Mishra MV, Srinivasan N. Exogenous attention intensifies perceived emotion expressions. Neurosci Conscious. 2017;2017(1):nix022. PMCID: PMC6007186. http://www.ncbi.nlm.nih.gov/pubmed/30042853
150. Bubl E, Kern E, Ebert D, Bach M, Tebartz van Elst L. Seeing gray when feeling blue? Depression can be measured in the eye of the diseased. Biol Psychiatry. 2010;68(2):205–8. PMID: 20359698. http://www.ncbi.nlm.nih.gov/pubmed/20359698
151. Barbot A, Carrasco M. Emotion and anxiety potentiate the way attention alters visual appearance. Sci Rep. 2018;8(1):5938. PMCID: PMC5897558. http://www.ncbi.nlm.nih.gov/pubmed/29651048.
152. Krajbich I. Accounting for attention in sequential sampling models of decision making. Curr Opin Psychol. 2019;29:6–11. PMID: 30368108. http://www.ncbi.nlm.nih.gov/pubmed/30368108
153. Shimojo S, Simion C, Shimojo E, Scheier C. Gaze bias both reflects and influences preference. Nat Neurosci. 2003;6(12):1317–22. PMID: 14608360. http://www.ncbi.nlm.nih.gov/pubmed/14608360
154. Saito T, Nouchi R, Kinjo H, Kawashima R. Gaze bias in preference judgments by younger and older adults. Front Aging Neurosci. 2017;9:285. PMCID: PMC5574931. http://www.ncbi.nlm.nih.gov/pubmed/28890696
155. Chelazzi L, Eštočinová J, Calletti R, Lo Gerfo E, Sani I, Della Libera C, Santandrea E. Altering spatial priority maps via reward-based learning. J Neurosci. 2014;34(25):8594–604. PMCID: PMC6608215. http://www.ncbi.nlm.nih.gov/pubmed/24948813
156. Leong YC, Radulescu A, Daniel R, DeWoskin V, Niv Y. Dynamic interaction between reinforcement learning and attention in multidimensional environments. Neuron. 2017;93(2):451–63. PMCID: PMC5287409. http://www.ncbi.nlm.nih.gov/pubmed/28103483
157. Niv Y, Daniel R, Geana A, Gershman SJ, Leong YC, Radulescu A, Wilson RC. Reinforcement learning in multidimensional environments relies on attention mechanisms. J Neurosci. 2015;35(21):8145–57. PMCID: PMC4444538. http://www.ncbi.nlm.nih.gov/pubmed/26019331
158. Huys QJM, Daw ND, Dayan P. Depression: a decision-theoretic analysis. Annu Rev Neurosci. 2015;38:1–23. PMID: 25705929. http://www.ncbi.nlm.nih.gov/pubmed/25705929
159. Negative Valence Systems – National Institute of Mental Health (NIMH)
160. Gotlib IH, Joormann J. Cognition and depression: current status and future directions. Annu Rev Clin Psychol. 2010;6:285–312. PMCID: PMC2845726. http://www.ncbi.nlm.nih.gov/pubmed/20192795
161. Lang PJ, Davis M. Emotion, motivation, and the brain: reflex foundations in animal and human research. Prog Brain Res.

2006;156:3–29. PMID: 17015072. http://www.ncbi.nlm.nih.gov/pubmed/17015072
162. Clasen PC, Wells TT, Ellis AJ, Beevers CG. Attentional biases and the persistence of sad mood in major depressive disorder. J Abnorm Psychol. 2013;122(1):74–85. PMCID: PMC3856951. http://www.ncbi.nlm.nih.gov/pubmed/22867117
163. Vanlessen N, De Raedt R, Koster EHW, Pourtois G. Happy heart, smiling eyes: a systematic review of positive mood effects on broadening of visuospatial attention. Neurosci Biobehav Rev. 2016;68:816–37. PMID: 27395341. http://www.ncbi.nlm.nih.gov/pubmed/27395341
164. Easterbrook JA. The effect of emotion on cue utilization and the organization of behavior. Psychol Rev. 1959;66(3):183–201. PMID: 13658305. http://www.ncbi.nlm.nih.gov/pubmed/13658305
165. Isen AM, Daubman KA, Nowicki GP. Positive affect facilitates creative problem solving. J Pers Soc Psychol. 1987;52(6):1122–31. PMID: 3598858. http://www.ncbi.nlm.nih.gov/pubmed/3598858
166. Motivating the focus of attention
167. The influence of affect on categorization
168. Corbetta M, Shulman GL. Control of goal-directed and stimulus-driven attention in the brain. Nat Rev Neurosci. 2002;3(3):201–15. PMID: 11994752. http://www.ncbi.nlm.nih.gov/pubmed/11994752
169. Kastner S, Pinsk MA, De Weerd P, Desimone R, Ungerleider LG. Increased activity in human visual cortex during directed attention in the absence of visual stimulation. Neuron. 1999;22(4):751–61. PMID: 10230795. http://www.ncbi.nlm.nih.gov/pubmed/10230795
170. Corbetta M. Frontoparietal cortical networks for directing attention and the eye to visual locations: identical, independent, or overlapping neural systems? Proc Natl Acad Sci U S A. 1998;95(3):831–838. PMCID: PMC33805. http://www.ncbi.nlm.nih.gov/pubmed/9448248.
171. Nobre AC, Sebestyen GN, Gitelman DR, Mesulam MM, Frackowiak RS, Frith CD. Functional localization of the system for visuospatial attention using positron emission tomography. Brain. 1997;120(Pt 3):515–33. PMID: 9126062. http://www.ncbi.nlm.nih.gov/pubmed/9126062
172. Falkenberg LE, Specht K, Westerhausen R. Attention and cognitive control networks assessed in a dichotic listening fMRI study. Brain Cogn. 2011;76(2):276–85. PMID: 21398015. http://www.ncbi.nlm.nih.gov/pubmed/21398015
173. Gu S, Pasqualetti F, Cieslak M, Telesford QK, Yu AB, Kahn AE, Medaglia JD, Vettel JM, Miller MB, Grafton ST, Bassett DS. Controllability of structural brain networks. Nat Commun. 2015;6:8414. PMCID: PMC4600713. http://www.ncbi.nlm.nih.gov/pubmed/26423222
174. Gu S, Betzel RF, Mattar MG, Cieslak M, Delio PR, Grafton ST, Pasqualetti F, Bassett DS. Optimal trajectories of brain state transitions. NeuroImage. 2017;148:305–17. PMCID: PMC5489344. http://www.ncbi.nlm.nih.gov/pubmed/28088484
175. Qin J, Wei M, Liu H, Yan R, Luo G, Yao Z, Lu Q. Abnormal brain anatomical topological organization of the cognitive-emotional and the frontoparietal circuitry in major depressive disorder. Magn Reson Med. 2014;72(5):1397–407. PMID: 24273210. http://www.ncbi.nlm.nih.gov/pubmed/24273210
176. Luo Q, Deng Z, Qin J, Wei D, Cun L, Qiu J, Hitchman G, Xie P. Frequency dependant topological alterations of intrinsic functional connectome in major depressive disorder. Sci Rep. 2015;5:9710. PMCID: PMC5155486. http://www.ncbi.nlm.nih.gov/pubmed/25856168
177. He Y, Lim S, Fortunato S, Sporns O, Zhang L, Qiu J, Xie P, Zuo XN. Reconfiguration of cortical networks in MDD uncovered by multiscale community detection with fMRI. Cereb Cortex. 2018;28(4):1383–95. PMCID: PMC6093364. http://www.ncbi.nlm.nih.gov/pubmed/29300840.
178. Fellrath J, Mottaz A, Schnider A, Guggisberg AG, Ptak R. Theta-band functional connectivity in the dorsal fronto-parietal network predicts goal-directed attention. Neuropsychologia. 2016;92:20–30. PMID: 27422540. http://www.ncbi.nlm.nih.gov/pubmed/27422540
179. Iwata M, Ota KT, Duman RS. The inflammasome: pathways linking psychological stress, depression, and systemic illnesses. Brain Behav Immun. 2013;31:105–14. PMCID: PMC4426992. http://www.ncbi.nlm.nih.gov/pubmed/23261775
180. Burke HM, Davis MC, Otte C, Mohr DC. Depression and cortisol responses to psychological stress: a meta-analysis. Psychoneuroendocrinology. 2005;30(9):846–56. PMID: 15961250. http://www.ncbi.nlm.nih.gov/pubmed/15961250
181. Sapolsky RM. Glucocorticoids and hippocampal atrophy in neuropsychiatric disorders. Arch Gen Psychiatry. 2000;57(10):925–35. PMID: 11015810. http://www.ncbi.nlm.nih.gov/pubmed/11015810
182. Wellman CL. Dendritic reorganization in pyramidal neurons in medial prefrontal cortex after chronic corticosterone administration. J Neurobiol. 2001;49(3):245–53. PMID: 11745662. http://www.ncbi.nlm.nih.gov/pubmed/11745662
183. Hyman JM, Zilli EA, Paley AM, Hasselmo ME. Working memory performance correlates with prefrontal-hippocampal theta interactions but not with prefrontal neuron firing rates. Front Integr Neurosci. 2010;4:2. PMCID: PMC2861479. http://www.ncbi.nlm.nih.gov/pubmed/20431726
184. Yu JY, Frank LM. Hippocampal-cortical interaction in decision making. Neurobiol Learn Mem. 2015;117:34–41. PMCID: PMC4133322. http://www.ncbi.nlm.nih.gov/pubmed/24530374
185. Cavanagh JF, Frank MJ. Frontal theta as a mechanism for cognitive control. Trends Cogn Sci. 2014;18(8):414–21. PMCID: PMC4112145. http://www.ncbi.nlm.nih.gov/pubmed/24835663
186. Belleau EL, Treadway MT, Pizzagalli DA. The impact of stress and major depressive disorder on hippocampal and medial prefrontal cortex morphology. Biol Psychiatry. 2019;85(6):443–53. PMCID: PMC6380948. http://www.ncbi.nlm.nih.gov/pubmed/30470559
187. Vertes RP. Interactions among the medial prefrontal cortex, hippocampus and midline thalamus in emotional and cognitive processing in the rat. Neuroscience. 2006;142(1):1–20. PMID: 16887277. http://www.ncbi.nlm.nih.gov/pubmed/16887277
188. Shilyansky C, Williams LM, Gyurak A, Harris A, Usherwood T, Etkin A. Effect of antidepressant treatment on cognitive impairments associated with depression: a randomised longitudinal study. Lancet. Psychiatry. 2016;3(5):425–35. PMCID: PMC4860142. http://www.ncbi.nlm.nih.gov/pubmed/26995298
189. Reppermund S, Zihl J, Lucae S, Horstmann S, Kloiber S, Holsboer F, Ising M. Persistent cognitive impairment in depression: the role of psychopathology and altered hypothalamic-pituitary-adrenocortical (HPA) system regulation. Biol Psychiatry. 2007;62(5):400–6. PMID: 17188252. http://www.ncbi.nlm.nih.gov/pubmed/17188252
190. Knorr U, Madsen JM, Kessing LV. The effect of selective serotonin reuptake inhibitors in healthy subjects revisited: a systematic review of the literature. Exp Clin Psychopharmacol. 2019;27(5):413–32. PMID: 30869982. http://www.ncbi.nlm.nih.gov/pubmed/30869982
191. Mahableshwarkar AR, Zajecka J, Jacobson W, Chen Y, Keefe RSE. A randomized, placebo-controlled, active-reference, double-blind, flexible-dose study of the efficacy of Vortioxetine on cognitive function in major depressive disorder. Neuropsychopharmacology. 2015;40(8):2025–37. PMCID: PMC4839526. http://www.ncbi.nlm.nih.gov/pubmed/25687662

192. Arnsten AFT. Catecholamine influences on dorsolateral prefrontal cortical networks. Biol Psychiatry. 2011;69(12):e89–99. PMCID: PMC3145207. http://www.ncbi.nlm.nih.gov/pubmed/21489408
193. Corp SA, Gitlin MJ, Altshuler LL. A review of the use of stimulants and stimulant alternatives in treating bipolar depression and major depressive disorder. J Clin Psychiatry. 2014;75(9):1010–8. PMID: 25295426. http://www.ncbi.nlm.nih.gov/pubmed/25295426
194. Gualtieri CT, Johnson LG. Bupropion normalizes cognitive performance in patients with depression. MedGenMed. 2007;9(1):22. PMCID: PMC1924979. http://www.ncbi.nlm.nih.gov/pubmed/17435629
195. Faraone SV, Biederman J, Spencer T, Michelson D, Adler L, Reimherr F, Seidman L. Atomoxetine and stroop task performance in adult attention-deficit/hyperactivity disorder. J Child Adolesc Psychopharmacol. 2005;15(4):664–70. PMID: 16190797. http://www.ncbi.nlm.nih.gov/pubmed/16190797
196. Tian Y, Du J, Spagna A, Mackie MA, Gu X, Dong Y, Fan J, Wang K. Venlafaxine treatment reduces the deficit of executive control of attention in patients with major depressive disorder. Sci Rep. 2016;6:28028. PMCID: PMC4910055. http://www.ncbi.nlm.nih.gov/pubmed/27306061
197. Taylor FB, Russo J. Comparing guanfacine and dextroamphetamine for the treatment of adult attention-deficit/hyperactivity disorder. J Clin Psychopharmacol. 2001;21(2):223–8. PMID: 11270920. http://www.ncbi.nlm.nih.gov/pubmed/11270920
198. Siepmann T, Mueck-Weymann M, Oertel R, Kirch W, Pittrow D, Siepmann M. The effects of venlafaxine on cognitive functions and quantitative EEG in healthy volunteers. Pharmacopsychiatry. 2008;41(4):146–50. PMID: 18651343. http://www.ncbi.nlm.nih.gov/pubmed/18651343
199. Rapoport JL, Buchsbaum MS, Weingartner H, Zahn TP, Ludlow C, Mikkelsen EJ. Dextroamphetamine. Its cognitive and behavioral effects in normal and hyperactive boys and normal men. Arch Gen Psychiatry. 1980;37(8):933–43. PMID: 7406657. http://www.ncbi.nlm.nih.gov/pubmed/7406657
200. MacQueen DA, Minassian A, Kenton JA, Geyer MA, Perry W, Brigman JL, Young JW. Amphetamine improves mouse and human attention in the 5-choice continuous performance test. Neuropharmacology. 2018;138:87–96. PMCID: PMC6340711. http://www.ncbi.nlm.nih.gov/pubmed/29859849
201. Servan-Schreiber D, Carter CS, Bruno RM, Cohen JD. Dopamine and the mechanisms of cognition: part II. D-amphetamine effects in human subjects performing a selective attention task. Biol Psychiatry. 1998;43(10):723–9. PMID: 9606525. http://www.ncbi.nlm.nih.gov/pubmed/9606525
202. Tamminga HGH, Reneman L, Huizenga HM, Geurts HM. Effects of methylphenidate on executive functioning in attention-deficit/hyperactivity disorder across the lifespan: a meta-regression analysis. Psychol Med. 2016;46(9):1791–807. PMID: 27019103. http://www.ncbi.nlm.nih.gov/pubmed/27019103
203. Linssen AMW, Sambeth A, Vuurman EFPM, Riedel WJ. Cognitive effects of methylphenidate in healthy volunteers: a review of single dose studies. Int J Neuropsychopharmacol. 2014;17(6):961–77. PMID: 24423151. http://www.ncbi.nlm.nih.gov/pubmed/24423151
204. Paton K, Hammond P, Barry E, Fitzgerald M, McNicholas F, Kirley A, Robertson IH, Bellgrove MA, Gill M, Johnson KA. Methylphenidate improves some but not all measures of attention, as measured by the TEA-Ch in medication-naïve children with ADHD. Child Neuropsychol. 2014;20(3):303–18. PMID: 23639119. http://www.ncbi.nlm.nih.gov/pubmed/23639119
205. ter Huurne N, Fallon SJ, van Schouwenburg M, van der Schaaf M, Buitelaar J, Jensen O, Cools R. Methylphenidate alters selective attention by amplifying salience. Psychopharmacology. 2015;232(23):4317–23. PMID: 26349753. http://www.ncbi.nlm.nih.gov/pubmed/26349753
206. Conners CK, Casat CD, Gualtieri CT, Weller E, Reader M, Reiss A, Weller RA, Khayrallah M, Ascher J. Bupropion hydrochloride in attention deficit disorder with hyperactivity. J Am Acad Child Adolesc Psychiatry. 1996;35(10):1314–21. PMID: 8885585. http://www.ncbi.nlm.nih.gov/pubmed/8885585
207. Acheson A, de Wit H. Bupropion improves attention but does not affect impulsive behavior in healthy young adults. Exp Clin Psychopharmacol. 2008;16(2):113–23. PMCID: PMC4270475. http://www.ncbi.nlm.nih.gov/pubmed/18489015
208. Cope ZA, Minassian A, Kreitner D, MacQueen DA, Milienne-Petiot M, Geyer MA, Perry W, Young JW. Modafinil improves attentional performance in healthy, non-sleep deprived humans at doses not inducing hyperarousal across species. Neuropharmacology. 2017;125:254–62. PMCID: PMC6472902. http://www.ncbi.nlm.nih.gov/pubmed/28774856
209. Ikeda Y, Funayama T, Tateno A, Fukayama H, Okubo Y, Suzuki H. Modafinil enhances alerting-related brain activity in attention networks. Psychopharmacology. 2017;234(14):2077–89. PMID: 28374089. http://www.ncbi.nlm.nih.gov/pubmed/28374089
210. Turner DC, Clark L, Dowson J, Robbins TW, Sahakian BJ. Modafinil improves cognition and response inhibition in adult attention-deficit/hyperactivity disorder. Biol Psychiatry. 2004;55(10):1031–40. PMID: 15121488 http://www.ncbi.nlm.nih.gov/pubmed/15121488
211. DeBattista C, Lembke A, Solvason HB, Ghebremichael R, Poirier J. A prospective trial of modafinil as an adjunctive treatment of major depression. J Clin Psychopharmacol. 2004;24(1):87–90. PMID: 14709953. http://www.ncbi.nlm.nih.gov/pubmed/14709953
212. Jung KY, Kim SM, Song JY, Lee BU, Lee C, Lee SK, Koo YS, Cho YW, Choi JW, Kim KH. Sternberg working memory performance following treatment with pramipexole in patients with moderate-to-severe restless legs syndrome. Sleep Med. 2015;16(6):703–8. PMID: 25934537. http://www.ncbi.nlm.nih.gov/pubmed/25934537
213. van Belkum SM, Bosker FJ, Kortekaas R, Beersma DGM, Schoevers RA. Treatment of depression with low-strength transcranial pulsed electromagnetic fields: a mechanistic point of view. Prog Neuro-Psychopharmacol Biol Psychiatry. 2016;71:137–43. PMID: 27449361. http://www.ncbi.nlm.nih.gov/pubmed/27449361
214. Marek S, Dosenbach NUF. The frontoparietal network: function, electrophysiology, and importance of individual precision mapping. Dialogues Clin Neurosci. 2018;20(2):133–40. PMCID: PMC6136121. http://www.ncbi.nlm.nih.gov/pubmed/30250390
215. Naim-Feil J, Bradshaw JL, Sheppard DM, Rosenberg O, Levkovitz Y, Dannon P, Fitzgerald PB, Isserles M, Zangen A. Neuromodulation of attentional control in major depression: a pilot DeepTMS Study. Neural Plast. 2016;2016:5760141. PMCID: PMC4707329. http://www.ncbi.nlm.nih.gov/pubmed/26823985.
216. Vanderhasselt MA, De Raedt R, Baeken C, Leyman L, D'Haenen H. A single session of rTMS over the left dorsolateral prefrontal cortex influences attentional control in depressed patients. World J Biol Psychiatry. 2009;10(1):34–42. PMID: 19673086. http://www.ncbi.nlm.nih.gov/pubmed/19673086
217. Levkovitz Y, Harel EV, Roth Y, Braw Y, Most D, Katz LN, Sheer A, Gersner R, Zangen A. Deep transcranial magnetic stimulation over the prefrontal cortex: evaluation of antidepressant and cognitive effects in depressive patients. Brain Stimul. 2009;2(4):188–200. PMID: 20633419. http://www.ncbi.nlm.nih.gov/pubmed/20633419
218. Loo CK, Alonzo A, Martin D, Mitchell PB, Galvez V, Sachdev P. Transcranial direct current stimulation for depression: 3-week, randomised, sham-controlled trial. Br J Psychiatry. 2012;200(1):52–9. PMID: 22215866. http://www.ncbi.nlm.nih.gov/pubmed/22215866

219. Iimori T, Nakajima S, Miyazaki T, Tarumi R, Ogyu K, Wada M, Tsugawa S, Masuda F, Daskalakis ZJ, Blumberger DM, Mimura M, Noda Y. Effectiveness of the prefrontal repetitive transcranial magnetic stimulation on cognitive profiles in depression, schizophrenia, and Alzheimer's disease: a systematic review. Prog Neuro-Psychopharmacol Biol Psychiatry. 2019;88:31–40. PMID: 29953934. http://www.ncbi.nlm.nih.gov/pubmed/29953934
220. Martin DM, McClintock SM, Forster J, Loo CK. Does therapeutic repetitive transcranial magnetic stimulation cause cognitive enhancing effects in patients with neuropsychiatric conditions? A systematic review and meta-analysis of randomised controlled trials. Neuropsychol Rev. 2016;26(3):295–309. PMCID: PMC5949868. http://www.ncbi.nlm.nih.gov/pubmed/27632386
221. Demirtas-Tatlidede A, Vahabzadeh-Hagh AM, Pascual-Leone A. Can noninvasive brain stimulation enhance cognition in neuropsychiatric disorders? Neuropharmacology. 2013;64:566–78. PMCID: PMC3725288. http://www.ncbi.nlm.nih.gov/pubmed/22749945
222. Chiesa A, Calati R, Serretti A. Does mindfulness training improve cognitive abilities? A systematic review of neuropsychological findings. Clin Psychol Rev. 2011;31(3):449–64. PMID: 21183265. http://www.ncbi.nlm.nih.gov/pubmed/21183265
223. Wielgosz J, Goldberg SB, Kral TRA, Dunne JD, Davidson RJ. Mindfulness meditation and psychopathology. Annu Rev Clin Psychol. 2019;15:285–316. PMCID: PMC6597263. http://www.ncbi.nlm.nih.gov/pubmed/30525995
224. Goldberg SB, Tucker RP, Greene PA, Davidson RJ, Kearney DJ, Simpson TL. Mindfulness-based cognitive therapy for the treatment of current depressive symptoms: a meta-analysis. Cogn Behav Ther. 2019;48(6):445–62. PMCID: PMC6687569. http://www.ncbi.nlm.nih.gov/pubmed/30732534
225. Kerr CE, Jones SR, Wan Q, Pritchett DL, Wasserman RH, Wexler A, Villanueva JJ, Shaw JR, Lazar SW, Kaptchuk TJ, Littenberg R, Hämäläinen MS, Moore CI. Effects of mindfulness meditation training on anticipatory alpha modulation in primary somatosensory cortex. Brain Res Bull. 2011;85(3–4):96–103. PMID: 21501665. http://www.ncbi.nlm.nih.gov/pubmed/21501665
226. Bhayee S, Tomaszewski P, Lee DH, Moffat G, Pino L, Moreno S, Farb NAS. Attentional and affective consequences of technology supported mindfulness training: a randomised, active control, efficacy trial. BMC Psychol. 2016;4(1):60. PMCID: PMC5127005. http://www.ncbi.nlm.nih.gov/pubmed/27894358
227. Deslandes AC, Moraes H, Alves H, Pompeu F a MS, Silveira H, Mouta R, Arcoverde C, Ribeiro P, Cagy M, Piedade R a M, Laks J, Coutinho ESF. Effect of aerobic training on EEG alpha asymmetry and depressive symptoms in the elderly: a 1-year follow-up study. Braz J Med Biol Res. 2010;43(6):585–92. PMID: 20464340. http://www.ncbi.nlm.nih.gov/pubmed/20464340
228. Kubesch S, Bretschneider V, Freudenmann R, Weidenhammer N, Lehmann M, Spitzer M, Grön G. Aerobic endurance exercise improves executive functions in depressed patients. J Clin Psychiatry. 2003;64(9):1005–12. PMID: 14628975. http://www.ncbi.nlm.nih.gov/pubmed/14628975
229. Vasques PE, Moraes H, Silveira H, Deslandes AC, Laks J. Acute exercise improves cognition in the depressed elderly: the effect of dual-tasks. Clinics (Sao Paulo). 2011;66(9):1553–7. PMCID: PMC3164403. http://www.ncbi.nlm.nih.gov/pubmed/22179158
230. Greer TL, Furman JL, Trivedi MH. Evaluation of the benefits of exercise on cognition in major depressive disorder. Gen Hosp Psychiatry. 2017;49:19–25. PMID: 28690019. http://www.ncbi.nlm.nih.gov/pubmed/28690019
231. Brondino N, Rocchetti M, Fusar-Poli L, Codrons E, Correale L, Vandoni M, Barbui C, Politi P. A systematic review of cognitive effects of exercise in depression. Acta Psychiatr Scand. 2017;135(4):285–95. PMID: 28110494. http://www.ncbi.nlm.nih.gov/pubmed/28110494
232. Anguera JA, Boccanfuso J, Rintoul JL, Al-Hashimi O, Faraji F, Janowich J, Kong E, Larraburo Y, Rolle C, Johnston E, Gazzaley A. Video game training enhances cognitive control in older adults. Nature. 2013;501(7465):97–101. PMCID: PMC3983066. http://www.ncbi.nlm.nih.gov/pubmed/24005416
233. Anguera JA, Gunning FM, Areán PA. Improving late life depression and cognitive control through the use of therapeutic video game technology: a proof-of-concept randomized trial. Depress Anxiety. 2017;34(6):508–17. PMCID: PMC6093618. http://www.ncbi.nlm.nih.gov/pubmed/28052513
234. Motter JN, Pimontel MA, Rindskopf D, Devanand DP, Doraiswamy PM, Sneed JR. Computerized cognitive training and functional recovery in major depressive disorder: a meta-analysis. J Affect Disord. 2016;189:184–91. PMID: 26437233. http://www.ncbi.nlm.nih.gov/pubmed/26437233
235. Arean PA, Hallgren KA, Jordan JT, Gazzaley A, Atkins DC, Heagerty PJ, Anguera JA. The use and effectiveness of Mobile apps for depression: results from a fully remote clinical trial. J Med Internet Res. 2016;18(12):e330. PMCID: PMC5209607. http://www.ncbi.nlm.nih.gov/pubmed/27998876
236. Linnoila VM, Virkkunen M. Aggression, suicidality, and serotonin. J Clin Psychiatry. 1992;53(Suppl):46–51. PMID: 1385390. http://www.ncbi.nlm.nih.gov/pubmed/1385390
237. Teismann T, Eimen JJ, Cwik JC. Misclassification of self-directed violence. Crisis. 2023;44(6):525–8. PMCID: PMC10658634. http://www.ncbi.nlm.nih.gov/pubmed/36636794
238. Fernandes H, Lima DV, Hino P, Taminato M, Okuno MFP. Self-inflicted violence and suicide in people living with HIV/AIDS: a systematic review. Rev Bras Enferm. 2022;75Suppl 3(Suppl 3):e20210768. PMID: 35703675. http://www.ncbi.nlm.nih.gov/pubmed/35703675
239. Liu RT, Walsh RFL, Sheehan AE, Cheek SM, Sanzari CM. Prevalence and correlates of suicide and nonsuicidal self-injury in children: a systematic review and meta-analysis. JAMA. Psychiatry. 2022;79(7):718–26. PMCID: PMC9134039. http://www.ncbi.nlm.nih.gov/pubmed/35612875
240. Bozzini AB, Bauer A, Maruyama J, Simões R, Matijasevich A. Factors associated with risk behaviors in adolescence: a systematic review. Braz J Psychiatry. 2021;43(2):210–21. PMCID: PMC8023154. http://www.ncbi.nlm.nih.gov/pubmed/32756805
241. Kaniuka AR, Bowling J. Suicidal self-directed violence among gender minority individuals: a systematic review. Suicide Life Threat Behav. 2021;51(2):212–9. PMID: 33876492. http://www.ncbi.nlm.nih.gov/pubmed/33876492
242. Bortolato M, Pivac N, Muck Seler D, Nikolac Perkovic M, Pessia M, Di Giovanni G. The role of the serotonergic system at the interface of aggression and suicide. Neuroscience. 2013;236:160–85. PMCID: PMC3657560. http://www.ncbi.nlm.nih.gov/pubmed/23333677.
243. Conner KR, Swogger MT, Houston RJ. A test of the reactive aggression-suicidal behavior hypothesis: is there a case for proactive aggression? J Abnorm Psychol. 2009;118(1):235–40. PMCID: PMC4861304. http://www.ncbi.nlm.nih.gov/pubmed/19222330
244. Conner KR, Cox C, Duberstein PR, Tian L, Nisbet PA, Conwell Y. Violence, alcohol, and completed suicide: a case-control study. Am J Psychiatry. 2001;158(10):1701–5. PMID: 11579005. http://www.ncbi.nlm.nih.gov/pubmed/11579005
245. Sutar R, Kumar A, Yadav V. Suicide and prevalence of mental disorders: a systematic review and meta-analysis of world data on case-control psychological autopsy studies. Psychiatry Res. 2023;329:115492. PMID: 37783094 http://www.ncbi.nlm.nih.gov/pubmed/37783094
246. Pfeffer CR, Jiang H, Kakuma T. Child-Adolescent Suicidal Potential Index (CASPI): a screen for risk for early onset suicidal

behavior. Psychol Assess. 2000;12(3):304–18. PMID: 11021154. http://www.ncbi.nlm.nih.gov/pubmed/11021154
247. O'Connor EA, Perdue LA, Coppola EL, Henninger ML, Thomas RG, Gaynes BN. Depression and suicide risk screening: updated evidence report and systematic review for the US preventive services task force. JAMA. 2023;329(23):2068–85. PMID: 37338873. http://www.ncbi.nlm.nih.gov/pubmed/37338873
248. O'Connor E, Henninger M, Perdue LA, Coppola EL, Thomas R, Gaynes BN. Screening for depression, anxiety, and suicide risk in adults: a systematic evidence review for the U.S. Preventive Services Task Force [Internet]. Rockville (MD): Agency for Healthcare Research and Quality (US); 2023 [cited 2025 Jan 16]. Available from: http://www.ncbi.nlm.nih.gov/books/NBK592805/ PMID: 37406149. http://www.ncbi.nlm.nih.gov/pubmed/37406149.
249. Arango V, Huang Y, yu, Underwood MD, Mann JJ. Genetics of the serotonergic system in suicidal behavior. J Psychiatr Res. 2003;37(5):375–86. PMID: 12849930. http://www.ncbi.nlm.nih.gov/pubmed/12849930
250. Plutchik R. Outward and inward directed aggressiveness: the interaction between violence and suicidality. Pharmacopsychiatry. 1995;28(Suppl 2):47–57. PMID: 8614701. http://www.ncbi.nlm.nih.gov/pubmed/8614701
251. Felthous AR, Masood Y, Kahlon C, Safari D, Rodgers E, Chennu N, Angly M. A classification of combined homicide-suicide: an update-part I: introduction and psychopathology. J Forensic Sci. 2024;69(1):222–30. PMID: 37919798. http://www.ncbi.nlm.nih.gov/pubmed/37919798
252. Gregory MJ, Milroy CM. Homicide and suicide in Yorkshire and the Humber: 1975–1992 and 1993–2007. Am J Forensic Med Pathol. 2010;31(1):58–63. PMID: 19935394. http://www.ncbi.nlm.nih.gov/pubmed/19935394
253. 9241594365_eng.pdf
254. Stacy M, Schulkin J. Suicide: Allostatic regulation and resilience. Psychoneuroendocrinology. 2022;139:105691. PMID: 35218982. http://www.ncbi.nlm.nih.gov/pubmed/35218982
255. Lipkind GM, Shashkov AS, Nechaev OA, Torgov VI, Shibaev VN, Kochetkov NK. Nuclear Overhauser effects and conformations of branched trisaccharide methyl beta-glycosides that contain a 2,3-disubstituted galactose residue. Carbohydr Res. 1989;195(1):27–37. PMID: 2636043. http://www.ncbi.nlm.nih.gov/pubmed/2636043
256. Robillard CL, Turner BJ, Helps CE. Testing a diathesis-stress model during the transition to university: associations between self-criticism, stress, and internalizing problems. J Am Coll Heal. 2023;71(6):1834–44. PMID: 34314640. http://www.ncbi.nlm.nih.gov/pubmed/34314640
257. O'Connor DB, Ferguson E, Green JA, O'Carroll RE, O'Connor RC. Cortisol levels and suicidal behavior: a meta-analysis. Psychoneuroendocrinology. 2016;63:370–9. PMID: 26555430. http://www.ncbi.nlm.nih.gov/pubmed/26555430
258. Docherty AR, Mullins N, Ashley-Koch AE, Qin X, Coleman JRI, Shabalin A, Kang J, Murnyak B, Wendt F, Adams M, Campos AI, DiBlasi E, Fullerton JM, Kranzler HR, Bakian AV, Monson ET, Rentería ME, Walss-Bass C, Andreassen OA, Behera C, Bulik CM, Edenberg HJ, Kessler RC, Mann JJ, Nurnberger JI, Pistis G, Streit F, Ursano RJ, Polimanti R, Dennis M, Garrett M, Hair L, Harvey P, Hauser ER, Hauser MA, Huffman J, Jacobson D, Madduri R, McMahon B, Oslin DW, Trafton J, Awasthi S, Berrettini WH, Bohus M, Chang X, Chen HC, Chen WJ, Christensen ED, Crow S, Duriez P, Edwards AC, Fernández-Aranda F, Galfalvy H, Gandal M, Gorwood P, Guo Y, Hafferty JD, Hakonarson H, Halmi KA, Hishimoto A, Jain S, Jamain S, Jiménez-Murcia S, Johnson C, Kaplan AS, Kaye WH, Keel PK, Kennedy JL, Kim M, Klump KL, Levey DF, Li D, Liao SC, Lieb K, Lilenfeld L, Marshall CR, Mitchell JE, Okazaki S, Otsuka I, Pinto D, Powers A, Ramoz N, Ripke S, Roepke S, Rozanov V, Scherer SW, Schmahl C, Sokolowski M, Starnawska A, Strober M, Su MH, Thornton LM, Treasure J, Ware EB, Watson HJ, Witt SH, Woodside DB, Yilmaz Z, Zillich L, Adolfsson R, Agartz I, Alda M, Alfredsson L, Appadurai V, Artigas MS, Van der Auwera S, Azevedo MH, Bass N, Bau CHD, Baune BT, Bellivier F, Berger K, Biernacka JM, Bigdeli TB, Binder EB, Boehnke M, Boks MP, Braff DL, Bryant R, Budde M, Byrne EM, Cahn W, Castelao E, Cervilla JA, Chaumette B, Corvin A, Craddock N, Djurovic S, Foo JC, Forstner AJ, Frye M, Gatt JM, Giegling I, Grabe HJ, Green MJ, Grevet EH, Grigoroiu-Serbanescu M, Gutierrez B, Guzman-Parra J, Hamshere ML, Hartmann AM, Hauser J, Heilmann-Heimbach S, Hoffmann P, Ising M, Jones I, Jones LA, Jonsson L, Kahn RS, Kelsoe JR, Kendler KS, Kloiber S, Koenen KC, Kogevinas M, Krebs MO, Landén M, Leboyer M, Lee PH, Levinson DF, Liao C, Lissowska J, Mayoral F, McElroy SL, McGrath P, McGuffin P, McQuillin A, Mehta D, Melle I, Mitchell PB, Molina E, Morken G, Nievergelt C, Nöthen MM, O'Donovan MC, Ophoff RA, Owen MJ, Pato C, Pato MT, Penninx BWJH, Potash JB, Power RA, Preisig M, Quested D, Ramos-Quiroga JA, Reif A, Ribasés M, Richarte V, Rietschel M, Rivera M, Roberts A, Roberts G, Rouleau GA, Rovaris DL, Sanders AR, Schofield PR, Schulze TG, Scott LJ, Serretti A, Shi J, Sirignano L, Sklar P, Smeland OB, Smoller JW, Sonuga-Barke EJS, Trzaskowski M, Tsuang MT, Turecki G, Vilar-Ribó L, Vincent JB, Völzke H, Walters JTR, Weickert CS, Weickert TW, Weissman MM, Williams LM, Wray NR, Zai CC, Agerbo E, Børglum AD, Breen G, Demontis D, Erlangsen A, Gelernter J, Glatt SJ, Hougaard DM, Hwu HG, Kuo PH, Lewis CM, Li QS, Liu CM, Martin NG, McIntosh AM, Medland SE, Mors O, Nordentoft M, Olsen CM, Porteous D, Smith DJ, Stahl EA, Stein MB, Wasserman D, Werge T, Whiteman DC, Willour V, VA Million Veteran Program (MVP), MVP Suicide Exemplar Workgroup, Suicide Working Group of the Psychiatric Genomics Consortium, Major Depressive Disorder Working Group of the Psychiatric Genomics Consortium, Bipolar Disorder Working Group of the Psychiatric Genomics Consortium, Schizophrenia Working Group of the Psychiatric Genomics Consortium, Eating Disorder Working Group of the Psychiatric Genomics Consortium, German Borderline Genomics Consortium, Coon H, Beckham JC, Kimbrel NA, Ruderfer DM. GWAS meta-analysis of suicide attempt: identification of 12 genome-wide significant loci and implication of genetic risks for specific health factors. Am J Psychiatry. 2023;180(10):723–38. PMCID: PMC10603363. http://www.ncbi.nlm.nih.gov/pubmed/37777856
259. Voracek M, Loibl LM. Genetics of suicide: a systematic review of twin studies. Wien Klin Wochenschr. 2007;119(15–16):463–75. PMID: 17721766. http://www.ncbi.nlm.nih.gov/pubmed/17721766
260. Tidemalm D, Runeson B, Waern M, Frisell T, Carlström E, Lichtenstein P, Långström N. Familial clustering of suicide risk: a total population study of 11.4 million individuals. Psychol Med. 2011;41(12):2527–34. PMCID: PMC3207221. http://www.ncbi.nlm.nih.gov/pubmed/21733212
261. McGuffin P, Marusic A, Farmer A. What can psychiatric genetics offer suicidology? Crisis. 2001;22(2):61–5. PMID: 11727895. http://www.ncbi.nlm.nih.gov/pubmed/11727895
262. McGuffin P, Perroud N, Uher R, Butler A, Aitchison KJ, Craig I, Lewis C, Farmer A. The genetics of affective disorder and suicide. Eur Psychiatry. 2010;25(5):275–7. PMID: 20462744. http://www.ncbi.nlm.nih.gov/pubmed/20462744
263. Baldessarini RJ, Hennen J. Genetics of suicide: an overview. Harv Rev Psychiatry. 2004;12(1):1–13. PMID: 14965851 http://www.ncbi.nlm.nih.gov/pubmed/14965851
264. Kim CD, Seguin M, Therrien N, Riopel G, Chawky N, Lesage AD, Turecki G. Familial aggregation of suicidal behavior: a fam-

ily study of male suicide completers from the general population. Am J Psychiatry. 2005;162(5):1017–9. PMID: 15863812. http://www.ncbi.nlm.nih.gov/pubmed/15863812
265. Bachmann S. Epidemiology of suicide and the psychiatric perspective. Int J Environ Res Public Health. 2018;15(7):1425. PMCID: PMC6068947. http://www.ncbi.nlm.nih.gov/pubmed/29986446
266. Spallek J, Reeske A, Norredam M, Nielsen SS, Lehnhardt J, Razum O. Suicide among immigrants in Europe–a systematic literature review. Eur J Pub Health. 2015;25(1):63–71. PMID: 25096258. http://www.ncbi.nlm.nih.gov/pubmed/25096258
267. Haas AP, Eliason M, Mays VM, Mathy RM, Cochran SD, D'Augelli AR, Silverman MM, Fisher PW, Hughes T, Rosario M, Russell ST, Malley E, Reed J, Litts DA, Haller E, Sell RL, Remafedi G, Bradford J, Beautrais AL, Brown GK, Diamond GM, Friedman MS, Garofalo R, Turner MS, Hollibaugh A, Clayton PJ. Suicide and suicide risk in lesbian, gay, bisexual, and transgender populations: review and recommendations. J Homosex. 2011;58(1):10–51. PMCID: PMC3662085 http://www.ncbi.nlm.nih.gov/pubmed/21213174
268. Tomoda A, Nishitani S, Takiguchi S, Fujisawa TX, Sugiyama T, Teicher MH. The neurobiological effects of childhood maltreatment on brain structure, function, and attachment. Eur Arch Psychiatry Clin Neurosci. 2024; PMID: 38466395. http://www.ncbi.nlm.nih.gov/pubmed/38466395
269. Bellis MA, Hughes K, Ford K, Ramos Rodriguez G, Sethi D, Passmore J. Life course health consequences and associated annual costs of adverse childhood experiences across Europe and North America: a systematic review and meta-analysis. Lancet. Public Health. 2019;4(10):e517–28. PMCID: PMC7098477. http://www.ncbi.nlm.nih.gov/pubmed/31492648
270. Bomysoad RN, Francis LA. Adverse childhood experiences and mental health conditions among adolescents. J Adolesc Health. 2020;67(6):868–70. PMID: 32576484. http://www.ncbi.nlm.nih.gov/pubmed/32576484
271. Daníelsdóttir HB, Aspelund T, Shen Q, Halldorsdottir T, Jakobsdóttir J, Song H, Lu D, Kuja-Halkola R, Larsson H, Fall K, Magnusson PKE, Fang F, Bergstedt J, Valdimarsdóttir UA. Adverse childhood experiences and adult mental health outcomes. JAMA Psychiatry. 2024;81(6):586–94. PMCID: PMC10918580. http://www.ncbi.nlm.nih.gov/pubmed/38446452
272. Li SM, Zhang C, Bi K, Chen MS. Longitudinal impacts of adverse childhood experiences on multidimensional health outcomes: predicting trajectories in mental, physical, and behavioral health. Child Abuse Negl. 2023:106543. PMID: 37980177. http://www.ncbi.nlm.nih.gov/pubmed/37980177
273. Petruccelli K, Davis J, Berman T. Adverse childhood experiences and associated health outcomes: a systematic review and meta-analysis. Child Abuse Negl. 2019;97:104127. PMID: 31454589. http://www.ncbi.nlm.nih.gov/pubmed/31454589
274. Gilgoff R, Singh L, Koita K, Gentile B, Marques SS. Adverse childhood experiences, outcomes, and interventions. Pediatr Clin N Am. 2020;67(2):259–73. PMID: 32122559. http://www.ncbi.nlm.nih.gov/pubmed/32122559
275. Bhutta ZA, Bhavnani S, Betancourt TS, Tomlinson M, Patel V. Adverse childhood experiences and lifelong health. Nat Med. 2023;29(7):1639–48. PMID: 37464047. http://www.ncbi.nlm.nih.gov/pubmed/37464047
276. Hogg B, Gardoki-Souto I, Valiente-Gómez A, Rosa AR, Fortea L, Radua J, Amann BL, Moreno-Alcázar A. Psychological trauma as a transdiagnostic risk factor for mental disorder: an umbrella meta-analysis. Eur Arch Psychiatry Clin Neurosci. 2023;273(2):397–410. PMID: 36208317. http://www.ncbi.nlm.nih.gov/pubmed/36208317
277. Arnold R, Ahmed F, Clarke A, Quinn N, Beenstock J, Holland P. The relationship between parental adverse childhood experiences and the health, well-being and development outcomes of their children: a systematic review. Public Health. 2023;219:146–53. PMID: 37186980. http://www.ncbi.nlm.nih.gov/pubmed/37186980
278. Švorcová J. Transgenerational epigenetic inheritance of traumatic experience in mammals. Genes (Basel). 2023;14(1):120. PMCID: PMC9859285. http://www.ncbi.nlm.nih.gov/pubmed/36672861
279. Dee G, Ryznar R, Dee C. Epigenetic changes associated with different types of stressors and suicide. Cells. 2023;12(9):1258. PMCID: PMC10177343. http://www.ncbi.nlm.nih.gov/pubmed/37174656.
280. Liu RT, Miller I. Life events and suicidal ideation and behavior: a systematic review. Clin Psychol Rev. 2014;34(3):181–92. PMID: 24534642. http://www.ncbi.nlm.nih.gov/pubmed/24534642
281. Brokke SS, Landrø NI, Haaland VØ. Impulsivity and aggression in suicide ideators and suicide attempters of high and low lethality. BMC Psychiatry. 2022;22(1):753. PMCID: PMC9714086. http://www.ncbi.nlm.nih.gov/pubmed/36457001
282. Gvion Y, Levi-Belz Y, Hadlaczky G, Apter A. On the role of impulsivity and decision-making in suicidal behavior. World J Psychiatry. 2015;5(3):255–9. PMCID: PMC4582302
283. Cameron S, Brown VJ, Dritschel B, Power K, Cook M. Understanding the relationship between suicidality, current depressed mood, personality, and cognitive factors. Psychol Psychother. 2017;90(4):530–49. PMID: 28296207. http://www.ncbi.nlm.nih.gov/pubmed/28296207
284. Mo Q, Ma Z, Wang G, Jia C, Niu L, Zhou L. The pattern of stressful life events prior to suicide among the older adults in rural China: a national case-control psychological autopsy study. BMC Geriatr. 2020;20(1):473. PMCID: PMC7670684. http://www.ncbi.nlm.nih.gov/pubmed/33198644
285. Cheung S, Woo J, Maes MS, Zai CC. Suicide epigenetics, a review of recent progress. J Affect Disord. 2020;(265):423–38. PMID: 32090769. http://www.ncbi.nlm.nih.gov/pubmed/32090769
286. Hughes K, Bellis MA, Hardcastle KA, Sethi D, Butchart A, Mikton C, Jones L, Dunne MP. The effect of multiple adverse childhood experiences on health: a systematic review and meta-analysis. Lancet Public Health. 2017;2(8):e356–66. PMID: 29253477. http://www.ncbi.nlm.nih.gov/pubmed/29253477
287. Angelakis I, Austin JL, Gooding P. Association of childhood maltreatment with suicide behaviors among young people: a systematic review and meta-analysis. JAMA Netw Open. 2020;3(8):e2012563. PMCID: PMC7407092. http://www.ncbi.nlm.nih.gov/pubmed/32756929
288. Kristof Z, Gal Z, Torok D, Eszlari N, Sutori S, Sperlagh B, Anderson IM, Deakin B, Bagdy G, Juhasz G, Gonda X. Embers of the past: early childhood traumas interact with variation in P2RX7 gene implicated in Neuroinflammation on markers of current suicide risk. Int J Mol Sci. 2024;25(2):865. PMCID: PMC10815854. http://www.ncbi.nlm.nih.gov/pubmed/38255938
289. Brent DA, Mann JJ. Familial pathways to suicidal behavior–understanding and preventing suicide among adolescents. N Engl J Med. 2006;355(26):2719–21. PMID: 17192535. http://www.ncbi.nlm.nih.gov/pubmed/17192535
290. Berardelli I, Serafini G, Cortese N, Fiaschè F, O'Connor RC, Pompili M. The involvement of hypothalamus-pituitary-adrenal (HPA) Axis in suicide risk. Brain Sci. 2020;10(9):653. PMCID: PMC7565104. http://www.ncbi.nlm.nih.gov/pubmed/32967089
291. Hoprekstad GE, Skrede S, Bartz-Johannessen C, Joa I, Reitan SK, Steen VM, Torsvik A, Johnsen E, Kroken RA, Rettenbacher M. Association between cytokines and suicidality in patients with psychosis: a multicentre longitudinal analysis. Brain Behav Immun. Health. 2024;37:100756. PMCID: PMC10973600. http://www.ncbi.nlm.nih.gov/pubmed/38549611

292. Liwinski T, Lang UE. Folate and its significance in depressive disorders and suicidality: a comprehensive narrative review. Nutrients. 2023;15(17):3859. PMCID: PMC10490031. http://www.ncbi.nlm.nih.gov/pubmed/37686891
293. Purselle DC, Nemeroff CB. Serotonin transporter: a potential substrate in the biology of suicide. Neuropsychopharmacology. 2003;28(4):613–9. PMID: 12655305. http://www.ncbi.nlm.nih.gov/pubmed/12655305
294. Bah J, Lindström M, Westberg L, Mannerås L, Ryding E, Henningsson S, Melke J, Rosén I, Träskman-Bendz L, Eriksson E. Serotonin transporter gene polymorphisms: effect on serotonin transporter availability in the brain of suicide attempters. Psychiatry Res. 2008;162(3):221–9. PMID: 18314311. http://www.ncbi.nlm.nih.gov/pubmed/18314311
295. Murphy DL, Moya PR. Human serotonin transporter gene (SLC6A4) variants: their contributions to understanding pharmacogenomic and other functional G×G and G×E differences in health and disease. Curr Opin Pharmacol. 2011;11(1):3–10. PMCID: PMC3487694. http://www.ncbi.nlm.nih.gov/pubmed/21439906
296. For neurological and psychiatric disorders. Adv Pharm Bull. 2019;9(3):374–81. PMCID: PMC6773935. http://www.ncbi.nlm.nih.gov/pubmed/31592064
297. Tirosh A, Nilubol N, Patel D, Kebebew E. Prognostic utility of 24-hour urinary 5-HIAA doubling time in patients with neuroendocrine tumors. Endocr Pract. 2018;24(8):710–7. PMCID: PMC8058621. http://www.ncbi.nlm.nih.gov/pubmed/30084688
298. Lenchner JR, Santos C. Biochemistry, 5 Hydroxyindoleacetic Acid. StatPearls [Internet]. Treasure Island (FL): StatPearls Publishing; 2025 [cited 2025 Jan 17]. Available from: http://www.ncbi.nlm.nih.gov/books/NBK551684/.; http://www.ncbi.nlm.nih.gov/pubmed/31869148
299. Asberg M, Träskman L. Studies of CSF 5-HIAA in depression and suicidal behaviour. Adv Exp Med Biol. 1981;133:739–52. PMID: 6172023. http://www.ncbi.nlm.nih.gov/pubmed/6172023
300. Beardsmore CS. Ethical aspects of respiratory research in infancy and early childhood. Pediatr Pulmonol. 1998;26(1):64–8. PMID: 9710280. http://www.ncbi.nlm.nih.gov/pubmed/9710280
301. Wang HQ, Wang ZZ, Chen NH. The receptor hypothesis and the pathogenesis of depression: genetic bases and biological correlates. Pharmacol Res. 2021;167:105542. PMID: 33711432. http://www.ncbi.nlm.nih.gov/pubmed/33711432
302. Nakamura M, Ueno S, Sano A, Tanabe H. The human serotonin transporter gene linked polymorphism (5-HTTLPR) shows ten novel allelic variants. Mol Psychiatry. 2000;5(1):32–8. PMID: 10673766. http://www.ncbi.nlm.nih.gov/pubmed/10673766
303. López-Echeverri YP, Cardona-Londoño KJ, Garcia-Aguirre JF, Orrego-Cardozo M. Effects of serotonin transporter and receptor polymorphisms on depression. Rev Colomb Psiquiatr (Engl Ed). 2023;52(2):130–8. PMID: 37453823. http://www.ncbi.nlm.nih.gov/pubmed/37453823
304. Sreeja V, Jose A, Patel S, Menon B, Athira KV, Chakravarty S. Pharmacogenetics of selective serotonin reuptake inhibitors (SSRI): a serotonin reuptake transporter (SERT)-based approach. Neurochem Int. 2024;173:105672. PMID: 38157886. http://www.ncbi.nlm.nih.gov/pubmed/38157886
305. Zhu JH, Bo HH, Liu BP, Jia CX. The associations between DNA methylation and depression: a systematic review and meta-analysis. J Affect Disord. 2023;327:439–50. PMID: 36717033. http://www.ncbi.nlm.nih.gov/pubmed/36717033
306. Mendlewicz J, Massat I, Souery D, Del-Favero J, Oruc L, Nöthen MM, Blackwood D, Muir W, Battersby S, Lerer B, Segman RH, Kaneva R, Serretti A, Lilli R, Lorenzi C, Jakovljevic M, Ivezic S, Rietschel M, Milanova V, Van Broeckhoven C. Serotonin transporter 5HTTLPR polymorphism and affective disorders: no evidence of association in a large European multicenter study. Eur J Hum Genet. 2004;12(5):377–82. PMID: 14735161. http://www.ncbi.nlm.nih.gov/pubmed/14735161
307. Culverhouse RC, Saccone NL, Horton AC, Ma Y, Anstey KJ, Banaschewski T, Burmeister M, Cohen-Woods S, Etain B, Fisher HL, Goldman N, Guillaume S, Horwood J, Juhasz G, Lester KJ, Mandelli L, Middeldorp CM, Olié E, Villafuerte S, Air TM, Araya R, Bowes L, Burns R, Byrne EM, Coffey C, Coventry WL, Gawronski K a B, Glei D, Hatzimanolis A, Hottenga JJ, Jaussent I, Jawahar C, Jennen-Steinmetz C, Kramer JR, Lajnef M, Little K, Zu Schwabedissen HM, Nauck M, Nederhof E, Petschner P, Peyrot WJ, Schwahn C, Sinnamon G, Stacey D, Tian Y, Toben C, Van der Auwera S, Wainwright N, Wang JC, Willemsen G, Anderson IM, Arolt V, Åslund C, Bagdy G, Baune BT, Bellivier F, Boomsma DI, Courtet P, Dannlowski U, de Geus EJC, Deakin JFW, Easteal S, Eley T, Fergusson DM, Goate AM, Gonda X, Grabe HJ, Holzman C, Johnson EO, Kennedy M, Laucht M, Martin NG, Munafò MR, Nilsson KW, Oldehinkel AJ, Olsson CA, Ormel J, Otte C, Patton GC, Penninx BWJH, Ritchie K, Sarchiapone M, Scheid JM, Serretti A, Smit JH, Stefanis NC, Surtees PG, Völzke H, Weinstein M, Whooley M, Nurnberger JI, Breslau N, Bierut LJ. Collaborative meta-analysis finds no evidence of a strong interaction between stress and 5-HTTLPR genotype contributing to the development of depression. Mol Psychiatry. 2018;23(1):133–142. PMCID: PMC5628077. http://www.ncbi.nlm.nih.gov/pubmed/28373689
308. Munafò MR, Durrant C, Lewis G, Flint J. Gene X environment interactions at the serotonin transporter locus. Biol Psychiatry. 2009;65(3):211–9. PMID: 18691701. http://www.ncbi.nlm.nih.gov/pubmed/18691701
309. Risch N, Herrell R, Lehner T, Liang KY, Eaves L, Hoh J, Griem A, Kovacs M, Ott J, Merikangas KR. Interaction between the serotonin transporter gene (5-HTTLPR), stressful life events, and risk of depression: a meta-analysis. JAMA. 2009;301(23):2462–71. PMCID: PMC2938776. http://www.ncbi.nlm.nih.gov/pubmed/19531786
310. Duncan LE, Keller MC. A critical review of the first 10 years of candidate gene-by-environment interaction research in psychiatry. Am J Psychiatry. 2011;168(10):1041–9. PMCID: PMC3222234. http://www.ncbi.nlm.nih.gov/pubmed/21890791
311. Moncrieff J, Cooper RE, Stockmann T, Amendola S, Hengartner MP, Horowitz MA. The serotonin theory of depression: a systematic umbrella review of the evidence. Mol Psychiatry. 2023;28(8):3243–56. PMCID: PMC10618090. http://www.ncbi.nlm.nih.gov/pubmed/35854107
312. Yohn CN, Gergues MM, Samuels BA. The role of 5-HT receptors in depression. Mol Brain 2017;10(1):28. PMCID: PMC5483313. http://www.ncbi.nlm.nih.gov/pubmed/28646910
313. Mechanisms of signal transduction by hormones and growth factors. Proceedings of the Second International Symposium on Cellular Endocrinology. Lake Placid, New York, September 8–11, 1986. Prog Clin Biol Res. 1987;249:1–321. PMID: 2823287. http://www.ncbi.nlm.nih.gov/pubmed/2823287
314. Kaufman J, DeLorenzo C, Choudhury S, Parsey RV. The 5-HT1A receptor in major depressive disorder. Eur Neuropsychopharmacol. 2016;26(3):397–410. PMCID: PMC5192019. http://www.ncbi.nlm.nih.gov/pubmed/26851834
315. Rojas PS, Neira D, Muñoz M, Lavandero S, Fiedler JL. Serotonin (5-HT) regulates neurite outgrowth through 5-HT1A and 5-HT7 receptors in cultured hippocampal neurons. J Neurosci Res. 2014;92(8):1000–9. PMID: 24752854. http://www.ncbi.nlm.nih.gov/pubmed/24752854
316. Popova NK, Tsybko AS, Naumenko VS. The implication of 5-HT receptor family members in aggression, depression and suicide: similarity and difference. Int J Mol Sci. 2022;23(15):8814. PMCID: PMC9369404. http://www.ncbi.nlm.nih.gov/pubmed/35955946

317. Amidfar M, Kim YK. Recent developments on future antidepressant-related serotonin receptors. Curr Pharm Des. 2018;24(22):2541–8. PMID: 30073919. http://www.ncbi.nlm.nih.gov/pubmed/30073919
318. Cowen PJ, Browning M. What has serotonin to do with depression? World Psychiatry. 2015;14(2):158–60. PMCID: PMC4471964 http://www.ncbi.nlm.nih.gov/pubmed/26043325
319. Harmer CJ, Duman RS, Cowen PJ. How do antidepressants work? New perspectives for refining future treatment approaches. Lancet. Psychiatry. 2017;4(5):409–18. PMCID: PMC5410405. http://www.ncbi.nlm.nih.gov/pubmed/28153641
320. Pilkington PD, Reavley NJ, Jorm AF. The Australian public's beliefs about the causes of depression: associated factors and changes over 16 years. J Affect Disord. 2013;150(2):356–62. PMID: 23688917. http://www.ncbi.nlm.nih.gov/pubmed/23688917
321. Pescosolido BA, Martin JK, Long JS, Medina TR, Phelan JC, Link BG. "A disease like any other"? A decade of change in public reactions to schizophrenia, depression, and alcohol dependence. Am J Psychiatry. 2010;167(11):1321–30. PMCID: PMC4429867. http://www.ncbi.nlm.nih.gov/pubmed/20843872
322. Demasi M, Gøtzsche PC. Presentation of benefits and harms of antidepressants on websites: a cross-sectional study. Int J Risk Saf Med. 2020;31(2):53–65. PMCID: PMC7369070. http://www.ncbi.nlm.nih.gov/pubmed/32144998
323. Read J, Renton J, Harrop C, Geekie J, Dowrick C. A survey of UK general practitioners about depression, antidepressants and withdrawal: implementing the 2019 Public Health England report. Ther Adv Psychopharmacol. 2020;10:2045125320950124. PMCID: PMC7457636. http://www.ncbi.nlm.nih.gov/pubmed/32922735
324. Healy D. Serotonin and depression. BMJ. 2015;350:h1771. PMID: 25900074. http://www.ncbi.nlm.nih.gov/pubmed/25900074
325. Jakobsen JC, Gluud C, Kirsch I. Should antidepressants be used for major depressive disorder? BMJ Evid Based Med. 2020;25(4):130. PMCID: PMC7418603. http://www.ncbi.nlm.nih.gov/pubmed/31554608.
326. Moncrieff J, Cohen D. Do antidepressants cure or create abnormal brain states? PLoS Med. 2006;3(7):e240. PMCID: PMC1472553. http://www.ncbi.nlm.nih.gov/pubmed/16724872
327. SLC6A4 solute carrier family 6 member 4 [Homo sapiens (human)] – Gene – NCBI
328. Bokor J, Krause S, Torok D, Eszlari N, Sutori S, Gal Z, Petschner P, Anderson IM, Deakin B, Bagdy G, Juhasz G, Gonda X. "Out, out, brief candle! Life's but a walking shadow": 5-HTTLPR Is Associated With Current Suicidal Ideation but Not With Previous Suicide Attempts and Interacts With Recent Relationship Problems. Front Psychiatry. 2020;11:567. PMCID: PMC7331851. http://www.ncbi.nlm.nih.gov/pubmed/32670107.
329. Sivaramakrishnan S, Venkatesan V, Paranthaman SK, Sathianathan R, Raghavan S, Pradhan P. Impact of serotonin pathway gene polymorphisms and serotonin levels in suicidal behavior. Med Princ Pract. 2023;32(4–5):250–9. PMCID: PMC10659705. http://www.ncbi.nlm.nih.gov/pubmed/37717578
330. Mullins N, Bigdeli TB, Børglum AD, Coleman JRI, Demontis D, Mehta D, Power RA, Ripke S, Stahl EA, Starnawska A, Anjorin A, M.R.C.Psych, Corvin A, Sanders AR, Forstner AJ, Reif A, Koller AC, Świątkowska B, Baune BT, Müller-Myhsok B, Penninx BWJH, Pato C, Zai C, Rujescu D, Hougaard DM, Quested D, Levinson DF, Binder EB, Byrne EM, Agerbo E, Dr.Med.Sc, Streit F, Mayoral F, Bellivier F, Degenhardt F, Breen G, Morken G, Turecki G, Rouleau GA, Grabe HJ, Völzke H, Jones I, Giegling I, Agartz I, Melle I, Lawrence J, M.R.C.Psych, Walters JTR, Strohmaier J, Shi J, Hauser J, Biernacka JM, Vincent JB, Kelsoe J, Strauss JS, Lissowska J, Pimm J, M.R.C.Psych, Smoller JW, Guzman-Parra J, Berger K, Scott LJ, Jones LA, Azevedo MH, Trzaskowski M, Kogevinas M, Rietschel M, Boks M, Ising M, Grigoroiu-Serbanescu M, Hamshere ML, Leboyer M, Frye M, Nöthen MM, Alda M, Preisig M, Nordentoft M, Boehnke M, O'Donovan MC, Owen MJ, Pato MT, Renteria ME, Budde M, Dipl.-Psych, Weissman MM, Wray NR, Bass N, M.R.C.Psych, Craddock N, Smeland OB, Andreassen OA, Mors O, Gejman PV, Sklar P, McGrath P, Hoffmann P, McGuffin P, Lee PH, Mortensen PB, Kahn RS, Ophoff RA, Adolfsson R, Van der Auwera S, Djurovic S, Kloiber S, Heilmann-Heimbach S, Jamain S, Hamilton SP, McElroy SL, Lucae S, Cichon S, Schulze TG, Hansen T, Werge T, Air TM, Nimgaonkar V, Appadurai V, Cahn W, Milaneschi Y, Major Depressive Disorder Working Group of the Psychiatric Genomics Consortium, Bipolar Disorder Working Group of the Psychiatric Genomics Consortium, Schizophrenia Working Group of the Psychiatric Genomics Consortium, Fanous AH, Kendler KS, McQuillin A, Lewis CM. GWAS of Suicide Attempt in Psychiatric Disorders and Association With Major Depression Polygenic Risk Scores. Am J Psychiatry 2019;176(8):651–660. PMCID: PMC6675659. http://www.ncbi.nlm.nih.gov/pubmed/31164008
331. Levey DF, Polimanti R, Cheng Z, Zhou H, Nuñez YZ, Jain S, He F, Sun X, Ursano RJ, Kessler RC, Smoller JW, Stein MB, Kranzler HR, Gelernter J. Genetic associations with suicide attempt severity and genetic overlap with major depression. Transl Psychiatry 2019;9(1):22. PMCID: PMC6336846. http://www.ncbi.nlm.nih.gov/pubmed/30655502
332. Sandberg JV, Hansson C, Göteson A, Joas E, Jakobsson J, Pålsson E, Landén M. Proteins associated with future suicide attempts in bipolar disorder: a large-scale biomarker discovery study. Mol Psychiatry. 2022;27(9):3857–63. PMCID: PMC9708594. http://www.ncbi.nlm.nih.gov/pubmed/35697758
333. Trepci A, Sellgren CM, Pålsson E, Brundin L, Khanlarkhani N, Schwieler L, Landén M, Erhardt S. Central levels of tryptophan metabolites in subjects with bipolar disorder. Eur Neuropsychopharmacol. 2021;43:52–62. PMID: 33339712. http://www.ncbi.nlm.nih.gov/pubmed/33339712
334. Mullins N, Kang J, Campos AI, Coleman JRI, Edwards AC, Galfalvy H, Levey DF, Lori A, Shabalin A, Starnawska A, Su MH, Watson HJ, Adams M, Awasthi S, Gandal M, Hafferty JD, Hishimoto A, Kim M, Okazaki S, Otsuka I, Ripke S, Ware EB, Bergen AW, Berrettini WH, Bohus M, Brandt H, Chang X, Chen WJ, Chen HC, Crawford S, Crow S, DiBlasi E, Duriez P, Fernández-Aranda F, Fichter MM, Gallinger S, Glatt SJ, Gorwood P, Guo Y, Hakonarson H, Halmi KA, Hwu HG, Jain S, Jamain S, Jiménez-Murcia S, Johnson C, Kaplan AS, Kaye WH, Keel PK, Kennedy JL, Klump KL, Li D, Liao SC, Lieb K, Lilenfeld L, Liu CM, Magistretti PJ, Marshall CR, Mitchell JE, Monson ET, Myers RM, Pinto D, Powers A, Ramoz N, Roepke S, Rozanov V, Scherer SW, Schmahl C, Sokolowski M, Strober M, Thornton LM, Treasure J, Tsuang MT, Witt SH, Woodside DB, Yilmaz Z, Zillich L, Adolfsson R, Agartz I, Air TM, Alda M, Alfredsson L, Andreassen OA, Anjorin A, Appadurai V, Soler Artigas M, Van der Auwera S, Azevedo MH, Bass N, Bau CHD, Baune BT, Bellivier F, Berger K, Biernacka JM, Bigdeli TB, Binder EB, Boehnke M, Boks MP, Bosch R, Braff DL, Bryant R, Budde M, Byrne EM, Cahn W, Casas M, Castelao E, Cervilla JA, Chaumette B, Cichon S, Corvin A, Craddock N, Craig D, Degenhardt F, Djurovic S, Edenberg HJ, Fanous AH, Foo JC, Forstner AJ, Frye M, Fullerton JM, Gatt JM, Gejman PV, Giegling I, Grabe HJ, Green MJ, Grevet EH, Grigoroiu-Serbanescu M, Gutierrez B, Guzman-Parra J, Hamilton SP, Hamshere ML, Hartmann A, Hauser J, Heilmann-Heimbach S, Hoffmann P, Ising M, Jones I, Jones LA, Jonsson L, Kahn RS, Kelsoe JR, Kendler KS, Kloiber S, Koenen KC, Kogevinas M, Konte B, Krebs MO, Landén M, Lawrence J, Leboyer M, Lee PH, Levinson DF, Liao C, Lissowska J, Lucae S, Mayoral F, McElroy SL, McGrath P, McGuffin P, McQuillin A, Medland

SE, Mehta D, Melle I, Milaneschi Y, Mitchell PB, Molina E, Morken G, Mortensen PB, Müller-Myhsok B, Nievergelt C, Nimgaonkar V, Nöthen MM, O'Donovan MC, Ophoff RA, Owen MJ, Pato C, Pato MT, Penninx BWJH, Pimm J, Pistis G, Potash JB, Power RA, Preisig M, Quested D, Ramos-Quiroga JA, Reif A, Ribasés M, Richarte V, Rietschel M, Rivera M, Roberts A, Roberts G, Rouleau GA, Rovaris DL, Rujescu D, Sánchez-Mora C, Sanders AR, Schofield PR, Schulze TG, Scott LJ, Serretti A, Shi J, Shyn SI, Sirignano L, Sklar P, Smeland OB, Smoller JW, Sonuga-Barke EJS, Spalletta G, Strauss JS, Świątkowska B, Trzaskowski M, Turecki G, Vilar-Ribó L, Vincent JB, Völzke H, Walters JTR, Shannon Weickert C, Weickert TW, Weissman MM, Williams LM, Wray NR, Zai CC, Ashley-Koch AE, Beckham JC, Hauser ER, Hauser MA, Kimbrel NA, Lindquist JH, McMahon B, Oslin DW, Qin X, Major Depressive Disorder Working Group of the Psychiatric Genomics Consortium, Bipolar Disorder Working Group of the Psychiatric Genomics Consortium, Eating Disorders Working Group of the Psychiatric Genomics Consortium, German Borderline Genomics Consortium, MVP Suicide Exemplar Workgroup, VA Million Veteran Program, Agerbo E, Børglum AD, Breen G, Erlangsen A, Esko T, Gelernter J, Hougaard DM, Kessler RC, Kranzler HR, Li QS, Martin NG, McIntosh AM, Mors O, Nordentoft M, Olsen CM, Porteous D, Ursano RJ, Wasserman D, Werge T, Whiteman DC, Bulik CM, Coon H, Demontis D, Docherty AR, Kuo PH, Lewis CM, Mann JJ, Rentería ME, Smith DJ, Stahl EA, Stein MB, Streit F, Willour V, Ruderfer DM. Dissecting the shared genetic architecture of suicide attempt, psychiatric disorders, and known risk factors. Biol Psychiatry. 2022;91(3):313–27. PMCID: PMC8851871. http://www.ncbi.nlm.nih.gov/pubmed/34861974

335. Meyer JH, Cervenka S, Kim MJ, Kreisl WC, Henter ID, Innis RB. Neuroinflammation in psychiatric disorders: PET imaging and promising new targets. Lancet. Psychiatry. 2020;7(12):1064–74. PMCID: PMC7893630. http://www.ncbi.nlm.nih.gov/pubmed/33098761
336. Bhattacharya A, Biber K. The microglial ATP-gated ion channel P2X7 as a CNS drug target. Glia. 2016;64(10):1772–87. PMID: 27219534. http://www.ncbi.nlm.nih.gov/pubmed/27219534
337. Sperlágh B, Illes P. P2X7 receptor: an emerging target in central nervous system diseases. Trends Pharmacol Sci. 2014;35(10):537–47. PMID: 25223574. http://www.ncbi.nlm.nih.gov/pubmed/25223574
338. Kristof Z, Eszlari N, Sutori S, Gal Z, Torok D, Baksa D, Petschner P, Sperlagh B, Anderson IM, Deakin JFW, Juhasz G, Bagdy G, Gonda X. P2RX7 gene variation mediates the effect of childhood adversity and recent stress on the severity of depressive symptoms. PLoS One. 2021;16(6):e0252766. PMCID: PMC8191953. http://www.ncbi.nlm.nih.gov/pubmed/34111150
339. Kristof Z, Gal Z, Torok D, Eszlari N, Sutori S, Erdelyi-Hamza B, Petschner P, Sperlagh B, Anderson IM, Deakin JFW, Bagdy G, Juhasz G, Gonda X. Variation along P2RX7 interacts with early traumas on severity of anxiety suggesting a role for neuroinflammation. Sci Rep. 2023;13(1):7757. PMCID: PMC10182087. http://www.ncbi.nlm.nih.gov/pubmed/37173368
340. Courtet P, Giner L, Seneque M, Guillaume S, Olie E, Ducasse D. Neuroinflammation in suicide: toward a comprehensive model. World J Biol Psychiatry. 2016;17(8):564–86. PMID: 26223957. http://www.ncbi.nlm.nih.gov/pubmed/26223957
341. Pastis I, Santos MG, Paruchuri A. Exploring the role of inflammation in major depressive disorder: beyond the monoamine hypothesis. Front Behav Neurosci. 2023;17:1282242. PMCID: PMC10829100. http://www.ncbi.nlm.nih.gov/pubmed/38299049
342. Brundin L, Bryleva EY, Thirtamara Rajamani K. Role of inflammation in suicide: from mechanisms to treatment. Neuropsychopharmacology. 2017;42(1):271–83. PMCID: PMC5143480. http://www.ncbi.nlm.nih.gov/pubmed/27377015
343. Ganança L, Oquendo MA, Tyrka AR, Cisneros-Trujillo S, Mann JJ, Sublette ME. The role of cytokines in the pathophysiology of suicidal behavior. Psychoneuroendocrinology. 2016;63:296–310. PMCID: PMC4910882. http://www.ncbi.nlm.nih.gov/pubmed/26546783
344. Beurel E, Toups M, Nemeroff CB. The bidirectional relationship of depression and inflammation: double trouble. Neuron. 2020;107(2):234–56. PMCID: PMC7381373. http://www.ncbi.nlm.nih.gov/pubmed/32553197
345. Caspani G, Green M, Swann JR, Foster JA. Microbe-immune crosstalk: evidence that T cells influence the development of the brain metabolome. Int J Mol Sci. 2022;23(6):3259. PMCID: PMC8952415. http://www.ncbi.nlm.nih.gov/pubmed/35328680.
346. Pronovost GN, Hsiao EY. Perinatal interactions between the microbiome, immunity, and neurodevelopment. Immunity. 2019;50(1):18–36. PMCID: PMC6447295. http://www.ncbi.nlm.nih.gov/pubmed/30650376
347. Dickerson F, Dilmore AH, Godoy-Vitorino F, Nguyen TT, Paulus M, Pinto-Tomas AA, Moya-Roman C, Zuniga-Chaves I, Severance EG, Jeste DV. The microbiome and mental health across the lifespan. Curr Top Behav Neurosci. 2023;61:119–40. PMID: 35947353. http://www.ncbi.nlm.nih.gov/pubmed/35947353
348. Corrigendum. Acta Psychiatr Scand. 2020;142(5):423. PMCID: PMC8097531. http://www.ncbi.nlm.nih.gov/pubmed/33164213
349. Jayashree B, Bibin YS, Prabhu D, Shanthirani CS, Gokulakrishnan K, Lakshmi BS, Mohan V, Balasubramanyam M. Increased circulatory levels of lipopolysaccharide (LPS) and zonulin signify novel biomarkers of proinflammation in patients with type 2 diabetes. Mol Cell Biochem. 2014;388(1–2):203–10. PMID: 24347174. http://www.ncbi.nlm.nih.gov/pubmed/24347174
350. Maes M, Kubera M, Leunis JC. The gut-brain barrier in major depression: intestinal mucosal dysfunction with an increased translocation of LPS from gram negative enterobacteria (leaky gut) plays a role in the inflammatory pathophysiology of depression. Neuro Endocrinol Lett. 2008;29(1):117–24. PMID: 18283240. http://www.ncbi.nlm.nih.gov/pubmed/18283240
351. Mitrea L, Nemeş SA, Szabo K, Teleky BE, Vodnar DC. Guts imbalance imbalances the brain: a review of gut microbiota association with neurological and psychiatric disorders. Front Med (Lausanne). 2022;9:813204. PMCID: PMC9009523. http://www.ncbi.nlm.nih.gov/pubmed/35433746.
352. Serafini G, Parisi VM, Aguglia A, Amerio A, Sampogna G, Fiorillo A, Pompili M, Amore M. A specific inflammatory profile underlying suicide risk? Systematic review of the main literature findings. Int J Environ Res Public Health. 2020;17(7):2393. PMCID: PMC7177217. http://www.ncbi.nlm.nih.gov/pubmed/32244611
353. Rohleder N. Stress and inflammation – the need to address the gap in the transition between acute and chronic stress effects. Psychoneuroendocrinology. 2019;105:164–71. PMID: 30826163. http://www.ncbi.nlm.nih.gov/pubmed/30826163
354. Hanisch UK. Microglia as a source and target of cytokines. Glia. 2002;40(2):140–55. PMID: 12379902. http://www.ncbi.nlm.nih.gov/pubmed/12379902
355. Brisch R, Wojtylak S, Saniotis A, Steiner J, Gos T, Kumaratilake J, Henneberg M, Wolf R. The role of microglia in neuropsychiatric disorders and suicide. Eur Arch Psychiatry Clin Neurosci. 2022;272(6):929–45. PMCID: PMC9388452. http://www.ncbi.nlm.nih.gov/pubmed/34595576
356. Réus GZ, Fries GR, Stertz L, Badawy M, Passos IC, Barichello T, Kapczinski F, Quevedo J. The role of inflammation and microglial activation in the pathophysiology of psychiatric disorders. Neuroscience. 2015;300:141–54. PMID: 25981208. http://www.ncbi.nlm.nih.gov/pubmed/25981208
357. Tay TL, Béchade C, D'Andrea I, St-Pierre MK, Henry MS, Roumier A, Tremblay ME. Microglia Gone Rogue: Impacts on psychiatric disorders across the lifespan. Front Mol Neurosci.

2017;10:421. PMCID: PMC5758507 http://www.ncbi.nlm.nih.gov/pubmed/29354029
358. Hong H, Kim BS, Im HI. Pathophysiological role of Neuroinflammation in neurodegenerative diseases and psychiatric disorders. Int Neurourol J. 2016;20(Suppl 1):S2–7. PMCID: PMC4895907 http://www.ncbi.nlm.nih.gov/pubmed/27230456
359. Brisch R, Steiner J, Mawrin C, Krzyżanowska M, Jankowski Z, Gos T. Microglia in the dorsal raphe nucleus plays a potential role in both suicide facilitation and prevention in affective disorders. Eur Arch Psychiatry Clin Neurosci. 2017;267(5):403–15. PMCID: PMC5509773. http://www.ncbi.nlm.nih.gov/pubmed/28229240
360. Baker KG, Halliday GM, Törk I. Cytoarchitecture of the human dorsal raphe nucleus. J Comp Neurol. 1990;301(2):147–61. PMID: 2262589. http://www.ncbi.nlm.nih.gov/pubmed/2262589
361. Stockmeier CA, Shapiro LA, Haycock JW, Thompson PA, Lowy MT. Quantitative subregional distribution of serotonin1A receptors and serotonin transporters in the human dorsal raphe. Brain Res. 1996;727(1–2):1–12. PMID: 8842377. http://www.ncbi.nlm.nih.gov/pubmed/8842377
362. Zhao H, Zhang BL, Yang SJ, Rusak B. The role of lateral habenula-dorsal raphe nucleus circuits in higher brain functions and psychiatric illness. Behav Brain Res. 2015;277:89–98. PMID: 25234226. http://www.ncbi.nlm.nih.gov/pubmed/25234226
363. Boldrini M, Underwood MD, Mann JJ, Arango V. More tryptophan hydroxylase in the brainstem dorsal raphe nucleus in depressed suicides. Brain Res. 2005;1041(1):19–28. PMID: 15804496. http://www.ncbi.nlm.nih.gov/pubmed/15804496
364. Bonkale WL, Murdock S, Janosky JE, Austin MC. Normal levels of tryptophan hydroxylase immunoreactivity in the dorsal raphe of depressed suicide victims. J Neurochem. 2004;88(4):958–64. PMID: 14756817. http://www.ncbi.nlm.nih.gov/pubmed/14756817
365. Bielau H, Mawrin C, Krell D, Agelink MW, Trübner K, Davis R, Gos T, Bogerts B, Bernstein HG, Baumann B. Differences in activation of the dorsal raphe nucleus depending on performance of suicide. Brain Res. 2005;1039(1–2):43–52. PMID: 15781045. http://www.ncbi.nlm.nih.gov/pubmed/15781045
366. Gos T, Krell D, Brisch R, Bielau H, Trübner K, Steiner J, Bernstein HG, Bogerts B. Demonstration of decreased activity of dorsal raphe nucleus neurons in depressed suicidal patients by the AgNOR staining method. J Affect Disord. 2008;111(2–3):251–60. PMID: 18423885. http://www.ncbi.nlm.nih.gov/pubmed/18423885
367. Krzyżanowska M, Steiner J, Karnecki K, Kaliszan M, Brisch R, Wiergowski M, Braun K, Jankowski Z, Gos T. Decreased ribosomal DNA transcription in dorsal raphe nucleus neurons differentiates between suicidal and non-suicidal death. Eur Arch Psychiatry Clin Neurosci. 2016;266(3):217–224. PMCID: PMC4819736. http://www.ncbi.nlm.nih.gov/pubmed/26590846
368. Albert PR, Benkelfat C. The neurobiology of depression–revisiting the serotonin hypothesis. II. Genetic, epigenetic and clinical studies. Philos Trans R Soc Lond Ser B Biol Sci. 2013;368(1615):20120535. PMCID: PMC3638388. http://www.ncbi.nlm.nih.gov/pubmed/23440469
369. Jasinska AJ, Lowry CA, Burmeister M. Serotonin transporter gene, stress and raphe-raphe interactions: a molecular mechanism of depression. Trends Neurosci. 2012;35(7):395–402. PMID: 22301434 http://www.ncbi.nlm.nih.gov/pubmed/22301434
370. Mann JJ. The serotonergic system in mood disorders and suicidal behaviour. Philos Trans R Soc Lond Ser B Biol Sci. 2013;368(1615):20120537. PMCID: PMC3638390. http://www.ncbi.nlm.nih.gov/pubmed/23440471
371. Hahn A, Haeusler D, Kraus C, Höflich AS, Kranz GS, Baldinger P, Savli M, Mitterhauser M, Wadsak W, Karanikas G, Kasper S, Lanzenberger R. Attenuated serotonin transporter association between dorsal raphe and ventral striatum in major depression. Hum Brain Mapp. 2014;35(8):3857–66. PMCID: PMC6868983 http://www.ncbi.nlm.nih.gov/pubmed/24443158
372. Arango V, Underwood MD, Boldrini M, Tamir H, Kassir SA, Hsiung S, Chen JJ, Mann JJ. Serotonin 1A receptors, serotonin transporter binding and serotonin transporter mRNA expression in the brainstem of depressed suicide victims. Neuropsychopharmacology. 2001;25(6):892–903. PMID: 11750182 http://www.ncbi.nlm.nih.gov/pubmed/11750182
373. Mann JJ. Neurobiology of suicidal behaviour. Nat Rev Neurosci. 2003;4(10):819–28. PMID: 14523381. http://www.ncbi.nlm.nih.gov/pubmed/14523381
374. Matthews PR, Harrison PJ. A morphometric, immunohistochemical, and in situ hybridization study of the dorsal raphe nucleus in major depression, bipolar disorder, schizophrenia, and suicide. J Affect Disord. 2012;137(1–3):125–34. PMCID: PMC3314923 http://www.ncbi.nlm.nih.gov/pubmed/22129767
375. Sullivan GM, Oquendo MA, Milak M, Miller JM, Burke A, Ogden RT, Parsey RV, Mann JJ. Positron emission tomography quantification of serotonin(1A) receptor binding in suicide attempters with major depressive disorder. JAMA Psychiatry. 2015;72(2):169–78. PMCID: PMC4329977. http://www.ncbi.nlm.nih.gov/pubmed/25549105
376. Wisłowska-Stanek A, Kołosowska K, Maciejak P. Neurobiological basis of increased risk for suicidal behaviour. Cells. 2021;10(10):2519. PMCID: PMC8534256. http://www.ncbi.nlm.nih.gov/pubmed/34685499
377. Thibaut F. Neuroinflammation: new vistas for neuropsychiatric research. Dialogues Clin Neurosci. 2017;19(1):3–4. PMCID: PMC5442362. http://www.ncbi.nlm.nih.gov/pubmed/28566942
378. Tian L, Hui CW, Bisht K, Tan Y, Sharma K, Chen S, Zhang X, Tremblay ME. Microglia under psychosocial stressors along the aging trajectory: consequences on neuronal circuits, behavior, and brain diseases. Prog Neuro-Psychopharmacol Biol Psychiatry. 2017;79(Pt A):27–39. PMID: 28095309. http://www.ncbi.nlm.nih.gov/pubmed/28095309
379. Calcia MA, Bonsall DR, Bloomfield PS, Selvaraj S, Barichello T, Howes OD. Stress and neuroinflammation: a systematic review of the effects of stress on microglia and the implications for mental illness. Psychopharmacology. 2016;233(9):1637–50. PMCID: PMC4828495. http://www.ncbi.nlm.nih.gov/pubmed/26847047
380. Klein RS, Garber C, Howard N. Infectious immunity in the central nervous system and brain function. Nat Immunol. 2017;18(2):132–41. PMCID: PMC5815515. http://www.ncbi.nlm.nih.gov/pubmed/28092376
381. Felger JC, Li Z, Haroon E, Woolwine BJ, Jung MY, Hu X, Miller AH. Inflammation is associated with decreased functional connectivity within corticostriatal reward circuitry in depression. Mol Psychiatry. 2016;21(10):1358–65. PMCID: PMC4862934. http://www.ncbi.nlm.nih.gov/pubmed/26552591
382. Neupane SP, Daray FM, Ballard ED, Galfalvy H, Itzhaky L, Segev A, Shelef A, Tene O, Rizk MM, Mann JJ, Zalsman G. Immune-related biomarkers and suicidal behaviors: a meta-analysis. Eur Neuropsychopharmacol. 2023;75:15–30. PMID: 37356288. http://www.ncbi.nlm.nih.gov/pubmed/37356288
383. Lombardo G. New frontiers in suicide vulnerability: immune system and sex hormones. Brain Behav Immun Health. 2021;18:100384. PMCID: PMC8607160. http://www.ncbi.nlm.nih.gov/pubmed/34841283
384. Jha MK, Cai L, Minhajuddin A, Fatt CC, Furman JL, Gadad BS, Mason BL, Greer TL, Hughes JL, Xiao G, Emslie G, Kennard B, Mayes T, Trivedi MH. Dysfunctional adaptive immune response in adolescents and young adults with suicide behavior. Psychoneuroendocrinology. 2020;111:104487. PMID: 31756521. http://www.ncbi.nlm.nih.gov/pubmed/31756521

385. Piras IS, Huentelman MJ, Pinna F, Paribello P, Solmi M, Murru A, Carpiniello B, Manchia M, Zai CC. A review and meta-analysis of gene expression profiles in suicide. Eur Neuropsychopharmacol. 2022;56:39–49. PMID: 34923210. http://www.ncbi.nlm.nih.gov/pubmed/34923210
386. Schiweck C, Valles-Colomer M, Arolt V, Müller N, Raes J, Wijkhuijs A, Claes S, Drexhage H, Vrieze E. Depression and suicidality: a link to premature T helper cell aging and increased Th17 cells. Brain Behav Immun. 2020;87:603–9. PMID: 32061905. http://www.ncbi.nlm.nih.gov/pubmed/32061905
387. Isaac V, Wu CY, Huang CT, Baune BT, Tseng CL, McLachlan CS. Elevated neutrophil to lymphocyte ratio predicts mortality in medical inpatients with multiple chronic conditions. Medicine (Baltimore). 2016;95(23):e3832. PMCID: PMC4907663. http://www.ncbi.nlm.nih.gov/pubmed/27281085.
388. Kayhan F, Gündüz Ş, Ersoy SA, Kandeğer A, Annagür BB. Relationships of neutrophil-lymphocyte and platelet-lymphocyte ratios with the severity of major depression. Psychiatry Res. 2017;247:332–5. PMID: 27978453. http://www.ncbi.nlm.nih.gov/pubmed/27978453
389. Demir S, Atli A, Bulut M, İbiloğlu AO, Güneş M, Kaya MC, Demirpençe Ö, Sır A. Neutrophil-lymphocyte ratio in patients with major depressive disorder undergoing no pharmacological therapy. Neuropsychiatr Dis Treat. 2015;11:2253–8. PMCID: PMC4556257. http://www.ncbi.nlm.nih.gov/pubmed/26347335
390. Mazza MG, Lucchi S, Tringali AGM, Rossetti A, Botti ER, Clerici M. Neutrophil/lymphocyte ratio and platelet/lymphocyte ratio in mood disorders: a meta-analysis. Prog Neuro-Psychopharmacol Biol Psychiatry. 2018;84(Pt A):229–36. PMID: 29535038 http://www.ncbi.nlm.nih.gov/pubmed/29535038
391. Ekinci O, Ekinci A. The connections among suicidal behavior, lipid profile and low-grade inflammation in patients with major depressive disorder: a specific relationship with the neutrophil-to-lymphocyte ratio. Nord J Psychiatry. 2017;71(8):574–80. PMID: 28800269. http://www.ncbi.nlm.nih.gov/pubmed/28800269
392. Ivković M, Pantović-Stefanović M, Dunjić-Kostić B, Jurišić V, Lačković M, Totić-Poznanović S, Jovanović AA, Damjanović A. Neutrophil-to-lymphocyte ratio predicting suicide risk in euthymic patients with bipolar disorder: moderatory effect of family history. Compr Psychiatry. 2016;66:87–95. PMID: 26995241. http://www.ncbi.nlm.nih.gov/pubmed/26995241
393. Velasco Á, Rodríguez-Revuelta J, Olié E, Abad I, Fernández-Peláez A, Cazals A, Guillaume S, de la Fuente-Tomás L, Jiménez-Treviño L, Gutiérrez L, García-Portilla P, Bobes J, Courtet P, Sáiz PA. Neutrophil-to-lymphocyte ratio: a potential new peripheral biomarker of suicidal behavior. Eur Psychiatry. 2020;63(1):e14. PMCID: PMC7315873. http://www.ncbi.nlm.nih.gov/pubmed/32093807.
394. Sha Q, Madaj Z, Keaton S, Escobar Galvis ML, Smart L, Krzyzanowski S, Fazleabas AT, Leach R, Postolache TT, Achtyes ED, Brundin L. Cytokines and tryptophan metabolites can predict depressive symptoms in pregnancy. Transl Psychiatry. 2022;12(1):35. PMCID: PMC8789799. http://www.ncbi.nlm.nih.gov/pubmed/35078975
395. Minnema LA, Giezen TJ, Souverein PC, Egberts TCG, Leufkens HGM, Gardarsdottir H. Exploring the association between monoclonal antibodies and depression and suicidal ideation and behavior: a VigiBase study. Drug Saf. 2019;42(7):887–95. PMCID: PMC6581921. http://www.ncbi.nlm.nih.gov/pubmed/30617497
396. Bender A, Hagan KE, Kingston N. The association of folate and depression: a meta-analysis. J Psychiatr Res. 2017;95:9–18. PMID: 28759846. http://www.ncbi.nlm.nih.gov/pubmed/28759846
397. Miller AL. The methylation, neurotransmitter, and antioxidant connections between folate and depression. Altern Med Rev. 2008;13(3):216–26. PMID: 18950248. http://www.ncbi.nlm.nih.gov/pubmed/18950248
398. Lewis SJ, Lawlor DA, Davey Smith G, Araya R, Timpson N, Day INM, Ebrahim S. The thermolabile variant of MTHFR is associated with depression in the British Women's Heart and Health Study and a meta-analysis. Mol Psychiatry. 2006;11(4):352–60. PMID: 16402130. http://www.ncbi.nlm.nih.gov/pubmed/16402130
399. Roberts E, Carter B, Young AH. Caveat emptor: folate in unipolar depressive illness, a systematic review and meta-analysis. J Psychopharmacol. 2018;32(4):377–84. PMID: 29442609. http://www.ncbi.nlm.nih.gov/pubmed/29442609
400. Dartois LL, Stutzman DL, Morrow M. L-methylfolate augmentation to antidepressants for adolescents with treatment-resistant depression: a case series. J Child Adolesc Psychopharmacol. 2019;29(5):386–91. http://www.ncbi.nlm.nih.gov/pubmed/31058543
401. Almeida OP, Ford AH, Flicker L. Systematic review and meta-analysis of randomized placebo-controlled trials of folate and vitamin B12 for depression. Int Psychogeriatr. 2015;27(5):727–37. PMID: 25644193. http://www.ncbi.nlm.nih.gov/pubmed/25644193
402. Booij L, Szyf M, Carballedo A, Frey EM, Morris D, Dymov S, Vaisheva F, Ly V, Fahey C, Meaney J, Gill M, Frodl T. DNA methylation of the serotonin transporter gene in peripheral cells and stress-related changes in hippocampal volume: a study in depressed patients and healthy controls. PLoS One. 2015;10(3):e0119061. PMCID: PMC4363605. http://www.ncbi.nlm.nih.gov/pubmed/25781010
403. Nemoda Z, Massart R, Suderman M, Hallett M, Li T, Coote M, Cody N, Sun ZS, Soares CN, Turecki G, Steiner M, Szyf M. Maternal depression is associated with DNA methylation changes in cord blood T lymphocytes and adult hippocampi. Transl Psychiatry. 2015;5(4):e545. PMCID: PMC4462598. http://www.ncbi.nlm.nih.gov/pubmed/25849984.
404. Zhu Y, Strachan E, Fowler E, Bacus T, Roy-Byrne P, Zhao J. Genome-wide profiling of DNA methylome and transcriptome in peripheral blood monocytes for major depression: a monozygotic discordant twin study. Transl Psychiatry. 2019;9(1):215. PMCID: PMC6718674. http://www.ncbi.nlm.nih.gov/pubmed/31477685
405. Hicks EM, Seah C, Cote A, Marchese S, Brennand KJ, Nestler EJ, Girgenti MJ, Huckins LM. Integrating genetics and transcriptomics to study major depressive disorder: a conceptual framework, bioinformatic approaches, and recent findings. Transl Psychiatry. 2023;13(1):129. PMCID: PMC10115809. http://www.ncbi.nlm.nih.gov/pubmed/37076454
406. Yuan M, Yang B, Rothschild G, Mann JJ, Sanford LD, Tang X, Huang C, Wang C, Zhang W. Epigenetic regulation in major depression and other stress-related disorders: molecular mechanisms, clinical relevance and therapeutic potential. Signal Transduct Target Ther. 2023;8(1):309. PMCID: PMC10465587. http://www.ncbi.nlm.nih.gov/pubmed/37644009
407. Murgatroyd C, Quinn JP, Sharp HM, Pickles A, Hill J. Effects of prenatal and postnatal depression, and maternal stroking, at the glucocorticoid receptor gene. Transl Psychiatry. 2015;5(5):e560. PMCID: PMC4471282. http://www.ncbi.nlm.nih.gov/pubmed/25942041
408. Maud C, Ryan J, McIntosh JE, Olsson CA. The role of oxytocin receptor gene (OXTR) DNA methylation (DNAm) in human social and emotional functioning: a systematic narrative review. BMC Psychiatry. 2018;18(1):154. PMCID: PMC5975530. http://www.ncbi.nlm.nih.gov/pubmed/29843655
409. Carlberg L, Scheibelreiter J, Hassler MR, Schloegelhofer M, Schmoeger M, Ludwig B, Kasper S, Aschauer H, Egger G, Schosser A. Brain-derived neurotrophic factor (BDNF)-epigenetic regulation in unipolar and bipolar affective disorder. J Affect Disord. 2014;168:399–406. PMID: 25106037. http://www.ncbi.nlm.nih.gov/pubmed/25106037

410. Tanaka M, Tóth F, Polyák H, Szabó Á, Mándi Y, Vécsei L. Immune influencers in action: metabolites and enzymes of the tryptophan-kynurenine metabolic pathway. Biomedicine. 2021;9(7):734. PMCID: PMC8301407. http://www.ncbi.nlm.nih.gov/pubmed/34202246
411. Franklin TB, Saab BJ, Mansuy IM. Neural mechanisms of stress resilience and vulnerability. Neuron. 2012;75(5):747–61. PMID: 22958817. http://www.ncbi.nlm.nih.gov/pubmed/22958817
412. Jiang S, Postovit L, Cattaneo A, Binder EB, Aitchison KJ. Epigenetic modifications in stress response genes associated with childhood trauma. Front Psychiatry. 2019;10:808. PMCID: PMC6857662. http://www.ncbi.nlm.nih.gov/pubmed/31780969
413. Li S, Papale LA, Kintner DB, Sabat G, Barrett-Wilt GA, Cengiz P, Alisch RS. Hippocampal increase of 5-hmC in the glucocorticoid receptor gene following acute stress. Behav Brain Res. 2015;286:236–40. PMCID: PMC4398338. http://www.ncbi.nlm.nih.gov/pubmed/25746451
414. Unternaehrer E, Luers P, Mill J, Dempster E, Meyer AH, Staehli S, Lieb R, Hellhammer DH, Meinlschmidt G. Dynamic changes in DNA methylation of stress-associated genes (OXTR, BDNF) after acute psychosocial stress. Transl Psychiatry. 2012;2(8):e150. PMCID: PMC3432191. http://www.ncbi.nlm.nih.gov/pubmed/22892716
415. Alasaari JS, Lagus M, Ollila HM, Toivola A, Kivimäki M, Vahtera J, Kronholm E, Härmä M, Puttonen S, Paunio T. Environmental stress affects DNA methylation of a CpG rich promoter region of serotonin transporter gene in a nurse cohort. PLoS One. 2012;7(9):e45813. PMCID: PMC3461019. http://www.ncbi.nlm.nih.gov/pubmed/23029256
416. Zhou A, Ancelin ML, Ritchie K, Ryan J. Childhood adverse events and BDNF promoter methylation in later-life. Front Psychiatry. 2023;14:1108485. PMCID: PMC9998928. http://www.ncbi.nlm.nih.gov/pubmed/36911114
417. Nagy C, Suderman M, Yang J, Szyf M, Mechawar N, Ernst C, Turecki G. Astrocytic abnormalities and global DNA methylation patterns in depression and suicide. Mol Psychiatry. 2015;20(3):320–8. PMCID: PMC5293540. http://www.ncbi.nlm.nih.gov/pubmed/24662927
418. Ropret S, Kouter K, Zupanc T, Videtic Paska A. BDNF methylation and mRNA expression in brain and blood of completed suicides in Slovenia. World J Psychiatry. 2021;11(12):1301–13. PMCID: PMC8717036. http://www.ncbi.nlm.nih.gov/pubmed/35070779
419. Haghighi F, Galfalvy H, Chen S, Huang YY, Cooper TB, Burke AK, Oquendo MA, Mann JJ, Sublette ME. DNA methylation perturbations in genes involved in polyunsaturated fatty acid biosynthesis associated with depression and suicide risk. Front Neurol. 2015;6:92. PMCID: PMC4412056. http://www.ncbi.nlm.nih.gov/pubmed/25972837
420. Kouter K, Zupanc T, Videtič Paska A. Genome-wide DNA methylation in suicide victims revealing impact on gene expression. J Affect Disord. 2019;253:419–25. PMID: 31103807. http://www.ncbi.nlm.nih.gov/pubmed/31103807
421. Lee A, Thuras P, Baller J, Jiao C, Guo B, Erbes CR, Polusny MA, Liu C, Wu B, Lim KO, Bishop JR. Serotonin transporter (SLC6A4) and FK506-binding protein 5 (FKBP5) genotype and methylation relationships with response to meditation in veterans with PTSD. Mol Neurobiol. 2024;61(11):9608–22. PMID: 38671329. http://www.ncbi.nlm.nih.gov/pubmed/38671329
422. Yehuda R, Daskalakis NP, Desarnaud F, Makotkine I, Lehrner AL, Koch E, Flory JD, Buxbaum JD, Meaney MJ, Bierer LM. Epigenetic biomarkers as predictors and correlates of symptom improvement following psychotherapy in combat veterans with PTSD. Front Psychiatry. 2013;4:118. PMCID: PMC3784793. http://www.ncbi.nlm.nih.gov/pubmed/24098286
423. Brown KM, Hui Q, Huang Y, Taylor JY, Prescott L, de Mendoza VB, Crusto C, Sun YV. Association between stress and coping with DNA methylation of blood pressure-related genes among African American women. Chronic Stress (Thousand Oaks). 2019;3:2470547019879088. PMCID: PMC7213592. http://www.ncbi.nlm.nih.gov/pubmed/32395678
424. Wilker S, Vukojevic V, Schneider A, Pfeiffer A, Inerle S, Pauly M, Elbert T, Papassotiropoulos A, de Quervain D, Kolassa IT. Epigenetics of traumatic stress: the association of NR3C1 methylation and posttraumatic stress disorder symptom changes in response to narrative exposure therapy. Transl Psychiatry. 2023;13(1):14. PMCID: PMC9852425. http://www.ncbi.nlm.nih.gov/pubmed/36658116
425. Ferioli M, Zauli G, Maiorano P, Milani D, Mirandola P, Neri LM. Role of physical exercise in the regulation of epigenetic mechanisms in inflammation, cancer, neurodegenerative diseases, and aging process. J Cell Physiol. 2019;234(9):14852–64. PMID: 30767204. http://www.ncbi.nlm.nih.gov/pubmed/30767204
426. Ieraci A, Mallei A, Musazzi L, Popoli M. Physical exercise and acute restraint stress differentially modulate hippocampal brain-derived neurotrophic factor transcripts and epigenetic mechanisms in mice. Hippocampus. 2015;25(11):1380–92. PMID: 25820928. http://www.ncbi.nlm.nih.gov/pubmed/25820928
427. Harkess KN, Ryan J, Delfabbro PH, Cohen-Woods S. Preliminary indications of the effect of a brief yoga intervention on markers of inflammation and DNA methylation in chronically stressed women. Transl Psychiatry. 2016;6(11):e965. PMCID: PMC5290356. http://www.ncbi.nlm.nih.gov/pubmed/27898068
428. Lewis CR, Tafur J, Spencer S, Green JM, Harrison C, Kelmendi B, Rabin DM, Yehuda R, Yazar-Klosinski B, Cahn BR. Pilot study suggests DNA methylation of the glucocorticoid receptor gene (NR3C1) is associated with MDMA-assisted therapy treatment response for severe PTSD. Front Psychiatry. 2023;14:959590. PMCID: PMC9939628. http://www.ncbi.nlm.nih.gov/pubmed/36815187
429. Son J, Shin J. Bimodal effects of sunlight on major depressive disorder. Compr Psychiatry. 2021;108:152232. PMID: 33905989. http://www.ncbi.nlm.nih.gov/pubmed/33905989
430. Munir S, Gunturu S, Abbas M. Seasonal Affective Disorder. StatPearls [Internet]. Treasure Island (FL): StatPearls Publishing; 2025 [cited 2025 Jan 17]. Available from: http://www.ncbi.nlm.nih.gov/books/NBK568745/. PMID: 33760504. http://www.ncbi.nlm.nih.gov/pubmed/33760504.
431. Foster RG, Hughes S, Peirson SN. Circadian Photoentrainment in mice and humans. Biology (Basel). 2020;9(7):180. PMCID: PMC7408241. http://www.ncbi.nlm.nih.gov/pubmed/32708259
432. Aranda ML, Schmidt TM. Diversity of intrinsically photosensitive retinal ganglion cells: circuits and functions. Cell Mol Life Sci. 2021;78(3):889–907. PMCID: PMC8650628. http://www.ncbi.nlm.nih.gov/pubmed/32965515
433. Wirz-Justice A, Skene DJ, Münch M. The relevance of daylight for humans. Biochem Pharmacol. 2021;191:114304. PMID: 33129807. http://www.ncbi.nlm.nih.gov/pubmed/33129807
434. Fisk AS, Tam SKE, Brown LA, Vyazovskiy VV, Bannerman DM, Peirson SN. Light and cognition: roles for circadian rhythms, sleep, and arousal. Front Neurol. 2018;9:56. PMCID: PMC5811463. http://www.ncbi.nlm.nih.gov/pubmed/37980177
435. Prayag AS, Münch M, Aeschbach D, Chellappa SL, Gronfier C. Light modulation of human clocks, wake, and sleep. Clocks Sleep. 2019;1(1):193–208. PMCID: PMC7185269. http://www.ncbi.nlm.nih.gov/pubmed/32342043.
436. Paul S, Brown T. Direct effects of the light environment on daily neuroendocrine control. J Endocrinol 2019;JOE-19-0302.R1. PMID: 31394505. http://www.ncbi.nlm.nih.gov/pubmed/31394505

437. Pollock NJ, Apok C, Concepcion T, Delgado RA, Rasmus S, Chatwood S, Collins PY. Global goals and suicide prevention in the Circumpolar North. Indian J Psychiatry. 2020;62(1):7–14. PMCID: PMC6964448. http://www.ncbi.nlm.nih.gov/pubmed/32001925
438. Bauer M, Glenn T, Achtyes ED, Alda M, Agaoglu E, Altınbaş K, Andreassen OA, Angelopoulos E, Ardau R, Vares EA, Aydin M, Ayhan Y, Baethge C, Bauer R, Baune BT, Balaban C, Becerra-Palars C, Behere AP, Behere PB, Belete H, Belete T, Belizario GO, Bellivier F, Belmaker RH, Benedetti F, Berk M, Bersudsky Y, Bicakci Ş, Birabwa-Oketcho H, Bjella TD, Brady C, Cabrera J, Cappucciati M, Castro AMP, Chen WL, Cheung EYW, Chiesa S, Crowe M, Cuomo A, Dallaspezia S, Del Zompo M, Desai P, Dodd S, Donix M, Etain B, Fagiolini A, Fellendorf FT, Ferensztajn-Rochowiak E, Fiedorowicz JG, Fountoulakis KN, Frye MA, Geoffroy PA, Gonzalez-Pinto A, Gottlieb JF, Grof P, Haarman BCM, Harima H, Hasse-Sousa M, Henry C, Høffding L, Houenou J, Imbesi M, Isometsä ET, Ivkovic M, Janno S, Johnsen S, Kapczinski F, Karakatsoulis GN, Kardell M, Kessing LV, Kim SJ, König B, Kot TL, Koval M, Kunz M, Lafer B, Landén M, Larsen ER, Lenger M, Lewitzka U, Licht RW, Lopez-Jaramillo C, MacKenzie A, Madsen HØ, Madsen SAKA, Mahadevan J, Mahardika A, Manchia M, Marsh W, Martinez-Cengotitabengoa M, Martiny K, Mashima Y, McLoughlin DM, Meesters Y, Melle I, Meza-Urzúa F, Ming MY, Monteith S, Moorthy M, Morken G, Mosca E, Mozzhegorov AA, Munoz R, Mythri SV, Nacef F, Nadella RK, Nakanotani T, Nielsen RE, O'Donovan C, Omrani A, Osher Y, Ouali U, Pantovic-Stefanovic M, Pariwatcharakul P, Petite J, Pfennig A, Ruiz YP, Pilhatsch M, Pinna M, Pompili M, Porter R, Quiroz D, Rabelo-da-Ponte FD, Ramesar R, Rasgon N, Ratta-Apha W, Ratzenhofer M, Redahan M, Reddy MS, Reif A, Reininghaus EZ, Richards JG, Ritter P, Rybakowski JK, Sathyaputri L, Scippa ÂM, Simhandl C, Severus E, Smith D, Smith J, Stackhouse PW, Stein DJ, Stilwell K, Strejilevich S, Su KP, Subramaniam M, Sulaiman AH, Suominen K, Tanra AJ, Tatebayashi Y, Teh WL, Tondo L, Torrent C, Tuinstra D, Uchida T, Vaaler AE, Veeh J, Vieta E, Viswanath B, Yoldi-Negrete M, Yalcinkaya OK, Young AH, Zgueb Y, Whybrow PC. Variations in seasonal solar insolation are associated with a history of suicide attempts in bipolar I disorder. Int J Bipolar Disord. 2021;9(1):26. PMCID: PMC8408297. http://www.ncbi.nlm.nih.gov/pubmed/34467430
439. Peng B, Wang R, Zuo W, Liu H, Deng C, Jing X, Hu H, Zhao W, Qin P, Dai L, Chen Z, Zhang Y, Liu XA. Distinct correlation network of clinical characteristics in suicide attempters having adolescent major depressive disorder with non-suicidal self-injury. Transl Psychiatry. 2024;14(1):134. PMCID: PMC10914800. http://www.ncbi.nlm.nih.gov/pubmed/38443348
440. Smith AR, Zuromski KL, Dodd DR. Eating disorders and suicidality: what we know, what we don't know, and suggestions for future research. Curr Opin Psychol. 2018;22:63–7. PMID: 28846874. http://www.ncbi.nlm.nih.gov/pubmed/28846874
441. Qin P. The impact of psychiatric illness on suicide: differences by diagnosis of disorders and by sex and age of subjects. J Psychiatr Res. 2011;45(11):1445–52. PMID: 21722920. http://www.ncbi.nlm.nih.gov/pubmed/21722920
442. López-Villatoro JM, De la Torre-Luque A, MacDowell KS, Galvez-Merlin A, Gómez Del Barrio A, Beato-Fernández L, Ruiz-Guerrero F, Mola-Cardenes P, Polo-Montes F, León-Velasco M, Castro-Fuentes L, Leza JC, Carrasco JL, Díaz-Marsá M. Transdiagnostic inflammatory and oxidative biomarkers with predictive capacity of self-injurious behavior in impulsive and unstable disorders. Prog Neuro-Psychopharmacol Biol Psychiatry. 2024;130:110927. PMID: 38151169. http://www.ncbi.nlm.nih.gov/pubmed/38151169
443. Steiger AE, Allemand M, Robins RW, Fend HA. Low and decreasing self-esteem during adolescence predict adult depression two decades later. J Pers Soc Psychol. 2014;106(2):325–38. PMID: 24467425. http://www.ncbi.nlm.nih.gov/pubmed/24467425
444. Park K, Yang TC. The long-term effects of self-esteem on depression: the roles of alcohol and substance uses during young adulthood. Sociol Q. 2017;58(3):429–46. PMCID: PMC5602593. http://www.ncbi.nlm.nih.gov/pubmed/28936002
445. Horvath S. Erratum to: DNA methylation age of human tissues and cell types. Genome Biol. 2015;16(1):96. PMCID: PMC4427927. http://www.ncbi.nlm.nih.gov/pubmed/25968125; http://www.ncbi.nlm.nih.gov/pubmed/24138928
446. Nixon MK, Levesque C, Preyde M, Vanderkooy J, Cloutier PF. The Ottawa self-injury inventory: evaluation of an assessment measure of nonsuicidal self-injury in an inpatient sample of adolescents. Child Adolesc Psychiatry Ment Health. 2015;9:26. PMCID: PMC4495629. http://www.ncbi.nlm.nih.gov/pubmed/26157482
447. Zheng D, Bi X, Zhang T, Han C, Ma T, Wang L, Sun M, Cui K, Yang L, Liu L. Epigenetic alterations of the promoter region of the POMC gene in adolescent depressive disorder patients with nonsuicidal self-injury behaviors. Psychol Res Behav Manag. 2020;13:997–1008. PMCID: PMC7678717. http://www.ncbi.nlm.nih.gov/pubmed/33235529
448. Xiao J, Kong T, McWhinnie CM, Yao S, Zhu X, Zhao S, Duan S. The tripartite model for assessing symptoms of depression and anxiety: psychometric properties of the Chinese version of the mood and anxiety symptoms questionnaire in patients with essential hypertension. J Cardiovasc Nurs. 2015;30(6):522–8. PMID: 25325368. http://www.ncbi.nlm.nih.gov/pubmed/25325368
449. Yao S, Yang H, Zhu X, Auerbach RP, Abela JRZ, Pulleyblank RW, Tong X. An examination of the psychometric properties of the Chinese version of the Barratt Impulsiveness Scale, 11th version in a sample of Chinese adolescents. Percept Mot Skills. 2007;104(3 Pt 2):1169–82. PMID: 17879649. http://www.ncbi.nlm.nih.gov/pubmed/17879649
450. Li J, Han ZR, Gao MM, Sun X, Ahemaitijiang N. Psychometric properties of the Chinese version of the Difficulties in Emotion Regulation Scale (DERS): factor structure, reliability, and validity. Psychol Assess. 2018;30(5):e1–9. PMID: 29756796. http://www.ncbi.nlm.nih.gov/pubmed/29756796
451. Bohus M, Kleindienst N, Limberger MF, Stieglitz RD, Domsalla M, Chapman AL, Steil R, Philipsen A, Wolf M. The short version of the Borderline Symptom List (BSL-23): development and initial data on psychometric properties. Psychopathology. 2009;42(1):32–9. PMID: 19023232 http://www.ncbi.nlm.nih.gov/pubmed/19023232
452. Bernstein DP, Stein JA, Newcomb MD, Walker E, Pogge D, Ahluvalia T, Stokes J, Handelsman L, Medrano M, Desmond D, Zule W. Development and validation of a brief screening version of the childhood trauma questionnaire. Child Abuse Negl. 2003;27(2):169–90. PMID: 12615092. http://www.ncbi.nlm.nih.gov/pubmed/12615092
453. Colledani D, Anselmi P, Robusto E. Using item response theory for the development of a new short form of the Eysenck personality questionnaire-revised. Front Psychol. 2018;9:1834. PMCID: PMC6190847. http://www.ncbi.nlm.nih.gov/pubmed/30356840
454. Scheibe VM, Brenner AM, de Souza GR, Menegol R, Almiro PA, da Rocha NS. The Eysenck Personality Questionnaire Revised – Abbreviated (EPQR-A): psychometric properties of the Brazilian Portuguese version. Trends Psychiatry Psychother. 2023;45:e20210342. PMCID: PMC9991414. http://www.ncbi.nlm.nih.gov/pubmed/34761882
455. Giovazolias T, Karagiannopoulou E, Mitsopoulou E. Can the factor structure of Defense Style Questionnaire (DSQ-40) contribute to our understanding of parental acceptance/rejection, bullying,

victimization and perceived well-being in Greek early adolescents? Eur J Psychol. 2017;13(2):269–85. PMCID: PMC5450984. http://www.ncbi.nlm.nih.gov/pubmed/28580026
456. Rosenberg M. The association between self-esteem and anxiety. J Psychiatr Res. 1962;1:135–52. PMID: 13974903. http://www.ncbi.nlm.nih.gov/pubmed/13974903
457. Miyamoto RH, Hishinuma ES, Nishimura ST, Nahulu LB, Andrade NN, Johnson RC, Makini GK, Yuen NY, Kim SP, Goebert DA, Carlton BS, Bell CK. Equivalencies regarding the measurement and constructs of self-esteem and major life events in an Asian/Pacific islander sample. Cultur Divers Ethnic Minor Psychol. 2001;7(2):152–63. PMID: 11381817. http://www.ncbi.nlm.nih.gov/pubmed/11381817
458. Oberdoerffer P, Sinclair DA. The role of nuclear architecture in genomic instability and ageing. Nat Rev Mol Cell Biol. 2007;8(9):692–702. PMID: 17700626. http://www.ncbi.nlm.nih.gov/pubmed/17700626
459. Campisi J, Vijg J. Does damage to DNA and other macromolecules play a role in aging? If so, how? J Gerontol A Biol Sci Med Sci. 2009;64(2):175–8. PMCID: PMC2655027. http://www.ncbi.nlm.nih.gov/pubmed/19228786
460. Bell JT, Tsai PC, Yang TP, Pidsley R, Nisbet J, Glass D, Mangino M, Zhai G, Zhang F, Valdes A, Shin SY, Dempster EL, Murray RM, Grundberg E, Hedman AK, Nica A, Small KS, MuTHER Consortium, Dermitzakis ET, McCarthy MI, Mill J, Spector TD, Deloukas P. Epigenome-wide scans identify differentially methylated regions for age and age-related phenotypes in a healthy ageing population. PLoS Genet. 2012;8(4):e1002629. PMCID: PMC3330116. http://www.ncbi.nlm.nih.gov/pubmed/22532803
461. Shiffman S, Stone AA, Hufford MR. Ecological momentary assessment. Annu Rev Clin Psychol. 2008;4:1–32. PMID: 18509902. http://www.ncbi.nlm.nih.gov/pubmed/18509902
462. Sedano-Capdevila A, Porras-Segovia A, Bello HJ, Baca-García E, Barrigon ML. Use of ecological momentary assessment to study suicidal thoughts and behavior: a systematic review. Curr Psychiatry Rep. 2021;23(7):41. PMID: 34003405. http://www.ncbi.nlm.nih.gov/pubmed/34003405
463. Torous J, Larsen ME, Depp C, Cosco TD, Barnett I, Nock MK, Firth J. Smartphones, Sensors, and machine learning to advance real-time prediction and interventions for suicide prevention: a review of current progress and next steps. Curr Psychiatry Rep 2018;20(7):51. PMID: 29956120. http://www.ncbi.nlm.nih.gov/pubmed/29956120
464. Singh V, Sarkar S, Gaur V, Grover S, Singh OP. Clinical practice guidelines on using artificial intelligence and gadgets for mental health and well-being. Indian J Psychiatry. 2024;66(Suppl 2):S414–9. PMCID: PMC10911327. http://www.ncbi.nlm.nih.gov/pubmed/38445270
465. Chi S, Lee MS. Personalized medicine using neuroimmunological biomarkers in depressive disorders. J Pers Med. 2021;11(2):114. PMCID: PMC7916349. http://www.ncbi.nlm.nih.gov/pubmed/33578686.
466. Ammerman BA, Law KC. Using intensive time sampling methods to capture daily suicidal ideation: a systematic review. J Affect Disord. 2022;299:108–17. PMID: 34718039. http://www.ncbi.nlm.nih.gov/pubmed/34718039
467. Gee BL, Han J, Benassi H, Batterham PJ. Suicidal thoughts, suicidal behaviours and self-harm in daily life: a systematic review of ecological momentary assessment studies. Digit Health. 2020;6:2055207620963958. PMCID: PMC7649887. http://www.ncbi.nlm.nih.gov/pubmed/33224516
468. Mann JJ, Apter A, Bertolote J, Beautrais A, Currier D, Haas A, Hegerl U, Lonnqvist J, Malone K, Marusic A, Mehlum L, Patton G, Phillips M, Rutz W, Rihmer Z, Schmidtke A, Shaffer D, Silverman M, Takahashi Y, Varnik A, Wasserman D, Yip P, Hendin H. Suicide prevention strategies: a systematic review. JAMA. 2005;294(16):2064–74. PMID: 16249421. http://www.ncbi.nlm.nih.gov/pubmed/16249421
469. Pompili M, Belvederi Murri M, Patti S, Innamorati M, Lester D, Girardi P, Amore M. The communication of suicidal intentions: a meta-analysis. Psychol Med. 2016;46(11):2239–53. PMID: 27239944. http://www.ncbi.nlm.nih.gov/pubmed/27239944
470. Czyz EK, King CA, Al-Dajani N, Zimmermann L, Hong V, Nahum-Shani I. Ecological momentary assessments and passive sensing in the prediction of short-term suicidal ideation in young adults. JAMA Netw Open 2023;6(8):e2328005. PMCID: PMC10410485. http://www.ncbi.nlm.nih.gov/pubmed/37552477
471. Miranda O, Fan P, Qi X, Yu Z, Ying J, Wang H, Brent DA, Silverstein JC, Chen Y, Wang L. DeepBiomarker: identifying important lab tests from electronic medical Records for the prediction of suicide-related events among PTSD patients. J Pers Med 2022;12(4):524. PMCID: PMC9025406. http://www.ncbi.nlm.nih.gov/pubmed/35455640
472. Martínez-Camblor P, Pérez-Fernández S, Díaz-Coto S. The area under the generalized receiver-operating characteristic curve. Int J Biostat. 2021;18(1):293–306. PMID: 33761578. http://www.ncbi.nlm.nih.gov/pubmed/33761578
473. Products – Data Briefs – Number 309 – June 2018
474. NCHS Data Brief, Number 362, April 2020
475. Key Substance Use and Mental Health Indicators in the United States: Results from the 2021 National Survey on Drug Use and Health
476. Suicide mortality in the United States, 2000–2020
477. Kleiman EM, Turner BJ, Fedor S, Beale EE, Huffman JC, Nock MK. Examination of real-time fluctuations in suicidal ideation and its risk factors: results from two ecological momentary assessment studies. J Abnorm Psychol. 2017;126(6):726–38. PMID: 28481571. http://www.ncbi.nlm.nih.gov/pubmed/28481571
478. Baryshnikov I, Rosenström T, Isometsä E. Predicting a short-term change of suicidal ideation in inpatients with depression: an ecological momentary assessment. J Affect Disord. 2024;350:1–6. PMID: 38232774. http://www.ncbi.nlm.nih.gov/pubmed/38232774
479. Nock MK, Borges G, Bromet EJ, Alonso J, Angermeyer M, Beautrais A, Bruffaerts R, Chiu WT, de Girolamo G, Gluzman S, de Graaf R, Gureje O, Haro JM, Huang Y, Karam E, Kessler RC, Lepine JP, Levinson D, Medina-Mora ME, Ono Y, Posada-Villa J, Williams D. Cross-national prevalence and risk factors for suicidal ideation, plans and attempts. Br J Psychiatry. 2008;192(2):98–105. PMCID: PMC2259024. http://www.ncbi.nlm.nih.gov/pubmed/18245022
480. Klonsky ED, May AM, Saffer BY. Suicide, suicide attempts, and suicidal ideation. Annu Rev Clin Psychol. 2016;12:307–30. PMID: 26772209. http://www.ncbi.nlm.nih.gov/pubmed/26772209
481. Suicide
482. Miller AB, Prinstein MJ. Adolescent suicide as a failure of acute stress-response systems. Annu Rev Clin Psychol. 2019;15:425–50. PMCID: PMC6953613. http://www.ncbi.nlm.nih.gov/pubmed/30786243
483. Nock MK, Green JG, Hwang I, McLaughlin KA, Sampson NA, Zaslavsky AM, Kessler RC. Prevalence, correlates, and treatment of lifetime suicidal behavior among adolescents: results from the National Comorbidity Survey Replication Adolescent Supplement. JAMA Psychiatry. 2013;70(3):300–10. PMCID: PMC3886236. http://www.ncbi.nlm.nih.gov/pubmed/23303463
484. Dobbertin M, Blair KS, Aloi J, Bajaj S, Bashford-Largo J, Mathur A, Zhang R, Carollo E, Schwartz A, Elowsky J, Ringle JL, Tyler P, Blair RJ. Neural correlates of automatic emotion regulation and their association with suicidal ideation in adolescents during the first 90-days of residential care. Transl Psychiatry.

2024;14(1):54. PMCID: PMC10806086. http://www.ncbi.nlm.nih.gov/pubmed/38263400
485. Kõlves K, de Leo D. Suicide methods in children and adolescents. Eur Child Adolesc Psychiatry. 2017;26(2):155–64. PMID: 27194156. http://www.ncbi.nlm.nih.gov/pubmed/27194156
486. Stanley IH. Advancements in the understanding of PTSD and suicide risk: introduction to a special section. Psychol Trauma. 2021;13(7):723–4. PMID: 34723566. http://www.ncbi.nlm.nih.gov/pubmed/34723566
487. Gilmore AK, Ward-Ciesielski EF, Smalling A, Limowski AR, Hahn CK, Jaffe AE. Managing post-sexual assault suicide risk. Arch Womens Ment Health. 2020;23(5):673–9. PMCID: PMC8104449. http://www.ncbi.nlm.nih.gov/pubmed/32623514
488. Chou PH, Ito M, Horikoshi M. Associations between PTSD symptoms and suicide risk: a comparison of 4-factor and 7-factor models. J Psychiatr Res. 2020;129:47–52. PMID: 32563777. http://www.ncbi.nlm.nih.gov/pubmed/32563777
489. Guidi J, Lucente M, Sonino N, Fava GA. Allostatic load and its impact on health: a systematic review. Psychother Psychosom. 2021;90(1):11–27. PMID: 32799204. http://www.ncbi.nlm.nih.gov/pubmed/32799204
490. Doering S, Probert-Lindström S, Ehnvall A, Wiktorsson S, Palmqvist Öberg N, Bergqvist E, Stefenson A, Fransson J, Westrin Å, Waern M. Anxiety symptoms preceding suicide: a Swedish nationwide record review. J Affect Disord. 2024;355:317–24. PMID: 38552915. http://www.ncbi.nlm.nih.gov/pubmed/38552915
491. Blasco-Fontecilla H, Delgado-Gomez D, Ruiz-Hernandez D, Aguado D, Baca-Garcia E, Lopez-Castroman J. Combining scales to assess suicide risk. J Psychiatr Res. 2012;46(10):1272–7. PMID: 22795298. http://www.ncbi.nlm.nih.gov/pubmed/22795298
492. Velupillai S, Hadlaczky G, Baca-Garcia E, Gorrell GM, Werbeloff N, Nguyen D, Patel R, Leightley D, Downs J, Hotopf M, Dutta R. Risk assessment tools and data-driven approaches for predicting and preventing suicidal behavior. Front Psychiatry. 2019;10:36. PMCID: PMC6381841. http://www.ncbi.nlm.nih.gov/pubmed/30814958
493. Blasco-Fontecilla H, Mendez-Bustos P, Lopez-Morinigo JD. Toward a biosignature of suicide reattempt. Curr Top Behav Neurosci. 2020;46:79–88. PMID: 32840862. http://www.ncbi.nlm.nih.gov/pubmed/32840862
494. Strimbu K, Tavel JA. What are biomarkers? Curr Opin HIV AIDS. 2010;5(6):463–6. PMCID: PMC3078627. http://www.ncbi.nlm.nih.gov/pubmed/20978388
495. Yuan N, Chen Y, Xia Y, Dai J, Liu C. Inflammation-related biomarkers in major psychiatric disorders: a cross-disorder assessment of reproducibility and specificity in 43 meta-analyses. Transl Psychiatry. 2019;9(1):233. PMCID: PMC6751188. http://www.ncbi.nlm.nih.gov/pubmed/31534116
496. Biomarkers In Risk Assessment: Validity And Validation (EHC 222, 2001)
497. Violence Prevention | Violence Prevention | CDC
498. Capuzzi E, Caldiroli A, Capellazzi M, Tagliabue I, Buoli M, Clerici M. Biomarkers of suicidal behaviors: a comprehensive critical review. Adv Clin Chem. 2020;96:179–216. PMID: 32362318. http://www.ncbi.nlm.nih.gov/pubmed/32362318
499. Kang HJ, Kim JW, Kim SW, Han JS, Lyoo IK, Kim JM. Peripheral markers of suicidal behavior: current findings and clinical implications. Clin Psychopharmacol Neurosci. 2023;21(4):650–64. PMCID: PMC10591170. http://www.ncbi.nlm.nih.gov/pubmed/37859438
500. Johnston JN, Campbell D, Caruncho HJ, Henter ID, Ballard ED, Zarate CA. Suicide biomarkers to predict risk, classify diagnostic subtypes, and identify novel therapeutic targets: 5 years of promising research. Int J Neuropsychopharmacol. 2022;25(3):197–214. PMCID: PMC8929755. http://www.ncbi.nlm.nih.gov/pubmed/34865007
501. Boudreaux ED, Rundensteiner E, Liu F, Wang B, Larkin C, Agu E, Ghosh S, Semeter J, Simon G, Davis-Martin RE. Applying machine learning approaches to suicide prediction using healthcare data: overview and future directions. Front Psychiatry. 2021;12:707916. PMCID: PMC8369059. http://www.ncbi.nlm.nih.gov/pubmed/34413800
502. Lamontagne SJ, Zabala PK, Zarate CA, Ballard ED. Toward objective characterizations of suicide risk: a narrative review of laboratory-based cognitive and behavioral tasks. Neurosci Biobehav Rev. 2023;153:105361. PMCID: PMC10592047. http://www.ncbi.nlm.nih.gov/pubmed/37595649
503. Khan NZ, Javed MA. Use of artificial intelligence-based strategies for assessing suicidal behavior and mental illness: a literature review. Cureus. 2022;14(7):e27225. PMCID: PMC9400551. http://www.ncbi.nlm.nih.gov/pubmed/36035036
504. Carson NJ, Mullin B, Sanchez MJ, Lu F, Yang K, Menezes M, Cook BL. Identification of suicidal behavior among psychiatrically hospitalized adolescents using natural language processing and machine learning of electronic health records. PLoS One. 2019;14(2):e0211116. PMCID: PMC6380543. http://www.ncbi.nlm.nih.gov/pubmed/30779800
505. Burke TA, Ammerman BA, Jacobucci R. The use of machine learning in the study of suicidal and non-suicidal self-injurious thoughts and behaviors: a systematic review. J Affect Disord. 2019;245:869–84. PMID: 30699872. http://www.ncbi.nlm.nih.gov/pubmed/30699872
506. D'Anci KE, Uhl S, Giradi G, Martin C. Treatments for the prevention and management of suicide: a systematic review. Ann Intern Med. 2019;171(5):334–42. PMID: 31450239. http://www.ncbi.nlm.nih.gov/pubmed/31450239
507. Gonda X, Serafini G, Dome P. Fight the fire: Association of Cytokine Genomic Markers and Suicidal Behavior May Pave the way for future therapies. J Pers Med. 2023;13(7):1078. PMCID: PMC10381806. http://www.ncbi.nlm.nih.gov/pubmed/37511694
508. Bryan CJ. Cognitive behavioral therapy for suicide prevention (CBT-SP): implications for meeting standard of care expectations with suicidal patients. Behav Sci Law. 2019;37(3):247–58. PMID: 31119794. http://www.ncbi.nlm.nih.gov/pubmed/31119794
509. Riblet NBV, Shiner B, Young-Xu Y, Watts BV. Strategies to prevent death by suicide: meta-analysis of randomised controlled trials. Br J Psychiatry. 2017;210(6):396–402. PMID: 28428338. http://www.ncbi.nlm.nih.gov/pubmed/28428338
510. Bergqvist E, Probert-Lindström S, Fröding E, Palmqvist-Öberg N, Ehnvall A, Sunnqvist C, Sellin T, Vaez M, Waern M, Westrin Å. Health care utilisation two years prior to suicide in Sweden: a retrospective explorative study based on medical records. BMC Health Serv Res. 2022;22(1):664. PMCID: PMC9115926. http://www.ncbi.nlm.nih.gov/pubmed/35581647
511. Ji JL, Kavanagh DJ, Holmes EA, MacLeod C, Di Simplicio M. Mental imagery in psychiatry: conceptual & clinical implications. CNS Spectr. 2019;24(1):114–26. PMID: 30688194. http://www.ncbi.nlm.nih.gov/pubmed/30688194
512. Pearson J, Naselaris T, Holmes EA, Kosslyn SM. Mental imagery: functional mechanisms and clinical applications. Trends Cogn Sci. 2015;19(10):590–602. PMCID: PMC4595480. http://www.ncbi.nlm.nih.gov/pubmed/26412097
513. Görgen SM, Joormann J, Hiller W, Witthöft M. The role of mental imagery in depression: negative mental imagery induces strong implicit and explicit affect in depression. Front. Psychiatry. 2015;6:94. PMCID: PMC4493655. http://www.ncbi.nlm.nih.gov/pubmed/26217240

514. Slofstra C, Nauta MH, Holmes EA, Bos EH, Wichers M, Batalas N, Klein NS, Bockting CLH. Exploring the relation between visual mental imagery and affect in the daily life of previously depressed and never depressed individuals. Cogn Emot. 2018;32(5):1131–8. PMID: 28818000. http://www.ncbi.nlm.nih.gov/pubmed/28818000
515. Hofstra E, van Nieuwenhuizen C, Bakker M, Özgül D, Elfeddali I, de Jong SJ, van der Feltz-Cornelis CM. Effectiveness of suicide prevention interventions: a systematic review and meta-analysis. Gen Hosp Psychiatry. 2020;63:127–40. PMID: 31078311. http://www.ncbi.nlm.nih.gov/pubmed/31078311
516. Becerra CY, Wells RK, Kunihiro BP, Lee RH, Umeda L, Allan NP, Rubas NC, McCracken TA, Nunokawa CKL, Lee MH, Pidlaoan FGS, Phankitnirondorn K, Dye CK, Yamamoto BY, Peres R, Juarez R, Maunakea AK. Examining the immunoepigenetic-gut microbiome axis in the context of self-esteem among Native Hawaiians and other Pacific Islanders. Front Genet. 2023;14:1125217. https://doi.org/10.3389/fgene.2023.1125217. PMID: 37152987; PMCID: PMC10154580. Examining the immunoepigenetic-gut microbiome axis in the context of self-esteem among Native Hawaiians and other Pacific Islanders – PubMed

Diet, Food, Supplements, and Depression

20

Franklin Sunzeri

Introduction

A variety of neuropsychiatric, neurodevelopmental, and neurodegenerative disorders have been associated with complex interactions among genetics and environmental factors including nutrition [1–3]. Nutrients modify gene expression through variable and individualized interactions with other environmental factors (such as infections and psychosocial stressors), alleles, mutations, noncoding RNAs, single-nucleotide polymorphisms, and copy number variants [4–6].

Nutrition affects neurogenesis, neurodevelopment, and functions of synapses and networks in multiple and specific areas of the brain [6–9]. As mentioned in many studies, deficiencies of various neurotransmitters are associated with depression [4, 10]. These include GABA [11], norepinephrine [12], serotonin [13–17], and dopamine [18]. Production of neurotransmitters is dependent upon the balance of nutrients, many of which are provided only from our diets.

Nutrients that are necessary for neurotransmission production include B vitamins (B6, B12, folic acid), amino acids (tryptophan, tyrosine, and glutamine), and minerals (zinc, copper, iron, and magnesium) [19]. Excellent and common sources of these nutrients are included in the *Mediterranean dietary eating pattern* [20]. The Mediterranean diet is low in meat and dairy products and high in fruits, vegetables, cereals, fish, and some poultry. These include vegetables such as cruciferous, alliaceous, dark green leafy ones, legumes, whole grains (source of copper, zinc, and magnesium), eggs, and yogurt (source of tyrosine, glutamine, magnesium, and zinc).

Many of the neurotransmitters rely upon dietary sources of the eight amino acids that cannot be synthesized by a human body [21, 22]. Tryptophan is the precursor to serotonin; tyrosine and phenylalanine are precursors to catecholamines dopamine, norepinephrine, and epinephrine. It has been suggested that depletion of tryptophan may decrease brain serotonin levels and aggravate depression [13, 23–29].

Tyrosine depletion has been associated with decreased catecholamine neurotransmission and adverse effects on mood and cognition [30]. Some patients with MDD have been reported to have low serum tyrosine levels [31–33].

In contradistinction to other neurotransmitter biosynthetic pathways, synthesis rates of catecholamines and serotonin in the brain are dependent upon local substrate concentrations within the normal ranges found in vivo [31]. As a result, there are functional effects of physiological factors such as diet that affect the brain pool concentrations of these amino acids and hence their rates of conversion to neurotransmitters. In the case of tyrosine, chronic or acutely increased intake increases tyrosine concentration and stimulates catecholamine synthesis, whereas decreased availability has the opposite effects [34, 35].

Mediterranean dietary patterns similar to those that are beneficial to cardiovascular disease [36] may be associated with prevention or amelioration of depression [37]. In addition, some of the substances that we take in from our diets appear to promote depression [19, 38]. However, these results are from cohort studies, so large randomized prevention trials, and interventions including folks at high risk for depression are still needed.

One of the large-scale questionnaire studies enrolled 9255 Adventists between 2002 and 2007 [39]. There were controls for age, gender, ethnicity, BMI, education, sleep, exercise, total caloric intake, alcohol, and time between the questionnaires. Foods often found in the Mediterranean diet associated with positive and lower negative affect. Western diets were associated with lower positive affect for both males and females. Red meat intake ($p < 0.001$) and fast-food frequency ($p < 0.001$) increased negative affect for females only. Significant results included: "Intake of vegetables, fruit, olive oil, nuts, and legumes were associated with positive affect. Sweets, desserts, soda and fast-food frequency were inversely associated with positive affect. Intake of sweets, desserts and fast-food frequency were associated with nega-

F. Sunzeri (✉)
Heather Hills Consulting, Coos Bay, OR, USA

J. Raber et al. (eds.), *Understanding and Treating Depressive Disorders*, https://doi.org/10.1007/978-3-032-14465-2_20

tive affect. Intake of vegetables, fruit and nuts were inversely associated with negative affect."

Another study published in 2009 analyzed data from 3486 participants (26.2% women, mean age 55.6 years) from the Whitehall II prospective cohort [40]. They found that participants who ate a "whole foods" diet (high amounts of vegetables, fruits, and fish) vs. those who had a "processed foods" diet had significantly fewer symptoms of depression 5 years later. In Spain, a higher risk of depression has been reported with consumption of fast foods and commercial baked goods [41]. In Australia, independent of age, socioeconomic status, education, or other health behaviors, a traditional dietary pattern similar to the Mediterranean pattern associated with less risk for major depression, dysthymia, and anxiety disorders vs. a "western" pattern with processed or fried foods, refined grains, surgery stuff, and beer [42].

However, a systematic review of all the studies published until 2012 concluded that the evidence for various dietary associations with depression is suggestive but not compelling [43]. It is also difficult to rule out reverse causality. Analyses of 25 studies from nine countries found limited but frequently positive evidence for an association between traditional diets (Mediterranean or Norwegian diets) and decreased depression. They found conflicting evidence for associations between a traditional Japanese diet and depression, a "healthy" diet and depression, a Western diet and depression, and individuals with depression and the likelihood of eating a less healthy diet. Prominent were heterogeneous definitions of "healthy diet" and wide variance in measurements of diet quality and patterns.

The conflicting level of evidence presented in the 2012 review is based upon two high-quality cohort and four cross-sectional studies that reported a healthy diet reduced the likelihood of depression, whereas one high-quality cohort and various cross-sectional studies reported no association. For example, one high-quality study showed that consumption of fish, vegetables, and cereals is more prevalent among people with low or moderate depression [44]. Another study found that those who had better quality diets were less likely to be depressed, and a higher intake of processed and unhealthy foods was associated with increased anxiety [45]. Several high-quality cross-sectional studies found significant relationships between healthy diets and reduced depression [40, 42, 45–47]. However, no associations were seen in the following studies. One cohort study did not substantiate clear associations between dietary patterns and the risk of postpartum depression [48]. One study found that folate administration ameliorated depression only in women [49]. Healthy diets in a Norwegian study were associated differentially between men and women relative to anxiety and depression [45].

A 2017 meta-analysis of dietary patterns and depression showed that healthy eating patterns may decrease the risk of depression and Western-style diets may increase the risk of depression [50].

A 2009 review of clinical trials on nutritional intervention in depression has shown considerable evidence for adjuvant rather than monotherapeutic benefits of nutrients [51]. Significant associations have been identified for adjuvant activity with antidepressants for folic acid, S-adenosyl-methionine, omega-3 fatty acids, and L-tryptophan. Difficulties with control fatty acids may have prevented proper interpretation of omega-3 benefits as a monotherapy. There was insufficient evidence of utility for inositol and L-tryptophan.

Although it has been accepted for some time that a high-fat diet can lead to a variety of problems [52], including depression [53–56], obesity [57], cardiovascular problems [58], and diabetes [59], a 2013 study has shed some new light on the molecular bases of the connections. It appears that at least in mice, a high-fat diet can lead to wholesale changes in the *circadian clock* [60].

Cellular metabolism is intimately linked to circadian rhythms [60]. High-fat diets can produce a striking reorganization of metabolic pathways that can generate an extensive remodeling of the hepatic clock. Moreover, high-fat diets cause a large-scale de novo oscillation of transcripts that reorganize coordinated oscillations between coherent transcripts and metabolites.

With mass spectrometry, the researchers identified 141 of 306 metabolites that normally oscillate in mice [60]. When the mice were fed a high-fat diet, 27% of those metabolites that normally do not oscillate began to oscillate. Others stopped oscillating, while still others shifted to a different phase. DNA analysis showed that of 2826 oscillating genes, 778 oscillated irrespective of diet, 1394 oscillated only on a normal diet and 654 oscillated only on a high-fat diet.

Underlying mechanisms involve compromising of the clock proteins CLOCK: BMAL1 chromatin recruitment and a prominent cyclic activation of surrogate pathways through the nuclear hormone receptor PPARγ a transcription regulator.

Chronic consumption of high-fat foods and obesity can induce neuroplastic changes in *mesolimbic reward circuitry* that is associated with depression [56]. In mice fed a high-fat diet, increased symptoms of depression were seen including increased immobility (interpreted as *behavioral despair*) in the forced swim test. In the high-fat-fed mice, increased corticosterone followed acute restraint stress, significantly higher D2 receptor, brain-derived neurotrophic factor (BDNF), and ΔFosB (a member of the Fos family of transcription factors), but reduced D1A receptor, and protein expression in the nucleus accumbens. A positive correlation was seen between behavioral despair and the expression of

BDNF in both the nucleus accumbens and dorsolateral striatum, and CREB (cAMP response element-binding protein is a cellular transcription factor) in the dorsolateral striatum.

Apparently, it is the nutritional challenge and not the obesity itself that is the culprit. In mice, the effects were seen within 3 days, long before obesity was manifest. After 10 weeks of the high-fat diet, the mice were returned to a normal diet for 2 weeks and the changes reversed. Therefore, the good news is that it appears the effects of the high-fat diet on the circadian clock are reversible.

Perhaps, due to the complexity of nutrition, studies on the influence of individual nutrients on depression have shown equivocal results, so overall patterns of overall dietary patterns and depression have begun to be investigated [42, 61–63]. A 2014 systematic review and meta-analysis of dietary patterns and depression in community-dwelling adults concluded that high intakes of fruit, vegetables, fish, and whole grains may be associated with a reduced depression risk [64]. Reduced odds of depression were significantly associated with a healthy diet (OR[1] = 0.84; 95% CI: 0.76–0.92; $p < 0.001$). The few studies that analyzed Western diet and depression (OR = 1.17; 95% CI: 0.97–1.68; $p = 0.094$) found insignificant associations. However, more high-quality RCTs were required to bolster these results.

A systematic review was published in 2014 of RCTs of dietary interventions that used depression and/or anxiety outcomes and sought to identify characteristics of program success [65]. They found a level of heterogeneity, but 47% of the studies reported a beneficial effect of diet on symptoms of depression. Characteristics of the successful interventions were based on a single delivery mode. They used a dietitian and were less likely to recommend reducing red meat intake, select leaner meat products, or follow a low-cholesterol diet. Only one study analyzed the effect of diet on clinical depression.

Results were published in 2017 of *SMILES*' (a 12-week, parallel-group, single blind, RCT), an adjunctive dietary intervention in the treatment of moderate to severe depression [66, 67]. The dietary intervention presented by a clinical dietician included dietary advice and nutritional counseling support, which included motivational interviewing, goal setting, and mindful eating. It was designed to be easy to follow, sustainable, palatable, and satiating. The diet is in this footnote.[2] The dietary support group had significantly greater improvement between baseline and 12 weeks on the *Montgomery–Åsberg Depression Rating Scale (MADRS)* than the social support control group, $t(60.7) = 4.38$, $p < 0.001$, Cohen's $d = -1.16$. Remission, defined as a MADRS score <10, was attained for 32.3% ($n = 10$) and 8.0% ($n = 2$) of the intervention and control groups, respectively ($\chi^2(1) = 4.84$, $p = 0.028$). The number needed to treat (NNT) based on remission scores was 4.1 (95% CI of NNT 2.3–27.8).

A 2017 meta-analysis found high intakes of fruit, vegetables, whole grain, fish, olive oil, low-fat dairy and antioxidants, and low intakes of animal foods were apparently associated with a decreased risk of depression. Whereas high consumption of red and/or processed meat, refined grains, sweets, high-fat dairy products, butter, potatoes and high-fat gravy, and low intakes of fruits and vegetables were associated with an increased risk of depression [50]. Of course, there could be many factors at work here.

A 2019 meta-analysis of 16 eligible RCTs were examined for the effects of diet on depression and anxiety [72]. Even though 15 of the samples were nonclinical depression, dietary interventions significantly reduced depressive symptoms. There was no effect of dietary interventions on anxiety. Significantly greater benefits from dietary interventions were seen in females for both depression and anxiety.

A 2019 brief 3-week dietary RCT intervention showed that young adults with elevated depression symptoms can engage in and adhere to a diet intervention resulting in significantly decreased symptoms of depression [73]. Compared to control, the diet group showed[3] CESD-R ($p = 0.007$, Cohen's $d = 0.65$) and DASS-21 depression subscale ($p = 0.002$, Cohen's $d = 0.75$). DASS-21 was $p = 0.009$ at 3 months post intervention.

[1]Odds ratio (OR) is a way to represent the odds that an outcome will result when a given exposure to a variable of interest occurs compared to when the exposure does not occur. OR quantifies the strength of the association between two events. An OR greater than 1 indicates a positive association or that exposure to that variable increases the odds of that outcome. An OR less than 1 indicates a negative relationship between two events. An OR of 1 suggests no relationship between two events. An OR is frequently accompanied by a 95% confidence interval (CI). CI is a measure of precision of the OR. The smaller the CI the higher precision as long as it does not overlap OR = 1. For more information, see the Chap. 4 on evidence basics in this text.

[2]This *ModiMedDiet* was based upon previous work in preventing depression [68] including *Australian Dietary Guidelines* [69] and the *Dietary Guidelines for Adults in Greece* [70]. Quoted from reference [66]: "The ModiMedDiet is based upon 12 key food groups (recommended servings in brackets): whole grains (5–8 servings per day); vegetables (6 per day); fruit (3 per day), legumes (3–4 per week); low-fat and unsweetened dairy foods (2–3 per day); raw and unsalted nuts (1 per day); fish (at least 2 per week); lean red meats (3–4 per week) [71], chicken (2–3 per week); eggs (up to 6 per week); and olive oil (3 tablespoons per day), whilst reducing intake of 'extras' foods, such as sweets, refined cereals, fried food, fast-food, processed meats and sugary drinks (no more than 3 per week). Red or white wine consumption beyond 2 standard drinks per day and all other alcohol (e.g., spirits, beer) were included within the 'extras' food group. Individuals were advised to select red wine preferably and only drink with meals. The dietary composition of the Mod*i*MedDiet was as follows: protein 18% of total energy (E); fat 40% of E; carbohydrates 37% of E; alcohol 2% of E; fiber/other 3% of E."

[3]Centre for Epidemiological Studies Depression Scale (CESD-R); and Depression Anxiety and Stress Scale–21 depression subscales (DASS-21-D).

Mental health problems typically emerge during adolescence [74]. According to the National Comorbidity Survey–Adolescent Supplement (NCS-A), the overall prevalence of anxiety disorders was 31.9%, behavioral disorders 19.1%, mood disorders 14.3%, and substance use disorders 11.4% [75]. Approximately 40% of adolescents had more than one mental health condition. Between the ages of 13 and 18, 22.2% were severely impaired by a mental health disorder. Of these, 11.2% had a mood disorder, 9.6% had a behavioral disorder, and 8.3% had an anxiety disorder. The median age of onset was 13 for mood disorders, 11 for behavioral disorders, 6 for anxiety disorders, and 15 for substance use disorders.

The role of healthy diets in decreasing and poor diets increasing prevalence of depression in children has been seen in several adolescent populations [76–79]. For example, a 2-year study of 3040 Australian adolescents, aged 11–18 years at baseline showed that improvements in diet quality associated with improvements in mental health during follow-up and deteriorating diet quality was associated with worse psychological functioning [77]. Reverse causality did not seem to be in play.

Although many people with classic depression are obese, only atypical depression[4] is associated with elevated risk of obesity compared to the overall population [54, 55, 78, 79]. Data from the *2001–2002 National Epidemiologic Survey on Alcohol and Related Conditions (NESARC)* identified 5092 US adults with past or current major depression based on DSM-IV-TR criteria and 1500 gender-matched controls. Based on core vegetative symptoms they were classified as classic, atypical, or undifferentiated depression. Atypical subtype of depression is characterized by increased appetite and weight gain, whereas classic depression is characterized by decreased appetite and weight loss.

Marked elevation was seen in subjects with atypical depression compared to population controls and to other subtypes (OR > 2.0: $p < 0.001$). Obesity rates in classic depression were not significantly different from non-depressed subjects.

Between the 1960s and 2010, the per capita caloric intake in the USA increased by about 28% [83, 84]. High-energy diets (excessive calories from fats and sugars) impair hippocampal-dependent memory apparently via decreased neuronal growth factors, neurogenesis, and synaptic plasticity [85].

It seems that relatively short indulgence in diets rich in sugar or rich in sugar and fats can compromise hippocampal-dependent place recognition memory but not perirhinal-dependent object recognition, even before weight increases [86]. A 2012 experiment in rats has suggested that oxidative stress and neuroinflammation may be involved in this decrement of memory [86]. Rats fed sucrose had both increased hippocampal inflammation (increased TNF-α and IL-1β mRNA) and oxidative stress (increased NRF1 mRNA).

Depression may interact with functional polymorphisms of the dopamine transporter (SLC6A3) to modify food intake. Such a relationship was investigated using the *National Longitudinal Study of Adolescent Health* [87]. The researchers examined interactions between symptoms of depression and functional polymorphisms of dopamine transporter (SLC6A3), monoamine oxidase A (MAOA), dopamine receptor D2 (DRD2), and dopamine receptor D4 (DRD4) on intake of high-calorie sweet, high-calorie non-sweet, and low-calorie foods. They found that females with high levels of depression and the SLC6A3 10/10 allele exhibited significantly greater intake of high-calorie sweet foods than those women with similar levels of depression who had any SLC6A3 9 allele ($p < 0.05$).

Omega-3 Fatty Acids

Fatty acids are vital to all cells providing structure of cell membranes, energy, and signaling.[5] Fatty acids compose a large part of the nervous system where they are intimately involved in functions such as neurogenesis, stimulation of gene expression, apoptosis, inflammation, and repair. And they are involved in dysfunctions such as mental disorders, neurodegeneration, and stroke. Fatty acids of different types have different properties. Unbalanced or excess of some of these have been implicated in various disorders [88]. See Fig. 20.1.

[4]Atypical depression (depression with atypical features) is characterized by a mood that can improve in response to positive events. Other symptoms include hypersomnia, increased appetite, feeling rejected, and feeling that arms or legs are heavy [80]. Atypical depression features such as overeating are frequently associated with inflammation and metabolic disorders [81]. HPA functions may relate to atypical vs typical depression symptoms [82].

[5]A 2013 discussion of fat in the brain, can be seen in reference [88]. In 2012, a special issue entitled Cognitive Enhancers was published in the journal *Neuropharmacology*. One of the articles covers the underlying biochemical and neurophysiological mechanisms by which n-3 PUFA mediate effects on cognition from childhood through old age [89]. It is a very good read for anyone wanting additional information.

Membrane lipid composition in the brain changes from 20 to 100 years of age in normal brains from folks who did not die an agonal death [90]. These changes are dependent upon the region of the brain and the tissue type (grey matter, white matter, and myelin) [91]. For example, in one study, myelin had much higher lipid content (7841% of the dry weight) than white matter (49–66%) or gray matter (36–400%). In addition, for each protein molecule in human myelin there are 186 lipid molecules, 111 of which are polar lipids and 75 of which consist of cholesterol. The molar ratio of amino acids to polar lipids in human myelin is 2.38 to 1.

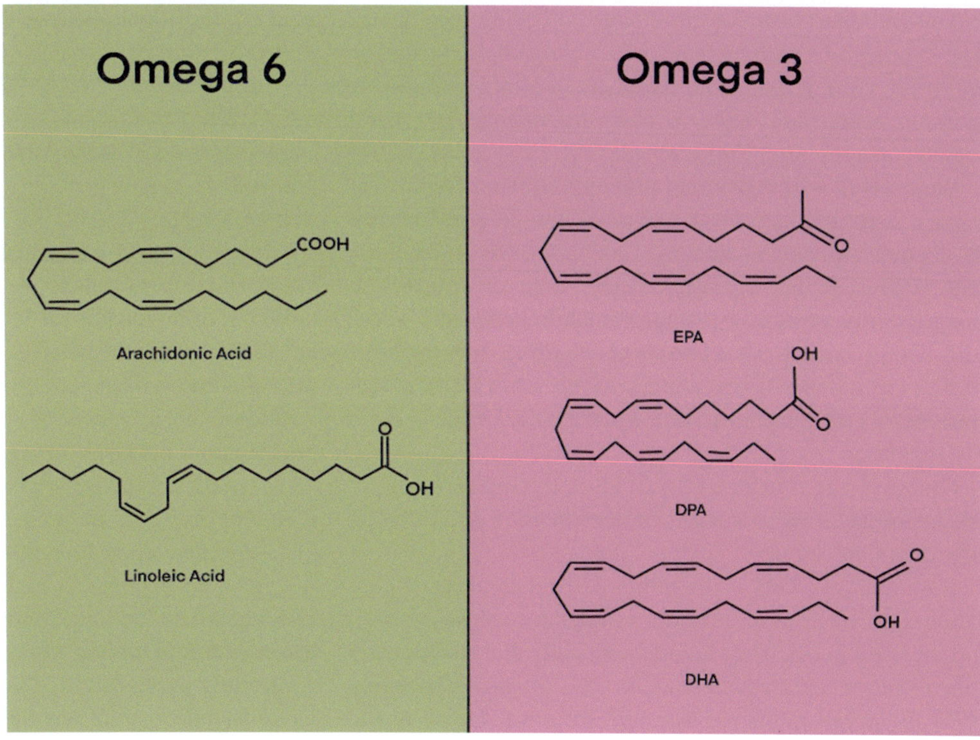

Fig. 20.1 Structural comparison of omega-6 and omega-3 polyunsaturated fatty acids. This figure illustrates the molecular structures of key omega-6 (arachidonic acid and linoleic acid) and omega-3 (eicosapentaenoic acid [EPA], docosapentaenoic acid [DPA], and docosahexaenoic acid [DHA]) fatty acids. These long-chain polyunsaturated lipids are distinguished by the position of their first double bond and play critical roles in cellular signaling, inflammation, and neurophysiology

A USDA list of dietary sources of omega-3 fatty acids and nutrient composition of foods can be found here [92, 93].

Omega-3 fatty acids (ω-3 fatty acids or n-3 fatty acids) are essential long-chain polyunsaturated fatty acids (PUFA) that human bodies cannot create. As such, they are derived from plant or marine dietary sources. These omega-3 fatty acids are composed of three groups. They are *α-Linolenic acid* (ALA) commonly found in seeds and nuts;[6] *Eicosapentaenoic acid* (EPA) which is found in algae and stored in fish that eat the algae [95]; and *Docosahexaenoic acid* (DHA) which is also derived from cold water aquatic microalgae and stored in bodies of consumers in the food chain [95, 96].

Human bodies convert ALA to EPA and DHA in hepatic pathways that are less efficient than obtaining them from a dietary source. Various stressors such as illness and aging, and consuming excessive quantities of omega-6 fatty acids can decrease this efficiency [97]. Estimates are less than 1% conversion from ALA to DHA [98, 99]. And about 5% of ALA is converted to EPA [99]. Females are more efficient than males are in converting EPA to DHA [100].

In the brain, DHA and eicosapentaenoic acid EPA appears to be the most active components of ω3-rich PUFA diets [101]. One study has shown that in mice a 2-month EPA/DHA dietary treatment increased EPA and DHA in the brain [101]. That regimen blocked inflammatory cytokines expression and changes in astrocytes morphology in the hippocampus. In addition, in aged mice, it restored spatial memory deficits and Fos-associated activation in the hippocampus.

DHA is highly concentrated in the nervous system especially in synaptic membranes and photoreceptors [102]. DHA is a vital structural component of the human brain, skin, and testes. DHA comprises more than 90% of the omega-3s in the human brain and makes up almost 25% of the total fat content of the brain [103].

It is essential to many functions including neuroprotection, memory, and successful aging. In contrast to several members of the omega-6 PUFAs, DHA is anti-inflammatory. *Neuroprotection D1 (NPD1)*, derived from DHA, is particularly involved in inflammatory balance.

It has been suggested that humans leapt ahead in producing the rapid expansion of grey matter in the cerebral cortex when shore-based dwellers discovered easily digested preformed sources of omega-3 fatty acids from coastal seafood and inland fresh waters [104]. In particular, DHA, which is not very efficiently produced in humans from the dietary ALA, has unique structural properties for cell membrane functions including being the precursor for *resolvins* and *protectins*. Along with our decreased intake of omega-3 fatty acids, excess consumption of omega-6 fatty acids displaces DHA from membrane phospholipids [104].

In the Western world, since the early part of the twentieth century, the dietary consumption of omega-3 fatty acids has declined sharply and been replaced by omega-6 fatty acids [105]. *Linoleic acid (LA)* is the principal omega 6. It is metabolized to *arachidonic acid (AA)*.

[6] *ALA* is *all-cis*-9,12,15-octadecatrienoic acid or 18:3(n-3); *EPA* is 20:5(n-3); *DHA* is *all-cis*-docosa-4,7,10,13,16,19-hexa-enoic acid, or 22:6(n-3) [94].

This trend has been fueled in large part using oils that are high in omega-6s with no omega-3s. For example, safflower, sunflower, corn, peanut, cottonseed, and sesame seed oils. In addition, using high omega-6 feeds for animals raised for human consumption [106].

We evolved with a diet that was high in fiber, fruits, vegetables, fish, and lean meat; hence, a low-fat diet that had about equal amounts of omega-3s and omega-6s [106]. It has been suggested that the ideal dietary ratio of omega-6 to omega-3 fatty acids is 1 to approximately between 1 and 2 [105–108]. Current ratios are about 20–25 to 1 in the West [105]. A minimum of 650 mg/day of EPA and DHA is recommended [109]. In North America, the daily intake is about 130 mg/day.

Omega-3 and omega-6 fatty acids are components of all cell membranes and influence gene expression and intercellular communication.

Both omega-3 fatty acids and omega-6 fatty acids in biomembranes are vital to function, maintenance, development, and integrity [110]. They are metabolically and functionally quite different and frequently are in physiological opposition [106]. Balanced ratios are essential for normal growth and development and largely the PUFA profile of cell membranes depends upon diet. Fatty acid derivatives interact with many signaling pathways [111, 112].

PUFAs constitute about 20% of the dry weight of the brain and are about 30% of the fatty acids in the brain [97]. It would seem therefore to be a reasonable hypothesis that for an individual without appropriate intake of omega-3s, there might be adverse neurological/neuropsychiatric consequences.

In addition, there is some evidence that fatty acids, especially polyunsaturated fatty acids, can modify the epigenome [113].

In order to study the essential fatty acids in the brain, it is necessary to use surrogate tissues. Two tissues that have been relatively easy to sample is blood (plasma and erythrocytes) and adipose tissue [114].

Correlations are significant but not absolute. Erythrocyte membranes reflect dietary fat intake within the past few weeks [115, 116]. For example, independent of dietary intake of EPA, in a study of 20 depressed folks, there was a significant correlation between the ratio of erythrocyte AA to EPA and severity of depression ($p < 0.05$) and depression ($p < 0.01$) [115, 117]. In erythrocyte membranes, there appears to be an association between depression and degree of esterification of serum cholesterol, an increased C20:4omega6/C20:5omega3 ratio and decreases in omega3 fractions reflecting a deficiency of omega-3s and a compensatory increase in medium chain unsaturated fatty and C22:5 omega-6 fatty acids [116]. Nonesterified fatty acid composition in plasma appears to be a good indicator of adipose fatty acid composition, because these plasma fatty acids are produced by lipolysis of adipose tissue [118].

Adipose tissue reflects dietary intake in the past 1–3 years [119, 120]. For example, adipose tissue samples of 63 survivors (mean age 84) of the *Greek Seven Countries Study* showed a negative relationship between C18:3n-3 and depression [121].

However, such relationships are not clear. In another study, when confounders of age, gender, body mass index, smoking and educational level were considered, a relationship was not found between depression and fatty acid content of adipose tissue or erythrocyte membranes [122].

Moreover, a couple of early studies showed an inverse relationship between omega-3s and depression [123]. A 1977 study found both plasma and erythrocyte EPA and DHA were higher in subjects with depression vs. controls [123]. A 1981 study found that subjects with endogenous but not reactive depression had significantly greater EPA and DHA and less LA than controls had in their plasma and to a lesser extent in their erythrocytes [124].

A study published in 2004 involving 90 adolescents from Crete found no significant association between adipose tissue levels of omega-3 or omega-6 polyunsaturated fatty acids and depression [121]. However, significant positive relationships with depression were seen between adipose tissue C20:3n-6/C18:3n-6 and (C20:3n-6 + C22:5n-3)/(C18:3n-6 + C20:5n-3) ratios. This data seems to point to an over expression of the gene encoding elongation of PUFA in adipose tissues of adolescents.

LA, among other things, favors oxidation of LDL cholesterol, stimulates immune system reactions, and platelet aggregation [106].

Proteins are either anchored within or float freely in the lipid bilayers of cell membranes. Their conformations are sensitive to the composition of surrounding lipids [110], which is critical to their functions as receptors and transporters [125–129]. Moreover, essential fatty acids can serve as precursors to second messengers involved in neuronal communication [130].

Omega fatty acids also appear to affect depression via inflammation modulation [131]. There are several mechanisms. These include via receptors and sensors that control inflammatory cell signaling and patterns of gene expressions that alter patterns of lipid and peptide mediator production. Some of these effects are related to cell membrane fatty acid composition that modifies membrane fluidity and formation of lipid rafts.

The role of cytokine mediation of depression has been discussed above. The cytokine hypothesis of depression suggests that pro-inflammatory cytokines, acting as neuromodulators, are the essential factors mediating the behavioral, neuroendocrine, and neurochemical attributes of depressive disorders [132]. Omega-3 fatty acids can reduce, whereas omega-6 fatty acids may increase, the expression of pro-inflammatory cytokines that may have indirect or direct effects on the brain [133]. The major cytokines include interleukin-1 beta (IL-1β), IL-2, IL-6, interferon-gamma, and tumor necrosis factor alpha (TNFα). Some of the effects on the brain include decrements in production and metabolism of neurotransmitters and increased activation of the HPA axis [134–136]. It is unclear, however, if cytokines are causes or epiphenomena related to depression [132].

In a circular fashion, negative moods can result in activation of peripheral pathways that increase systemic levels of inflammation [137]. In the reverse direction, the peripheral immune response may release mediators that tell the brain to make cognitive, affective, and behavioral changes of major depression.

Experiments have shown overexpression of monocyte-associated pro-inflammatory cytokines in men with mild to moderate depression compared to men with no or minimal symptoms [138].

Brain-derived neurotrophic factor (BDNF), which is negatively correlated with severity of depression, is enhanced by omega-3 fatty acids, antidepressant drugs, and voluntary exercise [139, 140]. BDNF is inhibited by psychological stress, diets high in sucrose and saturated fats.

Something fishy: There are a number of epidemiological studies that indicate a connection between declining seafood consumption and increased worldwide prevalence of depression [141]. Although they do not prove causality, it is interesting to contemplate decreased omega-3 consumption in the context of other psychosocial considerations.

Data from 23 countries (n = 14,532 subjects in 41 studies) revealed that both lower DHA content in mothers' milk [142–144] and lower seafood consumption were associated with higher rates of postpartum depression [145]. Data has also suggested that greater seafood consumption predicted lower lifetime prevalence rates of bipolar I disorder, bipolar II disorder, and bipolar spectrum disorder [146]. Fish consumption in Iceland seems to ward off seasonal affective disorder [147]. In a sample of 3204 Finnish adults, the probability of having depressive symptoms was significantly lower among frequent fish consumers than among infrequent consumers [148]. Cross-national data collected in the 1996/97 *New Zealand Health Survey* and 1997 Nutrition Survey of 4644 New Zealand adults aged 15 years and over indicated that fish consumption was significantly associated with higher self-reported mental health status [149].

However, other studies have not found such an association. For example, in a study of more than 15,000 older adults from seven low- and middle-income countries—the *10/66 study*, associations between fish consumption categories and depression were found only in Cuba (p for trend = 0.039) and China ($p < 0.001$) [150]. There were clear variations across these countries and depression seemed to be better explained by lifestyle and sociodemographics. A Finish study of 29,133 male smokers aged 50–69 years conducted from 1985 through 1988 showed that folks with anxiety or depressed mood had greater intake of both omega-3 and omega-6 fatty acids [151]. In the same Finish study, there was no correlation between omega-3 fatty acids or fish consumption and depressed mood, major depressive episodes, or suicide [152].

From the results of three cross-sectional data sets, the nationwide *Health 2000 Survey* (n = 5840), *the Fishermen Study on Finnish* fishermen and their family members (n = 1282) and the *Finntwin16 Study* on young adults (n = 4986), it appears that fish consumption or omega-3 PUFA intake is not associated with less psychological distress overall or in a population with high fish consumption [153].

As indicated above, these cases may also have introduced the confounder of increased omega-6. Moreover, there is considerable variation in toxins in species and locations of fish and shellfish. For example, mean values of the neurotoxin methyl mercury [154] concentrations for fish and shellfish species differ by greater than an order of magnitude [155–158].

On the positive side, it is possible that folks who consume more fish also have healthier lifestyles.

There is inconsistency in placebo-controlled case-report experiments designed to determine whether omega-3 supplementation is therapeutic and at what doses they might be effective in treating depression-related psychiatric conditions [159]. Some of the difficulty resides in doses ranging from recommended daily minimum up to three to four times that level and small sample sizes. What follows here are a few of the representative studies.

In the early 1980s, the first series of case reports were published where the connection between cognitive symptoms associated with the B vitamin deficiencies of pellagra and the lack of omega-3 substrates for prostaglandins was hypothesized [160–162]. Some early successes in these reports showed improvement of agoraphobia and bipolar depression with supplementation of linseed oil. One study showed that in one man who had treatment resistant depression and suicidal ideation, 4 g daily of pure EPA for 1 month not only eliminated his symptoms but MRI images also showed significant changes in increased brain cell volume in particular reduction in lateral ventricular volume [163].

Between 2006 and 2016, several meta-analyses have reviewed data on omega-3 fatty acids and depression symptoms. The results are briefly described below.

An RCT of omega-3 fatty acids as a treatment for perinatal depression found that there was no significant difference in depression scores between those receiving fish oil (800 mg/day DHA and 100 mg/day EPA) and those receiving the placebo (vegetable oil) [164].

An RCT of omega-3 fatty acids and supportive psychotherapy for perinatal depression did not find a benefit of omega-3 fatty acids over placebo [165]. All participants received psychotherapy. Participants in both groups had significant decreases in depression scores ($p < 0.0001$) from baseline.

Supplementation of 220 mg/day DHA or DHA + AA (220 mg/day each) did not prevent peri-partum depressive symptoms, in a population-based sample with low-background DHA intake [166].

The use of DHA-rich fish oil capsules (providing 800 mg/day of DHA) compared with vegetable oil capsules during pregnancy did not result in lower levels of postpartum depression in mothers or improved cognitive and language development in their offspring during early childhood [167].

An RCT compared omega-3 PUFAs (3.4 g/day) with placebo in 36 pregnant women with MDD [168]. No psychotropic agent was given 1 month prior to or during the study period. Women in the omega-3 group had significantly lower HAM-D scores at weeks 6 ($p = 0.001$) and 8 ($p = 0.019$), a significantly higher response rate (62% vs. 27%, $p = 0.03$), and a higher remission rate, although the latter did not reach statistical significance (38% vs. 18%, $p = 0.28$). At the study end, women in the omega-3 group also had significantly lower depression symptom ratings.

Several studies found beneficial results. In 2007, the *Omega-3 Fatty Acids Subcommittee, assembled by the Committee on Research on Psychiatric Treatments of the American Psychiatric Association (APA)*, showed the following [169]. The preponderance of epidemiologic and tissue compositional studies supports a protective effect of omega-3 EFA intake, particularly EPA and DHA, in mood disorders. Meta-analyses of RCTs indicated a statistically significant benefit in unipolar and bipolar depression ($p = 0.02$). Due to design and execution characteristics, the results were highly heterogeneous. They found less evidence of benefit in schizophrenia. They concluded, "EPA and DHA appear to have negligible risks and some potential benefit in major depressive disorder and bipolar disorder, but results remain inconclusive in most areas of interest in psychiatry."

In 2009, a meta-analysis suggested that there is more evidence for the benefit of EPA than for DHA in treating depression [170].

In a 2010 study of demographics of complementary and alternative medical (CAM) treatments including omega-3 EFA for MDD, meta-analysis indicated that both antidepressant and CAM monotherapy resulted in superior response rates compared with placebo [171]. Interestingly, they found that although participants had the same degree of severity, in CAM trials, they were more likely to be female and to have a lower placebo-response rate compared to those in standard antidepressant trials for MDD.

In 2010, reviewers found that despite considerable heterogeneity, there was increasing evidence of omega-3s benefit on depressed mood in individuals with diagnosed depressive illness but there was no evidence of any benefit in individuals without a diagnosis of depressive illness [172].

A 2007 analysis concluded that there was significant antidepressant benefit of omega-3 PUFAs; however, it was still premature to validate this finding due to publication bias and heterogeneity [173]. Overall beneficial antidepressant effects of omega-3 PUFAs was (ES = 0.61, $p = 0.003$) with clearly defined depression (ES = 0.69, $p = 0.002$) or with bipolar disorder (ES = 0.69, $p = 0.0009$).

In 2011, a meta-analysis tested the hypothesis that EPA is the effective component in PUFA treatment of major depressive episodes [174]. They concluded that supplements containing EPA $\geq$ 60% of total EPA + DHA, in a dose range of 200–2200 mg/day of EPA in excess of DHA, were effective against primary depression.

A 2012 meta-analysis concluded that there is strong evidence supporting the adjunctive use of omega-3 fatty acids to improve bipolar depressive symptoms, but not for attenuating manic symptoms [175].

Also in 2012, a meta-analysis was published that examined the heterogeneity in placebo-controlled trials of omega-3 fatty acid treatment of MDD [176]. They concluded, "Current published trials suggest a small, non-significant benefit of omega-3 FAs for major depression. Nearly all the treatment efficacy observed in the published literature may be attributable to publication bias." These conclusions, however, are disputed by other reviewers who find fault with their analyses [177, 178].

In 2013, a meta-analysis was performed to determine whether any psychological, pharmacological, or nutritional interventions could prevent or delay transition to psychotic disorders for people at high risk [179]. They identified 11 trials including 1246 participants with a median sample size of 81 (range 51–288). There was moderate quality evidence of an effect for CBT on reducing transition to psychosis at 12 months (risk ratio 0.54 (95% confidence interval 0.34–0.86); risk difference −0.07 (−0.14 to −0.01)). There was very low-quality evidence for omega-3 fatty acids and low to very low-quality evidence for integrated psychotherapy.

So, in terms of the evidence for therapeutic use of omega-3 fatty acids in treating depression, more large-scale, well-designed, randomized controlled trials are essential to determine the appropriate target subjects, therapeutic dose of EPA, and the composition of omega-3 fatty acids.

It should also be mentioned that indiscriminate use of EPA is not without risk [88]. For example, according to a study published in 2013, supplementation with dietary EPA

(300 mg/kg/day) in amyotrophic lateral sclerosis (ALS) may accelerate the disease progression [180]. There is some evidence that in a small percentage of individuals (<3%), high doses of omega-3 fatty acids, especially high doses of flax seed oil, may induce behavioral changes such as hypomania or mania [160, 181].

Trans-fatty Acids

Trans-fatty acid (TFA) intake appears to increase the risk for depression, whereas there is weaker evidence for a beneficial effect on depression of monounsaturated fatty acids, polyunsaturated fatty acids, and olive oil [182]. Further evidence for a detrimental association with TFAs comes from a study that looked at the quality of life assessed by *SF-36 Health Survey* [183]. It is, however, important to discriminate between natural and industrial TFAs.

TFAs are produced from natural ruminal hydrogenation and industrial partial catalytic hydrogenation [184]. These processes produce two types of TFAs with considerable differences between them. Although most of the TFAs in natural TFAs and to a lesser degree in industrial TFAs are isomers of the monounsaturated fat oleic acid (18:1), and most of the rest of the isomers are the same, their distributions are quite different. This difference appears to modify their effects. Natural TFAs are produced in ruminants (cows, sheep, and goats) by *biohydrogenation* of ingested unsaturated fats. This process occurs naturally at normal body temperature and pressure via bacterial enzymes found in the guts of these ruminants [185]. Industrial production of TFAs uses high pressure at high temperature and metal catalysts to transform liquid vegetable fats into solids. Until they became pervasive in the late 1940s, they did not exist or were found in only trace amounts in nature [185–187].

The industrial trans fatty acids found in partially hydrogenated vegetable fats have been implicated in cardiovascular disease, whereas the naturally occurring TFAs have not [143, 188]. Indeed, there is some evidence that the naturally occurring TFAs via conversion through vaccenic acid to linoleic acid may actually be beneficial in helping to lower the risk of breast cancer [144, 186, 189–191].

Dietary *trans-fatty acids (dTFA)* inhibit the production of omega-3 fatty acids. A clinical trial with 1018 subjects conducted between 1999 and 2004 demonstrated a strongly significant relationship between dTFA and greater aggression [192]. In addition, dTFA was the strongest predictor of aggression while considering cross-sectional and prospective confounders such as age, sex, and ethnicity.

In 2006, the FDA required trans fats to be labeled on all foods in which it was included [193].

Trans fatty acid intake has been seen to be predictive of depression symptoms 5 years later in middle-aged women enrolled in the Study of Women's Health Across the Nation (SWAN) [194].

Micronutrients

The World Health Organization states that more than two billion people worldwide suffer from vitamin and mineral deficiencies, primarily iodine, iron, vitamin A, and zinc, in both developing and in developed countries affecting people of all genders and ages, as well as particular risk groups [195–198]. Zinc, folic acid, selenium, and dietary antioxidants may also be relevant to MDD [199–204].

Zinc

In the developing world, it has been estimated that there are about two billion people deficient in zinc [205]. There are many diseases associated with zinc deficiency, including infections, growth retardation, delayed sexual maturity, and diarrhea. Zinc deficiency is associated with death of about 800,000 children per year [205–207].

A list of dietary sources of zinc can be found here [208].

Zinc is one of the essential micronutrients that has a variety of intracellular and extracellular roles to play in metabolism, apoptosis, cell differentiation, and cell growth [207, 209–211]. It is vital to regulation of neuronal, immunological, and endocrine functions [205, 212, 213]. Zinc is the reactive center in or a co-factor of more than 300 enzymes [206, 214, 215] and plays a central role in transcription, DNA and RNA metabolism, signal transduction, and hormone receptors [214–216]. In the body, zinc is the second most abundant divalent cation after calcium [217].

In the brain, zinc is found in the presynaptic vesicles of special neurons from which it is released into the synaptic cleft and is recycled back into the presynaptic terminal [218]. These neurons are found almost exclusively in the cerebral cortex and limbic structures, areas implicated in depression [219]. In its activity, it tonically modulates brain excitability through modulation of amino acid receptors. Excess zinc is associated with neurotoxicity of Alzheimer's disease and amyotrophic lateral sclerosis, epilepsy, and ischemia [219]. In this role, it participates in pathology of plaque deposition in Alzheimer's disease, exacerbating excitotoxic neuron injury [220], and strokes [221]. Zinc is an antagonist of the glutamate/*N*-methyl-D-aspartate (NMDA) receptor, induces brain derived neurotrophic factor (BDNF) gene expression, and increases the level of the hippocampal synaptic pool of zinc [222].

Zinc appears to function similar to calcium in that it is picked up by the postsynaptic cell. Areas of the brain such as the hippocampus are particularly sensitive to zinc deficiency

[211]. Deficiency of zinc can increase neuronal apoptosis and decrease neurogenesis; as such, it has been associated with learning and memory deficits [223]. Excellent reviews of zinc in brain functions can be found in previous works [224–226].

A systematic review examined genetic variations as modifying factors of dietary zinc requirements to determine whether recommendations for zinc intake could be made based on the genotype [227]. They confirmed a connection between genetics and zinc requirements; however, the direction and magnitude of the dietary modification for carriers of specific genotypes could not be defined.

Homeostatic control of zinc levels that normally prevents deficiency or excess of zinc involves different proteins participating in the uptake, excretion, and intracellular storage and trafficking of zinc. There is some evidence that suggests depression, Alzheimer's disease, and aging may involve derangements in that system [223].

Zinc is coreleased with glutamate from a subclass of glutamatergic neurons. It has been proposed that glucocorticoid–glutamatergic interactions may explain stress-mediated decline in hippocampal functions such as cognition and under chronic stress may lead to depressive symptoms [228].

It appears that the most important actions of zinc relative to depression that have been identified are modulating glutamatergic neurotransmission (via the *N*-methyl-D-aspartate (NMDA)/glutamatergic glutamate receptors), serotonergic transmission (especially via the 5-HT1A receptor), and regulation of brain-derived neurotrophic factor (BDNF) levels [229–231].

Significantly lower levels of serum zinc have been seen in subjects suffering from MDD or unipolar depression than people who are not depressed [232–238]. Severity of peripartum depression has also been seen to be negatively correlated with serum levels of zinc [239, 240]. Patients with treatment resistant depression vs. those who are not treatment resistant have demonstrated much lower levels of serum zinc [241].

As of 2013, we could find only two studies that have revealed no differences in serum zinc levels between non-depressed and depressed patients [239, 241]. The earlier study [239] did find significantly higher levels of zinc in patients who recovered from depression. The second study [242] found interesting significant results between fatty acid composition and zinc levels in depressed and non-depressed subjects. Higher stearic and AA concentrations were seen in depressed patients, and relative to their AA levels, their EPA and DHA concentrations were diminished compared to the general population. They concluded that zinc concentrations depended upon comorbid disorders, depression severity, and the apparent presence of diverging metabolic pathways as indicated by the different fatty acid profiles.

An interesting cross-sectional observational study has suggested an interaction ($p = 0.03$) with sex [236]. Zinc was associated with depressive symptoms in women but not men. Women with low dietary or supplemental zinc intake were more likely to have depressive symptoms and associations were stronger among women using antidepressant medications (p-trend = 0.0005). In a cross-sectional population-based Boston Area Community Health survey (2002–2005), low dietary or supplemental zinc was associated with depression symptoms among women, but not men [243].

Although these studies do not prove a link between depression and zinc, the data is highly suggestive. The next question would be, is there any evidence that zinc supplementation improves the clinical picture?

There are very few studies assessing relationships between dietary zinc intake and depression in humans. In these studies, it has been difficult to rule out reverse causality and confounders. A 2010 study of young university women found that those who were depressed ingested about two-thirds of the amount of zinc as women who were not depressed [236]. Their serum zinc levels mirrored their intake and the severity of depression correlated with the inverse of their serum zinc levels.

Another study conducted in a cohort of pregnant London women revealed an association of depression symptoms with social disadvantage, higher stress, and lower zinc intake [244]. Zinc intake moderated the association between stress and depressive symptoms such that higher intake buffered the effect of the stressors.

In a study of post-graduate students, an inverse relationship was seen between dietary intake of zinc and depression, independent of age, sex, years of education, smoking status, and physical activity [245].

In a large, randomly selected, population-based sample of women, an inverse association between the dietary intakes of magnesium, folate, and zinc and depressive illnesses were seen [246].

Zinc is also lipid protective and a constituent of fatty acid metabolism enzymes [242, 247]. One study has indicated that zinc concentrations are associated with different fatty acids in subjects with depression and without depression [242]. Depressed subjects had higher stearic and arachidonic acid (AA) concentrations, and their EPA/AA and DEA/AA ratios were significantly diminished compared to controls. Zinc supplementation (25 mg/day) for 2 months has been shown to significantly decrease saturated fats and increase omega-3 fatty acids in phospholipids [191].

There are several clinical trials for zinc supplementation in depression. The first clinical trial to demonstrate the benefit of zinc supplementation in antidepressant therapy showed in 2003 that zinc supplementation of 25 mg for 12 weeks significantly reduced Hamilton Depression Rating

Scale (HDRS) and Beck Depression Inventory (BDI) scores compared with placebo [248]. All the subjects received tricyclic antidepressants or selective serotonin reuptake inhibitors supplemented by zinc or a placebo.

In 2013, results of an RCT showed that zinc supplementation (25 mg for 12 weeks) of SSRIs significantly reduced BDI scores end of week 6 ($p < 0.01$) and 12 ($p < 0.001$) and compared to the placebo group at the end of 12th week ($p < 0.05$) [70].

In 2013, reported by the same group as, 25 mg/12 weeks zinc adjunct to antidepressant therapy significantly reduced HDRS compared to placebo ($p < 0.01$ at 12th week) [70]. They found no significant differences in plasma levels of IL-6, TNF-α, and BDNF-a between zinc-supplemented and placebo-supplemented group, which suggests that zinc effects do not seem to be mediated through the immune system.

An RCT in 2009 showed that the tricyclic antidepressant imipramine supplemented with zinc (25 mg/12 weeks) increased the efficacy and speed of the beginning of therapeutic response especially in subjects who were non-responsive to imipramine by itself [249].

A 2010 RCT conducted with young women in Japan compared multivitamins and zinc (7 mg/day) for 10 weeks [250]. Women who took the multivitamin and zinc had a significant reduction in anger-hostility scores ($p = 0.009$) and depression-dejection scores ($p = 0.011$) as assessed by the Profile of Moods State and a significant increase in serum zinc concentration ($p = 0.008$). Those women who took only the multivitamin did not show a change in the scores.

In 2012, results were published of six randomized controlled comparative treatment experiments in Chinese and Mexican American low-income children, aged 6–9 years, middle-income US adolescents, middle-income US premenopausal women, and middle-income US men [251]. The data seems to point to subclinical zinc deficiency-induced changes in brain functions and a remediation effect on utilization of zinc when an adequate omnivorous diet or a mixture of other micronutrients are added to the diets of those afflicted.

In 2006, results of a 6-month RCT comparing zinc supplementation (10 mg Zn daily, 5 days/week) with a placebo (10 mg glucose) in 674 Guatemalan children in grades 1–4 showed no difference in some measures of mental health between zinc-treated and placebo groups [252]. There was no difference from placebo in externalizing (i.e., hyperactivity and conduct disorder) problem behaviors and positive behaviors (i.e., socialization and leadership). Nevertheless, increases in serum zinc are associated with fewer symptoms of internalizing symptoms (depression and anxiety) and improvement in social skills.

In 2009, results were published of an RCT of 459 Guatemalan women who received weekly (5000 or 2800 mcg) or daily (400 or 200 mcg folic acid plus iron, zinc, and vitamin B12) for 12 weeks [253]. No associations were seen between depression and *serum* folate, homocysteine, vitamin B12, hemoglobin, ferritin, or zinc ($p > 0.05$). At baseline, low levels of *erythrocyte* folate are associated with depression. Mean depression scores decreased by 2.3 points after the intervention and depression prevalence decreased from 49.3% to 37.7%; however, there was no difference in amount of improvement among the four intervention groups ($p = 0.64$).

A cutting-edge diagnostic investigation (published in 2011) of the molecular signature of human zinc deficiency has applied a combination of transcriptome, cytokine, and microRNA analyses to a dietary zinc depletion/repletion protocol with young male human subjects [254]. They found the following results that are more sensitive than serum zinc.

- Changes in buccal and blood gene transcripts related to zinc homeostasis occurred with zinc depletion.
- Zinc-responsive genes were seen, particularly, those associated with cell cycle regulation and immunity.
- The diagnostic properties of specific serum microRNAs for dietary zinc deficiency were identified by acute responses to zinc depletion, which were reversible by subsequent zinc repletion.
- Depression of immune-stimulated TNFα secretion by blood cells was observed after low zinc consumption.
- Gene network analysis revealed potential clinical outcomes attributable to suboptimal zinc intake including immune function defects and predisposition to cancer.

Excessive consumption of zinc can cause copper deficiency, lethargy, and ataxia [238]. Indeed, an experiment in mice conducted in 2012 showed that high-dose zinc supplementation induces specific zinc deficiency in the hippocampus, which further impairs learning and memory due to decreased availability of synaptic zinc and BDNF deficits [255]. There is some evidence that high copper levels are associated with greater depression symptom severity [256]. It also seems that serum ratio of copper to zinc may be significantly higher in depressed individuals [257].

A 2018 comprehensive review of possible molecular mechanisms of zinc involvement in depression can be found in previous work [258].

Selenium

The primary source of selenium is the dietary consumption of grains which is dependent on the selenium content of the soils in which it is grown [259]. Suboptimal presence in regional soil may be the principal reason for the estimate that one in seven people have low dietary selenium intake. A list of dietary sources of selenium can be found here [260]. When selenium supply is deficient, the brain increases its retention [261].

Selenium interacts with multiple pathways that appear to be involved with depression such as inflammation [262], oxidative and nitrosative stress, and antioxidant levels [233, 263–267].

Depression is frequently accompanied by oxidative stress and depressed levels of antioxidants including glutathione and glutathione peroxidase enzyme. Selenoprotein P, a plasma protein that contains 10 selenocysteine residues per polypeptide and comprises 50% of the selenium in human plasma, protects against phospholipid hydroperoxide [267]. As part of the glutathione peroxidase system, selenium protects lipids in polyunsaturated membranes from oxidative degradation [268, 269]. The 25 selenoproteins in the form of the amino acid selenocysteine have functions that include redox regulation of intracellular signaling, redox homeostasis, and thyroid hormone metabolism [270].

A 2011 study concluded that in their sample, whole blood glutathione peroxidase (GPX) activity in depression was significantly lower ($p = 0.001$), but not in myalgic encephalomyelitis/chronic fatigue syndrome [271]. There was a significant negative correlation between Hamilton Depression Rating Scale score and autonomic symptoms. This lower GPX activity in depression contributes to the inflammatory and the oxidative and nitrosative pathways, and the comorbidity between depression and CAD.

A connection between selenium and lipids is suggested by an experiment where selenium deficiency in rats with adequate vitamin E and increased fish oil intake affected lipid concentration and fatty acid composition in the liver [272]. It was suggested that this change may reflect a deficiency of antioxidant selenoenzymes. Deficiency of selenium can decrease the conversion of ALA into EPA and DHA, thereby leading to an increase in the ratio of omega-6 to omega-3 fatty acids [272].

There are functional variants in the glutathione peroxidase (GPX) genes which may have a bearing on susceptibility to various diseases. GPX Glutathione peroxidase 1 (GPX1) is a key enzyme of the antioxidant system [4]. The Pro198Leu polymorphism c.599C>T SNP (aka, rs1050450) produces a variant protein that has been associated with cancers of the bladder, lung, prostate, and breast, alcohol consumption [273–276], intracerebral hemorrhage, and coronary artery disease [277, 278].

Analysis of groundwater selenium levels and decreased depression symptoms in a geriatric population has shown that selenium was most protective against depression among homozygous carriers of the C allele at the Pro198Leu [279].

Selenium is incorporated into iodothyronine deiodinases and is essential for thyroid synthesis, metabolism, and function [280]. Thyroid functioning is critical for appropriate neuropsychiatric functioning [280]. Selenium has significant modulatory effects on the dopaminergic, serotonergic, and noradrenergic systems [281]. For example, selenium and selenoprotein have a neuroprotective role in dopaminergic neurons vulnerable to oxidative stress [282].

A 2013 study examined relationships between oxidative imbalance, cellular immunity, and recurrent depressive disorder [283]. They found increased concentrations of malondialdehyde (MDA), and plasma H_2O_2, DNA damage, increased levels of the pro-inflammatory cytokine interleukin-6 and neopterin, and decreased hemoglobin and hematocrit in depressed patients. The study's authors suggested that a strong association between antioxidant defense, cytokine levels, and iron homeostasis represents a self-sustaining multi-pathway that may progressively worsen due to oxidative damage resulting in functional and structural consequences associated with depression.

In adolescents, alcohol and drug abuse are frequently comorbid with depression and suicide behavior. Alcohol abuse combined with lower selenium intake may decrease availability of selenium which through its role in selenoproteins would be protective for neurons [284]. As mentioned above, selenium deficiency is associated with depression, anxiety, and cognitive difficulties [285]. There is evidence that adolescence, a time of far-reaching structural and functional brain development, is a period of more susceptibility than adulthood to the long-term adverse effects of alcohol abuse [286, 287]. It has been suggested that the combination of alcohol abuse and decreased selenium may be a potent combination for depression and suicide.

Low levels of selenium have been associated with increased incidence of depression [285, 288], some forms of cancer, Alzheimer's disease, and cardiovascular disease [270, 289]. A nested case–control study of women found that compared with a high selenium intake, a low intake (<8.9 μg/MJ/day) was associated with an approximate trebling of the likelihood for developing a new case of MDD (OR = 2.95; 95% CI: 1.00–8.72) [288]. However, inconsistent results have been seen in other studies of associations of selenium with depression [258]. Decreased dietary levels of selenium and increased depression symptoms were seen in a geriatric population [279] and in women [288]. No association was seen in a geriatric population in China [290] or in a group of hemodialysis patients [291]. And high levels of selenium have been associated with increased depression symptoms in a population of young adults [292].

Supplementation with selenium has produced mixed results. A large-scale RCT (501 UK participants aged 60–74) published in 2006 found no evidence that selenium supplementation benefited mood or quality of life in that population [293]. In 2011, results of an RCT suggested that selenium supplementation during pregnancy might be an effective approach for the prevention of postpartum depression [294].

However, a search of the *Cochrane Pregnancy and Childbirth Group's Trials Register* (30 April 2013) to assess possible benefits of dietary supplements for preventing postnatal depression in the antenatal period, postnatal period, or both found that there is insufficient evidence to conclude that selenium, DHA, EPA, or any other dietary measure can prevent postnatal depression [295].

In young adults, an optimal range of serum selenium between ~82 and 85 μg/L has been associated with decreased risk of depressive symptoms [296]. This range is approximately the concentrations at which glutathione peroxidase is maximal.

Folate

Folate (vitamin B9) or its synthetic analogue folic acid is essential to many body functions. It is vital for synthesis, methylation, and repair of DNA and is a cofactor in a number of single-carbon-transfer reactions[7] [297–299]. Folate is necessary for the synthesis of monoamine neurotransmitters serotonin, epinephrine, and dopamine that are implicated in depression [300–302].

Folate is essential for synthesis of DNA nucleotides such as thymine and, by way of S-adenosylmethionine (SAM), it is necessary for maintenance of methylation of cytosine [303]. Methylation of cytosine is essential for control of gene expression and chromatin structure.

Although folate is therefore necessary for genetic stability in all cells, it is especially essential when there are high rates of cell division and growth such as in fetal development and infancy [304, 305]. Deficiencies of folate can damage DNA, both nuclear and mitochondrial, and decrease the ability to regenerate and repair cells.

The primary natural source of folate is fruits and fruit juices, nuts, beans, peas, dairy products, poultry and meat, eggs, seafood, and grains. However, in the Western world and parts of the developing world, folic acid–fortified flours and cereals have become the principal source [306].

Food processing can result in loss of up to 40% by cooking vegetables and up to 70% of folates can be destroyed by milling and baking grains and cereals [307–309].

Natural folates are polyglutamates that are enzymatically converted into folate monoglutamates by folate reductase in the jejunal mucosa to be absorbed [307, 308, 310]. Folic acid, on the other hand, is twice as well absorbed as natural folates [309].

Folates are active only after they are converted in the liver to dihydrofolic acid, which in turn is converted by dihydrofolate reductase (DHFR) in the liver to tetrahydrofolate and other derivatives [311]. The rate of this conversion is slow and in humans it varies at least fivefold [311]. Folate is transformed to L-methylfolate, a biologically active form of folate which crosses the blood–brain barrier.

Folate deficiency can result from inadequate intake, malabsorption [312, 313], or increased needs [314]. For example, folate deficiency is associated with alcohol consumption due to reduced dietary folate intake, intestinal malabsorption, decreased liver uptake and storage, and increased folate excretion in the urine [315, 316].

Symptoms of folate deficiency in developing embryos include neural tube defects and consequent central nervous system defects [317]. Folate deficiency during critical stages of fetal and infantile development affects both structural and functional fine-tuning of the brain [318]. Other symptoms include diarrhea, mental confusion, cognitive decline, headaches, irritability and behavioral problems, macrocytic anemia accompanied by weakness and shortness of breath, and peripheral neuropathies [319, 320].

A genetic variant of methylenetetrahydrofolate reductase gene 9 (MTHFR) (5,10) may make some people susceptible to folate deficiencies despite sufficient dietary intake [321]. However, C677T polymorphism of the MTHFR gene and the A2756G polymorphism of methionine synthase do not appear to significantly affect antidepressant response to fluoxetine treatment of MDD [322].

Folic acid supplementation without adequate intake of vitamin B12 can be problematic because supplementation with folic acid in dietary sources such as flours as opposed to natural folate (N5CH3HFGlu1) needs vitamin B12 to enter the cells and metabolic pathways [323]. In the elderly, this may result in subacute combined degeneration.

There is some evidence that low circulating levels of folate may increase the risk of breast, colon, and pancreatic cancers [324]. High levels of folic acid may increase the risk of breast cancer in postmenopausal women especially those who have a high intake of alcohol [325] and increase risk of prostate cancer [326]. Genetic polymorphisms with nutrient interactions [327] seem to be relevant to increasing risks of prostate cancer [328, 329] and other cancers [330–333].

There are some associations of folate and its derivatives with depressive disorders, both in terms of deficiencies [334] and therapeutics such as biopterins and synthesis of *S-adenosyl methionine (SAMe)* [335, 336]. Low levels of plasma and serum folate and vitamin B12 are frequently seen in depressed patients, especially those with recurrent mood disorders treated with lithium, and in patients who have a poor treatment response to antidepressants [337].

Folate may decrease levels of homocysteine, a sulfur containing amino acid that participates in one-carbon metabo-

[7] Some pathways of synthesis or modification need the transfer or addition of single carbons that are in a variety of oxidation states. These most common lower oxidation states are (–CHO, =CH–, –CH2, –CH3). CO2 is the most oxidized state of carbon.

lism [338]. Increased levels of homocysteine have been associated with geriatric multisystem problems such as cognitive impairment, dementia and depression, as well as a variety of diseases that relate to angiotoxicity, and inhibition of collagen cross-linking [338]. Homocysteine levels are frequently higher in men than in women and they tend to increase with age [339, 340].

The connection from folate to production of monoamine neurotransmitters passes through 5-methyltetrahydrofolate (5-MTHF, L-methylfolate) participates in re-methylation of the amino acid metabolite homocysteine, creating methionine, and then S-adenosylmethionine (SAMe) [301]. SAMe then participates in a variety of methyl donation reactions including those that form monoamine neurotransmitters. A deficiency of 5-MTHF decreases SAMe resulting in lower levels of neurotransmitters in the cerebrospinal fluid apparently contributing to depression [301].

Folic acid supplementation may inhibit noradrenergic receptors and stimulate serotonergic receptors in the brain [341, 342].

Supplementation with folate plus SSRI adjunctive treatment for depression has been suggested [343–345]. However, much of the evidence for the association of low folate level with depression comes from case–control and cross-sectional studies [346, 347]. A meta-analysis conducted in 2004 evaluated randomized controlled trials that compared treatment with folic acid or 5′-methyltetrahydrofolic acid to an alternative treatment for patients with a diagnosis of depressive disorder [319]. They found only two quality RCTs and concluded that there was some evidence that folate may have a role as a supplement to other depression treatments. Higher baseline blood levels of folate associated with a better response when combined with SSRIs and TCAs [348]. Low blood levels of folate associated with less response to antidepressant treatment [349].

Two multicenter RCT sequential parallel comparison design trials suggested that adjunctive L-methylfolate at 15 mg/day may be a suitable strategy for patients with MDD who have a partial response or no response to SSRIs [345, 350–352].

Differences in response to folate supplement have been seen in men vs. women. For example, supplemental folate produced less of an increase in plasma folate in men; plasma homocysteine was significantly decreased in women but not in men, and there was a significant improvement in fluoxetine plus folic acid but only in women ($p < 0.001$) [353].

Some but not all studies have reported an association of low folate levels and an increased risk of depression [253, 354, 355].

Folic acid supplementation appears to increase plasma concentration of DHA and EPA, which may in turn increase endothelial nitric oxide generation, enhancing brain acetylcholine levels, and suppressing the production of pro-inflammatory cytokines [356].

Connections of folate supplementation and PUFA have been demonstrated in rats where folate treatment did not significantly change omega-6 PUFA but did significantly increase omega-3 PUFA in plasma lipid fractions and in platelet, erythrocyte, and intestinal phospholipids [357]. Another study in rats fed a low amount of folic acid showed a significant decrease of omega-3 PUFA, increased oxidative stress indicated by increases in plasma lipid peroxidation products and an enhanced susceptibility of erythrocytes to free radicals, and increased total circulating homocysteine [358].

S-adenosyl-methionine (SAMe) naturally occurs in many tissues in humans, including in the brain [359]. SAMe is produced from the amino acid L-methionine through the one-carbon cycle using folate and vitamin B12.

Meta-analyses and RCTS have suggested that SAMe in doses of 200–1600 mg/day appears to be superior to placebo and is as effective as tricyclic antidepressants in treating MDD [360, 361]. SAMe may have a faster onset of action than conventional antidepressants and may potentiate the effect of tricyclic antidepressants. In addition, SAMe seems to be useful as an adjunct to SSRIs [362, 363].

A 2016 Cochrane reviewed evidence for SAMe use in depression [359]. They concluded that "With regard to all extractable measures of the acceptability of SAMe, the quality of the evidence was low to very low. SAMe was similar to placebo and established antidepressants. The exception was that compared to imipramine, fewer participants experienced troublesome adverse effects when treated with parenteral SAMe."

Magnesium

Magnesium is an intracellular cation that is a coenzyme or activator in more than 300 enzymatic pathways, including DNA replication, transcription, and translation, many of which are vital for appropriate brain functions [364, 365]. The primary diet source is fruits, whole grains, seeds, nuts, and green leafy vegetables [366]. It was estimated in 2005 that only 32% of people in the USA consume the RDA of magnesium [367].

Typically, over 84% of the magnesium found in whole wheat is removed in making refined flour, and magnesium has been removed from most drinking water supplies [368].

Imbalances of magnesium have been associated with depression, diabetes, stroke, migraines, Alzheimer's disease, hypertension, and ADHD [369].

Depression-like symptoms have been seen in mice who had magnesium-deficient diets [370–372]. Cross-sectional studies have shown an inverse relationship between magnesium levels and intake and depression symptoms [373–376]. On the other hand, in an RCT, no significant associations were seen between magnesium intake and risk of depression 10 years later [377]. And another study did not show an inverse relationship between magnesium intake and depression 6 years later [378].

An RCT of adults with mild to moderate depression who consumed 248 mg of magnesium per day for 6 weeks resulted in a clinically significant 6-point decrease in symptoms ($p < 0.001$) compared to placebo [365]. Another RCT of 60 individuals with depression and hypomagnesemia who received 500 mg daily for at least 8 weeks showed significant improvement of depression compared to those who did not receive the supplement [379]. Supplementation with 50 mg/day of MgCl2 in an elderly population of type 2 diabetics with hypomagnesemia was just as effective as imipramine in alleviating depression symptoms [380]. On the other hand, effects of zinc and magnesium supplements (27 mg zinc sulfate tablet or 320 mg magnesium sulfate tablet) on depressive symptoms and anxiety in postpartum women in an RCT found no significant difference between groups at 8 weeks after delivery [381].

Magnesium can modulate serotonergic, noradrenergic, and dopaminergic neurotransmission [382, 383], increase in BDNF [384], and increase in melatonin synthesis [385].

Magnesium deficiency can affect glutamatergic transmission in the limbic system and cerebral cortex [386]. Magnesium is an antagonist of NMDA glutamate receptor [387, 388]. Modulation of dietary intake may alter the function and signaling of GluN1-containing NMDA receptor complexes and several protein kinases in the amygdala and hypothalamus that appear to associate with depressive behavior in mice [389]. Depressive symptoms in mice can be reversed by NMDA receptor agonists [390].

Magnesium appears to function as an immunomodulator which suggests a possible role in an inflammatory relationship to depression [391–393]. Magnesium reduces the release of ACTH and can prevent over-action of the HPA axis that occurs in depression [394–397]. In so doing, magnesium may prevent the damage that excess glucocorticoids can do to the hippocampus [398, 399].

Magnesium intake has been inversely correlated with levels of the inflammatory mediators serum C-reactive protein, interleukin-6, and tumor necrosis factor-α receptor 2 [400, 401].

An interesting experiment showed a potentially "U"-shaped curve of magnesium and gut microbiome interaction [402]. Mice were fed a control or Mg-deficient diet (500 mg vs. 70 mg/kg) for 4 or 21 days. Compared with mice on the control diet, mice on the Mg-deficient diet for 4 days had a lower gut bifidobacteria content (−1.5 log). And there was a 36–50% lower mRNA content of factors controlling gut barrier function in the ileum and a higher mRNA content (by approximately twofold) in the liver and/or intestine of inflammatory molecules indicating cellular stress. Mice fed the Mg-deficient diet for 21 days had a higher cecal bifidobacteria content compared to the control group. In addition, inflammation markers decreased, and the intestinal barrier was restored.

Another experiment in mice suggests that a magnesium-deficient diet alters the gut microbiota (GM) and contributes to depression-like behavior [372]. In a forced swim test, the mice who were fed a magnesium-deficient diet for 6 weeks were less mobile which is interpreted as depression-like behavior. No difference was seen in a glucose tolerance test but changes in gut microbiota correlated positively with these behavioral changes and with hippocampal IL-6.

Tryptophan

Although true *tryptophan deficiency* is probably rare, experimentally depleted tryptophan can increase depression in susceptible folks such as in panic disorders [403]. For example, in a study of obsessive-compulsive folks who ingested low amounts of tryptophan containing foods for 24 h, depressive symptoms increased [404].

Another condition of tryptophan deficiency is associated with *post–partum blues* (transient decreased mood affecting many women a few days after delivery). It seems to be an interplay between psychosocial factors and nutritional and metabolic changes in the early post-partum [405]. In a group of 50 women, assessed between the day just before delivery and 3 days after delivery, the availability of tryptophan to the brain decreased 15% ($p < 0.01$) [405]. The availability of tryptophan was based upon competition with other amino acids for transportation across the blood–brain barrier. Even though the plasma concentration of tryptophan increased 19% during that same period, there was a concomitant dramatic increase in plasma levels of other amino acids (especially leucine, isoleucine, valine, and tyrosine). Intensity of post-partum blues significantly correlated with tryptophan availability ($p < 0.05$).

5 Hydroxytryptophan (5-HTP) and tryptophan easily cross the blood–brain barrier and are quickly decarboxylated to serotonin (5-hydroxytryptamine or 5-HT). Serotonin has a short half-life as it is quickly metabolized by monoamine oxidase. For tryptophan, there is little evidence that supplementation has any benefit [406]. Nevertheless, supplementation with 5-HTP and tryptophan are heavily marketed in the USA and Europe.

In this marketing, there are enthusiastic advocates who make unsupported claims for tryptophan effectiveness in treating depression and other serotonin-associated conditions. For example, the following retracted article [407]. Tryptophan supplementation-associated claims have been subjected to powerful meta-analysis [408, 409]. Despite a large number of studies, very few are of sufficient quality to warrant inclusion. Of these, the sample sizes are small and the evidence while suggestive of some benefit to depression over placebo is not conclusive. For example, a 2002 Cochrane systematic review found only 2 out of 108 trials with a total of 64 patients were of sufficient quality to meet inclusion criteria [409]. The evidence was low quality but there was indication that tryptophan treatments were better than placebo at alleviating depression (Peto odds ratio[8] 4.10; 95% confidence interval 1.28–13.15; RD 0.36; NNT 2.78).

For those who wish to ensure adequate supplies of tryptophan, there are many good dietary sources of tryptophan [411, 412].

Antioxidants

Lipid peroxidation concentration in 66 females 38–70 years of age showed significant positive correlation with depressive symptoms [413]. Lipid peroxidation is also seen in patients with obsessive compulsive disorder and is higher when depression is comorbid [414]. In rats, lipid peroxidation is decreased by supplementation with omega-3 fatty acids [415, 416].

Supplementation with antioxidants may be able to decrease the harmful effect of saturated fats on cognitive function and BDNF levels [417].

It is important to realize that oxidation may be beneficial in some conditions and harmful in others [418]. Oxidation participates in precise biochemical pathways with various requirements and constraints [419]. Different cell types and metabolic pathways respond differently to oxidants and antioxidants. For example, in the liver, PUFAs increase free oxygen radicals, which decrease secretion of atherogenic lipoprotein VLDL. On the other hand, antioxidants can prevent these effects at least in vitro [418].

Vitamin D

Systematic reviews and meta-analyses suggest that low vitamin D levels are associated with depression but additional RCTs of vitamin D for prevention and treatment of depression are needed [420]. A 2014 systematic review and meta-analysis concluded that vitamin D supplementation may be effective for reducing depressive symptoms in patients with clinically significant depression, but additional high-quality studies are necessary to resolve considerable heterogeneity [421].

Vitamin D is produced in our bodies by a multistep process that begins with previtamin D being converted from 7-dehydrocholesterol in the skin via ultraviolet B (UVB: 290–315 nm) radiation from the sun [422]. UVB from sunlight penetrates skin and is absorbed by proteins, DNA, RNA, and 7-dehydrocholesterol [423]. The majority of previtamin D3 is produced in the living epidermal cells and is retained there.

For a comprehensive review, see sunlight and vitamin D [422]. Previtamin D is isomerized to vitamin D3. Both absorb UVB radiation and are converted into products some of which have biological activities [424]. Sequential metabolism of vitamin D first in the liver and then the kidneys produce 25-hydroxyvitamin D which is a major serum form and then 1,25-dihydroxyvitamin D3 which is the biologically active form. 1,25-dihydroxyvitamin D3 is also called calcitriol. Metabolic pathways of vitamin D can be found here [425]. Synthesis and metabolism of vitamin D3 is nicely illustrated in the following reference [426].

In addition to production in the kidney, 1,25-dihydroxyvitamin D3 is produced in a variety of cells [425, 427, 428], The 1,25-dihydroxyvitamin D3 produces its effects via a nuclear receptor (VDR) [429]. Most cells of many tissues have VDRs [430–432].

D3 is most widely known for its functions in calcium and phosphate metabolism and bone health [433]. However, there are pleiotropic effects which we will mention a bit further on previous works [434–436].

Our ability to synthesize vitamin D3 is dependent upon latitude, season, time of day, skin exposure, aging, BMI, and skin pigment [437].

The stratosphere ozone layer efficiently absorbs UVB such that even at noon in the summer only about 1% of UVB reaches the surface of the earth [438, 439]. As the sun's rays travel a greater distance to where we are on earth, even fewer UVB photons reach us. Living above or below 33° latitude allows very little if any vitamin D3 to be produced in our skin during the winter [440]. In fact, folks living even farther from the equator cannot produce any vitamin D3 for up to 6 months [441]. At 42° North, no vitamin D3 is produced from November through February [442].

Human epidermis concentrations of 7-dehydrocholesterol concentrations vary inversely with age as is dose-dependent vitamin D3 production [443]. One small study demonstrated threefold higher vitamin levels from the same UVB exposure in adults aged 20–30 versus 62–80 [444].

UVB does not pass through glass or plastic, so we are also limited by spending time indoors. The higher the latitude, the less UVB is available; on the other hand, the higher the alti-

[8]For binary studies with rare events, the Peto odds ratio (POR) method is considered the relative effect estimator of choice [410]. For more, please see Chap. 4.

tude the greater the UVB is available [445]. Air pollution including nitrous oxide and ozone absorbs solar UVB [440]. Sunscreen with an SPF of 30 decreases the production of vitamin D3 by the same amount as it reduces the penetrance of UVB, in other words 95–98% [441]. Even a sunscreen with a low SPF could reduce vitamin D3 production [446, 447].

Melanin is our naturally evolved skin pigment that absorbs UV of wavelengths 290–700 nm [448]. Variations in skin pigment as humans migrated from Africa have reflected our ability to adapt to and utilize UVB that was less available further from the equator [449, 450].

Dose–response relationships for oral vitamin D3 supplementation and serum 25-hydroxyvitamin D depend upon BMI [451]. Consequently, *Clinical Practice Guidelines by the Endocrine Society* recommend vitamin D supplementation to be two to three times higher for obese subjects and 1.5 times higher for overweight subjects relative to normal weight subjects [452].

Vitamin D deficiency can be caused by several known factors [441]. These include reduced synthesis in the skin (e.g., sunscreen use, increased skin pigmentation, limited sunlight exposure, aging); decreased absorption (e.g., gastric bypass, cystic fibrosis, medication use); increased sequestration (BMI > 30); increased catabolism (e.g., glucocorticoids, anticonvulsants); breastfeeding without vitamin D supplementation; inherited disorders involving vitamin D resistance; reduced synthesis of 25-hydroxyvitamin D, as seen in hepatic failure; increased urinary loss of 25-hydroxyvitamin D, as in nephrotic proteinuria; and decreased synthesis of 1,25-dihydroxyvitamin D in chronic renal failure.

The CDC has estimated that vitamin D deficiency has become rampant due to obesity, lack of vitamin D fortified milk, spending more time indoors, and use of sunscreen [422, 453].

Because most of our cells have receptors for vitamin D and a variety of cells in different organs can produce 1,25-dihydroxyvitamin D, vitamin D is involved in a significant number of biological pathways that may be related to some of the vitamin D deficiency studies [422].

Vitamin D "deficiency" (circulating 25-hydroxyvitamin D concentration <30 nmol/L) has been claimed to be linked to an astounding array of chronic diseases, such as bone mineral disease [454], autoimmunity [455–457], respiratory infections [458], cancer [432, 459], diabetes [460], and cardiovascular events [461]. However, most of these studies are observational and may be statistically or otherwise challenged. Subclinical vitamin D deficiencies have also been suggested [251].

At least in a cohort of Norwegian elderly patients (greater than 64 yoa), vitamin D deficiency appears to be very common among psychogeriatric patients irrespective of diagnosis such as depression, bipolar disorders, psychosis, and dementia [462]. Differences of mean levels of plasma 25-hydroxyvitamin D between control and patients were significant ($p < 0.001$). Prevalence of vitamin D deficiency was significantly higher in the patients vs. controls (71.6% and 20.0%, respectively, $p < 0.001$). Independent of age, gender, season, body mass index, and smoking, being a patient remained significantly associated with vitamin D deficiency (OR = 12.95; 95% CI: 6.03–27.83, $p < 0.001$).

There is divergence in results of current systematic reviews and meta-analyses of vitamin D and disorders. For example, published in 2014, an umbrella review of systematic reviews and meta-analyses of observational studies of plasma 25-hydroxyvitamin D or 1,25-dihydroxyvitamin D concentrations and randomized controlled trials of vitamin D supplementation were conducted to evaluate breadth, validity, and biases of associations of vitamin D with various outcomes [463]. The reviewers found that there was no highly convincing evidence for the role of vitamin D in any outcome. Results did indicate probable associations between vitamin D concentrations and birth weight, dental caries in children, maternal vitamin D concentrations at term, and parathyroid hormone concentrations in patients with chronic kidney disease requiring dialysis. However, there was no compelling evidence that vitamin D supplementation increases bone mineral density, reduces the risk of fractures, or falls in older people. Critical comments on this review can be found in the following references [461, 464–466].

On the other hand, also published in 2014, a systematic review and meta-analysis of observational cohort and randomized intervention studies were conducted to evaluate the extent to which circulating biomarker and supplements of vitamin D are associated with mortality from cardiovascular disease, cancer, or other conditions, under a variety of circumstances [467]. Observational studies indicate inverse associations of circulating 25-hydroxyvitamin D with risks of death due to cardiovascular disease, cancer, and other causes. In addition, supplementation with vitamin D3 but not vitamin D2 significantly reduced overall mortality among older adults. Vitamin D3 given singly reduced mortality significantly by 11%. A comparison of the bottom third with the top third of baseline circulating 25-hydroxyvitamin D distribution revealed pooled relative risks of 1.35 (95% CI: 1.13–1.61) for death from cardiovascular disease, 1.14 (95% CI: 1.01–1.29) for death from cancer, 1.30 (95% CI: 1.07–1.59) for non-vascular, non-cancer death, and 1.35 (95% CI: 1.22–1.49) for all-cause mortality. Critical comments on this review can be seen in the following references [461, 468–470].

Additionally, metanalytical studies of UV exposure from sunlight in over 100 countries have shown strong inverse relationships with at least 15 types of cancer including bladder, breast, cervical, colon, endometrial, esophageal, gastric, lung, ovarian, pancreatic, rectal, renal, and vulvar cancer as well as Hodgkin's and non-Hodgkin's lymphoma [471, 472]. Weaker relationships were seen with nine other cancers (brain, gallbladder, laryngeal, oral/pharyngeal, prostate, and thyroid cancer; leukemia; melanoma; and multiple myeloma).

Vitamin D has an important role in cellular immunity [473]. When T and B lymphocytes are activated, they express vitamin D receptors and respond to immunomodulatory influence of 1, 25$(OH)_2$D [441, 474]. B-cell memory and immunoglobulin synthesis are downregulated by vitamin D, which may decrease production of autoantibodies in autoimmune diseases [475, 476]. Influences of 1, 25$(OH)_2$D on T cells include decreased T-cell proliferation [477–479], increased regulatory T-cell proliferation [475], and increased production of Th_2-Th_3 lymphocytes [480]. A direct influence of these effects on T cells is the upregulation of anti-inflammatory cytokines such as IL-10 and downregulation of pro-inflammatory cytokines such as IL-2, IL-4, IL-8, IL-12, tumor necrosis factor-α, and interferon-γ [475]. Resultant effects are modulation of the adaptive immune system while boosting the innate immune response of monocytes and macrophages to microbes [481].

Risk for autoimmune diseases increases with the distance from the equator [473, 482–485]. For example, the risk of multiple sclerosis increases by 100% for those who were born and lived the first 10 years at about 40° North vs. about 33° North [455, 486]. Correlations have been seen between high levels of serum 25-hydroxyvitamin D and lowered risk of multiple sclerosis [455, 487]. Vitamin D supplementation in 1-year-old children in Finland reduced their risk by 88% 31 years later of developing type I diabetes [487]. The risk for developing inflammatory bowel disease is significantly lower in the southern USA and southern Europe and is independent of ancestry or lifestyle factors [484, 488]. Risk of rheumatoid arthritis appears to be higher at higher latitudes [489, 490].

Vitamin D deficiency has been associated with a 50% increased risk of myocardial infarction and more than 100% increased risk of death from a heart attack [482, 491–494]. Highly significant associations between vitamin D deficiency with type 2 diabetes, hyperlipidemia, hypertension, and peripheral vascular disease may relate to coronary artery disease, heart failure, myocardial infarction, and stroke [495–498].

Vitamin D3 drives cellular differentiation and proliferation in muscle cells [499, 500]. Deficiency of D3 is significantly associated with decreased muscle function and performance, and increased frailty. Vitamin D supplementation can improve muscle strength and gait, especially in the elderly.

Less than adequate vitamin D and inadequate sunlight exposure has been associated with schizophrenia [501–503]. Scandinavian countries have a higher incidence of schizophrenia [501, 502]. Supplementation with vitamin D in Finish infants has been associated with a 77% reduction in risk of developing schizophrenia [503]. Winter births in Australia have been associated with developing schizophrenia [504].

Vitamin D receptors are expressed in the brain [505]. Vitamin D deficiency has been associated with increased risk for neurocognitive decline [426, 506, 507], Alzheimer's disease [508–510], epilepsy [510], and depression [421, 511–514]. It has been suggested that vitamin D_3 can stimulate amyloid-β phagocytosis and clearance by macrophages in Alzheimer patients [515].

Some caution has been advised in people with sarcoidosis and some lymphomas where poorly controlled conversion of 25(OH)D to 1,25$(OH)_2$D by activated macrophages within granulomas can create a hypersensitivity to supplemental vitamin D [516, 517]. However, a 2014 study found no association between hypercalcemia and vitamin D supplementation in people with sarcoidosis [518].

It has been estimated that exposure of the total human body to maximal natural sunlight provides equivalent of 10,000–20,000 IU [519, 520]. It appears that the relationship of vitamin D dose to serum 25-hydroxyvitamin D response is flat up to 250 μg (10,000 IU) vitamin D per day.

The amount of vitamin D produced by sunlight on our skin depends upon how much of our skin is exposed [521]. Each arm and the face accounts for 9% of the body surface. Each leg, the back, and the abdomen each is 18%. Very little vitamin D results from exposure of the face which is most sun-exposed and is the most susceptible to skin cancer [522, 523].

Excess vitamin D supplementation can be problematic [524, 525]. These data suggest that toxicity with hypercalcemia can occur with sustained intake of more than or equal to 40,000 IU per day. However, other information suggests a wide range of safety [519, 526].

Vitamin D3 produced in the skin lasts about two to three times longer in the circulation than that ingested [527]. Based upon experiments in chickens, it takes approximately 8 h for previtamin D produced in the skin to complete conversion to vitamin D3, and it takes time for the D3 produced in the skin to enter the circulation [527–529]. However, it appears that there are different concentrations of 7-dehydrocholesterol in different skin areas [527].

When vitamin D3 is produced in the skin, almost all of it is bound to vitamin D-binding protein which carries it to targets in the body [529]. On the other hand, when vitamin D3 is ingested, it is incorporated into chylomicrons which pass into the lymph and then into the venous blood where only about 60% is carried by the vitamin D-binding protein and the rest is eliminated [529].

Comparing ergocalciferol (vitamin D_2) and cholecalciferol (vitamin D_3) as ingested supplements, it seems that some studies indicate that both are absorbed as well [527–530]. However, there is evidence that after ingesting vitamin D_2, blood levels of 25[OH]D begin falling quickly after 3 days while levels achieved on vitamin D_3 are maintained for 2 weeks before gradually falling [528]. In addition, desirable physiological effects seem to be more readily achieved with vitamin D_3 than with vitamin D_2 [530–532].

Vitamin D toxicity is discussed in the following articles [185, 533–535]. Vitamin D drug interactions are reviewed in previous work [536]. Vitamin D toxicity will not occur from sunlight as excess vitamin D is degraded by sunlight [537].

A large clinical trial (*VITamin D and OmegA-3 TriaL (VITAL)*) of 25,875 men and women is examining the effects of vitamin D3 (2000 IU) or omega-3 fatty acids (Omacor® fish oil, 1 gram) on risks for developing cancer, heart disease, and stroke [538, 539]. Data will also be used to investigate effects on depression and other ancillary topics [540, 541].

The study found that *vitamin D supplementation* did not reduce the risk of cancer or major cardiovascular events (including heart attack, stroke, or cardiovascular death considered together), but it did appear to lower the risk of cancer-related mortality. *Omega-3 fatty acid supplementation* did not reduce risk of cancer and did not reduce risk of major cardiovascular events in the overall study population but did reduce risk of these events by 19% in people with low fish intake. It did reduce risk of heart attack by 28%, when heart attack was considered separately from other cardiovascular events; the benefit appeared strongest in African Americans. A 2019 update supported these conclusions [542].

Results for depression prevention found that there was no benefit to omega-3 supplementation in adults 50 years of older at baseline [543]. Over 5.3 years, there was a small but statistically significant increase in risk of depression or clinically relevant depressive symptoms, but no difference in mood scores.

Independent of vitamin D, *heliotherapy*, the use of sunlight in therapy, has been used to treat a range of chronic illnesses [184, 544]. These diseases include infections (e.g., tuberculosis [545]), and upper respiratory tract infections [546] psoriasis, vitiligo, atopic dermatitis, multiple sclerosis, and localized scleroderma. UVA can induce nitrous oxide which may decrease blood pressure and improve cardiovascular well-being [547].

As a response to UV, keratinocytes in the skin increase production of proopiomelanocortin (POMC), the precursor for adrenocorticotropic hormone, melanocyte-stimulating hormones, beta-lipotropic hormone (beta LPH), and beta endorphin [548]. These compounds are neurotransmitters, modulate immune responses, and affect melanogenesis [547]. Increased endorphins may enhance a feeling of well-being associated with sunlight.

One postulated connection between the multi-causality of seasonal variations of psychiatric problems [549–552] is the effects of sunshine on the skin [553, 554]. The human skin can generate serotonin in a relationship with sun exposure [555–557]. Seasonal variation in serotonin levels, serotonin receptor levels, and serotonin transporters in the brain seem to be statistically related to sunlight exposure [558]. Lower light levels have been associated with lower binding levels in the cortical and subcortical limbic regions [559] and the hypothalamus [560].

In addition, a tract between the retina and raphe nuclei might also be the source for the light-induced modulation of serotonin [561].

Psychobiotics

Modulation of human GI tract microbiota can influence brain function and change depression symptoms [562–566].

Psychobiotics is the term used to describe, "Exogenous interventions to effect changes in mental health via modulation of the gut microbiome" [567–569].

Some reviewers limit the definition of psychobiotics to living organisms [570]. Others include prebiotics, probiotics, diet, and exercise that influence the microbiome [571–573]. The *National Center for Complementary and Integrative Health* defines these as follows [574]. *Prebiotics* are nondigestible food components that selectively stimulate the growth or activity of desirable microorganisms. *Probiotics* are live microorganisms that are intended to have health benefits when consumed or applied to the body. *Synbiotics* are products that combine probiotics and prebiotics. See Fig. 20.2.

In rodent studies, depression-like symptoms have been reversed by administration of probiotics or restoration of a healthy microbiome [575–577]. Investigations of the effects of depression on microbiota have found disruptions in over representation of some bacteria. For example, too much Bacteroidales and too few Lachnospiraceae members [578].

There is preclinical evidence from RCT's in humans that supports the idea that probiotics may be beneficial for treatment of feelings of depression, stress, anxiety, and sad mood [562, 579, 580]. The first systematic review and meta-analysis with the goal of determining the effect of probiotics on depression in humans was published in 2016 [581]. They concluded that probiotics were associated with a significant reduction in depression. In particular, they found that probiotics significantly decreased the depression scale score (MD (depressive disorder) = −0.30, 95% CI: −0.51 to −0.09, $p = 0.005$) in the subjects. Probiotics had an effect on both the healthy population (MD = −0.25, 95% CI: −0.47 to −0.03, $p = 0.03$) and patients with major depressive disorder (MDD) (MD = −0.73, 95% CI: −1.37 to −0.09, $p = 0.03$). Probiotics had an effect on the population aged under 60 (MD = −0.43, 95% CI: −0.72 to −0.13, $p = 0.005$), while it had no effect on people aged over 65 (MD = −0.18, 95% CI: −0.47 to −0.11, $p = 0.22$).

A 2017 systematic review concluded, "The evidence for probiotics alleviating depressive symptoms is compelling

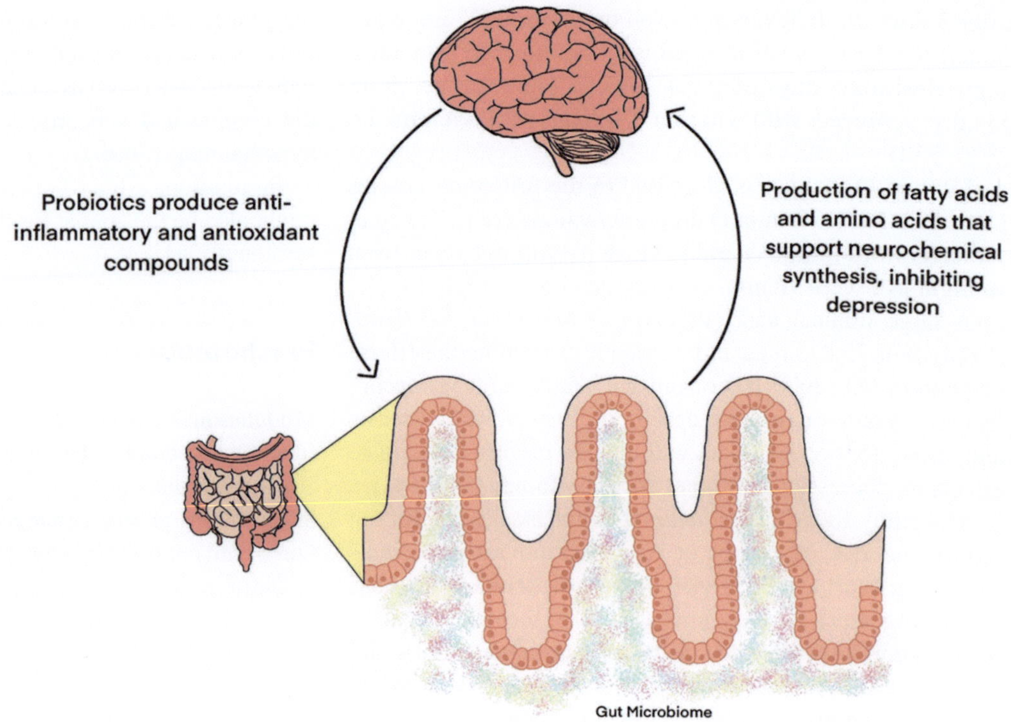

Fig. 20.2 Neuroprotective effects of probiotic metabolites. This figure illustrates how select probiotic strains produce anti-inflammatory and antioxidant compounds—such as short-chain fatty acids, polyphenols, and tryptophan metabolites—that modulate immune signaling, reduce oxidative stress, and support neurochemical synthesis. These actions collectively promote central nervous system homeostasis and may help mitigate depressive symptoms

but additional double-blind randomized control trials in clinical populations are warranted to further assess efficacy" [582]. A 2018 meta-analysis concluded, "Probiotic supplementation has an overall insignificant effect on mood. Future studies should be conducted on more patients with clinically diagnosed depression" [583].

A 2019 systematic review and meta-analysis of randomized controlled trials evaluating probiotics for the treatment of clinical depression concluded that evidence for efficacy remains limited. However, probiotics may exert a beneficial effect on depressive symptoms when used in conjunction with antidepressants [584]. While one stand-alone study was heterogeneous, two trials administering probiotics alongside antidepressants reported a significant improvement in depressive symptoms (standardized mean difference = 1.371; 95% CI: 0.130–2.613).

A promising approach to developing psychobiotic agents to treat depression is *pharmacomicrobiomics* which would match treatments based upon an individual's microbiome [585, 586].

Potpourri

Data from the *German Health Interview and Examination Survey and its Mental Health Supplement (GHS-MHS)* seems to indicate that vegetarians displayed elevated prevalence rates for depressive disorders, anxiety disorders, and somatoform disorders [587]. Sociodemographics were unclear. Although there was no suggestion of causality, the adoption of a vegetarian eating pattern tended to follow the onset of mental difficulties.

Traditional Iranian medicine prescribes and prohibits specific foods for patients who are depressed [588]. A 2015 review found that the highly nutrient rich recommended foods are in the vegetables group, spinach, lettuce, chicory, and squash, in the fruits and nuts group, pomegranate and almond and ultimately in the high-protein products group, trout. Prohibited foods are cabbage, eggplant, onion, garlic, broad beans, lentils, and beef.

There is some evidence that olive oil has neuroprotective effects by decreasing the levels of brain 5-HT (5-hydroxytryptamine), 5-HIAA (5-hydroxyindoleacetic acid), and levels of DA (dopamine) and increasing levels of the DA metabolite HVA (homovanillic acid) [589].

A comprehensive review of the impact of alcohol on the brain has revealed considerable quantitative structural abnormalities beginning in adolescents [287]. Adolescents (14–21 yoa) demonstrated hippocampal and prefrontal volume reductions; however, this was consistently observed only in females. In young adults (aged 21–40), grey matter deficits in the prefrontal cortex (PFC) in both sexes, and hippocampal volume reduction was reported in some subjects. Middle-aged or older alcohol abusers show a widespread loss of cortical grey and white matter, especially in the PFC. Adult women in particular show reduced corpus callosum area.

It appears there is a modest but consistent correlation between higher nutrient intake and higher levels of mental function [590]. This relationship was seen between Global

Assessment of Functioning (GAF) scores and energy, carbohydrates, fiber, total fat, linoleic acid, riboflavin, niacin, folate, vitamin B6, vitamin B12, pantothenic acid, calcium, phosphorus, potassium, and iron (all p values <0.05), as well as magnesium ($r = 0.41$, $p < 0.001$) and zinc ($r = 0.35$, $p < 0.001$). There were no consistent individual associations with generally mild or moderate depression and mania scores. Dietary supplements added to nutrient intake from food produced GAF scores that continued to be positively correlated with all dietary minerals.

In the elderly, depending on the dose, diets that are rich in some high-flavonoid foods may be associated with greater performance in some cognitive tasks [8]. For example, maximum effects in the study population were obtained from 10 g/day for chocolate and approximately 75–100 mL/day for wine, but approximately linear for tea. The most apparent improvement was seen with wine and a somewhat lower effect was seen with chocolate.

There is some evidence that caffeinated coffee may decrease the risk of depression. A study of middle-aged men in Finland found that coffee but neither tea nor caffeine intake associated with a decrease in depression [591]. In a large longitudinal study, depression risk was seen to decrease with increasing coffee consumption [592].

Oxidative stress and lipid peroxidation appear to be present in depressed patients [593]. An open-label randomized study conducted in India showed that there was a significant increase in serum superoxide dismutase (SOD), an antioxidant enzyme, serum malondialdehyde (MDA), a product of lipid peroxidation, and decrease in plasma ascorbic acid levels in patients who had MDD compared to controls. Treatment with fluoxetine and citalopram showed reduced oxidative stress and improved depression.

Brain-derived neurotrophic factor (BDNF) modulates synapsin I and CREB, both of which play critical roles in neuroplasticity underlying learning and memory [594]. Stress can decrease the expression of BDNF, and if chronic, it can lead to atrophy of the hippocampus [595]. In chronic depression, atrophy of the hippocampus and other areas of the limbic system are commonly seen. Expression of BDNF in the brain is increased by voluntary exercise [596, 597], intellectual stimulation, calorie restriction, glutamate, sleep deprivation [598], antidepressants [140], and electroconvulsive therapy [599]. Reversion of the hippocampal atrophy has been associated with this increased BDNF expression [600, 601].

High-saturated fat diets decrease BDNF and can impair neuroplasticity and cognition [417].

From the field of *nutriepigenomics*: It appears that there is a variety of natural chemo preventive agents that influence the activity or expression of DNA methyltransferases and histone modifying enzymes [602–604]. Here is a list from that review.

1. micronutrients (folate, retinoic acid, and selenium compounds)
2. butyrate
3. polyphenols from green tea, apples, coffee, black raspberries, and other dietary sources
4. genistein and soy isoflavones
5. curcumin
6. resveratrol
7. dihydrocoumarin
8. nordihydroguaiaretic acid (NDGA)
9. lycopene
10. anacardic acid
11. garcinol
12. constituents of Allium species and cruciferous vegetables, including indol-3-carbinol (I3C), diindolylmethane (DIM), sulforaphane, phenylethyl isothiocyanate (PEITC), phenylhexyl isothiocyanate (PHI), diallyldisulfide (DADS), and its metabolite allyl mercaptan (AM)
13. cambinol
14. relatively unexplored modulators of histone lysine methylation (chaetocin, polyamine analogs)

Summary

Genetics, environment, and nutrition interact to shape neuropsychiatric disorders. Many studies highlight neurotransmitter deficiencies like GABA, norepinephrine, serotonin, and dopamine in depression. Production of neurotransmitters is dependent upon appropriate nutrition. Many of the neurotransmitters rely upon dietary sources of the eight amino acids that cannot be synthesized by a human body. Tryptophan is the precursor to serotonin; tyrosine and phenylalanine are precursors to the catecholamines dopamine, norepinephrine, and epinephrine. Depletion of tryptophan may decrease brain serotonin levels and aggravate depression. Tyrosine depletion has been associated with decreased catecholamine neurotransmission and adverse effects on mood and cognition.

Nutrients impact gene expression, neurogenesis, and brain functions. Due to the complexity of nutrition, studies on the influence of individual nutrients on depression have shown equivocal results. Mediterranean diets, rich in such nutrients, may prevent depression, but conflicting evidence exists.

High-fat diets disrupt circadian rhythms, potentially leading to depression. Omega-3's efficacy for prevention and treatment of depression is suggestive but questionable. Vitamin and mineral deficiencies are linked to MDD. Tryptophan's role in depression treatment is inconclusive. A variety of micronutrients play as yet an undetermined role in depression. Microbiota modulation affects brain function and depression symptoms and is being investigated for treatment of depression.

Research, especially high-quality randomized trials, is needed for definitive conclusions on dietary associations with depression.

References

1. Dauncey MJ. Recent advances in nutrition, genes and brain health. Proc Nutr Soc. 2012;71(4):581–91. PMID: 22716958. http://www.ncbi.nlm.nih.gov/pubmed/22716958.
2. Gómez-Pinilla F. Brain foods: the effects of nutrients on brain function. Nat Rev Neurosci. 2008;9(7):568–78. PMCID: PMC2805706. http://www.ncbi.nlm.nih.gov/pubmed/18568016.
3. Dauncey MJ. New insights into nutrition and cognitive neuroscience. Proc Nutr Soc. 2009;68(4):408–15. PMID: 19698201. http://www.ncbi.nlm.nih.gov/pubmed/19698201.
4. Dauncey MJ. Genomic and epigenomic insights into nutrition and brain disorders. Nutrients. 2013;5(3):887–914. PMCID: PMC3705325. http://www.ncbi.nlm.nih.gov/pubmed/23503168.
5. Robinson S, Fall C. Infant nutrition and later health: a review of current evidence. Nutrients. 2012;4(8):859–74. PMCID: PMC3448076. http://www.ncbi.nlm.nih.gov/pubmed/23016121.
6. Dauncey MJ, Bicknell RJ. Nutrition and neurodevelopment: mechanisms of developmental dysfunction and disease in later life. Nutr Res Rev. 1999;12(2):231–53. PMID: 19087453. http://www.ncbi.nlm.nih.gov/pubmed/19087453.
7. Morris MS. The role of B vitamins in preventing and treating cognitive impairment and decline. Adv Nutr. 2012;3(6):801–12. PMCID: PMC3648704. http://www.ncbi.nlm.nih.gov/pubmed/23153734.
8. Nurk E, Refsum H, Drevon CA, Tell GS, Nygaard HA, Engedal K, Smith AD. Intake of flavonoid-rich wine, tea, and chocolate by elderly men and women is associated with better cognitive test performance. J Nutr. 2009;139(1):120–7. PMID: 19056649. http://www.ncbi.nlm.nih.gov/pubmed/19056649.
9. Park LK, Friso S, Choi SW. Nutritional influences on epigenetics and age-related disease. Proc Nutr Soc. 2012;71(1):75–83. PMID: 22051144. http://www.ncbi.nlm.nih.gov/pubmed/22051144.
10. Rush AJ. The varied clinical presentations of major depressive disorder. J Clin Psychiatry. 2007;68(Suppl 8):4–10. PMID: 17640152. http://www.ncbi.nlm.nih.gov/pubmed/17640152.
11. Petty F. GABA and mood disorders: a brief review and hypothesis. J Affect Disord. 1995;34(4):275–81. PMID: 8550953. http://www.ncbi.nlm.nih.gov/pubmed/8550953.
12. Leonard BE. The role of noradrenaline in depression: a review. J Psychopharmacol. 1997;11(4 Suppl):S39–47. PMID: 9438232. http://www.ncbi.nlm.nih.gov/pubmed/9438232.
13. Marazziti D, Baroni S, Picchetti M, Piccinni A, Silvestri S, Dell'Osso L. New developments on the serotonin hypothesis of depression: shunt of tryptophan. Riv Psichiatr. 2013;48(1):23–34. PMID: 23438698. http://www.ncbi.nlm.nih.gov/pubmed/23438698.
14. Firk C, Markus CR. Review: serotonin by stress interaction: a susceptibility factor for the development of depression? J Psychopharmacol. 2007;21(5):538–44. PMID: 17446201. http://www.ncbi.nlm.nih.gov/pubmed/17446201.
15. Brown GL, Ebert MH, Goyer PF, Jimerson DC, Klein WJ, Bunney WE, Goodwin FK. Aggression, suicide, and serotonin: relationships to CSF amine metabolites. Am J Psychiatry. 1982;139(6):741–6. PMID: 6177256. http://www.ncbi.nlm.nih.gov/pubmed/6177256.
16. Van Praag HM. Depression, suicide and the metabolism of serotonin in the brain. J Affect Disord. 1982;4(4):275–90. PMID: 6186712. http://www.ncbi.nlm.nih.gov/pubmed/6186712.
17. Stockmeier CA. Neurobiology of serotonin in depression and suicide. Ann N Y Acad Sci. 1997;836:220–32. PMID: 9616801. http://www.ncbi.nlm.nih.gov/pubmed/9616801.
18. Diehl DJ, Gershon S. The role of dopamine in mood disorders. Compr Psychiatry. 1992;33(2):115–20. PMID: 1347497. http://www.ncbi.nlm.nih.gov/pubmed/1347497.
19. Popa TA, Ladea M. Nutrition and depression at the forefront of progress. J Med Life. 2012;5(4):414–9. PMCID: PMC3539842. http://www.ncbi.nlm.nih.gov/pubmed/23346242.
20. Bonaccio M, Di Castelnuovo A, Bonanni A, Costanzo S, De Lucia F, Pounis G, Zito F, Donati MB, de Gaetano G, Iacoviello L, Moli-Sani Project Investigators*. Adherence to a Mediterranean diet is associated with a better health-related quality of life: a possible role of high dietary antioxidant content. BMJ Open. 2013;3(8):e003003. PMCID: PMC3752056. http://www.ncbi.nlm.nih.gov/pubmed/23943771.
21. Fernstrom JD. Aromatic amino acids and monoamine synthesis in the central nervous system: influence of the diet. J Nutr Biochem. 1990;1(10):508–17. PMID: 15539167. http://www.ncbi.nlm.nih.gov/pubmed/15539167.
22. Peters JC, Harper AE. Adaptation of rats to diets containing different levels of protein: effects on food intake, plasma and brain amino acid concentrations and brain neurotransmitter metabolism. J Nutr. 1985;115(3):382–98. PMID: 2857780. http://www.ncbi.nlm.nih.gov/pubmed/2857780.
23. Feder A, Skipper J, Blair JR, Buchholz K, Mathew SJ, Schwarz M, Doucette JT, Alonso A, Collins KA, Neumeister A, Charney DS. Tryptophan depletion and emotional processing in healthy volunteers at high risk for depression. Biol Psychiatry. 2011;69(8):804–7. PMCID: PMC3941748. http://www.ncbi.nlm.nih.gov/pubmed/21377656.
24. Kurz K, Schroecksnadel S, Weiss G, Fuchs D. Association between increased tryptophan degradation and depression in cancer patients. Curr Opin Clin Nutr Metab Care. 2011;14(1):49–56. PMID: 21076293. http://www.ncbi.nlm.nih.gov/pubmed/21076293.
25. Altman SE, Shankman SA, Spring B. Effect of acute tryptophan depletion on emotions in individuals with personal and family history of depression following a mood induction. Neuropsychobiology. 2010;62(3):171–6. PMID: 20664229. http://www.ncbi.nlm.nih.gov/pubmed/20664229.
26. Maes M, Leonard BE, Myint AM, Kubera M, Verkerk R. The new "5-HT" hypothesis of depression: cell-mediated immune activation induces indoleamine 2,3-dioxygenase, which leads to lower plasma tryptophan and an increased synthesis of detrimental tryptophan catabolites (TRYCATs), both of which contribute to the onset of depression. Prog Neuro-Psychopharmacol Biol Psychiatry. 2011;35(3):702–21. PMID: 21185346. http://www.ncbi.nlm.nih.gov/pubmed/21185346.
27. Young SN. Acute tryptophan depletion in humans: a review of theoretical, practical and ethical aspects. J Psychiatry Neurosci. 2013;38(5):294–305. PMCID: PMC3756112. http://www.ncbi.nlm.nih.gov/pubmed/23428157.
28. Friedman M. Analysis, nutrition, and health benefits of tryptophan. Int J Tryptophan Res. 2018;11:1178646918802282. PMCID: PMC6158605. http://www.ncbi.nlm.nih.gov/pubmed/30275700.
29. Poeggeler B, Singh SK, Pappolla MA. Tryptophan in nutrition and health. Int J Mol Sci. 2022;23(10):5455. PMCID: PMC9146092. http://www.ncbi.nlm.nih.gov/pubmed/35628285.
30. Leyton M, Young SN, Blier P, Baker GB, Pihl RO, Benkelfat C. Acute tyrosine depletion and alcohol ingestion in healthy women. Alcohol Clin Exp Res. 2000;24(4):459–64. PMID: 10798581. http://www.ncbi.nlm.nih.gov/pubmed/10798581.
31. Fernstrom JD, Fernstrom MH. Tyrosine, phenylalanine, and catecholamine synthesis and function in the brain. J Nutr. 2007;137(6 Suppl 1):1539S–47S; discussion 1548S. PMID: 17513421. http://www.ncbi.nlm.nih.gov/pubmed/17513421.

32. McLean A, Rubinsztein JS, Robbins TW, Sahakian BJ. The effects of tyrosine depletion in normal healthy volunteers: implications for unipolar depression. Psychopharmacology. 2004;171(3):286–97. PMID: 12955284. http://www.ncbi.nlm.nih.gov/pubmed/12955284.
33. Leyton M, Young SN, Pihl RO, Etezadi S, Lauze C, Blier P, Baker GB, Benkelfat C. Effects on mood of acute phenylalanine/tyrosine depletion in healthy women. Neuropsychopharmacology. 2000;22(1):52–63. PMID: 10633491. http://www.ncbi.nlm.nih.gov/pubmed/10633491.
34. Fernstrom MH, Fernstrom JD. Effect of chronic protein ingestion on rat central nervous system tyrosine levels and in vivo tyrosine hydroxylation rate. Brain Res. 1995;672(1–2):97–103. PMID: 7749758. http://www.ncbi.nlm.nih.gov/pubmed/7749758.
35. McTavish SF, Cowen PJ, Sharp T. Effect of a tyrosine-free amino acid mixture on regional brain catecholamine synthesis and release. Psychopharmacology. 1999;141(2):182–8. PMID: 9952043. http://www.ncbi.nlm.nih.gov/pubmed/9952043.
36. Mente A, de Koning L, Shannon HS, Anand SS. A systematic review of the evidence supporting a causal link between dietary factors and coronary heart disease. Arch Intern Med. 2009;169(7):659–69. PMID: 19364995. http://www.ncbi.nlm.nih.gov/pubmed/19364995.
37. Sanchez-Villegas A, Martínez-González MA. Diet, a new target to prevent depression? BMC Med. 2013;11:3. PMCID: PMC3570363. http://www.ncbi.nlm.nih.gov/pubmed/23286788.
38. Sánchez-Villegas A, Delgado-Rodríguez M, Alonso A, Schlatter J, Lahortiga F, Serra Majem L, Martínez-González MA. Association of the Mediterranean dietary pattern with the incidence of depression: the Seguimiento Universidad de Navarra/University of Navarra follow-up (SUN) cohort. Arch Gen Psychiatry. 2009;66(10):1090–8. PMID: 19805699. http://www.ncbi.nlm.nih.gov/pubmed/19805699.
39. Ford PA, Jaceldo-Siegl K, Lee JW, Youngberg W, Tonstad S. Intake of Mediterranean foods associated with positive affect and low negative affect. J Psychosom Res. 2013;74(2):142–8. PMCID: PMC3790574. http://www.ncbi.nlm.nih.gov/pubmed/23332529.
40. Akbaraly TN, Brunner EJ, Ferrie JE, Marmot MG, Kivimaki M, Singh-Manoux A. Dietary pattern and depressive symptoms in middle age. Br J Psychiatry. 2009;195(5):408–13. PMCID: PMC2801825. http://www.ncbi.nlm.nih.gov/pubmed/19880930.
41. Sánchez-Villegas A, Toledo E, de Irala J, Ruiz-Canela M, Pla-Vidal J, Martínez-González MA. Fast-food and commercial baked goods consumption and the risk of depression. Public Health Nutr. 2012;15(3):424–32. PMID: 21835082. http://www.ncbi.nlm.nih.gov/pubmed/21835082.
42. Jacka FN, Pasco JA, Mykletun A, Williams LJ, Hodge AM, O'Reilly SL, Nicholson GC, Kotowicz MA, Berk M. Association of Western and traditional diets with depression and anxiety in women. Am J Psychiatry. 2010;167(3):305–11. PMID: 20048020. http://www.ncbi.nlm.nih.gov/pubmed/20048020.
43. Quirk SE, Williams LJ, O'Neil A, Pasco JA, Jacka FN, Housden S, Berk M, Brennan SL. The association between diet quality, dietary patterns and depression in adults: a systematic review. BMC Psychiatry. 2013;13:175. PMCID: PMC3706241. http://www.ncbi.nlm.nih.gov/pubmed/23802679.
44. Mamplekou E, Bountziouka V, Psaltopoulou T, Zeimbekis A, Tsakoundakis N, Papaerakleous N, Gotsis E, Metallinos G, Pounis G, Polychronopoulos E, Lionis C, Panagiotakos D. Urban environment, physical inactivity and unhealthy dietary habits correlate to depression among elderly living in eastern Mediterranean islands: the MEDIS (MEDiterranean ISlands elderly) study. J Nutr Health Aging. 2010;14(6):449–55. PMID: 20617287. http://www.ncbi.nlm.nih.gov/pubmed/20617287.
45. Jacka FN, Mykletun A, Berk M, Bjelland I, Tell GS. The association between habitual diet quality and the common mental disorders in community-dwelling adults: the Hordaland Health study. Psychosom Med. 2011;73(6):483–90. PMID: 21715296. http://www.ncbi.nlm.nih.gov/pubmed/21715296.
46. Tangney CC, Young JA, Murtaugh MA, Cobleigh MA, Oleske DM. Self-reported dietary habits, overall dietary quality and symptomatology of breast cancer survivors: a cross-sectional examination. Breast Cancer Res Treat. 2002;71(2):113–23. PMID: 11881909. http://www.ncbi.nlm.nih.gov/pubmed/11881909.
47. Aihara Y, Minai J, Aoyama A, Shimanouchi S. Depressive symptoms and past lifestyle among Japanese elderly people. Community Ment Health J. 2011;47(2):186–93. PMID: 20455023. http://www.ncbi.nlm.nih.gov/pubmed/20455023.
48. Okubo H, Miyake Y, Sasaki S, Tanaka K, Murakami K, Hirota Y, Osaka Maternal and Child Health Study Group. Dietary patterns during pregnancy and the risk of postpartum depression in Japan: the Osaka Maternal and Child Health Study. Br J Nutr. 2011;105(8):1251–7. PMID: 21144112. http://www.ncbi.nlm.nih.gov/pubmed/21144112.
49. Beydoun MA, Fanelli Kuczmarski MT, Beydoun HA, Shroff MR, Mason MA, Evans MK, Zonderman AB. The sex-specific role of plasma folate in mediating the association of dietary quality with depressive symptoms. J Nutr. 2010;140(2):338–47. PMCID: PMC2806887. http://www.ncbi.nlm.nih.gov/pubmed/20032481.
50. Li Y, Lv MR, Wei YJ, Sun L, Zhang JX, Zhang HG, Li B. Dietary patterns and depression risk: a meta-analysis. Psychiatry Res. 2017;253:373–82. PMID: 28431261. http://www.ncbi.nlm.nih.gov/pubmed/28431261.
51. Sarris J, Schoendorfer N, Kavanagh DJ. Major depressive disorder and nutritional medicine: a review of monotherapies and adjuvant treatments. Nutr Rev. 2009;67(3):125–31. PMID: 19239627. http://www.ncbi.nlm.nih.gov/pubmed/19239627.
52. Schmid A. The role of meat fat in the human diet. Crit Rev Food Sci Nutr. 2011;51(1):50–66. PMID: 21229418. http://www.ncbi.nlm.nih.gov/pubmed/21229418.
53. Hammerton G, Thapar A, Thapar AK. Association between obesity and depressive disorder in adolescents at high risk for depression. Int J Obes. 2014;38(4):513–9. PMID: 23887062. http://www.ncbi.nlm.nih.gov/pubmed/23887062.
54. Levitan RD, Davis C, Kaplan AS, Arenovich T, Phillips DIW, Ravindran AV. Obesity comorbidity in unipolar major depressive disorder: refining the core phenotype. J Clin Psychiatry. 2012;73(8):1119–24. PMID: 22687640. http://www.ncbi.nlm.nih.gov/pubmed/22687640.
55. Chou KL, Yu KM. Atypical depressive symptoms and obesity in a national sample of older adults with major depressive disorder. Depress Anxiety. 2013;30(6):574–9. PMID: 23554014. http://www.ncbi.nlm.nih.gov/pubmed/23554014.
56. Sharma S, Fulton S. Diet-induced obesity promotes depressive-like behaviour that is associated with neural adaptations in brain reward circuitry. Int J Obes. 2013;37(3):382–9. PMID: 22508336. http://www.ncbi.nlm.nih.gov/pubmed/22508336.
57. Hariri N, Thibault L. High-fat diet-induced obesity in animal models. Nutr Res Rev. 2010;23(2):270–99. PMID: 20977819. http://www.ncbi.nlm.nih.gov/pubmed/20977819.
58. Dirkx E, Schwenk RW, Glatz JFC, Luiken JJFP, van Eys GJJM. High fat diet induced diabetic cardiomyopathy. Prostaglandins Leukot Essent Fatty Acids. 2011;85(5):219–25. PMID: 21571515. http://www.ncbi.nlm.nih.gov/pubmed/21571515.
59. Coelho DF, Pereira-Lancha LO, Chaves DS, Diwan D, Ferraz R, Campos-Ferraz PL, Poortmans JR, Lancha Junior AH. Effect of high-fat diets on body composition, lipid metabolism and insulin sensitivity, and the role of exercise on these parameters. Braz J Med Biol Res. 2011;44(10):966–72. PMID: 21876873. http://www.ncbi.nlm.nih.gov/pubmed/21876873.

60. Eckel-Mahan KL, Patel VR, de Mateo S, Orozco-Solis R, Ceglia NJ, Sahar S, Dilag-Penilla SA, Dyar KA, Baldi P, Sassone-Corsi P. Reprogramming of the circadian clock by nutritional challenge. Cell. 2013;155(7):1464–78. PMCID: PMC4573395. http://www.ncbi.nlm.nih.gov/pubmed/24360271.
61. O'Neil A, Quirk SE, Housden S, Brennan SL, Williams LJ, Pasco JA, Berk M, Jacka FN. Relationship between diet and mental health in children and adolescents: a systematic review. Am J Public Health. 2014;104(10):e31–42. PMCID: PMC4167107. http://www.ncbi.nlm.nih.gov/pubmed/25208008.
62. Jacka FN, Mykletun A, Berk M. Moving towards a population health approach to the primary prevention of common mental disorders. BMC Med. 2012;10:149. PMCID: PMC3534562. http://www.ncbi.nlm.nih.gov/pubmed/23186355.
63. Sarris J, Logan AC, Akbaraly TN, Amminger GP, Balanzá-Martínez V, Freeman MP, Hibbeln J, Matsuoka Y, Mischoulon D, Mizoue T, Nanri A, Nishi D, Ramsey D, Rucklidge JJ, Sanchez-Villegas A, Scholey A, Su KP, Jacka FN, International Society for Nutritional Psychiatry Research. Nutritional medicine as mainstream in psychiatry. Lancet Psychiatry. 2015;2(3):271–4. PMID: 26359904. http://www.ncbi.nlm.nih.gov/pubmed/26359904.
64. Lai JS, Hiles S, Bisquera A, Hure AJ, McEvoy M, Attia J. A systematic review and meta-analysis of dietary patterns and depression in community-dwelling adults. Am J Clin Nutr. 2014;99(1):181–97. PMID: 24196402. http://www.ncbi.nlm.nih.gov/pubmed/24196402.
65. Opie RS, O'Neil A, Itsiopoulos C, Jacka FN. The impact of whole-of-diet interventions on depression and anxiety: a systematic review of randomised controlled trials. Public Health Nutr. 2015;18(11):2074–93. PMCID: PMC10271872. http://www.ncbi.nlm.nih.gov/pubmed/25465596.
66. Jacka FN, O'Neil A, Opie R, Itsiopoulos C, Cotton S, Mohebbi M, Castle D, Dash S, Mihalopoulos C, Chatterton ML, Brazionis L, Dean OM, Hodge AM, Berk M. Correction to: A randomised controlled trial of dietary improvement for adults with major depression (the "SMILES" trial). BMC Med. 2018;16(1):236. PMCID: PMC6309070. http://www.ncbi.nlm.nih.gov/pubmed/30591046.
67. Jacka FN, O'Neil A, Opie R, Itsiopoulos C, Cotton S, Mohebbi M, Castle D, Dash S, Mihalopoulos C, Chatterton ML, Brazionis L, Dean OM, Hodge AM, Berk M. A randomised controlled trial of dietary improvement for adults with major depression (the "SMILES" trial). BMC Med. 2017;15(1):23. PMCID: PMC5282719. http://www.ncbi.nlm.nih.gov/pubmed/28137247.
68. Opie RS, Itsiopoulos C, Parletta N, Sanchez-Villegas A, Akbaraly TN, Ruusunen A, Jacka FN. Dietary recommendations for the prevention of depression. Nutr Neurosci. 2017;20(3):161–71. PMID: 26317148. http://www.ncbi.nlm.nih.gov/pubmed/26317148.
69. Martimianaki G, Peppa E, Valanou E, Papatesta EM, Klinaki E, Trichopoulou A. Today's Mediterranean diet in Greece: findings from the National Health and Nutrition Survey-HYDRIA (2013-2014). Nutrients. 2022;14(6):1193. PMCID: PMC8949101. http://www.ncbi.nlm.nih.gov/pubmed/35334847.
70. Ranjbar E, Kasaei MS, Mohammad-Shirazi M, Nasrollahzadeh J, Rashidkhani B, Shams J, Mostafavi SA, Mohammadi MR. Effects of zinc supplementation in patients with major depression: a randomized clinical trial. Iran J Psychiatry. 2013;8(2):73–9. PMCID: PMC3796297. http://www.ncbi.nlm.nih.gov/pubmed/24130605.
71. Jacka FN, Pasco JA, Williams LJ, Mann N, Hodge A, Brazionis L, Berk M. Red meat consumption and mood and anxiety disorders. Psychother Psychosom. 2012;81(3):196–8. PMID: 22433903. http://www.ncbi.nlm.nih.gov/pubmed/22433903.
72. The effects of dietary improvement on symptoms of depression and anxiety: a meta-analysis of randomized controlled trials: erratum. Psychosom Med. 2020;82(5):536. PMCID: PMC7515462. http://www.ncbi.nlm.nih.gov/pubmed/32310838.
73. Francis HM, Stevenson RJ, Chambers JR, Gupta D, Newey B, Lim CK. A brief diet intervention can reduce symptoms of depression in young adults – a randomised controlled trial. PLoS One. 2019;14(10):e0222768. PMCID: PMC6784975. http://www.ncbi.nlm.nih.gov/pubmed/31596866.
74. Kessler RC, Berglund P, Demler O, Jin R, Merikangas KR, Walters EE. Lifetime prevalence and age-of-onset distributions of DSM-IV disorders in the National Comorbidity Survey Replication. Arch Gen Psychiatry. 2005;62(6):593–602. PMID: 15939837. http://www.ncbi.nlm.nih.gov/pubmed/15939837.
75. Merikangas KR, He JP, Burstein M, Swanson SA, Avenevoli S, Cui L, Benjet C, Georgiades K, Swendsen J. Lifetime prevalence of mental disorders in U.S. adolescents: results from the National Comorbidity Survey Replication—Adolescent Supplement (NCS-A). J Am Acad Child Adolesc Psychiatry. 2010;49(10):980–9. PMCID: PMC2946114. http://www.ncbi.nlm.nih.gov/pubmed/20855043.
76. Weng TT, Hao JH, Qian QW, Cao H, Fu JL, Sun Y, Huang L, Tao FB. Is there any relationship between dietary patterns and depression and anxiety in Chinese adolescents? Public Health Nutr. 2012;15(4):673–82. PMID: 22115495. http://www.ncbi.nlm.nih.gov/pubmed/22115495.
77. Jacka FN, Kremer PJ, Berk M, de Silva-Sanigorski AM, Moodie M, Leslie ER, Pasco JA, Swinburn BA. A prospective study of diet quality and mental health in adolescents. PLoS One. 2011;6(9):e24805. PMCID: PMC3177848. http://www.ncbi.nlm.nih.gov/pubmed/21957462.
78. Oddy WH, Robinson M, Ambrosini GL, O'Sullivan TA, de Klerk NH, Beilin LJ, Silburn SR, Zubrick SR, Stanley FJ. The association between dietary patterns and mental health in early adolescence. Prev Med. 2009;49(1):39–44. PMID: 19467256. http://www.ncbi.nlm.nih.gov/pubmed/19467256.
79. Jacka FN, Kremer PJ, Leslie ER, Berk M, Patton GC, Toumbourou JW, Williams JW. Associations between diet quality and depressed mood in adolescents: results from the Australian Healthy Neighbourhoods Study. Aust N Z J Psychiatry. 2010;44(5):435–42. PMID: 20397785. http://www.ncbi.nlm.nih.gov/pubmed/20397785.
80. Łojko D, Rybakowski JK. Atypical depression: current perspectives. Neuropsychiatr Dis Treat. 2017;13:2447–56. PMCID: PMC5614762. http://www.ncbi.nlm.nih.gov/pubmed/29033570.
81. Sen ZD, Danyeli LV, Woelfer M, Lamers F, Wagner G, Sobanski T, Walter M. Linking atypical depression and insulin resistance-related disorders via low-grade chronic inflammation: integrating the phenotypic, molecular and neuroanatomical dimensions. Brain Behav Immun. 2021;93:335–52. PMID: 33359233. http://www.ncbi.nlm.nih.gov/pubmed/33359233.
82. Juruena MF, Bocharova M, Agustini B, Young AH. Atypical depression and non-atypical depression: is HPA axis function a biomarker? A systematic review. J Affect Disord. 2018;233:45–67. PMID: 29150144. http://www.ncbi.nlm.nih.gov/pubmed/29150144.
83. Greenthal E, Sorscher S, Pomeranz JL, Cash SB. Availability of calorie information on online menus from chain restaurants in the USA: current prevalence and legal landscape. Public Health Nutr. 2023;26:3239–46. https://www.cambridge.org/core/journals/public-health-nutrition/article/availability-of-calorie-information-on-online-menus-from-chain-restaurants-in-the-usa-current-prevalence-and-legal-landscape/40D83D5626951E8ABA4A9D4BA49D94B6
84. Lee JH, Duster M, Roberts T, Devinsky O. United States dietary trends since 1800: lack of association between saturated fatty acid consumption and non-communicable diseases. Front Nutr. 2022;8:748847. https://www.frontiersin.org/journals/nutrition/articles/10.3389/fnut.2021.748847/full

85. Ross AP, Darling JN, Parent MB. High energy diets prevent the enhancing effects of emotional arousal on memory. Behav Neurosci. 2013;127(5):771–9. PMID: 24128364. http://www.ncbi.nlm.nih.gov/pubmed/24128364.
86. Beilharz JE, Maniam J, Morris MJ. Short exposure to a diet rich in both fat and sugar or sugar alone impairs place, but not object recognition memory in rats. Brain Behav Immun. 2014;37:134–41. PMID: 24309633. http://www.ncbi.nlm.nih.gov/pubmed/24309633.
87. Agurs-Collins T, Fuemmeler BF. Dopamine polymorphisms and depressive symptoms predict foods intake. Results from a nationally representative sample. Appetite. 2011;57(2):339–48. PMCID: PMC3156384. http://www.ncbi.nlm.nih.gov/pubmed/21672565.
88. Hussain G, Schmitt F, Loeffler JP, Gonzalez de Aguilar JL. Fatting the brain: a brief of recent research. Front Cell Neurosci. 2013;7:144. PMCID: PMC3766822. shttp://www.ncbi.nlm.nih.gov/pubmed/24058332.
89. Luchtman DW, Song C. Cognitive enhancement by omega-3 fatty acids from child-hood to old age: findings from animal and clinical studies. Neuropharmacology. 2013;64:550–65. PMID: 22841917. http://www.ncbi.nlm.nih.gov/pubmed/22841917.
90. Svennerholm L, Boström K, Jungbjer B, Olsson L. Membrane lipids of adult human brain: lipid composition of frontal and temporal lobe in subjects of age 20 to 100 years. J Neurochem. 1994;63(5):1802–11. PMID: 7931336. http://www.ncbi.nlm.nih.gov/pubmed/7931336.
91. O'Brien JS, Sampson EL. Lipid composition of the normal human brain: gray matter, white matter, and myelin. J Lipid Res. 1965;6(4):537–44. PMID: 5865382. http://www.ncbi.nlm.nih.gov/pubmed/5865382.
92. USDA. New nutrient content information now online. 2019. https://www.usda.gov/about-usda/news/blog/new-nutrient-content-information-now-online.
93. National Agricultural Library. Food and Nutrition Information Center (FNIC). https://www.nal.usda.gov/programs/fnic.
94. Beare-Rogers J, Dieffenbacher A, Holm JV. Lexicon of lipid nutrition. Pure Appl Chem. 2001;73:685–744. http://www.iupac.org/publications/pac/2001/pdf/7304x0685.pdf
95. Martins DA, Custódio L, Barreira L, Pereira H, Ben-Hamadou R, Varela J, Abu-Salah KM. Alternative sources of n-3 long-chain polyunsaturated fatty acids in marine microalgae. Mar Drugs. 2013;11(7):2259–81. PMCID: PMC3736422. http://www.ncbi.nlm.nih.gov/pubmed/23807546.
96. de Carvalho CCCR, Caramujo MJ. Lipids of prokaryotic origin at the base of marine food webs. Mar Drugs. 2012;10(12):2698–714. PMCID: PMC3528120. http://www.ncbi.nlm.nih.gov/pubmed/23342392.
97. Bourre JM. Roles of unsaturated fatty acids (especially omega-3 fatty acids) in the brain at various ages and during ageing. J Nutr Health Aging. 2004;8(3):163–74. PMID: 15129302. http://www.ncbi.nlm.nih.gov/pubmed/15129302.
98. Domenichiello AF, Kitson AP, Bazinet RP. Is docosahexaenoic acid synthesis from α-linolenic acid sufficient to supply the adult brain? Prog Lipid Res. 2015;59:54–66. PMID: 25920364. http://www.ncbi.nlm.nih.gov/pubmed/25920364.
99. Plourde M, Cunnane SC. Extremely limited synthesis of long chain polyunsaturates in adults: implications for their dietary essentiality and use as supplements. Appl Physiol Nutr Metab. 2007;32(4):619–34. PMID: 17622276. http://www.ncbi.nlm.nih.gov/pubmed/17622276.
100. Giltay EJ, Gooren LJG, Toorians AWFT, Katan MB, Zock PL. Docosahexaenoic acid concentrations are higher in women than in men because of estrogenic effects. Am J Clin Nutr. 2004;80(5):1167–74. PMID: 15531662. http://www.ncbi.nlm.nih.gov/pubmed/15531662.
101. Labrousse VF, Nadjar A, Joffre C, Costes L, Aubert A, Grégoire S, Bretillon L, Layé S. Short-term long chain omega3 diet protects from neuroinflammatory processes and memory impairment in aged mice. PLoS One. 2012;7(5):e36861. PMCID: PMC3360741. http://www.ncbi.nlm.nih.gov/pubmed/22662127.
102. Bazan NG, Molina MF, Gordon WC. Docosahexaenoic acid signalolipidomics in nutrition: significance in aging, neuroinflammation, macular degeneration, Alzheimer's, and other neurodegenerative diseases. Annu Rev Nutr. 2011;31:321–51. PMCID: PMC3406932. http://www.ncbi.nlm.nih.gov/pubmed/21756134.
103. Guesnet P, Alessandri JM. Docosahexaenoic acid (DHA) and the developing central nervous system (CNS) – implications for dietary recommendations. Biochimie. 2011;93(1):7–12. PMID: 20478353. http://www.ncbi.nlm.nih.gov/pubmed/20478353.
104. Bradbury J. Docosahexaenoic acid (DHA): an ancient nutrient for the modern human brain. Nutrients. 2011;3(5):529–54. PMCID: PMC3257695. http://www.ncbi.nlm.nih.gov/pubmed/22254110.
105. Simopoulos AP. Importance of the ratio of omega-6/omega-3 essential fatty acids: evolutionary aspects. World Rev Nutr Diet. 2003;92:1–22. PMID: 14579680. http://www.ncbi.nlm.nih.gov/pubmed/14579680.
106. Simopoulos AP. Human requirement for N-3 polyunsaturated fatty acids. Poult Sci. 2000;79(7):961–70. PMID: 10901194. http://www.ncbi.nlm.nih.gov/pubmed/10901194.
107. Simopoulos AP, Leaf A, Salem N. Workshop on the essentiality of and recommended dietary intakes for omega-6 and omega-3 fatty acids. J Am Coll Nutr. 1999;18(5):487–9. PMID: 10511332. http://www.ncbi.nlm.nih.gov/pubmed/10511332.
108. Proceedings of a workshop on the essentiality of and recommended dietary intakes for omega-6 and omega-3 fatty acids. 7–9 April 1999, Bethesda, Maryland, USA. Prostaglandins Leukot Essent Fatty Acids. 2000;63(3):117–76. PMID: 10991763. http://www.ncbi.nlm.nih.gov/pubmed/10991763.
109. Holub BJ. Clinical nutrition: 4. Omega-3 fatty acids in cardiovascular care. CMAJ. 2002;166(5):608–15. PMCID: PMC99405. http://www.ncbi.nlm.nih.gov/pubmed/11898942.
110. Bourre JM, Dumont O, Piciotti M, Clément M, Chaudière J, Bonneil M, Nalbone G, Lafont H, Pascal G, Durand G. Essentiality of omega 3 fatty acids for brain structure and function. World Rev Nutr Diet. 1991;66:103–17. PMID: 2053331. http://www.ncbi.nlm.nih.gov/pubmed/2053331.
111. Logan AC. Neurobehavioral aspects of omega-3 fatty acids: possible mechanisms and therapeutic value in major depression. Altern Med Rev. 2003;8(4):410–25. PMID: 14653768. http://www.ncbi.nlm.nih.gov/pubmed/14653768.
112. Moullé VSF, Cansell C, Luquet S, Cruciani-Guglielmacci C. The multiple roles of fatty acid handling proteins in brain. Front Physiol. 2012;3:385. PMCID: PMC3460233. http://www.ncbi.nlm.nih.gov/pubmed/23060810.
113. Burdge GC, Lillycrop KA. Fatty acids and epigenetics. Curr Opin Clin Nutr Metab Care. 2014;17(2):156–61. PMID: 24322369. http://www.ncbi.nlm.nih.gov/pubmed/24322369.
114. Hodson L, Skeaff CM, Fielding BA. Fatty acid composition of adipose tissue and blood in humans and its use as a biomarker of dietary intake. Prog Lipid Res. 2008;47(5):348–80. PMID: 18435934. http://www.ncbi.nlm.nih.gov/pubmed/18435934.
115. Adams PB, Lawson S, Sanigorski A, Sinclair AJ. Arachidonic acid to eicosapentaenoic acid ratio in blood correlates positively with clinical symptoms of depression. Lipids. 1996;31(Suppl):S157–61. PMID: 8729112. http://www.ncbi.nlm.nih.gov/pubmed/8729112.
116. Peet M, Murphy B, Shay J, Horrobin D. Depletion of omega-3 fatty acid levels in red blood cell membranes of depressive patients. Biol Psychiatry. 1998;43(5):315–9. PMID: 9513745. http://www.ncbi.nlm.nih.gov/pubmed/9513745.
117. Maes M, Christophe A, Delanghe J, Altamura C, Neels H, Meltzer HY. Lowered omega3 polyunsaturated fatty acids in serum phos-

pholipids and cholesteryl esters of depressed patients. Psychiatry Res. 1999;85(3):275–91. PMID: 10333380. http://www.ncbi.nlm.nih.gov/pubmed/10333380.
118. Hellmuth C, Demmelmair H, Schmitt I, Peissner W, Blüher M, Koletzko B. Association between plasma nonesterified fatty acids species and adipose tissue fatty acid composition. PLoS One. 2013;8(10):e74927. PMCID: PMC3788793. http://www.ncbi.nlm.nih.gov/pubmed/24098359.
119. Mamalakis G, Tornaritis M, Kafatos A. Depression and adipose essential polyunsaturated fatty acids. Prostaglandins Leukot Essent Fatty Acids. 2002;67(5):311–8. https://doi.org/10.1054/plef.2002.0435. PMID: 12445491. https://pubmed.ncbi.nlm.nih.gov/12445491/.
120. Mamalakis G, Kalogeropoulos N, Andrikopoulos N, Hatzis C, Kromhout D, Moschandreas J, Kafatos A. Depression and long chain n-3 fatty acids in adipose tissue in adults from Crete. Eur J Clin Nutr. 2006;60(7):882–8. https://doi.org/10.1038/sj.ejcn.1602394. Epub 2006 Feb 8. PMID: 16465199. https://pubmed.ncbi.nlm.nih.gov/16465199/.
121. Mamalakis G, Kiriakakis M, Tsibinos G, Kafatos A. Depression and adipose polyunsaturated fatty acids in the survivors of the seven countries study population of Crete. Prostaglandins Leukot Essent Fatty Acids. 2004;70(6):495–501. PMID: 15120712. http://www.ncbi.nlm.nih.gov/pubmed/15120712.
122. Mamalakis G, Kiriakakis M, Tsibinos G, Jansen E, Cremers H, Strien C, Hatzis C, Moschandreas J, Linardakis M, Kromhout D, Kafatos A. Lack of an association of depression with n-3 polyunsaturated fatty acids in adipose tissue and serum phospholipids in healthy adults. Pharmacol Biochem Behav. 2008;89(1):6–10. PMID: 18023852. http://www.ncbi.nlm.nih.gov/pubmed/18023852.
123. Ellis FR, Sanders TA. Long chain polyunsaturated fatty acids in endogenous depression. J Neurol Neurosurg Psychiatry. 1977;40(2):168–9. PMCID: PMC492633. http://www.ncbi.nlm.nih.gov/pubmed/864481.
124. Fehily AM, Bowey OA, Ellis FR, Meade BW, Dickerson JW. Plasma and erythrocyte membrane long chain polyunsaturated fatty acids in endogenous depression. Neurochem Int. 1981;3(1):37–42. PMID: 20487806. http://www.ncbi.nlm.nih.gov/pubmed/20487806.
125. Heron DS, Shinitzky M, Hershkowitz M, Samuel D. Lipid fluidity markedly modulates the binding of serotonin to mouse brain membranes. Proc Natl Acad Sci USA. 1980;77(12):7463–7. PMCID: PMC350524. http://www.ncbi.nlm.nih.gov/pubmed/6938985.
126. Belokoneva OS, Zaĭtsev SV. The role of membrane lipids in regulating the function of neuromediator receptors. Biokhimiia. 1993;58(11):1685–708. PMID: 7903554. http://www.ncbi.nlm.nih.gov/pubmed/7903554.
127. Subczynski WK, Widomska J, Feix JB. Physical properties of lipid bilayers from EPR spin labeling and their influence on chemical reactions in a membrane environment. Free Radic Biol Med. 2009;46(6):707–18. PMCID: PMC2705953. http://www.ncbi.nlm.nih.gov/pubmed/19111611.
128. Yehuda S, Rabinovitz S, Mostofsky DI. Modulation of learning and neuronal membrane composition in the rat by essential fatty acid preparation: time-course analysis. Neurochem Res. 1998;23(5):627–34. PMID: 9566600. http://www.ncbi.nlm.nih.gov/pubmed/9566600.
129. Subczynski WK, Wisniewska A. Physical properties of lipid bilayer membranes: relevance to membrane biological functions. Acta Biochim Pol. 2000;47(3):613–25. PMID: 11310964. http://www.ncbi.nlm.nih.gov/pubmed/11310964.
130. Locke CA, Stoll AL. Omega-3 fatty acids in major depression. World Rev Nutr Diet. 2001;89:173–85. PMID: 11530734. http://www.ncbi.nlm.nih.gov/pubmed/11530734.
131. Calder PC. Fatty acids and inflammation: the cutting edge between food and pharma. Eur J Pharmacol. 2011;668(Suppl 1):S50–8. PMID: 21816146. http://www.ncbi.nlm.nih.gov/pubmed/21816146.
132. Schiepers OJG, Wichers MC, Maes M. Cytokines and major depression. Prog Neuro-Psychopharmacol Biol Psychiatry. 2005;29(2):201–17. PMID: 15694227. http://www.ncbi.nlm.nih.gov/pubmed/15694227.
133. Calder PC. Omega-3 fatty acids and inflammatory processes. Nutrients. 2010;2(3):355–74. PMCID: PMC3257651. http://www.ncbi.nlm.nih.gov/pubmed/22254027.
134. Müller N, Schwarz MJ. The immune-mediated alteration of serotonin and glutamate: towards an integrated view of depression. Mol Psychiatry. 2007;12(11):988–1000. PMID: 17457312. http://www.ncbi.nlm.nih.gov/pubmed/17457312.
135. Maes M, Smith RS. Fatty acids, cytokines, and major depression. Biol Psychiatry. 1998;43(5):313–4. PMID: 9513744. http://www.ncbi.nlm.nih.gov/pubmed/9513744.
136. Viljoen M, Panzer A. Proinflammatory cytokines: a common denominator in depression and somatic symptoms? Can J Psychiatr. 2005;50(2):128. PMID: 15807234. http://www.ncbi.nlm.nih.gov/pubmed/15807234.
137. Messay B, Lim A, Marsland AL. Current understanding of the bidirectional relationship of major depression with inflammation. Biol Mood Anxiety Disord. 2012;2:4. PMCID: PMC3384230. http://www.ncbi.nlm.nih.gov/pubmed/22738397.
138. Suarez EC, Krishnan RR, Lewis JG. The relation of severity of depressive symptoms to monocyte-associated proinflammatory cytokines and chemokines in apparently healthy men. Psychosom Med. 2003;65(3):362–8. PMID: 12764208. http://www.ncbi.nlm.nih.gov/pubmed/12764208.
139. Gomez-Pinilla F. Collaborative effects of diet and exercise on cognitive enhancement. Nutr Health. 2011;20(3–4):165–9. PMCID: PMC3258096. http://www.ncbi.nlm.nih.gov/pubmed/22141190.
140. Shimizu E, Hashimoto K, Okamura N, Koike K, Komatsu N, Kumakiri C, Nakazato M, Watanabe H, Shinoda N, Okada S-i, Iyo M. Alterations of serum levels of brain-derived neurotrophic factor (BDNF) in depressed patients with or without antidepressants. Biol Psychiatry. 2003;54(1):70–5. PMID: 12842310. http://www.ncbi.nlm.nih.gov/pubmed/12842310.
141. Hibbeln JR. Fish consumption and major depression. Lancet. 1998;351(9110):1213. PMID: 9643729. http://www.ncbi.nlm.nih.gov/pubmed/9643729.
142. Ratnayake WM, Chen ZY. Trans, n-3, and n-6 fatty acids in Canadian human milk. Lipids. 1996;31(Suppl):S279–82. PMID: 8729134. http://www.ncbi.nlm.nih.gov/pubmed/8729134.
143. Lock AL, Bauman DE. Modifying milk fat composition of dairy cows to enhance fatty acids beneficial to human health. Lipids. 2004;39(12):1197–206. PMID: 15736916. http://www.ncbi.nlm.nih.gov/pubmed/15736916.
144. Parodi PW. Cows' milk fat components as potential anticarcinogenic agents. J Nutr. 1997;127(6):1055–60. PMID: 9187617. http://www.ncbi.nlm.nih.gov/pubmed/9187617.
145. Hibbeln JR. Seafood consumption, the DHA content of mothers' milk and prevalence rates of postpartum depression: a cross-national, ecological analysis. J Affect Disord. 2002;69(1–3):15–29. PMID: 12103448. http://www.ncbi.nlm.nih.gov/pubmed/12103448.
146. Noaghiul S, Hibbeln JR. Cross-national comparisons of seafood consumption and rates of bipolar disorders. Am J Psychiatry. 2003;160(12):2222–7. PMID: 14638594. http://www.ncbi.nlm.nih.gov/pubmed/14638594.
147. Cott J, Hibbeln JR. Lack of seasonal mood change in Icelanders. Am J Psychiatry. 2001;158(2):328. PMID: 11156835. http://www.ncbi.nlm.nih.gov/pubmed/11156835.

148. Tanskanen A, Hibbeln JR, Tuomilehto J, Uutela A, Haukkala A, Viinamäki H, Lehtonen J, Vartiainen E. Fish consumption and depressive symptoms in the general population in Finland. Psychiatr Serv. 2001;52(4):529–31. PMID: 11274502. http://www.ncbi.nlm.nih.gov/pubmed/11274502.
149. Silvers KM, Scott KM. Fish consumption and self-reported physical and mental health status. Public Health Nutr. 2002;5(3):427–31. PMID: 12003654. http://www.ncbi.nlm.nih.gov/pubmed/12003654.
150. Albanese E, Lombardo FL, Dangour AD, Guerra M, Acosta D, Huang Y, Jacob KS, Llibre Rodriguez JDJ, Salas A, Schönborn C, Sosa AL, Williams J, Prince MJ, Ferri CP. No association between fish intake and depression in over 15,000 older adults from seven low and middle income countries--the 10/66 study. PLoS One. 2012;7(6):e38879. PMCID: PMC3378552. http://www.ncbi.nlm.nih.gov/pubmed/22723900.
151. Hakkarainen R, Partonen T, Haukka J, Virtamo J, Albanes D, Lönnqvist J. Food and nutrient intake in relation to mental well-being. Nutr J. 2004;3:14. PMCID: PMC519023. http://www.ncbi.nlm.nih.gov/pubmed/15363099.
152. Hakkarainen R, Partonen T, Haukka J, Virtamo J, Albanes D, Lönnqvist J. Is low dietary intake of omega-3 fatty acids associated with depression? Am J Psychiatry. 2004;161(3):567–9. PMID: 14992986. http://www.ncbi.nlm.nih.gov/pubmed/14992986.
153. Suominen-Taipale AL, Turunen AW, Partonen T, Kaprio J, Männistö S, Montonen J, Jula A, Tiittanen P, Verkasalo PK. Fish consumption and polyunsaturated fatty acids in relation to psychological distress. Int J Epidemiol. 2010;39(2):494–503. PMCID: PMC2846446. http://www.ncbi.nlm.nih.gov/pubmed/20156998.
154. Driscoll CT, Mason RP, Chan HM, Jacob DJ, Pirrone N. Mercury as a global pollutant: sources, pathways, and effects. Environ Sci Technol. 2013;47(10):4967–83. PMCID: PMC3701261. http://www.ncbi.nlm.nih.gov/pubmed/23590191.
155. Mahaffey KR, Clickner RP, Jeffries RA. Methylmercury and omega-3 fatty acids: co-occurrence of dietary sources with emphasis on fish and shellfish. Environ Res. 2008;107(1):20–9. PMID: 17996230. http://www.ncbi.nlm.nih.gov/pubmed/17996230.
156. Mahaffey KR. Fish and shellfish as dietary sources of methylmercury and the omega-3 fatty acids, eicosahexaenoic acid and docosahexaenoic acid: risks and benefits. Environ Res. 2004;95(3):414–28. PMID: 15220075. http://www.ncbi.nlm.nih.gov/pubmed/15220075.
157. Mahaffey KR, Sunderland EM, Chan HM, Choi AL, Grandjean P, Mariën K, Oken E, Sakamoto M, Schoeny R, Weihe P, Yan CH, Yasutake A. Balancing the benefits of n-3 polyunsaturated fatty acids and the risks of methylmercury exposure from fish consumption. Nutr Rev. 2011;69(9):493–508. PMCID: PMC3219437. http://www.ncbi.nlm.nih.gov/pubmed/21884130.
158. Ström S, Helmfrid I, Glynn A, Berglund M. Nutritional and toxicological aspects of seafood consumption--an integrated exposure and risk assessment of methylmercury and polyunsaturated fatty acids. Environ Res. 2011;111(2):274–80. PMID: 21211794. http://www.ncbi.nlm.nih.gov/pubmed/21211794.
159. De Croos PZ, Sangdee P, Stockwell BL, Kar L, Thompson EB, Johnson ME, Currie BL. Hemoglobin S antigelation agents based on 5-bromotryptophan with potential for sickle cell anemia. J Med Chem. 1990;33(12):3138–42. PMID: 2258900. http://www.ncbi.nlm.nih.gov/pubmed/2258900.
160. Rudin DO. The major psychoses and neuroses as omega-3 essential fatty acid deficiency syndrome: substrate pellagra. Biol Psychiatry. 1981;16(9):837–50. PMID: 7028146. http://www.ncbi.nlm.nih.gov/pubmed/7028146.
161. Lanska DJ. Chapter 30: Historical aspects of the major neurological vitamin deficiency disorders: the water-soluble B vitamins. Handb Clin Neurol. 2010;95:445–76. PMID: 19892133. http://www.ncbi.nlm.nih.gov/pubmed/19892133.
162. Rudin DO. The dominant diseases of modernized societies as omega-3 essential fatty acid deficiency syndrome: substrate beriberi. Med Hypotheses. 1982;8(1):17–47. PMID: 7062860. http://www.ncbi.nlm.nih.gov/pubmed/7062860.
163. Puri BK, Counsell SJ, Hamilton G, Richardson AJ, Horrobin DF. Eicosapentaenoic acid in treatment-resistant depression associated with symptom remission, structural brain changes and reduced neuronal phospholipid turnover. Int J Clin Pract. 2001;55(8):560–3. PMID: 11695079. http://www.ncbi.nlm.nih.gov/pubmed/11695079.
164. Rees AM, Austin MP, Parker GB. Omega-3 fatty acids as a treatment for perinatal depression: randomized double-blind placebo-controlled trial. Aust N Z J Psychiatry. 2008;42(3):199–205. PMID: 18247194. http://www.ncbi.nlm.nih.gov/pubmed/18247194.
165. Freeman MP, Davis M, Sinha P, Wisner KL, Hibbeln JR, Gelenberg AJ. Omega-3 fatty acids and supportive psychotherapy for perinatal depression: a randomized placebo-controlled study. J Affect Disord. 2008;110(1–2):142–8. PMCID: PMC5598081. http://www.ncbi.nlm.nih.gov/pubmed/18206247.
166. Doornbos B, van Goor SA, Dijck-Brouwer DAJ, Schaafsma A, Korf J, Muskiet FAJ. Supplementation of a low dose of DHA or DHA+AA does not prevent peripartum depressive symptoms in a small population based sample. Prog Neuro-Psychopharmacol Biol Psychiatry. 2009;33(1):49–52. PMID: 18955102. http://www.ncbi.nlm.nih.gov/pubmed/18955102.
167. Makrides M, Gibson RA, McPhee AJ, Yelland L, Quinlivan J, Ryan P, DOMInO Investigative Team. Effect of DHA supplementation during pregnancy on maternal depression and neurodevelopment of young children: a randomized controlled trial. JAMA. 2010;304(15):1675–83. PMID: 20959577. http://www.ncbi.nlm.nih.gov/pubmed/20959577.
168. Su KP, Huang SY, Chiu TH, Huang KC, Huang CL, Chang HC, Pariante CM. Omega-3 fatty acids for major depressive disorder during pregnancy: results from a randomized, double-blind, placebo-controlled trial. J Clin Psychiatry. 2008;69(4):644–51. PMID: 18370571. http://www.ncbi.nlm.nih.gov/pubmed/18370571.
169. Freeman MP, Hibbeln JR, Wisner KL, Davis JM, Mischoulon D, Peet M, Keck PE, Marangell LB, Richardson AJ, Lake J, Stoll AL. Omega-3 fatty acids: evidence basis for treatment and future research in psychiatry. J Clin Psychiatry. 2006;67(12):1954–67. PMID: 17194275. http://www.ncbi.nlm.nih.gov/pubmed/17194275.
170. Martins JG. EPA but not DHA appears to be responsible for the efficacy of omega-3 long chain polyunsaturated fatty acid supplementation in depression: evidence from a meta-analysis of randomized controlled trials. J Am Coll Nutr. 2009;28(5):525–42. PMID: 20439549. http://www.ncbi.nlm.nih.gov/pubmed/20439549.
171. Freeman MP, Mischoulon D, Tedeschini E, Goodness T, Cohen LS, Fava M, Papakostas GI. Complementary and alternative medicine for major depressive disorder: a meta-analysis of patient characteristics, placebo-response rates, and treatment outcomes relative to standard antidepressants. J Clin Psychiatry. 2010;71(6):682–8. PMID: 20573327. http://www.ncbi.nlm.nih.gov/pubmed/20573327.
172. Appleton KM, Rogers PJ, Ness AR. Updated systematic review and meta-analysis of the effects of n-3 long-chain polyunsaturated fatty acids on depressed mood. Am J Clin Nutr. 2010;91(3):757–70. PMID: 20130098. http://www.ncbi.nlm.nih.gov/pubmed/20130098.
173. Lin PY, Su KP. A meta-analytic review of double-blind, placebo-controlled trials of antidepressant efficacy of omega-3 fatty acids. J Clin Psychiatry. 2007;68(7):1056–61. PMID: 17685742. http://www.ncbi.nlm.nih.gov/pubmed/17685742.
174. Sublette ME, Ellis SP, Geant AL, Mann JJ. Meta-analysis of the effects of eicosapentaenoic acid (EPA) in clinical trials in

depression. J Clin Psychiatry. 2011;72(12):1577–84. PMCID: PMC3534764. http://www.ncbi.nlm.nih.gov/pubmed/21939614.
175. Sarris J, Mischoulon D, Schweitzer I. Omega-3 for bipolar disorder: meta-analyses of use in mania and bipolar depression. J Clin Psychiatry. 2012;73(1):81–6. PMID: 21903025. http://www.ncbi.nlm.nih.gov/pubmed/21903025.
176. Bloch MH, Hannestad J. Omega-3 fatty acids for the treatment of depression: systematic review and meta-analysis. Mol Psychiatry. 2012;17(12):1272–82. PMCID: PMC3625950. http://www.ncbi.nlm.nih.gov/pubmed/21931319.
177. Lin PY, Mischoulon D, Freeman MP, Matsuoka Y, Hibbeln J, Belmaker RH, Su KP. Are omega-3 fatty acids antidepressants or just mood-improving agents? The effect depends upon diagnosis, supplement preparation, and severity of depression. Mol Psychiatry. 2012;17(12):1161–3; author reply 1163–7. PMCID: PMC3504139. http://www.ncbi.nlm.nih.gov/pubmed/22824812.
178. Martins JG, Bentsen H, Puri BK. Eicosapentaenoic acid appears to be the key omega-3 fatty acid component associated with efficacy in major depressive disorder: a critique of Bloch and Hannestad and updated meta-analysis. Mol Psychiatry. 2012;17(12):1144–9; discussion 1163–7. PMID: 22488258. http://www.ncbi.nlm.nih.gov/pubmed/22488258.
179. Stafford MR, Jackson H, Mayo-Wilson E, Morrison AP, Kendall T. Early interventions to prevent psychosis: systematic review and meta-analysis. BMJ. 2013;346:f185. PMCID: PMC3548617. http://www.ncbi.nlm.nih.gov/pubmed/23335473.
180. Yip PK, Pizzasegola C, Gladman S, Biggio ML, Marino M, Jayasinghe M, Ullah F, Dyall SC, Malaspina A, Bendotti C, Michael-Titus A. The omega-3 fatty acid eicosapentaenoic acid accelerates disease progression in a model of amyotrophic lateral sclerosis. PLoS One. 2013;8(4):e61626. PMCID: PMC3631166. http://www.ncbi.nlm.nih.gov/pubmed/23620776.
181. Kinrys G. Hypomania associated with omega3 fatty acids. Arch Gen Psychiatry. 2000;57(7):715–6. PMID: 10891045. http://www.ncbi.nlm.nih.gov/pubmed/10891045.
182. Sánchez-Villegas A, Verberne L, De Irala J, Ruíz-Canela M, Toledo E, Serra-Majem L, Martínez-González MA. Dietary fat intake and the risk of depression: the SUN project. PLoS One. 2011;6(1):e16268. PMCID: PMC3027671. http://www.ncbi.nlm.nih.gov/pubmed/21298116.
183. Ruano C, Henriquez P, Bes-Rastrollo M, Ruiz-Canela M, del Burgo CL, Sánchez-Villegas A. Dietary fat intake and quality of life: the SUN project. Nutr J. 2011;10:121. PMCID: PMC3215177. http://www.ncbi.nlm.nih.gov/pubmed/22047452.
184. Menaa F, Menaa A, Tréton J, Menaa B. Technological approaches to minimize industrial trans fatty acids in foods. J Food Sci. 2013;78(3):R377–86. PMID: 23458752. http://www.ncbi.nlm.nih.gov/pubmed/23458752.
185. Holmqvist O. Trans fatty acids in hardened vegetable oils. Atherosclerosis. 1996;120(1–2):245–7. PMID: 8645366. http://www.ncbi.nlm.nih.gov/pubmed/8645366.
186. Przybylski R, McDonald BE. Chapter 3: Trans fatty acids in Canadian breast milk and diet. In: Przybylski R, McDonald BE, editors. Development and processing of vegetable oils for human nutrition. Champaign: AOCS Press; 1995. p. 20–35. https://www.semanticscholar.org/paper/Development-and-Processing-of-Vegetable-Oils-for-Przybylski-Mcdonald/bf315c1955af97f6225c5b7d9fb0f60ed2a3370a.
187. Willett WC, Ascherio A. Trans fatty acids: are the effects only marginal? Am J Public Health. 1994;84(5):722–4. PMCID: PMC1615057. http://www.ncbi.nlm.nih.gov/pubmed/8179036.
188. Stender S, Dyerberg J. Influence of trans fatty acids on health. Ann Nutr Metab. 2004;48(2):61–6. PMID: 14679314. http://www.ncbi.nlm.nih.gov/pubmed/14679314.
189. Turpeinen AM, Mutanen M, Aro A, Salminen I, Basu S, Palmquist DL, Griinari JM. Bioconversion of vaccenic acid to conjugated linoleic acid in humans. Am J Clin Nutr. 2002;76(3):504–10. PMID: 12197992. http://www.ncbi.nlm.nih.gov/pubmed/12197992.
190. Aro A, Männistö S, Salminen I, Ovaskainen ML, Kataja V, Uusitupa M. Inverse association between dietary and serum conjugated linoleic acid and risk of breast cancer in postmenopausal women. Nutr Cancer. 2000;38(2):151–7. PMID: 11525591. http://www.ncbi.nlm.nih.gov/pubmed/11525591.
191. Ascherio A, Katan MB, Zock PL, Stampfer MJ, Willett WC. Trans fatty acids and coronary heart disease. N Engl J Med. 1999;340(25):1994–8. PMID: 10379026. http://www.ncbi.nlm.nih.gov/pubmed/10379026.
192. Golomb BA, Evans MA, White HL, Dimsdale JE. Trans fat consumption and aggression. PLoS One. 2012;7(3):e32175. PMCID: PMC3293881. http://www.ncbi.nlm.nih.gov/pubmed/22403632.
193. Moss J. Labeling of trans fatty acid content in food, regulations and limits-the FDA view. Atheroscler Suppl. 2006;7(2):57–9. PMID: 16713387. http://www.ncbi.nlm.nih.gov/pubmed/16713387.
194. Li D, Zheng H, Tong Y, Li Y. Prospective association between trans fatty acid intake and depressive symptoms: results from the study of women's health across the nation. J Affect Disord. 2020;264:256–62. PMID: 32056759. http://www.ncbi.nlm.nih.gov/pubmed/32056759.
195. Tulchinsky TH. Micronutrient deficiency conditions: global health issues. Public Health Rev. 2010;32:243–55.
196. WHO. Preventing and controlling micronutrient deficiencies in populations affected by an emergency: multiple vitamin and mineral supplements for pregnant and lactating women, and for children aged 6 to 59 months. 2006. https://www.who.int/publications/m/item/WHO-WFP-UNICEF-statement-micronutrients-deficiencies-emergency.
197. Das JK, Salam RA, Kumar R, Bhutta ZA. Micronutrient fortification of food and its impact on woman and child health: a systematic review. Syst Rev. 2013;2:67. PMCID: PMC3765883. http://www.ncbi.nlm.nih.gov/pubmed/23971426.
198. Bodnar LM, Wisner KL. Nutrition and depression: implications for improving mental health among childbearing-aged women. Biol Psychiatry. 2005;58(9):679–85. PMCID: PMC4288963. http://www.ncbi.nlm.nih.gov/pubmed/16040007.
199. Huang Q, Liu H, Suzuki K, Ma S, Liu C. Linking what we eat to our mood: a review of diet, dietary antioxidants, and depression. Antioxidants (Basel). 2019;8(9):376. PMCID: PMC6769512. http://www.ncbi.nlm.nih.gov/pubmed/31491962.
200. Carnegie RE, Zheng J, Borges MC, Jones HJ, Wade KH, Sallis HM, Lewis SJ, Evans DM, Revez JA, The Major Depressive Disorder Working Group of the Psychiatric Genomics Consortium, Evans J, Martin RM. Micronutrients and major depression: a Mendelian randomisation study. Nutrients. 2024;16(21):3690. PMCID: PMC11547740. http://www.ncbi.nlm.nih.gov/pubmed/39519523.
201. Lin J, Zhou Y, Gu W. The synergistic effects of short interpregnancy interval and micronutrients deficiency on third-trimester depression. Front Nutr. 2022;9:949481. PMCID: PMC9554465. http://www.ncbi.nlm.nih.gov/pubmed/36245527.
202. Campisi SC, Zasowski C, Shah S, Shah A, Bradley-Ridout G, Korczak DJ, Szatmari P. Assessing the evidence of micronutrients on depression among children and adolescents: an evidence gap map. Adv Nutr. 2020;11(4):908–27. PMCID: PMC7360446. http://www.ncbi.nlm.nih.gov/pubmed/32193537.
203. Heaton JL, Campbell SA, Bradley HA, Mulder RT, Dixon L, Henderson J, Rucklidge JJ. Broad-spectrum micronutrients or antidepressants for antenatal depression: effect on maternal and infant birth outcomes in an observational secondary analysis of NUTRIMUM. J Clin Psychopharmacol. 2025;45(1):4–15. PMID: 39617974. http://www.ncbi.nlm.nih.gov/pubmed/39617974.
204. Campbell SA, Dys SP, Henderson JMT, Bradley HA, Rucklidge JJ. Exploring the impact of antenatal micronutrients used as a treatment for maternal depression on infant temperament

in the first year of life. Front Nutr. 2024;11:1307701. PMCID: PMC11073451. http://www.ncbi.nlm.nih.gov/pubmed/38711532.
205. Hambidge KM, Krebs NF. Zinc deficiency: a special challenge. J Nutr. 2007;137(4):1101–5. PMID: 17374687. http://www.ncbi.nlm.nih.gov/pubmed/17374687.
206. Maret W. Chapter 14: Zinc and the zinc proteome. In: Banci L, editor. Metallomics and the cell. Metal ions in life sciences, vol. 12. Springer; 2013. https://doi.org/10.1007/978-94-007-5561-10_14. ISBN 978-94-007-5560-4. electronic-book ISBN 978-94-007-5561-1 ISSN 1559-0836 electronic-ISSN 1868-0402. https://link.springer.com/chapter/10.1007/978-94-007-5561-1_14.
207. Prasad AS. Zinc deficiency. BMJ. 2003;326(7386):409–10. PMCID: PMC1125304. http://www.ncbi.nlm.nih.gov/pubmed/12595353.
208. NIH. Zinc – health professional fact sheet. https://ods.od.nih.gov/factsheets/Zinc-HealthProfessional/#h3.
209. Baddam S, Maxfield L, Shukla S, Crane JS. Zinc deficiency. In: StatPearls [Internet]. Treasure Island: StatPearls Publishing; 2025. https://www.ncbi.nlm.nih.gov/books/NBK493231/.
210. Truong-Tran AQ, Carter J, Ruffin RE, Zalewski PD. The role of zinc in caspase activation and apoptotic cell death. Biometals. 2001;14(3–4):315–30. PMID: 11831462. http://www.ncbi.nlm.nih.gov/pubmed/11831462.
211. Takeda A. Zinc signaling in the hippocampus and its relation to pathogenesis of depression. J Trace Elem Med Biol. 2012;26(2–3):80–4. PMID: 22560194. http://www.ncbi.nlm.nih.gov/pubmed/22560194.
212. Weismann K. The biological role of zinc in normal and pathological conditions: a survey. Dan Med Bull. 1976;23(3):146–52. PMID: 949920. http://www.ncbi.nlm.nih.gov/pubmed/949920.
213. Prasad AS. Clinical manifestations of zinc deficiency. Annu Rev Nutr. 1985;5:341–63. PMID: 3896271. http://www.ncbi.nlm.nih.gov/pubmed/3896271.
214. Stiles LI, Ferrao K, Mehta KJ. Role of zinc in health and disease. Clin Exp Med. 2024;24(1):38. PMCID: PMC10874324. http://www.ncbi.nlm.nih.gov/pubmed/38367035.
215. Takeda A. Movement of zinc and its functional significance in the brain. Brain Res Brain Res Rev. 2000;34(3):137–48. PMID: 11113504. http://www.ncbi.nlm.nih.gov/pubmed/11113504.
216. MacDonald RS. The role of zinc in growth and cell proliferation. J Nutr. 2000;130(5S Suppl):1500S–8S. PMID: 10801966. http://www.ncbi.nlm.nih.gov/pubmed/10801966.
217. Petrilli MA, Kranz TM, Kleinhaus K, Joe P, Getz M, Johnson P, Chao MV, Malaspina D. The emerging role for zinc in depression and psychosis. Front Pharmacol. 2017;8:414. PMCID: PMC5492454. http://www.ncbi.nlm.nih.gov/pubmed/28713269.
218. Frederickson CJ, Bush AI. Synaptically released zinc: physiological functions and pathological effects. Biometals. 2001;14(3–4):353–66. PMID: 11831465. http://www.ncbi.nlm.nih.gov/pubmed/11831465.
219. Bitanihirwe BKY, Cunningham MG. Zinc: the brain's dark horse. Synapse. 2009;63(11):1029–49. PMID: 19623531. http://www.ncbi.nlm.nih.gov/pubmed/19623531.
220. Frederickson CJ, Maret W, Cuajungco MP. Zinc and excitotoxic brain injury: a new model. Neuroscientist. 2004;10(1):18–25. PMID: 14987444. http://www.ncbi.nlm.nih.gov/pubmed/14987444.
221. Shuttleworth CW, Weiss JH. Zinc: new clues to diverse roles in brain ischemia. Trends Pharmacol Sci. 2011;32(8):480–6. PMCID: PMC3148334. http://www.ncbi.nlm.nih.gov/pubmed/21621864.
222. Nowak G, Szewczyk B, Pilc A. Zinc and depression. An update. Pharmacol Rep. 2005;57(6):713–8. PMID: 16382189. http://www.ncbi.nlm.nih.gov/pubmed/16382189.
223. Szewczyk B. Zinc homeostasis and neurodegenerative disorders. Front Aging Neurosci. 2013;5:33. PMCID: PMC3715721. http://www.ncbi.nlm.nih.gov/pubmed/23882214.
224. Prakash A, Bharti K, Majeed ABA. Zinc: indications in brain disorders. Fundam Clin Pharmacol. 2015;29(2):131–49. PMID: 25659970. http://www.ncbi.nlm.nih.gov/pubmed/25659970.
225. Nowak G. Zinc, future mono/adjunctive therapy for depression: mechanisms of antidepressant action. Pharmacol Rep. 2015;67(3):659–62. PMID: 25933983. http://www.ncbi.nlm.nih.gov/pubmed/25933983.
226. Marger L, Schubert CR, Bertrand D. Zinc: an underappreciated modulatory factor of brain function. Biochem Pharmacol. 2014;91(4):426–35. PMID: 25130547. http://www.ncbi.nlm.nih.gov/pubmed/25130547.
227. Day KJ, Adamski MM, Dordevic AL, Murgia C. Genetic variations as modifying factors to dietary zinc requirements-A systematic review. Nutrients. 2017;9(2):148. PMCID: PMC5331579. http://www.ncbi.nlm.nih.gov/pubmed/28218639.
228. Joshi M, Akhtar M, Najmi AK, Khuroo AH, Goswami D. Effect of zinc in animal models of anxiety, depression and psychosis. Hum Exp Toxicol. 2012;31(12):1237–43. PMID: 22549093. http://www.ncbi.nlm.nih.gov/pubmed/22549093.
229. Sowa-Kućma M, Legutko B, Szewczyk B, Novak K, Znojek P, Poleszak E, Papp M, Pilc A, Nowak G. Antidepressant-like activity of zinc: further behavioral and molecular evidence. J Neural Transm (Vienna). 2008;115(12):1621–8. PMID: 18766297. http://www.ncbi.nlm.nih.gov/pubmed/18766297.
230. Szewczyk B, Poleszak E, Sowa-Kućma M, Wróbel A, Słotwiński S, Listos J, Wlaź P, Cichy A, Siwek A, Dybała M, Gołembiowska K, Pilc A, Nowak G. The involvement of NMDA and AMPA receptors in the mechanism of antidepressant-like action of zinc in the forced swim test. Amino Acids. 2010;39(1):205–17. PMID: 19956994. http://www.ncbi.nlm.nih.gov/pubmed/19956994.
231. Cichy A, Sowa-Kućma M, Legutko B, Pomierny-Chamioło L, Siwek A, Piotrowska A, Szewczyk B, Poleszak E, Pilc A, Nowak G. Zinc-induced adaptive changes in NMDA/glutamatergic and serotonergic receptors. Pharmacol Rep. 2009;61(6):1184–91. PMID: 20081255. http://www.ncbi.nlm.nih.gov/pubmed/20081255.
232. Roozbeh J, Sharifian M, Ghanizadeh A, Sahraian A, Sagheb MM, Shabani S, Hamidian Jahromi A, Kashfi M, Afshariani R. Association of zinc deficiency and depression in the patients with end-stage renal disease on hemodialysis. J Ren Nutr. 2011;21(2):184–7. PMID: 21093288. http://www.ncbi.nlm.nih.gov/pubmed/21093288.
233. Maes M, Yirmyia R, Noraberg J, Brene S, Hibbeln J, Perini G, Kubera M, Bob P, Lerer B, Maj M. The inflammatory & neurodegenerative (I&ND) hypothesis of depression: leads for future research and new drug developments in depression. Metab Brain Dis. 2009;24(1):27–53. PMID: 19085093. http://www.ncbi.nlm.nih.gov/pubmed/19085093.
234. Szewczyk B, Kubera M, Nowak G. The role of zinc in neurodegenerative inflammatory pathways in depression. Prog Neuro-Psychopharmacol Biol Psychiatry. 2011;35(3):693–701. PMID: 20156515. http://www.ncbi.nlm.nih.gov/pubmed/20156515.
235. Swardfager W, Herrmann N, Mazereeuw G, Goldberger K, Harimoto T, Lanctôt KL. Zinc in depression: a meta-analysis. Biol Psychiatry. 2013;74(12):872–8. PMID: 23806573. http://www.ncbi.nlm.nih.gov/pubmed/23806573.
236. Amani R, Saeidi S, Nazari Z, Nematpour S. Correlation between dietary zinc intakes and its serum levels with depression scales in young female students. Biol Trace Elem Res. 2010;137(2):150–8. PMID: 20013161. http://www.ncbi.nlm.nih.gov/pubmed/20013161.
237. McLoughlin IJ, Hodge JS. Zinc in depressive disorder. Acta Psychiatr Scand. 1990;82(6):451–3. PMID: 2291414. http://www.ncbi.nlm.nih.gov/pubmed/2291414.
238. Plum LM, Rink L, Haase H. The essential toxin: impact of zinc on human health. Int J Environ Res Public Health.

2010;7(4):1342–65. PMCID: PMC2872358. http://www.ncbi.nlm.nih.gov/pubmed/20617034.
239. Narang RL, Gupta KR, Narang AP, Singh R. Levels of copper and zinc in depression. Indian J Physiol Pharmacol. 1991;35(4):272–4. PMID: 1812105. http://www.ncbi.nlm.nih.gov/pubmed/1812105.
240. Wójcik J, Dudek D, Schlegel-Zawadzka M, Grabowska M, Marcinek A, Florek E, Piekoszewski W, Nowak RJ, Opoka W, Nowak G. Antepartum/postpartum depressive symptoms and serum zinc and magnesium levels. Pharmacol Rep. 2006;58(4):571–6. PMID: 16963806. http://www.ncbi.nlm.nih.gov/pubmed/16963806.
241. Siwek M, Dudek D, Schlegel-Zawadzka M, Morawska A, Piekoszewski W, Opoka W, Zieba A, Pilc A, Popik P, Nowak G. Serum zinc level in depressed patients during zinc supplementation of imipramine treatment. J Affect Disord. 2010;126(3):447–52. PMID: 20493532. http://www.ncbi.nlm.nih.gov/pubmed/20493532.
242. Irmisch G, Schlaefke D, Richter J. Zinc and fatty acids in depression. Neurochem Res. 2010;35(9):1376–83. PMID: 20524151. http://www.ncbi.nlm.nih.gov/pubmed/20524151.
243. Maserejian NN, Hall SA, McKinlay JB. Low dietary or supplemental zinc is associated with depression symptoms among women, but not men, in a population-based epidemiological survey. J Affect Disord. 2012;136(3):781–8. PMCID: PMC3272121. http://www.ncbi.nlm.nih.gov/pubmed/22030131.
244. Roy A, Evers SE, Avison WR, Campbell MK. Higher zinc intake buffers the impact of stress on depressive symptoms in pregnancy. Nutr Res. 2010;30(10):695–704. PMID: 21056285. http://www.ncbi.nlm.nih.gov/pubmed/21056285.
245. Yary T, Aazami S. Dietary intake of zinc was inversely associated with depression. Biol Trace Elem Res. 2012;145(3):286–90. PMID: 21932045. http://www.ncbi.nlm.nih.gov/pubmed/21932045.
246. Jacka FN, Maes M, Pasco JA, Williams LJ, Berk M. Nutrient intakes and the common mental disorders in women. J Affect Disord. 2012;141(1):79–85. PMID: 22397891. http://www.ncbi.nlm.nih.gov/pubmed/22397891.
247. McClain CJ, Kasarskis EJ, Allen JJ. Functional consequences of zinc deficiency. Prog Food Nutr Sci. 1985;9(1–2):185–226. PMID: 3911268. http://www.ncbi.nlm.nih.gov/pubmed/3911268.
248. Nowak G, Siwek M, Dudek D, Zieba A, Pilc A. Effect of zinc supplementation on antidepressant therapy in unipolar depression: a preliminary placebo-controlled study. Pol J Pharmacol. 2003;55(6):1143–7. PMID: 14730113. http://www.ncbi.nlm.nih.gov/pubmed/14730113.
249. Siwek M, Dudek D, Paul IA, Sowa-Kućma M, Zieba A, Popik P, Pilc A, Nowak G. Zinc supplementation augments efficacy of imipramine in treatment resistant patients: a double blind, placebo-controlled study. J Affect Disord. 2009;118(1–3):187–95. PMID: 19278731. http://www.ncbi.nlm.nih.gov/pubmed/19278731.
250. Sawada T, Yokoi K. Effect of zinc supplementation on mood states in young women: a pilot study. Eur J Clin Nutr. 2010;64(3):331–3. PMID: 20087376. http://www.ncbi.nlm.nih.gov/pubmed/20087376.
251. Sandstead HH. Subclinical zinc deficiency impairs human brain function. J Trace Elem Med Biol. 2012;26(2–3):70–3. PMID: 22673824. http://www.ncbi.nlm.nih.gov/pubmed/22673824.
252. DiGirolamo AM, Ramirez-Zea M, Wang M, Flores-Ayala R, Martorell R, Neufeld LM, Ramakrishnan U, Sellen D, Black MM, Stein AD. Randomized trial of the effect of zinc supplementation on the mental health of school-age children in Guatemala. Am J Clin Nutr. 2010;92(5):1241–50. PMCID: PMC2954453. http://www.ncbi.nlm.nih.gov/pubmed/20881069.
253. Nguyen PH, Grajeda R, Melgar P, Marcinkevage J, DiGirolamo AM, Flores R, Martorell R. Micronutrient supplementation may reduce symptoms of depression in Guatemalan women. Arch Latinoam Nutr. 2009;59(3):278–86. PMID: 19886513. http://www.ncbi.nlm.nih.gov/pubmed/19886513.
254. Ryu MS, Langkamp-Henken B, Chang SM, Shankar MN, Cousins RJ. Genomic analysis, cytokine expression, and microRNA profiling reveal biomarkers of human dietary zinc depletion and homeostasis. Proc Natl Acad Sci USA. 2011;108(52):20970–5. PMCID: PMC3248538. http://www.ncbi.nlm.nih.gov/pubmed/22171008.
255. Yang Y, Jing XP, Zhang SP, Gu RX, Tang FX, Wang XL, Xiong Y, Qiu M, Sun XY, Ke D, Wang JZ, Liu R. High dose zinc supplementation induces hippocampal zinc deficiency and memory impairment with inhibition of BDNF signaling. PLoS One. 2013;8(1):e55384. PMCID: PMC3561272. http://www.ncbi.nlm.nih.gov/pubmed/23383172.
256. Russo AJ. Analysis of plasma zinc and copper concentration, and perceived symptoms, in individuals with depression, post zinc and anti-oxidant therapy. Nutr Metab Insights. 2011;4:19–27. PMCID: PMC3738484. http://www.ncbi.nlm.nih.gov/pubmed/23946658.
257. Russo AJ. Increased serum Cu/Zn SOD in individuals with clinical depression normalizes after zinc and anti-oxidant therapy. Nutr Metab Insights. 2010;3:37–42. PMCID: PMC3736885. http://www.ncbi.nlm.nih.gov/pubmed/23966790.
258. Wang J, Um P, Dickerman BA, Liu J. Zinc, magnesium, selenium and depression: a review of the evidence, potential mechanisms and implications. Nutrients. 2018;10(5):584. PMCID: PMC5986464. http://www.ncbi.nlm.nih.gov/pubmed/29747386.
259. UNICEF. Large-scale food fortification for the prevention of micronutrient deficiencies in children, women and communities. https://www.unicef.org/documents/large-scale-food-fortification-prevention-micronutrient-deficiencies-children-women-and.
260. NIH. Selenium – health professional fact sheet. https://ods.od.nih.gov/factsheets/Selenium-HealthProfessional/.
261. Zhang X, Liu RP, Cheng WH, Zhu JH. Prioritized brain selenium retention and selenoprotein expression: nutritional insights into Parkinson's disease. Mech Ageing Dev. 2019;180:89–96. PMID: 30998939. http://www.ncbi.nlm.nih.gov/pubmed/30998939.
262. Van Cauwenbergh R, Robberecht H, Van Vlaslaer V, Deelstra H. Comparison of the serum selenium content of healthy adults living in the Antwerp region (Belgium) with recent literature data. J Trace Elem Med Biol. 2004;18(1):99–112. PMID: 15487770. http://www.ncbi.nlm.nih.gov/pubmed/15487770.
263. Bai YZ, Zhang Y, Zhang SQ. New horizons for the role of selenium on cognitive function: advances and challenges. Metab Brain Dis. 2024;39(6):1255–68. PMID: 38963634. http://www.ncbi.nlm.nih.gov/pubmed/38963634.
264. Genchi G, Lauria G, Catalano A, Sinicropi MS, Carocci A. Biological activity of selenium and its impact on human health. Int J Mol Sci. 2023;24(3):2633. PMCID: PMC9917223. http://www.ncbi.nlm.nih.gov/pubmed/36768955.
265. Hariharan S, Dharmaraj S. Selenium and selenoproteins: it's role in regulation of inflammation. Inflammopharmacology. 2020;28(3):667–95. PMCID: PMC7222958. http://www.ncbi.nlm.nih.gov/pubmed/32144521.
266. Maes M, Galecki P, Chang YS, Berk M. A review on the oxidative and nitrosative stress (O&NS) pathways in major depression and their possible contribution to the (neuro)degenerative processes in that illness. Prog Neuro-Psychopharmacol Biol Psychiatry. 2011;35(3):676–92. PMID: 20471444. http://www.ncbi.nlm.nih.gov/pubmed/20471444.
267. Mostert V. Selenoprotein P: properties, functions, and regulation. Arch Biochem Biophys. 2000;376(2):433–8. PMID: 10775431. http://www.ncbi.nlm.nih.gov/pubmed/10775431.
268. Kodydková J, Vávrová L, Zeman M, Jirák R, Macásek J, Stanková B, Tvrzická E, Zák A. Antioxidative enzymes and increased oxidative stress in depressive women. Clin Biochem. 2009;42(13–14):1368–74. PMID: 19527700. http://www.ncbi.nlm.nih.gov/pubmed/19527700.

269. Ozcan ME, Gulec M, Ozerol E, Polat R, Akyol O. Antioxidant enzyme activities and oxidative stress in affective disorders. Int Clin Psychopharmacol. 2004;19(2):89–95. PMID: 15076017. http://www.ncbi.nlm.nih.gov/pubmed/15076017.
270. Papp LV, Holmgren A, Khanna KK. Selenium and selenoproteins in health and disease. Antioxid Redox Signal. 2010;12(7):793–5. PMID: 19905883. http://www.ncbi.nlm.nih.gov/pubmed/19905883.
271. Maes M, Mihaylova I, Kubera M, Uytterhoeven M, Vrydags N, Bosmans E. Lower whole blood glutathione peroxidase (GPX) activity in depression, but not in myalgic encephalomyelitis/chronic fatigue syndrome: another pathway that may be associated with coronary artery disease and neuroprogression in depression. Neuro Endocrinol Lett. 2011;32(2):133–40. PMID: 21552194. http://www.ncbi.nlm.nih.gov/pubmed/21552194.
272. Schäfer K, Kyriakopoulos A, Gessner H, Grune T, Behne D. Effects of selenium deficiency on fatty acid metabolism in rats fed fish oil-enriched diets. J Trace Elem Med Biol. 2004;18(1):89–97. PMID: 15487769. http://www.ncbi.nlm.nih.gov/pubmed/15487769.
273. Soerensen M, Christensen K, Stevnsner T, Christiansen L. The Mn-superoxide dismutase single nucleotide polymorphism rs4880 and the glutathione peroxidase 1 single nucleotide polymorphism rs1050450 are associated with aging and longevity in the oldest old. Mech Ageing Dev. 2009;130(5):308–14. PMCID: PMC2720516. http://www.ncbi.nlm.nih.gov/pubmed/19428448.
274. Ravn-Haren G, Olsen A, Tjønneland A, Dragsted LO, Nexø BA, Wallin H, Overvad K, Raaschou-Nielsen O, Vogel U. Associations between GPX1 Pro198Leu polymorphism, erythrocyte GPX activity, alcohol consumption and breast cancer risk in a prospective cohort study. Carcinogenesis. 2006;27(4):820–5. PMID: 16287877. http://www.ncbi.nlm.nih.gov/pubmed/16287877.
275. Chen J, Cao Q, Qin C, Shao P, Wu Y, Wang M, Zhang Z, Yin C. GPx-1 polymorphism (rs1050450) contributes to tumor susceptibility: evidence from meta-analysis. J Cancer Res Clin Oncol. 2011;137(10):1553–61. PMID: 21842217. http://www.ncbi.nlm.nih.gov/pubmed/21842217.
276. Cominetti C, de Bortoli MC, Purgatto E, Ong TP, Moreno FS, Garrido AB, Cozzolino SMF. Associations between glutathione peroxidase-1 Pro198Leu polymorphism, selenium status, and DNA damage levels in obese women after consumption of Brazil nuts. Nutrition. 2011;27(9):891–6. PMID: 21208780. http://www.ncbi.nlm.nih.gov/pubmed/21208780.
277. Pera J, Slowik A, Dziedzic T, Pulyk R, Wloch D, Szczudlik A. Glutathione peroxidase 1 C593T polymorphism is associated with lobar intracerebral hemorrhage. Cerebrovasc Dis. 2008;25(5):445–9. PMID: 18417962. http://www.ncbi.nlm.nih.gov/pubmed/18417962.
278. Tang NP, Wang LS, Yang L, Gu HJ, Sun QM, Cong RH, Zhou B, Zhu HJ, Wang B. Genetic variant in glutathione peroxidase 1 gene is associated with an increased risk of coronary artery disease in a Chinese population. Clin Chim Acta. 2008;395(1–2):89–93. PMID: 18541150. http://www.ncbi.nlm.nih.gov/pubmed/18541150.
279. Johnson LA, Phillips JA, Mauer C, Edwards M, Balldin VH, Hall JR, Barber R, Conger TL, Ho EJ, O'Bryant SE. The impact of GPX1 on the association of groundwater selenium and depression: a project FRONTIER study. BMC Psychiatry. 2013;13:7. PMCID: PMC3566946. http://www.ncbi.nlm.nih.gov/pubmed/23289525.
280. Köhrle J, Jakob F, Contempré B, Dumont JE. Selenium, the thyroid, and the endocrine system. Endocr Rev. 2005;26(7):944–84. PMID: 16174820. http://www.ncbi.nlm.nih.gov/pubmed/16174820.
281. Castaño A, Ayala A, Rodríguez-Gómez JA, Herrera AJ, Cano J, Machado A. Low selenium diet increases the dopamine turnover in prefrontal cortex of the rat. Neurochem Int. 1997;30(6):549–55. PMID: 9152996. http://www.ncbi.nlm.nih.gov/pubmed/9152996.
282. Solovyev ND. Importance of selenium and selenoprotein for brain function: from antioxidant protection to neuronal signalling. J Inorg Biochem. 2015;153:1–12. PMID: 26398431. http://www.ncbi.nlm.nih.gov/pubmed/26398431.
283. Rybka J, Kędziora-Kornatowska K, Banaś-Leżańska P, Majsterek I, Carvalho LA, Cattaneo A, Anacker C, Kędziora J. Interplay between the pro-oxidant and antioxidant systems and proinflammatory cytokine levels, in relation to iron metabolism and the erythron in depression. Free Radic Biol Med. 2013;63:187–94. PMID: 23707456. http://www.ncbi.nlm.nih.gov/pubmed/23707456.
284. Sher L. Depression and suicidal behavior in alcohol abusing adolescents: possible role of selenium deficiency. Minerva Pediatr. 2008;60(2):201–9. PMID: 18449137. http://www.ncbi.nlm.nih.gov/pubmed/18449137.
285. Hawkes WC, Hornbostel L. Effects of dietary selenium on mood in healthy men living in a metabolic research unit. Biol Psychiatry. 1996;39(2):121–8. PMID: 8717610. http://www.ncbi.nlm.nih.gov/pubmed/8717610.
286. Skala K, Walter H. Adolescence and alcohol: a review of the literature. Neuropsychiatrie. 2013;27(4):202–11. PMID: 23839238. http://www.ncbi.nlm.nih.gov/pubmed/23839238.
287. Welch KA, Carson A, Lawrie SM. Brain structure in adolescents and young adults with alcohol problems: systematic review of imaging studies. Alcohol Alcohol. 2013;48(4):433–44. PMID: 23632805. http://www.ncbi.nlm.nih.gov/pubmed/23632805.
288. Pasco JA, Jacka FN, Williams LJ, Evans-Cleverdon M, Brennan SL, Kotowicz MA, Nicholson GC, Ball MJ, Berk M. Dietary selenium and major depression: a nested case-control study. Complement Ther Med. 2012;20(3):119–23. PMID: 22500660. http://www.ncbi.nlm.nih.gov/pubmed/22500660.
289. Rayman MP. The importance of selenium to human health. Lancet. 2000;356(9225):233–41. PMID: 10963212. http://www.ncbi.nlm.nih.gov/pubmed/10963212.
290. Gao S, Jin Y, Unverzagt FW, Liang C, Hall KS, Cao J, Ma F, Murrell JR, Cheng Y, Li P, Bian J, Hendrie HC. Selenium level and depressive symptoms in a rural elderly Chinese cohort. BMC Psychiatry. 2012;12:72. PMCID: PMC3441866. http://www.ncbi.nlm.nih.gov/pubmed/22759565.
291. Ekramzadeh M, Mazloom Z, Sagheb M. Association of depression with selenium deficiency and nutritional markers in the patients with end-stage renal disease on hemodialysis. J Ren Nutr. 2015;25(4):381–7. PMID: 25680525. http://www.ncbi.nlm.nih.gov/pubmed/25680525.
292. Colangelo LA, He K, Whooley MA, Daviglus ML, Morris S, Liu K. Selenium exposure and depressive symptoms: the Coronary Artery Risk Development in Young Adults Trace Element Study. Neurotoxicology. 2014;41:167–74. PMCID: PMC4030293. http://www.ncbi.nlm.nih.gov/pubmed/24560993.
293. Rayman M, Thompson A, Warren-Perry M, Galassini R, Catterick J, Hall E, Lawrence D, Bliss J. Impact of selenium on mood and quality of life: a randomized, controlled trial. Biol Psychiatry. 2006;59(2):147–54. PMID: 16181615. http://www.ncbi.nlm.nih.gov/pubmed/16181615.
294. Mokhber N, Namjoo M, Tara F, Boskabadi H, Rayman MP, Ghayour-Mobarhan M, Sahebkar A, Majdi MR, Tavallaie S, Azimi-Nezhad M, Shakeri MT, Nematy M, Oladi M, Mohammadi M, Ferns G. Effect of supplementation with selenium on postpartum depression: a randomized double-blind placebo-controlled trial. J Matern Fetal Neonatal Med. 2011;24(1):104–8. PMID: 20528216. http://www.ncbi.nlm.nih.gov/pubmed/20528216.
295. Miller BJ, Murray L, Beckmann MM, Kent T, Macfarlane B. Dietary supplements for preventing postnatal depression. Cochrane Database Syst Rev. 2013;2013(10):CD009104. PMCID: PMC10166593. http://www.ncbi.nlm.nih.gov/pubmed/24158923.
296. Conner TS, Richardson AC, Miller JC. Optimal serum selenium concentrations are associated with lower depressive symptoms and negative mood among young adults. J Nutr. 2015;145(1):59–65. PMID: 25378685. http://www.ncbi.nlm.nih.gov/pubmed/25378685.

297. Ly A, Hoyt L, Crowell J, Kim YI. Folate and DNA methylation. Antioxid Redox Signal. 2012;17(2):302–26. PMID: 22332737. http://www.ncbi.nlm.nih.gov/pubmed/22332737.
298. Bhargava S, Tyagi SC. Nutriepigenetic regulation by folate-homocysteine-methionine axis: a review. Mol Cell Biochem. 2014;387(1–2):55–61. PMID: 24213682. http://www.ncbi.nlm.nih.gov/pubmed/24213682.
299. Ulrich CM, Reed MC, Nijhout HF. Modeling folate, one-carbon metabolism, and DNA methylation. Nutr Rev. 2008;66(Suppl 1):S27–30. PMID: 18673484. http://www.ncbi.nlm.nih.gov/pubmed/18673484.
300. Fava M, Mischoulon D. Evidence for folate in combination with antidepressants at initiation of therapy. J Clin Psychiatry. 2010;71(11):e31. PMID: 21114944. http://www.ncbi.nlm.nih.gov/pubmed/21114944.
301. Miller AL. The methylation, neurotransmitter, and antioxidant connections between folate and depression. Altern Med Rev. 2008;13(3):216–26. PMID: 18950248. http://www.ncbi.nlm.nih.gov/pubmed/18950248.
302. Stahl SM. L-methylfolate: a vitamin for your monoamines. J Clin Psychiatry. 2008;69(9):1352–3. PMID: 19193337. http://www.ncbi.nlm.nih.gov/pubmed/19193337.
303. Fenech M. Folate, DNA damage and the aging brain. Mech Ageing Dev. 2010;131(4):236–41. PMID: 20219521. http://www.ncbi.nlm.nih.gov/pubmed/20219521.
304. Morse NL. Benefits of docosahexaenoic acid, folic acid, vitamin D and iodine on foetal and infant brain development and function following maternal supplementation during pregnancy and lactation. Nutrients. 2012;4(7):799–840. PMCID: PMC3407995. http://www.ncbi.nlm.nih.gov/pubmed/22852064.
305. Pulikkunnel ST, Thomas SV. Neural tube defects: pathogenesis and folate metabolism. J Assoc Physicians India. 2005;53:127–35. PMID: 15847033. http://www.ncbi.nlm.nih.gov/pubmed/15847033.
306. NIH. Folate – health professional fact sheet. https://ods.od.nih.gov/factsheets/Folate-HealthProfessional/.
307. de Benoist B. Conclusions of a WHO Technical Consultation on folate and vitamin B12 deficiencies. Food Nutr Bull. 2008;29(2 Suppl):S238–44. PMID: 18709899. http://www.ncbi.nlm.nih.gov/pubmed/18709899.
308. Caudill MA. Folate bioavailability: implications for establishing dietary recommendations and optimizing status. Am J Clin Nutr. 2010;91(5):1455S–60S. PMCID: PMC2854911. http://www.ncbi.nlm.nih.gov/pubmed/20219964.
309. McNulty H, Scott JM. Intake and status of folate and related B-vitamins: considerations and challenges in achieving optimal status. Br J Nutr. 2008;99(Suppl 3):S48–54. PMID: 18598588. http://www.ncbi.nlm.nih.gov/pubmed/18598588.
310. Milman N, Byg KE, Hvas AM, Bergholt T, Eriksen L. Erythrocyte folate, plasma folate and plasma homocysteine during normal pregnancy and postpartum: a longitudinal study comprising 404 Danish women. Eur J Haematol. 2006;76(3):200–5. PMID: 16412135. http://www.ncbi.nlm.nih.gov/pubmed/16412135.
311. Bailey SW, Ayling JE. The extremely slow and variable activity of dihydrofolate reductase in human liver and its implications for high folic acid intake. Proc Natl Acad Sci USA. 2009;106(36):15424–9. PMCID: PMC2730961. http://www.ncbi.nlm.nih.gov/pubmed/19706381.
312. Milman N. Intestinal absorption of folic acid – new physiologic & molecular aspects. Indian J Med Res. 2012;136(5):725–8. PMCID: PMC3573592. http://www.ncbi.nlm.nih.gov/pubmed/23287118.
313. Malterre T. Digestive and nutritional considerations in celiac disease: could supplementation help? Altern Med Rev. 2009;14(3):247–57. PMID: 19803549. http://www.ncbi.nlm.nih.gov/pubmed/19803549.
314. Swain RA, St Clair L. The role of folic acid in deficiency states and prevention of disease. J Fam Pract. 1997;44(2):138–44. PMID: 9040515. http://www.ncbi.nlm.nih.gov/pubmed/9040515.
315. Medici V, Halsted CH. Folate, alcohol, and liver disease. Mol Nutr Food Res. 2013;57(4):596–606. PMCID: PMC3736728. http://www.ncbi.nlm.nih.gov/pubmed/23136133.
316. Ho E, Beaver LM, Williams DE, Dashwood RH. Dietary factors and epigenetic regulation for prostate cancer prevention. Adv Nutr. 2011;2(6):497–510. PMCID: PMC3226387. http://www.ncbi.nlm.nih.gov/pubmed/22332092.
317. Molloy AM, Kirke PN, Troendle JF, Burke H, Sutton M, Brody LC, Scott JM, Mills JL. Maternal vitamin B12 status and risk of neural tube defects in a population with high neural tube defect prevalence and no folic acid fortification. Pediatrics. 2009;123(3):917–23. PMCID: PMC4161975. http://www.ncbi.nlm.nih.gov/pubmed/19255021.
318. Ramaekers V, Sequeira JM, Quadros EV. Clinical recognition and aspects of the cerebral folate deficiency syndromes. Clin Chem Lab Med. 2013;51(3):497–511. PMID: 23314536. http://www.ncbi.nlm.nih.gov/pubmed/23314536.
319. Botez MI. Folate deficiency and neurological disorders in adults. Med Hypotheses. 1976;2(4):135–40. PMID: 958035. http://www.ncbi.nlm.nih.gov/pubmed/958035.
320. Bottiglieri T. Folate, vitamin B12, and neuropsychiatric disorders. Nutr Rev. 1996;54(12):382–90. PMID: 9155210. http://www.ncbi.nlm.nih.gov/pubmed/9155210.
321. Gilbody S, Lewis S, Lightfoot T. Methylenetetrahydrofolate reductase (MTHFR) genetic polymorphisms and psychiatric disorders: a HuGE review. Am J Epidemiol. 2007;165(1):1–13. PMID: 17074966. http://www.ncbi.nlm.nih.gov/pubmed/17074966.
322. Mischoulon D, Lamon-Fava S, Selhub J, Katz J, Papakostas GI, Iosifescu DV, Yeung AS, Dording CM, Farabaugh AH, Clain AJ, Baer L, Alpert JE, Nierenberg AA, Fava M. Prevalence of MTHFR C677T and MS A2756G polymorphisms in major depressive disorder, and their impact on response to fluoxetine treatment. CNS Spectr. 2012;17(2):76–86. PMCID: PMC4117348. http://www.ncbi.nlm.nih.gov/pubmed/22789065.
323. Weir DG, Scott JM. Brain function in the elderly: role of vitamin B12 and folate. Br Med Bull. 1999;55(3):669–82. PMID: 10746355. http://www.ncbi.nlm.nih.gov/pubmed/10746355.
324. Ulrich CM. Folate and cancer prevention: a closer look at a complex picture. Am J Clin Nutr. 2007;86(2):271–3. PMID: 17684194. http://www.ncbi.nlm.nih.gov/pubmed/17684194.
325. Stolzenberg-Solomon RZ, Chang SC, Leitzmann MF, Johnson KA, Johnson C, Buys SS, Hoover RN, Ziegler RG. Folate intake, alcohol use, and postmenopausal breast cancer risk in the Prostate, Lung, Colorectal, and Ovarian Cancer Screening Trial. Am J Clin Nutr. 2006;83(4):895–904. PMID: 16600944. http://www.ncbi.nlm.nih.gov/pubmed/16600944.
326. Tomaszewski JJ, Cummings JL, Parwani AV, Dhir R, Mason JB, Nelson JB, Bacich DJ, O'Keefe DS. Increased cancer cell proliferation in prostate cancer patients with high levels of serum folate. Prostate. 2011;71(12):1287–93. PMCID: PMC3120927. http://www.ncbi.nlm.nih.gov/pubmed/21308713.
327. Choi SW, Mason JB. Folate and carcinogenesis: an integrated scheme. J Nutr. 2000;130(2):129–32. PMID: 10720158. http://www.ncbi.nlm.nih.gov/pubmed/10720158.
328. Pieroth R, Paver S, Day S, Lammersfeld C. Folate and its impact on cancer risk. Curr Nutr Rep. 2018;7(3):70–84. PMCID: PMC6132377. http://www.ncbi.nlm.nih.gov/pubmed/30099693.
329. Ramos L, Henriksson M, Helleday T, Green AC. Targeting MTHFD2 to exploit cancer-specific metabolism and the DNA damage response. Cancer Res. 2024;84(1):9–16. PMID: 37922465. http://www.ncbi.nlm.nih.gov/pubmed/37922465.

330. Ma J, Stampfer MJ, Giovannucci E, Artigas C, Hunter DJ, Fuchs C, Willett WC, Selhub J, Hennekens CH, Rozen R. Methylenetetrahydrofolate reductase polymorphism, dietary interactions, and risk of colorectal cancer. Cancer Res. 1997;57(6):1098–102. PMID: 9067278. http://www.ncbi.nlm.nih.gov/pubmed/9067278.
331. Ulrich CM, Kampman E, Bigler J, Schwartz SM, Chen C, Bostick R, Fosdick L, Beresford SA, Yasui Y, Potter JD. Colorectal adenomas and the C677T MTHFR polymorphism: evidence for gene-environment interaction? Cancer Epidemiol Biomarkers Prev. 1999;8(8):659–68. PMID: 10744125. http://www.ncbi.nlm.nih.gov/pubmed/10744125.
332. Ulvik A, Evensen ET, Lien EA, Hoff G, Vollset SE, Majak BM, Ueland PM. Smoking, folate and methylenetetrahydrofolate reductase status as interactive determinants of adenomatous and hyperplastic polyps of colorectum. Am J Med Genet. 2001;101(3):246–54. PMID: 11424140. http://www.ncbi.nlm.nih.gov/pubmed/11424140.
333. Duthie SJ. Folic acid deficiency and cancer: mechanisms of DNA instability. Br Med Bull. 1999;55(3):578–92. PMID: 10746348. http://www.ncbi.nlm.nih.gov/pubmed/10746348.
334. Young SN. Folate and depression--a neglected problem. J Psychiatry Neurosci. 2007;32(2):80–2. PMCID: PMC1810582. http://www.ncbi.nlm.nih.gov/pubmed/17353937.
335. Paul RTP, McDonnell AP, Kelly CB. Folic acid: neurochemistry, metabolism and relationship to depression. Hum Psychopharmacol. 2004;19(7):477–88. PMID: 15378677. http://www.ncbi.nlm.nih.gov/pubmed/15378677.
336. Alpert JE, Papakostas G, Mischoulon D, Worthington JJ, Petersen T, Mahal Y, Burns A, Bottiglieri T, Nierenberg AA, Fava M. S-adenosyl-L-methionine (SAMe) as an adjunct for resistant major depressive disorder: an open trial following partial or nonresponse to selective serotonin reuptake inhibitors or venlafaxine. J Clin Psychopharmacol. 2004;24(6):661–4. PMID: 15538131. http://www.ncbi.nlm.nih.gov/pubmed/15538131.
337. Coppen A, Bolander-Gouaille C. Treatment of depression: time to consider folic acid and vitamin B12. J Psychopharmacol. 2005;19(1):59–65. PMID: 15671130. http://www.ncbi.nlm.nih.gov/pubmed/15671130.
338. Kuo HK, Sorond FA, Chen JH, Hashmi A, Milberg WP, Lipsitz LA. The role of homocysteine in multisystem age-related problems: a systematic review. J Gerontol A Biol Sci Med Sci. 2005;60(9):1190–201. PMID: 16183962. http://www.ncbi.nlm.nih.gov/pubmed/16183962.
339. Refsum H, Nurk E, Smith AD, Ueland PM, Gjesdal CG, Bjelland I, Tverdal A, Tell GS, Nygård O, Vollset SE. The Hordaland Homocysteine Study: a community-based study of homocysteine, its determinants, and associations with disease. J Nutr. 2006;136(6 Suppl):1731S–40S. PMID: 16702348. http://www.ncbi.nlm.nih.gov/pubmed/16702348.
340. Cappuccio FP, Bell R, Perry IJ, Gilg J, Ueland PM, Refsum H, Sagnella GA, Jeffery S, Cook DG. Homocysteine levels in men and women of different ethnic and cultural background living in England. Atherosclerosis. 2002;164(1):95–102. PMID: 12119198. http://www.ncbi.nlm.nih.gov/pubmed/12119198.
341. Gaweesh S, Ewies AAA. Folic acid supplementation cures hot flushes in postmenopausal women. Med Hypotheses. 2010;74(2):286–8. PMID: 19796883. http://www.ncbi.nlm.nih.gov/pubmed/19796883.
342. García-Miss MDR, Pérez-Mutul J, López-Canul B, Solís-Rodríguez F, Puga-Machado L, Oxté-Cabrera A, Gurubel-Maldonado J, Arankowsky-Sandoval G. Folate, homocysteine, interleukin-6, and tumor necrosis factor alfa levels, but not the methylenetetrahydrofolate reductase C677T polymorphism, are risk factors for schizophrenia. J Psychiatr Res. 2010;44(7):441–6. PMID: 19939410. http://www.ncbi.nlm.nih.gov/pubmed/19939410.
343. Roberts SH, Bedson E, Hughes D, Lloyd K, Menkes DB, Moat S, Pirmohamed M, Slegg G, Thome J, Tranter R, Whitaker R, Wilkinson C, Russell I. Folate augmentation of treatment – evaluation for depression (FolATED): protocol of a randomised controlled trial. BMC Psychiatry. 2007;7:65. PMCID: PMC2238748. http://www.ncbi.nlm.nih.gov/pubmed/18005429.
344. Morris DW, Trivedi MH, Rush AJ. Folate and unipolar depression. J Altern Complement Med. 2008;14(3):277–85. PMID: 18370582. http://www.ncbi.nlm.nih.gov/pubmed/18370582.
345. Papakostas GI, Shelton RC, Zajecka JM, Etemad B, Rickels K, Clain A, Baer L, Dalton ED, Sacco GR, Schoenfeld D, Pencina M, Meisner A, Bottiglieri T, Nelson E, Mischoulon D, Alpert JE, Barbee JG, Zisook S, Fava M. L-methylfolate as adjunctive therapy for SSRI-resistant major depression: results of two randomized, double-blind, parallel-sequential trials. Am J Psychiatry. 2012;169(12):1267–74. PMID: 23212058. http://www.ncbi.nlm.nih.gov/pubmed/23212058.
346. Gilbody S, Lightfoot T, Sheldon T. Is low folate a risk factor for depression? A meta-analysis and exploration of heterogeneity. J Epidemiol Community Health. 2007;61(7):631–7. PMCID: PMC2465760. http://www.ncbi.nlm.nih.gov/pubmed/17568057.
347. Sanhueza C, Ryan L, Foxcroft DR. Diet and the risk of unipolar depression in adults: systematic review of cohort studies. J Hum Nutr Diet. 2013;26(1):56–70. PMID: 23078460. http://www.ncbi.nlm.nih.gov/pubmed/23078460.
348. Alpert M, Silva RR, Pouget ER. Prediction of treatment response in geriatric depression from baseline folate level: interaction with an SSRI or a tricyclic antidepressant. J Clin Psychopharmacol. 2003;23(3):309–13. PMID: 12826993. http://www.ncbi.nlm.nih.gov/pubmed/12826993.
349. Papakostas GI, Petersen T, Mischoulon D, Ryan JL, Nierenberg AA, Bottiglieri T, Rosenbaum JF, Alpert JE, Fava M. Serum folate, vitamin B12, and homocysteine in major depressive disorder, part 1: predictors of clinical response in fluoxetine-resistant depression. J Clin Psychiatry. 2004;65(8):1090–5. PMID: 15323594. http://www.ncbi.nlm.nih.gov/pubmed/15323594.
350. Reynolds EH. Methylfolate as adjunctive treatment in major depression. Am J Psychiatry. 2013;170(5):560. PMID: 23632839. http://www.ncbi.nlm.nih.gov/pubmed/23632839.
351. Roberts SH, Tranter R. Higher dose L-methylfolate may be an effective adjunctive therapy for adults with major depression who have inadequate response to SSRIs. Evid Based Ment Health. 2013;16(3):75. PMID: 23625145. http://www.ncbi.nlm.nih.gov/pubmed/23625145.
352. Nelson JC. The evolving story of folate in depression and the therapeutic potential of l-methylfolate. Am J Psychiatry. 2012;169(12):1223–5. PMID: 23212050. http://www.ncbi.nlm.nih.gov/pubmed/23212050.
353. Coppen A, Bailey J. Enhancement of the antidepressant action of fluoxetine by folic acid: a randomised, placebo controlled trial. J Affect Disord. 2000;60(2):121–30. PMID: 10967371. http://www.ncbi.nlm.nih.gov/pubmed/10967371.
354. Kendrick T, Dunn N, Robinson S, Oestmann A, Godfrey K, Cooper C, Inskip H, Southampton Women's Survey Study Group. A longitudinal study of blood folate levels and depressive symptoms among young women in the Southampton Women's Survey. J Epidemiol Community Health. 2008;62(11):966–72. PMCID: PMC4558940. http://www.ncbi.nlm.nih.gov/pubmed/18854500.
355. Watanabe H, Ishida S, Konno Y, Matsumoto M, Nomachi S, Masaki K, Okayama H, Nagai Y. Impact of dietary folate intake on depressive symptoms in young women of reproductive age. J Midwifery Womens Health. 2012;57(1):43–8. PMID: 22251911. http://www.ncbi.nlm.nih.gov/pubmed/22251911.

356. Das UN. Folic acid and polyunsaturated fatty acids improve cognitive function and prevent depression, dementia, and Alzheimer's disease--but how and why? Prostaglandins Leukot Essent Fatty Acids. 2008;78(1):11–9. PMID: 18054217. http://www.ncbi.nlm.nih.gov/pubmed/18054217.
357. Pita ML, Delgado MJ. Folate administration increases n-3 polyunsaturated fatty acids in rat plasma and tissue lipids. Thromb Haemost. 2000;84(3):420–3. PMID: 11019965. http://www.ncbi.nlm.nih.gov/pubmed/11019965.
358. Durand P, Prost M, Blache D. Pro-thrombotic effects of a folic acid deficient diet in rat platelets and macrophages related to elevated homocysteine and decreased n-3 polyunsaturated fatty acids. Atherosclerosis. 1996;121(2):231–43. PMID: 9125297. http://www.ncbi.nlm.nih.gov/pubmed/9125297.
359. Galizia I, Oldani L, Macritchie K, Amari E, Dougall D, Jones TN, Lam RW, Massei GJ, Yatham LN, Young AH. S-adenosyl methionine (SAMe) for depression in adults. Cochrane Database Syst Rev. 2016;10(10):CD011286. PMCID: PMC6457972. http://www.ncbi.nlm.nih.gov/pubmed/27727432.
360. Mischoulon D, Fava M. Role of S-adenosyl-L-methionine in the treatment of depression: a review of the evidence. Am J Clin Nutr. 2002;76(5):1158S–61S. PMID: 12420702. http://www.ncbi.nlm.nih.gov/pubmed/12420702.
361. Bressa GM. S-adenosyl-l-methionine (SAMe) as antidepressant: meta-analysis of clinical studies. Acta Neurol Scand Suppl. 1994;154:7–14. PMID: 7941964. http://www.ncbi.nlm.nih.gov/pubmed/7941964.
362. Papakostas GI, Mischoulon D, Shyu I, Alpert JE, Fava M. S-adenosyl methionine (SAMe) augmentation of serotonin reuptake inhibitors for antidepressant nonresponders with major depressive disorder: a double-blind, randomized clinical trial. Am J Psychiatry. 2010;167(8):942–8. PMID: 20595412. http://www.ncbi.nlm.nih.gov/pubmed/20595412.
363. Levkovitz Y, Alpert JE, Brintz CE, Mischoulon D, Papakostas GI. Effects of S-adenosylmethionine augmentation of serotonin-reuptake inhibitor antidepressants on cognitive symptoms of major depressive disorder. J Affect Disord. 2012;136(3):1174–8. PMID: 21911258. http://www.ncbi.nlm.nih.gov/pubmed/21911258.
364. Kaplan BJ, Crawford SG, Field CJ, Simpson JSA. Vitamins, minerals, and mood. Psychol Bull. 2007;133(5):747–60. PMID: 17723028. http://www.ncbi.nlm.nih.gov/pubmed/17723028.
365. Altura BM, Altura BT. Role of magnesium in patho-physiological processes and the clinical utility of magnesium ion selective electrodes. Scand J Clin Lab Invest Suppl. 1996;224:211–34. PMID: 8865438. http://www.ncbi.nlm.nih.gov/pubmed/8865438.
366. NIH. Magnesium – health professional fact sheet. https://ods.od.nih.gov/factsheets/Magnesium-HealthProfessional/.
367. King DE, Mainous AG, Geesey ME, Woolson RF. Dietary magnesium and C-reactive protein levels. J Am Coll Nutr. 2005;24(3):166–71. PMID: 15930481. http://www.ncbi.nlm.nih.gov/pubmed/15930481.
368. Eby GA, Eby KL. Rapid recovery from major depression using magnesium treatment. Med Hypotheses. 2006;67(2):362–70. PMID: 16542786. http://www.ncbi.nlm.nih.gov/pubmed/16542786.
369. Gröber U, Schmidt J, Kisters K. Magnesium in prevention and therapy. Nutrients. 2015;7(9):8199–226. PMCID: PMC4586582. http://www.ncbi.nlm.nih.gov/pubmed/26404370.
370. Młyniec K, Davies CL, de Agüero Sánchez IG, Pytka K, Budziszewska B, Nowak G. Essential elements in depression and anxiety. Part I. Pharmacol Rep. 2014;66(4):534–44. PMID: 24948052. http://www.ncbi.nlm.nih.gov/pubmed/24948052.
371. Singewald N, Sinner C, Hetzenauer A, Sartori SB, Murck H. Magnesium-deficient diet alters depression- and anxiety-related behavior in mice--influence of desipramine and Hypericum perforatum extract. Neuropharmacology. 2004;47(8):1189–97. PMID: 15567428. http://www.ncbi.nlm.nih.gov/pubmed/15567428.
372. Winther G, Pyndt Jørgensen BM, Elfving B, Nielsen DS, Kihl P, Lund S, Sørensen DB, Wegener G. Dietary magnesium deficiency alters gut microbiota and leads to depressive-like behaviour. Acta Neuropsychiatr. 2015;27(3):168–76. PMID: 25690713. http://www.ncbi.nlm.nih.gov/pubmed/25690713.
373. Stanisławska M, Szkup-Jabłońska M, Jurczak A, Wieder-Huszla S, Samochowiec A, Jasiewicz A, Noceń I, Augustyniuk K, Brodowska A, Karakiewicz B, Chlubek D, Grochans E. The severity of depressive symptoms vs. serum Mg and Zn levels in postmenopausal women. Biol Trace Elem Res. 2014;157(1):30–5. PMCID: PMC3895221. http://www.ncbi.nlm.nih.gov/pubmed/24271492.
374. Gu Y, Zhao K, Luan X, Liu Z, Cai Y, Wang Q, Zhu B, He J. Association between serum magnesium levels and depression in stroke patients. Aging Dis. 2016;7(6):687–90. PMCID: PMC5198859. http://www.ncbi.nlm.nih.gov/pubmed/28053818.
375. Jacka FN, Overland S, Stewart R, Tell GS, Bjelland I, Mykletun A. Association between magnesium intake and depression and anxiety in community-dwelling adults: the Hordaland Health Study. Aust N Z J Psychiatry. 2009;43(1):45–52. PMID: 19085527. http://www.ncbi.nlm.nih.gov/pubmed/19085527.
376. Tarleton EK, Littenberg B. Magnesium intake and depression in adults. J Am Board Fam Med. 2015;28(2):249–56. PMID: 25748766. http://www.ncbi.nlm.nih.gov/pubmed/25748766.
377. Martínez-González MÁ, Sánchez-Villegas A. Magnesium intake and depression: the SUN cohort. Magnes Res. 2016;29(3):102–11. PMID: 27910807. http://www.ncbi.nlm.nih.gov/pubmed/27910807.
378. Derom ML, Martínez-González MA, Sayón-Orea MDC, Bes-Rastrollo M, Beunza JJ, Sánchez-Villegas A. Magnesium intake is not related to depression risk in Spanish university graduates. J Nutr. 2012;142(6):1053–9. PMID: 22513990. http://www.ncbi.nlm.nih.gov/pubmed/22513990.
379. Rajizadeh A, Mozaffari-Khosravi H, Yassini-Ardakani M, Dehghani A. Effect of magnesium supplementation on depression status in depressed patients with magnesium deficiency: a randomized, double-blind, placebo-controlled trial. Nutrition. 2017;35:56–60. PMID: 28241991. http://www.ncbi.nlm.nih.gov/pubmed/28241991.
380. Barragán-Rodríguez L, Rodríguez-Morán M, Guerrero-Romero F. Efficacy and safety of oral magnesium supplementation in the treatment of depression in the elderly with type 2 diabetes: a randomized, equivalent trial. Magnes Res. 2008;21(4):218–23. PMID: 19271419. http://www.ncbi.nlm.nih.gov/pubmed/19271419.
381. Fard FE, Mirghafourvand M, Mohammad-Alizadeh Charandabi S, Farshbaf-Khalili A, Javadzadeh Y, Asgharian H. Effects of zinc and magnesium supplements on postpartum depression and anxiety: a randomized controlled clinical trial. Women Health. 2017;57(9):1115–28. PMID: 27617502. http://www.ncbi.nlm.nih.gov/pubmed/27617502.
382. Cardoso CC, Lobato KR, Binfaré RW, Ferreira PK, Rosa AO, Santos ARS, Rodrigues ALS. Evidence for the involvement of the monoaminergic system in the antidepressant-like effect of magnesium. Prog Neuro-Psychopharmacol Biol Psychiatry. 2009;33(2):235–42. PMID: 19059299. http://www.ncbi.nlm.nih.gov/pubmed/19059299.
383. Poleszak E. Modulation of antidepressant-like activity of magnesium by serotonergic system. J Neural Transm (Vienna). 2007;114(9):1129–34. PMID: 17447000. http://www.ncbi.nlm.nih.gov/pubmed/17447000.
384. Pochwat B, Sowa-Kucma M, Kotarska K, Misztak P, Nowak G, Szewczyk B. Antidepressant-like activity of magnesium in the olfactory bulbectomy model is associated with the AMPA/BDNF

pathway. Psychopharmacology. 2015;232(2):355–67. PMCID: PMC4297308. http://www.ncbi.nlm.nih.gov/pubmed/25027582.
385. Billyard AJ, Eggett DL, Franz KB. Dietary magnesium deficiency decreases plasma melatonin in rats. Magnes Res. 2006;19(3):157–61. PMID: 17172005. http://www.ncbi.nlm.nih.gov/pubmed/17172005.
386. Kirkland AE, Sarlo GL, Holton KF. The role of magnesium in neurological disorders. Nutrients. 2018;10(6):730. PMCID: PMC6024559. http://www.ncbi.nlm.nih.gov/pubmed/29882776.
387. Coan EJ, Collingridge GL. Magnesium ions block an N-methyl-D-aspartate receptor-mediated component of synaptic transmission in rat hippocampus. Neurosci Lett. 1985;53(1):21–6. PMID: 2859558. http://www.ncbi.nlm.nih.gov/pubmed/2859558.
388. Murck H. Ketamine, magnesium and major depression--from pharmacology to pathophysiology and back. J Psychiatr Res. 2013;47(7):955–65. PMID: 23541145. http://www.ncbi.nlm.nih.gov/pubmed/23541145.
389. Ghafari M, Whittle N, Miklósi AG, Kotlowski C, Schmuckermair C, Berger J, Bennett KL, Singewald N, Lubec G. Dietary magnesium restriction reduces amygdala-hypothalamic GluN1 receptor complex levels in mice. Brain Struct Funct. 2015;220(4):2209–21. PMID: 24807818. http://www.ncbi.nlm.nih.gov/pubmed/24807818.
390. Poleszak E, Wlaź P, Kedzierska E, Nieoczym D, Wróbel A, Fidecka S, Pilc A, Nowak G. NMDA/glutamate mechanism of antidepressant-like action of magnesium in forced swim test in mice. Pharmacol Biochem Behav. 2007;88(2):158–64. PMID: 17825400. http://www.ncbi.nlm.nih.gov/pubmed/17825400.
391. Kiecolt-Glaser JK, Derry HM, Fagundes CP. Inflammation: depression fans the flames and feasts on the heat. Am J Psychiatry. 2015;172(11):1075–91. PMCID: PMC6511978. http://www.ncbi.nlm.nih.gov/pubmed/26357876.
392. Miller AH, Maletic V, Raison CL. Inflammation and its discontents: the role of cytokines in the pathophysiology of major depression. Biol Psychiatry. 2009;65(9):732–41. PMCID: PMC2680424. http://www.ncbi.nlm.nih.gov/pubmed/19150053.
393. Miller AH, Raison CL. The role of inflammation in depression: from evolutionary imperative to modern treatment target. Nat Rev Immunol. 2016;16(1):22–34. PMCID: PMC5542678. http://www.ncbi.nlm.nih.gov/pubmed/26711676.
394. Sartori SB, Whittle N, Hetzenauer A, Singewald N. Magnesium deficiency induces anxiety and HPA axis dysregulation: modulation by therapeutic drug treatment. Neuropharmacology. 2012;62(1):304–12. PMCID: PMC3198864. http://www.ncbi.nlm.nih.gov/pubmed/21835188.
395. Murck H, Steiger A. Mg2+ reduces ACTH secretion and enhances spindle power without changing delta power during sleep in men – possible therapeutic implications. Psychopharmacology. 1998;137(3):247–52. PMID: 9683002. http://www.ncbi.nlm.nih.gov/pubmed/9683002.
396. Ehlert U, Gaab J, Heinrichs M. Psychoneuroendocrinological contributions to the etiology of depression, posttraumatic stress disorder, and stress-related bodily disorders: the role of the hypothalamus-pituitary-adrenal axis. Biol Psychol. 2001;57(1–3):141–52. PMID: 11454437. http://www.ncbi.nlm.nih.gov/pubmed/11454437.
397. Guerry JD, Hastings PD. In search of HPA axis dysregulation in child and adolescent depression. Clin Child Fam Psychol Rev. 2011;14(2):135–60. PMCID: PMC3095794. http://www.ncbi.nlm.nih.gov/pubmed/21290178.
398. Lee AL, Ogle WO, Sapolsky RM. Stress and depression: possible links to neuron death in the hippocampus. Bipolar Disord. 2002;4(2):117–28. PMID: 12071509. http://www.ncbi.nlm.nih.gov/pubmed/12071509.
399. Uno H, Eisele S, Sakai A, Shelton S, Baker E, DeJesus O, Holden J. Neurotoxicity of glucocorticoids in the primate brain. Horm Behav. 1994;28(4):336–48. PMID: 7729802. http://www.ncbi.nlm.nih.gov/pubmed/7729802.
400. Dibaba DT, Xun P, He K. Dietary magnesium intake is inversely associated with serum C-reactive protein levels: meta-analysis and systematic review. Eur J Clin Nutr. 2014;68(4):510–6. PMCID: PMC3975661. http://www.ncbi.nlm.nih.gov/pubmed/24518747.
401. Chacko SA, Song Y, Nathan L, Tinker L, de Boer IH, Tylavsky F, Wallace R, Liu S. Relations of dietary magnesium intake to biomarkers of inflammation and endothelial dysfunction in an ethnically diverse cohort of postmenopausal women. Diabetes Care. 2010;33(2):304–10. PMCID: PMC2809271. http://www.ncbi.nlm.nih.gov/pubmed/19903755.
402. Pachikian BD, Neyrinck AM, Deldicque L, De Backer FC, Catry E, Dewulf EM, Sohet FM, Bindels LB, Everard A, Francaux M, Guiot Y, Cani PD, Delzenne NM. Changes in intestinal bifidobacteria levels are associated with the inflammatory response in magnesium-deficient mice. J Nutr. 2010;140(3):509–14. PMID: 20089787. http://www.ncbi.nlm.nih.gov/pubmed/20089787.
403. Maron E, Shlik J, Nutt DJ. Tryptophan research in panic disorder. Int J Tryptophan Res. 2008;1:3–12. PMCID: PMC3195213. http://www.ncbi.nlm.nih.gov/pubmed/22084577.
404. Barr LC, Goodman WK, McDougle CJ, Delgado PL, Heninger GR, Charney DS, Price LH. Tryptophan depletion in patients with obsessive-compulsive disorder who respond to serotonin reuptake inhibitors. Arch Gen Psychiatry. 1994;51(4):309–17. PMID: 8161291. http://www.ncbi.nlm.nih.gov/pubmed/8161291.
405. Baïlara KM, Henry C, Lestage J, Launay JM, Parrot F, Swendsen J, Sutter AL, Roux D, Dallay D, Demotes-Mainard J. Decreased brain tryptophan availability as a partial determinant of post-partum blues. Psychoneuroendocrinology. 2006;31(3):407–13. PMID: 16303256. http://www.ncbi.nlm.nih.gov/pubmed/16303256.
406. Meyers S. Use of neurotransmitter precursors for treatment of depression. Altern Med Rev. 2000;5(1):64–71. PMID: 10696120. http://www.ncbi.nlm.nih.gov/pubmed/10696120.
407. 5-HTP efficacy and contraindications [Retraction]. Neuropsychiatr Dis Treat. 2021;17:731. https://doi.org/10.2147/NDT.S308254. PMID: 33688195; PMCID: PMC7937375. https://pubmed.ncbi.nlm.nih.gov/33688195/.
408. Shaw K, Turner J, Del Mar C. Are tryptophan and 5-hydroxytryptophan effective treatments for depression? A meta-analysis. Aust N Z J Psychiatry. 2002;36(4):488–91. PMID: 12169147. http://www.ncbi.nlm.nih.gov/pubmed/12169147
409. Shaw K, Turner J, Del Mar C. Tryptophan and 5-hydroxytryptophan for depression. Cochrane Database Syst Rev. 2001;2002(3):CD003198. PMCID: PMC8711266. http://www.ncbi.nlm.nih.gov/pubmed/11687048.
410. Brockhaus AC, Bender R, Skipka G. The Peto odds ratio viewed as a new effect measure. Stat Med. 2014;33(28):4861–74. PMID: 25244540. http://www.ncbi.nlm.nih.gov/pubmed/25244540.
411. USDA FoodData Central. Food search. https://fdc.nal.usda.gov/food-search?component=1210.
412. National Academies. Protein and amino acids. In: Dietary reference intakes for energy, carbohydrate, fiber, fat, fatty acids, cholesterol, protein, and amino acids. The National Academies Press; 2005. https://nap.nationalacademies.org/read/10490/chapter/12#593.
413. Tsuboi H, Shimoi K, Kinae N, Oguni I, Hori R, Kobayashi F. Depressive symptoms are independently correlated with lipid peroxidation in a female population: comparison with vitamins and carotenoids. J Psychosom Res. 2004;56(1):53–8. PMID: 14987964. http://www.ncbi.nlm.nih.gov/pubmed/14987964.
414. Kuloglu M, Atmaca M, Tezcan E, Gecici O, Tunckol H, Ustundag B. Antioxidant enzyme activities and malondialdehyde levels in patients with obsessive-compulsive disorder. Neuropsychobiology. 2002;46(1):27–32. PMID: 12207144. http://www.ncbi.nlm.nih.gov/pubmed/12207144.

415. Erdogan H, Fadillioglu E, Ozgocmen S, Sogut S, Ozyurt B, Akyol O, Ardicoglu O. Effect of fish oil supplementation on plasma oxidant/antioxidant status in rats. Prostaglandins Leukot Essent Fatty Acids. 2004;71(3):149–52. PMID: 15253883. http://www.ncbi.nlm.nih.gov/pubmed/15253883.
416. Guelzim N, Huneau JF, Mathé V, Quignard-Boulangé A, Martin PG, Tomé D, Hermier D. Consequences of PPAR(α) invalidation on glutathione synthesis: interactions with dietary fatty acids. PPAR Res. 2011;2011:256186. PMCID: PMC3171156. http://www.ncbi.nlm.nih.gov/pubmed/21915176.
417. Wu A, Ying Z, Gomez-Pinilla F. The interplay between oxidative stress and brain-derived neurotrophic factor modulates the outcome of a saturated fat diet on synaptic plasticity and cognition. Eur J Neurosci. 2004;19(7):1699–707. PMID: 15078544. http://www.ncbi.nlm.nih.gov/pubmed/15078544.
418. Williams KJ, Fisher EA. Oxidation, lipoproteins, and atherosclerosis: which is wrong, the antioxidants or the theory? Curr Opin Clin Nutr Metab Care. 2005;8(2):139–46. PMID: 15716791. http://www.ncbi.nlm.nih.gov/pubmed/15716791.
419. Watson TA, Blake RJ, Callister R, Garg ML. Antioxidant-restricted diet reduces plasma nonesterified fatty acids in trained athletes. Lipids. 2005;40(4):433–5. PMID: 16028724 PubMed entry [Internet]. [cited 2025 Jan 19]. Available from: http://www.ncbi.nlm.nih.gov/pubmed/16028724.
420. Anglin RES, Samaan Z, Walter SD, McDonald SD. Vitamin D deficiency and depression in adults: systematic review and meta-analysis. Br J Psychiatry. 2013;202:100–7. PMID: 23377209. http://www.ncbi.nlm.nih.gov/pubmed/23377209.
421. Shaffer JA, Edmondson D, Wasson LT, Falzon L, Homma K, Ezeokoli N, Li P, Davidson KW. Vitamin D supplementation for depressive symptoms: a systematic review and meta-analysis of randomized controlled trials. Psychosom Med. 2014;76(3):190–6. PMCID: PMC4008710. http://www.ncbi.nlm.nih.gov/pubmed/24632894.
422. Wacker M, Holick MF. Sunlight and vitamin D: a global perspective for health. Dermatoendocrinol. 2013;5(1):51–108. PMCID: PMC3897598. http://www.ncbi.nlm.nih.gov/pubmed/24494042.
423. Holick MF. Vitamin D: a millenium perspective. J Cell Biochem. 2003;88(2):296–307. PMID: 12520530. http://www.ncbi.nlm.nih.gov/pubmed/12520530.
424. Dixon KM, Norman AW, Sequeira VB, Mohan R, Rybchyn MS, Reeve VE, Halliday GM, Mason RS. 1α,25$(OH)_2$-vitamin D and a nongenomic vitamin D analogue inhibit ultraviolet radiation-induced skin carcinogenesis. Cancer Prev Res (Phila). 2011;4(9):1485–94. PMID: 21733837. http://www.ncbi.nlm.nih.gov/pubmed/21733837.
425. Bikle DD. Vitamin D: production, metabolism and mechanisms of action. In: Endotext [Internet]. South Dartmouth: MDText.com, Inc.; 2000. https://www.ncbi.nlm.nih.gov/books/NBK278935/.
426. Schlögl M, Holick MF. Vitamin D and neurocognitive function. Clin Interv Aging. 2014;9:559–68. PMCID: PMC3979692. http://www.ncbi.nlm.nih.gov/pubmed/24729696.
427. Schwartz GG, Whitlatch LW, Chen TC, Lokeshwar BL, Holick MF. Human prostate cells synthesize 1,25-dihydroxyvitamin D3 from 25-hydroxyvitamin D3. Cancer Epidemiol Biomarkers Prev. 1998;7(5):391–5. PMID: 9610788. http://www.ncbi.nlm.nih.gov/pubmed/9610788.
428. Mawer EB, Hayes ME, Heys SE, Davies M, White A, Stewart MF, Smith GN. Constitutive synthesis of 1,25-dihydroxyvitamin D3 by a human small cell lung cancer cell line. J Clin Endocrinol Metab. 1994;79(2):554–60. PMID: 8045976. http://www.ncbi.nlm.nih.gov/pubmed/8045976.
429. DeLuca HF. Overview of general physiologic features and functions of vitamin D. Am J Clin Nutr. 2004;80(6 Suppl):1689S–96S. PMID: 15585789. http://www.ncbi.nlm.nih.gov/pubmed/15585789.
430. Dixon KM, Norman AW, Sequeira VB, Mohan R, Rybchyn MS, Reeve VE, Halliday GM, Mason RS. 1α,25$(OH)_2$-vitamin D and a nongenomic vitamin D analogue inhibit ultraviolet radiation-induced skin carcinogenesis. Cancer Prev Res (Phila). 2011;4(9):1485–94. PMID: 21733837. http://www.ncbi.nlm.nih.gov/pubmed/21733837.
431. Ooi JH, Chen J, Cantorna MT. Vitamin D regulation of immune function in the gut: why do T cells have vitamin D receptors? Mol Asp Med. 2012;33(1):77–82. PMCID: PMC3781946. http://www.ncbi.nlm.nih.gov/pubmed/22079836.
432. Narvaez CJ, Matthews D, LaPorta E, Simmons KM, Beaudin S, Welsh J. The impact of vitamin D in breast cancer: genomics, pathways, metabolism. Front Physiol. 2014;5:213. PMCID: PMC4055997. http://www.ncbi.nlm.nih.gov/pubmed/24982636.
433. Vaishya R, Vijay V, Agarwal AK, Jahangir J. Resurgence of vitamin D: old wine in new bottle. J Clin Orthop Trauma. 2015;6(3):173–83. PMCID: PMC4488032. http://www.ncbi.nlm.nih.gov/pubmed/26155053.
434. Colonese F, Laganà AS, Colonese E, Sofo V, Salmeri FM, Granese R, Triolo O. The pleiotropic effects of vitamin D in gynaecological and obstetric diseases: an overview on a hot topic. Biomed Res Int. 2015;2015:986281. PMCID: PMC4426767. http://www.ncbi.nlm.nih.gov/pubmed/26000308.
435. Jones G, Strugnell SA, DeLuca HF. Current understanding of the molecular actions of vitamin D. Physiol Rev. 1998;78(4):1193–231. PMID: 9790574. http://www.ncbi.nlm.nih.gov/pubmed/9790574.
436. Sebaaly A, Bachour F, Bayoud W, Adib G, Bedran F, Daher C, Maalouf G. The extraskeletal actions of vitamin D--myths and facts. J Med Liban. 2015;63(2):87–93. PMID: 26164977. http://www.ncbi.nlm.nih.gov/pubmed/26164977.
437. Holick MF. McCollum Award Lecture, 1994: vitamin D--new horizons for the 21st century. Am J Clin Nutr. 1994;60(4):619–30. PMID: 8092101. http://www.ncbi.nlm.nih.gov/pubmed/8092101.
438. Zepp RG, Erickson DJ, Paul ND, Sulzberger B. Interactive effects of solar UV radiation and climate change on biogeochemical cycling. Photochem Photobiol Sci. 2007;6(3):286–300. PMID: 17344963. http://www.ncbi.nlm.nih.gov/pubmed/17344963.
439. Caldwell MM, Flint SD. Stratospheric ozone reduction, solar UV-B radiation and terrestrial ecosystems. Clim Chang. 1994;28:375–94. https://link.springer.com/article/10.1007/BF01104080
440. Spina C, Tangpricha V, Yao M, Zhou W, Wolfe MM, Maehr H, Uskokovic M, Adorini L, Holick MF. Colon cancer and solar ultraviolet B radiation and prevention and treatment of colon cancer in mice with vitamin D and its Gemini analogs. J Steroid Biochem Mol Biol. 2005;97(1–2):111–20. PMID: 16154354. http://www.ncbi.nlm.nih.gov/pubmed/16154354.
441. Holick MF. Vitamin D deficiency. N Engl J Med. 2007;357(3):266–81. PMID: 17634462. http://www.ncbi.nlm.nih.gov/pubmed/17634462.
442. Ladizesky M, Lu Z, Oliveri B, San Roman N, Diaz S, Holick MF, Mautalen C. Solar ultraviolet B radiation and photoproduction of vitamin D3 in central and southern areas of Argentina. J Bone Miner Res. 1995;10(4):545–9. PMID: 7610924. http://www.ncbi.nlm.nih.gov/pubmed/7610924.
443. MacLaughlin J, Holick MF. Aging decreases the capacity of human skin to produce vitamin D3. J Clin Invest. 1985;76(4):1536–8. PMCID: PMC424123. http://www.ncbi.nlm.nih.gov/pubmed/2997282.
444. Holick MF, Matsuoka LY, Wortsman J. Age, vitamin D, and solar ultraviolet. Lancet. 1989;2(8671):1104–5. PMID: 2572832. http://www.ncbi.nlm.nih.gov/pubmed/2572832.
445. Holick MF, Chen TC, Lu Z, Sauter E. Vitamin D and skin physiology: a D-lightful story. J Bone Miner Res. 2007;22(Suppl 2):V28–33. PMID: 18290718. http://www.ncbi.nlm.nih.gov/pubmed/18290718.

446. Matsuoka LY, Ide L, Wortsman J, MacLaughlin JA, Holick MF. Sunscreens suppress cutaneous vitamin D3 synthesis. J Clin Endocrinol Metab. 1987;64(6):1165–8. PMID: 3033008. http://www.ncbi.nlm.nih.gov/pubmed/3033008.
447. Matsuoka LY, Wortsman J, Hanifan N, Holick MF. Chronic sunscreen use decreases circulating concentrations of 25-hydroxyvitamin D. A preliminary study. Arch Dermatol. 1988;124(12):1802–4. PMID: 3190255. http://www.ncbi.nlm.nih.gov/pubmed/3190255.
448. Jablonski NG, Chaplin G. The evolution of human skin coloration. J Hum Evol. 2000;39(1):57–106. PMID: 10896812. http://www.ncbi.nlm.nih.gov/pubmed/10896812.
449. Lalueza-Fox C, Römpler H, Caramelli D, Stäubert C, Catalano G, Hughes D, Rohland N, Pilli E, Longo L, Condemi S, de la Rasilla M, Fortea J, Rosas A, Stoneking M, Schöneberg T, Bertranpetit J, Hofreiter M. A melanocortin 1 receptor allele suggests varying pigmentation among Neanderthals. Science. 2007;318(5855):1453–5. PMID: 17962522. http://www.ncbi.nlm.nih.gov/pubmed/17962522.
450. Merewood A, Mehta SD, Chen TC, Bauchner H, Holick MF. Association between vitamin D deficiency and primary cesarean section. J Clin Endocrinol Metab. 2009;94(3):940–5. PMCID: PMC2681281. http://www.ncbi.nlm.nih.gov/pubmed/19106272.
451. Saliba W, Barnett-Griness O, Rennert G. The relationship between obesity and the increase in serum 25(OH)D levels in response to vitamin D supplementation. Osteoporos Int. 2013;24(4):1447–54. PMID: 22955311. http://www.ncbi.nlm.nih.gov/pubmed/22955311.
452. Ekwaru JP, Zwicker JD, Holick MF, Giovannucci E, Veugelers PJ. The importance of body weight for the dose response relationship of oral vitamin D supplementation and serum 25-hydroxyvitamin D in healthy volunteers. PLoS One. 2014;9(11):e111265. PMCID: PMC4220998. http://www.ncbi.nlm.nih.gov/pubmed/25372709.
453. Czarnecki D, Meehan CJ, Bruce F. The vitamin D status of Australian dermatologists. Clin Exp Dermatol. 2009;34(5):624–5. PMID: 19236420. http://www.ncbi.nlm.nih.gov/pubmed/19236420.
454. Reid IR, Bolland MJ, Grey A. Effects of vitamin D supplements on bone mineral density: a systematic review and meta-analysis. Lancet. 2014;383(9912):146–55. PMID: 24119980. http://www.ncbi.nlm.nih.gov/pubmed/24119980.
455. Munger KL, Levin LI, Hollis BW, Howard NS, Ascherio A. Serum 25-hydroxyvitamin D levels and risk of multiple sclerosis. JAMA. 2006;296(23):2832–8. PMID: 17179460. http://www.ncbi.nlm.nih.gov/pubmed/17179460.
456. Mahon BD, Gordon SA, Cruz J, Cosman F, Cantorna MT. Cytokine profile in patients with multiple sclerosis following vitamin D supplementation. J Neuroimmunol. 2003;134(1–2):128–32. PMID: 12507780. http://www.ncbi.nlm.nih.gov/pubmed/12507780.
457. Wallin MT, Page WF, Kurtzke JF. Multiple sclerosis in US veterans of the Vietnam era and later military service: race, sex, and geography. Ann Neurol. 2004;55(1):65–71. PMID: 14705113. http://www.ncbi.nlm.nih.gov/pubmed/14705113.
458. Sabetta JR, DePetrillo P, Cipriani RJ, Smardin J, Burns LA, Landry ML. Serum 25-hydroxyvitamin D and the incidence of acute viral respiratory tract infections in healthy adults. PLoS One. 2010;5(6):e11088. PMCID: PMC2885414. http://www.ncbi.nlm.nih.gov/pubmed/20559424.
459. Gandini S, Boniol M, Haukka J, Byrnes G, Cox B, Sneyd MJ, Mullie P, Autier P. Meta-analysis of observational studies of serum 25-hydroxyvitamin D levels and colorectal, breast and prostate cancer and colorectal adenoma. Int J Cancer. 2011;128(6):1414–24. https://doi.org/10.1002/ijc.25439. PMID: 20473927. https://pubmed.ncbi.nlm.nih.gov/20473927/.
460. Khan H, Kunutsor S, Franco OH, Chowdhury R. Vitamin D, type 2 diabetes and other metabolic outcomes: a systematic review and meta-analysis of prospective studies. Proc Nutr Soc. 2013;72(1):89–97. https://doi.org/10.1017/S0029665112002765. Epub 2012 Oct 30. PMID: 23107484. https://pubmed.ncbi.nlm.nih.gov/23107484/.
461. Welsh P, Sattar N. Vitamin D and chronic disease prevention. BMJ. 2014;348:g2280. PMID: 24690627. http://www.ncbi.nlm.nih.gov/pubmed/24690627.
462. Grønli O, Kvamme JM, Jorde R, Wynn R. Vitamin D deficiency is common in psychogeriatric patients, independent of diagnosis. BMC Psychiatry. 2014;14:134. PMCID: PMC4022542. http://www.ncbi.nlm.nih.gov/pubmed/24884774.
463. Theodoratou E, Tzoulaki I, Zgaga L, Ioannidis JPA. Vitamin D and multiple health outcomes: umbrella review of systematic reviews and meta-analyses of observational studies and randomised trials. BMJ. 2014;348:g2035. PMCID: PMC3972415. http://www.ncbi.nlm.nih.gov/pubmed/24690624.
464. Boucher BJ. Causal link between vitamin D deficiency and ill health still possible. BMJ. 2014;348:g2923. PMID: 24780246. http://www.ncbi.nlm.nih.gov/pubmed/24780246.
465. Theodoratou E, Ioannidis JPA. Authors' reply to Boucher. BMJ. 2014;348:g2927. PMID: 24780520. http://www.ncbi.nlm.nih.gov/pubmed/24780520.
466. Hill TR. Vitamin D status is poor in the UK. BMJ. 2014;348:g2818. PMID: 24755008. http://www.ncbi.nlm.nih.gov/pubmed/24755008.
467. Chowdhury R, Kunutsor S, Vitezova A, Oliver-Williams C, Chowdhury S, Kiefte-de-Jong JC, Khan H, Baena CP, Prabhakaran D, Hoshen MB, Feldman BS, Pan A, Johnson L, Crowe F, Hu FB, Franco OH. Vitamin D and risk of cause specific death: systematic review and meta-analysis of observational cohort and randomised intervention studies. BMJ. 2014;348:g1903. PMCID: PMC3972416. http://www.ncbi.nlm.nih.gov/pubmed/24690623.
468. Grant WB, Garland CF. Vitamin D has a greater impact on cancer mortality rates than on cancer incidence rates. BMJ. 2014;348:g2862. PMID: 24780390. http://www.ncbi.nlm.nih.gov/pubmed/24780390.
469. Kmietowicz Z. Vitamin D shows no clear evidence of benefits despite hundreds of studies. BMJ. 2014;348:g2489. PMID: 24692759. http://www.ncbi.nlm.nih.gov/pubmed/24692759.
470. Chowdhury R, Franco OH, Kunutsor S, Vitezova A, Oliver-Williams C, Chowdhury S, Kiefte-de-Jong JC, Khan H, Baena CP, Prabhakaran D, Hoshen MB, Feldman BS, Pan A, Johnson L, Crowe F, Hu FB. Authors' reply to Grant and Garland and to Bolland and colleagues. BMJ. 2014;348:g2931. PMID: 24780444. http://www.ncbi.nlm.nih.gov/pubmed/24780444.
471. Grant WB. Ecological studies of the UVB-vitamin D-cancer hypothesis. Anticancer Res. 2012;32(1):223–36. PMID: 22213311. http://www.ncbi.nlm.nih.gov/pubmed/22213311.
472. Grant WB. An estimate of premature cancer mortality in the U.S. due to inadequate doses of solar ultraviolet-B radiation. Cancer. 2002;94(6):1867–75. PMID: 11920550. http://www.ncbi.nlm.nih.gov/pubmed/11920550.
473. Antico A, Tampoia M, Tozzoli R, Bizzaro N. Can supplementation with vitamin D reduce the risk or modify the course of autoimmune diseases? A systematic review of the literature. Autoimmun Rev. 2012;12(2):127–36. PMID: 22776787. http://www.ncbi.nlm.nih.gov/pubmed/22776787.
474. Manolagas SC, Yu XP, Girasole G, Bellido T. Vitamin D and the hematolymphopoietic tissue: a 1994 update. Semin Nephrol. 1994;14(2):129–43. PMID: 8177980. http://www.ncbi.nlm.nih.gov/pubmed/8177980.
475. Bouillon R, Carmeliet G, Verlinden L, van Etten E, Verstuyf A, Luderer HF, Lieben L, Mathieu C, Demay M. Vitamin D and human health: lessons from vitamin D receptor null mice. Endocr

Rev. 2008;29(6):726–76. PMCID: PMC2583388. http://www.ncbi.nlm.nih.gov/pubmed/18694980.

476. Stoffels K, Overbergh L, Giulietti A, Verlinden L, Bouillon R, Mathieu C. Immune regulation of 25-hydroxyvitamin-D3-1alpha-hydroxylase in human monocytes. J Bone Miner Res. 2006;21(1):37–47. PMID: 16355272. http://www.ncbi.nlm.nih.gov/pubmed/16355272

477. Iho S, Takahashi T, Kura F, Sugiyama H, Hoshino T. The effect of 1,25-dihydroxyvitamin D3 on in vitro immunoglobulin production in human B cells. J Immunol. 1986;136(12):4427–31. PMID: 3519769. http://www.ncbi.nlm.nih.gov/pubmed/3519769.

478. Baeke F, Korf H, Overbergh L, van Etten E, Verstuyf A, Gysemans C, Mathieu C. Human T lymphocytes are direct targets of 1,25-dihydroxyvitamin D3 in the immune system. J Steroid Biochem Mol Biol. 2010;121(1–2):221–7. PMID: 20302932. http://www.ncbi.nlm.nih.gov/pubmed/20302932.

479. Chen S, Sims GP, Chen XX, Gu YY, Chen S, Lipsky PE. Modulatory effects of 1,25-dihydroxyvitamin D3 on human B cell differentiation. J Immunol. 2007;179(3):1634–47. PMID: 17641030. http://www.ncbi.nlm.nih.gov/pubmed/17641030.

480. Stio M, Bonanomi AG, d'Albasio G, Treves C. Suppressive effect of 1,25-dihydroxyvitamin D3 and its analogues EB 1089 and KH 1060 on T lymphocyte proliferation in active ulcerative colitis. Biochem Pharmacol. 2001;61(3):365–71. PMID: 11172742. http://www.ncbi.nlm.nih.gov/pubmed/11172742.

481. Liu PT, Stenger S, Li H, Wenzel L, Tan BH, Krutzik SR, Ochoa MT, Schauber J, Wu K, Meinken C, Kamen DL, Wagner M, Bals R, Steinmeyer A, Zügel U, Gallo RL, Eisenberg D, Hewison M, Hollis BW, Adams JS, Bloom BR, Modlin RL. Toll-like receptor triggering of a vitamin D-mediated human antimicrobial response. Science. 2006;311(5768):1770–3. PMID: 16497887. http://www.ncbi.nlm.nih.gov/pubmed/16497887.

482. Wacker M, Holick MF. Vitamin D – effects on skeletal and extraskeletal health and the need for supplementation. Nutrients. 2013;5(1):111–48. PMCID: PMC3571641. http://www.ncbi.nlm.nih.gov/pubmed/23306192

483. Grant WB. The prevalence of multiple sclerosis in 3 US communities: the role of vitamin D. Prev Chronic Dis. 2010;7(4):A89; author reply A90. PMCID: PMC2901587. http://www.ncbi.nlm.nih.gov/pubmed/20550847.

484. Schultz M, Butt AG. Is the north to south gradient in inflammatory bowel disease a global phenomenon? Expert Rev Gastroenterol Hepatol. 2012;6(4):445–7. PMID: 22928897. http://www.ncbi.nlm.nih.gov/pubmed/22928897.

485. Mohr SB, Garland CF, Gorham ED, Garland FC. The association between ultraviolet B irradiance, vitamin D status and incidence rates of type 1 diabetes in 51 regions worldwide. Diabetologia. 2008;51(8):1391–8. PMID: 18548227. http://www.ncbi.nlm.nih.gov/pubmed/18548227.

486. Crook M, Machin S, Crawford N. Electrokinetic properties and surface membrane sialic acid status of platelets in idiopathic thrombocytopenic purpura (ITP). Br J Haematol. 1991;77(2):209–14. PMID: 2004022. http://www.ncbi.nlm.nih.gov/pubmed/2004022.

487. Munger KL, Zhang SM, O'Reilly E, Hernán MA, Olek MJ, Willett WC, Ascherio A. Vitamin D intake and incidence of multiple sclerosis. Neurology. 2004;62(1):60–5. PMID: 14718698. http://www.ncbi.nlm.nih.gov/pubmed/14718698.

488. Ananthakrishnan AN, Khalili H, Higuchi LM, Bao Y, Korzenik JR, Giovannucci EL, Richter JM, Fuchs CS, Chan AT. Higher predicted vitamin D status is associated with reduced risk of Crohn's disease. Gastroenterology. 2012;142(3):482–9. PMCID: PMC3367959. http://www.ncbi.nlm.nih.gov/pubmed/22155183.

489. Vieira VM, Hart JE, Webster TF, Weinberg J, Puett R, Laden F, Costenbader KH, Karlson EW. Association between residences in U.S. northern latitudes and rheumatoid arthritis: a spatial analysis of the Nurses' Health Study. Environ Health Perspect. 2010;118(7):957–61. PMCID: PMC2920915. http://www.ncbi.nlm.nih.gov/pubmed/20338859.

490. Merlino LA, Curtis J, Mikuls TR, Cerhan JR, Criswell LA, Saag KG, Iowa Women's Health Study. Vitamin D intake is inversely associated with rheumatoid arthritis: results from the Iowa Women's Health Study. Arthritis Rheum. 2004;50(1):72–7. PMID: 14730601. http://www.ncbi.nlm.nih.gov/pubmed/14730601.

491. Pilz S, Tomaschitz A, März W, Drechsler C, Ritz E, Zittermann A, Cavalier E, Pieber TR, Lappe JM, Grant WB, Holick MF, Dekker JM. Vitamin D, cardiovascular disease and mortality. Clin Endocrinol. 2011;75(5):575–84. PMID: 21682758. http://www.ncbi.nlm.nih.gov/pubmed/21682758.

492. Grandi NC, Breitling LP, Brenner H. Vitamin D and cardiovascular disease: systematic review and meta-analysis of prospective studies. Prev Med. 2010;51(3–4):228–33. PMID: 20600257. http://www.ncbi.nlm.nih.gov/pubmed/20600257.

493. Vacek JL, Vanga SR, Good M, Lai SM, Lakkireddy D, Howard PA. Vitamin D deficiency and supplementation and relation to cardiovascular health. Am J Cardiol. 2012;109(3):359–63. PMID: 22071212. http://www.ncbi.nlm.nih.gov/pubmed/22071212.

494. Eaton CB, Young A, Allison MA, Robinson J, Martin LW, Kuller LH, Johnson KC, Curb JD, Van Horn L, McTiernan A, Liu S, Manson JE. Prospective association of vitamin D concentrations with mortality in postmenopausal women: results from the Women's Health Initiative (WHI). Am J Clin Nutr. 2011;94(6):1471–8. PMCID: PMC3252547. http://www.ncbi.nlm.nih.gov/pubmed/22030222.

495. Mandarino NR, Monteiro FDC Jr, Salgado JVL, Lages JS, Filho NS. Is vitamin D deficiency a new risk factor for cardiovascular disease? Open Cardiovasc Med J. 2015;9:40–9. PMCID: PMC4391213. http://www.ncbi.nlm.nih.gov/pubmed/25866591.

496. Pilz S, Dobnig H, Fischer JE, Wellnitz B, Seelhorst U, Boehm BO, März W. Low vitamin d levels predict stroke in patients referred to coronary angiography. Stroke. 2008;39(9):2611–3. PMID: 18635847. http://www.ncbi.nlm.nih.gov/pubmed/18635847.

497. Anderson JL, May HT, Horne BD, Bair TL, Hall NL, Carlquist JF, Lappé DL, Muhlestein JB, Intermountain Heart Collaborative (IHC) Study Group. Relation of vitamin D deficiency to cardiovascular risk factors, disease status, and incident events in a general healthcare population. Am J Cardiol. 2010;106(7):963–8. PMID: 20854958. http://www.ncbi.nlm.nih.gov/pubmed/20854958.

498. Wang TJ, Pencina MJ, Booth SL, Jacques PF, Ingelsson E, Lanier K, Benjamin EJ, D'Agostino RB, Wolf M, Vasan RS. Vitamin D deficiency and risk of cardiovascular disease. Circulation. 2008;117(4):503–11. PMCID: PMC2726624. http://www.ncbi.nlm.nih.gov/pubmed/18180395.

499. Ceglia L, Harris SS. Vitamin D and its role in skeletal muscle. Calcif Tissue Int. 2013;92(2):151–62. PMID: 22968766. http://www.ncbi.nlm.nih.gov/pubmed/22968766.

500. Halfon M, Phan O, Teta D. Vitamin D: a review on its effects on muscle strength, the risk of fall, and frailty. Biomed Res Int. 2015;2015:953241. PMCID: PMC4427016. http://www.ncbi.nlm.nih.gov/pubmed/26000306.

501. Kinney DK, Teixeira P, Hsu D, Napoleon SC, Crowley DJ, Miller A, Hyman W, Huang E. Relation of schizophrenia prevalence to latitude, climate, fish consumption, infant mortality, and skin color: a role for prenatal vitamin d deficiency and infections? Schizophr Bull. 2009;35(3):582–95. PMCID: PMC2669590. http://www.ncbi.nlm.nih.gov/pubmed/19357239.

502. Torrey EF. Prevalence studies in schizophrenia. Br J Psychiatry. 1987;150:598–608. PMID: 3307980. http://www.ncbi.nlm.nih.gov/pubmed/3307980.

503. McGrath J, Saari K, Hakko H, Jokelainen J, Jones P, Järvelin MR, Chant D, Isohanni M. Vitamin D supplementation during the first year of life and risk of schizophrenia: a Finnish birth cohort study.

Schizophr Res. 2004;67(2–3):237–45. PMID: 14984883. http://www.ncbi.nlm.nih.gov/pubmed/14984883.
504. Torrey EF, Miller J, Rawlings R, Yolken RH. Seasonality of births in schizophrenia and bipolar disorder: a review of the literature. Schizophr Res. 1997;28(1):1–38. PMID: 9428062. http://www.ncbi.nlm.nih.gov/pubmed/9428062.
505. Jande SS, Maler L, Lawson DE. Immunohistochemical mapping of vitamin D-dependent calcium-binding protein in brain. Nature. 1981;294(5843):765–7. PMID: 7033797. http://www.ncbi.nlm.nih.gov/pubmed/7033797.
506. Wilkins CH, Sheline YI, Roe CM, Birge SJ, Morris JC. Vitamin D deficiency is associated with low mood and worse cognitive performance in older adults. Am J Geriatr Psychiatry. 2006;14(12):1032–40. PMID: 17138809. http://www.ncbi.nlm.nih.gov/pubmed/17138809.
507. Llewellyn DJ, Lang IA, Langa KM, Muniz-Terrera G, Phillips CL, Cherubini A, Ferrucci L, Melzer D. Vitamin D and risk of cognitive decline in elderly persons. Arch Intern Med. 2010;170(13):1135–41. PMCID: PMC4053858. http://www.ncbi.nlm.nih.gov/pubmed/20625021.
508. Annweiler C, Llewellyn DJ, Beauchet O. Low serum vitamin D concentrations in Alzheimer's disease: a systematic review and meta-analysis. J Alzheimer's Dis. 2013;33(3):659–74. PMID: 23042216. http://www.ncbi.nlm.nih.gov/pubmed/23042216.
509. Banerjee A, Khemka VK, Ganguly A, Roy D, Ganguly U, Chakrabarti S. Vitamin D and Alzheimer's disease: neurocognition to therapeutics. Int J Alzheimers Dis. 2015;2015:192747. PMCID: PMC4553343. http://www.ncbi.nlm.nih.gov/pubmed/26351614.
510. Holló A, Clemens Z, Kamondi A, Lakatos P, Szűcs A. Correction of vitamin D deficiency improves seizure control in epilepsy: a pilot study. Epilepsy Behav. 2012;24(1):131–3. PMID: 22503468. http://www.ncbi.nlm.nih.gov/pubmed/22503468.
511. Hoogendijk WJG, Lips P, Dik MG, Deeg DJH, Beekman ATF, Penninx BWJH. Depression is associated with decreased 25-hydroxyvitamin D and increased parathyroid hormone levels in older adults. Arch Gen Psychiatry. 2008;65(5):508–12. PMID: 18458202. http://www.ncbi.nlm.nih.gov/pubmed/18458202.
512. Jorde R, Sneve M, Figenschau Y, Svartberg J, Waterloo K. Effects of vitamin D supplementation on symptoms of depression in overweight and obese subjects: randomized double blind trial. J Intern Med. 2008;264(6):599–609. PMID: 18793245. http://www.ncbi.nlm.nih.gov/pubmed/18793245
513. Bjelakovic G, Gluud LL, Nikolova D, Whitfield K, Wetterslev J, Simonetti RG, Bjelakovic M, Gluud C. Vitamin D supplementation for prevention of mortality in adults. Cochrane Database Syst Rev. 2014;2014(1):CD007470. PMCID: PMC11285307. http://www.ncbi.nlm.nih.gov/pubmed/24414552.
514. Spedding S. Vitamin D and depression: a systematic review and meta-analysis comparing studies with and without biological flaws. Nutrients. 2014;6(4):1501–18. PMCID: PMC4011048. http://www.ncbi.nlm.nih.gov/pubmed/24732019.
515. Masoumi A, Goldenson B, Ghirmai S, Avagyan H, Zaghi J, Abel K, Zheng X, Espinosa-Jeffrey A, Mahanian M, Liu PT, Hewison M, Mizwickie M, Cashman J, Fiala M. 1alpha,25-dihydroxyvitamin D3 interacts with curcuminoids to stimulate amyloid-beta clearance by macrophages of Alzheimer's disease patients. J Alzheimer's Dis. 2009;17(3):703–17. PMID: 19433889. http://www.ncbi.nlm.nih.gov/pubmed/19433889.
516. Berlin JL, Shantha GPS, Yeager H, Thomas-Hemak L. Serum vitamin D levels may not reflect tissue-level vitamin D in sarcoidosis. BMJ Case Rep. 2014;2014:bcr2014203759. PMCID: PMC3975517. http://www.ncbi.nlm.nih.gov/pubmed/24663253.
517. Donato J, Phillips CT, Gaffney AW, VanderLaan PA, Mouded M. A case of hypercalcemia secondary to hot tub lung. Chest. 2014;146(6):e186–9. PMID: 25451359. http://www.ncbi.nlm.nih.gov/pubmed/25451359.
518. Kamphuis LS, Bonte-Mineur F, van Laar JA, van Hagen PM, van Daele PL. Calcium and vitamin D in sarcoidosis: is supplementation safe? J Bone Miner Res. 2014;29(11):2498–503. PMID: 24753153. http://www.ncbi.nlm.nih.gov/pubmed/24753153.
519. Vieth R. Vitamin D supplementation, 25-hydroxyvitamin D concentrations, and safety. Am J Clin Nutr. 1999;69(5):842–56. PMID: 10232622. http://www.ncbi.nlm.nih.gov/pubmed/10232622.
520. Hollis BW. Circulating 25-hydroxyvitamin D levels indicative of vitamin D sufficiency: implications for establishing a new effective dietary intake recommendation for vitamin D. J Nutr. 2005;135(2):317–22. PMID: 15671234. http://www.ncbi.nlm.nih.gov/pubmed/15671234.
521. Holick MF. Vitamin D and sunlight: strategies for cancer prevention and other health benefits. Clin J Am Soc Nephrol. 2008;3(5):1548–54. PMCID: PMC4571149. http://www.ncbi.nlm.nih.gov/pubmed/18550652.
522. Warren R, Gartstein V, Kligman AM, Montagna W, Allendorf RA, Ridder GM. Age, sunlight, and facial skin: a histologic and quantitative study. J Am Acad Dermatol. 1991;25(5 Pt 1):751–60. PMID: 1802896. http://www.ncbi.nlm.nih.gov/pubmed/1802896.
523. Cleaver JE, Crowley E. UV damage, DNA repair and skin carcinogenesis. Front Biosci. 2002;7:d1024–43. PMID: 11897551.
524. Pandita KK, Razdan S, Kudyar RP, Beigh A, Kuchay S, Banday T. "Excess gooD can be Dangerous." A case series of iatrogenic symptomatic hypercalcemia due to hypervitaminosis D. Clin Cases Miner Bone Metab. 2012;9(2):118–20. PMCID: PMC3476516. http://www.ncbi.nlm.nih.gov/pubmed/23087723.
525. Hemachandar R, Shanmugam L, Malepati B, Venugopal S. Hyper vitaminosis D: are we overprescribing vitamin D? J Family Med Prim Care. 2014;3(4):464–6. PMCID: PMC4311368. http://www.ncbi.nlm.nih.gov/pubmed/25657969.
526. Balvers MGJ, Brouwer-Brolsma EM, Endenburg S, de Groot LCPGM, Kok FJ, Gunnewiek JK. Recommended intakes of vitamin D to optimise health, associated circulating 25-hydroxyvitamin D concentrations, and dosing regimens to treat deficiency: workshop report and overview of current literature. J Nutr Sci. 2015;4:e23. PMCID: PMC4463009. http://www.ncbi.nlm.nih.gov/pubmed/26090099.
527. Tian XQ, Chen TC, Lu Z, Shao Q, Holick MF. Characterization of the translocation process of vitamin D3 from the skin into the circulation. Endocrinology. 1994;135(2):655–61. PMID: 8033813. http://www.ncbi.nlm.nih.gov/pubmed/8033813.
528. Tian XQ, Holick MF. A liposomal model that mimics the cutaneous production of vitamin D3. Studies of the mechanism of the membrane-enhanced thermal isomerization of previtamin D3 to vitamin D3. J Biol Chem. 1999;274(7):4174–9. PMID: 9933613. http://www.ncbi.nlm.nih.gov/pubmed/9933613.
529. Haddad JG, Matsuoka LY, Hollis BW, Hu YZ, Wortsman J. Human plasma transport of vitamin D after its endogenous synthesis. J Clin Invest. 1993;91(6):2552–5. PMCID: PMC443317. http://www.ncbi.nlm.nih.gov/pubmed/8390483.
530. Tian XQ, Holick MF. Catalyzed thermal isomerization between previtamin D3 and vitamin D3 via beta-cyclodextrin complexation. J Biol Chem. 1995;270(15):8706–11. PMID: 7721775. http://www.ncbi.nlm.nih.gov/pubmed/7721775.
531. Holick MF. The D-lightful vitamin D for child health. JPEN J Parenter Enteral Nutr. 2012;36(1 Suppl):9S–19S. PMID: 22179524. http://www.ncbi.nlm.nih.gov/pubmed/22179524.
532. Holick MF, MacLaughlin JA, Doppelt SH. Regulation of cutaneous previtamin D3 photosynthesis in man: skin pigment is not an essential regulator. Science. 1981;211(4482):590–3. PMID: 6256855. http://www.ncbi.nlm.nih.gov/pubmed/6256855.
533. Chakraborty S, Sarkar AK, Bhattacharya C, Krishnan P, Chakraborty S. A nontoxic case of vitamin D toxicity. Lab Med. 2015;46(2):146–9; quiz e31. PMID: 25918194. http://www.ncbi.nlm.nih.gov/pubmed/25918194.

534. Alshahrani F, Aljohani N. Vitamin D: deficiency, sufficiency and toxicity. Nutrients. 2013;5(9):3605–16. PMCID: PMC3798924. http://www.ncbi.nlm.nih.gov/pubmed/24067388.
535. Schwalfenberg G. Not enough vitamin D: health consequences for Canadians. Can Fam Physician. 2007;53(5):841–54. PMCID: PMC1949171. http://www.ncbi.nlm.nih.gov/pubmed/17872747.
536. Robien K, Oppeneer SJ, Kelly JA, Hamilton-Reeves JM. Drug-vitamin D interactions: a systematic review of the literature. Nutr Clin Pract. 2013;28(2):194–208. PMCID: PMC5623087. http://www.ncbi.nlm.nih.gov/pubmed/23307906.
537. Mawer EB, Hann JT, Berry JL, Davies M. Vitamin D metabolism in patients intoxicated with ergocalciferol. Clin Sci (Lond). 1985;68(2):135–41. PMID: 3871380. http://www.ncbi.nlm.nih.gov/pubmed/3871380.
538. About the Vital Study. https://www.vitalstudy.org/.
539. Manson JE, Cook NR, Lee IM, Christen W, Bassuk SS, Mora S, Gibson H, Gordon D, Copeland T, D'Agostino D, Friedenberg G, Ridge C, Bubes V, Giovannucci EL, Willett WC, Buring JE, VITAL Research Group. Vitamin D supplements and prevention of cancer and cardiovascular disease. N Engl J Med. 2019;380(1):33–44. PMCID: PMC6425757. http://www.ncbi.nlm.nih.gov/pubmed/30415629.
540. Pradhan AD, Manson JE. Update on the vitamin D and omegA-3 trial (VITAL). J Steroid Biochem Mol Biol. 2016;155(Pt B):252–6. PMCID: PMC4600007. http://www.ncbi.nlm.nih.gov/pubmed/25864623.
541. Okereke OI, Reynolds CF, Mischoulon D, Chang G, Cook NR, Copeland T, Friedenberg G, Buring JE, Manson JE. The VITamin D and OmegA-3 TriaL-Depression Endpoint Prevention (VITAL-DEP): rationale and design of a large-scale ancillary study evaluating vitamin D and marine omega-3 fatty acid supplements for prevention of late-life depression. Contemp Clin Trials. 2018;68:133–45. PMCID: PMC5899680. http://www.ncbi.nlm.nih.gov/pubmed/29526608.
542. Manson JE, Bassuk SS, Buring JE, VITAL Research Group. Principal results of the VITamin D and OmegA-3 TriaL (VITAL) and updated meta-analyses of relevant vitamin D trials. J Steroid Biochem Mol Biol. 2020;198:105522. PMCID: PMC7089819. http://www.ncbi.nlm.nih.gov/pubmed/31733345.
543. Okereke OI, Vyas CM, Mischoulon D, Chang G, Cook NR, Weinberg A, Bubes V, Copeland T, Friedenberg G, Lee IM, Buring JE, Reynolds CF, Manson JE. Effect of long-term supplementation with marine omega-3 fatty acids vs placebo on risk of depression or clinically relevant depressive symptoms and on change in mood scores: a randomized clinical trial. JAMA. 2021;326(23):2385–94. PMCID: PMC8693224. http://www.ncbi.nlm.nih.gov/pubmed/34932079.
544. Nobel Prize. The Nobel Prize in Physiology or Medicine 1903. NobelPrize.org. https://www.nobelprize.org/prizes/medicine/1903/summary/.
545. Roelandts R. The history of phototherapy: something new under the sun? J Am Acad Dermatol. 2002;46(6):926–30. PMID: 12063493. http://www.ncbi.nlm.nih.gov/pubmed/12063493.
546. Albert MR, Ostheimer KG. The evolution of current medical and popular attitudes toward ultraviolet light exposure: part 2. J Am Acad Dermatol. 2003;48(6):909–18. PMID: 12789184. http://www.ncbi.nlm.nih.gov/pubmed/12789184.
547. Juzeniene A, Moan J. Beneficial effects of UV radiation other than via vitamin D production. Dermatoendocrinol. 2012;4(2):109–17. PMCID: PMC3427189. http://www.ncbi.nlm.nih.gov/pubmed/22928066.
548. Wintzen M, Yaar M, Burbach JP, Gilchrest BA. Proopiomelanocortin gene product regulation in keratinocytes. J Invest Dermatol. 1996;106(4):673–8. PMID: 8618003. http://www.ncbi.nlm.nih.gov/pubmed/8618003.
549. Oyane NMF, Bjelland I, Pallesen S, Holsten F, Bjorvatn B. Seasonality is associated with anxiety and depression: the Hordaland health study. J Affect Disord. 2008;105(1–3):147–55. PMID: 17573120. http://www.ncbi.nlm.nih.gov/pubmed/17573120.
550. Grimaldi S, Partonen T, Haukka J, Aromaa A, Lönnqvist J. Seasonal vegetative and affective symptoms in the Finnish general population: testing the dual vulnerability and latitude effect hypotheses. Nord J Psychiatry. 2009;63(5):397–404. PMID: 19363741. http://www.ncbi.nlm.nih.gov/pubmed/19363741.
551. Winthorst WH, Roest AM, Bos EH, Meesters Y, Penninx BWJH, Nolen WA, de Jonge P. Self-attributed seasonality of mood and behavior: a report from the Netherlands study of depression and anxiety. Depress Anxiety. 2014;31(6):517–23. PMID: 23695951. http://www.ncbi.nlm.nih.gov/pubmed/23695951.
552. Akhter A, Fiedorowicz JG, Zhang T, Potash JB, Cavanaugh J, Solomon DA, Coryell WH. Seasonal variation of manic and depressive symptoms in bipolar disorder. Bipolar Disord. 2013;15(4):377–84. PMCID: PMC3731411. http://www.ncbi.nlm.nih.gov/pubmed/23621686.
553. Lee KA, Hicks G, Nino-Murcia G. Validity and reliability of a scale to assess fatigue. Psychiatry Res. 1991;36(3):291–8. PMID: 2062970. http://www.ncbi.nlm.nih.gov/pubmed/2062970.
554. Gupta A, Sharma PK, Garg VK, Singh AK, Mondal SC. Role of serotonin in seasonal affective disorder. Eur Rev Med Pharmacol Sci. 2013;17(1):49–55. PMID: 23329523. http://www.ncbi.nlm.nih.gov/pubmed/23329523.
555. Slominski A, Wortsman J, Tobin DJ. The cutaneous serotoninergic/melatoninergic system: securing a place under the sun. FASEB J. 2005;19(2):176–94. PMID: 15677341. http://www.ncbi.nlm.nih.gov/pubmed/15677341.
556. Slominski A, Pisarchik A, Semak I, Sweatman T, Wortsman J, Szczesniewski A, Slugocki G, McNulty J, Kauser S, Tobin DJ, Jing C, Johansson O. Serotoninergic and melatoninergic systems are fully expressed in human skin. FASEB J. 2002;16(8):896–8. PMID: 12039872. http://www.ncbi.nlm.nih.gov/pubmed/12039872.
557. Fraikin GY, Strakhovskaya MG, Ivanova EV, Rubin AB. Near-UV activation of enzymatic conversion of 5-hydroxytryptophan to serotonin. Photochem Photobiol. 1989;49(4):475–7. PMID: 2786220. http://www.ncbi.nlm.nih.gov/pubmed/2786220.
558. Praschak-Rieder N, Willeit M, Wilson AA, Houle S, Meyer JH. Seasonal variation in human brain serotonin transporter binding. Arch Gen Psychiatry. 2008;65(9):1072–8. PMID: 18762593. http://www.ncbi.nlm.nih.gov/pubmed/18762593.
559. Spindelegger C, Stein P, Wadsak W, Fink M, Mitterhauser M, Moser U, Savli M, Mien LK, Akimova E, Hahn A, Willeit M, Kletter K, Kasper S, Lanzenberger R. Light-dependent alteration of serotonin-1A receptor binding in cortical and subcortical limbic regions in the human brain. World J Biol Psychiatry. 2012;13(6):413–22. PMID: 22111663. http://www.ncbi.nlm.nih.gov/pubmed/22111663.
560. Schulz KP, Newcorn JH, Schmeidler J, Halperin JM. Lack of seasonal rhythms in central serotonergic function in boys with ADHD. Psychoneuroendocrinology. 2002;27(4):463–73. PMID: 11911999. http://www.ncbi.nlm.nih.gov/pubmed/11911999.
561. Young SN. How to increase serotonin in the human brain without drugs. J Psychiatry Neurosci. 2007;32(6):394–9. PMCID: PMC2077351. http://www.ncbi.nlm.nih.gov/pubmed/18043762.
562. Benton D, Williams C, Brown A. Impact of consuming a milk drink containing a probiotic on mood and cognition. Eur J Clin Nutr. 2007;61(3):355–61. PMID: 17151594. http://www.ncbi.nlm.nih.gov/pubmed/17151594.
563. Messaoudi M, Violle N, Bisson JF, Desor D, Javelot H, Rougeot C. Beneficial psychological effects of a probiotic formulation (Lactobacillus helveticus R0052 and Bifidobacterium longum R0175) in healthy human volunteers. Gut Microbes. 2011;2(4):256–61. PMID: 21983070. http://www.ncbi.nlm.nih.gov/pubmed/21983070.

564. Steenbergen L, Sellaro R, van Hemert S, Bosch JA, Colzato LS. A randomized controlled trial to test the effect of multispecies probiotics on cognitive reactivity to sad mood. Brain Behav Immun. 2015;48:258–64. PMID: 25862297. http://www.ncbi.nlm.nih.gov/pubmed/25862297.
565. Allen AP, Hutch W, Borre YE, Kennedy PJ, Temko A, Boylan G, Murphy E, Cryan JF, Dinan TG, Clarke G. Bifidobacterium longum 1714 as a translational psychobiotic: modulation of stress, electrophysiology and neurocognition in healthy volunteers. Transl Psychiatry. 2016;6(11):e939. PMCID: PMC5314114. http://www.ncbi.nlm.nih.gov/pubmed/27801892.
566. Allen AP, Dinan TG, Clarke G, Cryan JF. A psychology of the human brain-gut-microbiome axis. Soc Personal Psychol Compass. 2017;11(4):e12309. PMCID: PMC5530613. http://www.ncbi.nlm.nih.gov/pubmed/28804508.
567. Lach G, Schellekens H, Dinan TG, Cryan JF. Anxiety, depression, and the microbiome: a role for gut peptides. Neurotherapeutics. 2018;15(1):36–59. PMCID: PMC5794698. http://www.ncbi.nlm.nih.gov/pubmed/29134359.
568. Bambury A, Sandhu K, Cryan JF, Dinan TG. Finding the needle in the haystack: systematic identification of psychobiotics. Br J Pharmacol. 2018;175(24):4430–8. PMCID: PMC6255950. http://www.ncbi.nlm.nih.gov/pubmed/29243233.
569. NCCIH. Towards psychobiotics: the microbiome as a key regulator of brain and behavior. https://www.nccih.nih.gov/training/videolectures/towards-psychobiotics.
570. Misra S, Mohanty D. Psychobiotics: a new approach for treating mental illness? Crit Rev Food Sci Nutr. 2019;59(8):1230–6. PMID: 29190117. http://www.ncbi.nlm.nih.gov/pubmed/29190117.
571. Sarkar A, Lehto SM, Harty S, Dinan TG, Cryan JF, Burnet PWJ. Psychobiotics and the manipulation of bacteria-gut-brain signals. Trends Neurosci. 2016;39(11):763–81. PMCID: PMC5102282. http://www.ncbi.nlm.nih.gov/pubmed/27793434.
572. Bermúdez-Humarán LG, Salinas E, Ortiz GG, Ramirez-Jirano LJ, Morales JA, Bitzer-Quintero OK. From probiotics to psychobiotics: live beneficial bacteria which act on the brain-gut axis. Nutrients. 2019;11(4):890. PMCID: PMC6521058. http://www.ncbi.nlm.nih.gov/pubmed/31010014.
573. Dinan TG, Stanton C, Cryan JF. Psychobiotics: a novel class of psychotropic. Biol Psychiatry. 2013;74(10):720–6. PMID: 23759244. http://www.ncbi.nlm.nih.gov/pubmed/23759244.
574. NCCIH. Probiotics: usefulness and safety. https://www.nccih.nih.gov/health/probiotics-usefulness-and-safety.
575. Rios AC, Maurya PK, Pedrini M, Zeni-Graiff M, Asevedo E, Mansur RB, Wieck A, Grassi-Oliveira R, McIntyre RS, Hayashi MAF, Brietzke E. Microbiota abnormalities and the therapeutic potential of probiotics in the treatment of mood disorders. Rev Neurosci. 2017;28(7):739–49. PMID: 28593878. http://www.ncbi.nlm.nih.gov/pubmed/28593878.
576. Bercik P, Denou E, Collins J, Jackson W, Lu J, Jury J, Deng Y, Blennerhassett P, Macri J, McCoy KD, Verdu EF, Collins SM. The intestinal microbiota affect central levels of brain-derived neurotropic factor and behavior in mice. Gastroenterology. 2011;141(2):599–609, 609.e1–3. PMID: 21683077. http://www.ncbi.nlm.nih.gov/pubmed/21683077.
577. Gareau MG, Wine E, Rodrigues DM, Cho JH, Whary MT, Philpott DJ, Macqueen G, Sherman PM. Bacterial infection causes stress-induced memory dysfunction in mice. Gut. 2011;60(3):307–17. PMID: 20966022. http://www.ncbi.nlm.nih.gov/pubmed/20966022.
578. Naseribafrouei A, Hestad K, Avershina E, Sekelja M, Linløkken A, Wilson R, Rudi K. Correlation between the human fecal microbiota and depression. Neurogastroenterol Motil. 2014;26(8):1155–62. PMID: 24888394. http://www.ncbi.nlm.nih.gov/pubmed/24888394.
579. Rao AV, Bested AC, Beaulne TM, Katzman MA, Iorio C, Berardi JM, Logan AC. A randomized, double-blind, placebo-controlled pilot study of a probiotic in emotional symptoms of chronic fatigue syndrome. Gut Pathog. 2009;1(1):6. PMCID: PMC2664325. http://www.ncbi.nlm.nih.gov/pubmed/19338686.
580. Gruenwald J, Graubaum HJ, Harde A. Effect of a probiotic multivitamin compound on stress and exhaustion. Adv Ther. 2002;19(3):141–50. PMID: 12201355. http://www.ncbi.nlm.nih.gov/pubmed/12201355.
581. Huang R, Wang K, Hu J. Effect of probiotics on depression: a systematic review and meta-analysis of randomized controlled trials. Nutrients. 2016;8(8):483. PMCID: PMC4997396. http://www.ncbi.nlm.nih.gov/pubmed/27509521.
582. Wallace CJK, Milev R. The effects of probiotics on depressive symptoms in humans: a systematic review. Ann General Psychiatry. 2017;16:14. PMCID: PMC5319175. http://www.ncbi.nlm.nih.gov/pubmed/28239408.
583. Ng QX, Peters C, Ho CYX, Lim DY, Yeo WS. A meta-analysis of the use of probiotics to alleviate depressive symptoms. J Affect Disord. 2018;228:13–9. PMID: 29197739. http://www.ncbi.nlm.nih.gov/pubmed/29197739.
584. Nikolova V, Zaidi SY, Young AH, Cleare AJ, Stone JM. Gut feeling: randomized controlled trials of probiotics for the treatment of clinical depression: systematic review and meta-analysis. Ther Adv Psychopharmacol. 2019;9:2045125319859963. PMCID: PMC6595633. http://www.ncbi.nlm.nih.gov/pubmed/31263542.
585. ElRakaiby M, Dutilh BE, Rizkallah MR, Boleij A, Cole JN, Aziz RK. Pharmacomicrobiomics: the impact of human microbiome variations on systems pharmacology and personalized therapeutics. OMICS. 2014;18(7):402–14. PMCID: PMC4086029. http://www.ncbi.nlm.nih.gov/pubmed/24785449.
586. Maldonado-Gómez MX, Martínez I, Bottacini F, O'Callaghan A, Ventura M, van Sinderen D, Hillmann B, Vangay P, Knights D, Hutkins RW, Walter J. Stable engraftment of Bifidobacterium longum AH1206 in the human gut depends on individualized features of the resident microbiome. Cell Host Microbe. 2016;20(4):515–26. PMID: 27693307. http://www.ncbi.nlm.nih.gov/pubmed/27693307.
587. Budick-Harmelin N, Anavi S, Madar Z, Tirosh O. Fatty acids-stress attenuates gluconeogenesis induction and glucose production in primary hepatocytes. Lipids Health Dis. 2012;11:66. PMCID: PMC3391994. http://www.ncbi.nlm.nih.gov/pubmed/22676303.
588. Tavakkoli-Kakhki M, Eslami S, Motavasselian M. Nutrient-rich versus nutrient-poor foods for depressed patients based on Iranian Traditional Medicine resources. Avicenna J Phytomed. 2015;5(4):298–308. PMCID: PMC4587607. http://www.ncbi.nlm.nih.gov/pubmed/26445711.
589. Perveen T, Hashmi BM, Haider S, Tabassum S, Saleem S, Siddiqui MA. Role of monoaminergic system in the etiology of olive oil induced antidepressant and anxiolytic effects in rats. ISRN Pharmacol. 2013;2013:615685. PMCID: PMC3725699. http://www.ncbi.nlm.nih.gov/pubmed/23936669.
590. Davison KM, Kaplan BJ. Nutrient intakes are correlated with overall psychiatric functioning in adults with mood disorders. Can J Psychiatr. 2012;57(2):85–92. PMID: 22340148. http://www.ncbi.nlm.nih.gov/pubmed/22340148.
591. Ruusunen A, Lehto SM, Tolmunen T, Mursu J, Kaplan GA, Voutilainen S. Coffee, tea and caffeine intake and the risk of severe depression in middle-aged Finnish men: the Kuopio Ischaemic Heart Disease Risk Factor Study. Public Health Nutr. 2010;13(8):1215–20. PMID: 20359377. http://www.ncbi.nlm.nih.gov/pubmed/20359377.
592. Lucas M, Mirzaei F, Pan A, Okereke OI, Willett WC, O'Reilly ÉJ, Koenen K, Ascherio A. Coffee, caffeine, and risk of depression among women. Arch Intern Med. 2011;171(17):1571–8. PMCID: PMC3296361. http://www.ncbi.nlm.nih.gov/pubmed/21949167.
593. Khanzode SD, Dakhale GN, Khanzode SS, Saoji A, Palasodkar R. Oxidative damage and major depression: the potential antioxidant action of selective serotonin re-uptake inhibitors. Redox Rep.

2003;8(6):365–70. PMID: 14980069. http://www.ncbi.nlm.nih.gov/pubmed/14980069.
594. Binder DK, Scharfman HE. Brain-derived neurotrophic factor. Growth Factors. 2004;22(3):123–31. PMCID: PMC2504526. http://www.ncbi.nlm.nih.gov/pubmed/15518235.
595. Warner-Schmidt JL, Duman RS. Hippocampal neurogenesis: opposing effects of stress and antidepressant treatment. Hippocampus. 2006;16(3):239–49. PMID: 16425236. http://www.ncbi.nlm.nih.gov/pubmed/16425236.
596. Russo-Neustadt AA, Beard RC, Huang YM, Cotman CW. Physical activity and antidepressant treatment potentiate the expression of specific brain-derived neurotrophic factor transcripts in the rat hippocampus. Neuroscience. 2000;101(2):305–12. PMID: 11074154. http://www.ncbi.nlm.nih.gov/pubmed/11074154.
597. Russo-Neustadt AA, Chen MJ. Brain-derived neurotrophic factor and antidepressant activity. Curr Pharm Des. 2005;11(12):1495–510. PMID: 15892658. http://www.ncbi.nlm.nih.gov/pubmed/15892658.
598. Gorgulu Y, Caliyurt O. Rapid antidepressant effects of sleep deprivation therapy correlates with serum BDNF changes in major depression. Brain Res Bull. 2009;80(3):158–62. PMID: 19576267. http://www.ncbi.nlm.nih.gov/pubmed/19576267.
599. Okamoto T, Yoshimura R, Ikenouchi-Sugita A, Hori H, Umene-Nakano W, Inoue Y, Ueda N, Nakamura J. Efficacy of electroconvulsive therapy is associated with changing blood levels of homovanillic acid and brain-derived neurotrophic factor (BDNF) in refractory depressed patients: a pilot study. Prog Neuro-Psychopharmacol Biol Psychiatry. 2008;32(5):1185–90. PMID: 18403081. http://www.ncbi.nlm.nih.gov/pubmed/18403081.
600. Drzyzga ŁR, Marcinowska A, Obuchowicz E. Antiapoptotic and neurotrophic effects of antidepressants: a review of clinical and experimental studies. Brain Res Bull. 2009;79(5):248–57. PMID: 19480984. http://www.ncbi.nlm.nih.gov/pubmed/19480984.
601. Schmidt HD, Duman RS. The role of neurotrophic factors in adult hippocampal neurogenesis, antidepressant treatments and animal models of depressive-like behavior. Behav Pharmacol. 2007;18(5–6):391–418. PMID: 17762509. http://www.ncbi.nlm.nih.gov/pubmed/17762509.
602. Nabavi SM, Daglia M, Braidy N, Nabavi SF. Natural products, micronutrients, and nutraceuticals for the treatment of depression: a short review. Nutr Neurosci. 2017;20(3):180–94. PMID: 26613119. http://www.ncbi.nlm.nih.gov/pubmed/26613119.
603. Kaelin WG, McKnight SL. Influence of metabolism on epigenetics and disease. Cell. 2013;153(1):56–69. PMCID: PMC3775362. http://www.ncbi.nlm.nih.gov/pubmed/23540690.
604. Gerhauser C. Cancer chemoprevention and nutriepigenetics: state of the art and future challenges. Top Curr Chem. 2013;329:73–132. PMID: 22955508. http://www.ncbi.nlm.nih.gov/pubmed/22955508.

Music and Depression

21

Franklin Sunzeri

Introduction

For some people who are depressed, verbal processing in psychotherapy may be difficult or not enough to ameliorate symptoms. Listening to music, active participation, and improvising can be a nonverbal, non-threatening self-expression that can facilitate catharsis, and change emotional states to escape from stress and pain [1–4, 8, 9].

A 2013 book by Ockelford (*Applied musicology using zygonic theory to inform music education, therapy, and psychology research*) is a fine resource for anyone who wishes to pursue more information about the possibilities of music as an adjunct to standard psychological interventions [5]. For a comprehensive review of the psychoneuroimmunological effects of music, we recommend a superbly rendered article *The psychoneuroimmunological effects of music: a systematic review and a new model* by Daisy Fancourt et al. in 2013 [10].

Music can be used in different ways and has a variety of attributes that may make a difference to the listener. Interaction with music may be passive, such as listening to live or recorded music, or it may be active, such as musical instruction, participation in groups, self-expression in therapy, or improvisation [5]. Music of any genre, tempo, or mode may have an influence on patients, often in a way that is based on individual preferences or that may produce a more universal reaction [10–15]. Faster, louder, erratic music may be arousing whereas slower, softer, and even-patterned music may be calming [14, 16]. Both peer perceptions and musical training may influence these preferences and reactions [12, 14].

As Fancourt has pointed out, music interacts with an individual both physically and psychosocially [10]. Physically, we perceive sound waves through auditory pathways; and when playing an instrument, our sensorimotor system becomes actively engaged. Emotionally, our responses to music are shaped by personal history and familiarity with specific genres. Psychosocially, engaging with others through music can foster social connection and open up a range of interpersonal opportunities. Emotional reactions to music may span from happiness—often cued by major modes in fast tempos—to sadness evoked by slow tempos in minor modes. However, it is also possible for a single song to evoke both happiness and sadness simultaneously, potentially due to modulations in tempo or mode, or conflicting cues such as fast songs in minor modes [17].

Music Therapy

Music therapy has the possibility to improve the condition of patients suffering with *depression*. One of the questions is who is most likely to respond to music-based interventions, and what interventions are most effective for which individuals. These are difficult questions.

Individual RCTs of the effect of music on depression are not always of high quality and are often measuring a small number of people. So, even though there is some evidence for improvement in mood, the results do not inspire confidence [19]. A stimulating overview of music and depression can be found on YouTube titled: *Music and the Brain: Depression and Creativity Symposium* [18]. There are additional videos on YouTube discussing various aspects of music and the brain.

In 2017, a Cochrane Review updated its 2008 meta-analysis [19] of music therapy for depression [20]. They found that music therapy provides short-term beneficial effects for people with depression. Music therapy added to treatment as usual (TAU) seems to improve depressive symptoms compared with TAU alone. There was no difference in adverse events compared to TAU alone. There was decreased anxiety levels and improved functioning of depressed individuals. They suggest that future trials should be based upon better design and larger samples of children and adolescents. Mechanisms of music therapy for depression should be

F. Sunzeri (✉)
Heather Hills Consulting, Coos Bay, OR, USA

J. Raber et al. (eds.), *Understanding and Treating Depressive Disorders*, https://doi.org/10.1007/978-3-032-14465-2_21

investigated. The music therapy, TAU, the comparator condition, and the profession of the person who delivers the intervention should be included for reproducibility and comparison purposes.

Several clinical methods have been used in music therapy [19, 21]. Communication skills for affecting changes in patients include listening, affirmation, vocal tone modulation, nonverbal communication, agreement, collaboration, acceptance, and validation [22]. The longer interventions are carried out, the greater and more lasting the improvement is [23].

Dance and movement therapy may decrease depression [24]. Music-movement therapy for 60 minutes three times per week for 8 weeks in stroke patients may significantly increase flexion and improve mood compared to standard care [25].

Group music therapy may be possible and effective as an adjunct therapy for PTSD patients who have not sufficiently responded to cognitive behavioral therapy [26].

A small sample of depressed Taiwanese outpatients engaged in guided imagery and music therapy [27]. Their experience showed that several themes emerged. These were (1) leisurely wandering in very natural surroundings, (2) creating surreal virtual surroundings, (3) recalling life experiences, (4) submerging in thematic music melodies, and (5) experiencing a variety of physical relaxation.

Patients may be better able to overcome inhibitions of verbal expression and express their emotions when listening to sad music instead of no music, angry, happy, or scary music. People with depression may be more likely to assign negative meaning to emotional stimuli, including interpersonal stimuli such as faces and voices and interpretation of music [28].

It appears that depressed folks demonstrate a judgment bias towards negative emotions [29]. A group of depressed individuals was exposed to music that portrayed clear examples of one of the emotional qualities of happiness, sadness, fear, anger, and tenderness. In direct proportion to the degree of depression or alexithymia, there was a moderate negative bias towards the amount of each one of those emotions perceived in the examples.

A 10-week RCT of group drumming showed that after 6 weeks, there was significant improvements in depression[1](−2.14 SE 0.50, CI: −3.16 to −1.11) and social resilience (7.69 SE 2.00, CI: 3.60 to 11.78) [30]. By 10 weeks, even more significant improvements were seen: (depression: −3.41 SE 0.62, CI: −4.68 to −2.15; social resilience: 10.59 SE 1.78, CI: 6.94 to 14.24). In addition, significant improvements were seen in anxiety (−2.21 SE 0.50, CI: −3.24 to −1.19) and mental well-being (6.14 SE 0.92, CI: 4.25 to 8.04). These changes persisted at 3-month follow-up. At the end of 10 weeks, a shift was noted away from pro-inflammatory to an anti-inflammatory immune system profile.

Ten weeks of passive and interactive music interventions in individuals with severe Alzheimer's disease created an improvement in emotional state and parasympathetic dominance [31]. Behavioral and psychological symptoms of dementia improved the most with the interactive intervention and persisted for 3 weeks. The individuals selected music from memorable times in their lives. Symptom improvements included decreased paranoid and delusional ideation, activity disturbances, and aggressiveness toward caregivers.

A meta-analysis of effects on behavioral and psychological symptoms of dementia showed that music therapy had moderate effects on anxiety and small effects on behavioral symptoms [32]. In studies lasting more than 3 months, music therapy had large effects on anxiety.

A mixed-effects meta-analysis model that analyzes the influence of study design, type of disorder, and number of sessions has been brought to bear on music therapy for folks with serious mental disorders [23]. As an adjunct to standard care, significant influences were seen on global state, general symptoms, negative symptoms, depression, anxiety, functioning, and musical engagement. Dose effects were significant for functioning, and general, depression, and negative symptoms. The greater the number of sessions, the greater the effect. Small effects were seen in as few as 3 to 10 sessions, and large effects were seen after 16 to 51 sessions.

Autonomic Functions

As of 2013, 16 studies had shown that relaxing music can change *autonomic functions* such as decrease respiration rate, blood pressure, and heart rate; reviewed in [10]. Valence and arousal are important in producing those effects [33]. Peaceful low-tempo music appears to be the most likely to achieve these results. In 207 patients, listening to relaxing recorded music was seen to be as effective as diazepam in reducing preoperative anxiety as measured by anxiety, cortisol level, heart rate, or blood pressure [34].

Decreased skin conductance associated with decreased sympathetic stimulation has been seen after engaging with peaceful music, but not with happy, sad, or agitated music [6]. Another experiment suggested that after a stressful situation skin conductance increases less in the presence of low-tempo music versus high-tempo music [7].

Effects of music on *neurotransmitter levels* appear to be a mixed bag; reviewed in previous work [10]. Most studies

[1] *Standard error of the mean (SE)* is the standard deviation divided by the square root of the number of people sampled. It measures the accuracy with which a sample distribution represents a population [138]. SE is the variation between the calculated mean of the population and one which is accepted as accurate. The SE tends to decrease with the more data points of the mean. For more information see Chap. 4 Evidence Basics.

with recorded music show no effect on norepinephrine, epinephrine, or dopamine. Fancourt found three studies that reported a decrease in norepinephrine and epinephrine in response to recorded music, and to music therapy.

As a response to imaging and relaxing classical music, levels of beta-endorphins have been reported to decrease [35].

Numerous articles indicate that both active participation in music and passive listening are associated with reduced cortisol levels (reviewed in [10]). Relaxing music selected by investigators was more likely to produce this effect than stimulating music. Participant-selected music may be more effective than investigator-selected music in lowering cortisol levels following day surgery [36]. Several reports suggest that listening to relaxing recorded music leads to decreases in state and trait anxiety scores, as well as cortisol levels (reviewed in [10]). However, a few other studies did not.

Fancourt identified two articles that indicated changes in cortisol levels. In one of these studies, patients undergoing gastroscopy were compared, and those in the music group exhibited smaller increases in cortisol and ACTH levels than the control group [40]. The other study showed less of an increase in salivary cortisol in the music group in patients undergoing colonoscopy [41].

Relaxing recorded music has increased oxytocin during bed rest after open heart surgery [42]. Dehydroepiandrosterone to cortisol ratios increased in a drumming group [37] and decreased accompanied by an increase in growth hormone in a group listening to recorded relaxing music [37]. Testosterone increased in men and decreased in women, while cortisol, ACTH, epinephrine, and norepinephrine were unchanged when they listened to participant-selected music [43].

Increases in serum noradrenaline, ACTH, cortisol, IL-6, and leptin levels elicited by an acute stressor in an RCT were moderated by an auditory mood-induction protocol with positive music during a 1-hour recovery period [44]. A more positive mood and stronger cortisol responses were seen.

Heart rate variability (HRV)[2] may be a result of responses to body stress [45, 46]. It is posited that decreased variability of heart rate in response to cues may reflect an overconsumption of body resources and a decrement in ability to sense environmental changes. Under environmental influences of acute time pressure, emotional strain (but not increased cognitive workload) and increased anxiety, HRV has been shown to decrease [47–49]. Increased frequency and duration of daily worry can increase heart rate and decrease HRV even carrying over into sleep [50].

In PTSD, HRV is decreased, whereas low-frequency changes are not, and there is blunted HRV and low-frequency reactivity to recall of trauma [51]. These changes are thought to reflect a hyperactive constant arousal response such that they are unable to summon a further response to stressors [51, 52].

Decreased HRV is associated with major depression, generalized anxiety disorder, social anxiety disorder, tobacco use, and cardiovascular disease [53–56]. Decreased HRV associations are especially prominent with sudden death, coronary artery disease, heart failure, and cardiovascular risk factors, including smoking, diabetes, hyperlipidemia, and hypertension [57].

It appears that autonomic responses are synchronized with music: there is physiological tracking of emphasis (such as crescendos) and rhythmic phrases [58]. An interesting study compared the relative effects on cardiovascular and respiratory systems induced by six different types of music in terms of tempo, rhythm, melodic structure, pause, individual preference, habituation, order effect of presentation, and previous musical training [59]. They began the experiment by taking a 5-minute baseline followed by a random order presentation of the six types of music for 2 and 4 minutes. This was followed by a randomly inserted pause in either sequence. Faster tempi and simpler rhythmic structures associated with increased ventilation, blood pressure, and heart rate, while mid cerebral artery flow and baroreflex decreased. There was no habituation. The random pause is associated with decreased ventilation, heart rate, and blood pressure below baseline. A progressive reduction in effect on mid-cerebral artery flow velocity independent of the style was seen with increased exposure. It appeared that music is arousing, especially with fast tempo. And slow or meditative music or pausing induces relaxation. Trained musicians appeared to be more attuned to the effects of tempo.

A comparison of endocrine, autonomic, and psychological stress responses in 60 young females after being exposed to three different conditions has demonstrated an impact of music on the psychobiological stress system [60]. Three groups received relaxing music (Miserere, Allegri), sound of rippling water, or rest without acoustic stimulation. Significant differences were seen in salivary cortisol responses between the groups; the relaxing music showed the highest response, and the rippling water showed the lowest response ($p = 0.025$). After the stress test, *salivary alpha-amylase*, a marker for psychological stress [61], returned to baseline significantly faster in the music group than in the silent group ($p = 0.026$). Psychological and heart rate measurements did not differ between the groups. These results suggest that music may have been related to a faster recovery.

[2]Although HRV mechanisms are well described [46], the popular polyvagal theory of HRV is controversial. A detailed discussion of the polyvagal theory can be found in discussions especially those represented in the literature by Porges and Grossman [64, 65].

Musical or verbal phrases of 10-second duration induce greater excursions of blood pressure and therefore heart rate resulting in triggering for more vagal induced slowing and sense of calm [62].

There is some evidence that music during exercise can induce relaxation of muscle tension, increase blood flow, and lactate production and clearance [63].

Autonomic nervous system effects (e.g., heart rate and heart rate variability) can be elicited not only by emotions in music but also the isochronous pulse (the principal accent or rhythmical beat) [66]. These effects are increases in sympathetic nervous system activity.

A critique of assessing music's impact on *well-being* suggests that standard quantitative instruments are biased, are devoid of relevance to individual experience, and produce artefactual data [67]. The author of the critique suggests that case studies are more appropriate to determine the impact on individuals.

Immunological Responses to Music

Quite a few studies have studied *immunological responses to music*; reviewed in [10]. Natural killer cells have been reported to either increase, decrease, or stay the same in response to music. Natural killer cells increased in response to drumming [37] and decreased in response to participant chosen music [36]. In a Chinese study, natural killer cells, CD3, CD4, and CD8 T cells stayed the same with participatory music therapy in tumor patients versus without music, they increased or decreased [68]. Listening to relaxing music increased μ-opiate receptors on mononuclear cells, some of circulating morphine converted to morphine 6 glucuronide, and IL-6 levels significantly decreased, whereas IL-1b, IL-10, and cortisol values did not change [69].

A group of Japanese college students listened to stimulating or relaxing recorded music after a stressful task [39]. Stimulating music tended to increase norepinephrine levels and liveliness and decrease depression. Plasma CD4 T cells increased, while CD8 T cells and other leukocytes and endocrine values stayed the same in response to stimulating music. Live music significantly increased CD8 T cells.

It appears that mood disorders and bipolar disorders are linked to artistic creativity and this association between psychopathology and creativity appears to be familial [70]. An analysis of unique triggers for manic or hypomanic episodes in bipolar individuals aged 18 to 30 have revealed that triggers can include falling in love, recreational stimulant use, starting a creative project, late-night partying, going on vacation, and listening to loud music [71]. Unique triggers for depression were stressful life events, general stress, fatigue, sleep deprivation, physical injury or illness, menstruation, and decreased physical exercise.

Age Differences

Elderly

There are a number of studies that suggest elderly folks may benefit by associating with music in several different ways.

In a sample of community-dwelling older adults, compared with non-exercising controls, a 6-month regimen of weekly music-based multitask training resulted in decreased anxiety and better cognition [72].

In one study, participants either received piano lessons and daily training for 4 months or participated in leisure activities such as physical exercise, computer lessons, and painting lessons [73]. Results suggest that playing the piano and learning to read music may decrease depression, improve psychological and physical quality of life, and enhance cognitive reserve in elderly folks. It seems that such a regimen integrates auditory, visual, motor, and somatosensory functions in a complex way.

The multisensory feedback system that is reinforced in musicians from an early age strengthens connections between auditory and motor regions while activating multimodal integration regions and can have a radiating effect on other cognitive and behavioral functions [74].

Music can be a simple, inexpensive, and non-invasive means of decreasing depression and improving the quality of life [75, 76]. A significant reduction in depression and increased sleep quality in elderly folks seems to be associated with listening to soft music; however, a comparison to a control group did not show a significant difference between the groups [75].

Music therapy in the form of 12 sessions of group music therapy (two 30-min sessions per week for 6 weeks) may improve depression in the elderly and delay deterioration of cognition [76].

A variety of complementary and alternative approaches for intervening in late-life depression, such as natural remedies, exercise, yoga, tai chi, massage therapy, music therapy, religion, and spirituality, were reviewed in 2013 [77]. This review is especially interesting because over-medication, side effects, and multiple drug–drug interactions are especially prominent in the elderly; consequently, adjunctive, or different therapies could be especially helpful.

An RCT in Hong Kong showed that listening to music in a community-dwelling elderly population resulted in a statistically significant decrease in depression ($p < 0.001$), blood pressure ($p = 0.001$), heart rate ($p < 0.001$), and respiratory rate ($p < 0.001$) after 1 month [78].

Attending live music or reading appears to increase quality of life and improve depression in the elderly [79, 80].

Even a single session of playing the piano may be able to produce a rapid and sustained improvement in mood and cognition of an elderly patient, or so found a single subject uncontrolled case study [81].

Improvements in depression and cognitive deficits were seen in elderly board and care residents who had been actively watching dance accompanied by music and passively listening to music; however, a greater improvement was seen in the actively watching group [82].

Youth

Relationships of youths with music have revealed some interesting associations. A large neurobehavioral study of depression in 106 adolescent Pittsburgh participants looked at associations between MDD and five types of media: television or movies, music, video games, Internet, and print media, such as magazines, newspapers, and books [83]. They found MDD was positively associated with popular music exposure and negatively associated with reading print media.

It seems that fans of different types of music may choose friends whose substance use patterns reinforce their own substance use tendencies. Or so it would appear from a study of 7324 Dutch school-going adolescents (aged 12–16) [84]. Preferences for eight genres of music segregated into four styles: Pop (chart music, Dutch pop), Adult (classical, jazz), Urban (rap/hip-hop, soul/R&B), and Hard (punk/hardcore, techno/hardhouse). Substance use was indicated by smoking, drinking, and cannabis use. The relationship of substance use and music preference was either completely or partly explained by perceived peer use.

Music and non-suicidal self-injury (NSSI) appear to serve as important means of emotional expression and protest for a subset of depressed individuals in a child and adolescent psychiatric unit [85]. In these adolescents who had participated in NSSI or suicide attempts in the last 3 months, music seemed to serve a self-regulatory function much as NSSI and might be self-protective. However, music in some instances appeared to be part of the NSSI ritual. However, there was no link seen between specific music preferences and NSSI or suicidality. The music and lyrics were associated with anti-dissociation, affect regulation, and interpersonal influences.

Online in-depth interviews of American college students who have been treated for depression have identified sources of stress and means of coping with them [86]. The most frequently cited sources of stress were roommate problems, academic problems, financial and career concerns, and family pressure. *The most frequent coping mechanisms* were exercise, talking to friends, self-talk, deep breathing, writing in a journal, marijuana use, and listening to music.

Mental health of fans of heavy metal music in France was examined using the Hospital Anxiety and Depression Scale (HADS) [87]. Fans of metal music identified in that study were mainly young adults (median age = 22.67, SD = 5.29) and male (87.85%). Despite the popular perception of an association between social problems such as suicide, self-destruction, and Satanism, the results showed that overall, metal music fans levels of anxiety and depression are similar to and lower than levels in the general population. Less than 5% showed pathological symptoms. And those that had higher levels of anxiety and depression had literary and/or arts backgrounds rather than scientific background, they wrote metal music lyrics, consumed alcohol, and practiced scarification.

Early adolescent music preferences may be powerful indicators of later delinquency (but not early delinquency) [88]. A 4-year longitudinal study of so-called *Music Marker Theory* involving 309 subjects indicated that rock (such as hard rock, heavy metal, gothic, punk), African-American music (rhythm and blues, hip-hop), and electronic dance music (trance, techno/hard house) favored an association with elevated minor delinquency concurrently and longitudinally. On the other hand, conventional pop or highbrow music (classic music and jazz) was not correlated with delinquency or was negatively correlated.

There may be a robust association between music preference and substance use. Substance use and music relationships have been studied among more than 18,000 fifteen-year-olds from 10 European countries [89]. Overall, in 2005–2006, preferences for mainstream pop-chart music, classical music, and jazz were negatively associated with substance use. Preferences for house/trance and techno/hardhouse were associated positively with substance use. In three of the countries, associations were seen between liking rock, heavy metal punk/hardcore, and gothic and substance use. There were mixed associations between hip-hop and R&B and substance use. They did not identify any gender differences in these associations.

Children

The *birthbeats project* is an evidence-based free web resource that was developed for parents and professionals to promote the use of music and explain how music can be beneficial during labor [90]. Music before labor and cesarean section can be emotionally calming [92].

Prenatal exposure to melodies may induce neural representations that may persist for several months [91–94]. Mothers who are depressed may produce infant-directed singing that lacks the sensitivity and emotional expression that infants require for affect regulation [95].

Preterm infants in the neonatal intensive care unit have been shown to significantly benefit from live music therapy, especially for pacification, reinforcement of sucking, and pacification as the basis for multilayered, multimodal stimulation [96].

Infant brains demonstrate right-hemispheric specializing in processing music as early as the first few prenatal hours [97]. These areas are related to the specific adult neural systems weighted toward the right hemisphere related to pitch, melody, and harmony.

Music therapy can assist the development of mutually responsive orientation behaviors of young children (aged 3–5) and their family members [98]. Harmonious communication can be facilitated by therapists encouraging and modeling musical interactions and by parent–child interactions encouraging, taking turns, being playful and joint attention.

Music and Illness

Music has been proposed as an adjunctive treatment to increase quality of life in cancer patients. Cancer is often accompanied by extensive emotional, physical, and social suffering. Music has been used in an attempt to decrease symptoms and alleviate side effects of treatment.

A 2011 meta-analysis of six English-language databases and three major Chinese-language databases was reviewed for quality RCTs that examined the effect of music interventions on psychological and physical outcome measures in cancer patients [99]. Out of 322 studies, they found 32 randomized trials with a total of 3181 participants that met appropriate quality standards. Several of these studies demonstrated significant reduction in anxiety and depression and decreased pain. Some studies suggest music decreases heart rate and respiratory rate. Two moderate quality studies suggested that music improved the quality of life. On the other hand, two moderate quality studies suggested that music increased fatigue.

Another meta-analysis conducted in 2010 of RCTs and quasi-RCTs in all available databases independent of language found 30 trials with a total of 1891 subjects that encompassed either formal music therapy ($n = 13$) or listening to prerecorded music ($n = 17$) [100]. It seems that a positive effect is possible on anxiety ($p = 0.009$ on the STAI-S scale and $p = 0.0007$ on other anxiety scales) and on mood ($p = 0.03$), but there was no evidence for depression. There were some reductions in heart rate, respiratory rate, and blood pressure, and a moderate effect on pain reduction ($p = 0.0003$), but no strong evidence for a benefit on fatigue or physical status. Two studies suggested a benefit on overall quality of life ($p = 0.00001$). The nature of the trials would not allow a comparison between music listening versus music therapy. It was not possible to draw conclusions about effects on distress, body image, oxygen saturation level, immunologic functioning, spirituality, and communication. Reviewers believed there was a significant risk of bias in most of the RCTs, so caution should be exercised in understanding the results.

A narrative review of music-based interventions of published literature between 1970 and 2012 revealed a positive influence on pain, anxiety, mood disturbance, and quality of life in cancer patients [101].

A 2011 Cochrane review cautiously indicated that musical interventions for people with cancer may be beneficial for anxiety, pain, mood, and quality of life [100]. Small effects were seen on heart rate, blood pressure, and respiratory rate.

Music therapy decreased State and Trait anxiety levels and systolic blood pressure in oncology patients who received 15 minutes of music therapy prior to radiation [102].

Music therapy has the potential to significantly improve depression and decrease hospital stay in women who have received radical mastectomy [103].

Music may improve the quality of life and mood in folks who suffer from a variety of physical ailments.

Eight-week structured music therapy and activity program can have a beneficial effect on behavioral and depressive symptoms in persons with dementia in a naturalistic setting ($p = 0.006$) [104].

A single-blind RCT of two daily music listening sessions for 90 days showed significant reduction in chronic pain ($p < 0.001$), anxiety/depression, and anxiolytics in subjects with lumbar pain, fibromyalgia, inflammatory disease, or neurological disease [105].

Listening to music of their choice in the perianesthesia period can produce a feeling of inner peace, detachment from reality, and decrease anxiety in patients undergoing surgery [106].

Music therapy may be beneficial for elevating mood in post-stroke patients [107].

Four weeks of listening to music once a day using two types of CDs produced significant reduction in pain in a group of patients with fibromyalgia [108].

Music therapy has the potential to significantly improve depression and decrease hospital stay in women who have received radical mastectomy [101].

People recovering from acute myocardial infarction may find psychological and physiological benefit of listening to music in a quiet restful environment [109]. A three-group ($n = 45$) repeated experimental design measures compared to 20 minutes of quiet restful environment and treatment as usual to listening to music. State anxiety was significantly decreased only in the music group. Significantly greater reductions in heart rate, respiratory rate, and myocardial oxygen demand immediately after the intervention were seen in the music group compared to the control group. The reductions in heart rate and respiratory rates remained significant for more than 1 hour. Immediately after the intervention, there were significantly greater increases in high-frequency heart rate variability in the musical and the quiet group compared to the control group. There were no differences in systolic blood pressure between the groups.

Neurobiological theories that attempt to explain relationships between music's effects on various mental illnesses are reviewed in reference [110]. There is some evidence that music therapy has been useful as an adjunct to conventional therapy for treating depression, anxiety, autism, schizophrenia, dementia, agitation, substance abuse, and sleeplessness [110].

Twenty minutes of listening to relaxing music compared to 20 minutes of bed rest in patients undergoing coronary angiography significantly decreased anxiety of state anxiety ($p = 0.006$), stress ($p = 0.001$), and depression ($p = 0.02$) [111].

Listening to music does not seem to significantly reduce pain for patients during sigmoidoscopy [112].

Music in the operating theater may be able to minimize distraction and annoyance and reduce stress and anxiety of patients and staff [113–116]. However, this feeling is not universal [117]. A systematic 2011 review of music in the theater found that music in the operating room had beneficial effects on patients in terms of decreased anxiety, stress, and demand for analgesia [118]. For surgeons, especially those who were musicians, heart rate, blood pressure, and muscle effort were reduced, while accuracy was increased, and tasks were completed faster. On the other hand, surgical staff found music distracting, including anesthesiologists who found difficulty in communication and providing a stable sedation level. In that review, the most appropriate music seemed to be classical.

Imaging Studies

In depressed folks, fMRI imaging of the reward-processing neurocircuitry when listening to music revealed less differences compared to controls in activation in medial orbital frontal cortex and nucleus accumbens/ventral striatum when listening to favorite versus neutral music [119]. Activity in the left medial prefrontal cortex was positively correlated with pleasure scores, while activity in the middle temporal cortex and globus pallidus was negatively correlated with pleasure. See Fig. 21.1.

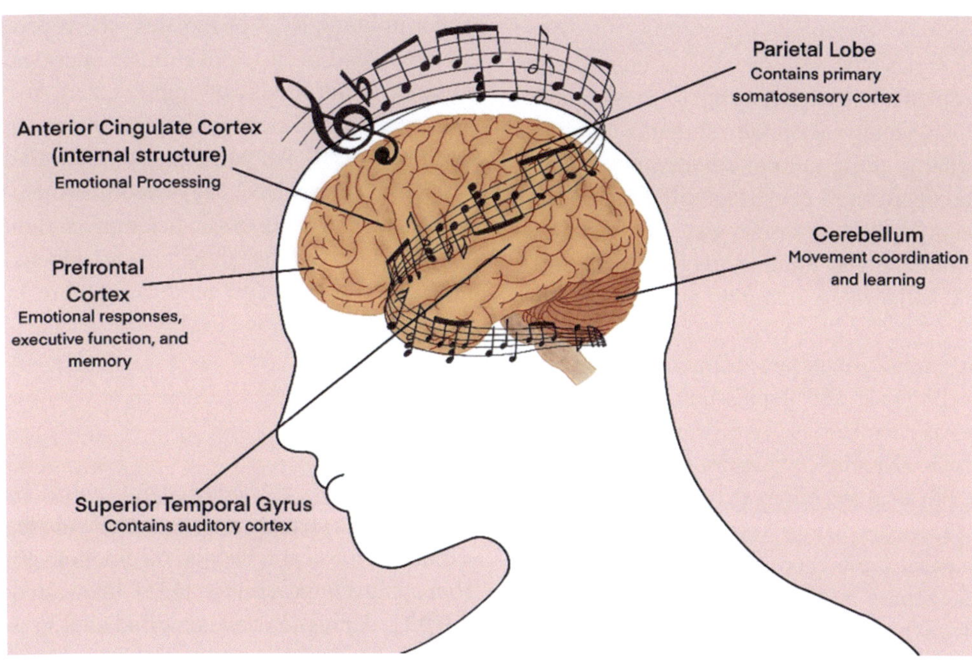

Fig. 21.1 This figure depicts key brain regions associated with musical perception, emotion, and cognition, including the anterior cingulate cortex (ACC), parietal lobe, prefrontal cortex, superior temporal gyrus, and cerebellum. These areas coordinate to support auditory-motor integration, emotional resonance, attention, and executive functions during music engagement

Musical Preferences

Personality dimensions are frequently associated with musical preferences that may reflect cultural differences. Results of such associations in Japanese college students revealed that openness to experience, especially aesthetic appreciation, was associated with preference for reflective music (jazz, classical, opera, gospel, enka[3]). The extraversion facet of sociability was associated with pop music preference [120].

It appears that we may project stereotypes about people relative to the music that we associate with them [121]. When both music therapy students and college students from the southeastern USA listened to the same script read over different genres of background music there was a decided difference in what the listeners thought about the personality of the reader. A good example is when a script was read over classical, jazz, or no music, the evaluation of the personality was rated significantly higher than when it was read over rap or country music.

In one study of 200 patients in a cardiac catheterization lab, participants were assigned to either listen to music of their choice (classical, relaxing modern music, or smooth jazz), receive no music, or be randomly assigned one of the genres [123]. Perhaps surprisingly, those who were randomly assigned music experienced a significantly greater reduction in anxiety compared to those who selected their own music. The group that received no music showed a markedly smaller reduction in anxiety relative to all music listeners.

Various singing styles have significantly different properties, which may influence their relationship to stress relief or induction. Perturbation analyses of jitter, shimmer, nonlinear dynamics, and signal to noise ratio of country, musical theater, jazz, soul, and opera show consistent differences [124]. For example, percent jitter and shimmer were low normal for country, whereas shimmer was significantly higher for opera. Opera was significantly more irregular and chaotic than other styles.

It appears that ethnic groups are different in their self-reported music experience and depression. Among Asian Americans, negative correlations have been seen between depression and Music Experience Questionnaire (MEQ) factor for Subjective/Physical Reactions to music and Affective Reactions scale [125].

A model of musical preferences that cuts across all cultures and musical genres has been proposed that reflects emotional and affective responses to music [126]. They suggest that these preferences are affected by social and auditory properties of the music. It is quoted as follows:

(a) *M*ellow factor comprising smooth and relaxing styles;
(b) *U*npretentious factor comprising a variety of different styles of sincere and rootsy music such as is often found in country and singer-songwriter genres;
(c) *S*ophisticated factor that includes classical, operatic, world, and jazz;
(d) *I*ntense factor defined by loud, forceful, and energetic music; and.
(e) *C*ontemporary factor defined largely by rhythmic and percussive music, such as is found in rap, funk, and acid jazz.

Several studies have suggested that in contrast to popular belief, the effect of music on calming autonomic responses occurs on a subconscious level that may be independent of the style of music [62, 127, 128]. For example, rhythmic patterns that involve breathing at six breaths per minute can induce favorable psychological and physiological effects through a synchronicity with cardiovascular rhythms [127]. This phenomenon relates to a 10-second rhythm of respiratory arterial blood pressure conversion into heart rate variability by a fast vagal (parasympathetic) baroreflex [128]. These cyclic changes are called *Mayer waves* that are products of oscillations in baroreceptor and chemoreceptor reflex controls [129]. These waves are seen in continuous blood pressure curves and in electrocardiograms. These waves are spontaneous, and their amplitude is enhanced during sympathetic activation, providing a surrogate marker for sympathetic activity.

An in-home RCT of females who received nursing presence/recorded music or live music intervention with nursing presence found significant improvement ($p < 0.05$) of depression, anxiety, and sleep quality as well as physiological measurements [130]. All participants preferred the live music.

Meta-analyses have suggested that there is no advantage of daily over weekly music listening, and that it is important that the intervention should be conducted repeatedly for more than 3 weeks to produce a more lasting benefit in decreasing depression [131].

Improvisation

Improvisational psychodynamic music therapy (IPMT) engages fronto-temporal areas of the brain that are involved in verbal and musical reflection on emotions and images arising from clinical improvisation [133]. In one study, after 3 months of IPMT, depression and comorbid anxiety were significantly reduced. Lasting changes were observed in resting EEG of the left fronto-temporal alpha and theta waves and in the left fronto-central and right temporoparietal areas [38].

At least in one case, a professional jazz musician was able to regain total musical ability after much of his left temporal

[3] A definition of enka can be seen in reference [122].

lobe was removed and he had completely lost musical interest and capabilities [132].

Musical improvisation can be used to deepen therapeutic relationships and decrease any inhibitions or limitations that may impede recovery [134].

Brain areas deactivated in musical improvisations are the same ones that are deactivated during dreaming and meditation, and areas that are activated include those controlling language and sensorimotor skills [135].

Improvised group singing may boost plasma oxytocin levels [136].

Although we commonly think about music performance as entertaining, relaxing, and pleasurable, professional musicians are often beset with stress and anxiety [137]. For example, a longitudinal study in Switzerland of first-year university music majors found increasing levels of fatigue, depression, and stage fright.

Summary

Music interacts with us both physically and psychosocially. Music therapy for depression may be active or passive. RCTs suggest that music therapy provides short-term beneficial effects for people with depression. Music therapy added to standard treatments seems to improve depressive symptoms. Decreased anxiety levels and improved functioning of depressed individuals are frequently seen. Individual and group interventions may provide benefits to diverse populations.

Relaxing music can change autonomic functions such as decrease respiration rate, blood pressure, and heart rate. Heart rate variability may be increased. Effects of music on neurotransmitter levels appear to be mixed. Sympathetic nervous system activation may be elicited by emotional content as well as rhythmicity of music.

Autonomic and immunological functions can be altered either in a positive or negative way by music. For example, natural killer cells have been reported to increase, decrease, or stay the same in response to music. Results are based upon musical preferences and age. Quality of life and mood may benefit by matching music types to desired effects on an individual.

In elderly people, playing the piano and learning to read music may decrease depression, improve psychological and physical quality of life, and enhance cognitive reserve. Such a regimen may integrate auditory, visual, motor, and somatosensory functions.

College students frequently use listening to music as a coping mechanism along with exercise, talking to friends, self-talk, deep breathing, writing in a journal, and marijuana use.

In adolescents, MDD may be positively associated with popular music exposure and negatively associated with reading print media. Fans of different types of music may choose friends whose substance use patterns reinforce their own substance use tendencies. Relationship of substance use, and music preference seems to be related to perceived peer use.

There is some evidence that early adolescent music preferences may be powerful indicators of later delinquency but not early delinquency. There may be a strong association between music preference and substance use. A large European study showed that preferences for mainstream pop-chart music, classical music, and jazz were negatively associated with substance use. Preferences for house/trance and techno/hardhouse were associated positively with substance use. In three of the countries, associations were seen between liking rock, heavy metal punk/hardcore, and gothic and substance use. There were mixed associations between hip-hop and R&B and substance use.

Prenatal exposure to melodies may induce neural representations that may last for several months. Preterm infants in the neonatal intensive care unit may significantly benefit from live music therapy. Infant brains demonstrate right-hemispheric specializing in processing music as early as the first few prenatal hours. These areas are related to the specific adult neural systems of the right hemisphere related to pitch, melody, and harmony.

Music may provide an adjunctive treatment to decrease pain, anxiety, and mood disturbance and increase quality of life in people with serious illnesses.

Imaging studies have shown differences in depressed individuals compared to controls in the reward processing areas of the brain when listening to music. Musical preferences that apply across all cultures and musical genres have been proposed that reflects emotional and affective responses to music. Effect of music on calming autonomic responses occurs on a subconscious level that may be independent of the style of music. Musical improvisation can deepen therapeutic relationships and decrease any inhibitions or limitations that may impede recovery.

References

1. De Backer J. Music and psychosis: a research report detailing the transition from sensorial play to musical form by psychotic patients. Nord J Music Ther. 2008;17:89–104.
2. Hadley S. Psychodynamic music therapy: an overview. In: Hadley S, editor. Psychodynamic music therapy: case studies. Barcelona Publishers; 2003. p. 1–22.
3. Erkkilä J. Musical improvisation and drawings as tools in the music therapy of children. Nord J Music Ther. 1997;6:112–20.
4. Erkkilä J. From signs to symbols, from symbols to words—about the relationship between music and language, music therapy and psychotherapy. Voices. 2004;4

5. Ockelford A. Applied musicology using zygonic theory to inform music education, therapy, and psychology research. Oxford University Press, Oxford 2013.
6. Sandstrom GM, Russo FA. Music hath charms: the effects of valence and arousal on recovery following an acute stressor. Music Med. 2010;2:137–43.
7. Yamamoto M, Naga S, Shimizu J. Positive musical effects on two types of negative stressful conditions. Psychol Music. 2007;35:249–75.
8. Gold C, Heldal TO, Dahle T, Wigram T. Music therapy for schizophrenia or schizophrenia-like illnesses. Cochrane Database Syst Rev. 2005;2:CD004025. PMID: 15846692 http://www.ncbi.nlm.nih.gov/pubmed/15846692
9. Erkkilä J, Punkanen M, Fachner J, Ala-Ruona E, Pöntiö I, Tervaniemi M, Vanhala M, Gold C. Individual music therapy for depression: randomised controlled trial. Br J Psychiatry. 2011;199(2):132–9. PMID: 21474494 http://www.ncbi.nlm.nih.gov/pubmed/21474494
10. Fancourt D, Ockelford A, Belai A. The psychoneuroimmunological effects of music: a systematic review and a new model. Brain Behav Immun. 2014;36:15–26. PMID: 24157429. PubMed entry [Internet]. [cited 2025 Jan 24]. Available from: http://www.ncbi.nlm.nih.gov/pubmed/24157429
11. Weninger F, Eyben F, Schuller BW, Mortillaro M, Scherer KR. On the acoustics of emotion in audio: what speech, music, and sound have in common. Front Psychol. 2013;4:292. PMCID: PMC3664314. http://www.ncbi.nlm.nih.gov/pubmed/23750144
12. Gold BP, Frank MJ, Bogert B, Brattico E. Pleasurable music affects reinforcement learning according to the listener. Front Psychol. 2013;4:541. PMCID: PMC3748532. http://www.ncbi.nlm.nih.gov/pubmed/23970875
13. Zentner M, Grandjean D, Scherer KR. Emotions evoked by the sound of music: characterization, classification, and measurement. Emotion. 2008;8(4):494–521. PMID: 18729581. http://www.ncbi.nlm.nih.gov/pubmed/18729581
14. Juslin PN. What does music express? Basic emotions and beyond. Front Psychol. 2013;4:596. PMCID: PMC3764399. http://www.ncbi.nlm.nih.gov/pubmed/24046758
15. Bigand E, Poulin-Charronnat B. Are we "experienced listeners"? A review of the musical capacities that do not depend on formal musical training. Cognition. 2006;100(1):100–30. PMID: 16412412. http://www.ncbi.nlm.nih.gov/pubmed/16412412
16. Laukka P, Eerola T, Thingujam NS, Yamasaki T, Beller G. Universal and culture-specific factors in the recognition and performance of musical affect expressions. Emotion. 2013;13(3):434–49. PMID: 23398579. http://www.ncbi.nlm.nih.gov/pubmed/23398579
17. Larsen JT, Stastny BJ. It's a bittersweet symphony: simultaneously mixed emotional responses to music with conflicting cues. Emotion. 2011;11(6):1469–73. PMID: 21707144. http://www.ncbi.nlm.nih.gov/pubmed/21707144
18. Music and the Brain: Depression and Creativity Symposium
19. Maratos AS, Gold C, Wang X, Crawford MJ. Music therapy for depression. Cochrane Database Syst Rev. 2008;1:CD004517. PMID: 18254052. http://www.ncbi.nlm.nih.gov/pubmed/18254052
20. Aalbers S, Fusar-Poli L, Freeman RE, Spreen M, Ket JC, Vink AC, Maratos A, Crawford M, Chen XJ, Gold C. Music therapy for depression. Cochrane Database Syst Rev. 2017;11(11):CD004517. PMCID: PMC6486188. http://www.ncbi.nlm.nih.gov/pubmed/29144545
21. Carr C, Odell-Miller H, Priebe S. A systematic review of music therapy practice and outcomes with acute adult psychiatric inpatients. PLoS One. 2013;8(8):e70252. PMCID: PMC3732280. http://www.ncbi.nlm.nih.gov/pubmed/23936399
22. Watanabe M, Aiso S, Hibi T, Watanabe N, Iwao Y, Yoshida T, Asakura H, Tsuru S, Tsuchiya M. Alteration of T cell maturation and proliferation in the mouse thymus induced by serum factors from patients with ulcerative colitis. Clin Exp Immunol. 1987;68(3):596–604. PMCID: PMC1542736. http://www.ncbi.nlm.nih.gov/pubmed/3498579
23. Gold C, Solli HP, Krüger V, Lie SA. Dose-response relationship in music therapy for people with serious mental disorders: systematic review and meta-analysis. Clin Psychol Rev. 2009;29(3):193–207. PMID: 19269725. http://www.ncbi.nlm.nih.gov/pubmed/19269725
24. Akandere M, Demir B. The effect of dance over depression. Coll Antropol. 2011;35(3):651–6. PMID: 22053537. http://www.ncbi.nlm.nih.gov/pubmed/22053537
25. Jun EM, Roh YH, Kim MJ. The effect of music-movement therapy on physical and psychological states of stroke patients. J Clin Nurs. 2013;22(1–2):22–31. PMID: 22978325. http://www.ncbi.nlm.nih.gov/pubmed/22978325
26. Carr C, d'Ardenne P, Sloboda A, Scott C, Wang D, Priebe S. Group music therapy for patients with persistent post-traumatic stress disorder–an exploratory randomized controlled trial with mixed methods evaluation. Psychol Psychother. 2012;85(2):179–202. PMID: 22903909. http://www.ncbi.nlm.nih.gov/pubmed/22903909
27. Chou MH, Lin MF. Exploring the listening experiences during guided imagery and music therapy of outpatients with depression. J Nurs Res. 2006;14(2):93–102. PMID: 16741859. http://www.ncbi.nlm.nih.gov/pubmed/16741859
28. Naranjo C, Kornreich C, Campanella S, Noël X, Vandriette Y, Gillain B, de Longueville X, Delatte B, Verbanck P, Constant E. Major depression is associated with impaired processing of emotion in music as well as in facial and vocal stimuli. J Affect Disord. 2011;128(3):243–51. PMID: 20663569. http://www.ncbi.nlm.nih.gov/pubmed/20663569
29. Punkanen M, Eerola T, Erkkilä J. Biased emotional recognition in depression: perception of emotions in music by depressed patients. J Affect Disord. 2011;130(1–2):118–26. PMID: 21071094. http://www.ncbi.nlm.nih.gov/pubmed/21071094
30. Fancourt D, Perkins R, Ascenso S, Carvalho LA, Steptoe A, Williamon A. Effects of group drumming interventions on anxiety, depression, social resilience and inflammatory immune response among mental health service users. PLoS One. 2016;11(3):e0151136. PMCID: PMC4790847. http://www.ncbi.nlm.nih.gov/pubmed/26974430
31. Sakamoto M, Ando H, Tsutou A. Comparing the effects of different individualized music interventions for elderly individuals with severe dementia. Int Psychogeriatr. 2013;25(5):775–84. PMCID: PMC3605862. http://www.ncbi.nlm.nih.gov/pubmed/23298693
32. Ueda T, Suzukamo Y, Sato M, Izumi SI. Effects of music therapy on behavioral and psychological symptoms of dementia: a systematic review and meta-analysis. Ageing Res Rev. 2013;12(2):628–41. PMID: 23511664. http://www.ncbi.nlm.nih.gov/pubmed/23511664
33. Russo FA, Vempala NN, Sandstrom GM. Predicting musically induced emotions from physiological inputs: linear and neural network models. Front Psychol. 2013;4:468. PMCID: PMC3737459. http://www.ncbi.nlm.nih.gov/pubmed/23964250
34. Berbel P, Moix J, Quintana S. Music versus diazepam to reduce preoperative anxiety: a randomized controlled clinical trial. Rev Esp Anestesiol Reanim. 2007;54(6):355–8. PMID: 17695946. http://www.ncbi.nlm.nih.gov/pubmed/17695946
35. McKinney CH, Tims FC, Kumar AM, Kumar M. The effect of selected classical music and spontaneous imagery on plasma beta-endorphin. J Behav Med. 1997;20(1):85–99. PMID: 9058181. http://www.ncbi.nlm.nih.gov/pubmed/9058181
36. Leardi S, Pietroletti R, Angeloni G, Necozione S, Ranalletta G, Del Gusto B. Randomized clinical trial examining the effect of music therapy in stress response to day surgery. Br J Surg.

2007;94(8):943–7. PMID: 17636513. http://www.ncbi.nlm.nih.gov/pubmed/17636513
37. Bittman BB, Berk LS, Felten DL, Westengard J, Simonton OC, Pappas J, Ninehouser M. Composite effects of group drumming music therapy on modulation of neuroendocrine-immune parameters in normal subjects. Altern Ther Health Med. 2001;7(1):38–47. PMID: 11191041. http://www.ncbi.nlm.nih.gov/pubmed/11191041
38. Field T, Martinez A, Nawrocki T, Pickens J, Fox NA, Schanberg S. Music shifts frontal EEG in depressed adolescents. Adolescence. 1998;33(129):109–16. PMID: 9583665. http://www.ncbi.nlm.nih.gov/pubmed/9583665
39. Hirokawa E, Ohira H. The effects of music listening after a stressful task on immune functions, neuroendocrine responses, and emotional states in college students. J Music Ther. 2003;40(3):189–211. PMID: 14567734. http://www.ncbi.nlm.nih.gov/pubmed/14567734
40. Escher J, Höhmann U, Anthenien L, Dayer E, Bosshard C, Gaillard RC. Music during gastroscopy. Schweiz Med Wochenschr. 1993;123(26):1354–8. PMID: 8393585. http://www.ncbi.nlm.nih.gov/pubmed/8393585
41. Uedo N, Ishikawa H, Morimoto K, Ishihara R, Narahara H, Akedo I, Ioka T, Kaji I, Fukuda S. Reduction in salivary cortisol level by music therapy during colonoscopic examination. Hepato-Gastroenterology. 2004;51(56):451–3. PMID: 15086180. http://www.ncbi.nlm.nih.gov/pubmed/15086180
42. Nilsson U. Soothing music can increase oxytocin levels during bed rest after open-heart surgery: a randomised control trial. J Clin Nurs. 2009;18(15):2153–61. PMID: 19583647. http://www.ncbi.nlm.nih.gov/pubmed/19583647
43. Migneault B, Girard F, Albert C, Chouinard P, Boudreault D, Provencher D, Todorov A, Ruel M, Girard DC. The effect of music on the neurohormonal stress response to surgery under general anesthesia. Anesth Analg. 2004;98(2):527–32. PMID: 14742400. http://www.ncbi.nlm.nih.gov/pubmed/14742400
44. Koelsch S, Boehlig A, Hohenadel M, Nitsche I, Bauer K, Sack U. The impact of acute stress on hormones and cytokines, and how their recovery is affected by music-evoked positive mood. Sci Rep. 2016;6:23008. PMCID: PMC4810374. http://www.ncbi.nlm.nih.gov/pubmed/27020850
45. Kim HG, Cheon EJ, Bai DS, Lee YH, Koo BH. Stress and heart rate variability: a meta-analysis and review of the literature. Psychiatry Investig. 2018;15(3):235–45. PMCID: PMC5900369. http://www.ncbi.nlm.nih.gov/pubmed/29486547
46. Immanuel S, Teferra MN, Baumert M, Bidargaddi N. Heart rate variability for evaluating psychological stress changes in healthy adults: a scoping review. Neuropsychobiology. 2023;82(4):187–202. PMCID: PMC10614455. http://www.ncbi.nlm.nih.gov/pubmed/37290411
47. Nickel P, Nachreiner F. Sensitivity and diagnosticity of the 0.1-Hz component of heart rate variability as an indicator of mental workload. Hum Factors. 2003;45(4):575–90. PMID: 15055455. http://www.ncbi.nlm.nih.gov/pubmed/15055455
48. Jönsson P. Respiratory sinus arrhythmia as a function of state anxiety in healthy individuals. Int J Psychophysiol. 2007;63(1):48–54. PMID: 16989914. http://www.ncbi.nlm.nih.gov/pubmed/16989914
49. Mujica-Parodi LR, Korgaonkar M, Ravindranath B, Greenberg T, Tomasi D, Wagshul M, Ardekani B, Guilfoyle D, Khan S, Zhong Y, Chon K, Malaspina D. Limbic dysregulation is associated with lowered heart rate variability and increased trait anxiety in healthy adults. Hum Brain Mapp. 2009;30(1):47–58. PMCID: PMC2993012. http://www.ncbi.nlm.nih.gov/pubmed/18041716
50. Brosschot JF, Van Dijk E, Thayer JF. Daily worry is related to low heart rate variability during waking and the subsequent nocturnal sleep period. Int J Psychophysiol. 2007;63(1):39–47. PMID: 17020787. http://www.ncbi.nlm.nih.gov/pubmed/17020787
51. Cohen H, Kotler M, Matar MA, Kaplan Z, Loewenthal U, Miodownik H, Cassuto Y. Analysis of heart rate variability in posttraumatic stress disorder patients in response to a trauma-related reminder. Biol Psychiatry. 1998;44(10):1054–9. PMID: 9821570. http://www.ncbi.nlm.nih.gov/pubmed/9821570
52. Dedert EA, Calhoun PS, Watkins LL, Sherwood A, Beckham JC. Posttraumatic stress disorder, cardiovascular, and metabolic disease: a review of the evidence. Ann Behav Med. 2010;39(1):61–78. PMCID: PMC3219414. http://www.ncbi.nlm.nih.gov/pubmed/20174903
53. Stapelberg NJ, Hamilton-Craig I, Neumann DL, Shum DHK, McConnell H. Mind and heart: heart rate variability in major depressive disorder and coronary heart disease – a review and recommendations. Aust N Z J Psychiatry. 2012;46(10):946–57. PMID: 22528974. http://www.ncbi.nlm.nih.gov/pubmed/22528974
54. Kemp AH, Quintana DS, Felmingham KL, Matthews S, Jelinek HF. Depression, comorbid anxiety disorders, and heart rate variability in physically healthy, unmedicated patients: implications for cardiovascular risk. PLoS One. 2012;7(2):e30777. PMCID: PMC3280258. http://www.ncbi.nlm.nih.gov/pubmed/22355326
55. Alvares GA, Quintana DS, Kemp AH, Van Zwieten A, Balleine BW, Hickie IB, Guastella AJ. Reduced heart rate variability in social anxiety disorder: associations with gender and symptom severity. PLoS One. 2013;8(7):e70468. PMCID: PMC3728204. http://www.ncbi.nlm.nih.gov/pubmed/23936207
56. Dinas PC, Koutedakis Y, Flouris AD. Effects of active and passive tobacco cigarette smoking on heart rate variability. Int J Cardiol. 2013;163(2):109–15. PMID: 22100604. http://www.ncbi.nlm.nih.gov/pubmed/22100604
57. Xhyheri B, Manfrini O, Mazzolini M, Pizzi C, Bugiardini R. Heart rate variability today. Prog Cardiovasc Dis. 2012;55(3):321–31. PMID: 23217437. http://www.ncbi.nlm.nih.gov/pubmed/23217437
58. Bernardi L, Porta C, Casucci G, Balsamo R, Bernardi NF, Fogari R, Sleight P. Dynamic interactions between musical, cardiovascular, and cerebral rhythms in humans. Circulation. 2009;119(25):3171–80. PMID: 19569263. http://www.ncbi.nlm.nih.gov/pubmed/19569263
59. Bernardi L, Porta C, Sleight P. Cardiovascular, cerebrovascular, and respiratory changes induced by different types of music in musicians and non-musicians: the importance of silence. Heart. 2006;92(4):445–452. PMCID: PMC1860846. http://www.ncbi.nlm.nih.gov/pubmed/16199412.
60. Thoma MV, La Marca R, Brönnimann R, Finkel L, Ehlert U, Nater UM. The effect of music on the human stress response. PLoS One. 2013;8(8):e70156. PMCID: PMC3734071. http://www.ncbi.nlm.nih.gov/pubmed/23940541
61. Noto Y, Sato T, Kudo M, Kurata K, Hirota K. The relationship between salivary biomarkers and state-trait anxiety inventory score under mental arithmetic stress: a pilot study. Anesth Analg. 2005;101(6):1873–6. PMID: 16301277. http://www.ncbi.nlm.nih.gov/pubmed/16301277
62. Sleight P. Cardiovascular effects of music by entraining cardiovascular autonomic rhythms music therapy update: tailored to each person, or does one size fit all? Neth Heart J. 2013;21(2):99–100. PMCID: PMC3547422. http://www.ncbi.nlm.nih.gov/pubmed/23225598
63. Szmedra L, Bacharach DW. Effect of music on perceived exertion, plasma lactate, norepinephrine and cardiovascular hemodynamics during treadmill running. Int J Sports Med. 1998;19(1):32–7. PMID: 9506797. http://www.ncbi.nlm.nih.gov/pubmed/9506797
64. Porges SW. The polyvagal theory: new insights into adaptive reactions of the autonomic nervous system. Cleve Clin J Med. 2009;76

Suppl 2(Suppl 2):S86–90. PMCID: PMC3108032. http://www.ncbi.nlm.nih.gov/pubmed/19376991
65. Grossman P. Fundamental challenges and likely refutations of the five basic premises of the polyvagal theory. Biol Psychol. 2023;180:108589. PMID: 37230290. http://www.ncbi.nlm.nih.gov/pubmed/37230290
66. Krabs RU, Enk R, Teich N, Koelsch S. Autonomic effects of music in health and Crohn's disease: the impact of isochronicity, emotional valence, and tempo. PLoS One. 2015;10(5):e0126224. PMCID: PMC4425535. http://www.ncbi.nlm.nih.gov/pubmed/25955253
67. DeNora T. "Time after time": a Quali-T method for assessing music's impact on well-being. Int J Qual Stud Health Well-being. 2013;8:20611. PMCID: PMC3740600. http://www.ncbi.nlm.nih.gov/pubmed/23930990
68. Cai GR, Li PW, Jiao LP. Clinical observation of music therapy combined with anti-tumor drugs in treating 116 cases of tumor patients. Zhongguo Zhong Xi Yi Jie He Za Zhi. 2001;21(12):891–4. PMID: 12575587. http://www.ncbi.nlm.nih.gov/pubmed/12575587
69. Stefano GB, Zhu W, Cadet P, Salamon E, Mantione KJ. Music alters constitutively expressed opiate and cytokine processes in listeners. Med Sci Monit. 2004;10(6):MS18–27. PMID: 15173680. http://www.ncbi.nlm.nih.gov/pubmed/15173680
70. Constant E. Music, composers and psychopathology: the psychiatrist's view. Bull Mem Acad R Med Belg. 2011;166(1–2):88–96. discussion 97–98. PMID: 22375492. http://www.ncbi.nlm.nih.gov/pubmed/22375492
71. Proudfoot J, Whitton A, Parker G, Doran J, Manicavasagar V, Delmas K. Triggers of mania and depression in young adults with bipolar disorder. J Affect Disord. 2012;143(1–3):196–202. PMID: 22884233. http://www.ncbi.nlm.nih.gov/pubmed/22884233
72. Hars M, Herrmann FR, Gold G, Rizzoli R, Trombetti A. Effect of music-based multitask training on cognition and mood in older adults. Age Ageing. 2014;43(2):196–200. PMID: 24212920. http://www.ncbi.nlm.nih.gov/pubmed/24212920
73. Seinfeld S, Figueroa H, Ortiz-Gil J, Sanchez-Vives MV. Effects of music learning and piano practice on cognitive function, mood and quality of life in older adults. Front Psychol. 2013;4:810. PMCID: PMC3814522. http://www.ncbi.nlm.nih.gov/pubmed/24198804
74. Wan CY, Schlaug G. Music making as a tool for promoting brain plasticity across the life span. Neuroscientist. 2010;16(5):566–77. PMCID: PMC2996135. http://www.ncbi.nlm.nih.gov/pubmed/20889966
75. Chan MF, Wong ZY, Onishi H, Thayala NV. Effects of music on depression in older people: a randomised controlled trial. J Clin Nurs. 2012;21(5–6):776–83. PMID: 22035368. http://www.ncbi.nlm.nih.gov/pubmed/22035368
76. Lee YY, Chan MF, Mok E. Effectiveness of music intervention on the quality of life of older people. J Adv Nurs. 2010;66(12):2677–87. PMID: 20831571. http://www.ncbi.nlm.nih.gov/pubmed/20831571
77. Chu H, Yang CY, Lin Y, Ou KL, Lee TY, O'Brien AP, Chou KR. The impact of group music therapy on depression and cognition in elderly persons with dementia: a randomized controlled study. Biol Res Nurs. 2014;16(2):209–17. PMID: 23639952. http://www.ncbi.nlm.nih.gov/pubmed/23639952
78. Nyer M, Doorley J, Durham K, Yeung AS, Freeman MP, Mischoulon D. What is the role of alternative treatments in late-life depression? Psychiatr Clin North Am. 2013;36(4):577–96. PMID: 24229658. http://www.ncbi.nlm.nih.gov/pubmed/24229658
79. Chan MF, Chan EA, Mok E, Kwan Tse FY. Effect of music on depression levels and physiological responses in community-based older adults. Int J Ment Health Nurs. 2009;18(4):285–94. PMID: 19594648. http://www.ncbi.nlm.nih.gov/pubmed/19594648
80. Cooke M, Moyle W, Shum D, Harrison S, Murfield J. A randomized controlled trial exploring the effect of music on quality of life and depression in older people with dementia. J Health Psychol. 2010;15(5):765–76. PMID: 20603300. http://www.ncbi.nlm.nih.gov/pubmed/20603300
81. Manalai G, Manalai P, Dutta R, Fegan G, Scrofani P. Rapid improvement of depressive symptoms and cognition in an elderly patient with a single session of piano playing: a clinical treatment report. Aging Clin Exp Res. 2012;24(3):278–80. PMID: 23114556. http://www.ncbi.nlm.nih.gov/pubmed/23114556
82. Cross K, Flores R, Butterfield J, Blackman M, Lee S. The effect of passive listening versus active observation of music and dance performances on memory recognition and mild to moderate depression in cognitively impaired older adults. Psychol Rep. 2012;111(2):413–23. PMID: 23234087. http://www.ncbi.nlm.nih.gov/pubmed/23234087
83. Primack BA, Silk JS, DeLozier CR, Shadel WG, Dillman Carpentier FR, Dahl RE, Switzer GE. Using ecological momentary assessment to determine media use by individuals with and without major depressive disorder. Arch Pediatr Adolesc Med. 2011;165(4):360–5. PMCID: PMC3074228. http://www.ncbi.nlm.nih.gov/pubmed/21464384
84. Mulder J, Ter Bogt TFM, Raaijmakers QAW, Nic Gabhainn S, Monshouwer K, Vollebergh WAM. Is it the music? Peer substance use as a mediator of the link between music preferences and adolescent substance use. J Adolesc. 2010;33(3):387–94. PMID: 19818488. http://www.ncbi.nlm.nih.gov/pubmed/19818488
85. Stegemann T, Brüggemann-Etchart A, Badorrek-Hinkelmann A, Romer G. The function of music in the context of non-suicidal self-injury. Prax Kinderpsychol Kinderpsychiatr. 2010;59(10):810–30. PMID: 21290852. http://www.ncbi.nlm.nih.gov/pubmed/21290852
86. Aselton P. Sources of stress and coping in American college students who have been diagnosed with depression. J Child Adolesc Psychiatr Nurs. 2012;25(3):119–23. PMID: 22830509. http://www.ncbi.nlm.nih.gov/pubmed/22830509
87. Recours R, Aussaguel F, Trujillo N. Metal music and mental health in France. Cult Med Psychiatry. 2009;33(3):473–88. PMID: 19521752. http://www.ncbi.nlm.nih.gov/pubmed/19521752
88. Ter Bogt TFM, Keijsers L, Meeus WHJ. Early adolescent music preferences and minor delinquency. Pediatrics. 2013;131(2):e380–9. PMID: 23296443. http://www.ncbi.nlm.nih.gov/pubmed/23296443
89. Ter Bogt TFM, Gabhainn SN, Simons-Morton BG, Ferreira M, Hublet A, Godeau E, Kuntsche E, Richter M, HBSC Risk Behavior and the HBSC Peer Culture Focus Groups. Dance is the new metal: adolescent music preferences and substance use across Europe. Subst Use Misuse. 2012;47(2):130–42. PMCID: PMC4121736. http://www.ncbi.nlm.nih.gov/pubmed/22217067
90. Beckett R. Birthbeats: music to your ears. Pract Midwife. 2012;15(5):32–4. PMID: 22788006. http://www.ncbi.nlm.nih.gov/pubmed/22788006
91. Partanen E, Kujala T, Tervaniemi M, Huotilainen M. Prenatal music exposure induces long-term neural effects. PLoS One. 2013;8(10):e78946. PMCID: PMC3813619. http://www.ncbi.nlm.nih.gov/pubmed/24205353
92. Kushnir J, Friedman A, Ehrenfeld M, Kushnir T. Coping with preoperative anxiety in cesarean section: physiological, cognitive, and emotional effects of listening to favorite music. Birth. 2012;39(2):121–7. PMID: 23281860. http://www.ncbi.nlm.nih.gov/pubmed/23281860
93. Granier-Deferre C, Bassereau S, Ribeiro A, Jacquet AY, Decasper AJ. A melodic contour repeatedly experienced by human near-term fetuses elicits a profound cardiac reaction one month after birth. PLoS One 2011;6(2):e17304. PMCID: PMC3044162.
94. Kisilevsky S, Hains SMJ, Jacquet AY, Granier-Deferre C, Lecanuet JP. Maturation of fetal responses to music. Dev Sci.

2004;7(5):550–9. PMID: 15603288. http://www.ncbi.nlm.nih.gov/pubmed/15603288

95. de l'Etoile SK, Leider CN. Acoustic parameters of infant-directed singing in mothers with depressive symptoms. Infant Behav Dev. 2011;34(2):248–56. PMID: 21255845. http://www.ncbi.nlm.nih.gov/pubmed/21255845
96. Standley J. Music therapy research in the NICU: an updated meta-analysis. Neonatal Netw. 2012;31(5):311–6. PMID: 22908052. http://www.ncbi.nlm.nih.gov/pubmed/22908052
97. Perani D, Saccuman MC, Scifo P, Spada D, Andreolli G, Rovelli R, Baldoli C, Koelsch S. Functional specializations for music processing in the human newborn brain. Proc Natl Acad Sci U S A. 2010;107(10):4758–63. PMCID: PMC2842045 http://www.ncbi.nlm.nih.gov/pubmed/20176953
98. Pasiali V. Supporting parent-child interactions: music therapy as an intervention for promoting mutually responsive orientation. J Music Ther. 2012;49(3):303–34. PMID: 23259232. http://www.ncbi.nlm.nih.gov/pubmed/23259232
99. Zhang JM, Wang P, Yao J xin, Zhao L, Davis MP, Walsh D, Yue GH. Music interventions for psychological and physical outcomes in cancer: a systematic review and meta-analysis. Support Care Cancer. 2012;20(12):3043–53. PMID: 23052912. http://www.ncbi.nlm.nih.gov/pubmed/23052912
100. Bradt J, Dileo C, Grocke D, Magill L. Music interventions for improving psychological and physical outcomes in cancer patients. Cochrane Database Syst Rev. 2011;8:CD006911. PMID: 21833957. http://www.ncbi.nlm.nih.gov/pubmed/21833957
101. Archie P, Bruera E, Cohen L. Music-based interventions in palliative cancer care: a review of quantitative studies and neurobiological literature. Support Care Cancer. 2013;21(9):2609–24. PMCID: PMC3728458. http://www.ncbi.nlm.nih.gov/pubmed/23715815
102. Chen LC, Wang TF, Shih YN, Wu LJ. Fifteen-minute music intervention reduces pre-radiotherapy anxiety in oncology patients. Eur J Oncol Nurs. 2013;17(4):436–41. PMID: 23218591. http://www.ncbi.nlm.nih.gov/pubmed/23218591
103. Zhou K-n, Li X-m, Yan H, Dang S-n, Wang D-l. Effects of music therapy on depression and duration of hospital stay of breast cancer patients after radical mastectomy. Chin Med J. 2011;124(15):2321–7. PMID: 21933563. http://www.ncbi.nlm.nih.gov/pubmed/21933563
104. Han P, Kwan M, Chen D, Yusoff SZ, Chionh HL, Goh J, Yap P. A controlled naturalistic study on a weekly music therapy and activity program on disruptive and depressive behaviors in dementia. Dement Geriatr Cogn Disord. 2010;30(6):540–6. PMID: 21252549. http://www.ncbi.nlm.nih.gov/pubmed/21252549
105. Guétin S, Giniès P, Siou DKA, Picot MC, Pommié C, Guldner E, Gosp AM, Ostyn K, Coudeyre E, Touchon J. The effects of music intervention in the management of chronic pain: a single-blind, randomized, controlled trial. Clin J Pain. 2012;28(4):329–37. PMID: 22001666. http://www.ncbi.nlm.nih.gov/pubmed/22001666
106. Sven-Olof Trängeberg Ö, Stomberg MW. Listening to music during regional anesthesia: patients' experiences and the effect on mood. J Perianesth Nurs. 2013;28(5):291–7. PMID: 24054454. http://www.ncbi.nlm.nih.gov/pubmed/24054454
107. Kim DS, Park YG, Choi JH, Im SH, Jung KJ, Cha YA, Jung CO, Yoon YH. Effects of music therapy on mood in stroke patients. Yonsei Med J. 2011;52(6):977–81. PMCID: PMC3220261. http://www.ncbi.nlm.nih.gov/pubmed/22028163
108. Onieva-Zafra MD, Castro-Sánchez AM, Matarán-Peñarrocha GA, Moreno-Lorenzo C. Effect of music as nursing intervention for people diagnosed with fibromyalgia. Pain Manag Nurs. 2013;14(2):e39–46. PMID: 23108015. http://www.ncbi.nlm.nih.gov/pubmed/23108015
109. White JM. Effects of relaxing music on cardiac autonomic balance and anxiety after acute myocardial infarction. Am J Crit Care. 1999;8(4):220–30. PMID: 10392221. http://www.ncbi.nlm.nih.gov/pubmed/10392221
110. Lin ST, Yang P, Lai CY, Su YY, Yeh YC, Huang MF, Chen CC. Mental health implications of music: insight from neuroscientific and clinical studies. Harv Rev Psychiatry. 2011;19(1):34–46. PMID: 21250895. http://www.ncbi.nlm.nih.gov/pubmed/21250895
111. Moradipanah F, Mohammadi E, Mohammadil AZ. Effect of music on anxiety, stress, and depression levels in patients undergoing coronary angiography. East Mediterr Health J. 2009;15(3):639–47. PMID: 19731780. http://www.ncbi.nlm.nih.gov/pubmed/19731780
112. Meeuse JJ, Koornstra JJ, Reyners AKL. Listening to music does not reduce pain during sigmoidoscopy. Eur J Gastroenterol Hepatol 2010;22(8):942–945. PMID: 20110821. http://www.ncbi.nlm.nih.gov/pubmed/20110821
113. Makama JG, Ameh EA, Eguma SA. Music in the operating theatre: opinions of staff and patients of a Nigerian teaching hospital. Afr Health Sci. 2010;10(4):386–9. PMCID: PMC3052799. http://www.ncbi.nlm.nih.gov/pubmed/21416041
114. Ullmann Y, Fodor L, Schwarzberg I, Carmi N, Ullmann A, Ramon Y. The sounds of music in the operating room. Injury. 2008;39(5):592–7. PMID: 16989832. http://www.ncbi.nlm.nih.gov/pubmed/16989832
115. Cunningham MF, Monson B, Bookbinder M. Introducing a music program in the perioperative area. AORN J. 1997;66(4):674–82. PMID: 9337469. http://www.ncbi.nlm.nih.gov/pubmed/9337469
116. George S, Ahmed S, Mammen KJ, John GM. Influence of music on operation theatre staff. J Anaesthesiol Clin Pharmacol. 2011;27(3):354–7. PMCID: PMC3161461. http://www.ncbi.nlm.nih.gov/pubmed/21897507
117. Hawksworth C, Asbury AJ, Millar K. Music in theatre: not so harmonious. A survey of attitudes to music played in the operating theatre. Anaesthesia. 1997;52(1):79–83. PMID: 9014553. http://www.ncbi.nlm.nih.gov/pubmed/9014553
118. Moris DN, Linos D. Music meets surgery: two sides to the art of "healing". Surg Endosc. 2013;27(3):719–23. PMID: 23052506. http://www.ncbi.nlm.nih.gov/pubmed/23052506
119. Lennings CJ. The Schalling sensation seeking and impulsivity scales: their relationship to time perspective and time awareness, a preliminary report. Psychol Rep. 1991;69(1):131–6. PMID: 1961780. http://www.ncbi.nlm.nih.gov/pubmed/1961780
120. Brown RA. Music preferences and personality among Japanese university students. Int J Psychol 2012;47(4):259–268. PMID: 22248342. http://www.ncbi.nlm.nih.gov/pubmed/22248342
121. Lastinger DL. The effect of background music on the perception of personality and demographics. J Music Ther. 2011;48(2):208–25. PMID: 21938892. http://www.ncbi.nlm.nih.gov/pubmed/21938892
122. Tears of Longing: Nostalgia and the Nation in Japanese Popular Song - Christine Reiko Yano – Google Books
123. Goertz W, Dominick K, Heussen N, vom Dahl J. Music in the cath lab: who should select it? Clin Res Cardiol. 2011;100(5):395–402. PMID: 21110034. http://www.ncbi.nlm.nih.gov/pubmed/21110034
124. Butte CJ, Zhang Y, Song H, Jiang JJ. Perturbation and nonlinear dynamic analysis of different singing styles. J Voice. 2009;23(6):647–52. PMCID: PMC3313593. http://www.ncbi.nlm.nih.gov/pubmed/18504114
125. Werner PD, Swope AJ, Heide FJ. Ethnicity, music experience, and depression. J Music Ther 2009;46(4):339–358. PMID: 20394134. http://www.ncbi.nlm.nih.gov/pubmed/20394134
126. Rentfrow PJ, Goldberg LR, Levitin DJ. The structure of musical preferences: a five-factor model. J Pers Soc Psychol 2011;100(6):1139–1157. PMCID: PMC3138530. http://www.ncbi.nlm.nih.gov/pubmed/21299309

127. Bernardi L, Sleight P, Bandinelli G, Cencetti S, Fattorini L, Wdowczyc-Szulc J, Lagi A. Effect of rosary prayer and yoga mantras on autonomic cardiovascular rhythms: comparative study. BMJ. 2001;323(7327):1446–9. PMCID: PMC61046. http://www.ncbi.nlm.nih.gov/pubmed/11751348
128. Sleight P, La Rovere MT, Mortara A, Pinna G, Maestri R, Leuzzi S, Bianchini B, Tavazzi L, Bernardi L. Physiology and pathophysiology of heart rate and blood pressure variability in humans: is power spectral analysis largely an index of baroreflex gain? Clin Sci Lond. 1995;88(1):103–9. PMID: 7677832. http://www.ncbi.nlm.nih.gov/pubmed/7677832
129. Julien C. The enigma of Mayer waves: facts and models. Cardiovasc Res. 2006;70(1):12–21. PMID: 16360130. http://www.ncbi.nlm.nih.gov/pubmed/16360130
130. Lai HL, Li YM, Lee LH. Effects of music intervention with nursing presence and recorded music on psycho-physiological indices of cancer patient caregivers. J Clin Nurs. 2012;21(5–6):745–56. PMID: 22098540. http://www.ncbi.nlm.nih.gov/pubmed/22098540
131. Chan MF, Wong ZY, Thayala NV. The effectiveness of music listening in reducing depressive symptoms in adults: a systematic review. Complement Ther Med 2011;19(6):332–348. PMID: 22036525. http://www.ncbi.nlm.nih.gov/pubmed/22036525
132. Galarza M, Isaac C, Pellicer O, Mayes A, Broks P, Montaldi D, Denby C, Simeone F. Jazz, guitar, and neurosurgery: the Pat Martino case report. World Neurosurg 2014;81(3–4):651.e1–651.e7. PMID: 24076057. http://www.ncbi.nlm.nih.gov/pubmed/24076057
133. Fachner J, Gold C, Erkkilä J. Music therapy modulates fronto-temporal activity in rest-EEG in depressed clients. Brain Topogr. 2013;26(2):338–54. PMID: 22983820. http://www.ncbi.nlm.nih.gov/pubmed/22983820
134. Tomaino CM. Creativity and improvisation as therapeutic tools within music therapy. Ann N Y Acad Sci. 2013;1303:84–6. PMID: 23944968. http://www.ncbi.nlm.nih.gov/pubmed/23944968
135. López-González M, Limb CJ. Musical creativity and the brain. Cerebrum 2012;2012:2. PMCID: PMC3574774. http://www.ncbi.nlm.nih.gov/pubmed/23447788
136. Keeler JR, Roth EA, Neuser BL, Spitsbergen JM, Waters DJM, Vianney JM. The neurochemistry and social flow of singing: bonding and oxytocin. Front Hum Neurosci 2015;9:518. PMCID: PMC4585277. http://www.ncbi.nlm.nih.gov/pubmed/26441614
137. Hildebrandt H, Nübling M, Candia V. Increment of fatigue, depression, and stage fright during the first year of high-level education in music students. Med Probl Perform Art 2012;27(1):43–48. PMID: 22543322. http://www.ncbi.nlm.nih.gov/pubmed/22543322
138. Standard Error (SE) Definition: Standard Deviation in Statistics Explained

22 Prescribed Interventions to Reduce Depression

Franklin Sunzeri

Introduction

In addition to pharmacotherapies and psychotherapies, other interventions can reduce the impact of depression. These include touch, exercise, light therapy, electromagnetic stimulation, and virtual reality.

Touch and Depression

Babies reach spontaneously for a hug. Parents cuddle their babies. Lovers hold hands, snuggle, and caress. Nurses touch their patients to ease their pain. Tired workers pay for massages. When relationships fall apart, loving touch is a casualty. When we are dying, human touch connects us to humanity [1]. Interpersonal touch is a powerful force in human interactions. See Fig. 22.1.

Touch is the first sense we develop. It is vital for acquiring information and manipulating our environment [2, 3]. Sensorimotor experiences in early life may create the platform upon which conceptual knowledge is built [4, 5]. Mental activity is based upon a physical substrate, wherein sensory and motor processing are necessary cognitive components [6]. Sensory and effector capabilities facilitate learning, communicating, and developing social bonds [7].

Candace Pert, the discoverer of the opioid receptor and former NIMH's section chief for brain biochemistry, has an interesting take on the *limbic system as the central control of emotions* [8]. She says that the limbic system has perhaps 40 times more neuropeptide receptors than other parts of the brain. Many of these emotion-related peptides can dynamically and quickly regulate blood flow to various areas of the brain and the rest of the body. She believes that blocking emotions can deprive blood flow to vital areas such as the frontal cortex. Touch modulates the limbic system.

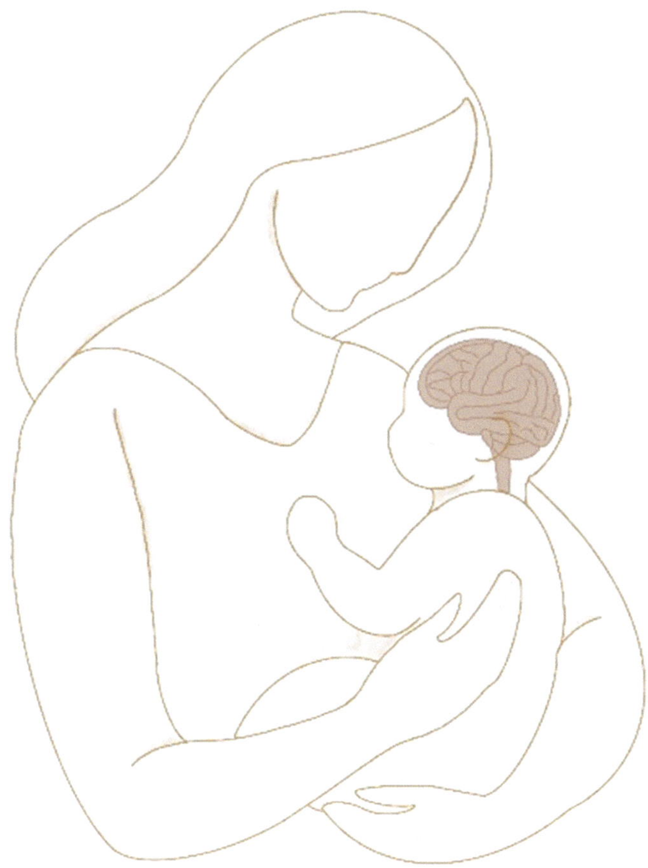

Fig. 22.1 Early maternal bonding and infant brain development. This illustration depicts a mother cradling her infant, emphasizing the intimate caregiving environment that supports neurodevelopment during early life. The infant's brain is shown undergoing rapid growth, reflecting the impact of warmth, attachment, and sensory stimulation on neural connectivity and cognitive maturation

She says, "Work that is both somatic and emotional fosters self-healing by giving patients access to the limbic system" [8, p. 193]. "In the case of treating mood disorders and other mental unwellness, the mainstream misses a lot by excluding touch, by ignoring the fact that the body really is a gateway to the mind, and by refusing to acknowledge the

F. Sunzeri (✉)
Heather Hills Consulting, Coos Bay, OR, USA

J. Raber et al. (eds.), *Understanding and Treating Depressive Disorders*, https://doi.org/10.1007/978-3-032-14465-2_22

importance of emotional release as a mind-body event with the potential to supplement or even sometimes replace talk cures and prescription pills" [8, p. 274]. "Your body is your unconscious mind, and you can't heal it by talk alone" [8, p. 306].

Research has identified the critical nature of touch in physiological and psychological regulation, development and maintenance of infants, children, and adults [9–15].

Emotional and physical health is strongly influenced by interpersonal touch [16–18]. Tactile sensations even when not accompanied by visual input can convey anger, fear, disgust, love, gratitude, happiness, sadness, and sympathy [19, 20]. However, one study suggests that there is a male or female bias in these perceptions [21]. For anger, at least one member of the communication dyad must be male. For sympathy, at least one member of the dyad must be female. For happiness, both members of the dyad must be female.

Bonding between infants and caregivers is more dependent upon physical touch than it is on feeding and can powerfully affect a person's relational style throughout life [22–28]. It has been said that abused, neglected, or touch-deprived children learn not to trust touch and have difficulty in forming reciprocally supportive adult relationships [22].

Deprivation of touch in infancy has been associated with failure to thrive [29, 30]. During the 1920s, death rates for institutionalized infants less than 1 year of age who did not receive adequate touch varied between 30% and 100% [31]. In addition, it is reported that in Bellevue Hospital in New York in the 1930s, the infant mortality rate dropped from 30% to 10% when increased touch was instituted [22].

Effects of skin-to-skin contact between mothers and preterm infants seem to benefit breast-feeding outcomes, cardiorespiratory stability, and decrease infant crying [32]. It appears that maternal bonding required for human infant survival is very important in regulating development in offspring [33]. Neurochemical systems such as oxytocin and vasopressin that regulate social behavior such as mothering are heavily influenced by nurturing received during infancy [33]. The quantity and quality of maternal care during infancy is associated with social competence as adults, ability to handle stress, aggression, and addictive behavior [33].

A social neurobiology hypothesis suggests that dysfunctional early life may result in a decrement in the capacity for rewarding interpersonal relationships and social bonding. When unconstrained by desire not to violate trusting relationships, other rewards such as drugs, sex, gangs, intimidation, and aggression may be more attractive.

There is some evidence that the more aggressive adolescents had received less physical affection, and more physical abuse from their parents and peers as preschoolers, and, as a result, they may have compensated by engaging in more self-stimulating behaviors [33, 34]. Higher levels of depression, use of illicit drugs, inferior academic performance, higher levels of anger and aggression have been seen in these adolescents independent of socioeconomic advantage.

Violent individuals appear to have an under aroused CNS with right EEG hypoactivation and lower norepinephrine, serotonin, and cortisol, and elevated dopamine and testosterone [33].

Massage therapy has been seen to decrease the aggressive behavior of violent adolescents and increase their empathy possibly by reducing their dopamine levels and increasing their serotonin levels [34].

It has been observed that when humans and other animals feel distressed or pain, they increase and intensify their activity, sometimes reaching levels where they inflicted self-injury [35]. Humans frequently become hyperactive and lack focus. Stress-related activity ranges from self-stimulation to binge eating [36], alcohol drinking [37], drug use, affiliation, and hyperactivity that depend upon the intensity of the stress, the situation, gender, and age [29, 38–41]. Intensity levels appear to vary with the severity of the stressful situation. At least in non-human animals, overeating, over drinking, and agitation are said to occur at lower levels, while higher levels provoke aggression or self-mutilation [42–45].

Moderating or calming influences on individuals that feel stressed or threatened can be brought to bear by physical closeness to loved ones or some types of stimulation [46–49]. For example, the almost immediate calming effect of vertical rocking at 60 cycles per second is more effective than an oral pacifier is for calming stressed babies [50]. Bowlby suggests that this is an evolutionary adaptation to the normal walking speed of primate mothers. He also suggests that loss of attachment figures and familiar environment can be some of the most stressful causes, and reunion and returning to familiar environments can be powerful in ending distress.

Self-esteem appears to modulate the experience of touch as it relates to existential concerns [51]. Four studies compared the reactions of people with low self-esteem to those with high self-esteem. In individuals with low self-esteem, a brief touch by a female decreased anxiety and more social connectedness after a death reminder. Reminders of death increased desire for touch. Holding a teddy bear instead of a cardboard box produced less defensive ethnocentrism. Touch had no effect on those who had high self-esteem.

Culture

Video recordings have shown differences between contact cultures of Italy and Greece, and the non-contact cultures of England, Scotland, Ireland, and Netherlands in terms of interpersonal distance, body orientation, and touch [13, 14, 52–55].

Montagu [13, 14] developed a continuum of tactility. People who derive their ethnicity from Mediterranean, Latin, and Third World stock tend to engage in touch that is more frequent. Those people from the Germanic or Anglo-Saxon ancestry tend to be the lowest in touch. Americans are slightly more inclined to touch. Scandinavians are in the middle.

Jourad counted the number of times that people from diverse cultures touched one another in casual conversations [54]. In London, it was 0; in the USA, it was 2; in Paris, it was 110; and in Puerto Rico, it was 180 times in 1 h.

Gender Related

A study of 67 women ages 20 through 37 found that positive physical couple interaction can reduce HPA and psychosocial stress [56]. Before exposure to the Trier Social Stress Test, the participants were divided into three groups to receive 10 min either of no partner interaction, verbal social support, or physical contact (standardized neck and shoulder massage).

The women who received positive physical contact showed significantly lower cortisol and heart rate responses to stress, but no different plasma oxytocin levels compared to the other two groups. There was no discernible reduced stress response to verbal social support.

In premenopausal women, more frequent hugs from partners and higher oxytocin levels have been associated with decreased blood pressure and heart rate [57]. A study evaluated self-reported frequency of partner hugs, plasma oxytocin, and blood pressure in 59 premenopausal women before and after warm contact with their husbands/partners ending with hugs. More frequent hugs seemed to partially mediate lower blood pressure and were associated with a higher baseline oxytocin level and lower heart rate ($P < 0.05$). Oxytocin levels during stress after contact were not related to hugs or blood pressure. Menstrual cycle phase had no effect on oxytocin levels.

For men and women, greater partner support is associated with higher oxytocin levels [46]. Influence of higher oxytocin on sympathetic nervous system activity (lower systolic blood pressure) and decreased norepinephrine may be more pronounced for women than for men [46].

A 4-week warm touch enhancement intervention for married couples aged 20–39 years of age enhanced oxytocin levels and reduced alpha amylase for both husbands and wives relative to controls [58]. Husbands achieved significantly lower 24-h systolic blood pressure than the control group.

A functional magnetic resonance imaging (fMRI) study has shown that the somatosensory cortices encode and are modulated by the visually perceived sex of the other person's caress [59]. In that study, heterosexual males believed that they were being caressed by either a man or a woman, when in fact the caress was delivered only by a female who was blind to the condition type.

Analysis showed that bus drivers who were touched accepted monetary requests more favorably but only when made by a female [60].

In a sample ($n = 95$) of mixed gender, 15 min of moderate-pressure massage of the upper back was shown to increase oxytocin and decrease adrenocorticotropic hormone (ACTH), nitric oxide (NO), and beta-endorphin (BE) [61].

Interpersonal closeness can increase salivary progesterone in females [62]. In addition, progesterone increase in a cohort of female college students was correlated with a willingness to sacrifice for the partner.

Affective and evaluative effects of interpersonal touch provide a valence that may modulate the subsequent sensory-affective processing of reward [63, 64]. An fMRI study of romantic partners found that anticipatory neural processes of active romantic caress are influenced by the intensity of the desire for affective contact based upon passionate feelings for the other [64]. Independent of the sensory-affective properties of the performed touch, right posterior insula activity anticipating a romantic caress significantly changed with the intensity of desire for union with the lover. This insular cluster communicated with areas related to sensory motor functions and processing and anticipation of reward.

It appears that touch between intimate partners creates a sense of strengthened bonds that enhances affect and well-being [65]. Partners completed an e-diary four times per day for 1 week. Touch enhanced intimacy and affect in both partners. Those participants who were touched more often during that study week described better psychological health 6 months after the study ended.

Amygdala

In healthy individuals, the amygdala is activated upon close personal proximity [66–69]. The amygdala in its role in social cognition and emotion (e.g., social approach and avoidance [70]) may be required for triggering emotional reactions to violations of personal space [71] and to regulate interpersonal distance in human beings [66, 72]. Apparently, when the amygdala is damaged, it may decrease the discomfort of what might otherwise have been a violation of personal space [73–75]. Of course, situational context, personal familiarity, and other factors probably mediated by the prefrontal cortex modify personal space.

Oxytocin

Physical touch appears to increase cooperation and sustain social bonds. Oxytocin facilitates social bonding, and it may be released by touch. Oxytocin is synthesized in the brain and many other places in the body including the heart, thymus, reproductive organs, and the gastrointestinal tract (reviewed in [76]). The oxytocin receptor system is even more widespread and changes during development and in response to external and internal cues in a complex sensitive biobehavioral system [77]. Salience, reward, and threats produce differential reactions in oxytocin pathways, including the HPA axis and the hypothalamic–pituitary–gonadal axis.

Oxytocin is also released by warmth, sound, taste, odors, and psychological triggers [78]. It may be involved in switching behavior from finding and eating food to reproducing [79]. Oxytocin is strongly anorexigenic, reducing duration of eating and food intake [23518828]. It may also selectively suppress sugar intake by inhibiting the reward pathway [80].

During the first 6 post-partum months, mother's and father's oxytocin levels are related to the amount of affectionate parenting behaviors [81]. For mom's, these include vocalizations, the expression of positive affect, and affectionate touch. Father's oxytocin levels are associated with degree of stimulatory parenting behaviors, such as proprioceptive contact, tactile stimulation, and object presentation. Another study that monitored oxytocin levels in mothers and fathers who interacted for 15 min of play and contact with their 4- to 6-month-old infants showed oxytocin increases only in those parents who engaged in high levels of affectionate contact [82].

In addition to stimulating positive social interactions, oxytocin can have anxiolytic and anti-stress effects including reducing cortisol, pain, and blood pressure [83–85]. Through its influence on other transmitter systems, it can promote healing and growth [85]. Oxytocin and arginine vasopressin are evolutionarily highly conserved mediators involved in regulating complex social cognition and behavior [86]. It has been suggested that positive social interaction involving touch, and types of psychotherapy that transfer support and empathy, may activate this system and its effects [85].

Childhood physical, sexual, and emotional abuses, as well as physical and emotional neglect, are known risk factors for onset of stress-related disorders such as depression and anxiety [86–89]. However, resilience of vulnerability factors seems to be in play because not all who had been abused develop mental disorders. It has been proposed that genetic and neurological factors that function in processing stress may be key resiliency and vulnerability factors [90]. One of those factors may be oxytocin.

Oxytocin is involved in trust, empathy, generosity, and emotional bonding between parents and infants, and it can reduce anxiety in stressful conditions [91–93].

Several factors mediate maternal transmission of depression to their offspring. One of the genetic factors appears to be oxytocin receptor gene (OXTR) polymorphism (rs53576) [94]. A community sample showed that youngsters with an A allele of OXTR who also had a history of maternal depression showed the highest levels of depressive symptoms at age 15. Another study of 90 men ages 18–56 showed that lower oxytocin levels were significantly associated with higher levels of early life stress ($P < 0.01$), and with depressive symptoms and trait anxiety (both $P < 0.05$) [95]. OXTR rs53576 has been associated with decreased trust, empathy, optimism, and social support seeking, components of coping with stressors [96].

Studies have shown that people differ in basal oxytocin levels and in oxytocin and oxytocin receptor gene polymorphisms. These polymorphisms are reflected in areas of the brain that process stress and emotions (hypothalamus, amygdala, and cingulate gyrus) [97].

There has not been much evidence to support any direct associations between OXTR gene polymorphisms and depressive disorders [98–100]. But, there is some evidence for associations between OXTR SNPs and personality or cognitive emotional characteristics that carry vulnerability for stress-related disorders [101–107].

Differential susceptibility to early life stressors in symptoms of depression and anxiety may be conferred by some OXTR SNPs [108]. In community samples, OXTR gene polymorphisms interacted with stressful life experiences in predicting levels of anxiety or depression [94, 108, 109]. In Caucasian adolescent females, OXTR SNP rs2254298 interacted with adverse parental environment to predict depression and anxiety symptoms [94]. OXTR SNP (rs53576) moderated associations between depression in adolescents and their early childhood exposure to maternal depression [94, 109].

As measured by the interpersonal perception task, social perception abilities and the rs2268498 polymorphism of the OXTR-gene are associated with social functioning ability [110]. T-allele carriers exhibit better performance in measures of social processing.

Three OXTR SNPs (rs2254298, rs53576, rs2268498) were examined in individuals from *the Netherlands Study of Depression and Anxiety* for possible interactions with childhood maltreatment in the development of clinically diagnosed depression and anxiety disorders [90]. They found these three OXTR gene SNPs did not interact with childhood maltreatment in predicting lifetime depression and anxiety diagnoses or sensitivity. Nevertheless, childhood maltreatment was highly associated with both lifetime depression and anxiety diagnoses, as well as with depression and anxiety sensitivity.

Associations between maternal depression, and mother and infant oxytocin receptor gene (OXTR_rs53576) polymorphisms [111]. GG in comparison with AG/AA mothers had higher depression scores. And for mothers of GG in comparison to AG/AA infants, infants', but not mothers', OXTR genotype predicted maternal depression scores. Their results suggest that GG infants have an enhanced capacity for processing both positive and negative socially meaningful contextual information, first amplifying and then differentially perpetuating negative affectivity in mothers who show depressive characteristics.

A 2019 study examined the interrelations of stressful life events, depression severity, and methylation of the promoter region of oxytocin (OXT) in 146 in-patients suffering from MDD [112]. They found significant negative associations of stressful life events with mean methylation and methylation status of single CpG sites in the OXT promotor. There was no association between depression severity and OXT methylation. However, women showed higher methylation rates than men, possibly indicating that OXT is less activated in females compared to males. This underscores the importance of sex as a factor when analyzing relationships of stress with depression.

Purposeful Touch

Tactile-Kinesthetic Stimulation may improve physical and behavioral development of low-birth-weight neonates [113–115] and premature infants [115]. However, a meta-analysis published in 2007 found that overall evidence of massage benefits for neonates is weak [114]. Nevertheless, since that time, other studies have shown positive results [113, 116]. For example, a 2010 RCT of massage therapy for preterm infants showed an association with higher NK cytotoxicity and more daily weight gain [117].

Deprivation of touch in infancy has also been associated with antisocial behavior and aggression in adults [34].

In recognition of the absence of tactile communication in technology-mediated remote communications (e.g., text-based messaging and Skype), attempts have been made to add physical contact to gain the benefits of interpersonal touch [118–122]. Two of these attempts are represented in the *Hug Shirt* [123] and *Tap Tap* that can record and playback human touch [124].

Human skin-to-skin interpersonal touch should not be confused with therapeutic touch [125]. *Therapeutic touch* is an alternative method of attempting to heal wounds. Practitioners place themselves in a meditative state, move their hands above a patient's body trying to sense, and correct a patient's "life energy" [126]. There is no scientific evidence that this energy exists. Meta-analyses have found high risk of bias in clinical trials [127]. Guidelines have been developed to improve reporting of biofield therapies such as therapeutic touch, healing touch, Reiki, and External Qigong [128].

Massage Therapy

Massage therapy is a way of manipulating by pressure and traction the soft tissues of the body. There are dozens of types of massage therapy [129, 130].

Effects of massage therapy were reviewed for their stress-relieving effects (decreased cortisol) and activating effects (increased serotonin and dopamine) in a number of different medical conditions and stressors [131]. The studies that were reviewed included depression, breast cancer, HIV infections, chronic fatigue, asthma, and pain, and stressors such as employment, aging, and pregnancy. Significant decreases in cortisol in either saliva or urine averaged 31%. Significant increases in serotonin averaged 28%, and for dopamine, it was 31%.

Massage may also reduce diastolic blood pressure, anxiety, and cortisol [132, 133]. In women who have been physically or sexually abused, massage therapy may be able to reduce depression, anxiety, and cortisol and reduce touch aversion [134].

Massage therapy has been reported to decrease depression, anxiety, cortisol and increase dopamine and serotonin levels in bulimic adolescent girls [135]. Massage therapy has decreased anxiety, depression, and stress hormones in children with PTSD who survived Hurricane Andrew [136]. Massage therapy has been reported to decrease aggression and hyperactivity [34, 137, 138], anxiety [139, 140], and depression [131, 139, 140].

However, a 2008 published systematic review that evaluated four RCTs for the effectiveness of multiple sessions of classical European (Swedish) message for treating depression found that there is a lack of evidence that massage is effective treatment of depression [141].

On the other hand, a 2010 meta-analysis that included data through 2008 of 17 moderate quality studies containing 786 persons found positive effect of massage therapy on depressed people [142]. The pooled standardized mean difference in fixed- and random-effects models was 0.76 (95% CI, 0.61–0.91) and 0.73 (95% CI, 0.52–0.93) for each of two independent reviewers. They found possible heterogeneity (tau (2) = 0.06, Cochran chi-squared (16) = 25.77, $P = 0.06$). They believe that standardized protocols and depression rating scales would make it easier to interpret results.

A comprehensive quantitative review of massage therapy on cortisol levels published in 2010 found that massage therapies' effects on cortisol are generally very small and, in most cases, not statistically different from zero [143]. They conclude that massage therapies well-established and statistically larger beneficial effects on anxiety, depression, and pain are due to other mechanisms. Interestingly, a multiple dose effect in children (based on only three studies and susceptible to file-drawer effect) showed a statistically significant larger effect ($d = 0.052$). The file-drawer effect is the practice of filing away or not publishing negative results or nonconfirmatory results.

An RCT that treated 68 persons with generalized anxiety disorder (GAD) with therapeutic massage, thermotherapy, or relaxing room therapy found equal improvements in GAD, depressive symptoms, worry, and disability [144].

Critical Illness

Interpersonal touch can be a powerful tool for caregivers of the critically ill. Results of 11 intervention studies indicated significant effects of nurse's interpersonal touch in included lowering systolic and diastolic blood pressure and respiratory rate, improving sleep, and decreasing pain [145]. Plasma cortisol and immune cell responses were variable. The amount of pressure, the body site, duration, and timing all produced different effects. Density of autonomic innervation of the body area being touched and the number of sessions make a difference. Light touch appeared to produce a sympathetic response while moderate pressure might produce a parasympathetic response. In those who are not critically ill, increases were seen in urinary dopamine and serotonin, natural killer cell cytotoxic activity, and salivary chromogranin.

A month of massage for gay men *infected with HIV* increased NK cell number, cytotoxicity, soluble CD8, and the cytotoxic CD8 cells [146]. However, no changes were seen in HIV disease progression markers (CD4, CD4/CD8 ratio, β-2 microglobulin, neopterin). Significant decreases in cortisol and anxiety were also seen. Increased relaxation was significantly correlated with increased NK cell number.

Pain

A systematic review and meta-analysis of RCTs up to June 2013 for massage therapy and *fibromyalgia* revealed that ≥5 weeks of massage therapy had significantly beneficial immediate effects on improving pain, anxiety, and depression [147].

It appears that some type of touch in conscious humans inhibits nociceptive transmission of heat stimulation into reflexive autonomic pathways independent of sensation and cognition [148]. In a cross-over double-blinded RCT, although participants barely perceived differences in the texture of touching materials, touch with a soft elastomeric brush vs. a flat disc significantly attenuated heat-induced autonomic responses while leaving subjective pain intensity unchanged.

A systematic review and multivariate meta-analysis of physical and mental health benefits of touch was published in 2024 [149]. There was small but significant study bias but results were suggestive. In newborns, they found that touch was particularly effective for regulating cortisol levels and increasing weight and parental touch was more beneficial than by a health care professional. For adults, touch intervention was effective for reducing pain, depression feelings, and state or trait anxiety. They found no difference in benefits if touch was applied by a health care provider or a familiar person. People with mental health concerns seemed to benefit from touch more than healthy individuals.

Cancer

In patients with advanced cancer, both massage and controls achieved significant immediate improvement in pain and mood [150]. Six 30-min massage or simple-touch sessions over 2 weeks were delivered to 380 adults who had advanced cancer and moderate-to-severe pain: 90% were enrolled in hospice. Massage was superior to controls for immediate pain and mood (mean difference, 0.90 and 0.61 points, respectively; $P < 0.001$). However, over time there was no between-group differences in sustained pain, worst pain, quality of life, symptom distress, or analgesic medications use. The effects of simple touch and attention cannot be excluded from these results.

A meta-analysis of massage therapy for supportive care of breast cancer up to December 2012 found that there are few rigorous trials, but that massage therapy does appear to provide useful support for symptomatic relief [151]. However, the risk of bias was considerable and meta-analyses failed to show favorable effects. One large RCT did show significant improvement in physical comfort [152].

Multimedia instruction in touch and massage may help family caregivers to provide comfort to cancer patients at home [153]. The RCT compared reading vs. massage for 4 weeks during which the intervention was practiced three times per week. Significant reduction in symptom severity and perceived stress, and improved quality of life and caregiver attitudes were seen in both interventions. Symptom severity and stress decreased 12–28% for the reading group and 29–44% for the massage intervention.

In a large study, a single session of massage was able to reduce symptom levels between 21% and 52% [154]. Massage and simple touch can both affect immediate and significant improvement in mood and pain in advanced cancer patients [150].

An uncontrolled, preliminary evaluation of healing by gentle touch in patients with cancer demonstrated statistically significant improvements in quality-of-life stress, relaxation, severe pain/discomfort, and depression/anxiety, especially in those who had the most severe baseline symptoms [155, 156]. Another uncontrolled study of gentle touch for self-reported impairments of psychological wellbeing or mental health reported decreased stress, anxiety, and depression scores and increased relaxation and ability to cope scores (all $P < 0.0004$) [157].

Cancer treatment centers, hospices, and other palliative care programs frequently use touch for comforting patients [158, 159].

Massaging cancer patients have shown significant improvements for the patients in perceived stress [160–162], in common symptoms of depression, anxiety, pain, sleeplessness, nausea, and fatigue [152, 163–166], and in quality of life [167–169].

For 5 weeks, women with breast cancer received massage therapy, practiced progressive muscle relaxation (PMR) for 30-min sessions three times a week, or received standard treatment [170]. Only the massage group reported being less depressed and less angry and feeling more vigorous. In addition, the massage group demonstrated increased dopamine levels, NK cells, and lymphocytes.

However, for many patients, the cost of massage and lack of insurance coverage make it difficult to obtain regular messages [157]. Family members and friends who want to improve the well-being of the patient can be trained to provide active hands-on therapy [171]. In addition, the self-efficacy and empowerment for the caregivers can also decrease their own distress [172, 173] and enhance the quality of their relationship with the patient [174, 175].

Gentle Touch

The touch that is described as "Gentle Touch is not derived from the techniques of Reiki, Therapeutic Touch or Massage. It is a light touch, with no greater pressure than one would exert in soothing a child's brow or laying a hand on a forehead to test temperature" [157, 176, 177]. Treatments are usually about 40 min during which informal conversation takes place regarding the health and well-being of the client and reports of any changes in the physical, mental, emotional, and spiritual conditions since the last session. Patients may talk, drowse, or sleep as they wish during the session, which ends with a 10-min rest.

Effectiveness and safety of healing by four sessions of gentle touch was seen in people who reported difficulties in their mental health [157]. Reductions were seen in stress, anxiety, and depression scores, as well as increases in relaxation and ability to cope scores (all p's < 0.0004). The greatest improvements were seen in those who originally had the most severe symptoms.

Two weeks of either Yakson (a type of massage therapy) or gentle human touch left preterm infants with a gestational age of less than or equal to 34 weeks in a more relaxed state [178]. However, Yakson touch aroused about half of the infants whereas the gentle human touch had no arousal effect.

Touch in Psychotherapy

Touch in psychotherapy by psychotherapists has been reviewed in the following publications [179–183]. Touch in psychotherapy is any physical contact between a patient and a psychotherapist [179].

Topics of special interest to touch include ethical considerations, historical and contemporary attitudes and practices of psychotherapists, cultural and individual client's perception of touch, context, types of touch, paradigms, and rationales for use.

An especially comprehensive review of touch in psychotherapy has been provided by Zur and Normarken in 2021 [179, 183, 184]. In addition, they offer an online CME course entitled Touch in Psychotherapy II: Advanced Standard of Care, Ethical and Clinical Explorations [183]. Among the topics of consideration are the impacts of touch and lack of touch on health, how physical touch has been used by therapists with their patients in traditional verbal psychotherapy and recommendations about the use of touch in today's therapy setting.

Bonitz in 2008 gives an excellent historical account of attitudes about touch and a very readable current review with practical suggestions for clinicians to consider in their practice [183].

A complex interrelationship of theoretical rationales, cultural and religious taboos, ethical and legal considerations has made this a controversial topic [179]. A diversity of literature supports its uses, benefits, effectiveness, and rationales, as well as prohibitions, contraindications, and cautions of using touch [181].

Powerful healing effects of touch in psychotherapy have been reported [31, 179, 185, 186]. A combination of physical contact between a psychotherapist and a patient in psychotherapy can significantly create a feeling of empathy, sympathy, comfort, calmness, comfort, and safety for the patient [31, 179]. Touch can increase the sense of being heard and acknowledged and can enhance the therapeutic alliance [52, 187, 188].

Touch can trigger a cascade of biochemical responses that may result in increased serotonin and dopamine levels and decreased urinary stress hormones (cortisol, catecholamines, norepinephrine, epinephrine) [11, 12, 189]. Although hugging may provide stress buffering support and modify susceptibility to upper respiratory infections and illness [190], direct effect of touch on immune responses is lacking. For example, a search of the literature up to 2025 did not find research on possible immune system boost that may be provided by increasing natural killer cells and killer cell activity or balancing the ratio of T4 cells and T8 cells.

Despite the significant use of touch in human interactions, Freud and other psychoanalysts believed that touch was an impediment to analysis and cure of neuroses [191]. Since that time, there has been a general suspicion of using touch in psychotherapy [31, 179, 182].

Later humanistic approaches believed that the taboo recreates a cold and distant environment that contributed to a client's dysfunction [191, 192]. These critics of the taboo say that it ignores the value of touch in therapy and the creation of a more open and intimate relationship between client and therapist [193, 194]. Touch as an adjunct to verbal psychotherapy [179] includes Reichian [195], Hakomi [196], Bioenergetics [196], and Somatic [197]. Formalized use of touch in psychotherapy includes Gestalt therapy [192], humanistic therapies [198], group therapies [199], and some child, family, feminist, dance, and movement therapies [187, 200].

Nevertheless, the potential for harm is real. These include sexual exploitation [201–204] reenactment of traumatic events [31], confusion, and imposition of societal power dynamics [203, 205, 206]. Sonne and Jochaie in 2014 provide a relevant review of romantic and sexual feelings, thoughts, and behaviors in psychotherapy [180].

There is, however, agreement in the very well-considered guidelines that Zur, Normarken, and Bonitz present. We highly recommend reading these guidelines [179, 182–184].

A bottom line as Zur sees it is:

> The meaning of touch can only be understood within the context of who the client is, the therapeutic relationship, and the therapeutic setting. Accordingly, before employing touch, it is essential that the clinician considers unique treatment elements for each client including factors, such as culture, history, presenting problem, diagnosis, gender, history, etc. One must also consider the therapists' education, training, theoretical orientations, and comfort with non-sexual touch. Systematic touch should be employed in therapy only when it is well thought out and is likely to have positive clinical effects.

Professional Caregivers

Since the advent of scientifically based medical practice touch has been a part of treatment [187].

A deeper inter-subjective clinical relationship that reaffirms a patient's dignity and worth can be achieved by empathetic touch as opposed to instrumental or philanthropic touch [207]. Dehumanization is a risk when we are ill, leaving us with feelings of isolation, powerlessness, and confusion that can be made worse by admission to a hospital [208]. Touch can be a bridge across the emotional and physical gap for physicians to demonstrate empathy and acknowledge suffering [208, 209]. Touch, of course, is part of physiotherapy, osteopathy, chiropractic, and acupressure and may be providing an added dimension to the healing process reinforcing patient trust and compliance or adding a placebo effect [210].

Perhaps, absence of touch is more common and problematic than objectifying touch [66, 80, 208–212]. Many health practitioners avoid the use of more personalized touch. There are several reasons why this may be true. Not the least of which is litigiousness [208]. Certainly, touch can also be misunderstood by the recipient or be perceived as inappropriate or invasive and so have a negative valence.

An observational sample conducted between January and March 2010 at a three-partner GP clinic in Britain found that 75% of males (56/75) and 83% of females (100/120) reported feeling comforted and reassured when touched by a male practitioner. In comparison, 77% of males (58/75) and 92% of females (110/120) expressed similar feelings when touched by a female practitioner [208].

There was little ethno-cultural or socioeconomic diversity in that study. The population was relatively socioeconomically deprived and ageing. Those who were uncomfortable most commonly said that they felt their personal space was invaded or they felt uncomfortable with the sex of the GP. No one gave religious, cultural, or familial beliefs as reasons for discomfort.

Most patients felt most comfortable with a more proximal position on the arm and secondarily with the back. More females than males felt being touched on the back was appropriate. The rest of the patients felt that the only place that was appropriate to be touched was on the hand or the arm.

A qualitative study has examined the perception of personal boundaries of physicians with respect to touch and spiritual care [213]. Some physicians never touched or explored spiritual care; others engaged in both. Still others varied their boundaries irrespective of their own beliefs when they believed that it was in the best interests of their patients.

Touch for physicians is either part of a procedure or expressive (i.e., unrelated to a procedure or examination) [212]. A qualitative study in urban and semi-rural areas of north-west England revealed that all patients and most physicians viewed expressive touch as an important part of communication. General practitioners were more comfortable with touching older folks, or those who were bereaved and who were the same sex as themselves. All the general practitioners were apprehensive that their touch could be misinterpreted, especially when a patient was distressed. Most of the patients believed that expressive touch was acceptable especially in times of distress. All the patients felt that touching the forearm or hand was appropriate.

Treatment of Sleep Disturbances

Treatment of sleep disturbances associated with depression includes CBT, pharmacotherapy, and manipulation of sleep–wake rhythms via light therapy, chronotherapy, cycles of sleep [214], and even sleep deprivation [215].

The impact of CPAP therapy on depression among obstructive sleep apnea patients is not clear: results are often conflicting [216, 217].

The *2016 Agency for Healthcare Research and Quality (AHRQ)* has written a comprehensive assessment of the efficacy, comparative effectiveness, and harms of treatments for insomnia disorder in the general adult population and older adults [218]. It would seem that CBT has the strongest evidence for treating various sleep disorders with the least amount of side effects.

If underlying disorders have been addressed, sleep experts generally recommend six ways to enhance sleep.

1. Keep to a regular sleep schedule.
2. Set the stage for sleep by performing a regular bedtime routine (e.g., teeth brushing, setting the alarm).
3. Make a bedroom environment that promotes sleep. For example, dark, quiet or mask disturbing noise, and cool. Do not use the bedroom for activities other than sleeping and sex.
4. Enjoy regular exercise, but not in the late evening before going to bed, as at that time it can stimulate the cardiovascular and nervous systems.
5. Use relaxation techniques such as reading, visual imagery, and warm baths.
6. Avoid taking stimulants and diuretics especially near bedtime.

A novel treatment for MDD is *therapeutic sleep deprivation* [214–222]. It has been claimed that within hours, sleep deprivation (SD) can dramatically decrease depression symptoms in 50–60% of patients with MDD [222]. The effects are transient, and the mood returns to baseline within 24 h [222]. It is hypothesized that by homeostatically enhancing cortical synaptic strength, SD shifts the initially deficient inducibility of associative synaptic long-term potentiation into a more favorable neural plastic state [223]. Proponents suggest combining SD with selective serotonin reuptake inhibitors and circadian-related interventions such as bright light and sleep phase advance would produce a powerful antidepressant effect [221, 224, 225].

A discussion of associations between hypertension and depression relative to sleep can be found in the chapter Depression and Hypertension.

There are several excellent on-line resources for sleep information for health professionals and health consumers. Among these are:

- The National Institutes of Health, National Center on Sleep Disorders Research [226]
- The Sleep Research Society [227]
- The American Academy of Sleep Medicine [228]
- Agency for Healthcare Research and Quality (AHRQ) [218]

Exercise and Depression

There is substantial interest in the relationship of exercise to mood disorders. For example, the National Library of Medicine cataloged 1400 systematic reviews from 2018 through 1/2025 on exercise and depression. These included 218 unique RCTs [229]. Contradictory results of various RCTs and some meta-analyses are common. These differences may be a result of factors such as bias, specific intervention characteristics relating to types of and duration of exercise, number of and demographics of study participants, monitoring and reporting characteristics, participant preferences for particular exercise, and comorbidities.

To present an accurate summary of the evidence on all sides of the issue, we will begin by reviewing information relative to mechanisms that might be involved with putative effects. Then we will present studies that have found varying degrees of positive effects, and that will be followed by articles that did not find these effects.

Possible Mechanisms

Therapeutic mechanisms for possible beneficial effects of physical exercise on depression are not fully worked out. It is thought that subtle variations in neuroimmune and neurobiological effects, based upon an individual's unique and shared central nervous system may be at work [45, 230, 231].

Eyre et al. argue that physical activity may benefit behavioral outcomes—such as reductions in depressive symptoms—through neurobiological mechanisms that enhance neuroplasticity, reduce oxidative stress, regulate serotonin, dopamine, and norepinephrine levels, and modulate glucocorticoid sensitivity [231].

Physical activity can increase monoamine neurotransmitter and endorphin levels in the brain [232–234]. In addition, regulation of the HPA axis [235] and reduction in oxidative stress in the hippocampus [236], increased hippocampal neuroplasticity [232, 233, 237], and increased hippocampal volume [238, 239] have been seen.

There is a wide variety of neuroimmune processes that are affected by physical activity [240, 241]. In particular, physical activity reduces pro-inflammatory cytokine levels in the brain of rodents [240] and in the periphery in humans [241, 242]. Increased levels of neuroprotective IL-6 [243], macrophage migration inhibitor factor [244], insulin-like growth factor-1[IGF-1] [245], and CX3CL1 [246] may be involved.

A 2013 comprehensive review of treating depression and depression-like behavior with physical activity found that there are beneficial neuroimmunomodulatory effects [231]. They concluded that there is evidence that physical exercise increases IL-10, IL-6 (acutely), macrophage migration inhibitory factor, central nervous system–specific autoreactive CD4+ T cells, M2 microglia, quiescent astrocytes, CX3CL1, and IGF-1. They also concluded that physical exercise appears to decrease harmful neuroimmune factors that include Th1/Th2 balance, pro-inflammatory cytokines, C-reactive protein, M1 microglia, and reactive astrocytes.

A meta-analysis examined evidence for the effect of exercise on resting concentrations of peripheral BDNF in MDD [247]. They did not find evidence that a chronic aerobic exercise intervention increases resting concentrations of BDNF in the blood of MDD patients, but there were not a lot of studies.

Stimulation-induced behavioral inhibition by sensory feedback is a process in which stress-induced behavior is part of a negative feedback system that modulates physiological arousal induced by a stressful stimulus [248, 249]. For example, physical activity is generally considered to be effective in reducing fear [250]. Aerobic exercise may reduce depression, anxiety, hostility, hunger, drug-seeking behavior, heart rate, and blood pressure [137, 251].

Although the human brain shrinks as we age, it is capable of significant plasticity even late in life [252]. One of the links to less cortical atrophy, better brain function, and enhanced cognitive function is physical activity [252, 253]. Effects of physical activity in the brain are widespread with prefrontal and hippocampal areas being the most neuroplastic. This effect may be one of the ways in which physical activity can influence neurocognitive disorders like depression and aging [254]. Brain-derived neurotrophic factor (BDNF), acting at the interface of metabolism and neuroplasticity, may be a critical component in this connection [255].

Increasing human cardiovascular fitness can improve attentional networks, processing speed, and executive functions in the brain when challenged with cognitive tasks [256–258]. Regular aerobic exercise can increase brain activation, synaptic connections [257], neurogenesis [259], and capillary supplies [238] potentially improving biological and cognitive fitness throughout our maturation and aging [258, 260, 261]. In particular, increased brain volumes in the hippocampus [237, 239] and frontal and parietal lobes can be seen [261, 262].

Neuropeptide Y (NPY) has been implicated in depression, emotional processing, and the stress response across both human and rat studies [263, 264]. One of the functional single-nucleotide polymorphisms (SNPs) that control *NPY*'s transcription has been shown to influence emotional processing [265, 266] and is affected by difficulties in early development [267]. Experiments in rats have indicated that a functional NPY SNP that may contribute depression-like characteristics can be epigenetically reprogrammed by physical exercise [268].

A 2018 systematic review and meta-analysis found that physical exercise promotes reduced cortisol levels in individuals with MDD [269]. Type of exercise, weekly frequency, and type of cortisol measurement influenced the results.

Acute and chronic biological responses to exercise in people with MDD were systematically reviewed in 2016 [270]. There were few studies and definite limitations that made it hard for them to draw definite conclusions. However, a single session of exercise increased atrial natriuretic peptide (ANP), brain natriuretic peptide (BNP), copepetin, and growth hormone among people with MDD. There were some indications that long-term adaptations of copeptin, thiobarbituric acid reactive species (TBARS), and total mean frequency (TMF) were promoted. Some evidence suggested that exercise promotes adaptations on neurogenesis, inflammation biomarkers, and brain structure. Improvement of depression symptoms was associated with hippocampal volume and IL-1β.

Regular physical activity, especially aerobic exercise, may not only decrease risks of age-related cognitive decline [271, 272], but also enhance recovery from strokes [273, 274], and decrease progression of Parkinson's [275–277] and Alzheimer's diseases [278–280].

Alterations in glucocorticoids, adipose-derived hormones, insulin, and inflammatory signaling that are typical of central obesity may be directly or indirectly implicated in the increased incidence of depression in obesity [281, 282]. In addition, depressed mood increases the risk of complications of obesity [283].

A narrative review of psychological and neurophysiological theories of exercise effects on mood and the central role of neuroplasticity in integrating these two theories is presented in previous work [284].

A review published in 2011 assesses the most effective methods of physical training for specific psychiatric symptoms [285].

In 2011, *The College of Sports Medicine (ACSM)* revised their Position Stand, "*The Recommended Quantity and Quality of Exercise for Developing and Maintaining Cardiorespiratory and Muscular Fitness, and Flexibility in Healthy Adults*" [286]. Exercises are designed to consider individual abilities and limitations and can include aerobics, resistance, neuromotor, and flexibility types. In the clinical environment, physical activity interventions have been defined as "planned, structured, and repetitive bodily movements done to improve or maintain one or more components of physical fitness" [286].[1]

Influence of exercise on epigenetics has been reviewed in reference [287]. Exerkines and epigenetics in depression related to exercise is reviewed in previous works [288–290].

Positive Effects

Physical activity may be a preventive or an early intervention treatment option in depression [231, 291]. For example, physical activity has been suggested to afford a level of prevention against MDD [292] and can stand alone [293] or augment other treatments for MDD [294].

In addition, physical activity is an appealing therapeutic approach for depression when one considers the added cardio-metabolic benefits [230, 232, 295, 296] on comorbid disorders such as heart disease, diabetes, and obesity [297, 298]. Among its attractions are improved cardiovascular metabolic risk factors including chronic inflammation, insulin sensitivity, glucose control, glucocorticoid sensitivity, and visceral fat that have an influence on psychological attributes of diseases [230, 232, 296, 298, 299].

Globally, physical inactivity is high and rising [299]. Estimates published in 2012 found that physical inactivity causes 6% of the burden of disease from coronary heart disease, 7% of type 2 diabetes, 10% of breast cancer, 10% of colon cancer, and 9% of premature mortality [300]. There is evidence suggesting an association of inactivity with depression [231, 292, 301].

Physical activity can improve self-esteem, has few adverse side effects, and can be adapted to individual needs and constraints [232, 286, 302]. In contrast, pharmacotherapy for depression has many side-effects and has a high failure rate [303, 304]. There is less stigma attached to physical exercise than there is for either antidepressants or psychotherapies for treatment of major depression [305, 306].

There is evidence that physical activity is clinically effective in treating major depressive disorder [302], anxiety disorders [307], impaired cognitive function [232, 233, 308, 309], and schizophrenia [310].

Comprehensive reviews on various aspects of physical activity effects on depression can be found in the works of HA Eyre [231, 310] and in the systematic review and network analysis of 2024 that is [229].

In a 2012 meta-analysis of participants 60 years of age and older, physical activity was significantly associated with lower severity of depression (SMD =[2] −0.34; 95% CI: −0.52 to −0.17) [311].

Several studies have found that for those with Alzheimer's disease, regular, moderate physical exercise can improve depression [231, 305]. These effects seem to be duration dependent [311]. One study found that the effects became significant only after 1 year of physical activity [312].

Exercise may be better than sertraline on improving executive functions but not working or verbal memory in sedentary adults 40 years of age and older who are suffering with MDD [313]. A 2010 meta-analysis showed that aerobic exercise can modestly improve attention and processing speed ($g = 0.158$; 95% CI: 0.055–0.260; $P = 0.003$), executive function ($g = 0.123$; 95% CI: 0.021–0.225; $P = 0.018$), and memory ($g = 0.128$; 95% CI: 0.015–0.241; $P = 0.026$) [256]. The meta-analyses covered RCTs where the mean age was greater than or equal to 18 years and duration of treatment >1 month, incorporated aerobic exercise components, supervised exercise training, and the presence of a non-aerobic-exercise control group.

The effect of exercise on depression severity in older people was assessed in a 2012 systematic review and meta-analysis of RCTs [314]. They found that older people with clinically meaningful symptoms of depression, who are prescribed structured exercise tailored to individual ability, will achieve decreased depression severity.

Several cardiovascular symptoms are accompanied by depression. For example, MDD affects 15–20% of patients with coronary heart disease (CHD) and elevated symptoms of depression without MDD can be found in an additional 20% of people with CHD [315]. It has been reported that up to 40% of patients with heart failure are depressed and up to 75% report elevated symptoms of depression [316].

Effects of exercise training on depressive symptoms in patients with chronic heart failure: the *HF-ACTION* randomized trial were presented in 2012 [316]. This multicenter RCT included 2322 stable patients treated for heart failure in the USA, Canada, and France who engaged in an aerobic exercise program under supervision for 1–3 months followed

[1] The ACSM recommends that most adults engage in moderate-intensity cardiorespiratory exercise training for ≥30 min·d on ≥5 d·wk for a total of ≥150 min·wk, vigorous-intensity cardiorespiratory exercise training for ≥20 min·d on ≥3 d·wk (≥75 min·wk), or a combination of moderate- and vigorous-intensity exercise to achieve a total energy expenditure of ≥500–1000 MET·min·wk.

On 2–3 d·wk, adults should also perform resistance exercises for each of the major muscle groups, and neuromotor exercise involving balance, agility, and coordination.

Crucial to maintaining joint range of movement, completing a series of flexibility exercises for each the major muscle-tendon groups (a total of 60 s per exercise) on ≥2 d·wk is recommended. [286]

[2] *Standardized mean difference (SMD)* is a measure of effect size in meta analyses when the studies all assess the same outcome but measure it in a variety of ways [2]. In systematic reviews, the SMD is the mean difference in depression score between the intervention and control groups divided by the pooled SD at follow-up. This gives a unit-free effect size. The conventional SMD effects sizes of 0.2 (small), 0.5 (medium), and 0.8 (large) are used. Dichotomous variables are usually expressed as risk ratio with a 95% CI. For more information, see Chap. 4.

up by exercising at home for 9 months, or education and usual heart failure care. During a median 30-month follow-up, 68% died or were hospitalized in the usual care group compared with 66% in the aerobic exercise group (HR = 0.89; 95% CI: 0.81–0.99; P = 0.03). Aerobic exercise achieved lower mean Beck Depression Inventory II scores at 3 months (difference, −0.76; 95% CI: −1.22 to −0.29; P = 0.002) and at 12 months (difference, −0.68; 95% CI: −1.20 to −0.16; P = 0.01).

Exercise and pharmacological treatment of depressive symptoms in patients with coronary heart disease were compared in the *UPBEAT (Understanding the Prognostic Benefits of Exercise and Antidepressant Therapy)* study [315]. Participants received 4 months of either aerobic exercise (3 times/week), sertraline (50–200 mg/day), or placebo. Depressive symptoms were equally reduced by exercise and sertraline (P = 0.607). Heart rate variability (a biomeasure of cardiac health) was improved by both, but exercise produced greater improvements in heart rate variability compared with sertraline (P = 0.093).

An RCT on the impact of moderate-intensity continuous aerobic exercise (MICAE) on the depression status of middle-aged patients with congestive heart failure found that 12 weeks of MICAE has positive effects on the depression status in patients with CHF [317].

There are several ways that exercise may produce a positive psychosocial effect. These include improved self-efficacy (a strong predictor of behavioral persistence) [318–320], self-esteem [306, 321], distraction from rumination and negative thoughts [231], and stress resiliency enhancement [306, 322]. Self-esteem and subjective well-being are strongly associated with good mental health [323, 324]. In addition, the social interaction provided by group exercise can decrease the stress of social isolation [302].

Indeed, in the population-based *MONICA/KORA* study, a synergistic effect of social isolation and depressed mood on inflammatory responses was seen in men but not in depressed women [325].

A 2012 systematic review and meta-analysis of RCTs was conducted on the effect of exercise training on depressive symptoms among patients with a chronic illness [326]. Exercise reduced depressive symptoms among patients with chronic illnesses. Those who had mild-to-moderate depression and gained improved functions had the largest antidepressant effects. A 2012 meta-analysis of 28 clinical trials showed a moderate clinical effect on MDD of physical activity compared with controls or no treatment [302]. This same meta-analysis found that physical activity had an initial treatment effect equal to antidepressants. Other studies have indicated that physical activity effects on MDD are slower [327] but had less tendency to relapse [328].

A 2016 meta-analysis adjusting for publication bias evaluated exercise as a treatment for depression [329]. Overall, they found that exercise had a large and statistically significant effect on depression (standardized mean difference [adjusted for publication bias] = 1.11; 95% CI: 0.79–1.43), with a fail-safe number of 1057. Most adjusted analyses suggested publication bias led to an underestimated SMD. For MDD, larger effects were found for use of aerobic exercise, at moderate and vigorous intensities, in a supervised and unsupervised format. Larger effects were also seen on MDD for moderate intensity, aerobic exercise, and interventions supervised by exercise professionals. They concluded that exercise has a large and significant antidepressant effect. They also suggested that previous meta-analyses may have underestimated the benefits of exercise due to publication bias. They strongly believe that exercise is an evidence-based treatment for depression.

A 2016 systematic review and meta-analysis of RCTs for treating depression with physical activity in adolescents and young adults made some tentative conclusions [330]. They suggested that the best current evidence is for supervised, aerobic-based activity of moderate-to-vigorous intensity, engaged in multiple times per week over 8 or more weeks may be the best.

A systematic review was published in 2018 on the effect of exercise versus CBT or no intervention on anxiety, depression, fitness, and quality of life in adults with previous methamphetamine dependency [331]. There was Level II evidence suggesting that exercise is effective in reducing anxiety and depression and improving fitness in previous methamphetamine users, and Level III-2 evidence that exercise is beneficial for improving quality of life in this group. Exercise was significantly better than CBT in improving depression and anxiety scores (P = 0.001). Balance, vital capacity, hand grip, and one-leg stands with eyes closed also significantly improved.

A systematic review and meta-analysis was published in 2019 of aerobic exercise for adult patients with MDD in mental health services [332]. They found large or moderate to large antidepressant effects (g = −0.79, 95% CI: −1.01 to −0.57, P < 0.00) for aerobic exercise (I^2 – ≤30%) among trials with lower risk of bias, trials with short-term interventions (up to 4 weeks), and trials involving individual preferences for exercise. They saw comparable effects for aerobic exercise across various settings and delivery formats, and in both outpatients and inpatients independent of symptom severity. Aerobic exercise was delivered on average for 45 min, at moderate intensity, three times/week, for 9.2 weeks. There were not very many trials, but there was no evidence of publication bias and low and non-statistically significant heterogeneity.

A systematic review and network meta-analysis of RCTs of comparative effectiveness of three exercise types to treat clinical depression in older adults was published in 2019

[333]. Compared with controls, mind-body exercise showed the largest improvement on depressive symptoms ($g = -0.87$ to -1.38), followed by aerobic exercise ($g = -0.51$ to -1.02), and resistance exercise ($g = -0.41$ to -0.92). No statistically significant differences were seen between exercise types or mind-body versus resistance. Encouragement of self-selection of type of exercise will likely result in higher levels of compliance [333].

A systematic review and meta-analysis of mind-body exercise for anxiety and depression in COPD patients was published in 2019 [334]. *Mind-body exercise was tai chi, health qigong, and yoga*. Significant benefits were seen in anxiety (SMD = −0.76, 95% CI: −0.91 to −0.60, $P = 0.04$, $I^2 = 47.4\%$) and depression (SMD = −0.86, 95% CI: −1.14 to −0.58, $P = 0.000$, $I^2 = 71.4\%$). Results indicated that for anxiety 30- to 60-min exercise sessions for 24 weeks of health qigong or yoga significantly benefited patients who had COPD who were more than 70 years old and had COPD for more than 10 years. For depression, two to three times a week, 30–60 min at a time of health qigong had a significant effect on patients with COPD patients who were more than 70 years old and had COPD less than 10 years.

Mindfulness-based Baduanjin exercise for depression and anxiety in people with physical or mental illnesses was examined in a systematic review and meta-analysis [335]. Baduanjin (also known as Eight Section Brocade) is a traditional Chinese mind-body exercise routine [336]. Like Tai Chi it uses slow, coordinative, sequential movements, but it is not as complex as Tai-Chi [337–339]. Significant benefits were seen of Baduanjin on anxiety (Hedges' $g = -0.99$; CI: −1.63 to −0.74) and depression (Hedges' $g = -1.07$; CI: −1.3 to −0.83). Meta-regression indicated a significant effect for total hours in Baduanjin practice ($\beta = -0.0053$; 95% CI: −0.009 to −0.0014; $P = 0.008$). And for depression, there was a significant effect for total sessions of Baduanjin practice ($\beta = -0.0023$; 95% CI: −0.006 to −0.0004; $P = 0.028$). There were, however, limitations in interpretation as there was a high risk of bias; Baduanjin combined with other behavioral interventions; and heterogeneity of control groups.

The *meditative movements* of *tai chi*, *qigong*, and *yoga* are safe and easily accessible. They are said to be the most popular complementary approaches for alleviating musculoskeletal pain, improving sleep quality, and reducing blood pressure [340]. A 2019 systematic review and meta-analysis was conducted on the effects of meditative movements on MDD [340]. Meta-analysis on 15 fair-to-high quality RCTs showed a significant benefit in favor of meditative movement on depression severity (SMD = −0.56, 95% CI: −0.76 to −0.37, $P < 0.001$, $I^2 = 35.76\%$) and on anxiety severity (SMD = −0.46, 95% CI: −0.71 to −0.21, $P < 0.001$, $I^2 = 1.17\%$). Meditative movement interventions showed significantly improved treatment remission rate (OR[3] = 6.7; 95% CI: 2.38–18.86, $P < 0.001$) and response rate (OR = 5.2; 95% CI: 1.73–15.59, $P < 0.001$) over passive controls.

There is some evidence that physical activity and yoga interventions during the perinatal period can be feasible, safe, acceptable, and effective in reducing depression in women [341].

One interesting type of exercise that has shown interesting results in treating depression is *bouldering* [342–344]. Bouldering is a type of climbing where a climber tries to master short but difficult climbing routes that are most often less than 12–15 feet high. Short term and longer term (at least 12 months) positive results have been documented [342, 344, 345]. It appears that reduction in depression symptoms may be independent of antidepressant medication, psychotherapy, and general level of physical activity [345].

A systematic review and meta-analysis suggests that physical activity during pregnancy appears to reduce the risk of post-partum depression [346]. However, significant heterogeneity in physical activity assessment was present, suggesting moderators that include intensity, frequency, and trimester of pregnancy or type of physical activity practiced. A systematic review and meta-analysis found that prenatal exercise reduced the odds and severity of prenatal depression [347]. However, prenatal exercise did not alter the odds of postpartum depression or the severity of depressive symptoms, nor anxiety or anxiety symptoms during or following pregnancy.

Some studies have suggested that general physical activity and antenatal aerobic exercise is associated with fewer depression symptoms during pregnancy [348–350]. Some studies did not find an association [351]. Exercise might be helpful in reducing post-partum depression [352–355].

A 2002 study analyzed effects of higher levels of physical activity on prevalent and incident depression with and without exclusion of disabled subjects in participants aged 50–94 years [356]. After adjusting for age, sex, ethnicity, financial strain, chronic conditions, disability, body mass index, alcohol consumption, smoking, and social relations, greater physical activity was protective for both prevalent depression (adjusted OR = 0.90; 95% CI: 0.79–1.01) and

[3]Odds ratio (OR) is a way to represent the odds that an outcome will result when a given exposure to a variable of interest occurs compared to when the exposure does not occur. OR quantifies the strength of the association between two events. An OR greater than 1 indicates a positive association or that exposure to that variable increases the odds of that outcome. An OR less than one indicates a negative relationship between two events. An OR of 1 suggests no relationship between two events. An OR is frequently accompanied by a 95% confidence interval (CI). CI is a measure of precision of the OR. The smaller the CI the higher precision as long as it does not overlap OR = 1. For more information, see the Chap. 4 on evidence basics in this text.

incident depression (adjusted OR = 0.83; 95% CI: 0.73–0.96) over 5 years.

A 2019 systematic review was published on the effects of exercise intensity, duration, and modality relative to therapeutic benefits of physical activity on mood [284]. Moderate-intensity anaerobic exercise was associated with greater mood improvements. There was a non-linear relationship between duration and mood: 10–30 min of exercise was sufficient to improve moods. Anaerobic exercise improved mood, but there was not enough information to judge the efficacy of aerobic and mindfulness-related exercises.

An RCT that consisted of a 12-week, home-based moderate exercise program of 30–45 min/day of walks, 5 days/week, improved depression, and functioning in treatment-resistant MDD patients and contributed to remission of 26% of these patients [357].

A 2024 systematic review and network meta-analysis of RCTs on the effects of exercise on depression found 218 unique RCTs [229]. They concluded that exercise is a moderately effective treatment for depression, with walking or jogging, yoga, and strength training more effective than other exercises, especially when they are intense. The effect was equal regardless of comorbidity and baseline depression levels. Strength training and yoga were particularly well tolerated. They also noted that seemed to have acceptably low risk of bias; however, only one study met the Cochrane criteria for low risk of bias. So, confidence in accordance with *CINeMA*[4] was low for walking or jogging and very low for other treatments.

Not So Positive Effects

Not all studies have found a positive effect of physical activity on depression [302]. It has been suggested that this lack of association may be due to inappropriate intensity or duration of physical activity [302]. Many researchers now suggest that in addition to tailoring the activity to the individual patient's functional status and other co-morbidities, activity should be moderately intense and last at least 8-weeks before assessment [294, 302, 359].

In the 2013 Cochrane meta-analysis to determine the effectiveness of exercise in the treatment of depression, six trials that compared physical exercise to cognitive behavioral therapy (CBT) found that the effect of exercise was not significantly different from CBT [302]. According to Cochrane meta-analysis in 2014, exercise is moderately more effective than control intervention in reducing depression symptoms [360]. Compared to pharmacological or psychological therapies, there was no evidence that exercise was more effective.

A 2018 systematic review of interventional studies for the influence of exercise on cognitive symptoms in depression found that overall, there was no impact of physical exercise on MDD [361]. Nevertheless, they did find that interventions that combined physical and cognitive activities had a positive impact on global cognition ($P = 0.048$). They stressed that there is a deficiency of high-quality data.

Treadmill exercise in rodents can reverse chronic unpredictable mild stress (CUMS) depression model-induced alteration of dendritic spines in the brain regions involved in mood [362].

A meta-analysis of RCTs for exercise in older adults found that adjusting for publication bias increased the beneficial effects of exercise [363].

A 2017 systematic review of cognitive effects of exercise in depression did not observe a substantial benefit of physical exercise on cognitive symptoms in depression [364].

A 2001 meta-analysis of exercise in managing depression concluded that there were not enough high-quality studies to reach a meaningful conclusion although there were suggestions that results might in the short term be equivalent to CBT [365].

A 2012 pragmatic RCT to evaluate the cost-effectiveness of a physical activity intervention as a treatment for depression [366]. The treating depression with physical activity (TREAD) trial was designed to encourage choice and autonomy in the adoption of physical activity. It consisted of up to three face-to-face and ten telephone contacts delivered by a trained physical activity facilitator over an 8-month period. Results showed that it was very unlikely to lead to any clinical benefit in depressive symptoms or cost-effectiveness. They suggested that the negative results may have been due to the increase in activity was not large enough to lead to a measurable influence; more vigorous activity might be beneficial; and previous studies that had shown positive results had recruited individuals with a pre-existing commitment to physical activity.

A 2011 systematic review and meta-analysis of RCTs on the effect of exercise in clinically depressed adults found little evidence of a long-term beneficial effect of exercise in patients with clinical depression [367].

A 2017 systematic review with meta-analysis and trial sequential analysis assessed the benefits and harms of exercise in patients with depression [368]. They included only participants diagnosed with depression according to a validated diagnostic system and they included only RCTS where patients had somatic comorbidity (e.g., cancer or diabetes).

[4] When evaluating confidence in the results from network meta-analyses when multiple interventions are compared, it is good practice to use *Confidence in Network Meta-Analysis (CINeMA)* [358]. CINeMA evaluates six domains: (i) within-study bias, (ii) reporting bias, (iii) indirectness, (iv) imprecision, (v) heterogeneity, and (vi) incoherence.

Based upon 35 RCTs and almost 2500 people, the effect of exercise versus control on depression severity was −0.66 standardized mean difference (SMD) (95%CI: −0.86 to −0.46; $P < 0.0010$). However, grading of recommendations assessment, development, and evaluation (GRADE) was *very low quality*. They found effect estimates were largely based on trials at high risk of bias and considerable heterogeneity. Considering the GRADE, they concluded, "trials with less risk of bias suggested no antidepressant effects of exercise and there were no significant effects of exercise on quality of life, depression severity or lack of remission during follow-up. Data for serious adverse events and adverse events were scarce not allowing conclusions for these outcomes."

A Perspective

A common problem with many of the reviews is that the population being assessed was not diagnosed by either DSM or ICD criteria [368]. Frequently, they were assessed based upon psychometric testing scales such as the HAM-D or the BDI.

The group who produced the tour de force 2018 systematic review with meta-analysis and trial sequential analysis of exercise for patients with major depression [369][5] have several recommendations for further study [368]. They are:

> Despite the large number of published trials, further trials with more robust methodology seem still required to establish progress in this field. Also, additional trials from outside North America and Europe may be required for results to be valid for patients in Asia, Africa and South America. To further elaborate on the current findings, we recommend that future trials must include blinded outcome assessors and outcomes assessing quality of life, metabolic effects, and long-term effects beyond the intervention. It is also important that future trials systematically collect and report data on death, suicide events, musculoskeletal injuries, and other potential adverse effects both in the intervention group and in the control group. Future trials ought to be designed according to the standard protocol items: recommendations for interventional trials (SPIRIT) guidelines and reported according to the consolidated standards for reporting of trials (CONSORT) guidelines and transparently report deidentified individual participant data enabling individual participant data meta-analyses.

[5]The Genome-wide association analyses identified 44 independent and significant risk variants and refined the genetic architecture of major depression [368]. They found important relationships of genetic risk for major depression with educational attainment, body mass, and schizophrenia: lower educational attainment and higher body mass were putatively causal; and major depression and schizophrenia reflected a partly shared biological etiology.

A Different Approach Noninvasive Neuromodulation Therapies

Noninvasive neuromodulation therapies involve transcranial application of electrical or magnetic stimulation to modulate cortical and subcortical brain activity [370–372]. An early noninvasive neuromodulation technique that was used for treating depression was electroconvulsive therapy [373, 374].

Between 1940 and 1980, treatment of depression centered on pharmaceuticals and psychotherapy [375]. Many patients with MDD get no benefit from either or are treatment resistant [304, 376–378]. As a response to this need, there has been a considerable increase in noninvasive neuromodulation therapies [379].

Noninvasive neuromodulation therapies can be classified relative to their spatial resolution (focal and nonfocal) and intensity (subthreshold, subconvulsive, and convulsive) [379]. Electroconvulsive therapy (ECT) and magnetic seizure therapy (MST) are convulsive. ECT is nonfocal, and MST is relatively focal. Transcranial magnetic stimulation (TMS), also known as repetitive transcranial magnetic stimulation (rTMS), is subconvulsive and relatively focal which depends on the coil type (dTMS, deep transcranial magnetic stimulation; sTMS, synchronized transcranial magnetic stimulation). Transcranial direct current stimulation (tDCS) is subthreshold and can be focal or nonfocal, depending on the electrode configuration (HD-tDCS, high-definition transcranial direct current stimulation).[6]

Transcranial magnetic stimulation (TMS) [380–382] and transcranial direct current stimulation (tDCS) [383, 384] seem to be promising treatments for MDD.

As of 2020 only ECT and TMS have FDA approval for treating depression [385, 386]. MST and tDCS are rated as investigational. ECT, vagus nerve stimulation, rTMS, and tDCS have been used as augmentations in depression, especially for treatment-resistant cases. Several TMS units have received FDA 510k clearance for use in treatment resistant MDD [387].

In 2013, a review of TMS and tDCS association with biological markers was conducted [380]. Positive associations with treatment were seen with functional magnetic resonance imaging, single-photon emission computed tomography, positron emission tomography, magnetic resonance spectroscopy, cortical excitability, and brain-derived neurotrophic factor (BDNF). BDNF was the best predictor of the probability of patients with MDD to respond to TMS or

[6]A 2019 review of clinical effects, neurocognitive effects, and possible mechanisms of action of noninvasive neuromodulation therapies, including ECT, transcranial magnetic stimulation, magnetic seizure therapy, and transcranial direct current stimulation are found in [379].

TDCS. However, confounders (e.g., sex, age, and family history), heterogeneous samples, and small sample sizes hampered the validation.

Repetitive Transcranial Magnetic Stimulation (rTMS)

In TMS, an electric coil that generates magnetic fields is held above the region of the brain that is the target [388]. The rapidly changing magnetic fields causes a depolarization of neurons which may either result in excitement or inhibition of brain activity. TMS is believed to work by directly or trans-synaptically exciting the pyramidal tract axons of neurons. Cortical excitability changes, long-term effects of rTMS, are thought to occur from induction of cortical plasticity via protein synthesis [389]. Processes similar to long-term potentiation and long-term depression may be the molecular mechanisms behind these long-term changes induced by TMS [390].

There are two types of TMS: repetitive TMS (rTMS) and single-pulse TMS [391]. Repetitive TMS is the only one that is used to produce a change that lasts longer than the impulse. A new TMS is synchronized TMS (sTMS) which is synchronized to alpha waves [392].

The FDA in 2018 approved theta-burst stimulation (TBS) for MDD [393–395]. TBS mimics the brain's endogenous theta rhythms, which may enhance synaptic long-term potentiation [396].

Besides depression, TMS has been used for treating a variety of CNS disturbances such as migraines [397], strokes [398], and schizophrenia [399].

Adverse effects of TMS are not common. They include fainting, seizures, short-term discomfort, pain, brief episodes of hypomania, cognitive change, hearing loss, and working memory difficulties [400, 401]. TMS is capable of interfering with cardiac pacemakers.

Convincing placebos are challenging to implement in RCTs of TMS [400, 402–404]. Blinding is quite difficult to achieve [405].

A 2019 systematic review of RCTs of rTMS in depression evaluated completeness of descriptions of rTMS as used in the interventions [406]. They found that rTMS interventions delivered in RCTs are incompletely reported, thereby preventing their evidence-based implementation in clinical practice. The researchers provide an adapted-to-rTMS *TIDieR* checklist that could help in reporting future trials. TMS generally targets the anterior cingulate cortex, the anterior limb of the capsula interna, the nucleus accumbens, and the medial forebrain bundle.

A systematic review and meta-analysis of rTMS for treatment-resistant depression found that rTMS for MDD patients with two or more antidepressant treatment failures is a reasonable, effective consideration [407].

A 2017 review of rTMS for adolescents with treatment-resistant depression found only ten multi-subject trials, all uncontrolled, and five case reports that met inclusion criteria [408]. Ten of the studies indicated that there might be some benefit. Most studies indicated that improvement took 2–8 weeks, and some long-term benefits might occur. Adverse events occurred included scalp pain, which was the most common, and seizures.

A systematic review and multiple-treatment meta-analysis compared efficacy and acceptability of electroconvulsive therapy (ECT) versus rTMS for MDD [409]. ECT was the most efficacious, but least tolerated. Right prefrontal -rTMS was the best tolerated treatment. Bilateral -rTMS seemed to be the best balance between efficacy and acceptability.

A 2018 systematic review and meta-analysis was conducted on placebo response to rTMS for depression trials [410]. Placebo response was large and associated with depression improvement of the active treatment group. Placebo response may be a component of therapeutic response to rTMS in MDD, and if placebo response increases over time, this may make for a better sham rTMS as a placebo.

A 2019 systematic review and meta-analysis of the efficacy and tolerability of *deep transcranial magnetic stimulation (dTMS)* for treatment-resistant depression concluded that dTMS is a safe and effective intervention in patients with treatment resistant depression [411]. Studies combining dTMS and antidepressant seemed to produce the best results.

A 2016 systematic review evaluated the effectiveness of rTMS in improving depression resulting from cerebrovascular disease including vascular depression and post-stroke depression [412]. Short-term rTMS appeared to be effective. But there were few studies, prominent heterogeneity of populations and variability in study design and protocol that made drawing conclusions difficult.

A 2019 systematic review and meta-analysis of rTMS for anxiety and trauma-related disorders found an overall treatment effect for both PTSD (ES = −0.88, 95% CI: −1.42 to −0.34) and GAD (ES = −2.06, 95% CI: −2.64 to −1.48) [413].

A 2019 review states that rTMS has been found to be safe and effective in pregnant patients and elderly patients, whereas use of either pharmacotherapy or ECT is challenging because of possible risk of adverse reactions.

A 2019 systematic review of the safety and effectiveness of rTMS in the treatment of peripartum depression found that most of data comes from sources with inherently higher risk of bias [414]. With that caveat, rTMS in the peripartum period appears to be efficacious, acceptable, and well tolerated.

A systematic review of the efficacy of rTMS in decreasing postnatal depression symptoms found that there are few reports, a lack of complete datasets and a serious/high risk of bias of the studies makes conclusions questionable [415].

A 2019 systematic review and network meta-analysis compared effectivity and acceptability of non-surgical brain stimulation for the acute treatment of MDD episodes in adults [416]. They concluded that non-surgical brain stimulation techniques are suitable as alternative or add-on treatments for adults with acute MDD. A 2016 systematic review and meta-analysis examined the antidepressant efficacy of rTMS in patients with treatment-resistant unipolar depression found that electroconvulsive therapy (ECT) was more beneficial for treatment of patients who are treatment-resistant [417]. A small short-term effect was seen for rTMS improving depression in comparison with sham. The small effect was unlikely to continue for longer periods.

A 2018 systematic review and meta-analysis of randomized sham-controlled trials found that there was not sufficient published data available to draw firm conclusions about the efficacy and acceptability of TBS and rTMS [418].

A systematic evaluation of the cognitive effects of rTMS on depression, schizophrenia, and Alzheimer's disease showed that prefrontal rTMS could have some pro-cognitive effects on executive function and attention in some patients with depression [419]. However, they found inconsistent effects in some cognitive domains especially in patients with schizophrenia and Alzheimer's disease.

Although rTMS is now widely available for the clinical treatment of depression, time and money considerations make it unappealing for many people [420]. *Accelerated TMS (aTMS)* may be able to increase the efficiency of rTMS. Meta-analysis suggested that aTMS may improve depressive symptom severity.

A 2019 systematic review and meta-analysis of the durability of antidepressant response to rTMS found sustained responder rates of 50% up to 1 year after a successful induction course of treatment [421]. A systematic review of potential predictors of depressive relapse following repetitive TMS found very few studies, and considerable inconsistency exists between studies [422]. So, only limited conclusions were able to be drawn.

A systematic review and meta-analysis of placebo-controlled clinical trials reviewed the safety, tolerability, and nocebo phenomena during TMS [423]. Active treatment vs. placebo showed estimated estimate of at least one episode of adverse reactions to be 29.3% (95% CI: 19.0–22.6%) and 13.6% (95% CI: 11.6–15.8%), respectively. The percentage of dropouts due to adverse events was 2.5% (95% CI: 1.9–3.2%) and 2.7% (95% CI: 2.0–3.5%), respectively. Odds for experiencing adverse events were 2.6 times higher in active treatment. HF-rTMS appears to be effective for post-stroke depression, but safety is a question [424].

Daily left prefrontal rTMS for MDD in a sham-controlled randomized trial showed remission was 4.2 times more likely with active rTMS than with sham (95% CI: 1.32–13.24) [425]. The NNT was 12. Low antidepressant treatment resistance characterized most of those who remitted.

In 2009, clinical predictors were analyzed in the outcome in a multisite, industry-sponsored RCT of daily left prefrontal rTMS in the acute treatment of MDD [426]. Degree of prior treatment resistance in the current episode predicted positive treatment outcome in both the controlled study and the open-label extension trial. In the RCT, shorter duration of current episode was also associated with a better outcome. In the open-label extension study, absence of anxiety disorder comorbidity was associated with better outcome, but duration of current episode was not associated. The number of prior treatment failures was the best predictor of a positive response to TMS.

Transcranial Direct Current Stimulation (tDCS)

Transcranial direct current stimulation (tDCS)[7] uses low direct current conducted to targeted areas of the brain via electrodes on the scalp [428–430]. At the anode, the current causes depolarization of the resting membrane potential of neurons nearby exciting them. At the cathode, hyperpolarization occurs, and the nearby neurons are inhibited. The intensity and duration of the stimulation determines the degree and duration of the effects. The effects can persist after the stimulation is removed [431]. So, it seems that tDCS promotes short and possibly long-term potentiation and short and possibly long-term depression [429, 432].

Improved mood in depressed patients takes several weeks of repeated treatments and there appears to be no mood effects in healthy subjects [433]. There is some evidence that neuroplastic changes occur especially in the serotonin system [434–437]. However, there does not appear to be any lasting cognitive benefits independent of mood effects [438].

In the EU, tDCS is approved for the treatment of pain and depression [427], However, in the USA, the FDA regulates tDCS as investigational which means that the FDA has not issued an opinion on it. Physicians can prescribe tDCS as an off-label treatment. The tDCS devices are easily available for personal and home use, but manufacturers cannot make any claims for their usefulness. Relative to other noninvasive neuromodulation antidepressant techniques tDCS costs less, is more portable, and may be safer [439, 440].

RCTs of tDCS have reported mixed results in diminishing depression symptoms [441]. A few RCTs have reported significant improvement [434, 442–445]. Others have not found positive effects compared to sham controls [446–449]. A

[7] Video presentations about tDCS can be found at [427].

single-center trial did not show noninferiority to escitalopram over a 10-week period and was associated with more adverse events [444]. Escitalopram and tDCS were both superior to placebo. Noninferiority of tDCS versus escitalopram was defined by a lower boundary of the confidence interval for the difference in the decreased score that was at least 50% of the difference in the scores with placebo versus escitalopram. Some newer techniques with tDCS may be better but the evidence still needs to be confirmed [450–453].

Electroconvulsive Therapy

Electroconvulsive therapy (ECT), formerly called electroshock therapy, uses electrical stimuli under general anesthesia to induce a therapeutic tonic-clonic convulsive seizure [454, 455]. ECT has been used for MDD, bipolar disorder, schizophrenia, and schizoaffective disorders.

In 2015, the FDA Office of Device Management proposed new rules for reclassifying ECT devices.

> Neurological Devices; Reclassification of Electroconvulsive Therapy Devices Intended for Use in Treating Severe Major Depressive Episode in Patients 18 Years of Age and Older Who Are Treatment Resistant or Require a Rapid Response; Effective Date of Requirement for Premarket Approval for Electroconvulsive Therapy for Certain Specified Intended Uses. [456, 457]

Limitations, indications, and warnings to be given to prospective patients and families are addressed. Among the salient points are reclassifying ECT devices into less restrictive category II for treating, "severe major depressive episode (MDE) associated with major depressive disorder (MDD) or bipolar disorder (BPD) in patients 18 years of age or older who are treatment-resistant or who require a rapid response due to the severity of their psychiatric or medical condition." For patients who are diagnosed with catatonia, schizophrenia, schizophreniform disorder, schizoaffective disorder, bipolar mania, or mixed states and for patients who are younger than 18 years of age, they propose leaving ECT devices in the more restrictive category of class III. Device labeling would have "special controls" that includes, "a precaution that describes the limitations of available information on the safety and effectiveness of long-term treatment with the ECT device, also known as maintenance ECT." A discussion of the FDA and ECT can be found here [458].

A 2018 in-depth look into recent advances in ECT technique and the evidence of ECT for managing depression in special populations and patients with comorbid medical problems can be found in previous work [455].

A 2003 systematic review and meta-analysis of the efficacy and safety of ECT in depressive disorders concluded that ECT is an effective short-term treatment for depression and is probably more effective than drug therapy [459]. Real ECT was significantly more effective than simulated ECT (six trials, 256 patients, standardized effect size (SES) −0.91, 95% CI: −1.27 to −0.54). Treatment with ECT was significantly more effective than pharmacotherapy (18 trials, 1144 participants, SES −0.80, 95% CI: −1.29 to −0.29).

Because of its spatially unfocused character and nonspecificity, the brain mechanisms underlying ECT effects on depression were still not clear as of 2019 [460, 461].

Virtual Reality for Managing Depression

Virtual Reality (VR) derives from the word virtual that has been used in the realm of computers since 1959 as "not physically existing but made to appear by software" [462]. In the late 1980s, Jaron Lanier of VPL Research began to use the term virtual reality [463].

Most simply and broadly VR can be defined as an interface between humans and computers, wherein users can interact with a computer-generated virtual environment in real time creating an immersive experience in that simulated world [464–466]. Various senses can be employed to generate that immersion. Typically, 3D visual near-eye displays [467, 468] are employed; smell, sound, and vibrations can also be used [469–473]. Several senses are engaged at the same time, permitting a user to hear and feel sensations that correlate with the visual display and allow an individual to dynamically interact real time with the virtual world and experience the virtual world reactions [474].

Typical VR setups include a computer proficient in providing interactive three-dimensional visualization, a controller to interact with the animations, a position tracker, and a head-mounted display (HMD) to see the visual output, headphones, and a hand-held controller [475, 476]. Trackers monitor the positions and orientation of a user in space and relay that information to the computer for real time updates for display [477, 478]. Based upon the degree of patient immersion, VR can be classified as (1) non-immersive performed through computers or game consoles and their devices; (2) semi-immersive, large screens with devices capable of interacting with the virtual environment while perceiving the real world; and (3) immersive, where the patient is inside the virtual environment with which they interact [479].

VR has been used to treat a variety of medical conditions including but not limited to depression, anxiety, pain [480], and fatigue [481–483].

VR in mental health was originally used for treating phobias, then anxiety and PTSD [473, 484]. VR is increasingly being used in mental health treatment of a variety of disorders [485]. These include various forms of anxiety [486–488], depression [484, 489–491], stress reactions [492], and feelings of loneliness [493]. VR work has shown promise on treating addictions such as eating disorders [494] and other cue-associated exposure problems [495–497]. Some studies have examined the use of VR for autism spectrum disorders [498–500], ADHD [501, 502], and psychosis [503–505].

VR provides a controlled and consistent safe space for experiencing realistic scenarios capable of triggering responses and facilitating therapy [476, 489, 506, 507]. Users can interact and respond to simulated real-world events, and psychotherapeutic interventions can take place [505].

One example of VR based therapy is *Virtual Reality Exposure Therapy (VRET)* that has been used to help reduce symptoms of depression, PTSD, phobias, anxiety, and loneliness [484, 493, 508]. VRET lets patients experience what stresses them or what triggers reactions in a safe environment where exposure intensity can be controlled, and a therapist can escort the patient in the treatment [473]. This form of exposure therapy can often be less stressful for the patient than experiencing the stressful situations in real life [473, 509]. VRET software and VR hardware are readily available at usually affordable prices [510, 511].

One downside of VRET is symptoms of what is known as *simulator sickness or cyber-sickness* in some users [512]. Symptoms of simulator related side effects can be dizziness and headaches [513–515]. However, these symptoms may not be caused directly using VR [514, 516, 517]. For example, one study of active-duty soldiers being treated for PTSD suggests that anxiety not the VR may be to blame [518].

A 2024 *PRISMA (Preferred Reporting Items for Systematic Reviews and Meta-Analyses)* framework across electronic databases presented an overview of benefits, limitations, and prospect for VR in neurotherapy and neurorehabilitation in basic/clinical and digital neuroscience [519].

Acceptance of VR for exposure focused therapy by potential users has been evaluated by the *Technology Acceptance Model (TAM)* [520]. Five possible barriers have been identified. These are (1) patient's concerns and misconceptions about consequences of prolonged exposure therapy such as cybersickness [520]; (2) limited time or access and therapist distress in using exposure focused therapy [521]; (3) distress about exposure based therapy among both the therapist and the patient; (4) limited number of mental health professionals trained in VR techniques [522]; and (5) confidentiality, privacy and other ethical concerns, and accessibility and controllability of the stimuli [523, 524].

A 2020 Systematic Review showed that VR intervention is more effective compared with the control (i.e., standard care) for anxiety, depression, fatigue, and pain [525]. As an emotion-focused distraction intervention, VR decreases the severity of these symptoms.

Those VR interventions are a type of cognitive behavioral therapy used for ameliorating symptoms by changing symptom-related thoughts, fading those beliefs that are exacerbating symptoms, and increasing personal perceptions of control over symptoms [507, 520]. Trials have shown that *virtual reality-assisted cognitive behavioral therapy (VRCBT)* in the treatment of anxiety and depression can have specific positive effects on anxiety and depression symptoms [520, 526–531].

Meta-analyses have demonstrated that VRET interventions in clinical settings can lead to significant decreases in anxiety- and depression-related symptoms [525, 529, 532]. Children preferred game-based interventions to distract from the medical environment, whereas adults preferred a variety of natural and relaxing virtual environments to choose from [525]. *Gamification*, applying elements commonly found in game design to non-game scenarios [533], has been used to enhance engagement, motivation, and behavior change in mental health treatment [534]. It has been suggested that persuasive gamification features harness cognitive and emotional elements of feedback, competition, and social influence to adopt positive behavior and sustain engagement [535].

Home-based VR techniques bring a sense of independence and self-improvement, and they have often been perceived as fun, immersive and enjoyable without many side effects [525, 532, 536–538]. Home-based VR can be empowering and can proceed at the users own pace and convenience without the necessity of a therapist being present [539].

Summary

Overall, the interventions described in this chapter offer diverse avenues for managing depression beyond traditional treatments, highlighting the importance of a multifaceted approach to mental health care.

Touch

Throughout our lives, we may encounter touch that can be gentle or violent and can have profound effects. Research has identified the critical nature of touch in physiological and psychological regulation, development and maintenance of infants, children, and adults. Touch modulates the limbic system and as such is the gateway to the mind. The limbic system is the central controller of emotions with many more neuropeptide receptors than other parts of the brain. It can dynamically and quickly regulate blood flow to areas of the brain and the rest of the body.

Emotional and physical health is strongly influenced by interpersonal touch. It has been said that emotionally, sexually or physically abused, neglected, or touch-deprived children learn not to trust touch, and have difficulty in forming reciprocally supportive adult relationships.

Studies suggest that more aggressive adolescents frequently received less physical affection, and more physical abuse from their parents and peers as preschoolers, and, as a result, they may have compensated by engaging in more self-stimulating behaviors. Independent of socioeconomic conditions, higher levels of depression, use of illicit drugs, inferior academic performance, higher levels of anger, and aggression have been seen in these adolescents. Violent individuals appear to have an under aroused CNS with right EEG hypoactivation and lower norepinephrine, serotonin, and cortisol, and elevated dopamine and testosterone.

Some forms of touching can trigger a cascade of biochemical responses that may result in increased serotonin and dopamine levels and decreased urinary stress hormones (cortisol, catecholamines, norepinephrine, and epinephrine). An immune system boost may increase natural killer cells and killer cell activity, balancing the ratio of T4 cells and T8 cells.

Moderating or calming influences on individuals that feel stressed or threatened can be brought to bear by physical closeness to loved ones or some types of stimulation. Self-esteem appears to modulate the experience of touch as it relates to existential concerns.

People who derive their ethnicity from Mediterranean, Latin, and Third World stock tend to engage in more frequent touching. People from the Germanic or Anglo-Saxon ancestry tend to be the lowest in touch. Americans are slightly more inclined to touch. Scandinavians are in the middle.

Affective and evaluative effects of interpersonal touch may modulate subsequent sensory-affective processing of reward. Positive physical interactions between couples can reduce activation of the HPA axis and alleviate psychosocial stress. Touch between intimate partners creates a sense of strengthened bonds that enhances affect and wellbeing. Interpersonal touch can be a powerful tool for caregivers of the critically ill. Nurse's interpersonal touch may result in lowering systolic and diastolic blood pressure and respiratory rate, improving sleep, and decreasing pain in their patients.

Massage therapies statistically beneficial effects on anxiety, depression, and pain may be due to other mechanisms that are not readily apparent. Massage therapy may have significantly beneficial immediate effects on improving pain, anxiety, and depression. Massaging cancer patients have shown significant improvements for the patients in perceived stress and in common symptoms of depression, anxiety, pain, sleeplessness, nausea, and fatigue. Meta-analyses of RCTs suggest that enthusiastic supporters of these therapies may have unintentionally biased gathering of data or interpreting results.

Use of touch in psychotherapy involves ethical considerations, historical and contemporary attitudes and practices of psychotherapists, cultural and individual client's perception of touch, context, types of touch, paradigms, and rationales for use. A complex interrelationship of theoretical rationales, cultural and religious taboos, ethical and legal considerations exist. A diversity of literature supports its uses, benefits, effectiveness, and rationales, as well as prohibitions, contraindications, and cautions of using touch. Touch has the potential to supplement or even sometimes replace talk cures and prescription pills.

Powerful healing effects of touch in psychotherapy have been reported. Physical contact between a psychotherapist and a patient in psychotherapy can significantly create a feeling of empathy, sympathy, comfort, calmness, comfort, and safety for the patient. Touch can increase the sense of being heard and acknowledged and can enhance the therapeutic alliance. Context and experience is an essential element when applying systematic touch in therapy.

Sleep

Treatment of sleep disturbances associated with depression includes CBT, pharmacotherapy, and manipulation of sleep–wake rhythms via light therapy, chronotherapy, cycles of sleep, and even sleep deprivation.

Exercise

There is substantial interest in the relationship of exercise to mood disorders. For example, the National Library of Medicine cataloged 168 systematic reviews from 2018 through 2/2020 on exercise and depression. Contradictory results of various RCTs and some meta-analyses are common. These differences may be a result of factors such as bias, specific intervention characteristics relating to types of and duration of exercise, number of and demographics of study participants, monitoring and reporting characteristics, participant preferences for particular exercise, and comorbidities.

On the positive side, physical activity may be a preventive or an early intervention treatment option in depression. For example, physical activity has been suggested to afford a level of prevention against MDD and can stand alone or augment other treatments for MDD. Therapeutic mechanisms for possible beneficial effects of physical exercise on depression are not fully worked out. It is thought that subtle variations in neuroimmune and neurobiological effects, based upon an individual's unique and shared central nervous system may be at work.

In addition, physical activity is an appealing therapeutic approach for depression when one considers the added cardio-metabolic benefits on comorbid disorders such as heart disease, diabetes, and obesity. Among its attractions are improved cardiovascular metabolic risk factors including chronic inflammation, insulin sensitivity, glucose control, glucocorticoid sensitivity, and visceral fat that have an influence on psychological attributes of diseases.

Not all studies have found a positive effect of physical activity on depression. It has been suggested that this lack of association may be due to inappropriate intensity or duration of physical activity. Many researchers now suggest that in addition to tailoring the activity to the individual patient's functional status and other co-morbidities, activity should be moderately intense and last at least 8 weeks before assessment.

Cochrane meta-analysis found there was no evidence that exercise was more effective than pharmacological or psychological therapies. A 2018 systematic review of interventional studies for the influence of exercise on cognitive symptoms in depression found that overall, there was no impact of physical exercise on MDD. Nevertheless, they did find that interventions that combined physical and cognitive activities had a positive impact on global cognition. They stressed that there is a deficiency of high-quality data.

Non-invasive Neuromodulation Therapies

Non-invasive neuromodulation therapies involve transcranial application of electrical or magnetic stimulation to modulate cortical and subcortical brain activity. Non-invasive neuromodulation therapies can be classified relative to their spatial resolution (focal and nonfocal) and intensity (subthreshold, subconvulsive, and convulsive). Electroconvulsive therapy (ECT) and magnetic seizure therapy (MST) are convulsive. ECT is nonfocal, and MST is relatively focal. Transcranial magnetic stimulation (TMS), also known as repetitive transcranial magnetic stimulation (rTMS), is subconvulsive and relatively focal which depends on the coil type (dTMS, deep transcranial magnetic stimulation; sTMS, synchronized transcranial magnetic stimulation). Transcranial direct current stimulation (tDCS) is subthreshold and can be focal or nonfocal, depending on the electrode configuration (HD-tDCS, high-definition transcranial direct current stimulation).

A systematic review and network meta-analysis comparing effectivity and acceptability of non-surgical brain stimulation for the acute treatment of MDD episodes in adults concluded that non-surgical brain stimulation techniques are suitable as alternative or add-on treatments for adults with acute MDD. A 2016 systematic review and meta-analysis examining the antidepressant efficacy of rTMS in patients with treatment-resistant unipolar depression found that electroconvulsive therapy (ECT) was more beneficial for treatment of patients who are treatment-resistant.

A 2003 systematic review and meta-analysis of the efficacy and safety of ECT in depressive disorders concluded that ECT is an effective short-term treatment for depression and is probably more effective than drug therapy. Real ECT was significantly more effective than simulated ECT. Treatment with ECT was significantly more effective than pharmacotherapy.

Virtual Reality

VR interventions are a type of cognitive behavioral therapy used for ameliorating symptoms by changing symptom-related thoughts, fading those beliefs that are exacerbating symptoms, and increasing personal perceptions of control over symptoms. Trials have shown that virtual reality-assisted cognitive behavioral therapy in the treatment of anxiety and depression can have specific positive effects on anxiety and depression symptoms.

A 2020 systematic review showed that VR intervention is more effective compared with standard care for anxiety, depression, fatigue, and pain. As an emotion-focused distraction VR decreases the severity of these symptoms.

Meta-analyses have demonstrated that VRET interventions in clinical settings can lead to significant decreases in anxiety- and depression-related symptoms.

References

1. Nicholls D, Chang E, Johnson A, Edenborough M. Touch, the essence of caring for people with end-stage dementia: a mental health perspective in Namaste Care. Aging Ment Health. 2013;17(5):571–8. PMID: 23323683. http://www.ncbi.nlm.nih.gov/pubmed/23323683.
2. Gibson JJ. Observations on active touch. Psychol Rev. 1962;69:477–91. PMID: 13947730. http://www.ncbi.nlm.nih.gov/pubmed/13947730.
3. Lederman SJ, Klatzky RL. Hand movements: a window into haptic object recognition. Cogn Psychol. 1987;19(3):342–68. PMID: 3608405. http://www.ncbi.nlm.nih.gov/pubmed/3608405.
4. Mandler JM. How to build a baby: II. Conceptual primitives. Psychol Rev. 1992;99(4):587–604. PMID: 1454900. http://www.ncbi.nlm.nih.gov/pubmed/1454900.
5. Williams LE, Huang JY, Bargh JA. The scaffolded mind: higher mental processes are grounded in early experience of the physical world. Eur J Soc Psychol. 2009;39(7):1257–67. PMCID: PMC2799930. http://www.ncbi.nlm.nih.gov/pubmed/20046813.
6. Niedenthal PM, Barsalou LW, Winkielman P, Krauth-Gruber S, Ric F. Embodiment in attitudes, social perception, and emotion. Personal Soc Psychol Rev. 2005;9(3):184–211. PMID: 16083360. http://www.ncbi.nlm.nih.gov/pubmed/16083360.
7. Ackerman JM, Nocera CC, Bargh JA. Incidental haptic sensations influence social judgments and decisions. Science. 2010;328(5986):1712–5. PMCID: PMC3005631. http://www.ncbi.nlm.nih.gov/pubmed/20576894.
8. Pert C. Molecules of emotion. New York: Scribner; 1997.

9. Bowlby J. Maternal care and mental health: a report on behalf of the World Health Organization. Geneva: World Health Organization; 1952.
10. Harlow H. Learning to love. New York: Albion; 1971. https://archive.org/details/learningtolove00harlrich.
11. Field T. Touch. Cambridge, MA: MIT Press; 2003.
12. Field T. Massage therapy effects. Am Psychol. 1998;53(12):1270–81.
13. Montagu A. Touching: the human significance of the skin. New York: Columbia University Press; 1971.
14. Montagu A. Touching: the human significance of the skin. 3rd ed. New York: Harper & Row; 1986.
15. Field T, Lasko D, Mundy P, Henteleff T, Kabat S, Talpins S, Dowling M. Brief report: autistic children's attentiveness and responsivity improve after touch therapy. J Autism Dev Disord. 1997;27(3):333–8. PMID: 9229263. http://www.ncbi.nlm.nih.gov/pubmed/9229263.
16. Field T. Touch for socioemotional and physical well-being: a review. Dev Rev. 2010;30:367–83. https://psycnet.apa.org/record/2011-06430-004.
17. Gallace A, Spence C. The science of interpersonal touch: an overview. Neurosci Biobehav Rev. 2010;34(2):246–59. PMID: 18992276. http://www.ncbi.nlm.nih.gov/pubmed/18992276.
18. Cohen S. Social relationships and health. Am Psychol. 2004;59(8):676–84. PMID: 15554821. http://www.ncbi.nlm.nih.gov/pubmed/15554821.
19. Hertenstein MJ, Holmes R, McCullough M, Keltner D. The communication of emotion via touch. Emotion. 2009;9(4):566–73. PMID: 19653781. http://www.ncbi.nlm.nih.gov/pubmed/19653781.
20. Hertenstein MJ, Keltner D, App B, Bulleit BA, Jaskolka AR. Touch communicates distinct emotions. Emotion. 2006;6(3):528–33. PMID: 16938094. http://www.ncbi.nlm.nih.gov/pubmed/16938094.
21. Hertenstein MJ, Keltner D. Gender and the communication of emotion via touch. Sex Roles. 2011;64(1–2):70–80. PMCID: PMC3016097. http://www.ncbi.nlm.nih.gov/pubmed/21297854.
22. Heller S. The vital touch. New York: Henry Holt and Company; 1997.
23. Ainsworth MD. Attachments beyond infancy. Am Psychol. 1989;44(4):709–16. PMID: 2729745. http://www.ncbi.nlm.nih.gov/pubmed/2729745.
24. Vicedo M. Playing the game: psychology textbooks speak out about love. Isis. 2012;103(1):111–25. PMID: 22655342. http://www.ncbi.nlm.nih.gov/pubmed/22655342.
25. Vicedo M. The evolution of Harry Harlow: from the nature to the nurture of love. Hist Psychiatry. 2010;21(82 Pt 2):190–205. PMID: 21877372. http://www.ncbi.nlm.nih.gov/pubmed/21877372.
26. van der Horst FCP, Leroy HA, van der Veer R. "When strangers meet": John Bowlby and Harry Harlow on attachment behavior. Integr Psychol Behav Sci. 2008;42(4):370–88. PMID: 18766423. http://www.ncbi.nlm.nih.gov/pubmed/18766423.
27. Barett H. Parents and children: facts and fallacies about attachment theory. J Fam Health Care. 2006;16(1):3–4. PMID: 16550805. http://www.ncbi.nlm.nih.gov/pubmed/16550805.
28. Harlow HF, Suomi SJ. Nature of love--simplified. Am Psychol. 1970;25(2):161–8. http://www.ncbi.nlm.nih.gov/pubmed/4984312.
29. Field TM, Schanberg SM, Scafidi F, Bauer CR, Vega-Lahr N, Garcia R, Nystrom J, Kuhn CM. Tactile/kinesthetic stimulation effects on preterm neonates. Pediatrics. 1986;77(5):654–8. PMID: 3754633. http://www.ncbi.nlm.nih.gov/pubmed/3754633.
30. Ardiel EL, Rankin CH. The importance of touch in development. Paediatr Child Health. 2010;15(3):153–6. PMCID: PMC2865952. http://www.ncbi.nlm.nih.gov/pubmed/21358895.
31. Hunter M, Struve J. The ethical use of touch in psychotherapy. Thousand Oaks: Sage Publications; 1998. https://psycnet.apa.org/record/1997-36467-000.
32. Moore ER, Anderson GC, Bergman N, Dowswell T. Early skin-to-skin contact for mothers and their healthy newborn infants. Cochrane Database Syst Rev. 2012;5(5):CD003519. PMCID: PMC3979156. http://www.ncbi.nlm.nih.gov/pubmed/22592691.
33. Pedersen CA. Biological aspects of social bonding and the roots of human violence. Ann N Y Acad Sci. 2004;1036:106–27. PMID: 15817733. http://www.ncbi.nlm.nih.gov/pubmed/15817733.
34. Field T. Violence and touch deprivation in adolescents. Adolescence. 2002;37(148):735–49. PMID: 12564826. http://www.ncbi.nlm.nih.gov/pubmed/12564826.
35. Hokanson JE. The physiological bases of motivation. New York: Wiley; 1969. p. 121. https://archive.org/details/physiologicalbas0000unse_d8f0.
36. Sulkowski ML, Dempsey J, Dempsey AG. Effects of stress and coping on binge eating in female college students. Eat Behav. 2011;12(3):188–91. PMID: 21741016. http://www.ncbi.nlm.nih.gov/pubmed/21741016.
37. Casement MD, Shaw DS, Sitnick SL, Musselman SC, Forbes EE. Life stress in adolescence predicts early adult reward-related brain function and alcohol dependence. Soc Cogn Affect Neurosci. 2015;10(3):416–23. PMCID: PMC4350480. http://www.ncbi.nlm.nih.gov/pubmed/24795442.
38. Hinde RA. Animal behavior. New York: McGraw-Hill; 1966. https://openlibrary.org/books/OL5986386M/Animal_behaviour.
39. Adesso VJ. Some correlates between cigarette smoking and alcohol use. Addict Behav. 1979;4(3):269–73. PMID: 495252. http://www.ncbi.nlm.nih.gov/pubmed/495252.
40. Sinha R, Jastreboff AM. Stress as a common risk factor for obesity and addiction. Biol Psychiatry. 2013;73(9):827–35. PMCID: PMC3658316. http://www.ncbi.nlm.nih.gov/pubmed/23541000.
41. Patterson TK, Craske MG, Knowlton BJ. The effect of early-life stress on memory systems supporting instrumental behavior. Hippocampus. 2013;23(11):1025–34. PMID: 23929764. http://www.ncbi.nlm.nih.gov/pubmed/23929764.
42. Koolhaas JM, Meerlo P, De Boer SF, Strubbe JH, Bohus B. The temporal dynamics of the stress response. Neurosci Biobehav Rev. 1997;21(6):775–82. PMID: 9415902. http://www.ncbi.nlm.nih.gov/pubmed/9415902.
43. Antelman SM, Szechtman H, Chin P, Fisher AE. Tail pinch-induced eating, gnawing and licking behavior in rats: dependence on the nigrostriatal dopamine system. Brain Res. 1975;99(2):319–37. PMID: 1182545. http://www.ncbi.nlm.nih.gov/pubmed/1182545.
44. Valenstein ES, Cox VC, Kakolewski JW. Reexamination of the role of the hypothalamus in motivation. Psychol Rev. 1970;77(1):16–31. PMID: 4908030. http://www.ncbi.nlm.nih.gov/pubmed/4908030.
45. Clemente CD, Chase MH. Neurological substrates of aggressive behavior. Annu Rev Physiol. 1973;35:329–56. PMID: 4581768. http://www.ncbi.nlm.nih.gov/pubmed/4581768.
46. Grewen KM, Girdler SS, Amico J, Light KC. Effects of partner support on resting oxytocin, cortisol, norepinephrine, and blood pressure before and after warm partner contact. Psychosom Med. 2005;67(4):531–8. PMID: 16046364. http://www.ncbi.nlm.nih.gov/pubmed/16046364.
47. Mawson AR. Understanding mass panic and other collective responses to threat and disaster. Psychiatry. 2005;68(2):95–113. PMID: 16247853. http://www.ncbi.nlm.nih.gov/pubmed/16247853.
48. Steptoe A, Dockray S, Wardle J. Positive affect and psychobiological processes relevant to health. J Pers. 2009;77(6):1747–76. PMCID: PMC2787693. http://www.ncbi.nlm.nih.gov/pubmed/19796062.

49. Thoits PA. Mechanisms linking social ties and support to physical and mental health. J Health Soc Behav. 2011;52(2):145–61. PMID: 21673143. http://www.ncbi.nlm.nih.gov/pubmed/21673143.
50. Bowlby J. Attachment and loss, vol. 1. London: Hogarth; 1969. p. 291–5. https://archive.org/details/attachmentlossvo00john.
51. Koole SL, Tjew A Sin M, Schneider IK. Embodied terror management: interpersonal touch alleviates existential concerns among individuals with low self-esteem. Psychol Sci. 2014;25(1):30–7. PMID: 24190907. http://www.ncbi.nlm.nih.gov/pubmed/24190907.
52. Phalan JE. Exploring the use of touch in the psychotherapeutic setting: a phenomenological review. Psychother Theory Res Pract Train. 2009;46(1):97–111.
53. Halbrook B, Duplechin R. Rethinking touch in psychotherapy: guidelines for practitioners. Psychother Priv Pract. 1994;13(3):43–53.
54. Jourard SM. An exploratory study of body-accessibility. Br J Soc Clin Psychol. 1966;5(3):221–31. PMID: 5975653. http://www.ncbi.nlm.nih.gov/pubmed/5975653.
55. Remland MS, Jones TS, Brinkman H. Interpersonal distance, body orientation, and touch: effects of culture, gender, and age. J Soc Psychol. 1995;135(3):281–97. PMID: 7650932. http://www.ncbi.nlm.nih.gov/pubmed/7650932.
56. Ditzen B, Neumann ID, Bodenmann G, von Dawans B, Turner RA, Ehlert U, Heinrichs M. Effects of different kinds of couple interaction on cortisol and heart rate responses to stress in women. Psychoneuroendocrinology. 2007;32(5):565–74. PMID: 17499441. http://www.ncbi.nlm.nih.gov/pubmed/17499441.
57. Light KC, Grewen KM, Amico JA. More frequent partner hugs and higher oxytocin levels are linked to lower blood pressure and heart rate in premenopausal women. Biol Psychol. 2005;69(1):5–21. PMID: 15740822. http://www.ncbi.nlm.nih.gov/pubmed/15740822.
58. Holt-Lunstad J, Birmingham WA, Light KC. Influence of a "warm touch" support enhancement intervention among married couples on ambulatory blood pressure, oxytocin, alpha amylase, and cortisol. Psychosom Med. 2008;70(9):976–85. PMID: 18842740. http://www.ncbi.nlm.nih.gov/pubmed/18842740.
59. Gazzola V, Spezio ML, Etzel JA, Castelli F, Adolphs R, Keysers C. Primary somatosensory cortex discriminates affective significance in social touch. Proc Natl Acad Sci USA. 2012;109(25):E1657–66. PMCID: PMC3382530. http://www.ncbi.nlm.nih.gov/pubmed/22665808.
60. Morhenn VB, Park JW, Piper E, Zak PJ. Monetary sacrifice among strangers is mediated by endogenous oxytocin release after physical contact. Evol Hum Behav. 2008;29:375–83. https://www.sciencedirect.com/science/article/abs/pii/S1090513808000482.
61. Morhenn V, Beavin LE, Zak PJ. Massage increases oxytocin and reduces adrenocorticotropin hormone in humans. Altern Ther Health Med. 2012;18(6):11–8. PMID: 23251939. http://www.ncbi.nlm.nih.gov/pubmed/23251939.
62. Brown SL, Fredrickson BL, Wirth MM, Poulin MJ, Meier EA, Heaphy ED, Cohen MD, Schultheiss OC. Social closeness increases salivary progesterone in humans. Horm Behav. 2009;56(1):108–11. PMCID: PMC2699766. http://www.ncbi.nlm.nih.gov/pubmed/19362559.
63. Fisher JD, Rytting M, Heslin R. Hands touching hands: affective and evaluative effects of an interpersonal touch. Sociometry. 1976;39(4):416–21. PMID: 1006362. http://www.ncbi.nlm.nih.gov/pubmed/1006362.
64. Ebisch SJ, Ferri F, Gallese V. Touching moments: desire modulates the neural anticipation of active romantic caress. Front Behav Neurosci. 2014;8:60. PMCID: PMC3937548. http://www.ncbi.nlm.nih.gov/pubmed/24616676.
65. Debrot A, Schoebi D, Perrez M, Horn AB. Touch as an interpersonal emotion regulation process in couples' daily lives: the mediating role of psychological intimacy. Personal Soc Psychol Bull. 2013;39(10):1373–85. PMID: 23885034. http://www.ncbi.nlm.nih.gov/pubmed/23885034.
66. Kennedy DP, Gläscher J, Tyszka JM, Adolphs R. Personal space regulation by the human amygdala. Nat Neurosci. 2009;12(10):1226–7. PMCID: PMC2753689. https://pmc.ncbi.nlm.nih.gov/articles/PMC2753689/pdf/nihms-131528.pdf.
67. Gupta R, Koscik TR, Bechara A, Tranel D. The amygdala and decision-making. Neuropsychologia. 2011;49(4):760–6. PMCID: PMC3032808. http://www.ncbi.nlm.nih.gov/pubmed/20920513.
68. Koscik TR, Tranel D. The human amygdala is necessary for developing and expressing normal interpersonal trust. Neuropsychologia. 2011;49(4):602–11. PMCID: PMC3056169. http://www.ncbi.nlm.nih.gov/pubmed/20920512.
69. Adolphs R. What does the amygdala contribute to social cognition? Ann N Y Acad Sci. 2010;1191(1):42–61. PMCID: PMC2871162. http://www.ncbi.nlm.nih.gov/pubmed/20392275.
70. Kluver H, Bucy PC. "Psychic blindness" and other symptoms following bilateral temporal lobectomy in Rhesus monkeys. Am J Physiol. 1937;119:352–3. https://psycnet.apa.org/record/1938-00651-001.
71. Hayduk LA. Personal space: an evaluative and orienting overview. Psychol Bull. 1978;85:117–34. https://psycnet.apa.org/record/1979-23561-001.
72. Hermann D, Weber-Fahr W, Sartorius A, Hoerst M, Frischknecht U, Tunc-Skarka N, Perreau-Lenz S, Hansson AC, Krumm B, Kiefer F, Spanagel R, Mann K, Ende G, Sommer WH. Translational magnetic resonance spectroscopy reveals excessive central glutamate levels during alcohol withdrawal in humans and rats. Biol Psychiatry. 2012;71(11):1015–21. PMID: 21907974. http://www.ncbi.nlm.nih.gov/pubmed/21907974.
73. Emery NJ, Capitanio JP, Mason WA, Machado CJ, Mendoza SP, Amaral DG. The effects of bilateral lesions of the amygdala on dyadic social interactions in rhesus monkeys (Macaca mulatta). Behav Neurosci. 2001;115(3):515–44. PMID: 11439444. http://www.ncbi.nlm.nih.gov/pubmed/11439444.
74. Mason WA, Capitanio JP, Machado CJ, Mendoza SP, Amaral DG. Amygdalectomy and responsiveness to novelty in rhesus monkeys (Macaca mulatta): generality and individual consistency of effects. Emotion. 2006;6(1):73–81. PMID: 16637751. http://www.ncbi.nlm.nih.gov/pubmed/16637751.
75. Adolphs R, Tranel D, Damasio AR. The human amygdala in social judgment. Nature. 1998;393(6684):470–4. PMID: 9624002. http://www.ncbi.nlm.nih.gov/pubmed/9624002.
76. Gordon I, Martin C, Feldman R, Leckman JF. Oxytocin and social motivation. Dev Cogn Neurosci. 2011;1(4):471–93. PMCID: PMC3185363. http://www.ncbi.nlm.nih.gov/pubmed/21984889.
77. Gimpl G, Fahrenholz F. The oxytocin receptor system: structure, function, and regulation. Physiol Rev. 2001;81(2):629–83. PMID: 11274341. http://www.ncbi.nlm.nih.gov/pubmed/11274341.
78. Bergquist F, Ludwig M. Dendritic transmitter release: a comparison of two model systems. J Neuroendocrinol. 2008;20(6):677–86. PMID: 18601689. http://www.ncbi.nlm.nih.gov/pubmed/18601689.
79. Leng G, Onaka T, Caquineau C, Sabatier N, Tobin VA, Takayanagi Y. Oxytocin and appetite. Prog Brain Res. 2008;170:137–51. PMID: 18655879. http://www.ncbi.nlm.nih.gov/pubmed/18655879.
80. Sabatier N, Leng G, Menzies J. Oxytocin, feeding, and satiety. Front Endocrinol (Lausanne). 2013;4:35. PMCID: PMC3603288. http://www.ncbi.nlm.nih.gov/pubmed/23518828.
81. Gordon I, Zagoory-Sharon O, Leckman JF, Feldman R. Oxytocin and the development of parenting in humans. Biol Psychiatry. 2010;68(4):377–82. PMCID: PMC3943240. http://www.ncbi.nlm.nih.gov/pubmed/20359699.

82. Feldman R, Gordon I, Schneiderman I, Weisman O, Zagoory-Sharon O. Natural variations in maternal and paternal care are associated with systematic changes in oxytocin following parent-infant contact. Psychoneuroendocrinology. 2010;35(8):1133–41. PMID: 20153585. http://www.ncbi.nlm.nih.gov/pubmed/20153585.
83. Lee HJ, Macbeth AH, Pagani JH, Young WS. Oxytocin: the great facilitator of life. Prog Neurobiol. 2009;88(2):127–51. PMCID: PMC2689929. http://www.ncbi.nlm.nih.gov/pubmed/19482229.
84. Insel TR. The challenge of translation in social neuroscience: a review of oxytocin, vasopressin, and affiliative behavior. Neuron. 2010;65(6):768–79. PMCID: PMC2847497. http://www.ncbi.nlm.nih.gov/pubmed/20346754.
85. Uvnas-Moberg K, Petersson M. Oxytocin, a mediator of anti-stress, well-being, social interaction, growth and healing. Z Psychosom Med Psychother. 2005;51(1):57–80. PMID: 15834840. http://www.ncbi.nlm.nih.gov/pubmed/15834840.
86. Meyer-Lindenberg A, Domes G, Kirsch P, Heinrichs M. Oxytocin and vasopressin in the human brain: social neuropeptides for translational medicine. Nat Rev Neurosci. 2011;12(9):524–38. PMID: 21852800. http://www.ncbi.nlm.nih.gov/pubmed/21852800.
87. de Graaf R, Bijl RV, ten Have M, Beekman ATF, Vollebergh WAM. Rapid onset of comorbidity of common mental disorders: findings from the Netherlands Mental Health Survey and Incidence Study (NEMESIS). Acta Psychiatr Scand. 2004;109(1):55–63. PMID: 14674959. http://www.ncbi.nlm.nih.gov/pubmed/14674959.
88. Hovens JGFM, Wiersma JE, Giltay EJ, van Oppen P, Spinhoven P, Penninx BWJH, Zitman FG. Childhood life events and childhood trauma in adult patients with depressive, anxiety and comorbid disorders vs. controls. Acta Psychiatr Scand. 2010;122(1):66–74. PMID: 19878136. http://www.ncbi.nlm.nih.gov/pubmed/19878136.
89. Keyes KM, Eaton NR, Krueger RF, McLaughlin KA, Wall MM, Grant BF, Hasin DS. Childhood maltreatment and the structure of common psychiatric disorders. Br J Psychiatry. 2012;200(2):107–15. PMCID: PMC3269653. http://www.ncbi.nlm.nih.gov/pubmed/22157798.
90. Sharma S, Powers A, Bradley B, Ressler KJ. Gene × environment determinants of stress- and anxiety-related disorders. Annu Rev Psychol. 2016;67:239–61. PMCID: PMC5739029. http://www.ncbi.nlm.nih.gov/pubmed/26442668.
91. Macdonald K, Macdonald TM. The peptide that binds: a systematic review of oxytocin and its prosocial effects in humans. Harv Rev Psychiatry. 2010;18(1):1–21. PMID: 20047458. http://www.ncbi.nlm.nih.gov/pubmed/20047458.
92. Heinrichs M, von Dawans B, Domes G. Oxytocin, vasopressin, and human social behavior. Front Neuroendocrinol. 2009;30(4):548–57. PMID: 19505497. http://www.ncbi.nlm.nih.gov/pubmed/19505497.
93. Carter CS. Oxytocin pathways and the evolution of human behavior. Annu Rev Psychol. 2014;65:17–39. PMID: 24050183. http://www.ncbi.nlm.nih.gov/pubmed/24050183.
94. Thompson SM, Hammen C, Starr LR, Najman JM. Oxytocin receptor gene polymorphism (rs53576) moderates the intergenerational transmission of depression. Psychoneuroendocrinology. 2014;43:11–9. PMCID: PMC3979470. http://www.ncbi.nlm.nih.gov/pubmed/24703166.
95. Opacka-Juffry J, Mohiyeddini C. Experience of stress in childhood negatively correlates with plasma oxytocin concentration in adult men. Stress. 2012;15(1):1–10. PMID: 21682649. http://www.ncbi.nlm.nih.gov/pubmed/21682649.
96. McInnis OA, McQuaid RJ, Matheson K, Anisman H. The moderating role of an oxytocin receptor gene polymorphism in the relation between unsupportive social interactions and coping profiles: implications for depression. Front Psychol. 2015;6:1133. PMCID: PMC4531231. http://www.ncbi.nlm.nih.gov/pubmed/26321972.
97. Kumsta R, Heinrichs M. Oxytocin, stress and social behavior: neurogenetics of the human oxytocin system. Curr Opin Neurobiol. 2013;23(1):11–6. PMID: 23040540. http://www.ncbi.nlm.nih.gov/pubmed/23040540.
98. Sullivan PF, de Geus EJC, Willemsen G, James MR, Smit JH, Zandbelt T, Arolt V, Baune BT, Blackwood D, Cichon S, Coventry WL, Domschke K, Farmer A, Fava M, Gordon SD, He Q, Heath AC, Heutink P, Holsboer F, Hoogendijk WJ, Hottenga JJ, Hu Y, Kohli M, Lin D, Lucae S, Macintyre DJ, Maier W, McGhee KA, McGuffin P, Montgomery GW, Muir WJ, Nolen WA, Nöthen MM, Perlis RH, Pirlo K, Posthuma D, Rietschel M, Rizzu P, Schosser A, Smit AB, Smoller JW, Tzeng JY, van Dyck R, Verhage M, Zitman FG, Martin NG, Wray NR, Boomsma DI, Penninx BWJH. Genome-wide association for major depressive disorder: a possible role for the presynaptic protein piccolo. Mol Psychiatry. 2009;14(4):359–75. http://www.ncbi.nlm.nih.gov/pubmed/19065144.
99. Major Depressive Disorder Working Group of the Psychiatric GWAS Consortium, Ripke S, Wray NR, Lewis CM, Hamilton SP, Weissman MM, Breen G, Byrne EM, Blackwood DHR, Boomsma DI, Cichon S, Heath AC, Holsboer F, Lucae S, Madden PAF, Martin NG, McGuffin P, Muglia P, Noethen MM, Penninx BP, Pergadia ML, Potash JB, Rietschel M, Lin D, Müller-Myhsok B, Shi J, Steinberg S, Grabe HJ, Lichtenstein P, Magnusson P, Perlis RH, Preisig M, Smoller JW, Stefansson K, Uher R, Kutalik Z, Tansey KE, Teumer A, Viktorin A, Barnes MR, Bettecken T, Binder EB, Breuer R, Castro VM, Churchill SE, Coryell WH, Craddock N, Craig IW, Czamara D, De Geus EJ, Degenhardt F, Farmer AE, Fava M, Frank J, Gainer VS, Gallagher PJ, Gordon SD, Goryachev S, Gross M, Guipponi M, Henders AK, Herms S, Hickie IB, Hoefels S, Hoogendijk W, Hottenga JJ, Iosifescu DV, Ising M, Jones I, Jones L, Jung-Ying T, Knowles JA, Kohane IS, Kohli MA, Korszun A, Landen M, Lawson WB, Lewis G, Macintyre D, Maier W, Mattheisen M, McGrath PJ, McIntosh A, McLean A, Middeldorp CM, Middleton L, Montgomery GM, Murphy SN, Nauck M, Nolen WA, Nyholt DR, O'Donovan M, Oskarsson H, Pedersen N, Scheftner WA, Schulz A, Schulze TG, Shyn SI, Sigurdsson E, Slager SL, Smit JH, Stefansson H, Steffens M, Thorgeirsson T, Tozzi F, Treutlein J, Uhr M, van den Oord EJCG, Van Grootheest G, Völzke H, Weilburg JB, Willemsen G, Zitman FG, Neale B, Daly M, Levinson DF, Sullivan PF. A mega-analysis of genome-wide association studies for major depressive disorder. Mol Psychiatry. 2013;18(4):497–511. PMCID: PMC3837431. http://www.ncbi.nlm.nih.gov/pubmed/19515497.
100. Costa B, Pini S, Gabelloni P, Abelli M, Lari L, Cardini A, Muti M, Gesi C, Landi S, Galderisi S, Mucci A, Lucacchini A, Cassano GB, Martini C. Oxytocin receptor polymorphisms and adult attachment style in patients with depression. Psychoneuroendocrinology. 2009;34(10):1506–14. PMID: 19515497. http://www.ncbi.nlm.nih.gov/pubmed/19515497.
101. Saphire-Bernstein S, Way BM, Kim HS, Sherman DK, Taylor SE. Oxytocin receptor gene (OXTR) is related to psychological resources. Proc Natl Acad Sci USA. 2011;108(37):15118–22. PMCID: PMC3174632. http://www.ncbi.nlm.nih.gov/pubmed/21896752.
102. Lucht MJ, Barnow S, Sonnenfeld C, Rosenberger A, Grabe HJ, Schroeder W, Völzke H, Freyberger HJ, Herrmann FH, Kroemer H, Rosskopf D. Associations between the oxytocin receptor gene (OXTR) and affect, loneliness and intelligence in normal subjects. Prog Neuro-Psychopharmacol Biol Psychiatry. 2009;33(5):860–6. PMID: 19376182. http://www.ncbi.nlm.nih.gov/pubmed/19376182.
103. Mileva-Seitz V, Steiner M, Atkinson L, Meaney MJ, Levitan R, Kennedy JL, Sokolowski MB, Fleming AS. Interaction between oxytocin genotypes and early experience predicts quality of mothering and postpartum mood. PLoS One. 2013;8(4):e61443.

PMCID: PMC3630168. http://www.ncbi.nlm.nih.gov/pubmed/23637833.
104. Kawamura Y, Liu X, Akiyama T, Shimada T, Otowa T, Sakai Y, Kakiuchi C, Umekage T, Sasaki T, Akiskal HS. The association between oxytocin receptor gene (OXTR) polymorphisms and affective temperaments, as measured by TEMPS-A. J Affect Disord. 2010;127(1–3):31–7. PMID: 20488544. http://www.ncbi.nlm.nih.gov/pubmed/20488544.
105. Lucas-Thompson RG, Holman EA. Environmental stress, oxytocin receptor gene (OXTR) polymorphism, and mental health following collective stress. Horm Behav. 2013;63(4):615–24. PMID: 23470776. http://www.ncbi.nlm.nih.gov/pubmed/23470776.
106. Wang J, Qin W, Liu B, Zhou Y, Wang D, Zhang Y, Jiang T, Yu C. Neural mechanisms of oxytocin receptor gene mediating anxiety-related temperament. Brain Struct Funct. 2014;219(5):1543–54. PMID: 23708061. http://www.ncbi.nlm.nih.gov/pubmed/23708061.
107. Montag C, Fiebach CJ, Kirsch P, Reuter M. Interaction of 5-HTTLPR and a variation on the oxytocin receptor gene influences negative emotionality. Biol Psychiatry. 2011;69(6):601–3. PMID: 21183159. http://www.ncbi.nlm.nih.gov/pubmed/21183159.
108. Myers AJ, Williams L, Gatt JM, McAuley-Clark EZ, Dobson-Stone C, Schofield PR, Nemeroff CB. Variation in the oxytocin receptor gene is associated with increased risk for anxiety, stress and depression in individuals with a history of exposure to early life stress. J Psychiatr Res. 2014;59:93–100. PMCID: PMC4252971. http://www.ncbi.nlm.nih.gov/pubmed/25262417.
109. McQuaid RJ, McInnis OA, Stead JD, Matheson K, Anisman H. A paradoxical association of an oxytocin receptor gene polymorphism: early-life adversity and vulnerability to depression. Front Neurosci. 2013;7:128. PMCID: PMC3721019. http://www.ncbi.nlm.nih.gov/pubmed/23898235.
110. Melchers M, Montag C, Felten A, Reuter M. The oxytocin receptor gene and social perception. Soc Neurosci. 2015;10(4):345–53. PMID: 25646574. http://www.ncbi.nlm.nih.gov/pubmed/25646574.
111. Asherin RM, Everhart KD, Stophaeros SL, Vogeli JM, Fowler J, Phiel CJ, Kaplan PS. Associations between maternal depression and mother and infant oxytocin receptor gene (OXTR_rs53576) polymorphisms. Dev Psychobiol. 2020;62(4):496–504. PMID: 31755553. http://www.ncbi.nlm.nih.gov/pubmed/31755553.
112. Sanwald S, Gahr M, Widenhorn-Müller K, Schönfeldt-Lecuona C, Richter K, Connemann BJ, Kammer T, Montag C, Kiefer M. Relation of promoter methylation of the oxytocin gene to stressful life events and depression severity. J Mol Neurosci. 2020;70(2):201–11. PMID: 31768943. http://www.ncbi.nlm.nih.gov/pubmed/31768943.
113. Akhavan Karbasi S, Golestan M, Fallah R, Golshan M, Dehghan Z. Effect of body massage on increase of low birth weight neonates growth parameters: a randomized clinical trial. Iran J Reprod Med. 2013;11(7):583–8. PMCID: PMC3941350. http://www.ncbi.nlm.nih.gov/pubmed/24639794.
114. Vickers A, Ohlsson A, Lacy JB, Horsley A. Massage for promoting growth and development of preterm and/or low birth-weight infants. Cochrane Database Syst Rev. 2004;2004(2):CD000390. PMCID: PMC6956667. http://www.ncbi.nlm.nih.gov/pubmed/15106151.
115. Field T, Diego M, Hernandez-Reif M. Preterm infant massage therapy research: a review. Infant Behav Dev. 2010;33(2):115–24. PMCID: PMC2844909. http://www.ncbi.nlm.nih.gov/pubmed/20137814.
116. Haley S, Beachy J, Ivaska KK, Slater H, Smith S, Moyer-Mileur LJ. Tactile/kinesthetic stimulation (TKS) increases tibial speed of sound and urinary osteocalcin (U-MidOC and unOC) in premature infants (29-32weeks PMA). Bone. 2012;51(4):661–6. PMCID: PMC3434881. http://www.ncbi.nlm.nih.gov/pubmed/22846674.
117. Ang JY, Lua JL, Mathur A, Thomas R, Asmar BI, Savasan S, Buck S, Long M, Shankaran S. A randomized placebo-controlled trial of massage therapy on the immune system of preterm infants. Pediatrics. 2012;130(6):e1549–58. PMCID: PMC3507248. http://www.ncbi.nlm.nih.gov/pubmed/23147978.
118. Haans A, IJsselsteijn W. Mediated social touch: a review of current research and future directions. Virtual Real. 2006;9:149–59. https://link.springer.com/article/10.1007/s10055-005-0014-2.
119. Stiehl W, Breazeal C. Design of a therapeutic robotic companion for relational, affective touch. In: Proceedings of the 14th IEEE international workshop on robot and human interactive communication. IEEE; 2005. p. 408–15. https://www.media.mit.edu/publications/design-of-a-therapeutic-robotic-companion-for-relational-affective-touch-2/.
120. Shibata T. An overview of human interactive robots for psychological enrichment. Proc IEEE. 2004;92:1749–58. https://www.researchgate.net/publication/2986368_Shibata_T_An_overview_of_human_interactive_robots_for_psychological_enrichment_Proc_of_the_IEEE_92_1749-1758.
121. Kanda T, Ishiguro H, Ono T, Imai M, Nakatsu R. Development, and evaluation of an interactive humanoid robot. In: Proceedings of the IEEE international conference on robotics and automation. IEEE; 2002. p. 1848–55. https://link.springer.com/chapter/10.1007/3-540-36460-9_12.
122. Sumioka H, Nakae A, Kanai R, Ishiguro H. Huggable communication medium decreases cortisol levels. Sci Rep. 2013;3:3034. PMCID: PMC3805974. http://www.ncbi.nlm.nih.gov/pubmed/24150186.
123. TIME. Amazing Embrace. Best Inventions 2006. https://web.archive.org/web/20100501160901/http:/www.time.com/time/specials/packages/article/0,28804,1939342_1939424_1939709,00.html.
124. Bonanni L, Vaumobilee C, Lieberman J, Zuckerman O. TapTap: a haptic wearable for asynchronous distributed touch therapy. Ext Abstr Hum Factors Computing Syst. 2006:580–5. https://www.media.mit.edu/publications/taptap-a-haptic-wearable-for-asynchronous-distributed-touch-therapy/.
125. Astin JA, Harkness E, Ernst E. The efficacy of "distant healing": a systematic review of randomized trials. Ann Intern Med. 2000;132(11):903–10. PMID: 10836918. http://www.ncbi.nlm.nih.gov/pubmed/10836918.
126. Winstead-Fry P, Kijek J. An integrative review and meta-analysis of therapeutic touch research. Altern Ther Health Med. 1999;5(6):58–67. PMID: 10550906. http://www.ncbi.nlm.nih.gov/pubmed/10550906.
127. Garrett B, Riou M. A rapid evidence assessment of recent therapeutic touch research. Nurs Open. 2021;8(5):2318–30. PMCID: PMC8363410. http://www.ncbi.nlm.nih.gov/pubmed/33742792.
128. Hammerschlag R, Sprengel ML, Baldwin AL. Biofield therapies: guidelines for reporting clinical trials. Explore (NY). 2024;20(2):196–205. PMID: 38307816. http://www.ncbi.nlm.nih.gov/pubmed/38307816.
129. Murillo-Muñoz F, Navarro-Cota C, Juárez-Ramírez R, Jiménez S, Nieto Hipólito JI, Molina AI, Vazquez-Briseno M. Characteristics of a persuasive educational system: a systematic literature review. Appl Sci. 2021;11(21):10089. https://www.researchgate.net/publication/367827110_Characteristics_of_a_Persuasive_Educational_System_A_Systematic_Literature_Review.
130. Natural Healers. 27 Types of massage therapy (session lengths & benefits). https://www.naturalhealers.com/massage-therapy/specialties/.
131. Field T, Hernandez-Reif M, Diego M, Schanberg S, Kuhn C. Cortisol decreases and serotonin and dopamine increase following massage therapy. Int J Neurosci. 2005;115(10):1397–413. PMID: 16162447. http://www.ncbi.nlm.nih.gov/pubmed/16162447.

132. Hernandez-Reif M, Field T, Krasnegor J, Theakston H, Hossain Z, Burman I. High blood pressure and associated symptoms were reduced by massage therapy. J Bodyw Mov Ther. 2000;4:31–8.
133. Moyer CA, Rounds J, Hannum JW. A meta-analysis of massage therapy research. Psychol Bull. 2004;130(1):3–18. PMID: 14717648. http://www.ncbi.nlm.nih.gov/pubmed/14717648.
134. Field T, Hernandez-Reif M, Hart S, Quintino O, Drose L, Field T, Kuhn C, Schanberg S. Sexual abuse effects are lessened by massage therapy. J Bodyw Mov Ther. 1997;1:65–6.
135. Field T, Schanberg S, Kuhn C, Field T, Fierro K, Henteleff T, Mueller C, Yando R, Shaw S, Burman I. Bulimic adolescents benefit from massage therapy. Adolescence. 1998;33(131):555–63. PMID: 9831872. http://www.ncbi.nlm.nih.gov/pubmed/9831872.
136. Field T, Seligman S, Scafidi F, Schanberg S. Alleviating posttraumatic stress in children following hurricane Andrew. J Appl Dev Psychol. 1996;17:37–50.
137. Taylor CB, Sallis JF, Needle R. The relation of physical activity and exercise to mental health. Public Health Rep. 1985;100(2):195–202. PMCID: PMC1424736. http://www.ncbi.nlm.nih.gov/pubmed/3920718.
138. Maddigan B, Hodgson P, Heath S, Dick B, St John K, McWilliam-Burton T, Snelgrove C, White H. The effects of massage therapy & exercise therapy on children/adolescents with attention deficit hyperactivity disorder. Can Child Adolesc Psychiatr Rev. 2003;12(2):40–3. PMCID: PMC2538473. http://www.ncbi.nlm.nih.gov/pubmed/19030480.
139. Field T. Massage therapy for infants and children. J Dev Behav Pediatr. 1995;16(2):105–11. PMID: 7790516. http://www.ncbi.nlm.nih.gov/pubmed/7790516.
140. Field T, Morrow C, Valdeon C, Larson S, Kuhn C, Schanberg S. Massage reduces anxiety in child and adolescent psychiatric patients. J Am Acad Child Adolesc Psychiatry. 1992;31(1):125–31. PMID: 1537763. http://www.ncbi.nlm.nih.gov/pubmed/1537763.
141. Coelho HF, Boddy K, Ernst E. Massage therapy for the treatment of depression: a systematic review. Int J Clin Pract. 2008;62(2):325–33. PMID: 18081800. http://www.ncbi.nlm.nih.gov/pubmed/18081800.
142. Hou WH, Chiang PT, Hsu TY, Chiu SY, Yen YC. Treatment effects of massage therapy in depressed people: a meta-analysis. J Clin Psychiatry. 2010;71(7):894–901. PMID: 20361919. http://www.ncbi.nlm.nih.gov/pubmed/20361919.
143. Moyer CA, Seefeldt L, Mann ES, Jackley LM. Does massage therapy reduce cortisol? A comprehensive quantitative review. J Bodyw Mov Ther. 2011;15(1):3–14. PMID: 21147413. http://www.ncbi.nlm.nih.gov/pubmed/21147413.
144. Sherman KJ, Ludman EJ, Cook AJ, Hawkes RJ, Roy-Byrne PP, Bentley S, Brooks MZ, Cherkin DC. Effectiveness of therapeutic massage for generalized anxiety disorder: a randomized controlled trial. Depress Anxiety. 2010;27(5):441–50. PMCID: PMC2922919. http://www.ncbi.nlm.nih.gov/pubmed/20186971.
145. Papathanassoglou EDE, Mpouzika MDA. Interpersonal touch: physiological effects in critical care. Biol Res Nurs. 2012;14(4):431–43. PMID: 22773451. http://www.ncbi.nlm.nih.gov/pubmed/22773451.
146. Ironson G, Field T, Scafidi F, Hashimoto M, Kumar M, Kumar A, Price A, Goncalves A, Burman I, Tetenman C, Patarca R, Fletcher MA. Massage therapy is associated with enhancement of the immune system's cytotoxic capacity. Int J Neurosci. 1996;84(1–4):205–17. PMID: 8707483. http://www.ncbi.nlm.nih.gov/pubmed/8707483.
147. Li Y, Wang F, Feng C, Yang X, Sun Y. Massage therapy for fibromyalgia: a systematic review and meta-analysis of randomized controlled trials. PLoS One. 2014;9(2):e89304. PMCID: PMC3930706. http://www.ncbi.nlm.nih.gov/pubmed/24586677.
148. Watanabe N, Miyazaki S, Mukaino Y, Hotta H. Effect of gentle cutaneous stimulation on heat-induced autonomic response and subjective pain intensity in healthy humans. J Physiol Sci. 2012;62(4):343–50. PMCID: PMC10717059. http://www.ncbi.nlm.nih.gov/pubmed/22614394.
149. Packheiser J, Hartmann H, Fredriksen K, Gazzola V, Keysers C, Michon F. A systematic review and multivariate meta-analysis of the physical and mental health benefits of touch interventions. Nat Hum Behav. 2024;8(6):1088–107. PMCID: PMC11199149. http://www.ncbi.nlm.nih.gov/pubmed/38589702.
150. Kutner JS, Smith MC, Corbin L, Hemphill L, Benton K, Mellis BK, Beaty B, Felton S, Yamashita TE, Bryant LL, Fairclough DL. Massage therapy versus simple touch to improve pain and mood in patients with advanced cancer: a randomized trial. Ann Intern Med. 2008;149(6):369–79. PMCID: PMC2631433. http://www.ncbi.nlm.nih.gov/pubmed/18794556.
151. Lee MS, Lee EN, Ernst E. Massage therapy for breast cancer patients: a systematic review. Ann Oncol. 2011;22(6):1459–61. PMID: 21543629. http://www.ncbi.nlm.nih.gov/pubmed/21543629.
152. Listing M, Reisshauer A, Krohn M, Voigt B, Tjahono G, Becker J, Klapp BF, Rauchfuss M. Massage therapy reduces physical discomfort and improves mood disturbances in women with breast cancer. Psychooncology. 2009;18(12):1290–9. PMID: 19189275. http://www.ncbi.nlm.nih.gov/pubmed/19189275.
153. Collinge W, Kahn J, Walton T, Kozak L, Bauer-Wu S, Fletcher K, Yarnold P, Soltysik R. Touch, caring, and cancer: randomized controlled trial of a multimedia caregiver education program. Support Care Cancer. 2013;21(5):1405–14. PMCID: PMC3612588. http://www.ncbi.nlm.nih.gov/pubmed/23262808.
154. Cassileth BR, Vickers AJ. Massage therapy for symptom control: outcome study at a major cancer center. J Pain Symptom Manag. 2004;28(3):244–9. PMID: 15336336. http://www.ncbi.nlm.nih.gov/pubmed/15336336.
155. Weze C, Leathard HL, Grange J, Tiplady P, Stevens G. Evaluation of healing by gentle touch in 35 clients with cancer. Eur J Oncol Nurs. 2004;8(1):40–9. PMID: 15003743. http://www.ncbi.nlm.nih.gov/pubmed/15003743.
156. Weze C, Leathard HL, Grange J, Tiplady P, Stevens G. Evaluation of healing by gentle touch. Public Health. 2005;119(1):3–10. PMID: 15560896. http://www.ncbi.nlm.nih.gov/pubmed/15560896.
157. Weze C, Leathard HL, Grange J, Tiplady P, Stevens G. Healing by gentle touch ameliorates stress and other symptoms in people suffering with mental health disorders or psychological stress. Evid Based Complement Alternat Med. 2007;4(1):115–23. PMCID: PMC1810357. http://www.ncbi.nlm.nih.gov/pubmed/17342249.
158. Demmer C. A survey of complementary therapy services provided by hospices. J Palliat Med. 2004;7(4):510–6. PMID: 15353094. http://www.ncbi.nlm.nih.gov/pubmed/15353094.
159. Kozak LE, Kayes L, McCarty R, Walkinshaw C, Congdon S, Kleinberger J, Hartman V, Standish LJ. Use of complementary and alternative medicine (CAM) by Washington State hospices. Am J Hosp Palliat Care. 2008;25(6):463–8. PMID: 19106280. http://www.ncbi.nlm.nih.gov/pubmed/19106280.
160. Listing M, Krohn M, Liezmann C, Kim I, Reisshauer A, Peters E, Klapp BF, Rauchfuss M. The efficacy of classical massage on stress perception and cortisol following primary treatment of breast cancer. Arch Womens Ment Health. 2010;13(2):165–73. PMID: 20169378. http://www.ncbi.nlm.nih.gov/pubmed/20169378.
161. Stringer J, Swindell R, Dennis M. Massage in patients undergoing intensive chemotherapy reduces serum cortisol and prolactin. Psychooncology. 2008;17(10):1024–31. PMID: 18300336. http://www.ncbi.nlm.nih.gov/pubmed/18300336.
162. Wilkinson S, Barnes K, Storey L. Massage for symptom relief in patients with cancer: systematic review. J Adv Nurs. 2008;63(5):430–9. PMID: 18727744. http://www.ncbi.nlm.nih.gov/pubmed/18727744.

163. Campeau MP, Gaboriault R, Drapeau M, Van Nguyen T, Roy I, Fortin B, Marois M, Nguyen-Tân PF. Impact of massage therapy on anxiety levels in patients undergoing radiation therapy: randomized controlled trial. J Soc Integr Oncol. 2007;5(4):133–8. PMID: 19087756. http://www.ncbi.nlm.nih.gov/pubmed/19087756.
164. Mehling WE, Jacobs B, Acree M, Wilson L, Bostrom A, West J, Acquah J, Burns B, Chapman J, Hecht FM. Symptom management with massage and acupuncture in postoperative cancer patients: a randomized controlled trial. J Pain Symptom Manag. 2007;33(3):258–66. PMID: 17349495. http://www.ncbi.nlm.nih.gov/pubmed/17349495.
165. Billhult A, Bergbom I, Stener-Victorin E. Massage relieves nausea in women with breast cancer who are undergoing chemotherapy. J Altern Complement Med. 2007;13(1):53–7. PMID: 17309378. http://www.ncbi.nlm.nih.gov/pubmed/17309378.
166. Weinrich SP, Weinrich MC. The effect of massage on pain in cancer patients. Appl Nurs Res. 1990;3(4):140–5. PMID: 2252400. http://www.ncbi.nlm.nih.gov/pubmed/2252400.
167. Sharp DM, Walker MB, Chaturvedi A, Upadhyay S, Hamid A, Walker AA, Bateman JS, Braid F, Ellwood K, Hebblewhite C, Hope T, Lines M, Walker LG. A randomised, controlled trial of the psychological effects of reflexology in early breast cancer. Eur J Cancer. 2010;46(2):312–22. PMID: 19906525. http://www.ncbi.nlm.nih.gov/pubmed/19906525.
168. Sturgeon M, Wetta-Hall R, Hart T, Good M, Dakhil S. Effects of therapeutic massage on the quality of life among patients with breast cancer during treatment. J Altern Complement Med. 2009;15(4):373–80. PMID: 19388859. http://www.ncbi.nlm.nih.gov/pubmed/19388859.
169. Billhult A, Stener-Victorin E, Bergbom I. The experience of massage during chemotherapy treatment in breast cancer patients. Clin Nurs Res. 2007;16(2):85–99; discussion 100–102. PMID: 17452429. http://www.ncbi.nlm.nih.gov/pubmed/17452429.
170. Hernandez-Reif M, Field T, Ironson G, Beutler J, Vera Y, Hurley J, Fletcher MA, Schanberg S, Kuhn C, Fraser M. Natural killer cells and lymphocytes increase in women with breast cancer following massage therapy. Int J Neurosci. 2005;115(4):495–510. PMID: 15809216. http://www.ncbi.nlm.nih.gov/pubmed/15809216.
171. Stephenson NLN, Swanson M, Dalton J, Keefe FJ, Engelke M. Partner-delivered reflexology: effects on cancer pain and anxiety. Oncol Nurs Forum. 2007;34(1):127–32. PMID: 17562639. http://www.ncbi.nlm.nih.gov/pubmed/17562639.
172. Poulin MJ, Brown SL, Ubel PA, Smith DM, Jankovic A, Langa KM. Does a helping hand mean a heavy heart? Helping behavior and well-being among spouse caregivers. Psychol Aging. 2010;25(1):108–17. PMCID: PMC2865132. http://www.ncbi.nlm.nih.gov/pubmed/20230132.
173. Kirschner-Hermanns R, Jakse G. Quality of life following radical prostatectomy. Crit Rev Oncol Hematol. 2002;43(2):141–51. PMID: 12191736. http://www.ncbi.nlm.nih.gov/pubmed/12191736.
174. McCorkle R, Pasacreta JV. Enhancing caregiver outcomes in palliative care. Cancer Control. 2001;8(1):36–45. PMID: 11252271. http://www.ncbi.nlm.nih.gov/pubmed/11252271.
175. Badr H, Bakhshaie J, Chhabria K. Dyadic interventions for cancer survivors and caregivers: state of the science and new directions. Semin Oncol Nurs. 2019;35(4):337–41. PMCID: PMC6660372. http://www.ncbi.nlm.nih.gov/pubmed/31248677.
176. Sehlstedt I, Ignell H, Backlund Wasling H, Ackerley R, Olausson H, Croy I. Gentle touch perception across the lifespan. Psychol Aging. 2016;31(2):176–84. PMID: 26950227. http://www.ncbi.nlm.nih.gov/pubmed/26950227.
177. Croy I, Sehlstedt I, Wasling HB, Ackerley R, Olausson H. Gentle touch perception: from early childhood to adolescence. Dev Cogn Neurosci. 2019;35:81–6. PMCID: PMC6968959. http://www.ncbi.nlm.nih.gov/pubmed/28927641.
178. Im H, Kim E, Cain KC. Acute effects of Yakson and gentle human touch on the behavioral state of preterm infants. J Child Health Care. 2009;13(3):212–26. PMID: 19713405. http://www.ncbi.nlm.nih.gov/pubmed/19713405.
179. Zur O, Nordmarken N. To touch or not to touch: exploring prohibition on touch in psychotherapy and counseling and the ethical considerations of touch. Zur Institute; 2021. https://drzur.com/touch-in-therapy/.
180. Sonne JL, Jochai D. The "vicissitudes of love" between therapist and patient: a review of the research on romantic and sexual feelings, thoughts, and behaviors in psychotherapy. J Clin Psychol. 2014;70(2):182–95. PMID: 24375472. http://www.ncbi.nlm.nih.gov/pubmed/24375472.
181. Phelan JE. Exploring the use of touch in the psychotherapeutic setting: a phenomenological review. Psychotherapy. 2009;46(1):97–111. PMID: 22122573. http://www.ncbi.nlm.nih.gov/pubmed/22122573.
182. Bonitz V. Use of physical touch in the "talking cure": a journey to the outskirts of psychotherapy. Psychotherapy. 2008;45(3):391–404. PMID: 22122498. http://www.ncbi.nlm.nih.gov/pubmed/22122498.
183. Zur O. To touch or not to touch: touch in psychotherapy. https://www.youtube.com/watch?v=j1UDtEoShC4.
184. Zur O. To touch or not to touch: clinical and ethical considerations in non-sexual touch in psychotherapy. https://drzur.com/clinical_updates/touch-in-therapy/.
185. Kertay L, Reviere SL. The use of touch in psychotherapy: theoretical and ethical considerations. Psychother Theory Res Pract Train. 1993;30(1):32–40. https://doi.org/10.1037/0033-3204.30.1.32.
186. Durana C. The use of touch in psychotherapy: ethical and clinical guidelines. Psychotherapy. 1998;35(2):269–80. PMID: 11658071. http://www.ncbi.nlm.nih.gov/pubmed/11658071.
187. Smith E, Clance PR, Imes S, editors. Touch in psychotherapy: theory, research and practice. New York: Guilford Press; 1998.
188. Lambert MJ. Implications of outcome research for psychotherapy integration. In: Norcross JC, Goldfried MR, editors. Handbook of psychotherapy integration. New York: Basic Books; 1992. p. 94–129.
189. Dreisoerner A, Junker NM, Schlotz W, Heimrich J, Bloemeke S, Ditzen B, van Dick R. Self-soothing touch and being hugged reduce cortisol responses to stress: a randomized controlled trial on stress, physical touch, and social identity. Compr Psychoneuroendocrinol. 2021;8:100091. PMCID: PMC9216399. http://www.ncbi.nlm.nih.gov/pubmed/35757667.
190. Cohen S, Janicki-Deverts D, Turner RB, Doyle WJ. Does hugging provide stress-buffering social support? A study of susceptibility to upper respiratory infection and illness. Psychol Sci. 2015;26(2):135–47. PMCID: PMC4323947. http://www.ncbi.nlm.nih.gov/pubmed/25526910.
191. Fosshage JL. The meanings of touch in psychoanalysis: a time for reassessment. Psychoanal Inq. 2000;20(1):21–43. Retrieved July 1, 2004 from: http://www.psychoanalyticinquiry.com/vol20no1.html.
192. Perls F. The gestalt approach and eye witness to therapy. Palo Alto: Science and Behavior Books; 1973.
193. Wilson JM. The value of touch in psychotherapy. Am J Orthopsychiatry. 1982;52(1):65–72.
194. Wilison BG, Masson RL. The role of touch in psychotherapy: an adjunct to communication. J Couns Dev. 1986;64:497–500.
195. Reich W. Character analysis. New York: Simon & Schuster; 1972.
196. Kurtz R. Body-centered psychotherapy: the Hakomi method. Mendocino: LifeRythm; 1990.
197. Caldwell C. Getting in touch: the guide to new body-centered therapies. Wheaton: Quest Books; 1997.
198. Rogers C. Carl Rogers on encounter groups. New York: Harper & Row; 1970.

199. Edwards DJA. The experience of interpersonal touch during a personal growth program: a factor analytic approach. Hum Relat. 1984;37(2):769–80.
200. Satir V. Peoplemaking. Palo Alto: Science and Behavior Books; 1972.
201. Stake JE, Oliver J. Sexual contact and touching between therapist and client: a survey of psychologists' attitudes and behavior. Prof Psychol Res Pract. 1991;22:1–11. https://psycnet.apa.org/record/1991-34546-001.
202. Brown LS, Borys DS, Brodsky AM, Gartrell NK, Bouhoutsos JC, Davidson VM, Feldman-Summers S, Gabbard GO, Herman JL, Olarte S. Psychotherapist-patient sexual contact after termination of treatment. Am J Psychiatry. 1992;149(7):979–80, author reply 987–9. PMID: 1472195. http://www.ncbi.nlm.nih.gov/pubmed/1472195.
203. Bouhoutsos J, Holroyd J, Lerman H, Forer BR, Greenberg M. Sexual intimacy between psychotherapists and patients. Prof Psychol Res Pr. 1983;14(2):185–96. PMID: 11653552. http://www.ncbi.nlm.nih.gov/pubmed/11653552.
204. Holroyd J, Bouhoutsos JC. Biased reporting of therapist-patient sexual intimacy. Prof Psychol Res Pr. 1985;16(5):701–9. PMID: 11658766. http://www.ncbi.nlm.nih.gov/pubmed/11658766.
205. Brown LS. Power, responsibility, boundaries: ethical concerns for the lesbian feminist therapist. Lesbian Ethics. 1985;1(3):30–45.
206. Brown LS. Boundaries in feminist therapy: a conceptual formulation. In: Gartrell NK, editor. Bringing ethics alive: feminist ethics in psychotherapy practice. New York: The Haworth Press; 1994. p. 29–38.
207. Gadow S. Touch and technology: two paradigms of patient care. J Relig Health. 1984;23(1):63–9. PMID: 24306940. http://www.ncbi.nlm.nih.gov/pubmed/24306940.
208. Singh C, Leder D. Touch in the consultation. Br J Gen Pract. 2012;62(596):147–8. PMCID: PMC3289810. http://www.ncbi.nlm.nih.gov/pubmed/22429421.
209. Elkiss ML, Jerome JA. Touch--more than a basic science. J Am Osteopath Assoc. 2012;112(8):514–7. PMID: 22904249. http://www.ncbi.nlm.nih.gov/pubmed/22904249.
210. Miller FG, Colloca L, Kaptchuk TJ. The placebo effect: illness and interpersonal healing. Perspect Biol Med. 2009;52(4):518–39. PMCID: PMC2814126. http://www.ncbi.nlm.nih.gov/pubmed/19855122.
211. Bennett PN. Use of the monographs on drugs. In: Bennett PN, editor. Drugs and human lactation. 2nd ed. London: Elsevier; 1996. p. 70–3. https://www.sciencedirect.com/science/article/abs/pii/B9780444819819500242.
212. Cocksedge S, George B, Renwick S, Chew-Graham CA. Touch in primary care consultations: qualitative investigation of doctors' and patients' perceptions. Br J Gen Pract. 2013;63(609):e283–90. PMCID: PMC3609476. http://www.ncbi.nlm.nih.gov/pubmed/23540485.
213. Cocksedge S, May C. Doctors' perceptions of personal boundaries to primary care interactions: a qualitative investigation. Commun Med. 2009;6(2):109–16. PMID: 20635548. http://www.ncbi.nlm.nih.gov/pubmed/20635548.
214. Luca A, Luca M, Calandra C. Sleep disorders and depression: brief review of the literature, case report, and nonpharmacologic interventions for depression. Clin Interv Aging. 2013;8:1033–9. PMCID: PMC3760296. http://www.ncbi.nlm.nih.gov/pubmed/24019746.
215. Wolf E, Kuhn M, Normann C, Mainberger F, Maier JG, Maywald S, Bredl A, Klöppel S, Biber K, van Calker D, Riemann D, Sterr A, Nissen C. Synaptic plasticity model of therapeutic sleep deprivation in major depression. Sleep Med Rev. 2016;30:53–62. PMID: 26803484. http://www.ncbi.nlm.nih.gov/pubmed/26803484.
216. BaHammam AS, Kendzerska T, Gupta R, Ramasubramanian C, Neubauer DN, Narasimhan M, Pandi-Perumal SR, Moscovitch A. Comorbid depression in obstructive sleep apnea: an under-recognized association. Sleep Breath. 2016;20(2):447–56. PMID: 26156890. http://www.ncbi.nlm.nih.gov/pubmed/26156890.
217. Gupta MA, Simpson FC, Lyons DCA. The effect of treating obstructive sleep apnea with positive airway pressure on depression and other subjective symptoms: a systematic review and meta-analysis. Sleep Med Rev. 2016;28:55–68. PMID: 26454823. http://www.ncbi.nlm.nih.gov/pubmed/26454823.
218. EHCP. AHRQ comparative effectiveness reviews. Rockville: Agency for Healthcare Research and Quality (US); 2005. https://www.ncbi.nlm.nih.gov/books/NBK42934/.
219. Benedetti F, Riccaboni R, Locatelli C, Poletti S, Dallaspezia S, Colombo C. Rapid treatment response of suicidal symptoms to lithium, sleep deprivation, and light therapy (chronotherapeutics) in drug-resistant bipolar depression. J Clin Psychiatry. 2014;75(2):133–40. PMID: 24345382. http://www.ncbi.nlm.nih.gov/pubmed/24345382.
220. Steinberg H, Hegerl U. Johann Christian August Heinroth on sleep deprivation as a therapeutic option for depressive disorders. Sleep Med. 2014;15(9):1159–64. PMID: 24994565. http://www.ncbi.nlm.nih.gov/pubmed/24994565.
221. Sahlem GL, Kalivas B, Fox JB, Lamb K, Roper A, Williams EN, Williams NR, Korte JE, Zuschlag ZD, El Sabbagh S, Guille C, Barth KS, Uhde TW, George MS, Short EB. Adjunctive triple chronotherapy (combined total sleep deprivation, sleep phase advance, and bright light therapy) rapidly improves mood and suicidality in suicidal depressed inpatients: an open label pilot study. J Psychiatr Res. 2014;59:101–7. PMCID: PMC4252537. http://www.ncbi.nlm.nih.gov/pubmed/25231629.
222. Wu JC, Bunney WE. The biological basis of an antidepressant response to sleep deprivation and relapse: review and hypothesis. Am J Psychiatry. 1990;147(1):14–21. PMID: 2403471. http://www.ncbi.nlm.nih.gov/pubmed/2403471.
223. Dallaspezia S, Benedetti F. Sleep deprivation therapy for depression. Curr Top Behav Neurosci. 2015;25:483–502. PMID: 25549913. http://www.ncbi.nlm.nih.gov/pubmed/25549913.
224. Dopierała E, Rybakowski J. Sleep deprivation as a method of chronotherapy in the treatment of depression. Psychiatr Pol. 2015;49(3):423–33. PMID: 26276912. http://www.ncbi.nlm.nih.gov/pubmed/26276912.
225. Echizenya M, Suda H, Takeshima M, Inomata Y, Shimizu T. Total sleep deprivation followed by sleep phase advance and bright light therapy in drug-resistant mood disorders. J Affect Disord. 2013;144(1–2):28–33. PMID: 22835846. http://www.ncbi.nlm.nih.gov/pubmed/22835846.
226. National Center on Sleep Disorders Research | NHLBI, NIH. https://www.nhlbi.nih.gov/about/divisions/division-lung-diseases/national-center-sleep-disorders-research.
227. Home – Sleep Research Society. https://sleepresearchsociety.org/.
228. American Academy of Sleep Medicine | AASM | Medical Society. https://aasm.org/.
229. Noetel M, Sanders T, Gallardo-Gómez D, Taylor P, Del Pozo Cruz B, van den Hoek D, Smith JJ, Mahoney J, Spathis J, Moresi M, Pagano R, Pagano L, Vasconcellos R, Arnott H, Varley B, Parker P, Biddle S, Lonsdale C. Effect of exercise for depression: systematic review and network meta-analysis of randomised controlled trials. BMJ. 2024;384:e075847. PMCID: PMC10870815. http://www.ncbi.nlm.nih.gov/pubmed/38355154.
230. Gleeson M, Bishop NC, Stensel DJ, Lindley MR, Mastana SS, Nimmo MA. The anti-inflammatory effects of exercise: mechanisms and implications for the prevention and treatment of disease. Nat Rev Immunol. 2011;11(9):607–15. PMID: 21818123. http://www.ncbi.nlm.nih.gov/pubmed/21818123.
231. Eyre HA, Papps E, Baune BT. Treating depression and depression-like behavior with physical activity: an immune perspective. Front

Psych. 2013;4:3. PMCID: PMC3562851. http://www.ncbi.nlm.nih.gov/pubmed/23382717.
232. Knöchel C, Oertel-Knöchel V, O'Dwyer L, Prvulovic D, Alves G, Kollmann B, Hampel H. Cognitive and behavioural effects of physical exercise in psychiatric patients. Prog Neurobiol. 2012;96(1):46–68. PMID: 22120173. http://www.ncbi.nlm.nih.gov/pubmed/22120173.
233. Lautenschlager NT, Cox K, Cyarto EV. The influence of exercise on brain aging and dementia. Biochim Biophys Acta. 2012;1822(3):474–81. PMID: 21810472. http://www.ncbi.nlm.nih.gov/pubmed/21810472.
234. Sarris J, Moylan S, Camfield DA, Pase MP, Mischoulon D, Berk M, Jacka FN, Schweitzer I. Complementary medicine, exercise, meditation, diet, and lifestyle modification for anxiety disorders: a review of current evidence. Evid Based Complement Alternat Med. 2012;2012:809653. PMCID: PMC3434451. http://www.ncbi.nlm.nih.gov/pubmed/22969831.
235. Eyre H, Baune BT. Neuroplastic changes in depression: a role for the immune system. Psychoneuroendocrinology. 2012;37(9):1397–416. PMID: 22525700. http://www.ncbi.nlm.nih.gov/pubmed/22525700.
236. Marosi K, Bori Z, Hart N, Sárga L, Koltai E, Radák Z, Nyakas C. Long-term exercise treatment reduces oxidative stress in the hippocampus of aging rats. Neuroscience. 2012;226:21–8. PMID: 22982624. http://www.ncbi.nlm.nih.gov/pubmed/22982624.
237. Erickson KI, Miller DL, Roecklein KA. The aging hippocampus: interactions between exercise, depression, and BDNF. Neuroscientist. 2012;18(1):82–97. PMCID: PMC3575139. http://www.ncbi.nlm.nih.gov/pubmed/21531985.
238. Pereira AC, Huddleston DE, Brickman AM, Sosunov AA, Hen R, McKhann GM, Sloan R, Gage FH, Brown TR, Small SA. An in vivo correlate of exercise-induced neurogenesis in the adult dentate gyrus. Proc Natl Acad Sci USA. 2007;104(13):5638–43. PMCID: PMC1838482. http://www.ncbi.nlm.nih.gov/pubmed/17374720.
239. Erickson KI, Voss MW, Prakash RS, Basak C, Szabo A, Chaddock L, Kim JS, Heo S, Alves H, White SM, Wojcicki TR, Mailey E, Vieira VJ, Martin SA, Pence BD, Woods JA, McAuley E, Kramer AF. Exercise training increases size of hippocampus and improves memory. Proc Natl Acad Sci USA. 2011;108(7):3017–22. PMCID: PMC3041121. http://www.ncbi.nlm.nih.gov/pubmed/21282661.
240. Eyre H, Baune BT. Neuroimmunological effects of physical exercise in depression. Brain Behav Immun. 2012;26(2):251–66. PMID: 21986304. http://www.ncbi.nlm.nih.gov/pubmed/21986304.
241. Rethorst CD, Toups MS, Greer TL, Nakonezny PA, Carmody TJ, Grannemann BD, Huebinger RM, Barber RC, Trivedi MH. Pro-inflammatory cytokines as predictors of antidepressant effects of exercise in major depressive disorder. Mol Psychiatry. 2013;18(10):1119–24. PMCID: PMC3511631. http://www.ncbi.nlm.nih.gov/pubmed/22925832.
242. Beavers KM, Brinkley TE, Nicklas BJ. Effect of exercise training on chronic inflammation. Clin Chim Acta. 2010;411(11–12):785–93. PMCID: PMC3629815. http://www.ncbi.nlm.nih.gov/pubmed/20188719.
243. Funk JA, Gohlke J, Kraft AD, McPherson CA, Collins JB, Jean HG. Voluntary exercise protects hippocampal neurons from trimethyltin injury: possible role of interleukin-6 to modulate tumor necrosis factor receptor-mediated neurotoxicity. Brain Behav Immun. 2011;25(6):1063–77. PMCID: PMC3138904. http://www.ncbi.nlm.nih.gov/pubmed/21435392.
244. Moon HY, Kim SH, Yang YR, Song P, Yu HS, Park HG, Hwang O, Lee-Kwon W, Seo JK, Hwang D, Choi JH, Bucala R, Ryu SH, Kim YS, Suh PG. Macrophage migration inhibitory factor mediates the antidepressant actions of voluntary exercise. Proc Natl Acad Sci USA. 2012;109(32):13094–9. PMCID: PMC3420190. http://www.ncbi.nlm.nih.gov/pubmed/22826223.
245. Duman CH, Schlesinger L, Terwilliger R, Russell DS, Newton SS, Duman RS. Peripheral insulin-like growth factor-I produces antidepressant-like behavior and contributes to the effect of exercise. Behav Brain Res. 2009;198(2):366–71. PMCID: PMC2729431. http://www.ncbi.nlm.nih.gov/pubmed/19056428.
246. Vukovic J, Colditz MJ, Blackmore DG, Ruitenberg MJ, Bartlett PF. Microglia modulate hippocampal neural precursor activity in response to exercise and aging. J Neurosci. 2012;32(19):6435–43. PMCID: PMC6621117. http://www.ncbi.nlm.nih.gov/pubmed/22573666.
247. Dinoff A, Herrmann N, Swardfager W, Gallagher D, Lanctôt KL. The effect of exercise on resting concentrations of peripheral brain-derived neurotrophic factor (BDNF) in major depressive disorder: a meta-analysis. J Psychiatr Res. 2018;105:123–31. PMID: 30219561. http://www.ncbi.nlm.nih.gov/pubmed/30219561.
248. Mawson AR. Stimulation-induced behavioral inhibition: a new model for understanding physical violence. Integr Physiol Behav Sci. 1999;34(3):177–97. PMID: 10534103. http://www.ncbi.nlm.nih.gov/pubmed/10534103.
249. Tops M, Boksem MAS, Luu P, Tucker DM. Brain substrates of behavioral programs associated with self-regulation. Front Psychol. 2010;1:152. PMCID: PMC3157933. http://www.ncbi.nlm.nih.gov/pubmed/21887146.
250. Rachman S. Fear and courage. San Francisco: W. H. Freeman & Company; 1978. https://openlibrary.org/books/OL17858354M/Fear_and_courage.
251. Biddle SJH, Asare M. Physical activity and mental health in children and adolescents: a review of reviews. Br J Sports Med. 2011;45(11):886–95. PMID: 21807669. http://www.ncbi.nlm.nih.gov/pubmed/21807669.
252. Erickson KI, Gildengers AG, Butters MA. Physical activity and brain plasticity in late adulthood. Dialogues Clin Neurosci. 2013;15(1):99–108. PMCID: PMC3622473. http://www.ncbi.nlm.nih.gov/pubmed/23576893.
253. Erickson KI, Weinstein AM, Lopez OL. Physical activity, brain plasticity, and Alzheimer's disease. Arch Med Res. 2012;43(8):615–21. PMCID: PMC3567914. http://www.ncbi.nlm.nih.gov/pubmed/23085449.
254. Smith GS. Aging and neuroplasticity. Dialogues Clin Neurosci. 2013;15(1):3–5. PMCID: PMC3622467. http://www.ncbi.nlm.nih.gov/pubmed/23576885.
255. Gomez-Pinilla F, Hillman C. The influence of exercise on cognitive abilities. Compr Physiol. 2013;3(1):403–28. PMCID: PMC3951958. http://www.ncbi.nlm.nih.gov/pubmed/23720292.
256. Smith PJ, Blumenthal JA, Hoffman BM, Cooper H, Strauman TA, Welsh-Bohmer K, Browndyke JN, Sherwood A. Aerobic exercise and neurocognitive performance: a meta-analytic review of randomized controlled trials. Psychosom Med. 2010;72(3):239–52. PMCID: PMC2897704. http://www.ncbi.nlm.nih.gov/pubmed/20223924.
257. Colcombe SJ, Kramer AF, Erickson KI, Scalf P, McAuley E, Cohen NJ, Webb A, Jerome GJ, Marquez DX, Elavsky S. Cardiovascular fitness, cortical plasticity, and aging. Proc Natl Acad Sci USA. 2004;101(9):3316–21. PMCID: PMC373255. http://www.ncbi.nlm.nih.gov/pubmed/14978288.
258. Burkhalter TM, Hillman CH. A narrative review of physical activity, nutrition, and obesity to cognition and scholastic performance across the human lifespan. Adv Nutr. 2011;2(2):201S–6S. PMCID: PMC3065760. http://www.ncbi.nlm.nih.gov/pubmed/22332052.
259. Voss MW, Erickson KI, Prakash RS, Chaddock L, Kim JS, Alves H, Szabo A, Phillips SM, Wójcicki TR, Mailey EL, Olson EA, Gothe N, Vieira-Potter VJ, Martin SA, Pence BD, Cook MD, Woods JA, McAuley E, Kramer AF. Neurobiological markers of exercise-related brain plasticity in older adults. Brain Behav Immun. 2013;28:90–9. PMCID: PMC3544982. http://www.ncbi.nlm.nih.gov/pubmed/23123199.

260. Thomas AG, Dennis A, Bandettini PA, Johansen-Berg H. The effects of aerobic activity on brain structure. Front Psychol. 2012;3:86. PMCID: PMC3311131. http://www.ncbi.nlm.nih.gov/pubmed/22470361.
261. Voss MW, Prakash RS, Erickson KI, Basak C, Chaddock L, Kim JS, Alves H, Heo S, Szabo AN, White SM, Wójcicki TR, Mailey EL, Gothe N, Olson EA, McAuley E, Kramer AF. Plasticity of brain networks in a randomized intervention trial of exercise training in older adults. Front Aging Neurosci. 2010;2:32. PMCID: PMC2947936. http://www.ncbi.nlm.nih.gov/pubmed/20890449.
262. Weinstein AM, Voss MW, Prakash RS, Chaddock L, Szabo A, White SM, Wojcicki TR, Mailey E, McAuley E, Kramer AF, Erickson KI. The association between aerobic fitness and executive function is mediated by prefrontal cortex volume. Brain Behav Immun. 2012;26(5):811–9. PMCID: PMC3321393. http://www.ncbi.nlm.nih.gov/pubmed/22172477.
263. Bosker FJ, Hartman CA, Nolte IM, Prins BP, Terpstra P, Posthuma D, van Veen T, Willemsen G, DeRijk RH, de Geus EJ, Hoogendijk WJ, Sullivan PF, Penninx BW, Boomsma DI, Snieder H, Nolen WA. Poor replication of candidate genes for major depressive disorder using genome-wide association data. Mol Psychiatry. 2011;16(5):516–32. PMID: 20351714. http://www.ncbi.nlm.nih.gov/pubmed/20351714.
264. Sommer WH, Lidström J, Sun H, Passer D, Eskay R, Parker SCJ, Witt SH, Zimmermann US, Nieratschker V, Rietschel M, Margulies EH, Palkovits M, Laucht M, Heilig M. Human NPY promoter variation rs16147:T>C as a moderator of prefrontal NPY gene expression and negative affect. Hum Mutat. 2010;31(8):E1594–608. PMCID: PMC2908962. http://www.ncbi.nlm.nih.gov/pubmed/20648632.
265. Zhou Z, Zhu G, Hariri AR, Enoch MA, Scott D, Sinha R, Virkkunen M, Mash DC, Lipsky RH, Hu XZ, Hodgkinson CA, Xu K, Buzas B, Yuan Q, Shen PH, Ferrell RE, Manuck SB, Brown SM, Hauger RL, Stohler CS, Zubieta JK, Goldman D. Genetic variation in human NPY expression affects stress response and emotion. Nature. 2008;452(7190):997–1001. PMCID: PMC2715959. http://www.ncbi.nlm.nih.gov/pubmed/18385673.
266. Domschke K, Dannlowski U, Hohoff C, Ohrmann P, Bauer J, Kugel H, Zwanzger P, Heindel W, Deckert J, Arolt V, Suslow T, Baune BT. Neuropeptide Y (NPY) gene: impact on emotional processing and treatment response in anxious depression. Eur Neuropsychopharmacol. 2010;20(5):301–9. PMID: 19854625. http://www.ncbi.nlm.nih.gov/pubmed/19854625.
267. Witt SH, Buchmann AF, Blomeyer D, Nieratschker V, Treutlein J, Esser G, Schmidt MH, Bidlingmaier M, Wiedemann K, Rietschel M, Laucht M, Wüst S, Zimmermann US. An interaction between a neuropeptide Y gene polymorphism and early adversity modulates endocrine stress responses. Psychoneuroendocrinology. 2011;36(7):1010–20. PMID: 21273004. http://www.ncbi.nlm.nih.gov/pubmed/21273004.
268. Melas PA, Lennartsson A, Vakifahmetoglu-Norberg H, Wei Y, Åberg E, Werme M, Rogdaki M, Mannervik M, Wegener G, Brené S, Mathé AA, Lavebratt C. Allele-specific programming of Npy and epigenetic effects of physical activity in a genetic model of depression. Transl Psychiatry. 2013;3(5):e255. PMCID: PMC3669918. http://www.ncbi.nlm.nih.gov/pubmed/23652932.
269. Beserra AHN, Kameda P, Deslandes AC, Schuch FB, Laks J, de Moraes HS. Can physical exercise modulate cortisol level in subjects with depression? A systematic review and meta-analysis. Trends Psychiatry Psychother. 2018;40(4):360–8. PMID: 30570106. http://www.ncbi.nlm.nih.gov/pubmed/30570106.
270. Schuch FB, Deslandes AC, Stubbs B, Gosmann NP, da Silva CTB, Fleck MPDA. Neurobiological effects of exercise on major depressive disorder: a systematic review. Neurosci Biobehav Rev. 2016;61:1–11. PMID: 26657969. http://www.ncbi.nlm.nih.gov/pubmed/26657969.
271. Angevaren M, Aufdemkampe G, Verhaar HJJ, Aleman A, Vanhees L. Physical activity and enhanced fitness to improve cognitive function in older people without known cognitive impairment. Cochrane Database Syst Rev. 2008;(2):CD005381. PMID: 18425918. http://www.ncbi.nlm.nih.gov/pubmed/18425918.
272. Karp A, Paillard-Borg S, Wang HX, Silverstein M, Winblad B, Fratiglioni L. Mental, physical and social components in leisure activities equally contribute to decrease dementia risk. Dement Geriatr Cogn Disord. 2006;21(2):65–73. PMID: 16319455. http://www.ncbi.nlm.nih.gov/pubmed/16319455.
273. Globas C, Becker C, Cerny J, Lam JM, Lindemann U, Forrester LW, Macko RF, Luft AR. Chronic stroke survivors benefit from high-intensity aerobic treadmill exercise: a randomized control trial. Neurorehabil Neural Repair. 2012;26(1):85–95. PMID: 21885867. http://www.ncbi.nlm.nih.gov/pubmed/21885867.
274. Ahlskog JE, Geda YE, Graff-Radford NR, Petersen RC. Physical exercise as a preventive or disease-modifying treatment of dementia and brain aging. Mayo Clin Proc. 2011;86(9):876–84. PMCID: PMC3258000. http://www.ncbi.nlm.nih.gov/pubmed/21878600.
275. Sasco AJ, Paffenbarger RS, Gendre I, Wing AL. The role of physical exercise in the occurrence of Parkinson's disease. Arch Neurol. 1992;49(4):360–5. PMID: 1558515. http://www.ncbi.nlm.nih.gov/pubmed/1558515.
276. Ahlskog JE. Does vigorous exercise have a neuroprotective effect in Parkinson disease? Neurology. 2011;77(3):288–94. PMCID: PMC3136051. http://www.ncbi.nlm.nih.gov/pubmed/21768599.
277. Verstynen TD, Lynch B, Miller DL, Voss MW, Prakash RS, Chaddock L, Basak C, Szabo A, Olson EA, Wojcicki TR, Fanning J, Gothe NP, McAuley E, Kramer AF, Erickson KI. Caudate nucleus volume mediates the link between cardiorespiratory fitness and cognitive flexibility in older adults. J Aging Res. 2012;2012:939285. PMCID: PMC3415086. http://www.ncbi.nlm.nih.gov/pubmed/22900181.
278. Lautenschlager NT, Cox KL, Flicker L, Foster JK, van Bockxmeer FM, Xiao J, Greenop KR, Almeida OP. Effect of physical activity on cognitive function in older adults at risk for Alzheimer disease: a randomized trial. JAMA. 2008;300(9):1027–37. PMID: 18768414. http://www.ncbi.nlm.nih.gov/pubmed/18768414.
279. Nouchi R, Taki Y, Takeuchi H, Hashizume H, Nozawa T, Sekiguchi A, Nouchi H, Kawashima R. Beneficial effects of short-term combination exercise training on diverse cognitive functions in healthy older people: study protocol for a randomized controlled trial. Trials. 2012;13:200. PMCID: PMC3495024. http://www.ncbi.nlm.nih.gov/pubmed/23107038.
280. Obisesan TO, Gillum RF, Johnson S, Umar N, Williams D, Bond V, Kwagyan J. Neuroprotection and neurodegeneration in Alzheimer's disease: role of cardiovascular disease risk factors, implications for dementia rates, and prevention with aerobic exercise in african americans. Int J Alzheimers Dis. 2012;2012:568382. PMCID: PMC3345220. http://www.ncbi.nlm.nih.gov/pubmed/22577592.
281. Hryhorczuk C, Sharma S, Fulton SE. Metabolic disturbances connecting obesity and depression. Front Neurosci. 2013;7:177. PMCID: PMC3791387. http://www.ncbi.nlm.nih.gov/pubmed/24109426.
282. Liu C, Lee S, Elmquist JK. Circuits controlling energy balance and mood: inherently intertwined or just complicated intersections? Cell Metab. 2014;19(6):902–9. PMCID: PMC4047152. http://www.ncbi.nlm.nih.gov/pubmed/24630814.
283. Shelton RC, Falola M, Li L, Zajecka J, Fava M, Papakostas GI. The pro-inflammatory profile of depressed patients is (partly) related to obesity. J Psychiatr Res. 2015;70:91–7. PMCID: PMC4734093. http://www.ncbi.nlm.nih.gov/pubmed/26424427.
284. Chan JSY, Liu G, Liang D, Deng K, Wu J, Yan JH. Special issue – therapeutic benefits of physical activity for mood: a systematic review on the effects of exercise intensity, duration, and modality.

J Psychol. 2019;153(1):102–25. PMID: 30321106. http://www.ncbi.nlm.nih.gov/pubmed/30321106.

285. Seikaly MG, Arant BS, Seney FD. Endogenous angiotensin concentrations in specific intrarenal fluid compartments of the rat. J Clin Invest. 1990;86(4):1352–7. PMCID: PMC296870. http://www.ncbi.nlm.nih.gov/pubmed/2212017.

286. Garber CE, Blissmer B, Deschenes MR, Franklin BA, Lamonte MJ, Lee IM, Nieman DC, Swain DP, American College of Sports Medicine. American College of Sports Medicine position stand. Quantity and quality of exercise for developing and maintaining cardiorespiratory, musculoskeletal, and neuromotor fitness in apparently healthy adults: guidance for prescribing exercise. Med Sci Sports Exerc. 2011;43(7):1334–59. PMID: 21694556. http://www.ncbi.nlm.nih.gov/pubmed/21694556.

287. Voisin S, Eynon N, Yan X, Bishop DJ. Exercise training and DNA methylation in humans. Acta Physiol (Oxf). 2015;213(1):39–59. PMID: 25345837. http://www.ncbi.nlm.nih.gov/pubmed/25345837.

288. Khoury R, Nagy C. Running from stress: a perspective on the potential benefits of exercise-induced small extracellular vesicles for individuals with major depressive disorder. Front Mol Biosci. 2023;10:1154872. PMCID: PMC10309045. http://www.ncbi.nlm.nih.gov/pubmed/37398548.

289. Chong MC, Shah AD, Schittenhelm RB, Silva A, James PF, Wu SSX, Howitt J. Acute exercise-induced release of innate immune proteins via small extracellular vesicles changes with aerobic fitness and age. Acta Physiol (Oxf). 2024;240(3):e14095. PMID: 38243724. http://www.ncbi.nlm.nih.gov/pubmed/38243724.

290. Kuznetsova M, Wilson C, Cheng L, Pang T, Li S, Roberts BR, Lago LC, Tran H, Hill AF, Hannan AJ, Renoir T. Serotonergic-dependent effects of exercise and elevated stress hormone on small non-coding RNA transcriptomics and proteomics in a mouse model of affective disorders. Neuropharmacology. 2025;265:110240. PMID: 39613253. http://www.ncbi.nlm.nih.gov/pubmed/39613253.

291. Berk M, Jacka F. Preventive strategies in depression: gathering evidence for risk factors and potential interventions. Br J Psychiatry. 2012;201(5):339–41. PMID: 23118032. http://www.ncbi.nlm.nih.gov/pubmed/23118032.

292. Pasco JA, Williams LJ, Jacka FN, Henry MJ, Coulson CE, Brennan SL, Leslie E, Nicholson GC, Kotowicz MA, Berk M. Habitual physical activity and the risk for depressive and anxiety disorders among older men and women. Int Psychogeriatr. 2011;23(2):292–8. PMID: 20863424. http://www.ncbi.nlm.nih.gov/pubmed/20863424.

293. Rethorst CD, Wipfli BM, Landers DM. The antidepressive effects of exercise: a meta-analysis of randomized trials. Sports Med. 2009;39(6):491–511. PMID: 19453207. http://www.ncbi.nlm.nih.gov/pubmed/19453207.

294. Trivedi MH, Greer TL, Church TS, Carmody TJ, Grannemann BD, Galper DI, Dunn AL, Earnest CP, Sunderajan P, Henley SS, Blair SN. Exercise as an augmentation treatment for nonremitted major depressive disorder: a randomized, parallel dose comparison. J Clin Psychiatry. 2011;72(5):677–84. PMCID: PMC9900872. http://www.ncbi.nlm.nih.gov/pubmed/21658349.

295. Hamer M, Sabia S, Batty GD, Shipley MJ, Tabák AG, Singh-Manoux A, Kivimaki M. Physical activity and inflammatory markers over 10 years: follow-up in men and women from the Whitehall II cohort study. Circulation. 2012;126(8):928–33. PMCID: PMC3890998. http://www.ncbi.nlm.nih.gov/pubmed/22891048.

296. Baune BT, Stuart M, Gilmour A, Wersching H, Heindel W, Arolt V, Berger K. The relationship between subtypes of depression and cardiovascular disease: a systematic review of biological models. Transl Psychiatry. 2012;2(3):e92. PMCID: PMC3309537. http://www.ncbi.nlm.nih.gov/pubmed/22832857.

297. Baune BT, Thome J. Translational research approach to biological and modifiable risk factors of psychosis and affective disorders. World J Biol Psychiatry. 2011;12(Suppl 1):28–34. PMID: 21905992. http://www.ncbi.nlm.nih.gov/pubmed/21905992.

298. Stuart MJ, Baune BT. Depression and type 2 diabetes: inflammatory mechanisms of a psychoneuroendocrine co-morbidity. Neurosci Biobehav Rev. 2012;36(1):658–76. PMID: 22020230. http://www.ncbi.nlm.nih.gov/pubmed/22020230.

299. Lim SS, Vos T, Flaxman AD, Danaei G, Shibuya K, Adair-Rohani H, Amann M, Anderson HR, Andrews KG, Aryee M, Atkinson C, Bacchus LJ, Bahalim AN, Balakrishnan K, Balmes J, Barker-Collo S, Baxter A, Bell ML, Blore JD, Blyth F, Bonner C, Borges G, Bourne R, Boussinesq M, Brauer M, Brooks P, Bruce NG, Brunekreef B, Bryan-Hancock C, Bucello C, Buchbinder R, Bull F, Burnett RT, Byers TE, Calabria B, Carapetis J, Carnahan E, Chafe Z, Charlson F, Chen H, Chen JS, Cheng ATA, Child JC, Cohen A, Colson KE, Cowie BC, Darby S, Darling S, Davis A, Degenhardt L, Dentener F, Des Jarlais DC, Devries K, Dherani M, Ding EL, Dorsey ER, Driscoll T, Edmond K, Ali SE, Engell RE, Erwin PJ, Fahimi S, Falder G, Farzadfar F, Ferrari A, Finucane MM, Flaxman S, Fowkes FGR, Freedman G, Freeman MK, Gakidou E, Ghosh S, Giovannucci E, Gmel G, Graham K, Grainger R, Grant B, Gunnell D, Gutierrez HR, Hall W, Hoek HW, Hogan A, Hosgood HD, Hoy D, Hu H, Hubbell BJ, Hutchings SJ, Ibeanusi SE, Jacklyn GL, Jasrasaria R, Jonas JB, Kan H, Kanis JA, Kassebaum N, Kawakami N, Khang YH, Khatibzadeh S, Khoo JP, Kok C, Laden F, Lalloo R, Lan Q, Lathlean T, Leasher JL, Leigh J, Li Y, Lin JK, Lipshultz SE, London S, Lozano R, Lu Y, Mak J, Malekzadeh R, Mallinger L, Marcenes W, March L, Marks R, Martin R, McGale P, McGrath J, Mehta S, Mensah GA, Merriman TR, Micha R, Michaud C, Mishra V, Mohd Hanafiah K, Mokdad AA, Morawska L, Mozaffarian D, Murphy T, Naghavi M, Neal B, Nelson PK, Nolla JM, Norman R, Olives C, Omer SB, Orchard J, Osborne R, Ostro B, Page A, Pandey KD, Parry CDH, Passmore E, Patra J, Pearce N, Pelizzari PM, Petzold M, Phillips MR, Pope D, Pope CA, Powles J, Rao M, Razavi H, Rehfuess EA, Rehm JT, Ritz B, Rivara FP, Roberts T, Robinson C, Rodriguez-Portales JA, Romieu I, Room R, Rosenfeld LC, Roy A, Rushton L, Salomon JA, Sampson U, Sanchez-Riera L, Sanman E, Sapkota A, Seedat S, Shi P, Shield K, Shivakoti R, Singh GM, Sleet DA, Smith E, Smith KR, Stapelberg NJC, Steenland K, Stöckl H, Stovner LJ, Straif K, Straney L, Thurston GD, Tran JH, Van Dingenen R, van Donkelaar A, Veerman JL, Vijayakumar L, Weintraub R, Weissman MM, White RA, Whiteford H, Wiersma ST, Wilkinson JD, Williams HC, Williams W, Wilson N, Woolf AD, Yip P, Zielinski JM, Lopez AD, Murray CJL, Ezzati M, AlMazroa MA, Memish ZA. A comparative risk assessment of burden of disease and injury attributable to 67 risk factors and risk factor clusters in 21 regions, 1990-2010: a systematic analysis for the Global Burden of Disease Study 2010. Lancet. 2012;380(9859):2224–60. PMCID: PMC4156511. http://www.ncbi.nlm.nih.gov/pubmed/23245609.

300. Lee IM, Shiroma EJ, Lobelo F, Puska P, Blair SN, Katzmarzyk PT, Lancet Physical Activity Series Working Group. Effect of physical inactivity on major non-communicable diseases worldwide: an analysis of burden of disease and life expectancy. Lancet. 2012;380(9838):219–29. PMCID: PMC3645500. http://www.ncbi.nlm.nih.gov/pubmed/22818936.

301. Pasco JA, Jacka FN, Williams LJ, Brennan SL, Leslie E, Berk M. Don't worry, be active: positive affect and habitual physical activity. Aust N Z J Psychiatry. 2011;45(12):1047–52. PMID: 22059484. http://www.ncbi.nlm.nih.gov/pubmed/22059484.

302. Rimer J, Dwan K, Lawlor DA, Greig CA, McMurdo M, Morley W, Mead GE. Exercise for depression. Cochrane Database Syst Rev. 2012;(7):CD004366. PMID: 22786489. http://www.ncbi.nlm.nih.gov/pubmed/22786489.

303. Rush AJ, Trivedi MH, Wisniewski SR, Nierenberg AA, Stewart JW, Warden D, Niederehe G, Thase ME, Lavori PW, Lebowitz BD, McGrath PJ, Rosenbaum JF, Sackeim HA, Kupfer DJ, Luther

J, Fava M. Acute and longer-term outcomes in depressed outpatients requiring one or several treatment steps: a STAR*D report. Am J Psychiatry. 2006;163(11):1905–17. PMID: 17074942. http://www.ncbi.nlm.nih.gov/pubmed/17074942.
304. Rush AJ, Trivedi MH, Wisniewski SR, Stewart JW, Nierenberg AA, Thase ME, Ritz L, Biggs MM, Warden D, Luther JF, Shores-Wilson K, Niederehe G, Fava M, STAR*D Study Team. Bupropion-SR, sertraline, or venlafaxine-XR after failure of SSRIs for depression. N Engl J Med. 2006;354(12):1231–42. PMID: 16554525. http://www.ncbi.nlm.nih.gov/pubmed/16554525.
305. Deslandes AC, Moraes H, Alves H, Pompeu FAMS, Silveira H, Mouta R, Arcoverde C, Ribeiro P, Cagy M, Piedade RAM, Laks J, Coutinho ESF. Effect of aerobic training on EEG alpha asymmetry and depressive symptoms in the elderly: a 1-year follow-up study. Braz J Med Biol Res. 2010;43(6):585–92. PMID: 20464340. http://www.ncbi.nlm.nih.gov/pubmed/20464340.
306. Salmon P. Effects of physical exercise on anxiety, depression, and sensitivity to stress: a unifying theory. Clin Psychol Rev. 2001;21(1):33–61. PMID: 11148895. http://www.ncbi.nlm.nih.gov/pubmed/11148895.
307. Asmundson GJG, Fetzner MG, Deboer LB, Powers MB, Otto MW, Smits JAJ. Let's get physical: a contemporary review of the anxiolytic effects of exercise for anxiety and its disorders. Depress Anxiety. 2013;30(4):362–73. PMID: 23300122. http://www.ncbi.nlm.nih.gov/pubmed/23300122.
308. Foster PP, Rosenblatt KP, Kuljiš RO. Exercise-induced cognitive plasticity, implications for mild cognitive impairment and Alzheimer's disease. Front Neurol. 2011;2:28. PMCID: PMC3092070. http://www.ncbi.nlm.nih.gov/pubmed/21602910.
309. Lee HB, Lyketsos CG. Depression in Alzheimer's disease: heterogeneity and related issues. Biol Psychiatry. 2003;54(3):353–62. PMID: 12893110. http://www.ncbi.nlm.nih.gov/pubmed/12893110.
310. Eyre HA, Baune BT. Assessing for unique immunomodulatory and neuroplastic profiles of physical activity subtypes: a focus on psychiatric disorders. Brain Behav Immun. 2014;39:42–55. PMID: 24269526. http://www.ncbi.nlm.nih.gov/pubmed/24269526.
311. Burgener SC, Yang Y, Gilbert R, Marsh-Yant S. The effects of a multimodal intervention on outcomes of persons with early-stage dementia. Am J Alzheimers Dis Other Dement. 2008;23(4):382–94. PMCID: PMC3014218. http://www.ncbi.nlm.nih.gov/pubmed/18453642.
312. Mahendra N, Arkin S. Effects of four years of exercise, language, and social interventions on Alzheimer discourse. J Commun Disord. 2003;36(5):395–422. PMID: 12927946. http://www.ncbi.nlm.nih.gov/pubmed/12927946.
313. Hoffman BM, Blumenthal JA, Babyak MA, Smith PJ, Rogers SD, Doraiswamy PM, Sherwood A. Exercise fails to improve neurocognition in depressed middle-aged and older adults. Med Sci Sports Exerc. 2008;40(7):1344–52. PMCID: PMC2745928. http://www.ncbi.nlm.nih.gov/pubmed/18580416.
314. Bridle C, Spanjers K, Patel S, Atherton NM, Lamb SE. Effect of exercise on depression severity in older people: systematic review and meta-analysis of randomised controlled trials. Br J Psychiatry. 2012;201(3):180–5. PMID: 22945926. http://www.ncbi.nlm.nih.gov/pubmed/22945926.
315. Blumenthal JA, Sherwood A, Babyak MA, Watkins LL, Smith PJ, Hoffman BM, O'Hayer CVF, Mabe S, Johnson J, Doraiswamy PM, Jiang W, Schocken DD, Hinderliter AL. Exercise and pharmacological treatment of depressive symptoms in patients with coronary heart disease: results from the UPBEAT (Understanding the Prognostic Benefits of Exercise and Antidepressant Therapy) study. J Am Coll Cardiol. 2012;60(12):1053–63. PMCID: PMC3498445. http://www.ncbi.nlm.nih.gov/pubmed/22858387.
316. Blumenthal JA, Babyak MA, O'Connor C, Keteyian S, Landzberg J, Howlett J, Kraus W, Gottlieb S, Blackburn G, Swank A, Whellan DJ. Effects of exercise training on depressive symptoms in patients with chronic heart failure: the HF-ACTION randomized trial. JAMA. 2012;308(5):465–74. PMCID: PMC3953459. http://www.ncbi.nlm.nih.gov/pubmed/22851113.
317. Abdelbasset WK, Alqahtani BA. A randomized controlled trial on the impact of moderate-intensity continuous aerobic exercise on the depression status of middle-aged patients with congestive heart failure. Medicine. 2019;98(17):e15344. PMCID: PMC6831310. http://www.ncbi.nlm.nih.gov/pubmed/31027110.
318. Rodgers WM, Murray TC, Selzler AM, Norman P. Development and impact of exercise self-efficacy types during and after cardiac rehabilitation. Rehabil Psychol. 2013;58(2):178–84. PMID: 23713728. http://www.ncbi.nlm.nih.gov/pubmed/23713728.
319. Barnett F. The effect of exercise on affective and self-efficacy responses in older and younger women. J Phys Act Health. 2013;10(1):97–105. PMID: 22396245. http://www.ncbi.nlm.nih.gov/pubmed/22396245.
320. Clum GA, Rice JC, Broussard M, Johnson CC, Webber LS. Associations between depressive symptoms, self-efficacy, eating styles, exercise and body mass index in women. J Behav Med. 2014;37(4):577–86. PMID: 23934179. http://www.ncbi.nlm.nih.gov/pubmed/23934179.
321. Fox K. The effects of exercise on self-perceptions and self-esteem. In: Biddle Sjh FK, editor. Physical activity and psychological well-being. London: Routledge; 2000. p. 88–117.
322. Knapen J, Sommerijns E, Vancampfort D, Sienaert P, Pieters G, Haake P, Probst M, Peuskens J. State anxiety and subjective well-being responses to acute bouts of aerobic exercise in patients with depressive and anxiety disorders. Br J Sports Med. 2009;43(10):756–9. PMID: 19019899. http://www.ncbi.nlm.nih.gov/pubmed/19019899.
323. Derdikman-Eiron R, Indredavik MS, Bratberg GH, Taraldsen G, Bakken IJ, Colton M. Gender differences in subjective well-being, self-esteem and psychosocial functioning in adolescents with symptoms of anxiety and depression: findings from the Nord-Trøndelag Health Study. Scand J Psychol. 2011;52(3):261–7. PMID: 21265857. http://www.ncbi.nlm.nih.gov/pubmed/21265857.
324. Diener E. Subjective well-being. Psychol Bull. 1984;95(3):542–75. PMID: 6399758. http://www.ncbi.nlm.nih.gov/pubmed/6399758.
325. Häfner S, Emeny RT, Lacruz ME, Baumert J, Herder C, Koenig W, Thorand B, Ladwig KH, KORA Study Investigators. Association between social isolation and inflammatory markers in depressed and non-depressed individuals: results from the MONICA/KORA study. Brain Behav Immun. 2011;25(8):1701–7. PMID: 21756997. http://www.ncbi.nlm.nih.gov/pubmed/21756997.
326. Herring MP, Puetz TW, O'Connor PJ, Dishman RK. Effect of exercise training on depressive symptoms among patients with a chronic illness: a systematic review and meta-analysis of randomized controlled trials. Arch Intern Med. 2012;172(2):101–11. PMID: 22271118. http://www.ncbi.nlm.nih.gov/pubmed/22271118.
327. Blumenthal JA, Babyak MA, Moore KA, Craighead WE, Herman S, Khatri P, Waugh R, Napolitano MA, Forman LM, Appelbaum M, Doraiswamy PM, Krishnan KR. Effects of exercise training on older patients with major depression. Arch Intern Med. 1999;159(19):2349–56. PMID: 10547175. http://www.ncbi.nlm.nih.gov/pubmed/10547175.
328. Babyak M, Blumenthal JA, Herman S, Khatri P, Doraiswamy M, Moore K, Craighead WE, Baldewicz TT, Krishnan KR. Exercise treatment for major depression: maintenance of therapeutic benefit at 10 months. Psychosom Med. 2000;62(5):633–8. PMID: 11020092. http://www.ncbi.nlm.nih.gov/pubmed/11020092.
329. Schuch FB, Vancampfort D, Richards J, Rosenbaum S, Ward PB, Stubbs B. Exercise as a treatment for depression: a meta-analysis adjusting for publication bias. J Psychiatr Res.

2016;77:42–51. PMID: 26978184. http://www.ncbi.nlm.nih.gov/pubmed/26978184.
330. Bailey AP, Hetrick SE, Rosenbaum S, Purcell R, Parker AG. Treating depression with physical activity in adolescents and young adults: a systematic review and meta-analysis of randomised controlled trials. Psychol Med. 2018;48(7):1068–83. PMID: 28994355. http://www.ncbi.nlm.nih.gov/pubmed/28994355.
331. Morris L, Stander J, Ebrahim W, Eksteen S, Meaden OA, Ras A, Wessels A. Effect of exercise versus cognitive behavioural therapy or no intervention on anxiety, depression, fitness and quality of life in adults with previous methamphetamine dependency: a systematic review. Addict Sci Clin Pract. 2018;13(1):4. PMCID: PMC5771022. http://www.ncbi.nlm.nih.gov/pubmed/29338767.
332. Morres ID, Hatzigeorgiadis A, Stathi A, Comoutos N, Arpin-Cribbie C, Krommidas C, Theodorakis Y. Aerobic exercise for adult patients with major depressive disorder in mental health services: a systematic review and meta-analysis. Depress Anxiety. 2019;36(1):39–53. PMID: 30334597. http://www.ncbi.nlm.nih.gov/pubmed/30334597.
333. Miller KJ, Gonçalves-Bradley DC, Areerob P, Hennessy D, Mesagno C, Grace F. Comparative effectiveness of three exercise types to treat clinical depression in older adults: a systematic review and network meta-analysis of randomised controlled trials. Ageing Res Rev. 2020;58:100999. PMID: 31837462. http://www.ncbi.nlm.nih.gov/pubmed/31837462.
334. Li Z, Liu S, Wang L, Smith L. Mind-body exercise for anxiety and depression in COPD patients: a systematic review and meta-analysis. Int J Environ Res Public Health. 2019;17(1):22. PMCID: PMC6981896. http://www.ncbi.nlm.nih.gov/pubmed/31861418.
335. Zou L, Yeung A, Quan X, Hui SSC, Hu X, Chan JSM, Wang C, Boyden SD, Sun L, Wang H. Mindfulness-based Baduanjin exercise for depression and anxiety in people with physical or mental illnesses: a systematic review and meta-analysis. Int J Environ Res Public Health. 2018;15(2):321. PMCID: PMC5858390. http://www.ncbi.nlm.nih.gov/pubmed/29439556.
336. Zou L, Pan Z, Yeung A, Talwar S, Wang C, Liu Y, Shu Y, Chen X, Thomas GA. A review study on the beneficial effects of Baduanjin. J Altern Complement Med. 2018;24(4):324–35. PMID: 29227709. http://www.ncbi.nlm.nih.gov/pubmed/29227709.
337. Zou L, Yeung A, Quan X, Boyden SD, Wang H. A systematic review and meta-analysis of mindfulness-based (Baduanjin) exercise for alleviating musculoskeletal pain and improving sleep quality in people with chronic diseases. Int J Environ Res Public Health. 2018;15(2):206. PMCID: PMC5858275. http://www.ncbi.nlm.nih.gov/pubmed/29370149.
338. Zou L, Wang H, Xiao Z, Fang Q, Zhang M, Li T, Du G, Liu Y. Tai chi for health benefits in patients with multiple sclerosis: a systematic review. PLoS One. 2017;12(2):e0170212. PMCID: PMC5300172. http://www.ncbi.nlm.nih.gov/pubmed/28182629.
339. Zou L, Wang C, Chen K, Shu Y, Chen X, Luo L, Zhao X. The effect of Taichi practice on attenuating bone mineral density loss: a systematic review and meta-analysis of randomized controlled trials. Int J Environ Res Public Health. 2017;14(9):1000. PMCID: PMC5615537. http://www.ncbi.nlm.nih.gov/pubmed/28862661.
340. Zou L, Yeung A, Li C, Wei GX, Chen KW, Kinser PA, Chan JSM, Ren Z. Effects of meditative movements on major depressive disorder: a systematic review and meta-analysis of randomized controlled trials. J Clin Med. 2018;7(8):195. PMCID: PMC6111244. http://www.ncbi.nlm.nih.gov/pubmed/30071662.
341. Eustis EH, Ernst S, Sutton K, Battle CL. Innovations in the treatment of perinatal depression: the role of yoga and physical activity interventions during pregnancy and postpartum. Curr Psychiatry Rep. 2019;21(12):133. PMID: 31802268. http://www.ncbi.nlm.nih.gov/pubmed/31802268.
342. Schwarz L, Dorscht L, Book S, Stelzer EM, Kornhuber J, Luttenberger K. Long-term effects of bouldering psychotherapy on depression: benefits can be maintained across a 12-month follow-up. Heliyon. 2019;5(12):e02929. PMCID: PMC6911955. http://www.ncbi.nlm.nih.gov/pubmed/31872117.
343. Dorscht L, Karg N, Book S, Graessel E, Kornhuber J, Luttenberger K. A German climbing study on depression: a bouldering psychotherapeutic group intervention in outpatients compared with state-of-the-art cognitive behavioural group therapy and physical activation – study protocol for a multicentre randomised controlled trial. BMC Psychiatry. 2019;19(1):154. PMCID: PMC6525374. http://www.ncbi.nlm.nih.gov/pubmed/31101097.
344. Luttenberger K, Stelzer EM, Först S, Schopper M, Kornhuber J, Book S. Indoor rock climbing (bouldering) as a new treatment for depression: study design of a waitlist-controlled randomized group pilot study and the first results. BMC Psychiatry. 2015;15:201. PMCID: PMC4548691. http://www.ncbi.nlm.nih.gov/pubmed/26302900.
345. Stelzer EM, Book S, Graessel E, Hofner B, Kornhuber J, Luttenberger K. Bouldering psychotherapy reduces depressive symptoms even when general physical activity is controlled for: a randomized controlled trial. Heliyon. 2018;4(3):e00580. PMCID: PMC5968135. http://www.ncbi.nlm.nih.gov/pubmed/29862344.
346. Nakamura A, van der Waerden J, Melchior M, Bolze C, El-Khoury F, Pryor L. Physical activity during pregnancy and postpartum depression: systematic review and meta-analysis. J Affect Disord. 2019;246:29–41. PMID: 30576955. http://www.ncbi.nlm.nih.gov/pubmed/30576955.
347. Davenport MH, McCurdy AP, Mottola MF, Skow RJ, Meah VL, Poitras VJ, Jaramillo Garcia A, Gray CE, Barrowman N, Riske L, Sobierajski F, James M, Nagpal T, Marchand AA, Nuspl M, Slater LG, Barakat R, Adamo KB, Davies GA, Ruchat SM. Impact of prenatal exercise on both prenatal and postnatal anxiety and depressive symptoms: a systematic review and meta-analysis. Br J Sports Med. 2018;52(21):1376–85. PMID: 30337464. http://www.ncbi.nlm.nih.gov/pubmed/30337464.
348. Artal R, O'Toole M. Guidelines of the American College of Obstetricians and Gynecologists for exercise during pregnancy and the postpartum period. Br J Sports Med. 2003;37(1):6–12; discussion 12. PMCID: PMC1724598. http://www.ncbi.nlm.nih.gov/pubmed/12547738.
349. Robledo-Colonia AF, Sandoval-Restrepo N, Mosquera-Valderrama YF, Escobar-Hurtado C, Ramírez-Vélez R. Aerobic exercise training during pregnancy reduces depressive symptoms in nulliparous women: a randomised trial. J Physiother. 2012;58(1):9–15. PMID: 22341377. http://www.ncbi.nlm.nih.gov/pubmed/22341377.
350. Da Costa D, Rippen N, Dritsa M, Ring A. Self-reported leisure-time physical activity during pregnancy and relationship to psychological well-being. J Psychosom Obstet Gynaecol. 2003;24(2):111–9. PMID: 12854395. http://www.ncbi.nlm.nih.gov/pubmed/12854395.
351. Songøygard KM, Stafne SN, Evensen KAI, Salvesen KÅ, Vik T, Mørkved S. Does exercise during pregnancy prevent postnatal depression? A randomized controlled trial. Acta Obstet Gynecol Scand. 2012;91(1):62–7. PMID: 21880023. http://www.ncbi.nlm.nih.gov/pubmed/21880023.
352. Norman E, Sherburn M, Osborne RH, Galea MP. An exercise and education program improves well-being of new mothers: a randomized controlled trial. Phys Ther. 2010;90(3):348–55. PMID: 20056720. http://www.ncbi.nlm.nih.gov/pubmed/20056720.
353. Heh SS, Huang LH, Ho SM, Fu YY, Wang LL. Effectiveness of an exercise support program in reducing the severity of postnatal depression in Taiwanese women. Birth. 2008;35(1):60–5. PMID: 18307489. http://www.ncbi.nlm.nih.gov/pubmed/18307489.
354. Armstrong K, Edwards H. The effects of exercise and social support on mothers reporting depressive symptoms: a pilot randomized

controlled trial. Int J Ment Health Nurs. 2003;12(2):130–8. PMID: 12956024. http://www.ncbi.nlm.nih.gov/pubmed/12956024.
355. Dritsa M, Da Costa D, Dupuis G, Lowensteyn I, Khalifé S. Effects of a home-based exercise intervention on fatigue in postpartum depressed women: results of a randomized controlled trial. Ann Behav Med. 2008;35(2):179–87. PMID: 18373127. http://www.ncbi.nlm.nih.gov/pubmed/18373127.
356. Strawbridge WJ, Deleger S, Roberts RE, Kaplan GA. Physical activity reduces the risk of subsequent depression for older adults. Am J Epidemiol. 2002;156(4):328–34. PMID: 12181102. http://www.ncbi.nlm.nih.gov/pubmed/12181102.
357. Mota-Pereira J, Silverio J, Carvalho S, Ribeiro JC, Fonte D, Ramos J. Moderate exercise improves depression parameters in treatment-resistant patients with major depressive disorder. J Psychiatr Res. 2011;45(8):1005–11. PMID: 21377690. http://www.ncbi.nlm.nih.gov/pubmed/21377690.
358. Nikolakopoulou A, Higgins JPT, Papakonstantinou T, Chaimani A, Del Giovane C, Egger M, Salanti G. CINeMA: an approach for assessing confidence in the results of a network meta-analysis. PLoS Med. 2020;17(4):e1003082. PMCID: PMC7122720. http://www.ncbi.nlm.nih.gov/pubmed/32243458.
359. Mead GE, Morley W, Campbell P, Greig CA, McMurdo M, Lawlor DA. Exercise for depression. Cochrane Database Syst Rev. 2008;(4):CD004366. PMID: 18843656. http://www.ncbi.nlm.nih.gov/pubmed/18843656.
360. Cooney GM, Dwan K, Greig CA, Lawlor DA, Rimer J, Waugh FR, McMurdo M, Mead GE. Exercise for depression. Cochrane Database Syst Rev. 2013;2013(9):CD004366. PMCID: PMC9721454. http://www.ncbi.nlm.nih.gov/pubmed/24026850.
361. Sun M, Lanctot K, Herrmann N, Gallagher D. Exercise for cognitive symptoms in depression: a systematic review of interventional studies. Can J Psychiatr. 2018;63(2):115–28. PMCID: PMC5788135. http://www.ncbi.nlm.nih.gov/pubmed/29186973.
362. Zhuang PC, Tan ZN, Jia ZY, Wang B, Grady JJ, Ma XM. Treadmill exercise reverses depression model-induced alteration of dendritic spines in the brain areas of mood circuit. Front Behav Neurosci. 2019;13:93. PMCID: PMC6509176. http://www.ncbi.nlm.nih.gov/pubmed/31130853.
363. Schuch FB, Vancampfort D, Rosenbaum S, Richards J, Ward PB, Veronese N, Solmi M, Cadore EL, Stubbs B. Exercise for depression in older adults: a meta-analysis of randomized controlled trials adjusting for publication bias. Braz J Psychiatry. 2016;38(3):247–54. PMCID: PMC7194268. http://www.ncbi.nlm.nih.gov/pubmed/27611903.
364. Brondino N, Rocchetti M, Fusar-Poli L, Codrons E, Correale L, Vandoni M, Barbui C, Politi P. A systematic review of cognitive effects of exercise in depression. Acta Psychiatr Scand. 2017;135(4):285–95. PMID: 28110494. http://www.ncbi.nlm.nih.gov/pubmed/28110494.
365. Lawlor DA, Hopker SW. The effectiveness of exercise as an intervention in the management of depression: systematic review and meta-regression analysis of randomised controlled trials. BMJ. 2001;322(7289):763–7. PMCID: PMC30551. http://www.ncbi.nlm.nih.gov/pubmed/11282860.
366. Chalder M, Wiles NJ, Campbell J, Hollinghurst SP, Searle A, Haase AM, Taylor AH, Fox KR, Baxter H, Davis M, Thorp H, Winder R, Wright C, Calnan M, Lawlor DA, Peters TJ, Sharp DJ, Turner KM, Montgomery AA, Lewis G. A pragmatic randomised controlled trial to evaluate the cost-effectiveness of a physical activity intervention as a treatment for depression: the treating depression with physical activity (TREAD) trial. Health Technol Assess. 2012;16(10):1–164, iii–iv. PMID: 22398106. http://www.ncbi.nlm.nih.gov/pubmed/22398106.
367. Krogh J, Nordentoft M, Sterne JAC, Lawlor DA. The effect of exercise in clinically depressed adults: systematic review and meta-analysis of randomized controlled trials. J Clin Psychiatry. 2011;72(4):529–38. PMID: 21034688. http://www.ncbi.nlm.nih.gov/pubmed/21034688.
368. Krogh J, Hjorthøj C, Speyer H, Gluud C, Nordentoft M. Exercise for patients with major depression: a systematic review with meta-analysis and trial sequential analysis. BMJ Open. 2017;7(9):e014820. PMCID: PMC5623558. http://www.ncbi.nlm.nih.gov/pubmed/28928174.
369. Wray NR, Ripke S, Mattheisen M, Trzaskowski M, Byrne EM, Abdellaoui A, Adams MJ, Agerbo E, Air TM, Andlauer TMF, Bacanu SA, Bækvad-Hansen M, Beekman AFT, Bigdeli TB, Binder EB, Blackwood DRH, Bryois J, Buttenschøn HN, Bybjerg-Grauholm J, Cai N, Castelao E, Christensen JH, Clarke TK, Coleman JIR, Colodro-Conde L, Couvy-Duchesne B, Craddock N, Crawford GE, Crowley CA, Dashti HS, Davies G, Deary IJ, Degenhardt F, Derks EM, Direk N, Dolan CV, Dunn EC, Eley TC, Eriksson N, Escott-Price V, Kiadeh FHF, Finucane HK, Forstner AJ, Frank J, Gaspar HA, Gill M, Giusti-Rodríguez P, Goes FS, Gordon SD, Grove J, Hall LS, Hannon E, Hansen CS, Hansen TF, Herms S, Hickie IB, Hoffmann P, Homuth G, Horn C, Hottenga JJ, Hougaard DM, Hu M, Hyde CL, Ising M, Jansen R, Jin F, Jorgenson E, Knowles JA, Kohane IS, Kraft J, Kretzschmar WW, Krogh J, Kutalik Z, Lane JM, Li Y, Li Y, Lind PA, Liu X, Lu L, MacIntyre DJ, MacKinnon DF, Maier RM, Maier W, Marchini J, Mbarek H, McGrath P, McGuffin P, Medland SE, Mehta D, Middeldorp CM, Mihailov E, Milaneschi Y, Milani L, Mill J, Mondimore FM, Montgomery GW, Mostafavi S, Mullins N, Nauck M, Ng B, Nivard MG, Nyholt DR, O'Reilly PF, Oskarsson H, Owen MJ, Painter JN, Pedersen CB, Pedersen MG, Peterson RE, Pettersson E, Peyrot WJ, Pistis G, Posthuma D, Purcell SM, Quiroz JA, Qvist P, Rice JP, Riley BP, Rivera M, Saeed Mirza S, Saxena R, Schoevers R, Schulte EC, Shen L, Shi J, Shyn SI, Sigurdsson E, Sinnamon GBC, Smit JH, Smith DJ, Stefansson H, Steinberg S, Stockmeier CA, Streit F, Strohmaier J, Tansey KE, Teismann H, Teumer A, Thompson W, Thomson PA, Thorgeirsson TE, Tian C, Traylor M, Treutlein J, Trubetskoy V, Uitterlinden AG, Umbricht D, Van der Auwera S, van Hemert AM, Viktorin A, Visscher PM, Wang Y, Webb BT, Weinsheimer SM, Wellmann J, Willemsen G, Witt SH, Wu Y, Xi HS, Yang J, Zhang F, eQTLGen, 23andMe, Arolt V, Baune BT, Berger K, Boomsma DI, Cichon S, Dannlowski U, de Geus ECJ, DePaulo JR, Domenici E, Domschke K, Esko T, Grabe HJ, Hamilton SP, Hayward C, Heath AC, Hinds DA, Kendler KS, Kloiber S, Lewis G, Li QS, Lucae S, Madden PFA, Magnusson PK, Martin NG, McIntosh AM, Metspalu A, Mors O, Mortensen PB, Müller-Myhsok B, Nordentoft M, Nöthen MM, O'Donovan MC, Paciga SA, Pedersen NL, Penninx BWJH, Perlis RH, Porteous DJ, Potash JB, Preisig M, Rietschel M, Schaefer C, Schulze TG, Smoller JW, Stefansson K, Tiemeier H, Uher R, Völzke H, Weissman MM, Werge T, Winslow AR, Lewis CM, Levinson DF, Breen G, Børglum AD, Sullivan PF, Major Depressive Disorder Working Group of the Psychiatric Genomics Consortium. Genome-wide association analyses identify 44 risk variants and refine the genetic architecture of major depression. Nat Genet. 2018;50(5):668–81. PMCID: PMC5934326. http://www.ncbi.nlm.nih.gov/pubmed/29700475.
370. Boes AD, Kelly MS, Trapp NT, Stern AP, Press DZ, Pascual-Leone A. Noninvasive brain stimulation: challenges and opportunities for a new clinical specialty. J Neuropsychiatry Clin Neurosci. 2018;30(3):173–9. PMID: 29685065. http://www.ncbi.nlm.nih.gov/pubmed/29685065.
371. Cook IA, Espinoza R, Leuchter AF. Neuromodulation for depression: invasive and noninvasive (deep brain stimulation, transcranial magnetic stimulation, trigeminal nerve stimulation). Neurosurg Clin N Am. 2014;25(1):103–16. PMID: 24262903. http://www.ncbi.nlm.nih.gov/pubmed/24262903.

372. Wagner T, Valero-Cabre A, Pascual-Leone A. Noninvasive human brain stimulation. Annu Rev Biomed Eng. 2007;9:527–65. PMID: 17444810. http://www.ncbi.nlm.nih.gov/pubmed/17444810.
373. Lisanby SH. Electroconvulsive therapy for depression. N Engl J Med. 2007;357(19):1939–45. PMID: 17989386. http://www.ncbi.nlm.nih.gov/pubmed/17989386.
374. Solomon JG. Electroconvulsive therapy: an overview. Va Med. 1979;106(5):280–2, 287–8. PMID: 441398. http://www.ncbi.nlm.nih.gov/pubmed/441398.
375. Holtzheimer PE, Mayberg HS. Stuck in a rut: rethinking depression and its treatment. Trends Neurosci. 2011;34(1):1–9. PMCID: PMC3014414. http://www.ncbi.nlm.nih.gov/pubmed/21067824.
376. Fekadu A, Wooderson S, Donaldson C, Markopoulou K, Masterson B, Poon L, Cleare AJ. A multidimensional tool to quantify treatment resistance in depression: the Maudsley staging method. J Clin Psychiatry. 2009;70(2):177–84. PMID: 19192471. http://www.ncbi.nlm.nih.gov/pubmed/19192471.
377. Trevino K, McClintock SM, McDonald Fischer N, Vora A, Husain MM. Defining treatment-resistant depression: a comprehensive review of the literature. Ann Clin Psychiatry. 2014;26(3):222–32. PMID: 25166485. http://www.ncbi.nlm.nih.gov/pubmed/25166485.
378. Akil H, Gordon J, Hen R, Javitch J, Mayberg H, McEwen B, Meaney MJ, Nestler EJ. Treatment resistant depression: a multi-scale, systems biology approach. Neurosci Biobehav Rev. 2018;84:272–88. PMCID: PMC5729118. http://www.ncbi.nlm.nih.gov/pubmed/28859997.
379. McClintock SM, Kallioniemi E, Martin DM, Kim JU, Weisenbach SL, Abbott CC. A critical review and synthesis of clinical and neurocognitive effects of noninvasive neuromodulation antidepressant therapies. Focus (Am Psychiatr Publ). 2019;17(1):18–29. PMCID: PMC6493152. http://www.ncbi.nlm.nih.gov/pubmed/31975955.
380. Fidalgo TM, Morales-Quezada JL, Muzy GSC, Chiavetta NM, Mendonca ME, Santana MVB, Goncalves OF, Brunoni AR, Fregni F. Biological markers in noninvasive brain stimulation trials in major depressive disorder: a systematic review. J ECT. 2014;30(1):47–61. PMCID: PMC4260176. http://www.ncbi.nlm.nih.gov/pubmed/23845938.
381. Schaller G, Sperling W, Richter-Schmidinger T, Mühle C, Heberlein A, Maihöfner C, Kornhuber J, Lenz B. Serial repetitive transcranial magnetic stimulation (rTMS) decreases BDNF serum levels in healthy male volunteers. J Neural Transm (Vienna). 2014;121(3):307–13. PMID: 24158279. http://www.ncbi.nlm.nih.gov/pubmed/24158279.
382. Lee JC, Blumberger DM, Fitzgerald PB, Daskalakis ZJ, Levinson AJ. The role of transcranial magnetic stimulation in treatment-resistant depression: a review. Curr Pharm Des. 2012;18(36):5846–52. PMID: 22681165. http://www.ncbi.nlm.nih.gov/pubmed/22681165.
383. Berlim MT, Van den Eynde F, Daskalakis ZJ. Clinical utility of transcranial direct current stimulation (tDCS) for treating major depression: a systematic review and meta-analysis of randomized, double-blind and sham-controlled trials. J Psychiatr Res. 2013;47(1):1–7. PMID: 23084964. http://www.ncbi.nlm.nih.gov/pubmed/23084964.
384. Kalu UG, Sexton CE, Loo CK, Ebmeier KP. Transcranial direct current stimulation in the treatment of major depression: a meta-analysis. Psychol Med. 2012;42(9):1791–800. PMID: 22236735. http://www.ncbi.nlm.nih.gov/pubmed/22236735.
385. McClintock SM, Reti IM, Carpenter LL, McDonald WM, Dubin M, Taylor SF, Cook IA, O'Reardon J, Husain MM, Wall C, Krystal AD, Sampson SM, Morales O, Nelson BG, Latoussakis V, George MS, Lisanby SH, National Network of Depression Centers rTMS Task Group, American Psychiatric Association Council on Research Task Force on Novel Biomarkers and Treatments. Consensus recommendations for the clinical application of repetitive transcranial magnetic stimulation (rTMS) in the treatment of depression. J Clin Psychiatry. 2018;79(1):16cs10905. PMCID: PMC5846193. http://www.ncbi.nlm.nih.gov/pubmed/28541649.
386. Somani A, Kar SK. Efficacy of repetitive transcranial magnetic stimulation in treatment-resistant depression: the evidence thus far. Gen Psychiatr. 2019;32(4):e100074. PMCID: PMC6738665. http://www.ncbi.nlm.nih.gov/pubmed/31552384.
387. Slotema CW, Blom JD, Hoek HW, Sommer IEC. Should we expand the toolbox of psychiatric treatment methods to include repetitive transcranial magnetic stimulation (rTMS)? A meta-analysis of the efficacy of rTMS in psychiatric disorders. J Clin Psychiatry. 2010;71(7):873–84. PMID: 20361902. http://www.ncbi.nlm.nih.gov/pubmed/20361902.
388. Deng ZD, Lisanby SH, Peterchev AV. Electric field depth-focality tradeoff in transcranial magnetic stimulation: simulation comparison of 50 coil designs. Brain Stimul. 2013;6(1):1–13. PMCID: PMC3568257. http://www.ncbi.nlm.nih.gov/pubmed/22483681.
389. Kamble N, Netravathi M, Pal PK. Therapeutic applications of repetitive transcranial magnetic stimulation (rTMS) in movement disorders: a review. Parkinsonism Relat Disord. 2014;20(7):695–707. PMID: 24726453. http://www.ncbi.nlm.nih.gov/pubmed/24726453.
390. Hallett M. Transcranial magnetic stimulation: a primer. Neuron. 2007;55(2):187–99. PMID: 17640522. http://www.ncbi.nlm.nih.gov/pubmed/17640522.
391. Groppa S, Oliviero A, Eisen A, Quartarone A, Cohen LG, Mall V, Kaelin-Lang A, Mima T, Rossi S, Thickbroom GW, Rossini PM, Ziemann U, Valls-Solé J, Siebner HR. A practical guide to diagnostic transcranial magnetic stimulation: report of an IFCN committee. Clin Neurophysiol. 2012;123(5):858–82. PMCID: PMC4890546. http://www.ncbi.nlm.nih.gov/pubmed/22349304.
392. Leuchter AF, Cook IA, Feifel D, Goethe JW, Husain M, Carpenter LL, Thase ME, Krystal AD, Philip NS, Bhati MT, Burke WJ, Howland RH, Sheline YI, Aaronson ST, Iosifescu DV, O'Reardon JP, Gilmer WS, Jain R, Burgoyne KS, Phillips B, Manberg PJ, Massaro J, Hunter AM, Lisanby SH, George MS. Efficacy and safety of low-field synchronized transcranial magnetic stimulation (sTMS) for treatment of major depression. Brain Stimul. 2015;8(4):787–94. PMID: 26143022. http://www.ncbi.nlm.nih.gov/pubmed/26143022.
393. Suppa A, Huang YZ, Funke K, Ridding MC, Cheeran B, Di Lazzaro V, Ziemann U, Rothwell JC. Ten years of theta burst stimulation in humans: established knowledge, unknowns and prospects. Brain Stimul. 2016;9(3):323–35. PMID: 26947241. http://www.ncbi.nlm.nih.gov/pubmed/26947241.
394. Blumberger DM, Vila-Rodriguez F, Thorpe KE, Feffer K, Noda Y, Giacobbe P, Knyahnytska Y, Kennedy SH, Lam RW, Daskalakis ZJ, Downar J. Effectiveness of theta burst versus high-frequency repetitive transcranial magnetic stimulation in patients with depression (THREE-D): a randomised non-inferiority trial. Lancet. 2018;391(10131):1683–92. PMID: 29726344. http://www.ncbi.nlm.nih.gov/pubmed/29726344.
395. Trevizol AP, Vigod SN, Daskalakis ZJ, Vila-Rodriguez F, Downar J, Blumberger DM. Intermittent theta burst stimulation for major depression during pregnancy. Brain Stimul. 2019;12(3):772–4. PMID: 30665752. http://www.ncbi.nlm.nih.gov/pubmed/30665752.
396. Chen L, Chung SW, Hoy KE, Fitzgerald PB. Is theta burst stimulation ready as a clinical treatment for depression? Expert Rev Neurother. 2019;19(11):1089–102. PMID: 31282224. http://www.ncbi.nlm.nih.gov/pubmed/31282224.
397. Lipton RB, Dodick DW, Silberstein SD, Saper JR, Aurora SK, Pearlman SH, Fischell RE, Ruppel PL, Goadsby PJ. Single-pulse transcranial magnetic stimulation for acute treatment of migraine with aura: a randomised, double-blind, parallel-group,

sham-controlled trial. Lancet Neurol. 2010;9(4):373–80. PMID: 20206581. http://www.ncbi.nlm.nih.gov/pubmed/20206581.
398. Hsu WY, Cheng CH, Liao KK, Lee IH, Lin YY. Effects of repetitive transcranial magnetic stimulation on motor functions in patients with stroke: a meta-analysis. Stroke. 2012;43(7):1849–57. PMID: 22713491. http://www.ncbi.nlm.nih.gov/pubmed/22713491.
399. Dougall N, Maayan N, Soares-Weiser K, McDermott LM, McIntosh A. Transcranial magnetic stimulation (TMS) for schizophrenia. Cochrane Database Syst Rev. 2015;2015(8):CD006081. PMCID: PMC9395125. http://www.ncbi.nlm.nih.gov/pubmed/26289586.
400. Rossi S, Hallett M, Rossini PM, Pascual-Leone A, Safety of TMS Consensus Group. Safety, ethical considerations, and application guidelines for the use of transcranial magnetic stimulation in clinical practice and research. Clin Neurophysiol. 2009;120(12):2008–39. PMCID: PMC3260536. http://www.ncbi.nlm.nih.gov/pubmed/19833552.
401. Dobek CE, Blumberger DM, Downar J, Daskalakis ZJ, Vila-Rodriguez F. Risk of seizures in transcranial magnetic stimulation: a clinical review to inform consent process focused on bupropion. Neuropsychiatr Dis Treat. 2015;11:2975–87. PMCID: PMC4670017. http://www.ncbi.nlm.nih.gov/pubmed/26664122.
402. Duecker F, Sack AT. Rethinking the role of sham TMS. Front Psychol. 2015;6:210. PMCID: PMC4341423. http://www.ncbi.nlm.nih.gov/pubmed/25767458.
403. Davis NJ, Gold E, Pascual-Leone A, Bracewell RM. Challenges of proper placebo control for non-invasive brain stimulation in clinical and experimental applications. Eur J Neurosci. 2013;38(7):2973–7. PMID: 23869660. http://www.ncbi.nlm.nih.gov/pubmed/23869660.
404. Lefaucheur JP, André-Obadia N, Antal A, Ayache SS, Baeken C, Benninger DH, Cantello RM, Cincotta M, de Carvalho M, De Ridder D, Devanne H, Di Lazzaro V, Filipović SR, Hummel FC, Jääskeläinen SK, Kimiskidis VK, Koch G, Langguth B, Nyffeler T, Oliviero A, Padberg F, Poulet E, Rossi S, Rossini PM, Rothwell JC, Schönfeldt-Lecuona C, Siebner HR, Slotema CW, Stagg CJ, Valls-Sole J, Ziemann U, Paulus W, Garcia-Larrea L. Evidence-based guidelines on the therapeutic use of repetitive transcranial magnetic stimulation (rTMS). Clin Neurophysiol. 2014;125(11):2150–206. PMID: 25034472. http://www.ncbi.nlm.nih.gov/pubmed/25034472.
405. Broadbent HJ, van den Eynde F, Guillaume S, Hanif EL, Stahl D, David AS, Campbell IC, Schmidt U. Blinding success of rTMS applied to the dorsolateral prefrontal cortex in randomised sham-controlled trials: a systematic review. World J Biol Psychiatry. 2011;12(4):240–8. PMID: 21426265. http://www.ncbi.nlm.nih.gov/pubmed/21426265.
406. Chantebel R, Chesneau A, Tavernier E, El-Hage W, Caille A. Completeness of descriptions of repetitive transcranial magnetic stimulation intervention: a systematic review of randomized controlled trials of rTMS in depression. J ECT. 2019;35(1):7–13. PMID: 30308571. http://www.ncbi.nlm.nih.gov/pubmed/30308571.
407. Gaynes BN, Lloyd SW, Lux L, Gartlehner G, Hansen RA, Brode S, Jonas DE, Swinson Evans T, Viswanathan M, Lohr KN. Repetitive transcranial magnetic stimulation for treatment-resistant depression: a systematic review and meta-analysis. J Clin Psychiatry. 2014;75(5):477–89; quiz 489. PMID: 24922485. http://www.ncbi.nlm.nih.gov/pubmed/24922485.
408. Magavi LR, Reti IM, Vasa RA. A review of repetitive transcranial magnetic stimulation for adolescents with treatment-resistant depression. Int Rev Psychiatry. 2017;29(2):79–88. PMID: 28306351. http://www.ncbi.nlm.nih.gov/pubmed/28306351.
409. Chen JJ, Zhao LB, Liu YY, Fan SH, Xie P. Comparative efficacy and acceptability of electroconvulsive therapy versus repetitive transcranial magnetic stimulation for major depression: a systematic review and multiple-treatments meta-analysis. Behav Brain Res. 2017;320:30–6. PMID: 27876667. http://www.ncbi.nlm.nih.gov/pubmed/27876667.
410. Razza LB, Moffa AH, Moreno ML, Carvalho AF, Padberg F, Fregni F, Brunoni AR. A systematic review and meta-analysis on placebo response to repetitive transcranial magnetic stimulation for depression trials. Prog Neuro-Psychopharmacol Biol Psychiatry. 2018;81:105–13. PMID: 29111404. http://www.ncbi.nlm.nih.gov/pubmed/29111404.
411. Hung YY, Yang LH, Stubbs B, Li DJ, Tseng PT, Yeh TC, Chen TY, Liang CS, Chu CS. Efficacy and tolerability of deep transcranial magnetic stimulation for treatment-resistant depression: a systematic review and meta-analysis. Prog Neuro-Psychopharmacol Biol Psychiatry. 2020;99:109850. PMID: 31863873. http://www.ncbi.nlm.nih.gov/pubmed/31863873.
412. McIntyre A, Thompson S, Burhan A, Mehta S, Teasell R. Repetitive transcranial magnetic stimulation for depression due to cerebrovascular disease: a systematic review. J Stroke Cerebrovasc Dis. 2016;25(12):2792–800. PMID: 27743927. http://www.ncbi.nlm.nih.gov/pubmed/27743927.
413. Cirillo P, Gold AK, Nardi AE, Ornelas AC, Nierenberg AA, Camprodon J, Kinrys G. Transcranial magnetic stimulation in anxiety and trauma-related disorders: a systematic review and meta-analysis. Brain Behav. 2019;9(6):e01284. PMCID: PMC6576151. http://www.ncbi.nlm.nih.gov/pubmed/31066227.
414. Cole J, Bright K, Gagnon L, McGirr A. A systematic review of the safety and effectiveness of repetitive transcranial magnetic stimulation in the treatment of peripartum depression. J Psychiatr Res. 2019;115:142–50. PMID: 31129438. http://www.ncbi.nlm.nih.gov/pubmed/31129438.
415. Ganho-Ávila A, Poleszczyk A, Mohamed MMA, Osório A. Efficacy of rTMS in decreasing postnatal depression symptoms: a systematic review. Psychiatry Res. 2019;279:315–22. PMID: 31196691. http://www.ncbi.nlm.nih.gov/pubmed/31196691.
416. Mutz J, Vipulananthan V, Carter B, Hurlemann R, Fu CHY, Young AH. Comparative efficacy and acceptability of non-surgical brain stimulation for the acute treatment of major depressive episodes in adults: systematic review and network meta-analysis. BMJ. 2019;364:l1079. PMCID: PMC6435996. http://www.ncbi.nlm.nih.gov/pubmed/30917990.
417. Magnezi R, Aminov E, Shmuel D, Dreifuss M, Dannon P. Comparison between neurostimulation techniques repetitive transcranial magnetic stimulation vs electroconvulsive therapy for the treatment of resistant depression: patient preference and cost-effectiveness. Patient Prefer Adherence. 2016;10:1481–7. PMCID: PMC4977067. http://www.ncbi.nlm.nih.gov/pubmed/27536079.
418. Mutz J, Edgcumbe DR, Brunoni AR, Fu CHY. Efficacy and acceptability of non-invasive brain stimulation for the treatment of adult unipolar and bipolar depression: a systematic review and meta-analysis of randomised sham-controlled trials. Neurosci Biobehav Rev. 2018;92:291–303. PMID: 29763711. http://www.ncbi.nlm.nih.gov/pubmed/29763711.
419. Iimori T, Nakajima S, Miyazaki T, Tarumi R, Ogyu K, Wada M, Tsugawa S, Masuda F, Daskalakis ZJ, Blumberger DM, Mimura M, Noda Y. Effectiveness of the prefrontal repetitive transcranial magnetic stimulation on cognitive profiles in depression, schizophrenia, and Alzheimer's disease: a systematic review. Prog Neuro-Psychopharmacol Biol Psychiatry. 2019;88:31–40. PMID: 29953934. http://www.ncbi.nlm.nih.gov/pubmed/29953934.
420. Sonmez AI, Camsari DD, Nandakumar AL, Voort JLV, Kung S, Lewis CP, Croarkin PE. Accelerated TMS for depression: a systematic review and meta-analysis. Psychiatry Res. 2019;273:770–81. PMCID: PMC6582998. http://www.ncbi.nlm.nih.gov/pubmed/31207865.
421. Senova S, Cotovio G, Pascual-Leone A, Oliveira-Maia AJ. Durability of antidepressant response to repetitive transcranial

magnetic stimulation: systematic review and meta-analysis. Brain Stimul. 2019;12(1):119–28. PMID: 30344109. http://www.ncbi.nlm.nih.gov/pubmed/30344109.

422. Miljevic A, Bailey NW, Herring SE, Fitzgerald PB. Potential predictors of depressive relapse following repetitive transcranial magnetic stimulation: a systematic review. J Affect Disord. 2019;256:317–23. PMID: 31201982. http://www.ncbi.nlm.nih.gov/pubmed/31201982.
423. Zis P, Shafique F, Hadjivassiliou M, Blackburn D, Venneri A, Iliodromiti S, Mitsikostas DD, Sarrigiannis PG. Safety, tolerability, and nocebo phenomena during transcranial magnetic stimulation: a systematic review and meta-analysis of placebo-controlled clinical trials. Neuromodulation. 2020;23(3):291–300. PMID: 30896060. http://www.ncbi.nlm.nih.gov/pubmed/30896060.
424. Liu C, Wang M, Liang X, Xue J, Zhang G. Efficacy and safety of high-frequency repetitive transcranial magnetic stimulation for poststroke depression: a systematic review and meta-analysis. Arch Phys Med Rehabil. 2019;100(10):1964–75. PMID: 31002813. http://www.ncbi.nlm.nih.gov/pubmed/31002813.
425. George MS, Lisanby SH, Avery D, McDonald WM, Durkalski V, Pavlicova M, Anderson B, Nahas Z, Bulow P, Zarkowski P, Holtzheimer PE, Schwartz T, Sackeim HA. Daily left prefrontal transcranial magnetic stimulation therapy for major depressive disorder: a sham-controlled randomized trial. Arch Gen Psychiatry. 2010;67(5):507–16. PMID: 20439832. http://www.ncbi.nlm.nih.gov/pubmed/20439832.
426. Lisanby SH, Husain MM, Rosenquist PB, Maixner D, Gutierrez R, Krystal A, Gilmer W, Marangell LB, Aaronson S, Daskalakis ZJ, Canterbury R, Richelson E, Sackeim HA, George MS. Daily left prefrontal repetitive transcranial magnetic stimulation in the acute treatment of major depression: clinical predictors of outcome in a multisite, randomized controlled clinical trial. Neuropsychopharmacology. 2009;34(2):522–34. PMID: 18704101. http://www.ncbi.nlm.nih.gov/pubmed/18704101.
427. What is tDCS? tDCS.com. https://tdcs.com/what-is-tdcs/.
428. Rosa MA, Lisanby SH. Somatic treatments for mood disorders. Neuropsychopharmacology. 2012;37(1):102–16. PMCID: PMC3238088. http://www.ncbi.nlm.nih.gov/pubmed/21976043.
429. Nitsche MA, Paulus W. Excitability changes induced in the human motor cortex by weak transcranial direct current stimulation. J Physiol. 2000;527 Pt3(Pt 3):633–9. PMCID: PMC2270099. http://www.ncbi.nlm.nih.gov/pubmed/10990547.
430. Nitsche MA, Paulus W. Sustained excitability elevations induced by transcranial DC motor cortex stimulation in humans. Neurology. 2001;57(10):1899–901. PMID: 11723286. http://www.ncbi.nlm.nih.gov/pubmed/11723286.
431. Utz KS, Dimova V, Oppenländer K, Kerkhoff G. Electrified minds: transcranial direct current stimulation (tDCS) and galvanic vestibular stimulation (GVS) as methods of non-invasive brain stimulation in neuropsychology--a review of current data and future implications. Neuropsychologia. 2010;48(10):2789–810. PMID: 20542047. http://www.ncbi.nlm.nih.gov/pubmed/20542047.
432. Chase HW, Boudewyn MA, Carter CS, Phillips ML. Transcranial direct current stimulation: a roadmap for research, from mechanism of action to clinical implementation. Mol Psychiatry. 2020;25(2):397–407. PMCID: PMC6981019. http://www.ncbi.nlm.nih.gov/pubmed/31455860.
433. Motohashi N, Yamaguchi M, Fujii T, Kitahara Y. Mood and cognitive function following repeated transcranial direct current stimulation in healthy volunteers: a preliminary report. Neurosci Res. 2013;77(1–2):64–9. PMID: 23811267. http://www.ncbi.nlm.nih.gov/pubmed/23811267.
434. Brunoni AR, Valiengo L, Baccaro A, Zanão TA, de Oliveira JF, Goulart A, Boggio PS, Lotufo PA, Benseñor IM, Fregni F. The sertraline vs. electrical current therapy for treating depression clinical study: results from a factorial, randomized, controlled trial. JAMA Psychiatry. 2013;70(4):383–91. PMID: 23389323. http://www.ncbi.nlm.nih.gov/pubmed/23389323.
435. Player MJ, Taylor JL, Weickert CS, Alonzo A, Sachdev PS, Martin D, Mitchell PB, Loo CK. Increase in PAS-induced neuroplasticity after a treatment course of transcranial direct current stimulation for depression. J Affect Disord. 2014;167:140–7. PMID: 24968188. http://www.ncbi.nlm.nih.gov/pubmed/24968188.
436. Lan MJ, Chhetry BT, Liston C, Mann JJ, Dubin M. Transcranial magnetic stimulation of left dorsolateral prefrontal cortex induces brain morphological changes in regions associated with a treatment resistant major depressive episode: an exploratory analysis. Brain Stimul. 2016;9(4):577–83. PMCID: PMC5554068. http://www.ncbi.nlm.nih.gov/pubmed/27017072.
437. Brunoni AR, Kemp AH, Shiozawa P, Cordeiro Q, Valiengo LCL, Goulart AC, Coprerski B, Lotufo PA, Brunoni D, Perez ABA, Fregni F, Benseñor IM. Impact of 5-HTTLPR and BDNF polymorphisms on response to sertraline versus transcranial direct current stimulation: implications for the serotonergic system. Eur Neuropsychopharmacol. 2013;23(11):1530–40. PMID: 23615118. http://www.ncbi.nlm.nih.gov/pubmed/23615118.
438. Martin DM, Moffa A, Nikolin S, Bennabi D, Brunoni AR, Flannery W, Haffen E, McClintock SM, Moreno ML, Padberg F, Palm U, Loo CK. Cognitive effects of transcranial direct current stimulation treatment in patients with major depressive disorder: an individual patient data meta-analysis of randomised, sham-controlled trials. Neurosci Biobehav Rev. 2018;90:137–45. PMID: 29660416. http://www.ncbi.nlm.nih.gov/pubmed/29660416.
439. Bikson M, Grossman P, Thomas C, Zannou AL, Jiang J, Adnan T, Mourdoukoutas AP, Kronberg G, Truong D, Boggio P, Brunoni AR, Charvet L, Fregni F, Fritsch B, Gillick B, Hamilton RH, Hampstead BM, Jankord R, Kirton A, Knotkova H, Liebetanz D, Liu A, Loo C, Nitsche MA, Reis J, Richardson JD, Rotenberg A, Turkeltaub PE, Woods AJ. Safety of transcranial direct current stimulation: evidence based update 2016. Brain Stimul. 2016;9(5):641–61. PMCID: PMC5007190. http://www.ncbi.nlm.nih.gov/pubmed/27372845.
440. Nikolin S, Huggins C, Martin D, Alonzo A, Loo CK. Safety of repeated sessions of transcranial direct current stimulation: a systematic review. Brain Stimul. 2018;11(2):278–88. PMID: 29169814. http://www.ncbi.nlm.nih.gov/pubmed/29169814.
441. Borrione L, Moffa AH, Martin D, Loo CK, Brunoni AR. Transcranial direct current stimulation in the acute depressive episode: a systematic review of current knowledge. J ECT. 2018;34(3):153–63. PMID: 29901497. http://www.ncbi.nlm.nih.gov/pubmed/29901497.
442. Fregni F, Boggio PS, Nitsche MA, Marcolin MA, Rigonatti SP, Pascual-Leone A. Treatment of major depression with transcranial direct current stimulation. Bipolar Disord. 2006;8(2):203–4. PMID: 16542193. http://www.ncbi.nlm.nih.gov/pubmed/16542193.
443. Boggio PS, Rigonatti SP, Ribeiro RB, Myczkowski ML, Nitsche MA, Pascual-Leone A, Fregni F. A randomized, double-blind clinical trial on the efficacy of cortical direct current stimulation for the treatment of major depression. Int J Neuropsychopharmacol. 2008;11(2):249–54. PMCID: PMC3372849. http://www.ncbi.nlm.nih.gov/pubmed/17559710.
444. Brunoni AR, Moffa AH, Sampaio-Junior B, Borrione L, Moreno ML, Fernandes RA, Veronezi BP, Nogueira BS, Aparicio LVM, Razza LB, Chamorro R, Tort LC, Fraguas R, Lotufo PA, Gattaz WF, Fregni F, Benseñor IM, ELECT-TDCS Investigators. Trial of electrical direct-current therapy versus escitalopram for depression. N Engl J Med. 2017;376(26):2523–33. PMID: 28657871. http://www.ncbi.nlm.nih.gov/pubmed/28657871.
445. Loo CK, Alonzo A, Martin D, Mitchell PB, Galvez V, Sachdev P. Transcranial direct current stimulation for depression: 3-week, randomised, sham-controlled trial. Br J Psychiatry.

2012;200(1):52–9. PMID: 22215866. http://www.ncbi.nlm.nih.gov/pubmed/22215866.
446. Loo CK, Sachdev P, Martin D, Pigot M, Alonzo A, Malhi GS, Lagopoulos J, Mitchell P. A double-blind, sham-controlled trial of transcranial direct current stimulation for the treatment of depression. Int J Neuropsychopharmacol. 2010;13(1):61–9. PMID: 19671217. http://www.ncbi.nlm.nih.gov/pubmed/19671217.
447. Loo CK, Husain MM, McDonald WM, Aaronson S, O'Reardon JP, Alonzo A, Weickert CS, Martin DM, McClintock SM, Mohan A, Lisanby SH, International Consortium of Research in tDCS (ICRT). International randomized-controlled trial of transcranial direct current stimulation in depression. Brain Stimul. 2018;11(1):125–33. PMID: 29111077. http://www.ncbi.nlm.nih.gov/pubmed/29111077.
448. Palm U, Schiller C, Fintescu Z, Obermeier M, Keeser D, Reisinger E, Pogarell O, Nitsche MA, Möller HJ, Padberg F. Transcranial direct current stimulation in treatment resistant depression: a randomized double-blind, placebo-controlled study. Brain Stimul. 2012;5(3):242–51. PMID: 21962978. http://www.ncbi.nlm.nih.gov/pubmed/21962978.
449. Bennabi D, Nicolier M, Monnin J, Tio G, Pazart L, Vandel P, Haffen E. Pilot study of feasibility of the effect of treatment with tDCS in patients suffering from treatment-resistant depression treated with escitalopram. Clin Neurophysiol. 2015;126(6):1185–9. PMID: 25454337. http://www.ncbi.nlm.nih.gov/pubmed/25454337.
450. Segrave RA, Arnold S, Hoy K, Fitzgerald PB. Concurrent cognitive control training augments the antidepressant efficacy of tDCS: a pilot study. Brain Stimul. 2014;7(2):325–31. PMID: 24486425. http://www.ncbi.nlm.nih.gov/pubmed/24486425.
451. Brunoni AR, Zanao TA, Vanderhasselt MA, Valiengo L, de Oliveira JF, Boggio PS, Lotufo PA, Benseñor IM, Fregni F. Enhancement of affective processing induced by bifrontal transcranial direct current stimulation in patients with major depression. Neuromodulation. 2014;17(2):138–42. PMID: 23710817. http://www.ncbi.nlm.nih.gov/pubmed/23710817.
452. Martin DM, Teng JZ, Lo TY, Alonzo A, Goh T, Iacoviello BM, Hoch MM, Loo CK. Clinical pilot study of transcranial direct current stimulation combined with Cognitive Emotional Training for medication resistant depression. J Affect Disord. 2018;232:89–95. PMID: 29477590. http://www.ncbi.nlm.nih.gov/pubmed/29477590.
453. Edwards D, Cortes M, Datta A, Minhas P, Wassermann EM, Bikson M. Physiological and modeling evidence for focal transcranial electrical brain stimulation in humans: a basis for high-definition tDCS. NeuroImage. 2013;74:266–75. PMCID: PMC4359173. http://www.ncbi.nlm.nih.gov/pubmed/23370061.
454. Frederikse M, Petrides G, Kellner C. Continuation and maintenance electroconvulsive therapy for the treatment of depressive illness: a response to the National Institute for Clinical Excellence report. J ECT. 2006;22(1):13–7. PMID: 16633200. http://www.ncbi.nlm.nih.gov/pubmed/16633200.
455. Hermida AP, Glass OM, Shafi H, McDonald WM. Electroconvulsive therapy in depression: current practice and future direction. Psychiatr Clin North Am. 2018;41(3):341–53. PMID: 30098649. http://www.ncbi.nlm.nih.gov/pubmed/30098649.
456. https://www.govinfo.gov/content/pkg/FR-2015-12-29/pdf/2015-32592.pdf.
457. FDA. Medical devices. https://www.fda.gov/medical-devices.
458. McDonald WM, Weiner RD, Fochtmann LJ, McCall WV. The FDA and ECT. J ECT. 2016;32(2):75–7. PMCID: PMC5137581. http://www.ncbi.nlm.nih.gov/pubmed/27191123.
459. UK ECT Review Group. Efficacy and safety of electroconvulsive therapy in depressive disorders: a systematic review and meta-analysis. Lancet. 2003;361(9360):799–808. PMID: 12642045. http://www.ncbi.nlm.nih.gov/pubmed/12642045.
460. Yrondi A, Péran P, Sauvaget A, Schmitt L, Arbus C. Structural-functional brain changes in depressed patients during and after electroconvulsive therapy. Acta Neuropsychiatr. 2018;30(1):17–28. PMID: 27876102. http://www.ncbi.nlm.nih.gov/pubmed/27876102.
461. Xu H, Zhao T, Luo F, Zheng Y. Dissociative changes in gray matter volume following electroconvulsive therapy in major depressive disorder: a longitudinal structural magnetic resonance imaging study. Neuroradiology. 2019;61(11):1297–308. PMID: 31410504. http://www.ncbi.nlm.nih.gov/pubmed/31410504.
462. Virtual. Search Online Etymology Dictionary. https://www.etymonline.com/search?q=virtual.
463. Firth N. Virtual reality: meet founding father Jaron Lanier. New Scientist. 2013. https://www.newscientist.com/article/mg21829226-000-virtual-reality-meet-founding-father-jaron-lanier/.
464. van der Meer RM, Willemsen MC, Smit F, Cuijpers P, Schippers GM. Effectiveness of a mood management component as an adjunct to a telephone counselling smoking cessation intervention for smokers with a past major depression: a pragmatic randomized controlled trial. Addiction. 2010;105(11):1991–9. PMID: 20735366. http://www.ncbi.nlm.nih.gov/pubmed/20735366.
465. Biocca F. Virtual reality technology: a tutorial. J Commun. 1992;42(4):23–72. https://psycnet.apa.org/record/1993-16916-001.
466. Serrano B, Baños RM, Botella C. Virtual reality and stimulation of touch and smell for inducing relaxation: a randomized controlled trial. Comput Human Behav. 2016;55:1–8. https://www.sciencedirect.com/science/article/abs/pii/S0747563215300856.
467. Lowood HE. Virtual reality. Definition, development, technology, examples, & facts. Britannica. 2025. https://www.britannica.com/technology/virtual-reality.
468. Microsoft Research. Holographic near-eye displays for virtual and augmented reality. 2017. https://www.microsoft.com/en-us/research/project/holographic-near-eye-displays-virtual-augmented-reality/.
469. Yasar K, Sheldon R. What is virtual reality? How it's used and how it will evolve. 2024. https://www.techtarget.com/whatis/definition/virtual-reality.
470. Flavián C, Ibáñez-Sánchez S, Orús C. The influence of scent on virtual reality experiences: the role of aroma-content congruence. J Bus Res. 2021;123:289–301. https://www.sciencedirect.com/science/article/pii/S0148296320306093.
471. Allen K. Simulating taste, touch, and smell is the final frontier for web 3.0. 2022. https://cloudwars.com/metaverse/simulating-taste-touch-and-smell-is-the-final-frontier-for-web-3-0/.
472. Liu Y, Yiu CK, Zhao Z, Park W, Shi R, Huang X, Zeng Y, Wang K, Wong TH, Jia S, Zhou J, Gao Z, Zhao L, Yao K, Li J, Sha C, Gao Y, Zhao G, Huang Y, Li D, Guo Q, Li Y, Yu X. Soft, miniaturized, wireless olfactory interface for virtual reality. Nat Commun. 2023;14(1):2297. PMCID: PMC10169775. http://www.ncbi.nlm.nih.gov/pubmed/37160931.
473. Wood DP, Murphy J, McLay R, Koffman R, Spira J, Obrecht RE, Pyne J, Wiederhold BK. Cost effectiveness of virtual reality graded exposure therapy with physiological monitoring for the treatment of combat related post traumatic stress disorder. Stud Health Technol Inform. 2009;144:223–9. PMID: 19592768. http://www.ncbi.nlm.nih.gov/pubmed/19592768.
474. Velez-Zea A, Barrera-Ramírez JF. Color multilayer holographic near-eye augmented reality display. Sci Rep. 2023;13(1):10651. PMCID: PMC10313800. http://www.ncbi.nlm.nih.gov/pubmed/37391489.
475. Slater M, Spanlang B, Sanchez-Vives MV, Blanke O. First person experience of body transfer in virtual reality. PLoS One. 2010;5(5):e10564. PMCID: PMC2868878. http://www.ncbi.nlm.nih.gov/pubmed/20485681.
476. Wiebe A, Kannen K, Selaskowski B, Mehren A, Thöne AK, Pramme L, Blumenthal N, Li M, Asché L, Jonas S, Bey K, Schulze M, Steffens M, Pensel MC, Guth M, Rohlfsen F, Ekhlas

M, Lügering H, Fileccia H, Pakos J, Lux S, Philipsen A, Braun N. Virtual reality in the diagnostic and therapy for mental disorders: a systematic review. Clin Psychol Rev. 2022;98:102213. PMID: 36356351. http://www.ncbi.nlm.nih.gov/pubmed/36356351.
477. Liszio S, Graf L, Masuch M. The relaxing effect of virtual nature: immersive technology provides relief in acute stress situations. Annu Rev Cyberther Telemed. 2018;16:87–93.
478. Caeiro-Rodríguez M, et al. A systematic review of commercial smart gloves: current status and applications. Sensors (Basel). 2021;21(8):2667. https://link.springer.com/article/10.1007/s10055-018-0374-z.
479. Salatino A, Zavattaro C, Gammeri R, Cirillo E, Piatti ML, Pyasik M, Serra H, Pia L, Geminiani G, Ricci R. Virtual reality rehabilitation for unilateral spatial neglect: a systematic review of immersive, semi-immersive and non-immersive techniques. Neurosci Biobehav Rev. 2023;152:105248. PMID: 37247829. http://www.ncbi.nlm.nih.gov/pubmed/37247829.
480. Hoffman HG, Patterson DR, Carrougher GJ. Use of virtual reality for adjunctive treatment of adult burn pain during physical therapy: a controlled study. Clin J Pain. 2000;16(3):244–50. PMID: 11014398. http://www.ncbi.nlm.nih.gov/pubmed/11014398.
481. Chirico A, Lucidi F, De Laurentiis M, Milanese C, Napoli A, Giordano A. Virtual reality in health system: beyond entertainment. a mini-review on the efficacy of VR during cancer treatment. J Cell Physiol. 2016;231(2):275–87. PMID: 26238976. http://www.ncbi.nlm.nih.gov/pubmed/26238976.
482. Llobera J, González-Franco M, Perez-Marcos D, Valls-Solé J, Slater M, Sanchez-Vives MV. Virtual reality for assessment of patients suffering chronic pain: a case study. Exp Brain Res. 2013;225(1):105–17. PMID: 23223781. http://www.ncbi.nlm.nih.gov/pubmed/23223781.
483. McCann RA, Armstrong CM, Skopp NA, Edwards-Stewart A, Smolenski DJ, June JD, Metzger-Abamukong M, Reger GM. Virtual reality exposure therapy for the treatment of anxiety disorders: an evaluation of research quality. J Anxiety Disord. 2014;28(6):625–31. PMID: 25093964. http://www.ncbi.nlm.nih.gov/pubmed/25093964.
484. Emmelkamp PMG, Meyerbröker K. Virtual reality therapy in mental health. Annu Rev Clin Psychol. 2021;17:495–519. PMID: 33606946. http://www.ncbi.nlm.nih.gov/pubmed/33606946.
485. Jingili N, Oyelere SS, Nyström MBT, Anyshchenko L. A systematic review on the efficacy of virtual reality and gamification interventions for managing anxiety and depression. Front Digit Health. 2023;5:1239435. PMCID: PMC10661329. http://www.ncbi.nlm.nih.gov/pubmed/38026832.
486. Kim H, Kim BH, Kim MK, Eom H, Kim JJ. Alteration of resting-state functional connectivity network properties in patients with social anxiety disorder after virtual reality-based self-training. Front Psych. 2022;13:959696. PMCID: PMC9530634. http://www.ncbi.nlm.nih.gov/pubmed/36203841.
487. Kim MK, Eom H, Kwon JH, Kyeong S, Kim JJ. Neural effects of a short-term virtual reality self-training program to reduce social anxiety. Psychol Med. 2022;52(7):1296–305. PMID: 32880252. http://www.ncbi.nlm.nih.gov/pubmed/32880252.
488. Rubin M, Muller K, Hayhoe MM, Telch MJ. Attention guidance augmentation of virtual reality exposure therapy for social anxiety disorder: a pilot randomized controlled trial. Cogn Behav Ther. 2022;51(5):371–87. PMCID: PMC9458616. http://www.ncbi.nlm.nih.gov/pubmed/35383544.
489. Jingili N, Oyelere SS, Ojwang F, Agbo FJ, Nyström MBT. Virtual reality for addressing depression and anxiety: a bibliometric analysis. Int J Environ Res Public Health. 2023;20(9):5621. PMCID: PMC10178384. http://www.ncbi.nlm.nih.gov/pubmed/37174141.
490. Wang Z, Li Y, An J, Dong W, Li H, Ma H, Wang J, Wu J, Jiang T, Wang G. Effects of restorative environment and presence on anxiety and depression based on interactive virtual reality scenarios. Int J Environ Res Public Health. 2022;19(13):7878. PMCID: PMC9266120. http://www.ncbi.nlm.nih.gov/pubmed/35805535.
491. Rowland DP, Casey LM, Ganapathy A, Cassimatis M, Clough BA. A decade in review: a systematic review of virtual reality interventions for emotional disorders. Psychosoc Interv. 2022;31(1):1–20. PMCID: PMC10268557. http://www.ncbi.nlm.nih.gov/pubmed/37362616.
492. Riches S, Jeyarajaguru P, Taylor L, Fialho C, Little J, Ahmed L, O'Brien A, van Driel C, Veling W, Valmaggia L. Virtual reality relaxation for people with mental health conditions: a systematic review. Soc Psychiatry Psychiatr Epidemiol. 2023;58(7):989–1007. PMCID: PMC9852806. http://www.ncbi.nlm.nih.gov/pubmed/36658261.
493. Baghaei N, Stemmet L, Hlasnik A, Emanov K, Hach S, Naslund JA, et al. Time to get personal: individualised virtual reality for mental health. In: Extended abstracts of the 2020 CHI conference on human factors in computing systems. ACM; 2020. p. 1–9. https://scholar.harvard.edu/jnaslund/publications/time-get-personal-individualised-virtual-reality-mental-health.
494. Ciążyńska J, Maciaszek J. Various types of virtual reality-based therapy for eating disorders: a systematic review. J Clin Med. 2022;11(17):4956. PMCID: PMC9456485. http://www.ncbi.nlm.nih.gov/pubmed/36078886.
495. Mazza M, Kammler-Sücker K, Leménager T, Kiefer F, Lenz B. Virtual reality: a powerful technology to provide novel insight into treatment mechanisms of addiction. Transl Psychiatry. 2021;11(1):617. PMCID: PMC8648903. http://www.ncbi.nlm.nih.gov/pubmed/34873146.
496. Segawa T, Baudry T, Bourla A, Blanc JV, Peretti CS, Mouchabac S, Ferreri F. Virtual reality (VR) in assessment and treatment of addictive disorders: a systematic review. Front Neurosci. 2019;13:1409. PMCID: PMC6965009. http://www.ncbi.nlm.nih.gov/pubmed/31998066.
497. Taubin D, Berger A, Greenwald D, Greenwald H, Burke C, Gongora DS, Wilens T. A systematic review of virtual reality therapies for substance use disorders: impact on secondary treatment outcomes. Am J Addict. 2023;32(1):13–23. PMCID: PMC10557052. http://www.ncbi.nlm.nih.gov/pubmed/36128667.
498. Shahmoradi L, Rezayi S. Cognitive rehabilitation in people with autism spectrum disorder: a systematic review of emerging virtual reality-based approaches. J Neuroeng Rehabil. 2022;19(1):91. PMCID: PMC9389666. http://www.ncbi.nlm.nih.gov/pubmed/35982460.
499. Skjoldborg NM, Bender PK, Jensen de López KM. The efficacy of head-mounted-display virtual reality intervention to improve life skills of individuals with autism spectrum disorders: a systematic review. Neuropsychiatr Dis Treat. 2022;18:2295–310. PMCID: PMC9586887. http://www.ncbi.nlm.nih.gov/pubmed/36281222.
500. Karami B, Koushki R, Arabgol F, Rahmani M, Vahabie AH. Effectiveness of virtual/augmented reality-based therapeutic interventions on individuals with autism spectrum disorder: a comprehensive meta-analysis. Front Psych. 2021;12:665326. PMCID: PMC8260941. http://www.ncbi.nlm.nih.gov/pubmed/34248702.
501. Romero-Ayuso D, Toledano-González A, Rodríguez-Martínez MDC, Arroyo-Castillo P, Triviño-Juárez JM, González P, Ariza-Vega P, González ADP, Segura-Fragoso A. Effectiveness of virtual reality-based interventions for children and adolescents with ADHD: a systematic review and meta-analysis. Children (Basel). 2021;8(2):70. PMCID: PMC7909839. http://www.ncbi.nlm.nih.gov/pubmed/33494272.
502. Corrigan N, Păsărelu CR, Voinescu A. Immersive virtual reality for improving cognitive deficits in children with ADHD: a systematic review and meta-analysis. Virtual Real. 2023:1–20. PMCID: PMC9938513. http://www.ncbi.nlm.nih.gov/pubmed/36845650.
503. Chan KCS, Hui CLM, Suen YN, Lee EHM, Chang WC, Chan SKW, Chen EYH. Application of immersive virtual reality for

assessment and intervention in psychosis: a systematic review. Brain Sci. 2023;13(3):471. PMCID: PMC10046161. http://www.ncbi.nlm.nih.gov/pubmed/36979281.

504. Riches S, Pisani S, Bird L, Rus-Calafell M, Garety P, Valmaggia L. Virtual reality-based assessment and treatment of social functioning impairments in psychosis: a systematic review. Int Rev Psychiatry. 2021;33(3):337–62. PMID: 34121587. http://www.ncbi.nlm.nih.gov/pubmed/34121587.
505. Monaghesh E, Samad-Soltani T, Farhang S. Virtual reality-based interventions for patients with paranoia: a systematic review. Psychiatry Res. 2022;307:114338. PMID: 34922239. http://www.ncbi.nlm.nih.gov/pubmed/34922239.
506. Anderson NC, Bischof WF, Kingstone A. Eye tracking in virtual reality. In: Maymon C, Grimshaw G, Wu YC, editors. Virtual reality in behavioral neuroscience: new insights and methods, Current topics in behavioral neurosciences, vol. 65. Cham: Springer; 2023. https://doi.org/10.1007/7854_2022_409. https://link.springer.com/chapter/10.1007/7854_2022_409.
507. Wu J, Sun Y, Zhang G, Zhou Z, Ren Z. Virtual reality-assisted cognitive behavioral therapy for anxiety disorders: a systematic review and meta-analysis. Front Psych. 2021;12:575094. PMCID: PMC8342859. http://www.ncbi.nlm.nih.gov/pubmed/34366904.
508. Ricciardi W, Pita Barros P, Bourek A, Brouwer W, Kelsey T, Lehtonen L, Expert Panel on Effective Ways of Investing in Health (EXPH). How to govern the digital transformation of health services. Eur J Public Health. 2019;29(Supplement_3):7–12. PMCID: PMC6859522. http://www.ncbi.nlm.nih.gov/pubmed/31738442.
509. Bas-Hoogendam JM. Commentary: gray matter structural alterations in social anxiety disorder: a voxel-based meta-analysis. Front Psych. 2019;10:1. PMCID: PMC6349716. http://www.ncbi.nlm.nih.gov/pubmed/30723425.
510. Soltani P. A SWOT analysis of virtual reality for seniors. In: Virtual and augmented reality in mental health treatment. IGI Global; 2019. p. 78–93. https://psycnet.apa.org/record/2018-38789-006.
511. Bun P, Gorski F, Grajewski D, Wichniarek R, Zawadzki P. Low–cost devices used in virtual reality exposure therapy. Procedia Comput Sci. 2017;104:445–51. https://www.researchgate.net/publication/313478976_Low_-_Cost_Devices_Used_in_Virtual_Reality_Exposure_Therapy.
512. Lundin RM, Yeap Y, Menkes DB. Adverse effects of virtual and augmented reality interventions in psychiatry: systematic review. JMIR Ment Health. 2023;10:e43240. PMCID: PMC10199391. http://www.ncbi.nlm.nih.gov/pubmed/37145841.
513. Bouchard S, Berthiaume M, Robillard G, Forget H, Daudelin-Peltier C, Renaud P, Blais C, Fiset D. Arguing in favor of revising the simulator sickness questionnaire factor structure when assessing side effects induced by immersions in virtual reality. Front Psych. 2021;12:739742. PMCID: PMC8604025. http://www.ncbi.nlm.nih.gov/pubmed/34803762.
514. Kim H, Kim DJ, Chung WH, Park KA, Kim JDK, Kim D, Kim K, Jeon HJ. Clinical predictors of cybersickness in virtual reality (VR) among highly stressed people. Sci Rep. 2021;11(1):12139. PMCID: PMC8190110. http://www.ncbi.nlm.nih.gov/pubmed/34108520.
515. Laessoe U, Abrahamsen S, Zepernick S, Raunsbaek A, Stensen C. Motion sickness and cybersickness – sensory mismatch. Physiol Behav. 2023;258:114015. PMID: 36323375. http://www.ncbi.nlm.nih.gov/pubmed/36323375.
516. Drazich BF, McPherson R, Gorman EF, Chan T, Teleb J, Galik E, Resnick B. In too deep? A systematic literature review of fully-immersive virtual reality and cybersickness among older adults. J Am Geriatr Soc. 2023;71(12):3906–15. PMID: 37560978. http://www.ncbi.nlm.nih.gov/pubmed/37560978.
517. Rmadi H, Maillot P, Artico R, Baudouin E, Hanneton S, Dietrich G, Duron E. Tolerance of immersive head-mounted virtual reality among older nursing home residents. Front Public Health. 2023;11:1163484. PMCID: PMC10394641. http://www.ncbi.nlm.nih.gov/pubmed/37538272.
518. Reger GM, Smolenski D, Edwards-Stewart A, Skopp NA, Rizzo AS, Norr A. Does virtual reality increase simulator sickness during exposure therapy for post-traumatic stress disorder? Telemed J E Health. 2019;25(9):859–61. PMID: 30379634. http://www.ncbi.nlm.nih.gov/pubmed/30379634.
519. Sokołowska B. Being in virtual reality and its influence on brain health: an overview of benefits, limitations and prospects. Brain Sci. 2024;14(1):72. PMCID: PMC10813118. http://www.ncbi.nlm.nih.gov/pubmed/38248287.
520. Hawajri O, Lindberg J, Suominen S. Virtual reality exposure therapy as a treatment method against anxiety disorders and depression – a structured literature review. Issues Ment Health Nurs. 2023;44(4):245–69. PMID: 37075308. http://www.ncbi.nlm.nih.gov/pubmed/37075308.
521. Pittig A, Kotter R, Hoyer J. The struggle of behavioral therapists with exposure: self-reported practicability, negative beliefs, and therapist distress about exposure-based interventions. Behav Ther. 2019;50(2):353–66. PMID: 30824251. http://www.ncbi.nlm.nih.gov/pubmed/30824251.
522. Botella C, Serrano B, Baños RM, Garcia-Palacios A. Virtual reality exposure-based therapy for the treatment of post-traumatic stress disorder: a review of its efficacy, the adequacy of the treatment protocol, and its acceptability. Neuropsychiatr Dis Treat. 2015;11:2533–45. PMCID: PMC4599639. http://www.ncbi.nlm.nih.gov/pubmed/26491332.
523. Ma L, Mor S, Anderson PL, Baños RM, Botella C, Bouchard S, Cárdenas-López G, Donker T, Fernández-Álvarez J, Lindner P, Mühlberger A, Powers MB, Quero S, Rothbaum B, Wiederhold BK, Carlbring P. Integrating virtual realities and psychotherapy: SWOT analysis on VR and MR based treatments of anxiety and stress-related disorders. Cogn Behav Ther. 2021;50(6):509–26. PMID: 34342251. http://www.ncbi.nlm.nih.gov/pubmed/34342251.
524. Maples-Keller JL, Bunnell BE, Kim SJ, Rothbaum BO. The use of virtual reality technology in the treatment of anxiety and other psychiatric disorders. Harv Rev Psychiatry. 2017;25(3):103–13. PMCID: PMC5421394. http://www.ncbi.nlm.nih.gov/pubmed/28475502.
525. Ioannou A, Papastavrou E, Avraamides MN, Charalambous A. Virtual reality and symptoms management of anxiety, depression, fatigue, and pain: a systematic review. SAGE Open Nurs. 2020;6:2377960820936163. PMCID: PMC7774450. http://www.ncbi.nlm.nih.gov/pubmed/33415290.
526. Lindner P, Hamilton W, Miloff A, Carlbring P. How to treat depression with low-intensity virtual reality interventions: perspectives on translating cognitive behavioral techniques into the virtual reality modality and how to make anti-depressive use of virtual reality-unique experiences. Front Psych. 2019;10:792. PMCID: PMC6836923. http://www.ncbi.nlm.nih.gov/pubmed/31736809.
527. van Loenen I, Scholten W, Muntingh A, Smit J, Batelaan N. The effectiveness of virtual reality exposure-based cognitive behavioral therapy for severe anxiety disorders, obsessive-compulsive disorder, and posttraumatic stress disorder: meta-analysis. J Med Internet Res. 2022;24(2):e26736. PMCID: PMC8874794. http://www.ncbi.nlm.nih.gov/pubmed/35142632.
528. Fodor LA, Coteț CD, Cuijpers P, Szamoskozi Ș, David D, Cristea IA. The effectiveness of virtual reality based interventions for symptoms of anxiety and depression: a meta-analysis. Sci Rep. 2018;8(1):10323. PMCID: PMC6037699. http://www.ncbi.nlm.nih.gov/pubmed/29985400.
529. Opriş D, Pintea S, García-Palacios A, Botella C, Szamosközi Ş, David D. Virtual reality exposure therapy in anxiety disorders: a quantitative meta-analysis. Depress Anxiety.

2012;29(2):85–93. PMID: 22065564. http://www.ncbi.nlm.nih.gov/pubmed/22065564.
530. Morina N, Ijntema H, Meyerbröker K, Emmelkamp PMG. Can virtual reality exposure therapy gains be generalized to real-life? A meta-analysis of studies applying behavioral assessments. Behav Res Ther. 2015;74:18–24. PMID: 26355646. http://www.ncbi.nlm.nih.gov/pubmed/26355646.
531. Powers MB, Emmelkamp PMG. Virtual reality exposure therapy for anxiety disorders: a meta-analysis. J Anxiety Disord. 2008;22(3):561–9. PMID: 17544252. http://www.ncbi.nlm.nih.gov/pubmed/17544252.
532. Beidel DC, Tuerk PW, Spitalnick J, Bowers CA, Morrison K. Treating childhood social anxiety disorder with virtual environments and serious games: a randomized trial. Behav Ther. 2021;52(6):1351–63. PMCID: PMC8531536. http://www.ncbi.nlm.nih.gov/pubmed/34656191.
533. Pedram S, Palmisano S, Perez P, Mursic R, Farrelly M. Examining the potential of virtual reality to deliver remote rehabilitation. Comput Human Behav. 2020;105:106223. https://psycnet.apa.org/record/2020-14656-001.
534. Deterding S, Dixon D, Khaled R, Nacke L. From game design elements to gamefulness: defining "gamification". In: Proceedings of the 15th international academic MindTrek conference: envisioning future media environments. ACM; 2011. p. 9–15. https://www.researchgate.net/publication/230854710_From_Game_Design_Elements_to_Gamefulness_Defining_Gamification.
535. Sailer M, Homner L. The gamification of learning: a meta-analysis. Educ Psychol Rev. 2020;32(1):77–112. https://link.springer.com/article/10.1007/s10648-019-09498-w.
536. Laurence E, Henderson L. Virtual reality therapy: how does it work? Forbes Health. 2024. https://www.forbes.com/health/mind/virtual-reality-therapy/.
537. Reichenberger J, Wechsler TF, Diemer J, Mühlberger A, Notzon S. Fear, psychophysiological arousal, and cognitions during a virtual social skills training in social anxiety disorder while manipulating gaze duration. Biol Psychol. 2022;175:108432. PMID: 36191863. http://www.ncbi.nlm.nih.gov/pubmed/36191863.
538. Pallavicini F, Orena E, di Santo S, Greci L, Caragnano C, Ranieri P, Vuolato C, Pepe A, Veronese G, Stefanini S, Achille F, Dakanalis A, Bernardelli L, Sforza F, Rossini A, Caltagirone C, Fascendini S, Clerici M, Riva G, Mantovani F. A virtual reality home-based training for the management of stress and anxiety among healthcare workers during the COVID-19 pandemic: study protocol for a randomized controlled trial. Trials. 2022;23(1):451. PMCID: PMC9161181. http://www.ncbi.nlm.nih.gov/pubmed/35655231.
539. Zainal NH, Chan WW, Saxena AP, Taylor CB, Newman MG. Pilot randomized trial of self-guided virtual reality exposure therapy for social anxiety disorder. Behav Res Ther. 2021;147:103984. PMCID: PMC8759454. http://www.ncbi.nlm.nih.gov/pubmed/34740099.

Self-medication in Depressed Individuals

23

Franklin Sunzeri

Introduction

To relieve symptoms of mood disorders, a review suggests that 24.1% of sufferers self-medicate with alcohol or drugs [28, 29]. Men were about twice as likely as women to self-medicate (OR[1] =2.18; 95% CI: 1.90 to 2.49). Comorbidity of anxiety and personality disorders were higher in this group who self-medicate when compared to those who do not self-medicate.

MDD is strongly linked with substance use disorders, which may influence specific depression symptoms [30, 31].

In 1990, the *National Institute of Mental Health Epidemiologic Catchment Area Program* surveyed the prevalence of comorbid alcohol, other drug, and mental disorders in the US total community and institutional populations [32]. They found the following (*directly quoted*).

- "The US population had lifetime prevalence rates of 22.5% for any non-substance abuse mental disorder, 13.5% for alcohol dependence-abuse, and 6.1% for other drug dependence abuse.
- Among those with a mental disorder, the odds ratio of having some addictive disorder was 2.7, with a lifetime prevalence of about 29% (including an overlapping 22% with an alcohol and 15% with another drug disorder).
- For those with either an alcohol or other drug disorder, the odds of having the other addictive disorder were seven times greater than in the rest of the population.
- Among those with an alcohol disorder, 37% had a comorbid mental disorder.
- The highest mental-addictive disorder comorbidity rate was found for those with drug (other than alcohol) disorders, among whom more than half (53%) were found to have a mental disorder with an odds ratio of 4.5.
- Individuals treated in specialty mental health and addictive disorder clinical settings have significantly higher odds of having comorbid disorders.
- Among the institutional settings, comorbidity of addictive and severe mental disorders was highest in the prison population, most notably with antisocial personality, schizophrenia, and bipolar disorders."

How rates have changed since then is unknown. Although this data is old, there is no truly comparable data available. However, the data from other more current large databased surveys underscores the basic relationships. For example, the *National Epidemiologic Survey on Alcohol and Related Conditions* data is not available as of 2024.[2] However, 2004–2005 data from NESARC Wave 2 indicates that 1-year incidence rates of DSM-IV substance, mood, and anxiety disorders were highest for alcohol abuse (1.02) alcohol dependence (1.70), major depressive disorder (MDD: 1.51), and generalized anxiety disorder (GAD: 1.12) [31]. The greatest incidence of all the disorders was in the youngest cohort, and incidence was greater among women than men for mood and anxiety disorders except bipolar disorder and

[1]Odds ratio (OR) is a way to represent the odds that an outcome will result when a given exposure to a variable of interest occurs compared to when the exposure does not occur. OR quantifies the strength of the association between two events. An OR greater than 1 indicates a positive association or that exposure to that variable increases the odds of that outcome. An OR less than one indicates a negative relationship between two events. An OR of 1 suggests no relationship between two events. An OR is frequently accompanied by a 95% confidence interval (CI). CI is a measure of precision of the OR. The smaller the CI the higher precision as long as it does not overlap OR = 1. For more information, see the Chap. 4 on evidence basics in this text.

[2]National Epidemiologic Survey on Alcohol and Related Conditions was sponsored, designed and directed by the *National Institute on Alcohol Abuse and Alcoholism* (NIAAA) [33].

F. Sunzeri (✉)
Heather Hills Consulting, Coos Bay, OR, USA

J. Raber et al. (eds.), *Understanding and Treating Depressive Disorders*, https://doi.org/10.1007/978-3-032-14465-2_23

social phobia. Incidence of substance use disorders was greater in men than in women.

NESARC data reveals that depressive disorders are the most common psychiatric disorders among people with alcohol use disorder [34]. Their cooccurrence is associated with worse prognosis, greater severity [35, 36], and increased risk of suicide [37]. Those people who have alcohol use disorder (AUD) vs. those who do not have AUD are 2.3 times more likely to have had MDD and 1.7 times more likely to have dysthymia in the previous year [38]. Racial and ethnic differences and disparities in health integrated mental health and substance disorder care seem to be common [39–41].

Both positive and negative reinforcing effects seem to be in play with alcohol and other drug use [42]. Dependence produces a negative emotional state that drives drug seeking by negative reinforcement [43]. During addiction, the negative emotional state develops from a decrease in reward circuit functions and an increase in antireward circuit functions. These brain stress and anti-stress systems seem to be involved in transition to and maintenance of drug dependence. This negative state makes it exceedingly difficult to cope with the stress and anxiety that occurs during abstinence.

Anti-stress reward systems are the *mesolimbic dopamine systems*. Drug-seeking behavior seems to particularly involve the dopamine neurons of the *ventral tegmental area* (VTA) [45] and the medium spiny neurons of the *nucleus accumbens* (NAc) [44]. However, other regions are also involved [46]. For example, the *bed nucleus of the stria terminalis* (BNST), which is part of the *extended amygdala* but not part of the classical reward network, is involved in regulating anxiety and stress [2, 27]. The extended amygdala includes the central nucleus of the amygdala, the bed nucleus of the stria terminalis, a transition area of the medial shell of the nucleus accumbens, and a major projection to the lateral hypothalamus [42]. Corticotropin-releasing hormone (CRH) in these areas appears to play a pivotal role [47] and regulates VTA dopamine firing [48]. Activity in the BNST has been implicated in various drugs of abuse [49, 50]. Brain anti-stress systems involve neuropeptide Y and nociceptin (orphanin FQ) [51]. See Fig. 23.1.

VTA-NAc is the primary reward detecting circuit that is tuned to respond to natural rewards including food, sex, and positive social interactions [52]. It also responds to rewards from drugs of abuse [53, 54]. When the VTA-NAc is activated, it motivates and incentivizes an individual to repeat the behavior that elicited the reward. In so doing, the VTA-NAc prompts memory of the details of the process and features of the reward.

The VTA-NAc communicates with and integrates with several areas of the brain. These include the amygdala, hippocampus, hypothalamus, prefrontal regions of the cerebral cortex, locus coeruleus, and the dorsal raphe.

The amygdala helps establish connections between environmental cues and the rewarding or aversive nature of the experience. The amygdala is highly associated with conditioned learning.

The hippocampus in collaboration with the amygdala is vital for remembering persons, places, or things that are associated with the rewards.

The hypothalamus integrates an interest in rewards with an individual's physiological needs.

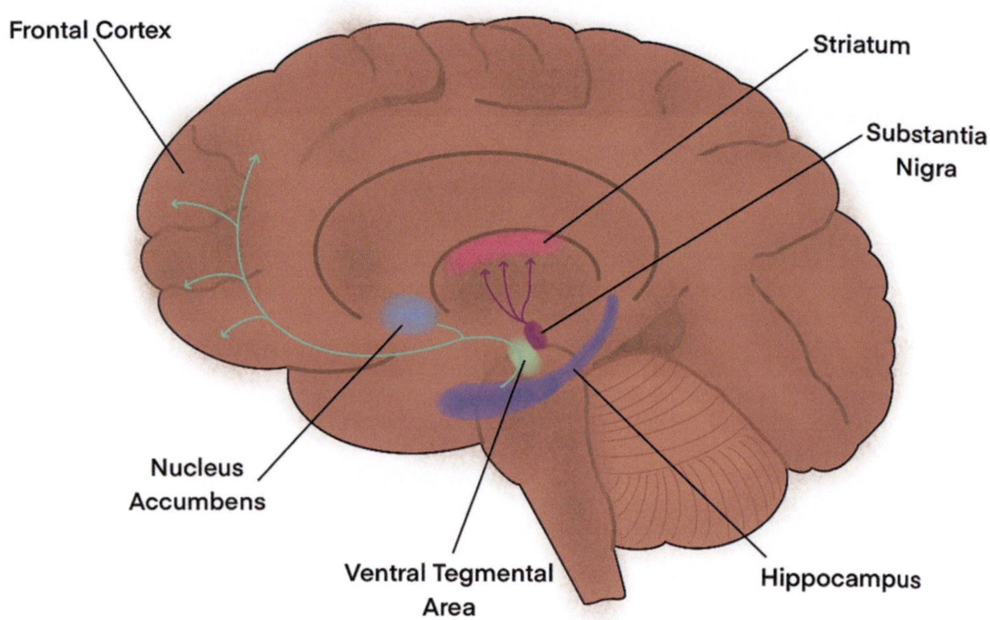

Fig. 23.1 Mesolimbic dopamine system and associated brain regions. This illustration highlights major components of the mesolimbic pathway, including the frontal cortex, ventral tegmental area (VTA), nucleus accumbens, hippocampus, substantia nigra, and striatum. Together, these interconnected regions orchestrate dopaminergic signaling that underlies reward processing, motivation, reinforcement learning, and mood regulation

The prefrontal regions (including the medial prefrontal cortex, anterior cingulate cortex, and orbitofrontal cortex) control the actual executive decision to seek a particular reward.

The locus coeruleus with its noradrenergic neurons regulates activation state and mood. *The dorsal raphe* is the principal location for serotonergic innervation in the brain, which also regulates activation state and mood. Acetylcholine from the pons modulates the motivation to seek the reward [55].

Motivational salience is a form of attention that regulates goal seeking strength, amount of risk taken, and the energy invested [56]. It also plays a significant role in persistence of memories that may or may not be adaptive. Prefrontal cortical norepinephrine transmission is necessary for motivational salience attribution to highly salient stimuli through dopamine modulation in the NAc [57, 58]. This prefrontal-accumbal catecholamine system is only active when the salience of the unconditioned stimulus is high enough to sustain catecholamine activation [57].

Transient increases in dopamine resulting from high-frequency firing of dopamine neurons in the VTA is accompanied by release of *endocannabinoids* from dopamine cell bodies [59]. The brain cannabinoid receptors (CB1 and CB2) and their endogenous ligands are important in regulating dopamine signaling during reinforcement processing [60, 61]. Endocannabinoids are formed on demand [62] and are retrograde messengers that bind to presynaptic CB1 receptors reducing presynaptic dopamine release to indirectly modulate excitability of the dopamine neurons [63]. Experiments have shown that disrupting endocannabinoid signaling significantly reduced cue-evoked dopamine concentrations and reward seeking, whereas augmenting levels of the endocannabinoid 2-arachidonoylglycerol (2AG) increased those behaviors [59].

The *antireward* concept is based upon the idea of systems that limit rewards [42]. These are sometimes characterized as *opponent systems* [64, 65]. It is engaged when there is excessive activation of the reward system. *Antireward systems include* the brain stress systems that involve CRH, norepinephrine, orexin (hypocretin), vasopressin, and dynorphin [51]. It corresponds to the deficit state of normal rewards produced by excessive drug taking [42].

The antireward system that goes into high gear during the process of addiction involves connections between the basal forebrain and the extrahypothalamic extended amygdala. It appears that cellular processes that sensitize these antireward systems may be influenced by genetic and developmental factors [51].

Although in the short term, drug taking can ameliorate the reward deficiency and suppress the antireward system, long-term use does the opposite. In a complex psychopathological process, often associated with comorbidities and polysubstance abuse, it seems that drug addiction involves decreased function of normal reward-related circuitry and persistent recruitment of anti-reward systems that may gradually worsen [42, 46, 64, 66]. It appears that counter-adaptive processes become an allostatic state by not returning to the normal homeostatic range. *Allostasis* is stability through change [7, 67]. It is a feed-forward mechanism rather than a homeostatic negative feedback system.

This *allostatic state* is characterized by decreased functioning of dopamine and opioids and increased corticotropin-releasing hormone (CRH) activity. CRH acts in both the brain and the periphery to coordinate the overall response of stress [68]. *Anxiety-causing effects of CRH* depend on type 1 CRH receptors (CRH-R1s), which are highly expressed in the cortex, hippocampus, amygdala, olfactory bulb, and pituitary cerebellum [69, 70]. CRH 1 in the central nucleus of the amygdala is highly involved in ethanol dependence and withdrawal [71, 72]. The result of this allostatic state may be reward-circuit dysregulation, and neurological and hormonal stress systems recruitment [46]. Although addiction vulnerability rests upon several areas of the reward and antireward systems, it appears that sensitization of brain stress networks is a key feature.

Caffeine

Caffeine is the most frequently consumed psychostimulant in the world [73]. A very large survey in 2014 reported that in the USA about 85% of the population consumes at least one caffeinated beverage each day [74]. This increases by age from 43% of children 2–4 years of age consuming caffeine daily until more than 90% of adults 35 and older consuming caffeine daily. Coffee has been by far the major source of caffeine in the USA followed by tea, soft drinks, and energy drinks [74].

The amount of caffeine in different beverages varies quite a bit [75]. Generally, an 8-ounce cup of coffee is 95–200 mg. A 12-ounce can of cola is 35–45 mg. An 8-ounce energy drink is 70–100 mg. And an 8-ounce cup of tea is 14–60 mg. In the 2014 survey, the mean daily intake was 165 ± 1 mg and the 90th percentile intake was 380 mg/day for all ages combined. Consumers aged 50–64 years averaged 226 ± 2 mg/day.

Daily doses of caffeine up to 400 mg are generally considered safe [102]. However, individuals may differ in their own level of sensitivity to caffeine [76, 77]. Usual intake varies by age, race/ethnicity, smoking status, and alcohol drinking [78].

In recent years, caffeinated sugar-sweetened beverages have declined while energy drinks have climbed [79, 80].

Caffeine affects fundamental processes, including sleep, arousal, cognition, learning, and memory [73]. Heightened arousal and tension increase with intake of caffeine [81].

Caffeine's psychoactive stimulation is based upon its ability to *temporarily reduce adenosine transmission in the brain.* When adenosine receptors are activated in the brain, they produce drowsiness. Caffeine and theophylline antagonize all four adenosine receptors (A1, A2a, A2b, and A3) [82]. These G protein-coupled receptors regulate heart rate, contraction, and relaxation of cardiac and smooth muscles, and neural signaling in the central nervous system [82]. Some research suggests caffeine's antagonism to the A_{2A} receptor may help control aberrant synaptic plasticity and may be able to reduce symptoms of depression [83].

Each of these receptors has a different function but there is some overlap [84]. A1 receptors and A2a regulate oxygen consumption and coronary blood flow, A2a receptors have broader anti-inflammatory effects in general, and A2a and A2b receptors have a variety of important roles in the brain [85]. A2a and A2b regulate the release of neurotransmitters in the CNS such as dopamine and glutamate [86–89].

At low doses, caffeine seems to improve anxiety and depression, and at high doses tends to exacerbate anxiety [90]. In people who have panic disorders, it is common for caffeine to increase anxiety-related symptoms. Mice that are deficient in A2a receptors appear to be more prone to anxiety-like behavior and less likely to express depression-like behavior [90]. Genetic polymorphisms in the A2a receptor gene (*ADORA2A*) and gene for the DRD_2 receptor (*DRD2*) polymorphisms can predict the subjective effects of caffeine [91, 92].

Twin studies of combined use of caffeine, alcohol, and tobacco suggest that a shared polysubstance use genetic factor may be involved in heritable effects [93, 94]. However, other twin studies suggest that caffeine and nicotine are independently genetically influenced [95, 96]. Genome-wide meta-analysis has identified six novel loci associated with habitual coffee consumption [97]. Of particular interest are SNP alleles near GCKR, MLXIPL, BDNF, and CYP1A2 that associated with higher coffee consumption are also associated with smoking initiation, higher adiposity and fasting insulin and glucose but lower blood pressure and favorable lipid, inflammatory, and liver enzyme profiles ($P < 5 \times 10(-8)$).

A 2024 systematic review found that several genes are involved in caffeine metabolism and reward with 3% to 32% effect size differences in the daily number of cups of caffeinated beverages [98]. Striking ethnic differences were seen in these associations.

Caffeine and nicotine share a common metabolic pathway, cytochrome P450 1A2 (CYP1A2), which is upregulated by their exposures [99]. So, it might not be surprising that current smokers tend to drink more coffee than former or never smokers.

Adult human behavioral effects from a moderate amount of caffeine include the following [100] (1). Increased alertness and reduction in fatigue especially in low arousal conditions. (2) Increased performance on simple tasks that require sustained vigilance, especially when alertness had been reduced. (3) Effects on more complex tasks are difficult to assess and may be a product of multiple factors. (4) Withdrawal from the effects of caffeine seems to dispose to a negative mood, but this is not clear. Otherwise, there seems to be few symptoms. Other studies cited below suggest that there are more symptoms. (5) Regular caffeine use appears to be beneficial. Folks who have higher consumption seem to have better mental functions. (6) Most people appear to be able to adjust their consumption to maximize the benefits. (7) Excessive consumption can lead to problems especially in particularly sensitive individuals. These include anxiety and sleep disturbances.

Caffeine consumption can trigger panic attacks [103, 104]. Polymorphisms in the A1 and A2a adenosine receptor genes associated with panic disorder are also associated with anxiogenic responses to caffeine [91]. Caffeine is known to exacerbate or induce psychosis, and mania, besides anxiety and panic attacks [100, 101, 105].

Caffeine competitively inhibits binding of benzodiazepines in brains and in chronic use involves up regulation of receptors and development of tolerance and dependence [106, 107].

Fun fact: Thigmotaxis [113] is enhanced at least in fish by caffeine [108].

According to a review article in the *Journal of Caffeine Research*, it appears that some caffeine users are dependent on caffeine and cannot reduce their intake despite knowing recurrent health problems associated with continued use [109]. Caffeine can produce behavioral and physiological effects similar to other drugs of dependence.

The World Health Organization recognizes a diagnosis of *Caffeine Dependence Syndrome* in the ICD-10. *Caffeine Use Disorder* is a condition for further study in the DSM-5 [109]. The central DSM-5 criteria for Caffeine Use Disorder are (1) persistent desire or unsuccessful efforts to cut down or control caffeine use; (2) continued caffeine use despite knowledge of having a persistent or recurrent physical or psychological problem that is likely to have been caused or exacerbated by caffeine; and (3) characteristic caffeine withdrawal syndrome or caffeine use to relieve or avoid withdrawal symptoms.

The DSM-5 also has diagnostic criteria for *Caffeine Intoxication* and *Caffeine Withdrawal* Prominent symptoms of *Caffeine Intoxication* may include restlessness, nervousness, excitement, insomnia, flushed face, and diuresis. gastrointestinal disturbance. muscle twitching rambling flow of thought and speech, tachycardia or cardiac arrhythmia periods of inexhaustibility, and psychomotor agitation.

Caffeine Withdrawal symptoms are real. For example, after 16 h of abstinence, using the *Caffeine Withdrawal*

Symptom Questionnaire, the following symptoms were reported in 213 caffeine consumers [110] (1). Fatigue/drowsiness, (2) Low alertness/difficulty concentrating, (3) Mood disturbances, (4) Low sociability/motivation to work, (5) Nausea/upset stomach, (6) Flu-like feelings, and (7) Headache.

Another study of men and women aged 20–29 identified 14 withdrawal symptoms, which were grouped into three factors: "fatigue and headache," "dysphoric mood," and "flu-like somatic" [111]. They found that increasing habitual caffeine consumption increased probability of reporting fatigue and headache and dysphoric mood symptoms, but not flu-like somatic symptoms.

Avoidance of caffeine withdrawal appears to be a powerful motivator for habitual caffeine consumption [112]. A critical review of the literature on caffeine withdrawal symptoms identified headache, fatigue, decreased energy/activeness, decreased alertness, drowsiness, decreased contentedness, depressed mood, difficulty concentrating, irritability, and foggy/not clearheaded [112]. Experimental studies indicated the incidence of headache was 50% and the incidence of clinically significant distress or functional impairment was 13%. Onset of symptoms usually occurred 12–24 h after abstinence, with peak intensity between 20 and 51 h, and lasted 2–9 days. Symptom severity increased with abstinence from higher doses, and they began with as low as 100 mg/day.

Coffee, tea, and chocolate are important dietary sources of polyphenols (flavanols and catechins) suggestive but not conclusive for reducing cardiovascular risk [114]. Indeed, coffee and tea have been both positively and negatively associated with cardiovascular disease [115]. Epidemiologically, black and green teas have been associated with a 10 to 20% reduction in cardiovascular disease. However, clinical trials and experiments sometimes show no benefit.

Controversy exists between coffee associations with hypercholesterolemia, hypertension, and myocardial infarction [116]. Genetic polymorphisms relating to metabolism and excretion of tea and coffee probably have an influence.

Adverse effects (e.g., an increase in plasma LDL-cholesterol and homocysteine levels) of caffeine and methylxanthines in general may be due to acute pressor effects either from high doses or lipids in non-filtered (e.g., boiled or French pressed) coffee [117, 118]. These are direct effects on vascular tone, myocardial contractility, and conduction, and on the sympathetic nervous system. Regular caffeine use may slightly increase blood pressure, by increasing total peripheral resistance and a slight decrease in heart rate. Some folks may be adversely susceptible to these hemodynamic and neurohumoral effects.

Protective effects are said to include effects on platelet function (adhesion and activation, aggregation, and clotting), vascular tone regulation, enhanced glucose metabolism (decreasing type II diabetes risk), increased reverse cholesterol transport and inhibition of foam cell formation, and inhibition of oxidative stress, and immunomodulation [115]. Meta-analysis of caffeine and cardiac affects suggests that irrespective of sex, baseline history of myocardial infarction or diabetes, compared with no consumption, the strongest inverse association was seen for four servings per day and a potentially higher risk at higher levels of consumption [119].

Inverse relations between coffee and a variety of diseases have been reported. These include total mortality [120, 121], depression [122, 123], liver cancer [124, 125], colorectal cancer [126–128], endometrial cancer [129, 130], melanoma [131–133], nonmelanoma skin cancer [134, 135], diabetes [136, 137], and Parkinson disease [138].

Energy drinks typically contain between 50 and 505 mg of caffeine—an amount sufficient to induce caffeine intoxication in some individuals [139]. A 2010 comprehensive review on health risks of energy drinks produced the following observations [140]. Adolescents' reports included jitteriness, nervousness, dizziness, inability to focus, difficulty concentrating, gastrointestinal upset, and insomnia. Health care providers noted dehydration, accelerated heart rates, anxiety, seizures, acute mania, and strokes.

Energy drink consumption has rapidly increased among children, adolescents, and young adults and so has adverse effects [141–143]. Consumption of energy drinks is associated with increased alcohol consumption and dependence [144, 145] and related risky behavior including sexual assault, physical injury, and increased marijuana use [146–148]. Energy drink consumption among college students is additionally associated with nonmedical use of prescription stimulants and analgesics [149, 150].

In 2013, after a comprehensive review, the *International Society of Sports Nutrition (ISSN)* produced a position statement of 9 points [151]. Among these points, they concluded, "(1) Consuming energy drinks 10–60 minutes before exercise can improve mental focus, alertness, anaerobic performance, and/or endurance performance. (2) Athletes should consider the impact of ingesting high glycemic load carbohydrates on metabolic health, blood glucose and insulin levels, as well as the effects of caffeine and other stimulants on motor skill performance. (3) Diabetics and individuals with pre-existing cardiovascular, metabolic, hepatorenal, and neurologic disease who are taking medications that may be affected by high glycemic load foods, caffeine, and/or other stimulants should avoid use of [energy drinks] ED and/or [energy stimulants] ES unless approved by their physician."

A study among participants ($n = 167$), who used caffeine in the last 7 days and who also reported using alcohol, nicotine, or illicit drugs within the past year, found that 35% met the DSM criteria for caffeine dependence [152]. Among the diagnostic criteria, 26% experienced withdrawal, 23% desired to cut down or control use, and 44% continued use despite harm. Thirty-four percent said they craved caffeine, 26% said they needed it to function, and 10% had talked to a physician about problems related to caffeine. A trend was seen between caffeine dependence and alcohol and nicotine dependence. In those who used alcohol, nicotine, and caffeine, 28% had caffeine dependence, 50% had alcohol dependence, and 80% had nicotine dependence.

Caffeine has been investigated in promoting better mental health especially on depressive mood and cognitive/attentional disorders [153], mental decline as in Alzheimer's [154–159]. Data from the 2005–2006 National Health and Nutrition Examination Survey (NHANES) suggests that caffeine's psychostimulant properties may offer protection against depressive symptoms; however, the authors note that prospective studies are needed to determine whether caffeine consumption can lead to a reduction in depressive symptoms [160]. One study that followed 50,739 US women (mean age 63) for 10 years suggests that depression risk decreases with increasing caffeinated coffee consumption [161].

Some studies suggest a moderate potential dose-dependent potential protective effect of moderate intake and others finding no significant effects [162].

Alcohol

About half of adults in the USA are frequent drinkers, while 14% are infrequent drinkers [163]. According to the National Epidemiologic Survey on Alcohol and Related Conditions (NESARC), 12-month prevalence in 2001–2002 of DSM-IV defined alcohol abuse and dependence were 4.65% and 3.81% [164].

Cooper's four-factor model of drinking motives is enhancement, socializing, conformity, and coping [1, 165–167].

Although there was considerable heterogeneity, a review of articles published between 1990 and 2004 indicated that most young people drink for social motives, some for enhancement motives, and a few for coping motives [168]. Social motives were associated with moderate alcohol use, enhancement with heavy drinking, and coping motives with alcohol-related problems. Adults who at baseline began to drink to reduce negative affect or to facilitate social interaction appear to be at a higher risk of alcohol dependence 10 years later if they had a family history of alcoholism [169].

Data from the Virginia Twin Study suggests a heritability of 23 to 48% of the individual differences in the drinking motives in women [170]. There was less effect in men.

Variance in drinking motivations may contribute to the covariance between personality (constraint, conscientiousness, neuroticism, and agreeableness) and alcohol abuse disorders [171, 172].

Depending upon multiple factors, anxiety sensitivity may predispose to alcohol dependence [173].

With initial ethanol use, the classical activation of the mesolimbic reward system usually produces an anxiolytic affect [42]. Following sustained ethanol use and/or when there is a preexisting anxiety disorder, negative reinforcing effects of ethanol may play an increasingly significant part in abusive drinking and relapse [66]. This may be conceptualized as a dysfunction of the reward system followed by recruitment of an anti-reward system [66, 174].

Separately and in combination with tobacco, alcohol may reduce anticipatory anxiety [175]. Alcohol produces selective *stress response dampening* (SRD) during uncertain but not certain threat [176]. Alcohol selectively reduces anxiety but not fear [177].

SRD differences between individuals are associated with a family history of alcoholism, personality traits, degree of self-consciousness, cognitive functioning, and gender. Situational effects on SRD are also seen. Depending upon attention allocated and disruption of appraisal, alcohol has a variable effect on SRD, e.g., distractions during a stressful situation and the timing of drinking and stress changes SRD [178].

Although alcohol may temporarily reduce stress, it may actually be a powerful anxiety-producing agent. Although acute exposure to low to moderate amounts of ethanol can be anxiolytic [179–181], repeat exposure and withdrawal appear to be associated with neuroadaptive modifications that may be conducive to long-lasting increase in a variety of anxiety symptoms [182–185].

There are three classical sets of cravings and relapse triggers for drug abuse [174]. Stress, re-exposure to environmental cues (people, places, and things associated with the drug), and re-exposure to addictive drugs. Each of these involves different areas of the brain: (1) stress involves the amygdala and CRH, and brain stem areas using norepinephrine; (2) cues involve the amygdala, the hippocampus, and glutamate; (3) drug triggers involve the nucleus accumbens and dopamine.

There are complex neurobiological mechanisms contributing to alcohol-stress–anxiety interactions [179, 182, 186, 187]. Neuroadaptive processes in the CNS that occur in the development of addiction and relapse appear to impair mechanisms that mediate positive reinforcement and emergence of anxiety, depression, and dysphoria that can occur during withdrawal [187]. Changes in dopamine and serotonin transmission in the nucleus accumbens and enhanced CRH release in the central nucleus of the amygdala appear to be involved in vulnerability to relapse. In addition, conditionally learned contextual environmental cues in eliciting drug-seeking behavior and stress have definite roles. The medial prefrontal cortex and the basolateral amygdala, along with opioid receptors, are involved.

Alcohol use disorders (especially alcohol dependence) and anxiety disorders show a reciprocal causal relationship over time, with anxiety disorders leading to alcohol dependence and vice versa [188].

Gamma-aminobutyric acid (GABA) and CRH appear to be involved in excessive alcohol intake that leads from social drinking to addiction [181]. It has been suggested that low doses of ethanol interact directly with proteins to produce ligand-gated receptor channels, such as the GABA receptor complex, to allosterically alter function. These specific areas include the ventral tegmental area, parts of the extended amygdala (including the central nucleus of the amygdala), and the globus pallidus. Chronic quantities of alcohol that are enough to create dependence and increased intake are associated with GABA release in the amygdala and increased sensitivity to GABA agonists. It is proposed that interaction of GABA with CRH in these areas may be a component of motivation to excess drinking.

In some people with preexisting anxiety disorders and/or prolonged exposure, there is a predisposition to abusive drinking and relapse [46].

Panic disorders with or without agoraphobia and alcohol abuse tend to occur in the same individuals [189]. Alcohol decreases anxious apprehension and in so doing decreases the probability of panic. However, alcohol increases sensitivity to CO2 and may promote panic. Familial transmission contributes to both.

Moderate and sustained alcohol abuse may increase anxiety and depression, and in one survey, about half of the persons presenting with anxiety, phobias, or panic disorder were found to have alcohol or benzodiazepines as the precipitating agent [190].

Dependence on alcohol, caffeine, and benzodiazepines may increase the severity of panic attacks [3, 191]. Upon withdrawal from alcohol addiction, it is common for anxiety to increase [4, 164, 192].

Heavy alcohol use in adolescents is associated with increased risk of comorbid psychopathology, including internalizing symptoms such as depression and anxiety [193].

Genome-wide association studies of comorbid major depression and alcohol dependence suggest that the comorbidity is partially influenced by genetic variants that do not affect alcohol dependence alone [194].

Stress, anxiety, depression, and alcohol abuse-related disorders appear to be regulated by cortisol releasing hormone receptors and urocortin (Ucn) peptides Ucn1, Ucn2, and Ucn3 [195]. It seems that high and low Ucn activity in a "U" shape pattern contributes to high-anxiety states. CRH seems to regulate dependence-induced drinking, binge drinking, and basal consumption of alcohol. Binge drinking and dependence-induced drinking relate to CRH influence on CRHR1 receptors and are inhibited by Ucns on CRHR2. Alcohol preference is related to Ucn1 influences on CRHR1 and CRHR2.

BDNF has a complex role to play in associations between anxiety, depression, and substance abuse [196]. For example, alcohol induced neurodegeneration in the brain may be related to decreased expression of BDNF or TrkB (BDNF receptor) malfunctions. Reduction in hippocampal BDNF seems to play a role in alcohol induced depression [350]. However, BDNF and associated signaling pathways are upregulated in anxiety, addiction, and homeostasis after exposure to alcohol.

Women metabolize alcohol differently compared to men [197]. As such, women of all ages are more susceptible to negative physical, psychological, and social consequences with higher alcohol consumption. This tendency is increased as women age. Any alcohol consumption in older women is associated with increased risk of breast cancer. In contrast, alcohol consumed at low levels may buffer declining hormonal levels effects of menopause on heart disease and osteoporosis.

Alcohol consumption may interact with a variety of medications [197]. Nicotine increases rewarding effects of alcohol and the motivation to consume it [198–202]. For example, in a survey of college students, smokers used more alcohol and reported greater effects from the simultaneous use of alcohol and tobacco [200].

Evidence suggests that about 90% of people who are dependent on alcohol are regular smokers, and less than 10% of them successfully quit smoking [203]. Indeed, this association may partly account for the statistic that more than half of alcoholic smokers die from a tobacco-related disease [204]. Quitting smoking, however, independent of sex, country, and amount smoked by itself does not lead to true changes in alcohol use [205].

Alcohol and tobacco, although differing in cellular and molecular mechanisms of activity, share common neural transmitters and neural pathways [206–208].

In a twin study in females of alcohol abuse and tobacco comorbidity, regular smokers were mostly motivated by coping, enhancement, and social motives, while non-regular smokers reported higher conformity motives [172]. Alcohol dependence was associated with higher scores on all motives, but coping was the most statistically significant [172].

A 2003 review of genetics of alcohol and nicotine dependence suggested that genetic components play a considerable role and are likely to be the result of a large number of genes, each contributing a small fraction of the overall risk [209].

Alcohol and tobacco together and separately increase the risk of several cancers, especially those involving the upper aero-digestive tract and liver [210].

The subjective effects of alcohol at levels that are consistent with alcohol intoxication appear to be due to glutamatergic and γ-aminobutyric acid neurotransmission [5, 6, 211]. When blood levels are rising in the early stages of intoxication, stimulatory effects including euphoria predominate. When blood levels are falling later in intoxication, sedative effects predominate. Excessive early alcohol intake over an extended period can induce tolerance.

Abrupt cessation can lead to overactivation of glutamatergic networks and under stimulation of the γ-aminobutyric acid system. Symptoms may include agitation, insomnia, irritability, anxiety, tremor, irritability, diaphoresis, instability of vital signs (such as hypertension, and tachycardia), seizures, alcoholic hallucinosis, delirium, and death [212]. According to a 2013 report, approximately 2–9% of the patients seen in family practice physician's offices in the USA are alcohol-dependent [212]. Benzodiazepines are the usual choice for moderating these effects [212, 213].

The *National Institute on Alcohol Abuse and Alcoholism* is a comprehensive resource for clinicians [214].

Cannabinoids

Cannabis is the most widely used illicit substance among individuals with depressive disorders [215].

About 9.5% of the adult US population used cannabis in 2015 according to *NIAAA's National Epidemiologic Survey on Alcohol and Related Conditions (NESARC)* [216] and 30% of the users met the criteria for a disorder. Dependence on cannabis was found to be twice as prevalent as dependence on any other illegal psychoactive substance; with a past-year cannabis abuse of ~1.1% and past-year dependence of 0.4% [7–10, 217]. These figures are likely to be rapidly out of date now that several states have made cannabis use legal.

A 2014 review found that for cannabis users, developing depression compared with controls was more likely with an OR = 1.17; 95% CI: 1.05 to 1.30). For heavy cannabis users, the likelihood of developing depression gave an OR = 1.62; 95% CI: 1.21 to 2.16), compared with non-users or light users [218]. There was no significant difference based on age and only marginal differences in effect that related to length of follow-up. There was, however, large heterogeneity between the studies.

A 2015 nationally representative sample of cannabis users who had depression found that quality of life (scored by the Short-Form 12 (SF-12) questionnaire) and Mental Component Summary score for women who regularly used cannabis was significantly lower than for non-users [215]. Women who used cannabis only occasionally showed no differences compared to non-users. Men who used cannabis regularly showed no difference in scores compared to occasional or non-users.

Amotivational syndrome (negative symptoms: combination of affective flattening and emotional reactivity) among depressed patients is significantly more severe in cannabis users (15.18 ± 2.25 versus 13.75 ± 2.44; t100 = 3.25 $p = 0.002$) [219].

Data from the *National Epidemiologic Survey of Alcohol and Related Conditions (NESARC)* indicated that alcohol use disorders (AUD) and cannabis use disorders (CUD) are positively and bidirectionally associated with MDD [10]. Cannabis dependence (OR = 6.61; 95% CI: 1.67 to 26.21) and co-occurring alcohol and cannabis dependence (OR = 2.34; 95% CI: 1.23 to 4.48) had the strongest association with MDD. MDD was strongly associated with new onset co-occurring alcohol and cannabis dependence (OR = 4 0.51; 95% CI: 1.31–15.60).

Simultaneous use of alcohol and cannabis is associated with greater social consequences, higher rates of alcohol dependence, and higher rates of depression compared to those who use only alcohol or only cannabis [223]. College students who use alcohol and cannabis appear to have more academic problems than those who use alcohol only [220].

Use of illicit drugs, education, family tension, place of upbringing, and alcohol confounds attempts to analyze associations between the increased relative risk for depression and anxiety that associates with cannabis use after adjusting for sex and age [221]. For female, but not male, users of 3,4-methylenedioxymethamphetamine (MDMA; ecstasy), lifetime use of cannabis was significantly associated with MDD [222].

Data from the *National Survey on Drug Use and Health (NSDUH)* indicates higher probability of arrest in White, African American, and Hispanic individuals who have co-occurring alcohol and cannabis use disorders [224]. MDD episodes within the past year are significantly more commonly reported by African American individuals who have co-occurring alcohol and cannabis use disorders [224]. A French study found that young adults who had parental history of both divorce and depression were more than twice as likely (OR = 2.38; 95% CI: 1.26 to 4.48) to be using cannabis as young adults whose parents were neither divorced nor depressed [225]. A study of Native American youths found that depression was more strongly associated with cannabis use by boys than by girls [226].

In the *Minnesota Twin Study*, consequences of *psychosocial failure* defined as educational failure (high school dropout), occupational failure (persistent unemployment), or engagement in crime were seen to partially account for association between early cannabis use and future MDD [227].

In a cohort of young Norwegians, exposure to cannabis by itself did not lead to depression but it did seem to be associated with later suicide thoughts and attempts [228].

Other studies have looked for an association between adolescent cannabis use and later depression but have not found it [229–231]. Associations between cannabis use and depression may be dependent upon other psychosocial factors [232].

One study suggests that people who have prior depression do not use cannabis for self-medication, but there is some evidence that they do use it as self-medication for aggression [233]. Depression, sadness, anxiety, and paranoia appear to be common in cannabis-dependent individuals when they are under the influence of cannabis [233]. Subjects who are cannabis-dependent and have difficulties in controlling violence frequently use cannabis to decrease aggression and suspiciousness, and to increase relaxation [233].

Cannabis use may make in-treatment alcohol recovery more difficult [234]. Association between early-onset cannabis use and other illicit drug use with depression and suicide appear to have overlapping genetic influences [235]. Although cannabis use rates are extremely high in people with psychotic disorders, it appears that there are no shared genetic etiologies [235].

The amygdala has a remarkably high concentration of CB1 cannabinoid receptors [235]. Cannabinoids may inhibit threat-related amygdala reactivity [236, 237]. Low doses of cannabis tend to be anxiolytics, whereas higher doses can be anxiety provoking or fear inducing [238, 239]. There is a great interindividual variation based on a wide variety of factors including genetics, environment, and differences in the concentrations of tetrahydrocannabinol and other alkaloids in the plant [239]. The brain's endogenous cannabinoid system modulates many cognitive and emotional processes and may have general (rather than specific) effects on the environmental influences on emotional and cognitive behavior [240].

Reviews of the adverse effects of cannabis can be found here [241, 242]. People with social anxiety are especially vulnerable to the adverse effects of cannabinoids [243].

During chronic cannabis use, the pattern of chronic intoxication during waking hours is followed by withdrawal that includes sleep disturbances, dysphoria, and irritability [51].

White matter maturation coincides with the age at which cannabis use is the highest [11, 12, 244, 245]. Regular cannabis use is associated with reduced white matter integrity in the frontolimbic area [246]. The *endocannabinoid system* which is highly invested in the frontolimbic area appears to regulate emotion-related memory, affective processing, stress response, and executive functioning [247–249]. This decrease in white matter has been linked to increased depressive and apathy symptoms in the cannabis users [246].

A discussion of the endocannabinoid system can be found in the Etiology chapter of this text.

Data from ALSPAC, a UK birth cohort study, found that both cannabis (unadjusted OR = 1.50; 95% CI: 1.26 to 1.80) and cigarette use (OR = 1.37; 95% CI: 1.16 to 1.61) increased the odds of developing depression [250].

Tobacco

There is a strong association between smoking and depression. Depressed individuals are about twice as likely to smoke as folks who are not depressed [16, 251–254]. Depression and smoking begin to be associated during adolescence [255, 256].

A strong positive association between smoking and depression has been reported by many [256–262] but not all [263–265] cross-sectional studies. A 2007 meta-analysis of many of the studies showed based upon 13–19 years of age that smoking predicted depression at a ratio of 1.73 (95% CI: 1.32 to 2.40; $p < 0.001$). Depression predicted smoking at 1.41 (95% CI: 1.21 to 1.63; $p < 0.001$).

Mechanisms that might explain the connection include shared genetic factors [254], shared environmental factors [254], self-medication [266], and bi-directional influences [17, 267].

It has been suggested that smoking cessation approaches for people who are depressed should be tailored to their characteristics that may be quite different from the non-smoking population [13–15, 268, 269].

Failure rates for quitting smoking are higher in those with depression compared to those without [18, 19, 270, 271] People with current depression may be less likely to be able to quit smoking than those who have recovered from depression [19].

For example, in a study conducted between 1980 and 1983 of 3213 people in the *St. Louis Epidemiologic Catchment Area Survey*, several interesting associations between depression and smoking were seen [272]. People who had experienced a major depressive episode vs. those who had not were more likely to have a history of regular smoking. The smokers who had experienced major depression had less success in quitting smoking. It also appears that when they did succeed in quitting, symptoms of depression, and serious major depression may have sometimes occurred. The gender difference in smoking that had been observed in the overall population was not found in those who had suffered from a major depression.

Typical smoking cessation interventions may be less effective for people with depression than they are for the general population [20–22, 273]. This may be due to depressed smokers being more likely to be susceptible to negative mood changes on withdrawal, to be more nicotine dependent, to be more likely to relapse, and to be at a heightened risk for morbidity and mortality.

Generally, smokers with depression do want to quit smoking [23, 269, 273–275]. Frequently though, health professionals do not urge them to quit because the providers fear that quitting may make depression worse [24, 25, 253]. However, the evidence actually suggests that depression symptoms may improve in individuals who remain abstinent [273, 276–279].

Smoking cessation techniques for smokers with depression have used standard smoking cessation counseling plus either an antidepressant or CBT [26, 269, 280–282].

Bright Light Therapy

Daily administration of light, or Bright Light Therapy (BLT), has been generally found to be an efficacious, first-line treatment for both seasonal and non-seasonal MDD [283]. BLT has also found use in experimental treatment for chronic depression, antepartum depression, premenstrual depression, bipolar depression, and disturbances of the sleep–wake cycle. BLT may be helpful for treating anorexia nervosa and bulimia nervosa [284] and delayed sleep phases in ADHD [285].

The DSM-5 does not include *seasonal affective disorder (SAD)* as a diagnosis separate from MDD or bipolar disorders, but the term SAD is still widely used [283]. SAD is defined as MDD with a seasonal pattern characterized by at least two consecutive years where the onset and offset of depressive symptoms occur at characteristic times with no non-seasonal episodes, a temporal relationship between onset of symptoms and time of year, a temporal relationship between remission of symptoms and time of year, and an outnumbering of seasonal compared to non-seasonal episodes throughout the lifetime of the patient [286, 287].

Hypersomnia, hyperphagia (especially carbohydrate craving), and weight gain are more frequent in SAD than in non-seasonal unipolar depression [288]. SAD is more common in winter than in summer [289].

The most well-accepted hypotheses for SAD are the *phase-shift hypothesis* and the *serotonin hypothesis* [283]. The phase-shift hypothesis suggests that an optimum relationship exists between alignment of the sleep–wake cycle and the endogenous circadian rhythm [290]. As the length of daylight shortens in autumn and winter, circadian rhythm starts drifting later relative to clock time and the sleep–wake cycle. This phase delay may instigate symptoms of depression in vulnerable people. Bright light therapy pulses a bright morning light to increase light exposure in an attempt to correct the misalignment of sleep and circadian rhythms [291].

The serotonin hypothesis posits that in autumn and winter there is greater binding potential at the pre-synaptic serotonin transporter than there is in summer [292, 293]. For people predisposed to SAD, there is more than normal binding capacity. With more binding to the serotonin transporter, there is less serotonin left in the synaptic cleft and less serotonin available to trigger post-synaptic firing. It is thought that BLT treatment in autumn and winter reduces transporter binding potential, hypothetically leading to less uptake, and more serotonin for possible use in the synapse [293, 294].

The suprachiasmatic nucleus is the primary oscillator in humans [295].[3] Indolamines (melatonin and serotonin) transduce light signals into cells and organisms and signal changing of the seasons. Melatonin is the central hormone in the internal clock circuits. Melatonin is synthesized via serotonin which modulates seasonal behaviors [297]. Melatonin is produced during darkness and is turned off in daylight. A light box is used in the early morning to provide a substitute for the "missing" daylight.[4] The use of low intensity narrow-band blue light appears to be equally effective as a treatment of depression as using bright white-light [296].

Interestingly, blue light, around 460–480 nm, which is emitted from LEDs used in the displays for most flat-panel televisions and computer monitors, smartphones, and tablet devices suppresses melatonin biosynthesis [298, 299]. At least one study in rodents suggests that there is a risk of depression symptoms with increased exposure to blue light. Blue light filtered white light induced depression-like symptoms and temporary spatial learning deficits in rats [300]. Evening use of light-emitting eReaders can negatively affect sleep, circadian timing, and next-morning alertness [301]. Subjects reading an LE-eBook took longer to fall asleep and experienced reduced evening sleepiness, reduced melatonin secretion, later timing of their circadian clock and reduced next-morning alertness than when reading a printed book.

A 2022 systematic review and meta-analysis of blue light therapy for seasonal and nonseasonal depression retrieved 582 articles and included nine RCTs [302]. They found no evidence for the efficacy of blue-light conditions compared to inactive conditions (mean difference [MD] = 2.43; 95% CI: −1.28 to 6.14, $p = 0.20$). Blue-light also showed no differences compared to active conditions (MD = −0.11; 95% CI: −2.38 to 2.16, p 0.93).

It is interesting to note that earlier analyses showed the following.

A 2020 updated meta-analysis in non-seasonal depression analyzed 23 RCTs [347]. The meta-analysis demonstrated light therapy was significantly more effective than comparative treatments and light therapy showed statistically significant mild to moderate treatment effect in reducing depressive symptoms. A 2016 meta-analysis found BLT appears to be efficacious when administered for 2–5 weeks (SMD = −0.78, $p < 0.001$, $I^2 = 0\%$), and as monotherapy (SMD = −0.71, $p < 0.001$, $I^2 = 18\%$) [303]. But studies of BLT for perinatal depression found statistically insignifi-

[3]A comprehensive review of bright light therapy can be found here [295].

[4]Light boxes are readily available.

cant improvement (SMD = −0.17, $p > 0.05$, $I^2 = 44\%$). They found moderate heterogeneity, participants were not adequately blinded, and sample size was small for certain subgroups. The long-term effect of BLT on depression symptoms was not addressed.

Conflicting results have been seen in using BLT for bipolar depression [304, 305]. However, a 2016 meta-analysis showed patients treated with either BLT monotherapy or in combination with other treatments had an effect size of −0.69, (95% CI: −0.90 to −0.48, $p < 0.001$) [306].

A 2007 case series involving women with bipolar disorder found that they are highly sensitive to morning bright light treatment, and that the induction of mixed states poses a substantial risk [307]. They recommended initiating treatment with a brief duration (15 min) of midday light for bipolar depression in women. A 2019 analysis underscores that suggestion [308]. They concluded that using BLT in BD is reasonable but requires concurrent antimanic treatment and careful clinical monitoring for response, safety, and mood polarity switch.

A 2002 open trial for BLT in antepartum depression was found after 3 weeks of treatment; the mean depression ratings improved by 49% [309]. Another study for antepartum depression indicated that BLT produced an effect size of 0.43, the same as antidepressants [310]. And a 2011 RCT found that for 5 weeks of BLT, remission was attained by 68.6% versus 36.4%, for placebo ($p < 0.05$) with minimal side effects for the mother and no known risk for the unborn child [311].

A 2016 systematic review and meta-analysis found that BLT of ≥5000 lux for ≥30 min improved results when augmenting standard antidepressant pharmacotherapy of MDD and BD without a seasonal pattern [312].

A 2015 critical review of the evidence for BLT found that methodological problems are present in most of the studies, and results of published meta-analyses are highly dependent on the study selection. Despite quality criteria in study selection, "when the results are carefully scrutinized, the evidence is not unequivocal" [291].

An interesting 2017 review discusses the history of SAD and BLT, the proposed pathophysiology of SAD and mechanisms of action of BLT in the treatment of SAD, and evidence supporting the efficacy of BLT in the treatment of non-seasonal unipolar major depression, bipolar depression, eating disorders, and ADHD [283].

A 2019 systematic review examined the management of BLT as a personalized and precision treatment in SAD, unipolar, and BD [313]. They concluded that BLT is an efficient antidepressant strategy in mono- or adjunct-therapy, which should be personalized according to the unipolar or bipolar subtype, the presence or absence of seasonal patterns, and its efficacy and tolerability.

Complementary and Alternative Treatment

Alternatives to pharmacological treatment for depression are numerous. For example, an Australian advocacy group of researchers at the Melbourne School of Population and Global Health, the Centre for Youth Mental Health and the Melbourne School of Psychological Sciences, The University of Melbourne, Victoria has produced a guide that lists dozens of complementary and alternative treatments of depression [314].

In 2012, in the USA, almost 59 million people spent more than 30 billion dollars out of pocket on CAM [315].

A nationally representative survey of 2055 respondents in 1997–1998 found that complementary and alternative therapies (CAT) were used more than conventional therapies by people with self-defined anxiety attacks and severe depression [316]. During that time, 53.6% of those with self-reported severe depression reported using CAT to treat their depression. And 66.7% of those seen by a conventional provider for severe depression also used CAT. Of those with severe depression 19.3% saw a CAT therapist. The respondents believed that the CATs were equally helpful to conventional treatments.

A 2007 review of CAM as the primary treatment for depression found no compelling evidence for efficacy in treating depression [317]. They did find *Grade 1 evidence*[5] on the use of St. John's wort, Tryptophan/5-Hydroxytryptophan, S-adenosyl methionine, folate, inositol, acupuncture, and exercise in depressive disorders, none of which was "conclusively positive." They found *Grade 2 level evidence* for use of saffron (herbal medicine), complex homoeopathy and relaxation training in depressive disorders, all of which showed "inconclusive results." Other RCTs gave "unequivocally negative results." Studies below that level gave "inconclusive or negative results." They believe that may be partly due to the incompatibility of RCTs and the "principles underlying many types of CAM."

Chai Hu Shu Gan San,[6] a traditional Chinese medicine, was analyzed in a systematic review and meta-analysis involving 42 RCTs (3234 patients) with depression in 15 diverse types of disease [318]. Their analyses showed better effects for Chai Hu Shu Gan San than for fluoxetine for pure depression (MD = −1.59, from −2.82 to −0.37, four trials, $I^2 = 26\%$), for post-stroke depression (MD = −4.20, from

[5] Oxford Centre for Evidence-Based Medicine [319].

[6] From reference [318]: "Chai Hu Shu Gan San is described in the Chinese ancient book Jing Yue Quan Shu • Gu Fang Ba Zhen • San Zhen, by Jingyue Zhang of the Ming dynasty. The primary constituent of this formula is Chai Hu (Bupleurum Chinese). The formula has two other constituents: Xiangfu (Cyperus rotundus) and Chuanxiong (Ligusticum chuanxiong). In China, a large number of clinical trial studies have indicated that Chai Hu Shu Gan San is widely used for treating all types of depression."

−6.20 to −2.19, seven trials, I^2[7] = 96%), and for postpartum depression (MD = −4.10, from −7.48 to −0.72, seven trials, I^2 = 86%). There were no reports of severe adverse events of oral administration of Chai Hu Shu Gan San and any adverse effects of using Chai Hu Shu Gan San alone were fewer than those of regular Western medicines.

Due to safety and risks of antidepressants in pregnancy and during lactation women often seek complementary and alternative treatments. One study indicated that over 25% of women used some form of CAM while pregnant [320].

There is insufficient evidence as of 2019 to recommend *acupuncture* for MDD treatment. One RCT did find benefit [321]. Response rates on intention to treat analyses were 72.0% and 18.2% ($p < 0.001$), for active laser, and placebo laser, respectively. Remission rates were 56.0% and 4.5% ($p < 0.001$) for active laser and placebo laser, respectively. A 2011 RCT found equal benefits of electroacupuncture and control acupuncture [322].

A 2022 review states that animal and human evidence suggests that acupuncture could increase hippocampal and network neuroplasticity and decrease brain inflammation potentially to alleviating depressive disorders, particularly milder cases [348]. Acupuncture, they believe, may be useful in management of post-stroke depression, pain-related depression, and postpartum depression both as an isolated and adjunct treatment. They believe that acupuncture combined with antidepressant pharmacological treatment enhanced improvement of primary and secondary depressive symptoms and reduced the side effects of the medical treatment. However, there were very few clinical trials to support that evidence.

A 2023 systematic review on acupuncture for depression was performed according to PRISMA (Preferred Reporting Items for Systematic Reviews and Meta-Analysis) guidelines [349]. Results suggested that electroacupuncture plus antidepressant was the best followed by manual acupuncture plus antidepressant and manual acupuncture.

A 2018 Cochrane found that.

"The reduction in severity of depression was less when acupuncture was compared with control acupuncture than when acupuncture was compared with no treatment control, although in both cases, results were rated as providing low-quality evidence. The reduction in severity of depression with acupuncture given alone or in conjunction with medication versus medication alone is uncertain owing to the very low quality of evidence. The effect of acupuncture compared with psychological therapy is unclear. The risk of adverse events with acupuncture is also unclear, as most trials did not report adverse events adequately. Few studies included follow-up periods or assessed important outcomes such as quality of life. High-quality randomized controlled trials are urgently needed to examine the clinical efficacy and acceptability of acupuncture, as well as its effectiveness, compared with acupuncture controls, medication, or psychological therapies." [323].

St. John's Wort

One of the folk remedies for depression as well as for other maladies is extracts of the plant *Hypericum perforatum* L. (popularly called St. John's wort). St John's wort is a popular herbal remedy frequently used in Traditional Chinese Medicine and widely prescribed for depression in many European countries [324, 325].

A 2019 scoping review about perceptions and use of St. John's wort for depression by general practitioners in clinical practice found that consumers drive St. John's wort use but often they do not disclose their use to their PCPs [326]. This raises concerns about safety. PCPs rarely recommend its use which may derive from lack of knowledge, especially regarding what preparations and dosages are supported by solid evidence, and lack of standardization of active ingredients.

A 2005 Cochrane review investigated to see if extracts of hypericum are more effective than placebo, if they are as effective as standard antidepressants in the treatment of depressive disorders in adults, and to see if they have less adverse effects than standard antidepressant drugs [327]. They concluded that current evidence regarding hypericum extracts is inconsistent and confusing. Some RCT trials suggest that the tested hypericum extracts have minimal beneficial effects, while other trials suggest that hypericum and standard antidepressants have similar beneficial effects. The reviewers stress that the results of their review apply only to the products tested in the included studies as preparations vary widely.

A 2015 systematic review and network meta-analysis efficacy and acceptability of pharmacological treatments for depressive disorders in primary care found that TCAs, SSRIs, an SNRI (venlafaxine), a low-dose serotonin antagonist and reuptake inhibitor (SARI; trazodone), and hypericum extracts were significantly superior to placebo, with estimated odds ratios between 1.69 and 2.03 [328]. No significant differences were seen between these drugs.

A 2016 systematic review found that St. John's wort for mild and moderate depression is superior to placebo in alleviating depression symptoms and not significantly different

[7] *I^2-statistic* is an indicator of heterogeneity in percentages. When the results from different studies on the same subject diverge or are conflicting, they are called *heterogeneous* A value of 0% indicates no observed heterogeneity, and larger values indicate increasing heterogeneity, with 25% as low, 50% as moderate, and 75% as high heterogeneity. A 95% confidence interval around I^2 is frequently used. Often the prediction interval is expressed, which indicates the range in which the true effect size of 95% of all populations will fall. For more information, see Chap. 4 Evidence Basics.

from antidepressant medication [329]. For severe depression, evidence was too heterogeneous, and there were too few studies to draw any conclusions. Similar results were seen in a 2017 meta-analysis [324]. They concluded that for patients with mild-to-moderate depression, St John's wort has comparable efficacy and safety when compared to SSRIs.

Nevertheless, a 2019 review of the evidence concluded that St. John's wort may exert potent antidepressant effects and is an efficacious and safe treatment [330].

There are several concerns regarding the use of Saint John's wort. Many of the assessments are limited by poor reporting of adverse events; there are very few data from primary care trials that considers long-term efficacy and safety (most studies are 4–12 weeks); there is little data on severe depression, suicidality, or suicide risk; much of the evidence on hypericum extracts is inconsistent and confusing; and the available preparations seem to vary considerably in pharmaceutical quality [328, 331, 332]. Hyperforin is a major active constituent of St. John's wort.[8]

Use of St. John's wort is frequently used by midwives for postpartum depression [334, 335]. There has been some concern over the possible presence of hypericin and hyperforin and flavonoids such as quercetin in breast milk [336, 337]. The issue of drug levels in lactation is discussed in the 2018 review [342]. Perinatal safety issues are discussed in previous works [338–341].

Pharmacokinetic interactions of drugs with St John's wort are reviewed in previous work [343]. The potential interaction of St John's wort with other drugs is a major safety concern.

It is worthy of quoting the following from the report:

- "St John's wort (Hypericum perforatum) is one of the most commonly used herbal antidepressants. St John's wort is a potent inducer of CYP 3A4 and P-glycoprotein (PgP), although it may inhibit or induce other CYPs, depending on the dose, route, and duration of administration.
- Data from human studies and case reports indicates that St John's wort decreased the blood concentrations of amitriptyline, cyclosporine, digoxin, fexofenadine, indinavir, methadone, midazolam, nevirapine, phenprocoumon, simvastatin, tacrolimus, theophylline, and warfarin, whereas it did not alter the pharmacokinetics of carbamazepine, dextromethorphan, mycophenolic acid, and pravastatin.
- St John's wort decreased the plasma concentration of the active metabolite SN-38 in cancer patients receiving irinotecan treatment. St John's wort did not alter the pharmacokinetics of tolbutamide but increased the incidence of hypoglycemia. Several cases have been reported that St John's wort decreased cyclosporine blood concentration leading to organ rejection.
- St John's wort caused breakthrough bleeding and unplanned pregnancies when used concomitantly with oral contraceptives.
- It also caused serotonin syndrome when coadministered with selective serotonin-reuptake inhibitors (e.g., sertraline and paroxetine)."

Useful resources to check for drug interactions can be found on the Internet. For example, [344–346].

Summary

Self-medication to relieve symptoms of mood disorders is common. Unfortunately, those self-medications are all too frequently dangerous and addictive. See Fig. 23.2.

To relieve symptoms of mood disorders, it appears that almost 25% of sufferers self-medicate with alcohol or drugs. Men may be about twice as likely as women to self-medicate. MDD is strongly linked with substance use disorders, which may influence specific depression symptoms. Depressive disorders are the most common psychiatric disorders among people with alcohol use disorder.

Positive and negative reinforcing effects are involved. Dependence produces a negative emotional state that drives drug seeking by negative reinforcement. The mesolimbic dopamine reward system works in opposition to the antireward systems which includes the brain stress systems that use CRH, norepinephrine, orexin, vasopressin, and dynorphin. The antireward state corresponds to the deficit state of normal rewards produced by excessive drug taking.

During addiction, an allostatic negative emotional state develops from a decrease in reward circuit functions and an increase in antireward circuit functions effecting transition to and maintenance of drug dependence. This negative state makes it exceedingly difficult to cope with the stress and anxiety that occurs during abstinence.

Changes in dopamine and serotonin transmission in the nucleus accumbens and enhanced CRH release in the central nucleus of the amygdala appear to be involved in vulnerability to relapse. In addition, conditionally learned contextual environmental cues in eliciting drug-seeking behavior and stress have definite roles. The medial prefrontal cortex and the basolateral amygdala, along with opioid receptors, are involved.

Caffeine addiction is considered to be relatively harmless. It affects basic processes including sleep, arousal, cognition, learning, and memory. Moderate amounts of caffeine may increase alertness and reduce fatigue. And it may increase performance on simple tasks that require sustained vigilance,

[8] Biotechnological production of hyperforin for pharmaceutical formulation [333].

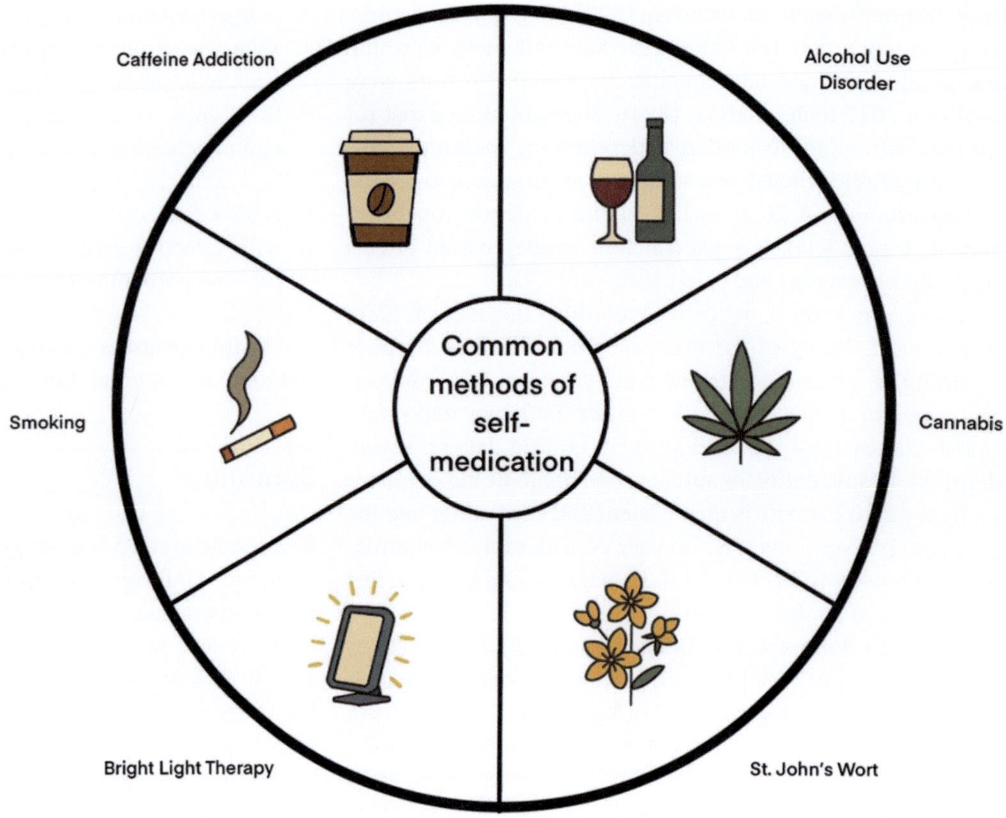

Fig. 23.2 Common self-medication strategies for depressive symptoms. This figure depicts widely used self-administered approaches for managing depressive symptoms, including caffeine, alcohol use, cannabis, St. John's wort supplementation, tobacco smoking, and bright light therapy. While some strategies may offer short-term mood enhancement or perceived relief, they vary in efficacy and carry distinct risks, with potential implications for neurochemical balance, addiction, and overall mental health

especially when alertness had been reduced. Folks who have higher consumption seem to have better mental functions. Effects on more complex tasks are difficult to assess.

Caffeine withdrawal may lead to fatigue and drowsiness; reduced alertness and difficulty concentrating; mood disturbances; decreased sociability and motivation to work; nausea and upset stomach; flu-like symptoms; and headache.

Most people appear to be able to adjust their consumption to maximize the benefits. Excessive consumption can lead to problems especially in particularly sensitive individuals. These include anxiety and sleep disturbances.

Nevertheless, some caffeine users are dependent on caffeine and cannot reduce their intake despite knowing recurrent health problems associated with continued use. Caffeine can produce behavioral and physiological effects similar to other drugs of dependence and caffeine use disorder.

Beneficial effects of coffee, tea, and chocolate are likely to be due to polyphenols and not caffeine. Effects of caffeine on the cardiovascular and immune system are not totally clear and are probably dose-dependent.

NESARC data reveals that depressive disorders are the most common psychiatric disorders among people with *alcohol use disorder*. Their cooccurrence is associated with worse prognosis, greater severity, and increased risk of suicide. Those people who have alcohol use disorder (AUD) versus those who do not have AUD are 2.3 times more likely to have had MDD and 1.7 times more likely to have dysthymia in the previous year.

Motives for drinking alcohol may be enhancement, socializing, conformity, and coping. Separately and in combination with tobacco, alcohol may reduce anticipatory anxiety. There are complex neurobiological mechanisms contributing to alcohol–stress–anxiety interactions.

Alcohol produces selective stress response dampening (SRD) during uncertain but not certain threat. Alcohol selectively reduces anxiety but not fear. SRD differences between individuals are associated with a family history of alcoholism, personality traits, degree of self-consciousness, cognitive functioning, and gender. Situational effects on SRD are also seen. Depending upon attention allocated and disruption of appraisal, alcohol has a variable effect on SRD.

Although alcohol may temporarily reduce stress, it may actually be a powerful anxiety-producing agent. Acute exposure to low to moderate amounts of ethanol can be anxiolytic, repeat exposure and withdrawal appear to be associated with neuroadaptive modifications that may be conducive to long lasting increase in a variety of anxiety symptoms. Heavy alcohol use in adolescents is associated with increased risk of comorbid psychopathology including internalizing symptoms such as depression and anxiety.

There are three classical sets of cravings and relapse triggers for drug abuse. Stress, re-exposure to environmental cues (people, places, and things associated with the drug), and re-exposure to addictive drugs. Neuroadaptive processes in the CNS that occur in the development of addiction and relapse appear to impair mechanisms that mediate positive reinforcement and emergence of anxiety, depression, and dysphoria that can occur during withdrawal.

Genome-wide association studies of comorbid major depression and alcohol dependence suggest that the comorbidity is partially influenced by genetic variants that do not affect alcohol dependence alone.

Dependence on alcohol, caffeine, and benzodiazepines may increase the severity of panic attacks. Upon withdrawal from alcohol addiction, it is common for anxiety to increase.

Cannabis is the most widely used illicit substance among individuals with depressive disorders. For cannabis users, developing depression compared with controls was more likely. For heavy cannabis users, have an increased likelihood of developing depression compared with non-users or light users. Data from the *NESARC* indicated that alcohol use disorders and cannabis use disorders are positively and bidirectionally associated with MDD. Cannabis dependence and co-occurring alcohol and cannabis dependence had the strongest association with MDD. MDD was strongly associated with new onset co-occurring alcohol and cannabis dependence.

Simultaneous use of alcohol and cannabis is associated with greater social consequences, higher rates of alcohol dependence, and higher rates of depression compared to those who use only alcohol or only cannabis. College students who use alcohol and cannabis appear to have more academic problems than those who use alcohol only.

Use of illicit drugs, education, family tension, place of upbringing, and alcohol confounds attempts to analyze associations between the increased relative risk for depression and anxiety that associates with cannabis use after adjusting for sex and age.

Psychosocial failure defined as educational failure (high school dropout), occupational failure (persistent unemployment), or engagement in crime partially accounts for association between early cannabis use and future MDD.

Some studies have looked for an association between adolescent cannabis use and later depression but have not found it. Associations between cannabis use and depression may be dependent upon other psychosocial factors.

Association between early-onset cannabis use and other illicit drug use with depression and suicide appear to have overlapping genetic influences.

The *endocannabinoid system* which is highly invested in the frontolimbic area appears to regulate emotion-related memory, affective processing, stress response, and executive functioning. The brain's endogenous cannabinoid system modulates many cognitive and emotional processes and may have general (rather than specific) effects on the environmental influences on emotional and cognitive behavior.

White matter maturation coincides with the age at which cannabis use is the highest. Regular cannabis use is associated with reduced white matter integrity in the frontolimbic area. This decrease in white matter has been linked to increased depressive and apathy symptoms in the cannabis users. Amygdalas have a remarkably high concentration of CB1 cannabinoid receptors. Cannabinoids may inhibit threat-related amygdala reactivity. Low doses of cannabis tend to be anxiolytics, whereas higher doses can be anxiety-provoking or fear-inducing.

There is a strong association between smoking and depression. Depressed individuals are about twice as likely to smoke as folks who are not depressed. Depression and smoking begin to be associated during adolescence.

A strong positive association between smoking and depression has been reported by many but not all cross-sectional studies. A 2007 meta-analysis of many of the studies showed based upon 13–19 years of age that smoking predicted depression at a ratio of 1.73. Depression predicted smoking at 1.41.

Mechanisms that might explain the connection include shared genetic factors, shared environmental factors, self-medication, and bi-directional influences.

It has been suggested that smoking cessation approaches for people who are depressed should be tailored to their characteristics that may be quite different from the non-smoking population.

Failure rates for quitting smoking are higher in those with depression compared to those without. People with current depression may be less likely to be able to quit smoking than those who have recovered from depression.

Daily administration of light, or *Bright Light Therapy* (BLT), has been generally found to be an efficacious, first-line treatment for both seasonal and non-seasonal MDD. BLT has also found use in experimental treatment for chronic depression, antepartum depression, premenstrual depression, bipolar depression, and disturbances of the sleep–wake cycle. Most studies have shown that BLT is effective in seasonal and non-seasonal depression as a primary treatment and as an adjunctive treatment where it might do better than antidepressants alone. On the other hand, a 2003 meta-analysis showed bright light as an adjunct to antidepressant pharmacotherapy for non-seasonal depression was not effective. They concluded that BLT is an efficient antidepressant strategy in mono- or adjunct-therapy, which should be personalized according to the unipolar or bipolar subtype, the presence or absence of seasonal patterns, and its efficacy and tolerability. The most well-accepted hypotheses for SAD are the *phase-shift hypothesis* and the *serotonin hypothesis.*

Alternatives to pharmacological treatment for depression are numerous. In 2012, in the USA almost 59 million people spent more than 30 billion dollars out of pocket on *complementary and alternative medicine* (CAM). A 2007 review of

CAM as the primary treatment for depression found no compelling evidence for efficacy in treating depression. There is insufficient evidence as of 2019 to recommend *acupuncture* for MDD treatment.

St. John's wort is a popular herbal remedy frequently used in Traditional Chinese Medicine and widely prescribed for depression in many European countries. Current evidence regarding hypericum extracts is inconsistent and confusing. Some RCT trials suggest that the tested hypericum extracts have minimal beneficial effects, while other trials suggest that hypericum and standard antidepressants have similar beneficial effects.

A 2015 systematic review and network meta-analysis efficacy and acceptability of pharmacological treatments for depressive disorders in primary care found that TCAs, SSRIs, an SNRI (venlafaxine), a low-dose serotonin antagonist and reuptake inhibitor (SARI; trazodone), and hypericum extracts were significantly superior to placebo, with estimated odds ratios between 1.69 and 2.03. No significant differences were seen between these drugs.

A 2016 systematic review found that St. John's wort for mild and moderate depression is superior to placebo in alleviating depression symptoms and not significantly different from antidepressant medication. For severe depression, evidence was too heterogeneous, and there were too few studies to draw any conclusions. Similar results were seen in a 2017 meta-analysis. They concluded that for patients with mild-to-moderate depression, St. John's wort has comparable efficacy and safety when compared to SSRIs.

Nevertheless, a 2019 review of the evidence concluded that St. John's wort may exert potent antidepressant effects and is an efficacious and safe treatment.

The potential interaction of St. John's wort with other drugs is a major safety concern. There is little data on severe depression, suicidality, or suicide risk; much of the evidence on hypericum extracts is inconsistent and confusing, and the available preparations seem to vary considerably in pharmaceutical quality.

References

1. Cooper ML. Motivations for alcohol use among adolescents: development and validation of a four-factor model. Psychol Assess. 1994;6(2):117.
2. Kluver H, Bucy PC. "Psychic blindness" and other symptoms following bilateral temporal lobectomy in Rhesus monkeys. Am J Physiol. 1937;119:352–3.
3. Aouizerate B, Martin-Guehl C, Tignol J. Neurobiology and pharmacotherapy of social phobia. Encephale. 2004; 30(4):301–13. PMID: 15538306. http://www.ncbi.nlm.nih.gov/pubmed/15538306.
4. Hinde RA. Animal behavior. New York, NY: McGraw-Hill; 1966. Animal behaviour; a synthesis of ethology and comparative psychology: Hinde, Robert A: Free Download, Borrow, and Streaming: Internet Archive.
5. Hermann D, Weber-Fahr W, Sartorius A, Hoerst M, Frischknecht U, Tunc-Skarka N, Perreau-Lenz S, Hansson AC, Krumm B, Kiefer F, Spanagel R, Mann K, Ende G, Sommer WH. Translational magnetic resonance spectroscopy reveals excessive central glutamate levels during alcohol withdrawal in humans and rats. Biol Psychiatry. 2012;71(11):1015–21. PMID: 21907974. http://www.ncbi.nlm.nih.gov/pubmed/21907974.
6. Gomez R, Behar KL, Watzl J, Weinzimer SA, Gulanski B, Sanacora G, Koretski J, Guidone E, Jiang L, Petrakis IL, Pittman B, Krystal JH, Mason GF. Intravenous ethanol infusion decreases human cortical γ-aminobutyric acid and N-acetylaspartate as measured with proton magnetic resonance spectroscopy at 4 tesla. Biol Psychiatry. 2012;71(3):239–46. PMCID: PMC3227760. http://www.ncbi.nlm.nih.gov/pubmed/21855054.
7. Sterling P, Eyer J. Allostasis: a new paradigm to explain arousal pathology. In: Fisher S, Reason J, editors. Handbook of life stress, cognition and health. Chichiester: Wiley; 1988. p. 629–49.
8. Substance Abuse and Mental Health Services Administration. National survey on drug use and health: summary of methodological studies, 1971–2014 [Internet]. Rockville: Substance Abuse and Mental Health Services Administration (US); 2014. [cited 2025 Jan 31]. Available from: http://www.ncbi.nlm.nih.gov/books/NBK519735/. PMID: 30199189.
9. Anthony JC, Warner LA, Kessler RC. Comparative epidemiology of dependence on tobacco, alcohol, controlled substance, and inhalants: basic findings from the National Comorbidity Survey. Comparative epidemiology of dependence on tobacco, alcohol, controlled substance, and inhalants: basic findings from the National Comorbidity Survey. Exp Clin Psychopharmacol. 1994;2:224–68.
10. Pacek LR, Martins SS, Crum RM. The bidirectional relationships between alcohol, cannabis, co-occurring alcohol and cannabis use disorders with major depressive disorder: results from a national sample. J Affect Disord. 2013;148(2–3):188–95. PMCID: PMC3608823. http://www.ncbi.nlm.nih.gov/pubmed/23260381.
11. Johnston LD, O'Malley PM, Bachman JG, Schulenburg JE, Miech RA. II. Institute for social research. Ann Arbor: The University of Michigan; 2014. p. 424. (Monitoring the future: National Survey Results on Drug Use, 1975–2011: College Students and Adults Ages 19–55). Monitoring the Future national survey results on drug use, 1975–2021: Overview, key findings on adolescent drug use.
12. Johnston LD, O'Malley PM, Bachman JG, Schulenberg JE. II. Institute for social research. Ann Arbor: University of Michigan; 2013. p. 400. (Monitoring the Future National Survey Results on Drug Use, 1975–2012: College Students and Adults Ages 19–50). Monitoring the Future national survey results on drug use, 1975–2021: Overview, key findings on adolescent drug use.
13. Borrelli B. Smoking cessation: next steps for special populations research and innovative treatments. J Consult Clin Psychol. 2010;78(1):1–12. PMID: 20099945. http://www.ncbi.nlm.nih.gov/pubmed/20099945.
14. Evins AE, Cather C, Laffer A. Treatment of tobacco use disorders in smokers with serious mental illness: toward clinical best practices. Harv Rev Psychiatry. 2015;23(2):90–8. PMCID: PMC4460830. http://www.ncbi.nlm.nih.gov/pubmed/25747922.
15. Hitsman B, Papandonatos GD, McChargue DE, DeMott A, Herrera MJ, Spring B, Borrelli B, Niaura R. Past major depression and smoking cessation outcome: a systematic review and meta-analysis update. Addiction. 2013;108(2):294–306. PMCID: PMC3593055. http://www.ncbi.nlm.nih.gov/pubmed/23072580.
16. Kalman D, Morissette SB, George TP. Co-morbidity of smoking in patients with psychiatric and substance use disorders. Am J

Addict. 2005;14(2):106–23. PMCID: PMC1199553. http://www.ncbi.nlm.nih.gov/pubmed/16019961.

17. Markou A, Kenny PJ. Neuroadaptations to chronic exposure to drugs of abuse: relevance to depressive symptomatology seen across psychiatric diagnostic categories. Neurotox Res. 2002;4(4):297–313. PMID: 12829420. http://www.ncbi.nlm.nih.gov/pubmed/12829420.
18. van der Meer RM, Willemsen MC, Smit F, Cuijpers P. Smoking cessation interventions for smokers with current or past depression. Cochrane Database Syst Rev. 2013;8:CD006102. PMID: 23963776. http://www.ncbi.nlm.nih.gov/pubmed/23963776.
19. Weinberger AH, Pilver CE, Desai RA, Mazure CM, McKee SA. The relationship of major depressive disorder and gender to changes in smoking for current and former smokers: longitudinal evaluation in the US population. Addiction. 2012;107(10):1847–56. PMCID: PMC3419319. http://www.ncbi.nlm.nih.gov/pubmed/22429388.
20. Bolam B, West R, Gunnell D. Does smoking cessation cause depression and anxiety? Findings from the ATTEMPT cohort. Nicotine Tob Res. 2011;13(3):209–14. PMID: 21330275. http://www.ncbi.nlm.nih.gov/pubmed/21330275.
21. Gierisch JM, Bastian LA, Calhoun PS, McDuffie JR, Williams JW. Smoking cessation interventions for patients with depression: a systematic review and meta-analysis. J Gen Intern Med. 2012;27(3):351–60. PMCID: PMC3286553. http://www.ncbi.nlm.nih.gov/pubmed/22038468.
22. Weinberger AH, Mazure CM, Morlett A, McKee SA. Two decades of smoking cessation treatment research on smokers with depression: 1990–2010. Nicotine Tob Res. 2013;15(6):1014–31. PMCID: PMC3693502. http://www.ncbi.nlm.nih.gov/pubmed/23100459.
23. Haukkala A, Uutela A, Vartiainen E, McAlister A, Knekt P. Depression and smoking cessation: the role of motivation and self-efficacy. Addict Behav. 2000;25(2):311–6. PMID: 10795958. http://www.ncbi.nlm.nih.gov/pubmed/10795958.
24. Hitsman B, Moss TG, Montoya ID, George TP. Treatment of tobacco dependence in mental health and addictive disorders. Can J Psychiatr. 2009;54(6):368–78. PMCID: PMC3632078. http://www.ncbi.nlm.nih.gov/pubmed/19527557.
25. Prochaska JJ. Failure to treat tobacco use in mental health and addiction treatment settings: a form of harm reduction? Drug Alcohol Depend. 2010;110(3):177–82. PMCID: PMC2916693. http://www.ncbi.nlm.nih.gov/pubmed/20378281.
26. van der Meer RM, Willemsen MC, Smit F, Cuijpers P, Schippers GM. Effectiveness of a mood management component as an adjunct to a telephone counselling smoking cessation intervention for smokers with a past major depression: a pragmatic randomized controlled trial. Addiction. 2010;105(11):1991–9. PMID: 20735366. http://www.ncbi.nlm.nih.gov/pubmed/20735366.
27. Lanska DJ. The Klüver-Bucy syndrome. Front Neurol Neurosci. 2018;41:77–89. PMID: 29145186. http://www.ncbi.nlm.nih.gov/pubmed/29145186.
28. Khantzian EJ. The self-medication hypothesis of substance use disorders: a reconsideration and recent applications. Harv Rev Psychiatry. 1997;4(5):231–44. PMID: 9385000. http://www.ncbi.nlm.nih.gov/pubmed/9385000.
29. Bolton JM, Robinson J, Sareen J. Self-medication of mood disorders with alcohol and drugs in the National Epidemiologic Survey on alcohol and related conditions. J Affect Disord. 2009;115(3):367–75. PMID: 19004504. http://www.ncbi.nlm.nih.gov/pubmed/19004504.
30. Moore AA, Neale MC, Silberg JL, Verhulst B. Substance use and depression symptomatology: measurement invariance of the Beck Depression Inventory (BDI-II) among non-users and frequent-users of alcohol, nicotine and cannabis. PLoS One. 2016;11(4):e0152118. PMCID: PMC4821457. http://www.ncbi.nlm.nih.gov/pubmed/27046165.
31. Grant BF, Goldstein RB, Chou SP, Huang B, Stinson FS, Dawson DA, Saha TD, Smith SM, Pulay AJ, Pickering RP, Ruan WJ, Compton WM. Sociodemographic and psychopathologic predictors of first incidence of DSM-IV substance use, mood and anxiety disorders: results from the wave 2 National Epidemiologic Survey on alcohol and related conditions. Mol Psychiatry. 2009;14(11):1051–66. PMCID: PMC2766434. http://www.ncbi.nlm.nih.gov/pubmed/18427559.
32. Regier DA, Farmer ME, Rae DS, Locke BZ, Keith SJ, Judd LL, Goodwin FK. Comorbidity of mental disorders with alcohol and other drug abuse. Results from the Epidemiologic Catchment Area (ECA) study. JAMA. 1990;264(19):2511–8. PMID: 2232018. http://www.ncbi.nlm.nih.gov/pubmed/2232018.
33. National Epidemiologic Survey on Alcohol and Related Conditions (NESARC) – III – Catalog.
34. McHugh RK, Weiss RD. Alcohol use disorder and depressive disorders. Alcohol Res. 2019;40(1):arcr.v40.1.01. PMCID: PMC6799954. http://www.ncbi.nlm.nih.gov/pubmed/31649834.
35. Greenfield SF, Weiss RD, Muenz LR, Vagge LM, Kelly JF, Bello LR, Michael J. The effect of depression on return to drinking: a prospective study. Arch Gen Psychiatry. 1998;55(3):259–65. PMID: 9510220. http://www.ncbi.nlm.nih.gov/pubmed/9510220.
36. Hasin D, Liu X, Nunes E, McCloud S, Samet S, Endicott J. Effects of major depression on remission and relapse of substance dependence. Arch Gen Psychiatry. 2002;59(4):375–80. PMID: 11926938. http://www.ncbi.nlm.nih.gov/pubmed/11926938.
37. Conner KR, Gamble SA, Bagge CL, He H, Swogger MT, Watts A, Houston RJ. Substance-induced depression and independent depression in proximal risk for suicidal behavior. J Stud Alcohol Drugs. 2014;75(4):567–72. PMCID: PMC9798469. http://www.ncbi.nlm.nih.gov/pubmed/24988255.
38. Grant BF, Stinson FS, Dawson DA, Chou SP, Dufour MC, Compton W, Pickering RP, Kaplan K. Prevalence and co-occurrence of substance use disorders and independent mood and anxiety disorders: results from the National Epidemiologic Survey on alcohol and related conditions. Arch Gen Psychiatry. 2004;61(8):807–16. PMID: 15289279. http://www.ncbi.nlm.nih.gov/pubmed/15289279.
39. Smith SM, Stinson FS, Dawson DA, Goldstein R, Huang B, Grant BF. Race/ethnic differences in the prevalence and co-occurrence of substance use disorders and independent mood and anxiety disorders: results from the National Epidemiologic Survey on alcohol and related conditions. Psychol Med. 2006;36(7):987–98. PMID: 16650344. http://www.ncbi.nlm.nih.gov/pubmed/16650344.
40. Hatzenbuehler ML, Keyes KM, Narrow WE, Grant BF, Hasin DS. Racial/ethnic disparities in service utilization for individuals with co-occurring mental health and substance use disorders in the general population: results from the national epidemiologic survey on alcohol and related conditions. J Clin Psychiatry. 2008;69(7):1112–21. PMCID: PMC2745048. http://www.ncbi.nlm.nih.gov/pubmed/18517286.
41. Nam E, Matejkowski J, Lee S. Racial/ethnic differences in contemporaneous use of mental health and substance use treatment among individuals experiencing both mental illness and substance use disorders. Psychiatr Q. 2017;88(1):185–98. PMID: 27271529. http://www.ncbi.nlm.nih.gov/pubmed/27271529.
42. Koob GF, Le Moal M. Plasticity of reward neurocircuitry and the "dark side" of drug addiction. Nat Neurosci. 2005;8(11):1442–4. PMID: 16251985. http://www.ncbi.nlm.nih.gov/pubmed/16251985.
43. Substance Abuse and Mental Health Services Administration. National survey on drug use and health: summary of methodological studies, 1971–2014 [Internet]. Rockville: Substance Abuse and Mental Health Services Administration (US); 2014. [cited 2025 Jan 31]. Available from: http://www.ncbi.nlm.nih.gov/

books/NBK519735/. PMID: 30199189 http://www.ncbi.nlm.nih.gov/pubmed/30199189.
44. Thomas MJ, Beurrier C, Bonci A, Malenka RC. Long-term depression in the nucleus accumbens: a neural correlate of behavioral sensitization to cocaine. Nat Neurosci. 2001;4(12):1217–23. PMID: 11694884. http://www.ncbi.nlm.nih.gov/pubmed/11694884.
45. Borgland SL, Taha SA, Sarti F, Fields HL, Bonci A. Orexin A in the VTA is critical for the induction of synaptic plasticity and behavioral sensitization to cocaine. Neuron. 2006;49(4):589–601. PMID: 16476667. http://www.ncbi.nlm.nih.gov/pubmed/16476667.
46. Koob GF, Le Moal M. Addiction and the brain antireward system. Annu Rev Psychol. 2008;59:29–53. PMID: 18154498. http://www.ncbi.nlm.nih.gov/pubmed/18154498.
47. Davis LL, Trivedi M, Choate A, Kramer GL, Petty F. Growth hormone response to the GABAB agonist baclofen in major depressive disorder. Psychoneuroendocrinology. 1997;22(3):129–40. PMID: 9203224. http://www.ncbi.nlm.nih.gov/pubmed/9203224.
48. Georges F, Aston-Jones G. Activation of ventral tegmental area cells by the bed nucleus of the stria terminalis: a novel excitatory amino acid input to midbrain dopamine neurons. J Neurosci. 2002;22(12):5173–87. PMCID: PMC6757737. http://www.ncbi.nlm.nih.gov/pubmed/12077212.
49. Carboni E, Silvagni A, Rolando MT, Di Chiara G. Stimulation of in vivo dopamine transmission in the bed nucleus of stria terminalis by reinforcing drugs. J Neurosci. 2000;20(20):RC102. PMCID: PMC6772858. http://www.ncbi.nlm.nih.gov/pubmed/11027253.
50. Eiler WJA, Seyoum R, Foster KL, Mailey C, June HL. D1 dopamine receptor regulates alcohol-motivated behaviors in the bed nucleus of the stria terminalis in alcohol-preferring (P) rats. Synapse. 2003;48(1):45–56. PMID: 12557272. http://www.ncbi.nlm.nih.gov/pubmed/12557272.
51. Koob GF. A role for brain stress systems in addiction. Neuron. 2008;59(1):11–34. PMCID: PMC2748830. http://www.ncbi.nlm.nih.gov/pubmed/18614026.
52. Baik JH. Dopamine signaling in reward-related behaviors. Front Neural Circuits. 2013;7:152. PMCID: PMC3795306. http://www.ncbi.nlm.nih.gov/pubmed/24130517.
53. Oleson EB, Cheer JF. A brain on cannabinoids: the role of dopamine release in reward seeking. Cold Spring Harb Perspect Med. 2012;2(8):a012229. PMCID: PMC3405830. http://www.ncbi.nlm.nih.gov/pubmed/22908200.
54. Salamone JD, Correa M. The mysterious motivational functions of mesolimbic dopamine. Neuron. 2012;76(3):470–85. PMCID: PMC4450094. http://www.ncbi.nlm.nih.gov/pubmed/23141060.
55. Mark GP, Shabani S, Dobbs LK, Hansen ST. Cholinergic modulation of mesolimbic dopamine function and reward. Physiol Behav. 2011;104(1):76–81. PMCID: PMC4495915. http://www.ncbi.nlm.nih.gov/pubmed/21549724.
56. Kim H, Nanavaty N, Ahmed H, Mathur VA, Anderson BA. Motivational salience guides attention to valuable and threatening stimuli: evidence from behavior and functional magnetic resonance imaging. J Cogn Neurosci. 2021;33(12):2440–60. PMCID: PMC8578406. http://www.ncbi.nlm.nih.gov/pubmed/34407195.
57. Puglisi-Allegra S, Ventura R. Prefrontal/accumbal catecholamine system processes high motivational salience. Front Behav Neurosci. 2012;6:31. PMCID: PMC3384081. http://www.ncbi.nlm.nih.gov/pubmed/22754514.
58. Wenzel JM, Rauscher NA, Cheer JF, Oleson EB. A role for phasic dopamine release within the nucleus accumbens in encoding aversion: a review of the neurochemical literature. ACS Chem Neurosci. 2015;6(1):16–26. PMCID: PMC5820768. http://www.ncbi.nlm.nih.gov/pubmed/25491156.
59. Oleson EB, Beckert MV, Morra JT, Lansink CS, Cachope R, Abdullah RA, Loriaux AL, Schetters D, Pattij T, Roitman MF, Lichtman AH, Cheer JF. Endocannabinoids shape accumbal encoding of cue-motivated behavior via CB1 receptor activation in the ventral tegmentum. Neuron. 2012;73(2):360–73. PMCID: PMC3269037. http://www.ncbi.nlm.nih.gov/pubmed/22284189.
60. Lupica CR, Riegel AC. Endocannabinoid release from midbrain dopamine neurons: a potential substrate for cannabinoid receptor antagonist treatment of addiction. Neuropharmacology. 2005;48(8):1105–16. PMID: 15878779. http://www.ncbi.nlm.nih.gov/pubmed/15878779.
61. Solinas M, Goldberg SR, Piomelli D. The endocannabinoid system in brain reward processes. Br J Pharmacol. 2008;154(2):369–83. PMCID: PMC2442437. http://www.ncbi.nlm.nih.gov/pubmed/18414385.
62. Freund TF, Katona I, Piomelli D. Role of endogenous cannabinoids in synaptic signaling. Physiol Rev. 2003;83(3):1017–66. PMID: 12843414. http://www.ncbi.nlm.nih.gov/pubmed/12843414.
63. Melis M, Pistis M, Perra S, Muntoni AL, Pillolla G, Gessa GL. Endocannabinoids mediate presynaptic inhibition of glutamatergic transmission in rat ventral tegmental area dopamine neurons through activation of CB1 receptors. J Neurosci. 2004;24(1):53–62. PMCID: PMC6729571. http://www.ncbi.nlm.nih.gov/pubmed/14715937.
64. Koob GF, Le Moal M. Drug abuse: hedonic homeostatic dysregulation. Science. 1997;278(5335):52–8. PMID: 9311926. http://www.ncbi.nlm.nih.gov/pubmed/9311926.
65. Solomon RL, Corbit JD. An opponent-process theory of motivation. I. Temporal dynamics of affect. Psychol Rev. 1974;81(2):119–45. PMID: 4817611. http://www.ncbi.nlm.nih.gov/pubmed/4817611.
66. Le Moal M, Koob GF. Drug addiction: pathways to the disease and pathophysiological perspectives. Eur Neuropsychopharmacol. 2007;17(6–7):377–93. PMID: 17169534. http://www.ncbi.nlm.nih.gov/pubmed/17169534.
67. Shaffer C, Westlin C, Quigley KS, Whitfield-Gabrieli S, Barrett LF. Allostasis, action, and affect in depression: insights from the theory of constructed emotion. Annu Rev Clin Psychol. 2022;18:553–80. PMCID: PMC9247744. http://www.ncbi.nlm.nih.gov/pubmed/35534123.
68. Chalmers DT, Lovenberg TW, Grigoriadis DE, Behan DP, De Souza EB. Corticotrophin-releasing factor receptors: from molecular biology to drug design. Trends Pharmacol Sci. 1996;17(4):166–72. PMID: 8984745. http://www.ncbi.nlm.nih.gov/pubmed/8984745.
69. Palchaudhuri MR, Wille S, Mevenkamp G, Spiess J, Fuchs E, Dautzenberg FM. Corticotropin-releasing factor receptor type 1 from Tupaia belangeri–cloning, functional expression and tissue distribution. Eur J Biochem. 1998;258(1):78–84. PMID: 9851694. http://www.ncbi.nlm.nih.gov/pubmed/9851694.
70. Potter E, Sutton S, Donaldson C, Chen R, Perrin M, Lewis K, Sawchenko PE, Vale W. Distribution of corticotropin-releasing factor receptor mRNA expression in the rat brain and pituitary. Proc Natl Acad Sci U S A. 1994;91(19):8777–81. PMCID: PMC44689. http://www.ncbi.nlm.nih.gov/pubmed/8090722.
71. Olive MF, Koenig HN, Nannini MA, Hodge CW. Elevated extracellular CRF levels in the bed nucleus of the stria terminalis during ethanol withdrawal and reduction by subsequent ethanol intake. Pharmacol Biochem Behav. 2002;72(1–2):213–20. PMCID: PMC11583329. http://www.ncbi.nlm.nih.gov/pubmed/11900791.
72. Rassnick S, Heinrichs SC, Britton KT, Koob GF. Microinjection of a corticotropin-releasing factor antagonist into the central nucleus of the amygdala reverses anxiogenic-like effects of ethanol withdrawal. Brain Res. 1993;605(1):25–32. PMID: 8467387. http://www.ncbi.nlm.nih.gov/pubmed/8467387.
73. Rivera-Oliver M, Díaz-Ríos M. Using caffeine and other adenosine receptor antagonists and agonists as therapeutic

tools against neurodegenerative diseases: a review. Life Sci. 2014;101(1–2):1–9. PMCID: PMC4115368. http://www.ncbi.nlm.nih.gov/pubmed/24530739.

74. Mitchell DC, Knight CA, Hockenberry J, Teplansky R, Hartman TJ. Beverage caffeine intakes in the U.S. Food Chem Toxicol. 2014;63:136–42. PMID: 24189158. http://www.ncbi.nlm.nih.gov/pubmed/24189158.
75. Fulgoni VL, Keast DR, Lieberman HR. Trends in intake and sources of caffeine in the diets of US adults: 2001–2010. Am J Clin Nutr. 2015;101(5):1081–7. PMID: 25832334. http://www.ncbi.nlm.nih.gov/pubmed/25832334.
76. Wikoff D, Welsh BT, Henderson R, Brorby GP, Britt J, Myers E, Goldberger J, Lieberman HR, O'Brien C, Peck J, Tenenbein M, Weaver C, Harvey S, Urban J, Doepker C. Systematic review of the potential adverse effects of caffeine consumption in healthy adults, pregnant women, adolescents, and children. Food Chem Toxicol. 2017;109(Pt 1):585–648. PMID: 28438661. http://www.ncbi.nlm.nih.gov/pubmed/28438661.
77. Doepker C, Franke K, Myers E, Goldberger JJ, Lieberman HR, O'Brien C, Peck J, Tenenbein M, Weaver C, Wikoff D. Key findings and implications of a recent systematic review of the potential adverse effects of caffeine consumption in healthy adults, pregnant women, adolescents, and children. Nutrients. 2018;10(10):1536. PMCID: PMC6212940. http://www.ncbi.nlm.nih.gov/pubmed/30340340.
78. Loftfield E, Freedman ND, Dodd KW, Vogtmann E, Xiao Q, Sinha R, Graubard BI. Coffee drinking is widespread in the United States, but usual intake varies by key demographic and lifestyle factors. J Nutr. 2016;146(9):1762–8. PMCID: PMC4997286. http://www.ncbi.nlm.nih.gov/pubmed/27489008.
79. Bailey RL, Saldanha LG, Dwyer JT. Estimating caffeine intake from energy drinks and dietary supplements in the United States. Nutr Rev. 2014;72(Suppl 1):9–13. PMCID: PMC4658518. http://www.ncbi.nlm.nih.gov/pubmed/25293539.
80. Kit BK, Fakhouri THI, Park S, Nielsen SJ, Ogden CL. Trends in sugar-sweetened beverage consumption among youth and adults in the United States: 1999–2010. Am J Clin Nutr. 2013;98(1):180–8. PMCID: PMC10401613. http://www.ncbi.nlm.nih.gov/pubmed/23676424.
81. Fredholm BB, Bättig K, Holmén J, Nehlig A, Zvartau EE. Actions of caffeine in the brain with special reference to factors that contribute to its widespread use. Pharmacol Rev. 1999;51(1):83–133. PMID: 10049999. http://www.ncbi.nlm.nih.gov/pubmed/10049999.
82. Fisone G, Borgkvist A, Usiello A. Caffeine as a psychomotor stimulant: mechanism of action. Cell Mol Life Sci. 2004;61(7–8):857–72. PMCID: PMC11138593. http://www.ncbi.nlm.nih.gov/pubmed/15095008.
83. Kaster MP, Machado NJ, Silva HB, Nunes A, Ardais AP, Santana M, Baqi Y, Müller CE, Rodrigues ALS, Porciúncula LO, Chen JF, Tomé ÂR, Agostinho P, Canas PM, Cunha RA. Caffeine acts through neuronal adenosine A2A receptors to prevent mood and memory dysfunction triggered by chronic stress. Proc Natl Acad Sci U S A. 2015;112(25):7833–8. PMCID: PMC4485143. http://www.ncbi.nlm.nih.gov/pubmed/26056314.
84. Gao ZG, Jacobson KA. Emerging adenosine receptor agonists. Expert Opin Emerg Drugs. 2007;12(3):479–92. PMID: 17874974. http://www.ncbi.nlm.nih.gov/pubmed/17874974.
85. Haskó G, Pacher P. A2A receptors in inflammation and injury: lessons learned from transgenic animals. J Leukoc Biol. 2008;83(3):447–55. PMCID: PMC2268631. http://www.ncbi.nlm.nih.gov/pubmed/18160539.
86. Popoli P, Pepponi R. Potential therapeutic relevance of adenosine A2B and A2A receptors in the central nervous system. CNS Neurol Disord Drug Targets. 2012;11(6):664–74. PMID: 22963436. http://www.ncbi.nlm.nih.gov/pubmed/22963436.
87. Fuxe K, Ferré S, Genedani S, Franco R, Agnati LF. Adenosine receptor-dopamine receptor interactions in the basal ganglia and their relevance for brain function. Physiol Behav. 2007;92(1–2):210–7. PMID: 17572452. http://www.ncbi.nlm.nih.gov/pubmed/17572452.
88. Schiffmann SN, Fisone G, Moresco R, Cunha RA, Ferré S. Adenosine A2A receptors and basal ganglia physiology. Prog Neurobiol. 2007;83(5):277–92. PMCID: PMC2148496. http://www.ncbi.nlm.nih.gov/pubmed/17646043.
89. Cunha RA, Ferré S, Vaugeois JM, Chen JF. Potential therapeutic interest of adenosine A2A receptors in psychiatric disorders. Curr Pharm Des. 2008;14(15):1512–24. PMCID: PMC2423946. http://www.ncbi.nlm.nih.gov/pubmed/18537674.
90. Yamada K, Kobayashi M, Kanda T. Involvement of adenosine A2A receptors in depression and anxiety. Int Rev Neurobiol. 2014;119:373–93. PMID: 25175973. http://www.ncbi.nlm.nih.gov/pubmed/25175973.
91. Alsene K, Deckert J, Sand P, de Wit H. Association between A2a receptor gene polymorphisms and caffeine-induced anxiety. Neuropsychopharmacology. 2003;28(9):1694–702. PMID: 12825092. http://www.ncbi.nlm.nih.gov/pubmed/12825092.
92. Childs E, Hohoff C, Deckert J, Xu K, Badner J, de Wit H. Association between ADORA2A and DRD2 polymorphisms and caffeine-induced anxiety. Neuropsychopharmacology. 2008;33(12):2791–800. PMCID: PMC2745641. http://www.ncbi.nlm.nih.gov/pubmed/18305461.
93. Swan GE, Carmelli D, Cardon LR. Heavy consumption of cigarettes, alcohol and coffee in male twins. J Stud Alcohol. 1997;58(2):182–90. PMID: 9065896. http://www.ncbi.nlm.nih.gov/pubmed/9065896.
94. Hettema JM, Corey LA, Kendler KS. A multivariate genetic analysis of the use of tobacco, alcohol, and caffeine in a population based sample of male and female twins. Drug Alcohol Depend. 1999;57(1):69–78. PMID: 10617315. http://www.ncbi.nlm.nih.gov/pubmed/10617315.
95. Kendler KS, Myers J, Prescott CA. Specificity of genetic and environmental risk factors for symptoms of cannabis, cocaine, alcohol, caffeine, and nicotine dependence. Arch Gen Psychiatry. 2007;64(11):1313–20. PMID: 17984400. http://www.ncbi.nlm.nih.gov/pubmed/17984400.
96. Kendler KS, Schmitt E, Aggen SH, Prescott CA. Genetic and environmental influences on alcohol, caffeine, cannabis, and nicotine use from early adolescence to middle adulthood. Arch Gen Psychiatry. 2008;65(6):674–82. PMCID: PMC2844891. http://www.ncbi.nlm.nih.gov/pubmed/18519825.
97. Coffee and Caffeine Genetics Consortium, Cornelis MC, Byrne EM, Esko T, Nalls MA, Ganna A, Paynter N, Monda KL, Amin N, Fischer K, Renstrom F, Ngwa JS, Huikari V, Cavadino A, Nolte IM, Teumer A, Yu K, Marques-Vidal P, Rawal R, Manichaikul A, Wojczynski MK, Vink JM, Zhao JH, Burlutsky G, Lahti J, Mikkilä V, Lemaitre RN, Eriksson J, Musani SK, Tanaka T, Geller F, Luan J, Hui J, Mägi R, Dimitriou M, Garcia ME, Ho WK, Wright MJ, Rose LM, Magnusson PK, Pedersen NL, Couper D, Oostra BA, Hofman A, Ikram MA, Tiemeier HW, Uitterlinden AG, van Rooij FJ, Barroso I, Johansson I, Xue L, Kaakinen M, Milani L, Power C, Snieder H, Stolk RP, Baumeister SE, Biffar R, Gu F, Bastardot F, Kutalik Z, Jacobs DR, Forouhi NG, Mihailov E, Lind L, Lindgren C, Michaëlsson K, Morris A, Jensen M, Khaw KT, Luben RN, Wang JJ, Männistö S, Perälä MM, Kähönen M, Lehtimäki T, Viikari J, Mozaffarian D, Mukamal K, Psaty BM, Döring A, Heath AC, Montgomery GW, Dahmen N, Carithers T, Tucker KL, Ferrucci L, Boyd HA, Melbye M, Treur JL, Mellström D, Hottenga JJ, Prokopenko I, Tönjes A, Deloukas P, Kanoni S, Lorentzon M, Houston DK, Liu Y, Danesh J, Rasheed A, Mason MA, Zonderman AB, Franke L, Kristal BS, International Parkinson's

Disease Genomics Consortium (IPDGC), North American Brain Expression Consortium (NABEC), UK Brain Expression Consortium (UKBEC), Karjalainen J, Reed DR, Westra HJ, Evans MK, Saleheen D, Harris TB, Dedoussis G, Curhan G, Stumvoll M, Beilby J, Pasquale LR, Feenstra B, Bandinelli S, Ordovas JM, Chan AT, Peters U, Ohlsson C, Gieger C, Martin NG, Waldenberger M, Siscovick DS, Raitakari O, Eriksson JG, Mitchell P, Hunter DJ, Kraft P, Rimm EB, Boomsma DI, Borecki IB, Loos RJ, Wareham NJ, Vollenweider P, Caporaso N, Grabe HJ, Neuhouser ML, Wolffenbuttel BH, Hu FB, Hyppönen E, Järvelin MR, Cupples LA, Franks PW, Ridker PM, van Duijn CM, Heiss G, Metspalu A, North KE, Ingelsson E, Nettleton JA, van Dam RM, Chasman DI. Genome-wide meta-analysis identifies six novel loci associated with habitual coffee consumption. Mol Psychiatry. 2015;20(5):647–56. PMCID: PMC4388784. http://www.ncbi.nlm.nih.gov/pubmed/25288136.
98. Low JJL, Tan BJW, Yi LX, Zhou ZD, Tan EK. Genetic susceptibility to caffeine intake and metabolism: a systematic review. J Transl Med. 2024;22(1):961. PMCID: PMC11515775. http://www.ncbi.nlm.nih.gov/pubmed/39438936.
99. Rodenburg EM, Eijgelsheim M, Geleijnse JM, Amin N, van Duijn CM, Hofman A, Uitterlinden AG, Stricker BH, Visser LE. CYP1A2 and coffee intake and the modifying effect of sex, age, and smoking. Am J Clin Nutr. 2012;96(1):182–7. PMID: 22648710. http://www.ncbi.nlm.nih.gov/pubmed/22648710.
100. Smith A. Effects of caffeine on human behavior. Food Chem Toxicol. 2002;40(9):1243–55. PMID: 12204388. http://www.ncbi.nlm.nih.gov/pubmed/12204388.
101. Spilling the Beans: How Much Caffeine is Too Much? | FDA.
102. Yang A, Palmer AA, de Wit H. Genetics of caffeine consumption and responses to caffeine. Psychopharmacology. 2010;211(3):245–57. PMCID: PMC4242593. http://www.ncbi.nlm.nih.gov/pubmed/20532872.
103. Nardi AE, Valença AM, Lopes FL, de-Melo-Neto VL, Freire RC, Veras AB, Nascimento I, King AL, Soares-Filho GL, Mezzasalma MA, Zin WA. Caffeine and 35% carbon dioxide challenge tests in panic disorder. Hum Psychopharmacol. 2007;22(4):231–40. PMID: 17407170. http://www.ncbi.nlm.nih.gov/pubmed/17407170.
104. Szpak A, Allen D. A case of acute suicidality following excessive caffeine intake. J Psychopharmacol. 2012;26(11):1502–10. PMID: 22472312. http://www.ncbi.nlm.nih.gov/pubmed/22472312.
105. Vilarim MM, Rocha Araujo DM, Nardi AE. Caffeine challenge test and panic disorder: a systematic literature review. Expert Rev Neurother. 2011;11(8):1185–95. PMID: 21797659. http://www.ncbi.nlm.nih.gov/pubmed/21797659.
106. Boulenger JP, Patel J, Post RM, Parma AM, Marangos PJ. Chronic caffeine consumption increases the number of brain adenosine receptors. Life Sci. 1983;32(10):1135–42. PMID: 6298543. http://www.ncbi.nlm.nih.gov/pubmed/6298543.
107. Mattila MJ. Interactions of benzodiazepines on psychomotor skills. Br J Clin Pharmacol. 1984;18(Suppl 1):21S–6S. PMCID: PMC1463358. http://www.ncbi.nlm.nih.gov/pubmed/6151848.
108. Schnörr SJ, Steenbergen PJ, Richardson MK, Champagne DL. Measuring thigmotaxis in larval zebrafish. Behav Brain Res. 2012;228(2):367–74. PMID: 22197677. http://www.ncbi.nlm.nih.gov/pubmed/22197677.
109. Meredith SE, Juliano LM, Hughes JR, Griffiths RR. Caffeine use disorder: a comprehensive review and research agenda. J Caffeine Res. 2013;3(3):114–30. PMCID: PMC3777290. http://www.ncbi.nlm.nih.gov/pubmed/24761279.
110. Juliano LM, Huntley ED, Harrell PT, Westerman AT. Development of the caffeine withdrawal symptom questionnaire: caffeine withdrawal symptoms cluster into 7 factors. Drug Alcohol Depend. 2012;124(3):229–34. PMID: 22341956. http://www.ncbi.nlm.nih.gov/pubmed/22341956.
111. Ozsungur S, Brenner D, El-Sohemy A. Fourteen well-described caffeine withdrawal symptoms factor into three clusters. Psychopharmacology. 2009;201(4):541–8. PMID: 18795265. http://www.ncbi.nlm.nih.gov/pubmed/18795265.
112. Juliano LM, Griffiths RR. A critical review of caffeine withdrawal: empirical validation of symptoms and signs, incidence, severity, and associated features. Psychopharmacology. 2004;176(1):1–29. PMID: 15448977. http://www.ncbi.nlm.nih.gov/pubmed/15448977.
113. Kallai J, Makany T, Csatho A, Karadi K, Horvath D, Kovacs-Labadi B, Jarai R, Nadel L, Jacobs JW. Cognitive and affective aspects of thigmotaxis strategy in humans. Behav Neurosci. 2007;121(1):21–30. PMID: 17324048. http://www.ncbi.nlm.nih.gov/pubmed/17324048.
114. Di Castelnuovo A, di Giuseppe R, Iacoviello L, de Gaetano G. Consumption of cocoa, tea and coffee and risk of cardiovascular disease. Eur J Intern Med. 2012;23(1):15–25. PMID: 22153525. http://www.ncbi.nlm.nih.gov/pubmed/22153525.
115. Bøhn SK, Ward NC, Hodgson JM, Croft KD. Effects of tea and coffee on cardiovascular disease risk. Food Funct. 2012;3(6):575–91. PMID: 22456725. http://www.ncbi.nlm.nih.gov/pubmed/22456725.
116. James JE. Critical review of dietary caffeine and blood pressure: a relationship that should be taken more seriously. Psychosom Med. 2004;66(1):63–71. PMID: 14747639. http://www.ncbi.nlm.nih.gov/pubmed/14747639.
117. Riksen NP, Smits P, Rongen GA. The cardiovascular effects of methylxanthines. Handb Exp Pharmacol. 2011;200:413–37. PMID: 20859806. http://www.ncbi.nlm.nih.gov/pubmed/20859806.
118. van Dam RM. Coffee consumption and risk of type 2 diabetes, cardiovascular diseases, and cancer. Appl Physiol Nutr Metab. 2008;33(6):1269–83. PMID: 19088789. http://www.ncbi.nlm.nih.gov/pubmed/19088789.
119. Mostofsky E, Rice MS, Levitan EB, Mittleman MA. Habitual coffee consumption and risk of heart failure: a dose-response meta-analysis. Circ Heart Fail. 2012;5(4):401–5. PMCID: PMC3425948. http://www.ncbi.nlm.nih.gov/pubmed/22740040.
120. Crippa A, Discacciati A, Larsson SC, Wolk A, Orsini N. Coffee consumption and mortality from all causes, cardiovascular disease, and cancer: a dose-response meta-analysis. Am J Epidemiol. 2014;180(8):763–75. PMID: 25156996. http://www.ncbi.nlm.nih.gov/pubmed/25156996.
121. Freedman ND, Park Y, Abnet CC, Hollenbeck AR, Sinha R. Association of coffee drinking with total and cause-specific mortality. N Engl J Med. 2012;366(20):1891–904. PMCID: PMC3439152. http://www.ncbi.nlm.nih.gov/pubmed/22591295.
122. Grosso G, Micek A, Castellano S, Pajak A, Galvano F. Coffee, tea, caffeine and risk of depression: a systematic review and dose-response meta-analysis of observational studies. Mol Nutr Food Res. 2016;60(1):223–34. PMID: 26518745. http://www.ncbi.nlm.nih.gov/pubmed/26518745.
123. Wang L, Shen X, Wu Y, Zhang D. Coffee and caffeine consumption and depression: a meta-analysis of observational studies. Aust N Z J Psychiatry. 2016;50(3):228–42. PMID: 26339067. http://www.ncbi.nlm.nih.gov/pubmed/26339067.
124. Sang LX, Chang B, Li XH, Jiang M. Consumption of coffee associated with reduced risk of liver cancer: a meta-analysis. BMC Gastroenterol. 2013;13:34. PMCID: PMC3598465. http://www.ncbi.nlm.nih.gov/pubmed/23433483.
125. Lai GY, Weinstein SJ, Albanes D, Taylor PR, McGlynn KA, Virtamo J, Sinha R, Freedman ND. The association of coffee intake with liver cancer incidence and chronic liver disease mortality in male smokers. Br J Cancer. 2013;109(5):1344–51. PMCID: PMC3778279. http://www.ncbi.nlm.nih.gov/pubmed/23880821.

126. Galeone C, Turati F, La Vecchia C, Tavani A. Coffee consumption and risk of colorectal cancer: a meta-analysis of case-control studies. Cancer Causes Control. 2010;21(11):1949–59. PMID: 20680435. http://www.ncbi.nlm.nih.gov/pubmed/20680435.
127. Je Y, Liu W, Giovannucci E. Coffee consumption and risk of colorectal cancer: a systematic review and meta-analysis of prospective cohort studies. Int J Cancer. 2009;124(7):1662–8. PMID: 19115212. http://www.ncbi.nlm.nih.gov/pubmed/19115212.
128. Sinha R, Cross AJ, Daniel CR, Graubard BI, Wu JW, Hollenbeck AR, Gunter MJ, Park Y, Freedman ND. Caffeinated and decaffeinated coffee and tea intakes and risk of colorectal cancer in a large prospective study. Am J Clin Nutr. 2012;96(2):374–81. PMCID: PMC3396445. http://www.ncbi.nlm.nih.gov/pubmed/22695871.
129. Je Y, Giovannucci E. Coffee consumption and risk of endometrial cancer: findings from a large up-to-date meta-analysis. Int J Cancer. 2012;131(7):1700–10. PMID: 22190017. http://www.ncbi.nlm.nih.gov/pubmed/22190017.
130. Gunter MJ, Schaub JA, Xue X, Freedman ND, Gaudet MM, Rohan TE, Hollenbeck AR, Sinha R. A prospective investigation of coffee drinking and endometrial cancer incidence. Int J Cancer. 2012;131(4):E530–6. PMCID: PMC3288610. http://www.ncbi.nlm.nih.gov/pubmed/22021096.
131. Yew YW, Lai YC, Schwartz RA. Coffee consumption and melanoma: a systematic review and meta-analysis of observational studies. Am J Clin Dermatol. 2016;17(2):113–23. PMID: 26547919. http://www.ncbi.nlm.nih.gov/pubmed/26547919.
132. Loftfield E, Freedman ND, Graubard BI, Hollenbeck AR, Shebl FM, Mayne ST, Sinha R. Coffee drinking and cutaneous melanoma risk in the NIH-AARP diet and health study. J Natl Cancer Inst. 2015;107(2):dju421. PMCID: PMC4311176. http://www.ncbi.nlm.nih.gov/pubmed/25604135.
133. Wu S, Han J, Song F, Cho E, Gao X, Hunter DJ, Qureshi AA. Caffeine intake, coffee consumption, and risk of cutaneous malignant melanoma. Epidemiology. 2015;26(6):898–908. PMCID: PMC4600068. http://www.ncbi.nlm.nih.gov/pubmed/26172864.
134. Ferrucci LM, Cartmel B, Molinaro AM, Leffell DJ, Bale AE, Mayne ST. Tea, coffee, and caffeine and early-onset basal cell carcinoma in a case-control study. Eur J Cancer Prev. 2014;23(4):296–302. PMCID: PMC4059399. http://www.ncbi.nlm.nih.gov/pubmed/24841641.
135. Song F, Qureshi AA, Han J. Increased caffeine intake is associated with reduced risk of basal cell carcinoma of the skin. Cancer Res. 2012;72(13):3282–9. PMID: 22752299. http://www.ncbi.nlm.nih.gov/pubmed/22752299.
136. Yao H, Li L, Wang X, Wang Z. Association of caffeine intake with all-cause and cardiovascular mortality in diabetes and prediabetes. Diabetol Metab Syndr. 2024;16(1):177. PMCID: PMC11282651. http://www.ncbi.nlm.nih.gov/pubmed/39061109.
137. Huxley R, Lee CMY, Barzi F, Timmermeister L, Czernichow S, Perkovic V, Grobbee DE, Batty D, Woodward M. Coffee, decaffeinated coffee, and tea consumption in relation to incident type 2 diabetes mellitus: a systematic review with meta-analysis. Arch Intern Med. 2009;169(22):2053–63. PMID: 20008687. http://www.ncbi.nlm.nih.gov/pubmed/20008687.
138. Liu R, Guo X, Park Y, Huang X, Sinha R, Freedman ND, Hollenbeck AR, Blair A, Chen H. Caffeine intake, smoking, and risk of Parkinson disease in men and women. Am J Epidemiol. 2012;175(11):1200–7. PMCID: PMC3370885. http://www.ncbi.nlm.nih.gov/pubmed/22505763.
139. Reissig CJ, Strain EC, Griffiths RR. Caffeinated energy drinks–a growing problem. Drug Alcohol Depend. 2009;99(1–3):1–10. PMCID: PMC2735818. http://www.ncbi.nlm.nih.gov/pubmed/18809264.
140. Pennington N, Johnson M, Delaney E, Blankenship MB. Energy drinks: a new health hazard for adolescents. J Sch Nurs. 2010;26(5):352–9. PMID: 20538866. http://www.ncbi.nlm.nih.gov/pubmed/20538866.
141. Rath M. Energy drinks: what is all the hype? The dangers of energy drink consumption. J Am Acad Nurse Pract. 2012;24(2):70–6. PMID: 22324861. http://www.ncbi.nlm.nih.gov/pubmed/22324861.
142. Sepkowitz KA. Energy drinks and caffeine-related adverse effects. JAMA. 2013;309(3):243–4. PMID: 23330171. http://www.ncbi.nlm.nih.gov/pubmed/23330171.
143. Curran CP, Marczinski CA. Taurine, caffeine, and energy drinks: reviewing the risks to the adolescent brain. Birth Defects Res. 2017;109(20):1640–8. PMCID: PMC5737830. http://www.ncbi.nlm.nih.gov/pubmed/29251842.
144. Arria AM, Caldeira KM, Kasperski SJ, Vincent KB, Griffiths RR, O'Grady KE. Energy drink consumption and increased risk for alcohol dependence. Alcohol Clin Exp Res. 2011;35(2):365–75. PMCID: PMC3058776. http://www.ncbi.nlm.nih.gov/pubmed/21073486.
145. Cobb CO, Nasim A, Jentink K, Blank MD. The role of caffeine in the alcohol consumption behaviors of college students. Subst Abus. 2015;36(1):90–8. PMID: 24965056. http://www.ncbi.nlm.nih.gov/pubmed/24965056.
146. McKetin R, Coen A, Kaye S. A comprehensive review of the effects of mixing caffeinated energy drinks with alcohol. Drug Alcohol Depend. 2015;151:15–30. PMID: 25861944. http://www.ncbi.nlm.nih.gov/pubmed/25861944.
147. Miller KE. Energy drinks, race, and problem behaviors among college students. J Adolesc Health. 2008;43(5):490–7. PMCID: PMC2575122. http://www.ncbi.nlm.nih.gov/pubmed/18848678.
148. O'Brien MC, McCoy TP, Rhodes SD, Wagoner A, Wolfson M. Caffeinated cocktails: energy drink consumption, high-risk drinking, and alcohol-related consequences among college students. Acad Emerg Med. 2008;15(5):453–60. PMID: 18439201. http://www.ncbi.nlm.nih.gov/pubmed/18439201.
149. Arria AM, Caldeira KM, Kasperski SJ, O'Grady KE, Vincent KB, Griffiths RR, Wish ED. Increased alcohol consumption, nonmedical prescription drug use, and illicit drug use are associated with energy drink consumption among college students. J Addict Med. 2010;4(2):74–80. PMCID: PMC2923814. http://www.ncbi.nlm.nih.gov/pubmed/20729975.
150. Arria AM, Caldeira KM, Bugbee BA, Vincent KB, O'Grady KE. Trajectories of energy drink consumption and subsequent drug use during young adulthood. Drug Alcohol Depend. 2017;179:424–32. PMCID: PMC5657439. http://www.ncbi.nlm.nih.gov/pubmed/28797805.
151. Campbell B, Wilborn C, La Bounty P, Taylor L, Nelson MT, Greenwood M, Ziegenfuss TN, Lopez HL, Hoffman JR, Stout JR, Schmitz S, Collins R, Kalman DS, Antonio J, Kreider RB. International Society of Sports Nutrition position stand: energy drinks. J Int Soc Sports Nutr. 2013;10(1):1. PMCID: PMC3538552. http://www.ncbi.nlm.nih.gov/pubmed/23281794.
152. Striley CLW, Griffiths RR, Cottler LB. Evaluating dependence criteria for caffeine. J Caffeine Res. 2011;1(4):219–25. PMCID: PMC3621326. http://www.ncbi.nlm.nih.gov/pubmed/24761264.
153. Lara DR. Caffeine, mental health, and psychiatric disorders. J Alzheimers Dis. 2010;20(Suppl 1):S239–48. PMID: 20164571. http://www.ncbi.nlm.nih.gov/pubmed/20164571.
154. Nila IS, Villagra Moran VM, Khan ZA, Hong Y. Effect of daily coffee consumption on the risk of Alzheimer's disease: a systematic review and meta-analysis. J Lifestyle Med. 2023;13(2):83–9. PMCID: PMC10630722. http://www.ncbi.nlm.nih.gov/pubmed/37970326.
155. Tira R, Viola G, Barracchia CG, Parolini F, Munari F, Capaldi S, Assfalg M, D'Onofrio M. Espresso coffee mitigates the

aggregation and condensation of Alzheimer's associated tau protein. J Agric Food Chem. 2023;71(30):11429–41. PMCID: PMC10401709. http://www.ncbi.nlm.nih.gov/pubmed/37466260.
156. Cunha RA, Agostinho PM. Chronic caffeine consumption prevents memory disturbance in different animal models of memory decline. J Alzheimers Dis. 2010;20(Suppl 1):S95–116. PMID: 20182043. http://www.ncbi.nlm.nih.gov/pubmed/20182043.
157. Arendash GW, Schleif W, Rezai-Zadeh K, Jackson EK, Zacharia LC, Cracchiolo JR, Shippy D, Tan J. Caffeine protects Alzheimer's mice against cognitive impairment and reduces brain beta-amyloid production. Neuroscience. 2006;142(4):941–52. PMID: 16938404. http://www.ncbi.nlm.nih.gov/pubmed/16938404.
158. Santos C, Costa J, Santos J, Vaz-Carneiro A, Lunet N. Caffeine intake and dementia: systematic review and meta-analysis. J Alzheimers Dis. 2010;20(Suppl 1):S187–204. PMID: 20182026. http://www.ncbi.nlm.nih.gov/pubmed/20182026.
159. Zheng YB, Sun J, Shi L, Su SZ, Chen X, Wang QW, Huang YT, Wang YJ, Zhu XM, Que JY, Zeng N, Lin X, Yuan K, Yan W, Deng JH, Shi J, Bao YP, Lu L. Association of Caffeine consumption and brain amyloid positivity in cognitively normal older adults. J Alzheimers Dis. 2023;93(2):483–93. PMCID: PMC10200149. http://www.ncbi.nlm.nih.gov/pubmed/37038808.
160. Iranpour S, Sabour S. Inverse association between caffeine intake and depressive symptoms in US adults: data from National Health and Nutrition Examination Survey (NHANES) 2005–2006. Psychiatry Res. 2019;271:732–9. PMID: 30791349. http://www.ncbi.nlm.nih.gov/pubmed/30791349.
161. Lucas M, Mirzaei F, Pan A, Okereke OI, Willett WC, O'Reilly ÉJ, Koenen K, Ascherio A. Coffee, caffeine, and risk of depression among women. Arch Intern Med. 2011;171(17):1571–8. PMCID: PMC3296361. http://www.ncbi.nlm.nih.gov/pubmed/21949167.
162. Meamar M, Raise-Abdullahi P, Rashidy-Pour A, Raeis-Abdollahi E. Coffee and mental disorders: how caffeine affects anxiety and depression. Prog Brain Res. 2024;288:115–32. PMID: 39168554. http://www.ncbi.nlm.nih.gov/pubmed/39168554.
163. Pleis JR, Lucas JW, Ward BW. Summary health statistics for U.S. adults: National Health Interview Survey, 2008. Vital Health Stat 10. 2009;242:1–157. PMID: 20821903. http://www.ncbi.nlm.nih.gov/pubmed/20821903.
164. Grant BF, Dawson DA, Stinson FS, Chou SP, Dufour MC, Pickering RP. The 12-month prevalence and trends in DSM-IV alcohol abuse and dependence: United States, 1991–1992 and 2001–2002. Drug Alcohol Depend. 2004;74(3):223–34. PMID: 15194200. http://www.ncbi.nlm.nih.gov/pubmed/15194200.
165. Cooper ML, Krull JL, Agocha VB, Flanagan ME, Orcutt HK, Grabe S, Dermen KH, Jackson M. Motivational pathways to alcohol use and abuse among black and white adolescents. J Abnorm Psychol. 2008;117(3):485–501. PMID: 18729604. http://www.ncbi.nlm.nih.gov/pubmed/18729604.
166. Ham LS, Zamboanga BL, Bacon AK, Garcia TA. Drinking motives as mediators of social anxiety and hazardous drinking among college students. Cogn Behav Ther. 2009;38(3):133–45. PMID: 19306146. http://www.ncbi.nlm.nih.gov/pubmed/19306146.
167. Lewis MA, Hove MC, Whiteside U, Lee CM, Kirkeby BS, Oster-Aaland L, Neighbors C, Larimer ME. Fitting in and feeling fine: conformity and coping motives as mediators of the relationship between social anxiety and problematic drinking. Psychol Addict Behav. 2008;22(1):58–67. PMID: 18298231. http://www.ncbi.nlm.nih.gov/pubmed/18298231.
168. Kuntsche E, Knibbe R, Gmel G, Engels R. Why do young people drink? A review of drinking motives. Clin Psychol Rev. 2005;25(7):841–61. PMID: 16095785. http://www.ncbi.nlm.nih.gov/pubmed/16095785.
169. Beseler CL, Aharonovich E, Keyes KM, Hasin DS. Adult transition from at-risk drinking to alcohol dependence: the relationship of family history and drinking motives. Alcohol Clin Exp Res. 2008;32(4):607–16. PMCID: PMC3850293. http://www.ncbi.nlm.nih.gov/pubmed/18341650.
170. Prescott CA, Cross RJ, Kuhn JW, Horn JL, Kendler KS. Is risk for alcoholism mediated by individual differences in drinking motivations? Alcohol Clin Exp Res. 2004;28(1):29–39. PMID: 14745300. http://www.ncbi.nlm.nih.gov/pubmed/14745300.
171. Littlefield AK, Agrawal A, Ellingson JM, Kristjansson S, Madden PAF, Bucholz KK, Slutske WS, Heath AC, Sher KJ. Does variance in drinking motives explain the genetic overlap between personality and alcohol use disorder symptoms? A twin study of young women. Alcohol Clin Exp Res. 2011;35(12):2242–50. PMCID: PMC3204320. http://www.ncbi.nlm.nih.gov/pubmed/21790670.
172. de Moor MHM, Vink JM, van Beek JHDA, Geels LM, Bartels M, de Geus EJC, Willemsen G, Boomsma DI. Heritability of problem drinking and the genetic overlap with personality in a general population sample. Front Genet. 2011;2:76. PMCID: PMC3268629. http://www.ncbi.nlm.nih.gov/pubmed/22303371.
173. DeMartini KS, Carey KB. The role of anxiety sensitivity and drinking motives in predicting alcohol use: a critical review. Clin Psychol Rev. 2011;31(1):169–77. PMID: 21074306. http://www.ncbi.nlm.nih.gov/pubmed/21074306.
174. Gardner EL. Addiction and brain reward and antireward pathways. Adv Psychosom Med. 2011;30:22–60. PMCID: PMC4549070. http://www.ncbi.nlm.nih.gov/pubmed/21508625.
175. Braun AR, Heinz AJ, Veilleux JC, Conrad M, Weber S, Wardle M, Greenstein J, Evatt D, Drobes D, Kassel JD. The separate and combined effects of alcohol and nicotine on anticipatory anxiety: a multidimensional analysis. Addict Behav. 2012;37(4):485–91. PMID: 22260966. http://www.ncbi.nlm.nih.gov/pubmed/22260966.
176. Hefner KR, Curtin JJ. Alcohol stress response dampening: selective reduction of anxiety in the face of uncertain threat. J Psychopharmacol. 2012;26(2):232–44. PMCID: PMC3413306. http://www.ncbi.nlm.nih.gov/pubmed/21937686.
177. Moberg CA, Curtin JJ. Alcohol selectively reduces anxiety but not fear: startle response during unpredictable versus predictable threat. J Abnorm Psychol. 2009;118(2):335–47. PMCID: PMC2756160. http://www.ncbi.nlm.nih.gov/pubmed/19413408.
178. Sayette MA. Does drinking reduce stress? Alcohol Res Health. 1999;23(4):250–5. PMCID: PMC6760384. http://www.ncbi.nlm.nih.gov/pubmed/10890821.
179. Silberman Y, Bajo M, Chappell AM, Christian DT, Cruz M, Diaz MR, Kash T, Lack AK, Messing RO, Siggins GR, Winder D, Roberto M, McCool BA, Weiner JL. Neurobiological mechanisms contributing to alcohol-stress-anxiety interactions. Alcohol. 2009;43(7):509–19. PMCID: PMC2814297. http://www.ncbi.nlm.nih.gov/pubmed/19913194.
180. Kushner MG, Abrams K, Thuras P, Thuras P, Hanson KL. Individual differences predictive of drinking to manage anxiety among non-problem drinkers with panic disorder. Alcohol Clin Exp Res. 2000;24(4):448–58. PMID: 10798580. http://www.ncbi.nlm.nih.gov/pubmed/10798580.
181. Koob GF. A role for GABA mechanisms in the motivational effects of alcohol. Biochem Pharmacol. 2004;68(8):1515–25. PMID: 15451394. http://www.ncbi.nlm.nih.gov/pubmed/15451394.
182. Roberts AJ, Heyser CJ, Cole M, Griffin P, Koob GF. Excessive ethanol drinking following a history of dependence: animal model of allostasis. Neuropsychopharmacology. 2000;22(6):581–94. PMID: 10788758. http://www.ncbi.nlm.nih.gov/pubmed/10788758.
183. Valdez GR, Roberts AJ, Chan K, Davis H, Brennan M, Zorrilla EP, Koob GF. Increased ethanol self-administration and anxiety-like behavior during acute ethanol withdrawal and protracted abstinence: regulation by corticotropin-releasing factor. Alcohol Clin Exp Res. 2002;26(10):1494–501. PMID: 12394282. http://www.ncbi.nlm.nih.gov/pubmed/12394282.

184. Kliethermes CL. Anxiety-like behaviors following chronic ethanol exposure. Neurosci Biobehav Rev. 2005;28(8):837–50. PMID: 15642625. http://www.ncbi.nlm.nih.gov/pubmed/15642625.
185. Santucci AC, Cortes C, Bettica A, Cortes F. Chronic ethanol consumption in rats produces residual increases in anxiety 4 months after withdrawal. Behav Brain Res. 2008;188(1):24–31. PMID: 18061285. http://www.ncbi.nlm.nih.gov/pubmed/18061285.
186. Piazza PV, Le Moal M. The role of stress in drug self-administration. Trends Pharmacol Sci. 1998;19(2):67–74. PMID: 9550944. http://www.ncbi.nlm.nih.gov/pubmed/9550944.
187. Weiss F, Ciccocioppo R, Parsons LH, Katner S, Liu X, Zorrilla EP, Valdez GR, Ben-Shahar O, Angeletti S, Richter RR. Compulsive drug-seeking behavior and relapse. Neuroadaptation, stress, and conditioning factors. Ann N Y Acad Sci. 2001;937:1–26. PMID: 11458532. http://www.ncbi.nlm.nih.gov/pubmed/11458532.
188. Kushner MG, Sher KJ, Erickson DJ. Prospective analysis of the relation between DSM-III anxiety disorders and alcohol use disorders. Am J Psychiatry. 1999;156(5):723–32. PMID: 10327905. http://www.ncbi.nlm.nih.gov/pubmed/10327905.
189. Cosci F, Schruers KRJ, Abrams K, Griez EJL. Alcohol use disorders and panic disorder: a review of the evidence of a direct relationship. J Clin Psychiatry. 2007;68(6):874–80. PMID: 17592911. http://www.ncbi.nlm.nih.gov/pubmed/17592911.
190. Cohen SI. Alcohol and benzodiazepines generate anxiety, panic and phobias. J R Soc Med. 1995;88(2):73–7. PMCID: PMC1295099. http://www.ncbi.nlm.nih.gov/pubmed/7769598.
191. Brady KT, Haynes LF, Hartwell KJ, Killeen TK. Substance use disorders and anxiety: a treatment challenge for social workers. Soc Work Public Health. 2013;28(3–4):407–23. PMCID: PMC3775646. http://www.ncbi.nlm.nih.gov/pubmed/23731428.
192. Bahji A. Navigating the complex intersection of substance use and psychiatric disorders: a comprehensive review. J Clin Med. 2024;13(4):999. PMCID: PMC10889170. http://www.ncbi.nlm.nih.gov/pubmed/38398311.
193. Saraceno L, Munafó M, Heron J, Craddock N, van den Bree MBM. Genetic and non-genetic influences on the development of co-occurring alcohol problem use and internalizing symptomatology in adolescence: a review. Addiction. 2009;104(7):1100–21. PMID: 19438423. http://www.ncbi.nlm.nih.gov/pubmed/19438423.
194. Edwards AC, Aliev F, Bierut LJ, Bucholz KK, Edenberg H, Hesselbrock V, Kramer J, Kuperman S, Nurnberger JI, Schuckit MA, Porjesz B, Dick DM. Genome-wide association study of comorbid depressive syndrome and alcohol dependence. Psychiatr Genet. 2012;22(1):31–41. PMCID: PMC3241912. http://www.ncbi.nlm.nih.gov/pubmed/22064162.
195. Ryabinin AE, Tsoory MM, Kozicz T, Thiele TE, Neufeld-Cohen A, Chen A, Lowery-Gionta EG, Giardino WJ, Kaur S. Urocortins: CRF's siblings and their potential role in anxiety, depression and alcohol drinking behavior. Alcohol. 2012;46(4):349–57. PMCID: PMC3358480. http://www.ncbi.nlm.nih.gov/pubmed/22444954.
196. Davis MI. Ethanol-BDNF interactions: still more questions than answers. Pharmacol Ther. 2008;118(1):36–57. PMCID: PMC2553254. http://www.ncbi.nlm.nih.gov/pubmed/18394710.
197. Epstein EE, Fischer-Elber K, Al-Otaiba Z. Women, aging, and alcohol use disorders. J Women Aging. 2007;19(1–2):31–48. PMID: 17588878. http://www.ncbi.nlm.nih.gov/pubmed/17588878.
198. Barrett SP, Tichauer M, Leyton M, Pihl RO. Nicotine increases alcohol self-administration in non-dependent male smokers. Drug Alcohol Depend. 2006;81(2):197–204. PMID: 16054779. http://www.ncbi.nlm.nih.gov/pubmed/16054779.
199. Kouri EM, McCarthy EM, Faust AH, Lukas SE. Pretreatment with transdermal nicotine enhances some of ethanol's acute effects in men. Drug Alcohol Depend. 2004;75(1):55–65. PMID: 15225889. http://www.ncbi.nlm.nih.gov/pubmed/15225889.
200. McKee SA, Hinson R, Rounsaville D, Petrelli P. Survey of subjective effects of smoking while drinking among college students. Nicotine Tob Res. 2004;6(1):111–7. PMID: 14982695. http://www.ncbi.nlm.nih.gov/pubmed/14982695.
201. Piasecki TM, Jahng S, Wood PK, Robertson BM, Epler AJ, Cronk NJ, Rohrbaugh JW, Heath AC, Shiffman S, Sher KJ. The subjective effects of alcohol-tobacco co-use: an ecological momentary assessment investigation. J Abnorm Psychol. 2011;120(3):557–71. PMCID: PMC3128190. http://www.ncbi.nlm.nih.gov/pubmed/21443289.
202. Piasecki TM, McCarthy DE, Fiore MC, Baker TB. Alcohol consumption, smoking urge, and the reinforcing effects of cigarettes: an ecological study. Psychol Addict Behav. 2008;22(2):230–9. PMCID: PMC6442476. http://www.ncbi.nlm.nih.gov/pubmed/18540720.
203. DiFranza JR, Guerrera MP. Alcoholism and smoking. J Stud Alcohol. 1990;51(2):130–5. PMID: 2308350. http://www.ncbi.nlm.nih.gov/pubmed/2308350.
204. Hurt RD, Offord KP, Croghan IT, Gomez-Dahl L, Kottke TE, Morse RM, Melton LJ. Mortality following inpatient addictions treatment. Role of tobacco use in a community-based cohort. JAMA. 1996;275(14):1097–103. PMID: 8601929. http://www.ncbi.nlm.nih.gov/pubmed/8601929.
205. Kahler CW, Borland R, Hyland A, McKee SA, O'Connor RJ, Fong GT, Cummings KM. Quitting smoking and change in alcohol consumption in the International Tobacco Control (ITC) four country survey. Drug Alcohol Depend. 2010;110(1–2):101–7. PMCID: PMC2885485. http://www.ncbi.nlm.nih.gov/pubmed/20227840.
206. Davis TJ, de Fiebre CM. Alcohol's actions on neuronal nicotinic acetylcholine receptors. Alcohol Res Health. 2006;29(3):179–85. PMCID: PMC6527039. http://www.ncbi.nlm.nih.gov/pubmed/17373406.
207. Dani JA, Harris RA. Nicotine addiction and comorbidity with alcohol abuse and mental illness. Nat Neurosci. 2005;8(11):1465–70. PMID: 16251989. http://www.ncbi.nlm.nih.gov/pubmed/16251989.
208. Drews E, Zimmer A. Modulation of alcohol and nicotine responses through the endogenous opioid system. Prog Neurobiol. 2010;90(1):1–15. PMID: 19800387. http://www.ncbi.nlm.nih.gov/pubmed/19800387.
209. Tyndale RF. Genetics of alcohol and tobacco use in humans. Ann Med. 2003;35(2):94–121. PMID: 12795339. http://www.ncbi.nlm.nih.gov/pubmed/12795339.
210. Pelucchi C, Gallus S, Garavello W, Bosetti C, La Vecchia C. Cancer risk associated with alcohol and tobacco use: focus on upper aero-digestive tract and liver. Alcohol Res Health. 2006;29(3):193–8. PMCID: PMC6527045. http://www.ncbi.nlm.nih.gov/pubmed/17373408.
211. Carton L, Auger F, Kyheng M, Pétrault M, Durieux N, Allorge D, Cottencin O, Jardri R, Bordet R, Rolland B. Dose-dependent metabolite changes after ethanol intoxication in rat prefrontal cortex using in vivo magnetic resonance spectroscopy. Sci Rep. 2019;9(1):10682. PMCID: PMC6650461. http://www.ncbi.nlm.nih.gov/pubmed/31337845.
212. Muncie HL, Yasinian Y, Oge' L. Outpatient management of alcohol withdrawal syndrome. Am Fam Physician. 2013;88(9):589–95. PMID: 24364635. http://www.ncbi.nlm.nih.gov/pubmed/24364635.
213. Cooper E, Vernon J. The effectiveness of pharmacological approaches in the treatment of alcohol withdrawal syndrome (AWS): a literature review. J Psychiatr Ment Health Nurs. 2013;20(7):601–12. PMID: 22989012. http://www.ncbi.nlm.nih.gov/pubmed/22989012.
214. Health Professionals & Communities | National Institute on Alcohol Abuse and Alcoholism (NIAAA).

215. Aspis I, Feingold D, Weiser M, Rehm J, Shoval G, Lev-Ran S. Cannabis use and mental health-related quality of life among individuals with depressive disorders. Psychiatry Res. 2015;230(2):341–9. PMID: 26388103. http://www.ncbi.nlm.nih.gov/pubmed/26388103.
216. Prevalence of Marijuana Use Among U.S. Adults Doubles Over Past Decade | National Institutes of Health (NIH).
217. Compton WM, Grant BF, Colliver JD, Glantz MD, Stinson FS. Prevalence of marijuana use disorders in the United States: 1991–1992 and 2001–2002. JAMA. 2004;291(17):2114–21. PMID: 15126440. http://www.ncbi.nlm.nih.gov/pubmed/15126440.
218. Lev-Ran S, Roerecke M, Le Foll B, George TP, McKenzie K, Rehm J. The association between cannabis use and depression: a systematic review and meta-analysis of longitudinal studies. Psychol Med. 2014;44(4):797–810. PMID: 23795762. http://www.ncbi.nlm.nih.gov/pubmed/23795762.
219. Bersani G, Bersani FS, Caroti E, Russo P, Albano G, Valeriani G, Imperatori C, Minichino A, Manuali G, Corazza O. Negative symptoms as key features of depression among cannabis users: a preliminary report. Eur Rev Med Pharmacol Sci. 2016;20(3):547–52. PMID: 26914132. http://www.ncbi.nlm.nih.gov/pubmed/26914132.
220. Shillington AM, Clapp JD. Substance use problems reported by college students: combined marijuana and alcohol use versus alcohol-only use. Subst Use Misuse. 2001;36(5):663–72. PMID: 11419493. http://www.ncbi.nlm.nih.gov/pubmed/11419493.
221. Danielsson AK, Lundin A, Agardh E, Allebeck P, Forsell Y. Cannabis use, depression and anxiety: a 3-year prospective population-based study. J Affect Disord. 2016;193:103–8. PMID: 26773900. http://www.ncbi.nlm.nih.gov/pubmed/26773900.
222. Durdle H, Lundahl LH, Johanson CE, Tancer M. Major depression: the relative contribution of gender, MDMA, and cannabis use. Depress Anxiety. 2008;25(3):241–7. PMID: 17345601. http://www.ncbi.nlm.nih.gov/pubmed/17345601.
223. Midanik LT, Tam TW, Weisner C. Concurrent and simultaneous drug and alcohol use: results of the 2000 National Alcohol Survey. Drug Alcohol Depend. 2007;90(1):72–80. PMCID: PMC2043125. http://www.ncbi.nlm.nih.gov/pubmed/17446013.
224. Pacek LR, Malcolm RJ, Martins SS. Race/ethnicity differences between alcohol, marijuana, and co-occurring alcohol and marijuana use disorders and their association with public health and social problems using a national sample. Am J Addict. 2012;21(5):435–44. PMCID: PMC3419382. http://www.ncbi.nlm.nih.gov/pubmed/22882394.
225. Sakyi KS, Melchior M, Chollet A, Surkan PJ. The combined effects of parental divorce and parental history of depression on cannabis use in young adults in France. Drug Alcohol Depend. 2012;126(1–2):195–9. PMID: 22682099. http://www.ncbi.nlm.nih.gov/pubmed/22682099.
226. Gilder DA, Ehlers CL. Depression symptoms associated with cannabis dependence in an adolescent American Indian community sample. Am J Addict. 2012;21(6):536–43. PMCID: PMC3498983. http://www.ncbi.nlm.nih.gov/pubmed/23082832.
227. Marmorstein NR, Iacono WG. Explaining associations between cannabis use disorders in adolescence and later major depression: a test of the psychosocial failure model. Addict Behav. 2011;36(7):773–6. PMCID: PMC3081975. http://www.ncbi.nlm.nih.gov/pubmed/21411234.
228. Pedersen W. Does cannabis use lead to depression and suicidal behaviours? A population-based longitudinal study. Acta Psychiatr Scand. 2008;118(5):395–403. PMID: 18798834. http://www.ncbi.nlm.nih.gov/pubmed/18798834.
229. Harder VS, Stuart EA, Anthony JC. Adolescent cannabis problems and young adult depression: male-female stratified propensity score analyses. Am J Epidemiol. 2008;168(6):592–601. PMCID: PMC2727198. http://www.ncbi.nlm.nih.gov/pubmed/18687663.
230. Brook JS, Cohen P, Brook DW. Longitudinal study of co-occurring psychiatric disorders and substance use. J Am Acad Child Adolesc Psychiatry. 1998;37(3):322–30. PMID: 9519638. http://www.ncbi.nlm.nih.gov/pubmed/9519638.
231. Fergusson DM, Horwood LJ. Early onset cannabis use and psychosocial adjustment in young adults. Addiction. 1997;92(3):279–96. PMID: 9219390. http://www.ncbi.nlm.nih.gov/pubmed/9219390.
232. Degenhardt L, Hall W, Lynskey M. Exploring the association between cannabis use and depression. Addiction. 2003;98(11):1493–504. PMID: 14616175. http://www.ncbi.nlm.nih.gov/pubmed/14616175.
233. Arendt M, Rosenberg R, Fjordback L, Brandholdt J, Foldager L, Sher L, Munk-Jørgensen P. Testing the self-medication hypothesis of depression and aggression in cannabis-dependent subjects. Psychol Med. 2007;37(7):935–45. PMID: 17202003. http://www.ncbi.nlm.nih.gov/pubmed/17202003.
234. Aharonovich E, Liu X, Samet S, Nunes E, Waxman R, Hasin D. Postdischarge cannabis use and its relationship to cocaine, alcohol, and heroin use: a prospective study. Am J Psychiatry. 2005;162(8):1507–14. PMID: 16055773. http://www.ncbi.nlm.nih.gov/pubmed/16055773.
235. Agrawal A, Lynskey MT. Cannabis controversies: how genetics can inform the study of comorbidity. Addiction. 2014;109(3):360–70. PMCID: PMC3943474. http://www.ncbi.nlm.nih.gov/pubmed/24438181.
236. Cornelius JR, Aizenstein HJ, Hariri AR. Amygdala reactivity is inversely related to level of cannabis use in individuals with comorbid cannabis dependence and major depression. Addict Behav. 2010;35(6):644–6. PMCID: PMC2841401. http://www.ncbi.nlm.nih.gov/pubmed/20189314.
237. Phan KL, Angstadt M, Golden J, Onyewuenyi I, Popovska A, de Wit H. Cannabinoid modulation of amygdala reactivity to social signals of threat in humans. J Neurosci. 2008;28(10):2313–9. PMCID: PMC2657360. http://www.ncbi.nlm.nih.gov/pubmed/18322078.
238. Moreira FA, Wotjak CT. Cannabinoids and anxiety. Curr Top Behav Neurosci. 2010;2:429–50. PMID: 21309120. http://www.ncbi.nlm.nih.gov/pubmed/21309120.
239. Tambaro S, Bortolato M. Cannabinoid-related agents in the treatment of anxiety disorders: current knowledge and future perspectives. Recent Pat CNS Drug Discov. 2012;7(1):25–40. PMCID: PMC3691841. http://www.ncbi.nlm.nih.gov/pubmed/22280339.
240. Zanettini C, Panlilio LV, Alicki M, Goldberg SR, Haller J, Yasar S. Effects of endocannabinoid system modulation on cognitive and emotional behavior. Front Behav Neurosci. 2011;5:57. PMCID: PMC3171696. http://www.ncbi.nlm.nih.gov/pubmed/21949506.
241. Adverse effects of cannabis. Prescrire Int. 2011;20(112):18–23. PMID: 21462790. http://www.ncbi.nlm.nih.gov/pubmed/21462790.
242. Greydanus DE, Hawver EK, Greydanus MM, Merrick J. Marijuana: current concepts(†). Front Public Health. 2013;1:42. PMCID: PMC3859982. http://www.ncbi.nlm.nih.gov/pubmed/24350211.
243. Buckner JD, Heimberg RG, Schmidt NB. Social anxiety and marijuana-related problems: the role of social avoidance. Addict Behav. 2011;36(1–2):129–32. PMCID: PMC2981690. http://www.ncbi.nlm.nih.gov/pubmed/20832947.
244. Saavedra MS, Thota P, Peresuodei TS, Gill A, Orji C, Reghefaoui M, Khan S. Neurocognitive impact of exposure to cannabis concentrates and cannabinoids including vaping in children and adolescents: a systematic review. Cureus. 2024;16(1):e52362. PMCID: PMC10867711. http://www.ncbi.nlm.nih.gov/pubmed/38361722.
245. Lichenstein SD, Shaw DS, Forbes EE. Cannabis, connectivity, and coming of age: associations between cannabis use and anterior

cingulate cortex connectivity during the transition to adulthood. Front Hum Neurosci. 2022;16:951204. PMCID: PMC9692120. http://www.ncbi.nlm.nih.gov/pubmed/36438638.

246. Shollenbarger SG, Price J, Wieser J, Lisdahl K. Poorer fronto-limbic white matter integrity is associated with chronic cannabis use, FAAH genotype, and increased depressive and apathy symptoms in adolescents and young adults. Neuroimage Clin. 2015;8:117–25. PMCID: PMC4473294. http://www.ncbi.nlm.nih.gov/pubmed/26106535.
247. Egerton A, Allison C, Brett RR, Pratt JA. Cannabinoids and prefrontal cortical function: insights from preclinical studies. Neurosci Biobehav Rev. 2006;30(5):680–95. PMID: 16574226. http://www.ncbi.nlm.nih.gov/pubmed/16574226.
248. Horder J, Cowen PJ, Di Simplicio M, Browning M, Harmer CJ. Acute administration of the cannabinoid CB1 antagonist rimonabant impairs positive affective memory in healthy volunteers. Psychopharmacology. 2009;205(1):85–91. PMID: 19337726. http://www.ncbi.nlm.nih.gov/pubmed/19337726.
249. Marco EM, Laviola G. The endocannabinoid system in the regulation of emotions throughout lifespan: a discussion on therapeutic perspectives. J Psychopharmacol. 2012;26(1):150–63. PMID: 21693551. http://www.ncbi.nlm.nih.gov/pubmed/21693551.
250. Gage SH, Hickman M, Heron J, Munafò MR, Lewis G, Macleod J, Zammit S. Associations of cannabis and cigarette use with depression and anxiety at age 18: findings from the Avon longitudinal study of parents and children. PLoS One. 2015;10(4):e0122896. PMCID: PMC4395304. http://www.ncbi.nlm.nih.gov/pubmed/25875443.
251. Ziedonis D, Hitsman B, Beckham JC, Zvolensky M, Adler LE, Audrain-McGovern J, Breslau N, Brown RA, George TP, Williams J, Calhoun PS, Riley WT. Tobacco use and cessation in psychiatric disorders: National Institute of Mental Health report. Nicotine Tob Res. 2008;10(12):1691–715. PMID: 19023823. http://www.ncbi.nlm.nih.gov/pubmed/19023823.
252. Lasser K, Boyd JW, Woolhandler S, Himmelstein DU, McCormick D, Bor DH. Smoking and mental illness: a population-based prevalence study. JAMA. 2000;284(20):2606–10. PMID: 11086367. http://www.ncbi.nlm.nih.gov/pubmed/11086367.
253. Hall SM, Prochaska JJ. Treatment of smokers with co-occurring disorders: emphasis on integration in mental health and addiction treatment settings. Annu Rev Clin Psychol. 2009;5:409–31. PMCID: PMC2718730. http://www.ncbi.nlm.nih.gov/pubmed/19327035.
254. Kendler KS, Neale MC, MacLean CJ, Heath AC, Eaves LJ, Kessler RC. Smoking and major depression. A causal analysis. Arch Gen Psychiatry. 1993;50(1):36–43. PMID: 8422220. http://www.ncbi.nlm.nih.gov/pubmed/8422220.
255. Park S, Romer D. Associations between smoking and depression in adolescence: an integrative review. Taehan Kanho Hakhoe Chi. 2007;37(2):227–41. PMID: 17435408. http://www.ncbi.nlm.nih.gov/pubmed/17435408.
256. Tercyak KP, Audrain J. Psychosocial correlates of alternate tobacco product use during early adolescence. Prev Med. 2002;35(2):193–8. PMID: 12200105. http://www.ncbi.nlm.nih.gov/pubmed/12200105.
257. Tercyak KP, Goldman P, Smith A, Audrain J. Interacting effects of depression and tobacco advertising receptivity on adolescent smoking. J Pediatr Psychol. 2002;27(2):145–54. PMID: 11821498. http://www.ncbi.nlm.nih.gov/pubmed/11821498.
258. Boys A, Farrell M, Taylor C, Marsden J, Goodman R, Brugha T, Bebbington P, Jenkins R, Meltzer H. Psychiatric morbidity and substance use in young people aged 13–15 years: results from the child and adolescent survey of mental health. Br J Psychiatry. 2003;182:509–17. PMID: 12777342. http://www.ncbi.nlm.nih.gov/pubmed/12777342.
259. Diego MA, Field TM, Sanders CE. Academic performance, popularity, and depression predict adolescent substance use. Adolescence. 2003;38(149):35–42. PMID: 12803452. http://www.ncbi.nlm.nih.gov/pubmed/12803452.
260. Kubik MY, Lytle LA, Birnbaum AS, Murray DM, Perry CL. Prevalence and correlates of depressive symptoms in young adolescents. Am J Health Behav. 2003;27(5):546–53. PMID: 14521250. http://www.ncbi.nlm.nih.gov/pubmed/14521250.
261. Haarasilta L, Marttunen M, Kaprio J, Aro H. Major depressive episode and health care use among adolescents and young adults. Soc Psychiatry Psychiatr Epidemiol. 2003;38(7):366–72. PMID: 12861442. http://www.ncbi.nlm.nih.gov/pubmed/12861442.
262. Albers AB, Biener L. The role of smoking and rebelliousness in the development of depressive symptoms among a cohort of Massachusetts adolescents. Prev Med. 2002;34(6):625–31. PMID: 12052023. http://www.ncbi.nlm.nih.gov/pubmed/12052023.
263. Koval JJ, Pederson LL, Mills CA, McGrady GA, Carvajal SC. Models of the relationship of stress, depression, and other psychosocial factors to smoking behavior: a comparison of a cohort of students in grades 6 and 8. Prev Med. 2000;30(6):463–77. PMID: 10901489. http://www.ncbi.nlm.nih.gov/pubmed/10901489.
264. Crisp AH, Halek C, Sedgewick P, Stravraki C, Williams E, Kiossis I. Smoking and pursuit of thinness in schoolgirls in London and Ottawa. Postgrad Med J. 1998;74(874):473–9. PMCID: PMC2360886. http://www.ncbi.nlm.nih.gov/pubmed/9926121.
265. Miller-Johnson S, Lochman JE, Coie JD, Terry R, Hyman C. Comorbidity of conduct and depressive problems at sixth grade: substance use outcomes across adolescence. J Abnorm Child Psychol. 1998;26(3):221–32. PMID: 9650628. http://www.ncbi.nlm.nih.gov/pubmed/9650628.
266. Fergusson DM, Goodwin RD, Horwood LJ. Major depression and cigarette smoking: results of a 21-year longitudinal study. Psychol Med. 2003;33(8):1357–67. PMID: 14672244. http://www.ncbi.nlm.nih.gov/pubmed/14672244.
267. Breslau N, Peterson EL, Schultz LR, Chilcoat HD, Andreski P. Major depression and stages of smoking. A longitudinal investigation. Arch Gen Psychiatry. 1998;55(2):161–6. PMID: 9477930. http://www.ncbi.nlm.nih.gov/pubmed/9477930.
268. Ranney L, Melvin C, Lux L, McClain E, Lohr KN. Systematic review: smoking cessation intervention strategies for adults and adults in special populations. Ann Intern Med. 2006;145(11):845–56. PMID: 16954352. http://www.ncbi.nlm.nih.gov/pubmed/16954352.
269. Hall SM, Muñoz RF, Reus VI. Cognitive-behavioral intervention increases abstinence rates for depressive-history smokers. J Consult Clin Psychol. 1994;62(1):141–6. PMID: 8034816. http://www.ncbi.nlm.nih.gov/pubmed/8034816.
270. Covey LS. Tobacco cessation among patients with depression. Prim Care. 1999;26(3):691–706. PMID: 10436294. http://www.ncbi.nlm.nih.gov/pubmed/10436294.
271. Glassman AH. Cigarette smoking: implications for psychiatric illness. Am J Psychiatry. 1993;150(4):546–53. PMID: 8465868. http://www.ncbi.nlm.nih.gov/pubmed/8465868.
272. Glassman AH, Helzer JE, Covey LS, Cottler LB, Stetner F, Tipp JE, Johnson J. Smoking, smoking cessation, and major depression. JAMA. 1990;264(12):1546–9. PMID: 2395194. http://www.ncbi.nlm.nih.gov/pubmed/2395194.
273. Tsoh JY, Humfleet GL, Muñoz RF, Reus VI, Hartz DT, Hall SM. Development of major depression after treatment for smoking cessation. Am J Psychiatry. 2000;157(3):368–74. PMID: 10698811. http://www.ncbi.nlm.nih.gov/pubmed/10698811.
274. Siru R, Hulse GK, Tait RJ. Assessing motivation to quit smoking in people with mental illness: a review. Addiction. 2009;104(5):719–33. PMID: 19413788. http://www.ncbi.nlm.nih.gov/pubmed/19413788.

275. Morozova M, Rabin RA, George TP. Co-morbid tobacco use disorder and depression: a re-evaluation of smoking cessation therapy in depressed smokers. Am J Addict. 2015;24(8):687–94. PMID: 26354720. http://www.ncbi.nlm.nih.gov/pubmed/26354720.
276. Blalock JA, Robinson JD, Wetter DW, Schreindorfer LS, Cinciripini PM. Nicotine withdrawal in smokers with current depressive disorders undergoing intensive smoking cessation treatment. Psychol Addict Behav. 2008;22(1):122–8. PMID: 18298238. http://www.ncbi.nlm.nih.gov/pubmed/18298238.
277. Kahler CW, Brown RA, Ramsey SE, Niaura R, Abrams DB, Goldstein MG, Mueller TI, Miller IW. Negative mood, depressive symptoms, and major depression after smoking cessation treatment in smokers with a history of major depressive disorder. J Abnorm Psychol. 2002;111(4):670–5. PMID: 12428781. http://www.ncbi.nlm.nih.gov/pubmed/12428781.
278. Prochaska JJ, Hall SM, Tsoh JY, Eisendrath S, Rossi JS, Redding CA, Rosen AB, Meisner M, Humfleet GL, Gorecki JA. Treating tobacco dependence in clinically depressed smokers: effect of smoking cessation on mental health functioning. Am J Public Health. 2008;98(3):446–8. PMCID: PMC2253568. http://www.ncbi.nlm.nih.gov/pubmed/17600251.
279. Thorsteinsson HS, Gillin JC, Patten CA, Golshan S, Sutton LD, Drummond S, Clark CP, Kelsoe J, Rapaport M. The effects of transdermal nicotine therapy for smoking cessation on depressive symptoms in patients with major depression. Neuropsychopharmacology. 2001;24(4):350–8. PMID: 11182530. http://www.ncbi.nlm.nih.gov/pubmed/11182530.
280. Brown RA, Kahler CW, Niaura R, Abrams DB, Sales SD, Ramsey SE, Goldstein MG, Burgess ES, Miller IW. Cognitive-behavioral treatment for depression in smoking cessation. J Consult Clin Psychol. 2001;69(3):471–80. PMCID: PMC1832078. http://www.ncbi.nlm.nih.gov/pubmed/11495176.
281. Hall SM, Muñoz RF, Reus VI, Sees KL, Duncan C, Humfleet GL, Hartz DT. Mood management and nicotine gum in smoking treatment: a therapeutic contact and placebo-controlled study. J Consult Clin Psychol. 1996;64(5):1003–9. PMID: 8916629. http://www.ncbi.nlm.nih.gov/pubmed/8916629.
282. Patten CA, Martin JE, Myers MG, Calfas KJ, Williams CD. Effectiveness of cognitive-behavioral therapy for smokers with histories of alcohol dependence and depression. J Stud Alcohol. 1998;59(3):327–35. PMID: 9598714. http://www.ncbi.nlm.nih.gov/pubmed/9598714.
283. Campbell PD, Miller AM, Woesner ME. Bright light therapy: seasonal affective disorder and beyond. Einstein J Biol Med. 2017;32:E13–25. PMCID: PMC6746555. http://www.ncbi.nlm.nih.gov/pubmed/31528147.
284. Daansen PJ, Haffmans J. Reducing symptoms in women with chronic anorexia nervosa. A pilot study on the effects of bright light therapy. Neuro Endocrinol Lett. 2010;31(3):290–6. PMID: 20588231. http://www.ncbi.nlm.nih.gov/pubmed/20588231.
285. Gruber R, Grizenko N, Joober R. Delayed sleep phase syndrome, ADHD, and bright light therapy. J Clin Psychiatry. 2007;68(2):337–8. PMID: 17335340. http://www.ncbi.nlm.nih.gov/pubmed/17335340.
286. Seasonal Affective Disorder – National Institute of Mental Health (NIMH).
287. Seasonal Affective Disorder: MedlinePlus.
288. Tam EM, Lam RW, Robertson HA, Stewart JN, Yatham LN, Zis AP. Atypical depressive symptoms in seasonal and non-seasonal mood disorders. J Affect Disord. 1997;44(1):39–44. PMID: 9186801. http://www.ncbi.nlm.nih.gov/pubmed/9186801.
289. Mersch PP, Middendorp HM, Bouhuys AL, Beersma DG, van den Hoofdakker RH. The prevalence of seasonal affective disorder in The Netherlands: a prospective and retrospective study of seasonal mood variation in the general population. Biol Psychiatry. 1999;45(8):1013–22. PMID: 10386184. http://www.ncbi.nlm.nih.gov/pubmed/10386184.
290. Lewy AJ, Lefler BJ, Emens JS, Bauer VK. The circadian basis of winter depression. Proc Natl Acad Sci U S A. 2006;103(19):7414–9. PMCID: PMC1450113. http://www.ncbi.nlm.nih.gov/pubmed/16648247.
291. Mårtensson B, Pettersson A, Berglund L, Ekselius L. Bright white light therapy in depression: a critical review of the evidence. J Affect Disord. 2015;182:1–7. PMID: 25942575. http://www.ncbi.nlm.nih.gov/pubmed/25942575.
292. Lam RW, Gorman CP, Michalon M, Steiner M, Levitt AJ, Corral MR, Watson GD, Morehouse RL, Tam W, Joffe RT. Multicenter, placebo-controlled study of fluoxetine in seasonal affective disorder. Am J Psychiatry. 1995;152(12):1765–70. PMID: 8526243. http://www.ncbi.nlm.nih.gov/pubmed/8526243.
293. Moscovitch A, Blashko CA, Eagles JM, Darcourt G, Thompson C, Kasper S, Lane RM, International Collaborative Group on Sertraline in the Treatment of Outpatients with Seasonal Affective Disorders. A placebo-controlled study of sertraline in the treatment of outpatients with seasonal affective disorder. Psychopharmacology. 2004;171(4):390–7. PMID: 14504682. http://www.ncbi.nlm.nih.gov/pubmed/14504682.
294. Lam RW, Levitt AJ, Levitan RD, Michalak EE, Cheung AH, Morehouse R, Ramasubbu R, Yatham LN, Tam EM. Efficacy of bright light treatment, fluoxetine, and the combination in patients with nonseasonal major depressive disorder: a randomized clinical trial. JAMA Psychiatr. 2016;73(1):56–63. PMID: 26580307. http://www.ncbi.nlm.nih.gov/pubmed/26580307.
295. Pail G, Huf W, Pjrek E, Winkler D, Willeit M, Praschak-Rieder N, Kasper S. Bright-light therapy in the treatment of mood disorders. Neuropsychobiology. 2011;64(3):152–62. PMID: 21811085. http://www.ncbi.nlm.nih.gov/pubmed/21811085.
296. Meesters Y, Duijzer WB, Hommes V. The effects of low-intensity narrow-band blue-light treatment compared to bright white-light treatment in seasonal affective disorder. J Affect Disord. 2018;232:48–51. PMID: 29477098. http://www.ncbi.nlm.nih.gov/pubmed/29477098.
297. Tordjman S, Chokron S, Delorme R, Charrier A, Bellissant E, Jaafari N, Fougerou C. Melatonin: pharmacology, functions and therapeutic benefits. Curr Neuropharmacol. 2017;15(3):434–43. PMCID: PMC5405617. http://www.ncbi.nlm.nih.gov/pubmed/28503116.
298. Brainard GC, Hanifin JP, Greeson JM, Byrne B, Glickman G, Gerner E, Rollag MD. Action spectrum for melatonin regulation in humans: evidence for a novel circadian photoreceptor. J Neurosci. 2001;21(16):6405–12. PMCID: PMC6763155. http://www.ncbi.nlm.nih.gov/pubmed/11487664.
299. Hatori M, Gronfier C, Van Gelder RN, Bernstein PS, Carreras J, Panda S, Marks F, Sliney D, Hunt CE, Hirota T, Furukawa T, Tsubota K. Global rise of potential health hazards caused by blue light-induced circadian disruption in modern aging societies. NPJ Aging Mech Dis. 2017;3:9. PMCID: PMC5473809. http://www.ncbi.nlm.nih.gov/pubmed/28649427.
300. Meng Q, Lian Y, Jiang J, Wang W, Hou X, Pan Y, Chu H, Shang L, Wei X, Hao W. Blue light filtered white light induces depression-like responses and temporary spatial learning deficits in rats. Photochem Photobiol Sci. 2018;17(4):386–94. PMID: 29404551. http://www.ncbi.nlm.nih.gov/pubmed/29404551.
301. Chang AM, Aeschbach D, Duffy JF, Czeisler CA. Evening use of light-emitting eReaders negatively affects sleep, circadian timing, and next-morning alertness. Proc Natl Acad Sci USA. 2015;112(4):1232–7. PMCID: PMC4313820. http://www.ncbi.nlm.nih.gov/pubmed/25535358.
302. Do A, Li VW, Huang S, Michalak EE, Tam EM, Chakrabarty T, Yatham LN, Lam RW. Blue-light therapy for seasonal and non-seasonal depression: a systematic review and meta-analysis of ran-

domized controlled trials. Can J Psychiatr. 2022;67(10):745–54. PMCID: PMC9511000. http://www.ncbi.nlm.nih.gov/pubmed/35522196.
303. Al-Karawi D, Jubair L. Bright light therapy for nonseasonal depression: meta-analysis of clinical trials. J Affect Disord. 2016;198:64–71. PMID: 27011361. http://www.ncbi.nlm.nih.gov/pubmed/27011361.
304. Dauphinais DR, Rosenthal JZ, Terman M, DiFebo HM, Tuggle C, Rosenthal NE. Controlled trial of safety and efficacy of bright light therapy vs. negative air ions in patients with bipolar depression. Psychiatry Res. 2012;196(1):57–61. PMID: 22424890. http://www.ncbi.nlm.nih.gov/pubmed/22424890.
305. Deltito JA, Moline M, Pollak C, Martin LY, Maremmani I. Effects of phototherapy on non-seasonal unipolar and bipolar depressive spectrum disorders. J Affect Disord. 1991;23(4):231–7. PMID: 1791269. http://www.ncbi.nlm.nih.gov/pubmed/1791269.
306. Tseng PT, Chen YW, Tu KY, Chung W, Wang HY, Wu CK, Lin PY. Light therapy in the treatment of patients with bipolar depression: a meta-analytic study. Eur Neuropsychopharmacol. 2016;26(6):1037–47. PMID: 26993616. http://www.ncbi.nlm.nih.gov/pubmed/26993616.
307. Sit D, Wisner KL, Hanusa BH, Stull S, Terman M. Light therapy for bipolar disorder: a case series in women. Bipolar Disord. 2007;9(8):918–27. PMID: 18076544. http://www.ncbi.nlm.nih.gov/pubmed/18076544.
308. Sit D, Haigh S. Use of "lights" for bipolar depression. Curr Psychiatry Rep. 2019;21(6):45. PMID: 31119407. http://www.ncbi.nlm.nih.gov/pubmed/31119407.
309. Oren DA, Wisner KL, Spinelli M, Epperson CN, Peindl KS, Terman JS, Terman M. An open trial of morning light therapy for treatment of antepartum depression. Am J Psychiatry. 2002;159(4):666–9. PMID: 11925310. http://www.ncbi.nlm.nih.gov/pubmed/11925310.
310. Epperson CN, Terman M, Terman JS, Hanusa BH, Oren DA, Peindl KS, Wisner KL. Randomized clinical trial of bright light therapy for antepartum depression: preliminary findings. J Clin Psychiatry. 2004;65(3):421–5. PMID: 15096083. http://www.ncbi.nlm.nih.gov/pubmed/15096083.
311. Wirz-Justice A, Bader A, Frisch U, Stieglitz RD, Alder J, Bitzer J, Hösli I, Jazbec S, Benedetti F, Terman M, Wisner KL, Riecher-Rössler A. A randomized, double-blind, placebo-controlled study of light therapy for antepartum depression. J Clin Psychiatry. 2011;72(7):986–93. PMID: 21535997. http://www.ncbi.nlm.nih.gov/pubmed/21535997.
312. Penders TM, Stanciu CN, Schoemann AM, Ninan PT, Bloch R, Saeed SA. Bright light therapy as augmentation of pharmacotherapy for treatment of depression: a systematic review and meta-analysis. Prim Care Companion CNS Disord. 2016;18(5) PMID: 27835725. http://www.ncbi.nlm.nih.gov/pubmed/27835725.
313. Maruani J, Geoffroy PA. Bright light as a personalized precision treatment of mood disorders. Front Psychiatry. 2019;10:85. PMCID: PMC6405415. http://www.ncbi.nlm.nih.gov/pubmed/30881318.
314. A guide to what works for depression: an evidence-based review: find an Expert: The University of Melbourne.
315. Nahin RL, Barnes PM, Stussman BJ. Expenditures on complementary health approaches: United States, 2012. Natl Health Stat Report. 2016;95:1–11. PMID: 27352222. http://www.ncbi.nlm.nih.gov/pubmed/27352222.
316. Kessler RC, Soukup J, Davis RB, Foster DF, Wilkey SA, Van Rompay MI, Eisenberg DM. The use of complementary and alternative therapies to treat anxiety and depression in the United States. Am J Psychiatry. 2001;158(2):289–94. PMID: 11156813. http://www.ncbi.nlm.nih.gov/pubmed/11156813.
317. Thachil AF, Mohan R, Bhugra D. The evidence base of complementary and alternative therapies in depression. J Affect Disord. 2007;97(1–3):23–35. PMID: 16926053. http://www.ncbi.nlm.nih.gov/pubmed/16926053.
318. Sun Y, Xu X, Zhang J, Chen Y. Treatment of depression with Chai Hu Shu Gan San: a systematic review and meta-analysis of 42 randomized controlled trials. BMC Complement Altern Med. 2018;18(1):66. PMCID: PMC5816377. http://www.ncbi.nlm.nih.gov/pubmed/29454341.
319. The Centre for Evidence-Based Medicine|Evidence Service to support the COVID-19 response.
320. Bishop JL, Northstone K, Green JR, Thompson EA. The use of complementary and alternative medicine in pregnancy: data from the Avon longitudinal study of parents and children (ALSPAC). Complement Ther Med. 2011;19(6):303–10. PMID: 22036522. http://www.ncbi.nlm.nih.gov/pubmed/22036522.
321. Quah-Smith I, Smith C, Crawford JD, Russell J. Laser acupuncture for depression: a randomised double blind controlled trial using low intensity laser intervention. J Affect Disord. 2013;148(2–3):179–87. PMID: 23337655. http://www.ncbi.nlm.nih.gov/pubmed/23337655.
322. Andreescu C, Glick RM, Emeremni CA, Houck PR, Mulsant BH. Acupuncture for the treatment of major depressive disorder: a randomized controlled trial. J Clin Psychiatry. 2011;72(8):1129–35. PMCID: PMC10536993. http://www.ncbi.nlm.nih.gov/pubmed/21672495.
323. Smith CA, Armour M, Lee MS, Wang LQ, Hay PJ. Acupuncture for depression. Cochrane Database Syst Rev. 2018;3(3):CD004046. PMCID: PMC6494180. http://www.ncbi.nlm.nih.gov/pubmed/29502347.
324. Ng QX, Venkatanarayanan N, Ho CYX. Clinical use of Hypericum perforatum (St John's wort) in depression: a meta-analysis. J Affect Disord. 2017;210:211–21. PMID: 28064110. http://www.ncbi.nlm.nih.gov/pubmed/28064110.
325. St. John's Wort: Usefulness and Safety | NCCIH.
326. Forsdike K, Pirotta M. St John's wort for depression: scoping review about perceptions and use by general practitioners in clinical practice. J Pharm Pharmacol. 2019;71(1):117–28. PMID: 28653745. http://www.ncbi.nlm.nih.gov/pubmed/28653745.
327. Linde K, Mulrow CD, Berner M, Egger M. St John's wort for depression. Cochrane Database Syst Rev. 2005;2:CD000448. PMID: 15846605. http://www.ncbi.nlm.nih.gov/pubmed/15846605.
328. Linde K, Kriston L, Rücker G, Jamil S, Schumann I, Meissner K, Sigterman K, Schneider A. Efficacy and acceptability of pharmacological treatments for depressive disorders in primary care: systematic review and network meta-analysis. Ann Fam Med. 2015;13(1):69–79. PMCID: PMC4291268. http://www.ncbi.nlm.nih.gov/pubmed/25583895.
329. Apaydin EA, Maher AR, Shanman R, Booth MS, Miles JNV, Sorbero ME, Hempel S. A systematic review of St. John's wort for major depressive disorder. Syst Rev. 2016;5(1):148. PMCID: PMC5010734. http://www.ncbi.nlm.nih.gov/pubmed/27589952.
330. Zirak N, Shafiee M, Soltani G, Mirzaei M, Sahebkar A. Hypericum perforatum in the treatment of psychiatric and neurodegenerative disorders: current evidence and potential mechanisms of action. J Cell Physiol. 2019;234(6):8496–508. PMID: 30461013. http://www.ncbi.nlm.nih.gov/pubmed/30461013.
331. Shelton RC. St John's wort (Hypericum perforatum) in major depression. J Clin Psychiatry. 2009;70(Suppl 5):23–7. PMID: 19909690. http://www.ncbi.nlm.nih.gov/pubmed/19909690.
332. Werneke U, Horn O, Taylor DM. How effective is St John's wort? The evidence revisited. J Clin Psychiatry. 2004;65(5):611–7. PMID: 15163246. http://www.ncbi.nlm.nih.gov/pubmed/15163246.
333. Biotechnological production of hyperforin for pharmaceutical formulation – ScienceDirect.

334. Allaire AD, Moos MK, Wells SR. Complementary and alternative medicine in pregnancy: a survey of North Carolina certified nurse-midwives. Obstet Gynecol. 2000;95(1):19–23. PMID: 10636495. http://www.ncbi.nlm.nih.gov/pubmed/10636495.
335. Dennehy C, Tsourounis C, Bui L, King TL. The use of herbs by California midwives. J Obstet Gynecol Neonatal Nurs. 2010;39(6):684–93. PMID: 21044150. http://www.ncbi.nlm.nih.gov/pubmed/21044150.
336. Klier CM, Schmid-Siegel B, Schäfer MR, Lenz G, Saria A, Lee A, Zernig G. St. John's wort (Hypericum perforatum) and breastfeeding: plasma and breast milk concentrations of hyperforin for 5 mothers and 2 infants. J Clin Psychiatry. 2006;67(2):305–9. PMID: 16566628. http://www.ncbi.nlm.nih.gov/pubmed/16566628.
337. Lee A, Minhas R, Matsuda N, Lam M, Ito S. The safety of St. John's wort (Hypericum perforatum) during breastfeeding. J Clin Psychiatry. 2003;64(8):966–8. PMID: 12927015. http://www.ncbi.nlm.nih.gov/pubmed/12927015.
338. Rayburn WF, Christensen HD, Gonzalez CL. Effect of antenatal exposure to Saint John's wort (Hypericum) on neurobehavior of developing mice. Am J Obstet Gynecol. 2000;183(5):1225–31. PMID: 11084570. http://www.ncbi.nlm.nih.gov/pubmed/11084570.
339. Dugoua JJ, Mills E, Perri D, Koren G. Safety and efficacy of St. John's wort (hypericum) during pregnancy and lactation. Can J Clin Pharmacol. 2006;13(3):e268–76. PMID: 17085775. http://www.ncbi.nlm.nih.gov/pubmed/17085775.
340. Gregoretti B, Stebel M, Candussio L, Crivellato E, Bartoli F, Decorti G. Toxicity of Hypericum perforatum (St. John's wort) administered during pregnancy and lactation in rats. Toxicol Appl Pharmacol. 2004;200(3):201–5. PMID: 15504456. http://www.ncbi.nlm.nih.gov/pubmed/15504456.
341. Moretti ME, Maxson A, Hanna F, Koren G. Evaluating the safety of St. John's Wort in human pregnancy. Reprod Toxicol. 2009;28(1):96–9. PMID: 19491000. http://www.ncbi.nlm.nih.gov/pubmed/19491000.
342. St. John's Wort – Drugs and Lactation Database (LactMed®) – NCBI Bookshelf.
343. Zhou S, Chan E, Pan SQ, Huang M, Lee EJD. Pharmacokinetic interactions of drugs with St John's wort. J Psychopharmacol. 2004;18(2):262–76. PMID: 15260917. http://www.ncbi.nlm.nih.gov/pubmed/15260917.
344. Drug Interaction Checker – Find Interactions Between Medications.
345. Drug Interactions Checker – Check Your Brand and Generic Drugs – RxList.
346. Drug Interaction Checker ← Quickly Check Your Meds.
347. Tao L, Jiang R, Zhang K, Qian Z, Chen P, Lv Y, Yao Y. Light therapy in non-seasonal depression: an update meta-analysis. Psychiatry Res. 2020;291:113247. PMID: 32622169. http://www.ncbi.nlm.nih.gov/pubmed/32622169.
348. Yang NN, Lin LL, Li YJ, Li HP, Cao Y, Tan CX, Hao XW, Ma SM, Wang L, Liu CZ. Potential mechanisms and clinical effectiveness of acupuncture in depression. Curr Neuropharmacol. 2022;20(4):738–50. PMCID: PMC9878952. http://www.ncbi.nlm.nih.gov/pubmed/35168522.
349. Chen B, Wang CC, Lee KH, Xia JC, Luo Z. Efficacy and safety of acupuncture for depression: a systematic review and meta-analysis. Res Nurs Health. 2023;46(1):48–67. PMCID: PMC10108109. http://www.ncbi.nlm.nih.gov/pubmed/36509453.
350. Hauser SR, Getachew B, Taylor RE, Tizabi Y. Alcohol induced depressive-like behavior is associated with a reduction in hippocampal BDNF. Pharmacol Biochem Behav. 2011;100(2):253–8. https://doi.org/10.1016/j.pbb.2011.08.014. Epub 2011 Sep 10. PMID: 21930150; PMCID: PMC3199315. Alcohol induced depressive-like behavior is associated with a reduction in hippocampal BDNF – PubMed.

Depression, Immune Mechanisms, and Anti-inflammatory Treatment Strategies

24

Jennifer M. Loftis

Introduction

Major depressive disorder (MDD) is a leading cause of disability, and chronic inflammation is a contributing factor to its onset, progression, and persistence. An appreciation and understanding of the role of the immune response in depression emerged, in large part, from the adverse side effects experienced by patients with cancer or chronic hepatitis C viral infection (HCV) who received cytokine-based immunotherapy (e.g., [1, 2]). Notably, interferon-alpha (IFN-α)-based therapies for HCV cause depression in 20–40% of patients [3–5]. Similar to MDD, IFN-α-induced depression is characterized by negative mood, fatigue, anhedonia, psychomotor retardation, loss of appetite, and cognitive deficits [6, 7]. Subsequent research has shown that the state of depression is associated with an increase in plasma levels of various cytokines and related immune factors [8]. Further, antidepressants can shift the cytokine network toward a decreased production of pro-inflammatory cytokines and an increased production of anti-inflammatory cytokines [9], as well as modify immune reactivity by acting on neural structures involved in neuroimmunomodulation [10].

While current first-line treatments for depression primarily target neurotransmitter imbalances, many patients do not experience full symptom resolution, underscoring the need for novel therapeutic approaches. Emerging evidence indicates that neuroinflammation, immune dysregulation, gut dysbiosis, and dysfunction of the hypothalamic-pituitary-adrenal (HPA) axis play significant roles in the pathophysiology of depression, often interacting bidirectionally with stress. This chapter integrates preclinical and clinical research findings to explore how chronic inflammation and alterations in neurotransmission may contribute to the emotional and cognitive symptoms of depression. The discussion highlights the complex interplay between peripheral immune responses, cytokine activity, and neurotransmitter systems. The involvement of the HPA axis, oxidative stress mechanisms, and systemic stress responses further illustrates the multifaceted nature of depression. Additionally, this chapter reviews how current and emerging pharmacological and non-pharmacological interventions may modulate inflammation and immune function. By advancing our understanding of these interconnected mechanisms, this chapter sets the stage for developing diagnostic biomarkers, novel anti-inflammatory approaches, and integrative therapeutic strategies that combine immune modulation with traditional depression treatments. For reviews, see [11, 12].

Immune Mechanisms and Biomarkers

Research shows that inflammatory immune factors contribute to the symptoms of depression by altering neurotransmission, neuroplasticity, and neuroendocrine processes. A variety of mechanisms are outlined herein and in Chaps. 7 and 10, indicating how inflammation may be involved in the pathogenesis, course, and treatment of MDD and depressive symptoms. This section highlights the inflammatory mechanisms (peripheral inflammation, gut dysbiosis, and neuroinflammation) involved in the pathophysiology of MDD (Fig. 24.1). Further, how inflammatory cytokines and other immune factors can be used as biomarkers of depression and potential predictors of treatment response is also discussed.

Research has identified a significant connection between psychological stress and MDD, with inflammation playing a central role in this relationship. Stress triggers a cascade of inflammatory signaling, leading to disruptions in neurotransmission, reduced synaptic plasticity, and alterations in neuroendocrine function. Studies have demonstrated that *peripheral immune changes* in individuals with MDD and in mouse models of stress are associated with depressive symp-

J. M. Loftis (✉)
VA Portland Health Care System, Portland, OR, USA

Departments of Psychiatry and Behavioral Neuroscience, Oregon Health & Science University, Portland, OR, USA
e-mail: jennifer.loftis2@va.gov; loftisj@ohsu.edu

J. Raber et al. (eds.), *Understanding and Treating Depressive Disorders*, https://doi.org/10.1007/978-3-032-14465-2_24

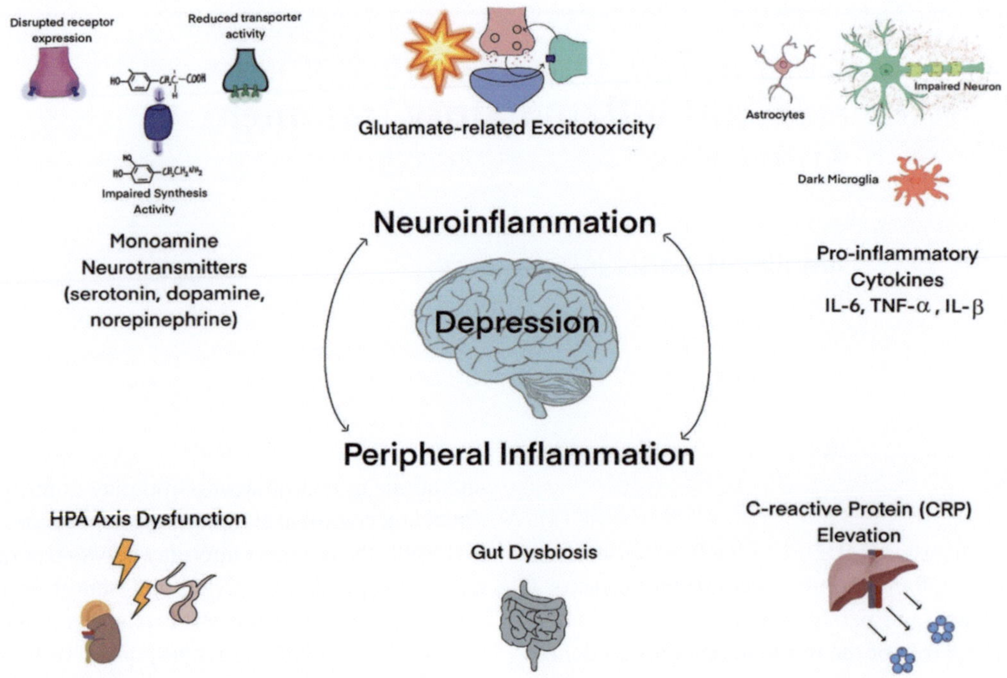

Fig. 24.1 Neuroimmune mechanisms linking early-life adversity to major depressive disorder (MDD). Early-life stressors—such as maltreatment, parental loss, and socioeconomic hardship—can prime peripheral immune and neuroendocrine systems toward a chronic pro-inflammatory state, increasing vulnerability to depression. The figure depicts bidirectional cross-talk between peripheral cytokines (e.g., IL-6, TNF-α, IL-β, CRP) and central neurotransmitter systems, including disrupted monoamine signaling, glutamate-related excitotoxicity, and impaired neuroplasticity. (Example of dopamine synthesis depicted in figure.) These interactions are mediated through neuroimmune pathways involving the HPA axis, gut–brain axis, and blood–brain barrier permeability. Cellular changes, such as astrocyte dysfunction and dark microglia activation, further illustrate how peripheral inflammation influences central nervous system function. Together, these mechanisms highlight how systemic inflammation and neural dysregulation converge to shape the emotional and cognitive symptoms of MDD

toms. These findings suggest that targeting peripheral immune factors could represent a novel approach for treating stress-related neuropsychiatric disorders, such as depression. Preclinical and clinical studies have identified specific immune factors that are elevated in the serum or plasma of patients with MDD and stress-exposed mice, indicating a mechanism by which peripheral immune responses can affect brain function and behavior. Furthermore, proteins, such as nuclear factor kappa-B (NF-κB), play a role in the regulation of stress hormones and are associated with depressive behaviors. For review, see [13].

Stress resulting from early-life adversities—such as childhood maltreatment, parental loss, and socioeconomic hardship—can sensitize immune and stress-regulation systems, promoting a pro-inflammatory state that increases vulnerability to depression later in life. Meta-analytic evidence shows that adverse childhood experiences significantly predict elevated inflammatory markers like C-reactive protein (CRP), interleukin-6 (IL-6), and tumor necrosis factor-alpha (TNF-α), which mediate the association between early adversity and adult depressive symptoms [14]. Longitudinal research further supports this linkage: for instance, childhood adversities measured prospectively (ages 1–8) are associated with higher IL-6 and CRP levels at ages 10 and 15, and in adolescents, high childhood adversity predicts depression accompanied by concurrent increases in CRP and IL-6 [15]. Adverse childhood experiences also foster maladaptive health behaviors (e.g., increased BMI and smoking) that further amplify chronic inflammation, thus exacerbating stress and mood dysregulation [16]. Overall, evidence from clinical, epidemiological, and preclinical studies converges on the model that inflammation is a key mechanistic mediator between early-life adversity and the later onset or persistence of depression. See also [17–19]. This is of consequence, as individuals with MDD and systemic inflammation appear to be biologically primed to respond more strongly to an inflammatory stimulus (e.g., lipopolysaccharide (LPS)), and psychologically, this sensitization impacts symptoms of depression [20].

Inflammation plays a prominent role in MDD, not only in the periphery but also in the *central nervous system (CNS)*. Inflammatory mediators impact brain regions involved in mood regulation, including the hippocampus, amygdala, and prefrontal cortex, and contribute to dysfunction across multiple cell types in the brain. Key neuroinflammatory mechanisms include glial cell activation, cytokine signaling, blood-brain barrier (BBB) disruption, and alterations in neurotransmitter systems. Inflammatory insults may "prime" microglia, increasing their sensitivity to stress, impairing synaptic plasticity, and promoting depressive symptoms [21]. Elevated pro-inflammatory cytokines, such as IL-1β, IL-6, IL-18, and TNF-α, have been observed in MDD and are associated with neuroinflammation, systemic inflammation, and gut microbiota dysbiosis—factors that contribute to disrupted neurotransmission [22–24]. Monoaminergic signaling modulates neuroinflammation by regulating CNS cytokine and chemokine expression, and this interaction is bidirectional: pro-inflammatory cytokines alter monoamine metabolism by influencing neurotransmitter synthesis, release, and reuptake [25]. For instance, studies of IFN-α-induced depression in individuals with HCV and animal models show that cytokines activate indoleamine 2,3-dioxygenase (IDO), leading to increased kynurenine pathway metabolites (e.g., kynurenic acid) and reduced serotonin synthesis, contributing to impaired neuroplasticity and glutamate-related excitotoxicity. For example, [26–28].

In addition to alterations in serotonergic signaling, cytokines and other immune factors also modulate dopaminergic neurotransmission by disrupting dopamine synthesis, release, and reuptake through multiple interlinked mechanisms. For example, pro-inflammatory cytokines such as IFN-α and IL-6 stimulate inducible nitric oxide synthase, elevating nitric oxide levels, which in turn oxidize tetrahydrobiopterin—a critical cofactor for tyrosine hydroxylase, the rate-limiting enzyme in dopamine synthesis. This pathway leads to diminished dopamine production. Chronic cytokine exposure reduces vesicular monoamine transporter 2 expression, impairing dopamine packaging into synaptic vesicles; the resulting cytosolic dopamine buildup can undergo auto-oxidation, increasing oxidative stress and dopamine neuron vulnerability. Moreover, cytokine-activated p38/MAPK signaling enhances dopamine transporter function, promoting dopamine reuptake and decreasing synaptic availability. Cytokine activation of IDO also has impacts on dopamine, as elevated kynurenic acid dampens glutamate-driven dopaminergic firing in the striatum, further suppressing dopamine release. Mechanisms are described in [29–31]. Collectively, these mechanisms contribute to inflammation-associated reductions in monoaminergic signaling and are correlated with depressive symptoms, including anhedonia, psychomotor slowing, and fatigue in humans and animal models.

The role of genetic contributions to inflammation and depression is beyond the scope of this chapter; however, Text Box 24.1 highlights a few key observations and provides references for additional information on this topic.

Text Box 24.1 Genetic Contributions to Depression via Immune Mechanisms

Converging evidence indicates that genetic risk factors for inflammation contribute to depression.

- Integrative genomic analysis identified GDP-mannose pyrophosphorylase B as a depression risk gene. This gene is active in brain regions critical to emotion (amygdala, anterior cingulate cortex) and may influence depression through inflammation-related glycosylation pathways [32].
- Genetic (CRP, IL-6, IL-6 receptor, soluble IL-6 receptor, and glycoprotein acetyls (GlycA)) links are found between inflammatory markers (CRP and GlycA) and negative affect, depression, and anxiety in over 55,000 individuals [33].
- Differential gene expression and co-expression network analyses of cortical and subcortical brain regions resulted in the identification of sex-specific genetic differences associated with MDD. A subset of genes associates with common symptomatic features in both sexes [34].
- A polygenic risk score for inflammation associates with MDD. Psychological resilience (optimism) reduces this genetic risk, and analyses highlight immune and brain-related gene pathways involved in MDD vulnerability [35].
- Gene signatures in peripheral blood immune cells related to insulin resistance and low tyrosine metabolism define a subtype of depression with high CRP and anhedonia [36].

These findings support a biologically meaningful link between immune-related genes and depression, particularly via inflammation. They also highlight potential protective factors (e.g., optimism) and molecular targets for future treatment.

Central and Peripheral Biomarkers of Inflammation in Depression

To date, brain inflammation is traceable in vivo with positron emission tomography (PET), through the quantification of the expression of 18-kDa *Translocator Protein (TSPO)* by active microglia. Results from a review of all in vivo PET imaging studies ($n = 9$) that evaluated microglia activation in MDD suggested the presence of TSPO upregulation in MDD, especially in the anterior cingulate cortex, prefrontal cortex, hippocampal formation, and insula. Notably, findings suggest that symptom amelioration, resulting from antidepressant medication and cognitive behavioral therapy, may be accompanied by reduced inflammatory status in the brain [37]. These studies support the role of neuroinflammation in MDD, suggesting that microgliosis may be an important pathophysiological mechanism for further investigation as a potential biomarker, as well as a target for treatment. In addition to increases in TSPO PET signal as a CNS marker of immune activation, inflammation-related depression can also be evaluated with biomarkers that measure structural changes, functional changes, trophic support, and neurotoxicity (Table 24.1). These neural biomarkers strengthen the understanding that inflammation can disrupt brain structure, function, and neurochemistry in depression.

In preclinical models, correlations of inflammatory cytokines between the hippocampus and blood indicate that assessing inflammatory damage (and treatment response) in the hippocampus could be done through blood tests of the signaling pathway and related cytokines [43]. More research is needed to validate these peripheral markers as reliable indicators of central inflammation and to clarify their specificity and sensitivity in reflecting hippocampal pathology. In the periphery, several biomarkers have been investigated for their potential utility as biomarkers for MDD symptoms and treatment response. Several of the more widely studied biomarkers are listed in Table 24.2 and summarized below.

C-reactive protein (CRP) is an acute-phase protein that is often elevated in MDD. CRP levels >3 mg/L can indicate heightened systemic inflammation [44]. Longitudinal data reveal that elevated CRP modestly predicts future depressive symptoms [45]. Elevated CRP also correlates with fatigue, atypical depression subtype, and treatment-resistant depression [46–48]. It has been suggested that to personalize antidepressant prescription, CRP-matched treatment assignment could be implemented in clinical practice with point-of-care fingerstick tests [49].

Complete blood count (CBC) parameters and inflammatory ratios can also be used as biomarkers of depression. Neutrophil/lymphocyte ratio (NLR), platelet/lymphocyte ratio (PLR), and monocyte/lymphocyte ratio (MLR) are inexpensive and reproducible biomarkers of inflammation [50]. Increased NLR, PLR, and MLR ratios are generally correlated with depression. While some studies show these ratios are elevated in individuals with depression compared to controls, others indicate varying degrees of significance and even conflicting results [51, 52]. In MDD, changes in CBC parameters and inflammatory ratios may be more closely related to the suicidality severity than depressive symptom severity [53].

Interleukin-1β (IL-1β) is associated with HPA axis dysfunction and reduced serotonin reuptake, linking it to depressive pathophysiology [54]. Meta-analyses confirm significantly higher peripheral IL-1β in depressed older adults, though TNF-α and CRP may not be elevated in all subgroups [55].

Interleukin-6 (IL-6) is a cytokine that is increased in MDD, showing strong positive associations with depression severity (e.g., anhedonia, lack of motivation) [44]. IL-6 has also been shown to be a longitudinal predictor of depressive

Table 24.1 Brain biomarkers associated with inflammation-linked depression

Biomarker type	Example	Significance	Reference
Immune activation	↑ TSPO PET signal	Microglial-driven neuroinflammation	[12, 37]
Structural changes	Gray matter reduction	Neurodegeneration in emotion/reward circuits	[38, 39]
Functional changes	Altered connectivity	Impaired reward, cognitive, and emotional processing	[40]
Trophic support	↓ BDNF	Reduced neuroplasticity	[41]
Neurotoxicity	↑ Quinolinic acid	Excitotoxic neuronal loss	[42]

Abbreviations: *BDNF* brain-derived neurotrophic factor, *PET* positron emission tomography, *TSPO* 18-kDa Translocator Protein

Table 24.2 Peripheral biomarkers associated with inflammation-linked depression

Biomarker	Direction in MDD	Clinical implication
CRP/hs-CRP	↑	Inflammation, severity, prognosis
IL-1β	↑ (especially in older adults)	HPA-axis dysregulation, serotonergic impact
IL-6	↑	Diagnosis, severity, treatment response
IL-8, sIL-2R	↑	Cognitive deficits, broad immune activation
TNF-α	↑ (variable with treatment)	Somatic symptoms, treatment-resistant depression, atypical depression
Leukocytes, haptoglobin	↑	Long-term risk marker
Kyn/trp ratio	↑	Tryptophan metabolism imbalance (neurotoxic)
Monocytes/T cells	↑ (pro-inflammatory subsets)	Cellular-level immune activation

See text for specific references

symptoms [45], and levels of IL-6 often decrease following antidepressant treatment [56].

Interleukin-8 (IL-8) is typically considered a pro-inflammatory cytokine, and its dysregulation is thought to play a role in the inflammation associated with depression, as well as cognitive deficits [57, 58]. Studies have shown that lower serum levels of IL-8 are correlated with higher depression scores in individuals with MDD [59]. Some studies indicate that lower baseline IL-8 levels and increases in IL-8 levels during treatment are associated with a better response to antidepressant treatments, particularly in females (e.g., [60]). While some studies show lower IL-8 levels in depressed individuals, others have found elevated levels, highlighting the complexity of the relationship [61].

Soluble IL-2 receptor (sIL-2R) is elevated in MDD and often mirrors CRP changes, indicating general immune activation [62]. While more research is needed to solidify the role of sIL-2R as a definitive biomarker, the evidence points to its potential as an indicator of immune system involvement in depression, particularly concerning somatic symptoms [63, 64].

Tumor necrosis factor-alpha (TNF-α) is elevated in many MDD cohorts and associated with somatic depressive symptoms and atypical depression [47]. TNF-α shows inconsistent changes with treatment; meta-analyses for antidepressant effects are mixed. In treatment-resistant depression, TNF-α emerges as one of the more distinguishing inflammatory markers [65].

Leukocyte count and haptoglobin. Large cohort studies find that elevated leukocytes and haptoglobin are associated with increased risk of depression (HR ≈ 1.1) up to 30 years before diagnosis [66].

Kynurenine pathway metabolites (kyn/trp ratio). The kyn/trp ratio reflects activation of indoleamine 2,3-dioxygenase (IDO), shifting tryptophan toward neuroactive kynurenines (e.g., quinolinic acid), which are tied to depressive symptoms [67–70].

Monocyte and T cell subsets are emerging biomarkers for depression. Patients with MDD and high levels of CRP show elevated pro-inflammatory monocyte ($CD14^+/CD16^+$) and T cell shifts; these cellular changes accompany anhedonia and may normalize with anti-inflammatory treatments [71].

Other potential peripheral indices of depression include the *uric acid/high-density lipoprotein cholesterol ratio (UHR)*—a new indicator of inflammation and metabolism that is associated with several chronic diseases, and recently, depression. In a large NHANES study (2005–2018) with 16,920 adults, elevated UHR levels were associated with a 52% higher risk of depression. A significant interaction with sex was found, but not with other demographic or lifestyle factors. Subgroup analyses revealed stronger associations in females, younger individuals, alcohol users, nonsmokers, those with higher education, cohabiters, individuals at both income extremes, and physically active participants. These findings suggest that UHR may serve as a useful peripheral indicator for early depression risk detection [72].

Apolipoprotein A4 (ApoA4) links lipid metabolism, inflammation, and depressive pathology and holds promise as a peripheral biomarker for depression. Genetic and proteomic evidence supports its relevance across age groups and clinical scenarios (e.g., identifying depressive states and severity; differentiating treatment responders versus non-responders [73–75]). However, conflicting findings necessitate validation before routine clinical implementation.

Heat shock protein 70 (HSP70) functions extracellularly as a danger-associated molecular pattern (DAMP), stimulating innate immune responses (e.g., macrophage activation). HSP70 is elevated in the serum from individuals with MDD and in the brain from rodents subjected to chronic mild stress [76, 77]. Thus, HSP70 shows promise as a peripheral biomarker for depression, reflecting underlying cellular stress, inflammation, and modulating treatment response. However, levels vary based on sample type (central vs. peripheral), timing, and clinical context; methodological refinement and clinical validation are needed before clinical adoption.

Oxidative stress and inflammation contribute to the pathophysiology of MDD. In a large study of 104 patients (drug-free) with an acute episode of MDD and 50 control participants, markers of oxidative stress and the Nrf2 antioxidant system were assessed before and after 12 weeks of antidepressant treatment. Compared to controls, MDD patients had lower levels of Nrf2, phospho-Nrf2, heme oxygenase-1 (HO-1), and superoxide dismutase, and higher levels of cyclooxygenase-2 (COX-2), phospholipase A2, and malondialdehyde. HO-1 levels varied by depression subtype, and lower Nrf2 levels were negatively correlated with somatic anxiety symptoms. Notably, COX-2 levels increased in non-remitters after treatment, but not in remitters [78]. These findings suggest that dysregulation of peripheral oxidative stress and the Nrf2 system may underlie specific MDD symptom profiles, with Nrf2 as a potential protective factor and COX-2 as a marker of treatment resistance.

Others suggest that *seasonal effects* on depressive symptoms may also involve the immune system and guide the selection of appropriate biomarkers. The immunoseasonal theory posits that seasonal immune shifts—specifically, a T-helper 1 (Th1)-dominant response in winter and a Th2-dominant response in summer—may influence psychiatric symptoms, with Th1 activity linked to worsened depression and anxiety, and Th2 activity associated with exacerbations of psychosis, mania, impulsivity, and suicide risk [79]. In a narrative review, immunological and psychiatric seasonality research are integrated, suggesting that immune biomarkers could help predict symptom fluctuations and guide personalized, seasonally adjusted treatments [80].

Taken together, these peripheral biomarkers—from acute-phase proteins and cytokines to metabolic by-products and immune-cell profiles—provide objective insight into inflammation-mediated depressive processes, help predict treatment responses, and suggest novel targets (e.g., IDO inhibitors, TNF blockers) for intervention. Thus, inflammatory biomarkers offer the potential to personalize antidepressant prescription as well as inform the development of mechanistically guided anti-inflammatory and antidepressant treatments. See also [81] for review of biomarkers that are relevant in the detection or treatment of MDD.

Of note, the development of biosensors may facilitate the utility of biomarkers in MDD. A range of depression biomarkers, including ApoA4 [82], HSP70 [83], BDNF [84], microRNAs [85], and combinatorial biomarker panels, have been detected via biosensor platforms. A recent review discusses the potential of electrochemical biosensors in combating depression [86]. By facilitating earlier and more accurate diagnoses, these biosensors can improve patient care and enhance treatment outcomes.

Anti-Inflammatory Treatment Strategies and Targets

Conventional treatments for MDD show limited efficacy, side effects, and delayed onset. Inflammation is one of the underlying causes for chronicity and treatment non-response in depression. Over a third of patients with MDD fail to respond to two or more antidepressant medications [87]. Cytokines interact with antidepressants and non-pharmacological antidepressive therapies, such as electroconvulsive therapy, deep brain stimulation, and physical activity [88]. In general, response to conventional antidepressants is associated with a decrease in inflammatory factors, whereas resistance to treatment is accompanied by an increase in inflammation. Given the suboptimal response and remission with monoaminergic antidepressants, anti-inflammatory therapies are proposed as an alternative way to treat depression and/or augment the antidepressant effect of monoaminergic antidepressants. Increasingly, studies are investigating the efficiency and efficacy of anti-inflammatory treatment strategies for MDD and depressive symptoms, particularly in the context of comorbid diseases. See also [89] for review of novel anti-inflammatory therapeutic approaches for MDD.

Several clinical trials have investigated the use of immunomodulatory agents in treating depression, including non-steroidal anti-inflammatory drugs (NSAIDs), minocycline, cytokine inhibitors, glycogen synthase kinase 3β (GSK-3β) inhibitors, ketamine, and statins [88, 90]. Monoclonal antibodies targeting pro-inflammatory cytokines such as IL-6, IL-17, and TNF-α have shown antidepressant effects in patients with chronic inflammatory conditions and co-occurring depressive symptoms. Other anti-inflammatory strategies involve blocking the impact of systemic inflammation on the brain [49]. A narrative review identified more than 45 prospective clinical trials, concluding that anti-inflammatory treatments can effectively reduce depressive symptoms as either standalone or adjunctive therapies. The review also proposed a clinical framework emphasizing the role of inflammation in depression, recommending the measurement of inflammatory biomarkers (e.g., CRP) at initial diagnosis. Specifically, patients with elevated CRP levels (>3 mg/L) may particularly benefit from adjunctive anti-inflammatory treatment, and such therapies should be considered in clinical guidelines for managing MDD [91].

Other research has found that in addition to antidepressant medications, physical exercise [92, 93], probiotics, nutritional therapy (e.g., omega-3 fatty acids, proteins) [94], nutraceuticals (e.g., agmatine, ascorbic acid, and vitamin D) [89], electroconvulsive therapy [95], and vagal nerve stimulation [96] possess anti-inflammatory effects that may contribute to their antidepressant properties. Ongoing and recently completed clinical trials evaluating anti-inflammatory treatment strategies for depression can be found at ClinicalTrials.gov. See also [97] for discussion on the utility and shortcomings of pharmacologic antidepressant treatment strategies focused on inflammatory pathways.

New(er) Therapeutic Targets

Complement System The complement system is an important component of the innate immune response and plays a key role in synaptic plasticity—a mechanism that is impaired in depression [98, 99]. An increase in complement component 3 (C3) expression was previously found in the prefrontal cortex of individuals with depression [100]. In a recent study of individuals with and without MDD, plasma levels of C3a and C4a, two key complement proteins implicated in synaptic plasticity, were measured. A significant diagnosis-by-sex interaction was observed for C3a but not C4a levels. These results suggest that treatment strategies targeting the complement pathway, such as ketamine, may yield fruitful insights and advances in treatment options for MDD [101].

Cyclooxygenase-2 (COX-2) The use of anti-inflammatory, COX-2 inhibitors may offer a new approach to treat MDD and depressive symptoms [102]. COX-2 inhibitors prevent the COX-2 enzyme from converting arachidonic acid into prostaglandins. By reducing prostaglandin production, COX-2 inhibitors help to decrease inflammation [103]. Although positive, anti-inflammatory effects of treatment with COX-2 inhibitors have been observed (e.g., [104]), further studies are needed to assess appropriate illness stage-related indications [105]. In addition to medications that target COX-2/prostaglandin signaling, other non-pharmacological approaches to depression treatment, such as rTMS, also appear to modulate this pathway, thereby reducing depression, inflammation, and the activation of astrocytes and microglia in brain [106].

Endocannabinoids Cannabinoid type 2 (CB2) receptors in treating depression—the CB2 receptor, encoded by the *CNR2* gene, plays a key role in modulating inflammatory activity. CB2 receptors are highly controlled at the epigenetic level, especially in response to stressful stimuli, positioning them between stress, neuroinflammation, and depression. A recent review addresses how epigenetic regulation of *CNR2* expression affects depression and the dissection, further, of molecular pathways driving neuroinflammation-related depressive states. The authors highlight the therapeutic potential of CB2 receptor agonists that selectively interact with activated microglia, which could facilitate a new strategy for the treatment of depression associated with neuroinflammation [107].

Fatty acid–binding protein 7 (FABP7) primarily expressed in astrocytes, is a key regulator of inflammatory responses and spinogenesis, the formation of dendritic spines crucial for neuronal communication [108]. Although its role in depressive disorders remains unclear, recent preclinical research using a chronic unpredictable mild stress (CUMS) model showed that CUMS reduced hippocampal FABP7 levels. Overexpressing FABP7 reversed depressive-like behaviors, upregulated caveolin-1, reduced IL-1β and IL-6 expression, and increased dendritic spine density. These findings suggest FABP7 may exert antidepressant effects by modulating inflammation and neuronal plasticity [109], highlighting it as a potential target for inflammation-related depression.

Glutamate receptors especially NMDA and metabotropic—are increasingly promising targets for depression treatments, going beyond classic monoamine-based drugs. Ketamine, a non-competitive NMDA antagonist, is a relatively new and rapid-acting antidepressant approved for therapy of treatment-resistant depression, which has a different mechanism of action than currently available antidepressant therapies [110]. There are several theories explaining how ketamine might reduce depressive symptoms, which have been described in detail; one of them is an immunomodulatory effect of ketamine. Preclinical and clinical studies have found ketamine to reduce inflammation, either directly or indirectly (e.g., by activating neuroprotective branches of the kynurenine pathway), among patients exhibiting higher levels of inflammation. Ketamine-associated changes in cytokine levels and number, ratio, and activity of various immune cell populations correlate with improvements in depressive symptoms (e.g., [111]). The relationships between the antidepressant effect of ketamine and its anti-inflammatory properties, and the resulting benefits in treatment-resistant depression have been comprehensively discussed and reviewed [112, 113].

IL-33/ST2-MyD88 Signaling Pathway The interleukin-33 (IL-33)/serum stimulation-2 (ST2)/myeloid differentiation factor 88 (MyD88) signaling pathway is an important component of the immune response, particularly in the context of inflammation and tissue repair. This pathway is being actively investigated for its potential therapy applications in various disorders, including depression [114]. A recent preclinical study examined how aerobic exercise affects the IL-33/ST2-MyD88 signaling pathway in mice with CUMS-induced depression. Results showed that mice in the exercise group had reduced signs of depression, accompanied by reduced serum and brain (hippocampal) levels of inflammatory factors IL-33, IL-1β, and NF-κB and a significant increase in the anti-inflammatory factor IL-10 [43]. Thus, aerobic exercise may counteract CUMS-induced depression in mice by regulating the IL-33/ST2-MyD88 signaling pathway.

Microglia Accumulating studies show that microglia, the primary resident immune cells of the brain, play a crucial role in the development and progression of depression [115]. While traditionally described as shifting between quiescent and active states, it is now recognized that microglia exist in a spectrum of functional states that are highly dynamic and context-dependent. One notable phenotype is the emergence of "dark" microglia—an ultrastructurally distinct and highly reactive form associated with chronic stress, neuroinflammation, and synaptic remodeling [116]. These cells exhibit condensed cytoplasm and nucleoplasm, increased mitochondrial density, and are often found in close association with synapses, suggesting a role in aberrant synaptic pruning during stress-induced neuropathology. Microglia respond to stress-triggered neuroinflammation, and through the release of pro-inflammatory cytokines and metabolic products, they influence the function of neurons and astrocytes, thereby contributing to depression pathophysiology. The diverse activation states of microglia; the correlative and causal evidence linking microglial dysfunction to depression; potential mechanisms by which microglia detect stress signals; and the impact of antidepressant therapies on microglial function are key areas of ongoing investigation. Understanding the nuanced roles of microglia—including the contribution of dark microglia—may shed light on novel therapeutic strategies for this debilitating mental illness, reviewed in [117, 118]. Indeed, studies suggest that certain classes of antidepressants may exert their effects, in part, by modulating microglial activation, particularly in individuals with elevated inflammation [119].

Mitochondria Mitochondrial function repair therapy is an emerging strategy for treating depression by targeting mitochondrial dysfunction, which is increasingly recognized as contributing to the disorder's pathogenesis. Abnormalities in mitochondrial dynamics—such as altered morphology, DNA damage, and impaired respiratory chain function—are linked to increased inflammation, oxidative stress, and neurotransmitter imbalance, all of which may worsen depressive symptoms [120]. Therapeutic approaches aimed at restoring mitochondrial function could enhance cellular energy production, reduce inflammation and oxidative damage, and alleviate depression symptoms [96, 120].

Toll-Like Receptors (TLRs) Elevated Toll-like receptor 4 (TLR4) levels have been observed in peripheral blood mononuclear cells (PBMCs) and postmortem brains of individuals with depression and suicidal behavior, suggesting abnormalities in TLR expression in depression. Antidepressant treatments and cognitive behavioral therapy have been shown to normalize TLR levels, supporting their potential as biomarkers for treatment response [121, 122]. Despite this, more clinical research is needed to assess the effects of targeting specific TLRs [88]. Preclinical studies show that TLR4 antagonists like TAK-242 and baicalin produce antidepressant-like effects in rodents [123]. Moreover, TLR signaling is modulated by microRNAs, which may contribute to MDD pathophysiology, though their value as therapeutic targets remains uncertain [124].

Plant-Derived Natural Compounds (Phytochemicals) and Formulations that Target Cascades of Inflammation Chemical ingredients of natural origin have been and are being investigated as new direct antidepressants or as adjuvants to improve the current treatment outcomes of existing antidepressant drugs [125–127]. Studies on plant-derived ingredients have highlighted alternative pathways that impact inflammation and modulate perturbed immunity and suggest strategies for treating depression—several of these studies are summarized below. For a comprehensive list of plant-derived compounds under investigation for the treatment of depression see [118].

Agarwood, the aromatic resin from the *Aquilaria* tree, has shown antidepressant potential through aromatherapy. A recent preclinical study using an LPS-induced inflammatory depression model in mice found that agarwood essential oil—administered via inhalation or injection—significantly reduced depression-like behaviors and lowered brain levels of pro-inflammatory cytokines (IL-1β, IL-6, TNF-α). It also inhibited the NF-κB/IκB-α inflammatory signaling pathway and activated the BDNF/TrkB/CREB neuroprotective pathway. These results support agarwood's potential as a neuroprotective and antidepressant agent, though further research is needed to clarify its active components and mechanisms [128].

The antidepressant effects of *arecoline*, a bioactive alkaloid derived from areca nuts, has been studied using a mouse model of depression induced by CUMS. Arecoline treatment alleviated depression-like behaviors, including anxiety, anhedonia, and despair, as evidenced by behavioral tests. Mechanistically, arecoline acts as an agonist at the muscarinic acetylcholine receptor, and treatment with arecoline restored serotonin and norepinephrine levels in the brain and serum, reduced pro-inflammatory markers such as IL-1β and LPS in the serum and colon, and enhanced neuroplasticity through increased BDNF and PSD-95 expression in the hippocampus. Moreover, arecoline modulated gut microbiota composition, particularly enriching beneficial species like *Bifidobacterium pseudolongum* and *Ligilactobacillus murinus*, and regulated serum metabolites associated with tryptophan metabolism, neurotransmitter synthesis, and oxidative stress. These findings demonstrate that arecoline exerts its antidepressant effects via a multitargeted approach involving the gut-brain axis, neurotransmitter modulation, and neuroplasticity enhancement [129].

Astragalin, a flavonoid glycoside found in edible plants and medicinal herbs, has shown antidepressant and neuroprotective effects in preclinical studies. It reduced LPS-induced inflammation in microglial and neuronal cells and alleviated depressive-like behaviors in mice by preserving BBB integrity and preventing inflammatory damage. Astragalin also inhibited glial cell activation and protected neuronal structures, including dendritic spines, synapses, and mitochondria. It lowered pro-inflammatory cytokines (TNF-α, IL-1β, IL-6) and normalized inflammatory signaling pathways such as RIPK1/RIPK3/MLKL and mTOR/NF-κB. These findings suggest astragalin may be a promising candidate for treating inflammation-related depression and protecting brain tissue during systemic inflammation [130].

Caffeine consumption has been inversely associated with depression in epidemiological studies and may influence gut microbiota. Given the link between gut health and depression, a preclinical study explored whether caffeine could prevent depression via the gut-brain axis. Mice subjected to chronic unpredictable stress showed depressive-like behaviors, reduced body weight, and impaired intestinal barrier markers (zonula occludens-1, claudin-1, and mucin2), along with elevated inflammatory markers (plasma LPS, NOD-like receptor thermal protein domain-associated protein 3; hippocampal TNF-α, IL-1β). These changes were not observed in mice pretreated with caffeine, whose behavioral and biological profiles resembled those of control mice. Findings suggest that early caffeine intervention may help prevent depression by modulating gut microbiota, preserving intestinal barrier integrity, and reducing neuroinflammation [131]. Notably, the antidepressant benefits of caffeine appear dose-dependent: a 2022 study reported reduced depression risk with caffeine intakes below 90 mg per day [132], while higher consumption has been linked to psychological distress [133]. This highlights the importance of identifying an optimal range of caffeine intake to support mental health.

Curcumin, a natural compound from *Curcuma longa*, has demonstrated antidepressant effects through multiple mechanisms, including restoring monoaminergic balance; regulating the HPA axis; reducing inflammation, oxidative stress, and nitrosative stress; and improving mitochondrial function. A comprehensive review summarized curcumin's mechanisms, preclinical findings, and clinical trial results, while also noting ongoing challenges in its therapeutic use [134]. To improve efficacy, curcumin analogues have been developed. Among them, the chlorine-containing compound CAK06 showed superior antidepressant effects in rodent models compared to fluoxetine after 28 days. CAK06 appeared to reduce inflammation and oxidative stress and enhance synaptic plasticity via the Nrf2-HO-1/BDNF-TrkB pathway, supporting its potential as a fast-acting, anti-inflammatory antidepressant [135].

Ershiwei Roudoukou Pills (ERP), a traditional Chinese herbal medicine, and its active compound *Macelignan* (from *Myristica fragrans*) demonstrated antidepressant effects in a CUMS mouse model. Both treatments significantly improved depression-like behaviors in behavioral tests and suppressed neuroinflammation by reducing IL-6, TNF-α, and microglial activation, while increasing the anti-inflammatory cytokine IL-10. They also enhanced synaptic plasticity by upregulating proteins such as PSD-95, MAP2, and synaptophysin, and activating the BDNF-TrkB pathway. ERP showed distinct anti-inflammatory effects compared to Macelignan, suggesting synergistic benefits from its multi-component formulation. These results highlight the multi-target potential of ERP and Macelignan for treating depression, particularly in treatment-resistant cases [136].

5-O-methylvisammioside, a flavonol compound from *Saposhnikovia divaricata*, has demonstrated anti-inflammatory, antioxidant, and neuroprotective properties. A recent preclinical study identified Src kinase and the nuclear factor kappa B (NF-κB) signaling pathway as key targets for its antidepressant effects. In a mouse model, 5-O-methylvisammioside alleviated LPS-induced depression-like behaviors, reduced microglial activation in the hippocampus, and inhibited Src phosphorylation and NF-κB activation—effects comparable to the Src inhibitor PP2. These findings suggest that 5-O-methylvisammioside may be a promising herbal treatment for depression via modulation of the Src/NF-κB pathway [137].

Fucosterol, a phytosterol from marine algae, was investigated in mouse models of depression induced by LPS and CUMS. Behavioral tests showed that fucosterol reduced depressive-like behaviors in both models. RNA sequencing analysis revealed that fucosterol suppressed microglial activation in the prefrontal cortex by inhibiting the MAPK/ERK1/2 signaling pathway, leading to reduced neuroinflammatory cytokine release. In primary microglial cultures, fucosterol also mitigated LPS-induced oxidative stress, proliferation, and inflammation, effects that were mirrored by the ERK1/2 inhibitor PD98059. These findings suggest that fucosterol may prevent or alleviate depression by modulating neuroinflammation, offering a promising natural compound for antidepressant development [138].

Luteolin, a flavonoid found in fruits and vegetables, has demonstrated antidepressant and neuroprotective properties in preclinical research. A systematic review of 17 preclinical studies, incorporating network pharmacology and molecular docking analyses, revealed that luteolin exerts its effects through multiple mechanisms. These include enhancing norepinephrine uptake, inhibiting serotonin reuptake, and modulating the expression of neuroprotective and antioxidant proteins such as BDNF, synaptophysin, superoxide dismutase, and glutathione S-transferase, while reducing markers of oxidative stress and apoptosis like malondialdehyde and caspase-3. Its mechanisms involve anti-inflammatory, antioxidant, anti-apoptotic actions, and regulation of the HPA axis and synaptic function. Despite promising findings, further clinical trials are needed to confirm luteolin's efficacy and direct molecular targets [139].

Mucuna pruriens is a tropical legume and candidate for treating depressive disorders. Preclinical studies provide evidence for the antidepressant effect of the *Mucuna pruriens* plant. This includes the mechanisms of action underlying its antidepressant activity, including effects on neurotransmitter systems (i.e., dopamine, serotonin, norepinephrine), reactive oxygen species, nitric oxide, cortisol, and inflammation. Clinical trials are needed to study the efficacy and safety of *Mucuna pruriens* for depression, reviewed in [140].

Oleanolic acid (OA) and ursolic acid (UA) are isomeric triterpenoids naturally found in a variety of medicinal plants, herbs, fruits, and vegetables [141]. These bioactives have anti-inflammatory properties (e.g., [142]) and have been investigated for their antidepressant-like effects in a maternal separation (MS) mouse model of depression [143]. Female MS-treated mice showed greater depressive-like behavior than males. OA significantly improved these behaviors, while UA primarily alleviated anxiety-like symptoms. Both compounds reduced microglial activation, TNF-α expression, and IDO1 mRNA levels, markers of neuroinflammation and altered tryptophan metabolism. Additionally, OA and UA restored synaptophysin expression, but only OA reversed the reduction in PSD-95, a key protein involved in synaptic plasticity. These results suggest that OA is more effective than UA in reversing MS-induced, female-specific depressive behaviors by targeting neuroinflammation, metabolic disruption, and synaptic plasticity. This aligns with earlier findings on OA's multi-target effects in mood regulation [144].

Rosa roxburghii Tratt, a traditional medicinal plant, has known neuroprotective effects, and its main active compound, *Kaji-ichigoside F1 (KF1)*, was recently studied for its antidepressant potential. Using an LPS-induced depression model in mice and an LPS-stimulated BV2 microglial cell model, researchers found that KF1 significantly reduced depression-like behaviors, neuronal damage, and apoptosis. It also suppressed pro-inflammatory cytokines (e.g., TNF-α, IL-6) and decreased inflammatory markers such as caspase-1, NF-κB, IL-1β, and NLRP3. Conversely, it increased antioxidant markers (e.g., HO-1, superoxide dismutase 1, Nrf2) and neuroprotective signaling proteins. Mechanistically, KF1 alleviated inflammation and oxidative stress by inhibiting the NF-κB/NLRP3 pathway and activating the PPARγ/CX3CR1/Nrf2 pathway, both in vivo and in vitro. These findings suggest that KF1 may be a promising therapeutic agent for inflammation-related depression [145].

The active *polyphenols in rosemary* (*Rosmarinus officinalis L.*) contain several pharmacological activities, including anti-inflammatory, antibacterial, and neuroprotective characteristics. A recent article reviewed the available reports and evidence on the use of polyphenols in rosemary as potential candidates for the treatment of depression. Authors conclude that the antidepressive effects of rosemary polyphenols are due to anti-inflammatory properties and a bidirectional relationship with gut microbiota, including inhibiting inflammatory pathways and cytokines (reducing pro-inflammation cytokines, suppressing NF-κB and NLRP3 inflammasomes, and upregulating Nrf2/HO-1 pathway), altering intestinal microbiota structure and metabolites (polyphenols-related microbial metabolites and biotransformation of polyphenols by microbiota) [146].

Related to the use of plant-based products, implementing an *anti-inflammatory diet* may help manage depressive symptoms, particularly through cost-effective strategies like dietary education. A randomized controlled trial evaluated the impact of a 12-week anti-inflammatory dietary education program in female patients with depression undergoing chemotherapy for breast cancer. Compared to routine care, the intervention group showed significantly reduced depressive symptoms, lower energy-adjusted dietary inflammatory index scores, and improved quality of life. Additionally, TNF-α and CRP levels decreased significantly only in the intervention group. These findings suggest that anti-inflammatory dietary education can reduce inflammation and improve both mood and well-being in this population [147].

Summary

Chronic inflammation contributes to a range of medical and psychiatric disorders, including MDD. Inflammatory stimuli can alter neurotransmitter systems and neural circuits, leading to symptoms such as anhedonia, fatigue, and psychomotor slowing. These depressive symptoms are often associated with elevated inflammatory biomarkers, which may also predict antidepressant treatment response. Only a subset of individuals with MDD exhibit increased inflammatory markers, suggesting the existence of an "inflammatory subtype" of depression with distinct symptom profiles and treatment outcomes. Identifying and characterizing this subgroup could inform the development of targeted immunotherapies and support a precision medicine approach [148].

The interactions between the immune system and the CNS (Fig. 24.1) not only influence behavior but also affect therapeutic response. In this context, inflammatory biomarkers may be useful tools for personalizing treatment strategies and refining diagnostic categories. Clinical evidence indicates that anti-inflammatory treatments can reduce depressive symptoms in both medically ill and individuals with depression. Preclinical research supports the development of new anti-inflammatory targets and treatment options, including plant-derived natural compounds that target cascades of inflammation. However, further research is needed to determine which individuals are most likely to benefit and to optimize the type, timing, and duration of treatment. Research with attention to safety, particularly during prolonged periods of anti-inflammatory treatments or co-treatments, will be important.

Note: This chapter primarily focused on adult depression. The findings and implications discussed may not generalize to childhood, adolescent, or late-life depression, which may involve different pathophysiological mechanisms. For example, children have lower baseline cortisol secretion and divergent responses in the HPA axis—unlike adults, who more commonly show hypercortisolemia [149]. *Adolescents often experience more vegetative symptoms (like appetite and sleep disturbances), while adults tend to present more anhedonia and cognitive complaints* [150]. *Further, greater prevalence of chronic diseases* (e.g., *cardiovascular, endocrine disorders) complicates the pathophysiology and treatment response in older adults compared to younger adults. Because childhood, adolescent, and late-life depression each involve distinct neurodevelopmental, neuroendocrine, immunological, and psychosocial pathways, findings from adult-only studies cannot be assumed to hold true across the lifespan. Clinical and research insights focused on adults should be generalized with caution—age-specific mechanisms influence depressive presentation, etiology, and treatment outcomes.*

Acknowledgements and Funding This book chapter was supported, in part, by the Department of Veterans Affairs, Veterans Health Administration, Office of Research and Development, Clinical Sciences Research and Development Merit Review Award I01 CX002668 (JML). Some work was conducted using facilities at Veterans Affairs Portland Health Care System (Portland, Oregon, United States). JML is a Research Scientist at the Veterans Affairs Portland Health Care System. The contents do not represent the views of the U.S. Department of Veterans Affairs or the United States Government.

References

1. Capuron L, Gumnick JF, Musselman DL, Lawson DH, Reemsnyder A, Nemeroff CB, et al. Neurobehavioral effects of interferon-α in cancer patients: phenomenology and paroxetine responsiveness of symptom dimensions. Neuropsychopharmacology. 2002;26:643–52. https://doi.org/10.1016/S0893-133X(01)00407-9.
2. Huckans M, Fuller B, Wheaton V, Jaehnert S, Ellis C, Kolessar M, et al. A longitudinal study evaluating the effects of interferon-alpha therapy on cognitive and psychiatric function in adults with chronic hepatitis C. J Psychosom Res. 2015:78. https://doi.org/10.1016/j.jpsychores.2014.07.020.
3. Dieperink E, Willenbring M, Ho SB. Neuropsychiatric symptoms associated with hepatitis C and interferon alpha: a review. Am J Psychiatry. 2000; https://doi.org/10.1176/appi.ajp.157.6.867.
4. Lotrich FE, Rabinovitz M, Gironda P, Pollock BG. Depression following pegylated interferon-alpha: characteristics and vulnerability. J Psychosom Res. 2007;63:131–5. https://doi.org/10.1016/j.jpsychores.2007.05.013.
5. Hauser P, Khosla J, Aurora H, Laurin J, Kling MA, Hill J, et al. A prospective study of the incidence and open-label treatment of interferon-induced major depressive disorder in patients with hepatitis C. Mol Psychiatry. 2002;7:942–7. https://doi.org/10.1038/SJ.MP.4001119.
6. Loftis JM, Patterson AL, Wilhelm CJ, McNett H, Morasco BJ, Huckans M, Morgan T, Saperstein S, Asghar A, Hauser P. Vulnerability to somatic symptoms of depression during interferon-alpha therapy for hepatitis C: a 16-week prospective study. J Psychosom Res. 2013;74(1):57–63. https://doi.org/10.1016/j.jpsychores.2012.10.012. Epub 2012 Nov 21.
7. Loftis JM, Hauser P. The phenomenology and treatment of interferon-induced depression. J Affect Disord. 2004:82. https://doi.org/10.1016/j.jad.2004.04.002.
8. Daray FM, Grendas LN, Arena ÁR, Tifner V, Álvarez Casiani RI, Olaviaga A, et al. Decoding the inflammatory signature of the major depressive episode: insights from peripheral immunophenotyping in active and remitted condition, a case–control study. Transl Psychiatry. 2024:14. https://doi.org/10.1038/S41398-024-02902-2.
9. Köhler CA, Freitas TH, Stubbs B, Maes M, Solmi M, Veronese N, et al. Peripheral alterations in cytokine and chemokine levels after antidepressant drug treatment for major depressive disorder: systematic review and meta-analysis. Mol Neurobiol. 2018;55:4195–206. https://doi.org/10.1007/S12035-017-0632-1.
10. Izumi Y, Reiersen AM, Lenze EJ, Mennerick SJ, Zorumski CF. SSRIs differentially modulate the effects of pro-inflammatory stimulation on hippocampal plasticity and memory via sigma 1 receptors and neurosteroids. Transl. Psychiatry. 2023:13. https://doi.org/10.1038/S41398-023-02343-3.
11. Hole C, Dhamsania A, Brown C, Ryznar R. Immune dysregulation in depression and anxiety: a review of the immune response in disease and treatment. Cells. 2025:14. https://doi.org/10.3390/CELLS14080607.
12. Sălcudean A, Bodo CR, Popovici RA, Cozma MM, Păcurar M, Crăciun RE, et al. Neuroinflammation—a crucial factor in the pathophysiology of depression—a comprehensive review. Biomolecules. 2025:15. https://doi.org/10.3390/BIOM15040502.
13. Liu Q, Nie B, Cui X, Wang W, Duan D. Inflammatory factors: a key contributor to stress-induced major depressive disorder. Cells. 2025;14:629. https://doi.org/10.3390/CELLS14090629.
14. Zagaria A, Fiori V, Vacca M, Lombardo C, Pariante CM, Ballesio A. Inflammation as a mediator between adverse childhood experiences and adult depression: a meta-analytic structural equation model. J Affect Disord. 2024;357:85–96. https://doi.org/10.1016/j.jad.2024.04.072.
15. Slopen N, Kubzansky LD, McLaughlin KA, Koenen KC. Childhood adversity and inflammatory processes in youth: a prospective study. Psychoneuroendocrinology. 2013;38:188–200. https://doi.org/10.1016/j.psyneuen.2012.05.013.
16. Raposa EB, Bower JE, Hammen CL, Najman JM, Brennan PA. A developmental pathway from early life stress to inflammation: the role of negative health behaviors. Psychol Sci. 2014;25:1268. https://doi.org/10.1177/0956797614530570.
17. Danese A, Moffitt TE, Pariante CM, Ambler A, Poulton R, Caspi A. Elevated inflammation levels in depressed adults with a history of childhood maltreatment. Arch Gen Psychiatry. 2008;65:409–16. https://doi.org/10.1001/archpsyc.65.4.409.
18. Baumeister D, Akhtar R, Ciufolini S, Pariante CM, Mondelli V. Childhood trauma and adulthood inflammation: a meta-analysis of peripheral C-reactive protein, interleukin-6 and tumour necrosis factor-α. Mol Psychiatry. 2016;21:642–9. https://doi.org/10.1038/MP.2015.67.
19. Flouri E, Francesconi M, Midouhas E, Lewis G. Prenatal and childhood adverse life events, inflammation and depressive symptoms across adolescence. J Affect Disord. 2020;260:577–82. https://doi.org/10.1016/j.jad.2019.09.024.
20. Savitz J, Figueroa-Hall LK, Teague TK, Yeh H-W, Zheng H, Kuplicki R, et al. Systemic inflammation and Anhedonic responses to an inflammatory challenge in adults with major depressive disorder: a randomized controlled trial. Am J Psychiatry. 2025; https://doi.org/10.1176/APPI.AJP.20240142.
21. Cao P, Chen C, Liu A, Shan Q, Zhu X, Jia C, et al. Early-life inflammation promotes depressive symptoms in adolescence via microglial engulfment of dendritic spines. Neuron. 2021;109:2573–2589.e9. https://doi.org/10.1016/j.neuron.2021.06.012.
22. Sharma VK. Diabetes-induced depression: unravelling the role of gut dysbiosis. J Diabetes Metab Disord. 2025:24. https://doi.org/10.1007/S40200-025-01643-3.
23. Luo K, Zhang M, Tu Q, Li J, Wang Y, Wan S, et al. From gut inflammation to psychiatric comorbidity: mechanisms and therapies for anxiety and depression in inflammatory bowel disease. J Neuroinflammation. 2025:22. https://doi.org/10.1186/S12974-025-03476-6.
24. Qiu X, Xu T, Huang Y, Wei C, Wang L, Wu B. Relationship between depression and oral microbiome diversity: analysis of NHANES data (2009–2012). BMC Oral Health. 2025:25. https://doi.org/10.1186/S12903-025-06274-X.
25. Saggu S, Pless A, Dew E, Ware D, Jiao K, Wang Q. Monoamine signaling and neuroinflammation: mechanistic connections and implications for neuropsychiatric disorders. Front Immunol. 2025;16 https://doi.org/10.3389/FIMMU.2025.1543730.
26. Maes M, Leonard BE, Myint AM, Kubera M, Verkerk R. The new "5-HT" hypothesis of depression: cell-mediated immune activation induces indoleamine 2,3-dioxygenase, which leads to lower plasma tryptophan and an increased synthesis of detrimental tryptophan catabolites (TRYCATs), both of which contribute to t. Prog Neuro-Psychopharmacol Biol Psychiatry. 2011;35:702–21. https://doi.org/10.1016/j.pnpbp.2010.12.017.

27. O'Connor JC, André C, Wang Y, Lawson MA, Szegedi SS, Lestage J, et al. Interferon-γ and tumor necrosis factor-α mediate the upregulation of indoleamine 2,3-dioxygenase and the induction of depressive-like behavior in mice in response to bacillus calmette-guérin. J Neurosci. 2009;29:4200–9. https://doi.org/10.1523/JNEUROSCI.5032-08.2009.
28. Loftis JM. Indolamine 2,3-dioxygenase regulation and neuropsychiatric symptoms. Psychoneuroendocrinology. 2013:38. https://doi.org/10.1016/j.psyneuen.2013.05.020.
29. Felger JC. The role of dopamine in inflammation-associated depression: mechanisms and therapeutic implications. Curr Top Behav Neurosci. 2017;31:199–220. https://doi.org/10.1007/7854_2016_13/FIGURES/1.
30. Felger JC, Miller AH. Cytokine effects on the basal ganglia and dopamine function: the subcortical source of inflammatory malaise. Front Neuroendocrinol. 2012;33:315. https://doi.org/10.1016/J.YFRNE.2012.09.003.
31. Miller AH, Timmie WP. Mechanisms of cytokine-induced behavioral changes: psychoneuroimmunology at the translational interface Norman cousins lecture. Brain Behav Immun. 2008;23:149. https://doi.org/10.1016/J.BBI.2008.08.006.
32. Du Y, Gao Y, Du X, An T, Zhang H, Wang B, et al. Further elucidation of GMPPB as a risk gene for depression through integrative multi-omics analyses. J Affect Disord. 2025;384:23–46. https://doi.org/10.1016/j.jad.2025.05.013.
33. Mac Giollabhui N, Slaney C, Hemani G, Foley ÉM, van der Most PJ, Nolte IM, et al. Role of inflammation in depressive and anxiety disorders, affect, and cognition: genetic and non-genetic findings in the lifelines cohort study. Transl Psychiatry. 2025:15. https://doi.org/10.1038/S41398-025-03372-W.
34. Mansouri S, Pessoni AM, Marroquín-Rivera A, Parise EM, Tamminga CA, Turecki G, et al. Transcriptional dissection of symptomatic profiles across the brain of men and women with depression. Nat Commun. 2023:14. https://doi.org/10.1038/S41467-023-42686-5.
35. Fischer IC, Overstreet C, Cabrera-Mendoza B, Qiu D, Krystal JH, Polimanti R, et al. Optimism moderates the relationship between inflammatory polygenic risk and major depressive disorder in U.S. Military veterans. World J Biol Psychiatry 2025:1–10. https://doi.org/10.1080/15622975.2025.2498352.
36. Bekhbat M, Treadway MT, Goldsmith DR, Woolwine BJ, Haroon E, Miller AH, et al. Gene signatures in peripheral blood immune cells related to insulin resistance and low tyrosine metabolism define a sub-type of depression with high CRP and anhedonia. Brain Behav Immun. 2020;88:161–5. https://doi.org/10.1016/j.bbi.2020.03.015.
37. Gritti D, Delvecchio G, Ferro A, Bressi C, Brambilla P. Neuroinflammation in major depressive disorder: a review of PET imaging studies examining the 18-kDa translocator protein. J Affect Disord. 2021;292:642–51. https://doi.org/10.1016/j.jad.2021.06.001.
38. Zheng H, Ford BN, Bergamino M, Kuplicki R, Aupperle R, Bodurka J, et al. A hidden menace? Cytomegalovirus infection is associated with reduced cortical gray matter volume in major depressive disorder. Mol Psychiatry. 2021;26:4234–44. https://doi.org/10.1038/S41380-020-00932-Y.
39. Colombo F, Calesella F, Bravi B, Fortaner-Uyà L, Monopoli C, Tassi E, et al. Multimodal brain-derived subtypes of major depressive disorder differentiate patients for anergic symptoms, immune-inflammatory markers, history of childhood trauma and treatment-resistance. Eur Neuropsychopharmacol. 2024;85:45–57. https://doi.org/10.1016/j.euroneuro.2024.05.015.
40. Han KM, Ham BJ. How inflammation affects the brain in depression: a review of functional and structural MRI studies. J Clin Neurol. 2021;17:503. https://doi.org/10.3988/JCN.2021.17.4.503.
41. Gholipour D, Shahraki M, Shakiba M, Shamsi-Goushki A. Supplementation of Omega-3 increases serum levels of brain-derived neurotrophic factor and decreases depression status in patients with bipolar disorder: a randomized, double-blind, placebo-controlled clinical trial. J Hum Nutr Diet. 2025:38. https://doi.org/10.1111/JHN.70076.
42. Bansal Y, Singh R, Parhar I, Kuhad A, Soga T. Quinolinic acid and nuclear factor erythroid 2-related factor 2 in depression: role in neuroprogression. Front Pharmacol. 2019:10. https://doi.org/10.3389/FPHAR.2019.00452.
43. Gao L, Liu R, Qu H, Qu H, Bai Q, Chen Y. Based on the IL-33/ST2-MyD88 signaling pathway to explore the mechanism of aerobic exercise in antagonizing the inflammatory response in depressive mice. Cytokine. 2025:191. https://doi.org/10.1016/j.cyto.2025.156956.
44. Paganin W, Signorini S. Inflammatory biomarkers in depression: scoping review. BJPsych Open. 2024;10:e165. https://doi.org/10.1192/BJO.2024.787.
45. Valkanova V, Ebmeier KP, Allan CL. CRP, IL-6 and depression: a systematic review and meta-analysis of longitudinal studies. J Affect Disord. 2013; https://doi.org/10.1016/j.jad.2013.06.004.
46. Chamberlain SR, Cavanagh J, De Boer P, Mondelli V, Jones DNC, Drevets WC, et al. Treatment-resistant depression and peripheral C-reactive protein. Br J Psychiatry. 2019;214:11. https://doi.org/10.1192/BJP.2018.66.
47. Křenek P, Hořínková J, Bartečků E. Peripheral inflammatory markers in subtypes and Core features of depression: a systematized review. Psychopathology. 2023;56:403–16. https://doi.org/10.1159/000528907.
48. Fellows E, Jones BDM, Hodsoll J, Husain N, Khoso AB, Young AH, et al. Associations between C-reactive protein and individual symptoms of depression in a lower-middle income country. BJPsych Open. 2024:10. https://doi.org/10.1192/BJO.2024.735.
49. Jha MK, Trivedi MH. Personalized antidepressant selection and pathway to novel treatments: clinical utility of targeting inflammation. Int J Mol Sci. 2018:19. https://doi.org/10.3390/IJMS19010233.
50. Mazza MG, Lucchi S, Tringali AGM, Rossetti A, Botti ER, Clerici M. Neutrophil/lymphocyte ratio and platelet/lymphocyte ratio in mood disorders: a meta-analysis. Prog Neuropsychopharmacol Biol Psychiatry. 2018;84:229–36. https://doi.org/10.1016/j.pnpbp.2018.03.012.
51. Cheng Y, Wang Y, Wang X, Jiang Z, Zhu L, Fang S. Neutrophil-to-lymphocyte ratio, platelet-to-lymphocyte ratio, and monocyte-to-lymphocyte ratio in depression: an updated systematic review and meta-analysis. Front Psychiatry. 2022:13. https://doi.org/10.3389/FPSYT.2022.893097/PDF.
52. Su M, Ouyang X, Song Y. Neutrophil to lymphocyte ratio, platelet to lymphocyte ratio, and monocyte to lymphocyte ratio in depression: a meta-analysis. J Affect Disord. 2022;308:375–83. https://doi.org/10.1016/j.jad.2022.04.038.
53. Puangsri P, Ninla-aesong P. Potential usefulness of complete blood count parameters and inflammatory ratios as simple biomarkers of depression and suicide risk in drug-naive, adolescents with major depressive disorder: simple peripheral markers for inflammation in drug-naive, adolescents with major depressive disorder. Psychiatry Res. 2021:305. https://doi.org/10.1016/j.psychres.2021.114216.
54. Qiu W, Cai X, Zheng C, Qiu S, Ke H, Huang Y. Update on the relationship between depression and neuroendocrine metabolism. Front Neurosci. 2021:15. https://doi.org/10.3389/FNINS.2021.728810.
55. Ng A, Tam WW, Zhang MW, Ho CS, Husain SF, McIntyre RS, et al. IL-1β, IL-6, TNF- α and CRP in elderly patients with depression or Alzheimer's disease: systematic review and meta-analysis. Sci Rep. 2018; https://doi.org/10.1038/s41598-018-30487-6.
56. Więdłocha M, Marcinowicz P, Krupa R, Janoska-Jaździk M, Janus M, Dębowska W, et al. Effect of antidepressant treatment on peripheral inflammation markers—a meta-analysis. Prog

Neuropsychopharmacol Biol Psychiatry. 2018;80:217–26. https://doi.org/10.1016/j.pnpbp.2017.04.026.
57. Teoh NSN, Gyanwali B, Lai MKP, Chai YL, Chong JR, Chong EJY, et al. Association of Interleukin-6 and Interleukin-8 with cognitive decline in an Asian memory clinic population. J Alzheimer's Dis. 2023;92:445–55. https://doi.org/10.3233/JAD-220971.
58. Chalmers RA, Cervin M, Choo C, Baune BT, Trollor JN, Numbers K, et al. Networks of inflammation, depression, and cognition in aging males and females. Aging Clin Exp Res. 2022;34:2387–98. https://doi.org/10.1007/S40520-022-02198-6/FIGURES/1.
59. Zhu ZH, Song XY, Man LJ, Chen P, Tang Z, Li RH, et al. Comparisons of serum Interleukin-8 levels in major depressive patients with drug-free versus SSRIs versus healthy controls. Front Psych. 2022;13:858675. https://doi.org/10.3389/FPSYT.2022.858675/FULL.
60. Kruse JL, Olmstead R, Hellemann G, Breen EC, Tye SJ, Brooks JO, et al. Interleukin-8 and lower severity of depression in females, but not males, with treatment-resistant depression. J Psychiatr Res. 2021;140:350. https://doi.org/10.1016/J.JPSYCHIRES.2021.06.009.
61. Islam S, Islam T, Nahar Z, Shahriar M, Islam SMA, Bhuiyan MA, et al. Altered serum adiponectin and interleukin-8 levels are associated in the pathophysiology of major depressive disorder: a case-control study. PLoS One. 2022;17:e0276619. https://doi.org/10.1371/JOURNAL.PONE.0276619.
62. Wang X-M, Zhang Y-G, Li A-L, Long Z-H, Wang D, Li X-X, et al. Relationship between levels of inflammatory cytokines in the peripheral blood and the severity of depression and anxiety in patients with Parkinson's disease. Eur Rev Med Pharmacol Sci. 2016;20:3853–6.
63. Nobis A, Zalewski D, Waszkiewicz N. Peripheral markers of depression. J Clin Med. 2020;9:3793. https://doi.org/10.3390/JCM9123793.
64. Euteneuer F, Schwarz MJ, Dannehl K, Hartung A, Westermann S, Rief W. Increased soluble interleukin-2 receptor levels are related to somatic but not to cognitive-affective features in major depression. Brain Behav Immun. 2012;26:1244–8. https://doi.org/10.1016/J.BBI.2012.06.007.
65. Mancuso E, Sampogna G, Boiano A, Della Rocca B, Di Vincenzo M, Lapadula MV, et al. Biological correlates of treatment resistant depression: a review of peripheral biomarkers. Front Psychiatry. 2023:14. https://doi.org/10.3389/FPSYT.2023.1291176.
66. Zeng Y, Chourpiliadis C, Hammar N, Seitz C, Valdimarsdóttir UA, Fang F, et al. Inflammatory biomarkers and risk of psychiatric disorders. JAMA Psychiatry. 2024;81:1118–29. https://doi.org/10.1001/JAMAPSYCHIATRY.2024.2185.
67. Dantzer R. Role of the kynurenine metabolism pathway in inflammation-induced depression: preclinical approaches. Curr Top Behav Neurosci. 2017:31. https://doi.org/10.1007/7854_2016_6.
68. Savitz J. Role of kynurenine metabolism pathway activation in major depressive disorders. Curr Top Behav Neurosci. 2017;31:249–68. https://doi.org/10.1007/7854_2016_12.
69. Strasser B, Sperner-Unterweger B, Fuchs D, Gostner JM. Mechanisms of inflammation-associated depression: immune influences on tryptophan and phenylalanine metabolisms. Curr Top Behav Neurosci. 2017:31. https://doi.org/10.1007/7854_2016_23.
70. Turner EH, Loftis JM, Blackwell AD. Serotonin a la carte: supplementation with the serotonin precursor 5-hydroxytryptophan. Pharmacol Ther. 2006:109. https://doi.org/10.1016/j.pharmthera.2005.06.004.
71. Bekhbat M, Ulukaya GB, Bhasin MK, Felger JC, Miller AH. Cellular and immunometabolic mechanisms of inflammation in depression: preliminary findings from single cell RNA sequencing and a tribute to Bruce McEwen. Neurobiol Stress. 2022:19. https://doi.org/10.1016/j.ynstr.2022.100462.
72. Liu L, Wang J, Hu S, Shao J, Ding F, Yu W. Association of uric acid/high-density lipoprotein cholesterol ratio (UHR) with depression risk in US adults: a cross-sectional study. J Affect Disord. 2025;383:53–8. https://doi.org/10.1016/j.jad.2025.04.151.
73. Guo QW, Si YJ, Shen YL, Chen X, Yang M, Fang DZ, et al. Depression augments plasma APOA4 without changes of plasma lipids and glucose in female adolescents carrying G allele of APOA4 rs5104. J Mol Neurosci. 2021;71:2060–70. https://doi.org/10.1007/S12031-020-01766-7.
74. Zhan Y, Yang YT, You HM, Cao D, Liu CY, Zhou CJ, et al. Plasma-based proteomics reveals lipid metabolic and immunoregulatory dysregulation in post-stroke depression. Eur Psychiatry. 2014;29:307–15. https://doi.org/10.1016/J.EURPSY.2014.03.004.
75. Mathew B, Srinivasan K, Pradeep J, Thomas T, Mandal AK. Plasma Apolipoprotein-AIV downregulated in patients with major depressive disorder having suicidal ideation compared to those without suicidal ideation. Curr Proteomics. 2022;19:226–31. https://doi.org/10.2174/1570164618666211104151005.
76. Bielawski A, Zelek-Molik A, Rafa-Zabłocka K, Kowalska M, Gruca P, Papp M, et al. Elevated expression of HSP72 in the prefrontal cortex and hippocampus of rats subjected to chronic mild stress and treated with imipramine. Int J Mol Sci. 2024:25. https://doi.org/10.3390/IJMS25010243.
77. Valiati FE, Feiten JG, Géa LP, Silveira Júnior É de M, Scotton E, Caldieraro MA, et al. Inflammation and damage-associated molecular patterns in major psychiatric disorders. Trends Psychiatry Psychother. 2023;45:e20220576. https://doi.org/10.47626/2237-6089-2022-0576.
78. Bai Y, Liu W, Zhang F, Zheng Y, Guo Q, Hu H, et al. Dysregulation of peripheral oxidative stress and the Nrf2 antioxidant system in major depressive disorder. J Affect Disord. 2025;382:336–45. https://doi.org/10.1016/j.jad.2025.04.066.
79. Waszkiewicz N. The Immunoseasonal theory of psychiatric disorders. J Clin Med. 2023:12. https://doi.org/10.3390/JCM12144615.
80. Modzelewski S, Naumowicz M, Suprunowicz M, Oracz AJ, Waszkiewicz N. The impact of seasonality on mental health disorders: a narrative review and extension of the Immunoseasonal theory. J Clin Med. 2025:14. https://doi.org/10.3390/JCM14041119.
81. Rimti FH, Shahbaz R, Bhatt K, Xiang A. A review of new insights into existing major depressive disorder biomarkers. Heliyon. 2023:9. https://doi.org/10.1016/j.heliyon.2023.e18909.
82. Fu Y, Xia P, Chen C, Wang C, Zhang C, Zhang G, et al. Miniaturized 3D-printed ratiometric electrochemical immunosensing platform for ultrasensitive detection of depression biomarker Apo-A4. Talanta. 2025:284. https://doi.org/10.1016/J.TALANTA.2024.127235.
83. Sun B, Cai J, Li W, Gou X, Gou Y, Li D, et al. A novel electrochemical immunosensor based on PG for early screening of depression markers-heat shock protein 70. Biosens Bioelectron. 2018;111:34–40. https://doi.org/10.1016/j.bios.2018.03.049.
84. Wei H, Sun B, Li YY, Wang Y, Chen Y, Guo M, et al. Electrochemical immunosensor AuNPs/NG-PANI/ITO-PET for the determination of BDNF in depressed mice serum. Microchim Acta 2023;190. https://doi.org/10.1007/S00604-023-05878-W,.
85. Guedes PHG, Brussasco JG, Moço ACR, Moraes DD, Segatto M, Flauzino JMR, et al. A highly reusable genosensor for late-life depression diagnosis based on microRNA 184 attomolar detection in human plasma. Talanta. 2023:258. https://doi.org/10.1016/j.talanta.2023.124342.
86. Asadi A, Ferdosi F, Anoosheh S, Kaveh M, Dadgostar E, Ehtiati S, et al. Electrochemical biosensors for depression: diagnosis and therapeutic monitoring. Clin Chim Acta. 2025:567. https://doi.org/10.1016/j.cca.2024.120091.
87. McIntyre RS, Alsuwaidan M, Baune BT, Berk M, Demyttenaere K, Goldberg JF, et al. Treatment-resistant depression: definition, prevalence, detection, management, and investigational interventions. World Psychiatry. 2023;22:394. https://doi.org/10.1002/WPS.21120.

88. Schmidt FM, Kirkby KC, Lichtblau N. Inflammation and immune regulation as potential drug targets in antidepressant treatment. Curr Neuropharmacol. 2016;14:674–87. https://doi.org/10.2174/1570159X14666160115130414.
89. Kouba BR, de Araujo Borba L, Borges de Souza P, Gil-Mohapel J, Rodrigues ALS. Role of inflammatory mechanisms in major depressive disorder: from etiology to potential pharmacological targets. Cells. 2024:13. https://doi.org/10.3390/cells13050423.
90. Duda P, Hajka D, Wójcicka O, Rakus D, Gizak A. GSK3β: a master player in depressive disorder pathogenesis and treatment responsiveness. Cells. 2020;9:727. https://doi.org/10.3390/CELLS9030727.
91. Su W-J, Hu T, Jiang C-L. Cool the inflamed brain: a novel anti-inflammatory strategy for the treatment of major depressive disorder. Curr Neuropharmacol. 2023;22:810–42. https://doi.org/10.2174/1570159X21666230809112028.
92. Hird EJ, Slanina-Davies A, Lewis G, Hamer M, Roiser JP. From movement to motivation: a proposed framework to understand the antidepressant effect of exercise. Transl. Psychiatry. 2024:14. https://doi.org/10.1038/S41398-024-02922-Y.
93. Zhang Z-X, Guo Q, Chen X-Y. Research progress in the anti-inflammatory effect of exercise in ameliorating Neuroinflammation-related depression. Zhongguo Yi Xue Ke Xue Yuan Xue Bao. 2025:47. https://doi.org/10.3881/J.ISSN.1000-503X.15991.
94. Ekong MB, Iniodu CF. Nutritional therapy can reduce the burden of depression management in low income countries: a review. IBRO Neurosci Rep. 2021;11:15–28. https://doi.org/10.1016/J.IBNEUR.2021.06.002.
95. Falhani N, Brunner L-M, Melchner D, Schwarzbach JV, Rupprecht R, Nothdurfter C. Electroconvulsive therapy changes peripheral blood neurotrophic and inflammatory markers in depressed patients. J ECT. 2025; https://doi.org/10.1097/YCT.0000000000001139.
96. Pope BS, Wood SK. Advances in understanding mechanisms and therapeutic targets to treat comorbid depression and cardiovascular disease. Neurosci Biobehav Rev. 2020;116:337–49. https://doi.org/10.1016/j.neubiorev.2020.06.031.
97. Adzic M, Brkic Z, Mitic M, Francija E, Jovicic MJ, Radulovic J, et al. Therapeutic strategies for treatment of inflammation-related depression. Curr Neuropharmacol. 2017;16 https://doi.org/10.2174/1570159X15666170828163048.
98. Innes S, Pariante CM, Borsini A. Microglial-driven changes in synaptic plasticity: a possible role in major depressive disorder. Psychoneuroendocrinology. 2019;102:236–47. https://doi.org/10.1016/j.psyneuen.2018.12.233.
99. Kuhn M, Höger N, Feige B, Blechert J, Normann C, Nissen C. Fear extinction as a model for synaptic plasticity in major depressive disorder. PLoS One. 2014:9. https://doi.org/10.1371/JOURNAL.PONE.0115280.
100. Crider A, Feng T, Pandya CD, Davis T, Nair A, Ahmed AO, et al. Complement component 3a receptor deficiency attenuates chronic stress-induced monocyte infiltration and depressive-like behavior. Brain Behav Immun. 2018;70:246–56. https://doi.org/10.1016/j.bbi.2018.03.004.
101. Quintanilla B, Greenstein D, Tripathi A, Bartosh A, Yuan P, Zarate CA, et al. Assessment of complement cascade components in patients with major depressive disorder. Brain Behav Immun. 2025;127:229–37. https://doi.org/10.1016/j.bbi.2025.03.009.
102. da Silva DMA, Sales ISL, Oliveira JVS, dos Santos Júnior MA, Rebouças M de O, Valentim JT, et al. Cyclooxygenase-2 inhibitors alleviated depressive and anxious-like behaviors in mice exposed to lipopolysaccharide: involvement of oxidative stress and neuroinflammation. Pharmacol Biochem Behav. 2024:240. https://doi.org/10.1016/j.pbb.2024.173778.
103. Mahboubi-Rabbani M, Abbasi M, Zarghi A. Natural-derived COX-2 inhibitors as anticancer drugs: a review of their structural diversity and mechanism of action. Anti Cancer Agents Med Chem. 2022;23:15–36. https://doi.org/10.2174/1389450123666220516153915.
104. Attwells S, Setiawan E, Rusjan PM, Xu C, Hutton C, Rafiei D, et al. Translocator protein distribution volume predicts reduction of symptoms during open-label trial of celecoxib in major depressive disorder. Biol Psychiatry. 2020;88:649–56. https://doi.org/10.1016/j.biopsych.2020.03.007.
105. Sharma V, Sharma P, Singh TG. Therapeutic potential of COX-2 inhibitors in neuropsychiatric disorders. J Neural Transm. 2025; https://doi.org/10.1007/S00702-025-02932-0.
106. Pei Y, Liu H, Lang J, Chen Y, Zhang F, Hao R, et al. rTMS ameliorates CUMS-induced anxiety-depression-like behaviour and cognitive dysfunction in rats by modulating the COX-2/PGE2 signalling pathway. J Psychiatr Res. 2025;186:116–28. https://doi.org/10.1016/j.jpsychires.2025.04.008.
107. Sharma P, Daksh R, Khanna S, Mudgal J, Lewis SA, Arora D, et al. Microglial cannabinoid receptor 2 and epigenetic regulation: implications for the treatment of depression. Eur J Pharmacol. 2025:995. https://doi.org/10.1016/j.ejphar.2025.177422.
108. Gan WB, Kasthuri N, Yang G. Spine plasticity. Encycl Neurosci. 2009:321–7. https://doi.org/10.1016/B978-008045046-9.00362-4.
109. Geng Z, Peng F, Cheng Z, Su J, Song J, Han X, et al. Astrocytic FABP7 alleviates depression-like behaviors of chronic unpredictable mild stress mice by regulating neuroinflammation and hippocampal Spinogenesis. FASEB J. 2025:39. https://doi.org/10.1096/FJ.202403417RR.
110. Sleigh J, Harvey M, Voss L, Denny B. Ketamine—more mechanisms of action than just NMDA blockade. Trends Anaesth Crit Care. 2014;4:76–81. https://doi.org/10.1016/J.TACC.2014.03.002.
111. Lin Z, Xu X, Zhang K, Wang T, Cao L, Wang Z, et al. Correlations between major depressive disorder, splenic morphology, and immune function. BMC Psychiatry. 2025;25:477. https://doi.org/10.1186/S12888-025-06853-W.
112. Jóźwiak-BeRbenista M, Sokołowska P, Wiktorowska-Owczarek A, Kowalczyk E, Sienkiewicz M. Ketamine—a new antidepressant drug with anti-inflammatory properties. J Pharmacol Exp Ther. 2024;388:134–44. https://doi.org/10.1124/JPET.123.001823.
113. Szałach ŁP, Lisowska KA, Słupski J, Włodarczyk A, Górska N, Szarmach J, et al. The immunomodulatory effect of ketamine in depression. Psychiatr Danub. 2019;31:252–7.
114. He P-Y, Wu M-Y, Zheng L-Y, Duan Y, Fan Q, Zhu X-M, Yao Y-M. Interleukin-33/serum stimulation-2 pathway: regulatory mechanisms and emerging implications in immune and inflammatory diseases. Cytokine Growth Factor Rev. 2024;76:112–26. https://doi.org/10.1016/J.CYTOGFR.2023.12.001.
115. Yirmiya R, Rimmerman N, Reshef R. Depression as a microglial disease. Trends Neurosci. 2015;38:637–58. https://doi.org/10.1016/j.tins.2015.08.001.
116. Di Paolo G, Lewcock JW. Stressed microglia turn to the dark side in Alzheimer's disease. Neuron. 2025;113:501–3. https://doi.org/10.1016/J.NEURON.2025.01.010.
117. Jia X, Gao Z, Hu H. Microglia in depression: current perspectives. Sci China Life Sci. 2021;64:911–25. https://doi.org/10.1007/S11427-020-1815-6.
118. Wang H, He Y, Sun Z, Ren S, Liu M, Wang G, et al. Microglia in depression: an overview of microglia in the pathogenesis and treatment of depression. J Neuroinflammation. 2022;19:132. https://doi.org/10.1186/S12974-022-02492-0.
119. Mariani N, Everson J, Pariante CM, Borsini A. Modulation of microglial activation by antidepressants. J Psychopharmacol. 2022;36:131–50. https://doi.org/10.1177/02698811211069110.
120. Chen W, Zhao H, Li Y. Mitochondrial dynamics in health and disease: mechanisms and potential targets. Signal

Transduct Target Ther. 2023:8. https://doi.org/10.1038/S41392-023-01547-9.

121. Redei EE, Andrus BM, Kwasny MJ, Seok J, Cai X, Ho J, et al. Blood transcriptomic biomarkers in adult primary care patients with major depressive disorder undergoing cognitive behavioral therapy. Transl Psychiatry. 2014:4. https://doi.org/10.1038/TP.2014.66.
122. Hung YY, Huang KW, Kang HY, Huang GYL, Huang TL. Antidepressants normalize elevated Toll-like receptor profile in major depressive disorder. Psychopharmacology. 2015;233:1707. https://doi.org/10.1007/S00213-015-4087-7.
123. Shirayama Y, Iwata M, Fujita Y, Oda Y, Hashimoto K. The Toll-like receptor 4 antagonist TAK-242 induces antidepressant-like effects in a rat learned helplessness model of depression through BDNF-TrkB signaling and AMPA receptor activation. Behav Brain Res. 2022;423:113769. https://doi.org/10.1016/J.BBR.2022.113769.
124. Figueroa-Hall LK, Paulus MP, Savitz J. Toll-like receptor signaling in depression. Psychoneuroendocrinology. 2020;121:104843. https://doi.org/10.1016/J.PSYNEUEN.2020.104843.
125. Trkulja V, Barić H. Current research on Complementary and Alternative Medicine (CAM) in the treatment of major depressive disorder: an evidence-based review. Adv Exp Med Biol. 2021;1305:375–427. https://doi.org/10.1007/978-981-33-6044-0_20.
126. Yeung KS, Hernandez M, Mao JJ, Haviland I, Gubili J. Herbal medicine for depression and anxiety: a systematic review with assessment of potential psycho-oncologic relevance. Phyther Res. 2018;32:865–91. https://doi.org/10.1002/PTR.6033.
127. Figueiredo Godoy AC, Frota FF, Araújo LP, Valenti VE, Pereira E de SBM, Detregiachi CRP, et al. Neuroinflammation and natural antidepressants: balancing fire with Flora. Biomedicine. 2025:13. https://doi.org/10.3390/BIOMEDICINES13051129.
128. Zhang S, Chen X, Wang C, Sun Y, Gong B, Li D, et al. Antidepressant activity of agarwood essential oil: a mechanistic study on inflammatory and neuroprotective signaling pathways. Pharmaceuticals. 2025;18:255. https://doi.org/10.3390/PH18020255.
129. Xu M, Li W, Hu X, Zhang J. Arecoline alleviates depression via gut-brain Axis modulation, neurotransmitter balance, neuroplasticity enhancement, and inflammation reduction in CUMS mice. J Agric Food Chem. 2025;73:10201–13. https://doi.org/10.1021/ACS.JAFC.4C11643.
130. Cao MM, Guo Z, Wang J, Ma HY, Qin XY, Hu Y, et al. Astragalin alleviates lipopolysaccharide-induced depressive-like behavior in mice by preserving blood-brain barrier integrity and suppressing neuroinflammation. Free Radic Biol Med. 2025;232:340–52. https://doi.org/10.1016/j.freeradbiomed.2025.03.014.
131. Wu W, Wang J, Chen J, Xie J, Xu K, Ren Y, et al. Caffeine plays a prevention role in stress-induced depression by modulating gut-brain axis function. Eur J Pharmacol. 2025;1000:177721. https://doi.org/10.1016/J.EJPHAR.2025.177721.
132. Bao J, Li P, Guo Y, Zheng Y, Smolinski M, He J. Caffeine is negatively associated with depression in patients aged 20 and older. Front Psychiatry. 2022:13. https://doi.org/10.3389/FPSYT.2022.1037579.
133. McIntosh HA, Borgas AJ, Aouira N, Mitchell BL, Crouse JJ, Medland SE, et al. Caffeine consumption, psychological distress, and insomnia in a cohort of individuals with depression. Complex Psychiatry. 2025;11:37–49. https://doi.org/10.1159/000545393.
134. Zhang Y, Li L, Zhang J. Curcumin in antidepressant treatments: An overview of potential mechanisms, pre-clinical/clinical trials and ongoing challenges. Basic Clin Pharmacol Toxicol. 2020;127:243–53. https://doi.org/10.1111/BCPT.13455.
135. Chen T, Yin S, Yue R, Pi C, Zuo Y, Jiang Y, et al. Novel chlorine-containing curcumin analogue CAK06 promotes neuroprotection and rapid antidepressant through Nrf2-induced anti-inflammatory and antioxidant effects. Neurotherapeutics. 2025:e00600. https://doi.org/10.1016/J.NEUROT.2025.E00600.
136. Wang YL, Chen L, Zhong XL, Liu QS, Li WQ, Cheng Y, et al. Antidepressant effects of ershiwei roudoukou pills and its active ingredient Macelignan: multiple mechanisms involving oxidative stress, neuroinflammation and synaptic plasticity. Transl Psychiatry. 2025:15. https://doi.org/10.1038/S41398-025-03378-4.
137. Zhu W, Li B, Cui R. 5-O-Methylvisammioside alleviates depression-like behaviors by inhibiting nuclear factor kappa B pathway activation via targeting SRC. Neural Regen Res. 2025; https://doi.org/10.4103/NRR.NRR-D-24-00714.
138. Huang L, Wang S, Zhang Q, Zhang J, Sun J. Fucosterol ameliorates depressive-like behaviours by suppressing microglial activation and neuroinflammation via inhibition the MAPK/ERK1/2 signaling pathway. Int Immunopharmacol. 2025:158. https://doi.org/10.1016/j.intimp.2025.114821.
139. Zhou J, Wu Z, Zhao P. Luteolin and its antidepressant properties: from mechanism of action to potential therapeutic application. J Pharm Anal. 2024;15:101097. https://doi.org/10.1016/j.jpha.2024.101097.
140. Mata-Bermudez A, Diaz-Ruiz A, Silva-García LR, Gines-Francisco EM, Noriega-Navarro R, Rios C, et al. Mucuna pruriens, a possible treatment for depressive disorders. Neurol Int. 2024;16:1509–27. https://doi.org/10.3390/NEUROLINT16060112.
141. Waheed A, Akram S, Mushtaq M, Adnan A. Oleanolic acid and ursolic acid. Centum Valuab Plant Bioact. 2021:93–115. https://doi.org/10.1016/B978-0-12-822923-1.00021-2.
142. Lee W, Yang EJ, Ku SK, Song KS, Bae JS. Anti-inflammatory effects of oleanolic acid on LPS-induced inflammation in vitro and in vivo. Inflammation. 2013;36:94–102. https://doi.org/10.1007/S10753-012-9523-9.
143. Kong CH, Park K, Kim DY, Kim JY, Kang WC, Jeon M, et al. Effects of oleanolic acid and ursolic acid on depression-like behaviors induced by maternal separation in mice. Eur J Pharmacol. 2023;956:175954. https://doi.org/10.1016/J.EJPHAR.2023.175954.
144. Fajemiroye JO, Galdino PM, Florentino IF, Da Rocha FF, Ghedini PC, Polepally PR, et al. Plurality of anxiety and depression alteration mechanism by oleanolic acid. J Psychopharmacol. 2014;28:923–34. https://doi.org/10.1177/0269881114536789.
145. Huang M, Chen F, Zhou L, Zhang Q, Wang L, Li L, et al. The antidepressant effects of kaji-ichigoside F1 via activating PPAR-γ/CX3CR1/Nrf2 signaling and suppressing NF-κB/NLRP3 signaling pathways. Front Pharmacol. 2025;16:1569888. https://doi.org/10.3389/FPHAR.2025.1569888.
146. Zhang L, Lu J. Combating depression with rosemary (Rosmarinus officinalis L.)-derived polyphenols: major phytochemicals, functional properties, and potential. Fitoterapia. 2025:183. https://doi.org/10.1016/j.fitote.2025.106563.
147. Cheng L, Chen Y, He J, Cheng X, Wang Y, Lin X, et al. Effects of 12-week anti-inflammatory dietary education on depressive symptoms among depressed patients with breast cancer undergoing adjuvant chemotherapy: a randomized controlled trial. Forum Nutr. 2025:17. https://doi.org/10.3390/NU17060957.
148. Miller AH. Advancing an inflammatory subtype of major depression. Am J Psychiatry. 2025; https://doi.org/10.1176/APPI.AJP.20250289.
149. Kaufman J, Martin A, King RA, Charney D. Are child-, adolescent-, and adult-onset depression one and the same disorder? Biol Psychiatry. 2001;49:980–1001. https://doi.org/10.1016/S0006-3223(01)01127-1.
150. Rice F, Riglin L, Lomax T, Souter E, Potter R, Smith DJ, et al. Adolescent and adult differences in major depression symptom profiles. J Affect Disord. 2019;243:175–81. https://doi.org/10.1016/j.jad.2018.09.015.

The Neurophysiology of Depression, Interactions Between the Brainstem and Cerebral Cortex

25

J. Wesson Ashford

Introduction

Depression has long been thought of as being a disorder of the frontal lobes. This perspective makes sense in the classic understanding of brain function since the frontal lobes generate movement, speech, thought, and planning dorso-laterally and emotions ventro-medially [1, 2]. See Fig. 25.1. If depression is seen with this view, depressive thoughts, lack of motivation, self-deprecating ruminations, and even suicidal ideation can be understood as generated by the frontal lobes. Even electroshock therapy and now trans-cranial magnetic stimulation target the frontal lobes with beneficial effect [3]. Further, special imaging of the frontal lobes has been used to find the most efficacious location for prefrontal targeting of transcranial magnetic stimulation [4]. Additionally, functional magnetic resonance imaging (fMRI) has shown distinct neurophysiological varieties (biotypes) of depression and specific symptoms involving the frontal lobes and limbic system, which can be categorized into four specific types of depression, defined by distinct patterns of dysfunctional connectivity in the limbic and frontostriatal networks[1] [5], and there are specific changes in the fronto-striatal salience network[2] found in individuals with depression [7].

Consider commonly used depression scales such as the *Hamilton Depression Rating Scale (HDRS)*[3] [10] and the *Geriatric Depression Scale (GDS)*[4] [12, 13], which list the most commonly recognized symptoms of depression. The items on these scales can be reviewed for estimating the neurological sources of depression-related symptoms.

HDRS Items:

- 1. Depressed Mood—sadness, hopeless, helpless, worthless
- 2. Work and Activities—thoughts and feelings of incapacity, fatigue, or weakness related to activities; work or hobbies
- 3. Social Withdrawal—loss of interest in activities
- 4. Genital Symptoms—loss of libido, menstrual disturbances
- 5. Somatic Symptoms—loss of appetite, GI symptoms
- 6–7. Weight—loss, gain
- 8–10. Appetite—increased eating, carbohydrate craving
- 11–14. Sleep Management: insomnia—early, middle, late, hypersomnia
- 15–16. Somatic Symptoms—heaviness, aches, loss of energy, fatigability

[1] In an endeavor to define depression subtypes, four biotypes have been suggested [5]. These are based upon fMRI data that attempts to correlate how distinct clinical symptom profiles might predict treatment responses as they relate to clustered patterns of dysfunctional connectivity. One of the goals is to use neuroimaging biomarkers to diagnose these subtypes.

[2] The frontostriatal salience network is involved in reward processing and the conscious integration of internal goals and environmental demands with autonomic responses and feedback [6]. It appears that the frontostriatal salience network is expanded almost two fold in the cortex of most individuals with depression [7, 8].

[3] There are several versions of the HDRS (aka Ham-D) varying from 17 to 29 questions. One of the limitations of the HDRS was the lack of assessing atypical symptoms. This version outlined here includes more of the symptoms such as increased eating. The HAM-D is considered to be a valid and sensitive clinimetric index [9].

[4] The GDS-15 scale referenced here is most accurate in screening for depression in older adults with normal cognitive functions vs. cognitively impaired [11].

J. W. Ashford (✉)
VA Palo Alto Health Care System, War Related Illness and Injury Study Center (WRIISC), Palo Alto, CA, USA

Department of Psychiatry, Stanford University, Palo Alto, CA, USA
e-mail: ashford@stanford.edu

J. Raber et al. (eds.), *Understanding and Treating Depressive Disorders*, https://doi.org/10.1007/978-3-032-14465-2_25

- 17. Feelings of Guilt—self-reproach, ideas of guilt or rumination
- 18. Suicide—feeling life is not worth living, death wishes, suicide ideation, plans, attempts
- 19–21. Anxiety—subjective tension and irritability, worrying, somatization, hypochondriasis
- 20. Anxiety—somatic
- 22. Insight—may deny being ill
- 23. Retardation—motor, speech, thought
- 24. Agitation—fidgetiness, cannot sit still, hand wringing

GDS Items:

1. Not feeling satisfied with life
2. Dropped many activities, interests
3. Feeling life is empty
4. Getting bored
5. Poor spirits most of the time
6. Afraid that something bad is going to happen
7. Feeling unhappy most of the time
8. Feeling helpless
9. Preferring to stay home
10. Concern about memory problems ("brain fog")
11. Not wishing to be alive
12. Feel worthless
13. Lacking energy
14. Feeling hopeless
15. Feeling not well off

These symptom lists have been developed from extensive experiences with depressed patients and selecting the items most consistently present in patients with depression. While many of the symptoms of the HDRS can be linked to frontal lobe function, there are many symptoms, including appetite, weight control, sleep, retardation, and even anxiety that can be related to brainstem function. The GDS items are much more clearly related to expressed feelings, but symptoms less clearly related to the frontal lobes develop, particularly no longer feeling full of energy, and the brainstem is the brain structure which regulates the energy of the body. See Fig. 25.1.

The most commonly prescribed medications for depression—antidepressants—primarily act on the neurotransmitters serotonin, norepinephrine, or both. The earliest antidepressants were mono-amine-oxidase inhibitors (MAOIs), which prevented oxidation of serotonin and norepinephrine and increased their effects at brain synapses. Later tri-cyclic antidepressant medications inhibit the reup-

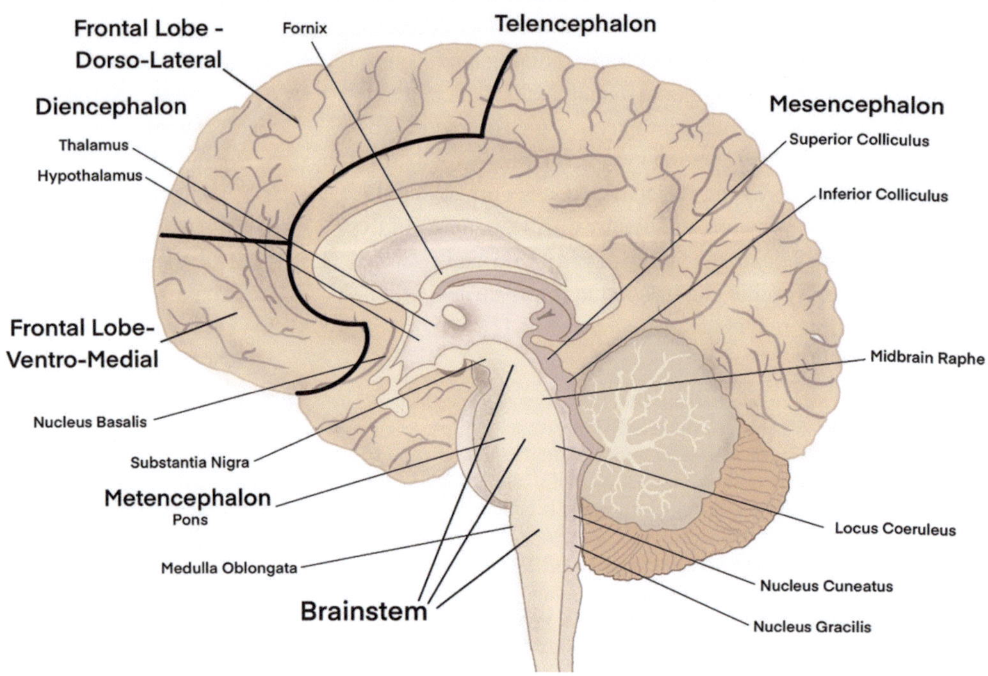

Fig. 25.1 Schematic representation of the human brain showing components of the brainstem and cerebral cortex

take of serotonin and norepinephrine to different degrees though with frequent side effects, mostly anti-cholinergic.[5] The more recent selective-reuptake inhibitors also increase the amount of serotonin (SSRIs) or norepinephrine (SNRIs) in synapses, though without the anti-cholinergic side effects. The relevant issue is that the cell bodies of the serotonin and norepinephrine systems are located in the brainstem—specifically, many serotonin neuronal cell bodies reside in the midbrain raphe nuclei, while norepinephrine neuronal cell bodies are situated in the midbrain locus coeruleus. See Fig. 25.1. Neurons from both of these groups have axons that project widely and diffusely throughout the cerebral neocortex, not just the frontal lobes [15, 16].

For understanding how the norepinephrine and serotonin neurons relate to depression, it is central to understand what their roles are in brain function. Serotonin neurons from the midbrain raphe nuclei are involved in the management of several vegetative functions, including energy management, appetite, temperature control,[6] and phases of sleep [18], as well as playing a role in mood regulation and sexual behavior. Of particular interest, the serotonin neurons have a major role in classical conditioning,[7] a fundamental learning mechanism in the brain and a major component of neuroplasticity [19]. A relevant sidenote is that serotonin neurons typically fire at a rate of approximately 1 to 5 times per second during wakefulness. While bursts of higher activity may occur in response to specific stimuli or environmental conditions, their firing rate decreases during slow-wave sleep and ceases altogether during REM sleep [20]. LSD toxicity causes a similar slowing and decreases of the firing of serotonin neurons [21], suggesting that serotonin neurons have a role in controlling thought processes and their encoding into memory.

Alternatively, norepinephrine neurons from the locus coeruleus have roles in regulating arousal, alertness, attention, cognitive function, and stress responses. In particular, the locus coeruleus has a role in generating anxiety. The locus coeruleus norepinephrine neurons also play a role in operant conditioning and reward-related learning [22], thus another important aspect of neuroplasticity.

A related consideration is the link between depression, apathy, and Alzheimer's disease (AD). Depression and apathy [23, 24] are both common in very early stages of AD. The earliest changes in AD are losses of brainstem norepinephrine neurons of the locus coeruleus [25–30] followed by the cortically projecting serotonin neurons of the midbrain raphe [31–34]. Both of these neurotransmitter systems project diffusely from the brainstem to the cerebral cortex, though therapies targeting these neurotransmitters have not been shown to have benefit in AD [35]. Since these are the same neuron groups related to depression, their demise may be the cause of depression frequently seen in early AD. There are still other considerations such as that losing one's memory and the onset of dementia are just depressing. However, given that AD is fundamentally an attack on neuroplasticity [36–38], this link supports the important consideration that impairment of neuroplasticity, learning, and memory are critical concerns for understanding, preventing, and treating depression.

Accordingly, both serotonin and norepinephrine significantly influence cerebral cortex activity, neuroplasticity, and the encoding of new information into memory. Given that these neurotransmitters—closely associated with depression—also play critical roles in neuroplasticity, psychotherapy may similarly support recovery by fostering the encoding of new insights and adaptive strategies for living. This neuroanatomical association thus provides a compelling basis for the therapeutic value of psychotherapy in treating depression.

Since it is then clear that two major brainstem nuclei are involved in depression, it is necessary to understand how these systems play a broader role in the brainstem, and how the brainstem functions with respect to overall brain activity [39]. The brainstem is the component of the brain which manages all vegetative functions, including the whole sleep–wake cycle, energy/fatigue, respirations, appetite, body temperature, and pain modulation, and through control of the autonomic nervous system, cardiovascular status and gastrointestinal and bowel activity. And all of these functions may be considered to be "energy management activities," and thus the brainstem controls the body and the rest of the brain to acquire and apportion energy resources. In this role, the brainstem can then be seen as managing the cerebral cortex, including overall activity (as it clearly does during sleep). Brainstem disruption is also seen in Gulf War Illness (GWI), particularly with regard to autonomic dysregulation, chronic pain intensity, and increased sleep difficulties [40], which are associated loss of brainstem volume and reduced integrity in brainstem-subcortical tracts [41].

[5] Anti-cholinergic symptoms that arise from blocking the acetylcholine neurotransmitter include peripheral and central effects [14]. Common central effects may include headaches, reduced cognitive functions, impaired memory, behavioral disturbances and anxiety. At higher doses confusion and agitation may occur. Peripheral symptoms may include such conditions as arrhythmias, flushing, constipation, urinary retention and dryness.

[6] Note about serotonin and temperature, unpublished observation made by J. Wesson Ashford in the laboratory of Michel Jouvet and Jacques Mouret (University of Lyon, France) in 1971: the drugs 6-chloro-tryptophan and 6-fluoro-tryptophan, short acting serotonin synthesis inhibitors (provided by Patrick McGeer, University of British Columbia), were injected intraperitoneally in rats [17]. Within 30 min their body temperature dropped by 2 degrees centigrade, then their temperature returned to normal within 4 h. When the injection was repeated 2–5 days later, the rats dropped their body temperature to ambient within an hour and did not recover, the rats dying 2–3 days later.

[7] Classical conditioning associates two stimuli to produce an automatic response. Operant conditioning associates a behavior with its consequence such as a reward or punishment to influence future behaviors.

The roof of the brainstem, the tectum (dorsal component), serves as a sentinel to detect relevant environmental events. The sensory sentinels of the tectum include the nuclei of Burdock and Gall (gracilis and cuneatus), which detect somatosensory stimuli; the auditory sentinel, the inferior colliculi; and the visual sentinel, the superior colliculi. See Fig. 25.1. The tectum is the initial manager of incoming information and is the first brain region to detect any tactile, auditory, or visual stimulus.

When a notable environmental stimulus is detected, the *reticular activating system (RAS)*[8] of the anterior brainstem is activated as well as the relevant thalamic relay nuclei, which in turn activate the cerebral cortex. When environmental stimuli are deemed novel or significant by the cerebrum (including regions such as the hippocampus and amygdala), the brainstem is engaged. It then sends projections back to the cerebrum, instructing relevant neurons to encode the new information via mechanisms such as the P300 evoked potential[9] [44–47]. In this way, the brainstem contributes to the regulation of awareness and consciousness. As noted above, many brainstem functions are mildly to severely disrupted in individuals with depression.

A related issue is post-traumatic stress disorder (PTSD), frequently accompanied by depression, which can be understood as a learned hyper-alert state, pointing to an important role of the tectum. When a notable environmental stimulus is detected, the RAS is activated as well as the relevant thalamic relay nuclei. However, the serotonin and norepinephrine systems are also activated. Importantly, certain antidepressant agents have been recommended for the treatment of PTSD—such as the SSRI sertraline and the atypical antidepressant trazodone—both of which modulate serotonin and norepinephrine systems [48, 49]. Also, the antihypertensive medication prazosin, which affects norepinephrine, has been recommended for the nightmares associated with PTSD [50, 51]. And PTSD can also be associated with neocortical damage related to the frontal lobes and connections back to the brainstem [52]. So, PTSD can also be understood as involving brainstem function or dysfunction.

Returning to the frontal lobe, it is important to consider the role of the *basal ganglia*, which generate movement in coordination with the motor cortex. The nucleus accumbens, at the rostral end of the basal ganglia, coordinates thought signals from the pre-frontal cortex. And the basal ganglia and nucleus accumbens are both managed by dopamine neuron projections from the brainstem, from the substantia nigra (see Fig. 25.1) and adjacent medial dopaminergic nuclei. Dopamine is involved both in the generating and pacing of movements and thoughts. Dopamine also has a role in reward-linked neuroplasticity and behavior, and unfortunately in addictive behavior as well [53]. These dopamine systems are involved in Parkinson's disease and schizophrenia. However, the dopaminergic medications used to treat these conditions, though speeding (e.g., stimulants, dopaminergic agonists, amphetamines) or slowing (e.g., neuroleptics) behavior and thought, are not particularly beneficial for treating mood disorders including depression.

Summary

Given the perspective of considering both frontal lobe and brainstem roles in depression, there needs to be more extensive understanding of the role of the brainstem, particularly the serotonin and norepinephrine projections to the cerebrum. Considering that both of these neurotransmitters are involved in neuroplasticity and depression, the issue to understand is that the brainstem is using these neurotransmitters to activate the frontal lobes to learn and retain information that is relevant for the energy management of the organism. If the brainstem is not set correctly, the thoughts encoded in the frontal lobes could be negative and lead to depression. Alternatively, an opposite brainstem activation of frontal lobe patterns could lead to manic behavior and explain manic-depressive illness. Of course, a tragic direction is perception that coping with the environment is hopeless, and suicidal ideation can lead to a self-perpetuating negative perception with a mortal consequence.

This perspective of brainstem function in affective disorder does lead to some very important considerations for prevention and management of depression. In addition to the interventions mentioned above, other preventive measures and interventions can be considered. Cultural exposure, music, art, exercise, sleep, and specific activities, including yoga and meditation [54], can help teach control of the brainstem and stabilization of mood, thus preventing depression. Psychotherapy and medications could be more effective if they are provided and prescribed with this focus on control of the brainstem. Further, appropriate encouragement to consider the positive aspects of life and caution to avoid thoughts of self-harm can help the frontal lobes to guide the direction from the brainstem to maintain a stable mood.

[8]The reticular activating system (RAS) is located in the most anterior segment of the brainstem [42]. The RAS coordinates sleep-wake cycles, attention, arousal, ability to focus and muscle tone. The RAS is composed of four main groups of nuclei. These are the locus coeruleus, raphe nuclei, posterior tuberomammillary hypothalamus, and pedunculopontine tegmentum. Each of these areas have characteristic neuropeptides that they release.

[9]The P300 wave is a positive deflection on an electroencephalogram that occurs about 300 msecs after a stimulus [43, 44]. The P300 is considered to be the results of cognitive processes including decision making and attention in response to unexpected or novel stimuli, but generated by cholinergic projections from the brainstem, Nucleus Basalis of Meynert (See Fig. 25.1) to the cerebral cortex.

References

1. Fuster JM. The prefrontal cortex, anatomy, physiology, and neuropsychology of the frontal lobe. 2nd ed. New York: Raven Press; 1989. The prefrontal cortex : anatomy, physiology, and neuropsychology of the frontal lobe: Fuster, Joaquin M: Free Download, Borrow, and Streaming: Internet Archive
2. Stuss DTBDF. The frontal lobes. New York: Raven Press; 1986. The frontal lobes: Stuss, Donald T: Free Download, Borrow, and Streaming: Internet Archive
3. Sunder K, Makale MT, Makale M, Bodhanapati J, Murphy KT, Dennen CA, Baron D, Thanos PK, Hanna C, Ashford JW, Lewandrowski KU, Blum K. Coupling Bio-Resonance Neurotechnology (BRNT) and dual hemispheric Repetitive Transcranial Magnetic Stimulation (rTMS) reduces comorbid Major Depressive Disorder (MDD) and Generalized Anxiety Disorder (GAD) as demonstrated by PHQ-9 and GAD-7: pilot case series. Psychol Res Behav Manag. 2025;18:225–40. https://doi.org/10.2147/PRBM.S482960. PMID: 39911857; PMCID: PMC11796452. Coupling Bio-Resonance Neurotechnology (BRNT) and Dual Hemispheric Repetitive Transcranial Magnetic Stimulation (rTMS) Reduces Comorbid Major Depressive Disorder (MDD) and Generalized Anxiety Disorder (GAD) as Demonstrated by PHQ-9 and GAD-7: Pilot Case Series – PubMed
4. Cardenas VA, Bhat JV, Horwege AM, Ehrlich TJ, Lavacot J, Mathalon DH, Glover GH, Roach BJ, Badran BW, Forman SD, George MS, Thase ME, Yesavage JA, Yurgelun-Todd D, Rosen AC. Anatomical and fMRI-network comparison of multiple DLPFC targeting strategies for repetitive transcranial magnetic stimulation treatment of depression. Brain Stimul. 2022;15(1):63–72. https://doi.org/10.1016/j.brs.2021.11.008. Epub 2021 Nov 10. PMID: 34767967; PMCID: PMC8900427. Anatomical and fMRI-network comparison of multiple DLPFC targeting strategies for repetitive transcranial magnetic stimulation treatment of depression – PubMed
5. Drysdale AT, Grosenick L, Downar J, Dunlop K, Mansouri F, Meng Y, Fetcho RN, Zebley B, Oathes DJ, Etkin A, Schatzberg AF, Sudheimer K, Keller J, Mayberg HS, Gunning FM, Alexopoulos GS, Fox MD, Pascual-Leone A, Voss HU, Casey BJ, Dubin MJ, Liston C. Resting-state connectivity biomarkers define neurophysiological subtypes of depression. Nat Med. 2017;23(1):28–38. https://doi.org/10.1038/nm.4246. Epub 2016 Dec 5. Erratum in: Nat Med. 2017 Feb 7;23(2):264. doi: 10.1038/nm0217-264d. PMID: 27918562; PMCID: PMC5624035. Resting-state connectivity biomarkers define neurophysiological subtypes of depression – PubMed
6. Seeley WW. The salience network: a neural system for perceiving and responding to homeostatic demands. J Neurosci. 2019;39(50):9878–82. https://doi.org/10.1523/JNEUROSCI.1138-17.2019. Epub 2019 Nov 1. PMID: 31676604; PMCID: PMC6978945. The Salience Network: A Neural System for Perceiving and Responding to Homeostatic Demands – PubMed
7. Lynch CJ, Elbau IG, Ng T, Ayaz A, Zhu S, Wolk D, Manfredi N, Johnson M, Chang M, Chou J, Summerville I, Ho C, Lueckel M, Bukhari H, Buchanan D, Victoria LW, Solomonov N, Goldwaser E, Moia S, Caballero-Gaudes C, Downar J, Vila-Rodriguez F, Daskalakis ZJ, Blumberger DM, Kay K, Aloysi A, Gordon EM, Bhati MT, Williams N, Power JD, Zebley B, Grosenick L, Gunning FM, Liston C. Frontostriatal salience network expansion in individuals in depression. Nature. 2024;633(8030):624–33. https://doi.org/10.1038/s41586-024-07805-2. Epub 2024 Sep 4. PMID: 39232159; PMCID: PMC11410656. Frontostriatal salience network expansion in individuals in depression – PubMed
8. Katharina Buehler S, Zhang R, Roiser J. A commentary on frontostriatal salience network expansion in individuals in depression. Psychoradiology. 2025;5:kkaf005. https://doi.org/10.1093/psyrad/kkaf005. PMID: 40160804; PMCID: PMC11949618. A commentary on frontostriatal salience network expansion in individuals in depression – PubMed
9. Carrozzino D, Patierno C, Fava GA, Guidi J. The Hamilton rating scales for depression: a critical review of clinimetric properties of different versions. Psychother Psychosom. 2020;89(3):133–50. https://doi.org/10.1159/000506879. Epub 2020 Apr 14. PMID: 32289809. The Hamilton Rating Scales for Depression: A Critical Review of Clinimetric Properties of Different Versions – PubMed
10. Hamilton M. A rating scale for depression. J Neurol Neurosurg Psychiatry. 1960;23(1):56–62. The dorsal raphe nucleus shows phospho-tau neurofibrillary changes before the transentorhinal region in Alzheimer's disease. A precocious onset? – PubMed
11. Park SH, Kwak MJ. Performance of the geriatric depression scale-15 with older adults aged over 65 years: an updated review 2000–2019. Clin Gerontol. 2021;44(2):83–96. https://doi.org/10.1080/07317115.2020.1839992. Epub 2020 Nov 7. PMID: 33164674. Performance of the Geriatric Depression Scale-15 with Older Adults Aged over 65 Years: An Updated Review 2000-2019 – PubMed
12. Yesavage JA, Brink TL, Rose TL, Lum O, Huang V, Adey M, Leirer VO. Development and validation of a geriatric depression screening scale: a preliminary report. J Psychiatr Res. 1982–1983;17(1):37–49. https://doi.org/10.1016/0022-3956(82)90033-4. PMID: 7183759. Development and validation of a geriatric depression screening scale: a preliminary report – PubMed.
13. Sheikh JI, Yesavage JA. Geriatric Depression Scale (GDS): recent evidence and development of a shorter version. Clin Gerontol J Aging Mental Health. 1986;5(1–2):165–73. https://doi.org/10.1300/J018v05n01_09. Geriatric Depression Scale (GDS): Recent evidence and development of a shorter version.
14. Ghossein N, Kang M, Lakhkar AD. Anticholinergic medications. 2023 May 8. In: StatPearls [Internet]. Treasure Island: StatPearls Publishing, PMID: 32310353. Anticholinergic Medications – PubMed; 2025.
15. Aston-Jones G, Waterhouse B. Locus coeruleus: from global projection system to adaptive regulation of behavior. Brain Res. 2016;1645:75–8. https://doi.org/10.1016/j.brainres.2016.03.001. Epub 2016 Mar 9. PMID: 26969408; PMCID: PMC4969192. Locus coeruleus: From global projection system to adaptive regulation of behavior – PubMed
16. Jacobs BL, Azmitia EC. Structure and function of the brain serotonin system. Physiol Rev. 1992;72(1):165–229. Distribution of Alzheimer's neurofibrillary changes in the brain stem and hypothalamus of senile dementia – PubMed
17. Pascalon A, Ashford W, Dansereau J, Mouret J. The effect of 6-chlorotryptophan on sleep in the rat. Life Sci. 1972;11(19, Part 1):893–903. ISSN 0024-3205 The effect of 6-chlorotryptophan on sleep in the rat – ScienceDirect
18. Jouvet M. Biogenic amines and the states of sleep. Science. 1969;163(3862):32–41. https://doi.org/10.1126/science.163.3862.32. PMID: 4303225. Biogenic amines and the states of sleep – PubMed
19. Kandel ER, Schwartz JH. Molecular biology of learning: modulation of transmitter release. Science. 1982;218(4571):433–43. https://doi.org/10.1126/science.6289442. PMID: 6289442. Molecular biology of learning: modulation of transmitter release – PubMed
20. McGinty DJ, Harper RM. Dorsal raphe neurons: depression of firing during sleep in cats. Brain Res. 1976;101(3):569–75. https://doi.org/10.1016/0006-8993(76)90480-7. PMID: 1244990. Dorsal raphe neurons: depression of firing during sleep in cats – PubMed
21. Aghajanian GK, Foote WE, Sheard MH. Lysergic acid diethylamide: sensitive neuronal units in the midbrain raphe. Science. 1968;161(3842):706–8. https://doi.org/10.1126/science.161.3842.706. PMID: 4874578. Lysergic acid diethylamide: sensitive neuronal units in the midbrain raphe – PubMed

22. Stein L, Wise CD. Release of norepinephrine from hypothalamus and amygdala by rewarding medial forebrain bundle stimulation and amphetamine. J Comp Physiol Psychol. 1969;67(2):189–98. https://doi.org/10.1037/h0026767. PMID: 4306672. Release of norepinephrine from hypothalamus and amygdala by rewarding medial forebrain bundle stimulation and amphetamine – PubMed
23. Benoit M, Berrut G, Doussaint J, Bakchine S, Bonin-Guillaume S, Frémont P, Gallarda T, Krolak-Salmon P, Marquet T, Mékiès C, Sellal F, Schuck S, David R, Robert P. Apathy and depression in mild Alzheimer's disease: a cross-sectional study using diagnostic criteria. J Alzheimers Dis. 2012;31(2):325–34. https://doi.org/10.3233/JAD-2012-112003. PMID: 22543849. Apathy and depression in mild Alzheimer's disease: a cross-sectional study using diagnostic criteria – PubMed
24. Robert PH, Berr C, Volteau M, Bertogliati C, Benoit M, Sarazin M, Legrain S, Dubois B, PréAL Study. Apathy in patients with mild cognitive impairment and the risk of developing dementia of Alzheimer's disease: a one-year follow-up study. Clin Neurol Neurosurg. 2006;108(8):733–6. https://doi.org/10.1016/j.clineuro.2006.02.003. Epub 2006 Mar 29. PMID: 16567037. Apathy in patients with mild cognitive impairment and the risk of developing dementia of Alzheimer's disease: a one-year follow-up study – PubMed
25. Bondareff W, Mountjoy CQ, Roth M. Selective loss of neurones of origin of adrenergic projection to cerebral cortex (nucleus locus coeruleus) in senile dementia. Lancet. 1981;1(8223):783–4. https://doi.org/10.1016/s0140-6736(81)92657-x. PMID: 6110985. Selective loss of neurones of origin of adrenergic projection to cerebral cortex (nucleus locus coeruleus) in senile dementia – PubMed
26. Braak H, Del Tredici K. Where, when, and in what form does sporadic Alzheimer's disease begin? Curr Opin Neurol. 2012;25(6):708–14. https://doi.org/10.1097/WCO.0b013e32835a3432. PMID: 23160422. Where, when, and in what form does sporadic Alzheimer's disease begin? – PubMed
27. Ghosh A, Torraville SE, Mukherjee B, Walling SG, Martin GM, Harley CW, Yuan Q. An experimental model of Braak's pretangle proposal for the origin of Alzheimer's disease: the role of locus coeruleus in early symptom development. Alzheimers Res Ther. 2019;11(1):59. https://doi.org/10.1186/s13195-019-0511-2. PMID: 31266535; PMCID: PMC6607586. An experimental model of Braak's pretangle proposal for the origin of Alzheimer's disease: the role of locus coeruleus in early symptom development – PubMed
28. Mann DM, Lincoln J, Yates PO, Stamp JE, Toper S. Changes in the monoamine containing neurones of the human CNS in senile dementia. Br J Psychiatry. 1980;136:533–41. https://doi.org/10.1192/bjp.136.6.533. PMID: 6155966. Changes in the monoamine containing neurones of the human CNS in senile dementia – PubMed
29. Matchett BJ, Grinberg LT, Theofilas P, Murray ME. The mechanistic link between selective vulnerability of the locus coeruleus and neurodegeneration in Alzheimer's disease. Acta Neuropathol. 2021;141(5):631–50. https://doi.org/10.1007/s00401-020-02248-1. Epub 2021 Jan 11. PMID: 33427939; PMCID: PMC8043919. The mechanistic link between selective vulnerability of the locus coeruleus and neurodegeneration in Alzheimer's disease – PubMed
30. Tomlinson BE, Irving D, Blessed G. Cell loss in the locus coeruleus in senile dementia of Alzheimer type. J Neurol Sci. 1981;49(3):419–28. https://doi.org/10.1016/0022-510x(81)90031-9. PMID: 7217992. Cell loss in the locus coeruleus in senile dementia of Alzheimer type – PubMed
31. Grinberg LT, Rüb U, Ferretti RE, Nitrini R, Farfel JM, Polichiso L, Gierga K, Jacob-Filho W, Heinsen H, Brazilian Brain Bank Study Group. The dorsal raphe nucleus shows phospho-tau neurofibrillary changes before the transentorhinal region in Alzheimer's disease. A precocious onset? Neuropathol Appl Neurobiol. 2009;35(4):406–16. https://doi.org/10.1111/j.1365--2990.2009.00997.x. PMID: 19508444. The dorsal raphe nucleus shows phospho-tau neurofibrillary changes before the transentorhinal region in Alzheimer's disease. A precocious onset? – PubMed
32. Ishii T. Distribution of Alzheimer's neurofibrillary changes in the brain stem and hypothalamus of senile dementia. Acta Neuropathol. 1966;6(2):181–7. https://doi.org/10.1007/BF00686763. PMID: 5963288
33. Michelsen KA, Prickaerts J, Steinbusch HW. The dorsal raphe nucleus and serotonin: implications for neuroplasticity linked to major depression and Alzheimer's disease. Prog Brain Res. 2008;172:233–64. https://doi.org/10.1016/S0079-6123(08)00912-6. PMID: 18772036
34. Theofilas P, Ehrenberg AJ, Nguy A, Thackrey JM, Dunlop S, Mejia MB, Alho AT, Paraizo Leite RE, Rodriguez RD, Suemoto CK, Nascimento CF, Chin M, Medina-Cleghorn D, Cuervo AM, Arkin M, Seeley WW, Miller BL, Nitrini R, Pasqualucci CA, Filho WJ, Rueb U, Neuhaus J, Heinsen H, Grinberg LT. Probing the correlation of neuronal loss, neurofibrillary tangles, and cell death markers across the Alzheimer's disease Braak stages: a quantitative study in humans. Neurobiol Aging. 2018;61:1–12. https://doi.org/10.1016/j.neurobiolaging.2017.09.007. Epub 2017 Sep 20. PMID: 29031088; PMCID: PMC5705284. Probing the correlation of neuronal loss, neurofibrillary tangles, and cell death markers across the Alzheimer's disease Braak stages: a quantitative study in humans – PubMed
35. Trillo L, Das D, Hsieh W, Medina B, Moghadam S, Lin B, Dang V, Sanchez MM, De Miguel Z, Ashford JW, Salehi A. Ascending monoaminergic systems alterations in Alzheimer's disease. Translating basic science into clinical care. Neurosci Biobehav Rev. 2013;37(8):1363–79. https://doi.org/10.1016/j.neubiorev.2013.05.008. Epub 2013 May 24. PMID: 23707776. Ascending monoaminergic systems alterations in Alzheimer's disease. translating basic science into clinical care – PubMed
36. Ashford JW. Neuroplasticity: the critical issue for Alzheimer's disease and links to obesity and depression. Am J Geriatr Psychiatry. 2023;31(10):867–75. https://doi.org/10.1016/j.jagp.2023.07.007. Epub 2023 Jul 15. PMID: 37481402. Neuroplasticity: The Critical Issue for Alzheimer's Disease and Links to Obesity and Depression – PubMed
37. Ashford JW, Jarvik L. Alzheimer's disease: does neuron plasticity predispose to axonal neurofibrillary degeneration? N Engl J Med. 1985;313(6):388–9. PMID: 4010760. Alzheimer's disease: does neuron plasticity predispose to axonal neurofibrillary degeneration? – PubMed
38. Oria RB, Smith CJ, Ashford JW, Vitek MP, Guerrant RL. Pros and cons of APOE4 homozygosity and effects on neuroplasticity, malnutrition, and infections in early life adversity, Alzheimer's disease, and Alzheimer's prevention. J Alzheimers Dis. 2024;100(s1):S179–85. The dorsal raphe nucleus and serotonin: implications for neuroplasticity linked to major depression and Alzheimer's disease – PubMed
39. Ashford JW, Coburn KL, Fuster JM. In: Parks RW, Levine DS, editors. Functional cognitive networks in primates. Fundamentals of neural networks: neuropsychology and cognitive neuroscience. Cambridge, MA: The MIT Press; 1998. (PDF) Functional cognitive networks in primates.
40. Bast E, Jester DJ, Palacio A, Krengel M, Reinhard M, Ashford JW. lf war illness: a historical review and considerations of a post-viral syndrome. Mil Med. 2025;usaf092. https://doi.org/10.1093/milmed/usaf092. Online ahead of print.
41. Zhang Y, Moore M, Jennings JS, Clark JD, Bayley PJ, Ashford JW, Furst AJ. The role of the brainstem in sleep disturbances and chronic pain of Gulf War and Iraq/Afghanistan veterans. Front Mol Neurosci. 2024;16:1266408. https://doi.org/10.3389/fnmol.2023.1266408. PMID: 38260809; PMCID: PMC10800562.

The role of the brainstem in sleep disturbances and chronic pain of Gulf War and Iraq/Afghanistan veterans – PubMed
42. Arguinchona JH, Tadi P. Neuroanatomy, reticular activating system. 2023. In: StatPearls [Internet]. Treasure Island: StatPearls Publishing; 2025. PMID: 31751025. Neuroanatomy, Reticular Activating System – PubMed.
43. Polich J. Updating P300: an integrative theory of P3a and P3b. Clin Neurophysiol. 2007;118(10):2128–48. https://doi.org/10.1016/j.clinph.2007.04.019. Epub 2007 Jun 18. PMID: 17573239; PMCID: PMC2715154. Updating P300: an integrative theory of P3a and P3b – PubMed
44. Ashford JW, Coburn KL, Rose TL, Bayley PJ. P300 energy loss in aging and Alzheimer's disease. J Alzheimers Dis. 2011;26(Suppl 3):229–38. https://doi.org/10.3233/JAD-2011-0061. PMID: 21971463. P300 energy loss in aging and Alzheimer's disease – PubMed
45. Donchin E. Presidential address, 1980. Surprise!... Surprise? Psychophysiology. 1981;18(5):493–513. https://doi.org/10.1111/j.1469-8986.1981.tb01815.x. PMID: 7280146. Presidential address, 1980. Surprise!...Surprise? – PubMed
46. Fabiani M, Karis D, Donchin E. P300 and recall in an incidental memory paradigm. Psychophysiology. 1986;23(3):298–308. https://doi.org/10.1111/j.1469-8986.1986.tb00636.x. PMID: 3749410. P300 and recall in an incidental memory paradigm – PubMed
47. Swick D, Pineda JA, Schacher S, Foote SL. Locus coeruleus neuronal activity in awake monkeys: relationship to auditory P300-like potentials and spontaneous EEG. Exp Brain Res. 1994;101(1):86–92. https://doi.org/10.1007/BF00243219. PMID: 7843306. Locus coeruleus neuronal activity in awake monkeys: relationship to auditory P300-like potentials and spontaneous EEG – PubMed
48. Ashford JW. Treatment of Alzheimer's disease: trazodone, sleep, serotonin, norepinephrine, and future directions. J Alzheimers Dis. 2019;67(3):923–30. https://doi.org/10.3233/JAD-181106. PMID: 30776014; PMCID: PMC6398534. Treatment of Alzheimer's Disease: Trazodone, Sleep, Serotonin, Norepinephrine, and Future Directions – PubMed
49. Ashford JW. Effect of trazodone on sleep in PTSD patients. J Contemp Psychother. 1996;26(3):221–33. Effects of trazodone on sleep in patients diagnosed with post-traumatic stress disorder (PTSD)
50. Raskind MA, Peskind ER. Prazosin for post-traumatic stress disorder. N Engl J Med. 2018;378(17):1649–50. https://doi.org/10.1056/NEJMc1803171. PMID: 29694817. Prazosin for Post-Traumatic Stress Disorder – PubMed
51. Raskind MA, Peskind ER, Chow B, Harris C, Davis-Karim A, Holmes HA, Hart KL, McFall M, Mellman TA, Reist C, Romesser J, Rosenheck R, Shih MC, Stein MB, Swift R, Gleason T, Lu Y, Huang GD. Trial of prazosin for post-traumatic stress disorder in military veterans. N Engl J Med. 2018;378(6):507–17. https://doi.org/10.1056/NEJMoa1507598. PMID: 29414272. Trial of Prazosin for Post-Traumatic Stress Disorder in Military Veterans – PubMed
52. Isaac L, Main KL, Soman S, Gotlib IH, Furst AJ, Kinoshita LM, Fairchild JK, Yesavage JA, Ashford JW, Bayley PJ, Adamson MM. The impact of depression on Veterans with PTSD and traumatic brain injury: a diffusion tensor imaging study. Biol Psychol. 2015;105:20–8. https://doi.org/10.1016/j.biopsycho.2014.12.011. Epub 2015 Jan 3. PMID: 25559772; PMCID: PMC11898798. The impact of depression on Veterans with PTSD and traumatic brain injury: a diffusion tensor imaging study – PubMed
53. Blum K, Ashford JW, Kateb B, Sipple D, Braverman E, Dennen CA, Baron D, Badgaiyan R, Elman I, Cadet JL, Thanos PK, Hanna C, Bowirrat A, Modestino EJ, Yamamoto V, Gupta A, McLaughlin T, Makale M, Gold MS. Dopaminergic dysfunction: role for genetic & epigenetic testing in the new psychiatry. J Neurol Sci. 2023;453:120809. https://doi.org/10.1016/j.jns.2023.120809. Epub 2023 Sep 23. PMID: 37774561. Dopaminergic dysfunction: Role for genetic & epigenetic testing in the new psychiatry – PubMed
54. Ashford JW, Mahoney L, Burkett T. A role for complementary and integrative medicine in Alzheimer's disease prevention. J Alzheimers Dis. 2015;48(1):13–4. https://doi.org/10.3233/JAD-150505. PMID: 26401924. A Role for Complementary and Integrative Medicine in Alzheimer's Disease Prevention – PubMed

Epilogue

26

Franklin Sunzeri

Mutatis Mutandis As mentioned in the introduction to this monograph, our goal has been to present the strongest evidence for the changes individuals can make to treat their depression. Equally important in that pursuit is identifying ways to prevent depression from occurring.

We have seen that environment plays at least an equal part with genetics in determining many of our characteristics including depression [1–3] and that dysfunctional families may have had pathological influences in our formative years on our self-image, perception of stress, and our coping mechanisms [4, 5].

Although telomere length and associated psychiatric disorders [6–9] are influenced by perceived stress, childhood adversities, educational attainment, physical activity, and sleep duration, even these telomeric changes may be reversible through behavioral modifications [10, 11].

Our experiences, emotions, expectations, physical limitations, language abilities, and intelligence, all combine to make us varying degrees of changeable individuals. In addition, the choices we make are often constrained by our mobility, physical limitations, monetary resources, the attitudes, and social mores of the society or even the country in which we were born or live.

So, where in the Gordian knot of depression can we find a thread to pull to unravel the disorder?

We have seen that therapeutic and psychotherapeutic interventions do not produce universal results. Different responses appear to be based upon our biopsychobehavioral individuality. A salient question based upon this individuality is: Are some individuals more likely to benefit from psychotherapy, antidepressant pharmacotherapy, adjunctive treatments, alternative treatments, or combinations of these?

It is exceedingly difficult to generalize what is the best treatment. The characteristics of study participants may vary greatly. The variables of age (children, adolescents, adults, and elderly), patients with different forms of depression, combinations of psychological and physical conditions, depression and substance abuse, severity of symptoms, history of prior treatments, remissions and recurrence, and motivational characteristics can influence treatment resistance vs. non-treatment resistance [12–14]. And, of course, epigenetic and genetic considerations may have direct and indirect impact upon treatment outcome.

As discussed in the first chapter of this work, *stratified medicine* begins by identifying subgroups of patients who have distinct disease mechanisms or specific responses to treatments. Then it categorizes a population into the most biologically appropriate groupings to determine the optimal therapeutic response.

Precision medicine relies on a more discriminating subclassification of disease, adding repeated monitoring of disease markers to enable designing and modifying treatment to fit individual responses.

Personalized medicine recognizes the unique characteristics of each individual. That is the individual phenotype profile (i.e., genetics, epigenetics, clinical symptoms, observable biomarker changes, and environmental factors) [15]. It incorporates precision and stratification along with patient participation and preference to both treat and prevent disease [16].

The goal of personalized medicine is to identify which characteristics of an individual best predict the best match for a specific treatment. To that end, published in 2012, reviewers performed a meta-analysis of RCTs that directly compared two treatments in a group of patients with a spe-

F. Sunzeri (✉)
Heather Hills Consulting, Coos Bay, OR, USA

J. Raber et al. (eds.), *Understanding and Treating Depressive Disorders*, https://doi.org/10.1007/978-3-032-14465-2_26

cific characteristic [17]. Their search identified 52 studies with 4734 depressed participants. They examined 20 characteristics in trials that compared "(1) medication with psychotherapy, (2) medication with combined treatment, and (3) psychotherapy with combined treatment, in specific target groups (a) with a predefined sociodemographic characteristic, (b) a specific type of depression, (c) a comorbid mental or somatic disorder, or (d) from a specific setting (outpatients, primary care)." Sociodemographics included age, economic status, education, living alone, and ethnicity. Types of depression were dysthymia, atypical depression, chronic depression, postnatal depression, minor depression, high cognitive dysfunction, and bereavement-related depression. The settings were primary care and outpatients.

There were some indications that combined treatments are more effective in depressed outpatients and older adults, and antidepressants might be better for dysthymia. However, they found that not enough studies had been conducted to examine the 20 characteristics in these three categories. They estimated that 254 studies would be needed to show an effect size of $g = 0.5$.

An important concept in personalized medicine is to realize that even though different treatments may appear to be equally effective, this is not necessarily true for all classes of patients [or individuals] [18]. For example, an examination of differential effects of CBT vs. treatment as usual in specific subpopulations of patients found that four different trajectory classes could be identified over a 1.5-year follow-up [18]. On average, patients improved significantly with no difference between the treatments. This held true for those patients who were classified as having the lowest depression scores at baseline (31 and 33% of the total sample). However, for the classes that had the more severe depression scores at baseline (10% and 26% of the total sample), CBT was significantly more effective than treatment as usual.

Multivariate prediction models, such as the *Personalized Advantage Index (PAI)*, may point the way toward optimal depression treatment [19–21].

Typically, in the PAI, the variables comprise information from structured interviews, self-report questionnaires, and demographic forms, any of which can easily be obtained in a routine clinical setting.

These variables are either prognostic [22, 23] predicting the post-intervention Hamilton Rating Scale for Depression scores (HRSD) or prescriptive [24–28]. In the original PLOS paper, they were "(1) pre-treatment HRSD, where higher scores predicted higher end-HRSD scores; (2) Chronic versus Non-chronic course of major depressive disorder, where chronicity was associated with poorer outcome; (3) age, where older patients fared more poorly [26]; and (4) low (<100), middle (>=100 and <115), or high (>=115) scores on the *Shipley Institute of Living Scale*, a brief measure of intellectual functioning [29], where higher scores predicted better outcomes." The prescriptive variables predicted different outcomes based upon the treatment received.

In that original PLOS study, a comparison was made between antidepressant medications (ADM) versus CBT. The variables were the following "(1) presence (favoring ADM) versus absence (favoring CBT) of comorbid personality disorder [25]; (2) married or cohabiting (favoring CBT) versus single; (3) employed or not expected to work versus unemployed (favoring CBT); (4) number of stressful life events (more events favoring CBT) [26]; (5) number of prior antidepressant trials, capped at 2 trials (more trials favored CBT)." Higher end-HRSD scores were predicted by having a personality disorder or having had a larger number of prior medication attempts. Lower end-HRSD scores were predicted by being married, employed, or having a higher number of life events.

An example of the PAI in use is an RCT that compared cognitive therapy to interpersonal therapy for MDD [23]. After using a two-step machine learning approach, predictors and moderators were selected and combined into a cross-validated algorithm to make PAI predictions. Results of predictions were then compared to actual therapeutic outcomes. Parental alcohol abuse (a predictor) and recent life events and childhood maltreatment (two moderators) were used to assign the PAI suggested treatment. Those who received the PAI assigned treatment had lower follow-up depression severity than the non-PAI assigned individuals. Significant differences were seen in those whose PAI score was in the upper 60%, and those whose PAI indicated cognitive therapy, irrespective of magnitude. There was no substantial overlap between acute predictions and long-term predictions.

For these early trials, although patients randomized to their PAI optimized treatment tended to fare better than those who were randomized to their non-optimized treatment, there is much more that needs to be explored [21]. For example, attempts at external validation across two different RCTs showed that PAI had only modest results, demonstrated between-study differences, and presented many other challenges [30].

If we might be permitted to indulge our desire to predict the future of personalized depression treatment, it might be to incorporate evidence gained in pursuit of putative treatment influencing factors such as the 20 clinical symptoms and sociodemographic factors outlined above by Pim Cuijpers [17] and by multivariate prediction models, such as the PAI [19]. As more evidence accumulates, it might be possible to screen for relevant genetic and epigenetic profiles, and observable biomarker changes. And, as will be discussed below, neural circuit biotypes [31].

As discussed before, up to a third of depressed patients do not respond to pharmacotherapy and there are mixed results for non-pharmacological approaches [32]. It is likely that differential responses are due to heterogeneity of biological factors underlying psychopathology symptoms [33].

Typical diagnosis and classification of mental illness relies upon patient's self-reporting and behavioral observations. However, in attempting to find the best approach to treat an individual, it might be necessary to understand how psychiatric illnesses develop from behavioral traits underpinned by psychobiological processes [33]. To arrive at that understanding, complex longitudinal data is needed. There are several datasets presently acquiring that multimodal data across different behavioral and biological realms.

During adolescence, there are considerable physical, neurobiological, and social changes. Half of the lifetime burden of mental disorders emerges by the mid-teens and three quarters by mid-20s [34–36]. To identify prenatal, perinatal, and childhood influences on physical, behavioral, and cognitive development, prospective birth cohort databases have been developed. These include the *Avon Longitudinal Study of Parents and Children* [37] and the *Generation R* study [38]. The *Adolescent Brain Cognitive Development [ABCD)* study [39] targets ages 5 to 25. Since 2015, the ABCD has been repeatedly assessing physical and mental health, neuroimaging, cognition, substance use, culture/environment, and samples for DNA, hormones, substance use and toxin exposures. It is the largest long-term study of brain development in the USA.

Longitudinal twin studies are gathering genetic and environmental information. These include *Twins Early Development Study (TEDS)* [40] and the *Environmental Risk Longitudinal Twin Study (E-Risk)* [41].

The *Global Imaging Genetics of Adolescents initiative (GIGA)* is a "collaboration between several major cohorts in the UK, Europe, the USA, China, and India who investigate health outcomes in children and adolescents via behavioral and imaging genetic studies. Its aim is to enable comparative research on brain development and behavior in diverse cultures, environments, and ethnic groups, both in industrialized nations and low- and medium-income countries" [42].

The *IMAGEN* study is a longitudinal neuro**ima**ging-**gen**etics study of adolescents focusing on reinforcement behaviors (impulsivity, reward sensitivity, and emotional processing) in normal development and psychopathology [44]. The participants submit to repeated biological sample collection, including neuroimaging, genotyping, DNA methylation analysis, and gene expression, as well as behavioral and cognitive assessments [43]. Results from the IMAGEN study have revealed, "… functional and structural neural networks, often stratified by genetics, which are common and distinct among psychiatric symptom clusters and traditional diagnostic disorders" [33].

In 2015, President Obama launched the *Precision Medicine Initiative.*[1] The goal is to *"leverage existing research and clinical networks and build on innovative research models that enable patients to be active participants and partners"* [46]. Precision psychiatry is part of this initiative [47–49]. An introduction to precision psychiatry can be found in [50].

The *neurobiological taxonomy of depression* holds promising implications for treatment [51–53]. Mental illness involving the most complex and nuanced human functions including cognition, emotions, abstract reasoning, and social interactions are exceedingly difficult to measure. While signs and symptoms are the basics of diagnosis and treatment in psychiatric disorders, their perspective is at best imprecise relative to the workings of the brain. Modern brain imaging techniques now have sufficient spatial and temporal resolution to quantify neural connections in vivo and to home in on mental disorders as neural circuit dysfunctions [31]. The National Institute of Mental Health and the American Psychological Association used discoveries in neuroscience to provide a stronger support for diagnostic criteria in the DSM-5 [54]. The *Brain Research through Advancing Innovative Neurotechnologies* initiative is aimed at revolu-

[1]Obama B. Video and transcript: President Obama: Speech on the Precision Medicine Initiative. January 30, 2015. Available at: [45].

Creation of a voluntary national research cohort: NIH, in collaboration with other agencies and stakeholders, will launch a national, patient-powered research cohort of one million or more Americans who volunteer to participate in research. Participants will be involved in the design of the Initiative and will have the opportunity to contribute diverse sources of data—including medical records; profiles of the patient's genes, metabolites (chemical makeup), and microorganisms in and on the body; environmental and lifestyle data; patient-generated information; and personal device and sensor data. Privacy will be rigorously protected. This ambitious project will leverage existing research and clinical networks and build on innovative research models that enable patients to be active participants and partners. The cohort will be broadly accessible to qualified researchers and will have the potential to inspire scientists from multiple disciplines to join the effort and apply their creative thinking to generate new insights. The ONC [Office of the National Coordinator for Health Information Technology] will develop interoperability standards and requirements to ensure secure data exchange with patients' consent, to empower patients and clinicians and advance individual, community, and population health. National Institutes of Health. Creation of a voluntary national research cohort. Available at [46].

tionizing our understanding of the human brain [55].[2] In an attempt to develop neurobiologically valid classifications for mental disorders, the National Institute of Mental Health is funding the *Research Domain Criteria* project [56–60].

Variations in neural circuitry, inherited or acquired, seem to be the matrix for important individual differences in thought, feeling, and action patterns [61]. There is a strong relationship between intrinsic resting-state functional connectivity and task-evoked functional connectivity areas of the brain [62, 63]. Task-driven brain neuronal activation and behavior reflects a dynamic, continuous, functional organization of the brain [64]. There is a widely distributed diametrically opposed system of circuits that are task-related activated, while there are others that are task-related deactivated.

Neuroscience-based tools are generally not available for clinicians to use in making treatment decisions despite considerable efforts [31]. One of the impediments to implementing these neuroscience-based advances is the lack of a coherent taxonomy relatable to clinical observations. Advances in precision imaging and analysis techniques, such as used in the *Human Connectome Project* have afforded a closer look at associations with symptoms [65–67].

In attempting to develop such a new taxonomy to deal with the burgeoning data from the neuroscience projects, Leann Williams has formulated a broad hypothesis that specific dysfunctions in the functional and structural connectivity of large-scale circuits in the brain that govern emotional, cognitive, and self-reflective functions define unique biotypes of depression and anxiety [31]. She focuses on six circuits that have been implicated in dysfunctions expressed in depression and anxiety: default mode, salience, negative affect, positive affect (reward), attention, and cognitive control. These large-scale intrinsic and task-evoked circuits are diagrammed in [100].

She follows that up with a proposal for eight putative biotypes of dysfunction that might explain the natural heterogeneity of depression and anxiety [101]. The eight biotypes are rumination, anxious avoidance, negative bias, threat dysregulation, anhedonia, context insensitivity, inattention, and cognitive dyscontrol. She relates each of these biotypes to the six underlying circuits that seem to be involved. For each of the biotypes, functions and connectivity of each of the parts within these circuits may be hyper, typical, or hypo.

Here are a few examples. For *rumination* in depression, the default mode has shown a consistent profile of functional overactivation and hyperconnectivity [68]. For *anxious avoidance*, the salience circuit components may be hyper, hypo, or typical. Connections between the salience and default circuit may be hyper and between the salience and attention circuit may be hyper or hypo depending upon the nature of interoceptive or exteroceptive stimuli. For *threat dysregulation*, the negative affect circuit is central. In depressive disorder [69], generalized anxiety disorder [70], generalized social phobia–anxiety disorder [71], specific phobia [72], and panic disorder, the amygdala is hyperreactive. In generalized anxiety disorder [73] and generalized social anxiety [73], the anterior cerebral cortex is hypoactive. In task context-dependent anxiety disorders, the anterior cerebral cortex is hyperactive [74].

Williams believes that these neural circuit biotypes could be used to help guide choice of interventions [102]. She suggests the following interventions for remediating depression and anxiety problems within each of the six neural circuit biotypes. Default mode: mindfulness and self-context therapies. Salience: SSRI's and deep brain stimulation. Negative affect: cognitive behavioral therapies. Positive affect: DNRI's. Attention: attention training and stimulants. Cognitive control: cognitive training and transcranial magnetic stimulation.

Using a *methylome-wide association study*,[3] attempts have been made to identify methylation signatures in blood that could be indirectly associated with future MDD status [75]. Epigenetic states are metastable and change in response to environmental and behavioral stressors and those states may be reflected in the brain as well as the blood [76–80]. Methylation marks in the blood may be useful as they are stable and easily accessible with very little risk to the patient.

Researchers from the *Center for Biomarker Research and Precision Medicine* [81] used a sequencing-based methylation assay that provided almost complete coverage of all 28 million CpGs in the human genome [82, 83]. They analyzed blood DNA methylation of 581 patients at baseline and 6 years later [75]. Results showed a highly significant association between methylation profiles in blood at baseline and future disease status ($P = 2.0 \times 10^{-16}$).

Methylation enrichment was seen in specific pathways that overlapped with genes identified in GWASs of MDD, autoimmune disease, and inflammation. Enrichment co-localized with cis expression quantitative trait loci

[2] *The Brain Research through Advancing Innovative Neurotechnologies® (BRAIN) Initiative* is aimed at revolutionizing our understanding of the human brain. By accelerating the development and application of innovative technologies, researchers will be able to produce a revolutionary new dynamic picture of the brain that, for the first time, shows how individual cells and complex neural circuits interact in both time and space. Long desired by researchers seeking new ways to treat, cure, and even prevent brain disorders, this picture will fill major gaps in our current knowledge and provide unprecedented opportunities for exploring exactly how the brain enables the human body to record, process, utilize, store, and retrieve vast quantities of information, all at the speed of thought.

[3] Also known as *epigenome wide association study* [84–88].

(*cis-eQTLs*)[4] in two brain regions[5] and whole blood, and regulatory sites of transcription sites in brain and blood. The main pathways that seem to be most highly associated are cellular responses to stress and signaling mechanisms linked to immune cell migration and inflammation.

The researchers developed a *methylation risk score (MRS)* for predicting MDD status 6 years in the future. They found an *AUC*[6] of 0.724 for their MRS. This was higher than risk scores created using a "set of five putative MDD biomarkers, genome-wide SNP data, and 27 clinical, demographic and lifestyle variables." They believe that these results could lend themselves to generating prediction algorithms to improve MDD treatment.

Data from physiology, brain images, biosocial and environmental exposures, genomics, epigenomics, transcriptomics, proteomics, metabolomics, metagenomics, and lipidomics [96, 97] when combined and analyzed in systems biology computations have led to exciting progress in revealing biological pathways in psychiatric disorders [98, 99].

The goal is that armed with data from these collaborations, environmental, behavioral, pharmacological, and other interventions can be created and implemented earlier in the development of mental illnesses. In that way, depression may be precisely treated if not prevented by changing those things which needed to be changed.

Nevertheless, superimposed upon all these factors will be the willingness and ability of any individual to change. Helping to make that change may be the biggest challenge to the art and experience of the skilled practitioner.

References

1. Bierut LJ, Heath AC, Bucholz KK, Dinwiddie SH, Madden PA, Statham DJ, Dunne MP, Martin NG. Major depressive disorder in a community-based twin sample: are there different genetic and environmental contributions for men and women? Arch Gen Psychiatry. 1999;56(6):557–63. PMID: 10359473 http://www.ncbi.nlm.nih.gov/pubmed/10359473
2. Schumann G, Benegal V, Yu C, Tao S, Jernigan T, Heinz A, Araya R, Yu L, Calhoun V. Precision medicine and global mental health. The Lancet Global Health [Internet]. Elsevier; 2019. [cited 2024 Dec 17];7(1):e32. Available from: https://doi.org/10.1016/S2214-109X(18)30406-6
3. Kendler KS, Prescott CA. A population-based twin study of lifetime major depression in men and women. Arch Gen Psychiatry. 1999;56(1):39–44. PMID: 9892254 http://www.ncbi.nlm.nih.gov/pubmed/9892254
4. Mullen PE, Martin JL, Anderson JC, Romans SE, Herbison GP. The effect of child sexual abuse on social, interpersonal and sexual function in adult life. Br J Psychiatry. 1994;165(1):35–47. PMID: 7953055 http://www.ncbi.nlm.nih.gov/pubmed/7953055
5. Szili I, György S. The role of mother-child relationship in development of self-image, dysfunctional attitudes and coping strategies. Psychiatr Hung. 2005;20(2):126–40. PMID: 16389782 http://www.ncbi.nlm.nih.gov/pubmed/16389782
6. Starkweather AR, Alhaeeri AA, Montpetit A, Brumelle J, Filler K, Montpetit M, Mohanraj L, Lyon DE, Jackson-Cook CK. An integrative review of factors associated with telomere length and implications for biobehavioral research. Nurs Res. 2014;63(1):36–50. PMCID: PMC4112289 http://www.ncbi.nlm.nih.gov/pubmed/24335912
7. Hanssen LM, Schutte NS, Malouff JM, Epel ES. The relationship between childhood psychosocial stressor level and telomere length: a meta-analysis. Health Psychol Res. 2017;5(1):6378. PMCID: PMC5452631 http://www.ncbi.nlm.nih.gov/pubmed/28603779
8. Boccardi M, Boccardi V. Psychological wellbeing and healthy aging: focus on telomeres. Geriatrics (Basel). 2019;4(1):25. PMCID: PMC6473912 http://www.ncbi.nlm.nih.gov/pubmed/31023993
9. Chilton W, O'Brien B, Charchar F. Telomeres, aging and exercise: guilty by association? Int J Mol Sci. 2017;18(12):2573. PMCID: PMC5751176 http://www.ncbi.nlm.nih.gov/pubmed/29186077
10. Epel E. How "reversible" is telomeric aging? Cancer Prev Res (Phila). 2012;5(10):1163–8. PMID: 23041472 http://www.ncbi.nlm.nih.gov/pubmed/23041472
11. Conklin QA, Crosswell AD, Saron CD, Epel ES. Meditation, stress processes, and telomere biology. Curr Opin Psychol. 2019;28:92–101. PMCID: PMC6526075 http://www.ncbi.nlm.nih.gov/pubmed/30553080
12. Lesko CR, Buchanan AL, Westreich D, Edwards JK, Hudgens MG, Cole SR. Generalizing study results: a potential outcomes perspective. Epidemiology. 2017;28(4):553–61. PMCID: PMC5466356 http://www.ncbi.nlm.nih.gov/pubmed/28346267
13. Westreich D, Edwards JK, Lesko CR, Cole SR, Stuart EA. Target validity and the hierarchy of study designs. Am J Epidemiol. 2019;188(2):438–43. PMCID: PMC6357801 http://www.ncbi.nlm.nih.gov/pubmed/30299451
14. Remes O, Mendes JF, Templeton P. Biological, psychological, and social determinants of depression: a review of recent literature. Brain Sci. 2021;11(12):1633. PMCID: PMC8699555 http://www.ncbi.nlm.nih.gov/pubmed/34942936
15. Ozomaro U, Wahlestedt C, Nemeroff CB. Personalized medicine in psychiatry: problems and promises. BMC Med. 2013;11:132. PMCID: PMC3668172 http://www.ncbi.nlm.nih.gov/pubmed/23680237
16. Day S, Coombes RC, McGrath-Lone L, Schoenborn C, Ward H. Stratified, precision or personalised medicine? Cancer services in the "real world" of a London hospital. Sociol Health Illn. 2017;39(1):143–58. PMID: 27460935 http://www.ncbi.nlm.nih.gov/pubmed/27460935
17. Cuijpers P, Reynolds CF, Donker T, Li J, Andersson G, Beekman A. Personalized treatment of adult depression: medication, psychotherapy, or both? A systematic review. Depress Anxiety. 2012;29(10):855–64. PMID: 22815247 http://www.ncbi.nlm.nih.gov/pubmed/22815247
18. Cuijpers P, van Lier PAC, van Straten A, Donker M. Examining differential effects of psychological treatment of depressive

[4]In analyzing variations in genomic function relative to genomic expression levels, extensive use has been made of studies on expression quantitative trait loci (eQTLs) [89].

[5]These are Brodmann area 9 and 24. Brodmann area 9 is a region of the frontal cortex involved in processes such as short-term memory and interpreting the intentions of others [90]. Brodmann area 24 is the associational part of the cingulate cortex and has been described as the seat of free will due to its involvement in motivation [90–94].

[6]*AUC (Area Under The Curve) ROC (Receiver Operating Characteristics)* curve is used extensively for measuring performance in machine learning. An AUC near to 1 would be an excellent model with a good measure of separability. An AUC near to 0 would indicate that the model is reciprocating the result. An AUC of 0.5 indicates that the model has no separation ability [95].

disorder: an application of trajectory analyses. J Affect Disord. 2005;89(1–3):137–46. PMID: 16274750 http://www.ncbi.nlm.nih.gov/pubmed/16274750

19. Friedl N, Berger T, Krieger T, Caspar F, Grosse HM. Using the Personalized Advantage Index for individual treatment allocation to cognitive behavioral therapy (CBT) or a CBT with integrated exposure and emotion-focused elements (CBT-EE). Psychother Res. 2020;30(6):763–75. PMID: 31507250 http://www.ncbi.nlm.nih.gov/pubmed/31507250
20. Lopez-Gomez I, Lorenzo-Luaces L, Chaves C, Hervas G, DeRubeis RJ, Vazquez C. Predicting optimal interventions for clinical depression: moderators of outcomes in a positive psychological intervention vs. cognitive-behavioral therapy. Gen Hosp Psychiatry. 2019;61:104–10. PMID: 31395363 http://www.ncbi.nlm.nih.gov/pubmed/31395363
21. DeRubeis RJ, Cohen ZD, Forand NR, Fournier JC, Gelfand LA, Lorenzo-Luaces L. The Personalized Advantage Index: translating research on prediction into individualized treatment recommendations. A demonstration. PLoS One. 2014;9(1):e83875. PMCID: PMC3885521 http://www.ncbi.nlm.nih.gov/pubmed/24416178
22. Senger K, Schröder A, Kleinstäuber M, Rubel JA, Rief W, Heider J. Predicting optimal treatment outcomes using the Personalized Advantage Index for patients with persistent somatic symptoms. Psychother Res. 2022;32(2):165–78. PMID: 33910487 http://www.ncbi.nlm.nih.gov/pubmed/33910487
23. van Bronswijk SC, DeRubeis RJ, Lemmens LHJM, Peeters FPML, Keefe JR, Cohen ZD, Huibers MJH. Precision medicine for long-term depression outcomes using the Personalized Advantage Index approach: cognitive therapy or interpersonal psychotherapy? Psychol Med. 2021;51(2):279–89. PMCID: PMC7893512 http://www.ncbi.nlm.nih.gov/pubmed/31753043
24. Leykin Y, Amsterdam JD, DeRubeis RJ, Gallop R, Shelton RC, Hollon SD. Progressive resistance to a selective serotonin reuptake inhibitor but not to cognitive therapy in the treatment of major depression. J Consult Clin Psychol. 2007;75(2):267–76. PMID: 17469884 http://www.ncbi.nlm.nih.gov/pubmed/17469884
25. Fournier JC, DeRubeis RJ, Shelton RC, Gallop R, Amsterdam JD, Hollon SD. Antidepressant medications v. cognitive therapy in people with depression with or without personality disorder. Br J Psychiatry. 2008;192(2):124–9. PMCID: PMC2682552 http://www.ncbi.nlm.nih.gov/pubmed/18245030
26. Fournier JC, DeRubeis RJ, Shelton RC, Hollon SD, Amsterdam JD, Gallop R. Prediction of response to medication and cognitive therapy in the treatment of moderate to severe depression. J Consult Clin Psychol. 2009;77(4):775–87. PMCID: PMC2810269 http://www.ncbi.nlm.nih.gov/pubmed/19634969
27. Wade B, Pindale R, Camprodon J, Luccarelli J, Li S, Meisner R, Seiner S, Henry M. Individual prediction of optimal treatment allocation between electroconvulsive therapy or ketamine using the Personalized Advantage Index. Res Sq. 2023:rs.3.rs-3682009. PMCID: PMC10705694 http://www.ncbi.nlm.nih.gov/pubmed/38077094
28. Webb CA, Hirshberg MJ, Davidson RJ, Goldberg SB. Personalized prediction of response to smartphone-delivered meditation training: Randomized Controlled Trial. J Med Internet Res. 2022;24(11):e41566. PMCID: PMC9682449 http://www.ncbi.nlm.nih.gov/pubmed/36346668
29. Zachary RA, Shipley WC. Shipley institute of living scale: revised manual. WPS, Western Psychological Services; 1986. Shipley Institute of Living Scale | SpringerLink
30. van Bronswijk SC, Bruijniks SJE, Lorenzo-Luaces L, Derubeis RJ, Lemmens LHJM, Peeters FPML, Huibers MJH. Cross-trial prediction in psychotherapy: external validation of the Personalized Advantage Index using machine learning in two Dutch randomized trials comparing CBT versus IPT for depression. Psychother Res. 2021;31(1):78–91. PMID: 32964809 http://www.ncbi.nlm.nih.gov/pubmed/32964809
31. Williams LM. Precision psychiatry: a neural circuit taxonomy for depression and anxiety. Lancet Psychiatry. 2016;3(5):472–80. PMCID: PMC4922884 http://www.ncbi.nlm.nih.gov/pubmed/27150382
32. Schlaepfer TE, Agren H, Monteleone P, Gasto C, Pitchot W, Rouillon F, Nutt DJ, Kasper S. The hidden third: improving outcome in treatment-resistant depression. J Psychopharmacol. 2012;26(5):587–602. PMID: 22236505 http://www.ncbi.nlm.nih.gov/pubmed/22236505
33. Quinlan EB, Banaschewski T, Barker GJ, ALW B, Bromberg U, Büchel C, Desrivières S, Flor H, Frouin V, Garavan H, Heinz A, Brühl R, Martinot JL, Paillère Martinot ML, Nees F, Orfanos DP, Paus T, Poustka L, Hohmann S, Smolka MN, Fröhner JH, Walter H, Whelan R, Schumann G, IMAGEN Consortium. Identifying biological markers for improved precision medicine in psychiatry. Mol Psychiatry. 2020;25(2):243–53. PMCID: PMC6978138 http://www.ncbi.nlm.nih.gov/pubmed/31676814
34. Kessler RC, Amminger GP, Aguilar-Gaxiola S, Alonso J, Lee S, Ustün TB. Age of onset of mental disorders: a review of recent literature. Curr Opin Psychiatry. 2007;20(4):359–64. PMCID: PMC1925038 http://www.ncbi.nlm.nih.gov/pubmed/17551351
35. de Girolamo G, Dagani J, Purcell R, Cocchi A, McGorry PD. Age of onset of mental disorders and use of mental health services: needs, opportunities and obstacles. Epidemiol Psychiatr Sci. 2012;21(1):47–57. PMID: 22670412 http://www.ncbi.nlm.nih.gov/pubmed/22670412
36. Child and adolescent mental and brain health
37. Avon Longitudinal Study of Parents and Children | Avon Longitudinal Study of Parents and Children | University of Bristol
38. Researchers - Generation R
39. Adolescent Brain Cognitive Development ABCD Study
40. Twins Early Development Study Home
41. Environmental Risk (E-Risk) Longitudinal Twin Study eriskstudy.com
42. Schumann G, Benegal V, Yu C, Tao S, Jernigan T, Heinz A, Araya R, Yu L, Calhoun V. Global Imaging Genetics in Adolescents Consortium. Precision medicine and global mental health. Lancet Glob Health. 2019;7(1):e32. PMCID: PMC7313318 http://www.ncbi.nlm.nih.gov/pubmed/30554758
43. Mascarell Maričić L, Walter H, Rosenthal A, Ripke S, Quinlan EB, Banaschewski T, Barker GJ, Bokde ALW, Bromberg U, Büchel C, Desrivières S, Flor H, Frouin V, Garavan H, Itterman B, Martinot JL, Martinot MLP, Nees F, Orfanos DP, Paus T, Poustka L, Hohmann S, Smolka MN, Fröhner JH, Whelan R, Kaminski J, Schumann G, Heinz A, IMAGEN Consortium. The IMAGEN study: a decade of imaging genetics in adolescents. Mol Psychiatry. 2020;25(11):2648–71. PMCID: PMC7577859 http://www.ncbi.nlm.nih.gov/pubmed/32601453
44. Schumann G, Loth E, Banaschewski T, Barbot A, Barker G, Büchel C, Conrod PJ, Dalley JW, Flor H, Gallinat J, Garavan H, Heinz A, Itterman B, Lathrop M, Mallik C, Mann K, Martinot JL, Paus T, Poline JB, Robbins TW, Rietschel M, Reed L, Smolka M, Spanagel R, Speiser C, Stephens DN, Ströhle A, Struve M, IMAGEN Consortium. The IMAGEN study: reinforcement-related behaviour in normal brain function and psychopathology. Mol Psychiatry. 2010;15(12):1128–39. PMID: 21102431 http://www.ncbi.nlm.nih.gov/pubmed/21102431
45. http://www.shallownation.com/2015/01/30/president-obama-speech-precision-medicine-initiative-jan-30-2015-white-house/
46. All of Us Research Program | National Institutes of Health (NIH)
47. Terry SF. Obama's precision medicine initiative. Genet Test Mol Biomarkers. 2015;19(3):113–4. PMCID: PMC4361161 http://www.ncbi.nlm.nih.gov/pubmed/25751403

48. Collins FS, Varmus H. A new initiative on precision medicine. N Engl J Med. 2015;372(9):793–5. PMCID: PMC5101938 http://www.ncbi.nlm.nih.gov/pubmed/25635347
49. Vieta E. Personalised medicine applied to mental health: Precision psychiatry. Rev Psiquiatr Salud Ment. 2015;8(3):117–8. PMID: 25959401 http://www.ncbi.nlm.nih.gov/pubmed/25959401
50. Fernandes BS, Williams LM, Steiner J, Leboyer M, Carvalho AF, Berk M. The new field of "precision psychiatry". BMC Med. 2017;15(1):80. PMCID: PMC5390384 http://www.ncbi.nlm.nih.gov/pubmed/28403846
51. aan het Rot M, Mathew SJ, Charney DS. Neurobiological mechanisms in major depressive disorder. CMAJ. 2009;180(3):305–13. PMCID: PMC2630359 http://www.ncbi.nlm.nih.gov/pubmed/19188629
52. Ferrari F, Villa RF. The neurobiology of depression: an integrated overview from biological theories to clinical evidence. Mol Neurobiol. 2017;54(7):4847–65. PMID: 27510505 http://www.ncbi.nlm.nih.gov/pubmed/27510505
53. DeYoung CG, Blain SD, Latzman RD, Grazioplene RG, Haltigan JD, Kotov R, Michelini G, Venables NC, Docherty AR, Goghari VM, Kallen AM, Martin EA, Palumbo IM, Patrick CJ, Perkins ER, Shackman AJ, Snyder ME, Tobin KE. The hierarchical taxonomy of psychopathology and the search for neurobiological substrates of mental illness: a systematic review and roadmap for future research. J Psychopathol Clin Sci. 2024;133(8):697–715. PMCID: PMC11529694 http://www.ncbi.nlm.nih.gov/pubmed/39480338
54. Kupfer DJ, Regier DA. Neuroscience, clinical evidence, and the future of psychiatric classification in DSM-5. Am J Psychiatry. 2011;168(7):672–4. PMID: 21724672 http://www.ncbi.nlm.nih.gov/pubmed/21724672
55. Home | BRAIN Initiative
56. Insel T, Cuthbert B, Garvey M, Heinssen R, Pine DS, Quinn K, Sanislow C, Wang P. Research domain criteria (RDoC): toward a new classification framework for research on mental disorders. Am J Psychiatry. 2010;167(7):748–51. PMID: 20595427 http://www.ncbi.nlm.nih.gov/pubmed/20595427
57. Cuthbert BN. Research Domain Criteria: toward future psychiatric nosologies. Dialogues Clin Neurosci. 2015;17(1):89–97. PMCID: PMC4421905 http://www.ncbi.nlm.nih.gov/pubmed/25987867
58. Cuthbert BN. The RDoC framework: facilitating transition from ICD/DSM to dimensional approaches that integrate neuroscience and psychopathology. World Psychiatry. 2014;13(1):28–35. PMCID: PMC3918011 http://www.ncbi.nlm.nih.gov/pubmed/24497240
59. Cuthbert BN, Insel TR. Toward the future of psychiatric diagnosis: the seven pillars of RDoC. BMC Med. 2013;11:126. PMCID: PMC3653747 http://www.ncbi.nlm.nih.gov/pubmed/23672542
60. Morris SE, Cuthbert BN. Research Domain Criteria: cognitive systems, neural circuits, and dimensions of behavior. Dialogues Clin Neurosci. 2012;14(1):29–37. PMCID: PMC3341647 http://www.ncbi.nlm.nih.gov/pubmed/22577302
61. Seeley WW, Menon V, Schatzberg AF, Keller J, Glover GH, Kenna H, Reiss AL, Greicius MD. Dissociable intrinsic connectivity networks for salience processing and executive control. J Neurosci. 2007;27(9):2349–56. PMCID: PMC2680293 http://www.ncbi.nlm.nih.gov/pubmed/17329432
62. Cole MW, Bassett DS, Power JD, Braver TS, Petersen SE. Intrinsic and task-evoked network architectures of the human brain. Neuron. 2014;83(1):238–51. PMCID: PMC4082806 http://www.ncbi.nlm.nih.gov/pubmed/24991964
63. Power JD, Cohen AL, Nelson SM, Wig GS, Barnes KA, Church JA, Vogel AC, Laumann TO, Miezin FM, Schlaggar BL, Petersen SE. Functional network organization of the human brain. Neuron. 2011;72(4):665–78. PMCID: PMC3222858 http://www.ncbi.nlm.nih.gov/pubmed/22099467
64. Fox MD, Snyder AZ, Vincent JL, Corbetta M, Van Essen DC, Raichle ME. The human brain is intrinsically organized into dynamic, anticorrelated functional networks. Proc Natl Acad Sci U S A. 2005;102(27):9673–8. PMCID: PMC1157105 http://www.ncbi.nlm.nih.gov/pubmed/15976020
65. Barch DM, Burgess GC, Harms MP, Petersen SE, Schlaggar BL, Corbetta M, Glasser MF, Curtiss S, Dixit S, Feldt C, Nolan D, Bryant E, Hartley T, Footer O, Bjork JM, Poldrack R, Smith S, Johansen-Berg H, Snyder AZ, Van Essen DC, WU-Minn HCP Consortium. Function in the human connectome: task-fMRI and individual differences in behavior. Neuroimage. 2013;80:169–89. PMCID: PMC4011498 http://www.ncbi.nlm.nih.gov/pubmed/23684877
66. Van Essen DC, Smith SM, Barch DM, Behrens TEJ, Yacoub E, Ugurbil K, WU-Minn HCP Consortium. The WU-Minn Human Connectome Project: an overview. Neuroimage. 2013;80:62–79. PMCID: PMC3724347 http://www.ncbi.nlm.nih.gov/pubmed/23684880
67. Williams LM. Defining biotypes for depression and anxiety based on large-scale circuit dysfunction: a theoretical review of the evidence and future directions for clinical translation. Depress Anxiety. 2017;34(1):9–24. PMCID: PMC5702265 http://www.ncbi.nlm.nih.gov/pubmed/27653321
68. Hamilton JP, Farmer M, Fogelman P, Gotlib IH. Depressive rumination, the default-mode network, and the dark matter of clinical neuroscience. Biol Psychiatry. 2015;78(4):224–30. PMCID: PMC4524294 http://www.ncbi.nlm.nih.gov/pubmed/25861700
69. Jaworska N, Yang XR, Knott V, MacQueen G. A review of fMRI studies during visual emotive processing in major depressive disorder. World J Biol Psychiatry. 2015;16(7):448–71. PMID: 24635551 http://www.ncbi.nlm.nih.gov/pubmed/24635551
70. Fonzo GA, Ramsawh HJ, Flagan TM, Sullivan SG, Letamendi A, Simmons AN, Paulus MP, Stein MB. Common and disorder-specific neural responses to emotional faces in generalised anxiety, social anxiety and panic disorders. Br J Psychiatry. 2015;206(3):206–15. PMCID: PMC4345308 http://www.ncbi.nlm.nih.gov/pubmed/25573399
71. Phan KL, Fitzgerald DA, Nathan PJ, Tancer ME. Association between amygdala hyperactivity to harsh faces and severity of social anxiety in generalized social phobia. Biol Psychiatry. 2006;59(5):424–9. PMID: 16256956 http://www.ncbi.nlm.nih.gov/pubmed/16256956
72. Killgore WDS, Britton JC, Schwab ZJ, Price LM, Weiner MR, Gold AL, Rosso IM, Simon NM, Pollack MH, Rauch SL. Cortico-limbic responses to masked affective faces across ptsd, panic disorder, and specific phobia. Depress Anxiety. 2014;31(2):150–9. PMCID: PMC4593618 http://www.ncbi.nlm.nih.gov/pubmed/23861215
73. Blair KS, Geraci M, Smith BW, Hollon N, DeVido J, Otero M, Blair JR, Pine DS. Reduced dorsal anterior cingulate cortical activity during emotional regulation and top-down attentional control in generalized social phobia, generalized anxiety disorder, and comorbid generalized social phobia/generalized anxiety disorder. Biol Psychiatry. 2012;72(6):476–82. PMCID: PMC3424322 http://www.ncbi.nlm.nih.gov/pubmed/22592057
74. Etkin A, Prater KE, Hoeft F, Menon V, Schatzberg AF. Failure of anterior cingulate activation and connectivity with the amygdala during implicit regulation of emotional processing in generalized anxiety disorder. Am J Psychiatry. 2010;167(5):545–54. PMCID: PMC4367202 http://www.ncbi.nlm.nih.gov/pubmed/20123913
75. Clark SL, Hattab MW, Chan RF, Shabalin AA, Han LKM, Zhao M, Smit JH, Jansen R, Milaneschi Y, Xie LY, van Grootheest G, Penninx BWJH, Aberg KA, van den Oord EJCG. A methylation study of long-term depression risk. Mol Psychiatry.

2020;25(6):1334–43. PMCID: PMC7061076 http://www.ncbi.nlm.nih.gov/pubmed/31501512
76. Sun YV. The influences of genetic and environmental factors on methylome-wide association studies for human diseases. Curr Genet Med Rep. 2014;2(4):261–70. PMCID: PMC4239213 http://www.ncbi.nlm.nih.gov/pubmed/25422794
77. Aberg KA, Shabalin AA, Chan RF, Zhao M, Kumar G, van Grootheest G, Clark SL, Xie LY, Milaneschi Y, Penninx BWJH, van den Oord EJCG. Convergence of evidence from a methylome-wide CpG-SNP association study and GWAS of major depressive disorder. Transl Psychiatry. 2018;8(1):162. PMCID: PMC6105579 http://www.ncbi.nlm.nih.gov/pubmed/30135428
78. Bonasio R, Tu S, Reinberg D. Molecular signals of epigenetic states. Science. 2010;330(6004):612–6. PMCID: PMC3772643 http://www.ncbi.nlm.nih.gov/pubmed/21030644
79. Vialou V, Feng J, Robison AJ, Nestler EJ. Epigenetic mechanisms of depression and antidepressant action. Annu Rev Pharmacol Toxicol. 2013;53:59–87. PMCID: PMC3711377 http://www.ncbi.nlm.nih.gov/pubmed/23020296
80. Murgatroyd C, Patchev AV, Wu Y, Micale V, Bockmühl Y, Fischer D, Holsboer F, Wotjak CT, Almeida OFX, Spengler D. Dynamic DNA methylation programs persistent adverse effects of early-life stress. Nat Neurosci. 2009;12(12):1559–66. PMID: 19898468 http://www.ncbi.nlm.nih.gov/pubmed/19898468
81. Home – Center for Biomarker Research & Precision Medicine
82. Chan RF, Shabalin AA, Xie LY, Adkins DE, Zhao M, Turecki G, Clark SL, Aberg KA, van den Oord EJCG. Enrichment methods provide a feasible approach to comprehensive and adequately powered investigations of the brain methylome. Nucleic Acids Res. 2017;45(11):e97. PMCID: PMC5499761 http://www.ncbi.nlm.nih.gov/pubmed/28334972
83. Aberg KA, Chan RF, Shabalin AA, Zhao M, Turecki G, Staunstrup NH, Starnawska A, Mors O, Xie LY, van den Oord EJ. A MBD-seq protocol for large-scale methylome-wide studies with (very) low amounts of DNA. Epigenetics. 2017;12(9):743–50. PMCID: PMC5739096 http://www.ncbi.nlm.nih.gov/pubmed/28703682
84. Rakyan VK, Down TA, Balding DJ, Beck S. Epigenome-wide association studies for common human diseases. Nat Rev Genet. 2011;12(8):529–41. PMCID: PMC3508712 http://www.ncbi.nlm.nih.gov/pubmed/21747404
85. Wheater ENW, Stoye DQ, Cox SR, Wardlaw JM, Drake AJ, Bastin ME, Boardman JP. DNA methylation and brain structure and function across the life course: A systematic review. Neurosci Biobehav Rev. 2020;113:133–56. PMCID: PMC7237884 http://www.ncbi.nlm.nih.gov/pubmed/32151655
86. Nemoda Z, Szyf M. Epigenetic alterations and prenatal maternal depression. Birth Defects Res. 2017;109(12):888–97. PMID: 28714605 http://www.ncbi.nlm.nih.gov/pubmed/28714605
87. Stonawski V, Frey S, Golub Y, Moll GH, Heinrich H, Eichler A. Epigenetic modifications in children associated with maternal emotional stress during pregnancy. Z Kinder Jugendpsychiatr Psychother. 2018;46(2):155–67. PMID: 28256157 http://www.ncbi.nlm.nih.gov/pubmed/28256157
88. Januar V, Saffery R, Ryan J. Epigenetics and depressive disorders: a review of current progress and future directions. Int J Epidemiol. 2015;44(4):1364–87. PMID: 25716985 http://www.ncbi.nlm.nih.gov/pubmed/25716985
89. Nica AC, Dermitzakis ET. Expression quantitative trait loci: present and future. Philos Trans R Soc Lond B Biol Sci. 2013;368(1620):20120362. PMCID: PMC3682727 http://www.ncbi.nlm.nih.gov/pubmed/23650636
90. Cerebral cortex cytoarchitecture and layers | Kenhub
91. Brodmann Areas of the Brain: Anatomy and Functions
92. Brodmann Area 24 – an overview | ScienceDirect Topics
93. Bijanki KR, Matsui JT, Mayberg HS, Magnotta VA, Arndt S, Johnson HJ, Nopoulos P, Paradiso S, McCormick LM, Fiedorowicz JG, Epping EA, Moser DJ. Depressive symptoms related to low fractional anisotropy of white matter underlying the right ventral anterior cingulate in older adults with atherosclerotic vascular disease. Front Hum Neurosci. 2015;9:408. PMCID: PMC4502350 http://www.ncbi.nlm.nih.gov/pubmed/26236221
94. Cano-Astorga N, Plaza-Alonso S, DeFelipe J, Alonso-Nanclares L. 3D synaptic organization of layer III of the human anterior cingulate and temporopolar cortex. Cereb Cortex. 2023;33(17):9691–708. PMCID: PMC10472499 http://www.ncbi.nlm.nih.gov/pubmed/37455478
95. Understanding AUC – ROC Curve | by Sarang Narkhede | Towards Data Science
96. Yang K, Han X. Lipidomics: techniques, applications, and outcomes related to biomedical sciences. Trends Biochem Sci. 2016;41(11):954–69. PMCID: PMC5085849 http://www.ncbi.nlm.nih.gov/pubmed/27663237
97. Wang J, Wang C, Han X. Tutorial on lipidomics. Anal Chim Acta. 2019;1061:28–41. PMCID: PMC7375172 http://www.ncbi.nlm.nih.gov/pubmed/30926037
98. Kitano H. Systems biology: a brief overview. Science. 2002;295(5560):1662–4. PMID: 11872829 http://www.ncbi.nlm.nih.gov/pubmed/11872829
99. Tretter F, Gebicke-Haerter PJ. Systems biology in psychiatric research: from complex data sets over wiring diagrams to computer simulations. Methods Mol Biol. 2012;829:567–92. PMID: 22231839 http://www.ncbi.nlm.nih.gov/pubmed/22231839
100. https://www.ncbi.nlm.nih.gov/pmc/articles/PMC4922884/figure/F1/
101. https://www.ncbi.nlm.nih.gov/pmc/articles/PMC4922884/figure/F2/
102. https://www.ncbi.nlm.nih.gov/pmc/articles/PMC4922884/figure/F3/

Index

J. Raber et al. (eds.), *Understanding and Treating Depressive Disorders*, https://doi.org/10.1007/978-3-032-14465-2

C

D

E

Q

R

MIX
Papier aus verantwortungsvollen Quellen
Paper from responsible sources
FSC® C105338

If you have any concerns about our products,
you can contact us on
ProductSafety@springernature.com

In case Publisher is established outside the EU,
the EU authorized representative is:
Springer Nature Customer Service Center GmbH
Europaplatz 3, 69115 Heidelberg, Germany

Printed by Libri Plureos GmbH
in Hamburg, Germany